Fields
VIROLOGY

VOLUME 1: Emerging Viruses

SEVENTH
EDITION

Fields
VIROLOGY
VOLUME 1: Emerging Viruses

EDITORS-IN-CHIEF

Peter M. Howley, MD

Shattuck Professor of Pathological Anatomy
Department of Immunology
Harvard Medical School
Boston, Massachusetts

David M. Knipe, PhD

Higgins Professor of Microbiology and Molecular
  Genetics
Department of Microbiology
Chair, Harvard Program in Virology
Harvard Medical School
Boston, Massachusetts

VOLUME ASSOCIATE EDITOR

Sean P. J. Whelan, PhD

Marvin A. Brennecke Distinguished Professor
Chair, Molecular Microbiology
Washington University in Saint Louis, School of Medicine
Saint Louis, Missouri

ASSOCIATE EDITORS

Jeffrey I. Cohen, MD

Chief, Laboratory of Infectious Diseases
National Institute of Allergy and Infectious Diseases
National Institutes of Health
Bethesda, Maryland

Lynn Enquist, PhD

Henry L. Hillman Professor of Molecular Biology
Department of Molecular Biology
Princeton University
Princeton, New Jersey

Blossom Damania, PhD

Boshamer Distinguished Professor and Vice Dean
  for Research, School of Medicine
Department of Microbiology and Immunology
University of North Carolina at Chapel Hill
Chapel Hill, North Carolina

Eric O. Freed, PhD

Director
HIV Dynamics and Replication Program Center
  for Cancer Research
National Cancer Institute
Frederick, Maryland

Wolters Kluwer

Philadelphia • Baltimore • New York • London
Buenos Aires • Hong Kong • Sydney • Tokyo

Acquisitions Editor: Nicole Dernoski
Development Editor: Ariel Winter
Senior Editorial Coordinator: David Murphy
Marketing Manager: Phyllis Hitner
Production Project Manager: Sadie Buckallew
Design Coordinator: Stephen Druding
Senior Manufacturing Coordinator: Beth Welsh
Prepress Vendor: SPi Global

Seventh Edition

Cataloging-in-Publication Data available on request from the Publisher
ISBN: 978-1-9751-1254-7

Contributors

Gaya K. Amarasinghe, PhD
Professor
Department of Pathology and Immunology
Washington University School of Medicine
St. Louis, Missouri

John N. Barr, PhD
Associate Professor
Faculty of Biological Sciences
University of Leeds
Leeds, United Kingdom

Ralf Bartenschlager, PhD
Division Head and Group Leader
Department of Infectious Diseases, Molecular Virology
Heidelberg University
Heidelberg, Baden-Württemberg, Germany

Dennis A. Bente, DVM, PhD
Associate Professor
Department of Microbiology & Immunology
University of Texas Medical Branch/Galveston National Laboratory
Galveston, Texas

Christopher C. Broder, PhD
Professor and Chair
Department of Microbiology and Immunology
Uniformed Services University of the Health Sciences
Bethesda, Maryland

Michael J. Buchmeier, PhD
Professor
Department of Medicine
University of California, Irvine
Irvine, California

Carolyn B. Coyne, PhD
Professor of Pediatrics
Department of Pediatrics
Children's Hospital of Pittsburgh of UPMC
Pittsburgh, Pennsylvania

Juan Carlos de la Torre, PhD
Professor
Department of Immunology and Microbiology
The Scripps Research Institute
La Jolla, California

Michael S. Diamond, MD, PhD
The Herbert S. Gasser Professor
Departments of Medicine, Molecular Microbiology, Pathology & Immunology
Associate Director
The Andrew M. and Jane M. Bursky Center for Human Immunology and Immunotherapy Programs
Washington University School of Medicine
St. Louis, Missouri

Jemma L. Geoghegan, PhD
Lecturer
Department of Biological Sciences
Macquarie University
Sydney, New South Wales, Australia

Kim Y. Green, PhD
Senior Investigator
Department of NIAID
National Institutes of Health
Rockville, Maryland

Diane E. Griffin, MD, PhD
Professor
Department of Molecular Microbiology and Immunology
Bloomberg School of Public Health
Johns Hopkins University
Baltimore, Maryland

Edward C. Holmes, PhD
ARC Australian Laureate Fellow and Professor
School of Life and Environmental Sciences and Sydney Medical School
University of Sydney
Sydney, New South Wales, Australia

Yoshihiro Kawaoka, DVM, PhD
Professor
Influenza Research Institute
Department of Pathobiological Sciences
School of Veterinary Medicine
University of Wisconsin–Madison
Madison, Wisconsin

Florian Krammer, PhD
Professor
Department of Microbiology
Icahn School of Medicine at Mount Sinai
New York, New York

Jens H. Kuhn, MD, PhD, PhD, MS
Virology Lead
Integrated Research Facility at Fort Detrick
Division of Clinical Research
National Institute of Allergy and Infectious Diseases
National Institutes of Health
Frederick, Maryland

Richard J. Kuhn, PhD
Professor
Department of Biological Sciences
Purdue University
West Lafayette, Indiana

Robert A. Lamb, PhD
Professor
Department of Molecular Biosciences
Northwestern University
Evanston, Illinois

Helen M. Lazear, PhD
Assistant Professor
Department of Microbiology and Immunology
University of North Carolina at Chapel Hill
Chapel Hill, North Carolina

Benhur Lee, MD
Ward-Coleman Chair in Microbiology
Department of Microbiology
Icahn School of Medicine at Mount Sinai
New York, New York

Brett D. Lindenbach, PhD
Associate Professor
Department of Microbial Pathogenesis
Yale University School of Medicine
New Haven, Connecticut

Paul S. Masters, PhD
Chief
Laboratory of Viral Replication and Vector Biology
Division of Infectious Diseases
Wadsworth Center
New York State Department of Health
Albany, New York

Gabriele Neumann, PhD
Research Professor, Distinguished Scientist
Department of Pathobiological Sciences
Influenza Research Institute
School of Veterinary Medicine
University of Wisconsin–Madison
Madison, Wisconsin

M. Steven Oberste, PhD
Chief, Polio and Picornavirus Laboratory Branch
Division of Viral Diseases
Centers for Disease Control and Prevention
Atlanta, Georgia

Peter Palese, PhD
Professor and Chair
Department of Microbiology
Icahn School of Medicine at Mount Sinai
New York, New York

Mark A. Pallansch, PhD
Director
Division of Viral Diseases
Centers for Disease Control and Prevention
Atlanta, Georgia

Stanley Perlman, MD, PhD
Professor
Department of Microbiology and Immunology
Department of Pediatrics
University of Iowa
Iowa City, Iowa

Donna L. Perry, DVM, PhD
Integrated Research Facility at Fort Detrick
Division of Clinical Research
National Institute of Allergy and Infectious Diseases
National Institutes of Health
Frederick, Maryland

Theodore C. Pierson, PhD
Senior Investigator
Chief, Laboratory of Viral DiseasesNational Institute of Allergy and
    Infectious Diseases
National Institutes of Health
Bethesda, Maryland

Richard K. Plemper, PhD
Professor
Institute for Biomedical Sciences
Georgia State University
Atlanta, Georgia

Vincent R. Racaniello, PhD
Professor of Microbiology & Immunology
Department of Microbiology & Immunology
Columbia University Vagelos College of Physicians and Surgeons
New York, New York

Sheli R. Radoshitzky, PhD
Principal Investigator
Countermeasures Division
United States Army Medical Research Institute of Infectious Diseases
Frederick, Maryland

Glenn Randall, PhD
Associate Professor
Department of Microbiology
University of Chicago Medical Center
Chicago, Illinois

Charles M. Rice, PhD
Maurice R. and Corinne P. Greenberg Professor
Laboratory for Virology and Infectious Disease
Rockefeller University
New York, New York

Amy B. Rosenfeld, PhD
Research Scientist
Department of Microbiology & Immunology
Columbia University Vagelos College of Physicians and Surgeons
New York, New York

Connie S. Schmaljohn, PhD
Senior Research Scientist
Department of Infectious Diseases
United States Army Medical Research Institute of Infectious Diseases
Fredrick, Maryland

Christina F. Spiropoulou, PhD
Deputy Branch Chief
Viral Special Pathogens Branch
Centers for Disease Control and Prevention
Atlanta, Georgia

John J. Treanor, MD
Professor Emeritus
University of Rochester Medical Center
Rochester, New York

Christopher Walker, PhD
Professor
Department of Vaccines & Immunity
Research Institute at Nationwide Children's Hospital
Columbus, Ohio

Lin-Fa Wang, PhD
Professor and Director
Programme in Emerging Infectious Diseases
Duke-NUS Medical School
Singapore, Singapore

Scott C. Weaver, PhD
Professor
Department of Microbiology and Immunology
University of Texas Medical Branch at Galveston
Galveston, Texas

Friedemann Weber, PhD
Professor and Head of Institute
Institute of Virology
Veterinary Medicine
Justus-Liebig University
Giessen, Germany

Christiane E. Wobus, PhD
Associate Professor
Department of Microbiology and Immunology
University of Michigan
Ann Arbor, Michigan

Preface

In the early 1980s, Bernie Fields originated the idea of a virology reference textbook that combined the molecular aspects of viral replication with the medical features of viral infections. This broad view of virology reflected Bernie's own research, which applied molecular and genetic analyses to the study of viral pathogenesis, providing an important part of the foundation for the field of molecular pathogenesis. Bernie led the publication of the first three editions of *Virology*, but he unfortunately died soon after the third edition went into production. The third edition became *Fields Virology* in his memory, and it is fitting that the book continues to carry his name.

A number of changes and enhancements are being introduced with the seventh edition of *Fields Virology*. The publication format of *Fields Virology* has been changed from a once every 5 to 6 years, two volume book to an annual publication that comprises approximately one-fourth of the chapters organized by category. The annual publication will be both a physical book volume and importantly an eBook with an improved platform. Using an eBook format, our expectation is that individual chapters can be easily updated when major advances, outbreaks, etc., occur. The editorial board organized a four-volume series for the seventh edition consisting of volumes on Emerging Viruses, DNA Viruses, RNA Viruses, and Fundamental Virology, which will be published on an annual basis, with the expectation that the topics will then cycle every 4 years creating an annualized, up-to-date publication. Each volume will contain approximately 20 chapters.

The first volume of this seventh edition of *Fields Virology*, entitled *Emerging Viruses*, has been edited principally by Sean Whelan. There have been continued rapid advances in virology since the previous edition 6 years ago, and all of the chapters in the *Emerging Viruses* volume are either completely new or have been significantly updated to reflect these advances. In this seventh edition, we have chosen to highlight updated lists of references while maintaining older classics. The main emphasis continues to be on viruses of medical importance and interest, but other viruses are described in specific cases where more is known about their mechanisms of replication or pathogenesis.

We wish to thank Patrick Waters of Harvard Medical School and all of the editorial staff members of Lippincott Williams & Wilkins for all their important contributions to the preparation of this book.

David M. Knipe, PhD
Peter M. Howley, MD
Jeffrey I. Cohen, MD
Blossom Damania, PhD
Lynn Enquist, PhD
Eric Freed, PhD
Sean Whelan, PhD

Contents

Virus Evolution

Jemma L. Geoghegan • Edward C. Holmes

INTRODUCTION

Although Charles Darwin preempted many of the great questions in evolutionary biology, he wrote little about viruses. Of course, viruses were not formally identified until a full decade after Darwin's death and, aside from some brief discussion of the origins of yellow fever, his writings make scant reference to what we now know are diseases caused by viruses. This is a great historical shame because it seems certain that Darwin would have held viruses up as some of the best exemplars of evolution by natural selection, with the evolutionary process sometimes so rapid that it can be effectively followed in "real time" by observant researchers.[91,100,236]

Although evolutionary analysis arrived relatively late in the science of virology, the study of virus evolution has become one of the most rapidly growing and successful aspects of modern microbiology. The blossoming of evolutionary virology is largely due to two developments. First, viruses, and especially those that possess RNA genomes, have become remarkably powerful research tools for the study of evolutionary processes. The utility of RNA viruses in this respect is a function of the fact that they usually evolve extremely rapidly, they are easy to

manipulate *in vitro* and *in vivo*, mutations in their genomes can have large and measurable effects on phenotype, and they possess such small genomes that the mutations associated with any phenotypic change can sometimes be determined relatively easily.[68,247] It is therefore no surprise that a growing number of evolutionary researchers are turning to viruses as model systems. For example, studies of viruses represent one of the few cases in which biologists have been able to achieve two of the great aims of modern evolutionary genetics: to measure the fitness effects of individual mutations,[3,227,248] and to determine the nature of the epistatic interactions between these mutations.[228] Second, the rapidity of virus evolution has acted as a direct stimulus for the development of phylogenetic methods that are able to incorporate information on the exact time of sampling of the sequences in question, allowing the spread of viruses through populations to be carefully tracked and in turn revolutionizing molecular epidemiology.[53,100,152] Similarly, many of the computer programs designed for the evolutionary analysis of genome sequence data were first applied to viruses, such that determining the origin and pathways of spread of specific viruses over epidemiologic time has become a relatively exact science with a myriad of potential applications. The advent of next-generation sequencing and metagenomics promises even more rapid advances in this area, potentially enabling the analysis of many thousands of sequences with detailed associated clinical and epidemiological metadata.[115] An important spin-off from these studies has been new insights into the patterns and processes of virus evolution.[110] In sum, although their focus is very different, the combination of experimental analyses of model viruses as a means to understand the intricacies of the evolutionary process and studies of molecular epidemiology and phylogeography based on the comparative analysis of virus genome sequence data to document patterns of virus spread has told us a great deal about the nature of virus evolution (Fig. 1.1). Evolutionary virology has blossomed into a well-developed science.

Despite advances on multiple fronts, some fundamental aspects of viral evolution remain unknown, contentious, or both, which will be highlighted in this chapter. There are still major debates over some of the key mechanisms of evolutionary change in viruses, particularly the exact roles and frequency of mutation, natural selection, genetic drift and recombination as forces of evolutionary change.[110] Similarly, although we know a great deal more about the origin of viruses than we did

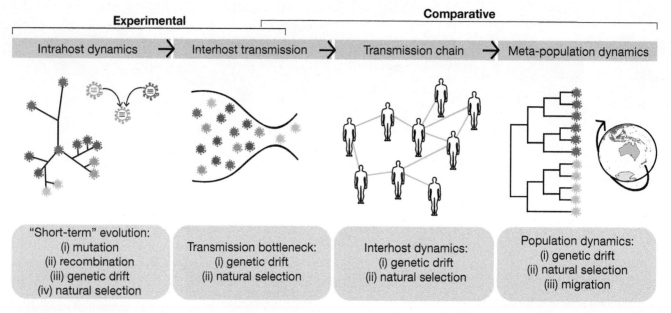

FIGURE 1.1 The different scales over which studies of virus evolution can be performed, using both experimental and comparative (i.e., largely phylogenetic) approaches, and the evolutionary processes that occur at each scale. These range from analyzing short-term intrahost evolution, through the interhost transmission bottleneck, to analyses of the initial host contact network within an infected population, and finally out to the meta-population scale, representing long-term virus evolution as often considered in the fields of molecular epidemiology and phylogeography.

a generation ago, particularly through the analysis of highly conserved protein structures, exactly when and how viruses first evolved, whether this occurred before or after the appearance of the first cellular organisms, what a precellular world might have looked like, and even if viruses should be classified as living are sources of major debate.[81,141,162,184] In part, this debate highlights our profound ignorance of the total universe of viruses—the virosphere. For example, does the apparent absence of RNA viruses in *Archaea* (besides a single highly debatable case[23]) mean that they never existed in these organisms, that they have been selectively removed, or that they are too divergent in sequence to detect using the standard sequence-similarity searching methods like BLAST? We also remain ignorant of a number of key aspects of the patterns and processes of DNA virus evolution, particularly whether common principles can be applied to DNA viruses that differ so fundamentally in size and genome structure and which likely have different origins, and even how large the genome sizes of the largest DNA viruses can be. It is hoped that the rise of metagenomics will enable us to sample far more of the virosphere, and it has already led to the discovery of a multitude of diverse viruses and a changing view of the fundamental patterns and processes of virus evolution.[240,241] Finally, the time scale of evolutionary history in many viruses is unclear, with very different inferences drawn from the study of virus distributions among hosts and of endogenous viruses, which are usually indicative of ancient origins,[239] or the molecular clock analysis of recently sampled and often rapidly evolving viral genomes, which usually paint a picture of very recent origins.[95,111] Fortunately, metagenomics has already provided important insights into this area (see below).

Aside from their ability to inform on evolutionary processes, there are a variety of practical reasons why the study of

virus evolution matters. It is likely that a better understanding of the exact processes of evolutionary change in viruses will assist in the development of improved strategies for their treatment and control and for understanding the origin and spread of newly emerged pathogens. For example, knowledge of the factors that impact how viruses diffuse at the epidemiologic scale represents useful information for any emergent virus,[115] while knowing whether natural selection or genetic drift largely controls how mutations spread through a population is essential to understanding the likelihood and rate that a specific drug resistance mutation will become established.[150] Similarly, it is likely that a better understanding of the origin of viruses will be essential to obtaining a more precise picture of the earliest events in the early history of life on earth, including the genesis of both RNA and DNA, as it seems reasonable to suppose that some of the earliest replicators resemble what we now know as viruses.

The future of evolutionary virology is strong. The development and continued refinement of next-generation sequencing and metagenomic methods will doubtless provide unprecedented amounts of data for evolutionary study and stimulate the development of new analytical methods for use in all genetic systems. Innovations in experimental studies of virus evolution will continue, addressing ever more intricate questions, increasingly considering *in vivo* systems, and providing broad-scale evolutionary insights particularly when linked with comparative data. Metagenomic studies of the virosphere will give a powerful new perspective on virus biodiversity and evolution, providing important new information on virus ecology, origins, and cross-species transmission and emergence. It therefore seems easy to predict that our understanding of viral evolution a decade from now will be very different, and more complete, than it is today.

THE ORIGINS OF VIRUSES AND PATTERNS OF VIRUS EVOLUTION

The Origins of Viruses

Of all topics in the study of virus evolution, determining exactly how and when viruses first evolved is perhaps the most challenging. The main hindrance to progress in this area is that viruses likely originated so long ago, perhaps even before the first cellular species, that the signal of ancient evolutionary history that can be recovered through phylogenetic analysis has largely been eroded. This is particularly true for RNA viruses in which rapid rates of evolutionary change ensure that phylogenetic signal is quickly lost. Accordingly, each individual amino acid and nucleotide site in a viral genome has accumulated so many substitutions since its origin that accurate phylogenetic inference, and hence establishing evolutionary links, becomes a highly challenging, if not impossible, task. For this reason, sequence-based phylogenies have proven to be blunt tools for the study of viral origins, although signs of common ancestry may still reside in aspects of protein structure.

Despite the inherent limitations to understanding viral origins, a number of important theories have been proposed for the genesis of both RNA and DNA viruses, which continue to be debated to this day. Two such theories currently dominate discussions in this area; first, that viruses have a precellular origin, such that they are billions of years old, and may have even contributed to some of the fundamental architecture of the first cells; second, that viruses evolved after the first cellular organisms as "escaped genes" that acquired capsid proteins and the ability to replicate autonomously[110] (Fig. 1.2). Although a third hypothesis—that viruses are regressed copies of cellular species that have shed those genes whose functions are provided by the host—has also been proposed, most notably in the case of the giant mimiviruses of amoeba,[13,144] this hypothesis does not appear to be of general applicability. For example, the gene contents of RNA viruses and cellular species have almost no overlap, whereas under the regressive theory, virus genes should have their ancestries in cellular genomes. In addition, although often discussed as such, these theories of viral origins are not mutually exclusive, and it is plausible that while some viruses predate the appearance of the first cells, others appeared more recently.

For many years, the escaped gene theory dominated discussions on virus origins.[110,162,185] Support for this theory was often based on the idea that as viruses are, by definition, obligate parasites of host cells now, they must have always been so, such that cells must have evolved before viruses. However, this idea is easy to refute. Because it is commonly thought that the first replicating molecules resided in an "RNA world" that existed before the evolution of DNA,[78] it is easy to believe that the lineages that gave rise to modern RNA viruses originated from such ancient self-replicating RNA molecules and parasitized cells at a later date. Important evidence for the existence of an RNA world is that ribonucleotides can be synthesized *de novo* under conditions that might replicate those of early Earth.[210] In most cases, the escaped gene theory was also taken to mean that viruses could have escaped from host cells on multiple occasions. This is an attractive idea given the huge (and growing) phylogenetic and phenotypic diversity seen in viruses and that there is no one gene that characterizes all viruses. For example, an early idea was that eukaryotic viruses had escaped

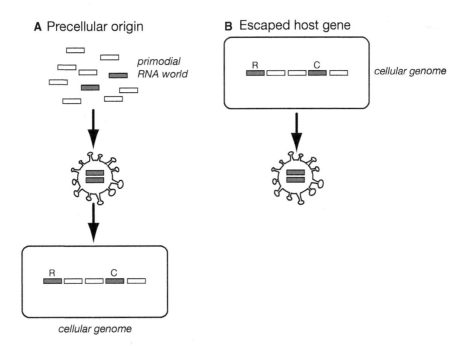

A Precellular origin

primodial RNA world

cellular genome

B Escaped host gene

cellular genome

FIGURE 1.2 Schematic representation of two competing models for the origin of viruses. A: The precellular origin theory, in this case depicting the origin of RNA viruses. **B:** The escaped gene theory. Cellular genomes are represented by *rounded rectangles*, and the simplest model virus is shown here to comprise replicase (R) and capsid (C) genes only. (Adapted from Holmes EC. *The Evolution and Emergence of RNA Viruses.* Oxford: Oxford University Press, 2009, by permission of Oxford University Press.)

from eukaryotic cells, while bacteriophages had escaped from bacterial cells.[211] Similarly, it is possible that RNA, DNA, and perhaps retroviruses represent independent episodes of host gene escape, and it is clear that small ssDNA and large dsDNA viruses have little in common, strongly suggestive of independent origins.

However many different origins are postulated, the same general mechanisms are thought to have occurred: that a host gene that possessed or acquired the ability to self-replicate escaped from the cell, acquiring a protein coat on the way, eventually evolving into an autonomously replicating entity. For example, RNA viruses, particularly those with single-strand positive-sense RNA (ssRNA+) genomes, might be descended from escaped cellular messenger RNA (mRNA) molecules that either possessed or evolved RNA polymerase activity, while DNA viruses could be descended from DNA transposable elements or bacterial plasmids. It is also the case that all forms of the escaped gene theory make two important predictions: first, that most virus genes, including the capsid and replicase proteins, ultimately have their ancestries in cellular genomes, and second, because escape events could have occurred multiple times, viruses do not have a single (i.e., monophyletic) origin. In other words, there is no single phylogeny linking all types of virus, as is easily argued from the huge diversity of viruses described today. In theory, both of these predictions are testable, although in practice this is greatly inhibited by the enormous sequence divergence among viruses.

A number of pieces of data have been used to support the idea that viruses had multiple origins after the appearance of cells. At the level of primary amino acid sequence, there is currently no robust sequence-based phylogeny for either RNA or DNA viruses, nor any gene that contains statistically significant sequence similarity at such vast evolutionary distances. Although there have been attempts to infer the evolutionary history of RNA viruses based on phylogenetic analyses of the RNA-dependent RNA polymerase (RdRp), the phylogenies in question are highly uncertain at the deepest branches, such as those linking the different orders of ssRNA+ and ssRNA− viruses, where there is often no more sequence similarity than expected by chance alone, greatly compromising these analyses including reliable sequence alignment.[113,272] Importantly, however, lack of phylogenetic resolution is not the same thing as an absence of common ancestry, and it is more likely that the inability to accurately infer the evolutionary history of all RNA viruses simply reflects extreme levels of sequence divergence. Indeed, it is striking that the RdRp sequences assigned to different RNA virus families still share a number of short, signature, amino acid motifs (such as a highly conserved GDD motif), some of which are also found in the RT protein used by retroviruses.[96,139] Such conservation, albeit fragmentary, suggests that these replicatory proteins are distantly related. Unfortunately, these motifs are too short to allow the inference of robust phylogenetic trees. Even more notable is that recent analyses of protein structures have revealed strong similarities between viruses that exhibit no primary sequence similarity,[71] including between RNA and DNA viruses, that again argues for their common ancestry (see later).

In the case of RNA viruses, early phylogenetic analyses of RdRp sequences combined with information on gene order and content were used to construct higher level classification schemes encompassing multiple viral families. For example, one such early study suggested that RNA viruses be classified into the alpha-like, carmo-like, corona-like, flavi-like, picorna-like, and sobemo-like "supergroups," each of which is characterized by a conserved gene order, distinctive 5′ and 3′ genome structures, and clustered together in RdRp phylogenies.[96] Similarly, there is now considerable effort devoted to establishing orders and even higher level taxonomic ranks in viruses, although how these relate to each other is far less certain because of the huge genetic distances involved. Indeed, all-encompassing RdRp phylogenies are of debatable validity.[113,270] For example, the ssRNA viruses are now classed as a phylum (the *Negarnaviricota*), containing subphyla, classes, and multiple orders (such as the *Mononegavirales*). Unfortunately, it is also difficult to infer phylogenetic trees using aspects of genome composition like gene order and content because these characteristics differ so dramatically among viral families and in the case of RNA viruses contain too few genes to be informative. Because of these inherent difficulties, deep interorder phylogenies of RNA viruses have in reality told us little about their origins.

In contrast, interfamily phylogenetic analyses of DNA viruses have generally proven more successful, in large part because the reliance on high-fidelity DNA polymerases for replication means that dsDNA viruses exhibit lower rates of nucleotide substitution and hence preserve the phylogenetic signal for longer time periods. For example, a number of families of large dsDNA viruses (i.e., those with genomes >100 kb) clearly possess common ancestry such that they can be classified as nucleocytoplasmic large DNA viruses (NCLDVs), currently comprising ascoviruses, asfarviruses, iridoviruses, marselleviruses, mimiviruses, phycodnaviruses, and poxviruses, with newly identified viruses such as pandoraviruses, pithoviruses, and molliviruses, also likely to be classified as new families.[86,124] In other DNA viruses, elements of capsid protein structure have been used to link herpesviruses with tailed bacteriophages,[173] while there are clear evolutionary links between the *Papillomaviridae* and *Polyomaviridae* families of small dsDNA viruses.[268] However, there is no single phylogeny that encompasses both single- and double-stranded DNA viruses, which again reflects the great divergence between these very different types of virus that share no genes in common and differ massively in genome size. More starkly, it is even difficult to infer phylogenetic trees that link all the large dsDNA viruses that infect eukaryotes.[125]

The second component of the escaped gene theory—that most virus proteins ultimately have a host origin—is equally difficult to resolve. The two most important proteins in this respect, as they essentially define viruses, are the polymerase (a defining feature of all RNA viruses that carry an RdRp or RT) and those that make up the capsid (a defining feature of viruses). The case of the DNA polymerases used by DNA viruses is the easiest to discuss in this context as these enzymes are of the same form, and hence ancestry, as those used by cellular species (i.e., they are classified within the same polymerase families), and small DNA viruses utilize the host DNA polymerases for replication. However, while it is clear that these host and virus DNA polymerases are related,[72,123] the position of the root and therefore the direction of evolutionary change, in phylogenetic trees of DNA polymerases is uncertain. Hence, it is difficult to determine whether DNA polymerases are ultimately of host or viral origin,[233] particularly as DNA polymerases may also have been involved in ancient lateral gene transfer (LGT) events.[73]

A similar discussion can be mounted in the case of RT. Proteins that function as RT are a common component of cellular genomes in the form of telomerase, the group II (self-replicating) introns observed in a variety of bacterial species, not to mention the abundant retroelements found in many cellular species, as well as a variety of other genetic elements. Importantly, there are recognizable sequence similarities between the RTs of viruses and those that reside in host genomes, such that it is possible to infer phylogenetic trees containing both.[34,62] These trees have revealed a number of interesting features, including a major division between the long terminal repeat (LTR) and non-LTR retrotransposons, with retroviruses most closely related to the LTR retrotransposons, and that hepadnaviruses and caulimoviruses (small dsDNA viruses that utilize RT) have independent origins and are probably from LTR retrotransposons. However, as with the case of the DNA polymerases, the lack of an outgroup makes the rooting of these phylogenies uncertain, so whether viral RT genes preceded those present in cells or vice versa is difficult to determine.[63]

The situation is far more complex when it comes to the origin of the RdRp used by RNA viruses. Although the cells of some eukaryotic species contain proteins that function as RdRps, particularly those involved in the production of microRNAs, these exhibit little similarity with the RdRps encoded by viruses, even at the structural level.[126] Similarly, cellular DNA polymerase (Pol) II, which catalyzes the synthesis of RNA from DNA, possesses RdRp activity[149] yet shares little similarity with the RdRp utilized by RNA viruses, such that their evolutionary origins are currently impossible to resolve. Clearly, determining the evolutionary relationships among these highly diverse polymerase proteins represents a major technical challenge.

Another challenge for the escaped gene theory is that there is little evidence of its defining process—host gene escape. A highly informative example concerns the HDV agent, the ribozyme of which shows sequence similarity to the CPEB3 ribozyme found in a human intron sequence.[223] That HDV was until recently only found in humans and thought to always require hepatitis B virus (HBV) for replication suggested that its origins lay with the human genome.[223] However, it has now been shown that viruses other than HBV can act as helpers for HDV replication,[206] and close relatives of HDV have recently been discovered in both ducks and snakes with no evidence of HBV coinfection.[107,266] These results indicate that HDV has a far longer history as an exogenous replicating virus and hence poses a major challenge to the escape gene theory.

There has also been considerable debate over the significance of the giant DNA viruses for understanding viral origins, particularly those from the families *Mimiviridae* and *Pandoraviridae*. For example, although phylogenetic analysis has shown that a small proportion (<1%) of mimivirus genes are of host origin, which has been used as support for the idea that viruses are "gene pickpockets" that originated after cellular species,[183,184] at least 25% of the approximately 1,000 genes in mimivirus clearly link it to the NCLDV group of large DNA viruses,[125] while an even larger set of genes (~70% at the time of writing) have no known homologs in either viral or cellular genomes.[72] A similar proportion of family-unique genes have

been reported in the *Pandoraviridae* which are proposed to have arisen through a process of *de novo* creation within these viruses.[148]

Finally, it is striking that, at the time of writing, there is no clear-cut evidence for the presence of RNA viruses in *Archaea* (although there is one disputed case[23]). This could mean that either RNA viruses arose as escaped genes after the divergence of *Archaea* from other cellular species or that temperature constraints have led to a major reduction in the frequency of RNA viruses in hyperthermophilic *Archaea*,[273] although this does not explain their absence in nonthermophiles. An alternative, and perhaps more likely, explanation is that RNA viruses do exist in *Archaea* but have simply not been detected as yet, perhaps in large part because they are so divergent in sequence as to be "invisible" in metagenomic studies that rely on simple sequence comparisons.

The competing theory for the origin of viruses, for which there is growing evidence and making it the most likely, is that viruses originated before the last universal cellular ancestor (LUCA) and represent the modern descendants of the earliest time in earth's history. Hence, modern RNA viruses would be descendants of replicating elements from the RNA world, while DNA viruses would be remnants of the first DNA replicators, and retroviruses perhaps descendants of the first molecules that made the transition from RNA to DNA. For example, because they lack protein-coding regions, possess ribozyme activity, exhibit complex secondary structures, and mutate very rapidly, viroids have been suggested to be potential candidates for extant descendants of the RNA world.[67] However, although the earliest RNA replicators may share some features with contemporary viroids, because viroids are currently only seen in plants and likely replicate with the assistance of host cellular DNA Pol II makes it more likely that they represent escaped host genes or introns that never acquired protein coats. Whether metagenomic studies will identify viroid-like sequences in host organisms other than plants is obviously a key topic for the future.

There are a number of ideas for what the pre-LUCA world may have looked like, although all reasonably assume that this precellular stage of evolutionary history contained genetic elements less complex than the viruses we see today. One theory is that there was an *ancient virus world* of primordial replicators that existed before any cellular organisms and that both RNA (first) and DNA (later) viruses originated at this time.[141] These ancient "viruses" may even have provided some of the features that characterized the first cellular organisms. For example, it has been proposed that the eukaryotic cell nucleus is derived from a virus envelope (the so-called viral eukaryogenesis hypothesis).[15] An alternative theory for the pre-LUCA world is that RNA cells existed before the LUCA, that RNA viruses parasitized these hypothetical RNA cells, and that DNA evolved later as a way of escaping host cell responses.[80] Although fascinating, such theories are unfortunately extremely difficult to test.

As sequence-based phylogenetic trees cannot provide insights into the pre-LUCA world, the main evidence for the precellular theory of virus origins is the presence of conserved genes, and more notably protein structures, among divergent viruses. In fact, arguably one of the most important advances in viral evolution has been the discovery of protein structures that are conserved among diverse viruses that possess little, if any, primary sequence similarity.[14] For example, a conserved palm subdomain protein structure, consisting of a four-stranded antiparallel β-sheet and two α-helices, is found in both RNA-dependent and DNA-dependent polymerases.[99] A more important case in point concerns the jelly-roll capsid, a tightly structured protein barrel that forms the major capsid subunit of virions with an icosahedral structure. Remarkably, the jelly-roll capsid is found in the virions of both RNA and DNA viruses, including such diverse groups as herpesviruses (dsDNA), picornaviruses (ssRNA+), and birnaviruses (dsRNA).[14,43] Such conservation is strongly suggestive of an ancient common ancestry. Other highly conserved capsid architectures that strongly argue for ancient origins include the PRD1-adenovirus lineage, which is characterized by a double β-barrel fold and found in dsDNA viruses as diverse as bacteriophage PRD1, human adenovirus, and a variety of archaean viruses; the BTV-like lineage, which is found in some dsRNA viruses including members of the *Reoviridae* and *Totiviridae*; and the HK97-like lineage, which encompasses tailed dsDNA viruses that infect archaea, bacteria, and eukaryotes.[19,20,142] Finally, a common virion architecture has been proposed for some viruses that do not possess an icosahedral capsid, including the archaean virus *Halorubrum* pleomorphic virus type 1 (HRPV-1).[209]

Although such structural conservation seems to provide a compelling argument for the antiquity of viruses, it has been suggested that any similarities in protein structure could have arisen more recently due to either strong convergent evolution or LGT.[184] While it is theoretically possible that convergent evolution may occur relatively frequently in viral capsid proteins that may be subject to strong selection to be small and perhaps of a specific shape, such large-scale convergence seems highly unlikely given that the similarity in capsid structure covers a huge range of viral taxa. As a consequence, multiple convergent events need to be invoked from very different starting points, and the more convergent evolution that is required, the less likely it becomes. Although metagenomic data have provided greater evidence that LGT occurs more frequently in viruses than previously thought (see below), it seems unlikely that such a fundamental trait as the viral capsid would move so freely horizontally, although this view may change with increased sample size. In conclusion, the presence of structural similarities among highly divergent viruses currently constitutes the strongest evidence that viruses have a precellular origin.

The Time Scale of Virus Evolution

While our understanding of viral origins is vague, rather more is known about the antiquity of those families of viruses that circulate today. Although viruses lack a fossil record, a growing number of studies of the host distribution of viral families have provided important insights into how long they have been in existence, which in many cases means times of origin hundreds of millions of years ago.[242]

There are four ways in which the evolutionary history of viruses has been placed on a chronological scale. First, if there is a general correspondence between the phylogenetic tree of viruses and that of their hosts, such that they have *codiverged* through evolutionary history, then it is possible to use the divergence times of hosts to calibrate the time scale of virus evolution. Second, for viruses that evolve rapidly such that there is *measurable evolution* (i.e., mutations are fixed in viral populations during the time frame of human observation),

which has been clearly demonstrated in both RNA viruses and ssDNA viruses, as well as some larger dsDNA viruses following complete genome sequencing,[53] it is possible to determine the number of nucleotide or amino acid substitutions that have occurred between viruses sampled at known times (i.e., "heterochronous" samples) and use this information to calibrate the time scale of virus evolution under the assumption of a molecular clock (i.e., that there is an approximately constant rate of nucleotide or amino acid fixation). Third, for viruses where endogenous genome copies are present in the host, it is possible to use the substitution rate of the host to determine when these genome integration events occurred, especially if the endogenous sequences also codiverge with their host species.[130] Finally, in a limited number of cases, including some poxviruses,[60] hepadnaviruses,[187,202] and parvoviruses[188] it is possible to use virus sequences obtained from archival samples (i.e., ancient DNA) to date virus evolution. All four approaches have limitations and can lead to wildly different interpretations of evolutionary time scales, such that all should be used with caution.

Dating the time scale of virus evolution through the use of host divergence times (i.e., codivergence) is perhaps the simplest and most robust approach to this form of molecular archaeology. This approach has been successful in the study of DNA virus evolution, and metagenomic studies of families of animal RNA viruses have suggested that these may be as old as the animals they infect, so that they likely have origins with the earliest metazoans.[242] Specific examples of its utility are the dating of herpesvirus evolution through an examination of the phylogenetic relationships of their vertebrate hosts, in which virus–host codivergence may extend to some 400 million years[172,173]; of the animal iridoviruses[128]; of the baculoviruses of insects[106]; and of the papillomaviruses sampled from a number of vertebrates including humans.[22] Clearly, although each of these virus families can be considered "ancient," they are in no way of sufficient age to inform on the question of virus origins. In addition, in some other large DNA viruses, with the poxviruses a good example, frequent host jumping and limited sampling means that patterns of host–virus codivergence can be difficult to infer, so that the times of origin of key human pathogens like variola virus (VARV; the agent of smallpox) are still the source of considerable debate.[60,156,238] A compelling example of virus–host codivergence being used to date the origin of a number of RNA viruses and retroviruses concerns the retrovirus simian foamy virus (SFV). Here, a statistically significant match between the phylogenetic trees of host and virus may extend to at least 30 million years,[160,250] and the analysis of endogenous foamy viruses places their evolutionary history in mammals to over 100 million years,[132] with a likely origin early in vertebrate evolution.[102] More recently, metagenomic analyses have revealed a general correspondence between different classes of vertebrate and the RNA viruses they carry (although with frequent host jumping), which again points to ancestries dating back hundreds of millions of years.[90,239]

While *bona fide* examples of virus–host codivergence constitute a powerful way to date the age of specific viruses, it is also the case that the resemblance of between host and virus phylogeny could occur by chance alone or because related host species are more likely to share their pathogens.[37] Given that cross-species transmission is a very common mode of virus macroevolution,[90] it can be dangerous to construct a time scale of virus evolution without strong evidence for codivergence. Overall, there is a growing view that virus evolution represents a complex interplay between codivergence and cross-species transmission, with both processes commonly co-occurring in many virus families (see below).[90] Although these broad-scale patterns have provided important insights into the timescale of virus evolution, such complexity can make dating the ancestry of individual viruses very difficult.

Using heterochronous samples to calibrate the virus molecular clock is an extremely powerful and increasingly popular way to study the time scale of virus evolution in the recent past (i.e., on time scales no more than a few hundred years) and is commonly used with RNA viruses where measurable sequence evolution is a routine observation. Because large numbers of gene sequences where the precise date of sampling is known are now available, and because virus evolution is often relatively clock-like, it is a straightforward exercise to date the age of samples of genetic diversity if performed with care.[53] In some cases, divergence times estimated in this manner can be very accurate. For example, an analysis of heterochronous samples of human influenza A virus was able to accurately reconstruct the seasonal peaks and troughs in the population size of this virus.[214] However, while these molecular clock approaches can work well for recent virus evolution, they are prone to error at deeper divergence times, providing a picture of virus evolution that is too recent, particularly given the time-dependent nature of virus evolution in which rate estimates are elevated toward to present (see below).[56] An important example of this effect is provided by

the case of the SIVs. While molecular clock studies of SIV evolution using heterochronous samples place this on a time scale of hundreds of years, a calibration based on the biogeographic separation of Bioko Island from the coast of West Africa gave dates of at least 32,000, and perhaps over 100,000 years.[269]

In a number of cases, the time scale of virus evolution can be inferred using the sequences of endogenous viral sequences that are a common component of eukaryotic genomes. Endogenous genomic copies of exogenous viruses that have entered the germ line are particularly commonplace in retroviruses, and it is estimated that approximately 5% to 8% of the human genome is composed of endogenous retrovirus, comprising many distinct families.[133] In addition, there is a growing list of endogenous RNA and small DNA viruses, also referred to as endogenous viral elements (EVEs), that usually comprise partial virus genome sequences and are commonly found following the sequencing of host genomes.[5,111,130] Endogenous viruses also represent a sort of "fossil record" of past viral infections: once integrated into host genomes, they cease to evolve like viruses and instead assume the low rates of nucleotide substitution that characterize their hosts, replicating using high-fidelity host DNA polymerases and likely experiencing fewer replications per unit time (Fig. 1.3). Consequently, if the mutational differences between endogenous viruses are known to occur postintegration, such as those observed between the LTRs of a single endogenous retrovirus, between duplicated EVEs, or when there is clear evidence for codivergence, then divergence times can be estimated in a relatively straightforward manner using host substitution rates.

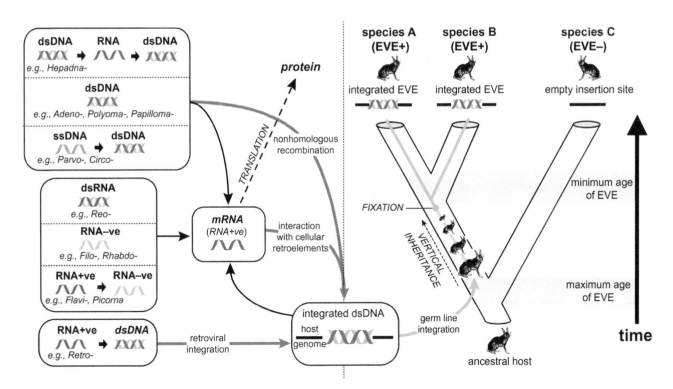

FIGURE 1.3 How endogenous virus elements (EVEs) are generated and can be used to estimate the age of viral families. Examples of different types of mammalian RNA and DNA viruses are shown. The presence of EVEs in related host species A and B and integrated into the same genomic position indicates that this integration event occurred prior to the divergence of these two species, such that its minimum age can be estimated if it is known when the host species diverged. (From Katzourakis A, Gifford RJ. Endogenous viral elements in animal genomes. *PLoS Genet* 2010;6:e1001191. Original figure kindly provided by Dr. Rob Gifford.)

Molecular clock dating using EVEs suggests that the exogenous ancestors of some human retroviruses may have diversified relatively early on in mammalian evolution.[133] Most dramatic are cases of when both exogenous and endogenous copies of the same virus exist: these have generally resulted in a radically different picture of the time scale of viral evolution than using clock estimates based on heterochronous samples. For example, estimates of the age of primate lentiviruses based on the use of heterochronous sequences generally result in time scales of thousands of years at most,[237] while the presence of endogenous lentiviruses in lemurs suggests that these viruses have circulated in primates for at least several million years.[131] The same is true of endogenous viruses that are not retroviruses. A compelling example is provided by the avian hepadnaviruses, in which the observation of EVEs integrated at the same genomic positions in bird species that diverged at least 19 million years ago strongly suggests that hepadnaviruses are at least of the same age,[95] and endogenous hepadnaviruses are now increasingly observed in the genomes of birds[46] and other vertebrates.[249] The same phenomenon has been proposed for a variety of other RNA viruses, including bornaviruses and filoviruses,[17,118,132] and help to calibrate the timescale of virus evolution when combined with comparative studies of exogenous viruses,[239] as well as ssDNA viruses of the families *Circoviridae* and *Parvoviridae*.[18,129,159] In each case, integrated copies of these viruses are observed in diverse host species, for example comprising both placental and marsupial mammals in the case of the filoviruses, and sometimes showing virus–host codivergence indicating that they are millions of years old.[130] As more host genomes are sequenced, it is certain that more EVEs will be discovered, which in turn will shed new light on the true time scale of virus evolution.

The final way in which a timescale has been placed on virus evolution has been through the use of so-called ancient DNA, in which evolutionary analyses are performed on viruses sampled from archival material. Because of its greater preservation, this approach has been more successful in the case of DNA than RNA viruses, with variola virus (VARV),[60] human papillomavirus,[38] HBV,[187,202] human T-cell lymphotropic virus,[157] and B19 parvovirus[188] constituting important examples. Although there have been a number of reports of ancient RNA viruses, including the compelling case of a plant virus recovered from a caribou feces frozen on permafrost dating to 700 years ago,[194] in many other instances it is difficult to exclude the issue of contamination that plagues studies of ancient DNA, particularly as the ancient samples possess sequences that are closely related to modern variants.[207] In addition, in the case of human RNA viruses, there is currently little evidence for the preservation of viruses older than the influenza A virus associated with the global pandemic of 1918–1919.[251] However, with *bona fide* samples, the analysis of ancient DNA can provide important insights into virus evolution. For example, in the case of HBV the ancient samples showed not only that modern viral genotypes have been associated with human populations for at least 7,000 years but also that the ancient geographic distributions of genotypes are different to those observed today.[187] This has important implications for theories of HBV origin and spread, and shows that rates of evolutionary change in this virus are lower than those observed using heterochronous samples.[187] Similarly, the analysis of VARV samples dating to the 17th century has shown that the diversification of smallpox virus to generate the lineages present during the 20th century occurred more recently than previously imagined.[60] Importantly, however, while ancient DNA is an increasingly valuable tool to study virus evolution on the time scales of thousands of years at most, it will not be informative on the deep origins and evolution of viruses as a whole.

Codivergence and Cross-Species Transmission in Virus Evolution

Emerging infectious diseases are often characterized by "host switching" events, in which a pathogen jumps from its original host to infect a novel species. Indeed, the cross-species transmission of viruses is responsible for the majority of emerging infections and can profoundly affect human and animal health. More fundamentally, cross-species transmission is also one of the key processes of virus evolution.[90] Although most emerging diseases seemingly result from such a process of cross-species transmission, it is also the case that some viruses seem to rarely jump the species barrier and instead codiverge with their hosts over long stretches of evolutionary time. For example, long-term virus–host codivergence has been suggested to play a key role in the evolution of vertebrate herpesviruses over periods of approximately 400 million years[172] and insect baculoviruses over a timescale of approximately 310 million years.[253] In fact, a number of families of DNA viruses have clearly codiverged with their hosts over long evolutionary timescales,[110,260] and do so more frequently than do RNA viruses.[90] This may, in part, be due to the fact that many RNA viruses are characterized by short durations of infection that will limit the opportunities for virus–host codivergence, although there is also growing evidence for host codivergence among families of RNA viruses.[240,241] Similarly, the high rates of evolutionary change that characterize RNA viruses should confer more rapid adaptation to new environments, which, coupled with the frequency of exposure to new hosts, will facilitate host switching.

Most attention has been directed to RNA viruses, and these often seem to evolve through a combination of codivergence and host switching. While phylogenetic trees for some RNA viruses, such as particular retroviruses, are similar with those from their hosts suggesting that there has been long-term codivergence,[127] for others, such as coronaviruses, flaviviruses, and picornaviruses, host jumping appears to be relatively frequent.[90,138] The situation appears to be even more complex in cases such as the hantaviruses, where the respective contributions of codivergence and host jumping can be difficult to determine.[116]

Although host jumping is commonplace, it is also the case that many emerging diseases are in reality transient "spill-over" infections, in which onward transmission between members of a new host species is limited and extinction of any novel virus occurs rapidly. This is to be expected as viruses must overcome a variety of evolutionary and ecological barriers to successfully establish themselves in new hosts.[92,93] Nevertheless, it is possible that an increased sampling of hosts and their viruses, particularly through novel virus discovery via metagenomics, will reveal even further instances of cross-species transmission. As a case in point, although there is strong evidence that hepadnaviruses have codiverged with their vertebrate hosts over hundreds of millions of years,[249] the recent identification of hepadnaviruses in fish and amphibians has revealed more instances of cross-species transmission, potentially including that from aquatic to terrestrial vertebrates[49,89] (Fig. 1.4).

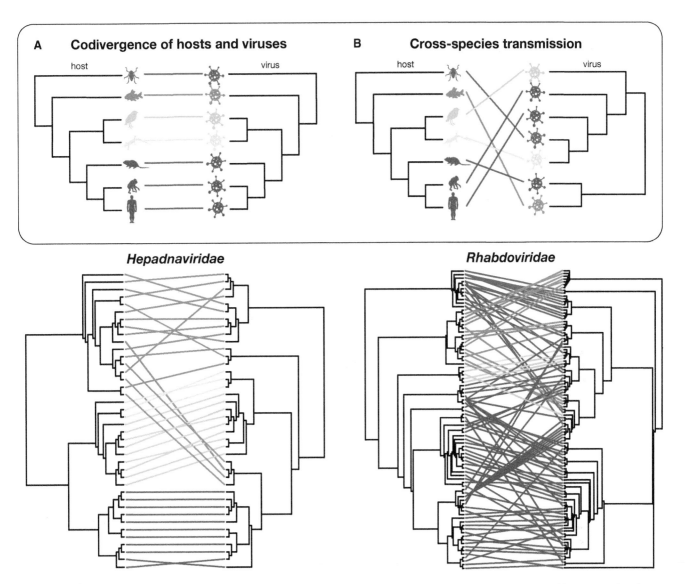

A   Codivergence of hosts and viruses

host   virus

B   Cross-species transmission

host   virus

Hepadnaviridae

Rhabdoviridae

FIGURE 1.4 The contrasting processes of virus–host codivergence and virus cross-species transmission to novel hosts. A: When host populations diverge and speciate, often over periods of millions of years, viruses may evolve with them through codivergence and hence the phylogenies for viruses and hosts will have similar topologies (i.e., exhibit congruence). **B:** Conversely, if viruses evolve by jumping to new hosts, then the phylogenetic relationships among viruses and their hosts will mismatch (i.e., exhibit incongruence). Real data examples are shown in the bottom part of the figure, in which the match between the virus and host phylogenies are shown for the *Hepadnaviridae* and the *Rhabdoviridae*. Cross-species transmission is relatively common in both cases, especially the *Rhabdoviridae*.

To understand the basic mechanisms of virus evolution and disease emergence, it is obviously important to identify the relative frequencies of codivergence and cross-species transmission among viruses and their hosts. In particular, this information will help determine whether some virus families have a greater propensity to jump hosts than do others and, if so, even reveal what factors may govern this pattern. This can be achieved using a "co-phylogenetic" analysis that assesses the degree of phylogenetic congruence (i.e., similarity) between hosts and their parasites.[127] That is, a clear congruence between the host and virus phylogenies provides strong evidence for a history of codivergence, whereas phylogenetic incongruence (i.e., discord) is compatible with cross-species transmission (Fig. 1.4).

It is also likely that successful cross-species transmission occurs more frequently among phylogenetically related hosts, a

process termed "preferential host switching."[37] This is because it is easier for a virus to infect and replicate in genetically similar hosts that share less divergent cell receptors.[201] In addition, related hosts may often inhabit the same geographic region, increasing the probability of cross-species transmission through more frequent exposure.[190] Hence, the closer the phylogenetic relationship between hosts, then, given appropriate exposure, the more likely that a pathogen will be able to jump between them.

Finally, it is important to note that cross-species transmission events revealed through such co-phylogenetic analyses have likely occurred over very long evolutionary timescales, and that many of the viral families that present frequent host switching have done so for many millions of years. Therefore, the observation that many viruses can frequently jump species boundaries over evolutionary timescales[198] provides no assistance in predicting what happens over shorter timescales that govern epidemiological processes relevant to epidemics.[91]

Metagenomics and Virus Evolution

Metagenomics is transforming studies of virus evolution, with a massive amount of new genetic diversity revealed in DNA bacteriophage[105] and RNA viruses.[240,241] Indeed, it is a safe bet that our view of the virosphere and the evolutionary processes that shape it will be very different in this edition of Field's virology and the next.

Before the advent of DNA sequencing, new viruses were discovered using a variety of approaches, including filtration, cell culture, electron microscopy, and serology. Many of these techniques remain important,[151] and the gold standard for virus discovery is still the propagation of viruses in cells, accompanied by the visualization of virus particles by electron microscopy and the successful replication of infection in animal models. However, the enormous time and effort required for work of this kind, and the sheer scale of the virosphere, means that this is often practically impossible. In addition, most viruses are not culturable, and there are not enough cell lines to meet the diversity of viruses.

A more modern approach to virus discovery, which is transforming our understanding of virus diversity and evolution, is through a coupling of metagenomics and high-throughput sequencing. Indeed, metagenomics has revolutionized virus discovery in terms of speed, accuracy, sensitivity, and the amount of information generated.[77] Among the various metagenomics approaches that are available, meta-transcriptomics, based on total RNA sequencing, has recently come to the fore in the case of RNA viruses. This approach involves gathering total transcriptome information from a host sample, often after depletion of ribosomal (r) RNA as this is the dominant component of host transcriptomes. Previous methodologies were often based on removing as much nucleic acid outside viral particles as possible by filtering, centrifugation, lysis, and nuclease treatment, although this seldom results in a complete depletion of host RNA and may bias against the detection of particular types of virus.[76,181] In contrast, in meta-transcriptomics total RNA is directly extracted from untreated homogenates and used for library preparation without filtering, capture, or enrichment, thereby providing an unbiased picture of host viromes, although what viruses are found strongly depends on the depth of sequencing coverage. Metagenomics based on shotgun DNA sequencing may still be the most profitable approach for the study of DNA viruses, although to date less effort has been devoted to describing new DNA viruses in animal hosts.

The most obvious evolutionary insight from metagenomics is that the number of undetected viruses is enormous such that we are still only scratching the surface of the virosphere, particularly when compared with the number and diversity of viruses that can be revealed through other approaches such as cell culture and consensus PCR (Fig. 1.5). This, in turn, suggests that we still have a great deal to learn about virus diversity and evolution. As well as revealing an abundance of new virus

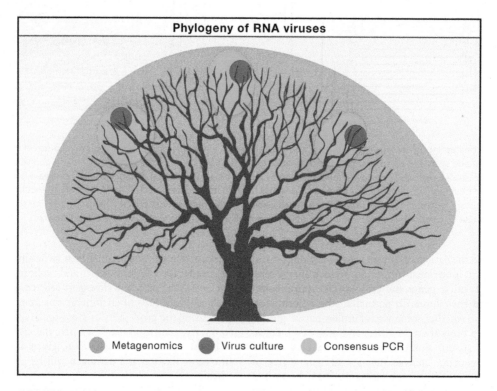

FIGURE 1.5 Different analytical techniques to explore the virosphere. A schematic tree is used to represent the total phylogenic diversity of RNA viruses (although the same scheme also applies to DNA viruses). The *colored circles* depict the extent of viral diversity that can be discovered using cell culture (*red*), consensus PCR (*blue*), and metagenomics, such as RNA sequencing (meta-transcriptomics, *orange*). (From Zhang YZ, Shi M, Holmes EC. Using metagenomics to characterize an expanding virosphere. *Cell* 2018;172:1168–1172, by permission of Cell Press.)

taxa, and determining the evolutionary processes that have shaped this diversity, it is undoubtedly the case that viruses exist in hosts that have not yet been screened for viruses or that are so divergent in sequence that they cannot readily be detected by standard homology-based methods (such as Blast) or included in phylogenetic analyses.[242] If the nature of this "dark matter" can be resolved, it will doubtless shed new light on the ultimate origins of viruses as well as their deep phylogenetic relationships, and perhaps even on the origins and evolution of the first replicating systems. In particular, it is of critical importance to characterize the unknown biodiversity of viruses in prokaryotes (both archaea and bacteria) and basal eukaryotes that may possess highly divergent genome sequences that are currently difficult to identify. Unfortunately, this will also require the development of new computational methods to extract sequence information from highly divergent genome sequences.

The rise of metagenomics has also made it clear that our knowledge of the evolutionary processes that have generated the diversity of the virosphere has been strongly skewed by a focus on those viruses that act as agents of disease in economically important animals and plants as well as those that can be easily cultured. In particular, recent work has shown that animals, and invertebrates in particular, harbor enormous uncharacterized viral diversity, only some of which has been associated with disease.[158,240] Key questions for future research that can be addressed with metagenomic data include (a) determining the processes that shape virus ecosystems, particularly the factors that assist or inhibit the flow of viruses between hosts; (b) revealing the mechanisms of long-term virus macroevolution, particularly the rates and causes of virus lineage birth and death, and (c) revealing the mechanisms and evolutionary processes that are responsible for the diverse array of virus genome structures, and how these genome structures are connected to each other in evolutionary space.[242] Finally, there is a growing realization that metagenomic data provide both important opportunities and challenges for virus classification,[244] and that a combination of metagenomics and phylogenetics will soon become the standard means to address issues of virus taxonomy.

PROCESSES OF VIRUS EVOLUTION

One of the strongest arguments that viruses are alive is that they are subject to the same forces that shape the evolution seen in cellular species: mutation, natural selection, genetic drift, recombination (and reassortment), and migration. We will discuss the first four of these processes in this chapter. Migration, in the guise of viral epidemiology, is discussed elsewhere in this volume.

Mutation and Nucleotide Substitution in Viruses

The simplest way to examine the role of mutation in virus evolution is to measure the rate of its occurrence. Indeed, understanding the factors that shape the speed at which genetic variation is generated in viruses is central to understanding their evolution. For RNA viruses, mutation can in some ways be thought of as their defining evolutionary feature, as it occurs at a pace that greatly exceeds that observed in other organisms and determines much of their evolutionary "behavior."

Although mutation is the ultimate source of genetic variation, the pace of evolutionary change can be measured in two rather different ways. One method is to estimate, experimentally, the rate at which mutations are generated *de novo*. Such rates have usually been presented as the number of mutations per nucleotide or per genome, per replication. However, because of the inherent complexities and biases in making these estimates, it has been suggested that estimates of mutation rate per nucleotide, per cell infection may be more informative.[229] For example, one important complicating factor is that some viruses employ so-called stamping machine replication, in which a single virus acts as the template for all progeny genomes, so that mutations accumulate linearly, while others utilize "geometric" replication, in which some of the early progeny genomes are used as templates to produce further progeny, in turn increasing the rate of mutation accumulation.[59]

The importance of mutation rate estimates is that they reveal the intrinsic error dynamics of the RNA or DNA polymerases used in viral replication and in theory allow a count of each type of mutation—advantageous, neutral, or deleterious—before they have been shaped by natural selection, although it is always difficult to accurately count the number of lethal mutations that are rapidly removed by purifying selection. A detailed compilation of mutation rate estimates for 27 viruses, and accounting for many of the complexities inherent in analyses of this kind, revealed that these rates vary from averages of 1.6×10^{-6} to 1.5×10^{-4} mutations/nucleotide/cell infection for RNA viruses, from 1.6×10^{-5} to 4.4×10^{-3} mutations/nucleotide/cell infection for retrotranscribing viruses, and 5.9×10^{-8} to 1.1×10^{-6} mutations/nucleotide/cell infection for DNA viruses (Fig. 1.6).[226,229] For RNA viruses that replicate with a RdRp, an enzyme that lacks a proofreading or repair function, this equates to mutation rates that are usually around one per genome, per replication.[51,52,57] Similarly, the lower mutation rates observed in large DNA viruses clearly reflect the higher fidelity of the DNA polymerases employed

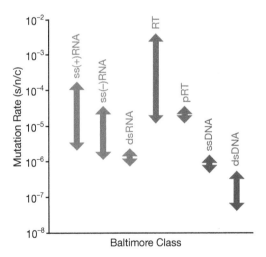

FIGURE 1.6 The large-scale variation in mutation rates among viruses. The range of variation in mutation rates is shown for the seven classes of viruses classified under the Baltimore scheme. ss, single-strand; ds, double-strand; +/− genome polarity; RT, retroviruses; pRT, para-retroviruses. (From Sanjuán R, Domingo-Calap P. Mechanisms of viral mutation. *Cell Mol Life Sci* 2016;7:4433–4448, by permission of Springer Nature.)

in their replication cycle. Of particular note is that mutation rate estimates in ssDNA viruses (a maximum of 1.1×10^{-6}, although only two estimates are available) are higher than those of large dsDNA viruses (which range from 5.9×10^{-8} to 5.4×10^{-7}),[226] even though ssDNA viruses have such small genomes that they use host DNA polymerases for replication. Although it remains to be determined, it is possible that the higher mutation rates in ssDNA viruses reflect less efficient proofreading and excision repair on ssDNA and/or frequent deamination.[58] The study of Sanjuán and Domingo-Calap[226] was also of note in that it revealed that retroviruses such as HIV have error rates that often higher than those of RdRp-utilizing viruses, even though earlier studies suggested that RT exhibits higher fidelity than does RdRp.[51,52,166]

From a broader perspective, these estimates of mutation rate are compatible with the idea that there is a strongly inverse relationship between mutation rate and genome size that applies to all living systems (Fig. 1.7).[85,112] It also seems likely that the systematic difference in mutation rate and genome size between RNA and DNA viruses is associated with many of the main evolutionary distinctions between these two types of infectious agents that are discussed throughout this chapter.[110]

Although they utilize related DNA polymerases, mutation rates in large DNA viruses are higher than those of bacteria and eukaryotes, which may reflect an absence of the full set of repair enzymes and pathways. There are, however, two possible exceptions to this rule. First, there is currently no estimate of mutation rates in the giant DNA viruses, although these are expected to fall within the bacterial range (as the genome sizes of these viruses overlap with those of bacteria), and hence lower than that observed in any virus to date. Although a higher rate of nucleotide substitution was estimated in the case of the giant pandoraviruses,[154] which would imply a high background mutation rate, this was later shown to be questionable and it is

clear that more data are required.[55] Second, we similarly lack an estimate of mutation rate in the small dsDNA viruses, such as the papillomaviruses. Although the relationship depicted in Figures 1.6 and 1.7 implies that these viruses will mutate rapidly, most estimates of substitution rate in papillomaviruses are in a similar range to those of large DNA viruses.[76,216] This implies that papillomaviruses similarly mutate relatively slowly, which would break the simple relationship between mutation rate and genome size. Whether any of the new viruses discovered by metagenomic surveys will similarly break the proposed association between mutation rate and genome size is a key research question.

The relationship between mutation rate and genome size is of twofold importance. First, because it incorporates genetic systems ranging from viroids to eukaryotes, it covers at least eight orders of magnitude of both genome size and mutation rate, and few things in biology encompass such diversity. Second, it implies that mutation rates that are either too high or too low are selected against.[112] With respect to the latter, a popular idea is that viral mutation rates, particularly the high mutation rates of RNA viruses, are the result of an evolutionary trade-off, either between replication rate and replication fidelity[84] or between the rates of deleterious and advantageous mutation.[59,247] Data can be cited in support of both relationships,[110,167,259] with a recent study showing that the evolution of mutation rates may reflect an evolutionary trade-off between replication speed and fidelity; that is, rapid replication is selectively advantageous for a virus but comes at the cost of lower replication fidelity.[79] However, it is also likely that this evolutionary trade-off will vary depending on virus type and the duration of infection, differing, for example, between viruses associated with either acute or chronic infections.

It is also possible that there is trade-off between the rates of deleterious and advantageous mutation in viruses. On the one hand, as viruses will be commonly exposed to changing environments (i.e., different hosts, a variety of cell types, frequent immune pressure), the generation of some genetic variation via mutation is likely to be selectively advantageous. This idea also has experimental support: RNA polymerases with lower fidelity and that generate more diversity are sometimes selectively favored over those with higher fidelity.[110,167,259] On the other hand, there must be an upper limit on the mutation rates experienced by viruses (and all living systems), as excessive error will result in major fitness losses. Powerful evidence for this ceiling on mutation rates is provided by experiments invoking *lethal mutagenesis* (see later), in which artificially increasing error rates with mutagens such as 5-fluorouracil and ribavirin result in an excessive mutational load.[30] It is therefore likely that RNA viruses exist close to their maximum tolerable mutation rates, which in turn imposes an upper limit on genome size. However, it is also likely that RNA viruses are mechanistically unable to reduce their error rates to the levels associated with DNA polymerases. A higher-fidelity RNA polymerase would need to be more complex, and hence longer, than those that currently exist, yet this cannot evolve because by increasing genome length too many deleterious mutations will accumulate. This evolutionary conundrum is commonly referred to as *Eigen's paradox* and is a key element in theories for the early evolution of genomic complexity.[109]

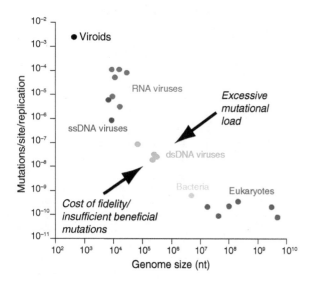

FIGURE 1.7 Relationship between mutation rate and genome size in diverse organisms including RNA and DNA viruses and viroids. The competing evolutionary forces that might be responsible for the limited range of observed mutation rates and genome sizes are shown. See also Figure 1.6. (From Holmes EC. What does virus evolution tell us about virus origins? *J Virol* 2011;85:5247–5251, by permission of the American Society for Microbiology.)[108]

The second measure of the pace of virus evolution is the rate of nucleotide substitution per nucleotide site, per year (subs/site/year). As this measure reflects the *population* success of any mutation, it by necessity incorporates the action of natural selection. Accordingly, deleterious mutations that have been removed by purifying selection will not be counted, while advantageous mutations will be fixed more rapidly than neutral ones. Because they only involve sequence comparisons, nucleotide substitution rates are usually far easier to estimate than mutation rates and so provide a simple and powerful means to compare patterns of virus evolution.

As with rates of mutation, rates of nucleotide substitution vary markedly among viruses. Across RNA and DNA viruses as a whole, nucleotide substitution rates vary by over five orders of magnitude, in large part reflecting the differences in background mutation rate described earlier.[57,114] Hence, most substitution rates in RNA viruses fall within an order of magnitude of a value of 1×10^{-3} subs/site/year,[110,114] while the rates in many dsDNA viruses are closer to 1×10^{-8} subs/site/year.[104,168,172,216] Undoubtedly, our understanding of viral substitution rates would be improved by reliable measures of evolutionary dynamics in the smallest (i.e., viroids) and largest (i.e., pandoravirus) viral systems.

Most of the variance in the substitution rates in both RNA and DNA viruses likely reflects virus-specific differences in rates of mutation, replication, or both. Mutation rates have been discussed earlier. Although few direct estimates of replication rate are available, they likewise clearly play a major role in shaping substitution rates. For example, although the retrovirus SFV likely has an RT-associated error rate that is similar to those of other retroviruses, its codivergence with primates for over 30 million years leads to estimates of the substitution rate of only 1.7×10^{-8} subs/site/year.[250] This most likely reflects a low rate of replication in the long term, although this merits further investigation. Similarly, replication rates appear to be low in papillomaviruses, in which virus replication occurs simultaneously with the division of host epithelial cells, at approximately 10 to 100 generations per year,[22] which likely contributes to the low substitution rates estimated in this virus. In contrast, that DNA viruses often replicate more rapidly than do their hosts may in part explain why virus substitution rates are higher than host substitution rates even though they utilize similar polymerases. For example, the Bo17 protein of bovine herpesvirus 4 represents a viral capture of the mammalian 2β-1,6-*N*-acetylglucosaminyltransferase-mucin protein.[168] As a phylogenetic analysis revealed that this gene was captured from the host after the split between cattle and African buffalo approximately 1.5 million years ago, it was possible to estimate that the viral gene had evolved 20 to 30 times faster than its cellular homolog.[168] Finally, for persistently infecting viruses, substitution rates may also differ between periods of intra- and interhost evolution. For example, HIV-1 substitution rates are higher within than among hosts.[165] This may be because intrahost HIV evolution is dominated by the positive selection of immune escape mutations or because some of the mutations that occur within hosts are purged at interhost transmission, thereby reducing the substitution rate. As noted earlier, it is also the case that substitution rates in viruses are strongly time dependent, such that they are elevated in the recent past because of the presence of transient deleterious mutations that have yet to be purged by purifying (negative) selection.[56] When comparing substitution rates among viruses, it is therefore critical to base studies on those sampled over approximately the same time frame.

Although most estimates of substitution rates suggest a fundamental division in virus evolution in which RNA viruses evolve rapidly and DNA viruses evolve slowly, there are a number of important exceptions (although there is currently no convincing evidence for anomalously slowly evolving RNA viruses). Most notably, most ssDNA viruses seem to exhibit substitution rates—often in the realm of 10^{-5} to 10^{-6} subs/site/year—that are lower than those of RNA viruses but more rapid than those of large DNA viruses and likely reflect the specifics of their background rates of mutation and replication. Such rate estimates have now been provided for carnivore[235] and human[196,234] parvoviruses, including involving comparisons utilizing ancient sequences sampled many hundreds of years before the present,[188] in some circoviruses,[75] and in plant geminiviruses.[58,257]

Nucleotide substitution rates also exhibit marked variation within large DNA viruses with some, particularly poxviruses, exhibiting such relatively high rates that they can be readily measured over the timescale of human observation and which likely reflects high background rates of mutation and replication. A case in point is VARV, in which estimates of the substitution rate fall between 10^{-6} and 10^{-5} subs/site/year, and hence are far higher than those observed in other large DNA viruses (particularly the herpesviruses) where evolutionary rates have been inferred.[60,76,238] VARV evolution is also characterized by a strongly linear relationship between genetic distance and time of sampling (i.e., measurable evolution) that is indicative of both a relatively constant molecular clock and a high substitution rate.[60,76] A similar picture can be painted for myxoma virus (MYXV). Sampling over 50 years in both Australia and Europe has revealed usually highly clock-like evolution on both continents, with substitution rates again in the realm of 10^{-5} subs/site/year.[136]

Natural Selection and Genetic Drift in Virus Evolution

Despite long-standing and continuing debates over whether natural selection or genetic drift is the more important process of evolutionary change at the molecular level, there is little doubt that viruses provide some of the very best examples of natural selection in action. The available literature contains numerous examples of natural selection for such properties as immune evasion (of antibody, T-cell, or innate responses), antiviral resistance, and the adaptation to new cell types and host species. The strength of these selection pressures is readily apparent in the fact that the genomes of large DNA viruses such as poxviruses and herpesviruses contain many genes dedicated to immune evasion, and that host genes that provide the strongest evidence for adaptive evolution are those involved in antiviral responses.[176] The frequency with which positive (i.e., Darwinian) selection is identified should come as no surprise as virus and host are locked in an evolutionary arms race.[231]

As there are numerous examples of positive selection for both RNA and DNA viruses, and since they are generally not contentious, we will not discuss them here. A more pressing question is what proportion of all the mutations that arise and are fixed in viral genomes are entirely free of natural selection and hence evolve in a strictly neutral manner, compared to the proportion that are fixed because they are selectively advantageous. Simple population genetic theory predicts that natural selection should be a potent force in viral evolution because of their often very large population sizes. Specifically, natural selection dominates molecular evolution when $Nes \gg 1$, where Ne is the effective population size, and s the selection coefficient (i.e., the fitness of the mutation in question). However, estimating these parameters is usually extremely difficult, such that the measures obtained are often only approximate. As a consequence, conclusively determining the role of natural selection versus genetic drift in viral evolution is inherently complex, although a number of important generalities can be made.

In the case of RNA viruses, and likely small DNA viruses, it is probable that few amino acid mutations are strictly neutral (i.e., $s = 0$), with most clearly deleterious. In particular, the small genomes of RNA viruses ensure there is extensive pleiotropy, epistasis, and multifunctionality such that there is little evolutionary elbow room. For example, mutagenesis studies of vesicular stomatitis virus (VSV) revealed that nearly 40% of random mutations are lethal, another 29% deleterious, a further 27% neutral, and only 4% beneficial.[227] A similar preponderance of deleterious compared to beneficial mutations was observed in poliovirus (Fig. 1.8).[3] Importantly, however, these estimates only relate to fitness effects in a single cell and a far larger proportion of mutations are expected to be deleterious

(or lethal) when considering the entirety of the virus life cycle. The same is also likely to be true of ssDNA viruses, which are also characterized by very small genome sizes. Accordingly, most estimates of the ratio of nonsynonymous (d_N) to synonymous (d_S) nucleotide substitutions per site (ratio d_N/d_S, a common measure of selection pressures, with $d_N/d_S = 1$ indicative of selective neutrality) in RNA and ssDNA viruses indicate that purifying selection is the most common evolutionary force (i.e., $d_N/d_S < 1$).[110,121] However, the case of large DNA viruses is far less clear, in large part because relatively few studies of their molecular evolution have been undertaken. One comparative study of d_N/d_S revealed weaker purifying selection in DNA than RNA viruses,[121] suggesting that the former may possess a class of neutrally evolving amino acid sites. Although the explanation for this effect is unclear, it may be a function of the large genome sizes in large dsDNA viruses, which allow more genetic redundancy through the presence of duplicated genes (see later). Alternatively, it may be indicative of greater levels of positive selection in DNA viruses, as also suggested by the high rates of nucleotide substitution documented in some cases.[76] Determining the exact nature of the selection pressures acting on large DNA viruses, including the fitness of individual mutations, is clearly an area where a combination of experimental study and evolutionary analysis will be of fundamental importance. Finally, in the same way that substitution rates are time dependent in viruses, so are inferences of selection pressures based on estimates of d_N/d_S.[56] In particular, the presence of transient deleterious mutations will tend to inflate

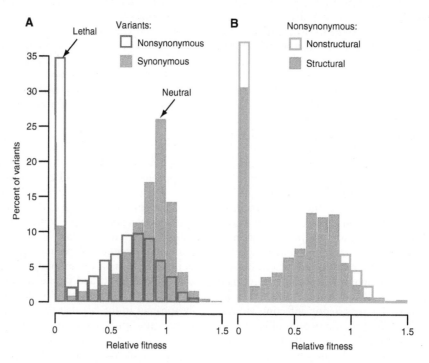

FIGURE 1.8 The distributions of fitness values among mutations in poliovirus revealed by a next-generation sequencing approach. A: The overall fitness of synonymous (*gray*) and nonsynonymous (*red*) mutations. **B:** The fitness of nonsynonymous mutations in structural (*gray*) and nonstructural (*blue*) genes. Note that the great majority of mutations fall into the deleterious class. (Adapted from Acevedo A, Brodsky L, Andino R. Mutational and fitness landscapes of an RNA virus revealed through population sequencing. *Nature* 2014;505:686–690, by permission of Springer Nature. Original figure kindly provided by Dr. Raul Andino.)

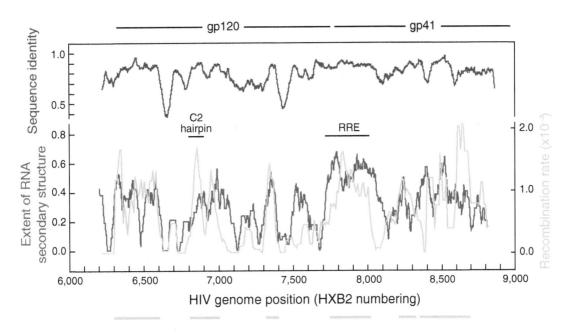

FIGURE 1.9 The relationship between recombination rate, sequence similarity, and RNA secondary structure in the *env* (envelope) gene of human immunodeficiency virus type 1 (HIV-1). Recombination rates are shown in *light blue*, conserved RNA structures in *dark blue*, and sequence similarity (identity) in *brown*. The location of recombination hotspots are marked by *light blue bars* at the bottom of the figure. (Adapted from Simon-Loriere E, Martin DP, Weeks KM, et al. RNA structures facilitate recombination-mediated gene swapping in HIV-1. *J Virol* 2010;84:12675–12682, which should be consulted for more details; by permission of the American Society for Microbiology. Figure kindly provided by Etienne Simon-Loriere.)

estimates of d_N/d_S toward the present, such that sequence comparisons should again only utilize sequences sampled over the time spans.

Obviously, the most likely class of neutral sites in viral genomes are those that do not code for proteins. For RNA viruses it is debatable how many nucleotide sites fall into this category, particularly as these viruses contain very few, if any, clear-cut examples of "functionless" noncoding RNA, such as pseudogenes and introns, and where RNA secondary structure may also impose selective constraints (Fig. 1.9). A similar story can be told for small DNA viruses, either single or double stranded, which can be considered as exemplars of genomic efficiency. Indeed, many small DNA viruses, such as circoviruses, parvoviruses, and hepadnaviruses, contain extensive overlapping reading frames, suggesting that they are under strong selective pressure to maximize the phenotypic diversity they can produce from a restricted genomic space.[39] Importantly, the existence of overlapping reading frames changes the selective regime acting on many nucleotide sites. In particular, synonymous sites in one reading frame are likely to be nonsynonymous in another, such that they must be subject to some sort of purifying selection. Similarly, although some pseudogenes are present in the genomes of large DNA viruses,[87] there are relatively few gene overlaps, and it is unclear whether they contain stretches of purely nonfunctional DNA. For example, although the genomes of herpesviruses and poxviruses contain many regions that do not code for protein (~5%–15% of the genome in the case of poxviruses), these may still encode promoters, transcription termination signals, functional RNA molecules, or other functional elements. One candidate for truly

nonfunctional sequences is the imperfect tandem repeat seen in the intergenic regions of some poxviruses and that exhibit various deletions and duplications. Understanding the potential functions, if any, of these noncoding regions is an important goal for the future.

Intra- and Interhost Diversity and Transmission Bottlenecks

After the selective coefficient of mutations, the second factor that determines the respective roles of natural selection and genetic drift in virus evolution is the effective population size (*Ne*), which is usually far lower than the census population size, *N*. Available data indicate that *Ne* fluctuates dramatically during the life cycle of most viruses. For all exogenous viruses, large values of *Ne* are most likely observed within an individual host following multiple rounds of replication and at the epidemiologic scale. Natural selection is expected to be an efficient force in these cases. For example, perhaps 10^{10} virions are produced by HIV-1 replication per day in every infected individual,[205] with some 10^7 human hosts HIV infected on a global scale. In addition, the burst sizes of many acute viruses will be large, such that within-host values of *Ne* are expected to be high for at least some parts of the virus life cycle. The exception to this rule may be latent viruses, in which effective population sizes are often likely to be relatively small, reflecting a lack of active replication.

Conversely, low values of *Ne*, reflecting the time when genetic drift is strongest and perhaps overriding the action of natural selection, will generally occur at interhost transmission. At this point in the virus life cycle, a major population bottleneck may be a common occurrence, although this is also likely to be at least in part determined by the mode of transmission and hence the infecting dose; for example, vertical transmission (wide bottleneck) might be expected to be associated with the transfer of more viruses between hosts than sexual transmission (narrow bottleneck).[155] In some cases, including HIV-1 and influenza virus, it is possible that the transmission bottleneck is so extensive that new infections are initiated by a single virus particle,[2,79] which would obviously result in a major stochastic effect on virus genetic diversity. Similarly, experimental studies of plant viruses have commonly revealed the existence of extensive population bottlenecks, both at interhost transmission and as the virus moves through an individual plant[6,221] and which may also be true of vector-borne viruses of animals.[246] In these cases, the stochastic effects of genetic drift are expected to be strong, even to the extent of allowing many slightly deleterious mutations to rise to appreciable frequencies, although there have been few experiments to address this issue. Interestingly, other sequencing studies have suggested that interhost transmission might be associated with relatively wide population bottlenecks. For example, multiple viral lineages passed among horses during experimental transmissions with equine influenza virus,[189] while the occurrence of mixed infections in viruses such as influenza[94] and dengue[1] also suggests that transmission bottlenecks might be relatively broad in some cases. Overall, it is evident that a great deal more work is needed to fully understand the nature and scale of population bottlenecks in viruses, particularly those that accompany interhost transmission, and what this means for the relative frequencies of natural selection versus genetic drift, and for evolutionary processes like complementation (see below) that require the transmission of multiple virus particles (Fig. 1.10).

Evolutionary Interactions: Epistasis, Defecting Interfering Particles, and Complementation

A common assumption in many evolutionary studies is that nucleotide sites evolve independently. However, this assumption is often highly simplistic as epistatic interactions among mutations are a regular occurrence in viral genomes. Not only might such epistasis be of great functional importance, such as that resulting from RNA or protein secondary structure (see Fig. 1.9), but it may also tell us a great deal about the basic mechanics of virus evolution.

Epistatic effects can be antagonistic (positive), in which case they reduce the effect of combined mutations on fitness, or synergistic (negative), in which case they increase this effect. Although determining the nature of epistasis represents a major technical challenge because it entails a precise measurement of the combined fitness effects of multiple mutations, there is strong evidence for epistasis in viruses, and particularly in RNA viruses where experimental studies are rather easier to perform. Importantly, most of the epistatic interactions determined to date in RNA viruses are antagonistic rather than synergistic,[24,143,228] which has major implications for understanding why recombination evolved in viruses (see later). Similar epistatic effects have been observed in small ssDNA viruses.[204]

It is useful to discuss the extent of epistasis in the context of mutational robustness, which is a way in which phenotypes can be "protected" against the adverse effects of deleterious mutation pressure. Robustness can be generated in a number of ways, including through genetic redundancies such as duplicated genes, through the creation of neutral spaces as might be contained in RNA or protein secondary structure, or by

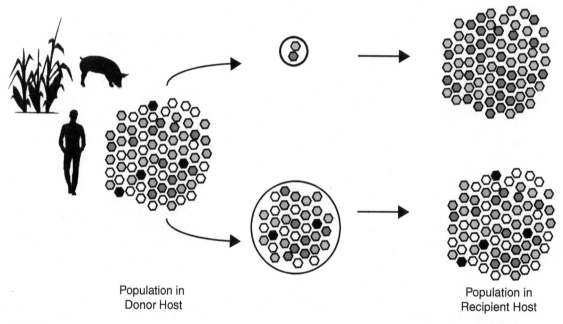

Population in Donor Host

Population in Recipient Host

FIGURE 1.10 The effect of transmission bottlenecks on viral diversity. In a variety of hosts (with the examples of humans, pigs, plant shown here), severe population bottlenecks (*top*) limit the size and diversity of a virus population and hence greatly alter their composition. In contrast, the relatively large populations that pass through looser bottlenecks (*bottom*) allow for the transmission of rarer variants, thereby impacting onward virus evolution, and facilitate virus–virus interactions. (From McCrone JT, Lauring AS. Genetic bottlenecks in intraspecies virus transmission. *Curr Opin Virol* 2018;28:20–25, by permission of Elsevier.)

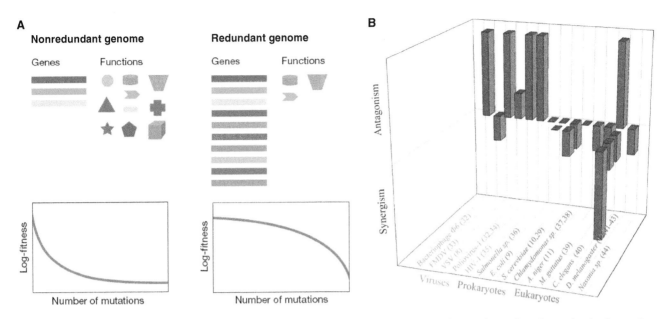

FIGURE 1.11 Redundancy and epistasis in viruses. A: Differing properties of robust (redundant) and nonrobust (nonredundant) genetic systems. In robust genetic systems that contain many genes, which may include large DNA viruses, the presence of genetic redundancy means that individual mutations have weak fitness effects and interact through synergistic epistasis. In contrast, in nonrobust systems such as RNA viruses and single-stranded DNA (ssDNA) viruses, there are few genes, and hence little genetic redundancy, so that single genes have multiple functions and single mutations have strong fitness effects. This results in antagonistic epistasis. (From Elena SF, Carrasco P, Daròs JA, et al. Mechanisms of genetic robustness in RNA viruses. *EMBO Rep* 2006;7:168–173, by permission of EMBO Press.) **B:** The type of epistasis seen in a variety of organisms: long bars, significant epistasis; short bars, nonsignificant epistasis; flat bars, no evidence for epistasis. For details see reference[225]. (From Sanjuán R, Elena SF. Epistasis correlates to genomic complexity. *Proc Natl Acad Sci U S A* 2006;103:14402–14405, by permission of the US National Academy of Sciences.)

complementation.[48,182] There is a strong relationship between the level of genetic redundancy and epistasis, such that antagonistic epistasis is most common in genomes that are characterized by little redundancy and weak robustness, as is the case for RNA and ssDNA viruses (Fig. 1.11).[66,224] Hence, when mutations occur in viruses with small genomes, which contain many overlapping reading frames and functions, they will tend to repeatedly damage the same functions, leading to antagonistic epistasis.[264] Conversely, synergistic epistasis is more commonplace in larger DNA-based organisms that exhibit a greater level of genetic redundancy and robustness, of which duplicated genes are a good example, which allows them to tolerate a certain number of deleterious mutations (Fig. 1.11). Where large DNA viruses fall on this spectrum is uncertain, as there have been no experimental measures of the rate and sign of epistasis in these organisms to date. However, that multigene families are a common occurrence in large DNA viruses, resulting in a level of genetic redundancy, suggests that most of the epistatic interactions that occur in these viruses will be synergistic.

While individual mutations in viruses can interact through epistasis, whole virus genomes can interact through the presence of defective interfering (DI) particles and complementation.[256] DI particles are a common observation in many virus families[119] and have been implicated in a number of virological traits, including persistence.[219] DI particles often harbor large genomic deletions and compete with fully functional viruses during replication because they are able to replicate faster. DI particles have a number of interesting evolutionary consequences, although these will usually be short term. First, the high frequency of DI particles further illustrates the high rate

at which deleterious mutations are produced in virus populations, including large-scale deletions. Second, as noted later, the polymerase error process that generates DI particles also has important implications for the evolution of recombination in viruses. Third, because they are able to replicate more rapidly than full-length viral genomes, DI particles may theoretically inhibit the spread of the advantageous mutations that are present on full-length viral genomes, if only transiently.

DI particles are likely to be maintained in virus populations through complementation, which is predicted to be a common occurrence at high multiplicity of infection (i.e., in the absence of large-scale transmission bottlenecks), and which has been relatively frequently documented in both RNA[88,256] and DNA viruses.[40,174,222] Perhaps the most interesting evolutionary consequence of complementation is that it allows deleterious mutations to persist for extended periods.[83] Traditionally, the evidence for complementation came from *in vitro* studies, such that DI particles were thought to survive for just a few generations and therefore had little long-term evolutionary consequence. However, it is now clear that complementation may be frequent in nature[82] and may extend over very long time periods.[1,134] As a consequence, complementation may play more of a role in virus evolution than is usually envisioned,[153] particularly in the context of how deleterious and advantageous mutations interact with each other, although this will evidently require further study.

The Evolution of Viral Recombination
A combination of comparative genomics and experimental study has provided growing evidence for the importance

of recombination, and its sister process reassortment, in viral genomes, although recombination rates vary substantially among viruses. At the sequence level recombination is commonly observed and displayed as incongruent phylogenetic trees, in which phylogenies inferred on either side of a recombination breakpoint differ significantly in topology, reflecting the contrasting evolutionary histories of these gene regions. Although such phylogenetic approaches can be biased in two ways—false positives caused by mixed infection or experimental error[25] and that tree-based methods only detect recombination when there is measurable sequence diversity—they represent a simple means to detect recombination in a wide range of viruses.

Mechanisms of recombination differ markedly between viruses, reflecting the very different types of replication strategy employed, although all require co-infection of a single cell by two or more viruses and it is likely that rates of cellular co-infection vary markedly among viruses. In the case of dsDNA viruses, recombination likely occurs in a manner analogous to that observed in other DNA-based organisms, although the precise mechanisms of recombination are not known in all cases. Hence, recombination will involve the occurrence and repair of double-stranded breaks and, in the case of large dsDNA viruses, the presence of multiple recombination enzymes.[125] Recombination appears to be particularly commonplace in poxviruses, an apparent outcome of the form of DNA strand invasion used in replication,[70,72] as well as in herpesviruses.[27] Recombination in large DNA viruses can be both homologous, in that it occurs at regions exhibiting strong sequence identity, and nonhomologous, involving divergent gene sequences (usually occurring as LGT) and can occur at the intra- and interspecific levels.[254] It therefore plays a major role in shaping genomic architecture.[175] For example, in poxviruses recombination may be more commonplace at the extremities of the genome, as these contain most of the species-specific genes, than in the central genomic regions that are conserved among viruses.[69,175] Less is known about the mechanics of recombination in ssDNA viruses, although it is likely to occur as a consequence of the rolling circle replication employed by these viruses,[232] which may both determine the distribution of recombination breakpoints[258] and result in frequent genome rearrangements, as in the case of Torque teno (TT) virus.[153]

Evolutionary aspects of recombination are better studied in RNA viruses. Recombination in this case occurs by two rather different mechanisms. The first, sometimes called RNA recombination, occurs when two viruses co-infect a single host cell and a hybrid molecule is produced, most likely through a process of *copy-choice replication*,[146] although other mechanisms have been proposed. Under the copy-choice model, the viral polymerase is thought to jump templates during negative strand synthesis, generating a chimeric RNA molecule.[146] Although this process is usually homologous, template switching can also occur among genomic regions that do not share sequence similarity. In theory, RNA recombination can occur in any type of RNA virus, irrespective of their genome structure or orientation, although rates vary substantially among viruses (see later). The second process of recombination in RNA viruses is reassortment, which only occurs in RNA viruses that possess segmented genomes, such that a progeny virus packages segments with different ancestries. Rates of reassortment also vary markedly among RNA viruses, from very frequent in the case of influenza A virus,[161] in which it is likely to be a common occurrence during individual infections, while the process is far less so in the case of hantaviruses.[193]

Clearly, recombination can be of great evolutionary importance for viruses[245] and has been associated with such features as the evasion of host immunity,[164] the development of antiviral resistance,[195] the ability to infect new hosts,[117] escape from RNAi,[4] increases in virulence,[137] and even the creation of new viruses.[262] As a consequence, it is important to document cases of viral recombination and reveal the determinants of this process. However, the occasional occurrence of beneficial traits arising from recombination, including those documented in experimental studies focusing on single systems, does not necessarily mean that recombination evolved for this purpose, as recombination is as likely to break up beneficial genotypic configurations as create them. Indeed, explaining why recombination evolved in general is one of the outstanding questions in evolutionary biology.

For viruses, clues for the reasons underlying the evolution of recombination are provided by the huge variation in recombination rates, from effectively clonal (i.e., asexual) as seen in some single-stranded ssRNA− viruses,[245] to cases in which the recombination rate per nucleotide exceeds that of mutation. This extensive rate variation is particularly true of RNA viruses. The most common theory for the evolution of recombination across living systems as a whole is that it functions as a form of sexual reproduction in viruses and as such has been selectively optimized to either create advantageous genetic configurations or remove deleterious mutations (Fig. 1.12). However, this seems unlikely as high rates of recombination are only seen in some viruses, with picornaviruses a good example, such that high recombination rates cannot be universally advantageous.[245] This rather patchy distribution sits in marked contrast to theories for the evolution of sex in eukaryotes, the aim of which is to explain common recombination and sporadic asexuality.[218] Similarly, the patchy distribution of recombination means that it is unlikely to universally have evolved as a form of repair.[178]

It is obvious that recombination allows viruses to create potentially beneficial genetic configurations more rapidly than asexual populations, and there are many documented cases in viruses in which recombination has been associated with the generation of advantageous characteristics, such as drug-resistant genotypes. However, there are a number of viruses where rates of recombination are very low but where adaptive evolution is extremely common, with hepatitis C virus (HCV) a good case in point.[217] Hence, it may be that many RNA viruses are able to create a sufficient number of beneficial genotypes through mutation alone to offset the need for recombination.

As well as generating advantageous genotypes, recombination disassociates advantageous from linked deleterious mutations,[218] and prevents *clonal interference*. The latter describes a competition between beneficial mutations as they go to fixation in asexual populations, such that their rate of adaptation is retarded compared to that of sexual populations. Although both these processes are likely to occur in virus populations,[180] their overall importance is unclear.

The second advantage of recombination over purely clonal evolution is that it facilitates the efficient removal of deleterious mutations. This is often called the *mutational deterministic hypothesis* and is a much debated theory for the evolution of sex

Evolutionary Benefit of Recombination

(1) Creation of beneficial genotypes:

Recombination increases the rate of adaptive evolution compared to clonal evolution. It also disassociates advantageous from deleterious mutations, allowing the former to spread.

(2) Purging of deleterious mutations:

Recombination enables deleterious mutations to be placed into a single genome which can be removed by purifying selection. This can be selectively favored if deleterious mutations occur at a high rate (i.e., $U > 1$) and interact through synergistic epistasis.

Schematic Representation

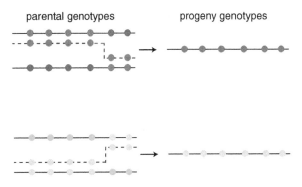

FIGURE 1.12 Potential evolutionary benefits of viral recombination (and reassortment) that might be favored by natural selection and that are commonly invoked in discussions of the evolution of sex. Accordingly, recombination can either (1) create advantageous genetic configurations (*red circles*), and also disassociate advantageous from deleterious mutations, or (2) purge deleterious mutations (*green circles*) by placing them in a single individual, which can be removed by purifying selection. In both cases, the *dashed line* denotes the recombination event. The rate of deleterious mutations per genome replication is denoted U. (Adapted from Simon-Loriere E, Holmes EC. Why do RNA viruses recombine? *Nat Rev Microbiol* 2011;9:617–626, which should be consulted for more details, by permission of Springer Nature.)

in a wide range of species.[135] The central idea is that rather than many individuals (or genomes) carrying deleterious mutations, which would have a major negative impact on fitness, recombination allows these injurious mutations to be placed in a single individual whose selective removal greatly reduces fitness costs. A related theory is that of Muller's ratchet, which describes a progressive decrease in fitness due to the gradual accumulation of deleterious mutations in asexual populations of finite size and where genetic drift accelerates the loss of mutation-free individuals. Muller's ratchet has been observed in laboratory populations of RNA viruses[35,36,54] and may play some role when clonal viruses experience small population sizes, such as during transmission bottlenecks, although its effects are likely to be negated when viruses reach large population sizes. Importantly, sequence comparisons suggest that the burden of deleterious mutation is high for all RNA viruses studied, irrespective of background recombination rate.[212] Hence, it is not recombination that saves RNA viruses from an excessive mutational load as predicted under the deleterious mutation hypothesis, but their large population sizes that provide a form of *population robustness* that offsets the effects of deleterious mutation.[66]

An opposing theory for the evolutionary origin of viral recombination is that rather than being optimized by natural selection as a form of sexual reproduction, it is in fact a mechanistic by-product of differing types of genome architecture, replication strategy, and polymerase processivity.[245] Importantly, however, this does not exclude recombination rates then being selectively optimized in individual viruses to increase other aspects of viral fitness.[271] The main evidence for this theory is that there is an apparent association between recombination frequency and virus genome structure. Hence, recombination is relatively frequent in some retroviruses, and as reassortment in viruses with segmented genomes. Far more variable recombination rates are observed in ssRNA+ viruses; for example, frequently in coronaviruses and picornaviruses, sporadically in flaviviruses, and currently not documented in the *Leviviridae* and *Narnaviridae* (although this may simply be a function of sample size). Finally, recombination is far less common in ssRNA– viruses. An informative example of the disparity of recombination rates is provided by a comparison of HIV-1 and HCV. In the former, recombination rates have been estimated at between 1.38×10^{-4} and 1.4×10^{-5} recombination events per site, per generation,[192,243] while the equivalent estimates for HCV are only 4×10^{-8}.[217] Most DNA viruses studied to date seem to experience relatively high levels of recombination (including through LGT in the case of large DNA viruses), although there have been few attempts to estimate rates of recombination relative to those of mutation.[27]

In each case described previously, the frequency of recombination seems to reflect the genome structure of the virus in question.[245] Hence, the high recombination rates of retroviruses are likely a function of the fact that their virions carry two RNA molecules, such that *heterozygous* progeny will be produced when viruses with different ancestries are packaged together. Copy-choice recombination, which is common in RNA viruses, may then produce genetically distinct progeny during reverse transcription. That heterozygous viral progeny cannot be produced when the genomic material is present as a single molecule obviously acts to reduce recombination rates in most RNA viruses. However, in some cases specific genome organizations can facilitate frequent recombination. Case in point are the coronaviruses, such as murine hepatitis virus (MHV), where up to 25% of the progeny of coinfected cells may be recombinant. Such a high recombination rate reflects the mechanisms controlling gene expression in coronaviruses, in which discontinuous transcription leads to the production of subgenomic RNAs through a copy-choice mechanism.[230] An even more dramatic example of how replication strategy and genome organization may shape recombination rate occurs in the ssRNA– viruses, in which recombination is relatively infrequent. In these viruses the genomic and antigenomic RNA molecules are quickly bound to multiple nucleoprotein subunits, as well as to other proteins, to form ribonucleoprotein (RNP) complexes from which viral replication and transcription can proceed.

This tight complex of RNA and protein necessarily limits the probability of hybridization of complementary sequences between the nascent and acceptor nucleic acid molecules, and hence the probability of template switching.[245] This likely explains why phylogenetic studies undertaken to date have revealed relatively few cases of recombination in ssRNA− viruses.[10,267]

The RNA Virus Quasispecies

One of the most debated issues in the study of virus evolution is whether RNA viruses evolve according to a particular population genetic model known as the *quasispecies*.[110] In some respects, this merely reflects a semantic point about how best to describe the intrahost genetic variation commonly seen in RNA viruses. However, a far more important issue, and the true essence of the quasispecies debate, is how natural selection acts on virus genomes.

Quasispecies theory was originally developed by Manfred Eigen and colleagues as a model of the evolution of self-replicating RNA molecules that are strong candidates for the first replicators on earth.[64,65] The theory was first applied to RNA viruses after genetic variation was observed in a number of experimental systems, beginning with the bacteriophage Qβ.[50] Since this time, the quasispecies has become a popular and common descriptor of intrahost RNA virus evolution, particularly because widespread gene sequencing has uncovered abundant genetic diversity. However, because the theory is based on high mutation rates (see later), it should not be applied to large DNA viruses where error frequencies are lower and hence there is no evidence for quasispecies evolution.

Although commonly used simply as a synonym for genetic variation, the quasispecies in fact describes a specific mutation–selection balance. Mutation–selection balances are commonly invoked in population genetics and describe an evolutionary equilibrium between the generation of new mutations and their removal by purifying selection.[91] The mutation–selection balance in quasispecies theory is based on the occurrence of an extremely high mutation rate, which ensures that the frequency of any variant in the virus population is a function of both its individual fitness *plus* the frequency at which it is produced by the erroneous replication of other variants in the population that are linked to it in mutational (i.e., sequence) space. This *mutational coupling* (which should be distinguished from complementation) means that viral genomes are not independent entities, such that natural selection favors the entire population as opposed to individual variants. In this manner the group, rather than the individual, becomes the unit of selection.[9,65]

The central tenet of quasispecies theory is thus that natural selection acts on the viral population as a whole, rather than on individual variants. As a consequence, the entire quasispecies evolves to maximize its average fitness, rather than that of individual variants as is the case in other population genetic models. The most interesting outcome of this particular evolutionary process is that low-fitness variants can sometimes outcompete those of higher individual fitness if the former are surrounded by beneficial mutational neighbors. This is sometimes referred to as the *quasispecies effect* or the *survival of the flattest*,[265] and describes a situation in which a population whose component mutants have a similar mean fitness can outcompete a population that has a lower average fitness even

though it contains variants of higher individual fitness. Under classic *survival of the fittest* population genetic models, the individual high-fitness variants are selectively favored, whereas under *survival of the flattest* (i.e., quasispecies) models, the flatter population is selectively superior as it possesses a higher mean fitness (Fig. 1.13). This can also be thought of as a form of mutational robustness.

A key component of quasispecies theory is that intrahost populations of RNA viruses harbor abundant genetic diversity. There is no doubt that this specific aspect of quasispecies theory is correct, and even so for short-term acute infections, as intrahost genetic variation is commonly observed in RNA viruses.[110] In particular, deep sequencing studies of individual virus populations have revealed extensive genetic diversity, with HIV-1,[33] HCV,[177] foot-and-mouth disease virus (FMDV),[270] dengue virus,[199,200] and influenza virus[171] serving as good examples, although a multitude now exist. Importantly, however, although the observation of intrahost genetic variation is a necessary criterion for an RNA virus population to be thought of as a quasispecies, it is not sufficient in itself as intrahost genetic diversity is expected under any evolutionary model where mutation rates are high. Hence, the quasispecies is not simply another word for intrahost genetic variation.

Both *in silico* and *in vitro* studies have provided some evidence for the existence of quasispecies dynamics defined correctly. As an example of the former, computational studies using *digital organisms* revealed that the survival of the flattest could be induced at very high mutation rates.[42,265] However, as the mutation rates involved were always higher than one mutation per genome replication, it is uncertain whether such mutation rates could ever be attained for sustained periods in RNA viruses in nature. Similar results have been obtained from some experimental analyses of RNA virus evolution. Studies using both viroids of plants and VSV showed that viral populations with lower replication rates were able to outcompete those with higher replication rates, as expected under the quasispecies model, although this again requires the elevation of mutation rate (by either chemical mutagens or ultraviolet C light) to levels that may not commonly occur in RNA viruses in nature.[41,225] Additional experimental evidence for the existence of RNA virus quasispecies was the observation that high-fitness clones of bacteriophage ϕf6 evolved to a lower mean fitness because their mutational neighbors were of low fitness.[31] More controversial evidence was that strains of poliovirus that possessed higher fidelity than the wild type, such that the virus population carried less genetic diversity, were unable to infect the full range of tissues that are associated with severe disease.[259] While this was suggested to mean that quasispecies dynamics might be a central determinant of viral pathogenesis,[259] it has also been suggested that this observation more likely reflects a trade-off between replication speed and fidelity.[79]

Another class of experimental studies that have been cited in support of the quasispecies model involves lethal mutagenesis. This entails treating virus populations with mutagens, such as 5-fluorouracil and ribavirin, that increase the error rate to the extent that so many deleterious mutations are produced that fit genotypes are never able to regenerate themselves. Although lethal mutagenesis can clearly result in virus extinction, especially if mutagens are used in combination with more standard antiviral inhibitors,[8] the basis of this effect is more

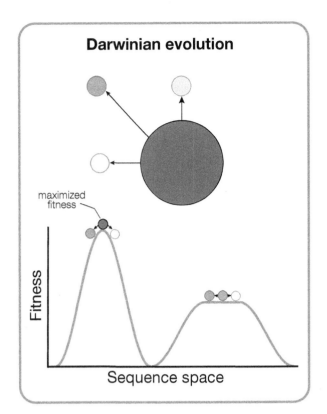
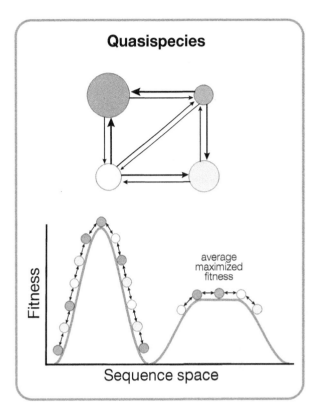

FIGURE 1.13 Comparing "Darwinian" and quasispecies models of RNA virus evolution. In the Darwinian virus population, natural selection favors the single variant with the highest individual fitness (*circle shown in red*). Genetic variants of lower fitness (*colored blue, green, and yellow*) are produced by mutation at a relatively low rate. In contrast, under the quasispecies model, very high mutation rates mean that individual variants (represented by different colors) experience a mutational coupling. This, in turn, means that the viral population will evolve as a single unit, with natural selection acting on the population as a whole (rather than on individual variants), maximizing mean fitness. Accordingly, the mutational landscape greatly impacts virus evolution. In the top part of the figure the circle sizes represent relative fitness values, whereas they are drawn to equivalent sizes in the bottom part of the figure. (From Geoghegan JL, Holmes EC. Evolutionary virology at 40. *Genetics* 2018;210(4):1151–1162. https://doi.org/10.1534/genetics.118.301556)

complex. Quasispecies theory predicts that virus extinction in this instance occurs because of an *error catastrophe*, which is the point at which the fittest genotype suffers so many deleterious mutations that it cannot sustain itself in the population (i.e., it has breached an *error threshold*). However, another interpretation is that the virus has instead crossed an *extinction threshold*, the point at which deleterious mutations accumulate faster than they can be eliminated by natural selection, which will also lead to population extinction.[30] Importantly, error catastrophe requires a fundamental shift in viral genotype that is independent of population size, whereas extinction threshold entails a major decline in viral population size.

Studies of RNA virus evolution based on the comparative analysis of gene sequence data have provided less support for the existence of quasispecies. Indeed, there is currently no clear evidence from comparative genomics that selection acts on groups rather than individual variants in natural populations of RNA viruses, although this may reflect the fact that even with the most sophisticated tools of gene sequence analysis it is difficult to discern the effects of all but the most strongly favored and disfavored variants. For example, the deep sequencing of intra- and interhost diversity in dengue virus provided strong evidence for host adaptation, with the same virus mutations appearing independently across multiple patients.[200] Importantly,

however, there was no evidence for the quasispecies expectation that fitness was impacted by mutational neighborhood and hence no evidence for quasispecies dynamics. In other cases, such as influenza virus, the adaptive evolution required under quasispecies theory appears to be of limited importance within individual hosts, with random genetic drift and large-scale population bottlenecks playing a more important role.[170] Again, though, it is arguable that natural selection is so strong in these cases as to obscure any quasispecies effect, and that the latter model is a far better description of mutations subject to weaker positive selection as most natural selection will be in nature. This is clearly a major area for further study.

Given a sufficiently high mutation rate, quasispecies is a viable and interesting evolutionary model that has undoubtedly helped introduce evolutionary ideas into virology. However, it is less clear whether the quasispecies concept can be successfully applied to RNA viruses in nature, where to date there has been no convincing evidence for its occurrence. This does not necessarily mean that the quasispecies model is wrong, but rather that too few RNA viruses have been studied in sufficient detail through a combination of deep sequencing and precise fitness assays to determine whether they form quasispecies, exemplified by a process of natural selection acting on the virus population as a whole.

PATTERNS AND PROCESSES OF VIRAL GENOME EVOLUTION

The Evolution of Virus Genome Size

Viruses possess a remarkable range of genome sizes (Fig. 1.14). This is especially so in the case of DNA viruses in which genome sizes range from less than 2,000 nt in circoviruses (ssDNA) to a remarkable 2,473,870 nt (comprising 2,394 ORFs) in the case of *Pandoravirus salinus* (dsDNA),[148,208] hence covering over three orders of magnitude, although all ssDNA viruses have genomes less than 11,000 nt in length. A far narrower range of genome sizes is observed in RNA viruses. The smallest RNA virus currently known is HDV at only about 1,700 nt, while the largest RNA viruses are from the order *Nidovirales*, and can possess genome sizes over 40,000 nt,[220] and it is possible that ongoing metagenomic surveys will eventually uncover far larger viruses. Interestingly, there does not appear to be a major difference in genome size between segmented and unsegmented RNA viruses,[110] with, for example, the unsegmented *Nidovirales* possessing larger genomes than all segmented RNA viruses, and metagenomic studies have shown that invertebrate viruses often possess longer genomes than do their vertebrate counterparts.[240,241] This strongly suggests that genome segmentation has not evolved as a way to increase virus genome sizes. Similarly, metagenomic studies have revealed that in the case of some RNA virus families such as the *Flaviviridae,* the genomes of viruses are longer and more complex than those of their vertebrate counterparts,[241] although the reasons why are again unclear.

A variety of theories have been proposed to explain the evolution of genome sizes in viruses. One theory is that virus genome sizes are constrained by the maximum size of the genetic material that can be contained within a single capsid protein,[274] and there does appear to be a strong allometric relationship between genome and virion sizes in viruses, although what drives what is difficult to resolve.[45] However, the huge range of genome sizes, especially in DNA viruses, argues against this. The genome content of large DNA viruses in part reflects often frequent LGT and gene duplication (see later). In particular, the central part of the genome of many large DNA viruses is composed of a set of core genes that control basic biochemical functions, including replication, while the outer, flanking genes distinguish individual viruses and are often responsible for modulating immunity, host range, and virulence, and it is

these that have often been captured from host genomes. This process of gene birth and depth has resulted in a great variation in genome sizes, with, for example, a massive increase in genome size from the ancestral NCLDV to those circulating today.[125] This evolutionary process, combined with the discovery of the giant viruses of algae and amoeba, suggests that there are unlikely to be strict constraints against genome sizes in large DNA viruses. Similarly, that bacteriophages are able to transiently carry large parts of bacterial genomes, which evidently plays a key role in LGT among bacterial species,[197] also argues against strict constraints on genome size.

However, it is also the case that certain structural features must constrain genome sizes to some extent. First, longer viral genomes are expected to cause an increase in replication times, which may be disadvantageous. Second, in the case of RNA viruses, it is possible that the difficulty in unwinding potentially long regions of dsRNA during replication inhibits the maximum genome size attainable.[215] For example, it has been argued that the unwinding of dsRNA in RNA viruses with genomes greater than 6,000 nt is controlled by the presence of a helicase (HEL) domain,[98] the evolution of which allowed RNA viruses to greatly increase their genome size.[97]

A more plausible explanation for the range of viral genome sizes is that they reflect background mutation rates. As noted previously, there is a fundamental relationship between mutation rate and genome size that seemingly applies to all living systems (Fig. 1.7). Accordingly, dsDNA viruses with relatively low mutation rates will be able to attain relatively large genome sizes, while the small genomes observed in RNA and ssDNA viruses reflect the higher error rates seen in these systems. Perhaps paradoxically, the idea that mutation rates set genome size can be extended to explain the very large (by RNA virus standards) genomes seen in the *Nidovirales*. The major part of the genomes of these families is composed of a large (>20,000 nt) replicase gene that contains an ExoN domain encoding a 3′ to 5′ exoribonuclease. As this ExoN domain is homologous to cellular proteins of the DEDD superfamily of exonucleases that are involved in proofreading and repair,[179] it is possible that *Nidovirales* reduce their error rate through some sort of proofreading activity of the 3′ to 5′ exoribonucleases.[61] This, in turn, will reduce mutational load and allow larger genome sizes.

A final important difference between RNA and dsDNA viruses with respect to genome size is that the former (as well as ssDNA viruses) frequently utilize overlapping open reading frames, whereas these are less common in the latter (although, e.g., the M065R and M066R genes of the poxvirus myxoma virus overlap by ~100 bp). Belshaw et al.[16] noted 819 cases of gene overlap among 701 RNA virus genomes; 56% of the viruses examined possessed some degree of overlap, which nearly always involved a +1 or −1 frame shift. In addition, RNA viruses with longer genomes tend to show less gene overlap than do those with shorter genomes.[16] Although the exact evolutionary processes responsible for the evolution of overlapping reading frames are uncertain, they clearly allow an increase in the number of proteins and hence the amount of protein diversity encoded by a single nucleotide sequence.

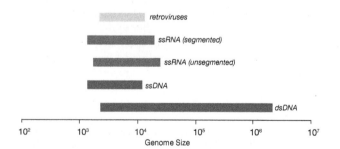

FIGURE 1.14 Currently known distribution of genome sizes (bp) in RNA and DNA viruses. Note the similarity in (small) genome sizes between RNA viruses, retroviruses, and single-stranded DNA (ssDNA) viruses.

The Evolution of Genome Organization

It is arguable that viruses contain a greater diversity of genome structures and organizations than any other group of organisms. As well as the obvious division into RNA viruses, DNA viruses, and retroviruses, distinct genome structures include viruses in positive and negative sense orientations, those with single or double strands of the nucleic acid, those with single or multiple segments (which are usually multicomponent in the case of ssRNA+ viruses from plants), those that utilize subgenomic RNAs, and those like the coronaviruses that utilize ribosomal frame shifting. A key challenge for evolutionary virologists is therefore to explain why such a diverse array of structures exists.

One of the most debated issues with respect to the evolution of genome structures in RNA viruses is why some are segmented and others not. As noted previously, one theory for the evolution of segmentation is that it evolved as a way of facilitating reassortment, although this seems unlikely.[245] Similarly, there is no good evidence that segmentation allows the evolution of longer genomes. Another possibility is that genome segmentation, particularly in the case of multicomponent viruses, resulted from the intracellular selection for smaller RNAs that, because they are shorter, would have had a replication advantage over their full-length counterparts.[191] However, this theory cannot easily explain why multicomponent viruses are nearly all restricted to plants (although this may change with more extensive sampling).

A competing theory for the evolution of genome segmentation is that it allows greater control over gene expression.

Clearly, all RNA viruses need to control the levels of each protein they produce. For many ssRNA+ viruses such control occurs at the level of translation as this is necessarily the first step in the virus life cycle. Additional constraints faced by viruses of this type are that eukaryotic ribosomes only recognize the 5' regions of mRNA molecules, so that internal start codons are not utilized, and mRNAs are usually monocistronic.[110] Many ssRNA+ viruses therefore simply translate a single polyprotein that is proteolytically cleaved into individual protein products, which may represent the ancestral type of genome organization in ssRNA viruses. Although this genomic structure allows efficient replication, similar amounts of each protein product are produced, so that there is relatively little control over gene expression. As a consequence, other ssRNA+ viruses have evolved a variety of more complex ways to control gene expression, all of which can be envisioned as ways of dividing the viral genome into individual *transcriptional units*, within which transcription (and translation) can occur at different rates. Such a division can involve the creation of multiple genome segments, the utilization of subgenomic RNAs, and the use of a −1 ribosomal frameshift to produce multiple open reading frames as in the case of the *Nidovirales*[110] (Fig. 1.15).

The situation is rather different in the case of ssRNA− viruses. Because ssRNA− viruses by necessity transcribe their

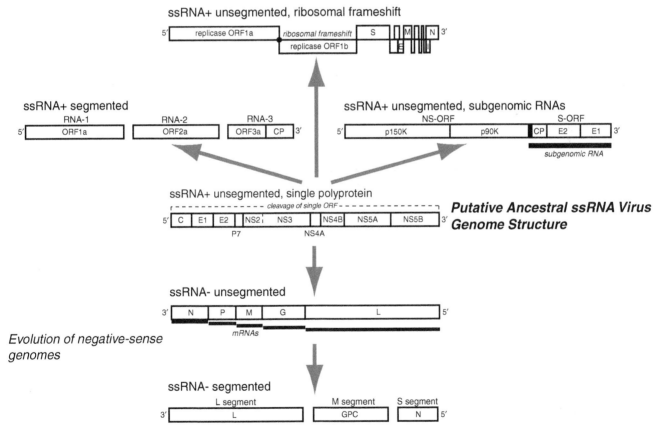

FIGURE 1.15 Schematic representation of the major types of genome organization and replication strategy in RNA viruses and a scenario for their evolutionary origin. Each of these organizations results in a different way to control gene expression, although they should not be considered as mutually exclusive. Unsegmented single-stranded RNA-positive (ssRNA+) viruses that produce a single polyprotein are considered here to be the ancestral type, although this is debatable. Gene and segment sizes are drawn approximately to scale within each of the six organizations, but not among them, and the 5' and 3' terminal sequences have been excluded for ease of presentation. (From Holmes EC. *The Evolution and Emergence of RNA Viruses*. Oxford: Oxford University Press, 2009, by permission of Oxford University Press.)

genomes before translating them, some control over gene expression can occur at the level of transcription; multiple mRNAs can be produced and there will be a transcriptional gradient from the first (i.e., 3′) mRNA, of which most is produced, to the last (5′) mRNA, of which least is produced. It is therefore possible that the ability to better control gene expression, itself through the control of transcription, represents the reason that negative-sense genomes evolved in the first instance. In this respect, it is significant that the genomes of unsegmented ssRNA– viruses possess a highly conserved gene order, cluster together on polymerase phylogenies, and can easily be classified within the *Mononegavirales*. Moreover, this genome order seems to be a function of the amount of each protein product required, such that the 3′ gene encodes the nucleocapsid while the 5′ gene encodes the RNA polymerase, again suggesting that it is an adaptation to facilitate the control of gene expression.

It is also possible that some of the variation in the genome sizes of RNA viruses reflects the action of gene duplication. Indeed, gene duplication is one of the most important processes of genome evolution in eukaryotes and is a simple way to create new genes that, following subsequent mutation and adaptation, can exhibit different but related functions, which often appear as multigene families. However, it is striking how rarely this process has been observed in RNA viruses,[110] although more examples are being recovered from expansive metagenomic studies and highly divergent gene duplicates may be very difficult to detect. Only occasionally have gene duplication events been described that produce multiple complete (and sometimes tandemly repeated) genes,[28,261] although improvements in computational analysis are likely to reveal more. For example, phylogenetic analysis revealed that three proteins within the Flanders virus genome arose by gene duplication rather than simply being pseudogenes as previously reported.[7] The difficulties in analyzing highly divergent sequences notwithstanding, there are good reasons for the relative rareness of gene duplication in RNA (and ssDNA) viruses. In particular, given the size limit on virus genome discussed throughout this chapter, increasing genome size through gene duplication is likely to result in major fitness losses through an increase in the load of deleterious mutations.

The situation is very different in large dsDNA viruses, where cases of gene duplication, as well as gene loss, are a common observation and are evidently responsible for some of the size variations among viruses[120,233] (Fig. 1.16). Gene duplication can occur in both the core and species-specific genes of large DNA viruses as signified by the presence of related gene pairs and multigene families.[173] For example, gene duplication has been commonplace in the E4 region of some adenoviruses[47] and in the terminal inverted repeats of the poxvirus myxoma virus,[145] although many other examples exist. The process of gene duplication may also be related to that of recombination. For example, in some poxviruses recombination seems to have resulted in the duplication, inversion, and transposition of genes to opposite ends of the genome.[186] Finally, the analysis of protein structure suggests that some of these gene duplication events may have occurred in the distant past and assisted in the production of very distinct proteins, such as the head–tail connector protein and tail tube protein of bacteriophage lambda.[32]

Lateral Gene Transfer and Modular Evolution

A major way for bacteria to create evolutionary novelty is through lateral (or horizontal) gene transfer (LGT), which can sometimes result in genes being transferred for large phylogenetic distances.[197] Both recombination and LGT are also important because they pose a major challenge to current phylogenetic protocols and may require a new computational tool kit.[122,140] As LGT will also result in an increase in virus genome size, unless the original gene is directly replaced by the invading gene (which is unlikely unless an exact excision is made, as faulty excision will result in deleterious mutants), it might be expected that it should only occur sporadically in RNA viruses. Although this initially appeared to be the case,[110] more recent metagenomic studies have now revealed multiple examples of this process, including the capture of some host genes.[240] For example, LGT from the host genome was responsible for the appearance of two exoribonucleases in two RNA viruses found in the sea-slater, an invertebrate.[240] Another well-documented case of LGT in an RNA virus involves the acquisition by influenza C virus of the hemagglutinin-esterase (*HE*) gene of coronaviruses.[163] In reality, however, there are few reports of the stable integration of cellular sequences into the genomes of RNA viruses, although more are likely to be documented following more intensive metagenomic studies.

The capture of host genes is very well documented in the case of large DNA viruses, including those from both bacteria[203] and eukaryotes,[125] although the complex phylogenetic shadows cast by gene birth and gene loss means that it is sometimes difficult to determine from which host species and when these gene transfer events occurred. The poxviruses have been very well studied in this respect, with the interleukin-10 (*IL-10*) gene family and the vertebrate vascular endothelial growth factor (*VEGFA*) genes, which are distributed among both poxviruses and a range of vertebrates, as well as the DNA ligases, acting as good examples (and the IL-10 family is also observed in herpesviruses).[29,120,175] In fact, LGT is a common occurrence in all NCLDVs and covers an enormous taxonomic range of hosts.[74,125] For example, it has been suggested that mimivirus acquired some 10% of its total gene content from bacterial species, including a number of mobile genetic elements.[72] In poxviruses, gene content seems to change more rapidly than gene order, reflecting the fact that species-specific genes tend to get added to the extremities of genomes (Fig. 1.16). That the flanking genes of large DNA viruses are often the ones captured by the host in turn suggests that internal gene orders are optimized to the extent that disrupting them may result in major fitness losses. Similarly, human herpesviruses contain homologs to such important immune genes as those that encode cytokines, chemokines, and complement system proteins, as well as those of the immunoglobulin superfamily.[168,213] These genes may modulate the immune response of the host, often by interfering or mimicking their cellular homologs. However, it is not only host immune genes that are acquired by dsDNA viruses. As a case in point, iridoviruses encode a number of cellular proteins that seem essential for virus replication.[255]

It is also the case that LGT has occurred among large DNA viruses and is particularly well documented in bacteriophage, where it appears to be a common mode of molecular evolution (see below)[101] (and phage-mediated LGT is of course a key

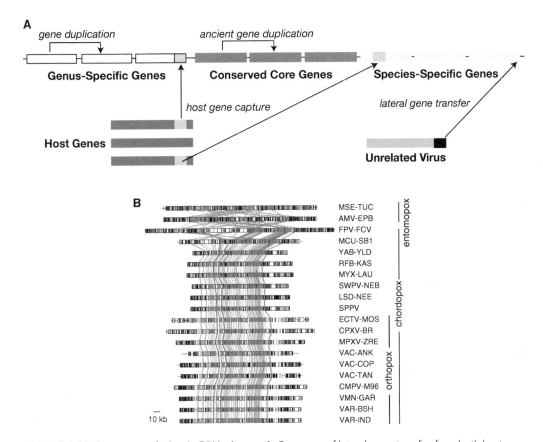

FIGURE 1.16 Genome evolution in DNA viruses. A: Processes of lateral gene transfer, from both hosts and other viruses, and gene duplication in large double-stranded DNA (dsDNA) viruses. Core viral genes, which are conserved across divergent taxa, are shown in *red* and often located in the central part of the genome. Genus and species-specific genes are shown as *white* and *yellow*, respectively, and more often located at the terminal regions of the genome. (Adapted from Shackelton LA, Holmes EC. The evolution of large DNA viruses: combining genomic information of viruses and their hosts. *Trends Microbiol* 2004;12:458–465, by permission of Cell Press.) **B:** Specific example of the comparative genomics of poxviruses. The figure shows a comparison of 92 gene families from 20 different poxviruses. Genes present in all the poxviruses analyzed are shown in *red* and are located in the central genomic regions. Those genes present in chordopox viruses only are shown in *blue*, while those present in orthopoxviruses only are shown in *yellow*. Vertical lines link orthologous genes. Horizontal differences are drawn proportional to genetic distances. (From McLysaght A, Baldi PF, Gaut BS. Extensive gene gain associated with adaptive evolution of poxviruses. *Proc Natl Acad Sci U S A* 2003;100:14960–14965, by permission of the US National Academy of Sciences. Figure kindly provided by Dr. Aoife McLysaght.)

process of bacteria evolution,[197] as well as in a number of eukaryotic viruses,[47] including the giant viruses from the *Mimiviridae* and *Pandoraviridae*.[148] As another example, the entomopoxvirus *Amsacta moorei* virus (AMV) contains a number of genes that have been acquired from baculoviruses.[125] However, as with the case of LGT among viruses and hosts, it is often hard to pinpoint the exact origin and direction of any gene transfer event.

Less clear is exactly how viruses capture host genes. Although such an event could obviously occur through direct recombination, this would require entry into the nucleus and would result in virus genes containing introns. An alternative possibility is that complementary DNA (cDNA) copies of spliced cellular mRNAs, which do not contain introns, have been inserted into virus genomes, perhaps utilizing the RTs present in cellular retroelements.[233] On the other hand, LGT that occurs among viruses, or between viruses and bacteria, most likely occurs during host co-infections.

One of the most interesting developments in studies of virus evolution in recent years has been the observation of segments of RNA virus genomes incorporated into host cellular genomes. For retroviruses that make dsDNA and enter the cell nucleus, as well as small ssDNA viruses that are so restricted in size that they do not carry their own polymerase genes and similarly must enter the cell nucleus, the presence of these integrated virus genes is perhaps not a surprise. Indeed, it has been known for many years that much of the eukaryotic genome was composed of endogenous retroviruses.[21,263] More surprising was the discovery that RNA viruses, which do not make a DNA genomic copy and often replicate in the cytoplasm, could also become integrated into host genomes (in the form of EVEs; see earlier). The first clear-cut case of virus-to-host LGT to be documented involved sequences closely related to those of insect flaviviruses and found to be integrated into the genomes of *Aedes* mosquitoes.[44] Since this time, a number of other examples have been discovered, including bornavirus,[118] filoviruses,[252] and rhabdoviruses,[130] often comprising a very wide range of hosts.[110,240] Similarly, EVEs have also been documented in a number of small DNA viruses, including circoviruses, parvoviruses,[12,18,129,159] and hepadnaviruses.[95,249]

As noted at the start of this chapter, the presence of these endogenous virus elements has changed our perspective of the time scale of virus evolution, providing important evidence that some virus families are older than previously anticipated. However, these sequences raise other interesting questions, most notably by what mechanisms single-stranded RNA is converted into double-stranded DNA. The most plausible answer involves interaction with the cellular retroelements that are an abundant component of eukaryotic genomes, with the L1 long interspersed nucleotide elements a notable example[118] (Fig. 1.3). In addition, some EVEs appear to be more conserved than expected if they were evolving in a strictly neutral manner, free of all selective constraints.[130] As such, some of these endogenous virus copies may be of functional importance, perhaps because they confer resistance against related exogenous viruses.[11]

Finally, one process of genome evolution that is mechanistically similar to that of LGT, and that has been of great historical importance in studies of virus evolution, is that of *modular evolution*.[26] This theory posits that viral genomes can be thought of as comprising a series of functional modules, such as those containing the capsid and the polymerase, that can be exchanged through recombination, and in doing so sometimes create entirely new viruses. For example, it has been suggested that some RNA viruses were created through a process of modular evolution,[103] and evidence that this is the case has increased through metagenomic studies.[240] Indeed, interfamily phylogenetic trees based on RdRp sequences are often markedly different to those derived from viral capsids, indicative of relatively widespread recombination and LGT which would drive modular evolution. In addition, it has been proposed that extensive sharing among diverse taxa dominates the evolution of DNA viruses.[140] Finally, there is evidence that recombination may occasionally reflect aspects of genome modularity in some small DNA viruses,[147,169] as well as some RNA viruses, which is compatible with a form of modular evolution.

REFERENCES

1. Aaskov J, Buzacott K, Thu HM, et al. Long-term transmission of defective RNA viruses in humans and *Aedes* mosquitoes. *Science* 2006;311:236–238.
2. Abel S, Abel zur Wiesch P, Davis BM, et al. Analysis of bottlenecks in experimental models of infection. *PLoS Pathog* 2015;11:e1004823.
3. Acevedo A, Brodsky L, Andino R. Mutational and fitness landscapes of an RNA virus revealed through population sequencing. *Nature* 2014;505:686–690.
4. Aguado LC, Jordan TX, Hsieh E, et al. Homologous recombination is an intrinsic defense against antiviral RNA interference. *Proc Natl Acad Sci U S A* 2018;115:E9211–E9219.
5. Aiewsakun P, Katzourakis A. Endogenous viruses: connecting recent and ancient viral evolution. *Virology* 2015;479–480:26–37.
6. Ali A, Li H, Schneider WL, et al. Analysis of genetic bottlenecks during horizontal transmission of *Cucumber mosaic virus*. *J Virol* 2006;80:8345–8350.
7. Allison AB, Mead DG, Palacios GF, et al. Gene duplication and phylogeography of North American members of the Hart Park serogroup of avian rhabdoviruses. *Virology* 2014;448:284–292.
8. Anderson JP, Daifuku R, Loeb LA. Viral error catastrophe by mutagenic nucleosides. *Annu Rev Microbiol* 2004;58:183–205.
9. Andino R, Domingo E. Viral quasispecies. *Virology* 2015;479–480:46–51.
10. Archer AM, Rico-Hesse R. High genetic divergence and recombination in arenaviruses from the Americas. *Virology* 2002;304:274–281.
11. Arnaud F, Caporale M, Varela M, et al. A paradigm for virus-host coevolution: sequential counter-adaptations between endogenous and exogenous retroviruses. *PLoS Pathog* 2007;3:e170.
12. Arriagada G, Gifford RJ. Parvovirus-derived endogenous viral elements in two South American rodent genomes. *J Virol* 2014;88:12158–12162.
13. Arslan D, Legendre M, Seltzer V, et al. Distant mimivirus relative with a larger genome highlights the fundamental features of *Megaviridae*. *Proc Natl Acad Sci U S A* 2011;108:17486–17491.
14. Bamford DH, Grimes JM, Stuart DI. What does structure tell us about viral evolution? *Curr Op Struct Biol* 2005;15:1–9.
15. Bell PJ. The viral eukaryogenesis hypothesis: a key role for viruses in the emergence of eukaryotes from a prokaryotic world environment. *Ann N Y Acad Sci* 2009;1178:91–105.
16. Belshaw R, Pybus OG, Rambaut A. The evolution of genome compression in RNA viruses. *Genome Res* 2007;17:1496–1504.
17. Belyi VA, Levine AJ, Skalka AM. Unexpected inheritance: multiple integrations of ancient bornavirus and ebolavirus/marburgvirus sequences in vertebrate genomes. *PLoS Pathog* 2010;6:e1001030.
18. Belyi VA, Levine AJ, Skalka AM. Sequences from ancestral single-stranded DNA viruses in vertebrate genomes: the *Parvoviridae* and *Circoviridae* are more than 40 to 50 million years old. *J Virol* 2010;84:12458–12462.
19. Benson SD, Bamford JKH, Bamford DH, et al. Viral evolution revealed by bacteriophage PRD1 and human adenovirus coat protein structures. *Cell* 1999;98:825–833.
20. Benson SD, Bamford JKH, Bamford DH, et al. Does common architecture reveal a viral lineage spanning all three domains of life. *Mol Cell* 2004;16:673–685.
21. Benveniste RE, Todaro GJ. Evolution of C-type viral genes: inheritance of exogenously acquired viral genes. *Nature* 1974;252:456–459.
22. Bernard H-U, Calleja-Macias IE, Dunn ST. Genome variation of human papillomavirus types: phylogenetic and medical implications. *Int J Cancer* 2006;118:1071–1076.
23. Bolduc B, Shaughnessy DP, Wolf YI, et al. Identification of novel positive-strand RNA viruses by metagenomic analysis of Archaea-dominated Yellowstone hot springs. *J Virol* 2012;86:5562–5573.
24. Bonhoeffer S, Chappey C, Parkin NT, et al. Evidence for positive epistasis in HIV-1. *Science* 2004;306:1547–1550.
25. Boni MF, de Jong MD, van Doorn HR, et al. Guidelines for identifying homologous recombination events in influenza A virus. *PLoS One* 2010;5:e10434.
26. Botstein D. A theory of modular evolution for bacteriophages. *Ann N Y Acad Sci* 1980;354:484–490.
27. Bowden R, Sakaoka H, Donnelly P, et al. High recombination rate in herpes simplex virus type 1 natural populations suggests significant co-infection. *Infect Genet Evol* 2004;4:115–123.
28. Boyko VP, Karasev AV, Agranovsky AA, et al. Coat protein gene duplication in a filamentous RNA virus of plants. *Proc Natl Acad Sci U S A* 1992;89:9156–9160.
29. Bratke KA, McLysaght A. Identification of multiple independent horizontal gene transfer events into poxviruses using a comparative genomics approach. *BMC Evol Biol* 2008;8:67.
30. Bull JJ, Sanjuan R, Wilke CO. Theory of lethal mutagenesis for viruses. *J Virol* 2007;81:2930–2939.
31. Burch CL, Chao L. Evolvability of an RNA virus is determined by its mutational neighbourhood. *Nature* 2000;406:625–628.
32. Cardarelli L, Pell LG, Neudecker P, et al. Phages have adapted the same protein fold to fulfill multiple functions in virion assembly. *Proc Natl Acad Sci U S A* 2010;107:14384–14389.
33. Chabria SB, Gupta S, Kozal MJ. Deep sequencing of HIV: clinical and research applications. *Annu Rev Genomics Hum Genet* 2014;15:295–325.
34. Chang GS, Hoon Y, Ko KD, et al. Phylogenetic profiles reveal evolutionary relationships within the 'twilight zone' of sequence similarity. *Proc Natl Acad Sci U S A* 2008;105:13474–13479.
35. Chao L. Fitness of RNA virus decreased by Muller's ratchet. *Nature* 1990;348:454–455.
36. Chao L, Tran TT, Tran TT. The advantage of sex in the RNA virus φphi6. *Genetics* 1997;147:953–959.
37. Charleston MA, Robertson DL. Preferential host switching by primate lentiviruses can account for phylogenetic similarity with the primate phylogeny. *Syst Biol* 2002;51:528–535.
38. Chen Z, Ho WCS, Boon SS, et al. Ancient evolution and dispersion of human papillomavirus 58 variants. *J Virol* 2017;91:e01285-17.
39. Chirico N, Vianelli A, Belshaw R. Why genes overlap in viruses. *Proc R Soc B* 2010;277:3809–3817.
40. Cicin-Sain L, Podlech J, Messerle M, et al. Frequent coinfection of cells explains functional in vivo complementation between cytomegalovirus variants in the multiply infected host. *J Virol* 2005;79:9492–9502.
41. Codoñer FM, Daros JA, Sole RV, et al. The fittest versus the flattest: experimental confirmation of the quasispecies effect with subviral pathogens. *PLoS Pathog* 2006;2:e136.
42. Comas I, Moya A, Gonzalez-Candelas F. Validating viral quasispecies with digital organisms: a re-examination of the critical mutation rate. *BMC Evol Biol* 2005;5:5.
43. Coulibaly F, Chevalier C, Gutsche I, et al. The birnavirus crystal structure reveals structural relationships among icosahedral viruses. *Cell* 2005;120:761–772.
44. Crochu S, Cook S, Attoui H, et al. Sequences of flavivirus-related RNA viruses persist in DNA form integrated in the genome of *Aedes* spp. mosquitoes. *J Gen Virol* 2004;85:1971–1980.
45. Cui J, Schlub T, Holmes EC. An allometric relationship between the genome length and virion volume of viruses. *J Virol* 2014;88:6403–6410.
46. Cui J, Zhao W, Huang Z, et al. Low frequency of paleoviral infiltration across the avian phylogeny. *Genome Biol* 2014;15:539.
47. Davison AJ, Telford EA, Watson MS, et al. The DNA sequence of adenovirus type 40. *J Mol Biol* 1993;234:1308–1316.
48. de Visser JA, Hermisson J, Wagner GP, et al. Evolution and detection of genetic robustness. *Evolution* 2003;57:1959–1972.
49. Dill JA, Camus AC, Leary JH, et al. Distinct viral lineages of hepadnavirus from fish and amphibians reveal the complex evolutionary history of hepadnaviruses. *J Virol* 2016;90:7920–7933.
50. Domingo E, Sabo D, Taniguchi T, et al. Nucleotide sequence heterogeneity of an RNA phage population. *Cell* 1978;13:735–744.
51. Drake JW. Rates of spontaneous mutation among RNA viruses. *Proc Natl Acad Sci U S A* 1993;90:4171–4175.

52. Drake JW, Charlesworth B, Charlesworth D, et al. Rates of spontaneous mutation. *Genetics* 1998;148:1667–1686.
53. Drummond AJ, Pybus OG, Rambaut A, et al. Measurably evolving populations. *Trends Ecol Evol* 2003;18:481–488.
54. Duarte E, Clarke D, Moya A, et al. Rapid fitness losses in mammalian RNA virus clones due to Muller's ratchet. *Proc Natl Acad Sci U S A* 1992;89:6015–6019.
55. Duchêne S, Holmes EC. Estimating evolutionary rates in giant viruses using ancient genomes. *Virus Evol* 2018;4:vey006.
56. Duchêne S, Holmes EC, Ho SYW. Analyses of evolutionary dynamics in viruses are hindered by a time-dependent bias in rate estimates. *Proc R Soc B* 2014;281:20140732.
57. Duffy S. Why are RNA virus mutation rates so damn high? *PLoS Biol* 2018;16:e3000003.
58. Duffy S, Holmes EC. Phylogenetic evidence for rapid rates of molecular evolution in the single-stranded DNA begomovirus Tomato Yellow Leaf Curl Virus. *J Virol* 2008;82:957–965.
59. Duffy S, Shackelton LA, Holmes EC. Rates of evolutionary change in viruses: patterns and determinants. *Nat Rev Genet* 2008;9:267–276.
60. Duggan AT, Perdomo MF, Piombino-Mascali D, et al. 17th century variola virus reveals the recent history of smallpox. *Curr Biol* 2016;26:3407–3412.
61. Eckerle LD, Lu X, Sperry SM, et al. High fidelity of murine hepatitis virus replication is decreased in nsp14 exoribonuclease mutants. *J Virol* 2007;81:12135–12144.
62. Eickbush TH. Origin and evolutionary relationships of retroelements. In: Morse SS, ed. *The Evolutionary Biology of Viruses.* New York: Raven Press; 1994:121–157.
63. Eickbush TH. Telomerase and retrotransposons: which came first? *Science* 1997;277:911–912.
64. Eigen M. Self-organization of matter and the evolution of biological macromolecules. *Naturwissenschaften* 1971;58:465–523.
65. Eigen M. *Steps Towards Life.* New York: Oxford University Press; 1996.
66. Elena SF, Carrasco P, Daròs JA, et al. Mechanisms of genetic robustness in RNA viruses. *EMBO Rep* 2006;7:168–173.
67. Elena SF, Dopazo J, Flores R, et al. Phylogeny of viroids, viroidlike satellite RNAs, and the viroidlike domain of hepatitis δ virus RNA. *Proc Natl Acad Sci U S A* 1991;88:5631–5634.
68. Elena SF, Lenski RE. Evolution experiments with microorganisms: the dynamics and genetic bases of adaptation. *Nat Rev Genet* 2003;4:457–470.
69. Esposito JJ, Sammons SA, Frace AM, et al. Genome sequence diversity and clues to the evolution of variola (smallpox) virus. *Science* 2006;313:807–812.
70. Evans DH, Stuart D, McFadden G. High levels of genetic recombination among cotransfected plasmid DNAs in poxvirus-infected mammalian cells. *J Virol* 1988;62:367–375.
71. Fédry J, Liu Y, Péhau-Arnaudet G, et al. The ancient gamete fusogen HAP2 is a eukaryotic class II fusion protein. *Cell* 2017;168:904–915.
72. Filée J, Chandler M. Gene exchange and the origin of giant viruses. *Intervirology* 2010;53:354–361.
73. Filée J, Forterre P, Sen-Lin T, et al. Evolution of DNA polymerase families: evidences for multiple gene exchange between cellular and viral proteins. *J Mol Evol* 2002;54:763–773.
74. Filée J, Pouget N, Chandler M. Phylogenetic evidence for extensive lateral acquisition of cellular genes by nucleocytoplasmic large DNA viruses. *BMC Evol Biol* 2008;8:320.
75. Firth C, Charleston MA, Duffy S, et al. Insights into the evolutionary history of an emerging livestock pathogen: porcine circovirus 2. *J Virol* 2009;83:12813–12821.
76. Firth C, Kitchen A, Shapiro B, et al. Using time-structured data to estimate evolutionary rates of double-stranded DNA viruses. *Mol Biol Evol* 2010;27:2038–2051.
77. Firth C, Lipkin WI. The genomics of emerging pathogens. *Annu Rev Genom Human Genet* 2013;14:281–300.
78. Fisher S. Are RNA viruses vestiges of an RNA world? *J Gen Philos Sci* 2010;41:212–141.
79. Fitzsimmons WJ, Woods RJ, McCrone JT, et al. A speed–fidelity trade-off determines the mutation rate and virulence of an RNA virus. *PLoS Biol* 2018;16:e2006459.
80. Forterre P. The two ages of the RNA world, and the transition to the DNA world: a story of viruses and cells. *Biochimie* 2005;87:793–803.
81. Forterre P, Prangishvili D. The origin of viruses. *Res Microbiol* 2009;160:466–472.
82. Froissart R, Michalakis Y, Blanc S. Helper component-transcomplementation in the vector transmission of plant viruses. *Phytopathology* 2002;92:576–579.
83. Froissart R, Wilke CO, Montville R, et al. Co-infection weakens selection again epistatic mutations in RNA viruses. *Genetics* 2004;168:9–19.
84. Furió V, Moya A, Sanjuan R. The cost of replication fidelity in an RNA virus. *Proc Natl Acad Sci U S A* 2005;102:10233–10237.
85. Gago S, Elena SF, Flores R, et al. Extremely high mutation rate of a hammerhead viroid. *Science* 2009;323:1308.
86. Gallot-Lavallée L, Blanc G. A glimpse of nucleo-cytoplasmic large DNA virus biodiversity through the eukaryotic genomics window. *Viruses* 2017;9:17.
87. Garcel A, Crance JM, Drillien R, et al. Genomic sequence of a clonal isolate of the vaccinia virus Lister strain employed for smallpox vaccination in France and its comparison to other orthopoxviruses. *J Gen Virol* 2007;88:1906–1916.
88. García-Arriaza J, Manrubia SC, Toja M, et al. Evolutionary transition toward defective RNAs that are infectious by complementation. *J Virol* 2004;78:11678–11685.
89. Geoghegan JL, Di Giallonardo F, Cousins K, et al. Hidden diversity and evolution of viruses in market fish. *Virus Evol* 2018;4:vey031.
90. Geoghegan JL, Duchêne S, Holmes EC. Comparative analysis estimates the relative frequencies of co-divergence and cross-species transmission within viral families. *PLoS Pathog* 2017;13:e1006215.
91. Geoghegan JL, Holmes EC. Evolutionary virology at 40. *Genetics* 2018;210:1151–1162.
92. Geoghegan JL, Senior AM, Di Giallonardo F, et al. Virological factors that increase the transmissibility of emerging human viruses. *Proc Natl Acad Sci U S A* 2016;113:4170–4175.
93. Geoghegan JL, Senior AM, Holmes EC. Pathogen population bottlenecks and adaptive landscapes: overcoming the barriers to disease emergence. *Proc R Soc B* 2016;283:20160727.
94. Ghedin E, Fitch A, Boyne A, et al. Mixed infection and the genesis of influenza diversity. *J Virol* 2009;83:8832–8841.
95. Gilbert C, Feschotte C. Genomic fossils calibrate the long-term evolution of hepadnaviruses. *PLoS Biol* 2010;8:e1000495.
96. Goldbach R, de Haan P. RNA viral supergroups and evolution of RNA viruses. In: Morse SS, ed. *The Evolutionary Biology of Viruses.* New York: Raven Press; 1994:105–119.
97. Gorbalenya AE, Enjuanes L, Ziebuhr J, et al. Nidovirales: evolving the largest RNA virus genome. *Virus Res* 2006;117:17–37.
98. Gorbalenya AE, Koonin EV. Viral proteins containing the purine NTP-binding sequence pattern. *Nucleic Acids Res* 1989;17:8413–8440.
99. Gorbalenya AE, Pringle FM, Zeddam JL, et al. The palm subdomain-based active site is internally permuted in viral RNA-dependent RNA polymerases of an ancient lineage. *J Mol Biol* 2002;324:47–62.
100. Grubaugh ND, Ladner JT, Lemey P, et al. Tracking virus epidemics in the twenty-first century. *Nat Micro* 2019;4:10–19.
101. Hambly E, Suttle CA. The viriosphere, diversity, and genetic exchange within phage communities. *Curr Opin Microbiol* 2005;8:444–450.
102. Han G-Z, Worobey M. An endogenous foamy-like viral element in the coelacanth genome. *PLoS Pathog* 2012;8:e1002790.
103. Haseloff J, Goelet P, Zimmern D, et al. Striking similarities in amino acid sequence among nonstructural proteins encoded by RNA viruses that have dissimilar genomic organization. *Proc Natl Acad Sci U S A* 1984;81:4358–4362.
104. Hatwell JN, Sharp PM. Evolution of human polyomavirus JC. *J Gen Virol* 2000;81:1191–1200.
105. Hayes S. Mahony J, Nauta A, et al. Metagenomic approaches to assess bacteriophages in various environmental niches. *Viruses* 2017;9:127.
106. Herniou EA, Olszewski JA, O'Reilly DR, et al. Ancient coevolution of baculoviruses and their insect hosts. *J Virol* 2004;78:3244–3251.
107. Hetzel U, Sironen T, Laurinmäki P, et al. Identification of a novel deltavirus in boa constrictors. *mBio* 2019;10:e00014-19.
108. Holmes EC. Molecular clocks and the puzzle of RNA virus origins. *J Virol* 2003;77:3893–3897.
109. Holmes EC. On being the right size. *Nat Genet* 2005;37:923–924.
110. Holmes EC. *The Evolution and Emergence of RNA Viruses.* Oxford: Oxford University Press; 2009.
111. Holmes EC. The evolution of endogenous viral elements. *Cell Host Microbe* 2011;10:368–377.
112. Holmes EC. What does virus evolution tell us about virus origins? *J Virol* 2011;85:5247–5251.
113. Holmes EC, Duchêne S. Can sequence phylogenies safely infer the origin of the global virome? *mBio* 2009;10:e00289-19.
114. Holmes EC, Dudas G, Rambaut A, et al. The evolution of Ebola virus: Insights from the 2013–2016 epidemic. *Nature* 2016;358:193–200.
115. Holmes EC, Grenfell BT. Discovering the phylodynamics of RNA viruses. *PLoS Comput Biol* 2009;5:e1000505.
116. Holmes EC, Zhang Y-Z. The evolution and emergence of hantaviruses. *Curr Opin Virol* 2015;10:27–33.
117. Hon CC, Lam TY, Shi ZL, et al. Evidence of the recombinant origin of a bat severe acute respiratory syndrome (SARS)-like coronavirus and its implications on the direct ancestor of SARS coronavirus. *J Virol* 2008;82:1819–1826.
118. Horie M, Honda T, Suzuki Y, et al. Endogenous non-retroviral RNA virus elements in mammalian genomes. *Nature* 2010;463:84–87.
119. Huang AS, Baltimore D. Defective viral particles and viral disease processes. *Nature* 1970;226:325–327.
120. Hughes AL, Friedman R. Poxvirus genome evolution by gene gain and loss. *Mol Phylogenet Evol* 2005;35:186–195.
121. Hughes AL, Hughes MA. More effective purifying selection on RNA viruses than in DNA viruses. *Gene* 2007;404:117–125.
122. Iranzo J, Krupovic M, Koonin EV. The double-stranded DNA virosphere as a modular hierarchical network of gene sharing. *mBio* 2016;7:e00978-16.
123. Ito J, Braithwaite DK. Compilation and alignment of DNA polymerase sequences. *Nucleic Acids Res* 1991;19:4045–4057.
124. Iyer LM, Aravind L, Koonin EV. Common origin of four diverse families of large eukaryotic viruses. *J Virol* 2001;75:11720–11734.
125. Iyer LM, Balaji S, Koonin EV, et al. Evolutionary genomics of nucleo-cytoplasmic large DNA viruses. *Virus Res* 2006;117:156–184.
126. Iyer LM, Koonin EV, Aravind L. Evolutionary connection between the catalytic subunits of DNA-dependent RNA polymerases and eukaryotic RNA-dependent RNA polymerases and the origin of RNA polymerases. *BMC Struct Biol* 2003;3:1.
127. Jackson AP, Charleston MA. A cophylogenetic perspective of RNA-virus evolution. *Mol Biol Evol* 2004;21:45–57.
128. Jancovich JK, Bremont M, Touchman JW, et al. Evidence for multiple recent host species shifts among the Ranaviruses (family Iridoviridae). *J Virol* 2010;84:2636–2647.
129. Kapoor A, Simmonds P, Lipkin WI. Discovery and characterization of mammalian endogenous parvoviruses. *J Virol* 2010;84:12628–12635.
130. Katzourakis A, Gifford RJ. Endogenous viral elements in animal genomes. *PLoS Genet* 2010;6:e1001191.
131. Katzourakis A, Gifford RJ, Tristem M, et al. Macroevolution of complex retroviruses. *Science* 2009;325:1512.
132. Katzourakis A, Tristem M. Phylogeny of human endogenous and exogenous retroviruses. In: Sverdlov ED, ed. *Retroviruses and Primate Genome Evolution.* Austin: Landes Bioscience; 2005:186–203.
133. Katzourakis A, Tristem M, Pybus OG, et al. Discovery and analysis of the first endogenous lentivirus. *Proc Natl Acad Sci U S A* 2007;104:6261–6265.
134. Ke R, Aaskov J, Holmes EC, et al. Phylodynamic analysis of the emergence and epidemiological impact of transmissible defective dengue viruses. *PLoS Pathog* 2013;9:e1003193.
135. Keightley PD, Eyre-Walker A. Deleterious mutations and the evolution of sex. *Science* 2000;290:331–333.
136. Kerr PJ, Ghedin E, DePasse JV, et al. Evolutionary history and attenuation of myxoma virus on two continents. *PLoS Pathogens* 2012;8:e1002950.

137. Khatchikian D, Orlich M, Rott R. Increased viral pathogenicity after insertion of a 28S ribosomal RNA sequence into the haemagglutinin gene of an influenza virus. *Nature* 1989;340:156–157.
138. Kitchen A, Shackelton L, Holmes EC. Family level phylogenies reveal modes of macroevolution in RNA viruses. *Proc Natl Acad Sci USA* 2011;108:238–243.
139. Koonin EV. The phylogeny of RNA-dependent RNA polymerases of positive-strand RNA viruses. *J Gen Virol* 1991;72:2197–2206.
140. Koonin EV, Dolja VV. Virus world as an evolutionary network of viruses and capsidless selfish elements. *Microbiol Mol Biol Rev* 2014;78:278–303.
141. Koonin EV, Senkevich TG, Dolja VV. The ancient virus world and evolution of cells. *Biol Direct* 2006;1:29.
142. Krupovic M, Bamford DH. Virus evolution: how far does the double beta-barrel viral lineage extend? *Nat Rev Microbiol* 2008;6:941–948.
143. Kryazhimskiy S, Dushoff J, Bazykin GA, et al. Prevalence of epistasis in the evolution of influenza A surface proteins. *PLoS Genet* 2011;7:e1001301.
144. La Scola B, Audic S, Robert C, et al. A giant virus in amoebae. *Science* 2003;299:2033.
145. Labudovic A, Perkins H, van Leeuwen B, et al. Sequence mapping of the Californian MSW strain of Myxoma virus. *Arch Virol* 2004;149:553–570.
146. Lai MMC. RNA recombination in animal and plant viruses. *Microbiol Rev* 1992;56:61–79.
147. Lefeuvre P, Lett JM, Reynaud B, et al. Avoidance of protein fold disruption in natural virus recombinants. *PLoS Pathog* 2007;3:e181.
148. Legendre M, Fabre E, Poirot O, et al. Diversity and evolution of the emerging *Pandoraviridae* family. *Nat Commun* 2018;9:2285.
149. Lehmann E, Brueckner F, Cramer P. Molecular basis of RNA-dependent RNA polymerase II activity. *Nature* 2007;450:445–459.
150. Leigh Brown AJ, Richman DD. HIV-1: Gambling on the evolution of drug resistance? *Nat Med* 1997;3:268–271.
151. Leland DS, Ginocchio CC. Role of cell culture for virus detection in the age of technology. *Clin Microbiol Rev* 2007;20:49–59.
152. Lemey P, Rambaut A, Drummond AJ, et al. Bayesian phylogeography finds its roots. *PLoS Comput Biol* 2009;9:e1000520.
153. Leppik L, Gunst K, Lehtinen M, et al. *In vivo* and *in vitro* intragenomic rearrangement of TT viruses. *J Virol* 2007;81:9346–9356.
154. Levasseur A, Andreani J, Delerce J, et al. Comparison of a modern and fossil pithovirus reveals its genetic conservation and evolution. *Genome Biol Evol* 2016;8:2333–2339.
155. Li H, Bar KJ, Wang S, et al. High multiplicity infection by HIV-1 in men who have sex with men. *PLoS Pathog* 2010;6:e1000890.
156. Li Y, Carroll DS, Gardner SN, et al. On the origin of smallpox: correlating variola phylogenics with historical smallpox records. *Proc Natl Acad Sci U S A* 2007;104: 15787–15792.
157. Li HC, Fujiyoshi T, Lou H, et al. The presence of ancient human T-cell lymphotropic virus type I provirus DNA in an Andean mummy. *Nat Med* 1999;5:1428–1432.
158. Li C-X, Shi M, Tian JH, et al. Unprecedented genomic diversity of RNA viruses in arthropods reveals the ancestry of negative-sense RNA viruses. *eLife* 2015;4:e05378.
159. Liu H, Fu Y, Xie J, et al. Widespread endogenization of densoviruses and parvoviruses in animal and human genomes. *J Virol* 2011;85:9863–9876.
160. Liu W, Worobey M, Li Y, et al. Molecular ecology and natural history of simian foamy virus infection in wild-living chimpanzees. *PLoS Pathog* 2008;4:e1000097.
161. Lowen AC. Constraints, drivers, and implications of influenza A virus reassortment. *Annu Rev Virol* 2017;4:105–121.
162. Ludmir EB, Enquist LW. Viral genomes are part of the phylogenetic tree of life. *Nat Rev Microbiol* 2009;7:615.
163. Luytjes W, Bredenbeek PJ, Noten AF, et al. Sequence of mouse hepatitis virus A59 mRNA 2: indications for RNA recombination between coronaviruses and influenza C virus. *Virology* 1988;166:415–422.
164. Malim MH, Emerman M. HIV-1 sequence variation: drift, shift, and attenuation. *Cell* 2001;104:469–472.
165. Maljkovic Berry I, Ribeiro R, Kothari M, et al. Unequal evolutionary rates in the human immunodeficiency virus type 1 (HIV-1) pandemic: the evolutionary rate of HIV-1 slows down when the epidemic rate increases. *J Virol* 2007;81:10625–10635.
166. Mansky LM. Retrovirus mutation rates and their role in genetic variation. *J Gen Virol* 1998;79:1337–1345.
167. Mansky LM, Cunningham KS. Virus mutators and antimutators: roles in evolution, pathogenesis and emergence. *Trends Genet* 2000;16:512–517.
168. Markine-Goriaynoff N, Georgin JP, Goltz M, et al. The core 2 β-1,6-N-acetylglucosaminyltransferase-mucin encoded by bovine herpesvirus 4 was acquired from an ancestor of the African buffalo. *J Virol* 2003;77:1784–1992.
169. Martin DP, van der Walt E, Posada D, et al. The evolutionary value of recombination is constrained by genome modularity. *PLoS Genet* 2005;51:475–479.
170. McCrone JT, Lauring AS. Genetic bottlenecks in intraspecies virus transmission. *Curr Opin Virol* 2018;28:20–25.
171. McCrone JT, Woods RJ, Martin ET, et al. 2018 Stochastic processes constrain the within and between host evolution of influenza virus. *eLife* 2018;7:e35962.
172. McGeoch DJ, Gatherer D. Integrating reptilian herpesviruses into the family Herpesviridae. *J Virol* 2005;79:725–731.
173. McGeoch DJ, Rixon FJ, Davison AJ. Topics in herpesvirus genomics and evolution. *Virus Res* 2006;117:90–104.
174. McGregor A, Choi KY, Schleiss MR. Guinea pig cytomegalovirus GP84 is a functional homolog of the human cytomegalovirus (HCMV) UL84 gene that can complement for the loss of UL84 in a chimeric HCMV. *Virology* 2011;410:76–87.
175. McLysaght A, Baldi PF, Gaut BS. Extensive gene gain associated with adaptive evolution of poxviruses. *Proc Natl Acad Sci U S A* 2003;100:14960–14965.
176. McTaggart SJ, Obbard DJ, Conlon C, et al. Immune genes undergo more adaptive evolution than non-immune system genes in *Daphnia pulex*. *BMC Evol Biol* 2012;12:63.
177. McWilliam Leitch EC, McLauchlan J. Determining the cellular diversity of hepatitis C virus quasispecies by single-cell viral sequencing. *J Virol* 2013;87:12648–12655.
178. Michod RE, Bernstein H, Nedelcu AM. Adaptive value of sex in microbial pathogens. *Infect Genet Evol* 2008;8:267–285.
179. Minskaia E, Hertzig T, Gorbalenya AE, et al. Discovery of an RNA virus 3'->5' exoribonuclease that is critically involved in coronavirus RNA synthesis. *Proc Natl Acad Sci U S A* 2006;103:5108–5113.
180. Miralles R, Gerrish PJ, Moya A, et al. Clonal interference and the evolution of RNA viruses. *Science* 1999;285:1745–1747.
181. Mokili JL, Rohwer F, Dutilh BE. Metagenomics and future perspectives in virus discovery. *Curr Opin Virol* 2012;2:63–77.
182. Montville R, Froissart R, Remold SK, et al. Evolution of mutational robustness in an RNA virus. *PLoS Biol* 2005;3:e381.
183. Moreira D, López-Garcia P. Comment on 'The 1.2-megabase genome sequence of mimivirus'. *Science* 2005;308:1114a.
184. Moreira D, López-Garcia P. Ten reasons to exclude viruses from the tree of life. *Nat Rev Microbiol* 2009;7:306–311.
185. Morse SS. Toward an evolutionary biology of viruses. In: Morse SS, ed. *The Evolutionary Biology of Viruses*. New York: Raven Press; 1994:1–28.
186. Moyer RW, Graves RL, Rothe CT. The white pock (mu) mutants of rabbit poxvirus. III. Terminal DNA sequence duplication and transposition in rabbit poxvirus. *Cell* 1980;22:545–553.
187. Mühlemann B, Jones TC, Damgaard PB, et al. Ancient hepatitis B viruses from the Bronze Age to the Medieval period. *Nature* 2018;557:418–423.
188. Mühlemann B, Margaryan A, Damgaard PB, et al. Ancient human parvovirus B19 in Eurasia reveals its long-term association with humans. *Proc Natl Acad Sci U S A* 2018;115:7557–7562.
189. Murcia PR, Baillie GJ, Daley J, et al. The intra- and inter-host evolutionary dynamics of equine influenza virus. *J Virol* 2010;84:6943–6954.
190. Murthy S, Couacy-Hymann E, Metzger S, et al. Absence of frequent herpesvirus transmission in a nonhuman primate predator-prey system in the wild. *J Virol* 2013;87:10651–10659.
191. Nee S. The evolution of multicompartmental genomes in viruses. *J Mol Evol* 1987;25:277–281.
192. Neher RA, Leitner T. Recombination rate and selection strength in HIV intra-patient evolution. *PLoS Comput Biol* 2010;6:e1000660.
193. Nemirov K, Vapalahti O, Lundkvist A, et al. Isolation and characterization of Dobrava hantavirus carried by the striped field mouse (*Apodemus agrarius*) in Estonia. *J Gen Virol* 1999;80:371–379.
194. Ng TFF, Chen LF, Zhou Y, et al. Ancient viral genomes in 700-y-old feces. *Proc Natl Acad Sci U S A* 2014;111:16842–16847.
195. Nora T, Charpentier C, Tenaillon O, et al. Contribution of recombination to the evolution of human immunodeficiency viruses expressing resistance to antiretroviral treatment. *J Virol* 2007;81:7620–7628.
196. Norja P, Eis-Hübinger AM, Söderlund-Venermo M, et al. Rapid sequence change and geographical spread of human parvovirus B19: comparison of B19 virus evolution in acute and persistent infections. *J Virol* 2008;82:6427–6433.
197. Ochman H, Lawrence JG, Groisman EA. Lateral gene transfer and the nature of bacterial innovation. *Nature* 2000;405:299–304.
198. Olival KJ, Hosseini PR, Zambrana-Torrelio C, et al. Host and viral traits predict zoonotic spillover from mammals. *Nature* 2017;546:646–650.
199. Parameswaran P, Charlebois P, Tellez Y, et al. Genome-wide patterns of intrahuman dengue virus diversity reveal associations with viral phylogenetic clade and interhost diversity. *J Virol* 2012;86:8546–8558.
200. Parameswaran P, Wang C, Trivedi SB, et al. Intrahost selection pressures drive rapid dengue virus microevolution in acute human infections. *Cell Host Microbe* 2017;22:400–410.
201. Parrish CR, Holmes EC, Morens DM, et al. Cross-species virus transmission and the emergence of new epidemic diseases. *Microbiol Mol Biol Rev* 2008;72:457–470.
202. Patterson Ross Z, Klunk J, Fornaciari G, et al. The paradox of HBV evolution as revealed from a 16th century mummy. *PLoS Pathog* 2018;14:e1006750.
203. Pedulla ML, Ford ME, Houtz JM, et al. Origins of highly mosaic mycobacteriophage genomes. *Cell* 2003;113:171–182.
204. Pepin KM, Wichman HA. Variable epistatic effects between mutations at host recognition sites in phiX174 bacteriophage. *Evolution* 2007;61:1710–1724.
205. Perelson AS, Neumann AU, Markowitz M, et al. HIV-1 dynamics in vivo: virion clearance rate, infected cell life-span, and viral generation time. *Science* 1996;271:1582–1586.
206. Perez-Vargas J, Amirache F, Boson B, et al. Enveloped viruses distinct from HBV induce dissemination of hepatitis D virus in vivo. *Nat Comm* 2019;10:2098.
207. Peyambari M, Warner S, Stoler N, et al. A 1000 year-old RNA virus. *J Virol* 2019;93:e01188-18.
208. Philippe N, Legendre M, Doutre G, et al. Pandoraviruses: amoeba viruses with genomes up to 2.5 Mb reaching that of parasitic eukaryotes. *Science* 2013;341:281–286.
209. Pietilä MK, Roine E, Paulin L, et al. An ssDNA virus infecting archaea: a new lineage of viruses with a membrane envelope. *Mol Microbiol* 2009;72:307–319.
210. Powner MW, Gerland B, Sutherland JD. Synthesis of activated pyrimidine ribonucleotides in prebiotally plausible conditions. *Nature* 2009;459:239–242.
211. Prangishvili D, Forterre P, Garrett RA. Viruses of the Archaea: a unifying view. *Nat Rev Microbiol* 2006;4:837–848.
212. Pybus OG, Rambaut A, Freckleton RP, et al. Phylogenetic evidence for deleterious mutation load in RNA viruses and its contribution to viral evolution. *Mol Biol Evol* 2007;24:845–852.
213. Raftery M, Müller A, Schönrich G. Herpesvirus homologues of cellular genes. *Virus Genes* 2000;21:65–75.
214. Rambaut A, Pybus OG, Nelson MI, et al. The genomic and epidemiological dynamics of human influenza A virus. *Nature* 2008;453:615–619.
215. Reanney DC. The evolution of RNA viruses. *Annu Rev Microbiol* 1982;36:47–73.
216. Rector A, Lemey P, Tachezy R, et al. Ancient papillomavirus-host co-speciation in *Felidae*. *Genome Biol* 2007;8:R57.

217. Reiter J, Pérez-Vilaró G, Scheller N, et al. Hepatitis C virus RNA recombination in cell culture. *J Hepatol* 2011;55:777–783.

218. Rice WR. Experimental tests of the adaptive significance of sexual recombination. *Nat Rev Genet* 2002;3:241–251.

219. Robinson RA, Vance RB, O'Callaghan DJ. Oncogenic transformation by equine herpesviruses. II. Coestablishment of persistent infection and oncogenic transformation of hamster embryo cells by equine herpesvirus type 1 preparations enriched for defective interfering particles. *J Virol* 1980;36:204–219.

220. Saberi A, Gulyaeva AA, Brubacher JL, et al. A planarian nidovirus expands the limits of RNA genome size. *PLoS Pathog* 2018;14:e1007314.

221. Sacristán S, Malpica JM, Fraile A, et al. Estimation of population bottlenecks during systemic movement of Tobacco mosaic virus in tobacco plants. *J Virol* 2004;77:9906–9911.

222. Saira K, Lin X, DePasse JV, Halpin R, et al. Sequence analysis of *in vivo* defective-interfering (DI)-like RNA of influenza A H1N1 pandemic virus. *J Virol* 2013;87:8064–8074.

223. Salehi-Ashtiani K, Lupták A, Litovchick A, et al. A genomewide search for ribozymes reveals an HDV-like sequence in the human CPEB3 gene. *Science* 2006;313:1788–1792.

224. Sanjuán R, Elena SF. Epistasis correlates to genomic complexity. *Proc Natl Acad Sci U S A* 2006;103:14402–14405.

225. Sanjuán R, Cuevas JM, Furió V, et al. Selection for robustness in mutagenesized RNA viruses. *PLoS Genet* 2007;3:e93.

226. Sanjuán R, Domingo-Calap P. Mechanisms of viral mutation. *Cell Mol Life Sci* 2016;73:4433–4448.

227. Sanjuán R, Moya A, Elena SF. The distribution of fitness effects caused by single-nucleotide substitutions in an RNA virus. *Proc Natl Acad Sci U S A* 2004;101:8396–8401.

228. Sanjuán R, Moya A, Elena SF. The contribution of epistasis to the architecture of fitness in an RNA virus. *Proc Natl Acad Sci U S A* 2004;101:15376–15379.

229. Sanjuán R, Nebot MR, Chirico N, et al. Viral mutation rates. *J Virol* 2010;84:9733–9748.

230. Sawicki SG, Sawicki DL, Siddell SG. A contemporary view of coronavirus transcription. *J Virol* 2007;81:20–29.

231. Sawyer SL, Emerman M, Malik HS. Ancient adaptive evolution of the primate antiviral DNA-editing enzyme APOBEC3G. *PLoS Biol* 2004;2:e275.

232. Shackelton LA, Hoelzer K, Parrish CR, et al. Comparative analysis reveals frequent recombination in the parvoviruses. *J Gen Virol* 2007;88:3294–3301.

233. Shackelton LA, Holmes EC. The evolution of large DNA viruses: combining genomic information of viruses and their hosts. *Trends Microbiol* 2004;12:458–465.

234. Shackelton LA, Holmes EC. Phylogenetic evidence for the rapid evolution of human B19 erythrovirus. *J Virol* 2006;80:3666–3669.

235. Shackelton LA, Parrish CR, Truyen U, et al. High rate of viral evolution associated with the emergence of canine parvoviruses. *Proc Natl Acad Sci U S A* 2005;102:379–384.

236. Sharp PM. Origins of human virus diversity. *Cell* 2002;108:305–312.

237. Sharp PM, Bailes E, Chaudhuri RR, et al. The origins of acquired immune deficiency syndrome viruses: where and when? *Phil Trans Roy Lond B* 2001;356:867–876.

238. Shchelkunov SN. How long ago did smallpox virus emerge? *Arch Virol* 2009;154:1865–1871.

239. Shi M, Lin XD, Chen X, et al. The evolutionary history of vertebrate RNA viruses. *Nature* 2018;556:197–202.

240. Shi M, Lin XD, Tian JH, et al. Redefining the invertebrate RNA virosphere. *Nature* 2016;540:539–543.

241. Shi M, Lin X-D, Vasilakis N, et al. Divergent viruses discovered in arthropods and vertebrates revise the evolutionary history of the *Flaviviridae* and related viruses. *J Virol* 2016;90:659–669.

242. Shi M, Zhang Y-Z, Holmes EC. Meta-transcriptomics and the evolutionary biology of RNA viruses. *Virus Res* 2018;243:83–90.

243. Shriner D, Rodrigo AG, Nickle DC, et al. Pervasive genomic recombination of HIV-1 in vivo. *Genetics* 2004;167:1573–1583.

244. Simmonds P, Adams MJ, Shakhnovich M, et al. Consensus statement: virus taxonomy in the age of metagenomics. *Nat Rev Microbiol* 2017;15:161–168.

245. Simon-Loriere E, Holmes EC. Why do RNA viruses recombine? *Nat Rev Microbiol* 2011;9:617–626.

246. Smith DR, Adams AP, Kenney JL, et al. Venezuelan equine encephalitis virus in the mosquito vector *Aedes taeniorhynchus:* infection initiated by a small number of susceptible epithelial cells and a population bottleneck. *Virology* 2008;372:176–186.

247. Sniegowski PD, Gerrish PJ, Johnson T, et al. The evolution of mutation rates: separating causes from consequences. *BioEssays* 2000;22:1057–1066.

248. Stern A, Yeh MT, Zinger T, et al. The evolutionary pathway to virulence of an RNA virus. *Cell* 2017;169:35–46.

249. Suh A, Weber CC, Kehlmaier C, et al. Early Mesozoic coexistence of amniotes and *Hepadnaviridae*. *PLoS Genet* 2014;10:e1004559.

250. Switzer WM, Salemi M, Shanmugam V, et al. Ancient co-speciation of simian foamy viruses and primates. *Nature* 2005;434:376–380.

251. Taubenberger JK, Reid AH, Frafft AE, et al. Initial genetic characterization of the 1918 "Spanish" influenza virus. *Science* 1997;275:1793–1796.

252. Taylor DJ, Leach RW, Bruenn J. Filoviruses are ancient and integrated into mammalian genomes. *BMC Evol Biol* 2010;10:193.

253. Thézé J, Bézier A, Periquet G, et al. Paleozoic origin of insect large dsDNA viruses. *Proc Natl Acad Sci U S A* 2011;108:15931–15935.

254. Thiry E, Muylkens B, Meurens F, et al. Recombination in the alphaherpesvirus bovine herpesvirus 1. *Vet Microbiol* 2006;113:171–177.

255. Tidona CA, Darai G. Iridovirus homologues of cellular genes—implications for the molecular evolution of large DNA viruses. *Virus Genes* 2000;21:77–81.

256. Tzeng WP, Frey TK. Complementation of a deletion in the rubella virus p150 nonstructural protein by the viral capsid protein. *J Virol* 2003;77:9502–9510.

257. van der Walt E, Martin DP, Varsani A, et al. Experimental observations of rapid Maize streak virus evolution reveal a strand-specific nucleotide substitution bias. *Virol J* 2008;5:104.

258. van der Walt E, Rybicki EP, Varsani A, et al. Rapid host adaptation by extensive recombination. *J Gen Virol* 2009;90:734–746.

259. Vignuzzi M, Stone JK, Arnold JJ, et al. Quasispecies diversity determines pathogenesis through cooperative interactions in a viral population. *Nature* 2005;439:344–348.

260. Villarreal LP, Defilippis VR, Gottlieb KA. Acute and persistent viral life strategies and their relationship to emerging diseases. *Virology* 2000;272:1–6.

261. Walker PJ, Byrne KA, Riding GA, et al. The genome of bovine ephemeral fever rhabdovirus contains two related glycoprotein genes. *Virology* 1992;191:49–61.

262. Weaver SC. Evolutionary influences in arboviral disease. *Curr Top Microbiol Immunol* 2006;299:285–314.

263. Weiss RA, Mason WS, Vogt PK. Genetic recombinants and heterozygotes derived from endogenous and exogenous avian RNA tumor viruses. *Virology* 1973;52:535–552.

264. Wilke CO, Lenski RE, Adami C. Compensatory mutations cause excess of antagonistic epistasis in RNA secondary structure folding. *BMC Evol Biol* 2003;3:3.

265. Wilke CO, Wang JL, Ofria C, et al. Evolution of digital organisms at high mutation rates leads to survival of the flattest. *Nature* 2001;412:331–333.

266. Wille M, Netter HJ, Littlejohn M, et al. A divergent hepatitis D-like agent in birds. *Viruses* 2018;10:720.

267. Wittmann TJ, Biek R, Hassanin A, et al. Isolates of Zaire ebolavirus from wild apes reveal genetic lineage and recombinants. *Proc Natl Acad Sci U S A* 2007;104:17123–17127.

268. Woolford L, Rector A, Van Ranst M, et al. A novel virus detected in papillomas and carcinomas of the endangered western barred bandicoot (*Perameles bougainville*) exhibits genomic features of both the *Papillomaviridae* and *Polyomaviridae*. *J Virol* 2007;81:13280–13290.

269. Worobey M, Telfer P, Souquière S, et al. Island biogeography reveals the deep history of SIV. *Science* 2010;329:1487.

270. Wright CF, Morelli MJ, Thébaud G, et al. Beyond the consensus: dissecting within-host viral population diversity of foot-and-mouth disease virus by using next-generation genome sequencing. *J Virol* 2011;85:2266–2275.

271. Xiao Y, Rouzine IM, Bianco S, et al. RNA Recombination enhances adaptability and is required for virus spread and virulence. *Cell Host Microbe* 2016;19:493–503.

272. Zanotto PM, Gibbs MJ, Gould EA, et al. A reevaluation of the higher taxonomy of viruses based on RNA polymerases. *J Virol* 1996;70:6083–6096.

273. Zeldovich KB, Chen P, Shakhnovich EI. Protein stability imposes limits on organism complexity and speed of molecular evolution. *Proc Natl Acad Sci U S A* 2007;104:16152–16157.

274. Zhang Z, Kottadiel VI, Vafabakhsh R, et al. A promiscuous DNA packaging machine from bacteriophage T4. *PLoS Biol* 2011;9:e1000592.

Picornaviridae: The Viruses and Their Replication

Amy B. Rosenfeld • Vincent R. Racaniello

Viruses in the family *Picornaviridae* comprise nonenveloped particles with a single-stranded RNA (ssRNA) genome of positive polarity. Among the many members of this family are numerous important human and animal pathogens, such as poliovirus, hepatitis A virus, foot-and-mouth disease virus (FMDV), enteroviruses, coxsackieviruses, and rhinoviruses. The name of the virus family was intended to convey the small size of the viruses (pico, a small unit of measurement [10^{-12}]) and the type of nucleic acid that constitutes the viral genome (RNA).

Picornaviruses have played important roles in the development of modern virology. FMDV was the first animal virus

to be discovered, by Loeffler and Frosch in 1898.[422] Poliovirus was isolated 10 years later,[393] a discovery spurred by the emergence of epidemic poliomyelitis at the turn of the 20th century. The discovery in 1949 that poliovirus could be propagated in cells in culture led to studies of viral replication.[183] The plaque assay, an essential method for quantification of viral infectivity, was developed using poliovirus.[176] The first RNA-dependent RNA polymerase identified was that of mengovirus,[38] a picornavirus, and the synthesis of a precursor polyprotein from which viral proteins are derived by proteolytic processing was first identified in poliovirus-infected cells.[668] The first infectious DNA clone of an animal RNA virus was that of poliovirus,[581] and the first three-dimensional structures of animal viruses determined by x-ray crystallography were those of poliovirus[303] and rhinovirus.[607] Poliovirus RNA was the first messenger RNA (mRNA) shown to lack a 5′ cap structure.[295,508] This observation was subsequently explained by the finding that the genome RNA of poliovirus, and other picornaviruses, is translated by internal ribosome binding.[330,543] Because they cause serious diseases, poliovirus and FMDV have been the best-studied picornaviruses. Research on poliovirus has produced two effective vaccines, and it is likely that poliomyelitis will be eradicated from the globe in the near future. The World Health Organization (WHO) has established a future goal of cessation of vaccination, at which time all poliovirus stocks must be destroyed. When this historic event takes place, all research on this virus will cease, as has already been the case for type 2 poliovirus, which has been declared eradicated by the WHO.[229] Consequently, other picornaviruses have become the focus of research on fundamental mechanisms of reproduction.

CLASSIFICATION

The family *Picornaviridae* is part of the order *Picornavirales* and comprises 40 genera (Table 2.1), all of which contain viruses that infect vertebrates.[314] The number of new picornaviruses has seen a stunning increase in the past 5 years, mainly due to metagenomic analysis. In many cases, classification is based only on genome sequences, and no virus isolates are available. It is therefore unknown if replication occurs in the hosts from which these nucleic acids were isolated. Some of the best-studied picornaviruses are described below.

TABLE 2.1   Members of the family *Picornaviridae*

Genus	Species
Aalivirus *Ampivirus* *Aphthovirus*	*Aalivirus A* *Ampivirus A* *Foot-and-mouth disease virus* *Equine rhinitis A virus* *Bovine rhinitis A virus*
Aquamavirus *Avihepatovirus*	*Aquamavirus A* *Avihepatovirus A*
Avisivirus *Bopivirus* *Cardiovirus*	*Avisivirus A* *Bopivirus A* *Cardiovirus A* (encephalomyocarditis viruses 1–2, Theiler murine encephalomyelitis virus) *Cardiovirus B* (Vilyuisk human encephalomyelitis virus, Saffold viruses 1–11) *Cardiovirus C*
Cosavirus *Crohivirus* *Dicipivirus* *Enterovirus*	*Cosavirus A–F* *Crohivirus A, B* *Cadicivirus A* *Enterovirus A* (coxsackievirus, enterovirus) *Enterovirus B* (coxsackievirus, echovirus, enterovirus) *Enterovirus C* (poliovirus, coxsackievirus, enterovirus) *Enterovirus D* (enterovirus) *Enterovirus E* (group A bovine enteroviruses) *Enterovirus F* (group B bovine enteroviruses) *Enterovirus G* (porcine enteroviruses) *Enterovirus H* (simian enteroviruses) *Enterovirus I* (camel enterovirus) *Enterovirus J* (simian enteroviruses) *Enterovirus K* (rodent enterovirus) *Enterovirus L* (monkey enterovirus) *Rhinovirus A* *Rhinovirus B* *Rhinovirus C*
Erbovirus	*Erbovirus A*
Gallivirus *Harkavirus* *Hepatovirus*	*Gallivirus A* *Harkavirus A* *Hepatovirus A* (hepatitis A virus) *Hepatovirus B–I*
Hunnivirus *Kobuvirus*	*Hunnivirus A* *Aichivirus A–F*
Kunsagivirus *Limnipivirus* *Megrivirus* *Mischivirus* *Mosavirus* *Orivirus* *Oscivirus* *Parechovirus*	*Kunsagivirus A–C* *Limnipivirus A–C* *Megrivirus A–E* *Mischivirus A–C* *Mosavirus A* *Orivirus A* *Oscivirus A* *Parechovirus A–D*
Pasivirus *Passerivirus* *Potampivirus* *Rabovirus* *Rosavirus* *Sakubovirus* *Salivirus* *Sapelovirus*	*Pasivirus A* *Passerivirus A* *Potampivirus A* *Rabovirus A* *Rosavirus A* *Sakubovirus A* *Salivirus A* *Avian sapelovirus* *Sapelovirus A, B*
Senecavirus	*Senecavirus A*
Shanbavirus *Sicinivirus* *Teschovirus* *Torchivirus* *Tremovirus*	*Shanbavirus A* *Sicinivirus A* *Teschovirus A* *Torchivirus A* *Tremovirus A*

The genus *Aphthovirus* consists of four species: *foot-and-mouth disease virus* (FMDV), *bovine rhinitis A* virus, *bovine rhinitis B virus*, and *equine rhinitis A virus*. FMDV infects cloven-footed animals (e.g., cattle, goats, pigs, and sheep), primarily via the upper respiratory tract, and has been isolated from at least 70 species of mammals. Seven serotypes of FMDV have been identified, and within each serotype, there are many subtypes. These viruses are highly labile and rapidly lose infectivity at pH values of less than 6.8.

There are three species within the genus *Cardiovirus*: *Cardiovirus A, Cardiovirus B, and Cardiovirus C*. Isolates of *Cardiovirus A* include encephalomyocarditis viruses (EMCV) 1 to 2 and Theiler murine encephalomyelitis virus. These are murine viruses, which can also infect many other hosts, including humans, monkeys, pigs, elephants, and squirrels. *Cardiovirus B* includes Vilyuisk human encephalomyelitis virus and Saffold viruses 1 to 11.

There are 15 species in the *Enterovirus* genus: *Enterovirus A to L and Rhinovirus A to C*. Common members of this genus include polioviruses (3 serotypes), coxsackieviruses (28 serotypes), echoviruses (28 serotypes), human enteroviruses (53 serotypes), and many nonhuman viruses. There are 78, 30, and 51 types of *Rhinoviruses A, B,* and *C*, respectively.[522] Enteroviruses such as poliovirus and some coxsackieviruses replicate in the alimentary tract and are resistant to low pH. The acid-labile rhinoviruses (so named because they replicate in the nasopharynx) are important agents of the common cold. Rhinoviruses may also replicate in the lower respiratory tract; human rhinovirus C have been associated with severe lower respiratory tract disease.[452] Enterovirus D68 is unusual in that it shares genetic and biochemical properties of poliovirus and rhinovirus. This acid-labile virus replicates in both the upper and lower respiratory tracts and may be associated with a polio-like acute flaccid paralysis.[32,250,360,394,437,462,464–466,552,658,659]

The genus *Hepatovirus* with nine species has one human pathogen, *Hepatovirus A*, hepatitis A virus. Other members of this genus infect bats, hedgehogs, and shrews. Hepatitis A virus particles are highly stable and resistant to acid pH and high temperatures (60°C for 10 minutes). The virus infects epithelial cells of the small intestine and hepatocytes. An unusual feature of hepatitis A virus is the acquisition of a lipid envelope during nonlytic release from cells.[187]

The *Parechovirus* genus contains four species, *Parechovirus A to D*. The 16 different types of *Parechovirus A* are etiologic agents of respiratory and gastrointestinal disease. Proteins of parechoviruses are substantially diverged from those of other picornaviruses, with no greater than 30% amino acid identity. Ljungan virus is a virus of rodents within *Parechovirus B*.

The *Erbovirus* genus consists of one species, *Erbovirus A*, with three types of equine rhinitis B virus. These viruses cause upper respiratory tract disease in horses that is associated with viremia and fecal shedding of virus particles. The *Kobuvirus* genus contains six species, *Aichivirus A to F*, which cause gastroenteritis in humans and possibly in other animals. The *Teschovirus* genus consists of *Teschovirus A* with 13 types of porcine teschovirus. Some isolates can cause polioencephalitis in pigs, also called Teschen/Talfan disease or teschovirus encephalomyelitis. There are three species in the *Sapelovirus* genus: *Avian sapelovirus* and *Sapelovirus A and B*. Porcine sapelovirus, classified in *Sapelovirus A*, is a ubiquitous virus of pigs first isolated in the 1950s. The sole species in the genus

Senecavirus is *Senecavirus A* whose members are found in pigs throughout the United States, Brazil, and China. Virus infection causes blisters on the snout and hoofs,[12,188] though the prototype isolate, Seneca Valley virus 001, is nonpathogenic in both pigs and humans. This trait has been exploited for the clinical development of Seneca Valley virus as a safe and effective oncolytic agent for treating human tumors.[101,611]

The picornavirus family will continue to expand, as hundreds of genome sequences of these viruses have been determined but not yet assigned to either a species or genus.[377]

VIRION STRUCTURE

Physical Properties

Picornavirus particles are spherical with a diameter of about 30 nm and consist of a protein shell surrounding the naked RNA genome (Fig. 2.1A). Infectivity is insensitive to organic solvents as the particles lack a membrane. Cardioviruses, enteroviruses (except enterovirus D viruses), hepatoviruses, and parechoviruses are acid stable and retain infectivity at pH values of 3.0 and lower. In contrast, rhinoviruses and aphthoviruses are labile at pH values of less than 6.0. Differences in pH stability reflect the sites of replication of the virus. For example, rhinoviruses and aphthoviruses replicate in the respiratory tract and need not be acid stable. Because they are acid labile, they cannot replicate in the alimentary tract. Cardioviruses, enteroviruses, hepatoviruses, and parechoviruses pass through the stomach to gain access to the intestine and, therefore, must be resistant to low pH. The structural basis for the acid lability of FMDV and enterovirus D68 is partly understood (see *Entry into Cells*).

The buoyant densities of picornaviruses are quite different (Table 2.2). Cardioviruses and enteroviruses have a buoyant density of 1.34 g/mL, that of FMDV is 1.45 g/mL, and rhinoviruses have an intermediate value (1.40 g/mL). The reason for the difference lies in the permeability of the viral capsid to cesium. The capsid of poliovirus does not allow cesium to reach the RNA interior; hence, the virus sediments at an abnormally light buoyant density.[201] In contrast, *Aphthovirus* capsids contain pores that allow cesium to enter.[1] The rhinovirus capsid is permeable to cesium, but the presence of polyamines in the capsid interior limits the amount of cesium that can enter, which provides a possible explanation for the intermediate buoyant density value of these viruses.[201]

Ratio of Particles to Infectious Viruses

The ratio of particles to infectious virus is determined by dividing the number of virus particles in a sample (determined by electron microscopy or spectrophotometric measurements) by the plaque titer, yielding the particle–to–plaque-forming unit (pfu) ratio. This ratio is a measurement of the fraction of virus particles that can complete an infectious cycle. The particle-to-pfu ratio of poliovirus ranges from 30 to 1,000, and that of other picornaviruses is in the same range. The high particle-to-pfu ratio may be caused by the presence of lethal mutations in the viral genome. This explanation, however, probably does not apply to all picornaviruses; it has been shown that the infectivity of *Aphthovirus* RNA approaches one infectious unit per molecule.[69] An alternative explanation is that all viruses do not successfully complete an infectious cycle because they fail

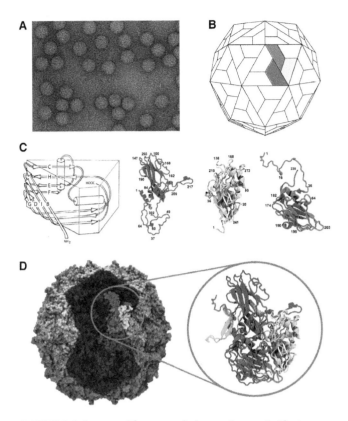

FIGURE 2.1 Structural features of picornaviruses. A: Electron micrograph of negatively stained poliovirus (×270,000 magnification). **B:** Schematic of the picornavirus capsid, showing the pseudo-equivalent packing arrangement of VP1 (*blue*), VP2 (*yellow*), and VP3 (*red*). VP4 (*green*) is on the interior of the capsid. A single biologic protomer is colored. **C:** The topology of the polypeptide chain in β-barrel jelly roll, which composes the core of the three capsid proteins, VP1, VP2, and VP3. The β-strands, named by the letters B to I, form two antiparallel sheets juxtaposed in a wedge-shaped–like structure. The loops that connect β-strands are denoted by two letters reflecting those they connect. Individual capsid proteins VP1, VP2, VP3, and VP4 are shown as cartoon representations of the alpha carbon backbone. **D:** Model of poliovirus type 1, Mahoney, based on x-ray crystallographic structure determined at 2.9 Å. Two adjacent pentamers aligned at the twofold axis of symmetry are shaded *dark gray*. A single protomer is colored and also expanded at right as a cartoon of the alpha carbon backbone; capsid proteins are color coded according to **(B)**.

at one of several essential steps, including attachment, entry, replication, and assembly. For additional discussion of the role of mutation in the particle–to–plaque-forming unit ratio, see *Origins of Diversity*.

High-Resolution Structure of the Virus Particle

The capsids of picornaviruses are composed of three structural proteins: VP1, VP2, and VP3. All but hepatoviruses and kobuviruses have a fourth protein, VP4, in the capsid interior, which is the N-terminal cleavage product of the VP2 precursor, VP0. The results of x-ray diffraction studies, electron microscopic observations, and biochemical studies of virus particles and their dissociation products led to the hypothesis that the picornavirus capsid contains 60 structural units composed of three virus-specific proteins arranged into an icosahedral lattice.[612] Our understanding of the architecture of picornaviruses was substantially advanced in 1985 when the atomic structures of poliovirus type 1[303] and human rhinovirus type 14[607] were determined by x-ray crystallography. Since then, the high-resolution structures of over 200 picornaviruses have been determined.

The smallest structural unit of the picornavirus capsid is the protomer, which is built with one copy of each capsid protein (Fig. 2.1B, C). Five protomers form the pentamer, and 60 pentamers form the characteristic icosahedral capsid of this family of viruses. The virus particles are described as a pseudo T = 3 structure because they are constructed with three different polypeptides.

VP1, VP2, and VP3, which compose the outside of the shell of the particle, have no sequence homology, yet all three proteins have the same topology: they form an eight-stranded, antiparallel β-barrel (also called a β-barrel jelly roll or a Swiss-roll β-barrel) (Fig. 2.1C). The picornavirus particle is therefore composed of 180 β-barrels: 60 β-barrels each of VP1, VP2, and VP3.

The β-barrel is a wedge-shaped structure made up of two antiparallel β-sheets (Fig. 2.1C). One β-sheet forms the wall of the wedge, and the second, which has a bend in the center, forms both a wall and the floor. The wedge shape facilitates the packing of structural units to form a dense, rigid protein shell. Packing of the β-barrel domains is strengthened by a network of protein–protein contacts on the interior of the capsid, particularly around the fivefold axes, generating a pentamer.

TABLE 2.2   Physical properties of some picornaviruses

Genus	pH Stability	Virion Buoyant Density	Sedimentation Coefficient
Aphthovirus	Labile, <6.8	1.43–1.45	142–146S
Cardiovirus	Stable, 3–9	1.33–1.34	160S
Enterovirus Enteroviruses Rhinoviruses	Stable, 3–9 Labile, <6	1.34 1.40	160S 160S
Hepatovirus	Stable	1.32–1.34	160S
Parechovirus	Stable	1.36	160S
Kobuvirus	Stable, >4	1.25–1.30	140–165S
Teschovirus	Stable	1.35	

This network, which is formed by the N-terminal extensions of VP1 to VP3 as well as VP4, is essential for the stability of the virus particle. The increased length of VP4 in kobuviruses leads to the "bow and arrow" shape of the protein, allowing more extensive interactions between VP4 and the other protomers of a pentamer and formation of an extensive network at the inner surface of the capsid. Despite these interactions, stability of kobuvirus particles is very similar to that of other enteroviruses. The lack of extensive interactions between pentamers in the *Aphthovirus* capsid renders these virions the least stable of all picornaviruses.

A different organization in the structure of hepatitis A virus is caused by a flip in the torsion angle of the peptide at VP2 residue 53, which sends the chain across the interpentamer boundary. The consequence is that neighboring protomers of one pentamer are linked together via the adjacent pentamer. Such an arrangement is not seen in other picornaviruses but does occur in insect picorna-like viruses. Together with properties of the pocket (see below), these observations suggest that hepatitis A virus is a primordial picornavirus.

The antiparallel β-sheets of each capsid protein are connected to each other via the BC, HI, DE, FG, GH, and CD loops (Fig. 2.1C). These loops confer the main structural differences among VP1, VP2, and VP3: their amino acid sequences and length give each picornavirus its distinct morphology and antigenicity. The N- and C-terminal sequences of each protein extend from the β-barrel domain. The C-termini of the proteins are located on the surface of the virion, and the N-termini are in the interior, indicating that significant rearrangement of the P1 precursor occurs on proteolytic cleavage (see *Assembly of Virus Particles*).

Resolution of the structures of poliovirus and rhinovirus revealed that the β-barrel domains are strikingly similar in structure to those of plant viruses such as southern bean mosaic virus and tomato bushy stunt virus. The capsid proteins of these viruses bear no sequence homology with those of the picornaviruses. It has since become apparent that similar protein topology is found in the capsid proteins of many plant, insect, and vertebrate positive-strand RNA viruses as well as in the DNA-containing polyomaviruses and adenoviruses. These findings suggest that either the polypeptides evolved from a common ancestor or the β-barrel domain is one of the few ways to allow proteins to pack to form a sphere.

VP4 lies on the inner capsid surface and differs significantly from the other three proteins in that it has an extended conformation (Fig. 2.1D). This protein is similar in position and conformation to the NH₂-terminal sequences of VP1 and VP3 and functions as a detached NH₂-terminal extension of VP2 rather than an independent capsid protein. In some viruses, such as the kobuviruses and parechoviruses, VP0 remains uncleaved. In the Aichi virus capsid, the consequence is a unique extended "bow and arrow" structure described above. In kobuviruses, uncleaved VP4 is approximately 30 to 50 amino acids longer than in other picornaviruses,[781] while in hepatitis A virus VP4 is very small.

Surface of the Virus Particle

Resolution of the structures of poliovirus, rhinovirus, and mengovirus revealed that the surfaces of these viruses have a corrugated topography: a prominent, star-shaped plateau (mesa) and solvent-filled channel at the fivefold axis of symmetry, surrounded by a deep depression (canyon) and another protrusion (three-bladed propellers) at the threefold axis (Fig. 2.2). The spike-like protrusions on the external surface of the capsid reflect the length and amino acid composition of the loops. Despite VP1 being the most external and antigenic capsid protein of picornaviruses, the majority of residues that line the canyon are derived from the core of VP1, while the loops form the star-shaped mesa. The unstructured ends of VP1 are found at the fivefold axes. In contrast, the unstructured ends of VP2 and VP3 are found at the threefold axes, while the cores of these proteins are woven together to form the hubs of the propellers. The propeller blades are made up by the EF loop of VP2 and supported by the GH loop of VP1 and the C-terminus extensions of VP1 and VP2. The north wall of the canyon lies near the fivefold axis and is composed of two N-terminal loops of VP1,

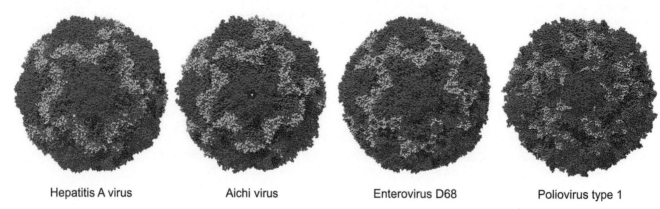

| Hepatitis A virus | Aichi virus | Enterovirus D68 | Poliovirus type 1 |

FIGURE 2.2 Structures of four different picornavirus virus particles. In all panels, VP1 is *blue*, VP2 is *yellow*, and VP3 is *deep pink*. Surface view of the 3 Å structure of the hepatitis A virus particle, which lacks both a canyon and a VP1 hydrophobic pocket, determined by x-ray crystallography of purified virions [4QPI]. The smooth surface of the particle is due to woven interactions between pentamers that prevent formation of the canyon that surrounds the fivefold axes of symmetry. Surface view of the 3.7 Å structure of the Aichi virus virion, which lacks a VP1 hydrophobic pocket but deep pits are found at the fivefold axes, determined by cryo-EM reconstruction [5GKA]. Surface view of the 2 Å structure of the enterovirus D68 (Fermon) particle, has a shallow canyon and ill-formed VP1 hydrophobic pocket filled with a C12 cell lipid, determined by x-ray crystallography of purified virions [4WM8]. Surface view of the 2.2 Å structure of the poliovirus type 1 particle, possess both a deep canyon and VP1 hydrophobic pocket occupied by a C16 cell lipid, determined by x-ray crystallography of purified virions [1HXS].

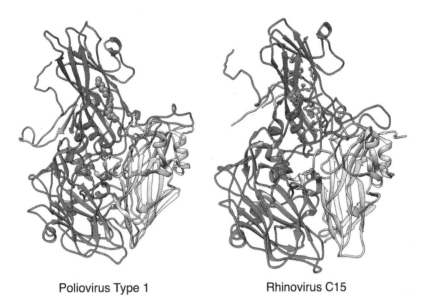

Poliovirus Type 1   Rhinovirus C15

FIGURE 2.3 The hydrophobic pocket in the picornavirus capsid. VP1 is *blue*, VP2 is *yellow*, VP3 is *deep pink*, and VP4 is *green*. Cellular lipid bound in the hydrophobic pocket of poliovirus type 1. Top view of the poliovirus protomer, consisting of one copy each of VP1, VP2, VP3, and VP4. RNA is below, and the fivefold axis of symmetry is at the upper left. *Orange spheres* represent what is believed to be a molecule of sphingosine bound in the hydrophobic pocket. The lipid is just below the canyon floor [1HXS]. Top view of the rhinovirus C15 protomer, consisting of one copy each of VP1, VP2, and VP3. RNA is below, and the fivefold axis of symmetry is at the upper left. Capsid proteins are colored as in panel A. In *orange* are amino acids of VP1 GH loop (V1156, I1130, F1132, F1167, I1120, V118, I1169, M1116, W1080, F1096, M1180, Y1178, I1094) and one within VP3 (I3024) that occlude the hydrophobic pocket, inhibiting binding of the cellular lipid and activity of pocket-binding antiviral compounds [5KOU].

the BC and DE loops. The C-terminal GH loop of VP1 as well as parts of VP2 and VP3 form the south wall and floor of the canyon. The GH loop of VP1 also forms the entrance to and defines the VP1 hydrophobic pocket (Fig. 2.3). Additionally, the C-terminus of VP3 decorates the north side of the canyon. The GH loop of VP0/VP2 forms the antigenic "puff." The remaining loops of VP0/VP2 and VP3 are not long enough to deform the particle surface. However, the b β-sheet of VP3 is fractured, leaving a long hairpin loop, "the knob," to extend from the surface of the virion. The internalized N-termini of VP3, a parallel β-tube, together with a three-stranded β-sheet of the myristylated N-termini of VP4, compose the plug of the solvent channel.

The presence of the canyon prompted the hypothesis that this depression is the receptor-binding site, which has been proved for a number of enteroviruses. Not all picornaviruses have canyons: the surface of cardioviruses and senecaviruses bears a series of depressions or "pits," which are involved in receptor binding, while the surface of FMDV, echoviruses, enterovirus D68, hepatitis A virus, and kobuviruses is much smoother (Fig. 2.2). The pits around the fivefold axes of cardioviruses are filled by the CD loop of VP1, and the VP2 "puff" is subdivided into two, puff A and puff B. The VP3 "knob" is the most prominent projection of the capsid and is composed of two β-strands. Also, within the CD loop of VP3, which is close to the knob, is a disulfide bond between cysteines that are separated by one amino acid. This disulfide bond introduces

a sharp bend, which when disrupted results in a decrease of virus infectivity and increase in particle stability.[489] As will be discussed later, a flexible loop that projects from the capsid surface binds to the cellular receptor for FMDV and cardioviruses. Unlike the canyon of enteroviruses and other parechoviruses, the canyon of human parechovirus 3 is wide and shallow.[632]

Interior of the Virus Particle

A network formed by the N-termini on the interior of the capsid contributes significantly to the stability of the virion. For the majority of picornaviruses, the N-terminus of VP1 lines the interior of the virus particle along the fivefold axis, where the N-termini of five VP3 molecules form a cylindrically parallel β-sheet. This structure is surrounded by five three-stranded β-sheets formed by the N-termini of VP4 and VP1. The crystal structure of enterovirus A71, however, revealed an alternative organization of the interior of the capsid. Underneath the αA helices of VP2 and adjacent to the twofold axes and across the protomer lies the very N-terminus of VP1, while VP4 forms a loose spiral beneath VP1[739] (Fig. 2.4). For picornaviruses such as human parechoviruses, in which VP0 is not cleaved, the N-terminus does not surround the fivefold axis; instead, it straddles the adjacent threefold axes forming a loop, which stabilizes VP0 of the neighboring pentamer.[632] The myristate group attached to the N-terminus of VP4 mediates the interaction between the VP3 cylinder and the three-stranded β-sheet of VP4 and VP1.[125] Interactions among pentamers are stabilized

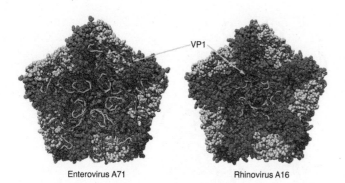

FIGURE 2.4 The unique inner organization of the enterovirus A71 particle. VP1 is *blue*, VP2 is *yellow*, VP3 is *deep pink*, and VP4 is *green*. *Turquoise arrows* point to N-terminus of VP1. Interior of the enterovirus A71 pentamer showing amino acids 1 to 26 of VP1 as a ribbon. This part of VP1 lays across the protomer underneath the αA helices of VP2 next to the twofold axes, while the loose spiral of VP4 (shown as a *ribbon*) is beneath VP1 [3VBS]. Interior of human rhinovirus 16 pentamer illustrates the more typical organization of amino acids of 1 to 28 of VP1 (shown as *ribbon*), which fold toward the fivefold axis and the five N-termini of VP4, which form five three-stranded β-sheets (shown as *ribbon*) [1AYN].

by a seven-stranded β-sheet, composed of four β-strands of the VP3 β-barrel and one strand from the N-terminus of VP1 that surround a two-stranded β-sheet made from the N-terminus of VP2 from a neighboring pentamer.[192]

Poliovirus genomes containing an extra 1,250 nucleotides (17%) can be successfully packaged, indicating that the interior of the capsid is not fully occupied.[9] For some picornaviruses, it has been possible to visualize the RNA genome, which is highly condensed and may be evenly packed into the particle at a concentration of 800 mg/mL.[173,388] The RNA is arranged in multiple layers approximately 18 Å apart, with a similar distance between the most external layer and inner capsid shell. For some picornaviruses such as Coxsackievirus A16, the RNA is more condensed and arranged so that a 15-Å gap exists between the genome and the capsid.[589] In cardioviruses, the inner and outer edges of the RNA genome are located 35 and 95 Å away from the center, respectively.[489]

It has been suggested that picornaviral capsids are stabilized by interactions with the RNA genome, based on findings with bean pod mottle virus, which is related to picornaviruses. In this virus, ordered RNA can be observed at the threefold axis, and packaging of viral RNA stabilizes subunit interactions.[119,409] Several nucleotides have been tentatively identified in a similar location in the structures of P3/Sabin and rhinovirus type 14.[29,192] In the atomic structure of poliovirus P2/Lansing, RNA bases have been observed stacking with conserved aromatic residues of VP4.[404] The structures of rhinovirus 2, Seneca Valley virus, and Coxsackievirus A10 also revealed the arrangement of the RNA within the capsid.[557,719,779] Much of the nucleic acid contacts the inner surface of the capsid, particularly near the twofold axes under VP2. The RNA forms a shell that contacts both VP2 and VP4 and which could serve as a scaffold for capsid assembly or might contribute to virion stability. A basic motif at the N-terminus of Ljungan virus VP3 around the fivefold axes interacts with 15 bases of ordered genomic RNA.[780] The basic amino acids constitute a positively charged environment that counters the negative charge of the RNA phosphate moieties. Approximately 900 bases, or 12% of the viral genome, are ordered within the capsid. The Coxsackievirus A10 virion is distinct in that the N-terminus of VP4 lies under the adjacent protomer and is of the opposite charge. The reversed orientation of the charge reveals a novel interaction between the inner capsid proteins and the tightly compacted RNA genome.[779] Additionally, amino acids of VP1 and VP3 that lie beneath the base of the canyon also interact with the RNA genome, suggesting that transmission of a signal is necessary for uncoating. Furthermore, the majority of the RNA within the particle does not exhibit icosahedral symmetry; instead, the RNA takes on a spherical shape with pseudo-fivefold symmetry. Analysis of the human parechovirus 3 structure determined that 25% of the genome is ordered and takes on a "finger-like" structure contacting the βIC terminus of VP1 and the N-terminus of VP3 around the 60 vertices. Interaction between the N-terminus of VP3 and two RNA stem–loops was also observed.[632]

Hydrophobic Pocket

Lipids in the Virus Particle

Within the core of VP1, just beneath the canyon floor of many picornaviruses, is a hydrophobic tunnel or pocket (Fig. 2.3). Electron density observed in this area has been interpreted to be cell-derived lipids called "pocket factors" that regulate the conformational states of the virus during cell entry. Members of *Enteroviruses A*, *B*, and *C* have a well-formed pocket factor with a long aliphatic chain. In poliovirus types 1 and 3, the pocket factor is the C18 sphingosine[192] (Fig. 2.3). A C12 lipid occupies the pocket of human rhinoviruses types A16 and A2, a C16 lipid sits within the pocket of Coxsackievirus B3,[268,364,487] and Coxsackievirus A21 is believed to carry myristic acid.[759] A mixture of palmitic and myristic acid is present in the pocket of bovine enterovirus,[644] and a branched, elongated lipid is found in the pocket of Coxsackievirus A24 and swine vesicular disease virus.[721,782] In the enterovirus A71 virus particle, the C18 pocket factor is partly exposed on the floor of the canyon.[566] The pocket of some isolates of enterovirus D68, including the prototype Fermon, is shallow and ill-formed and contains a C10 lipid,[417] while in other isolates, the pocket is fully collapsed and unable to accommodate the lipid.[418] This trait, the absence of pocket factor, has also been recognized for rhinoviruses types B3 and B14, in which the pocket is empty and not well formed.[29] In rhinovirus C15, the pocket is collapsed but filled with bulky hydrophobic amino acids and cannot accommodate a lipid[416] (Fig. 2.3). The results of introducing amino acid changes in the pocket of rhinovirus 16 suggest that the hydrophobic pocket, and not the pocket factor, is important for maintaining capsid dynamics.[355] Additionally, kobuviruses, including Aichi virus, have a shallow and narrow depression, not a canyon around the fivefold axes; consequently, these virus particles lack a hydrophobic pocket and a pocket factor.[781] Viruses that lack canyons, such as hepatitis A virus and parechoviruses, do not have pockets or pocket factors[740] and may be a link between primitive and modern (e.g., with pocket factors) picornaviruses. Furthermore, the absence of a canyon suggests there must be at least two mechanisms by which receptor binding, internalization, and uncoating occur.

Myristate

Myristic acid (*n*-tetradecanoic acid) is covalently linked to glycine at the amino terminus of VP4 of most picornaviruses.[125,536]

This fatty acid is an integral part of the viral capsid. The N-termini of VP4 and VP3 cluster together at the fivefold axis of symmetry where they intertwine and form a twisted tube of parallel β-structure.[303] The five myristyl groups extend to cradle this twisted tube by interacting with amino acid side chains of VP4 and VP3.[125] The study of viruses with amino acid substitutions within VP4 has revealed a role for myristic acid modification in virus assembly and in the stability of the capsid.[20,439,440,481] However, inhibition of myristoylation modestly inhibits infectivity of enterovirus A71.[676] For most picornaviruses, particle *breathing* occurs at physiological temperatures, allowing for partial exit of VP4 including the N-terminal myristic acid. The presence of myristic acid facilitates membrane permeability by VP4 at high and low pH, both requirements for virus entry and uncoating.[526] These observations cast additional doubt that myristic acid is needed for virion stability.[406,410,652]

Myristic acid is added to VP0, the precursor to VP4+VP2, by cellular N-myristoyltransferases. Inhibitors of these enzymes suppress rhinovirus, poliovirus, Coxsackievirus B3 and FMDV replication by blocking particle assembly, RNA encapsidation, and inhibiting the cleavage between VP2 and VP4 that is necessary for particle maturation.[20,136,385] Infectivity of parechoviruses and Aichi viruses is resistant to myristoyltransferase inhibitors, likely because VP0 of these viruses does not undergo this maturation cleavage.[136] Myristoyltransferase inhibitors may be developed as antipicornavirus drugs against those viruses that require cleavage between VP2 and VP4 for mature particle formation.[136,486] (See *Assembly of Virus Particles*.)

Neutralizing Antigenic Sites

Viral serotype is determined by the connecting loops and C-termini of the capsid proteins that decorate the outer surface of the virus particle. These contain the major neutralization antigenic sites of the virus, the amino acid sequences that are recognized by antibodies that block viral infectivity. The identification of mutations that confer resistance to neutralization with murine monoclonal antibodies directed against rhinovirus and poliovirus particles have defined four enterovirus neutralization antigenic sites.[468,469,636] Human sera contain antibodies directed against poliovirus antigenic sites identified in mice.[590] The major antigenic site for many picornaviruses is a linear stretch of 10 amino acids within the BC loop of VP1. Five neutralization antigenic sites have been identified in FMDV serotype O.[147,370] Eleven different neutralizing antibodies directed against porcine teschovirus 1 recognize three antigenic sites on the virus particle.[347] Neutralizing antibodies against hepatitis A virus protect against infection by acting as a receptor mimic, leading to destabilization of the particle in a fashion that is independent of virion expansion.[741] In contrast, two neutralizing antibodies generated against the empty capsid of enterovirus A71 are able to induce virion alteration and genome release.[565]

The capsids of rhinovirus, poliovirus, and other picornaviruses are dynamic, leading to transient display of the buried N-termini of VP1 on the particle surface.[336,354,410,576,602,621] Antibodies to this sequence of VP1 neutralize viral infectivity.

GENOME STRUCTURE AND ORGANIZATION

The genome of picornaviruses is a single positive-strand RNA molecule ranging in length from 6.7 to 10.1 kb (Fig. 2.5). The viral RNA is infectious because it is translated on entry into the cell to produce all the proteins required for viral reproduction. Picornavirus genomic RNA is unique because it is covalently linked at the 5′ end to a protein called *VPg* (virion protein, genome linked)[195,402] that is covalently joined to the 5′-uridylylate moiety of the viral RNA by an O4-(5′-uridylyl)-tyrosine linkage. The tyrosine that is linked to the viral RNA

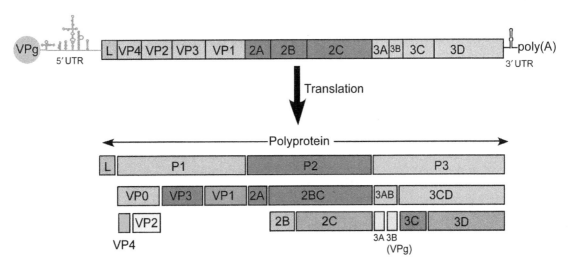

FIGURE 2.5 Organization of a picornavirus genome. Top: Schematic of the viral RNA genome, with the genome-linked protein VPg at the 5′ end, the 5′-untranslated region containing the IRES, the protein-coding region, the 3′ untranslated region containing a pseudoknot, and the poly(A) tail. L is a leader protein encoded in the genomes of erboviruses, cardioviruses, and aphthoviruses but not in other picornaviruses. Coding regions for the viral proteins are indicated. **Bottom:** Processing pattern of picornavirus polyprotein. Some genomes encode multiple copies of protein-coding regions, for example, there are three VPgs in the FMDV genome, two 2A motifs in Ljungan virus and three 2A motifs in the duck hepatitis A virus genome.

is always the third amino acid from the N-terminus. VPg of different picornaviruses varies in length from 22 to 24 amino acid residues and is present in one copy except in the genome of FMDV, which encodes three VPg proteins.[200] The absence of VPg differentiates poliovirus mRNA from virion RNA. Furthermore, VPg is not required for infectivity of poliovirus RNA. If VPg is removed from viral RNA by treatment with proteinase, the specific infectivity of the viral RNA is not reduced. VPg is not found on poliovirus mRNA that is associated with cellular ribosomes and undergoing translation; these mRNAs contain only uridine 5′-phosphate (pU) at their 5′ ends.[507,547] It is not known whether removal of VPg is a prerequisite for association with ribosomes or is a result of that association, though its removal must occur as the genome is released into the cytoplasm.[13,725] Despite the fact that VPg-linked RNA can be translated in cell-free extracts, in the infected cell it is possible that VPg is rapidly cleaved from the RNA such that only RNAs lacking VPg are translated.[232,475,724] Furthermore, removal of VPg from CVB3 RNA is not necessary for translation or replication of the incoming genome, as determined by the introduction of a noncleavable bond between VPg and RNA.[395] VPg is present on nascent RNA chains of the replicative intermediate RNA and on negative-strand RNA, which has led to the suggestion that VPg is a primer for poliovirus RNA synthesis[506,547] (see *Viral RNA Synthesis*). These observations distinguish picornavirus VPg from that of calicivirus, in that it predominantly coordinates genome replication and does not participate in virus protein synthesis. The role of VPg in viral RNA synthesis is discussed in subsequent sections.

VPg is removed from virion RNA by a host protein originally called *unlinking enzyme*[14] and subsequently identified as the DNA repair enzyme TDP2 (5′ tyrosyl-DNA phosphodiesterase 2).[725] This predominantly nuclear enzyme, which cleaves the 5′-tyrosine-phosphodiester bond of DNA linked to topoisomerase, is relocalized to the cytoplasm during picornaviral infection. However, the results of infecting cells lacking the gene encoding TDP2 reveal that the VPg unlinking activity is not essential for the replication of enteroviruses and cardioviruses. Its absence affects replication efficiency to different extents, depending on the virus.[434,435] Late in infection, TDP2 is sequestered away from sites of viral replication, possibly to avoid removal of VPg from newly synthesized genomes destined for packaging into new virus particles. Why removal of VPg is required earlier in infection for efficient replication is not known.

Nucleotide sequence analysis of many picornavirus genomes has revealed a common organizational pattern (Fig. 2.5). The 5′-noncoding regions of picornaviruses are long (192–1,500 bases) and highly structured. This region of the genome contains sequences that control genome replication and translation. Removal of several nucleotides from the 5′ end of the genome ablates the infectivity of the viral RNA of some picornaviruses such as hepatitis A virus, but for others, including poliovirus, the loss of two nucleotides from the 5′ end only reduces its infectivity.[281,290] Within the 5′-noncoding region is the internal ribosome entry site (IRES), which directs initiation of mRNA translation by internal ribosome binding. The 5′-noncoding regions of aphthoviruses and cardioviruses contain a poly(C) tract that varies in length among different virus strains (80–250 nucleotides in cardioviruses,

40–400 nucleotides in aphthoviruses). Among cardioviruses, longer poly(C) length is associated with higher virulence in animals.[175,270]

A second characteristic of the 5′-noncoding region is the presence of multiple AUG codons, which vary in number among picornaviruses. Initially, these AUG codons were not thought to be physiologically relevant as deletion or alteration of these codons had no effect on picornavirus replication in HeLa cells, an assumption that is no longer correct. A small upstream open reading frame (uORF) encoding a polypeptide of approximately 56 to 76 amino acids with a predicted transmembrane domain has been identified within the 5′ end of type 1 poliovirus and enterovirus 7 that initiates from the sixth AUG.[428] The encoded polypeptide is thought to function during virus release from intestinal cells. A shorter ORF is present within the 5′-noncoding region of type 2 poliovirus; alteration of this AUG leads to a small plaque phenotype.[541] Bioinformatic analysis has identified uORFs initiating at the analogous AUG within the genome of viruses in the enterovirus A, B, C, E, F, and G species, as well as other picornavirus genera that infect the gut such as hunniviruses, lyssaviruses, rosaviruses B and C, siniviruses, and cosaviruses.[428] No similar polypeptide was found to be encoded and initiating from this AUG within the 5′-noncoding region of rhinoviruses or enterovirus D viruses. Though no uORF has been identified within the 5′-noncoding region of cardioviruses, an alternative reading frame has been identified within the mRNA of Theiler murine encephalomyelitis virus (TMEV), which promotes the production of two different leader (L)* proteins, p18 and p15, in certain isolates such as DA.[709] Production of the smaller polypeptide begins at an AUG codon internal to and out of frame with the large polyprotein.[384,604] L* is thought to be produced during persistent infection by neurotropic isolates of TMEV.

The 3′-noncoding regions of picornaviruses vary in length from 14 to 795 nucleotides (Fig. 2.5). This region may also contain secondary structure, including a pseudoknot, that has been implicated in controlling viral RNA synthesis[328] and stem–loops. The 3′-noncoding regions of parechoviruses and pasiviruses are short and hypothesized to fold into one stem–loop, while that of FMDV and other picornaviruses are longer and may fold into multiple stem–loops[89] (reviewed in Ref.[375]). The entire 3′-noncoding region of poliovirus and rhinovirus is not required, however, for infectivity.[97,685] Removal of part of the 3′-noncoding region, including sequence between the two stem–loops and the 5′ end of stem–loop 2 from the FMDV genome, renders the RNA noninfectious.[81] Additionally, bioinformatic analysis of the 3′-noncoding region of the megrivirus turkey hepatitis virus 1 and multiple chicken megriviruses suggest the presence of a short ORF.[90]

Both virion RNA and mRNA contain a 3′ stretch of poly(A).[769] This stretch of poly(A) varies in length, for example, from 50 to 125 nucleotides in poliovirus RNA,[5,657] and is required for genome replication. Viral RNA from which the poly(A) tract is removed is noninfectious.[651] Negative-strand RNA contains a 5′ stretch of poly(U), which is copied to form poly(A) of the positive strand.[768]

The results of early biochemical studies of poliovirus-infected cells had predicted the presence of a single, long ORF on the viral RNA that is processed to form individual viral proteins.[668] This hypothesis was supported by determination of the nucleotide sequence of the poliovirus genome, which revealed that the viral RNA encodes a single ORF.[369,582] The polyprotein is cleaved during translation, so that the full-length product is not observed. Processing is carried out by virus-encoded proteinases to yield 11 to 15 final cleavage products. Some of the uncleaved precursors also have functions during replication. A similar strategy for viral protein production occurs during the replication of all picornaviruses except those within the genus *Dicipivirus*. The genome of these viruses encodes two ORFs.

To unify the nomenclature of picornavirus proteins, the polyprotein has been divided into three regions: P1, P2, and P3 (Fig. 2.5). The genomes of some picornaviruses encode an L protein before the P1 region. It was once thought that many L proteins had protease and autocatalytic activities; however, L protein of kobuviruses possesses neither.[619] The P1 region encodes the viral capsid proteins, whereas the P2 and P3 regions encode proteins involved in protein processing (2A, 3C^{pro}, 3CD^{pro}) and genome replication (2B, 2C, 3AB, 3B^{VPg}, 3CD^{pro}, 3D^{pol}). For many picornaviruses such as EMCV, FMDV, and kobuviruses, the 2A protein lacks protease activity; for others such as poliovirus, rhinovirus, and hepatitis A, 2A is a serine protease. The genome of Ljungan virus, a parechovirus, may encode two unrelated 2A proteins,[338] that of duck hepatitis A virus in the genus *Avihepatovirus* encodes three 2A motifs, and the genome of *Aalivirus* may encode for up to six 2A proteins.[737]

Genetics

Infectious DNA Clones of Picornavirus Genomes

Recombinant DNA techniques allow the introduction of mutations anywhere within a gene or genome. Generation of an infectious DNA clone—a double-stranded DNA copy of a viral genome within a bacterial plasmid—or RNA transcripts derived by *in vitro* transcription of a DNA copy of the genome, can be introduced into cultured cells by transfection to recover infectious virus. The first infectious DNA clone of an animal RNA virus was that of poliovirus.[581] The infectivity of cloned poliovirus DNA (10^3 pfu/μg) is much lower than that of genomic RNA (10^6 pfu/μg). The development of plasmid vectors incorporating promoters for bacteriophage SP6, T7, or T3 RNA polymerase for the production of RNA transcripts *in vitro* enabled the production of infectious picornavirus RNA from cloned DNA.[706] Such RNA transcripts have an infectivity approaching that of genomic RNA. A similar approach has been adopted for the recovery of many other picornaviruses from cloned DNA copies of the viral genome.

Replicons

Development of infectious DNA clones of picornavirus genomes has facilitated studies to understand the mechanism of virus reproduction. One result of such studies has been the production of replicons and viral vectors. Picornaviral replicons can consist of defective genomes or genomes lacking specific proteins (subgenomic replicons), with the complementary or missing genes encoded within separate plasmids or transcripts. Introduction of mutant genomes together with plasmids encoding the unaltered gene can lead to the production of infectious virus lacking the mutation. The use of poliovirus subgenomic replicons demonstrated that the P1 region, which encodes the capsid proteins, is not necessary for translation or replication of the viral genome. However, these subgenomic replicons may interfere with production of infectious virus.[350] Furthermore, subgenomic replicons of picornaviruses allow for the production

of exogenous proteins in cells.[544] Replicons have been used to study genetic and protein requirements for the replication of multiple picornaviruses.

Gene Editing

The manipulation of DNA *in vitro* once solely depended upon restriction enzymes and other modifying enzymes such as DNA ligases. With the identification and elucidation of the mechanism of CRISPR/Cas9 (clustered regularly interspaced short palindromic repeats/CRISPR-associated nuclease 9) methodology, a DNA copy of the viral genome can be easily modified to encode desired mutations and also encode for exogenous genes.

STAGES OF REPLICATION

Replication of all picornaviruses occurs in the cell cytoplasm. The first step is attachment to a cell receptor (Fig. 2.6). The RNA genome is then uncoated, a process that involves structural changes in the particle. Once the positive-strand viral RNA enters the cytoplasm, it is translated to provide viral proteins essential for genome replication and the production of new virus particles. The viral proteins are synthesized from a polyprotein precursor, which is cleaved nascently. Cleavages are carried out mainly by two viral proteinases, 2A^{pro} and 3C^{pro} or 3CD^{pro}. Among the proteins synthesized are the viral RNA–dependent RNA polymerase and accessory proteins required for genome replication and mRNA synthesis and the capsid precursor. The first step in genome replication is copying of the positive-strand RNA to form a negative-strand intermediate; this step is followed by the production of additional positive strands. These events occur on small membranous vesicles that are induced by several virus proteins. Once the pool of capsid proteins is sufficiently large, encapsidation begins. The precursor P1 is cleaved to produce an immature protomer, which then assembles into pentamers. Newly synthesized, positive-strand RNA associates with pentamers to form the infectious virus. Empty capsids that are found in infected cells are likely to be a storage form of pentamers.

The entire time required for a single replication cycle ranges from 5 to 10 hours, depending on many variables, including the particular virus, temperature, pH, host cell, and multiplicity of infection. Analysis of poliovirus replication in single cells reveals differences that are not apparent when infections are done in populations of cells.[262] For example, replication start times vary widely, and the production of infectious virus may begin later than predicted by population measurements. However, when multiple single-cell reproductive cycles are averaged, the result approximates the kinetics observed in populations of cells. Many picornaviruses are released as the cell loses its integrity and lyses. Other picornaviruses (e.g., hepatitis A virus) are released from cells in the absence of cytopathic effect within membranous vesicles.

Attachment

Cellular Receptors and Coreceptors

Like many viruses, picornaviruses initiate infection of cells by first attaching to a receptor on the host cell plasma membrane. The nature of picornavirus receptors remained obscure until 1989, when the receptors for poliovirus and the major group rhinoviruses were identified.[251,460,656] Receptors for many other

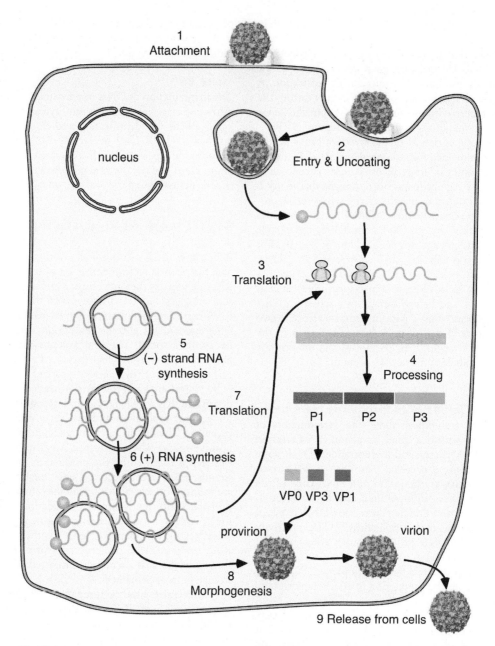

FIGURE 2.6 Overview of the picornavirus replication cycle. Virus binds to a cellular receptor (*1*) and the genome is uncoated (*2*). VPg (virion protein, genome linked) is removed from the viral RNA, which is then translated (*3*). The polyprotein is cleaved nascently to produce individual viral proteins (*4*). RNA synthesis occurs on membrane vesicles induced by viral proteins (not drawn to scale). Viral (+) strand RNA is copied by the viral RNA polymerase to form full-length (−) strand RNAs (*5*), which are then copied to produce additional (+) strand RNA (*6*). Early in infection, newly synthesized (+) strand RNA is translated to produce additional viral proteins (*7*). Later in infection, the (+) strands enter the morphogenetic pathway (*8*). Newly synthesized virus particles are released from the cell by lysis (*9*).

members of this virus family have since been determined (Table 2.3). Different types of cell surface molecules serve as cellular receptors for picornaviruses, and some are shared among picornaviruses and members of other virus families. For example, the cell surface protein CD55 is a receptor for certain Coxsackieviruses, echoviruses, and enterovirus 70, and the poliovirus receptor, CD155, is a receptor for alpha-herpesviruses. For some picornaviruses (e.g., poliovirus and

rhinovirus), a single type of receptor is sufficient for entry of viruses into cells. For other viruses, cell entry requires more than one molecule.

One Type of Receptor Molecule for Virus Binding and Entry

Picornaviruses for which a single type of receptor molecule is sufficient for virus binding and entry include poliovirus

TABLE 2.3   Some cell receptors for picornaviruses

Genus/Virus	Virus Receptor	Type of Receptor	Second Receptor	References
Aphthovirus				
Foot-and-mouth disease virus (cell culture adapted)	Heparan sulfate	Glycosaminoglycan		323
Foot-and-mouth disease virus	$\alpha_v\beta_1$, $\alpha_v\beta_3$, $\alpha_v\beta_6$, $\alpha_v\beta_8$	Integrin		322,326,495
Equine rhinitis A virus	Sialic acid	Carbohydrate		660
Cardiovirus				
Encephalomyocarditis virus	Vcam-1	Ig-like		309
	Sialylated glycophorin A (for hemagglutination only) Sialic acid	Carbohydrate Carbohydrate		266
	ADAM9 (a disintegrin and metalloproteinase domain)	Metalloproteinase		60
Theiler murine encephalomyelitis virus				415
Low-neurovirulence strains	Sialic acid	Carbohydrate		
High-neurovirulence strains	Heparin sulfate	Proteoglycan		
Enterovirus				
Bovine enterovirus	Sialic acid	Carbohydrate		774
Coxsackievirus A9	$\alpha_v\beta_3$, $\alpha_v\beta_6$	Integrin	β_2-microglobulin, GRP78, MHC-1	601,694,696,754
Coxsackievirus A2–A6, A10, A12	KREMEN 1	Signaling receptor		653
Coxsackieviruses A13, A18, A21	Icam-1 (CD)	Ig-like		132
Coxsackievirus A16	P-selectin glycoprotein ligand-1 (PSGL-1), scavenger receptor class B (SCARB2)	Mucin-like	Heparan sulfate glycosaminoglycans	505,766
Coxsackievirus A21	Decay-accelerating factor (CD55)	SCR-like (complement cascade)	Icam-1	630
Coxsackievirus A24	Icam-1			36
Coxsackievirus A24 (variant)	Icam-1 α2,6-Sialic acid–containing, O-linked glycoconjugates	Carbohydrate		470,504
Coxsackieviruses B1–B6	Car (Coxsackievirus–adenovirus receptor)	Ig-like		71
Coxsackievirus B1, B3, B5	Decay-accelerating factor (CD55)	SCR-like (complement cascade)	$\alpha_v\beta_6$ integrin (CVB1) CAR (CVB3)	4,629,631
Echovirus 1, 8	$\alpha_2\beta_1$-Integrin (Vla-2)	Integrin	β_2-microglobulin	72,743
Echovirus 3, 6, 7, 11–13, 20, 21, 24, 29, 30, 33	Decay-accelerating factor (CD55)	SCR-like (complement cascade)	β_2-microglobulin, CD59 (E7)	70,238,574,608,743,743
Echovirus 5, 9, 11, 13, 25, 29, 30, 31, 32	FcRn		β_2-microglobulin	477,778
Echovirus 5	Heparan sulfate	Proteoglycan		320

(continued)

TABLE 2.3 Some cell receptors for picornaviruses (*Continued*)

Genus/Virus	Virus Receptor	Type of Receptor	Second Receptor	References
Echovirus 9	$\alpha_v\beta_3$-Integrin	Integrin		496
Enterovirus D68	$\alpha2,6$-Sialic acid–containing, O-linked glycoconjugates ICAM-5	Carbohydrate Ig-like		318,746
Enterovirus 70	Decay-accelerating factor (CD55) sialic acid	SCR-like (complement cascade) Carbohydrate		8,353
Enterovirus 71	P-selectin glycoprotein ligand-1 (PSGL-1), scavenger receptor class B (SCARB2) Annexin II	Mucin-like	Heparan sulfate Vimentin	505,766
Parechovirus 1	$\alpha_v\beta_1$, $\alpha_v\beta_3$, $\alpha_v\beta_6$	Integrin		695
Hepatitis A virus	HAVcr-1	T-cell Ig-like, mucin-like (TIM)		351
Polioviruses 1–3	PVR (CD155)	Ig-like		460
Rhinoviruses (major group, 91 serotypes)	Icam-1	Ig-like		251,656,688
Rhinoviruses (minor group, 10 serotypes)	Low-density lipoprotein receptor protein family	Signaling receptor		302
Rhinoviruses species C	CDHR3	Cadherin related		85
Porcine sapelovirus	$\alpha2,3$-Linked sialic acid GD1a	Ganglioside		365
Seneca Valley virus	Anthrax toxin receptor 1/ TEM 8	Signaling receptor		332

Ig, immunoglobulin; SCR, short consensus repeat.

(PVR/CD155) (Fig. 2.7), rhinoviruses (ICAM-1, low-density lipoprotein receptor [LDLR], LDLR-related protein, very-low-density lipoprotein receptor, CDHR3, cadherin-related family membrane 3), and Seneca Valley virus (TEM 8).

The poliovirus receptor is a type I transmembrane protein and a member of the immunoglobulin (Ig) superfamily of proteins, with three extracellular Ig-like domains: a membrane-distal V-type domain followed by two C2-type domains.[460] Domain 1 of PVR binds to the virus. Production of PVR in mice is sufficient to overcome the lack of susceptibility of this species to poliovirus infection.[380,586] Because *PVR* transgenic mice develop paralysis after inoculation with poliovirus by different routes, they have proved to be a valuable model for studying the pathogenesis of poliomyelitis.[580] *PVR* transgenic mice are not susceptible to infection by the oral route, the natural route of infection in humans, unless the gene encoding type I interferon receptors has been deleted.[516,776] PVR is synthesized in many tissues in transgenic mice, yet the main sites of poliovirus replication are the brain and spinal cord.[380,588] This restricted tropism is regulated by the interferon (IFN)-α/β response, which limits viral replication in extraneural organs.[315]

Production of PVR on cells in culture derived from different animal species leads to susceptibility to poliovirus infection. Therefore, it is likely that PVR is the only molecule required for poliovirus binding and entry. The observation that a monoclonal antibody directed against the lymphocyte homing receptor, CD44, blocks poliovirus binding to cells suggested that this protein might be a second receptor for poliovirus entry.[634,635] It was subsequently shown that CD44 is not a receptor for poliovirus and is not required for poliovirus infection of cells that produce PVR.[93,204] It seems likely that PVR and CD44 are associated in the cell membrane[205] and that anti-CD44 antibodies block poliovirus attachment by blocking the virus-binding sites on PVR.

Orthologs of the *PVR* gene are present in the genomes of a number of mammals, including those not susceptible to poliovirus infection.[316] The amino acid sequence of domain 1 of PVR varies extensively among the nonsusceptible mammals, especially in the regions known to contact poliovirus. The absence of a poliovirus-binding site on these PVR molecules, therefore, explains why infection is restricted to simians.

PVR is an adhesion molecule that participates in the formation of adherens junctions through interaction with nectin-3, a related immunoglobulin-like protein.[488] It is also a recognition molecule for natural killer (NK) cells and interacts with CD226 and CD96 on NK cells to stimulate their cytotoxic activity.[92,209] PVR also interacts with T-cell Ig and ITIM domain membrane protein (TIGIT), a protein involved in regulating T-cell function.[426] The UL141 protein of cytomegalovirus (CMV) blocks display of PVR on the cell surface, leading to evasion of NK cell–mediated killing.[687]

The cell surface receptor for many human rhinoviruses (species A and B) was identified by using monoclonal antibodies directed against the cellular binding site to isolate the receptor protein from susceptible cells. Amino acid sequence

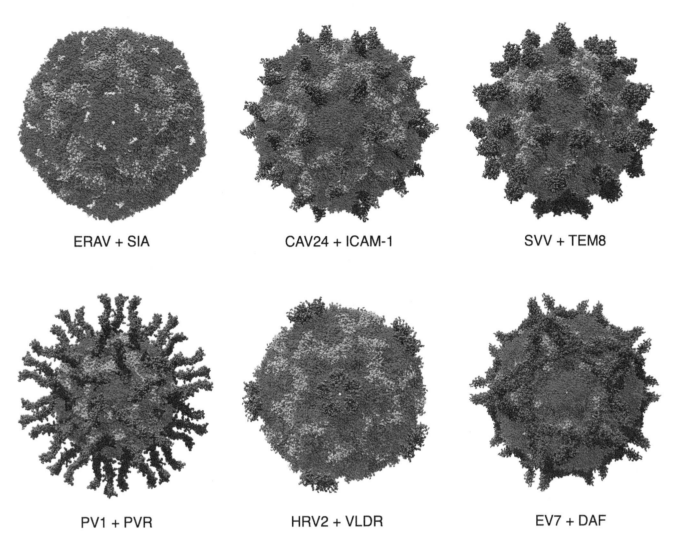

ERAV + SIA   CAV24 + ICAM-1   SVV + TEM8

PV1 + PVR   HRV2 + VLDR   EV7 + DAF

FIGURE 2.7 Interactions of six different picornaviruses with cellular receptors. VP1 is *blue*, VP2 is *yellow*, and VP3 is *deep pink*. Proteinaceous receptors are shown in *gray*. The 4 Å structure determined by x-ray crystallography of the cell receptor sialic acid bound to equine rhinitis A virus. The sugar moiety sialic acid (*white*) attaches to the rim of the capsid pit [2XBO]. The 3.9 Å structure determined by cryo-EM of domains 1 and 2 of the cell receptor ICAM-1 bound to Coxsackievirus A21. The immunoglobulin-like receptor binds at the pseudo threefold axes of the capsid [6EIT]. The 3.8 Å structure determined by cryo-EM of the cell receptor anthrax toxin receptor 1/TEM 8 bound to Seneca Valley virus (SVV). The single-chain transmembrane domain protein binds in a crown-like arrangement around the fivefold axis of the icosahedron [6CX1]. The 4.0 Å structure determined by cryo-EM of the cell receptor PVR (CD155) bound to poliovirus type 1. The immunoglobulin-like protein binds within the canyon of the capsid [3J8F]. The 3.6 Å structure determined by x-ray crystallography of the cell receptor low-density lipoprotein receptor bound to rhinovirus 2. The single pass transmembrane protein binds on the plateau at the fivefold axis [2XBO]. The 7.2 Å structure determined by cryo-EM of the cell receptor DAF (CD55) bound to echovirus 7. The complement protein binds echovirus 7 near the twofold icosahedral axes [3IYP].

analysis of the purified protein revealed that it is ICAM-1, a type I transmembrane protein with five immunoglobulin-like domains.[251,656,688] The normal cellular functions of ICAM-1 are to bind its ligand, lymphocyte function–associated antigen 1 (LFA-1), on the surface of lymphocytes and to promote a wide range of immunologic functions.[704] ICAM-1 is expressed on the surfaces of many tissues, including the nasal epithelium, which is the entry site for rhinoviruses.

Three members of the low-density lipoprotein receptor family are receptors for other species of A and B rhinoviruses (10 serotypes) (Fig. 2.7). These proteins consist of 7 LDLR, 8 VLDLR, or 31 LRP ligand-binding repeats, transmembrane, and cytoplasmic domains.

Bioinformatic comparison of susceptible and permissive cells with nonsusceptible but permissive cells leads to the identification of cadherin-related family member 3 (CDHR3) as a cellular receptor for rhinovirus C species.[85] These viruses are more likely to cause wheezing illnesses and asthma exacerbations than rhinoviruses A and B. It is hypothesized that a single amino acid change, Y529 within CDHR3, a transmembrane protein of unknown biological function, but found on the surface of lung tissue and bronchial epithelial cells, and associated with asthma severity, also promotes rhinovirus C infection and may explain the association of virus infection with enhanced respiratory distress.[85] Most humans today have the nonrisk allele C529; however, Y529 is found in the genome of

Neanderthals and Denisovans, indicating that it was initially present and then replaced with C529 by selection imposed by virus infection.[85] After an outbreak of lethal rhinovirus C infection in a chimpanzee population of Uganda, sequence analysis of the CDHR3 encoding locus revealed chimpanzees to be homozygous for Y529.[625] This observation suggests that rhinovirus C is only rarely transmitted from humans to chimpanzees; therefore, there has been little selection pressure for spread of the C529 amino acid change in apes.

Identification of virus receptors has been accelerated by the use of novel gene editing methodologies such as CRISPR/Cas9 and reagents including a collection of haploid human cells harboring retroviral gene insertions. Anthrax toxin receptor 1/TEM 8 and KREMEN 1 were determined to be the cellular receptors for Seneca Valley virus (Fig. 2.7) and Coxsackieviruses A2 to A6, A10, and A12, respectively, via these technologies.[467,653] These methodologies however do not distinguish between molecules necessary for cell surface attachment and those necessary for particle internalization and uncoating. Anthrax toxin receptor 1/TEM 8 is sufficient for Seneca Valley virus attachment to the cell surface but not for the conformational changes necessary for uncoating.[332]

Many picornaviruses bind integrins, which are dimeric cell adhesion receptors with α and β subunits. Integrin receptors recognize the tripeptide Arg-Gly-Asp (RGD) whose presence in the viral capsid suggests interaction with this type of receptor. A number of integrins can serve as entry receptors for FMDV (Table 2.3) although all may not be utilized during infection of animals. Although integrins are sufficient for FMDV infection, their interaction with the viral capsid does not lead to uncoating (see *Entry into Cells*). Enteroviruses that bind integrins typically require a coreceptor for cell entry. For CAV9, it has been suggested that β_2-microglobulin,[697] GRP78, and MHC-1[694] might fulfill this role.

The carbohydrate sialic acid is thought to function as the cellular receptor for numerous picornaviruses including enterovirus D68, bovine enterovirus, equine rhinitis virus A (Fig. 2.7), and a variant of Coxsackievirus A24.[36,318,504,660,661] Sialic acid interacts with different picornavirus capsids at diverse sites. It binds within a shallow groove near the outer edge of the EF loop of VP1 of the adjacent protomer on the equine rhinitis virus A capsid.[208] Though the interactions between Coxsackievirus A24 (CAV24) and equine rhinitis virus with sialic acid are similar, it functions as an attachment molecule for CAV24, allowing for an increased concentration of virus on the cell surface. This binding facilitates the interaction between the entry receptor ICAM-1 and enhances infection and transmission.[36] Sialic acid binds within the VP1 pocket of enterovirus D68. Despite being able to evict the C10 lipid found in the pocket of enterovirus D68, binding of sialic acid does not lead to uncoating[417] indicating that another cell surface molecule is required for entry of this virus.

Two Receptors Required for Infection

Many enteroviruses bind to decay-accelerating factor (DAF, or CD55), a member of the complement cascade (Table 2.3); it is composed of four extracellular short consensus repeat modules (SCR1–SCR4) and is attached to the plasma membrane by a glycosylphosphatidylinositol (GPI) anchor (Fig. 2.7). Its ability to function as the receptor of viruses such as echovirus 6, 7, 11, 12, 13, 20, 21, 29, and 33 was defined not only by the use of antibodies generated against DAF that inhibit virus infection but also by conferring susceptibility to virus infection of nonsusceptible cells by production of the protein from a plasmid.[70,742] However, for most of these viruses, interaction with DAF is not sufficient for infection. Binding to DAF does not cause conformational changes and internalization; therefore, interaction between DAF and the virion does not lead to uncoating. Instead, DAF is an attachment receptor, facilitating virus adsorption, and a second receptor is necessary for conformational changes, internalization of the particle, and uncoating.[564,574] For example, Coxsackievirus A21 binds to DAF, but infection does not occur unless ICAM-1 is also bound.[630] In this case, ICAM-1 inserts into the canyon where it triggers capsid uncoating.[758] Coxsackievirus B3 also binds DAF, but virion uncoating does not occur unless CAR (coxsackievirus–adenovirus receptor; see below) binds in the canyon.[287] Despite being able to bind mouse CAR, production of human DAF within the alimentary tract of mice, either immunocompetent or deficient in the IFN-α/β receptor, still does not allow for enteral infection by Coxsackievirus B3.[524] However, for other echoviruses, the absence of Fc receptors, antibodies against β2-microglobulin, or class I human leukocyte antigen (HLA) inhibited productive infection despite virus attachment to the cell surface being unaffected.[121,477,573] The requirement for binding to DAF for echoviruses to attach to the cell surface appears not only to be isolate specific but to be controlled by the cells in which the virus is passaged. The D'Amori-derived strain of echovirus 6, serially passaged in human rhabdomyosarcoma cells, weakly interacts with DAF, while the same isolate cultured in HeLa cells may attach to the cell surface in a DAF-independent manner.[573] Enzymatic removal of heparin sulfate impaired infection by both isolates suggesting a role for this extracellular matrix component in cell surface attachment of echoviruses.[239] Taken together, these observations suggest that a large protein complex that includes DAF, HLA, FcR, and β2-microglobulin may mediate echovirus cell surface attachment, internalization, and uncoating.

How two receptors collaborate in virus entry is illustrated by Coxsackievirus B3 infections of polarized epithelial cells.[139] The coxsackievirus and adenovirus receptor, CAR, mediates cell entry of all Coxsackie B viruses.[71] CAR is not present on the apical surface of epithelial cells that line the intestinal and respiratory tracts but is a component of the tight junction and is inaccessible to virus entry. Coxsackie B viruses first bind an attachment receptor, DAF, which is present on the apical surface of epithelial cells. Virus binding to DAF activates Abl kinase, which in turn triggers Rac-dependent actin rearrangements leading to virus movement to the tight junction where it can bind CAR and enter cells.[139]

Alternative Receptors

Some viruses bind to different cell surface receptors, depending on the virus isolate or the cell line (Table 2.3). Clinical isolates of FMDV bind to integrin receptors, but passage in cell culture can select for viruses that bind to heparin sulfate, a sulfated glycan.[323,445,614] Cell culture passage may also produce a virus that infects cells independent of heparin sulfate and integrins.[43]

How Picornaviruses Attach to Cell Receptors

Among the picornavirus members, the four capsid proteins are arranged similarly, but the surface architecture varies. These differences account for both the diverse serotypes and the varied modes of interaction with cell receptors. For example, the capsids of enteroviruses have a groove, or canyon, surrounding each fivefold axis of symmetry. In contrast, cardioviruses, aphthoviruses, and senecaviruses have a sharp pit.

The canyons of multiple enteroviruses are the sites of interaction with Ig-like cell receptors. The results of genetic and structural experiments demonstrate that the first Ig-like domain contains the site that binds poliovirus. Cells producing the first Ig-like domain of PVR, either alone or as a hybrid with other Ig-like proteins, are susceptible to infection with poliovirus.[379,479,627,628] Amino acid changes in the first Ig-like domain of PVR interfere with poliovirus binding.[21,74,478] Mutagenesis of ICAM-1 DNA has revealed that the binding site for rhinovirus is located in the first Ig-like domain.[450,585,655] Models of the interaction of poliovirus, rhinovirus, and Coxsackieviruses A and B with their cellular receptors have been produced from cryoelectron microscopy and x-ray crystallographic data (Fig. 2.7).[36,63,64,109,110,286,381,518,520,763] These models reveal that only domain 1 of PVR or ICAM-1 penetrates the canyon of the respective virus and the alteration induced, pivoting of VP1 away from the fivefold axes, leads to the expulsion of pocket factor, which facilitates particle expansion, and destabilization.[662] Alterations that affect receptor binding map to the virion–receptor interface as determined by these structural studies. Change of amino acids that line the canyons of poliovirus and rhinovirus can alter the affinity of binding to receptors.[133–135,279,411] Despite also binding in the canyon and having the similar footprint to that of PVR and ICAM-1 on their respective viruses, CAR does not interact with the south canyon rim nor the floor of the canyon of the Coxsackievirus B3 virion.[520]

Although the capsids of some rhinoviruses possess a canyon around the fivefold axes, it is not the binding site for their cell receptor, members of the low-density lipoprotein receptor family (Fig. 2.7). Rather, the LDL receptor binds close to the fivefold axis, on the star-shaped mesa that is surrounded by the canyon.[294,579,583,720] In this way, multiple low-affinity interactions are combined to yield a high avidity virus–receptor complex.

Domain 1 of cadherin-related family member 3 (CDHR3), the cell receptor for members of *Rhinovirus C*, is sufficient to bind virus particles. Peptides that encompass this domain block attachment of virus to cells.[745] Molecular modeling suggests that the linear tandem repeat extracellular domains of CDHR3 occur as rod-like molecules that lie across the twofold axis of adjacent protomers, with domain 1 interacting just outside of the fivefold axis of symmetry.[85]

Sequence and structural comparisons have revealed how rhinoviruses bind either ICAM-1 or LDL. A lysine at position 224 of VP1, which is conserved in all minor group rhinoviruses, is the key amino acid that interacts with a negatively charged cluster of LDLR.[720] The electrostatic attraction between Lys1224 and the acidic cluster in LDLR might initiate contact between virus and receptor. Neighboring hydrophobic and basic residues in VP1 could then lead to tight binding between virus and receptor. The conserved lysine is not present in VP1 of rhinoviruses that bind ICAM-1, providing an explanation for failure of these viruses to bind LDLR. An exception is rhinovirus 85 that has the conserved lysine; presumably, it does not bind LDLR because of other amino acid differences in neighboring hydrophobic and basic VP1 residues.

It was originally hypothesized that the picornavirus canyons were too deep and narrow to allow penetration by antibody molecules, which contain adjacent immunoglobulin domains.[606] This physical barrier was thought to hide amino acids crucial for receptor binding from the immune system. Structural studies of a rhinovirus–antibody complex, however, revealed that antibody does penetrate deep into the canyon, as does ICAM-1.[641] The shape of the picornavirus canyon, therefore, is not likely to play a role in concealing virus from the immune system.

In contrast to the Ig-like receptors that bind the canyons of enteroviruses, the binding sites for DAF on the virion are diverse. For example, five amino acids of DAF interact with the VP2 puff region of Coxsackievirus B3 in an area that lies between the icosahedral threefold, twofold, and fivefold axes and away from the twofold axis.[564] In contrast, the binding sites of DAF on echovirus 7 (Fig. 2.7) and 12 are completely different, far from the canyon, at the edge of the depression at the twofold icosahedral axis.[548,564] There is no overlap between surfaces on echoviruses 7 and 12 and Coxsackievirus B3 that interact with DAF.

Integrin-binding picornaviruses attach to cell receptors through surface loops. In FMDV, an Arg-Gly-Asp sequence in the flexible, exposed βG–βH loop of the capsid protein VP1 is recognized by integrin receptors on cells.[162,203,423] Arg-Gly-Asp–containing peptides block attachment of FMDV,[55] and alteration of this sequence interferes with virus binding.[448] In Coxsackievirus A9, the Arg-Gly-Asp sequence is present in a 17–amino acid extension of the C-terminus of VP1 and is also the site of attachment to cell receptors.[114,601] Alteration of this sequence does not abolish binding to some cell lines but blocks infectivity in A549 cells (human lung carcinoma), suggesting that the virus can bind to another cell surface receptor.[310] In susceptible cells, $\beta 2M$ and HSPA5 (heat shock 70-kDa protein 5, also known as BiP or glucose-regulated protein 78 kDa, GRP78) are sufficient for infection by Coxsackievirus A9 with an altered Arg-Gly-Asp sequence.[288] Echovirus 1 is unusual in that it binds the RGD-independent integrin $\alpha_2\beta_1$ in the canyon.[762]

As discussed, FMDV binds alternative receptors, either integrin or heparan sulfate, depending on the virus isolate. The binding site for heparan sulfate on cell culture–adapted FMDV is a shallow depression on the virion surface, where the three major capsid proteins, VP1, VP2, and VP3, are located.[207] Binding specificity is controlled by two preformed sulfate-binding sites on the capsid. Residue 56 of VP3 is a critical regulator of receptor recognition. In field isolates of the virus, this amino acid is histidine. Adaptation to cell culture selects for viruses with an arginine at this position, which forms the high-affinity, heparan sulfate–binding site.

While the Seneca Valley virus particle is similar to that of cardioviruses lacking a canyon, structure of the virus bound to anthrax toxin receptor 1/TEM 8, a type I transmembrane protein, revealed that the protein binds the virion in a crown-like arrangement around the fivefold axis of the icosahedron (Fig. 2.7). TEM 8 is composed of an N-terminal integrin–like fold, an Ig-like domain followed by the transmembrane domain and cytoplasmic tail. The high-affinity interaction between TEM 8 and Seneca Valley virus occurs between helices $\alpha 4$ and $\alpha 3$ of the integrin-like fold and loops $\alpha 2$–$\alpha 3$ and $\beta 2$–$\beta 3$ of the Ig-like domain and the BC loop and loop II of VP1, the puff of VP2, and the knob of VP3 of the virus.[332]

Kinetics and Affinity of the Virus–Receptor Interaction

The affinity and kinetics of picornaviruses binding to soluble forms of their receptors (sPVR, sICAM, sCAR) and antibodies have been studied by surface plasmon resonance. Two classes of receptor-binding sites, with distinct binding affinities, exist on the capsids of poliovirus and rhinovirus.[110,451,763] The association rates for the two binding classes are 25 and 13 times higher for the poliovirus–sPVR interaction than for the rhinovirus 3 or 16–sICAM interaction at 20°C; though the first association rate of rhinoviruses 3 and 16–sICAM was highly similar, the second association rate for rhinovirus 16 is slower.[763] The greater association rate of poliovirus and sPVR may be caused, in part, by differences in the extent of contact between virus and receptor. However, the association rate for receptor binding to the virion is slower than that for antibody binding. This observation supports the hypothesis that a conformational change in the virus particle is required for receptor function.[110] In contrast, whereas two dissociation rate constants exist for the poliovirus–sPVR and coxsackievirus–sCAR interactions, only one has been reported for the rhinovirus 3–sICAM interaction.[108,110,451] The dissociation rates for the poliovirus–sPVR interaction are 1.5 and 2.0 times faster than for the rhinovirus–sICAM interaction, indicating greater instability of the former complex. The affinity constants for the poliovirus–sPVR interaction are 19 and 6 times greater than those reported for the rhinovirus–sICAM-1 complex. Despite lacking interaction with the south wall and floor of the canyon, the binding affinity for the monomeric sCAR–Coxsackievirus B3 interaction is similar to that for the poliovirus–sPVR and rhinovirus–sICAM interactions even though the dissociation rate for the sCAR–Coxsackievirus B3 is much lower than for poliovirus–sPVR.[237,520]

In contrast to the observations with poliovirus and rhinovirus, a single class of binding site was found on echovirus 11 for a soluble form of its receptor, CD55.[400] The affinity of this interaction is at least fourfold lower than either of the binding sites on poliovirus for sPVR. The association rate for the interaction between echovirus 11 and sCD55 is faster than that of poliovirus–sPVR and rhinovirus–sICAM-1. One explanation for these findings is that the contact between echovirus 11 and sCD55 is more extensive than that of the other two virus–receptor complexes. The binding site for CD55 on echovirus 11 may also be more accessible than those of PVR and ICAM-1. The dissociation rate for the echovirus–sCD55 interaction is at least 97 times faster than that of either the poliovirus–sPVR or the rhinovirus–sICAM-1 interaction. These findings are consistent with a more accessible binding site for CD55 on echovirus 11, compared with the receptor-binding sites on poliovirus and rhinovirus. Atomic interactions between CD55 and echovirus 11 may be weaker than between the other two viruses and their receptors. The faster dissociation rate of the echovirus 11–sCD55 complex may be related to the finding that the interaction does not lead to structural changes of the virus particle,[574] as occurs with poliovirus and rhinovirus. In general, there is a higher affinity for virions of receptors that can uncoat particles ("unzippers"—poliovirus/PVR, HRV/ICAM-1, CVB3/CAR) compared with attachment receptors (E6, E7, E11, E12, CVB3 with DAF). This difference may reflect the energy necessary to release the viral RNA.

Why do poliovirus, rhinovirus, and Coxsackievirus B have two classes of receptor-binding sites? For poliovirus and rhinovirus, the receptors for both viruses make contacts at two major sites on the virus surface, one in a cleft on the south rim of the canyon and a second on the side of the mesa on the north rim. These two contact sites may correspond to the two classes of binding sites. Two classes of binding sites may also be a consequence of the structural flexibility exhibited by both viruses, which may cause exposure of different binding sites. Normally, internal parts of the capsid proteins of many picornaviruses including poliovirus, swine vesicular disease virus, and rhinovirus have been shown to be transiently displayed on the virion surface, a process called *breathing*.[336,406,410,577,621] As discussed later, the interaction of poliovirus and rhinovirus with their cellular receptors leads to irreversible and more extensive structural changes of the particle. In contrast to the findings with poliovirus and rhinovirus, binding of echovirus 11 with CD55 can be described by a simple 1:1 binding model. Such behavior, which would be expected for the interaction of two preformed binding sites, is consistent with the fact that CD55 is an attachment molecule and the echovirus–CD55 interaction does not result in detectable structural changes in the capsid.[574,666] Instead, secondary factors may contribute to internalization and uncoating the virus.

Entry into Cells

Once picornaviruses have attached to their cellular receptor, the viral capsid is brought into the cell by an endocytic pathway, followed by genome release into the cytoplasm, the site of picornavirus replication. For some picornaviruses, interaction with a cell receptor serves only to concentrate virus on the cell surface; release of the genome is a consequence of low pH or perhaps the activity of a second receptor. For other picornaviruses, the cell receptor is also an unzipper and initiates conformational changes in the virus that lead to release of the genome. In some cases, only one cell surface molecule functions as the cellular receptor, and the requirements for entry are determined by the cell type infected; the identity of the receptor may change according to how the virus is passaged, thereby changing the entry route.

Entry by Clathrin-Mediated Endocytosis

Several lines of evidence indicate that clinical isolates of FMDV, which bind multiple $\alpha_v\beta$ integrins to attach to the cell surface, enter cells by clathrin-mediated endocytosis.[322] Infection is inhibited by sucrose, which eliminates clathrin-coated pits and induces clathrin to polymerize into empty cages, by synthesis of a dominant negative form of the clathrin coat assembly protein AP180 that is needed for assembly of clathrin cages, or by chlorpromazine treatment of cells prior to infection; all treatments decreased FMDV internalization and replication.[75,276] Confocal microscopy also revealed that FMDV enters cells via a clathrin-dependent mechanism through colocalization of FMDV with the early endosome protein EEA1.[514] There is also some evidence that entry is dependent upon cholesterol in the plasma membrane, a requirement generally observed for lipid rafts.[442] While cholesterol may be required for clathrin-induced membrane curving and budding of the plasma membrane, it is also required for macropinocytosis.[252,596] Another *Aphthovirus*, equine rhinitis A virus, binds sialic acid–containing receptors but also enters into cells via clathrin-mediated endocytosis.[254] However, the cellular receptor for serially passaged isolates of FMDV is heparin sulfate; these viruses are thought to enter the cell via macropinocytosis, a pathway taken by echovirus 1, Coxsackievirus B, and Coxsackievirus A9.

LDLR family members that are receptors for some HRVs possess C-terminal cytoplasmic domains with tyrosine- and di-leucine–based internalization signals that lead to clustering of the receptors in clathrin-coated pits.[540] Evidence for HRV entry via this pathway includes the inhibition of infection in cells producing dominant negative inhibitors of the clathrin pathway.[57,645] Cholesterol depletion also significantly impairs entry of LDLR binding rhinoviruses.[645] Despite ceramide-mediated inhibition of entry of LDLR–rhinovirus 2 complexes, lipid rafts do not directly participate in rhinovirus entry. It is thought that ceramide inhibits receptor clustering instead.[248] There is little genetic or biochemical evidence that ICAM-1–binding rhinoviruses enter cells via clathrin-mediated endocytosis despite transmission electron microscopy, which shows virions in clathrin-coated pits and vesicles 5 minutes after infection.[257] Entry of ICAM-1–binding rhinoviruses is not inhibited by sucrose, chlorpromazine, nystatin, cholesterol depletion or dominant negative forms of AP180, or the endosome adaptor Eps15.[490] Additionally, the internalized rhinovirus vesicles take on a unique morphology including alignment as "beads on a string." Though a dominant negative dynamin inhibits infection,[159] dynamin also participates in non–clathrin-mediated entry. HRV infection also activates signaling pathways with links to the endocytic machinery. The cytoplasmic domain of ICAM-1 binds the adaptor protein ezrin, which links the receptor to Syk, a tyrosine kinase.[736] When HRV binds ICAM-1, Syk is recruited from the cytoplasm to the plasma membrane together with clathrin. Functional Syk is required for HRV entry via ICAM-1.[397]

When virions enter cells by clathrin-dependent endocytosis, they encounter low pH, which triggers release of the viral RNA from the capsid. A role for low pH in infection can be demonstrated by determining the effect on entry of compounds that block acidification, such as weak bases (ammonium chloride, chloroquine, methylamine), ionophores (monensin, nigericin, X537A), or inhibitors of the vacuolar proton ATPase (concanamycin A, bafilomycin A). The pH of early endosomes is 6.5; as these vesicles mature to late endosomes, the pH drops to 5.5. Endosomal maturation is dependent not only upon vacuolar ATPases but also upon microtubules and membrane GTPases of the Rab family. Early to late endosome maturation can be inhibited by drugs that depolymerize microtubules (nocodazole), dominant negative Rabs, or inhibitors of PI3K signaling (wortmannin). In this way, it is possible to determine if viral entry occurs from early or late endosomes.

Uncoating by FMDV clearly requires low pH because concanamycin A, monensin, and ammonium chloride all inhibit infection.[54,75,514,730] Entry occurs from the early endosome as determined by experiments with dominant negative Rab proteins.[339] FMDV that bind heparan sulfate enter cells via a caveolae-dependent route, but low pH is still required for infection.[513] Consistent with this mechanism of uncoating, FMDV that has been coated with antibody can bind to, and infect, cells that produce Fc receptors, in contrast to poliovirus, which cannot productively infect cells via this pathway.[446] Cell receptors for FMDV are, therefore, *hooks*: they do not induce

uncoating-related changes in the virus particle but rather serve only to tether the virus to the cell and bring it into the endocytic pathway.

The range of pH at which rhinoviruses uncoat depends on the serotype and receptor bound by the virus. For LDLR interacting rhinoviruses such rhinovirus 2, the receptor is thought to only be required for trafficking the virus to the late endosome; downstream events are acid induced. Upon acidification of the virus-containing vesicle, LDLR dissociates from the virion, simultaneously pocket factor is released, and a hinge movement around the VP1 pocket facilitates a shift of VP2 and VP3, leading to particle expansion and formation of pores at the base of the canyon and twofold axes. VP4 is released and the amphipathic N-terminus of VP1 is relocalized to the surface of the virion.[58,79,214,383,497,512,575] Similar alterations have been observed between the native and empty capsids of enterovirus A71.[739] Infection by LDLR interacting rhinoviruses is inhibited by monensin, bafilomycin A1, nocodazole, and wortmannin.[73,95,497] Uncoating of ICAM-1–binding rhinoviruses, such as rhinovirus 14, is also sensitive to bafilomycin and monensin, but at too low a pH, the particle dissociates, suggesting that higher pH of the early endosome is sufficient for uncoating.[58] Although the receptor for enterovirus D68 is not known, low pH has been shown to lead to uncoating of multiple viral isolates. Analysis of cryo-EM reconstructions of acid-treated particles unveiled the structure of the expanded particle (E1), a transition intermediate between native and altered (Fig. 2.8). This newly described E1 particle retains the ordered structure of the N-terminal amino acids of VP1 and the ordered structure of VP4 despite expansion of the particle. Furthermore, pentameric interactions are weakened by disruption of the interpentamer β-sheets, and the capsid shell is thinner possibly allowing the influx of protons into the interior of the capsid needed to disrupt the stability of the N-terminus of VP1 within the E1 particle.[418]

Echovirus 7, which binds DAF, enters cells by clathrin-mediated endocytosis, and trafficking into late endosomes is required.[362] However, infection does not appear to require low pH, and therefore the trigger for uncoating and its intracellular location remains in question.

Entry by Caveolin-Mediated Endocytosis

As discussed above, CVB3 binds DAF, a GPI-linked protein localized within lipid rafts on the apical surface of polarized cells. The virus–DAF complex then moves to tight junctions (TJ) where it engages CAR. The virus is then internalized along with the TJ protein occludin by caveolin-1–dependent endocytosis.[142] The role of occludin is not known but it could provide a scaffold for recruiting other molecules. Within 60 minutes, the virus is within caveolin-1–containing vesicles (caveolae and caveosomes). Phosphorylation of caveolin-1 by tyrosine kinases is required for CVB3 entry, but the role of this modification is not known. Dynamin is not required for uptake of this virus, suggesting that other routes of entry are involved. Inhibitors of micropinocytosis (rottlerin and dominant negative Rab34) block infection, indicating a role for this type of uptake.

Echovirus 1, which binds the integrin $\alpha_2\beta_1$, is taken into the cell by the caveolin-mediated endocytic pathway. The receptor is present in raft-like membrane domains that do not contain caveolin. Internalization of the virus does not depend on dynamin, but components of the macropinocytosis pathway,

Native   Expanded

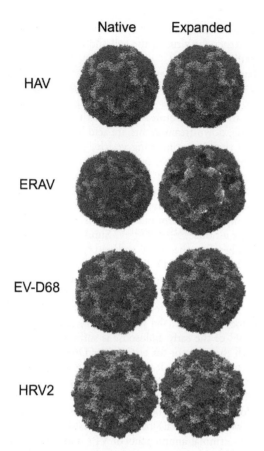

HAV

ERAV

EV-D68

HRV2

FIGURE 2.8 Structures of the native and altered particle of four different picornaviruses. VP1 is *blue*, VP2 is *yellow*, and VP3 is *deep pink*. Hepatitis A virus (HAV) native [4QPI] and empty [4QPG] capsids, equine rhinitis A virus (ERAV) native [4CTF] and acid-induced expanded capsids [4CTG], enterovirus D68 (EV-D68) native [4WM8] and acid-induced expanded capsids [6CS5], and rhinovirus 2 (HRV2) native [1FPN] and empty B capsids [3TN9].

such as PKC, Pak1, and Rac1, are involved. By 30 minutes after infection, the virus appears in vesicular structures that may be caveolae.[441] These vesicles fuse with caveosomes, delivering the virus and its receptor to the perinuclear region.[558] The resulting compartment may be a novel type of multivesicular body; virus transport to them appears to depend upon ESCRT proteins.[352]

Caveolin- and Clathrin-Independent Endocytosis

In HeLa cells, poliovirus is taken up into cells by an endocytic pathway that is dependent on actin, ATP, and a tyrosine kinase but independent of clathrin, caveolin, flotillin, microtubules, and pinocytosis.[96] Only after the conversion from the native to altered particle is poliovirus internalized.[96] These virus-containing endocytic vesicles lack signature characteristics of either the early or late endosome. Within the endosome, transition to the altered particle occurs. This alteration significantly reduces the affinity of PVR for the virion, suggesting that infectivity is independent of the receptor.[149] Subsequent work showed that within the endosomal vesicle, the altered particle is released from PVR but remains tethered to the membrane via insertion of the N-terminus of VP1.[253] RNA released from the particle into the lumen of the vesicle occurs rapidly and

within 100 to 200 nm of the cell surface. Entry was different in a highly polarized human brain microvascular endothelial cell line.[142] Poliovirus enters these cells very slowly via dynamin-dependent caveolar endocytosis. Virus binding to PVR induces tyrosine phosphorylation of the receptor cytoplasmic domain, which in turn recruits and activates SHP-2, which is required for infection. These observations emphasize that virus entry pathways are likely to differ substantially according to cell type.

Uncoating

The interaction of enteroviruses and ICAM-1–binding rhinoviruses with susceptible cells leads to the conversion of virions to a more slowly sedimenting form (135S vs. 160S for native particles) (Fig. 2.7).[146,341] The resulting particles, called *altered*, or *A, particles*, contain the viral RNA but have lost the internal capsid protein VP4. In addition, the N-terminus of VP1, which is normally on the interior of the capsid, is on the surface of the A particle, externalized via a pore found at the pseudo threefold axes at the base of the canyon, binding the rearranged GH loop of VP3 and the top surface of VP2.[103,294,405,413,418] Conversion from the native particle to the altered particle typically includes a 4% increase in the diameter of the virion and creation of pores within protomers by movement of the β-barrel cores of VP1, VP2, and VP3 at the twofold axes[64,293,294,418] (Fig. 2.9). Physiological temperatures can spontaneously induce the reversible conversion between native and altered particles at a slow rate; however, upon receptor binding or the presence of low pH for poliovirus and rhinovirus, respectively, the conversion is irreversible.[406,410] This tectonic rearrangement of the physical particle ends with formation of an amphipathic helix composed of VP4 and the N-terminus of VP1 inserted into the membrane of the endosome through which the viral RNA can travel to the cytoplasm (Fig. 2.9).[152,206,293,294,525,526,664,689,701] A variant of poliovirus containing an amino acid change at position 28 of VP4 can bind to cells and be converted to A particles, but these are blocked at a subsequent step in virus entry.[482] Additional genetic studies demonstrated that VP4 variants at position 28 lost the ability to form ion channels *in vitro* and delayed genome release.[152] Ectopic production of myristoylated rhinovirus VP4 can lead to the formation of membrane multimeric pores, which are similar in size to those necessary for RNA translocation.[154,526] Receptor binding (poliovirus) or low pH (rhinoviruses, cardioviruses, aphthoviruses, enterovirus D) are therefore the catalysts that lower the energy barrier for the irreversible conversion to the A particle necessary for uncoating and genome delivery to the cell.[418,575]

The initial model describing picornavirus uncoating and release of the RNA genome into the cytoplasm implied formation of a wide channel at the fivefold axes, displacing the solvent channel plug, and VP4, the N-termini of VP1 and RNA all exiting at this axis from a symmetric particle.[226,381] The initial cryo-EM reconstructions of the poliovirus 135S and 80S particles or those of the rhinovirus 2 80S particle do not support this model. This work did not reveal openings at the fivefold axes, which could allow for release of the viral genome, nor was removal of the solvent channel plug observed. Instead, this work leads to the suggestion that VP4 and the amino terminus of VP1 are externalized from the base of the canyon; the amphipathic helix bridges the canyon, binding to the EF loop of VP2 at the tip of the propeller near the threefold axes and at the twofold axes; and the RNA genome exits from the threefold

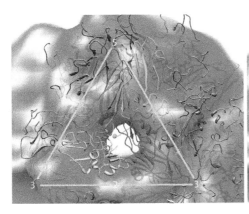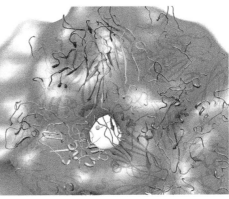

FIGURE 2.9 Hypothetical site for translocation of poliovirus RNA out of the capsid. Stereo views of the 80S pseudoatomic model superimposed on a map produced from 206 135S particles made by incubation of native virus particles with receptor-decorated liposomes.[664] These particles have a pore in the capsid that is thought to be the exit channel for RNA. The pore lies above Gln-68 in the N-terminal extension of VP1 from the adjacent protomer (*green ball*). VP1 is *blue*, VP2 is *yellow*, and VP3 is *magenta*. Exposed N-terminus of VP1 is colored *cyan*. (Courtesy of Michael Strauss, McGill University, and James M. Hogle, Harvard Medical School.)

axes[64,99,192,294,405,413,418,761] (Fig. 2.9). This hypothesis is further supported and refined by the finding that VP4 of rhinoviruses forms oligomers upon extrusion and exits near the twofold axis, based on the observation that insertion of a cysteine in the N-terminus of VP4 leads to disulfide linking upon breathing.[354] Cryo-EM reconstruction of the E1 and A particles of enterovirus D68 as well as the cryo-EM reconstruction of the poliovirus 135S and the rhinovirus 2 80S particle further support this model; hinge-like movement of the VP1 β-barrel flattening the top and temporarily moving through pores at the twofold axes is generated by the internalization of the C-termini of VP2 and expelling VP4. The GH loops of VP1 are rearranged to form a radially oriented hairpin. Together with VP2, a hole at a quasi-threefold axis is formed, and the tips of the propeller blades disappear (Fig. 2.9). By disordering the loops of VP1 and VP2, externalization of the N-terminus of VP1 through the two-loop gates that separate holes at the twofold and pseudo threefold axes at the base of the canyon occurs. Once through the pore at the pseudo threefold axes, the N-terminus of VP1 is locked into place by interacting with the rearranged and exposed GH loops of VP3 and VP1 and binding the tips of the VP2 propellers.[103,294,418] The result of these structural alterations is tethering of an asymmetric particle to the vesicular membrane, the formation of an asymmetric channel, an umbilicus at the pseudo threefold axes necessary for RNA translocation into the cytosol on only the surface near where VP4 has inserted into the vesicular membrane in order to tether the virion.[103,403,664] However, the structural rearrangement of capsid proteins upon ICAM-1 binding of rhinovirus 14 is different. Analysis of the rhinovirus 14 80S particles revealed that the N-termini of VP1 exit through pores between neighboring VP1 molecules on the north rim of the canyon, not at the pseudo threefold axes, due to rearrangement of the N-termini of VP3 induced by ICAM-1 binding.[293]

Cryo-EM reconstructions of 80S particles of HRV2,[294] HRV14,[293] and poliovirus[405] also revealed a minimum of two classes of particles: those with partial or no electron density and particles surrounded by electron density, inside and out (presumably RNA). Analysis of these particles indicates that portions of VP1, which are not critical for the core structure of the virion, are no longer icosahedrally constrained, while the mesa found at the fivefold axes remains intact. The large pores between pentamers at the twofold axes also form during "breathing." Moreover, the cryo-EM reconstructions divulged the presence of a highly structured RNA genome inside the virion; poliovirus genomic RNA is knobby and highly branched, while that of rhinovirus 2 is a well-ordered layer condensed into a rod under the protein shell oriented toward the twofold axes.[91,96,285,413,626] Analysis of the crystal structure of the enterovirus A71 73S particle, the empty capsid, unveiled a 5-degree counterclockwise rotation of the promoter around VP3 at the threefold axes, which pulls VP0 away from and leads to formation of pores at the twofold axes, as well as collapse of the external walls of the VP1 pocket including that formed by the GH loop of VP1.[739] Moreover, x-ray crystallography and cryo-EM reconstruction of the rhinovirus 2 native and altered particles highlighted specific changes in contacts between the RNA and the interior of the capsid that are thought to help maintain the protein network between promoters. In particular, the VP2 contact with the genome is maintained during alteration, but expulsion of the N-terminus of VP1 breaks the RNA–VP1 interface promoting formation of a new interaction between the N-terminal β-tubes of VP3 and the RNA at the fivefold axes.[557] Consequently, exit of the RNA genome cannot occur at the fivefold axes; instead, the viral RNA gradually exits via a ratchet-like mechanism from an asymmetric site at the base of the canyon near the twofold axes as a single strand lacking any secondary structures. The interior of the capsid may function as rails that conduct the RNA toward the pore.[91,96,214] Annealing of complementary fluorescently labeled oligonucleotides to the ends of the rhinovirus 2 genome revealed that egress of the RNA begins with the poly(A) tail–3′ end in a tightly coordinated process to avoid tangling and steric hindrance of the capsid.[285]

Despite not knowing the cell molecule that functions as the receptor for Saffold virus, the energy required to facilitate A particle formation can be mimicked by heating the virus. Heating to 42 degrees and cooling induce particle alteration as well as dissociation into 14S pentamers. Similar observations have been made during mengovirus uncoating.[272] Cryo-EM reconstruction of the heat-induced A particle revealed that transition from the native to altered particle of cardioviruses follows a path similar to that described for enteroviruses: particle expansion of 4% and formation of large pores at the fivefold and threefold axes. Unlike enteroviruses, ordered residues of VP4 begin near the fivefold axes and end near the threefold axes of the same promoter, and no pore is observed at the twofold axes.[489] Further analysis of the A particle found that the RNA density was uniformly distributed at the center of the particle independent of any contact with the capsid.[489]

While enterovirus capsids are stable at low pH and maintain icosahedral symmetry during uncoating due to the presence of extra β-sheet interactions in VP1, the acid-labile aphthoviruses dissociate into pentamers at low pH, as the viral RNA is released.[75,107,192,376,436,442–444,716] A mechanism by which low pH causes disassembly of the FMDV capsid has been illuminated by structural and genetic studies. Examination of the atomic structure of the virus revealed a high density of histidine residues lining the pentamer interfaces, which are stabilized by β-sheet interactions.[1] These residues confer stability to the capsid; because the pK_a of histidine is 6.8, close to the pH at which the virus dissociates, protonation of the side chains of the histidines might cause electrostatic repulsion, leading to disassembly.[148] To test this hypothesis, a histidine residue at position 142 of VP3 was changed to aspartic acid or phenylalanine. The resulting capsids were more stable at low pH than wild-type capsids,[181] supporting the proposed role of the histidine residue in acid-catalyzed disassembly. A single amino acid change of an alanine to valine in VP3 near the interpentameric interface enhances acid lability of the virus, while alterations of asparagine 17 in VP1 and histidine 145 in VP2 enhance acid stability of the capsid. These observations suggest that acid sensitivity is mediated by not only the pentameric interface of VP3 but also the N-terminus of VP1.[107,443,718] These data imply that the initial model may have oversimplified the mechanism of acid-induced RNA and VP4 release during *Aphthovirus* infection. Accounting for function of nonhistidine residues and cryo-EM reconstruction of the native and acid-treated virions, it has been proposed that protonation of two histidine residues within the interpentameric face of VP3 introduces an electrostatic repulsion with the dipole of the α-helix of the neighboring pentamer, which initiates uncoating, while the N-terminus of VP1 modulates the pH threshold necessary for uncoating and dissociating into pentamer subunits.[107] Uncoating of these viruses ends with the pentamers in an "inside-out" conformation as interactions at the midpoint between the two- and threefold axes remain intact.[436] How FMDV breaches the endosome membrane is not known; it does not have a hydrophobic VP1 N-terminus, and A particles are not produced. Despite the acid lability of equine rhinitis A virus and the absence of a hydrophobic N-terminus of VP1, this particle still undergoes acid-induced structural arrangement, VP4 expulsion, and gross expansion[37,702] (Fig. 2.8). Changes among all adjacent pentamers as well as disruption of the electrostatic interactions occur at low pH. The interface between pentamers is significantly smaller, hydrophobic, and built upon a ring stacking interaction between two VP2 proteins across the twofold axes, leading to formation of pores at the threefold axes of no less than 45 Å in diameter.[37]

Considering the various mechanisms for uncoating, the central problem is the same, how does the intact RNA genome transverse the protein shell and the vesicular membrane and enter the cytoplasm when its surrounding environment contains RNases and ions known to damage long molecules of RNA. Using fluorescent dyes, which only bind ssRNA, *in vitro* experiments of heated receptor-decorated liposomes bound with poliovirus further supported the hypothesis that the RNA genome traverses the lipid membrane into the lumen of the vesicle as a linear molecule. A similar amount of intraluminal fluorescence was observed when the same receptor-decorated liposome–virus complexes were heated in the presence of RNase A. This observation suggests that the RNA genome is protected from degradation during uncoating and release.[253] Immunofluorescence assays of HeLa cells infected with poliovirus in the presence of RNase A confirmed the observation that the RNA genome is protected from degradation even though the RNase is taken up with the virion. Using this same assay, it was found that infection of equine rhinitis A virus was also refractory to the presence of RNase A and the genome remained protected from degradation.[253]

Regulation of Uncoating by Cellular Molecules

The majority of studies examining picornavirus attachment, entry, internalization, and uncoating were based upon the assumption that all that was necessary for these processes was the cellular receptor, formation of an endosome, and acidification of the endosome. Viral proteins perforated the membrane, formed the pore, and protected the genome as it was released as a single unstructured strand via a ratcheting motion. However, a perforated endocytic vesicle is generally marked and targeted for autophagic degradation. Consequently, cell proteins may participate in the later steps of picornavirus uncoating in order to circumvent premature degradation of the virus-containing vesicle and allow for genome release. The recent identification of the host lipid–modifying protein PLA2G16 as a modulator of enterovirus infection supports the need for cell proteins during virus entry.[654] PLA2G16 is a phospholipase, catalyzing the conversion of phospholipids to fatty acids. When PLA2G16 is absent from the cell, both poliovirus and rhinovirus replications are impaired. Specifically, it is thought that the recruitment of PLA2G16 to the surface of the virus-containing endosome may block autophagic degradation of these vesicles by preventing their detection by the glycan-binding LGALS8, a protein known to participate in the clearance of damaged vesicles.[182,654] Several picornavirus 2A proteins lack enzymatic activity, including those of kobuviruses, parechoviruses, and tremoviruses, but are homologs of PLA2G16.[654] It remains unknown if these proteins participate in viral uncoating as they are not found within the incoming virion.

Beneath the canyon floor is a hydrophobic pocket that opens at the base of the canyon and extends toward the fivefold axis of symmetry. For many picornaviruses, this pocket is filled with a lipid of varied length. The icosahedral symmetry of the capsid therefore would allow each virion to contain up to 60 lipid molecules. It was originally thought that the presence of lipids in the hydrophobic pocket contributed to the stability of the native virus particle by locking the capsid and preventing conformational changes. This hypothesis comes from the study of antiviral drugs, such as the WIN compounds (first identified by Sterling-Winthrop, Inc.) and others including 3-(4-pyridyl)-2-imidazolidinone (GPP3), which displace the lipid and bind tightly in the hydrophobic pocket (Fig. 2.10).[156,643] These

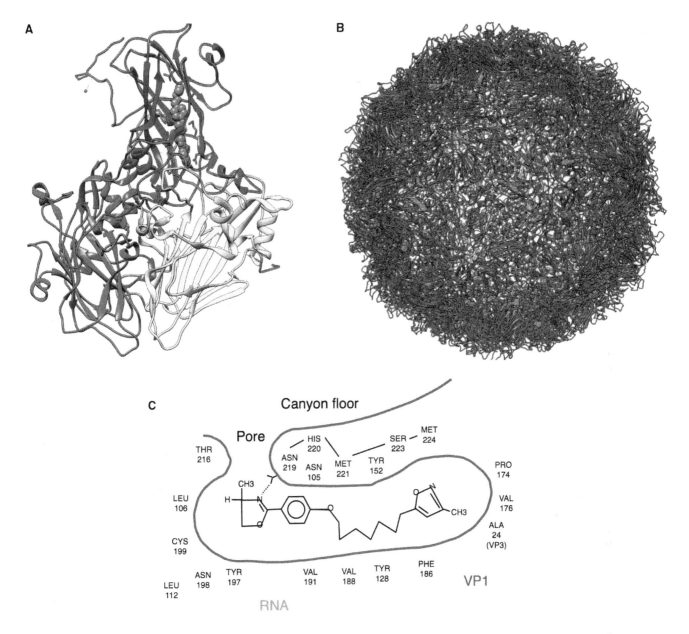

FIGURE 2.10 Mechanism of antiviral activity of compounds that bind within the hydrophobic VP1 pocket. A: Top view of a protomer, consisting of one copy of VP1 (*blue*), VP2 (*yellow*), VP3 (*deep pink*), and VP4 (*green*). *Orange spheres* represent one molecule of the pocket-binding compound 3-(4-pyridyl)-2-imidazolidinone (GPP3) bound in the hydrophobic VP1 pocket. **B:** GPP3 bound in the Coxsackievirus A16 capsid. The drug is the *small orange* molecule at the base of the canyon. **C:** WIN52084 bound in the hydrophobic pocket. These drugs displace the lipid from the pocket, thereby blocking infectivity. Amino acids of VP1 that line the pocket are indicated.

antiviral compounds block breathing of the picornavirus capsid.[406] For instance, binding of WIN compounds to rhinoviruses 14 and 16 causes conformational changes in the canyon that prevent attachment to cells.[550] Inhibition of virus attachment to the cell surface by these compounds is probably not a consequence of altering the receptor-binding site but rather the result of preventing conformational changes required for receptor binding. In contrast, drug binding to rhinoviruses 1A, 3, and 16, poliovirus, enterovirus A71, and Coxsackievirus A16 can cause small or negligible structural changes in the capsid.[155,156,247,267,298] Polioviruses containing bound WIN compounds can bind to cells, but the interaction with PVR does not result in the production of A particles.[202,455,775] WIN

compounds appear to inhibit poliovirus infectivity by preventing PVR-mediated conformational alterations that are required for uncoating. Additional support for the role of lipids in uncoating comes from the analysis of poliovirus mutants that cannot replicate unless WIN compounds are present.[485] Such WIN-dependent mutants spontaneously convert to altered particles at 37°C, without the cell receptor, probably because of the absence of lipid in the hydrophobic pocket. Moreover, drug-dependent mutants of poliovirus are thermolabile and spontaneously lose infectivity in the absence of drug at 37°C, probably because they do not contain stabilizing lipid in the pocket.[485] Domain 1 of PVR penetrates the canyon of poliovirus and induces several dramatic structural arrangements, the pivoting of VP1 away from the fivefold axes, expulsion of pocket factor, and expansion of the particle.[662] Presence of the lipid in the hydrophobic pocket may therefore be a critical regulator of the receptor-induced structural transitions of enteroviruses. Removal of the lipid is therefore necessary to provide the capsid with sufficient flexibility to undergo the changes that permit the RNA to leave the shell. The results of computational modeling and kinetic studies suggest that stabilization of virus particles by drugs that replace the lipid is a consequence of increased compressibility rather than increased rigidity.[555,652,698] In some picornaviruses (e.g., rhinovirus types 3 and 14, rhinovirus C), however, the pockets appear to be empty, and these viruses are not inhibited by pocket-binding drugs.[29,777]

Several of these pocket-binding drugs have been evaluated in clinical trials, such as pleconaril for treatment of common colds caused by rhinoviruses[551] and for enteroviral sepsis syndrome.[501] Such drugs are ineffective against picornaviruses for which the VP1 is collapsed or are filled such as rhinovirus C (Fig. 2.3) and human parechovirus 3.[53,632]

Translation of the Viral RNA

Internal Ribosome Binding: The Internal Ribosome Entry Site

Once the picornavirus positive-strand genomic RNA is released into the cell cytoplasm, it must be translated because it cannot be copied by any cellular RNA polymerase and no viral enzymes are brought into the cell within the viral capsid. Several experimental findings led to the hypothesis that translation of the picornavirus genome was accomplished by an unusual mechanism. The positive-strand RNA genomes lack 5′-terminal cap structures; although virion RNA is linked to the viral protein VPg, this protein is removed by the cellular *unlinking* enzyme TDP2[13,725] on entry of the RNA into the cell. Furthermore, picornavirus genomes are efficiently translated in infected cells despite inhibition of cellular mRNA translation. Determination of the nucleotide sequence of poliovirus positive-strand RNA revealed a 741-nucleotide 5′-noncoding region that contains seven AUG codons.[369,582] Similar 5′-noncoding regions were subsequently found in other picornaviruses and shown to contain highly ordered RNA structures.[594,640] Removal of an internal sequence of 300 nucleotides from the poliovirus 5′-noncoding region abrogates viral protein production,[542] while an internal sequence from the 5′-noncoding region of EMCV promoted translation initiation.[330] These findings led to the suggestion that ribosomes do not scan through picornaviral 5′-noncoding regions but rather bind to an internal sequence. The 5′-noncoding region of poliovirus positive-strand RNA was subsequently shown to contain a sequence that promotes internal binding of the 40S ribosomal subunit, and it was called the *internal ribosome entry site* (IRES) (Fig. 2.11).

All picornavirus RNAs contain an IRES, as do other viral mRNAs.[432] Viral IRESs have been placed in eight groups, based on a variety of criteria, including primary sequence, secondary structure, location of the initiation codon, and activity in different cell types.[389] In the type I IRES (found in the genomes of enteroviruses and rhinoviruses) and the type III IRES (hepatitis A virus), the initiation codon is located 50 to 100 nucleotides beyond the 3′ end of the IRES, whereas it is located at the 3′ end of a type II IRES (cardioviruses and aphthoviruses)

(Fig. 2.12). Avihepatoviruses, teschoviruses, tremoviruses, and members of the *Kobuvirus* genus harbor a type V IRES.

There is little nucleotide sequence conservation among different IRES elements. The picornavirus IRES contains extensive regions of RNA secondary structure (Fig. 2.12) that are not strictly conserved but are crucial for ribosome binding. One sequence motif that is conserved among picornavirus IRESs is a GNRA sequence (G, guanine; N, any nucleotide; R, purine; A, adenine) in stem–loop IV of the type I IRES and in stem–loop I of the type II IRES. Another conserved element is an Yn-Xm-AUG motif, in which Yn is a pyrimidine-rich region and Xm is a 15- to 25-nucleotide spacer followed by an AUG codon. Translation initiation mediated by a type I IRES involves binding of the 40S ribosomal subunit to the RNA and scanning of the subunit to the AUG initiation codon. The 40S subunit probably binds at the AUG initiation codon of a type II IRES.

The type III IRES has little homology with type I and type II IRES except for the Yn-Xm-AUG motif. It is structurally distinct, consisting of two major domains, and in addition requires intact eIF4F complex[10] (Fig. 2.12). The type V IRES functions in a prokaryotic-like manner. The secondary structures of these RNA elements facilitate direct interaction with the small 40S ribosome.[196,197,329,650] These interactions place a portion of the RNA within the P-site of the 40S ribosomal subunit as observed by *in vitro* toeprinting and structural analyses of RNA–protein complexes. Initiation of translation mediated by the type V IRES is therefore independent of all canonical translation initiation proteins including the ternary complex of eIF2α-GTP-met-tRNA$_i$. The only initiation protein required is DHX29, necessary to unwind secondary structure surrounding the initiation codon.[563,773] No Met-tRNA$_i$ is required as the first amino acid of this polyprotein is glycine.[329] Translation initiation mediated by the type V IRES may be also independent of all canonical translation initiation proteins as under stress conditions, the Met-tRNA$_i$ may bind directly to the ribosome.

The IRES of kobuviruses is distinct from the type I, II, and III IRES.[773] Domain I is not related to elements found in any other IRES. Domain J consists of a long interrupted basal helix and an apical four-way helical junction, similar to but smaller than domain IV in the type I IRES. Its apical subdomain (Jb) also includes a GNRA tetraloop, which is essential for the function of the type I and type II IRES. The apex of domain K contains an element identical to an apical motif in domain J of the type II IRES that is essential for specific interaction with eIF4G.[52,128] These domains are otherwise unrelated. An equivalent domain K of the type II IRES is also absent. Finally, the initiation codon is preceded by a Yn motif as in the type I/II IRES, but in contrast, it is sequestered in a long, stable hairpin, explaining why this IRES requires the DExH-box protein DHX29.

Mechanism of Internal Ribosome Binding

Different sets of translation initiation proteins are needed for internal initiation. Internal ribosome binding via the type IV IRES requires all of the initiation proteins, including eIF4E. A subset of translation initiation proteins is required for the activity of most picornavirus IRES.

Translation initiation via a type I IRES involves binding of the 40S ribosomal subunit to the IRES, followed by scanning of the subunit to the initiation codon. In cells infected with enteroviruses, eIF4G, the large scaffold protein, which binds

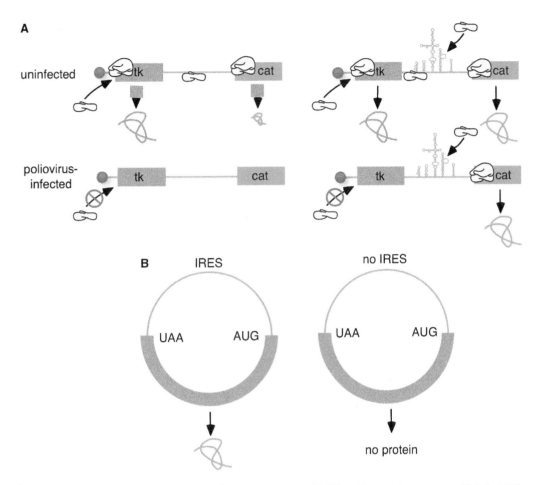

FIGURE 2.11 Discovery of the internal ribosome entry site (IRES). A: Bicistronic messenger RNA (mRNA) assay used to discover the IRES. Plasmids were constructed that encode two reporter molecules, thymidine kinase (tk) and chloramphenicol acetyl transferase (cat), separated by an IRES or a spacer. After introduction into mammalian cells, the plasmids give rise to mRNA of the structure shown in the figure. In uninfected cells (*top line*), both reporter molecules can be detected, although cat synthesis is inefficient without an IRES and is probably caused by reinitiation. In poliovirus-infected cells, 5′-end–dependent initiation is inhibited, and no proteins are detected without an IRES, demonstrating internal ribosome binding. **B:** Circular mRNA assay for an IRES. Circular mRNAs were constructed and translated *in vitro* in cell extracts. In the absence of an IRES, no protein is observed because 5′-end initiation requires a free 5′ end. Inclusion of an IRES allows protein translation from the circular mRNA, demonstrating internal ribosome binding.

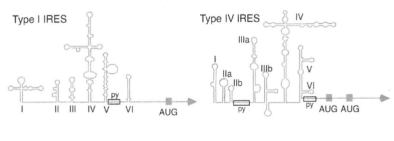

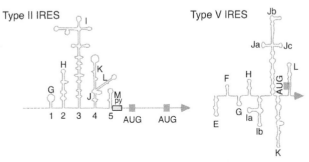

FIGURE 2.12 Four major types of picornaviral internal ribosome entry sites (IRES). The type I IRES is found in the genomes of enteroviruses. The genomes of cardioviruses and aphthoviruses contain a type II IRES. The IRES of hepatitis A virus is type IV, and the type V IRES is represented by porcine teschovirus 1 and kobuvirus.

5′-end dependent

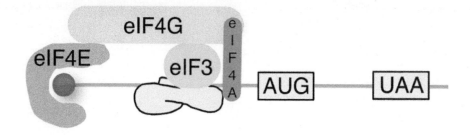

IRES-dependent

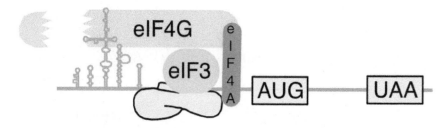

FIGURE 2.13 Models for translation initiation complex formation. In 5′ end–dependent initiation, the 40S subunit is recruited to the messenger RNA (mRNA) through its interaction with eIF3, which binds eIF4G. The latter initiation factor is part of eIF4F, which also contains eIF4A, a helicase to unwind RNA secondary structure, and eIF4E, the cap-binding protein. Binding of eIF4E to the cap thus positions eIF4E at the 5′ end and positions the 40S subunit on the mRNA. In IRES-dependent translation, a 5′ end is not required. The eIF3–40S complex is believed to be recruited to the RNA by the interaction of eIF4G with the IRES.

eIF4E, eIF4A, eIF3, and poly(A)–binding protein (Pabp), is cleaved, inactivating the translation of most cellular mRNA (Fig. 2.13). This observation led to the hypothesis that full-length eIF4G is not required for function of the IRES of poliovirus and other type I IRESs and that mRNA translation initiates when the 40S ribosomal subunit is recruited to the IRES through interaction with eIF3 bound to the C-terminal domain of eIF4G, which binds directly to the RNA. Addition of the C-terminal fragment of eIF4G to *in vitro* translation reactions stimulates activity of the poliovirus and other type I IRESs (Fig. 2.13).[100,517] These data are explained by the observation that the C-terminal fragment of eIF4G stimulates the helicase activity of eIF4A, which is necessary for initiation dependent upon the type I IRES, as the 40S ribosomal subunit is loaded on the RNA upstream of the initiating codon and must scan to the AUG.[31] It also explains why type I IRES activity is enhanced in cells in which the poliovirus protease 2A[pro] is produced.[31,274] Protease 2A[pro] is the picornaviral proteinase responsible for cleavage of eIF4G. Although the IRES of many picornaviruses functions with cleaved eIF4G, the type II and IV IRESs require intact eIF4G.[88] While the 40S ribosomal subunit binds at or near the AUG initiation codon of the type II IRES and no scanning occurs, eIF4G is required to induce conformational changes around the initiating codon necessary for recruitment of the 40S subunit and placement of the initiation codon in the ribosomal A site.[382] Independent of the IRES type,

the efficiency of translation initiation is also dependent upon the interaction between eIF4G and Pabp. This interaction is thought to form a closed loop of mRNA, which is necessary for the efficient return of translating ribosomes to the 5′ end.

The poliovirus IRES functions poorly in reticulocyte lysates, in which capped mRNA can be translated efficiently. Addition of a cytoplasmic extract to reticulocyte lysates restores efficient translation from this IRES. These observations led to the suggestion that ribosome binding to the IRES requires cell proteins other than the canonical initiation proteins. Such proteins have been identified by their ability to bind the IRES and restore internal initiation in reticulocyte lysates (reviewed in[193]). One host protein identified by this approach is the La protein, which binds to the 3′ end of the poliovirus IRES.[456] This protein is associated with the 3′-termini of newly synthesized small RNAs, including transcripts made by cellular RNA polymerase III. La protein is present in low amounts in reticulocyte lysates; addition of the protein to such lysates stimulates the activity of the poliovirus IRES.[456] La is a nuclear protein that is relocalized to the cytoplasm in poliovirus-infected cells.[638] La protein is also required for efficient function of the EMCV IRES.[363]

Polypyrimidine tract–binding (PTB) protein is composed of four RNA-binding domains and functions as a regulator of pre–mRNA splicing. It binds the poliovirus IRES[289] and is required by the type I, II, IV, and V IRES.[312] Removal of this protein from a cell extract with an RNA affinity column inhibits the function of the FMDV IRES[503,559] and that of EMCV, but does not affect translation by 5'-end–dependent initiation.[348] The deficiency in the function of these IRESs is restored by adding the purified protein back to the lysate. The depleted lysate, however, still supports the function of the IRES from Theiler murine encephalomyocarditis virus. It was subsequently shown that the requirement for PTB by the EMCV IRES depends on the nature of the reporter and the size of an A-rich bulge in the IRES.[349] It is thought that PTB facilitates initiation via the type I IRES by modulating binding of eIF4G to the viral RNA, through the interaction between the RNA-binding motifs 1 and 2 of PTB, the bottom of domain V, and the RNA-binding motifs 3 and 4 within the single-stranded region of the viral RNA surrounding domain V of the IRES.[346] Unlike the type I IRES, multiple copies of PTB are required to bind the FMDV, EMCV, and other type II IRES. RNA-binding domains 1 and 2 of one PTB molecule bind domain F of the IRES, and RNA-binding domains 3 and 4 bind domains D and E of the IRES. RNA-binding domains 1 and 2 of a second molecule of PTB bind domain K of the IRES, and RNA-binding domains 3 and 4 interact with IRES domains H, I, and L, all with lower affinity.[345]

HeLa cell extracts also contain unr, an RNA-binding protein with five cold-shock domains that is required for IRES function.[311] Recombinant unr stimulates the function of the rhinovirus IRES in the reticulocyte lysate and acts synergistically with recombinant PTB protein to stimulate translation mediated by the rhinovirus IRES *in vitro*. However, the poliovirus IRES inefficiently mediates translation initiation in *unr*[-/-] cells even though PTB is present.[94]

Ribosome-associated poly r(C)–binding proteins bind at multiple sites within the poliovirus IRES.[83,211] One binding site for these proteins has been identified within stem–loop IV of the poliovirus IRES.[83] Mutations in this region that abolish binding of poly r(C)–binding proteins cause decreased translation *in vitro*. Furthermore, depletion of poly r(C)–binding proteins from HeLa cell translation extracts results in inhibition of poliovirus IRES function.[84] When this assay was used to survey a wide range of picornaviral IRES elements, it was found that poly r(C)–binding proteins are required for function of the type I, but not the type II, IRES.[731] A second binding site for poly r(C)–binding proteins has been identified within a cloverleaf RNA structure that forms within the first 108 nucleotides of the positive-strand poliovirus RNA genome.[211,529] The interaction of poly r(C)–binding proteins with this part of the RNA has been proposed to regulate whether a positive-strand RNA molecule is translated or replicated.

The nucleocytoplasmic protein SRp20 functions with poly r(C)–binding protein 2 to promote initiation on poliovirus mRNA.[62] SRp20 binds to the KH3 domain of poly r(C)–binding protein 2. Depletion of SRp20 from cellular lysates by monoclonal antibodies or from cells by short interfering RNAs reduced IRES-mediated translation by 50%. Polysome analysis of infected cells by sucrose gradient fractionation demonstrated that both SRp20 and poly r(C)–binding protein 2 are at least partly associated with translation initiation complexes bound to stem–loop V of the poliovirus 5'-UTR.[194]

Murine proliferation–associated protein 1 (Mpp-1) is required for the function of the FMDV IRES. This protein binds to a central domain of the viral IRES and acts synergistically with PTB to increase the binding of eIF4F. It has been suggested that Mpp-1 may determine the tissues in which the

IRES functions. To test this hypothesis, a recombinant virus was constructed by replacing the IRES of Theiler virus with that of FMDV. Theiler virus replicates in the mouse brain, but the recombinant virus cannot, possibly because of the absence of Mpp-1 in this organ.[559]

The DExH-box helicase DHX29 is necessary for the activity of the type V IRES.[773] Initially, this protein was identified because it enabled efficient 48S preinitiation complex formation on cellular mRNAs possessing highly structured 5'-noncoding regions.[563] It is believed to be required for proper placement of the ribosome on RNAs possessing prokaryotic-like IRES elements, such as those of the flavivirus classical swine fever virus and the intergenic IRES of cricket paralysis virus, member of the *Dicistroviridae*.[563]

Two proteins that function during vesicular trafficking between the endoplasmic reticulum and Golgi apparatus, Rab1b and ARF5, modulate the activity of the FMDV IRES. By interacting with the RNA, Rab1b may facilitate RNA localization to the rough endoplasmic reticulum and promote protein synthesis, while ARF5 binding to the RNA on the surface of the trans-Golgi may prevent mRNA translation from occurring in the wrong cellular compartment.[189]

Several cell proteins have been identified that inhibit virus protein production, including double-stranded RNA-binding protein 76 (DRBP76), K homology–type RNA splicing regulatory protein (KHSRP), and AU-rich element degradation factor 1 (AUF1). These proteins were identified as binding the 5'-noncoding regions of different picornaviruses, and many inhibit mRNA translation[703] (reviewed in Ref.[401]).

No single cellular protein has been identified that is essential for the function of all viral IRESs. It has been suggested that the small ribosomal protein RPS25 may be an exception, as it appears to be required for translation from the IRES of poliovirus and the type IV IRES of the flavivirus hepatitis C virus, but not for 5' end–dependent translation.[292] How RPS25 functions during internal ribosome entry has not been determined. A common property of some cellular proteins needed for IRES activity is that they are RNA-binding proteins that can form multimers with the potential to contact the IRES at multiple points. This observation has led to the hypothesis that such proteins may act as RNA chaperones, maintaining the IRES in a structure that permits it to bind directly to the translational machinery.[325] IRESs that do not require such chaperones may fold properly without the need for cellular proteins.

Processing of the Viral Polyprotein
Cleavage Cascades
Picornavirus proteins are synthesized by the translation of a single, long ORF encoded by the viral positive-strand RNA genome, followed by cleavage of the polyprotein by virus-encoded proteinases (Figs. 2.5 and 2.14). This strategy allows the synthesis of multiple protein products from a single RNA genome. The polyprotein is not observed in infected cells because it is processed as soon as the protease-coding sequences have been translated. The polyprotein precursor is processed cotranslationally by intramolecular reactions (in *cis*) in what are called *primary cleavages*, followed by secondary processing in *cis* or in *trans* (intermolecular). All picornavirus genomes encode at least one proteinase, 3C[pro]/3CD[pro], and some encode two others: L[pro] and 2A[pro].

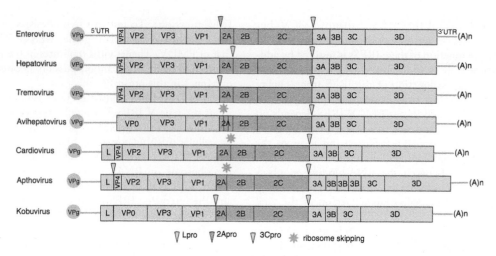

FIGURE 2.14 Primary cleavages of picornavirus polyprotein. In all viruses shown, the P2–P3 cleavage is carried out by 3C[pro] (*green triangle*). In some picornaviruses, the P1–P2 cleavage is carried out by 2A[pro] (*magenta triangle*) or 3C[pro]; in others, the 2A/2B bond is separated by ribosome skipping (*orange asterisk*). The L[pro] proteinase (*blue triangle*) of aphthoviruses catalyzes its release from VP4.

L Proteinase

The first protein encoded in the genome of aphthoviruses, cardioviruses, erboviruses, and sapeloviruses is the L protein (Figs. 2.14 and 2.15). The L protein of aphthoviruses and erboviruses (and possibly that of avian sapelovirus) is a proteinase that releases itself from the polyprotein by cleaving between its C-terminus and the N-terminus of VP4.[297,665] Based on sequence analysis, it was suggested that FMDV L[pro] is related to thiol proteases.[243] This prediction was supported by the results of site-directed mutagenesis, which showed that Cys-51 and

His-148 are the active site amino acids.[556,595] The atomic structure of L[pro] reveals that it consists of two domains, with a topology related to that of papain, a thiol proteinase[260] (Fig. 2.15). The active site His is located at the top of the central α-helix, and substrate binds in the groove between the two domains. Besides releasing itself from the polyprotein, L[pro] also cleaves the translation initiation protein eIF4G, causing inhibition of cellular translation, and G3BP1 and G3BP2, preventing stress granule formation.[160,726] Independent of its protease activity, L[pro] may have deubiquitinase and deISGylase activities.[673,733]

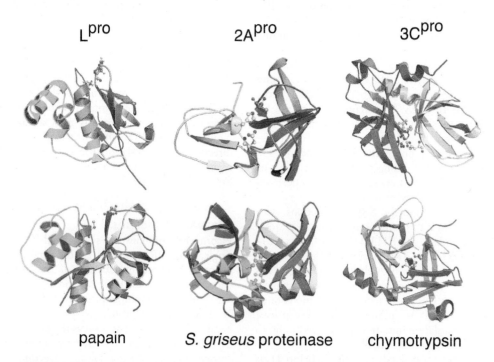

FIGURE 2.15 Three-dimensional structures of L[pro] of foot-and-mouth disease virus, rhinovirus 2A[pro], and hepatitis A virus 3C[pro]. Below each is the cellular proteinase that is structurally similar to each viral enzyme. Catalytic residues are drawn as *balls* and *sticks*. Images drawn with MacPymol using the following pdb files: [2SGA, 2HRV, 2JQG, 1PIP, 1HAV, 5CHA].

L^{pro} also is an antagonist of the innate immune response. By cleaving eIF4G, L^{pro} prevents synthesis of many IFN-stimulated gene products, but it also cleaves the Rig-I–like receptor laboratory of genetics and physiology 2 (LGP2) by impairing the positive feedback loop regulating interferon production.[599]

The cardiovirus and senecavirus L proteins, which do not have proteolytic activity, are released from the P1 precursor by 3C^{pro}[523] (Fig. 2.14). They are small polypeptides with an N-terminal CHCC zinc-finger motif and interact with the cellular GTPase Ran, inhibiting many cellular processes dependent upon GTP/GDP cycling.[549,570] L protein is necessary for assembly of the virion and stimulates translation of the viral mRNA.[35,177] Although the proteins lack enzymatic activity, L proteins are potent antagonists of the innate immune response by inhibiting transcription of cytokine-encoding genes and iron/ferritin–mediated activation of the transcription protein NF-κB as well as modulating nucleocytoplasmic trafficking.[570,708,715,783] The range of cell processes affected by L protein may allow for persistent infections by cardioviruses.

2A Protease

In cells infected with enteroviruses (and possibly sapeloviruses), the primary cleavage between P1 and P2 is mediated by 2A^{pro} (Fig. 2.14). Cellular proteins are also cleaved by 2A^{pro}, including eIF4GI, eIF4GII, Pabp, heart muscle dystrophin, and nucleoporins.[34,112,245,246,264,265,337,359,387,527] In the protein precursor of rhinovirus, poliovirus, and some other enteroviruses, the cleavage site for 2A^{pro} is between tyrosine and glycine. Other sites cleaved by 2A^{pro} include threonine–glycine and phenylalanine–glycine in certain coxsackieviruses and echoviruses.

The relative resistance of poliovirus to IFN has been ascribed to 2A^{pro}, as a single amino acid change from Y to L at amino acid 88 renders the virus sensitive to inhibition by this cytokine.[480] Additional support for the role of 2A^{pro} in countering IFN comes from experiments in which the proteinase-coding sequence was added to the genome of the IFN-sensitive EMCV. The production of 2A^{pro} during EMCV infection confers IFN resistance to the recombinant virus.[480]

Based on sequence alignments, it was suggested that the structure of 2A^{pro} would resemble that of small bacterial chymotrypsin-like proteinases (e.g., *Streptomyces griseus* proteinase A) and would possess a catalytic triad consisting of His-20, Asp-38, and an active site nucleophile of Cys-109 rather than serine.[59] The results of site-directed mutagenesis and the resolution of the atomic structure of rhinovirus and Coxsackievirus B4 2A^{pro} confirm that these residues comprise the active site and that the fold of 2A^{pro} is very similar to that of *Streptomyces griseus* proteinase A[56,546,647,772] (Fig. 2.15). However, 2A^{pro} differs from all known chymotrypsin-like proteinases in that the N-terminal domain is not a β-barrel but rather a four-stranded antiparallel β-sheet. The larger C-terminal domain contains a six-stranded antiparallel β-barrel. The active site catalytic triad is located in a cleft between the two domains. Another unusual feature of 2A^{pro} is a tightly bound zinc ion located at the beginning of the C-terminal domain. Biochemical and structural studies indicate that zinc is essential for the structure of the enzyme.[546,646,729]

The 2A/2B junction of aphthoviruses, avihepatoviruses, cardioviruses, erboviruses, senecaviruses, teschoviruses, Ljungan virus, and duck hepatitis virus is cleaved not by proteolysis but by an unusual mechanism called ribosomal skipping[167] (Fig. 2.14). Changes within the conserved amino acid sequence Asp-(Val/Ile)-Glu-X-Asn-Pro-Gly-Pro, which contains the cleavage site Gly-Pro, disrupt cleavage.[523] The cleavage reaction occurs within the ribosomal peptidyl transferase (P-) site. Despite the Pro-encoding codon at the end of the 2A-coding sequence being within the aminoacyl (A-) site, the translating ribosome pauses. This "stop," together with the conformational constraint of the added proline and the α-helix formed by upstream amino acids occluding the exit tunnel of the translating ribosome, impairs peptide bond formation between the Gly and Pro. These events lead the eukaryotic release factor 1 to enter the A-site, followed by release of the synthesized peptide chain. Mutation of the Pro codon inhibits ribosomal skipping, confirming that insertion of proline is essential for the stop and release of the synthesized polypeptide, not the codon sequence.[171,371,372] Consequently, the first amino acid of 2B is always a proline. Impairment of ribosomal skipping negatively impacts cleavage at the L-P1-2A boundaries by 3C^{pro}.[271] The ability of the 2A sequence to yield two proteins from a single open reading frame, without proteinase activity, has led to its use in many research and biomedical applications.[609]

Because only enteroviruses and possibly sapeloviruses have proteolytically active 2A^{pro}, in cells infected with other picornaviruses, the VP1-2A cleavage is either carried out by 3C^{pro}[333,523,623,624] or in Ljungan virus–infected cells by a NPG/P sequence following the VP1 protein[338] (Fig. 2.14).

The polyprotein of Aichi virus, a member of the *Kobuvirus* genus, is unusual because the L and 2A proteins are not proteinases and there is no NPG/P motif at the 2A/2B junction. The only active proteinase encoded in the genome of this virus is 3C^{pro} and 3CD^{pro}, which can process all cleavage sites in the polyprotein, including the VP1/2A site[618] (Fig. 2.14). Efficient cleavage of the VP1/2A site requires tight binding of 3CD^{pro} to the 2A region of the substrate.

3C Protease

All picornaviruses encode 3C^{pro}, which carries out a primary cleavage between 2C and 3A (Fig. 2.14). Unlike the other picornavirus proteinases, 3C^{pro} may also carry out secondary cleavages of the P1 and P2 precursors. Poliovirus 3C^{pro} cleaves only at the Gln-Gly dipeptide; however, 3C^{pro} of other picornaviruses has less strict cleavage specificities and cleaves at other sites, including Gln-Ser, Gln-Ile, Gln-Asn, Gln-Ala, Gln-Thr, and Gln-Val. Clearly, other determinants of cleavage exist because not all such dipeptides in picornavirus polyproteins are cleaved by 3C^{pro}. Additional determinants include accessibility of the cleavage site to the enzyme, recognition of secondary and tertiary structures in the substrate by the enzyme, and amino acid sequences surrounding the cleavage site. For example, efficient cleavage of poliovirus Gln-Gly pairs requires an Ala at the P4 position (Gln is residue P1, numbering is toward the N-terminus).[82]

Sequence comparisons with cellular proteinases led to the prediction that 3C^{pro} folds similarly to the chymotrypsin-like serine proteinases, in particular *Staphylococcus aureus* proteinase.[59,240–242] The putative catalytic triad was believed to consist of His-40, Asp-71 (aphthoviruses and cardioviruses) or Glu-71 (enteroviruses and rhinoviruses), and Cys-147 as the nucleophilic residue, in contrast to serine in cellular serine proteinases. These predictions have been confirmed by site-directed mutagenesis and by resolution of the atomic structures of rhinovirus, hepatitis A virus, poliovirus, FMDV, and enterovirus 71 3C^{pro}.[116,255,275,356,449,483,546,732] The viral enzyme folds into two equivalent β-barrels like chymotrypsin (Fig. 2.15) but differs in some of the connecting loops, in the orientation of the catalytic residues, and in areas needed for transition-state stabilization. The acidic member of the catalytic triad, Glu or Asp, points away from the active site His and, therefore, is not believed to assist in catalysis. However, 3C^{pro} also binds viral RNA (see discussion of genome replication and mRNA synthesis), and this binding site is distal from the active site of the enzyme. Despite the distance between the enzymatic active site and the RNA-binding motif, protease activity of 3C^{pro} is regulated by RNA binding, and the ability to bind RNA is modulated by protease activity.[113] The presence of this RNA-binding site imposes evolutionary constraints on 3C^{pro} that are not found in other proteinases.

Both 3C^{pro} and 2A^{pro} are active in the nascent polypeptide and release themselves from the polyprotein by self-cleavage. After the proteinases have been released, they cleave the polyprotein in *trans*. The cascade of processing events varies for different picornaviruses (Fig. 2.14). In cells infected with rhinovirus and enteroviruses, the initial event in the processing cascade is the release of the P1 precursor from the nascent P2–P3 protein by 2A^{pro}. The activity of 2A^{pro} does not depend on whether it is cleaved from the precursor,[275] but further processing of P1 by 3CD^{pro} does not occur unless 2A^{pro} is released from P1.[502,771] Next, 3CD^{pro} is released from the P3 precursor by autocatalytic cleavage. This proteinase, which contains the entire sequence of the viral RNA polymerase, carries out secondary cleavage of glutamine–glycine dipeptides in poliovirus P1 far more efficiently than 3C^{pro}.[342,770] Both 3C^{pro} and 3CD^{pro} process proteins of the P2 and P3 regions with similar efficiency. The 3D^{pol} sequence within 3CD^{pro} may be required to recognize structural motifs in properly folded P1, allowing efficient processing by the 3C^{pro} part of the enzyme. The presence of multiple activities in a single protein is not found among eukaryotic proteinases and is an example of how the coding capacity of small viral genomes can be maximized. Not all picornaviruses require 3CD^{pro} to process P1; aphthoviruses, cardioviruses, and hepatoviruses produce 3C^{pro} that can cleave P1 without additional viral protein sequence.

An advantage of the polyprotein strategy is that expression can be controlled by the rate and extent of proteolytic processing. Alternative use of cleavage sites can also produce proteins with different activities. For example, because 3CD^{pro} is required for processing of the poliovirus capsid protein precursor P1, the extent of capsid protein processing can be controlled by regulating the amount of 3CD^{pro} that is produced. Because 3CD^{pro} does not possess RNA polymerase activity, some of it must be cleaved to allow RNA replication. Cleavage of 3CD^{pro} releasing 3D^{pol} is regulated by cholesterol.[317]

A final processing step occurs during maturation, when VP0 is cleaved to form VP4 and VP2. This event is discussed later.

Viral RNA Synthesis

In the 1950s, it was believed that the genome of RNA viruses was replicated by the cellular DNA-dependent RNA polymerase, through an intermediate DNA strand. The replication of RNA viruses, therefore, was thought to occur entirely in the cell nucleus. In the early 1960s, studies of mengovirus showed that virus infection results in the induction of a cytoplasmic enzyme that can synthesize viral RNA in the presence of actinomycin D.[39] This observation suggested that viral genome replication occurred through a virus-specific RNA-dependent RNA polymerase because cellular RNA synthesis is DNA dependent; it occurs in the nucleus and is sensitive to actinomycin D. A similar cytoplasmic, actinomycin D–resistant genome replication system was discovered in poliovirus-infected cells.[39]

In poliovirus-infected cells, the positive-strand genome is amplified to about 50,000 copies per cell through a negative-strand intermediate. Three forms of viral RNA have been identified in the cell: ssRNA, replicative intermediate (RI), and replicative form (RF). ssRNA, the most abundant form, is exclusively positive-strand; free negative strands have never been detected in infected cells. RI is a full-length RNA from which six to eight nascent strands are attached. RI is largely of positive polarity with nascent negative strands, although the opposite configuration has been detected. RF is a double-stranded structure, consisting of one full-length copy of the positive and negative strands. Viral RNA synthesis is asymmetric; the synthesis of positive strands is 30 to 70 times greater than the synthesis of negative strands.[223,509]

Viral RNA–Dependent RNA Polymerase, 3D^{pol}

The first evidence for a viral RNA–dependent RNA polymerase activity came from experiments in which lysates from cells infected with mengovirus or poliovirus were assayed for viral RNA polymerase activity by the incorporation of a radioactive nucleotide into viral RNA.[38] Initial experiments demonstrated that the viral RNA polymerase is associated with a cellular membrane fraction, subsequently shown to be comprised of smooth membranes, which was called the RNA replication complex.[227] A major component of the replication complex was a viral protein that migrated at 63 kD on polyacrylamide gels (therefore, called p63), which was suggested to be the viral RNA–dependent RNA polymerase. Other viral and host proteins, including 2BC, 2C, 3AB, and 3C^{pro}, however, were detected in the RNA replication complexes.

A limitation of this early work was that replication complexes only copied viral RNA already present in the complex and did not respond to added RNA. Attempts were made, therefore, to purify a template-dependent enzyme from membrane fractions of infected cells, using a poly(A) template and an oligo(U) primer. A poly(U) polymerase activity was purified from poliovirus-infected cells, which could also copy poliovirus RNA in the presence of an oligo(U) primer. Highly purified preparations contained only p63, the major viral protein found in membranous replication complexes.[195,707] This protein is the poliovirus RNA polymerase, now known as 3D^{pol}. In the absence of an oligo(U) primer, 3D^{pol} cannot copy poliovirus RNA. Recombinant 3D^{pol} purified from bacteria or insect cells also requires the presence of an oligo(U) primer to copy poliovirus RNA.[498,568] 3D^{pol}, therefore, is a template- and primer-dependent enzyme that can copy poliovirus RNA. Its molecular weight predicted from the amino acid sequence is 53 kD.

The structures of all four types of polymerases, DNA-dependent DNA polymerase, DNA-dependent RNA polymerase, RNA-dependent DNA polymerase (reverse transcriptase), and RNA-dependent RNA polymerase, are characterized by analogy with a right hand, consisting of a palm, fingers, and thumb. The palm domain contains the active site of the enzyme. The picornavirus RNA polymerase 3D^{pol} is produced by cleavage of a precursor protein, 3CD^{pro}, which is highly active as a proteinase, and binds *cre* (see below). The precursor 3CD^{pro} has no polymerase activity, nor does it take on the hand-like structure of a polymerase.[283] The hand-like structure of a viral RNA–dependent RNA polymerase was first observed when that of poliovirus 3D^{pol} was determined at 2.6 Å resolution by x-ray crystallography.[277] Additional structures of 3D^{pol} from poliovirus, three rhinovirus serotypes, FMDV, EMCV, and Coxsackievirus B3, provide resolution of virtually all amino acids in the protein, offering a complete picture of this monomeric enzyme.[22,105,191,234,424,683] While the picornavirus polymerase has the same overall shape as other polymerases, the fingers and thumb differ (Fig. 2.16). The palm domain contains four conserved amino acid motifs (B, C, D, E) that are found in other RNA-dependent polymerases. Amino acids 1 to 68 of the index finger rise from the palm domain before forming a loop that contacts the thumb domain by reaching across the palm. This loop traps the ring finger underneath it, leading it to form the top of the channel through which

nucleotide triphosphates enter. The channel includes conserved motif F that is important for interacting with the triphosphates. This interaction also forms a large pore between the thumb and pinky through which the template–product RNA duplex exits, with the thumb domain stuck in the RNA major groove. The template and product are of reverse complementarity and anneal together such that no strand separation can be physically observed. Yet, mutations in the thumb domain can alter the length of the poly(A) tail, implying that slippage between the stands in the absence of detectable strand separation occurs in order to generate a tail of varied length, which is not fully templated.[357] *In vitro* RNA transcription by picornavirus polymerases occurs via a duplex template suggesting that 3D^{pol} must have an inherent strand separation function.[122] Together with data from structures of the elongating polymerase–RNA complex, the footprint of 3D^{pol} bound to the RNA duplex has been determined to include eight nucleotides of the elongating RNA and three base pairs downstream on the template.[233]

It was suggested that processing of 3CD affected the location of the N-terminal glycine of 3D^{pol}, which is buried in a

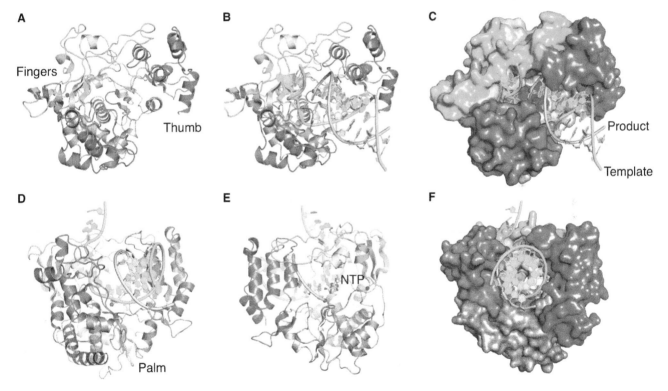

FIGURE 2.16 Three-dimensional structure of poliovirus 3D^{pol}. Structure of poliovirus 3D^{pol} polymerase and its elongation complex with primer-template RNA. The polymerase structure can be described by analogy to a cupped right hand, consisting of palm (*gray*) and thumb (*blue*) domains and finger domains with four discrete structural elements known as the index (*green*), middle (*orange*), ring (*yellow*), and pinky (*red*) fingers. The structure of the elongation complex shows the path of the RNA as the template strand (*cyan*) enters the polymerase from the top and of the template–product (*gold*) duplex as it exits the polymerase between the pinky finger and thumb structures.[300] **A–C:** Views from the top of the polymerase looking down into the active site (*magenta*) of 3D^{pol} in the absence of RNA **(A)**, the 3D^{pol} elongation complex with bound RNA **(B)**, and the elongation complex with a surface representation of the polymerase to show how the product RNA duplex is clamped in place between the pinky finger and thumb structures **(C)**. **D:** Front view of the elongation complex showing the path template and product RNA strands. **E:** Back view of the elongation complex showing the NTP entry channel with the priming 3′ OH (*red sphere*) positioned above the active site and a bound di-deoxy-CTP (*green ball-and-stick* with phosphate groups in *red* and *yellow*). **F:** Surface representation of the elongation complex looking down the axis of the exiting RNA duplex. 3D^{pol} from poliovirus and closely related picornaviruses is activated upon cleavage from the viral polyprotein, resulting in a newly created N-terminus that becomes buried in a pocket at the base of the finger domain that is ≈15 Å away from the active site itself (*blue sphere* in **A** and **E**). (Courtesy of Olve Peersen, Colorado State University.)

pocket at the base of the fingers domain, in order to position Asp238 slightly away from the active site of the polymerase. On proteolysis, the N-terminal Gly was believed to push Asp-238 a distance of 1.4 Å into the catalytic site. This slight shift in position would allow for hydrogen bonding between the Asp and both the 2'- and 3'-ribose hydroxyl groups of the incoming NTP, a reaction critical for discriminating between rNTPs and dNTPs[230,234,308] and active site closure. Furthermore, it correctly coordinates Asp233 and two magnesium ions, which are necessary for polymerization.[234] Resolution of the structure of the Coxsackievirus B3 3D[pol] reveals an unusual conformation for residue 5, which is located at a distortion within a β-strand near the exit of the RNA channel and is conserved in all known 3D[pol] structures.[105] Substitution of more hydrophobic residues, such as tryptophan at this position, results in higher enzymatic activity. Alterations at this position primarily change the temporal stability of the postinitiation elongation complex but may also affect the processivity of the enzyme and virus replication.[300]

The catalytic cycle is composed of six structural states beginning with paused polymerase bound to the template stacked upon the RNA duplex and poised for the incoming NTP and an unstructured active site. Nucleotides enter the catalytic site via a large opening on the backside of 3D[pol]. Upon selection, the nucleotide is positioned by the lysine and arginine residues that line the entrance. Base pairing between the template base and the incoming nucleotide triggers movement of the palm, facilitating rearrangement between the motif A-motif C- and the 2'OH of the triphosphate such that when the active site is closed, the triphosphate is correctly placed with the required magnesium ions coordinated to promote bond formation. Addition of the new base to the growing strand opens the active site, independent of movement of the fingers domain. Translocation of the RNA duplex one nucleotide occurs by "Brownian motion" and places the next templating base within the active site. The lack of movement in the fingers domain during polymerization is another unique feature of 3D[pol].

What sets apart the picornavirus RNA polymerase from all others is that the templating nucleotide is prepositioned right above the active site stacked with the first base pair of the elongating strand and is ready for catalysis even in the absence of a bound nucleotide.[234] Consequently, there is negligible RNA movement during phosphodiester bond formation. Moreover, there are little to no changes when compared with the protein structure in the absence of RNA. The simplicity of this nucleotide selection mechanism greatly influences polymerase fidelity.

The first poliovirus 3D[pol] structure also revealed that the polymerase molecules interacted in a head-to-tail manner and formed fibers; subsequently, the protein was shown to form a lattice.[429] The implication was that RNA would be replicated as it moved along the lattice, rather than the polymerase moving on the template. The head-to-tail fibers were formed by interface I, which involves more than 23 amino acid side chains between the thumb of one polymerase and the back of the palm of another. Amino acid changes in the back of the thumb that disrupt this interface impaired replication.[161,301] Repetition of this interaction in a head-to-tail fashion results in long fibers of polymerase molecules 50 Å in diameter. A similar interface was observed in crystals of 3D[pol] of rhinovirus 14 but not rhinoviruses 16 or 1b.[424] Interface II is formed by N-terminal polypeptide segments, which may lead to a network of polymerase fibers in combination with interactions at interface I. These N-terminal polypeptide segments may originate from different polymerase molecules.

The N-terminus of 3D[pol] is required for enzyme activity, which would support the idea that interface II interactions are of functional consequence. Furthermore, intermolecular cross-linking has been observed between cysteines engineered at Ala-29 and Ile-441 of poliovirus 3D[pol],[301] and disruption of these interactions leads to lethality.[680] Polymerase-containing oligomeric structures resembling those seen with purified 3D[pol] were observed on the surface of vesicles isolated from poliovirus-infected cells.[429] Because picornavirus RNA synthesis occurs on membranous vesicles, the concept of a flat, catalytic lattice is mechanistically attractive.

Viral Accessory Proteins

The poliovirus capsid proteins are not required for viral RNA synthesis; the region of the viral genome that encodes these proteins can be deleted without affecting the ability of viral RNA to replicate in cells.[350] The capsid-coding regions of rhinovirus, Theiler virus, and mengovirus, however, contain a cis-acting RNA sequence required for genome replication.[421,453,454] A cis-acting RNA sequence required for RNA replication has also been identified in the poliovirus protein 2C–coding region.[236] Genetic and biochemical studies implicate most proteins of the P2 and P3 regions of the genome in RNA synthesis.

2A Protein

As discussed above, 2A[pro] protein is necessary for proteolytic cleavage of the polyprotein. The protein also appears to have a role in RNA replication. A deletion within the 2A[pro]-coding sequence severely inhibits replication of subgenomic replicons, which lack the capsid region and are not dependent on proteolytic activity of 2A[pro] to release the P1 region.[131] In another approach, a second IRES element was placed in the poliovirus genome before the 2A[pro]-coding region, effectively alleviating the need for the processing activity of the enzyme. Such viruses are viable.[474] Deletion of part of the coding region for 2A[pro] is lethal, however. By using a cell-free replication system, it was possible to determine the effect of 2A[pro] on each step of the replication cycle.[343] The results show that 2A[pro] stimulates the initiation of negative-strand synthesis, but has no effect on positive-strand synthesis. How 2A[pro] achieves this affect is not known, but it has been suggested that the proteinase might modify a cellular protein required for negative-strand RNA synthesis.[343]

2B Protein

The 2B protein is a small, membrane-associated protein that is involved at an early step of viral RNA synthesis. Protein 2B has been called a viroporin, a protein that oligomerizes and inserts into membranes to create channels.[2,235] Alterations of the 2B protein of poliovirus and coxsackievirus lead to viruses with defects in RNA synthesis.[340,710] Adaptation of rhinoviruses to mouse cells is mediated in part by amino acid changes in 2B, which allow viral RNA synthesis in this host cell.[282] The structure and mechanisms by which 2B is membrane-associated varies among picornaviruses. Enterovirus 2B proteins, which are 97 to 99 amino acids long, are predicted to possess two small hydrophobic domains, the first is a cationic amphiphilic α-helix, while the second is a fully hydrophobic helix,[530,713] while that of hepatitis A virus is 274 amino acids. Membrane pores induced by 2B proteins of enteroviruses are thought to result from protein oligomerization and assembly of tetrameric bundles that insert into the membrane. While the 2B protein of hepatitis A virus associates with membranes and induces the formation of tube-shaped vesicles, it does not oligomerize nor does it form a transmembrane pore. The structure of the soluble region of hepatitis A virus 2B protein including the C-terminus as determined by x-ray crystallography reiterated these differences. This region of the hepatitis A virus 2B protein is a curved five-stranded antiparallel β-sheet of striking similarity to the β-barrel domain of 2A[pro] followed by a helical bundle.[727] The crystal structure also unveiled that 2B self-associates into a fiber- and amyloid-like structure that can act as platform for the recruitment of cellular and viral proteins necessary for replication.

The role of protein 2B in RNA synthesis, however, is not known. Synthesis of the protein leads to an inhibition of protein secretion from the Golgi apparatus[45,165] and permeabilization of membranes,[2,6,616,711,712] which may play a role in release of virus from cells. Protein 2B is also partly responsible for the proliferation of membranous vesicles in infected cells, which are the sites of viral RNA replication. Because protein 3A has the same effect, it is not clear whether altered membrane proliferation is responsible for the RNA-defective phenotype in 2B mutants.

2C Protein

Protein 2C is a highly conserved protein with membrane-, RNA-, and NTP-binding regions.[178,597,598,711,712] The structure of 2C suggests that it contains three domains, with amphipathic α-helices at both the N- and C-termini that mediate peripheral association with membranes[386,681] and a central region with NTP-binding domains. Mutations responsible for resistance of poliovirus and echovirus to guanidine hydrochloride, which blocks viral RNA replication, are located in the 2C protein.[373,560,561] This compound has been shown to inhibit specifically the initiation of negative-stranded RNA synthesis and has no effect on initiation of positive-strand RNA synthesis or on elongation on either strand.[50] The nucleoside triphosphatase (NTPase) activity of protein 2C is inhibited by guanidine.[554] Protein 2C shares amino acid homology with known RNA helicases, proteins encoded by most positive-strand RNA viruses with large genomes. These enzymes are believed to be necessary to unwind double-stranded RNA structures that form during RNA replication. Purified protein 2C, however, does not have RNA helicase activity.[597] Alteration of conserved amino acids within the NTPase domain of 2C results in loss of viral infectivity; the protein may therefore have two functions during viral RNA synthesis: as an NTPase and directing replication complexes to cell membranes. Synthesis of 2C causes disassembly of the Golgi apparatus and endoplasmic reticulum, and formation of vesicular structures similar, but not identical to, those that constitute the replication complex.[7,123]

2BC Protein

Much of protein 2BC, the precursor to 2B and 2C, remains uncleaved during infection, and its presence is critical to viral replication.[123] Synthesis of 2BC causes membrane permeabilization to a greater degree than 2B synthesis alone[6] and leads to the formation of vesicles that are more similar to those formed during viral infection than does protein 2C.[7,123] The C-terminus of

2B and the N-terminus of 2C may interact intramolecularly in 2BC, and protein cleavage may cause a conformational change that alters the properties of 2B and 2C individually.[45,713] Larger 2BC-containing precursors are also required for certain steps of replication,[344] although an intact 2C–3A junction is not strictly required.[533]

3AB, 3A, and 3B Proteins

A strongly hydrophobic region in the C-terminus of 3A mediates the association of 3A and its precursor, 3AB, with membranes,[164,663,691] thereby orienting the protein such that the majority of it is on the cytosolic side of the vesicle.[124] Amino acid changes in the hydrophobic region of 3A yield replication-defective viruses.[221,390] Changes in viral host range have been mapped to 3A protein.[61,282,390,511] The efficiency of cleavage 3ABCD into 3ABC, 3AB, 3CD, 3A, 3B, 3C, and 3D[pol] varies among picornaviruses. This series of cleavages occurs more efficiently during poliovirus infection than during Aichi or hepatitis A virus.[284,492,624] The solution structure of 3A demonstrates that it is a homodimer, with the dimer interface located in the central region of the protein.[663] The requirement for 3A dimerization during infection has not been explored. Protein 3B, also known as VPg, plays an indispensable role in viral replication by acting as a protein primer for viral RNA synthesis (see below). Protein 3AB is believed to anchor VPg in membranes for the priming step of RNA synthesis. The purified protein greatly stimulates 3D[pol] activity *in vitro*[532,567,591] as well as the proteolytic activity of 3CD[pro].[473] 3AB interacts with 3D[pol] and 3CD[pro] in infected cells and with 3D[pol] in the yeast two-hybrid system.[306] Amino acid changes in 3D[pol] that disrupt its interaction with 3AB result in viruses with defects in protein processing and viral RNA synthesis.[221,222] A complex of 3AB and 3CD[pro] also binds the cloverleaf at the 5′ end of the genome forming a RNA–protein complex that interacts with the poly(A) tail via interaction with Pabp.[284,757] Aichi virus replication, particularly negative-strand synthesis, may be dependent upon formation of a closed loop.[492] A complex of 3AB and 3CD[pro] also binds 3′-terminal sequences of poliovirus RNA.

Cellular Accessory Proteins

Early studies of poliovirus replication using purified components suggested that a host cell protein is required for copying the viral RNA by 3D[pol] in the absence of an oligo(U) primer.[153] Although this protein was never identified, the concept of a host factor required for poliovirus replication endured, largely because an ample precedent was seen for the participation of host cell components in a viral RNA polymerase. The best-studied example is the RNA polymerase of the bacteriophage Qβ, which is a multisubunit enzyme consisting of a 65-kD virus-encoded protein and three host proteins: ribosomal protein S1 and translation factors EF-Tu and EF-Ts.[278] The 65-kD viral protein has no RNA polymerase activity in the absence of the host proteins but has sequence similarity with known RNA-dependent RNA polymerases. A subunit of the translation initiation protein eIF3 is part of the polymerase from brome mosaic virus.[578] Two different experimental systems have been used to provide additional evidence that poliovirus RNA synthesis requires host cell components.

When purified poliovirus RNA is incubated *in vitro* with a cytoplasmic extract prepared from cultured, permissive cells, the viral RNA is translated, the resulting protein is proteolytically processed, and the genome is replicated and assembled into new infectious virus particles.[475] If guanidine, an inhibitor of poliovirus RNA synthesis, is included in the reaction, complexes are formed, but elongation cannot occur.[48] The preinitiation complexes can be isolated free of guanidine, and, when added to new cytoplasmic extracts, RNA synthesis occurs. In the absence of cytoplasmic extract, preinitiation complexes do not synthesize viral RNA.[47] These results indicate that one or more soluble cellular components are required for the initiation of viral RNA replication. A similar conclusion comes from studies in which poliovirus RNA is injected into oocytes derived from the African clawed toad, *Xenopus laevis*. Poliovirus RNA cannot replicate in *Xenopus* oocytes unless it is coinjected with a cytoplasmic extract from human cells.[210]

Cellular poly r(C)–binding proteins are required for poliovirus RNA synthesis. These proteins bind to a cloverleaf secondary structure, also called stem–loop I, that forms in the first 108 nucleotides of positive-strand RNA (Fig. 2.17). Binding of poly r(C)–binding protein to the cloverleaf is necessary for the efficient binding of viral protein 3CD[pro] to the opposite side of the same cloverleaf.[17,19,211,529] Formation of a ribonucleoprotein complex composed of the 5′ cloverleaf, 3CD[pro], and a cellular protein is essential for the initiation of viral RNA synthesis.[17] The human cell protein required for replication of poliovirus RNA in *Xenopus* oocytes has also been identified as poly r(C)–binding protein.[211] A model of how these interactions lead to viral RNA synthesis is shown in Figure 2.17. The ternary complex with stem–loop I may also function during positive-strand RNA synthesis.[728]

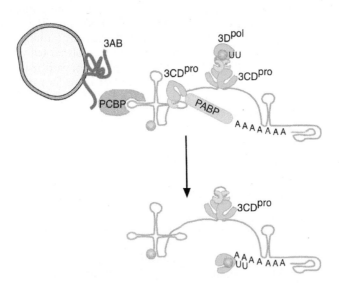

FIGURE 2.17 Model for the synthesis of poliovirus (–) strand RNA. The (+) strand template is shown in *green* with the 5′-cloverleaf structure, the internal *cre* sequence, and the 3′ pseudoknot. A ribonucleoprotein complex is formed when poly r(C)–binding protein (PCBP) and 3CD[pro] bind the cloverleaf structure. The ribonucleoprotein complex interacts with Pabp1, which is bound to the 3′-poly(A) sequence, producing a circular template. Protease 3CD[pro] cleaves membrane-bound 3AB to produce VPg and 3A. The cre sequence binds 3D[pol], 3CD[pro], and VPg. VPg-pUpU is synthesized by 3D[pol] using the sequence AAACA of *cre* as template. The complex is transferred to the 3′ end of the genome, and 3D[pol] uses VPg-pUpU to prime RNA synthesis.

Another candidate for a host protein that is essential for poliovirus RNA synthesis is poly(A)–binding protein 1. This protein interacts with poly r(C)–binding protein, 3CD[pro], and the 3′-poly(A) tail of poliovirus RNA, circularizing the genome[50,291] (Fig. 2.17). The mechanism for negative-strand RNA synthesis is hypothesized to include formation of a circular ribonucleoprotein complex.

Even though infectious poliovirus and other picornaviruses can be produced from viruses that lack the 3′-noncoding region, replication is inefficient.[98,615,684,714] Binding of heterogeneous nuclear ribonucleoprotein C is necessary to bring both the 5′ and 3′ ends of the negative-strand RNA together forming a closed loop of RNA, necessary to stabilize interactions between the two ends to promote 3C/3CD binding to the replicative intermediate. The absence of the 3′-noncoding region abolishes the closed loop needed. Consequently, initiation of positive-strand synthesis is compromised.[184]

Protein-Primed RNA Synthesis

As discussed, poliovirus 3D[pol] is a primer-dependent enzyme that will not copy poliovirus RNA *in vitro* without an oligo(U) primer. The discovery of VPg linked to poliovirus genome RNA, as well as to the 5′ end of newly synthesized positive- and negative-strand RNA, suggested that VPg might be involved in the initiation of RNA synthesis. This hypothesis was supported by the finding that both VPg and a uridylylated form of the protein, VPg-pUpU, can be found in infected cells.[143] Furthermore, VPg-pUpU can be synthesized *in vitro* in a membrane fraction from poliovirus-infected cells.[675] Additional evidence that VPg can serve as a primer for poliovirus RNA synthesis comes from experiments in which synthetic VPg is first uridylylated *in vitro* and then added to an *in vitro* polymerase reaction containing a poly(A) template and 3D[pol].[537] The labeled, uridylylated VPg is extended to form poly(U). This evidence shows that poliovirus RNA replication is primed by a genome-linked protein, a mechanism also involved in adenovirus DNA replication. A model for VPg priming of poliovirus RNA synthesis is shown in Figure 2.16.

The unprocessed P3 precursors 3BC and 3BCD, though minor products of P3 processing, can be uridylylated *in vitro* and bind the RNA stem–loop where RNA replication is initiated with greater affinity than VPg. Moreover, the presence of 3BC facilitates recruitment and retention of 3D[pol] for VPg and RNA.[531] Although no protein larger than VPg has been detected linked to nascent RNA strands during virus infection, the use of a subgenomic replicon with an uncleavable bond between 3B and 3C (Gly-Gly instead of Gln-Gly) demonstrated that processing of 3BC is not necessary for genome replication as 3BC could be linked to the nascent RNA strand. In fact, 3BC has a higher affinity for RNA than 3B.

The template for uridylylation of VPg is an RNA hairpin, the cis-acting replication element, *cre*, located in the coding region of many picornaviruses[535,593,767] (Fig. 2.17). The cre for FMDV replication is located within the 5′-noncoding region.[447] The *cre* functions independent of position in the genome, and its location differs among viruses. Within all *cre* elements is a conserved sequence, GXXXAAAXXXXXA, of which only [5]AAA[7] is essential for the reaction. VPg and two molecules of 3D[pol] bind the RNA hairpin, placing [5]A within the palm domain of one molecule of polymerase. Uridylylation occurs within the active site of the second molecule of 3D[pol].[669]

The addition of two uracils to Tyr3 of VPg is templated by the ^{5}A, suggesting that uridylylation occurs via a "slide-back" mechanism.[538]

Results of genetic analysis suggested that the interaction of VPg with 3D^{pol} occurs on the surface of the enzyme near conserved motif E, on the back side of the palm near the base of the thumb, which is distant from the catalytic site, and are not consistent with structural data or the observation that alterations within the proposed 3AB binding site impair the reaction.[22,190,256,430,669] Instead, the crystal structures of the VPg-3D^{pol} of FMDV, rhinovirus, enterovirus 71, and Coxsackievirus B3 suggest that the VPg contact sites on 3D^{pol} may vary among picornaviruses; VPg binds motif F and the thumb on FMDV 3D^{pol} placing VPg within the catalytic site and facilitating the *cis* mechanism of uridylylation, while VPg binds the end of the palm of Coxsackievirus B virus 3D^{pol}, and the addition of UMP to tyrosine 3 occurs in *trans*.[22,190,256,680]

Cellular Site of RNA Synthesis

Remodeling of Cell Membranes

Picornaviral RNA synthesis, like that of most RNA viruses, occurs in the cytoplasm of the cell. Virus infection leads to the proliferation and rearrangement of intracellular membranes in infected cells, first described by electron microscopy studies done in the 1960s.[151] The single- and double-membraned vesicles, replication organelles (RO), are primarily derived from the ER, Golgi apparatus, and lysosomes, and *de novo* synthesized lipids eventually fill the cytoplasm.[307,484] Two distinct types of ROs have been identified, as vesicles with numerous separate invaginations at the boundary between the RO and host organelle with RNA synthesis taking place inside the folds or as a membrane protrusion from the cell organelle creating a tubular and/or vesicular structure and genome replication occurring on their surfaces. Both structures serve as platforms for viral replication by increasing the local concentration of proteins necessary for virus reproduction as well as hiding intermediates and preventing sensing by the innate immune response. Consequently, networks of single-membrane vesicles are the site of virus replication.

Rearrangement of the secretory pathway components ER, Golgi apparatus, and lysosomes begins early during picornavirus infection.[307] At 2 hours postinfection, dramatic alterations of cytoplasm can be seen, comprising an increased number of ribosomes along the ER and nuclear membrane and formation of single-membrane tubules with interior density.[78,180] Furthermore, trafficking of secretory cargo is also impaired. Electron tomography experiments revealed that poliovirus 3A–associated RO originates from the GM130-positive cis-Golgi apparatus as an intertwining network of clusters of single-membrane branched tubular structures in a porous sponge-like arrangement.[67,77,215,458,476,622] These observations support earlier data in which the RNA RF of the Coxsackievirus B3 genome in combination with the 3A and 3D^{pol} proteins and the Golgi-specific proteins Arf1, a small Ras-family GTPase, and GBF1, a guanine nucleotide exchange factor, were found to colocalize on the surface of the Golgi apparatus.[307] However, no component of the RO of cardioviruses colocalizes with Golgi-specific markers; instead, these structures are thought to be derived from the ER.[168] For those picornaviruses whose RO originates from the Golgi apparatus, the ER is a source of phosphatidylinositol-4-phosphate (PI4P)-rich membranes.

Membrane contact sites are critical regulators of lipid homeostasis in both the infected and uninfected cell. They facilitate the nonvesicular exchange of lipids, cholesterol, and phosphatidylinositol-4-phosphate (PI4P) between organelles and are particularly crucial for movement of the molecules between the ER and Golgi apparatus. Proteins found within membrane contact sites include oxysterol-binding protein (OSBP) 1 and 2, a sterol-binding protein, which responds to levels of free intracellular cholesterol and PI4kα/β, phosphatidylinositol-4-kinase IIIα/β, which catalyzes production of PI4P in addition to regulating membrane fluidity. OSBP facilitates the trafficking of cholesterol from the ER to the Golgi and PI4P from the Golgi to ER,[461] ensuring a continuous flux of cholesterol toward the Golgi. During picornavirus infection, the membrane-bound 3A protein recruits both OSBP and PI4KIIIβ to the RO, creating contact points between the RO and either the Golgi (for enteroviruses and kobuviruses) or ER (for cardioviruses). Via activity of OSBP and PI4K, the lipid composition of the RO is unique, enriched for both PI4P and cholesterol.[493] 3A protein also interacts with ACBD3, acyl–coenzyme A–binding domain–containing 3 protein, aiding in the recruitment of PI4KIIIβ to the RO and to the surface of the Golgi apparatus. However, the need for ACBD3 to recruit PI4KIIIβ to the surface of the RO may be virus specific.[26,27,158,169,170,249,319,617,705] Furthermore, RO formation during hepatitis A virus and *Aphthovirus* infection is independent of PI4K and OSBP.[65,66,68,145,215,249,396,667] While modulation of the lipid composition of the RO may be necessary to ensure proper processing of the viral polypeptide,[24,25,199,459] the mechanisms by which the RO forms and how its lipid composition is achieved may reflect an evolutionary relationship among picornaviruses.

Although the ER is rearranged during picornavirus infection and vesicular trafficking proteins COPII and COPI, which mediate traffic between the ER and Golgi apparatus, associate with the replication structures of some picornaviruses such as echovirus and poliovirus and replication of these viruses is sensitive to BFA, a compound that inhibits GBF1 activity, the ER does not seem to be a source of membranes for enterovirus or kobuvirus RO generation as once thought.[120,215,307,613,693] The ER protein calnexin does not colocalize with 3A or other viral proteins needed for replication, COPII vesicle formation increases only early during infection, and the presence of inactive Sar1, an ER-resident GTPase known to function during ER to Golgi trafficking, has little effect on Coxsackievirus B3 replication. Moreover, neither poliovirus nor Coxsackievirus B3 replication was rescued by the production of catalytically inactive GBF1 in the presence of BFA, and production of poliovirus 3A and 2C led to membrane arrangement indistinguishable from that observed during infection in the presence of BFA. Replication of a poliovirus variant with amino acid changes in 2C and 3A was not altered in the presence BFA despite the requirement for GBF1. Furthermore, Aichi virus replication is BFA insensitive and neither protein is necessary for cardiovirus replication. Moreover, reorganization of the membrane network and vesicle formation during virus infection does not rely on the vesicle budding machinery.[65,412] These data further support the notion that the requirement for proteins of the secretory and lipid-modulating pathways is virus specific. GBF1 and Arf1 instead may be needed for PI4KIIIβ and/or OSBP recruitment or functions of the RO during RNA synthesis.

Membranes for picornavirus ROs may also come from the ER–Golgi intermediate compartment (ERGIC). These membranes are enriched for PI4P, phosphatidylcholine, and phosphatidylinositol-4,5-bisphosphate (PIP2). Generation of RO from this membrane source is dependent upon 3CD instead of 3A. The results of numerous biochemical experiments describing replication of several picornaviruses, including poliovirus and coxsackievirus, indicate dependence upon GBF1. In this model, 3CD recruits GBF1 as well as Arf1 and GTP to the surface of the RO. The complex may in part be anchored by 3AB. Formation of a complex consisting of 3CD-GBF1-Arf1 promotes PI4Kβ recruitment, activation, and *de novo* synthesis of PI4P in the absence of Golgi destruction. The 3CD-anchored complex allows 3AB to inhibit GBF1 or PI4Kβ such that PI4P is removed from the Golgi membrane, and all PI4P biosynthesis would depend upon 3CD. Variants of poliovirus resistant to the PIK93, a compound that inhibits PI4P biosynthesis, were found to have amino acid changes within the 3AB protein. The increase in PIP2 concentration may aid in transiting the single-membrane RO to double-membraned and the autophagosome by recruiting ATG14, lipidated LC3, and proteins of the early autophagy pathway.[41]

Independent of the source of the membranes used to construct the RO, there is a continuous need for new membranes and lipids including cholesterol and PI4P lipids.[249,307,317,617] Picornavirus infection stimulates *de novo* phospholipid synthesis, enhances uptake of long-chain fatty acids, and increases activity of acyl–CoA synthetase, elevating levels of intracellular free cholesterol and the rerouting of triglycerides to phosphatidylcholine synthesis.[261,317,494,723] Synthesis of 2BC protein stimulates clathrin-mediated endocytosis of cholesterol early during infection, while 2A^{pro}, independent of its catalytic activity, is required for the import of long-chain fatty acids.[494] In addition, picornavirus infection triggers the relocalization of many enzymes, including those that participate in *de novo* lipid synthesis such as CCTα, from the nucleus to the RO, and the hydrolysis of neutral fatty acids.[723]

In enterovirus-infected cells, membrane contacts with lipid droplets are also essential for the formation of the RO.[398] The viral proteins 2C and 2BC on the surface of lipid droplets and the RO interact, tethering the two together. Furthermore, 2C interacts with the host lipolysis machinery to provide lipids needed for RO formation. Disruption of the membrane contacts or inhibition of lipolysis blocks RO biogenesis and interferes with viral replication.

Despite being morphologically distinct from the double-membraned vesicles, which fill the cytosol late during virus infection, the early single-membrane vesicles, sites of the exponential phase of RNA replication, are the precursors for these later vesicles.[67] The transition from single- to double-membraned vesicles may reflect the production of sites of encapsidation and particle maturation.

Vesicular maturation occurs via a bending mechanism, during which the single-membrane structures increase in size, become irregular in shape, and collapse inward facilitating membrane pairing and promoting fusion of the ends of the single-membrane structure engulfing some cytoplasm[412] (Fig. 2.18). The resulting double-membraned vesicles, autophagosomes, are decorated with lipidated LC3 protein, an autophagy protein sensor, late endosomal protein LAMP-1, and lysosomal cathepsin but lack the adaptor SQSTM1/

p62. They have a deflated, crumpled exterior and an electron-dense interior.[137,324,392,472,493,637,678,679] Some virus-containing double-membraned vesicles will fuse with the lysosome prior to virus release. Fusion of the autophagosome with either the late endosome or lysosome is mediated by SNARE complexes composed of STX17, VAMP8, SNAP 29 on the surface of the autophagosome, SNAP 47 that associates with the late endosome,[305] and the adaptor PLEKHM1.[321,335] By merging with the lysosome, the interior of the autophagosome is acidified. The influx of protons stimulates cleavage of VP0, a maturation step for many picornaviruses, releasing VP4 into the interior of the capsid as well as destruction of the outer membrane of the autophagosome. This step facilitates acquisition of and release of an enveloped virion.[80,592] Inhibition of autophagosome formation impairs RNA replication and virus release, but blocking acidification only impairs the cleavage of VP0 into VP2 and VP4.[592] During Coxsackievirus B3 and enterovirus D68 infection, 3C^{pro} cleaves proteins that mediate autophagosome maturation and flux including SNAP 29, SNAP 47, SQSTM1, and PLEKHM1.[137,472] Poliovirus infection also prevents induction of the mTOR–ULK1/ULK2 canonical autophagy pathway (reviewed in Ref.[534]). Inhibition of autophagosome maturation may favor picornavirus replication by augmenting the amount of cytoplasmic membranes for RO assembly and preventing RNA and/or protein degradation, as the intracellular virus concentration has been shown to significantly increase but extracellular virus titers decrease by a similar amount. How and when these membranes would be incorporated into the RO remains unknown as recycling of membranes is not observed during virus replication and infection up-regulates *de novo* phospholipid synthesis for this purpose.[261,317,494,723]

Nonlytic release of hepatitis A virus occurs independent of autophagy. Similar to retrovirus release, which is dependent upon a stretch of 4 amino acids PPXY, P(S/T)AP, or (L)YPX$_{1/3}$L within the "L" domain of the Gag polypeptide to recruit the Endosomal Sorting Complexes Required for Transport (ESCRT) machinery via the adaptor ALIX, two "L"-like domains can be found within the hepatitis A virus VP2 protein.[187,313,587] These domains are on the surface of the particle and promote recruitment of ALIX, which in turn assembles the ESCRT complex. Together with ALIX–ESCRT, virus particles are trafficked to the plasma membrane and enveloped and bud into the extracellular environment.[187] The ROs of other enteroviruses such as poliovirus, Coxsackievirus B3, and rhinovirus have been found to be adjacent to sites of capsid synthesis. The colocalization of RNA synthesis with capsid formation suggests that RO may also be a platform for particle assembly, enabling for particles to be encapsidated in phosphatidylserine, a core component of RO membranes.[117]

Translation and Replication of the Same RNA Molecule

The genomic RNA of picornaviruses is not only mRNA but also the template for synthesis of negative-strand RNA. How does the viral polymerase, traveling in a $3'$ to $5'$ direction on the positive strand, avoid collisions with ribosomes translating in the opposite direction? It is thought that a mechanism exists to avoid the two processes occurring simultaneously. *In vitro* experiments using inhibitors of protein synthesis demonstrate that, when ribosomes are frozen on the viral RNA, replication of the RNA is inhibited. In contrast, when ribosomes are

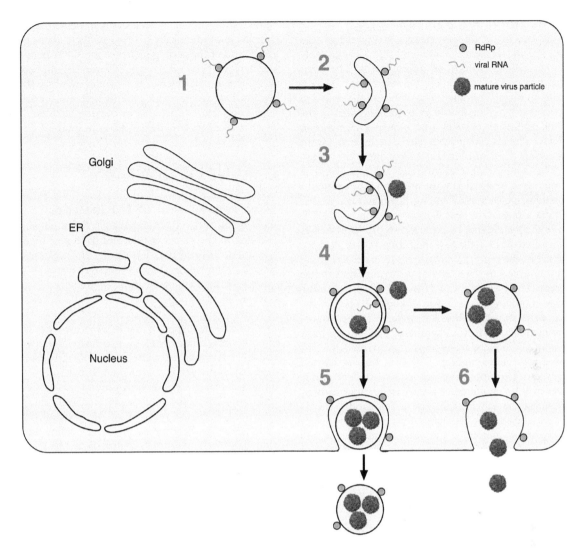

FIGURE 2.18 Schematic diagram of membrane rearrangement during picornavirus infection. *1.* Early during infection, virus-specific 3A protein is recruited to the surface of the cis-Golgi apparatus, bringing along 3D^{pol}, 3CD^{pro}, and the viral RNA. In addition, 3A stimulates relocalization of the Golgi proteins Arf1, GBF1, and PI4KIIIβ. *2.* As infection proceeds, an intertwined network of single-membrane tubular vesicles form, which are the predominant sites of virus replication. *3.* During the course of infection, the vesicles begin to collapse and invaginate inward, generating a double-membraned vesicle. *4.* As the ends fuse, cytosol is included within the lumen of the vesicle, giving it an electron density. Genome replication and particle assembly occur on the inside and outside of the vesicle. *5.* Some vesicles will become preautophagosomal and recruit the lipidated form of LC3. The autophagosomal vesicles predominate. As these vesicles traffic toward the plasma membrane, they become acidified stimulating virion maturation. At the plasma membrane, the virus-filled autophagosomal vesicles fuse with the membrane, releasing virus into the extracellular environment in a nonlytic manner. *6.* Other vesicles remain single-membrane that, when filled with viral progeny, lyse and release the virion into the external environment.

released from the viral RNA, its replication is increased.[49] These results suggest that replication and translation cannot occur on the same template simultaneously.

A mechanism for regulating viral RNA translation and replication involves cleavage of poly r(C)–binding protein. This protein functions in IRES-dependent translation by binding stem–loop IV[83,211] (Fig. 2.12) and in viral RNA synthesis by binding stem–loop I[213,529] (Fig. 2.17). Poly r(C)–binding protein is cleaved by viral 3C^{pro}; the cleaved protein can no longer stimulate IRES-dependent protein synthesis but is competent to participate in the initiation of viral RNA replication.[545] Another mechanism involves binding of 3CD to stem–loop I, which increases the affinity of poly r(C)–binding

protein for stem–loop I and decreases it for stem–loop IV.[212] Cleavage of PTB by 3C^{pro} also leads to reduced viral translation.[33] The consequence of these modifications is that viral IRES-dependent translation is down-regulated and ribosomes are cleared from the viral mRNA, allowing unimpeded transit of RNA polymerase.

Experimental evidence indicates that some ribosome and RNA polymerase collisions do occur. This conclusion is based on the isolation of a poliovirus variant whose genome contains an insertion of a 15 nucleotide sequence from 28S ribosomal RNA (rRNA).[115] Apparently, the RNA polymerase collided with a ribosome, copied 15 nucleotides of rRNA, and then returned to the viral RNA template.

Discrimination of Viral and Cellular RNA

The RNA-dependent RNA polymerases of picornaviruses are template-specific enzymes. Poliovirus 3D^{pol} copies only viral RNA, not cellular mRNA, in infected cells. The purified enzyme, however, will copy any polyadenylated RNA if provided with an oligo(U) primer. This observation has led to the suggestion that template specificity probably resides in the interaction of replication proteins with sequence elements in the viral RNA. The cis-acting RNA elements located within the coding region of picornaviruses, which direct the uridylylation of VPg, are binding sites for 3CD^{pro} (Fig. 2.17). The 3′-noncoding region of the viral positive-strand RNA contains an RNA pseudoknot conserved among picornaviruses that is believed to play a role in the specificity of copying by 3D^{pol}.[328] Disruption of the pseudoknot by mutagenesis produces viruses that have impaired RNA synthesis, indicating the importance of the structure in the synthesis of negative-strand RNA. 3D^{pol} or 3CD^{pro} cannot bind to the 3′ end of poliovirus RNA unless 3AB is present. The interaction of 3AB–3D^{pol} may determine the specificity of binding to the 3′ pseudoknot.

Despite experimental results that underscore the importance of the pseudoknot in RNA synthesis, polioviruses from which the entire 3′-noncoding region of the viral RNA has been removed are able to replicate.[97,685] This finding has led to the suggestion that template specificity imparted by terminal structures of RNA might be of greater importance early in infection. During the initiation phases of replication, the 3′ pseudoknot structure might facilitate template selection when few viral polymerase molecules are available and membrane association has not yet provided high concentrations of replication components. Later, determinants of template selection by the polymerase might include the membrane association of the RNA polymerase. Template specificity may also be conferred by the position of the 3D^{pol} gene at the very 3′ end of the viral RNA; translation places the polymerase at the 3′ end of the genome, ready for initiation.

A cloverleaf-like structure that forms in the 5′-noncoding region also plays an important role in template specificity (Fig. 2.17). The finding that a mutation in a cloverleaf structure in the 5′-noncoding region that affects RNA synthesis could be complemented by a suppressor mutation in 3C^{pro} led to the suggestion that 3C^{pro} might bind the cloverleaf and play a role in viral RNA replication.[19] It was subsequently found that 3CD^{pro} binds the cloverleaf structure in the positive strand, together with a cellular protein, now known to be poly r(C)–binding protein, that is required for complex formation.[17,18,529] The RNA-binding domain of 3CD^{pro} is contained within the 3C^{pro} portion of the protein, on the opposite face of the molecule from the site involved in proteolysis. Mutations within this domain abolish complex formation and RNA replication without affecting viral protein processing. 3CD^{pro}, therefore, plays an important role in viral RNA synthesis by participating in formation of a ribonucleoprotein complex at the 5′ end of the positive-strand RNA. A structural model of rhinovirus 3C^{pro} bound to stem–loop I shows that RNA binding induces changes in the proteinase active site, although their effect on catalytic activity is not known.[126] A role for these interactions in viral RNA replication is suggested in the model in Figure 2.17.

While the tertiary structures of the cre, IRES, and 3′-UTR of the picornavirus RNA are the best characterized and functionally understood, structural features can be found throughout the open reading frame. Several of these elements have been predicted bioinformatically.[755] Two of these elements are within the 3′ end of the coding sequence for 3D^{pol}. Both elements are needed for efficient RNA replication as determined by recoding and reporter experiments.[102,649] Mutations of the RNA sequence within these elements are able to suppress alterations of 3C^{pro} suggesting that a functional interaction between the RNA and 3C^{pro} is necessary for efficient RNA replication.[102]

ORIGINS OF DIVERSITY

Misincorporation of Nucleotides

As with all other RNA-dependent RNA polymerases, those encoded in picornavirus genomes have very high error rates, because of misincorporation during chain elongation and the lack of proofreading ability in these enzymes. With error frequencies as high as one misincorporation per 10^3 to 10^4 nucleotides, RNA virus populations exist as quasispecies or mixtures of many different genome sequences.[166]

It has been suggested that RNA viruses exist on the threshold of error catastrophe, to maximize diversity and adaptability.[166] A moderate increase in error frequency would be expected to destroy the virus population. In one study, it was estimated that each poliovirus genome synthesized after multiple rounds of replication in an infected cell contains two point mutations.[144] In the presence of the antiviral drug ribavirin, each poliovirus genome contained 15 point mutations, and viral yields were 0.00001% of untreated cells. Similar observations have been made with FMDV[258] and Coxsackievirus B3.[244] These findings demonstrate that RNA viruses do exist at the error threshold and that ribavirin is an RNA virus mutagen that inhibits virus replication by increasing the RNA polymerase error rate beyond the threshold.

High RNA virus error rates are believed to be necessary to enable persistence of the virus population under selective pressure. Consequently, viruses with less error-prone RNA polymerases should be at a competitive disadvantage in complex environments such as an infected animal. To test this hypothesis, a poliovirus mutant resistant to the antiviral effects of ribavirin was isolated.[553,722] Resistance to ribavirin was conferred by a single amino acid change, G64S, in 3D^{pol} that reduces errors during replication. The high-fidelity mutant virus replicated and spread poorly in mice and was unable to compete with a low-fidelity virus. The results indicate that mutations, and the formation of a diverse quasispecies, benefit viral populations, particularly in an infected animal. Analysis of a ribavirin-resistant mutant of FMDV reveals no restriction of the viral quasispecies.[23] This apparent paradox is explained by the observation that the RNA polymerase mutation increased the frequency of misincorporation of natural nucleotides while decreasing the frequency of the incorporation of ribavirin.

Recombination

Recombination, the exchange of nucleotide sequences among different RNA molecules, was first discovered in cells infected with poliovirus and was subsequently found to occur during infection with other positive-strand RNA viruses. It can occur by two different mechanisms: nonreplicative, the nonhomologous end joining of two different RNA molecules, or replicative, switching of templates. Nonreplicative recombination is highly inefficient and thought to minimally influence virus evolution.

Replicative recombination mainly occurs between nucleotide sequences of the two parental genome RNA strands that have a high percentage of nucleotide identity. This mechanism of RNA recombination is coupled with the process of genome RNA replication: it occurs by template switching during negative-strand synthesis, as first demonstrated in poliovirus-infected cells[368] and subsequently in cell-free extracts.[174,677] The RNA polymerase first copies the 3′ end of one parental positive strand, then switches templates, and continues synthesis at the corresponding position on a second parental positive strand. Template switching in poliovirus-infected cells occurs predominantly during negative-strand synthesis because the concentration of positive-strand acceptors for template switching is 30 to 70 times higher than that of negative-strand acceptors. A prediction of the replicative mechanism is that recombination frequencies should be lower between different poliovirus serotypes, a prediction that has been verified experimentally. For example, recombination between poliovirus types 1 and 2 occurs about 100 times less frequently than among type 1 polioviruses (the poliovirus serotypes differ by about 15% in their nucleotide sequences).[366] This mechanism of genetic recombination is polymerase dependent and biphasic and drives virus evolution. It reflects the low fidelity of an RNA-dependent RNA polymerase as well as the absence of proofreading and repair enzymes.

Replicative recombination can be assessed experimentally in cell culture by infecting with viruses whose genomes contain with two different known lethal mutations[304,358,425] (Fig. 2.19). All progeny viruses will lack both mutations. The resolved x-ray crystal structure of elongating poliovirus 3D[pol] identified amino acids within the thumb domain that directly interact with the RNA duplex. Alteration of these residues to alanine identified Leu 420 as critical for replicative recombination. The alanine substitution dramatically diminished genomic recombination by reducing the stability of 3D[pol] elongation complexes without substantially affecting fidelity.[358]

The frequency of replicative recombination, which is calculated by dividing the yield of recombinant virus by the sum of the yields of parental viruses, can be relatively high. In one study of poliovirus and FMDV, the genomic recombination frequency was 0.9%, leading to the estimation that 10% to 20% of the viral genomes recombine in one growth cycle. When poliovirus recombination is studied by quantitative polymerase chain reaction, obviating the necessity to select for viable viruses, the recombination frequency for marker loci 600 nucleotides apart is 2×10^{-3}, similar to estimates obtained using selectable markers.[331] RNA recombination also occurs in natural infections. For example, intertypic recombinants among the three serotypes of Sabin poliovirus vaccine strains are readily isolated from the intestines of vaccinees; some recombinants contain sequences from all three serotypes.[104] The significance of these recombinants is unknown, but it has been suggested that such viruses are selected for their improved ability to replicate in the human alimentary tract compared with the parental viruses. However, results from studies in which PVR transgenic mice were infected with a variant of poliovirus sensitive to the innate immune response demonstrated the efficiency by which replicative recombination influences virus evolution and ultimately pathogenesis.[760] Recombination in nature has also been demonstrated among nonpolio enteroviruses[639] (reviewed in Ref.[427]).

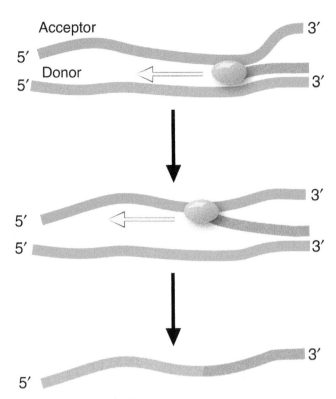

FIGURE 2.19 Schematic diagram of RNA recombination in picornavirus-infected cells by template switching or copy choice. Two parental genomes, the acceptor and donor, are shown. The RNA polymerase (*blue*) is shown copying the 3′ end of donor RNA and switching to the acceptor genome (*middle*). As a result of this template switch, the recombinant RNA shown is formed (*bottom*).

Codon Usage

Redundancy of the genetic code allows for most amino acids to be specified by multiple codons. Not all codons are used at the same frequency, and the regularity at which they are used is cell and virus specific. The under- or overrepresentation of a codon suggests that there is a bias for how an amino acid is encoded. Most vertebrate and plant RNA viruses have low CpG and UpA dinucleotide frequencies, as do the mRNAs of their host cells. For RNA viruses such as picornaviruses, this bias may influence not only translation rates but stability of critical structures that modulate RNA metabolism, replication, genome packaging, and particle stability.

When the frequency of CpG and UpA dinucleotides in the viral genome is increased by mutagenesis, viral replication is impaired. An example is echovirus 7: engineering of viruses with increased frequencies of CpG and UpA in an approximately 1-kb region of the genome reduced viral replication efficiency.[30] A similar effect is observed for human immunodeficiency virus type 1; the replication deficiency is reversed by knockout of the cell gene encoding the zinc-finger antiviral protein, ZAP.[674] The implication is that ZAP identifies non–self RNA by its higher CpG composition, possibly targeting it for degradation. Whether ZAP is involved in restricting replication of echovirus 7 or other picornaviruses that have been modified to have higher CpG/UpA dinucleotides remains to be determined.

Alteration of codon pair frequencies of capsid-coding regions has been used to produce polioviruses with attenuated pathogenicity. Such attenuated viruses might be safe vaccine candidates as the hundreds of changes introduced into the viral genome are not likely to revert.[129] It has been suggested that alterations of codon pair frequency have the unintended consequence of increasing CpG and UpA frequencies, which would also attenuate viral replication.[700]

The generation of polioviruses with altered codon pair frequencies has made it possible to study how codon usage affects mutational robustness and evolutionary capacity.[399] A comparison of wild-type poliovirus with a variant harboring hundreds of synonymous mutations in the capsid-coding region revealed that changing the position of a virus in sequence space affects its mutant spectrum, evolutionary trajectory, and virulence. Similar experiments with other viruses have led to the principle that the sequence space occupied by a virus population is important for its ability to adapt to new environments.

ASSEMBLY OF VIRUS PARTICLES

Morphogenesis of picornaviruses has been studied extensively because the 60-subunit capsid is relatively simple, and the assembly intermediates can be readily detected in infected cells (Fig. 2.20). During the synthesis of the P1 protein, the capsid protein precursor, the central β-barrel domains form, and intramolecular interactions among the surfaces of these domains lead to formation of the structural units. Once P1 is released from the P2 protein, the VP0–VP3 and VP3–VP1 bonds are cleaved by proteinase 3CD^{pro}. These cleavage sites are located in flexible regions between the β-barrels; considerable movement of the amino termini and carboxyl termini occurs after cleavage, but the contacts between β-barrels are not disturbed.[303] In the mature capsid, the carboxyl termini of VP1, VP2, and VP3 are on the outer surface of the capsid, whereas the amino termini are on the interior, where they participate in an extensive network of interactions among protomers. This process produces the first assembly intermediate in the poliovirus pathway, the 5S protomer, the immature structural unit consisting of one copy each of VP0, VP3, and VP1.

Five protomers then assemble to form a pentamer, which sediments at 14S. Based upon *in vitro* experiments, it was thought that the protomers self-assembled into pentamers and no cell proteins function during this process; however, the addition of L-buthionine sulfoximine, a compound that selectively inhibits glutathione synthesis, significantly decreases the production of infectious rhinovirus, poliovirus, coxsackievirus, and other enterovirus C viruses.[431,642,682] The observed replication impairment can be overcome with the addition of glutathione. The decrease in the formation of mature virus particles was found to be independent of protein synthesis and RNA replication, suggesting that glutathione may function during particle assembly. Glutathione, a small non–protein thiol reducing agent found within the cell, helps maintain the redox state of the cell by either functioning as a cofactor for reactions catalyzed by glutathione peroxidases and glutathione S-transferases or directly interacting with cysteine residues.[457,569] Maintenance of the proper oxidative state of the protomers is necessary for their structure, conformation, and ability to self-assemble into pentamers. Viruses that are resistant to the depletion of glutathione or the presence of L-buthionine sulfoximine were found to have amino acid substitutions in both VP1 and

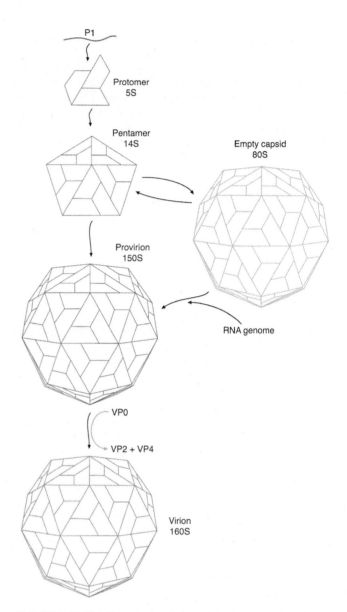

FIGURE 2.20 Morphogenesis of picornaviruses. The capsid protein precursor, P1, folds nascently, is cleaved from P2, and then is further cleaved to VP0 + VP3 + VP1 by 3CD^{pro}. Protomers (5S) self-assemble into 14S pentamers, and pentamers assemble into 80S empty capsids. Glutathione is necessary for assembly of 14S pentamers into 150S provirions. In one model of encapsidation, RNA is threaded into the empty capsid, producing a 150S provirion in which VP0 is uncleaved. Another possibility is that pentamers assemble around the RNA genome and that empty capsids are storage depots for pentamers. Cleavage of VP0 is the final morphogenetic step that produces the infectious 160S virion. The proteinase responsible for the cleavage of VP0 is unknown.

VP3, along surfaces at the protomer interface. These variants are also resistant to heat inactivation, suggesting that glutathione may function to stabilize protomer–protomer and/or pentamer–pentamer interactions necessary for assembly of the 14S pentamer and production of infectious virus.[431,682]

Cleavage of P1 is required for assembly of the pentamer.[521] This conclusion is supported by examination of the virion structure. The β-cylinder at the fivefold axis of symmetry is formed from the N-termini of neighboring VP3 molecules; the cylinder is surrounded by a bundle composed of the amino termini of VP0 and VP1. The cell chaperone proteins Hsp 70, Hsp 90, and p23 are required for both precursor processing and protomer and pentamer assembly of many picornaviruses including cardioviruses, enteroviruses, and FMDV; however, no chaperone protein is thought to be required for cleavage of the P1 region of the hepatitis A virus polyprotein. Hsp 90 and p23 interact with unprocessed P1, protecting the polypeptide from misfolding and proteasomal degradation. Pharmacologic inhibition of Hsp 90 reduces the assembly of infectious particles by preventing the first cleavage event necessary for protomer formation between P1-2A and assembly of pentamer subunits. Virus variants resistant to inhibitors of Hsp 90 have never been identified, suggesting that complexity of capsid folding precludes the emergence of alternate folding pathways.[217,218,378,408,433,491,499,600,699,717,735] A second interpretation of the data is that Hsp 90 can act as a chaperone at both the protein and RNA levels, to overcome the evolutionary constraints imposed by protein stability, aggregation, and rate of synthesis.[216]

Pentamers are structurally important intermediates in the assembly of all picornaviruses.[86,603] They can self-assemble *in vitro* or *in vivo* into 80S empty capsids (Fig. 2.20). The structure of this particle reveals differences in the network formed by the N-terminal extensions of the capsid proteins on the inner surface of the shell, compared with the native virion.[51] In empty capsids, VP4 and the entire N-terminal extensions of VP1 and VP2 are disordered, and many stabilizing interactions that are present in the mature virion are not present. The final morphogenetic step involves cleavage of most of the VP0 molecules to VP4 + VP2. The proteinase that carries out this final maturation cleavage has not been identified. The VP0 scissile bond is located on the interior of empty capsids and mature virions and is inaccessible to viral or cellular proteinases. The presence of a conserved serine in VP2 near one of the cleaved termini led to a model that cleavage occurs by a novel autocatalytic serine protease-like mechanism in which basic viral RNA groups serve as proton abstracters during the cleavage reaction.[28] Replacement of serine 10, however, does not impair VP0 cleavage.[280] In another hypothesis, a conserved histidine in VP2 is involved in catalysis, together with the viral RNA.[51,150] Substitution of this histidine with different amino acids lead to lack of infectivity or highly unstable particles, supporting the involvement of VP2 histidine 195 in mediating VP0 cleavage during assembly.[296] Cleavage of VP0 establishes the ordered N-terminal network, an interlocking seven-stranded β-sheet formed by residues from adjacent pentamers. This network results in an increase in particle stability and the acquisition of infectivity.

During its synthesis, the P1 capsid protein precursor is linked to myristic acid at the amino-terminal glycine residue of VP4 that is exposed after removal of the initiation Met residue.[125] The myristate groups, which form part of a network of interactions between subunits that form when protomers assemble into pentamers, cluster around the fivefold axis of symmetry and stabilize the β-cylinder that is made by the amino termini of five copies of VP3. The results of mutagenesis indicate that the myristate group plays a role in stabilizing pentamers and, therefore, virions.[20,438–440,481]

How the RNA genome is encapsidated remains an unsolved problem. Packaging motor proteins encapsidated the genomes of many bacteriophages into preassembled procapsids. While no picornavirus protein is known to have packaging motor activity, one model of assembly could include the introduction of newly synthesized viral RNA into these partially assembled particles to form the provirion,[327] in which the capsid protein VP0 remains uncleaved. This assembly model would seemingly require an opening in the empty capsid through which the RNA can enter. Examination of the high-resolution x-ray crystallographic structure of these particles does not provide evidence for such an opening.[51] This finding does not exclude this morphogenetic pathway because the pore might be dynamic and not observed in the crystals. In an alternative morphogenesis pathway, 14S pentamers assemble with virion RNA to form provirions. In this model, for which there is some experimental support,[511] the empty capsids found in infected cells serve as storage depots for 14S pentamers.

The RNA genomes of plant viruses are encapsidated via protein–protein and RNA–protein interactions.[111,198] This mechanism does not appear to be the means by which picornaviruses acquire their genomes.[334] The picornavirus encapsidation process is highly specific with only VPg-conjugated positive-strand RNA, and not viral mRNA, negative-strand viral RNA, or any cellular RNA incorporated into the virion.[507,509] Yet, VPg is probably not an encapsidation signal because VPg-containing negative-strand RNA is not packaged despite the observation that genomic RNA lacking VPg is never encapsidated.[507,510] No packaging signal, structure, or sequence has been identified within the picornavirus genome. The coupling of encapsidation to viral RNA synthesis may explain the selective packaging of viral positive-strand RNA. In infected cells, newly synthesized RNA is packaged into virions within 5 minutes, whereas incorporation of capsid proteins in virions requires at least 20 minutes.[40] The pool of viral RNA available for packaging, therefore, is small, and the pool of capsid proteins is large. If capsid formation is inhibited with *p*-fluorophenylalanine, the accumulated RNA cannot be packaged after removal of the inhibitor.[273] These results suggest that packaging of the viral genome is linked to RNA synthesis and would explain why only RNA containing VPg are encapsidated. This conclusion is questioned by findings showing that inhibition of virion assembly by hydantoin, which targets the 2C protein, does not affect genome replication. Furthermore, when hydantoin is removed from infected cells after RNA synthesis is complete, and in the presence of an inhibitor of replication, normal levels of virions are produced.[515] Yet, a temperature-sensitive alteration in 2C protein allows for uncoating to occur at low temperature.[407] These results suggest that RNA encapsidation is dependent upon interactions between 2C protein and VP1 and VP3.[419,734,738] For Aichi virus, the L protein, instead of 2C protein, participates in RNA encapsidation. Removal of the C-terminal 50 amino acids of L protein of Aichi virus prevents the transition of empty capsids to mature virions.[619]

Cryo-EM reconstruction of the Ljungan virus particle revealed that the RNA genome maintains an ordered structure of within the virion: 15 nucleotides associating with the N-terminus of VP3 near the fivefold axes. This observation suggests that the Ljungan genome may be encapsidated via a mechanism similar to that observed for insect picorna-like viruses in which a capsid protein functions as an RNA chaperone. Compaction of the genome occurs via electrostatic interactions between short regions of the RNA, in a sequence-independent manner, and 20 highly basic residues found at

N-termini of VP3 that line the interior surface. A condensed structure of nucleic acid with icosahedral symmetry results. This model is supported by the observation that empty capsids are not found during parechovirus infection. A similar model has been proposed for the encapsidation of the hepatitis A virus genome but is contrary to the model based upon interaction between structural and nonstructural proteins in the RNA replication complex as proposed for poliovirus and the identification of a packaging signal in the Aichi virus genome.[419,620] Experimental data in which poliovirus was recoded to enhance the number of underrepresented synonymous codon pairs suggest that acquisition of the genome and assembly may occur via a two-step assembly mechanism that combines the ideas above: (a) interaction between capsid protein and the replication structure, including proteins and newly synthesized genomes and (b) a coordinate condensing of the genome resulting in an array of hairpin structures to promote RNA–protein interactions to complete the assembly and promote stability of the particle.[648]

EFFECTS OF VIRAL REPRODUCTION ON THE HOST CELL

Inhibition of 5′ End–Dependent mRNA Translation

In cultured mammalian cells, poliovirus infection results in inhibition of cellular protein synthesis. By 2 hours after infection, polyribosomes are disrupted, and translation of nearly all cellular mRNA stops and is replaced by viral mRNA translation (Fig. 2.21). Poliovirus mRNA, but not capped mRNA, can be translated in extracts from infected cells. In such extracts, the eIF4GI/eIF4GII component of the translation initiation complex eIF4F has been cleaved.[185,605,692] Cleavage of eIF4G separates the N-terminal eIF4E–binding domain of eIF4G (p100) from the C-terminal fragment (Fig. 2.22). The assumption that the C-terminal fragment of eIF4G cannot support the translation of capped mRNA has been proven incorrect.[11] It is now thought that picornavirus-induced translational inhibition is not solely due to the inability of p100 to support capped mRNA translation but to the viral RNA outcompeting host cell mRNA for the limiting concentration of p100. Optimal function of the IRES does require the C-terminal fragment of eIF4G, which, as discussed previously, is necessary to anchor 40S ribosomal subunits to the IRES. Although both eIF4GI and eIF4GII are cleaved in poliovirus- and rhinovirus-infected cells, the kinetics of shutoff of host translation correlates with cleavage of eIF4GII and not eIF4GI.[245,671]

Both forms of eIF4G are cleaved by protease 2A[pro] of poliovirus and rhinovirus.[245,671] *In vitro* cleavage of eIF4G by purified 2A[pro] of rhinovirus is inefficient unless eIF4G is bound to eIF4E.[269] This finding indicates that eIF4G is cleaved not as an individual polypeptide but rather as part of the eIF4F complex. Binding of eIF4E to eIF4G may induce conformational changes in eIF4G that make it a more efficient substrate for the protease. Poliovirus 2A[pro] efficiently cleaves eIF4GI, but not eIF4GII, consistent with the differential cleavage of these proteins during virus infection.[245] The L[pro] protein cleaves eIF4GI in cells infected with FMDV. The cleavage sites in eIF4GI for the two proteinases are different: L[pro] cleaves between Gly-479 and Arg-480, whereas 2A[pro] cleaves between Arg-486 and Gly-487.[367,391]

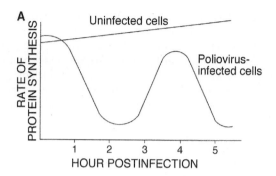

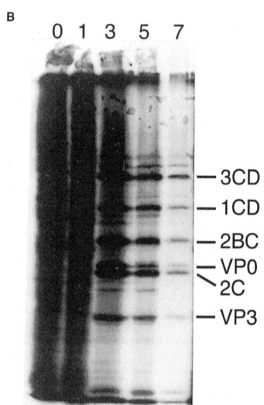

FIGURE 2.21 Inhibition of cellular translation in cells infected with poliovirus. A: Protein synthesis in poliovirus-infected and uninfected cells at different times after infection. Poliovirus infection results in inhibition of host cell translation beginning about 1 hour after infection. The increase in translation beginning 3 hours after infection is caused by the synthesis of viral proteins. **B:** Polyacrylamide gel showing inhibition of cellular translation. At different times after infection (top of each lane), cells were incubated with ^{35}S-methionine for 15 minutes; the cell extracts were then fractionated on an SDS-polyacrylamide gel. By 5 hours after infection, host translation is markedly inhibited and replaced by the synthesis of viral proteins, identified at the right.

Modulation of eIF4F Activity

Three related low molecular weight cell proteins, 4E-BP1, 4E-BP2, and 4E-BP3, bind to eIF4E and inhibit translation by 5′-end–dependent scanning, but not by internal ribosome entry (Fig. 2.22).[539] 4E-BP1 is identical to a protein called PHAS-I (phosphorylated heat- and acid-stable protein regulated by insulin), which was previously known to be an important phosphorylation substrate in cells treated with insulin and

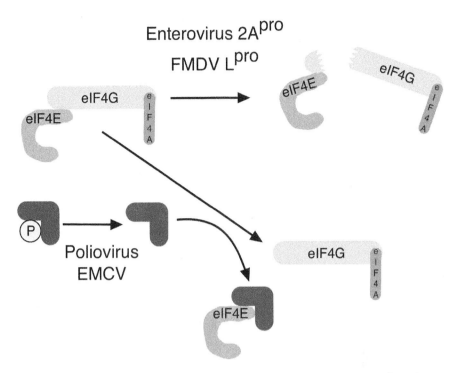

FIGURE 2.22 Two mechanisms for regulating eIF4F activity in picornavirus-infected cells. The proteins 4E-BP1 and 4E-BP1 bind eIF4E and prevent it from interacting with eIF4G. 4E-BP1 binds eIF4E when it is dephosphorylated, an event that occurs in cells infected with poliovirus and EMCV. Cleavage of eIF4G takes place in cells infected with poliovirus, rhinovirus, and foot-and-mouth disease virus, among others. Cleavage reduces the efficiency of translation of capped messenger RNA (mRNA). 5′ End–dependent initiation is inhibited because capped mRNA cannot compete with viral mRNA for the translation machinery.

growth factors.[414] Phosphorylation of 4E-BP1 *in vitro* blocks its association with eIF4E. Binding of either 4E-BP1 or 4E-BP2 to eIF4E does not prevent it from interacting with the 5′ cap but does inhibit binding to eIF4G. Consequently, active eIF4F is not formed. eIF4G and the 4E-BP have a common sequence motif that binds eIF4E. Treatment of cells with hormones and growth factors leads to the phosphorylation of 4E-BP1 and its release from eIF4E. Those mRNAs with extensive secondary structure in the 5′-noncoding region, which are translated poorly, are preferentially sensitive to the phosphorylation state of 4E-BP1. As expected, translation by internal ribosome binding is not affected when 4E-BP1 is dephosphorylated. Binding of extracellular ligands leads to phosphorylation of 4E-BP through a signaling pathway that includes the mammalian target of rapamycin.[756]

Infection with several picornaviruses causes alteration of the phosphorylation state of 4E-BP1 and 4E-BP2 (Fig. 2.22). Infection of cells with EMCV causes inhibition of cellular translation, but in contrast to the shutoff that occurs in poliovirus-infected cells, shutoff of cellular protein synthesis occurs late in infection and is not mediated by cleavage of eIF4G. Infection with EMCV induces dephosphorylation of 4E-BP1, which then binds eIF4E to prevent it from forming eIF4F.[179] Translation of cellular mRNA is inhibited, but that of the viral RNA is not because it contains an IRES. Dephosphorylation of 4E-BP1 also occurs late in cells infected with poliovirus, but this event does not coincide with inhibition of cellular translation, which occurs earlier in infection.[225] Inhibition of translation by dephosphorylation of 4E-BP1 also influences the ability

of the cell to productively combat viral infection by reducing production of type I IFN.[130]

Efficient translation initiation is hypothesized to be dependent upon formation of a closed loop of mRNA. Circularization of the RNA is mediated by the interaction of eIF4G bound at 5′ end of the RNA and poly(A)–binding protein bound to the poly(A) tail at the 3′ end. The initial synthesis of picornavirus-specific proteins is stimulated by the interaction of eIF4G with poly(A)–binding protein.[463,672] Like eIF4G, poly(A)–binding protein is cleaved during enterovirus infection by viral proteinases 2A^pro and 3C^pro; however, the kinetics of poly(A)–binding protein cleavage are slower than those of eIF4G.[337] Cleavage of poly(A)–binding protein is necessary but not sufficient for efficient inhibition of cellular translation; instead, cleavage of this protein is believed to participate in the switch from RNA translation to replication (see *Translation and replication of the same RNA molecule*).[87] The effect of poly(A)–binding protein cleavage during this switch is controversial, as depletion of poly(A)–binding protein from cell lysates did not reduce virus production.[670] The cellular polyadenylation factor CstF-64 is cleaved by enterovirus 71 3C^pro proteinase, impairing the addition of poly(A) to host cell mRNAs.[748]

Formation of the eIF4F complex can also be regulated by miRNAs. During enterovirus infection, transcription of miR-141 is enhanced. Because multiple binding sites for this miRNA are found within the 3′-noncoding region of eIF4E mRNA, levels of eIF4E and consequently the eIF4F complex are reduced, and cellular protein synthesis is impaired.[299] Viral translation is unaffected as it does not require eIF4E.

The production of double-stranded RNA during infection with many viruses leads to activation of PKR, phosphorylation of eIF2α, and inhibition of translation. It occurs very late in the replication cycle of poliovirus.[519] Like most cellular mRNAs, the polyprotein begins with a methionine encoded by an AUG codon, and early in infection, initiation of protein synthesis requires the ternary complex of eIF2-GTP-met-tRNA$_i$. Late in infection, phosphorylation of serine 52 of the alpha subunit of eIF2 prevents the recycling of the ternary complex after initiation. However, poliovirus-specific protein synthesis continues throughout infection. It is thought that initiation of translation late during infection occurs independently of eIF2.[747,753] The exact mechanism for this mode of initiation is not well understood but is thought to be dependent upon the generation of a fragment of eIF5 that functions in a similar manner as eIF2 in recruiting the initiating tRNA to the small 40S ribosomal subunit while bound to the mRNA.[753] The proteolytic activity of 2A^{pro} is believed to be required to enable poliovirus mRNA translation in the absence of eIF2.[584]

Stress-Associated RNA Granules

Sequestering of mRNA away from the translation apparatus in processing (P) bodies and stress granules is another mechanism by which cellular mRNA translation can be impaired.[16] P bodies and stress granules are two nonmembranous cytoplasmic aggregates composed of RNA and protein, including many proteins involved in mRNA translation. These granules are believed to form when translation is inhibited in the presence of intracellular and extracellular stresses, including viral infection. When stress conditions are alleviated, the mRNAs found in these aggregates can either be deadenylated and degraded or returned to the pool of actively translated RNAs.

Stress granules are thought to be nucleated upon two cellular proteins, T-cell–restricted intracellular antigen-1 (TIA-1) and the RasGAP SH3 domain–binding protein 1 (G3BP). Reduction of either protein impairs formation of stress granules, and overproduction of either component stimulates formation of these aggregates.[224,690] Stalled translation complexes consisting of mRNA, eIF4E, eIF4G, eIF4A, eIF3, poly(A)–binding protein, and phosphorylated eIF2α are found within these granules. The presence of phosphorylated eIF2α is a hallmark of stress granules. Formation of stress granules is enhanced during early picornavirus infection and correlates with the inhibition of cellular translation but is independent of eIF2α phosphorylation. Late in infection, the viral proteinase 3C^{pro} cleaves RasGAP SH3 domain–binding protein 1la, disassembling stress granules, an event required for efficient viral replication. The presence of an altered form of cleaved RasGAP SH3 domain–binding protein 1^{Q326E} prevents the disassembly of stress granules and impairs viral replication.[751] Instead, a noncanonical form of stress granules remains, an aggregate containing only TIA-1.[562,752] The opposite is observed during infection with members of the *Discistroviridae*: cricket paralysis virus infection prohibits stress granule formation as defined by foci of the *Drosophila* homologs of TIA-1 and RasGAP SH3 domain–binding protein 1, Rox8 and Rin. Addition of potent inducers of stress granules such as arsenite and pateamine A to the culture medium is unable to overcome viral inhibition.[361]

Processing (P-) bodies are a second type of non–membrane-bound aggregate found in the cytoplasm. These aggregates, which are the sites of RNA deadenylation and mRNA repression, are composed of proteins such as the decapping enzymes Dcp1a and Dcp2 and proteins that mediate mRNA deadenylation including Pan3, the CCR4/Not 1 complex, Xrn-1, a 5′-3′ RNA exonuclease, and the DEAD-box helicase p54/Rck. In uninfected cells, P-bodies are the consequence of micro-RNA (miRNA)–mediated repression.[186] Ultrastructural analysis of these granules suggests that there is an anchoring core composed of proteins required for repression with proteins mediating decay on the periphery. The protein that bridges between the two regions of the aggregate is p54/Rck.[138] P-bodies are found in proximity to both the ribosome and mitochondria. Although cellular mRNA translation is inhibited during picornavirus infection, the RNA is not degraded, possibly due to inhibition of P-body formation. The 3C^{pro} proteinase of poliovirus cleaves several P-body components including Xrn1, Dcp1a, and Pan 3, disrupting P-body formation.[172]

Inhibition of Cellular RNA Synthesis

Infection of cells with picornaviruses leads to a rapid inhibition of host cell RNA synthesis catalyzed by all three classes of DNA-dependent RNA polymerase. RNA polymerases I, II, and III from poliovirus-infected cells are enzymatically active, suggesting that accessory proteins may be the target of transcriptional inhibition. Studies of *in vitro* systems have demonstrated the inhibition of specific transcription factors required by each of the three RNA polymerases. The RNA polymerase factor TFIID, which is a multiprotein complex, is inactivated in poliovirus-infected cells.[374] This inactivation appears to be caused, at least in part, by cleavage of a subunit of TFIID, the TATA-binding protein, by protease 3C^{pro}.[764] A pol III DNA–binding transcription factor, TFIIC, is also cleaved and inactivated by 3C^{pro}.[127] The target of 3C^{pro} is a subunit of TFIIIC, which contacts the pol III promoter. The pol I transcription factors SL-1 (selectivity factor) and UBF (upstream binding factor) are inactivated in poliovirus-infected cells by 3C^{pro}, resulting in inhibition of pol I transcription.[42,610]

Because poliovirus replication occurs in the cytoplasm, cleavage of RNA polymerase transcription factors requires that the viral proteinase 3C^{pro} enters the nucleus. 3C^{pro} lacks a nuclear localization signal (NLS), but the precursor 3CD^{pro} enters the nucleus by virtue of an NLS in protein 3D^{pol}. Transcription factors in the nucleus are then cleaved by either 3CD^{pro} or 3C^{pro} that is released by autocatalysis.[633] Rhinovirus 16 3CD^{pro} has also been shown to enter the nucleus.[15]

Inhibition of Nucleocytoplasmic Trafficking

Infection of cells with picornaviruses leads to the disruption of nucleocytoplasmic trafficking. One mechanism by which this is achieved is the proteolysis of nucleoporins, proteins that constitute the nuclear pore complex. In cells infected with poliovirus, two protein components of the nuclear pore complex are cleaved, Nup153 and Nup62.[264,265] The proteinase responsible for cleavage of Nup62 in rhinovirus-infected cells is 2A^{pro}.[528] This cleavage results in the cytoplasmic accumulation of nuclear proteins, some of which, such as La protein[638] and SRp20,[194] are required for viral mRNA translation. The rates and processing profiles of Nups by 2A^{pro} proteinases of different rhinoviruses vary widely.[744] The rhinovirus 3C^{pro} and its precursor 3CD^{pro} are imported into the nucleus, leading to the degradation of nuclear pore components.[220]

Another mechanism of disruption of nucleocytoplasmic trafficking involves the L protein of cardioviruses (the 2A protein of these viruses is not a proteinase). The L protein binds directly to the Ran-GTPase, a key regulator of nucleocytoplasmic transport.[570] Infection also leads to phosphorylation of nucleoporins Nup62, Nup153, and Nup214.[572] Staurosporine, a broad-spectrum protein kinase inhibitor, and ERK and p38 MAP kinase inhibitors block Nup phosphorylation and restore normal nuclear trafficking.[571] Inhibition of Nup activity is therefore achieved by phosphorylation in cardiovirus-infected cells and by proteolysis in cells infected with enteroviruses.

The disruption of nucleocytoplasmic trafficking by picornaviruses not only provides cytoplasmic access to nuclear proteins needed for viral replication but blocks the export of cell mRNAs with antiviral activity produced as part of the innate immune response.

Inhibition of Protein Secretion

Transport of both secretory and plasma membrane proteins is blocked in picornavirus-infected cells.[165] The 2B and 2BC proteins block protein secretion from the Golgi apparatus, and the 3A protein blocks vesicular traffic from the ERGIC to the Golgi complex.[44,76,164,616] Inhibition of protein secretion by poliovirus protein 3A is not required for viral growth in cell culture.[163] Protein 3A inhibits protein transport by binding to and inhibiting GBF1, a guanine exchange protein that is needed for activity of Arf1 and is required for the transport through the secretory pathway.[65] Cells infected with the poliovirus mutant 3A-2, which has a single amino acid change in the protein, have reduced inhibition of protein transport.[164] This amino acid change abrogates binding of 3A to GBF1 and therefore does not inhibit activity of the protein.[749,750] Because the 3A protein prevents secretion of cytokines[163] and major histocompatibility complex I (MHC-I)–dependent antigen presentation,[157] it is likely to modulate the innate and adaptive immune responses of the host and, therefore, the outcome of infection. Consistent with this hypothesis, when the 3A mutation is introduced into the genome of Coxsackievirus B3, the variant is less pathogenic in mice, although the mechanism of attenuation is not known.[750] Inhibition of protein secretion in cells infected by FMDV is caused not by protein 3A but by protein 2BC.[471]

Metabolic Reprogramming

Virus are obligate intracellular parasites and their reproduction cycles require the host metabolic machineries, as no known viral genome encodes all components, including the ribosome, necessary for their replication. Consequently, the production of infectious virus is dependent upon the cell's biosynthetic pathways supplying macromolecules, which in turn leads to dramatic elevations in the bioenergetic demands of cell. To adjust for these demands, the metabolic pathways of the cell are altered. As discussed in *Cellular site of RNA synthesis*, picornavirus infection stimulates the uptake of fatty acids and *de novo* phospholipid synthesis. Infection also enhances sugar uptake and the reprogramming of anabolic pathways such as glycolysis and oxidative phosphorylation, as well as gluconeogenesis needed to enhance amino acid, enhance nucleotide synthesis, and maintain energetic homeostasis of the infected cell. Consequently, rhinovirus infection is impaired in the presence of the glycolysis inhibitor 2-deoxyglucose.[259]

Cell Death and Virus Release

When cells are productively infected with poliovirus, they develop the characteristic morphologic changes known as *cytopathic effects*. These include condensation of chromatin, nuclear blebbing, proliferation of membranous vesicles, changes in membrane permeability, leakage of intracellular components, and shriveling of the entire cell. The cause of cytopathic effects is unknown. One hypothesis is that leakage of lysosomal contents is partly responsible.[263] Although cellular RNA, protein, and DNA synthesis are inhibited during the first few hours of infection, they cannot account for cytopathic effects.

When poliovirus reproduction is hindered by certain drugs or other restrictive conditions, cell death occurs through induction of apoptosis.[686] Although certain manifestations of cytopathic effects and apoptosis are similar (e.g., chromatin condensation and nuclear deformation), the pathways leading to their induction differ.[3] During productive infections of cultured cells with poliovirus, apoptosis is blocked by a virus-encoded inhibitor.[686] Viral replication and central nervous system injury in mice infected with poliovirus, however, are associated with apoptosis.[228] Viral inducers of apoptosis include proteins 2C, 2A[pro], and 3C[pro],[46,231,420] and inhibitors of apoptosis include L[pro], 2B, and 3A.[106,163,219,500,765] The ability of different strains of Theiler murine encephalomyelitis virus to induce apoptosis may be a determinant of disease. The TO strain of Theiler virus, which causes a persistent demyelinating disease in mice, encodes an additional protein, L*.[118] This protein is produced by initiation from an AUG that is 13 nucleotides downstream from the initiator AUG of the polyprotein, in a different reading frame. In contrast, nondemyelinating isolates of the virus (e.g., GDVII) do not encode L*. It was subsequently found that L* has antiapoptotic properties in macrophages and is critical for virus persistence[219] and prevents antiviral cytotoxic T-cell activation.[765] The ability of L* to inhibit apoptosis may be a key factor in determining whether infection of mice results in acute disease or persistence and demyelination.

PERSPECTIVES

Since the identification in 1908 of poliovirus as the etiologic agent of poliomyelitis, research on the virus has waxed and waned. With each lull in activity, questions were raised about whether it was productive to continue research on the virus. Each time, new technologies emerged that allowed the field to advance and become active once again. Today, research on poliovirus continues, as the difficulties have been encountered in the effort to globally eradicate this virus. Nevertheless, work on other picornaviruses has become highly productive, and research on a wide range of cardioviruses, aphthoviruses, enteroviruses, and members of many other genera flourishes. Many questions remain about nearly every stage of the replicative cycle, and an unprecedented array of experimental techniques and reagents are available to address them. Genome-wide editing screens are being applied to picornaviruses and have already identified hundreds of cell genes that not only are required for picornavirus infection but regulate replication.[140,141] It can be anticipated that cellular genes will be identified whose products participate in all aspects of the picornaviral replication cycle, from receptor binding and entry to macromolecular synthesis, assembly of new virus particles, and release. Studies of these processes will contribute to understanding questions about how the viral RNA is released from the capsid, whether RNA synthesis proceeds in infected cells as has been learned from *in vitro* systems, how replication complexes are produced in infected cells, and how the viral RNA enters the virion and becomes folded to fit in a very small space. Because poliovirus is a model system, its study provides a unique opportunity to address fundamental questions in virology. The polio eradication program has made impressive gains—as of this writing in July 2019, there have been fewer cases of poliomyelitis than there were of enterovirus D68–associated paralytic disease. When the time comes when research on poliovirus must cease, the picornavirus field will be ready to move on to other fascinating subjects. As viral discovery in general has greatly accelerated in the past 5 years, the size of the *Picornaviridae* has grown remarkably. With this growth come new opportunities to study fascinating new viral systems, one of which might someday become the next model system for this virus family.

REFERENCES

1. Acharya R, Fry E, Stuart D, et al. The three-dimensional structure of foot-and-mouth disease virus at 2.9 Å resolution. *Nature* 1989;337:709–716.
2. Agirre A, Barco A, Carrasco L, et al. Viroporin-mediated membrane permeabilization. Pore formation by nonstructural poliovirus 2B protein. *J Biol Chem* 2002;277(43):40434–40441.
3. Agol VI, Belov GA, Bienz K, et al. Two types of death of poliovirus-infected cells: caspase involvement in the apoptosis but not cytopathic effect. *Virology* 1998;252(2):343–353.
4. Agrez MV, Shafren DR, Gu X, et al. Integrin alpha v beta 6 enhances coxsackievirus B1 lytic infection of human colon cancer cells. *Virology* 1997;239(1):71–77.
5. Ahlquist P, Kaesberg P. Determination of the length distribution of poly(A) at the 3′ terminus of the virion RNAs of EMC virus, poliovirus, rhinovirus, RAV-61 and CPMV and of mouse globin mRNA. *Nucleic Acids Res* 1979;7(5):1195–1204.
6. Aldabe R, Barco A, Carrasco L. Membrane permeabilization by poliovirus proteins 2B and 2BC. *J Biol Chem* 1996;271(38):23134–23137.
7. Aldabe R, Carrasco L. Induction of membrane proliferation by poliovirus proteins 2C and 2BC. *Biochem Biophys Res Commun* 1995;206(1):64–76.
8. Alexander DA, Dimock K. Sialic acid functions in enterovirus 70 binding and infection. *J Virol* 2002;76(22):11265–11272.
9. Alexander L, Lu HH, Wimmer E. Polioviruses containing picornavirus type 1 and/or type 2 internal ribosomal entry site elements: genetic hybrids and the expression of a foreign gene. *Proc Natl Acad Sci U S A* 1994;91(4):1406–1410.
10. Ali IK, McKendrick L, Morley SJ, et al. Activity of the hepatitis A virus IRES requires association between the cap-binding translation initiation factor (eIF4E) and eIF4G. *J Virol* 2001;75(17):7854–7863.
11. Ali IK, McKendrick L, Morley SJ, et al. Truncated initiation factor eIF4G lacking an eIF4E binding site can support capped mRNA translation. *EMBO J* 2001;20(15):4233–4242.
12. Amass SF, Abvp D, Schneider JL, et al. Idiopathic vesicular disease in a swine herd in Indiana. *J Swine Health Prod* 2004;12:192–196.
13. Ambros V, Baltimore D. Purification and properties of a HeLa cell enzyme able to remove the 5′-terminal protein from poliovirus RNA. *J Biol Chem* 1980;255(14):6739–6744.
14. Ambros V, Pettersson RF, Baltimore D. An enzymatic activity in uninfected cells that cleaves the linkage between poliovirion RNA and the 5′ terminal protein. *Cell* 1978;15(4):1439–1446.
15. Amineva SP, Aminev AG, Palmenberg AC, et al. Rhinovirus 3C protease precursors 3CD and 3CD′ localize to the nuclei of infected cells. *J Gen Virol* 2004;85(Pt 10):2969–2979.
16. Anderson P, Kedersha N. RNA granules: post-transcriptional and epigenetic modulators of gene expression. *Nat Rev Mol Cell Biol* 2009;10(6):430–436.
17. Andino R, Rieckhof GE, Achacoso PL, et al. Poliovirus RNA synthesis utilizes an RNP complex formed around the 5′-end of viral RNA. *EMBO J* 1993;12(9):3587–3598.
18. Andino R, Rieckhof GE, Baltimore D. A functional ribonucleoprotein complex forms around the 5′ end of poliovirus RNA. *Cell* 1990;63(2):369–380.
19. Andino R, Rieckhof GE, Trono D, et al. Substitutions in the protease (3Cpro) gene of poliovirus can suppress a mutation in the 5′ noncoding region. *J Virol* 1990;64(2):607–612.
20. Ansardi DC, Luo M, Morrow CD. Mutations in the poliovirus P1 capsid precursor at arginine residues VP4-ARG34, VP3-ARG223, and VP1-ARG129 affect virus assembly and encapsidation of genomic RNA. *Virology* 1994;199(1):20–34.
21. Aoki J, Koike S, Ise I, et al. Amino acid residues on human poliovirus receptor involved in interaction with poliovirus. *J Biol Chem* 1994;269(11):8431–8438.
22. Appleby TC, Luecke H, Shim JH, et al. Crystal structure of complete rhinovirus RNA polymerase suggests front loading of protein primer. *J Virol* 2005;79(1):277–288.
23. Arias A, Arnold JJ, Sierra M, et al. Determinants of RNA-dependent RNA polymerase (in)fidelity revealed by kinetic analysis of the polymerase encoded by a foot-and-mouth disease virus mutant with reduced sensitivity to ribavirin. *J Virol* 2008;82(24):12346–12355.
24. Arita M. Phosphatidylinositol-4 kinase III beta and oxysterol-binding protein accumulate unesterified cholesterol on poliovirus-induced membrane structure. *Microbiol Immunol* 2014;58(4):239–256.
25. Arita M. Mechanism of poliovirus resistance to host phosphatidylinositol-4 kinase III beta inhibitor. *ACS Infect Dis* 2016;2(2):140–148.
26. Arita M, Kojima H, Nagano T, et al. Phosphatidylinositol 4-kinase III beta is a target of enviroxime-like compounds for antipoliovirus activity. *J Virol* 2011;85(5):2364–2372.
27. Arita M, Wakita T, Shimizu H. Cellular kinase inhibitors that suppress enterovirus replication have a conserved target in viral protein 3A similar to that of enviroxime. *J Gen Virol* 2009;90(Pt 8):1869–1879.
28. Arnold E, Luo M, Vriend G, et al. Implications of the picornavirus capsid structure for polyprotein processing. *Proc Natl Acad Sci U S A* 1987;84(1):21–25.
29. Arnold E, Rossmann MG. Analysis of the structure of a common cold virus, human rhinovirus 14, refined at a resolution of 3.0 A. *J Mol Biol* 1990;211(4):763–801.
30. Atkinson NJ, Witteveldt J, Evans DJ, et al. The influence of CpG and UpA dinucleotide frequencies on RNA virus replication and characterization of the innate cellular pathways underlying virus attenuation and enhanced replication. *Nucleic Acids Res* 2014;42(7):4527–4545.
31. Avanzino BC, Fuchs G, Fraser CS. Cellular cap-binding protein, eIF4E, promotes picornavirus genome restructuring and translation. *Proc Natl Acad Sci U S A* 2017;114(36):9611–9616.
32. Ayscue P, Van Haren K, Sheriff H, et al. Acute flaccid paralysis with anterior myelitis—California, June 2012–June 2014. *MMWR Morb Mortal Wkly Rep* 2014;63(40):903–906.
33. Back SH, Kim YK, Kim WJ, et al. Translation of polioviral mRNA is inhibited by cleavage of polypyrimidine tract-binding proteins executed by polioviral 3C(pro). *J Virol* 2002;76(5):2529–2542.
34. Badorff C, Lee GH, Lamphear BJ, et al. Enteroviral protease 2A cleaves dystrophin: evidence of cytoskeletal disruption in an acquired cardiomyopathy. *Nat Med* 1999;5(3):320–326.
35. Badshah C, Calenoff MA, Rundell K. The leader polypeptide of Theiler's murine encephalomyelitis virus is required for the assembly of virions in mouse L cells. *J Virol* 2000;74(2):875–882.
36. Baggen J, Hurdiss DL, Zocher G, et al. Role of enhanced receptor engagement in the evolution of a pandemic acute hemorrhagic conjunctivitis virus. *Proc Natl Acad Sci U S A* 2018;115(2):397–402.
37. Bakker SE, Groppelli E, Pearson AR, et al. Limits of structural plasticity in a picornavirus capsid revealed by a massively expanded equine rhinitis A virus particle. *J Virol* 2014;88(11):6093–6099.
38. Baltimore D, Franklin RM. A new ribonucleic acid polymerase appearing after mengovirus infection of L-cells. *J Biol Chem* 1963;238:3395–3400.
39. Baltimore D, Eggers HJ, Franklin RM, et al. Poliovirus-induced RNA polymerase and the effects of virus-specific inhibitors on its production. *Proc Natl Acad Sci U S A* 1963;49:843–849.
40. Baltimore D, Girard M, Darnell JE. Aspects of the synthesis of poliovirus RNA and the formation of virus particles. *Virol* 1966;29:179–189.
41. Banerjee S, Aponte-Diaz D, Yeager C, et al. Hijacking of multiple phospholipid biosynthetic pathways and induction of membrane biogenesis by a picornaviral 3CD protein. *PLoS Pathog* 2018;14(5):e1007086.
42. Banerjee R, Weidman MK, Navarro S, et al. Modifications of both selectivity factor and upstream binding factor contribute to poliovirus-mediated inhibition of RNA polymerase I transcription. *J Gen Virol* 2005;86(Pt 8):2315–2322.
43. Baranowski E, Ruiz-Jarabo CM, Sevilla N, et al. Cell recognition by foot-and-mouth disease virus that lacks the RGD integrin-binding motif: flexibility in aphthovirus receptor usage. *J Virol* 2000;74(4):1641–1647.
44. Barco A, Carrasco L. A human virus protein, poliovirus protein 2BC, induces membrane proliferation and blocks the exocytic pathway in the yeast *Saccharomyces cerevisiae*. *EMBO J* 1995;14(14):3349–3364.
45. Barco A, Carrasco L. Identification of regions of poliovirus 2BC protein that are involved in cytotoxicity. *J Virol* 1998;72(5):3560–3570.
46. Barco A, Feduchi E, Carrasco L. Poliovirus protease 3C(pro) kills cells by apoptosis. *Virology* 2000;266(2):352–360.
47. Barton DJ, Black EP, Flanegan JB. Complete replication of poliovirus in vitro: preinitiation RNA replication complexes require soluble cellular factors for the synthesis of VPg-linked RNA. *J Virol* 1995;69(9):5516–5527.
48. Barton DJ, Flanegan JB. Synchronous replication of poliovirus RNA: initiation of negative-strand RNA synthesis requires the guanidine-inhibited activity of protein 2C. *J Virol* 1997;71(11):8482–8489.
49. Barton DJ, Morasco BJ, Flanegan JB. Translating ribosomes inhibit poliovirus negative-strand RNA synthesis. *J Virol* 1999;73(12):10104–10112.
50. Barton DJ, O'Donnell BJ, Flanegan JB. 5′ cloverleaf in poliovirus RNA is a cis-acting replication element required for negative-strand synthesis. *EMBO J* 2001;20(6):1439–1448.
51. Basavappa R, Syed R, Flore O, et al. Role and mechanism of the maturation cleavage of VP0 in poliovirus assembly: structure of the empty capsid assembly intermediate at 2.9 A resolution. *Protein Sci* 1994;3(10):1651–1669.
52. Bassili G, Tzima E, Song Y, et al. Sequence and secondary structure requirements in a highly conserved element for foot-and-mouth disease virus internal ribosome entry site activity and eIF4G binding. *J Gen Virol* 2004;85(Pt 9):2555–2565.
53. Basta HA, Ashraf S, Sgro JY, et al. Modeling of the human rhinovirus C capsid suggests possible causes for antiviral drug resistance. *Virology* 2014;448:82–90.
54. Baxt B. Effect of lysosomotropic compounds on early events in foot-and-mouth disease virus replication. *Virus Res* 1987;7(3):257–271.
55. Baxt B, Becker Y. The effect of peptides containing the arginine-glycine-aspartic acid sequence on the adsorption of foot-and-mouth disease virus to tissue culture cells. *Virus Genes* 1990;4(1):73–83.
56. Baxter NJ, Roetzer A, Liebig HD, et al. Structure and dynamics of coxsackievirus B4 2A proteinase, an enzyme involved in the etiology of heart disease. *J Virol* 2006;80(3):1451–1462.
57. Bayer N, Schober D, Huttinger M, et al. Inhibition of clathrin-dependent endocytosis has multiple effects on human rhinovirus serotype 2 cell entry. *J Biol Chem* 2001;276(6):3952–3962.
58. Bayer N, Schober D, Prchla E, et al. Effect of bafilomycin A1 and nocodazole on endocytic transport in HeLa cells: implications for viral uncoating and infection. *J Virol* 1998;72(12):9645–9655.

59. Bazan JF, Fletterick RJ. Viral cysteine proteases are homologous to the trypsin-like family of serine proteases: structural and functional implications. *Proc Natl Acad Sci U S A* 1988;85(21):7872–7876.
60. Bazzone LE, King M, MacKay CR, et al. A disintegrin and metalloproteinase 9 domain (ADAM9) is a major susceptibility factor in the early stages of encephalomyocarditis virus infection. *MBio* 2019;10(1):e02734-18.
61. Beard CW, Mason PW. Genetic determinants of altered virulence of Taiwanese foot-and-mouth disease virus. *J Virol* 2000;74(2):987–991.
62. Bedard KM, Daijogo S, Semler BL. A nucleo-cytoplasmic SR protein functions in viral IRES-mediated translation initiation. *EMBO J* 2007;26(2):459–467.
63. Bella J, Kolatkar PR, Marlor CW, et al. The structure of the two amino-terminal domains of human ICAM-1 suggests how it functions as a rhinovirus receptor and as an LFA-1 integrin ligand. *Proc Natl Acad Sci U S A* 1998;95(8):4140–4145.
64. Belnap DM, Filman DJ, Trus BL, et al. Molecular tectonic model of virus structural transitions: the putative cell entry states of poliovirus. *J Virol* 2000;74(3):1342–1354.
65. Belov GA, Feng Q, Nikovics K, et al. A critical role of a cellular membrane traffic protein in poliovirus RNA replication. *PLoS Pathog* 2008;4(11):e1000216.
66. Belov GA, Kovtunovych G, Jackson CL, et al. Poliovirus replication requires the N-terminus but not the catalytic Sec7 domain of ArfGEF GBF1. *Cell Microbiol* 2010;12(10):1463–1479.
67. Belov GA, Nair V, Hansen BT, et al. Complex dynamic development of poliovirus membranous replication complexes. *J Virol* 2012;86(1):302–312.
68. Belov GA, Sztul E. Rewiring of cellular membrane homeostasis by picornaviruses. *J Virol* 2014;88(17):9478–9489.
69. Belsham GJ, Bostock CJ. Studies on the infectivity of foot-and-mouth disease virus RNA using microinjection. *J Gen Virol* 1988;69 (Pt 2):265–274.
70. Bergelson JM, Chan M, Solomon KR, et al. Decay-accelerating factor (CD55), a glycosylphosphatidylinositol-anchored complement regulatory protein, is a receptor for several echoviruses. *Proc Natl Acad Sci U S A* 1994;91(13):6245–6248.
71. Bergelson JM, Cunningham JA, Droguett G, et al. Isolation of a common receptor for Coxsackie B viruses and adenoviruses 2 and 5. *Science* 1997;275(5304):1320–1323.
72. Bergelson JM, Shepley MP, Chan BM, et al. Identification of the integrin VLA-2 as a receptor for echovirus 1. *Science* 1992;255(5052):1718–1720.
73. Berka U, Khan A, Blaas D, et al. Human rhinovirus type 2 uncoating at the plasma membrane is not affected by a pH gradient but is affected by the membrane potential. *J Virol* 2009;83(8):3778–3787.
74. Bernhardt G, Harber J, Zibert A, et al. The poliovirus receptor: identification of domains and amino acid residues critical for virus binding. *Virology* 1994;203(2):344–356.
75. Berryman S, Clark S, Monaghan P, et al. Early events in integrin alphavbeta6-mediated cell entry of foot-and-mouth disease virus. *J Virol* 2005;79(13):8519–8534.
76. Beske O, Reichelt M, Taylor MP, et al. Poliovirus infection blocks ERGIC-to-Golgi trafficking and induces microtubule-dependent disruption of the Golgi complex. *J Cell Sci* 2007;120(Pt 18):3207–3218.
77. Bienz K, Egger D, Pfister T, et al. Structural and functional characterization of the poliovirus replication complex. *J Virol* 1992;66(5):2740–2747.
78. Bienz K, Egger D, Rasser Y, et al. Kinetics and location of poliovirus macromolecular synthesis in correlation to virus-induced cytopathology. *Virology* 1980;100(2):390–399.
79. Bilek G, Matscheko NM, Pickl-Herk A, et al. Liposomal nanocontainers as models for viral infection: monitoring viral genomic RNA transfer through lipid membranes. *J Virol* 2011;85(16):8368–8375.
80. Bird SW, Maynard ND, Covert MW, et al. Nonlytic viral spread enhanced by autophagy components. *Proc Natl Acad Sci U S A* 2014;111(36):13081–13086.
81. Biswal JK, Subramaniam S, Ranjan R, et al. Partial deletion of stem-loop 2 in the 3′ untranslated region of foot-and-mouth disease virus identifies a region that is dispensable for virus replication. *Arch Virol* 2016;161(8):2285–2290.
82. Blair WS, Semler BL. Role for the P4 amino acid residue in substrate utilization by the poliovirus 3CD proteinase. *J Virol* 1991;65(11):6111–6123.
83. Blyn LB, Swiderek KM, Richards O, et al. Poly(rC) binding protein 2 binds to stem-loop IV of the poliovirus RNA 5′ noncoding region: identification by automated liquid chromatography-tandem mass spectrometry. *Proc Natl Acad Sci U S A* 1996;93(20):11115–11120.
84. Blyn LB, Towner JS, Semler BL, et al. Requirement of poly(rC) binding protein 2 for translation of poliovirus RNA. *J Virol* 1997;71(8):6243–6246.
85. Bochkov YA, Watters K, Ashraf S, et al. Cadherin-related family member 3, a childhood asthma susceptibility gene product, mediates rhinovirus C binding and replication. *Proc Natl Acad Sci U S A* 2015;112(17):5485–5490.
86. Boege U, Ko DS, Scraba DG. Toward an in vitro system for picornavirus assembly: purification of mengovirus 14S capsid precursor particles. *J Virol* 1986;57(1):275–284.
87. Bonderoff JM, Larey JL, Lloyd RE. Cleavage of poly(A)-binding protein by poliovirus 3C proteinase inhibits viral internal ribosome entry site-mediated translation. *J Virol* 2008;82(19):9389–9399.
88. Borman AM, Kean KM. Intact eukaryotic initiation factor 4G is required for hepatitis A virus internal initiation of translation. *Virology* 1997;237(1):129–136.
89. Boros A, Fenyvesi H, Pankovics P, et al. Secondary structure analysis of swine pasivirus (family Picornaviridae) RNA reveals a type-IV IRES and a parechovirus-like 3′ UTR organization. *Arch Virol* 2015;160(5):1363–1366.
90. Boros A, Pankovics P, Knowles NJ, et al. Comparative complete genome analysis of chicken and Turkey megriviruses (family picornaviridae): long 3′ untranslated regions with a potential second open reading frame and evidence for possible recombination. *J Virol* 2014;88(11):6434–6443.
91. Bostina M, Levy H, Filman DJ, et al. Poliovirus RNA is released from the capsid near a twofold symmetry axis. *J Virol* 2011;85(2):776–783.
92. Bottino C, Castriconi R, Pende D, et al. Identification of PVR (CD155) and Nectin-2 (CD112) as cell surface ligands for the human DNAM-1 (CD226) activating molecule. *J Exp Med* 2003;198(4):557–567.
93. Bouchard MJ, Racaniello VR. CD44 is not required for poliovirus replication. *J Virol* 1997;71(4):2793–2798.
94. Boussadia O, Niepmann M, Creancier L, et al. Unr is required in vivo for efficient initiation of translation from the internal ribosome entry sites of both rhinovirus and poliovirus. *J Virol* 2003;77(6):3353–3359.
95. Brabec M, Blaas D, Fuchs R. Wortmannin delays transfer of human rhinovirus serotype 2 to late endocytic compartments. *Biochem Biophys Res Commun* 2006;348(2):741–749.
96. Brandenburg B, Lee LY, Lakadamyali M, et al. Imaging poliovirus entry in live cells. *PLoS Biol* 2007;5(7):e183.
97. Brown DM, Cornell CT, Tran GP, et al. An authentic 3′ noncoding region is necessary for efficient poliovirus replication. *J Virol* 2005;79(18):11962–11973.
98. Brown DM, Kauder SE, Cornell CT, et al. Cell-dependent role for the poliovirus 3′ noncoding region in positive-strand RNA synthesis. *J Virol* 2004;78(3):1344–1351.
99. Bubeck D, Filman DJ, Cheng N, et al. The structure of the poliovirus 135S cell entry intermediate at 10-angstrom resolution reveals the location of an externalized polypeptide that binds to membranes. *J Virol* 2005;79(12):7745–7755.
100. Buckley B, Ehrenfeld E. The cap-binding protein complex in uninfected and poliovirus-infected HeLa cells. *J Biol Chem* 1987;262(28):13599–13606.
101. Burke MJ, Ahern C, Weigel BJ, et al. Phase I trial of Seneca Valley Virus (NTX-010) in children with relapsed/refractory solid tumors: a report of the Children's Oncology Group. *Pediatr Blood Cancer* 2015;62(5):743–750.
102. Burrill CP, Westesson O, Schulte MB, et al. Global RNA structure analysis of poliovirus identifies a conserved RNA structure involved in viral replication and infectivity. *J Virol* 2013;87(21):11670–11683.
103. Butan C, Filman DJ, Hogle JM. Cryo-electron microscopy reconstruction shows poliovirus 135S particles poised for membrane interaction and RNA release. *J Virol* 2014;88(3):1758–1770.
104. Cammack N, Phillips A, Dunn G, et al. Intertypic genomic rearrangements of poliovirus strains in vaccinees. *Virology* 1988;167(2):507–514.
105. Campagnola G, Weygandt M, Scoggin K, et al. Crystal structure of coxsackievirus B3 3Dpol highlights the functional importance of residue 5 in picornavirus polymerases. *J Virol* 2008;82(19):9458–9464.
106. Campanella M, de Jong AS, Lanke KW, et al. The coxsackievirus 2B protein suppresses apoptotic host cell responses by manipulating intracellular Ca2+ homeostasis. *J Biol Chem* 2004;279(18):18440–18450.
107. Caridi F, Vazquez-Calvo A, Sobrino F, et al. The pH stability of foot-and-mouth disease virus particles is modulated by residues located at the pentameric interface and in the N terminus of VP1. *J Virol* 2015;89(10):5633–5642.
108. Carson SD. Kinetic models for receptor-catalyzed conversion of coxsackievirus B3 to A-particles. *J Virol* 2014;88(19):11568–11575.
109. Casasnovas JM, Bickford JK, Springer TA. The domain structure of ICAM-1 and the kinetics of binding to rhinovirus. *J Virol* 1998;72(7):6244–6246.
110. Casasnovas JM, Springer TA. Kinetics and thermodynamics of virus binding to receptor. Studies with rhinovirus, intercellular adhesion molecule-1 (ICAM-1), and surface plasmon resonance. *J Biol Chem* 1995;270(22):13216–13224.
111. Casjens SR. The DNA-packaging nanomotor of tailed bacteriophages. *Nat Rev Microbiol* 2011;9(9):647–657.
112. Castello A, Alvarez E, Carrasco L. The multifaceted poliovirus 2A protease: regulation of gene expression by picornavirus proteases. *J Biomed Biotechnol* 2011;2011:369648.
113. Chan YM, Moustafa IM, Arnold JJ, et al. Long-range communication between different functional sites in the picornaviral 3C protein. *Structure* 2016;24(4):509–517.
114. Chang KH, Day C, Walker J, et al. The nucleotide sequences of wild-type coxsackievirus A9 strains imply that an RGD motif in VP1 is functionally significant. *J Gen Virol* 1992;73(Pt 3):621–626.
115. Charini WA, Todd S, Gutman GA, et al. Transduction of a human RNA sequence by poliovirus. *J Virol* 1994;68(10):6547–6552.
116. Cheah KC, Leong LE, Porter AG. Site-directed mutagenesis suggests close functional relationship between a human rhinovirus 3C cysteine protease and cellular trypsin-like serine proteases. *J Biol Chem* 1990;265(13):7180–7187.
117. Chen YH, Du W, Hagemeijer MC, et al. Phosphatidylserine vesicles enable efficient en bloc transmission of enteroviruses. *Cell* 2015;160(4):619–630.
118. Chen HH, Kong WP, Zhang L, et al. A picornaviral protein synthesized out of frame with the polyprotein plays a key role in a virus-induced immune-mediated demyelinating disease. *Nat Med* 1995;1(9):927–931.
119. Chen ZG, Stauffacher C, Li Y, et al. Protein-RNA interactions in an icosahedral virus at 3.0 A resolution. *Science* 1989;245(4914):154–159.
120. Cherry S, Kunte A, Wang H, et al. COPI activity coupled with fatty acid biosynthesis is required for viral replication. *PLoS Pathog* 2006;2(10):e102.
121. Chevaliez S, Balanant J, Maillard P, et al. Role of class I human leukocyte antigen molecules in early steps of echovirus infection of rhabdomyosarcoma cells. *Virology* 2008;381(2):203–214.
122. Cho MW, Richards OC, Dmitrieva TM, et al. RNA duplex unwinding activity of poliovirus RNA-dependent RNA polymerase 3Dpol. *J Virol* 1993;67(6):3010–3018.
123. Cho MW, Teterina N, Egger D, et al. Membrane rearrangement and vesicle induction by recombinant poliovirus 2C and 2BC in human cells. *Virology* 1994;202(1):129–145.
124. Choe SS, Kirkegaard K. Intracellular topology and epitope shielding of poliovirus 3A protein. *J Virol* 2004;78(11):5973–5982.
125. Chow M, Newman JF, Filman D, et al. Myristoylation of picornavirus capsid protein VP4 and its structural significance. *Nature* 1987;327(6122):482–486.
126. Claridge JK, Headey SJ, Chow JY, et al. A picornaviral loop-to-loop replication complex. *J Struct Biol* 2009;166(3):251–262.
127. Clark ME, Lieberman PM, Berk AJ, et al. Direct cleavage of human TATA-binding protein by poliovirus protease 3C in vivo and in vitro. *Mol Cell Biol* 1993;13:1232–1237.
128. Clark AT, Robertson ME, Conn GL, et al. Conserved nucleotides within the J domain of the encephalomyocarditis virus internal ribosome entry site are required for activity and for interaction with eIF4G. *J Virol* 2003;77(23):12441–12449.
129. Coleman JR, Papamichail D, Skiena S, et al. Virus attenuation by genome-scale changes in codon pair bias. *Science* 2008;320(5884):1784–1787.

130. Colina R, Costa-Mattioli M, Dowling RJ, et al. Translational control of the innate immune response through IRF-7. *Nature* 2008;452(7185):323–328.
131. Collis PS, O'Donnell BJ, Barton DJ, et al. Replication of poliovirus RNA and subgenomic RNA transcripts in transfected cells. *J Virol* 1992;66(11):6480–6488.
132. Colonno RJ, Callahan PL, Long WJ. Isolation of a monoclonal antibody that blocks attachment of the major group of human rhinoviruses. *J Virol* 1986;57(1):7–12.
133. Colonno RJ, Condra JH, Mizutani S, et al. Evidence for the direct involvement of the rhinovirus canyon in receptor binding. *Proc Natl Acad Sci U S A* 1988;85(15):5449–5453.
134. Colston E, Racaniello VR. Soluble receptor-resistant poliovirus mutants identify surface and internal capsid residues that control interaction with the cell receptor. *EMBO J* 1994;13(24):5855–5862.
135. Colston EM, Racaniello VR. Poliovirus variants selected on mutant receptor-expressing cells identify capsid residues that expand receptor recognition. *J Virol* 1995;69(8):4823–4829.
136. Corbic Ramljak I, Stanger J, Real-Hohn A, et al. Cellular N-myristoyltransferases play a crucial picornavirus genus-specific role in viral assembly, virion maturation, and infectivity. *PLoS Pathog* 2018;14(8):e1007203.
137. Corona AK, Saulsbery HM, Corona Velazquez AF, et al. Enteroviruses remodel autophagic trafficking through regulation of host SNARE proteins to promote virus replication and cell exit. *Cell Rep* 2018;22(12):3304–3314.
138. Cougot N, Cavalier A, Thomas D, et al. The dual organization of P-bodies revealed by immunoelectron microscopy and electron tomography. *J Mol Biol* 2012;420(1–2):17–28.
139. Coyne CB, Bergelson JM. Virus-induced Abl and Fyn kinase signals permit coxsackievirus entry through epithelial tight junctions. *Cell* 2006;124(1):119–131.
140. Coyne CB, Bozym R, Morosky SA, et al. Comparative RNAi screening reveals host factors involved in enterovirus infection of polarized endothelial monolayers. *Cell Host Microbe* 2011;9(1):70–82.
141. Coyne CB, Cherry S. RNAi screening in mammalian cells to identify novel host cell molecules involved in the regulation of viral infections. *Methods Mol Biol* 2011;721:397–405.
142. Coyne CB, Kim KS, Bergelson JM. Poliovirus entry into human brain microvascular cells requires receptor-induced activation of SHP-2. *EMBO J* 2007;26(17):4016–4028.
143. Crawford NM, Baltimore D. Genome-linked protein VPg of poliovirus is present as free VPg and VPg-pUpU in poliovirus-infected cells. *Proc Natl Acad Sci U S A* 1983;80:7452–7455.
144. Crotty S, Maag D, Arnold JJ, et al. The broad-spectrum antiviral ribonucleoside ribavirin is an RNA virus mutagen. *Nat Med* 2000;6(12):1375–1379.
145. Crotty S, Saleh MC, Gitlin L, et al. The poliovirus replication machinery can escape inhibition by an antiviral drug that targets a host cell protein. *J Virol* 2004;78(7):3378–3386.
146. Crowell RL, Philipson L. Specific alterations of coxsackievirus B3 eluted from HeLa cells. *J Virol* 1971;8(4):509–515.
147. Crowther JR, Farias S, Carpenter WC, et al. Identification of a fifth neutralizable site on type O foot-and-mouth disease virus following characterization of single and quintuple monoclonal antibody escape mutants. *J Gen Virol* 1993;74 (Pt 8):1547–1553.
148. Curry S, Abrams CC, Fry E, et al. Viral RNA modulates the acid sensitivity of foot-and-mouth disease virus capsids. *J Virol* 1995;69(1):430–438.
149. Curry S, Chow M, Hogle JM. The poliovirus 135S particle is infectious. *J Virol* 1996;70(10):7125–7131.
150. Curry S, Fry E, Blakemore W, et al. Dissecting the roles of VP0 cleavage and RNA packaging in picornavirus capsid stabilization: the structure of empty capsids of foot-and-mouth disease virus. *J Virol* 1997;71(12):9743–9752.
151. Dales S, Eggers HJ, Tamm I, et al. Electron microscopic study of the formation of poliovirus. *Virology* 1965;26:379–389.
152. Danthi P, Tosteson M, Li QH, et al. Genome delivery and ion channel properties are altered in VP4 mutants of poliovirus. *J Virol* 2003;77(9):5266–5274.
153. Dasgupta A, Zabel P, Baltimore D. Dependence of the activity of the poliovirus replicase on a host cell protein. *Cell* 1980;19:423–429.
154. Davis MP, Bottley G, Beales LP, et al. Recombinant VP4 of human rhinovirus induces permeability in model membranes. *J Virol* 2008;82(8):4169–4174.
155. De Colibus L, Wang X, Spyrou JAB, et al. More-powerful virus inhibitors from structure-based analysis of HEV71 capsid-binding molecules. *Nat Struct Mol Biol* 2014;21(3):282–288.
156. De Colibus L, Wang X, Tijsma A, et al. Structure elucidation of coxsackievirus A16 in complex with GPP3 informs a systematic review of highly potent capsid binders to enteroviruses. *PLoS Pathog* 2015;11(10):e1005165.
157. Deitz SB, Dodd DA, Cooper S, et al. MHC I-dependent antigen presentation is inhibited by poliovirus protein 3A. *Proc Natl Acad Sci U S A* 2000;97(25):13790–13795.
158. DeLong DC, Reed SE. Inhibition of rhinovirus replication in organ culture by a potential antiviral drug. *J Infect Dis* 1980;141(1):87–91.
159. DeTulleo L, Kirchhausen T. The clathrin endocytic pathway in viral infection. *EMBO J* 1998;17(16):4585–4593.
160. Devaney MA, Vakharia VN, Lloyd RE, et al. Leader protein of foot-and-mouth disease virus is required for cleavage of the p220 component of the cap-binding protein complex. *J Virol* 1988;62(11):4407–4409.
161. Diamond SE, Kirkegaard K. Clustered charged-to-alanine mutagenesis of poliovirus RNA-dependent RNA polymerase yields multiple temperature-sensitive mutants defective in RNA synthesis. *J Virol* 1994;68(2):863–876.
162. Dicara D, Burman A, Clark S, et al. Foot-and-mouth disease virus forms a highly stable, EDTA-resistant complex with its principal receptor, integrin alphavbeta6: implications for infectiousness. *J Virol* 2008;82(3):1537–1546.
163. Dodd DA, Giddings TH Jr, Kirkegaard K. Poliovirus 3A protein limits interleukin-6 (IL-6), IL-8, and beta interferon secretion during viral infection. *J Virol* 2001;75(17):8158–8165.
164. Doedens JR, Giddings TH Jr, Kirkegaard K. Inhibition of endoplasmic reticulum-to-Golgi traffic by poliovirus protein 3A: genetic and ultrastructural analysis. *J Virol* 1997;71(12):9054–9064.
165. Doedens JR, Kirkegaard K. Inhibition of cellular protein secretion by poliovirus proteins 2B and 3A. *EMBO J* 1995;14(5):894–907.
166. Domingo E, Holland JJ. RNA virus mutations and fitness for survival. *Annu Rev Microbiol* 1997;51:151–178.
167. Donnelly ML, Gani D, Flint M, et al. The cleavage activities of aphthovirus and cardiovirus 2A proteins. *J Gen Virol* 1997;78(Pt 1):13–21.
168. Dorobantu CM, Albulescu L, Harak C, et al. Modulation of the host lipid landscape to promote RNA virus replication: the picornavirus encephalomyocarditis virus converges on the pathway used by hepatitis C virus. *PLoS Pathog* 2015;11(9):e1005185.
169. Dorobantu CM, Ford-Siltz LA, Sittig SP, et al. GBF1- and ACBD3-independent recruitment of PI4KIIIbeta to replication sites by rhinovirus 3A proteins. *J Virol* 2015;89(3):1913–1918.
170. Dorobantu CM, van der Schaar HM, Ford LA, et al. Recruitment of PI4KIIIbeta to coxsackievirus B3 replication organelles is independent of ACBD3, GBF1, and Arf1. *J Virol* 2014;88(5):2725–2736.
171. Doronina VA, Wu C, de Felipe P, et al. Site-specific release of nascent chains from ribosomes at a sense codon. *Mol Cell Biol* 2008;28(13):4227–4239.
172. Dougherty JD, White JP, Lloyd RE. Poliovirus-mediated disruption of cytoplasmic processing bodies. *J Virol* 2011;85(1):64–75.
173. Dubra MS, La Torre JL, Scodeller EA, et al. Cores in foot-and-mouth disease virus. *Virology* 1982;116(1):349–353.
174. Duggal R, Cuconati A, Gromeier M, et al. Genetic recombination of poliovirus in a cell-free system. *Proc Natl Acad Sci U S A* 1997;94(25):13786–13791.
175. Duke GM, Osorio JE, Palmenberg AC. Attenuation of Mengo virus through genetic engineering of the 5′ noncoding poly(C) tract. *Nature* 1990;343(6257):474–476.
176. Dulbecco R. Production of plaques in monolayer tissue cultures by single particles of an animal virus. *Proc Natl Acad Sci U S A* 1952;38:747–752.
177. Dvorak CM, Hall DJ, Hill M, et al. Leader protein of encephalomyocarditis virus binds zinc, is phosphorylated during viral infection, and affects the efficiency of genome translation. *Virology* 2001;290(2):261–271.
178. Echeverri A, Banerjee R, Dasgupta A. Amino-terminal region of poliovirus 2C protein is sufficient for membrane binding. *Virus Res* 1998;54(2):217–223.
179. Echeverri AC, Dasgupta A. Amino terminal regions of poliovirus 2C protein mediate membrane binding. *Virology* 1995;208(2):540–553.
180. Egger D, Bienz K. Intracellular location and translocation of silent and active poliovirus replication complexes. *J Gen Virol* 2005;86(Pt 3):707–718.
181. Ellard FM, Drew J, Blakemore WE, et al. Evidence for the role of His-142 of protein 1C in the acid-induced disassembly of foot-and-mouth disease virus capsids. *J Gen Virol* 1999;80(Pt 8):1911–1918.
182. Elling U, Wimmer RA, Leibbrandt A, et al. A reversible haploid mouse embryonic stem cell biobank resource for functional genomics. *Nature* 2017;550(7674):114–118.
183. Enders JF, Weller TH, Robbins FC. Cultivation of the Lansing strain of poliomyelitis virus in cultures of various human embryonic tissues. *Science* 1949;109:85–87.
184. Ertel KJ, Brunner JE, Semler BL. Mechanistic consequences of hnRNP C binding to both RNA termini of poliovirus negative-strand RNA intermediates. *J Virol* 2010;84(9):4229–4242.
185. Etchison D, Milburn SC, Edery I, et al. Inhibition of HeLa cell protein synthesis following poliovirus infection correlates with the proteolysis of a 220,000-dalton polypeptide associated with eucaryotic initiation factor 3 and a cap binding protein complex. *J Biol Chem* 1982;257(24):14806–14810.
186. Eulalio A, Behm-Ansmant I, Schweizer D, et al. P-body formation is a consequence, not the cause, of RNA-mediated gene silencing. *Mol Cell Biol* 2007;27(11):3970–3981.
187. Feng Z, Hensley L, McKnight KL, et al. A pathogenic picornavirus acquires an envelope by hijacking cellular membranes. *Nature* 2013;496(7445):367–371.
188. Fernandes MHV, Maggioli MF, Joshi LR, et al. Pathogenicity and cross-reactive immune responses of a historical and a contemporary Senecavirus A strains in pigs. *Virology* 2018;522:147–157.
189. Fernandez-Chamorro J, Francisco-Velilla R, Ramajo J, et al. Rab1b and ARF5 are novel RNA-binding proteins involved in FMDV IRES-driven RNA localization. *Life Sci Alliance* 2019;2(1).
190. Ferrer-Orta C, Arias A, Agudo R, et al. The structure of a protein primer-polymerase complex in the initiation of genome replication. *EMBO J* 2006;25(4):880–888.
191. Ferrer-Orta C, Arias A, Perez-Luque R, et al. Structure of foot-and-mouth disease virus RNA-dependent RNA polymerase and its complex with a template-primer RNA. *J Biol Chem* 2004;279(45):47212–47221.
192. Filman DJ, Syed R, Chow M, et al. Structural factors that control conformational transitions and serotype specificity in type 3 poliovirus. *EMBO J* 1989;8(5):1567–1579.
193. Fitzgerald KD, Semler BL. Bridging IRES elements in mRNAs to the eukaryotic translation apparatus. *Biochim Biophys Acta* 2009;1789(9–10):518–528.
194. Fitzgerald KD, Semler BL. Re-localization of cellular protein SRp20 during poliovirus infection: bridging a viral IRES to the host cell translation apparatus. *PLoS Pathog* 2011;7(7):e1002127.
195. Flanegan JB, Petterson RF, Ambros V, et al. Covalent linkage of a protein to a defined nucleotide sequence at the 5′-terminus of virion and replicative intermediate RNAs of poliovirus. *Proc Natl Acad Sci U S A* 1977;74(3):961–965.
196. Fletcher SP, Ali IK, Kaminski A, et al. The influence of viral coding sequences on pestivirus IRES activity reveals further parallels with translation initiation in prokaryotes. *RNA* 2002;8(12):1558–1571.
197. Fletcher SP, Jackson RJ. Pestivirus internal ribosome entry site (IRES) structure and function: elements in the 5′ untranslated region important for IRES function. *J Virol* 2002;76(10):5024–5033.
198. Ford RJ, Barker AM, Bakker SE, et al. Sequence-specific, RNA-protein interactions overcome electrostatic barriers preventing assembly of satellite tobacco necrosis virus coat protein. *J Mol Biol* 2013;425(6):1050–1064.
199. Ford Siltz LA, Viktorova EG, Zhang B, et al. New small-molecule inhibitors effectively blocking picornavirus replication. *J Virol* 2014;88(19):11091–11107.
200. Forss S, Schaller H. A tandem repeat gene in a picornavirus. *Nucleic Acids Res* 1982;10(20):6441–6450.
201. Fout GS, Medappa KC, Mapoles JE, et al. Radiochemical determination of polyamines in poliovirus and human rhinovirus 14. *J Biol Chem* 1984;259:3639–3643.

202. Fox MP, Otto MJ, McKinlay MA. Prevention of rhinovirus and poliovirus uncoating by WIN 51711, a new antiviral drug. *Antimicrob Agents Chemother* 1986;30(1):110–116.
203. Fox G, Parry NR, Barnett PV, et al. The cell attachment site on foot-and-mouth disease virus includes the amino acid sequence RGD (arginine-glycine-aspartic acid). *J Gen Virol* 1989;70(Pt 3):625–637.
204. Freistadt MS, Eberle KE. CD44 is not required for poliovirus replication in cultured cells and does not limit replication in monocytes. *Virology* 1996;224(2):542–547.
205. Freistadt MS, Eberle KE. Physical association between CD155 and CD44 in human monocytes. *Mol Immunol* 1997;34(18):1247–1257.
206. Fricks CE, Hogle JM. Cell-induced conformational change in poliovirus: externalization of the amino terminus of VP1 is responsible for liposome binding. *J Virol* 1990;64(5):1934–1945.
207. Fry EE, Lea SM, Jackson T, et al. The structure and function of a foot-and-mouth disease virus- oligosaccharide receptor complex. *EMBO J* 1999;18(3):543–554.
208. Fry EE, Tuthill TJ, Harlos K, et al. Crystal structure of equine rhinitis A virus in complex with its sialic acid receptor. *J Gen Virol* 2010;91(Pt 8):1971–1977.
209. Fuchs A, Cella M, Giurisato E, et al. Cutting edge: CD96 (tactile) promotes NK cell-target cell adhesion by interacting with the poliovirus receptor (CD155). *J Immunol* 2004;172(7):3994–3998.
210. Gamarnik AV, Andino R. Replication of poliovirus in Xenopus oocytes requires two human factors. *EMBO J* 1996;15(21):5988–5998.
211. Gamarnik AV, Andino R. Two functional complexes formed by KH domain containing proteins with the 5′ noncoding region of poliovirus RNA. *RNA* 1997;3(8):882–892.
212. Gamarnik AV, Andino R. Switch from translation to RNA replication in a positive-stranded RNA virus. *Genes Dev* 1998;12(15):2293–2304.
213. Gamarnik AV, Andino R. Interactions of viral protein 3CD and Poly(rC) binding protein with the 5′ untranslated region of the poliovirus genome [In Process Citation]. *J Virol* 2000;74(5):2219–2226.
214. Garriga D, Pickl-Herk A, Luque D, et al. Insights into minor group rhinovirus uncoating: the X-ray structure of the HRV2 empty capsid. *PLoS Pathog* 2012;8(1):e1002473.
215. Gazina EV, Mackenzie JM, Gorrell RJ, et al. Differential requirements for COPI coats in formation of replication complexes among three genera of Picornaviridae. *J Virol* 2002;76(21):11113–11122.
216. Geller R, Pechmann S, Acevedo A, et al. Hsp90 shapes protein and RNA evolution to balance trade-offs between protein stability and aggregation. *Nat Commun* 2018;9(1):1781.
217. Geller R, Taguwa S, Frydman J. Broad action of Hsp90 as a host chaperone required for viral replication. *Biochim Biophys Acta* 2012;1823(3):698–706.
218. Geller R, Vignuzzi M, Andino R, et al. Evolutionary constraints on chaperone-mediated folding provide an antiviral approach refractory to development of drug resistance. *Genes Dev* 2007;21(2):195–205.
219. Ghadge GD, Ma L, Sato S, et al. A protein critical for a Theiler's virus-induced immune system-mediated demyelinating disease has a cell type-specific antiapoptotic effect and a key role in virus persistence. *J Virol* 1998;72(11):8605–8612.
220. Ghildyal R, Jordan B, Li D, et al. Rhinovirus 3C protease can localize in the nucleus and alter active and passive nucleocytoplasmic transport. *J Virol* 2009;83(14):7349–7352.
221. Giachetti C, Hwang S-S, Semler BL. cis-Acting lesions targeted to the hydrophobic domain of a poliovirus membrane protein involved in RNA replication. *J Virol* 1992;66:6045–6057.
222. Giachetti C, Semler BL. Molecular genetic analysis of poliovirus RNA replication by mutagenesis of a VPg precursor polypeptide. In: Brinton MA, Heinz FX, eds. *New Aspects of Positive-Strand RNA Viruses*. Washington, DC: American Society for Microbiology; 1990:83–93.
223. Giachetti C, Semler BL. Role of a viral membrane polypeptide in strand-specific initiation of poliovirus RNA synthesis [published errata appear in J Virol 1991 Jul;65(7):3972 and 1991 Oct;65(10):5653]. *J Virol* 1991;65(5):2647–2654.
224. Gilks N, Kedersha N, Ayodele M, et al. Stress granule assembly is mediated by prion-like aggregation of TIA-1. *Mol Biol Cell* 2004;15(12):5383–5398.
225. Gingras AC, Svitkin Y, Belsham GJ, et al. Activation of the translational suppressor 4E-BP1 following infection with encephalomyocarditis virus and poliovirus. *Proc Natl Acad Sci U S A* 1996;93(11):5578–5583.
226. Giranda VL, Heinz BA, Oliveira MA, et al. Acid-induced structural changes in human rhinovirus 14: possible role in uncoating. *Proc Natl Acad Sci U S A* 1992;89(21):10213–10217.
227. Girard M, Baltimore D, Darnell JE. The poliovirus replication complex: sites for synthesis of poliovirus RNA. *J Mol Biol* 1967;24:59–74.
228. Girard S, Couderc T, Destombes J, et al. Poliovirus induces apoptosis in the mouse central nervous system. *J Virol* 1999;73(7):6066–6072.
229. Global polio eradication: progress towards containment of poliovirus type 2, worldwide 2017. *Wkly Epidemiol Rec* 2017;92(25):350–356.
230. Gohara DW, Crotty S, Arnold JJ, et al. Poliovirus RNA-dependent RNA polymerase (3Dpol): structural, biochemical, and biological analysis of conserved structural motifs A and B. *J Biol Chem* 2000;275(33):25523–25532.
231. Goldstaub D, Gradi A, Bercovitch Z, et al. Poliovirus 2A protease induces apoptotic cell death. *Mol Cell Biol* 2000;20(4):1271–1277.
232. Golini F, Semler BL, Dorner AJ, et al. Protein-linked RNA of poliovirus is competent to form an initiation complex of translation in vitro. *Nature* 1980;287(5783):600–603.
233. Gong P, Kortus MG, Nix JC, et al. Structures of coxsackievirus, rhinovirus, and poliovirus polymerase elongation complexes solved by engineering RNA mediated crystal contacts. *PLoS One* 2013;8(5):e60272.
234. Gong P, Peersen OB. Structural basis for active site closure by the poliovirus RNA-dependent RNA polymerase. *Proc Natl Acad Sci U S A* 2010;107(52):22505–22510.
235. Gonzalez ME, Carrasco L. Viroporins. *FEBS Lett* 2003;552(1):28–34.
236. Goodfellow I, Chaudhry Y, Richardson A, et al. Identification of a cis-acting replication element within the poliovirus coding region. *J Virol* 2000;74(10):4590–4600.
237. Goodfellow IG, Evans DJ, Blom AM, et al. Inhibition of coxsackie B virus infection by soluble forms of its receptors: binding affinities, altered particle formation, and competition with cellular receptors. *J Virol* 2005;79(18):12016–12024.
238. Goodfellow IG, Powell RM, Ward T, et al. Echovirus infection of rhabdomyosarcoma cells is inhibited by antiserum to the complement control protein CD59. *J Gen Virol* 2000;81(Pt 5):1393–1401.
239. Goodfellow IG, Sioofy AB, Powell RM, et al. Echoviruses bind heparan sulfate at the cell surface. *J Virol* 2001;75(10):4918–4921.
240. Gorbalenya AE, Blinov VM, Donchenko AP. Poliovirus-encoded proteinase 3C: a possible evolutionary link between cellular serine and cysteine proteinase families [published erratum appears in FEBS Lett 1986 May 26;201(1):179]. *FEBS Lett* 1986;194(2): 253–257.
241. Gorbalenya AE, Donchenko AP, Blinov VM, et al. Cysteine proteases of positive strand RNA viruses and chymotrypsin-like serine proteases. A distinct protein superfamily with a common structural fold. *FEBS Lett* 1989;243(2):103–114.
242. Gorbalenya AE, Koonin EV, Blinov VM, et al. Sobemovirus genome appears to encode a serine protease related to cysteine proteases of picornaviruses. *FEBS Lett* 1988;236(2):287–290.
243. Gorbalenya AE, Koonin EV, Lai MM. Putative papain-related thiol proteases of positive-strand RNA viruses. Identification of rubi- and aphthovirus proteases and delineation of a novel conserved domain associated with proteases of rubi-, alpha- and coronaviruses. *FEBS Lett* 1991;288(1–2):201–205.
244. Graci JD, Gnadig NF, Galarraga JE, et al. Mutational robustness of an RNA virus influences sensitivity to lethal mutagenesis. *J Virol* 2012;86(5):2869–2873.
245. Gradi A, Svitkin YV, Imataka H, et al. Proteolysis of human eukaryotic translation initiation factor eIF4GII, but not eIF4GI, coincides with the shutoff of host protein synthesis after poliovirus infection. *Proc Natl Acad Sci U S A* 1998;95(19):11089–11094.
246. Gradi A, Svitkin YV, Sommergruber W, et al. Human rhinovirus 2A proteinase cleavage sites in eukaryotic initiation factors (eIF) 4GI and eIF4GII are different. *J Virol* 2003;77(8):5026–5029.
247. Grant RA, Hiremath CN, Filman DJ, et al. Structures of poliovirus complexes with antiviral drugs: implications for viral stability and drug design. *Curr Biol* 1994;4(9):784–797.
248. Grassme H, Riehle A, Wilker B, et al. Rhinoviruses infect human epithelial cells via ceramide-enriched membrane platforms. *J Biol Chem* 2005;280(28):26256–26262.
249. Greninger AL, Knudsen GM, Betegon M, et al. The 3A protein from multiple picornaviruses utilizes the golgi adaptor protein ACBD3 to recruit PI4KIIIbeta. *J Virol* 2012;86(7):3605–3616.
250. Greninger AL, Naccache SN, Messacar K, et al. A novel outbreak enterovirus D68 strain associated with acute flaccid myelitis cases in the USA (2012–14): a retrospective cohort study. *Lancet Infect Dis* 2015;15(6):671–682.
251. Greve JM, Davis G, Meyer AM, et al. The major human rhinovirus receptor is ICAM-1. *Cell* 1989;56:839–847.
252. Grimmer S, van Deurs B, Sandvig K. Membrane ruffling and macropinocytosis in A431 cells require cholesterol. *J Cell Sci* 2002;115(Pt 14):2953–2962.
253. Groppelli E, Levy HC, Sun E, et al. Picornavirus RNA is protected from cleavage by ribonuclease during virion uncoating and transfer across cellular and model membranes. *PLoS Pathog* 2017;13(2):e1006197.
254. Groppelli E, Tuthill TJ, Rowlands DJ. Cell entry of the aphthovirus equine rhinitis A virus is dependent on endosome acidification. *J Virol* 2010;84(12):6235–6240.
255. Grubman MJ, Zellner M, Bablanian G, et al. Identification of the active-site residues of the 3C proteinase of foot- and-mouth disease virus. *Virology* 1995;213(2):581–589.
256. Gruez A, Selisko B, Roberts M, et al. The crystal structure of coxsackievirus B3 RNA-dependent RNA polymerase in complex with its protein primer VPg confirms the existence of a second VPg binding site on Picornaviridae polymerases. *J Virol* 2008;82(19):9577–9590.
257. Grunert HP, Wolf KU, Langner KD, et al. Internalization of human rhinovirus 14 into HeLa and ICAM-1-transfected BHK cells. *Med Microbiol Immunol* 1997;186(1):1–9.
258. Gu CJ, Zheng CY, Zhang Q, et al. An antiviral mechanism investigated with ribavirin as an RNA virus mutagen for foot-and-mouth disease virus. *J Biochem Mol Biol* 2006;39(1):9–15.
259. Gualdoni GA, Mayer KA, Kapsch AM, et al. Rhinovirus induces an anabolic reprogramming in host cell metabolism essential for viral replication. *Proc Natl Acad Sci U S A* 2018;115(30):E7158–E7165.
260. Guarne A, Tormo J, Kirchweger R, et al. Structure of the foot-and-mouth disease virus leader protease: a papain-like fold adapted for self-processing and eIF4G recognition. *EMBO J* 1998;17(24):7469–7479.
261. Guinea R, Carrasco L. Phospholipid biosynthesis and poliovirus genome replication, two coupled phenomena. *EMBO J* 1990;9(6):2011–2016.
262. Guo F, Li S, Caglar MU, et al. Single-cell virology: on-chip investigation of viral infection dynamics. *Cell Rep* 2017;21(6):1692–1704.
263. Guskey LE, Smith PC, Wolff DA. Patterns of cytopathology and lysosomal enzyme release in poliovirus- infected HEp-2 cells treated with either 2-(alpha-hydroxybenzyl)-benzimidazole or guanidine HCl. *J Gen Virol* 1970;6(1):151–161.
264. Gustin KE, Sarnow P. Effects of poliovirus infection on nucleo-cytoplasmic trafficking and nuclear pore complex composition. *EMBO J* 2001;20(1–2):240–249.
265. Gustin KE, Sarnow P. Inhibition of nuclear import and alteration of nuclear pore complex composition by rhinovirus. *J Virol* 2002;76(17):8787–8796.
266. Guy M, Chilmonczyk S, Cruciere C, et al. Efficient infection of buffalo rat liver-resistant cells by encephalomyocarditis virus requires binding to cell surface sialic acids. *J Gen Virol* 2009;90(Pt 1):187–196.
267. Hadfield AT, Diana GD, Rossmann MG. Analysis of three structurally related antiviral compounds in complex with human rhinovirus 16. *Proc Natl Acad Sci U S A* 1999;96(26):14730–14735.
268. Hadfield AT, Lee W, Zhao R, et al. The refined structure of human rhinovirus 16 at 2.15 A resolution: implications for the viral life cycle. *Structure* 1997;5(3):427–441.
269. Haghighat A, Svitkin Y, Novoa I, et al. The eIF4G-eIF4E complex is the target for direct cleavage by the rhinovirus 2A proteinase. *J Virol* 1996;70(12):8444–8450.
270. Hahn H, Palmenberg AC. Encephalomyocarditis viruses with short poly(C) tracts are more virulent than their mengovirus counterparts. *J Virol* 1995;69(4):2697–2699.

271. Hahn H, Palmenberg AC. Mutational analysis of the encephalomyocarditis virus primary cleavage. *J Virol* 1996;70(10):6870–6875.
272. Hall L, Rueckert RR. Infection of mouse fibroblasts by cardioviruses: premature uncoating and its prevention by elevated pH and magnesium chloride. *Virology* 1971;43(1):152–165.
273. Halperen S, Eggers HJ, Tamm I. Evidence for uncoupled synthesis of viral RNA and viral capsids. *Virology* 1964;24:36–46.
274. Hambidge SJ, Sarnow P. Translational enhancement of the poliovirus 5′ noncoding region mediated by virus-encoded polypeptide 2A. *Proc Natl Acad Sci U S A* 1992;89:10272–10276.
275. Hammerle T, Hellen CU, Wimmer E. Site-directed mutagenesis of the putative catalytic triad of poliovirus 3C proteinase. *J Biol Chem* 1991;266(9):5412–5416.
276. Han SC, Guo HC, Sun SQ, et al. Productive entry of foot-and-mouth disease virus via macropinocytosis independent of phosphatidylinositol 3-kinase. *Sci Rep* 2016;6:19294.
277. Hansen JL, Long AM, Schultz SC. Structure of the RNA-dependent RNA polymerase of poliovirus. *Structure* 1997;5(8):1109–1122.
278. Happe M, Jockusch H. Phage Qbeta replicase: cell-free synthesis of the phage-specific subunit and its assembly with host subunits to form active enzyme. *Eur J Biochem* 1975;58(2):359–366.
279. Harber J, Bernhardt G, Lu H-H, et al. Canyon rim residues, including antigenic determinants, modulate serotype-specific binding of polioviruses to mutants of the poliovirus receptor. *Virology* 1995;214:559–570.
280. Harber JJ, Bradley J, Anderson CW, et al. Catalysis of poliovirus VP0 maturation cleavage is not mediated by serine 10 of VP2. *J Virol* 1991;65(1):326–334.
281. Harmon SA, Richards OC, Summers DF, et al. The 5′-terminal nucleotides of hepatitis A virus RNA, but not poliovirus RNA, are required for infectivity. *J Virol* 1991;65(5):2757–2760.
282. Harris JR, Racaniello VR. Amino acid changes in proteins 2B and 3A mediate rhinovirus type 39 growth in mouse cells. *J Virol* 2005;79(9):5363–5373.
283. Harris KS, Reddigari SR, Nicklin MJ, et al. Purification and characterization of poliovirus polypeptide 3CD, a proteinase and a precursor for RNA polymerase. *J Virol* 1992;66(12):7481–7489.
284. Harris KS, Xiang W, Alexander L, et al. Interaction of poliovirus polypeptide 3CDpro with the 5′ and 3′ termini of the poliovirus genome. Identification of viral and cellular cofactors needed for efficient binding. *J Biol Chem* 1994;269(43):27004–27014.
285. Harutyunyan S, Kumar M, Sedivy A, et al. Viral uncoating is directional: exit of the genomic RNA in a common cold virus starts with the poly-(A) tail at the 3′-end. *PLoS Pathog* 2013;9(4):e1003270.
286. He Y, Bowman VD, Mueller S, et al. Interaction of the poliovirus receptor with poliovirus. *Proc Natl Acad Sci U S A* 2000;97(1):79–84.
287. He Y, Chipman PR, Howitt J, et al. Interaction of coxsackievirus B3 with the full length coxsackievirus-adenovirus receptor. *Nat Struct Biol* 2001;8(10):874–878.
288. Heikkila O, Merilahti P, Hakanen M, et al. Integrins are not essential for entry of coxsackievirus A9 into SW480 human colon adenocarcinoma cells. *Virol J* 2016;13(1):171.
289. Hellen CU, Witherell GW, Schmid M, et al. A cytoplasmic 57-kDa protein that is required for translation of picornavirus RNA by internal ribosomal entry is identical to the nuclear pyrimidine tract-binding protein. *Proc Natl Acad Sci U S A* 1993;90(16):7642–7646.
290. Herold J, Andino R. Poliovirus requires a precise 5′ end for efficient positive-strand RNA synthesis. *J Virol* 2000;74(14):6394–6400.
291. Herold J, Andino R. Poliovirus RNA replication requires genome circularization through a protein-protein bridge. *Mol Cell* 2001;7(3):581–591.
292. Hertz MI, Landry DM, Willis AE, et al. Ribosomal protein S25 dependency reveals a common mechanism for diverse internal ribosome entry sites and ribosome shunting. *Mol Cell Biol* 2013;33(5):1016–1026.
293. Hewat EA, Blaas D. Cryoelectron microscopy analysis of the structural changes associated with human rhinovirus type 14 uncoating. *J Virol* 2004;78(6):2935–2942.
294. Hewat EA, Neumann E, Blaas D. The concerted conformational changes during human rhinovirus 2 uncoating. *Mol Cell* 2002;10(2):317–326.
295. Hewlett MJ, Rose JK, Baltimore D. 5′-terminal structure of poliovirus polyribosomal RNA is pUp. *Proc Natl Acad Sci U S A* 1976;73:327–330.
296. Hindiyeh M, Li QH, Basavappa R, et al. Poliovirus mutants at histidine 195 of VP2 do not cleave VP0 into VP2 and VP4. *J Virol* 1999;73(11):9072–9079.
297. Hinton TM, Ross-Smith N, Warner S, et al. Conservation of L and 3C proteinase activities across distantly related aphthoviruses. *J Gen Virol* 2002;83(Pt 12):3111–3121.
298. Hiremath CN, Grant RA, Filman DJ, et al. The binding of the anti-viral drug WIN51711 to the Sabin strain of type 3 poliovirus: structural comparison with drug binding to rhinovirus 14. *Acta Crystallogr D Biol Crystallogr* 1995;51(Pt 4):473–489.
299. Ho BC, Yu SL, Chen JJ, et al. Enterovirus-induced miR-141 contributes to shutoff of host protein translation by targeting the translation initiation factor eIF4E. *Cell Host Microbe* 2011;9(1):58–69.
300. Hobdey SE, Kempf BJ, Steil BP, et al. Poliovirus polymerase residue 5 plays a critical role in elongation complex stability. *J Virol* 2010;84(16):8072–8084.
301. Hobson SD, Rosenblum ES, Richards OC, et al. Oligomeric structures of poliovirus polymerase are important for function. *EMBO J* 2001;20(5):1153–1163.
302. Hofer F, Gruenberger M, Kowalski H, et al. Members of the low density lipoprotein receptor family mediate cell entry of a minor-group common cold virus. *Proc Natl Acad Sci U S A* 1994;91(5):1839–1842.
303. Hogle JM, Chow M, Filman DJ. Three-dimensional structure of poliovirus at 2.9 A resolution. *Science* 1985;229(4720):1358–1365.
304. Holmblat B, Jegouic S, Muslin C, et al. Nonhomologous recombination between defective poliovirus and coxsackievirus genomes suggests a new model of genetic plasticity for picornaviruses. *MBio* 2014;5(4):e01119-14.
305. Holt M, Varoqueaux F, Wiederhold K, et al. Identification of SNAP-47, a novel Qbc-SNARE with ubiquitous expression. *J Biol Chem* 2006;281(25):17076–17083.
306. Hope DA, Diamond SE, Kirkegaard K. Genetic dissection of interaction between poliovirus 3D polymerase and viral protein 3AB. *J Virol* 1997;71(12):9490–9498.
307. Hsu NY, Ilnytska O, Belov G, et al. Viral reorganization of the secretory pathway generates distinct organelles for RNA replication. *Cell* 2010;141(5):799–811.
308. Huang Y, Eckstein F, Padilla R, et al. Mechanism of ribose 2′-group discrimination by an RNA polymerase. *Biochemistry* 1997;36(27):8231–8242.
309. Huber SA. VCAM-1 is a receptor for encephalomyocarditis virus on murine vascular endothelial cells. *J Virol* 1994;68(6):3453–3458.
310. Hughes PJ, Horsnell C, Hyypia T, et al. The coxsackievirus A9 RGD motif is not essential for virus viability. *J Virol* 1995;69(12):8035–8040.
311. Hunt SL, Hsuan JJ, Totty N, et al. unr, a cellular cytoplasmic RNA-binding protein with five cold-shock domains, is required for internal initiation of translation of human rhinovirus RNA. *Genes Dev* 1999;13(4):437–448.
312. Hunt SL, Jackson RJ. Polypyrimidine-tract binding protein (PTB) is necessary, but not sufficient, for efficient internal initiation of translation of human rhinovirus-2 RNA. *RNA* 1999;5(3):344–359.
313. Hurley JH. The ESCRT complexes. *Crit Rev Biochem Mol Biol* 2010;45(6):463–487.
314. ICTV. *International Committee for the Taxonomy of Viruses.* 2018. Available at: https://talk.ictvonline.org
315. Ida-Hosonuma M, Iwasaki T, Yoshikawa T, et al. The alpha/beta interferon response controls tissue tropism and pathogenicity of poliovirus. *J Virol* 2005;79(7):4460–4469.
316. Ida-Hosonuma M, Sasaki Y, Toyoda H, et al. Host range of poliovirus is restricted to simians because of a rapid sequence change of the poliovirus receptor gene during evolution. *Arch Virol* 2003;148(1):29–44.
317. Ilnytska O, Santiana M, Hsu NY, et al. Enteroviruses harness the cellular endocytic machinery to remodel the host cell cholesterol landscape for effective viral replication. *Cell Host Microbe* 2013;14(3):281–293.
318. Imamura T, Okamoto M, Nakakita S, et al. Antigenic and receptor binding properties of enterovirus 68. *J Virol* 2014;88(5):2374–2384.
319. Ishikawa-Sasaki K, Sasaki J, Taniguchi K. A complex comprising phosphatidylinositol 4-kinase IIIbeta, ACBD3, and Aichi virus proteins enhances phosphatidylinositol 4-phosphate synthesis and is critical for formation of the viral replication complex. *J Virol* 2014;88(12):6586–6598.
320. Israelsson S, Gullberg M, Jonsson N, et al. Studies of Echovirus 5 interactions with the cell surface: heparan sulfate mediates attachment to the host cell. *Virus Res* 2010;151(2):170–176.
321. Itakura E, Kishi-Itakura C, Mizushima N. The hairpin-type tail-anchored SNARE syntaxin 17 targets to autophagosomes for fusion with endosomes/lysosomes. *Cell* 2012;151(6):1256–1269.
322. Jackson T, Clark S, Berryman S, et al. Integrin alphavbeta8 functions as a receptor for foot-and-mouth disease virus: role of the beta-chain cytodomain in integrin-mediated infection. *J Virol* 2004;78(9):4533–4540.
323. Jackson T, Ellard FM, Ghazaleh RA, et al. Efficient infection of cells in culture by type O foot-and-mouth disease virus requires binding to cell surface heparan sulfate. *J Virol* 1996;70(8):5282–5287.
324. Jackson WT, Giddings TH Jr, Taylor MP, et al. Subversion of cellular autophagosomal machinery by RNA viruses. *PLoS Biol* 2005;3(5):e156.
325. Jackson RJ, Hunt SL, Reynolds JE, et al. Cap-dependent and cap-independent translation—operational distinctions and mechanistic interpretations. *Curr Top Microbiol Immunol* 1995;203:1–29.
326. Jackson T, Mould AP, Sheppard D, et al. Integrin alphavbeta1 is a receptor for foot-and-mouth disease virus. *J Virol* 2002;76(3):935–941.
327. Jacobson MF, Baltimore D. Morphogenesis of poliovirus I. Association of the viral RNA with coat protein. *J Mol Biol* 1968;3:369–378.
328. Jacobson SJ, Konings DA, Sarnow P. Biochemical and genetic evidence for a pseudoknot structure at the 3′ terminus of the poliovirus RNA genome and its role in viral RNA amplification. *J Virol* 1993;67(6):2961–2971.
329. Jan E, Sarnow P. Factorless ribosome assembly on the internal ribosome entry site of cricket paralysis virus. *J Mol Biol* 2002;324(5):889–902.
330. Jang SK, Krausslich H-G, Nicklin MJH, et al. A segment of the 5′ nontranslated region of encephalomyocarditis virus RNA directs internal entry of ribosomes during in vitro translation. *J Virol* 1988;62:2636–2643.
331. Jarvis TC, Kirkegaard K. Poliovirus RNA recombination: mechanistic studies in the absence of selection. *EMBO J* 1992;11(8):3135–3145.
332. Jayawardena N, Burga LN, Easingwood RA, et al. Structural basis for anthrax toxin receptor 1 recognition by Seneca Valley virus. *Proc Natl Acad Sci U S A* 2018;115(46):E10934–E10940.
333. Jia XY, Summers DF, Ehrenfeld E. Primary cleavage of the HAV capsid protein precursor in the middle of the proposed 2A coding region. *Virology* 1993;193(1):515–519.
334. Jiang P, Liu Y, Ma HC, et al. Picornavirus morphogenesis. *Microbiol Mol Biol Rev* 2014;78(3):418–437.
335. Jiang P, Nishimura T, Sakamaki Y, et al. The HOPS complex mediates autophagosome-lysosome fusion through interaction with syntaxin 17. *Mol Biol Cell* 2014;25(8):1327–1337.
336. Jimenez-Clavero MA, Douglas A, Lavery T, et al. Immune recognition of swine vesicular disease virus structural proteins: novel antigenic regions that are not exposed in the capsid. *Virology* 2000;270(1):76–83.
337. Joachims M, Van Breugel PC, Lloyd RE. Cleavage of poly(A)-binding protein by enterovirus proteases concurrent with inhibition of translation in vitro. *J Virol* 1999;73(1):718–727.
338. Johansson S, Niklasson B, Maizel J, et al. Molecular analysis of three Ljungan virus isolates reveals a new, close-to-root lineage of the Picornaviridae with a cluster of two unrelated 2A proteins. *J Virol* 2002;76(17):8920–8930.
339. Johns HL, Berryman S, Monaghan P, et al. A dominant-negative mutant of rab5 inhibits infection of cells by foot-and-mouth disease virus: implications for virus entry. *J Virol* 2009;83(12):6247–6256.
340. Johnson KL, Sarnow P. Three poliovirus 2B mutants exhibit noncomplementable defects in viral RNA amplification and display dosage-dependent dominance over wild-type poliovirus. *J Virol* 1991;65(8):4341–4349.
341. Joklik WK, Darnell JE Jr. The adsorption and early fate of purified poliovirus in HeLa cells. *Virology* 1961;13:439–447.
342. Jore J, De Geus B, Jackson RJ, et al. Poliovirus protein 3CD is the active protease for processing of the precursor protein P1 in vitro. *J Gen Virol* 1988;69(Pt 7):1627–1636.

343. Jurgens CK, Barton DJ, Sharma N, et al. 2Apro is a multifunctional protein that regulates the stability, translation and replication of poliovirus RNA. *Virology* 2006;345(2):346–357.

344. Jurgens C, Flanegan JB. Initiation of poliovirus negative-strand RNA synthesis requires precursor forms of p2 proteins. *J Virol* 2003;77(2):1075–1083.

345. Kafasla P, Morgner N, Poyry TA, et al. Polypyrimidine tract binding protein stabilizes the encephalomyocarditis virus IRES structure via binding multiple sites in a unique orientation. *Mol Cell* 2009;34(5):556–568.

346. Kafasla P, Morgner N, Robinson CV, et al. Polypyrimidine tract-binding protein stimulates the poliovirus IRES by modulating eIF4G binding. *EMBO J* 2010;29(21):3710–3722.

347. Kaku Y, Murakami Y, Sarai A, et al. Antigenic properties of porcine teschovirus 1 (PTV-1) Talfan strain and molecular strategy for serotyping of PTVs. *Arch Virol* 2007;152(5):929–940.

348. Kaminski A, Hunt SL, Patton JG, et al. Direct evidence that polypyrimidine tract binding protein (PTB) is essential for internal initiation of translation of encephalomyocarditis virus RNA. *RNA* 1995;1(9):924–938.

349. Kaminski A, Jackson RJ. The polypyrimidine tract binding protein (PTB) requirement for internal initiation of translation of cardiovirus RNAs is conditional rather than absolute. *RNA* 1998;4(6):626–638.

350. Kaplan G, Racaniello VR. Construction and characterization of poliovirus subgenomic replicons. *J Virol* 1988;62(5):1687–1696.

351. Kaplan G, Totsuka A, Thompson P, et al. Identification of a surface glycoprotein on African green monkey kidney cells as a receptor for hepatitis A virus. *EMBO J* 1996;15(16):4282–4296.

352. Karjalainen M, Rintanen N, Lehkonen M, et al. Echovirus 1 infection depends on biogenesis of novel multivesicular bodies. *Cell Microbiol* 2011;13(12):1975–1995.

353. Karnauchow TM, Tolson DL, Harrison BA, et al. The HeLa cell receptor for enterovirus 70 is decay-accelerating factor (CD55). *J Virol* 1996;70(8):5143–5152.

354. Katpally U, Fu TM, Freed DC, et al. Antibodies to the buried N terminus of rhinovirus VP4 exhibit cross-serotypic neutralization. *J Virol* 2009;83(14):7040–7048.

355. Katpally U, Smith TJ. Pocket factors are unlikely to play a major role in the life cycle of human rhinovirus. *J Virol* 2007;81(12):6307–6315.

356. Kean KM, Teterina NL, Marc D, et al. Analysis of putative active site residues of the poliovirus 3C protease. *Virology* 1991;181(2):609–619.

357. Kempf BJ, Kelly MM, Springer CL, et al. Structural features of a picornavirus polymerase involved in the polyadenylation of viral RNA. *J Virol* 2013;87(10):5629–5644.

358. Kempf BJ, Peersen OB, Barton DJ. Poliovirus Polymerase Leu420 Facilitates RNA Recombination and Ribavirin Resistance. *J Virol* 2016;90(19):8410–8421.

359. Kerekatte V, Keiper BD, Badorff C, et al. Cleavage of Poly(A)-binding protein by coxsackievirus 2A protease in vitro and in vivo: another mechanism for host protein synthesis shutoff? *J Virol* 1999;73(1):709–717.

360. Khetsuriani N, Lamonte-Fowlkes A, Oberst S, et al.; Centers for Disease Control and Prevention. Enterovirus surveillance—United States, 1970–2005. *MMWR Surveill Summ* 2006;55(8):1–20.

361. Khong A, Jan E. Modulation of stress granules and P bodies during dicistrovirus infection. *J Virol* 2011;85(4):1439–1451.

362. Kim C, Bergelson JM. Echovirus 7 entry into polarized intestinal epithelial cells requires clathrin and rab7. *MBio* 2012;3(2):e00304-11.

363. Kim YK, Jang SK. La protein is required for efficient translation driven by encephalomyocarditis virus internal ribosomal entry site. *J Gen Virol* 1999;80(Pt 12):3159–3166.

364. Kim SS, Smith TJ, Chapman MS, et al. Crystal structure of human rhinovirus serotype 1A (HRV1A). *J Mol Biol* 1989;210(1):91–111.

365. Kim DS, Son KY, Koo KM, et al. Porcine sapelovirus uses alpha2,3-linked sialic acid on GD1a ganglioside as a receptor. *J Virol* 2016;90(8):4067–4077.

366. King AM. Preferred sites of recombination in poliovirus RNA: an analysis of 40 intertypic cross-over sequences. *Nucleic Acids Res* 1988;16(24):11705–11723.

367. Kirchweger R, Ziegler E, Lamphear BJ, et al. Foot-and-mouth disease virus leader proteinase: purification of the Lb form and determination of its cleavage site on eIF-4 gamma. *J Virol* 1994;68(9):5677–5684.

368. Kirkegaard K, Baltimore D. The mechanism of RNA recombination in poliovirus. *Cell* 1986;47(3):433–443.

369. Kitamura N, Semler BL, Rothberg PG, et al. Primary structure, gene organization and polypeptide expression of poliovirus RNA. *Nature* 1981;291:547–553.

370. Kitson JD, McCahon D, Belsham GJ. Sequence analysis of monoclonal antibody resistant mutants of type O foot and mouth disease virus: evidence for the involvement of the three surface exposed capsid proteins in four antigenic sites. *Virology* 1990;179(1):26–34.

371. Kjaer J, Belsham GJ. Modifications to the foot-and-mouth disease virus 2A peptide: influence on polyprotein processing and virus replication. *J Virol* 2018;92(8):e02218-17.

372. Kjaer J, Belsham GJ. Selection of functional 2A sequences within foot-and-mouth disease virus; requirements for the NPGP motif with a distinct codon bias. *RNA* 2018;24(1):12–17.

373. Klein M, Hadaschik D, Zimmermann H, et al. The picornavirus replication inhibitors HBB and guanidine in the echovirus-9 system: the significance of viral protein 2C. *J Gen Virol* 2000;81(Pt 4):895–901.

374. Kliewer S, Dasgupta A. An RNA polymerase II transcription factor inactivated in poliovirus-infected cells copurified with transcription factor TFIID. *Mol Cell Biol* 1988;8:3175–3182.

375. Kloc A, Rai DK, Rieder E. The roles of picornavirus untranslated regions in infection and innate immunity. *Front Microbiol* 2018;9:485.

376. Knipe T, Rieder E, Baxt B, et al. Characterization of synthetic foot-and-mouth disease virus provirions separates acid-mediated disassembly from infectivity. *J Virol* 1997;71(4):2851–2856.

377. Knowles NJ. The Picornavirus Pages. 2018. Available at: http://www.picornaviridae.com/unassigned/unassigned.htm

378. Knox C, Luke GA, Blatch GL, et al. Heat shock protein 40 (Hsp40) plays a key role in the virus life cycle. *Virus Res* 2011;160(1–2):15–24.

379. Koike S, Ise I, Nomoto A. Functional domains of the poliovirus receptor. *Proc Natl Acad Sci U S A* 1991;88:4104–4108.

380. Koike S, Taya C, Kurata T, et al. Transgenic mice susceptible to poliovirus. *Proc Natl Acad Sci U S A* 1991;88(3):951–955.

381. Kolatkar PR, Bella J, Olson NH, et al. Structural studies of two rhinovirus serotypes complexed with fragments of their cellular receptor. *EMBO J* 1999;18(22):6249–6259.

382. Kolupaeva VG, Lomakin IB, Pestova TV, et al. Eukaryotic initiation factors 4G and 4A mediate conformational changes downstream of the initiation codon of the encephalomyocarditis virus internal ribosomal entry site. *Mol Cell Biol* 2003;23(2):687–698.

383. Konecsni T, Berka U, Pickl-Herk A, et al. Low pH-triggered beta-propeller switch of the low-density lipoprotein receptor assists rhinovirus infection. *J Virol* 2009;83(21):10922–10930.

384. Kong WP, Roos RP. Alternative translation initiation site in the DA strain of Theiler's murine encephalomyelitis virus. *J Virol* 1991;65(6):3395–3399.

385. Krausslich HG, Holscher C, Reuer Q, et al. Myristoylation of the poliovirus polyprotein is required for proteolytic processing of the capsid and for viral infectivity. *J Virol* 1990;64(5):2433–2436.

386. Kusov YY, Probst C, Jecht M, et al. Membrane association and RNA binding of recombinant hepatitis A virus protein 2C. *Arch Virol* 1998;143(5):931–944.

387. Kuyumcu-Martinez NM, Joachims M, Lloyd RE. Efficient cleavage of ribosome-associated poly(A)-binding protein by enterovirus 3C protease. *J Virol* 2002;76(5):2062–2074.

388. Kuznetsov YG, Daijogo S, Zhou J, et al. Atomic force microscopy analysis of icosahedral virus RNA. *J Mol Biol* 2005;347(1):41–52.

389. Kwan T, Thompson SR. Noncanonical translation initiation in eukaryotes. *Cold Spring Harb Perspect Biol* 2019;11(4).

390. Lama J, Sanz MA, Carrasco L. Genetic analysis of poliovirus protein 3A: characterization of a non-cytopathic mutant virus defective in killing Vero cells. *J Gen Virol* 1998;79 (Pt 8):1911–1921.

391. Lamphear BJ, Yan R, Yang F, et al. Mapping the cleavage site in protein synthesis initiation factor eIF-4 gamma of the 2A proteases from human Coxsackievirus and rhinovirus. *J Biol Chem* 1993;268(26):19200–19203.

392. Landajuela A, Hervas JH, Anton Z, et al. Lipid geometry and bilayer curvature modulate LC3/GABARAP-mediated model autophagosomal elongation. *Biophys J* 2016;110(2):411–422.

393. Landsteiner K, Popper E. Mikroscopische präparate von einem menschlichen und zwei affentückermarker. *Wien Klin Wochenschr* 1908;21:1930.

394. Lang M, Mirand A, Savy N, et al. Acute flaccid paralysis following enterovirus D68 associated pneumonia, France, 2014. *Euro Surveill* 2014;19(44).

395. Langereis MA, Feng Q, Nelissen FH, et al. Modification of picornavirus genomic RNA using 'click' chemistry shows that unlinking of the VPg peptide is dispensable for translation and replication of the incoming viral RNA. *Nucleic Acids Res* 2014;42(4):2473–2482.

396. Lanke KH, van der Schaar HM, Belov GA, et al. GBF1, a guanine nucleotide exchange factor for Arf, is crucial for coxsackievirus B3 RNA replication. *J Virol* 2009;83(22):11940–11949.

397. Lau C, Wang X, Song L, et al. Syk associates with clathrin and mediates phosphatidylinositol 3-kinase activation during human rhinovirus internalization. *J Immunol* 2008;180(2):870–880.

398. Laufman O, Perrino J, Andino R. Viral generated inter-organelle contacts redirect lipid flux for genome replication. *Cell* 2019;178(2):275–289.e16.

399. Lauring AS, Acevedo A, Cooper SB, et al. Codon usage determines the mutational robustness, evolutionary capacity, and virulence of an RNA virus. *Cell Host Microbe* 2012;12(5):623–632.

400. Lea SM, Powell RM, McKee T, et al. Determination of the affinity and kinetic constants for the interaction between the human virus echovirus 11 and its cellular receptor, CD55. *J Biol Chem* 1998;273(46):30443–30447.

401. Lee KM, Chen CJ, Shih SR. Regulation mechanisms of viral IRES-driven translation. *Trends Microbiol* 2017;25(7):546–561.

402. Lee YF, Nomoto A, Detjen BM, et al. A protein covalently linked to poliovirus genome RNA. *Proc Natl Acad Sci U S A* 1977;74(1):59–63.

403. Lee H, Shingler KL, Organtini LJ, et al. The novel asymmetric entry intermediate of a picornavirus captured with nanodiscs. *Sci Adv* 2016;2(8):e1501929.

404. Lentz KN, Smith AD, Geisler SC, et al. Structure of poliovirus type 2 Lansing complexed with antiviral agent SCH48973: comparison of the structural and biological properties of three poliovirus serotypes. *Structure* 1997;5(7):961–978.

405. Levy HC, Bostina M, Filman DJ, et al. Catching a virus in the act of RNA release: a novel poliovirus uncoating intermediate characterized by cryo-electron microscopy. *J Virol* 2010;84(9):4426–4441.

406. Lewis JK, Bothner B, Smith TJ, et al. Antiviral agent blocks breathing of the common cold virus. *Proc Natl Acad Sci U S A* 1998;95(12):6774–6778.

407. Li JP, Baltimore D. An intragenic revertant of a poliovirus 2C mutant has an uncoating defect. *J Virol* 1990;64(3):1102–1107.

408. Li J, Buchner J. Structure, function and regulation of the hsp90 machinery. *Biomed J* 2013;36(3):106–117.

409. Li T, Chen Z, Johnson JE, et al Conformations, interactions, and thermostabilities of RNA and proteins in bean pod mottle virus: investigation of solution and crystal structures by laser Raman spectroscopy. *Biochemistry* 1992;31(29):6673–6682.

410. Li Q, Yafal AG, Lee YM, et al. Poliovirus neutralization by antibodies to internal epitopes of VP4 and VP1 results from reversible exposure of these sequences at physiological temperature. *J Virol* 1994;68(6):3965–3970.

411. Liao S, Racaniello V. Allele-specific adaptation of poliovirus VP1 B-C loop variants to mutant cell receptors. *J Virol* 1997;71(12):9770–9777.

412. Limpens RW, van der Schaar HM, Kumar D, et al. The transformation of enterovirus replication structures: a three-dimensional study of single- and double-membrane compartments. *MBio* 2011;2(5):e00166-11.

413. Lin J, Cheng N, Chow M, et al. An externalized polypeptide partitions between two distinct sites on genome-released poliovirus particles. *J Virol* 2011;85(19):9974–9983.

414. Lin TA, Kong X, Haystead TA, et al. PHAS-I as a link between mitogen-activated protein kinase and translation initiation [see comments]. *Science* 1994;266(5185):653–656.

415. Lipton HL, Kumar AS, Hertzler S, et al. Differential usage of carbohydrate co-receptors influences cellular tropism of Theiler's murine encephalomyelitis virus infection of the central nervous system. *Glycoconj J* 2006;23(1–2):39–49.

416. Liu Y, Hill MG, Klose T, et al. Atomic structure of a rhinovirus C, a virus species linked to severe childhood asthma. *Proc Natl Acad Sci U S A* 2016;113(32):8997–9002.

417. Liu Y, Sheng J, Fokine A, et al. Structure and inhibition of EV-D68, a virus that causes respiratory illness in children. *Science* 2015;347(6217):71–74.

418. Liu Y, Sheng J, Rossmann MG. Molecular basis for the acid initiated uncoating of human enterovirus D68. *Proc Natl Acad Sci U S A* 2018;115(52):E12209–E12217.

419. Liu Y, Wang C, Mueller S, et al. Direct interaction between two viral proteins, the nonstructural protein 2C and the capsid protein VP3, is required for enterovirus morphogenesis. *PLoS Pathog* 2010;6(8):e1001066.

420. Liu J, Wei T, Kwang J. Avian encephalomyelitis virus nonstructural protein 2C induces apoptosis by activating cytochrome c/caspase-9 pathway. *Virology* 2004;318(1):169–182.

421. Lobert PE, Escriou N, Ruelle J, et al. A coding RNA sequence acts as a replication signal in cardioviruses. *Proc Natl Acad Sci U S A* 1999;96(20):11560–11565.

422. Loeffler F, Frosch P. Report of the Commission for Research on foot-and-mouth disease. In: Hahon N, ed. *Selected Papers on Virology.* Englewood Cliffs: Prentice-Hall; 1964:64–68.

423. Logan D, Abu-Ghazaleh R, Blakemore W, et al. Structure of a major immunogenic site on foot-and-mouth disease virus. *Nature* 1993;362(6420):566–568.

424. Love RA, Maegley KA, Yu X, et al. The crystal structure of the RNA-dependent RNA polymerase from human rhinovirus: a dual function target for common cold antiviral therapy. *Structure* 2004;12(8):1533–1544.

425. Lowry K, Woodman A, Cook J, et al. Recombination in enteroviruses is a biphasic replicative process involving the generation of greater-than genome length 'imprecise' intermediates. *PLoS Pathog* 2014;10(6):e1004191.

426. Lozano E, Dominguez-Villar M, Kuchroo V, et al. The TIGIT/CD226 axis regulates human T cell function. *J Immunol* 2012;188(8):3869–3875.

427. Lukashev AN. Recombination among picornaviruses. *Rev Med Virol* 2010;20(5):327–337.

428. Lulla V, Dinan AM, Hosmillo M, et al. An upstream protein-coding region in enteroviruses modulates virus infection in gut epithelial cells. *Nat Microbiol* 2018;4(2):280–292.

429. Lyle JM, Bullitt E, Bienz K, et al. Visualization and functional analysis of RNA-dependent RNA polymerase lattices. *Science* 2002;296(5576):2218–2222.

430. Lyle JM, Clewell A, Richmond K, et al. Similar structural basis for membrane localization and protein priming by an RNA-dependent RNA polymerase. *J Biol Chem* 2002;277(18):16324–16331.

431. Ma HC, Liu Y, Wang C, et al. An interaction between glutathione and the capsid is required for the morphogenesis of C-cluster enteroviruses. *PLoS Pathog* 2014;10(4):e1004052.

432. Macejak DG, Sarnow P. Internal initiation of translation mediated by the 5′ leader of a cellular mRNA. *Nature* 1991;353:90–94.

433. Macejak DG, Sarnow P. Association of heat shock protein 70 with enterovirus capsid precursor P1 in infected human cells. *J Virol* 1992;66(3):1520–1527.

434. Maciejewski S, Nguyen JH, Gomez-Herreros F, et al. Divergent requirement for a DNA repair enzyme during enterovirus infections. *MBio* 2015;7(1):e01931-15.

435. Maciejewski S, Ullmer W, Semler BL. VPg unlinkase/TDP2 in cardiovirus infected cells: re-localization and proteolytic cleavage. *Virology* 2018;516:139–146.

436. Malik N, Kotecha A, Gold S, et al. Structures of foot and mouth disease virus pentamers: insight into capsid dissociation and unexpected pentamer reassociation. *PLoS Pathog* 2017;13(9):e1006607.

437. Maloney JA, Mirsky DM, Messacar K, et al. MRI findings in children with acute flaccid paralysis and cranial nerve dysfunction occurring during the 2014 enterovirus D68 outbreak. *AJNR Am J Neuroradiol* 2015;36(2):245–250.

438. Marc D, Drugeon G, Haenni AL, et al. Role of myristoylation of poliovirus capsid protein VP4 as determined by site-directed mutagenesis of its N-terminal sequence. *EMBO J* 1989;8(9):2661–2668.

439. Marc D, Girard M, van der Werf S. A Gly1 to Ala substitution in poliovirus capsid protein VP0 blocks its myristoylation and prevents viral assembly. *J Gen Virol* 1991;72(Pt 5):1151–1157.

440. Marc D, Masson G, Girard M, et al. Lack of myristoylation of poliovirus capsid polypeptide VP0 prevents the formation of virions or results in the assembly of noninfectious virus particles. *J Virol* 1990;64(9):4099–4107.

441. Marjomaki V, Pietiainen V, Matilainen H, et al. Internalization of echovirus 1 in caveolae. *J Virol* 2002;76(4):1856–1865.

442. Martin-Acebes MA, Gonzalez-Magaldi M, Sandvig K, et al. Productive entry of type C foot-and-mouth disease virus into susceptible cultured cells requires clathrin and is dependent on the presence of plasma membrane cholesterol. *Virology* 2007;369(1):105–118.

443. Martin-Acebes MA, Rincon V, Armas-Portela R, et al. A single amino acid substitution in the capsid of foot-and-mouth disease virus can increase acid lability and confer resistance to acid-dependent uncoating inhibition. *J Virol* 2010;84(6):2902–2912.

444. Martin-Acebes MA, Vazquez-Calvo A, Rincon V, et al. A single amino acid substitution in the capsid of foot-and-mouth disease virus can increase acid resistance. *J Virol* 2011;85(6):2733–2740.

445. Martinez MA, Verdaguer N, Mateu MG, et al. Evolution subverting essentiality: dispensability of the cell attachment Arg-Gly-Asp motif in multiply passaged foot-and-mouth disease virus. *Proc Natl Acad Sci U S A* 1997;94(13):6798–6802.

446. Mason PW, Baxt B, Brown F, et al. Antibody-complexed foot-and-mouth disease virus, but not poliovirus, can infect normally insusceptible cells via the Fc receptor. *Virology* 1993;192:568–577.

447. Mason PW, Bezborodova SV, Henry TM. Identification and characterization of a cis-acting replication element (cre) adjacent to the internal ribosome entry site of foot-and-mouth disease virus. *J Virol* 2002;76(19):9686–9694.

448. Mason PW, Rieder E, Baxt B. RGD sequence of foot-and-mouth disease virus is essential for infecting cells via the natural receptor but can be bypassed by an antibody-dependent enhancement pathway. *Proc Natl Acad Sci U S A* 1994;91(5):1932–1936.

449. Matthews DA, Smith WW, Ferre RA, et al. Structure of human rhinovirus 3C protease reveals a trypsin-like polypeptide fold, RNA-binding site, and means for cleaving precursor polyprotein. *Cell* 1994;77(5):761–771.

450. McClelland A, deBear J, Yost SC, et al. Identification of monoclonal antibody epitopes and critical residues for rhinovirus binding in domain 1 of ICAM-1. *Proc Natl Acad Sci U S A* 1991;88:7993–7997.

451. McDermott BM Jr, Rux AH, Eisenberg RJ, et al. Two distinct binding affinities of poliovirus for its cellular receptor. *J Biol Chem* 2000;275(30):23089–23096.

452. McErlean P, Shackelton LA, Andrews E, et al. Distinguishing molecular features and clinical characteristics of a putative new rhinovirus species, human rhinovirus C (HRV C). *PLoS One* 2008;3(4):e1847.

453. McKnight KL, Lemon SM. Capsid coding sequence is required for efficient replication of human rhinovirus 14 RNA. *J Virol* 1996;70(3):1941–1952.

454. McKnight KL, Lemon SM. The rhinovirus type 14 genome contains an internally located RNA structure that is required for viral replication. *RNA* 1998;4(12):1569–1584.

455. McSharry JJ, Caliguiri LA, Eggers HJ. Inhibition of uncoating of poliovirus by arildone, a new antiviral drug. *Virology* 1979;97(2):307–315.

456. Meerovitch K, Svitkin YV, Lee HS, et al. La autoantigen enhances and corrects aberrant translation of poliovirus RNA in reticulocyte lysate. *J Virol* 1993;67(7):3798–3807.

457. Meister A, Anderson ME. Glutathione. *Annu Rev Biochem* 1983;52:711–760.

458. Melia CE, van der Schaar HM, de Jong AWM, et al. The origin, dynamic morphology, and PI4P-independent formation of encephalomyocarditis virus replication organelles. *MBio* 2018;9(2):e00420-18.

459. Melia CE, van der Schaar HM, Lyoo H, et al. Escaping host factor PI4KB inhibition: enterovirus genomic RNA replication in the absence of replication organelles. *Cell Rep* 2017;21(3):587–599.

460. Mendelsohn CL, Wimmer E, Racaniello VR. Cellular receptor for poliovirus: molecular cloning, nucleotide sequence, and expression of a new member of the immunoglobulin superfamily. *Cell* 1989;56(5):855–865.

461. Mesmin B, Bigay J, Moser von Filseck J, Lacas-Gervais S, et al. A four-step cycle driven by PI(4)P hydrolysis directs sterol/PI(4)P exchange by the ER-Golgi tether OSBP. *Cell* 2013;155(4):830–843.

462. Messacar K, Schreiner TL, Maloney JA, et al. A cluster of acute flaccid paralysis and cranial nerve dysfunction temporally associated with an outbreak of enterovirus D68 in children in Colorado, USA. *Lancet* 2015;385(9978):1662–1671.

463. Michel YM, Borman AM, Paulous S, et al. Eukaryotic initiation factor 4G-poly(A) binding protein interaction is required for poly(A) tail-mediated stimulation of picornavirus internal ribosome entry segment-driven translation but not for X-mediated stimulation of hepatitis C virus translation. *Mol Cell Biol* 2001;21(13):4097–4109.

464. Midgley SE, Christiansen CB, Poulsen MW, et al. Emergence of enterovirus D68 in Denmark, June 2014 to February 2015. *Euro Surveill* 2015;20(17):21105.

465. Midgley CM, Jackson MA, Selvarangan R, et al. Severe respiratory illness associated with enterovirus D68—Missouri and Illinois, 2014. *MMWR Morb Mortal Wkly Rep* 2014;63(36):798–799.

466. Midgley CM, Watson JT, Nix WA, et al. Severe respiratory illness associated with a nationwide outbreak of enterovirus D68 in the USA (2014): a descriptive epidemiological investigation. *Lancet Respir Med* 2015;3(11):879–887.

467. Miles LA, Burga LN, Gardner EE, et al. Anthrax toxin receptor 1 is the cellular receptor for Seneca Valley virus. *J Clin Invest* 2017;127(8):2957–2967.

468. Minor PD, Ferguson M, Evans DM, et al. Antigenic structure of polioviruses of serotypes 1, 2 and 3. *J Gen Virol* 1986;67(Pt 7):1283–1291.

469. Minor PD, Schild GC, Bootman J, et al. Location and primary structure of a major antigenic site for poliovirus neutralization. *Nature* 1983;301(5902):674–679.

470. Mistry N, Inoue H, Jamshidi F, et al. Coxsackievirus A24 variant uses sialic acid-containing O-linked glycoconjugates as cellular receptors on human ocular cells. *J Virol* 2011;85(21):11283–11290.

471. Moffat K, Howell G, Knox C, et al. Effects of foot-and-mouth disease virus nonstructural proteins on the structure and function of the early secretory pathway: 2BC but not 3A blocks endoplasmic reticulum to Golgi transport. *J Virol* 2005;79(7):4382–4395.

472. Mohamud Y, Shi J, Qu J, et al. Enteroviral infection inhibits autophagic flux via disruption of the SNARE complex to enhance viral replication. *Cell Rep* 2018;22(12):3292–3303.

473. Molla A, Harris KS, Paul AV, et al. Stimulation of poliovirus proteinase 3Cpro-related proteolysis by the genome-linked protein VPg and its precursor 3AB. *J Biol Chem* 1994;269(43):27015–27020.

474. Molla A, Paul AV, Schmid M, et al. Studies on dicistronic polioviruses implicate viral proteinase 2Apro in RNA replication. *Virology* 1993;196(2):739–747.

475. Molla A, Paul AV, Wimmer E. Cell-free, de novo synthesis of poliovirus. *Science* 1991;254:1647–1651.

476. Monaghan P, Cook H, Jackson T, et al. The ultrastructure of the developing replication site in foot-and-mouth disease virus-infected BHK-38 cells. *J Gen Virol* 2004;85(Pt 4):933–946.

477. Morosky S, Wells AI, Lemon K, et al. The neonatal Fc receptor is a pan-echovirus receptor. *Proc Natl Acad Sci U S A* 2019;116(9):3758–3763.

478. Morrison ME, He YJ, Wien MW, et al. Homolog-scanning mutagenesis reveals poliovirus receptor residues important for virus binding and replication. *J Virol* 1994;68(4):2578–2588.

479. Morrison ME, Racaniello VR. Molecular cloning and expression of a murine homolog of the human poliovirus receptor gene. *J Virol* 1992;66(5):2807–2813.

480. Morrison JM, Racaniello VR. Proteinase 2Apro is essential for enterovirus replication in type I interferon-treated cells. *J Virol* 2009;83(9):4412–4422.

481. Moscufo N, Chow M. Myristate-protein interactions in poliovirus: interactions of VP4 threonine 28 contribute to the structural conformation of assembly intermediates and the stability of assembled virions. *J Virol* 1992;66(12):6849–6857.

482. Moscufo N, Yafal AG, Rogove A, et al. A mutation in VP4 defines a new step in the late stages of cell entry by poliovirus. *J Virol* 1993;67(8):5075–5078.

483. Mosimann SC, Cherney MM, Sia S, et al. Refined X-ray crystallographic structure of the poliovirus 3C gene product. *J Mol Biol* 1997;273(5):1032–1047.

484. Mosser AG, Caliguiri LA, Tamm I. Incorporation of lipid precursors into cytoplasmic membranes of poliovirus-infected HeLa cells. *Virology* 1972;47(1):39–47.

485. Mosser AG, Rueckert RR. WIN 51711-dependent mutants of poliovirus type 3: evidence that virions decay after release from cells unless drug is present. *J Virol* 1993;67(3): 1246–1254.
486. Mousnier A, Bell AS, Swieboda DP, et al. Fragment-derived inhibitors of human N-myristoyltransferase block capsid assembly and replication of the common cold virus. *Nat Chem* 2018;10(6):599–606.
487. Muckelbauer JK, Kremer M, Minor I, et al. The structure of coxsackievirus B3 at 3.5 A resolution. *Structure* 1995;3(7):653–667.
488. Mueller S, Wimmer E. Recruitment of nectin-3 to cell-cell junctions through trans-heterophilic interaction with CD155, a vitronectin and poliovirus receptor that localizes to alpha(v)beta3 integrin-containing membrane microdomains. *J Biol Chem* 2003;278(33):31251–31260.
489. Mullapudi E, Novacek J, Palkova L, et al. Structure and genome release mechanism of the human cardiovirus saffold virus 3. *J Virol* 2016;90(17):7628–7639.
490. Muro S, Wiewrodt R, Thomas A, et al. A novel endocytic pathway induced by clustering endothelial ICAM-1 or PECAM-1. *J Cell Sci* 2003;116(Pt 8):1599–1609.
491. Mutsvunguma LZ, Moetlhoa B, Edkins AL, et al. Theiler's murine encephalomyelitis virus infection induces a redistribution of heat shock proteins 70 and 90 in BHK-21 cells, and is inhibited by novobiocin and geldanamycin. *Cell Stress Chaperones* 2011;16(5):505–515.
492. Nagashima S, Sasaki J, Taniguchi K. Interaction between polypeptide 3ABC and the 5′-terminal structural elements of the genome of Aichi virus: implication for negative-strand RNA synthesis. *J Virol* 2008;82(13):6161–6171.
493. Nagy PD, Strating JR, van Kuppeveld FJ. Building viral replication organelles: close encounters of the membrane Types. *PLoS Pathog* 2016;12(10):e1005912.
494. Nchoutmboube JA, Viktorova EG, Scott AJ, et al. Increased long chain acyl-Coa synthetase activity and fatty acid import is linked to membrane synthesis for development of picornavirus replication organelles. *PLoS Pathog* 2013;9(6):e1003401.
495. Neff S, Sa-Carvalho D, Rieder E, et al. Foot-and-mouth disease virus virulent for cattle utilizes the integrin alpha(v)beta3 as its receptor. *J Virol* 1998;72(5):3587–3594.
496. Nelsen-Salz B, Eggers HJ, Zimmermann H. Integrin alpha(v)beta3 (vitronectin receptor) is a candidate receptor for the virulent echovirus 9 strain Barty. *J Gen Virol* 1999;80 (Pt 9):2311–2313.
497. Neubauer C, Frasel L, Kuechler E, et al. Mechanism of entry of human rhinovirus 2 into HeLa cells. *Virology* 1987;158(1):255–258.
498. Neufeld KL, Richards OC, Ehrenfeld E. Purification, characterization and comparison of poliovirus RNA polymerase from native and recombinant sources. *J Biol Chem* 1991;266:24212–24219.
499. Newman J, Asfor AS, Berryman S, et al. The cellular chaperone heat shock protein 90 is required for foot-and-mouth disease virus capsid precursor processing and assembly of capsid pentamers. *J Virol* 2018;92(5):e01415-17.
500. Neznanov N, Kondratova A, Chumakov KM, et al. Poliovirus protein 3A inhibits tumor necrosis factor (TNF)-induced apoptosis by eliminating the TNF receptor from the cell surface. *J Virol* 2001;75(21):10409–10420.
501. NIAID. Pleconaril Enteroviral Sepsis Syndrome. 2002. Available at: http://clinicaltrials.gov/ct2/show/NCT00031512?term=pleconaril&rank=1
502. Nicklin MJ, Krausslich HG, Toyoda H, et al. Poliovirus polypeptide precursors: expression in vitro and processing by exogenous 3C and 2A proteinases. *Proc Natl Acad Sci U S A* 1987;84(12):4002–4006.
503. Niepmann M. Porcine polypyrimidine tract-binding protein stimulates translation initiation at the internal ribosome entry site of foot-and-mouth-disease virus. *FEBS Lett* 1996;388(1):39–42.
504. Nilsson EC, Jamshidi F, Johansson SM, et al. Sialic acid is a cellular receptor for coxsackievirus A24 variant, an emerging virus with pandemic potential. *J Virol* 2008;82(6): 3061–3068.
505. Nishimura Y, Shimojima M, Tano Y, et al. Human P-selectin glycoprotein ligand-1 is a functional receptor for enterovirus 71. *Nat Med* 2009;15(7):794–797.
506. Nomoto A, Detjen B, Pozzatti R, et al. The location of the polio genome protein in viral RNAs and its implication for RNA synthesis. *Nature* 1977;268(5617):208–213.
507. Nomoto A, Kitamura N, Golini F, et al. The 5′-terminal structures of poliovirion RNA and poliovirus mRNA differ only in the genome-linked protein VPg. *Proc Natl Acad Sci U S A* 1977;74(12):5345–5349.
508. Nomoto A, Lee YF, Wimmer E. The 5′ end of poliovirus mRNA is not capped with m7G(5′)ppp(5′)np. *Proc Natl Acad Sci U S A* 1976;73:375–380.
509. Novak JE, Kirkegaard K. Improved method for detecting poliovirus negative strands used to demonstrate specificity of positive-strand encapsidation and the ratio of positive to negative strands in infected cells. *J Virol* 1991;65:3384–3387.
510. Nugent CI, Johnson KL, Sarnow P, et al. Functional coupling between replication and packaging of poliovirus replicon RNA. *J Virol* 1999;73(1):427–435.
511. Nunez JI, Baranowski E, Molina N, et al. A single amino acid substitution in nonstructural protein 3A can mediate adaptation of foot-and-mouth disease virus to the guinea pig. *J Virol* 2001;75(8):3977–3983.
512. Nurani G, Lindqvist B, Casasnovas JM. Receptor priming of major group human rhinoviruses for uncoating and entry at mild low-pH environments. *J Virol* 2003;77(22): 11985–11991.
513. O'Donnell V, Larocco M, Baxt B. Heparan sulfate-binding foot-and-mouth disease virus enters cells via caveola-mediated endocytosis. *J Virol* 2008;82(18):9075–9085.
514. O'Donnell V, LaRocco M, Duque H, et al. Analysis of foot-and-mouth disease virus internalization events in cultured cells. *J Virol* 2005;79(13):8506–8518.
515. Oh HS, Pathak HB, Goodfellow IG, et al. Insight into poliovirus genome replication and encapsidation obtained from studies of 3B-3C cleavage site mutants. *J Virol* 2009;83(18):9370–9387.
516. Ohka S, Igarashi H, Nagata N, et al. Establishment of a poliovirus oral infection system in human poliovirus receptor-expressing transgenic mice that are deficient in alpha/beta interferon receptor. *J Virol* 2007;81(15):7902–7912.
517. Ohlmann T, Rau M, Morley SJ, et al. Proteolytic cleavage of initiation factor eIF-4 gamma in the reticulocyte lysate inhibits translation of capped mRNAs but enhances that of uncapped mRNAs. *Nucleic Acids Res* 1995;23(3):334–340.
518. Olson NH, Kolatkar PR, Oliveira MA, et al. Structure of a human rhinovirus complexed with its receptor molecule. *Proc Natl Acad Sci U S A* 1993;90:507–511.
519. O'Neill RE, Racaniello VR. Inhibition of translation in cells infected with a poliovirus 2Apro mutant correlates with phosphorylation of the alpha subunit of eucaryotic initiation factor 2. *J Virol* 1989;63(12):5069–5075.
520. Organtini LJ, Makhov AM, Conway JF, et al. Kinetic and structural analysis of coxsackievirus B3 receptor interactions and formation of the A-particle. *J Virol* 2014;88(10):5755–5765.
521. Palmenberg AC. In vitro synthesis and assembly of picornaviral capsid intermediate structures. *J Virol* 1982;44(3):900–906.
522. Palmenberg AC, Gern JE. Classification and evolution of human rhinoviruses. *Methods Mol Biol* 2015;1221:1–10.
523. Palmenberg AC, Parks GD, Hall DJ, et al. Proteolytic processing of the cardioviral P2 region: primary 2A/2B cleavage in clone-derived precursors. *Virology* 1992;190(2):754–762.
524. Pan J, Zhang L, Odenwald MA, et al. Expression of human decay-accelerating factor on intestinal epithelium of transgenic mice does not facilitate infection by the enteral route. *J Virol* 2015;89(8):4311–4318.
525. Panjwani A, Asfor AS, Tuthill TJ. The conserved N-terminus of human rhinovirus capsid protein VP4 contains membrane pore-forming activity and is a target for neutralizing antibodies. *J Gen Virol* 2016;97(12):3238–3242.
526. Panjwani A, Strauss M, Gold S, et al. Capsid protein VP4 of human rhinovirus induces membrane permeability by the formation of a size-selective multimeric pore. *PLoS Pathog* 2014;10(8):e1004294.
527. Park N, Katikaneni P, Skern T, et al. Differential targeting of nuclear pore complex proteins in poliovirus-infected cells. *J Virol* 2008;82(4):1647–1655.
528. Park N, Skern T, Gustin KE. Specific cleavage of the nuclear pore complex protein Nup62 by a viral protease. *J Biol Chem* 2010;285(37):28796–28805.
529. Parsley TB, Towner JS, Blyn LB, et al. Poly (rC) binding protein 2 forms a ternary complex with the 5′-terminal sequences of poliovirus RNA and the viral 3CD proteinase. *RNA* 1997;3(10):1124–1134.
530. Patargias G, Barke T, Watts A, et al. Model generation of viral channel forming 2B protein bundles from polio and coxsackie viruses. *Mol Membr Biol* 2009;26(5):309–320.
531. Pathak HB, Oh HS, Goodfellow IG, et al. Picornavirus genome replication: roles of precursor proteins and rate-limiting steps in oriI-dependent VPg uridylylation. *J Biol Chem* 2008;283(45):30677–30688.
532. Paul AV, Cao X, Harris KS, et al. Studies with poliovirus polymerase 3Dpol. Stimulation of poly(U) synthesis in vitro by purified poliovirus protein 3AB. *J Biol Chem* 1994;269(46):29173–29181.
533. Paul AV, Mugavero J, Molla A, et al. Internal ribosomal entry site scanning of the poliovirus polyprotein: implications for proteolytic processing. *Virology* 1998;250(1):241–253.
534. Paul P, Munz C. Autophagy and mammalian viruses: roles in immune response, viral replication, and beyond. *Adv Virus Res* 2016;95:149–195.
535. Paul AV, Rieder E, Kim DW, et al. Identification of an RNA hairpin in poliovirus RNA that serves as the primary template in the in vitro uridylylation of VPg. *J Virol* 2000;74(22):10359–10370.
536. Paul AV, Schultz A, Pincus SE, et al. Capsid protein VP4 of poliovirus is N-myristoylated. *Proc Natl Acad Sci U S A* 1987;84(22):7827–7831.
537. Paul AV, van Boom JH, Filippov D, et al. Protein-primed RNA synthesis by purified poliovirus RNA polymerase. *Nature* 1998;393(6682):280–284.
538. Paul AV, Yin J, Mugavero J, et al. A "slide-back" mechanism for the initiation of protein-primed RNA synthesis by the RNA polymerase of poliovirus. *J Biol Chem* 2003;278(45):43951–43960.
539. Pause A, Belsham GJ, Gingras AC, et al. Insulin-dependent stimulation of protein synthesis by phosphorylation of a regulator of 5′-cap function [see comments]. *Nature* 1994;371(6500):762–767.
540. Pearse BM. Receptors compete for adaptors found in plasma membrane coated pits. *EMBO J* 1988;7(11):3331–3336.
541. Pelletier J, Flynn ME, Kaplan G, et al. Mutational analysis of upstream AUG codons of poliovirus RNA. *J Virol* 1988;62(12):4486–4492.
542. Pelletier J, Kaplan G, Racaniello VR, et al. Cap-independent translation of poliovirus mRNA is conferred by sequence elements within the 5′ noncoding region. *Mol Cell Biol* 1988;8(3):1103–1112.
543. Pelletier J, Sonenberg N. Internal initiation of translation of eukaryotic mRNA directed by a sequence derived from poliovirus RNA. *Nature* 1988;334(6180):320–325.
544. Percy N, Barclay WS, Sullivan M, et al. A poliovirus replicon containing the chloramphenicol acetyltransferase gene can be used to study the replication and encapsidation of poliovirus RNA. *J Virol* 1992;66(8):5040–5046.
545. Perera R, Daijogo S, Walter BL, et al. Cellular protein modification by poliovirus: the two faces of poly(rC)-binding protein. *J Virol* 2007;81(17):8919–8932.
546. Petersen JF, Cherney MM, Liebig HD, et al. The structure of the 2A proteinase from a common cold virus: a proteinase responsible for the shut-off of host-cell protein synthesis. *EMBO J* 1999;18(20):5463–5475.
547. Pettersson RF, Ambros V, Baltimore D. Identification of a protein linked to nascent poliovirus RNA and to the polyuridylic acid of negative-strand RNA. *J Virol* 1978;27(2): 357–365.
548. Pettigrew DM, Williams DT, Kerrigan D, et al. Structural and functional insights into the interaction of echoviruses and decay-accelerating factor. *J Biol Chem* 2006;281(8):5169–5177.
549. Petty RV, Palmenberg AC. Guanine-nucleotide exchange factor RCC1 facilitates a tight binding between the encephalomyocarditis virus leader and cellular Ran GTPase. *J Virol* 2013;87(11):6517–6520.
550. Pevear DC, Fancher MJ, Felock PJ, et al. Conformational change in the floor of the human rhinovirus canyon blocks adsorption to HeLa cell receptors. *J Virol* 1989;63(5):2002–2007.
551. Pevear DC, Hayden FG, Demenczuk TM, et al. Relationship of pleconaril susceptibility and clinical outcomes in treatment of common colds caused by rhinoviruses. *Antimicrob Agents Chemother* 2005;49(11):4492–4499.

552. Pfeiffer HC, Bragstad K, Skram MK, et al. Two cases of acute severe flaccid myelitis associated with enterovirus D68 infection in children, Norway, autumn 2014. *Euro Surveill* 2015;20(10):21062.
553. Pfeiffer JK, Kirkegaard K. Increased fidelity reduces poliovirus fitness and virulence under selective pressure in mice. *PLoS Pathog* 2005;1(2):e11.
554. Pfister T, Wimmer E. Characterization of the nucleoside triphosphatase activity of poliovirus protein 2C reveals a mechanism by which guanidine inhibits poliovirus replication. *J Biol Chem* 1999;274(11):6992–7001.
555. Phelps DK, Post CB. Molecular dynamics investigation of the effect of an antiviral compound on human rhinovirus. *Protein Sci* 1999;8(11):2281–2289.
556. Piccone ME, Zellner M, Kumosinski TF, et al. Identification of the active-site residues of the L proteinase of foot- and-mouth disease virus. *J Virol* 1995;69(8):4950–4956.
557. Pickl-Herk A, Luque D, Vives-Adrian L, et al. Uncoating of common cold virus is preceded by RNA switching as determined by X-ray and cryo-EM analyses of the subviral A-particle. *Proc Natl Acad Sci U S A* 2013;110(50):20063–20068.
558. Pietiainen V, Marjomaki V, Upla P, et al. Echovirus 1 endocytosis into caveosomes requires lipid rafts, dynamin II, and signaling events. *Mol Biol Cell* 2004;15(11):4911–4925.
559. Pilipenko EV, Pestova TV, Kolupaeva VG, et al. A cell cycle-dependent protein serves as a template-specific translation initiation factor. *Genes Dev* 2000;14(16):2028–2045.
560. Pincus SE, Diamond DC, Emini EA, et al. Guanidine-selected mutants of poliovirus: mapping of point mutations to polypeptide 2C. *J Virol* 1986;57(2):638–646.
561. Pincus SE, Wimmer E. Production of guanidine-resistant and -dependent poliovirus mutants from cloned cDNA: mutations in polypeptide 2C are directly responsible for altered guanidine sensitivity. *J Virol* 1986;60(2):793–796.
562. Piotrowska J, Hansen SJ, Park N, et al. Stable formation of compositionally unique stress granules in virus-infected cells. *J Virol* 2010;84(7):3654–3665.
563. Pisarev VP, Pisarev AV, Komar AA, et al. Translation initiation on mammalian mRNAs with structured 5'UTRs requires DExH-box protein DHX29. *Cell* 2008;135(7):1237–1250.
564. Plevka P, Hafenstein S, Harris KG, et al. Interaction of decay-accelerating factor with echovirus 7. *J Virol* 2010;84(24):12665–12674.
565. Plevka P, Lim PY, Perera R, et al. Neutralizing antibodies can initiate genome release from human enterovirus 71. *Proc Natl Acad Sci U S A* 2014;111(6):2134–2139.
566. Plevka P, Perera R, Cardosa J, et al. Crystal structure of human enterovirus 71. *Science* 2012;336(6086):1274.
567. Plotch SJ, Palant O. Poliovirus protein 3AB forms a complex with and stimulates the activity of the viral RNA polymerase, 3Dpol [published erratum appears in J Virol 1996 Jan;70(1):682]. *J Virol* 1995;69(11):7169–7179.
568. Plotch SJ, Palant O, Gluzman Y. Purification and properties of poliovirus RNA polymerase expressed in Escherichia coli. *J Virol* 1989;63:216–225.
569. Pompella A, Visvikis A, Paolicchi A, et al. The changing faces of glutathione, a cellular protagonist. *Biochem Pharmacol* 2003;66(8):1499–1503.
570. Porter FW, Bochkov YA, Albee AJ, et al. A picornavirus protein interacts with Ran-GTPase and disrupts nucleocytoplasmic transport. *Proc Natl Acad Sci U S A* 2006;103(33):12417–12422.
571. Porter FW, Brown B, Palmenberg AC. Nucleoporin phosphorylation triggered by the encephalomyocarditis virus leader protein is mediated by mitogen-activated protein kinases. *J Virol* 2010;84(24):12538–12548.
572. Porter FW, Palmenberg AC. Leader-induced phosphorylation of nucleoporins correlates with nuclear trafficking inhibition by cardioviruses. *J Virol* 2009;83(4):1941–1951.
573. Powell RM, Schmitt V, Ward T, et al. Characterization of echoviruses that bind decay accelerating factor (CD55): evidence that some haemagglutinating strains use more than one cellular receptor. *J Gen Virol* 1998;79(Pt 7):1707–1713.
574. Powell RM, Ward T, Evans DJ, et al. Interaction between echovirus 7 and its receptor, decay-accelerating factor (CD55): evidence for a secondary cellular factor in A-particle formation. *J Virol* 1997;71(12):9306–9312.
575. Prchla E, Kuechler E, Blaas D, et al. Uncoating of human rhinovirus serotype 2 from late endosomes. *J Virol* 1994;68(6):3713–3723.
576. Pulli T, Lankinen H, Roivainen M, et al. Antigenic sites of coxsackievirus A9. *Virology* 1998;240(2):202–212.
577. Pulli T, Roivainen M, Hovi T, et al. Induction of neutralizing antibodies by synthetic peptides representing the C terminus of coxsackievirus A9 capsid protein VP1. *J Gen Virol* 1998;79 (Pt 9):2249–2253.
578. Quadt R, Kao CC, Browning KS, et al. Characterization of a host protein associated with brome mosaic virus RNA-dependent RNA polymerase. *Proc Natl Acad Sci U S A* 1993;90(4):1498–1502.
579. Querol-Audi J, Konecsni T, Pous J, et al. Minor group human rhinovirus-receptor interactions: geometry of multimodular attachment and basis of recognition. *FEBS Lett* 2009;583(1):235–240.
580. Racaniello VR. One hundred years of poliovirus pathogenesis. *Virology* 2006;344(1):9–16.
581. Racaniello VR, Baltimore D. Cloned poliovirus complementary DNA is infectious in mammalian cells. *Science* 1981;214(4523):916–919.
582. Racaniello VR, Baltimore D. Molecular cloning of poliovirus cDNA and determination of the complete nucleotide sequence of the viral genome. *Proc Natl Acad Sci U S A* 1981;78(8):4887–4891.
583. Rankl C, Kienberger F, Wildling L, et al. Multiple receptors involved in human rhinovirus attachment to live cells. *Proc Natl Acad Sci U S A* 2008;105(46):17778–17783.
584. Redondo N, Sanz MA, Welnowska E, et al. Translation without eIF2 promoted by poliovirus 2A protease. *PLoS One* 2011;6(10):e25699.
585. Register RB, Uncapher CR, Naylor AM, et al. Human-murine chimeras of ICAM-1 identify amino acid residues critical for rhinovirus and antibody binding. *J Virol* 1991;65:6589–6596.
586. Ren R, Costantini FC, Gorgacz EJ, et al. Transgenic mice expressing a human poliovirus receptor: a new model for poliomyelitis. *Cell* 1990;63:353–362.
587. Ren X, Hurley JH. VHS domains of ESCRT-0 cooperate in high-avidity binding to polyubiquitinated cargo. *EMBO J* 2010;29(6):1045–1054.
588. Ren R, Racaniello V. Human poliovirus receptor gene expression and poliovirus tissue tropism in transgenic mice. *J Virol* 1992;66:296–304.
589. Ren J, Wang X, Hu Z, et al. Picornavirus uncoating intermediate captured in atomic detail. *Nat Commun* 2013;4:1929.
590. Rezapkin G, Neverov A, Cherkasova E, et al. Repertoire of antibodies against type 1 poliovirus in human sera. *J Virol Methods* 2010;169(2):322–331.
591. Richards OC, Ehrenfeld E. Effects of poliovirus 3AB protein on 3D polymerase-catalyzed reaction. *J Biol Chem* 1998;273(21):12832–12840.
592. Richards AL, Jackson WT. Intracellular vesicle acidification promotes maturation of infectious poliovirus particles. *PLoS Pathog* 2012;8(11):e1003046.
593. Rieder E, Paul AV, Kim DW, et al. Genetic and biochemical studies of poliovirus cis-acting replication element cre in relation to VPg uridylylation. *J Virol* 2000;74(22):10371–10380.
594. Rivera V, Welsh J, Maizel JJ. Comparative sequence analysis of the 5'-noncoding region of the enteroviruses and rhinoviruses. *Virology* 1988;165:42–50.
595. Roberts PJ, Belsham GJ. Identification of critical amino acids within the foot-and-mouth disease virus leader protein, a cysteine protease. *Virology* 1995;213(1):140–146.
596. Rodal SK, Skretting G, Garred O, et al. Extraction of cholesterol with methyl-beta-cyclodextrin perturbs formation of clathrin-coated endocytic vesicles. *Mol Biol Cell* 1999;10(4):961–974.
597. Rodriguez PL, Carrasco L. Poliovirus protein 2C has ATPase and GTPase activities. *J Biol Chem* 1993;268(11):8105–8110.
598. Rodriguez PL, Carrasco L. Poliovirus protein 2C contains two regions involved in RNA binding activity. *J Biol Chem* 1995;270(17):10105–10112.
599. Rodriguez Pulido M, Sanchez-Aparicio MT, Martinez-Salas E, et al. Innate immune sensor LGP2 is cleaved by the Leader protease of foot-and-mouth disease virus. *PLoS Pathog* 2018;14(6):e1007135.
600. Rohl A, Rohrberg J, Buchner J. The chaperone Hsp90: changing partners for demanding clients. *Trends Biochem Sci* 2013;38(5):253–262.
601. Roivainen M, Hyypia T, Piirainen L, et al. RGD-dependent entry of coxsackievirus A9 into host cells and its bypass after cleavage of VP1 protein by intestinal proteases. *J Virol* 1991;65(9):4735–4740.
602. Roivainen M, Piirainen L, Rysa T, et al. An immunodominant N-terminal region of VP1 protein of poliovirion that is buried in crystal structure can be exposed in solution. *Virology* 1993;195(2):762–765.
603. Rombaut B, Vrijsen R, Boeye A. New evidence for the precursor role of 14 S subunits in poliovirus morphogenesis. *Virology* 1990;177(1):411–414.
604. Roos RP, Kong WP, Semler BL. Polyprotein processing of Theiler's murine encephalomyelitis virus. *J Virol* 1989;63(12):5344–5353.
605. Rose JK, Trachsel H, Leong K, et al. Inhibition of translation by poliovirus: inactivation of a specific initiation factor. *Proc Natl Acad Sci U S A* 1978;75(6):2732–2736.
606. Rossmann MG. The canyon hypothesis. Hiding the host cell receptor attachment site on a viral surface from immune surveillance. *J Biol Chem* 1989;264(25):14587–14590.
607. Rossmann MG, Arnold E, Erickson JW, et al. Structure of a human common cold virus and functional relationship to other picornaviruses. *Nature* 1985;317:145–153.
608. Rothe D, Werk D, Niedrig S, et al. Antiviral activity of highly potent siRNAs against echovirus 30 and its receptor. *J Virol Methods* 2009;157(2):211–218.
609. Rothwell DG, Crossley R, Bridgeman JS, et al. Functional expression of secreted proteins from a bicistronic retroviral cassette based on foot-and-mouth disease virus 2A can be position dependent. *Hum Gene Ther* 2010;21(11):1631–1637.
610. Rubinstein SJ, Hammerle T, Wimmer E, et al. Infection of HeLa cells with poliovirus results in modification of a complex that binds to the rRNA promoter. *J Virol* 1992;66:3062–3068.
611. Rudin CM, Poirier JT, Senzer NN, et al. Phase I clinical study of Seneca Valley Virus (SVV-001), a replication-competent picornavirus, in advanced solid tumors with neuroendocrine features. *Clin Cancer Res* 2011;17(4):888–895.
612. Rueckert RR, Dunker AK, Stoltzfus CM. The structure of mouse-Elberfeld virus: a model. *Proc Natl Acad Sci U S A* 1969;62(3):912–919.
613. Rust RC, Landmann L, Gosert R, et al. Cellular COPII proteins are involved in production of the vesicles that form the poliovirus replication complex. *J Virol* 2001;75(20):9808–9818.
614. Sa-Carvalho D, Rieder E, Baxt B, et al. Tissue culture adaptation of foot-and-mouth disease virus selects viruses that bind to heparin and are attenuated in cattle. *J Virol* 1997;71(7):5115–5123.
615. Saiz M, Gomez S, Martinez-Salas E, et al. Deletion or substitution of the aphthovirus 3' NCR abrogates infectivity and virus replication. *J Gen Virol* 2001;82(Pt 1):93–101.
616. Sandoval IV, Carrasco L. Poliovirus infection and expression of the poliovirus protein 2B provoke the disassembly of the Golgi complex, the organelle target for the antipoliovirus drug Ro-090179. *J Virol* 1997;71(6):4679–4693.
617. Sasaki J, Ishikawa K, Arita M, et al. ACBD3-mediated recruitment of PI4KB to picornavirus RNA replication sites. *EMBO J* 2012;31(3):754–766.
618. Sasaki J, Ishikawa K, Taniguchi K. 3CD, but not 3C, cleaves the VP1/2A site efficiently during Aichi virus polyprotein processing through interaction with 2A. *Virus Res* 2012;163(2):592–598.
619. Sasaki J, Nagashima S, Taniguchi K. Aichi virus leader protein is involved in viral RNA replication and encapsidation. *J Virol* 2003;77(20):10799–10807.
620. Sasaki J, Taniguchi K. The 5'-end sequence of the genome of Aichi virus, a picornavirus, contains an element critical for viral RNA encapsidation. *J Virol* 2003;77(6):3542–3548.
621. Sauter P, Chehadeh W, Lobert PE, et al. A part of the VP4 capsid protein exhibited by coxsackievirus B4 E2 is the target of antibodies contained in plasma from patients with type 1 diabetes. *J Med Virol* 2008;80(5):866–878.
622. Schlegel A, Giddings TH Jr, Ladinsky MS, et al. Cellular origin and ultrastructure of membranes induced during poliovirus infection. *J Virol* 1996;70(10):6576–6588.
623. Schultheiss T, Emerson SU, Purcell RH, et al. Polyprotein processing in echovirus 22: a first assessment. *Biochem Biophys Res Commun* 1995;217(3):1120–1127.
624. Schultheiss T, Kusov YY, Gauss-Muller V. Proteinase 3C of hepatitis A virus (HAV) cleaves the HAV polyprotein P2- P3 at all sites including VP1/2A and 2A/2B. *Virology* 1994;198(1):275–281.
625. Scully EJ, Basnet S, Wrangham RW, et al. Lethal respiratory disease associated with human rhinovirus C in wild chimpanzees, Uganda, 2013. *Emerg Infect Dis* 2018;24(2):267–274.

626. Seal LA, Jamison RM. Evidence for secondary structure within the virion RNA of echovirus 22. *J Virol* 1984;50(2):641–644.

627. Selinka H-C, Zibert A, Wimmer E. Poliovirus can enter and infect mammalian cells by way of an intercellular adhesion molecule 1 pathway. *Proc Natl Acad Sci U S A* 1991;88:3598–3602.

628. Selinka H-C, Zibert A, Wimmer E. A chimeric poliovirus/CD4 receptor confers susceptibility to poliovirus on mouse cells. *J Virol* 1992;66:2523–2526.

629. Shafren DR, Bates RC, Agrez MV, et al. Coxsackieviruses B1, B3, and B5 use decay accelerating factor as a receptor for cell attachment. *J Virol* 1995;69(6):3873–3877.

630. Shafren DR, Dorahy DJ, Ingham RA, et al. Coxsackievirus A21 binds to decay-accelerating factor but requires intercellular adhesion molecule 1 for cell entry. *J Virol* 1997;71(6):4736–4743.

631. Shafren DR, Williams DT, Barry RD. A decay-accelerating factor-binding strain of coxsackievirus B3 requires the coxsackievirus-adenovirus receptor protein to mediate lytic infection of rhabdomyosarcoma cells. *J Virol* 1997;71(12):9844–9848.

632. Shakeel S, Westerhuis BM, Domanska A, et al. Multiple capsid-stabilizing interactions revealed in a high-resolution structure of an emerging picornavirus causing neonatal sepsis. *Nat Commun* 2016;7:11387.

633. Sharma R, Raychaudhuri S, Dasgupta A. Nuclear entry of poliovirus protease-polymerase precursor 3CD: implications for host cell transcription shut-off. *Virology* 2004;320(2):195–205.

634. Shepley MP, Racaniello VR. A monoclonal antibody that blocks poliovirus attachment recognizes the lymphocyte homing receptor CD44. *J Virol* 1994;68(3):1301–1308.

635. Shepley MP, Sherry B, Weiner HL. Monoclonal antibody identification of a 100-kDa membrane protein in HeLa cells and human spinal cord involved in poliovirus attachment. *Proc Natl Acad Sci U S A* 1988;85:7743–7747.

636. Sherry B, Mosser AG, Colonno RJ, et al. Use of monoclonal antibodies to identify four neutralization immunogens on a common cold picornavirus, human rhinovirus 14. *J Virol* 1986;57(1):246–257.

637. Shi J, Wong J, Piesik P, et al. Cleavage of sequestosome 1/p62 by an enteroviral protease results in disrupted selective autophagy and impaired NFKB signaling. *Autophagy* 2013;9(10):1591–1603.

638. Shiroki K, Isoyama T, Kuge S, et al. Intracellular redistribution of truncated La protein produced by poliovirus 3Cpro-mediated cleavage. *J Virol* 1999;73(3):2193–2200.

639. Simmonds P, Welch J. Frequency and dynamics of recombination within different species of human enteroviruses. *J Virol* 2006;80(1):483–493.

640. Skinner MA, Racaniello VR, Dunn G, et al. New model for the secondary structure of the 5′ non-coding RNA of poliovirus is supported by biochemical and genetic data that also show that RNA secondary structure is important in neurovirulence. *J Mol Biol* 1989;207(2):379–392.

641. Smith TJ, Chase ES, Schmidt TJ, et al. Neutralizing antibody to human rhinovirus 14 penetrates the receptor-binding canyon. *Nature* 1996;383(6598):350–354.

642. Smith AD, Dawson H. Glutathione is required for efficient production of infectious picornavirus virions. *Virology* 2006;353(2):258–267.

643. Smith TJ, Kremer MJ, Luo M, et al. The site of attachment in human rhinovirus 14 for antiviral agents that inhibit uncoating. *Science* 1986;233(4770):1286–1293.

644. Smyth M, Pettitt T, Symonds A, et al. Identification of the pocket factors in a picornavirus. *Arch Virol* 2003;148(6):1225–1233.

645. Snyers L, Zwickl H, Blaas D. Human rhinovirus type 2 is internalized by clathrin-mediated endocytosis. *J Virol* 2003;77(9):5360–5369.

646. Sommergruber W, Casari G, Fessl F, et al. The 2A proteinase of human rhinovirus is a zinc containing enzyme. *Virology* 1994;204(2):815–818.

647. Sommergruber W, Seipelt J, Fessl F, et al. Mutational analyses support a model for the HRV2 2A proteinase. *Virology* 1997;234(2):203–214.

648. Song Y, Gorbatsevych O, Liu Y, et al. Limits of variation, specific infectivity, and genome packaging of massively recoded poliovirus genomes. *Proc Natl Acad Sci U S A* 2017;114(41):E8731–E8740.

649. Song Y, Liu Y, Ward CB, et al. Identification of two functionally redundant RNA elements in the coding sequence of poliovirus using computer-generated design. *Proc Natl Acad Sci U S A* 2012;109(36):14301–14307.

650. Spahn CM, Kieft JS, Grassucci RA, et al. Hepatitis C virus IRES RNA-induced changes in the conformation of the 40s ribosomal subunit. *Science* 2001;291(5510):1959–1962.

651. Spector DH, Baltimore D. Requirement of 3′-terminal poly(adenylic acid) for the infectivity of poliovirus RNA. *Proc Natl Acad Sci U S A* 1974;71(8):2983–2987.

652. Speelman B, Brooks BR, Post CB. Molecular dynamics simulations of human rhinovirus and an antiviral compound. *Biophys J* 2001;80(1):121–129.

653. Staring J, van den Hengel LG, Raaben M, et al. KREMEN1 Is a Host Entry Receptor for a Major Group of Enteroviruses. *Cell Host Microbe* 2018;23(5):636–643 e635.

654. Staring J, von Castelmur E, Blomen VA, et al. PLA2G16 represents a switch between entry and clearance of Picornaviridae. *Nature* 2017;541(7637):412–416.

655. Staunton DE, Dustin ML, Erickson HP, et al. The arrangement of the immunoglobulin-like domains of ICAM-1 and the binding sites for LFA-1 and rhinovirus. *Cell* 1990;61:243–254.

656. Staunton DE, Merluzzi VJ, Rothlein R, et al. A cell adhesion molecule, ICAM-1, is the major surface receptor for rhinoviruses. *Cell* 1989;56:849–853.

657. Steil BP, Kempf BJ, Barton DJ. Poly(A) at the 3′ end of positive-strand RNA and VPg-linked poly(U) at the 5′ end of negative-strand RNA are reciprocal templates during replication of poliovirus RNA. *J Virol* 2010;84(6):2843–2858.

658. Stephenson J. CDC to clinicians: be alert for children with poliolike illness. *JAMA* 2014;312(16):1623.

659. Stephenson J. CDC tracking enterovirus D-68 outbreak causing severe respiratory illness in children in the Midwest. *JAMA* 2014;312(13):1290.

660. Stevenson RA, Huang JA, Studdert MJ, et al. Sialic acid acts as a receptor for equine rhinitis A virus binding and infection. *J Gen Virol* 2004;85(Pt 9):2535–2543.

661. Stoner GD, Williams B, Kniazeff A, et al. Effect of neuraminidase pretreatment on the susceptibility of normal and transformed mammalian cells to bovine enterovirus 261. *Nature* 1973;245(5424):319–320.

662. Strauss M, Filman DJ, Belnap DM, et al. Nectin-like interactions between poliovirus and its receptor trigger conformational changes associated with cell entry. *J Virol* 2015;89(8):4143–4157.

663. Strauss DM, Glustrom LW, Wuttke DS. Towards an understanding of the poliovirus replication complex: the solution structure of the soluble domain of the poliovirus 3A protein. *J Mol Biol* 2003;330(2):225–234.

664. Strauss M, Levy HC, Bostina M, et al. RNA transfer from poliovirus 135S particles across membranes is mediated by long umbilical connectors. *J Virol* 2013;87(7):3903–3914.

665. Strebel K, Beck E. A second protease of foot-and-mouth disease virus. *J Virol* 1986;58(3):893–899.

666. Stuart AD, McKee TA, Williams PA, et al. Determination of the structure of a decay accelerating factor-binding clinical isolate of echovirus 11 allows mapping of mutants with altered receptor requirements for infection. *J Virol* 2002;76(15):7694–7704.

667. Suhy DA, Giddings TH Jr, Kirkegaard K. Remodeling the endoplasmic reticulum by poliovirus infection and by individual viral proteins: an autophagy-like origin for virus-induced vesicles. *J Virol* 2000;74(19):8953–8965.

668. Summers DF, Maizel JV. Evidence for large precursor proteins in poliovirus synthesis. *Proc Natl Acad Sci U S A* 1968;59:966–971.

669. Sun Y, Wang Y, Shan C, et al. Enterovirus 71 VPg uridylation uses a two-molecular mechanism of 3D polymerase. *J Virol* 2012;86(24):13662–13671.

670. Svitkin YV, Costa-Mattioli M, Herdy B, et al. Stimulation of picornavirus replication by the poly(A) tail in a cell-free extract is largely independent of the poly(A) binding protein (PABP). *RNA* 2007;13(12):2330–2340.

671. Svitkin YV, Gradi A, Imataka H, et al. Eukaryotic initiation factor 4GII (eIF4GII), but not eIF4GI, cleavage correlates with inhibition of host cell protein synthesis after human rhinovirus infection. *J Virol* 1999;73(4):3467–3472.

672. Svitkin YV, Imataka H, Khaleghpour K, et al. Poly(A)-binding protein interaction with eIF4G stimulates picornavirus IRES-dependent translation. *RNA* 2001;7(12):1743–1752.

673. Swatek KN, Aumayr M, Pruneda JN, et al. Irreversible inactivation of ISG15 by a viral leader protease enables alternative infection detection strategies. *Proc Natl Acad Sci U S A* 2018;115(10):2371–2376.

674. Takata MA, Goncalves-Carneiro D, Zang TM, et al. CG dinucleotide suppression enables antiviral defence targeting non-self RNA. *Nature* 2017;550(7674):124–127.

675. Takegami T, Kuhn RJ, Anderson CW, et al. Membrane-dependent uridylylation of the genome-linked protein VPg of poliovirus. *Proc Natl Acad Sci U S A* 1983;80(24):7447–7451.

676. Tan YW, Hong WJ, Chu JJ. Inhibition of enterovirus VP4 myristoylation is a potential antiviral strategy for hand, foot and mouth disease. *Antiviral Res* 2016;133:191–195.

677. Tang RS, Barton DJ, Flanegan JB, et al. Poliovirus RNA recombination in cell-free extracts. *RNA* 1997;3(6):624–633.

678. Taylor MP, Burgon TB, Kirkegaard K, et al. Role of microtubules in extracellular release of poliovirus. *J Virol* 2009;83(13):6599–6609.

679. Taylor MP, Kirkegaard K. Potential subversion of autophagosomal pathway by picornaviruses. *Autophagy* 2008;4(3):286–289.

680. Tellez AB, Wang J, Tanner EJ, et al. Interstitial contacts in an RNA-dependent RNA polymerase lattice. *J Mol Biol* 2011;412(4):737–750.

681. Teterina NL, Gorbalenya AE, Egger D, et al. Poliovirus 2C protein determinants of membrane binding and rearrangements in mammalian cells. *J Virol* 1997;71(12):8962–8972.

682. Thibaut HJ, van der Linden L, Jiang P, et al. Binding of glutathione to enterovirus capsids is essential for virion morphogenesis. *PLoS Pathog* 2014;10(4):e1004039.

683. Thompson AA, Peersen OB. Structural basis for proteolysis-dependent activation of the poliovirus RNA-dependent RNA polymerase. *EMBO J* 2004;23(17):3462–3471.

684. Todd S, Semler BL. Structure-infectivity analysis of the human rhinovirus genomic RNA 3′ non-coding region. *Nucleic Acids Res* 1996;24(11):2133–2142.

685. Todd S, Towner JS, Brown DM, et al. Replication-competent picornaviruses with complete genomic RNA 3′ noncoding region deletions. *J Virol* 1997;71(11):8868–8874.

686. Tolskaya EA, Romanova LI, Kolesnikova MS, et al. Apoptosis-inducing and apoptosis-preventing functions of poliovirus. *J Virol* 1995;69(2):1181–1189.

687. Tomasec P, Wang EC, Davison AJ, et al. Downregulation of natural killer cell-activating ligand CD155 by human cytomegalovirus UL141. *Nat Immunol* 2005;6(2):181–188.

688. Tomassini JE, Graham D, DeWitt CM, et al. cDNA cloning reveals that the major group rhinovirus receptor on HeLa cells is intercellular adhesion molecule 1. *Proc Natl Acad Sci U S A* 1989;86:4907–4911.

689. Tosteson MT, Chow M. Characterization of the ion channels formed by poliovirus in planar lipid membranes. *J Virol* 1997;71(1):507–511.

690. Tourriere H, Chebli K, Zekri L, et al. The RasGAP-associated endoribonuclease G3BP assembles stress granules. *J Cell Biol* 2003;160(6):823–831.

691. Towner JS, Ho TV, Semler BL. Determinants of membrane association for poliovirus protein 3AB. *J Biol Chem* 1996;271(43):26810–26818.

692. Trachsel H, Sonenberg N, Shatkin AJ, et al. Purification of a factor that restores translation of vesicular stomatitis virus mRNA in extracts from poliovirus-infected HeLa cells. *Proc Natl Acad Sci U S A* 1980;77(2):770–774.

693. Trahey M, Oh HS, Cameron CE, et al. Poliovirus infection transiently increases COPII vesicle budding. *J Virol* 2012;86(18):9675–9682.

694. Triantafilou K, Fradelizi D, Wilson K, et al. GRP78, a coreceptor for coxsackievirus A9, interacts with major histocompatibility complex class I molecules which mediate virus internalization. *J Virol* 2002;76(2):633–643.

695. Triantafilou K, Triantafilou M, Takada Y, et al. Human parechovirus 1 utilizes integrins alphavbeta3 and alphavbeta1 as receptors. *J Virol* 2000;74(13):5856–5862.

696. Triantafilou K, Triantafilou M, Wilson KM, et al. Intracellular and cell surface heterotypic associations of human leukocyte antigen-DR and human invariant chain. *Hum Immunol* 1999;60(11):1101–1112.

697. Triantafilou M, Triantafilou K, Wilson KM, et al. Involvement of beta2-microglobulin and integrin alphavbeta3 molecules in the coxsackievirus A9 infectious cycle. *J Gen Virol* 1999;80 (Pt 10):2591–2600.

698. Tsang SK, Danthi P, Chow M, et al. Stabilization of poliovirus by capsid-binding antiviral drugs is due to entropic effects. *J Mol Biol* 2000;296(2):335–340.

699. Tsou YL, Lin YW, Chang HW, et al. Heat shock protein 90: role in enterovirus 71 entry and assembly and potential target for therapy. *PLoS One* 2013;8(10):e77133.

700. Tulloch F, Atkinson NJ, Evans DJ, et al. RNA virus attenuation by codon pair deoptimisation is an artefact of increases in CpG/UpA dinucleotide frequencies. *Elife* 2014;3:e04531.

701. Tuthill TJ, Bubeck D, Rowlands DJ, et al. Characterization of early steps in the poliovirus infection process: receptor-decorated liposomes induce conversion of the virus to membrane-anchored entry-intermediate particles. *J Virol* 2006;80(1):172–180.

702. Tuthill TJ, Harlos K, Walter TS, et al. Equine rhinitis A virus and its low pH empty particle: clues towards an aphthovirus entry mechanism? *PLoS Pathog* 2009;5(10):e1000620.

703. Ullmer W, Semler BL. Direct and indirect effects on viral translation and RNA replication are required for AUF1 restriction of enterovirus infections in human cells. *MBio* 2018;9(5):e01669-18.

704. van de Stolpe A, van der Saag PT. Intercellular adhesion molecule-1. *J Mol Med* 1996;74(1):13–33.

705. van der Schaar HM, van der Linden L, Lanke KH, et al. Coxsackievirus mutants that can bypass host factor PI4KIIIbeta and the need for high levels of PI4P lipids for replication. *Cell Res* 2012;22(11):1576–1592.

706. van der Werf S, Bradley J, Wimmer E, et al. Synthesis of infectious poliovirus RNA by purified T7 RNA polymerase. *Proc Natl Acad Sci U S A* 1986;83(8):2330–2334.

707. Van Dyke TA, Flanegan JB. Identification of poliovirus polypeptide p63 as a soluble RNA-dependent RNA polymerase. *J Virol* 1980;35:732–740.

708. van Eyll O, Michiels T. Influence of the Theiler's virus L* protein on macrophage infection, viral persistence, and neurovirulence. *J Virol* 2000;74(19):9071–9077.

709. van Eyll O, Michiels T. Non-AUG-initiated internal translation of the L* protein of Theiler's virus and importance of this protein for viral persistence. *J Virol* 2002;76(21):10665–10673.

710. van Kuppeveld FJ, Galama JM, Zoll J, et al. Genetic analysis of a hydrophobic domain of coxsackie B3 virus protein 2B: a moderate degree of hydrophobicity is required for a cis-acting function in viral RNA synthesis. *J Virol* 1995;69(12):7782–7790.

711. van Kuppeveld FJ, Hoenderop JG, Smeets RL, et al. Coxsackievirus protein 2B modifies endoplasmic reticulum membrane and plasma membrane permeability and facilitates virus release. *EMBO J* 1997;16(12):3519–3532.

712. van kuppeveld FJ, Melchers WJ, Kirkegaard K, Doedens JR. Structure-function analysis of coxsackie B3 virus protein 2B. *Virology* 1997;227(1):111–118.

713. van Kuppeveld FJ, van den Hurk PJ, Zoll J, et al. Mutagenesis of the coxsackie B3 virus 2B/2C cleavage site: determinants of processing efficiency and effects on viral replication. *J Virol* 1996;70(11):7632–7640.

714. van Ooij MJ, Polacek C, Glaudemans DH, et al. Polyadenylation of genomic RNA and initiation of antigenomic RNA in a positive-strand RNA virus are controlled by the same cis-element. *Nucleic Acids Res* 2006;34(10):2953–2965.

715. van Pesch V, van Eyll O, Michiels T. The leader protein of Theiler's virus inhibits immediate-early alpha/beta interferon production. *J Virol* 2001;75(17):7811–7817.

716. van Vlijmen HW, Curry S, Schaefer M, et al. Titration calculations of foot-and-mouth disease virus capsids and their stabilities as a function of pH. *J Mol Biol* 1998;275(2):295–308.

717. Vashist S, Urena L, Gonzalez-Hernandez MB, et al. Molecular chaperone Hsp90 is a therapeutic target for noroviruses. *J Virol* 2015;89(12):6352–6363.

718. Vazquez-Calvo A, Caridi F, Sobrino F, et al. An increase in acid resistance of foot-and-mouth disease virus capsid is mediated by a tyrosine replacement of the VP2 histidine previously associated with VP0 cleavage. *J Virol* 2014;88(5):3039–3042.

719. Venkataraman S, Reddy SP, Loo J, et al. Structure of Seneca Valley virus-001: an oncolytic picornavirus representing a new genus. *Structure* 2008;16(10):1555–1561.

720. Verdaguer N, Fita I, Reithmayer M, et al. X-ray structure of a minor group human rhinovirus bound to a fragment of its cellular receptor protein. *Nat Struct Mol Biol* 2004;11(5):429–434.

721. Verdaguer N, Jimenez-Clavero MA, Fita I, et al. Structure of swine vesicular disease virus: mapping of changes occurring during adaptation of human coxsackie B5 virus to infect swine. *J Virol* 2003;77(18):9780–9789.

722. Vignuzzi M, Stone JK, Arnold JJ, et al. Quasispecies diversity determines pathogenesis through cooperative interactions in a viral population. *Nature* 2006;439(7074):344–348.

723. Viktorova EG, Nchoutmboube JA, Ford-Siltz LA, et al. Phospholipid synthesis fueled by lipid droplets drives the structural development of poliovirus replication organelles. *PLoS Pathog* 2018;14(8):e1007280.

724. Villa-Komaroff L, Guttman N, Baltimore D, et al. Complete translation of poliovirus RNA in a eukaryotic cell-free system. *Proc Natl Acad Sci U S A* 1975;72(10):4157–4161.

725. Virgen-Slane R, Rozovics JM, Fitzgerald KD, et al. An RNA virus hijacks an incognito function of a DNA repair enzyme. *Proc Natl Acad Sci U S A* 2012;109(36):14634–14639.

726. Visser LJ, Medina GN, Rabouw HH, et al. Foot-and-mouth disease virus leader protease cleaves G3BP1 and G3BP2 and inhibits stress granule formation. *J Virol* 2019;93(2):e00922-18.

727. Vives-Adrian L, Garriga D, Buxaderas M, et al. Structural basis for host membrane remodeling induced by protein 2B of hepatitis A virus. *J Virol* 2015;89(7):3648–3658.

728. Vogt DA, Andino R. An RNA element at the 5′-end of the poliovirus genome functions as a general promoter for RNA synthesis. *PLoS Pathog* 2010;6(6):e1000936.

729. Voss T, Meyer R, Sommergruber W. Spectroscopic characterization of rhinoviral protease 2A: Zn is essential for the structural integrity. *Protein Sci* 1995;4(12):2526–2531.

730. Wachsman MB, Castilla V, Coto CE. Inhibition of foot and mouth disease virus (FMDV) uncoating by a plant-derived peptide isolated from Melia azedarach L leaves. *Arch Virol* 1998;143(3):581–590.

731. Walter BL, Nguyen JH, Ehrenfeld E, et al. Differential utilization of poly(rC) binding protein 2 in translation directed by picornavirus IRES elements. *RNA* 1999;5(12):1570–1585.

732. Wang J, Fan T, Yao X, et al. Crystal structures of enterovirus 71 3C protease complexed with rupintrivir reveal the roles of catalytically important residues. *J Virol* 2011;85(19):10021–10030.

733. Wang D, Fang L, Li P, et al. The leader proteinase of foot-and-mouth disease virus negatively regulates the type I interferon pathway by acting as a viral deubiquitinase. *J Virol* 2011;85(8):3758–3766.

734. Wang C, Jiang P, Sand C, et al. Alanine scanning of poliovirus 2CATPase reveals new genetic evidence that capsid protein/2CATPase interactions are essential for morphogenesis. *J Virol* 2012;86(18):9964–9975.

735. Wang RY, Kuo RL, Ma WC, et al. Heat shock protein-90-beta facilitates enterovirus 71 viral particles assembly. *Virology* 2013;443(2):236–247.

736. Wang X, Lau C, Wiehler S, et al. Syk is downstream of intercellular adhesion molecule-1 and mediates human rhinovirus activation of p38 MAPK in airway epithelial cells. *J Immunol* 2006;177(10):6859–6870.

737. Wang X, Liu N, Wang F, et al. Genetic characterization of a novel duck-origin picornavirus with six 2A proteins. *J Gen Virol* 2014;95(Pt 6):1289–1296.

738. Wang C, Ma HC, Wimmer E, et al. A C-terminal, cysteine-rich site in poliovirus 2C(ATPase) is required for morphogenesis. *J Gen Virol* 2014;95(Pt 6):1255–1265.

739. Wang X, Peng W, Ren J, et al. A sensor-adaptor mechanism for enterovirus uncoating from structures of EV71. *Nat Struct Mol Biol* 2012;19(4):424–429.

740. Wang X, Ren J, Gao Q, et al. Hepatitis A virus and the origins of picornaviruses. *Nature* 2015;517(7532):85–88.

741. Wang X, Zhu L, Dang M, et al. Potent neutralization of hepatitis A virus reveals a receptor mimic mechanism and the receptor recognition site. *Proc Natl Acad Sci U S A* 2017;114(4):770–775.

742. Ward T, Pipkin PA, Clarkson NA, et al. Decay-accelerating factor CD55 is identified as the receptor for echovirus 7 using CELICS, a rapid immuno-focal cloning method. *EMBO J* 1994;13(21):5070–5074.

743. Ward T, Powell RM, Pipkin PA, et al. Role for beta2-microglobulin in echovirus infection of rhabdomyosarcoma cells. *J Virol* 1998;72(7):5360–5365.

744. Watters K, Palmenberg AC. Differential processing of nuclear pore complex proteins by rhinovirus 2A proteases from different species and serotypes. *J Virol* 2011;85(20):10874–10883.

745. Watters K, Palmenberg AC. CDHR3 extracellular domains EC1–3 mediate rhinovirus C interaction with cells and as recombinant derivatives, are inhibitory to virus infection. *PLoS Pathog* 2018;14(12):e1007477.

746. Wei W, Guo H, Chang J, et al. ICAM-5/Telencephalin is a functional entry receptor for enterovirus D68. *Cell Host Microbe* 2016;20(5):631–641.

747. Welnowska E, Sanz MA, Redondo N, et al. Translation of viral mRNA without active eIF2: the case of picornaviruses. *PLoS One* 2011;6(7):e22230.

748. Weng KF, Li ML, Hung CT, et al. Enterovirus 71 3C protease cleaves a novel target CstF-64 and inhibits cellular polyadenylation. *PLoS Pathog* 2009;5(9):e1000593.

749. Wessels E, Duijsings D, Lanke KH, et al. Molecular determinants of the interaction between coxsackievirus protein 3A and guanine nucleotide exchange factor GBF1. *J Virol* 2007;81(10):5238–5245.

750. Wessels E, Duijsings D, Lanke KH, et al. Effects of picornavirus 3A proteins on protein transport and GBF1-dependent COP-I recruitment. *J Virol* 2006;80(23):11852–11860.

751. White JP, Cardenas AM, Marissen WE, et al. Inhibition of cytoplasmic mRNA stress granule formation by a viral proteinase. *Cell Host Microbe* 2007;2(5):295–305.

752. White JP, Lloyd RE. Poliovirus unlinks TIA1 aggregation and mRNA stress granule formation. *J Virol* 2011;85(23):12442–12454.

753. White JP, Reineke LC, Lloyd RE. Poliovirus switches to an eIF2-independent mode of translation during infection. *J Virol* 2011;85(17):8884–8893.

754. Williams CH, Kajander T, Hyypia T, et al. Integrin alpha v beta 6 is an RGD-dependent receptor for coxsackievirus A9. *J Virol* 2004;78(13):6967–6973.

755. Witwer C, Rauscher S, Hofacker IL, et al. Conserved RNA secondary structures in Picornaviridae genomes. *Nucleic Acids Res* 2001;29(24):5079–5089.

756. Wullschleger S, Loewith R, Hall MN. TOR signaling in growth and metabolism. *Cell* 2006;124(3):471–484.

757. Xiang W, Harris KS, Alexander L, et al. Interaction between the 5′-terminal cloverleaf and 3AB/3CDpro of poliovirus is essential for RNA replication. *J Virol* 1995;69(6):3658–3667.

758. Xiao C, Bator CM, Bowman VD, et al. Interaction of coxsackievirus A21 with its cellular receptor, ICAM-1. *J Virol* 2001;75(5):2444–2451.

759. Xiao C, Bator-Kelly CM, Rieder E, et al. The crystal structure of coxsackievirus A21 and its interaction with ICAM-1. *Structure* 2005;13(7):1019–1033.

760. Xiao Y, Dolan PT, Goldstein EF, et al. Poliovirus intrahost evolution is required to overcome tissue-specific innate immune responses. *Nat Commun* 2017;8(1):375.

761. Xing L, Casasnovas JM, Cheng RH. Structural analysis of human rhinovirus complexed with ICAM-1 reveals the dynamics of receptor-mediated virus uncoating. *J Virol* 2003;77(11):6101–6107.

762. Xing L, Huhtala M, Pietiainen V, et al. Structural and functional analysis of integrin alpha2I domain interaction with echovirus 1. *J Biol Chem* 2004;279(12):11632–11638.

763. Xing L, Tjarnlund K, Lindqvist B, et al. Distinct cellular receptor interactions in poliovirus and rhinoviruses. *EMBO J* 2000;19(6):1207–1216.

764. Yalamanchili P, Banerjee R, Dasgupta A. Poliovirus-encoded protease 2APro cleaves the TATA-binding protein but does not inhibit host cell RNA polymerase II transcription in vitro. *J Virol* 1997;71(9):6881–6886.

765. Yamasaki K, Weihl CC, Roos RP. Alternative translation initiation of Theiler's murine encephalomyelitis virus. *J Virol* 1999;73(10):8519–8526.

766. Yamayoshi S, Yamashita Y, Li J, et al. Scavenger receptor B2 is a cellular receptor for enterovirus 71. *Nat Med* 2009;15(7):798–801.

767. Yin J, Paul AV, Wimmer E, et al. Functional dissection of a poliovirus cis-acting replication element [PV-cre(2C)]: analysis of single- and dual-cre viral genomes and proteins that bind specifically to PV-cre RNA. *J Virol* 2003;77(9):5152–5166.

768. Yogo Y, Teng MH, Wimmer E. Poly(U) in poliovirus minus RNA is 5′-terminal. *Biochem Biophys Res Commun* 1974;61(4):1101–1109.

769. Yogo Y, Wimmer E. Polyadenylic acid at the 3′-terminus of poliovirus RNA. *Proc Natl Acad Sci U S A* 1972;69(7):1877–1882.

770. Ypma-Wong MF, Filman DJ, Hogle JM, et al. Structural domains of the poliovirus polyprotein are major determinants for proteolytic cleavage at Gln-Gly pairs. *J Biol Chem* 1988;263(33):17846–17856.

771. Ypma-Wong MF, Semler BL. In vitro molecular genetics as a tool for determining the differential cleavage specificities of the poliovirus 3C proteinase. *Nucleic Acids Res* 1987;15(5):2069–2088.

772. Yu SF, Lloyd RE. Identification of essential amino acid residues in the functional activity of poliovirus 2A protease. *Virology* 1991;182(2):615–625.

773. Yu Y, Sweeney TR, Kafasla P, et al. The mechanism of translation initiation on Aichivirus RNA mediated by a novel type of picornavirus IRES. *EMBO J* 2011;30(21):4423–4436.

774. Zajac I, Crowell R. Location and regeneration of enterovirus receptors of HeLa cells. *J Bacteriol* 1965;89:1097–1100.

775. Zeichhardt H, Otto MJ, McKinlay MA, et al. Inhibition of poliovirus uncoating by disoxaril (WIN 51711). *Virology* 1987;160(1):281–285.

776. Zhang S, Racaniello VR. Expression of the poliovirus receptor in intestinal epithelial cells is not sufficient to permit poliovirus replication in the mouse gut. *J Virol* 1997;71(7):4915–4920.

777. Zhao R, Pevear DC, Kremer MJ, et al. Human rhinovirus 3 at 3.0 A resolution. *Structure* 1996;4(10):1205–1220.

778. Zhao X, Zhang G, Liu S, et al. Human neonatal Fc receptor is the cellular uncoating receptor for enterovirus B. *Cell* 2019;177(6):1553–1565 e1516.

779. Zhu L, Sun Y, Fan J, et al. Structures of Coxsackievirus A10 unveil the molecular mechanisms of receptor binding and viral uncoating. *Nat Commun* 2018;9(1):4985.

780. Zhu L, Wang X, Ren J, et al. Structure of Ljungan virus provides insight into genome packaging of this picornavirus. *Nat Commun* 2015;6:8316.

781. Zhu L, Wang X, Ren J, et al. Structure of human Aichi virus and implications for receptor binding. *Nat Microbiol* 2016;1(11):16150.

782. Zocher G, Mistry N, Frank M, et al. A sialic acid binding site in a human picornavirus. *PLoS Pathog* 2014;10(10):e1004401.

783. Zoll J, Melchers WJ, Galama JM, et al. The mengovirus leader protein suppresses alpha/beta interferon production by inhibition of the iron/ferritin-mediated activation of NF-kappa B. *J Virol* 2002;76(19):9664–9672.

CHAPTER 3

Enteroviruses: Polioviruses, Coxsackieviruses, Echoviruses, and Newer Enteroviruses

Carolyn B. Coyne • M. Steven Oberste • Mark A. Pallansch

HISTORY

The history of enteroviruses (EVs) is very much the history of poliovirus (PV). In fact, many of the PV milestones are landmarks in the study of EV and, in fact, all of virology.

Poliomyelitis is believed to be an ancient disease. It has been suggested that the depiction of a young man with an atrophic limb on an Egyptian stele from the second millennium b.c. represents a sequela of poliomyelitis.[243] The first clinical descriptions of poliomyelitis were made in the 1800s, with reports of cases of paralysis with fever. In 1840, von Heine[190] published a monograph more specifically describing the affliction. His contributions and those published later by Medin from Sweden[335] led to paralytic poliomyelitis being referred to as *Heine-Medin disease*. Another early report, by Charcot and Joffroy,[80] described the pathologic changes in the anterior horn motor neurons of the spinal cord in poliomyelitis.

The 1900s began a new era in poliomyelitis investigations, and the beginning of an understanding of the infectious nature of this disease. Wickman[514] and others recognized the communicable nature of poliomyelitis, the importance of asymptomatic infected individuals in transmission of PV, and the role of enteric infection in disease pathogenesis. The role of the gastrointestinal tract in the initiation and spread of PV infection was later confirmed by Trask et al.[485] In a classic study, Viennese investigators Landsteiner and Popper[297] proved the infectious nature of poliomyelitis by successfully transmitting the clinical disease and its pathology to monkeys following inoculation of CNS tissue homogenates from human cases.

Despite this progress, a number of unfortunate misconceptions emerged about poliomyelitis that initially confused scientists and misdirected efforts for control. These misconceptions included a belief that the virus was exclusively neurotropic, that the nasopharynx was a major site for virus entry into the CNS, and that the virus spread to the nervous system before viremia and by way of the olfactory nerve. As a result of these misconceptions and the failure of several poorly conceived immunization attempts, some with rather disastrous results,[401] an atmosphere of pessimism existed by the middle of the 20th century concerning the eventual control of poliomyelitis, even among scientists working in the field. In 1945, Burnet[60] wrote, "The practical problem of preventing infantile paralysis has not been solved. It is even doubtful whether it ever will be solved." The eventual realization that virus entered via the oral–gastrointestinal route and that CNS disease followed a viremia did much to boost hopes for effective immunization.[50]

Building on studies of others, Enders et al.[128] performed a landmark study showing that PV could be propagated in non-neural tissue culture. These investigations had implications for all of virology because they indicated, first, that PV grew in various tissue culture cells that did not correspond to the tissues infected during the human disease and, second, that PV destroyed cells with a specific cytopathic effect. Neutralization tests showed that PV has three serotypes,[51] and serologic tests[29] confirmed that most infected individuals do not manifest clinical disease. These investigations laid a critical framework for the development of a vaccine, and they clarified a host of confusing data, such as the apparent presence of second attacks of poliomyelitis.

A variety of vaccines were subsequently produced, with the most well known being the Salk inactivated polio vaccine (IPV) delivered via the intramuscular route (licensed in 1955 in the United States) and the Sabin live, attenuated vaccine (oral polio vaccine [OPV]) delivered via the oral route (licensed in 1961–1962). The importance of these vaccines and the individuals who produced them can begin to be realized by noting that more Americans knew the name of Jonas Salk than the President of the United States. The real impact of these vaccines will ultimately be felt with the complete global eradication of poliomyelitis. The eradication will undoubtedly provide a fitting dramatic finale to the compelling story of poliomyelitis.

PV work has had a continuing significant impact on the field of molecular virology. PV was the first animal virus completely cloned and sequenced,[277,411] the first RNA animal virus for which an infectious clone was constructed,[412] and the first human virus that had its three-dimensional structure solved by x-ray crystallography.[201] In 1989, Mendelsohn et al.[342] identified the PV receptor, CD155, a finding that was followed by the generation of mice carrying CD155 as a transgene.[284,421]

Coxsackieviruses (group A) were first isolated during poliomyelitis outbreaks in 1947 from the feces of paralyzed children in Coxsackie, New York.[108] These isolates were obtained by inoculation of suckling mice, the pathogenicity in mice clearly differentiating these viruses from PV that did not paralyze mice. In the following year, the first coxsackievirus (CV) group B was isolated from cases of aseptic meningitis.[339] The original CV group A (CVA) isolates produced myositis with flaccid hind limb paralysis in newborn mice, whereas the coxsackievirus group B (CVB) produced a spastic paralysis and generalized infection in newborn mice, with myositis as well as involvement of the brain, pancreas, heart, and brown fat.

In 1951, echoviruses were first isolated from the stool of asymptomatic individuals.[426] Echoviruses received their name because they were *e*nteric isolates, *c*ytopathogenic in tissue culture, isolated from *h*umans, and *o*rphans (i.e., unassociated with a known clinical disease). Subsequent studies have shown that echoviruses, in fact, do cause a variety of human diseases including aseptic meningitis, hepatitis, and orchitis, among others. After this period of rapid growth in the number of enteroviruses, there were several decades where new enteroviruses were uncommonly identified. This changed with the introduction of molecular detection methods, and the last 15 years have seen a rapid expansion in the number of recognized enteroviruses. This period of discovery is still in progress.

INFECTIOUS AGENTS

Physical and Chemical Properties

Enteroviruses are distinguished from other picornaviruses on the basis of physical properties, such as buoyant density in cesium chloride and stability in weak acid. Many aspects of enteroviral pathology, transmission, and general epidemiology are directly related to the biophysical properties and their cytolytic life cycle. The infectious virus is relatively resistant to many common laboratory disinfectants, including 70% ethanol, isopropanol, dilute Lysol, and quaternary ammonium compounds. The virus is insensitive to lipid solvents, including ether and chloroform, and it is stable in many detergents at ambient temperature. Formaldehyde, glutaraldehyde, strong acid, sodium hypochlorite, and free residual chlorine inactivate enteroviruses. Concentration, pH, extraneous organic materials, and contact time affect the degree of inactivation by these compounds. Similar inactivation is achieved when virus is present on fomites, although conditions may not be exactly comparable.[2] In general, most reagents that inactivate EV depend on active chemical modification of the virion, whereas most extractive solvents have no effect.

Enteroviruses are relatively thermostable, but less so than hepatitis A virus. Most enteroviruses are readily inactivated at 42°C, although some sulfhydryl-reducing agents and magnesium cations can stabilize viruses so that they are relatively stable at 50°C.[10,121] The relative sensitivity to modest elevations in temperature makes it possible to use pasteurization to inactivate EV in many biologically active preparations.[197]

As with other infectious agents, ultraviolet light can be used to inactivate EV, particularly on surfaces. In addition, the process of drying on surfaces significantly reduces virus titers. The degree of virus loss by drying is related to porosity of the surfaces and the presence of organic material.[1] Many studies of EV inactivation have been conducted using PV as a model EV. A report describing strain-specific differences for glutaraldehyde inactivation among echovirus 25 isolates implies, however, that the assumption that PV is representative of all EV may not be valid.[77] The inactivation of infectivity may not be directly related to the destruction of the viral genome, because the polymerase chain reaction (PCR) can be used to amplify viral RNA, even after inactivation of virus has occurred.[321] This would suggest that reactivation of infectivity may be possible in some circumstances. In fact, some examples of recovered infectivity have been reported through increased multiplicity of infection in cell culture,[455,543] but the practical significance of these observations is not clear.

Antigenic Characteristics and Taxonomy

As described in Chapter 2, the picornaviruses are among the simplest RNA viruses, having a highly structured capsid with little place for elaboration. Yet, despite the limited genetic material and structural constraints, evolution within the picornaviruses has resulted in a large number of readily distinguishable members. This variability has been categorized antigenically as serotype.

In the case of human enteroviruses, each of the serotypes correlates with the immunologic response of the human host, protection from disease, receptor usage, and, to a lesser extent, the spectrum of clinical disease. These correlations, however, have only a partial relationship with the original classification of enteroviruses into polioviruses, coxsackie A or B viruses, and echoviruses, based on biological activity and disease: human CNS disease with flaccid paralysis (poliomyelitis); flaccid paralysis in newborn mice, human CNS disease, and herpangina (coxsackie A viruses); spastic paralysis in newborn mice and human CNS and cardiac disease (coxsackie B viruses); and no disease in mice and (originally) no human disease (echoviruses). Within each of these groups, isolates can be readily distinguished on the basis of antigenicity as measured with antisera raised in animals. The original classification scheme broke down with the identification of viruses antigenically identical to known echoviruses that were found to cause disease in mice and humans. This and other inconsistencies led to the numbering of new EV serotypes starting with EV68 (now termed EV-D68). These antigenic groupings, which define the

serotypes, became increasingly more complicated as the number of different viruses grew. Despite these limitations, the serotype remains the single most important physical and immunologic property that distinguishes the different EV. Most of the prototype EV strains are maintained in the American Type Culture Collection, Manassas, Virginia, and in many of the WHO collaborating reference laboratories.

Despite the importance of the antigenic properties, the introduction of molecular typing methods and a reassessment of the limitations of the old classification scheme led to the development of the current classification system that divides the members of the EV genus into species on the basis of genome organization and sequence similarity as well as biological properties (see Tables 3.1 and 3.4 to 3.6).

TABLE 3.1   Picornavirus genera, species[a], and (sero)types with members known to infect humans

Genus and Species	No. of Types	Comments
Genus *Enterovirus*[b]		
Enterovirus A	25	5 types have been found only in nonhuman primates
Enterovirus B	63	4 types have been found only in nonhuman primates
Enterovirus C	23	
Enterovirus D	5	1 type has been found only in nonhuman primates
Rhinovirus A	80	
Rhinovirus B	25	
Rhinovirus C	56	
Genus *Parechovirus*[c]		
Parechovirus A	19	
Genus *Cardiovirus*[d]		
Cardiovirus A	2	Additional viruses not assigned to type
Cardiovirus B	14	
Genus *Cosavirus*[e]		
Cosavirus A	24	
Cosavirus B	?	
Cosavirus D	?	
Cosavirus E	?	
Cosavirus F	?	
Genus *Hepatovirus*[f]		
Hepatovirus A	1	Hepatitis A virus; also known to infect nonhuman primates
Genus *Kobuvirus*[g]		
Aichivirus A	1	
Genus *Salivirus*		
Salivirus A	1	Additional viruses not assigned to type
40 additional genera infecting mammals, birds, amphibians, reptiles, and fish		

[a]The classification scheme shown is from the Picornavirus Study Group of the International Committee on Taxonomy of Viruses (https://talk.ictvonline.org/ictv-reports/ictv_online_report/positive-sense-rna-viruses/picornavirales/w/picornaviridae; additional details from http://www.picornaviridae.com).
[b]*Enterovirus*: Eight additional species infect mammals other than humans. The types that constitute *Enterovirus A* through *Enterovirus D* are listed in Tables 3.4 to 3.6.
[c]*Parechovirus*: Two additional species infect mammals other than humans. PeV-A1 and PeV-A2 were formerly classified as echoviruses 22 and 23, respectively.
[d]*Cardiovirus*: One additional species infects mammals other than humans.
[e]Establishment of *Cosavirus C* is pending due to incomplete virus sequences. Types not established in species other than *Cosavirus A*.
[f]Eight additional species infect mammals other than humans.
[g]Two additional species infect mammals other than humans.

The human enteroviruses are now classified into four species: *Enterovirus A* (EV-A), EV-B, EV-C, and EV-D. In this system, members within an EV species

> "share (i) a significant degree of amino acid identity of the P1, 2C, 3C and 3D proteins; (ii) monophyly in phylogenetic trees; and (iii) essentially identical genome maps."[280,548]

Coding for the capsid proteins, the P1 region provides a reliable correlation between sequence relatedness and the traditional definition of serotype. This also appears to be true for the various individual capsid protein regions, with the exception of VP4; the VP4 sequence does not always correlate with serotype and, therefore, is not reliable for serotype identification.

The molecular studies have also provided a framework in which the EV antigenic relationships can be better understood. These studies suggest that the nucleotide sequence of VP1 can function as an excellent surrogate for the reference antigenic typing methods that use neutralization tests in order to distinguish EV serotypes. VP1 nucleotide sequence identity of at least 75% (85% aa identity) between an isolate and a serotype prototype strain suggests that the isolate is serotypically identical to the prototype (assuming that the next highest identity with other prototype strains is <70%). For example, a capsid sequence identity of 85.4% aa between CVA3 and A8 compared with a mean sequence identity among prototype strains of 71.5% confirmed the antigenic relationships that had previously been described, and suggested that these two viruses probably derived relatively recently from a common ancestor.[386] Similarly, capsid sequences with more than 96% identity confirmed the antigenic relationships between CVA11 and A15 and between A13 and A18[58]; as a result, CVA15 and A18 have been reclassified as A11 and A15, respectively. In this way, the use of VP1 sequencing studies has supported and clarified early serologic data and led to proposals regarding the classification of isolates into new EV serotypes.[387,388]

No general correlation is found, however, between sequence similarities with serotype in genome segments outside of the capsid region because of frequent recombination in the noncapsid regions. For example, sequencing studies have shown that phylogenetic trees constructed from sequences from varying genome regions of members of EV-C and *poliovirus* have incongruities between the capsid region and noncapsid regions,[58] suggesting that viruses with a PV capsid may recombine with these CV nonstructural protein coding regions to acquire different nonstructural protein sequences and, similarly, viruses with a CV capsid protein sequence may recombine to acquire different nonstructural protein sequences.[315,438] These findings imply that recombination occurs between PV and other EV-C viruses within the nonstructural protein coding regions and this interchange of different nonstructural protein coding regions may lead to strains that become dominant due to selective advantages. The frequency of recombination in the noncapsid region supports the idea that serotype is defined by the capsid region and that limited correlations likely exist between the serotype of isolates and other phenotypic characteristics not associated with the capsid proteins. The findings also demonstrated that the phylogenetic clustering of prototype strains changes, depending on the nonstructural region that is analyzed.

Recombination within the nonstructural proteins was also found among EV-A and EV-B prototype members with other members of the same species, consistent with their classification into two separate species.[378,386] An analysis of multiple isolates within several EV-B serotypes[381] found relatively frequent interserotypic recombination of the noncoding regions, which appeared to occur at least once every 6 years for the isolates that were analyzed. Although no evidence was found of interserotypic recombination within the capsid (perhaps, because of structural constraints specific for a particular serotype), intraserotypic recombination within this region appeared to occur.

Additional sequencing studies showed that the 5'-untranslated region (UTR) of enteroviruses forms two clusters: the viruses of EV-C and EV-D constitute cluster I, whereas EV-A and EV-B constitute cluster II.[58,232]

Sequencing studies have also demonstrated significant similarities between human rhinoviruses and the human enteroviruses, resulting in a reclassification of the human rhinoviruses as members of three different species within the genus *Enterovirus*.[280]

In addition to the genetic relatedness, many different EV serotypes share some antigenicity. For example, PV1 and PV2 share a common antigen, and antigenic relationships also exist between coxsackieviruses A3 and A8, A16 and EV71, and A24 and EV70 and between echoviruses 6 and 30 and 12 and 29. When virions are disrupted by heating, particularly in the presence of detergent, nonsurface antigens are exposed that are shared broadly among many EVs.[343]

Despite this lack of understanding of molecular variation in virus structure as measured by polyclonal antibodies, high-resolution studies of the virion surface have been particularly useful in identifying the targets of neutralization of EV by monoclonal antibodies.[202,400] Other less-investigated antigenic sites elicit immune responses that are not neutralizing but, nevertheless, contribute to serotype identity. The observed structure of some antigenic sites has been shown to span noncontinuous polypeptide chains, providing an explanation for why antigenicity of the virus is destroyed by disruption of the virion structure.

Antisera raised in animals to each of the enteroviruses are largely type specific and are used to determine serotype in a neutralization assay. The PV neutralizing antibody response is serotype specific, with the exception of some minor cross-reaction between PV1 and PV2. A monoclonal antibody has been described that reacts with this shared site that is not found on PV3.[492] As noted, heat-disrupted virions, particularly those heated in the presence of detergent, induce antibodies that react with many EVs.[343] These broadly reacting antibodies are generally not neutralizing, and at least one of these epitopes has been mapped to the amino-terminal region of capsid protein VP1.[441] Although measurable *in vitro* differences are found in antigenic properties among strains within a serotype, the significance of these differences during natural infection has not been determined. Several PV isolated during outbreaks have demonstrated different antigenic properties when compared with the reference vaccine strains.[175,228] In all cases, however, immunity derived from vaccination has been sufficient to provide protection and control of these strains.[54] In addition, even in the face of massive immunization campaigns, no antigenic escape mutants resistant to neutralization have ever been observed, and successive genotypes of PV have been eliminated. Natural antigenic variants have also been identified with panels of monoclonal antibodies for several nonpolio EVs.[184,402]

Propagation and Assay in Cell Culture

One of the prominent characteristics of enteroviruses is the cytolytic nature of growth in cell culture. For many years, PV was the prototype of a lytic viral infection. At the microscopic level, infection is usually manifest within 1 to 7 days, and sometimes within mere hours, by the appearance of a characteristic cytopathic effect, which features visible rounding, shrinking, nuclear pyknosis, refractility, and cell degeneration (Fig. 3.1). The earliest effects can often be seen in less than 24 hours, often as soon as in 4 hours, if the inoculum contains many infectious particles. With fewer virions, however, visible changes are not generally recognizable for several days, although a sufficient number of cells are infected. In addition, some EVs either do not cause cytopathic effect at all or do so only after several passages. In general, once focal cytopathic effect is detected, infection spreads rapidly throughout the cell sheet with total destruction of the monolayer.

All known EVs can be propagated either in cell culture or in suckling mice, though for many of the newer EV, attempts to propagate have been limited and suckling mice are now seldom used. Most of the serotypes can be grown in at least one human or primate continuous cell culture. No cell line, however, can support the growth of all cultivable EVs. Even after many years of experimentation, a few serotypes (e.g., CVA19) can be propagated only in suckling mice. The typical host range of human EV in cell cultures or animals is shown in a broad, generalized way in Table 3.2 and is not clearly associated specifically with a given virus species. Infection of target cells depends on viruses binding to specific receptors on the cell surface. Collectively,

the EVs use many different receptors. A practical adaptation resulting from the identification and genetic cloning of EV receptors is the introduction of the receptor into animals and cells that do not normally permit virus infection. This approach has resulted in both advances in understanding the pathogenesis of PV infection in a nonprimate animal model system and its practical application in the diagnostic laboratory. The L20B cells, which are murine cells that express CD155, are now used routinely to selectively isolate PV (see *Diagnosis*) as part of the global PV laboratory network supporting the poliomyelitis eradication initiative.[406]

Major advances in the isolation and propagation of human-derived primary cells are beginning to advance our understanding of the possible interactions of EV with human cells *in vivo*. For example, the use of primary airway epithelia isolated from human nasal polyps grown at an air–liquid interface (ALI) has shown that EV-D68 alters mucociliary clearance and induces significant cytotoxicity in the epithelium.[130] Similarly, the isolation of human intestinal crypts, which can be propagated in the presence of growth factors that induced the differentiation of intestinal stem cells into all of the major cell types present in the gastrointestinal tract, has been used to study the impact of EV infection on intestinal structure and function.[125,163] These studies have revealed that different EVs target distinct cell types in the human GI epithelium and exhibit differences in their ability to dysregulate barrier function. The continued development and application of these models to *in vitro* studies of EVs will likely provide important insights into a number of facets of EV biology.

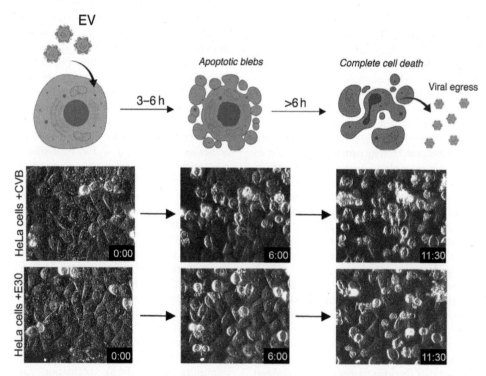

FIGURE 3.1 Enteroviruses commonly induce apoptosis, which is induced in cell culture models within 3 to 6 hours postinfection, with complete cell lysis by greater than 6 hours postinfection. Top, Schematic of the morphological changes induce by enterovirus infections, which can include cell blebbing and eventual cell lysis, which facilitates viral egress. **Bottom,** time-lapse imaging of HeLa cells infected with CVB or echovirus 30 demonstrates the timing and magnitude of EV-induced cell death over a span of 11.5 hours post-infection. Time stamp at bottom right denotes hours post-infection. (Video 3.1, Video 3.2)

TABLE 3.2   Usual host range of human enteroviruses: animal and tissue culture spectrum[a]

Virus	Antigenic Types[b]	Cytopathic Effect		Illness and Pathology	
		Monkey Kidney Tissue Culture	Human Tissue Culture	Suckling Mouse	Monkey
Polioviruses	1–3	+	+	−	+
Coxsackieviruses, group A	1–22, 24	±	±	+	−
Coxsackieviruses, group B	1–6	+	+	+	−
Echoviruses	1–33	+	±	−	−
Enteroviruses	68–121	+	+	−	−

[a]Many enteroviral strains have been isolated that do not conform to these categories.
[b]New types, beginning with type 68, are now assigned enterovirus type numbers instead of coxsackievirus or echovirus numbers. Types 68 to 121 have been identified.

Infection in Experimental Animals: Host Range

The natural host for all human enteroviruses is the human. Although serologically distinct picornaviruses with the same physical properties as those of human EV have been found in many animals, human beings do not usually have recognizable infections with these animal EVs. On the other hand, some animals are susceptible to experimental infection with human EV. These include nonhuman primates and CD155-transgenic mice for polioviruses, mice and some monkeys for coxsackieviruses A and B, monkeys for echoviruses, mice for EV-D68, and mice and monkeys for EV-A71. In some cases, mouse models of EV require ablation of host innate immune signaling through the deletion or inhibition of antiviral type I interferon (IFN) signaling. Human EV can infect nonhuman primates, perhaps related to the homology that several simian EVs share with human viruses, but the infections appear to be largely subclinical.[379,409] Among higher primates, chimpanzees and gorillas appear to be able to acquire PV infection and develop disease from humans through natural exposure.[122] CVB5 is closely related antigenically to the porcine EV causing swine vesicular disease, with about 50% genetic identity over the entire genome. Genetic studies of a number of strains of swine vesicular disease virus, as well as epidemiologic information gleaned from outbreaks, strongly suggest that a human CVB5 was specifically introduced into swine decades ago and led to establishment in this new host.[551]

Although most coxsackie A viruses have been successfully grown in various cell culture systems, isolation from clinical specimens is sometimes unsuccessful, necessitating the inoculation of suckling mice. Inoculation of suckling mice and subsequent virus identification is a process analogous to that of cell culture inoculation. A blind passage in mice may be necessary if the inoculum is of very low titer or, possibly, because passage of the virus is needed for it to adapt to growth in mice. The two groups of coxsackieviruses can be distinguished by the distinct pathology that they cause in mice. With CVA infection, newborn mice develop flaccid paralysis and severe, extensive degeneration of skeletal muscle (sparing the tongue, heart, and CNS), and they may have renal lesions. Death usually occurs within a week. CVB infection proceeds more slowly and is characterized by spastic paralysis and tremors associated with encephalomyelitis, focal myositis, necrosis of brown fat pads, myocarditis, hepatitis, and acinar cell pancreatitis. Echoviruses, except for some isolates of echovirus type 9, do not generally cause disease in mice, but disease can be induced in neonatal mice expressing human homologs of echovirus receptors.[223,354] The expression of the human homolog of the EV71 receptor SCARB2 also sensitizes mice to EV71 infection, with disease resembling that observed in humans (including paralysis and death).[150,311]

Other Human Picornaviruses

In addition to the enteroviruses, rhinoviruses, and hepatitis A virus, other picornaviruses that infect humans have been recently discovered or previously considered to be enteroviruses and are now reclassified as a separate genus (Table 3.1). These genera are genetically distinct from the EV genus (Fig. 3.2), but share some physical and structural similarity with EV. On the basis of a very low genetic relationship, differences in viral proteins and processing, and a novel 2A protease, echoviruses 22 and 23 were reclassified as a new genus, *Parechovirus*. Additional members of this genus exist, including additional serotypes of human parechovirus (HPeV),[236] as well as a separate species first isolated in Swedish bank voles, Ljungan virus; Ljungan virus has been associated with diabetes in its natural host and has been postulated to have a role in human disease.[370] The human parechoviruses (PeV-A; 19 types) cause a similar spectrum of illnesses as the EV and can often be detected in cerebrospinal fluid (CSF) from meningitis cases at a frequency similar to that of the EV.[499,518] Serologic studies suggest that HPeV infection occurs at an early age, as most children were seropositive by the age of 2 years.[3,244,471] HPeV3 has been associated with sepsis-like illness and central nervous system disease in infants.[41,52]

Another distinct picornavirus genus associated with human infection is *Kobuvirus*.[531] Although little is known about this virus, it appears that it is often associated with gastroenteritis in young children and infection is common, and distinct types cause diarrhea in cats and dogs.[65,307] Members of the genus *Cardiovirus* have also been associated with disease in humans, but they do not appear to be a major cause of human illness.[367,389] Viruses in the genus, *Salivirus*, are related to kobuviruses and have also been associated with gastroenteritis in humans.[205,306] Cosaviruses (genus *Cosavirus*) have been detected at a relatively high frequency in stool and have been isolated from children

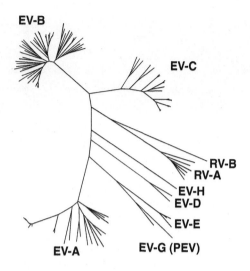

FIGURE 3.2 Dendrogram of genus _Enterovirus_. The figure illustrates the phylogenetic relationship among the prototype strains (see Tables 3.4 to 3.6) within the genus _Enterovirus_ and the distinct grouping of isolates into each of the species of viruses that affects humans and other related animal enteroviruses based on the amino acid sequence of the P1 (capsid) coding region of the genomes. Species: EV-A (formerly human enterovirus A), EV-B (formerly human enterovirus B), EV-C (formerly human enterovirus C), EV-D (formerly human enterovirus D), RV-A (formerly human rhinovirus A), RV-B (formerly human rhinovirus B), EV-E (formerly bovine enterovirus), EV-G (formerly porcine enterovirus B), and EV-H (formerly simian enterovirus B). Not shown: EV-F (bovine enterovirus 2), EV-J (simian virus 6 and related viruses), and RV-C.

with diarrhea or gastroenteritis.[204,271,368] What is notable about all of these newer genera is that the molecular reagents for the detection of EV do not detect these viruses (see _Diagnosis_).

PATHOGENESIS AND PATHOLOGY

Entry into the Host
Virus infection normally requires that the virion attaches to the cell surface, and it was long imagined that each virus would have a single receptor. For PV, at least, this may be the case: the virus binds to the PV receptor (PVR[342]; now named CD155), a transmembrane glycoprotein in the immunoglobulin superfamily that mediates adhesion of NK cells and triggers their effector functions. PVR (human CD155) appears to be the major factor regulating the natural host range of PV, which is limited to humans and old world primates. CD155 homologs/orthologs have been identified and characterized in mice[355] and in new world monkeys; the extracellular domains share approximately 70% amino acid homology with hCD155, and these homologs do not support efficient PV binding or infection. Several laboratories have generated transgenic mice that express PVR, and, in many of the resulting models, PV was shown to induce neurological disease and paralysis following parenteral administration.[101,145,233,285,342,360,419–421,549] However, oral administration did not cause disease even when the PVR transgene was regulated by a promoter that drove protein expression in enterocytes and M cells; PV appeared to bind to the intestinal cells, but productive infection was not observed following oral

inoculation of greater than 10^8 PFU of virus.[549] These findings are consistent with studies of humans and susceptible primates, in which hCD155 expression has been identified in many tissues, but productive infection is limited largely to the CNS. In mice, deletion of the receptor required for antiviral type I IFN signaling (the interferon-α/β receptor, IFNAR) permits PV entry into the CNS following inoculation by the intramuscular or intraperitoneal routes.[292,296] Thus, factors other than PVR expression play a key role in determining _in vivo_ tropism, which may differ between species.

It is now generally accepted that some viruses, or viral strains, may have more than one receptor, perhaps expanding their potential host range. EV71, most frequently associated with hand-foot-and-mouth disease in children but capable of causing devastating neurological pathology,[465] has at least two receptors: scavenger receptor B2, SCARB2,[532] and P-selectin glycoprotein ligand-1, PSGL-1.[371] However, although EV71 binds with greater efficiency to PSGL-1, this binding may not be sufficient to induce genome release, which requires both SCARB2 and endosomal low pH.[533] EV-D68 may also utilize two cellular receptors, with some isolates binding to sialic acid[32] and all binding to the neuronal-specific intercellular adhesion molecule 5 (ICAM5).[510] Many CVA viruses appear to share a single receptor, KREMIN1, the murine homology of which is required for _in vivo_ infection.[466]

Indeed, some viruses appear to interact with two different surface molecules on a single cell, perhaps in series, with one protein acting as the binding moiety, before "handing over" the virus to a second protein that facilitates its entry into the cell. This is thought to occur for some CVBs that bind to decay-accelerating factor (DAF, CD55) but then must interact with another protein, the _c_oxsackievirus and _a_denovirus _r_eceptor (CAR), in order to enter the cell.[99] DAF also serves as an attachment factor for other EVs, including several echoviruses,[42] but similar to CVB, this binding is not sufficient to induce genome release. Instead, echoviruses utilize the neonatal Fc receptor (FcRn) as a primary receptor, but the precise role of this receptor in echovirus entry remains unclear.[354]

Site of Primary Replication
Human enteroviruses are spread by the fecal–oral route and respiratory droplets, so systemic infection requires the virus to cross the gastrointestinal wall, most of which is lined with epithelial cells that form a barrier to invasion. Perhaps surprisingly, given the many years of study, the primary site of PV infection and replication in the intestine remains unknown. PV has been identified in lymphoid tissues such as the tonsils[50] and in lymphoid aggregates, commonly termed Peyer patches (PP), that are present in the ileum of the small intestine. PP are overlaid with a specialized follicle-associated epithelium (FAE) that contains microfold (M) cells, which can transport certain molecules from the gastrointestinal lumen, across the epithelial layer, and into cells in the PP. Some studies suggest that PV may replicate within these epithelial cells and lymphoid cells,[251] while others suggest that the virus may be transcytosed through the M cell, subsequently establishing infection in an unidentified cell in the PP.[459] The cells in which CVB initially replicates are also uncertain; this issue is further clouded by the predominant use, in mouse models, of the intraperitoneal route of infection. As discussed above, the application of human stem cell–derived models of the intestinal epithelial (often referred

to as "organoids" or "enteroids") has provided some insights into the cell-type–specific nature of EV infection within the GI epithelium. Utilizing this model, it has been shown that echovirus 11 preferentially infected enterocytes, with infection also observed in enteroendocrine cells, but that mucus-secreting goblet cells were not permissive to infection.[125] Consistent with this, echovirus 11 infection induces profound loss of epithelial barrier integrity.[163] In contrast, EV71 infection of stem cell–derived GI epithelial monolayers does not induce any loss of epithelial barrier function, which might be attributed to its preferential infection of goblet cells.[163] However, given that the intestinal microbiome may be an important mediator of EV-GI epithelial attachment and infection, which is missing from these models, whether this specificity exists *in vivo* is unknown.[293,427]

HRV infects epithelial cells of the airways. Infection of the nasal epithelium causes few detectable pathological changes, even if rhinitis is quite severe, and—as is true for many virus-induced diseases—many of the symptoms appear to be caused by the host response, rather than by direct virus-mediated tissue damage.[516,517] In contrast to HRV, EV-D68 infection induces pronounced cytotoxicity in primary airway cells.[130]

Spread in the Host

Following replication in the GI tract, PV enters the blood, thereby potentially gaining access to all tissues. However, in most hosts, viral replication is highly restricted, being readily detected mainly in the CNS.[50] PV can enter the CNS in two ways. First, PV can access from the blood, where it cross the blood–brain barrier (BBB), perhaps independently of CD155.[534] Second, the virus (apparently in the form of an intact virion) can traffic by retrograde axonal transport, ascending the neuronal axon, perhaps in endosomes, with uncoating beginning once the virus reaches the cell body.[394–396] This may underpin provocation poliomyelitis, a phenomenon in which a traumatized limb is more susceptible to paralytic polio. The trauma may be directly associated with the virus, as reported in 1935, when it was noted that paralysis first appeared in (or was most severe in) the limb that had received an intramuscular inoculation of "pre-Salk" polio vaccine.[299] Such inoculation poliomyelitis also was observed in the "Cutter incident," when an incompletely inactivated Salk vaccine was administered.[362] However, provocation poliomyelitis does not require that trauma and virus be administered to the same limb; when PV was administered intravascularly to monkeys that had received innocuous injections into one limb, paralysis was more likely to develop in the injected muscles.[49] Provocation poliomyelitis also has been reproduced in a mouse model.[174] Mechanisms other than retrograde axonal transport may also contribute to this phenomenon. For example, the peripheral trauma may increase vascular permeability locally, in the region that innervates the injured muscle; this could explain why provocation poliomyelitis still occurs in traumatized limbs despite scission of the ipsilateral peroneal muscle.[361] In contrast, dissemination of CVB and other enteroviruses appears to occur largely by the hematogenous route given that viremia is frequently found.

Cell and Tissue Tropism

EVs exhibit broad cell and tissue tropism (Fig. 3.3). It has been proposed that the observed *in vivo* tropism of PV for the CNS may result from differing efficiencies of viral internal ribosome entry site (IRES) utilization by various host cell types.

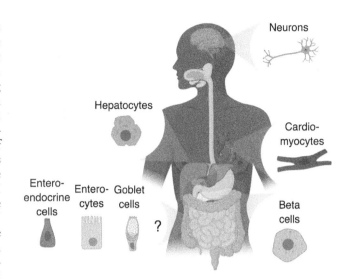

FIGURE 3.3 EVs exhibit broad cell and tissue tropism. The neuronal complications associated with EV infections can include direct infection of neurons. In the heart and pancreas, viruses like CVB replicate specifically in cardiomyocytes and β-cells, respectively. The cellular tropism at other tissue sites is less clear, but some evidence suggests specific cell types (including enterocytes, goblet cells, and enteroendocrine cell) could be targeted by EVs in the gastrointestinal tract. Other common tissues include the liver, with evidence that some EVs may preferentially replicate in hepatocytes, although the specific cell tropism remains unclear.

However, this explanation appears to be incorrect; the PV IRES is equally functional in many cell types *in vivo*, including those that do not support virus replication *in vivo*.[259] A key driver of PV tropism likely lies in the ability of a given cell type to induce antiviral signaling and respond to these signals. For example, CD155-transgenic mice lacking type I IFN signaling due to the deletion of IFNAR developed severe lesions not only in the CNS but also in the liver, spleen, and pancreas.[234] Thus, the absence of PV-induced damage and disease in immunocompetent mice expressing CD155 supports a model whereby type I IFN signaling directly limits PV neurotropism.

CVB3 can cause pancreatitis, myocarditis, and meningoencephalitis. Enteroviruses, and especially CVB, have been implicated in up to one-third of human pancreatitis cases.[24,399,493] In the mouse model, the pancreas appears to be a major site of CVB3 replication.[340,341] CVB4 also causes pancreatitis,[415,416,496] the severity of which depends on the virus isolate that is used; a single amino acid change in VP1 appears to be largely responsible for switching the phenotype from mild pancreatitis to a more severe form.[64,178] In mice, CVB has been found in acinar cells, but not in the islets of Langerhans[434,498,501] by immunohistochemistry[25,496] and by *in situ* hybridization.[25,498,501] Expression of the CVB primary receptor CAR correlates with the observed pathology—the receptor mRNA is expressed at very high levels in acinar cells, but not in the pancreatic ducts or the islets of Langerhans,[250] consistent with the observation that CVB-infected mice do not develop hyperglycemia.[341,418] Deletion of CAR specifically from the pancreas in mice confers substantial, albeit incomplete, protection against organ damage during CVB3 infection,[250] suggesting that CAR expression is an important determinant of CVB-associated pancreatic dysfunction. In addition to receptor expression, the potency of antiviral signaling in pancreatic cell types may also explain the cellular tropism of CVBs in the pancreas. For example, α cells induce more potent antiviral signaling than do β cells in response to CVB infection, which might explain their ability to resist infection and evade autoimmune responses during infection.[329]

CVB has long been considered one of the principal causes of viral myocarditis[100] and this view has been confirmed in several reports.[19,129,324,326,328] CAR is expressed at high levels in cardiomyocytes,[375] where it is involved in heart development and cardiac function in mice.[26,82,120,314] Notably, CAR is expressed at high levels in neonatal rat cardiomyocytes but is expressed at low levels in adult rat cardiomyocytes.[257] This spatiotemporal expression has been speculated to explain the enhanced susceptibility of neonates to CVB-induced cardiac complications. *In vivo*, CAR expression on cardiomyocytes is required for CVB-induced myocarditis as mice lacking CAR specifically in these cells are protected from cardiac infection and disease.[250]

Several mechanisms have been proposed to explain CVB-mediated cardiomyocyte destruction. The first is direct virus-mediated damage. Human cardiomyocytes can be infected *in vitro*,[189,253] and infected cells are rapidly lysed.[195] These *in vitro* findings are corroborated by *in vivo* ultrastructural studies of myocardial tissue, which show clear evidence of virus infection of cardiac muscle cells and cell death in mice.[161,200,278] The second is immunopathological damage. The inflammatory infiltrate contains CD8[+] T cells, natural killer cells, and macrophages,[81,159,193,452] and other studies have implicated $\gamma\delta$ T cells in CVB pathogenesis.[215,216,220,221] Finally, studies have implicated autoimmunity in CVB-triggered myocarditis.[215,364,432,433] One potential means by which this could occur is *via* molecular mimicry, that is, immunological cross-reactivity between viral and heart proteins, and there is evidence that this occurs at both the antibody[151,152] and T-cell[214,215,219] levels. Virus replication in the heart is a prerequisite for myocardial destruction, and this is difficult to reconcile with molecular mimicry; these data do not, of course, exclude a role for autoimmunity induced by other means, for example, by virus-driven exposure of sequestered cardiac antigens or to genetic factors that might predispose individuals to cardiac complications.

Although a rare polymorphism in the dsRNA sensor toll-like receptor 3 (TLR3) was identified in a patient who developed CVB-associated myocarditis,[164] and mice lacking TLR3 or are deficient in type I IFN signaling are more susceptible to CVB-induced cardiac dysfunction,[116,363] genetic variants in TLR3 or other IFN-associated factors are not commonly found in patients with viral-associated myocarditis.[36] Instead, many of these patients have homozygous variants in genes associated with inherited cardiomyopathies, suggesting that a genetic predisposition to cardiac dysfunction may sensitize individuals to CVB-induced myocarditis.

Most EVs are neurotropic and are associated with severe neurological outcomes including aseptic meningitis and acute flaccid myelitis. However, the specific factors that drive this tropism remain largely unclear. The receptors for many neurotropic EVs are expressed on diverse cell types within the CNS, suggesting that receptor expression is likely to play a role. In some cases, EV receptors are uniquely expressed in the CNS, such as ICAM5, which is a primary receptor for EV-D68[510] and is expressed almost exclusively in the CNS.[542] Given that expression of the human homologs of many EV receptors is sufficient to promote CNS infection and disease in mice,[150,223]

neuronal tropism is likely influenced largely by receptor expression and/or localization. However, other factors, such as the degree of viremia, host immune response, etc., also likely play important roles in this tropism given that neuronal complications are not observed in every infection.

The liver is also a primary site of EV-associated disease, with hepatitis and acute liver failure observed in infected infants and children. Hepatocytes are highly permissive to CVB infection when type I IFN signaling is inhibited or ablated *in vivo* or in human primary cells.[281] Like cardiomyocytes, this hepatic tropism has also been attributed to age-related changes in CAR expression, with hepatocytes from neonatal animals exhibiting higher levels of CAR expression and enhanced sensitivity to infection.[316] Echoviruses, in particular, are commonly associated with liver disease in infected neonates.[44] The mediators for the hepatic tropism of echoviruses are unclear, particularly given that few *in vivo* models exist to study this aspect of infection, but recent work in neonatal mice expressing the echovirus receptor FcRn recapitulates echovirus 11 infection in the liver.[354] In adult mice lacking IFN signaling, echoviruses replicate to high levels in the liver and induce apoptotic cell death (Fig. 3.4).

Immune Response

Innate Immunity

The innate immune response plays a central role in regulating virus infection, as illustrated above by the important role that this pathway plays in regulating EV tissue tropism and pathogenesis in animal models. RNA viruses may trigger one (or more) of at least three pattern recognition receptors (PRRs): TLRs, RIG-I–like receptors (RLRs), and NOD-like receptors (NLRs, some of which assemble into larger structures termed inflammasomes). The interactions between enteroviruses and PRRs have been extensively studied with TLRs and RLRs, with fewer studies focused on enteroviruses and NLRs. The detection of "nonself" pathogen-associated molecular patterns (PAMPs) triggers the PRR-mediated expression of hundreds of genes, including a variety of cytokines, chemokines, and other proteins, some of which can directly counter virus infection (e.g., *p*rotein *k*inase regulated by *R*NA [PKR, discussed below] and IFNs), while others may regulate the development of the adaptive antiviral immune response. The roles of cell-surface and endosomal TLRs during EV infections have been evaluated in several *in vitro* and *in vivo* models (Fig. 3.5). Despite being considered primarily a bacterial sensor, given that it binds to lipopolysaccharide, TLR4 on human pancreatic cells is triggered by CVB4.[486] However, TLR4KO mice infected with CVB3 show reduced virus titers and myocarditis,[134] which suggests that TLR4 does not play a protective role in CVB3 infections of the heart, but its signaling exacerbates disease. A comparison of male and female mice confirmed that TLR4 signaling was correlated with the severity of myocarditis.[146] However, the administration of TLR4 stimulants such as LPS greatly increased the severity of CVB-induced myocarditis, suggesting that CVB-mediated triggering of TLR4 *in vivo* is likely to be submaximal.[298,423] The endosomal TLRs, TLR3, TLR7, and TLR8, have been implicated in the detection of CVB infection, and mice expressing a loss of function mutation in Unc93b, the ER-localized molecule required for the trafficking of these TLRs to the endosome, are more permissive

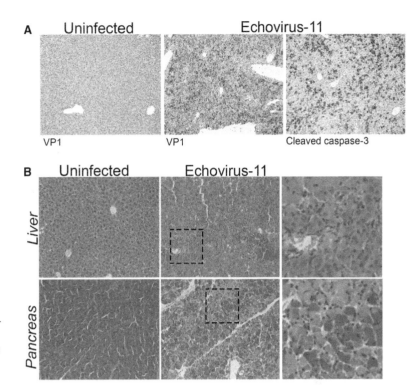

FIGURE 3.4 In adult mice lacking IFN signaling, echoviruses replicate to high levels in the liver and induce apoptotic cell death, as evidenced by immunohistochemistry for VP1 and cleaved caspase-3 in these animals **(A)**. Echoviruses also replicate to high levels in the pancreas of these animals and induce damage to acinar cells **(B)**.

to CVB3-induced tissue damage and infection.[295] TLR3 senses dsRNA molecules that are commonly produced during EV replication.[14] One study of CVB4 infection of TLR3-deficient mice suggested that TLR3 was almost indispensable for the innate response to this virus,[424] and, when compared to wild-type mice, TLR3KO mice showed increased mortality and developed more severe myocarditis following CVB3 infection.[363,511] Genomic screening of patients diagnosed with enteroviral myocarditis or dilated cardiomyopathy (DCM) revealed two TLR3 sequence variants, both of which showed reduced responsiveness to ligand,[149] suggesting that a strong TLR3-triggered response may protect against enteroviral myocarditis. In addition, a rare polymorphism in TLR3 was identified in a patient who developed CVB-associated myocarditis.[164] However, another study reported that genetic variants in TLR3 are not commonly found in patients with viral-associated myocarditis,[36] who were instead homozygous for variants in genes associated with inherited cardiomyopathies, suggesting that a genetic predisposition to cardiac dysfunction may sensitize individuals to CVB-induced myocarditis. Other endosomal TLRs also can contribute to the control of CVB infections. For example, human cardiac inflammatory responses to CVB are reported to be dependent largely on TLR7 and TLR8,[487] both of which recognize ssRNA and other small molecules.[188] Contrary to the reported beneficial effects of a strong TLR3 response to enteroviruses, a strong TLR8 response may be associated with adverse outcomes in patients with EV-associated DCM.[445] In addition to canonical antiviral signaling, autophagy is also up-regulated by TLRs, and the most potent pro-autophagic effects are mediated by ssRNA/TLR7 signaling.[110] Autophagy functions in the clearance of damaged organelles to maintain normal homeostasis but can function in an antiviral capacity in some settings by delivering viral particles to the lyso-

somes, which are subsequently destroyed by cellular proteases. However, autophagy appears to function in a proviral manner during most EV infections. Early electron microscopy (EM) studies of PV-infected cells revealed an association between PV and double-membraned intracellular vesicles,[107] subsequently shown to be autophagy related.[449] Extensive membrane remodeling occurs in a PV-infected cell, mediated by the viral 2BC and 3A proteins,[468] and the resulting vesicles carry several autophagosome-related proteins.[478,479] A similar relationship between CVB and autophagic vesicles has been reported,[167] and there is a marked increase in double-membraned structures within CVB-infected cells, both in tissue culture[520,540] and *in vivo*.[263] *In vitro*, the proviral effects of autophagy on EV replication are relatively modest with PV,[238] CVB3,[520] CVB4,[540] or EV71,[213] with inhibition of this pathway reducing production of each of these viruses by approximately 1.5- to 4-fold. *In vivo*, the proviral impact of autophagy is striking, and mice with targeted deficiency in the required autophagy factor Atg5 in pancreatic acinar cells exhibit approximately 2,000-fold lower CVB3 titers in the pancreas, with corresponding reductions in pancreatic inflammation and damage.[16] In addition to replication, autophagy has also been proposed to facilitate the nonlytic release of enteroviruses.[45] However, given that this has only been evaluated using *in vitro* cell culture models, the relevance of this *in vivo* is unclear.

Three RLRs have been identified: RIG-I, MDA5, and LGP2 (retinoic acid–inducible gene I, melanoma differentiation–associated gene 5, and laboratory of genetics and physiology 2, respectively). Unlike TLRs, these proteins are expressed in most cell types. All are activated by nucleic acids and are primarily cytosolic. Although RIG-I and MDA5 both detect dsRNA, they differ in their interactions with specific moieties on this RNA. Whereas the C-terminal domain of RIG-I binds

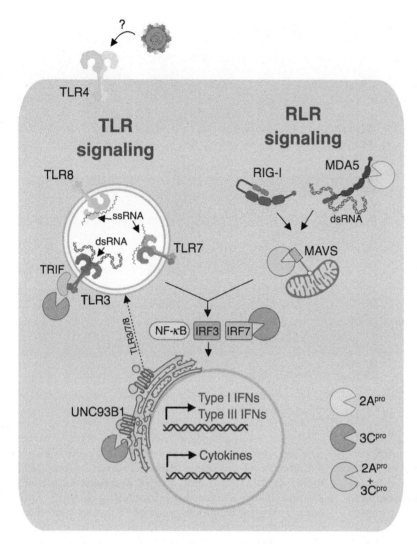

FIGURE 3.5 EV innate immune sensing and antagonism. EVs rely on their virally encoded 2A^{pro} and 3C^{pro} proteases to cleave essential components of the host innate immune response. These include key pattern recognition receptors (PRRs) such as MDA5, essential components for PRR trafficking and function such as UNC93B1, and essential adaptors for downstream signaling including TRIF, MAVS, and IRF7.

to 5′-triphosphate or 5′-diphosphate groups,[166,207,407] MDA5 RNA recognition relies on RNA length and secondary structure, with long dsRNA serving as a primary determinant.[527] Once activated, both RIG-I and MDA5 signal to a shared downstream adaptor localized to the mitochondrial membrane, mitochondrial antiviral-signaling protein (MAVS). Many RNA viruses produce abundant dsRNA and ssRNA with 5′-ppp and, therefore, strongly activate RIG-I. In the absence of RIG-I, the innate response to several RNA virus families is abrogated.[318] The 5′ terminus of an enteroviral RNA lacks the 5′-triphosphate moiety, instead bearing a modified protein (VPg), and, for this reason, these viruses do not stimulate RIG-I. Infected cells appear to rely largely on MDA5 to alert them to the presence of picornaviral RNA. This sensor is activated by the cardiovirus EMCV,[158,258] and two publications using MDA5 knockout mice suggest that enteroviruses, too, trigger MDA5 signaling.[225,507]

In addition to PRR-mediated induction of antiviral signaling, several innate immune cell types, which can include dendritic cells, macrophages, and natural killer (NK) cells, also play roles in restricting EV infection. NK cells, which are part of the innate response to many viral infections, are important in protecting against CVB-induced pancreatitis in the mouse model[497] and have been implicated in age-related

susceptibly to EV71 infection in neonatal versus adult mice.[553] The importance of NK cells in combating human enteroviral infections is unknown, but human NK cells can produce IFNγ in response to CVB-infected cells.[224] Many cells—exemplified by macrophages and dendritic cells—are phagocytic and engulf dead or dying cells. Thus, although human DCs cannot be productively infected by CVB,[290] these cells can consume debris from CVB-infected cells, thereby potentially introducing viral materials to the cytosolic and intravesicular sensors, potentially inducing an antiviral state in the DCs.[291]

Effectors of the Innate Immune Response

As discussed above, the key role of type I IFNs in the control of enteroviral infections is supported by extensive *in vivo* data demonstrating that ablation of this pathway greatly enhances EV replication and influences tissue tropism and spread. In addition to type I IFNs (which include 13 IFN-α subtypes and a single IFN-β subtype), it is likely that other IFNs, most notably type III IFNs, are also important in the control of enteroviruses. Type III IFNs include IFN-λ1, IFN-λ2, and IFN-λ3 (also known as interleukin IL-29, IL-28A, and IL-28B[50,60]). Although a fourth type III IFN, IFN-λ4, exists, it is nonfunctional in a large subset of the world's human population due to a single nucleotide polymorphism (SNP) that causes a frameshift in the gene.[51,128] IFN-λs have emerged as key antiviral effectors that are preferentially induced in and detected by "barrier" cell types, including those of the gastrointestinal and respiratory tracts, the placenta, and the BBB.[512] Unlike the ubiquitous expression of the receptor for type I IFNs (IFNAR), the receptor for type III IFNs is largely restricted to cells at mucosal and other barrier surfaces.[201] The tropism of enteroviruses for barrier surfaces suggests that IFN-λs will likely influence important aspects of their pathogenesis. In support of this, recent studies in primary human stem cell–derived intestinal cells show that IFN-λs, but not IFN-β, are preferentially induced by EV71 and echovirus 11 infection and that inhibition of this pathway enhances viral replication.[163] In addition, CVB-infected primary hepatocytes induce type III IFNs, which confer a protective state.[312]

Once produced, type I and III IFNs induce hundreds of antiviral effectors called interferon-stimulated genes (ISGs) following receptor engagement. These effectors are directly antiviral, are often cytotoxic, and function to restrict viral replication. Several ISGs directly target enteroviruses by nonredundant mechanisms. High-throughput screening of hundreds of known ISGs identified many that restrict CVB infection.[450] The complete spectrum of ISGs that restrict EV replication, particularly *in vivo* and in relevant cell types, remains to be elucidated.

Antagonism of the Innate Immune Response

Perhaps not surprisingly given their prevalence, enteroviruses are adept at attenuating antiviral signaling pathways to promote their replication (Fig. 3.5). They accomplish this antagonism through a number of mechanisms, most commonly utilizing the encoded proteases 2A and 3C to alter the ability of PRRs to sense them and/or activate signals downstream of this sensing. MDA5 and RIG-I are degraded in EV-infected cells *in vitro*, most commonly studied in HeLa cells, which interferes with the ability of these sensors to bind viral RNA.[33,136,439] Enteroviruses also target MAVS, the adaptor for both RIG-I and MDA5, further disabling this pathway.[136,358,508] Similarly, enteroviruses also attenuate TLR-mediated signaling by directed proteolysis of TLRs themselves or by targeting downstream adaptors, such as the TLR3 adaptor TRIF.[301,358,529] Accordingly, many cell culture models induce very little to no IFNs when infected with enteroviruses. However, the observation that EV replication is markedly enhanced in animal models lacking components of the innate immune sensing pathways and that primary cell–based models induce IFNs in response to infection suggests that this antagonism may be less efficient *in vivo*.

Adaptive Immunity

Antibodies and CD8[+] T cells together provide a strong antigen-specific barrier against virus infections. Under normal circumstances, these two arms of the adaptive response complement each other. However, members of the EV species appear to be an exception to this general rule. Patients with X-linked agammaglobulinemia are highly susceptible to enteroviral infections,[347] and, after receiving live PV vaccine, such individuals may continue to shed virulent PV for up to approximately 20 years.[268,330] The near-absolute requirement for antibodies in protecting against enteroviruses has been confirmed in an animal model of CVB3 infection, using B-cell knockout (BcKO) mice; these mice cannot eradicate the virus, and high titers are present in many organs.[340] The above observations suggest that,

for agammaglobulinemic hosts infected with an EV, there may be some deficit in the backup system that, for most viruses, is provided by CD8[+] T-cell responses. This may, in part, explain why most studies of enteroviral infections, in mouse and in humans, have identified strong antibody responses, while CD8[+] T-cell responses—so easily detected in most virus infections—are weak (if detected at all). The *Enterovirus* genus is large, and the adaptive responses to only a select few enteroviral species will be discussed below.

Human enterovirus A

The best-studied pathogen in this species is enterovirus 71 (EV71). The virus triggers an IgM response that is detectable as early as 2 days postinfection,[488] as well as a strong neutralizing IgG response that recognizes epitopes in the N-terminal segment of VP1.[473] Neutralizing antibodies, when transferred to uninfected neonatal recipient mice, are able to protect against a lethal challenge infection.[546] Studies of knockout mice showed that B cells, in particular, were important for survival following EV71 infection and B-cell–deficient mice treated with virus-specific antibody either before or during EV71 infection had lower virus titers, less severe disease, and lower mortality.[310] Memory Th1 CD4[+] T-cell responses specific for three epitopes in VP1 have been identified in EV71[+] individuals,[143] but no CD8[+] T-cell epitopes have been reported.

Human enterovirus B

CVBs are the best-studied pathogens in this species and, as described above, can trigger severe acute and chronic diseases including myocarditis, DCM, pancreatitis, and aseptic meningitis. Infection by these viruses triggers a rapid and strong neutralizing antibody response. Virus-specific IgM appears during the first week of infection, followed by a strong neutralizing IgG response. The CVB3-specific IgM titer wanes over time, but IgG antibodies persist.[317] Work in T-cell–deficient (nude) mice indicates that at least some of the CVB-specific antibody response is T-cell independent,[187,444,522] although some studies suggest that CD4[+] T cells may be important for the induction of strong neutralizing antibody responses.[302] B cells appear to be targeted by CVB[340] and may provide a reservoir for the virus during persistent CVB infection. Viral RNA[+] cells, probably B cells, can be found in the splenic follicles and germinal centers[17,240,254,279,340]; approximately 1% of B cells are infected with CVB3 *in vivo*, and these cells may accelerate the systemic distribution of virus.[340] T cells can help control CVB infection, although much less effectively than antibodies. *In vivo* analysis of CVB-specific T cells has been challenging because these viruses, despite replicating to high titers in mice, induce remarkably weak CD8[+] T-cell responses.[262,462] Nevertheless, some responses can be identified, exemplified by CD4[+] T-cell responses against epitopes expressed by CVB4.[177,179] CD8[+] T-cell responses are particularly meager. Epitopes in several viral proteins have been identified in human studies, but their detection required approximately 2 weeks of *in vitro* peptide antigen restimulation.[511]

Human enterovirus C

This species contains a number of coxsackie A viruses, but the most studied pathogen is PV, which induces a strong neutralizing antibody response that is necessary to control the infection. Virus infection and vaccination induce strong and long-lasting humoral responses,[97] but the immunity is not sterilizing and secondary infections of the gut can occur. Susceptibility to such reinfections, and subsequent shedding of PV, may be controlled by IgA.[59] PV-driven T-cell proliferation has been observed in infant vaccinees, and the responses appear to be cross-reactive across different enteroviruses.[248] However, PV-specific T-cell responses in OPV-vaccinated infants may be weaker than those in adults.[495] OPV induces MHC class II–restricted memory CD4[+] T-cell response targeted to epitopes in all four capsid proteins.[461] CD8[+] T-cell responses to PV vaccination are long-lived but—as is true for most CVB-specific responses—they became detectable only after several rounds of *in vitro* restimulation, suggesting that T-cell numbers *in vivo* were low.[504] Mice are not naturally infected by PV, but PVR-Tg animals have allowed the analysis of T- and B-cell responses and their roles in antiviral protection. Adoptive transfer of PV-primed B cells together with a VP4-specific CD4[+] T-cell clone protected PVR-Tg mice against a lethal challenge of PV, but neither cell population alone was protective, indicating that the virus-specific B cells required T-cell help.[327]

Release from Host

Virion assembly and RNA packaging of enteroviruses remain very poorly understood. In most cell culture systems, enteroviruses are highly lytic and induce pronounced cell death signaling through both apoptotic and nonapoptotic pathways such as necrosis. The lytic nature of enteroviruses accompanies infection on both cell lines, in which cell blebbing and lysis can be observed within several hours of infection, and in primary cells. *In vivo*, enteroviruses induce profound cellular damage and the generation of cleaved caspase-3, a marker of apoptosis. Although enteroviruses are generally considered to be highly lytic—and, therefore, released from cells upon their lysis—early evidence from cell culture studies was consistent with PV release by non-lytic means.[403,490] It has been proposed that autophagy-mediated release of enteroviruses may occur, permitting the virus to exit a cell in a noncytolytic manner[238]; this proposed mechanism has been termed AWOL (*a*utophagy-mediated exit *without l*ysis).[480] The release of enteroviruses into extracellular vesicles has now been documented for several enteroviruses including PV, CVB, and EV71.[45,84,482] Extracellular vesicles include microvesicles (100 nm to 1 μm in size), apoptotic blebs or bodies (50 nm to 5 μm in size), and exosomes (30–100 nm in size). These vesicles can be distinguished based upon size, cargo composition, and their intracellular site of origin. In cultured cells, enteroviruses have been detected both in large vesicles and in smaller exosomes. Some studies have even suggested that progeny virions are released in very large vesicles that can contain up to dozens of viral particles.[443] This method of egress would not only shield released particles from possible neutralizing antibodies but would also dampen signals that might induce inflammation, such as through the release of danger-associated molecular patterns (DAMPs) from lysed cells. It remains unclear whether the nonlytic release of enteroviruses occurs *in vivo* or plays any role in pathogenesis as all of the studies to date have been performed in cell culture systems.

Virulence

Viral virulence is a complex interplay between virus and host, and some of the contributing elements, such as receptor distribution and host responses, have been discussed above. Here, we shall focus on selected enteroviral sequences and proteins and their contributions to a virulent phenotype. Wild-type PV is more neurovirulent than the attenuated viruses that constitute the oral vaccine, and studies have identified, in all three PV serotypes, changes in the 5' noncoding region that can alter neurovirulence. For example, sequence comparison between the attenuated Sabin 3 virus and revertants from cases of vaccine-associated poliomyelitis showed that a single U-C change in the viral IRES, at position 472, conferred a growth advantage in the human intestine and resulted in increased neurovirulence although, on its own, the change was insufficient to confer full neurovirulence[133]; a second change, leading to an amino acid substitution in VP3, almost completely restored virulence.[513] Mutations in the IRES of PV types 1 and 2 also modulate the neurovirulent phenotype.[260,322,323] The *in vivo* neuroattenuating phenotype imposed by changes in the IRES, together with tissue culture studies showing apparent cell-specific effects of the IRES mutations,[181] led to the proposal that neuroattenuation might be explained by a neuron-specific reduction in usage of the mutated IRES. However, *in vivo* analyses have demonstrated that, while the Sabin 3 IRES sequence is indeed less effectively utilized in neurons, this defect also is observed in other cells and tissues.[260] Thus, another explanation was sought; the importance of type I IFNs in modulating PV neurovirulence *in vivo* has been described above. Cardiovirulence in CVB3 also has been mapped to various locations in the 5' NTR, approximately 80 to 240 bases from the 5' end of the genome,[78,127,489] although the capsid region, too, plays a part.[484] In contrast to the extensive mapping of the limits of, and functional domains within, the PV IRES, analysis of the CVB IRES has been limited.

Persistence

Although both PV and CVB are rapidly cytolytic in many of the cell types that they infect, both viruses can establish persistent or chronic infection in some tissue culture systems.[96,148,332,404] In neuroblastoma cells, PV persistence is associated with accrual of mutations in the capsid region,[403] and, for both PV and CVB, moving from cytolytic to persistent phenotype in cell culture may be inversely related to the capacity of the virus to adsorb to the receptor and/or to the level of receptor expression.[66,272,294] It has been reported that, during persistent infection of cultured cells that express low levels of CAR, CVB accumulated changes in the capsid that allow the variant virus to bind to novel (non-DAF, non-CAR) molecules, and this more promiscuous activity conferred a replicative advantage upon the variant.[67] Cellular factors contribute to the establishment of PV persistence.[157] Cell cycle status may play a role in the case of CVB that does not replicate efficiently in tissue culture cells rendered quiescent by drugs or by serum starvation but undergoes productive and cytolytic replication when the cell cycle is triggered.[137,139]

Enteroviral persistent infections can take place under two general scenarios. *First*, a chronic productive EV infection can occur in immunocompromised hosts. As noted above, agammaglobulinemic individuals who received OPV may retain, and excrete, the virus for many years. One study of individuals with primary immunodeficiency who had developed vaccine-associated paralytic poliomyelitis found that approximately 1 in 5 secreted vaccine-derived PV at 6 months after their last OPV dose, but this frequency declined to 0%

when the interval was 10 years.[272] The low prevalence of the underlying condition means that such persons are rare; only approximately 40 such individuals have been identified.[525] Fortunately, a more common potential cause of immunosuppression, HIV infection, seems not to correlate with PV persistence/shedding.[27,194] *Second*, immunocompetent hosts may carry virus (or, at least, viral RNA) for many years. Given the frequency of enteroviral infections, it is reasonable to suppose that this is the more common of the two types of EV persistence. In the vast majority of cases in which "enteroviral persistence *in vivo*" has been reported in immunocompetent hosts, infectious virus was not identified; rather, viral materials (most commonly, RNA) were reported and infectious particles, if sought, were not found. CVB RNA has frequently been detected by PCR in many analyses of cardiac biopsies from individuals with DCM[22,23,56,283] or inflammatory peripheral myopathy.[25] From results obtained in a murine model of polymyositis, the authors concluded that the RNA was maintained in double-stranded form, with little indication of virus mutation/evolution.[472] However, analyses of CVB3 genomes isolated from the hearts of persistently infected mice suggest that CVB persistence *in vivo* may be dependent upon the deletion of nucleotides at the 5′ end of the genome.[276] Several deletions were reported, some extending to nucleotide 49 and all affecting the 5′ cloverleaf structure that is considered vital for RNA replication. Importantly, the materials were infectious; although replicating very slowly, they could be maintained in culture and do not require a helper virus. The VPg protein was present on several of the deletion mutant genomes, and, notably, approximately 25% of RNA encapsidated into virions was negative sense. The authors proposed that the encapsidation of negative strands might occur because the terminal deletions, by altering RNA replication, markedly reduced the ratio of positive to negative strands. Similar 5′-terminal deletion variants subsequently were identified in CVB3 that had been passed in primary tissue culture cells[59] and, critically, in a CVB2 genome isolated from the heart of a human who had succumbed to enteroviral myocarditis.[79] The poor infectivity of these mutated viruses may explain why infectious virus was not identified in the vast majority of previous studies in which EV RNA was found. To date, there is no evidence to suggest that these terminally deleted variants can be transmitted under normal circumstances.

EPIDEMIOLOGY

Demographics

Despite the nearly ubiquitous nature of EV infections and the wide variety of clinical presentations, the demographics of the various infections and diseases have some consistent characteristics. In particular, several factors, including age, sex and socioeconomic status, have largely predictable effects.

One of the most important determinants of EV infection outcome is age. Different age groups have different susceptibilities to infection, severity of illness, clinical manifestations, and prognoses following EV infection. Understanding these age effects on outcome of infection is complicated by the widely divergent prior history of infection and resulting immunity. Nevertheless, it is possible to make certain generalizations.

The largest amount and duration of virus shedding occur on primary infection with a given EV serotype. Because infection is so common, most primary infections occur during childhood. For these reasons, young children are probably the most important transmitters of EV, particularly within households. The greater exposure of children to virus during infection may make them more likely to have significant clinical symptoms. For example, in outbreaks of meningitis, children typically have higher rates of disease than adults.[167,235] Most studies, however, do not separately determine age-specific infection rates and disease rates, and the relative rates at which adults are infected are not generally known.

The incidence of poliomyelitis is relatively low for the first 4 to 6 months of life in countries in which control through vaccination has not yet been achieved, because of the frequent presence of protective maternal antibodies. In these countries, an increased incidence is seen of paralytic disease in children older than 6 months compared with children in wealthier developed countries, presumably related to an earlier exposure to virus as a result of poor sanitary conditions. Ironically, areas with improved hygiene may have a decrease in infant exposure, leaving an older (unexposed) population susceptible to epidemic disease, with high rates of paralytic disease during an outbreak.[410] Adults are more likely to be severely affected in both developing and developed countries, tending to acquire paralytic poliomyelitis rather than nonparalytic CNS disease (i.e., aseptic meningitis), abortive illness, or asymptomatic infection.[71,72,208] The reason for the increase in severity later in life is unknown. A possible reason relates to the finding that fast axonal flow, which appears important in the spread of PV within the CNS,[246] increases with age. In addition, it may be that receptor expression or host factors important in replication change with age, as has been speculated to play a role with CVB.

Severity of a number of enteroviral diseases besides poliomyelitis may be strikingly age related. An indirect indication is that a delay in first infection with a number of EV increases risk of more severe disease. For example, exanthema associated with CVA and echoviruses is for the most part milder in children than in adults. On the other hand, some EVs cause more severe disease in newborns than in older children and adults, possibly inducing a fulminant *viral sepsis* with myocarditis, encephalitis, hepatitis, and sometimes death (see *Clinical Features, Neonate and Infant Disease*).[85,239] Outbreaks of hand-foot-and-mouth disease caused by EV-A71 have been associated with a significant CNS complication, fatal brainstem encephalitis, that was restricted largely to young children (see *Clinical Features: Meningitis and Encephalitis*).[286,320] In addition, EV-D68 has been associated with large outbreaks of serious acute respiratory illness (see Clinical Features: *Respiratory Infections*) and with cases of acute flaccid myelitis (see Clinical Features: *Acute Flaccid Myelitis*).

In general, encephalitis and aseptic meningitis caused by EV appear to be most frequent among those 5 to 14 years of age rather than those older or younger. In a 10-year surveillance summary from the United States,[340] adults tended to be overrepresented among cases of severe disease (paralysis, encephalitis, meningitis, carditis) when compared with the age distribution of the EV-infected population as a whole. In another study, the mean age among patients with CVB meningitis (7.7 years) or pericarditis (9.9 years) was greater than the mean age of patients with CVB gastroenteritis (1.3 years).[117]

EV infections are more prevalent among persons of lower socioeconomic status and those living in urban areas.[180,241] In a study utilizing active surveillance of healthy children for EV infections in West Virginia during 1951–1953, the rate of isolations among children in a lower socioeconomic setting was two- to sevenfold higher than among children in a higher socioeconomic setting.[206] A similar study in Ghana during 1971–1973 further indicated that EV isolations were significantly more frequent among children in areas with poorer sanitation and in urban areas during both rainy and dry seasons.[398]

Paradoxically, poliomyelitis and possibly other EV diseases tend to be *diseases of development*. In the case of poliomyelitis, improvement in a country's hygienic and socioeconomic conditions (before vaccination programs) successfully reduces the incidence of paralysis caused by PV and leads to a transitional period in which there is a delay in age of first infection with a subsequent temporary increase in the paralysis-to-infection ratio. Before the introduction of the PV vaccine in the United States and other developed countries, paralytic poliomyelitis was disproportionately a disease of the middle and upper socioeconomic classes; this disease distribution was a result of infection at an older age, when paralysis was a more frequent complication. Ironically, the delay was a result of improved hygiene. The infant mortality rate, a general indicator of a country's level of health development, may be inversely correlated with the age-specific incidence of poliomyelitis.[337]

EV diseases, and possibly also EV infections, occur more frequently in males than in females,[162,352] although some exceptions have been described.[113] In numerous reports, the male-to-female ratio appears generally to range between about 1.2 and 2.5:1; that is, approximately 55% to 70% of such diseases occur in males. Male predominance tends to be greater for the more severe diseases (e.g., CNS disease or carditis) than for less severe disease (e.g., pleurodynia, hand-foot-and-mouth disease, respiratory disease, acute hemorrhagic conjunctivitis, rash, or undifferentiated febrile illness).

The apparent predominance of enteroviral infections among males may have both sociologic and biologic explanations. Population-based measurements of infection (e.g., sero-surveys), which should be gender neutral, have not consistently demonstrated a higher infection rate for males. Several additional explanations for the male predominance have been proposed on the basis of studies of infections in healthy children[153]: A longer duration of virus excretion occurs in males than in females (leading to increased chance of identifying infected males); a higher virus titer occurs in the feces of males (leading to a similar increase in diagnosis). Another possibility is that, indeed, more frequent infections occur in males because of a greater exposure to the pathogen, perhaps because of differences in the parental treatment and play habits of younger boys, and because of greater activity among older boys. An additional possibility is that males are more likely to develop a serious illness from a given EV infection than females. For example, the reason that human myopericarditis is more common in adolescent and adult males than in females (except in pregnant and postpartum women)[519] could be caused by sex-related endocrine effects leading to differences in disease susceptibility. The skewing of EV-related complications in males has also been observed in animals *in vivo*, where male mice exhibit higher levels of CVB replication in their intestines, which were proposed to be related to sex hormone– and type I IFN-related differences.[428]

Transmission

Enteroviruses can be isolated from both the lower and upper alimentary tracts and can be transmitted by both fecal–oral and respiratory routes. Fecal–oral transmission may predominate in areas with poor sanitary conditions, whereas respiratory transmission may be important in more developed areas.[209] The relative importance of the different modes of transmission probably varies with the particular EV and environmental setting. It is believed that almost all EVs, except possibly EV-D70, can be transmitted by the fecal–oral route; however, it is not known whether most can also be transmitted by the respiratory route. EV70 and CVA24 variant, the agents that cause acute hemorrhagic conjunctivitis, are seldom isolated from the respiratory tract or stool specimens and are probably primarily spread by direct or indirect contact with eye secretions.[287] Enteroviruses that cause a vesicular exanthema presumably can be spread by direct or indirect contact with vesicular fluid, which contains infectious virus.

It is likely that EVs are transmitted in the same manner as are other viruses causing the common cold—that is, by hand contact with secretions (e.g., on the hand of another person) and autoinoculation to the mouth, nose, or eyes. Direct bloodstream inoculation, usually by laboratory accidents (e.g., needle sticks), can result in EV infection; however, neither blood transfusion nor mosquito or other insect bite appears to be a significant route of transmission. The isolation of EV from flies has led to a suspicion that houseflies (*Musca domestica*) and various filth flies may be vehicles of mechanical transmission.[170,229] No evidence indicates that venereal transmission is important.

Transmission within households has been well studied for both PV and nonpolio EV. Small children generally introduce EV into the family, although young adults make up the majority of index cases in some outbreaks of acute hemorrhagic conjunctivitis.[446] Intrafamily transmission can be rapid and relatively complete, depending on duration of virus excretion, household size, number of siblings, socioeconomic status, immune status of household members, and other risk factors.[180] Transmission has been generally found to be greatest in large families of lower socioeconomic status with a greater number of children 5 to 9 years of age and with no evidence of serologic immunity to the virus type. Not surprisingly, infections in different family members can result in different clinical manifestations.

Observations of household transmission of various EVs have documented that many infected contacts do not become ill and that the extent of secondary transmission varies with different EVs. Household secondary attack rates in susceptible members may be greatest for the agents of acute hemorrhagic conjunctivitis (EV-D70 and CVA24 variant) and for PV and of lesser magnitude for the coxsackieviruses and echoviruses. In some studies, secondary attack rates may be 90% or greater, although they are typically lower. New York Virus Watch data indicate that EV infections were more frequent among children 2 to 9 years of age and that secondary CV infections were more frequent in mothers (78%) than in fathers (47%).[282] In the same study, coxsackieviruses spread to 76% of exposed susceptible persons versus 25% of exposed persons who had detectable antibody to the infecting type; echoviruses infected 43% of those who were susceptible and only one person with antibody. The greater spread of polioviruses and coxsackieviruses may derive from longer periods of virus excretion.

Transmission occurs within the neighborhood and community, particularly where people congregate. In addition, as with many other viruses, EV can be rapidly transmitted within institutions when circumstances permit (e.g., crowding, poor hygiene, or contaminated water). School teams or activity groups and institutionalized ambulatory retarded children or adults may be at special risk.[12] Despite crowding, EV transmission is not usually accelerated to a noticeable degree in institutions where good sanitation is found.

EV transmission has also been observed *in utero* and has led to EVs being classified as members of the "TORCH" family of pathogens. TORCH pathogens include *Toxoplasma gondii*, *Others* (*Listeria monocytogenes*, parvovirus B19, varicella zoster virus, and enteroviruses), *Rubella*, *Cytomegalovirus*, and *Herpesvirus*. EV infections during early pregnancy have been associated with miscarriage and other pregnancy complications. Adverse pregnancy outcomes have been observed for CVA,[392,545] CVB,[28,34,89,230,288] and echoviruses.[34,242,245,366,477] EVs have been recovered from both placental and fetal specimens in cases of fetal death, and women who experienced miscarriages had higher levels of CVB antibody levels,[40,147] supporting that *in utero* transmission and teratogenicity may occur during the context of a maternal infection. However, given that data on the prevalence of EV infections during pregnancy and the impact of these infections on the fetus are largely unknown, the impact of vertical transmission *in utero* remains to be fully explored or perhaps appreciated.

As a result of widespread but incomplete PV immunization, rare PV-susceptible enclaves have arisen. These usually consist of unvaccinated religious groups in countries with an otherwise high prevalence of PV immunity. Despite the barrier of millions of immune persons, PV outbreaks have occurred in some of these enclaves.[397] The frequency and ease of international travel may result in the continuous introduction of wild-type PV in all regions of the world, indicating that a large proportion of the population must be vaccinated if poliomyelitis epidemics are to be prevented. This suggests that herd immunity may be of only limited value in protecting groups of susceptible persons who have regular contact with outside populations, and it raises questions about the risks that such groups may pose to the community at large.

Nosocomial transmission of various CVA and CVB and the echoviruses has also been well documented, typically in newborn nurseries. Hospital staff may have been involved in mediating transmission in some of these outbreaks. EV-D70, as well as CVA24 variant, is highly transmissible and can cause outbreaks in ophthalmology clinics when instruments are inadequately cleaned between patients. An apparent outbreak of CVA1, which included some fatal cases, has been reported in bone marrow transplant recipients.[483]

Although human EVs have been isolated from various environmental sources, humans are thought to constitute the only important natural reservoir.[123,135] Survival beyond a few weeks does not generally occur, although EV can survive for months in favorable environmental conditions; these favorable conditions include neutral pH, moisture, and low temperatures, especially in the presence of organic matter, which protects against inactivation. Simian enteroviruses have been identified that are closely related to a number of human viruses,[185,374,377,390,409] and human enteroviruses have been detected in free-living nonhuman primates,[391] but it is not known whether primates can serve as a reservoir for human infection.

Although little evidence suggests that EVs found in the environment are of public health importance, concern has been expressed about possible dangers of contaminated sources of water. Recreational swimming water has been investigated in several studies, and EVs have been isolated from swimming and wading pools in the absence of fecal coliforms and in the presence of *recommended* levels of free residual chlorine. CVB5 was isolated from an unchlorinated lake swimming area during an outbreak at a boy's camp in Vermont, although the outbreak itself was explained by person-to-person transmission. In one study, the relative risk of EV infection among children was found to be significantly higher for beach swimmers, especially for those less than 4 years of age.[103] These reports suggest that swallowing of contaminated pool or lake water may theoretically account for transmission, but no proof exists that this type of transmission is significant in recreational settings.

Enteroviruses have been found in surface and ground waters throughout the world. In the tropics, virus survival is more prolonged in groundwater because it is cooler than surface water. As in the case with swimming pools, EV can be found in these waters even after chlorination and even in the absence of fecal coliforms. In industrialized countries, EV transmission from potable water is apparently uncommon, but is a constant source of concern for public health investigators, because the usual conditions under which city drinking water is chlorinated may be insufficient to completely inactivate enteroviruses.

Enteroviruses have been isolated from raw or partly cooked mollusks and crustacea and their overlying waters.[167] Shellfish rapidly concentrate many viruses, including EV. These viruses can survive in oysters for 3 weeks at temperatures of 1°C to 21°C. To date, no outbreak of EV disease has been attributed to consumption of shellfish. Other foodborne transmission has been documented but is thought to be uncommon. A 1976 outbreak of aseptic meningitis attributed to echovirus type 4 was apparently caused by consumption of contaminated coleslaw at a large picnic (Centers for Disease Control and Prevention [CDC], unpublished data, 1976).

Enteroviruses, especially polioviruses, are regularly found in sewage. Enteroviruses are more prevalent in sewage from areas with low socioeconomic conditions or with large proportions of young children. In addition, sewage workers have been shown to have a higher prevalence of serum antibodies to EV than highway maintenance workers, which is consistent with an occupational risk.[93]

Soil and crops also provide conditions favorable to EV. Enteroviruses survive well in sludge and remain on the surface of sludge-treated soil and even on crops. Air samples from aerosolized spray irrigants using contaminated effluents have also been found to contain EV.[351] Survival of EV on vegetable food crops exposed to contaminated water or fertilizer has not been proved to be associated with virus transmission.

Prevalence and Disease Incidence

Incidence data about diseases caused by particular EV types can be derived from prospective longitudinal surveillance of a defined population or from a sample of the population in which the occurrence of disease or infection can be reliably determined. The Virus Watch program in the 1960s in US cities exemplifies this type of surveillance study, in which specimens from subject children were obtained every 2 weeks for virologic evaluation.[98,282,467] Although difficult and extremely expensive, such prospective cohort studies avoid many of the pitfalls of passive surveillance, and they allow interpretations about both infection and disease incidence.

Less-useful information is based on passive case finding. Ascertainment may be incomplete because the surveillance system is likely to identify a case only if it is easily recognizable and diagnosed by someone who decides to report it. Because such data indicate neither how many ill persons were not reported nor how many ill persons had negative laboratory tests, the information is mostly of qualitative value; however, it may be useful in indicating trends. Despite these limitations, occasional reports do appear.[37,273]

In the United States, EV surveillance data are collected and analyzed by the CDC. The data have been reported irregularly since the beginning of the program in 1961.[273,350,353] In the United States, the only notifiable enteroviral diseases are poliomyelitis and encephalitis. These are reportable by diagnosis only (e.g., encephalitis) and not etiology (e.g., echovirus encephalitis). Such disease-based surveillance is the most accessible but least representative of all surveillance data.

EV excretion does not necessarily imply association with disease, because most such excretion is asymptomatic. This applies particularly to developing countries where EVs are ubiquitous and childhood infections commonplace and characteristically silent.

EV activity in populations can be either sporadic or epidemic, and certain EV types are associated with both sporadic and epidemic disease occurrences. The reported incidence or prevalence of a given EV disease may actually or artifactually be increased in an outbreak situation when sudden focus of attention improves diagnosis and reporting of cases, but this may also increase reporting of *noncases*. In addition, there may be a tendency for other strains to be excluded when a particular strain is predominant in a community; however, large communities with summer enteroviral disease typically support cocirculation of several different types simultaneously and in no particular pattern.

An important concept in understanding the epidemiology of the EV is variation: by serotype, by time, by geographic location, and by disease. This concept is illustrated in surveillance studies of nonpolio EV infections. For example, Figure 3.6 summarizes the data for the years from 1970 to 1998 for CVB3, echovirus 11, and echovirus 30 isolates in the United States collected and analyzed by the CDC. These data illustrate endemic and epidemic patterns of EV prevalence. The epidemic pattern, as typified by E11 and E30, is characterized by peaks in numbers of isolations followed by periods with few isolations.[273] These peaks may be sharp (1- or 2-year) or broad (multiyear) periods of increased virus isolations. For example, during the study period, several major epidemics occurred of echovirus 30 in the United States: outbreaks from 1981 to 1982, 1990 to 1994, and 1997 to 1998. By contrast, endemic viruses (e.g., CVB3) are isolated nearly every year and in similar numbers each year. Even with endemic viruses, larger outbreaks do occasionally occur, as with CVB3 in 1980. Similar endemic and epidemic patterns are seen for the other echoviruses and coxsackie A viruses.

Variation by location is also a major characteristic of EV. Outbreaks can be restricted to small groups (e.g., schools and day care centers) or to select communities, or they may become widespread at the regional, national, or even international level.

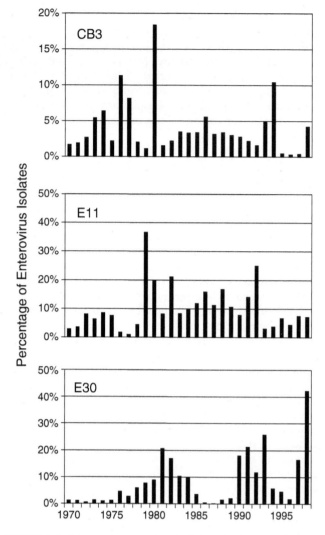

FIGURE 3.6 Reported enterovirus isolations in the United States, 1970–1998. The graphs represent the percentage of total enterovirus isolations in a given year for each of three common serotypes, CVB3 (CB3), echovirus 11 (E11), and echovirus 30 (E30). Note that full scale for the CVB3 panel is 20%, whereas it is 50% for both of the echoviruses.

Outbreaks in small groups can sometimes be linked epidemiologically to a breakdown in hygiene practices. Even during national outbreaks of a specific serotype, the location of virus activity may not be uniform. During the period of 1990–1993, echovirus 30 was the most commonly isolated EV in the United States (Fig. 3.7). As can be seen in the figure, not all parts of the country had echovirus 30 isolates during the entire period. Some areas, such as the New England states, had extensive circulation in only 1 year, whereas other areas, such as the entire western United States, had extensive virus circulation for 3 or more of the 4 years. It is important to note, therefore, that aggregate national data can obscure significant regional and local variation in viral prevalence.

In temperate climates, EVs are characteristically found during the summer and early autumn, although outbreaks can continue into the winter. In fact, naturally occurring EVs have a distinct seasonal pattern of circulation that varies by

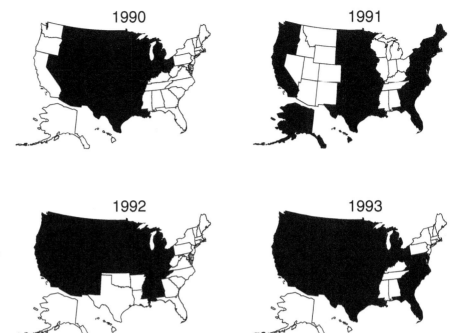

FIGURE 3.7 Geographic distribution of echovirus 30 isolates in the United States, 1990–1993. Maps represent regions of the United States where echovirus 30 was one of the three most common enterovirus isolates for the given year. States are *shaded* on a regional basis, because not all states report enterovirus isolation data.

geographic area; in contrast, live attenuated PV (mostly vaccine strains) are isolated year-round, reflecting the routine administration of poliomyelitis vaccine to children. In tropical and semitropical areas, circulation tends to be year-round or associated with the rainy season. In the United States, 23 years of surveillance indicated that 78% of EV isolations were made during the five summer or fall months of June to October.[273] In a 6-year study of viral CNS disease, 85% of enteroviral disease, compared with 12% to 26% of diseases caused by other viral agents, occurred between June and November.[350]

Many studies have examined the prevalence of antibodies to the EV in specific populations, as has been reviewed elsewhere,[338,348] with several important conclusions. First, the number of persons who have neutralizing antibody to any given EV is large, indicating a high incidence of past infection. A high incidence of recent infection is also suggested by surveys of IgM antibodies to EV, which typically show 4% to 6% positivity. Second, infections with one serotype of EV can boost antibody titers to other EV serotypes as measured by either IgM or neutralization. The pattern of the heterotypic response varies by serotype and among individuals. The nature of this heterotypic response has been explored through the identification of specific epitopes using monoclonal antibodies and peptide antisera.[176,441,530] Third, the pattern of antibody prevalence by serotype varies by geographic location, time, and age. Thus, prevalence data from different years and locations are not directly comparable. These three points must be considered when interpreting the findings of serologic studies of associations between EV infection and disease.

Molecular Epidemiology

Study of the molecular variation of viral proteins or nucleic acid may contribute significant epidemiologic information on viral diseases (see *Diagnosis*). Molecular epidemiologic studies have helped in our understanding of EV including the following: providing the opportunity for unequivocal strain identification, providing insights into EV classification and taxonomy, clarifying the origins of outbreaks, and allowing identification of strains transmitted between outbreaks. For the EV, and in particular PV, the primary method used to generate epidemiologic information is direct analysis of genomic variation using nucleic acid sequencing. Previously, both monoclonal antibodies and oligonucleotide fingerprinting were also used to study variation in PV and EV; however, these approaches are limited by their ability to show similarities and small differences only among relatively closely related viruses. Neither technique, however, is able to readily detect any patterns among seemingly unrelated virus isolates. The introduction of the technique of genomic nucleic acid sequencing and its application to the study of wild PV isolates from different parts of the world has significantly extended the epidemiologic power of molecular studies.[425] By analyzing the random mutations that occur in the genome of different PV, closely related viruses were easily detected, and, in addition, more distantly related viruses were clustered into distinct geographic groupings of endemic circulation. This approach allowed epidemiologic links to be extended beyond those identified with other techniques.

Nucleic acid sequencing technology has been most comprehensively applied to studies of PV, where the information has proved valuable for supporting the global PV eradication program.[264,266,267] From these studies, it is possible to determine (a) if an isolated PV is related to vaccine virus, (b) similarities among isolates in an epidemic, and (c) differences among isolates from different geographic areas. By comparing the changes that are observed between virus strains, the geographic and temporal origin of a virus can be determined. Building on a nucleic acid sequence database of PV strains worldwide, it has been possible to develop rapid approaches to tracking wild PV strains.[11,313,359,425,552]

Studies on the molecular epidemiology of nonpolio EV have focused on the evolutionary inference derived from the comparison of virus isolates within a serotype over time, as well as the comparison of isolates from different serotypes and even between different genera within the *Picornaviridae*. Molecular epidemiologic studies using sequencing have been reported for CVB1, CVB5, echovirus 30, and EV71.[57,124,289,382,555] One of the studies of CVB5 isolates examined the pattern of genetic changes over three separate outbreaks in the United States. The nucleotide sequence from multiple isolates from the epidemics showed that each of the epidemics was caused by a single genotype. The genotype of CVB5 observed in the 1967 epidemic showed more similarity to the virus observed in the 1983 epidemic than to viruses isolated during the intervening years,[289] suggesting discontinuous transmission of epidemic CVB5 in the United States during this time. In an analogous manner, echovirus 30 genotypes have demonstrated an overlapping succession among the isolates characterized in the United States.[382] More than one genotype may be found in certain periods, and the displaced genotype can be found in other parts of the world after isolations have ceased in the United States for many years. In studies of EV71 isolates, three distinct genotypes have been characterized.[57] Unlike the situation with echovirus 30 and more similar to the CVB5 example, the transition from one genotype to another occurred during a single year, 1987, and the older genotype has not been isolated since in the United States despite isolation in other parts of the world.

CLINICAL FEATURES

Most EV infections are asymptomatic. On the other hand, these viruses can cause a spectrum of clinically distinct syndromes when they lead to disease. Tables 3.3 to 3.6 list the prototype EV strains and the illness, if any, in the person from whom the prototype virus was isolated. Individual serotypes generally lead to varied symptomatology and disease processes. Similarly, individual clinical disorders can generally be caused by a number of different EVs. On occasion, however, particular syndromes are associated with specific EV (Table 3.7). For example, acute hemorrhagic conjunctivitis is usually caused by the CVA24 variant or EV-D70. Acute flaccid paralysis (AFP) is usually caused by PV or EV-A71. The occasional isolates from cases of diabetes are usually CVB serotypes.

Poliomyelitis

As is true for nonpolio EV, infection of most patients with PV does not result in disease or lead to any symptomatology. The most common symptomatic disease caused by PV, known as *abortive poliomyelitis*, is a mild febrile illness with or without gastrointestinal signs that occurs in 4% to 8% of individuals. The incubation period from infection to the onset of abortive

---

TABLE 3.3 *Enterovirus A (EV-A)*

Type	Prototype Strain	Geographic Origin	Illness or Source Prototype Virus	Accession Number
CVA2	Fleetwood	Delaware	Poliomyelitis	AY421760
CVA3	Olson	New York	Meningitis	AY421761
CVA4	High Point	North Carolina	Sewage of community with polio	AY421762
CVA5	Swartz	New York	Poliomyelitis	AY421763
CVA6	Gdula	New York	Meningitis	AY421764
CVA7	Parker	New York	Meningitis	AY421765
CVA8	Donovan	New York	Poliomyelitis	AY421766
CVA10	Kowalik	New York	Meningitis	AY421767
CVA12	Texas-12	Texas	Files in community with polio	AY421768
CVA14	G-14	South Africa	None	AY421769
CVA16	G-10	South Africa	None	U05876
EV-A71	BrCr	California	Meningitis[a]	U22521
EV-A76	10226	France	Gastroenteritis	AY697458
EV-A89	10359	Bangladesh	Acute flaccid paralysis	AY697459
EV-A90	10399	Bangladesh	Acute flaccid paralysis	AY697460
EV-A91	10406	Bangladesh	Acute flaccid paralysis	AY697461
EV-A114	11610	Bangladesh	Acute flaccid paralysis	KU355876
EV-A120	MAD-2741-11	Madagascar	None	LK021688
EV-A121	V13-0682/IND/2013	India	None	KU787153

[a]An identical strain was isolated from the brain of a fatal encephalitis case in the same local outbreak of central nervous system disease.
NA, information not available.

TABLE 3.4 *Enterovirus B (EV-B)*[a]

Type	Prototype Strain	Geographic Origin	Illness Yielding Prototype Virus	Accession Number
CVA9	Bozek	New York	Meningitis	D00627
CVB1	Conn-5	Connecticut	Meningitis	M16560
CVB2	Ohio-1	Ohio	Summer grippe	AF085363
CVB3	Nancy	Connecticut	Minor febrile illness	M16572
CVB4	JVB	New York	Chest and abdominal pain	X05690
CVB5	Faulkner	Kentucky	Mild paralytic disease with atrophy	AF114383
CVB6	Schmidt	Philippine Islands	None	AF105342
E1	Farouk	Egypt	None	AF029859
E2	Cornelis	Connecticut	Meningitis	AY302545
E3	Morrisey	Connecticut	Meningitis	AY302553
E4	Pesascek	Connecticut	Meningitis	AY302557
E5	Noyce	Maine	Meningitis	AF083069
E6	D'Amori	Rhode Island	Meningitis	AY302558
E7	Wallace	Ohio	None	AY302559
E9	Hill	Ohio	None	X84981
E11	Gregory	Ohio	None	X80059
E12	Travis	Philippine Islands	None	X79047
E13	Del Carmen	Philippine Islands	None	AY302539
E14	Tow	Rhode Island	Meningitis	AY302540
E15	CH 96-51	West Virginia	None	AY302541
E16	Harrington	Massachusetts	Meningitis	AY302542
E17	CHHE-29	Mexico City	None	AY302543
E18	Metcalf	Ohio	Diarrhea	AF317694
E19	Burke	Ohio	Diarrhea	AY302544
E20	JV-1	Washington, DC	Fever	AY302546
E21	Farina	Massachusetts	Meningitis	AY302547
E24	DeCamp	Ohio	Diarrhea	AY302548
E25	JV-4	Washington, DC	Diarrhea	AY302549
E26	Coronel	Philippine Islands	None	AY302550
E27	Bacon	Philippine Islands	None	AY302551
E29	JV-10	Washington, DC	None	AY302552
E30	Bastianni	New York	Meningitis	AF162711
E31	Caldwell	Kansas	Meningitis	AY302554
E32	PR-10	Puerto Rico	Meningitis	AY302555
E33	Toluca-3	Mexico	None	AY302556
EV-B69	Toluca-1	Mexico	None	AY302560
EV-B73	CA55-1988	California	Unknown	AF241359
EV-B74	10213	California	Unknown	AY556057
EV-B75	10219	Oklahoma	Unknown	AY556070
EV-B77	CF496-99	France	Unknown	AJ493062
EV-B78	W137-126/99	France	Unknown	AY208120
EV-B79	10384	California	Unknown	AY843297
EV-B80	10387	California	Unknown	AY843298
EV-B81	10389	California	Unknown	AY843299
EV-B82	10390	California	Unknown	AY843300

(continued)

TABLE 3.4   Enterovirus B (EV-B)[a] (Continued)

Type	Prototype Strain	Geographic Origin	Illness Yielding Prototype Virus	Accession Number
EV-B83	10392	California	Unknown	AY843301
EV-B84	10603	Côte d'Ivoire	None	DQ902712
EV-B85	10353	Bangladesh	Acute flaccid paralysis	AY843303
EV-B86	10354	Bangladesh	Acute flaccid paralysis	AY843304
EV-B87	10396	Bangladesh	Acute flaccid paralysis	AY843305
EV-B88	10398	Bangladesh	Acute flaccid paralysis	AY843306
EV-B93	38-03	DR Congo	Acute flaccid paralysis	EF127244
EV-B97	10355	Bangladesh	Acute flaccid paralysis	AY843307
EV-B98	T92-1499	Thailand	Gastroenteritis	AB426608
EV-B100	10500	Bangladesh	Acute flaccid paralysis	DQ902713
EV-B101	10361	Côte d'Ivoire	None	AY843308
EV-B106	10634	Bangladesh	Acute flaccid paralysis	NA[b]
EV-B107	TN94-0349	Thailand	Gastroenteritis	AB266609
EV-B111	Q0011/XZ/CHN/2000	China	Acute flaccid paralysis	KF312882

[a]Echovirus types 1 and 8 share antigens, type 1 having the broader spectrum. Type 10 was soon excluded from this group: it turned out to be a larger RNA virus and was reclassified as a prototypic reovirus. Type 28 was reclassified as rhinovirus type 1. Types 22 and 23 have been reclassified as members of the genus *Parechovirus* and are named parechoviruses 1 and 2; these viruses along with Ljungan virus represent the only members of this new genus. Type 34, DN-19, is now considered a prime strain of CVA24, rather than a distinct echovirus. Additional newer serotypes (EV73 and higher) are proposed new types defined on the basis of genetic sequence information.
[b]NA, information not available.

TABLE 3.5   Enterovirus C (EV-C)

Type	Prototype Strain	Geographic Origin	Illness in Person with Prototype	Accession Number
CVA1	Tompkins	Coxsackie, NY	Poliomyelitis	AF499635
CVA11	Belgium-1	Belgium	Epidemic myalgia	AF499636
CVA13	Flores	Mexico	None	AF499637
CVA17	G-12	South Africa	None	AF499639
CVA19	NIH-8663	Japan	Guillain-Barré syndrome	AF499641
CVA20	IH-35	New York	Infectious hepatitis	AF499642
CVA21	Kuykendall; Coe	California	Poliomyelitis, mild respiratory diseases	AF546702
CVA22	Chulman	New York	Vomiting and diarrhea	AF499643
CVA24	Joseph	South Africa	None	D90457
PV1	Brunhilde	Maryland	Paralytic poliomyelitis	AY560657
PV2	Lansing	Michigan	Fatal paralytic poliomyelitis	AY082680
PV3	Leon	California	Fatal paralytic poliomyelitis	K01392
EV-C96	10358	Bangladesh	Acute flaccid paralysis	EF015886
EV-C99	10461	Bangladesh	Acute flaccid paralysis	EF555644
EV-C102	10424	Bangladesh	Acute flaccid paralysis	EF555645
EV-C104	CL-1231094	Switzerland	Acute respiratory illness	EU840733
EV-C105	TW/NTU07	NA[a]	NA	NA
EV-C109	NICA08-4327	Nicaragua	Acute respiratory illness	GQ865517
EV-C116	126/Russia/2010	Russia	Gastroenteritis	JQ446368
EV-C117	LIT22	Lithuania	Pneumonia	JQ446368
EV-C118	ISR10	Israel	Acute otitis media and pneumonia	JX961708

[a]NA, information not available.

TABLE 3.6 *Enterovirus D* (EV-D)

Type	Prototype Strain	Geographic Origin	Illness in Person with Prototype	Accession Number
EV-D68	Fermon	California	Lower respiratory illness	AY426531
EV-D70	J670/71	Japan and Singapore	Acute hemorrhagic conjunctivitis	D00820
EV-D94	E210	Egypt	Detected in sewage	DQ916376
EV-D111	KK2640	Cameroon	None[a]	JF416935

[a]The prototype strain was detected in a chimpanzee, but another strain of EV111 was detected in a human with acute flaccid paralysis in Democratic Republic of the Congo.

TABLE 3.7 Clinical syndromes associated with infections by enteroviruses

Polioviruses, types 1–3
  Paralysis (complete to slight muscle weakness)
  Aseptic meningitis
  Undifferentiated febrile illness, particularly during the summer

Coxsackieviruses, group A, types 1–24
  Herpangina
  Acute lymphatic or nodular pharyngitis
  Aseptic meningitis
  Paralysis
  Exanthema
  Hand-foot-and-mouth disease (A10, A16)
  Pneumonitis of infants
  "Common cold"
  Hepatitis
  Infantile diarrhea
  Acute hemorrhagic conjunctivitis (type A24 variant)

Coxsackieviruses, group B, types 1–6
  Pleurodynia
  Aseptic meningitis
  Paralysis (infrequently)
  Severe systemic infection in infants, meningoencephalitis, and
    myocarditis
  Pericarditis, myocarditis
  Upper respiratory illness and pneumonia
  Rash
  Hepatitis
  Undifferentiated febrile illness

Echoviruses, types 1–33
  Aseptic meningitis
  Paralysis
  Encephalitis, ataxia, or Guillain-Barré syndrome
  Exanthema
  Respiratory disease
  Others: Diarrhea
  Pericarditis and myocarditis
  Hepatic disturbance

Numbered enteroviruses[a]
  Pneumonia and bronchiolitis
  Acute hemorrhagic conjunctivitis (EV-D70)
  Paralysis (EV-D68, EV-A71)[b]
  Meningoencephalitis (EV-D70, EV-A71)
  Hand-foot-and-mouth disease (EV-A71)

[a]Since 1969, new enterovirus types have been assigned enterovirus type numbers rather than being subclassified as coxsackieviruses or echoviruses. The vernacular names of the previously identified enteroviruses have been retained.
[b]Numerous additional types have been identified in stool from acute flaccid paralysis cases, but an etiologic link has not been confirmed.

poliomyelitis is usually 1 to 3 days, although symptoms can be seen as late as 5 days after infection. Less frequently, PV infection results in aseptic meningitis. This nonparalytic illness has the typical features of viral meningitis, with fever, headache, and meningeal signs but an absence of signs of CNS parenchymal involvement. The meningitis has a self-limited course and lasts for a few days to 2 weeks.

On average, only about 1 in 200 PV infections in a fully susceptible population results in the paralytic disease known as *poliomyelitis*. The incubation period from infection to the onset of paralysis is usually 4 to 10 days, although it can be as short as 3 days or longer than a month. The paralysis generally occurs 2 to 5 days after headaches occur and peaks within a few days. Usually, a prodrome occurs with sensory complaints and shooting or aching pains in muscle. The muscle pains may reflect replication of the virus in this tissue, which is known to occur. In children, it can be seen as a biphasic or *dromedary* course of neurologic involvement, and paralysis can occur as the initial symptom.

Paralysis is classified as either spinal or bulbar, depending on whether the spinal cord or brainstem, respectively, is involved. Not infrequently, the spinal form becomes associated with the bulbar form during the course of the disease, resulting in so-called bulbospinal polio. Spinal polio is usually asymmetric, flaccid, and limited to the extremities and trunk and varies from mild weakness to quadriplegia. Only about 10% to 15% of poliomyelitis cases are bulbar, a term indicating involvement of the motor cranial nerves or medullary centers controlling respiration and the vasomotor system. Involvement of cranial nerves IX and X, those most affected, leads to paralysis of the pharyngeal and laryngeal muscles with resultant difficulty swallowing and talking. Involvement of other cranial nerves can lead to weakness of the face (VII) and tongue (XII). Most dreaded is involvement of the brainstem reticular formation, resulting in respiratory compromise, potentially requiring ventilatory support. Also seen is autonomic involvement, which manifests as abnormalities of sweating, urination, defecation, and blood pressure control. Recovery can be delayed significantly. Not infrequently, one extremity is left severely weak and atrophic, with a relatively normal contralateral limb.

The pathology of poliomyelitis is one of inflammation and destruction of the gray matter of the CNS, especially of the spinal cord. Motor neurons up and down the neuraxis can be infected, including upper motor neurons located rostrally in the brainstem and cerebral hemispheres in addition to the anterior horn lower motor neurons in the spinal cord. The widespread nature of the gray matter infection demonstrates that the disease is frequently a polioencephalomyelitis (i.e., inflammation of the gray matter of the brain and spinal cord) rather than merely a poliomyelitis (inflammation of the gray matter of the spinal cord). Interestingly, perivascular mononuclear inflammatory cells can persist for months, although virus is difficult to culture from the spinal cord after a week.[48] Although the focus of pathology in the spinal cord is in the anterior horn, abnormalities also occur outside the motor system in the posterior horn and intermediolateral column. Similarly, the brainstem shows involvement of a number of sensory cranial nerve nuclei and of the reticular formation in addition to the motor cranial nerve nuclei. Neurons die with evidence of chromatolysis followed by neuronophagia. Investigations of CD155-transgenic mice have reported that spinal cord neurons die by apoptosis.[156]

Poliomyelitis or AFP can occur as a result of infection with EV other than PV. EV-A71 emerged an important virulent neurotropic EV during the poliomyelitis eradication period. This virus causes epidemics of poliomyelitis-type disease, including bulbar disease.[90] In an EV-A71 epidemic in Bulgaria in 1975, a paralytic disease occurred in as many as 21% of approximately 700 patients, with a case fatality rate approaching 30%.[457] EV-A71 is also associated with epidemic encephalitis and meningitis (see *Clinical Features: Meningitis and Encephalitis*). EV-D70, a cause of epidemics of acute hemorrhagic conjunctivitis, can lead to a severe and acute paralytic disease.[502] The incidence of paralysis is probably 1 of 10,000 infections.[243] These patients can also have cranial nerve palsies, autonomic abnormalities, and sensory signs. Sometimes, EV-D70 infections cause isolated cranial nerve palsies, most commonly involving the facial nerve. The eye disease is usually spread by direct or indirect contamination of the eye rather than the fecal–oral route. Some echoviruses and coxsackieviruses have also been associated with AFP (e.g., CVA7).[172]

Postpolio Syndrome and Amyotrophic Lateral Sclerosis

Patients with postpolio syndrome complain of new weakness, fatigue, and pain decades after paralytic poliomyelitis. One subgroup of this syndrome, called *postpoliomyelitis progressive muscular atrophy*, is an uncommon primary neurologic disorder manifested by slowly progressive atrophy of muscles with evidence of ongoing motor nerve damage.[68] Some investigators have reported a persistent PV infection in the spinal fluid or CNS tissue from patients with postpoliomyelitis progressive muscular atrophy,[304,305,356,406,454] but others have failed to confirm these findings.[247,336,440] One of the groups that originally reported EV genome in patients with postpolio syndrome later claimed that both patients and controls had evidence of enteroviral genome in the CNS.[357] Although the PV genome of a mouse-adapted mutant PV has been reported to persist at low levels following experimental infection of mice,[118] the only consistent evidence for persistent PV infection in humans has been found in individuals who are immunocompromised. We await more convincing data demonstrating that a persistent infection underlies the postpolio syndrome.

The issue of whether PV can persist in postpoliomyelitis progressive muscular atrophy has raised questions about whether PV or another EV is involved in amyotrophic lateral sclerosis, a chronic progressive weakening disease of unknown cause associated with death of motor neurons. A possible role for EV in amyotrophic lateral sclerosis seems unlikely given the immunocompetence of these patients and the noninflammatory pathology of the disease. Although some studies have reported enteroviral genomic sequences in tissues of patients with amyotrophic lateral sclerosis and motor neuron diseases, a more investigation using a very sensitive molecular detection method failed to find evidence to support this hypothesis.[373]

Acute Flaccid Myelitis

Coincident with a large outbreak of EV-D68–associated severe respiratory illness in children in 2014, cases of what was later termed acute flaccid myelitis (AFM) were identified in multiple states.[15,451] Since 2014, AFM case numbers have peaked every other year.[333] EV-D68 has been implicated in a number of AFM cases, but virus has not been consistently detected in sterile-site specimens and the prevalence of other enteroviruses in non–sterile-site specimens nearly equals that of EV-D68.[333,451] The clinical spectrum, epidemiology, possible mechanisms of pathogenesis of AFM, as well as the role of EV-D68 and other enteroviruses remain under investigation.

Meningitis and Encephalitis

Aseptic meningitis is a nonbacterial inflammation of the meninges associated with fever, headache, photophobia, and meningeal signs in the absence of signs of brain parenchymal involvement.[437] The syndrome is the most common CNS infection, with 7,000 cases of aseptic meningitis reported per year in the United States and an actual incidence believed to be 10-fold higher.[435]

Enteroviruses are the main recognized cause of aseptic meningitis in both children and adults in developed countries. Enteroviruses were identified in 85% to 95% of cases in which a specific pathogen was cultured.[437] In one study, 62% of infants less than 3 months of age with aseptic meningitis had CVB as the etiologic agent.[255] Of note, aseptic meningitis is the most common clinical syndrome caused by EV that results in medical attention.

Enteroviruses should be suspected as the causative agent for aseptic meningitis occurring in the summer and fall in temperate zones. The seasonal increase in incidence of enteroviral aseptic meningitis is largely related to climate[408] and may result because the fecal–oral route of transmission is facilitated in warm periods when less clothing is worn.[243] Fever is common in patients with EV-induced aseptic meningitis, as with most cases of aseptic meningitis. At times, the fever has a biphasic pattern, initially associated with constitutional symptoms and then returning with meningeal signs. One may see nonneurologic abnormalities associated with enteroviral meningitis (e.g., rash), which may be helpful in the diagnosis and identification of the particular enteroviral serotype.[243] For example, rashes have been associated with CNS disease caused by CVA5, CVA6, CVA9, and CVA16 and echoviruses 4, 6, 9, and 16. The rash associated with echovirus 9 meningitis can be petechial, resembling that seen with meningococcemia.

Encephalitis signifies that the brain parenchyma is infected and is not infrequently associated with a disturbed state of consciousness, focal neurologic signs, and seizures. The distinction between aseptic meningitis and encephalitis is important because the absence of parenchymal involvement in aseptic meningitis suggests a more benign condition and more favorable prognosis. Encephalitis is usually associated with aseptic meningitis, usually resulting in a meningoencephalitis.

Although a specific virus is not usually identified in most cases of encephalitis, and the number of cases in which an EV has been identified as the cause of encephalitis is low, EVs nevertheless rank second to herpes simplex virus and comparable to arboviruses as a recognized cause of encephalitis in the United States.[144,154] The New York State Department of Health found evidence of EV genome by PCR in the spinal fluid of 3 of 41 cases of encephalitis over the period from July 1997 to November 1998[212]; herpes simplex virus genome and arbovirus genome were each found in 5 cases.

Patients with EV encephalitis usually have a global neurologic depression in function, although occasionally seen are focal neurologic signs, resembling herpes simplex virus encephalitis.[344,349] Cases associated with an acute cerebellar ataxia have been reported in children infected with various EVs, including PV, echoviruses 6 and 9, and coxsackieviruses A2 and A9.[243] Other uncommon clinical manifestations reported include acute hemiplegia, opsoclonus–myoclonus, movement disorders, and Guillain-Barré syndrome.[243]

The meningeal syndrome is usually self-limited and benign, with evidence of improvement in days to a week. Deaths have been reported, however, following infection with a number of enteroviruses, including CVB1 and echoviruses 9, 17, and 21.[243] Morbidity and mortality are also increased in the neonate. The neonate's disease tends to be especially severe when the disease appears soon after birth, perhaps reflecting perinatal spread of virus to the fetus from the mother, as discussed above. Mortality is increased in the neonate partly because the aseptic meningitis can be associated with systemic disease (e.g., hepatitis and myocarditis), as well as encephalitis. The largest study of recovered patients failed to find any neurodevelopmental abnormalities above levels seen in controls.[431]

Isolation of EV from CSF may be unsuccessful because a particular EV may grow poorly in cell culture or because inhibitory factors (e.g., neutralizing antibody) may be present in the spinal fluid. With the use of RT-PCR, EV genome may be found in a significant number of culture-negative spinal fluid samples from cases of aseptic meningitis. The potential usefulness of RT-PCR can be seen in a report of a Swiss epidemic of aseptic meningitis caused by echovirus 30, when the EV genome was identified using this technique in 42 of 50 spinal fluid cultures (84%) that were negative for virus isolation.[165]

In some areas of the world, epidemics of EV-A71[5,90,457,506,536] have been associated with a high incidence of aseptic meningitis as well as CNS parenchymal involvement; the CNS infection has caused AFP as well as a more varied clinical symptomatology.[337] As noted, EV-A71 is emerging as one of the most significant neurotropic EVs in some areas of the world. This virus circulates in the United States, and 26% of adults tested in a seroepidemiologic study in New York in 1972 had antibody.[114] An epidemic of EV-A71 infection in 1998 in Taiwan caused frequent CNS disease and more than 100,000 reports of hand-foot-and-mouth disease or herpangina (see *Respiratory Infections, Herpangina, and Hand-Foot-and-Mouth Disease*), which may correspond to 1 million actual cases of EV infection.[198] The patients with hand-foot-and-mouth disease had vesicular lesions on their hands, feet, mouth, and, at times, buttocks, whereas the patients with herpangina had vesicular lesions of the palate and pharynx. Of special concern was the finding of 405 severe cases with associated complications, 78 of which were fatal. Among the more severe cases, the case fatality rate in different areas ranged from 7.7% to 31.0%. Most of the hospitalized cases (80%) and the deaths (91%) were in chil-

dren younger than 5 years of age. The most frequent complication was encephalitis. Other serious complications, which were associated at times with encephalitis, included aseptic meningitis, myocarditis, and pulmonary edema and hemorrhage. It is unclear whether the pulmonary signs were related to viral invasion of the lungs or to brain injury from the viral encephalitis.

A review[212] of 41 hospitalized children with neurologic complications and culture-confirmed EV-A71 infection during the Taiwan epidemic in 1998 demonstrated an unusual and rather distinctive neurologic manifestation, brainstem encephalitis, or rhombencephalitis. The mean age of the 41 children was 2.5 years (with a range from 3 months to 8.2 years). There was frequently an associated condition: hand-foot-and-mouth disease in 68% or herpangina in 15%. The neurologic disease usually followed the initial illness of fever and skin or mucosal lesions, and it was manifested as rhombencephalitis (37 patients), aseptic meningitis (3 patients), and AFP (associated with the disease in 4 patients and following rhombencephalitis in 3 of the 4). At times, breathing difficulties and coma were seen in the patients with rhombencephalitis, progressing to death in 5 patients. The brainstem and spinal cord pathology was presumably related to direct viral injury, because virus was cultured from the spinal cord and brainstem of the 1 patient who underwent autopsy. Five of the patients who survived had neurologic sequelae. EV-A71 brainstem involvement was also seen during an epidemic in Malaysia in 1997, but not in earlier epidemics. In contrast, hand-foot-and-mouth disease and herpangina did not occur during the previous epidemics in Bulgaria and Hungary. It is not clear whether the changes in EV-A71 disease phenotype represent the emergence (or reemergence) of a more virulent strain or whether it is related to the serologic status of the at-risk populations.

The presence of immunodeficiency predisposes to a syndrome of EV-induced aseptic meningitis or meningoencephalitis, at times producing a persistent CNS infection. McKinney et al.[334] reviewed more than 40 cases of chronic enteroviral meningoencephalitis in patients with congenital immunodeficiencies, most commonly X-linked agammaglobulinemia. Clinical features were remarkably varied and included headaches, seizures, ataxia, a disturbed state of consciousness, motor deficits, personality changes with cognitive decline, and sensory disturbances. At times, patients had other associated abnormalities, such as a dermatomyositis syndrome (in 21 of 41 patients; see *Clinical Features, Muscle Disease*), rashes (16 of 35 cases), edema (20 of 40 cases), and hepatitis (15 of 32 patients). Although some cases started abruptly, most tended to be slowly progressive, at times lasting years, and with a frequent fatal outcome. Most patients had a spinal fluid mononuclear cell pleocytosis with an increase in protein. Some cases at autopsy had evidence of inflammatory infiltrates in the heart, lungs, kidneys, adrenal glands, thyroid, and pancreas, in addition to the CNS. Immunosuppression of B-cell function with monoclonal antibody drugs can also lead to chronic enteroviral infection, with potentially serious consequences.[171]

Cardiac Disease

Myocarditis is an inflammation of the myocardium associated with damage that is unrelated to an ischemic injury. Myocarditis is frequently self-limited and subclinical, with few if any sequelae. On the other hand, the acute disease can lead to significant morbidity and even death. On the basis of well-established criteria, one study found evidence of myocarditis in approximately 1% of autopsies.[169]

In some cases, myocardial inflammation may persist, producing a chronic myocarditis that can progress to DCM.[76,252,432] In DCM, the heart is enlarged, with impaired function and evidence of heart failure but with little or no inflammation. The incidence of DCM in the United States has been reported to be 6 per 100,000 cases,[95] with approximately 100,000 new cases each year. Because of the high mortality of DCM, patients are frequent recipients of heart transplants, making up perhaps 50% of all cardiac transplant patients. Of note is the observation that nonpolio EVs, especially CVB3, cause acute and chronic myocarditis in experimental animals and that a contribution from the immune system to the chronic disease has been proposed (see *Pathogenesis*).

Acute Cardiac Disease

CVB has long been considered one of the principal causes of viral myocarditis[100] and this view has been confirmed in several recent reports.[19,129,324,326,328] Epidemiological and other studies suggest that 70% of the general public will be exposed to cardiotropic viruses and half of these individuals will develop acute viral myocarditis.[376] It is believed that 1.5% of enteroviral infections, including 3.2% of CVB infections, result in overt cardiac signs or symptoms.[172] Myocarditis is a frequent autopsy finding in children who die of overwhelming CV infection.[255] The peak age group in which myocarditis caused by coxsackieviruses of the B group occurs is young adults, primarily between the ages of 20 and 39 years, with a higher prevalence among men.[521]

However, even the larger group of symptom-free individuals are at risk; collapse and death of young and vigorous individuals, especially during exertion, can result from catastrophic dysfunction of the electrical pathways in the heart, as a consequence of unsuspected acute viral myocarditis.[39,509] A remarkably high prevalence of asymptomatic myocarditis has been shown by necropsy studies of victims of violent or accidental deaths; in this relatively random human population, approximately 1% had active myocarditis.[169]

A summary of data from varied sources shows that the prevalence of enteroviral infection in acute myocarditis on the basis of serologic studies is 34% (214 positives in 636 patients) compared with 4% (44 of 1,139) of controls (199). However, these serologic studies demonstrating seroconversion with an EV do not prove that EV caused the cardiomyopathy, as they may result merely from an unrelated EV infection. In addition, evidence suggests that multiple EV can circulate at the time of an epidemic, so that isolation of an EV does not prove its role in a disease; for example, more than 10 EVs were recovered from the community during an echovirus 9 epidemic.[243]

A meta-analysis of data obtained from molecular studies (slot blot hybridization, *in situ* hybridization, and RT-PCR) published in 12 reports found 23% of cases (68 of 289) and 6% of controls (14 of 216) had evidence of EV genome in heart tissue, giving an odds ratio of 4.4 with a 95% confidence interval of 2.4 to 8.2.[30] These data, coupled with reports of positive virus isolations from the heart, indicate that EV may represent a common cause of acute myocarditis. The surprisingly large number of positive findings in controls is presumed to result from difficulties in obtaining appropriately controlled heart tissue.

Chronic Cardiac Disease

Human DCM has multiple causes, both inherited and sporadic. A prior history of enteroviral infection of the heart, especially with CVB, has been implicated in sporadic human DCM.[31,467] Although the majority of patients with symptoms recover well from acute myocarditis, the disease can have serious long-term sequelae; some 10% to 20% of people with symptoms (i.e., ~20,000–40,000 patients per year in the United States) will develop chronic disease, progressing over time to DCM.[376,464] A summary of serologic data from multiple sources found that the prevalence of EV in DCM was 25% (64 of 260) compared to 10% of controls (26 of 255).[331] These serologic data suffer from the same drawbacks that are noted above.

In contrast to acute myocarditis, no reports are found of isolation of EV from chronic DCM, suggesting that the virus may have a restricted expression or disappear following the acute infection; however, some reports exist of EV VP1 antigen in the heart of patients with DCM and chronic coronary disease.[18]

The difficulty in isolating infectious virus led to studies probing affected tissues for persistent enteroviral genome. A meta-analysis of data from molecular studies described in 17 published reports found 23% of the patients and 7% of controls had evidence of enteroviral genome, giving an odds ratio of 3.8 with a 95% confidence interval of 2.1 to 4.6.[30] The meta-analysis data support an association between EV infection and chronic cardiac disease; however, it remains a possibility that RNA from other laboratory-based enteroviral studies contaminated test samples in the highly sensitive PCR studies. Most of the hybridization and PCR studies did not include sequencing of the viral genome and, therefore, failed to prove more directly that an EV was involved. In a few cases, however, partial sequencing was done of the RNA found in clinical samples; for example, Archard et al.[23] identified the amplified sequence as CVB. One proposed mechanism of viral persistence in chronic cardiomyopathies is 5′-terminal deletion of the genome, leading to chronic, low-level expression.[55,79]

Not all the viral genomic studies have been positive. One investigation involving a nested PCR failed to find evidence of EV RNA in 287 heart biopsy specimens from 38 patients with DCM and 39 patients with heart failure of unknown cause.[111] At least two other studies have also resulted in negative findings.[308,453] The lack of consistent, reproducible results regarding the presence of enteroviral genome in tissue from patients with cardiomyopathy indicates that further studies are needed under careful, blinded conditions.

Muscle Disease Including Pleurodynia

The relationship of EV to inflammatory muscle diseases was initially recognized because of the myotropism of coxsackieviruses in suckling mice. This observation was fueled by the association of these viruses with epidemic pleurodynia on the Danish island of Bornholm. The latter disease, called *Bornholm disease*, is an acute febrile illness with myalgia, especially involving the chest and abdomen, but without muscle weakness. It has occurred as an epidemic and also sporadically in various locales. Relapses can occur. CVB3 and CVB5 are the most frequently recognized causative agents, although other EVs have also been isolated.[547] The limited information from muscle biopsy findings suggests that the inflammation in this disease may be confined to the endomysial part of the muscle and, therefore, is not a true myositis.[106]

Enteroviruses have been implicated in acute and chronic inflammatory muscle disease. The acute diseases, which are usually called acute polymyositis or myositis, are characterized by fever with myalgia, elevated muscle enzymes, and, at times, myoglobinuria. Chronic inflammatory muscle diseases, which are generally classified as polymyositis, dermatomyositis, or inclusion body myositis, have a subacute to chronic progressive weakness with a distinctive pathology on muscle biopsy. Dermatomyositis is distinguished from the other two inflammatory myopathies because it is associated with a characteristic rash.

The causes of chronic inflammatory myopathy are generally unknown. Hypotheses concerning the etiology of polymyositis and dermatomyositis include a direct virus infection, especially an EV infection, or an autoimmune process in which the virus infection triggers a reaction against muscle (see *Pathogenesis*). That coxsackieviruses cause acute and chronic inflammatory myopathy in experimental animals provides additional support for their involvement in human inflammatory muscle diseases. Investigations of these model systems may help clarify the pathogenesis of these diseases in humans.

Enteroviruses have been isolated from cases of inflammatory myopathies, but these isolations have generally been rare and from single cases with acute[43] or atypical clinical pictures.[475] The inability to isolate virus from cases of chronic inflammatory myopathy has raised the possibility of a restricted expression of the virus with little infectious virus present. For this reason, investigators have probed muscle tissue from patients with inflammatory myopathy for picornaviral genome. Some reports involving slot blot or *in situ* hybridization studies of muscle tissues from patients with inflammatory myopathies have shown positive results using EV-specific probes.[544] In some cases, the product amplified in a RT-PCR has been identified as CV group B sequence.[22] In contrast, other studies using RT-PCR and nucleic acid hybridization have found negative results.[300,303,401] It remains a possibility that an EV could trigger an autoimmune inflammatory muscle disease and then disappear. Studies regarding the possible role of EV in chronic fatigue syndrome have similarly failed to find reproducible evidence of EV involvement.[106]

Of special interest with respect to the issue of EV involvement in inflammatory muscle disease is the observation that patients with immunodeficient states can manifest a disease similar to dermatomyositis with an accompanying persistent echovirus infection.[503,515] It should be noted, however, that questions have been raised whether these patients had a true myositis (i.e., inflammation of the muscle) or a fasciitis with interstitial inflammation in the endomysium.[106] The inflammatory muscle disease is associated with a chronic encephalomyelitis as well as a more disseminated disease in which EV, especially echoviruses, can be cultured from the spinal fluid (see *Clinical Features: Meningitis and Encephalitis*).[554] Although virus has occasionally been isolated from affected muscle, it remains unclear whether the dermatomyositis syndrome in patients who are immunodeficient is a result of direct virus invasion of the muscle or an immune-mediated disease associated with virus persistence. The existence of this syndrome similar to dermatomyositis demonstrates that echoviruses, and perhaps other EVs, can produce a chronic myositis in humans that is associated with persistent infection and chronic inflammation.

Diabetes

Both genetic and environmental factors, including EV infection, have been implicated in the cause of insulin-dependent diabetes (type 1 diabetes, T1D). A number of epidemiologic and serologic studies have demonstrated a relationship between EV infection and the development of diabetes. D'Alessio[103] found that 15 of 84 cases (17.8%) of newly diagnosed T1D patients had evidence of IgM antibody against CVB, compared with 5 of 71 controls (7.0%). The individuals with IgM antibody were especially common in association with HLA antigen-DR3 positivity. A prospective study in Finland found a greater incidence of seroconversion of EV antibodies among children who developed T1D than among those who did not.[231] The antibody present in the prediabetic period was directed against a number of different EV serotypes, including CVA9, CVB1, CVB2, CVB3, and CVB5.[430] At times, the EV antibodies are associated with autoantibodies to GAD_{65} and other important targets.

Rare, but well-documented, isolations of CVB4 have come from the pancreas of patients with acute-onset as well as fatal cases of insulin-dependent diabetes.[417,422] Some of the isolates have been demonstrated to be diabetogenic when inoculated into certain mouse strains[540] and nonhuman primates.[541] Patients dying from coxsackieviral myocarditis can have an associated pancreatitis, including islitis. More recent investigations have involved probing tissues from patients for evidence of EV genome. An *in situ* hybridization study showed evidence of EV genome: in the islets of autopsy pancreases from 7 of 12 newborn infants who died of fulminant CV infection (and 6 of the 7 had islitis), in the islets of autopsy pancreases of 4 of 65 adults with T1D, and in 1 of the pancreatic control tissues from 40 nondiabetic patients.[539]

Although it is likely that EVs are capable of causing diabetes mellitus in animals and humans, it remains unclear how often this occurs in humans and what if any immune mechanisms are involved.

Several studies have implicated antibody or T-cell cross-reactivity between CVB and host proteins to explain many of the observed correlations.[132,217,218,364,365,432] However, *in vivo* mouse studies appeared to clarify these seeming discrepancies and suggested that virus-mediated damage and inflammation were directly responsible for CVB-induced T1D.[210] Pancreatic tissues from three of six T1D patients were found to contain CVB4-infected β cells, which was isolated and could infect β cells from normal patient samples (Dotta, 2007). Some studies have even suggested that *in utero* infection with CVB predisposes the fetus to the eventual development of T1D postnatally.[500]

In addition to direct infection, the innate immune system also may play a role in EV-induced T1D (recently reviewed by Rodriguez-Calvo [Rodriguez-Calvo, 2019]). Human genome-wide analyses for nonsynonymous SNPs between healthy individuals and T1D patients identified the double-stranded RNA sensor melanoma differentiation–associated protein 5 (MDA5) as a T1D susceptibility locus.[463] MDA5 has been proposed to act as a key host sensor of CVB infection.[507] Consistent with a role for innate immune-mediated antiviral signaling in CVB-induced diabetes in a mouse model, β cells lacking functional type I IFN signaling through genetic deletion of the IFN-α receptor enhance CVB4-induced infection and T1D.[140]

However, despite many years of study, a causal role for CVB (or any EV) in T1D has not been directly demonstrated in humans, and the issue remains controversial. It is possible that, as has been proposed for pancreatitis, EVs are a cofactor in T1D, very rarely initiating disease in healthy islets, but tipping the balance in individuals who—unbeknownst to them—have ongoing islet inflammation and are in a prediabetic status.

Eye Infections

Acute hemorrhagic conjunctivitis is characterized by a short incubation period of 24 to 48 hours preceding a rapid onset of uniocular or binocular symptoms and signs. Patients manifest excessive lacrimation, pain, periorbital swelling, and redness of the conjunctiva (from subconjunctival petechiae to frank hemorrhages).[537] Keratitis with accompanying pain and possible visual impairment as well as anterior uveitis may be seen. The epidemic disease can also be associated with non-ophthalmic symptoms and signs, such as neurologic dysfunction (see *Clinical Features*) and respiratory and gastrointestinal disturbances. The disease usually resolves without sequelae in 1 to 2 weeks.

The first pandemic of acute hemorrhagic conjunctivitis was recognized in 1969 in Africa. Within 2 years, two EVs, a new antigenic variant of CVA24 and a previously unknown EV serotype designated EV70 (now EV-D70), were implicated as causative agents responsible for the epidemics of this disease.[309] During the first pandemic from 1969 to 1971, hundreds of millions of people were likely to have been infected. Subsequent epidemics of acute hemorrhagic conjunctivitis have continued in various locations throughout the world. Other EVs have also been recognized as causes of acute hemorrhagic conjunctivitis (e.g., echovirus type 7)[442] and as causes of sporadic conjunctivitis and keratoconjunctivitis.[261] The ocular disease caused by EV is often indistinguishable from acute hemorrhagic conjunctivitis caused by various adenovirus serotypes.

Respiratory Infections

Enteroviruses are a common cause of respiratory illnesses. Enteroviruses were isolated in 1.7% of 3,119 respiratory specimens submitted for viral culture from 1983 to 1994[86] and constituted 6.4% of all the viruses that were isolated from these specimens (54 of 838). Respiratory illness occurred in 15% of EV infections collected by the WHO from 1967 to 1974[172] and 21% of cases from the CDC obtained from 1970 to 1979.[20] The EV implicated in these respiratory infections included CVA (12.4%), CVB (20.3%), and echoviruses (12.6%).[172]

Enteroviral respiratory infections are more frequently associated with upper respiratory infections (e.g., the common cold, croup, and epiglottitis) than with lower respiratory infections (e.g., pneumonia). The infections are frequently subclinical, but if they cause clinical disease, it tends to be self-limited and mild, with a short incubation period of 1 to 3 days. More severe lower respiratory infections may be related to a higher dose of virus in the inoculum. In a series of infants with CVB infections, 30 of 77 patients had marked abnormalities (e.g., interstitial inflammation and hemorrhage), and 12 had virus isolated from the lung.[255]

EV-D68 was originally isolated in 1962 from children with bronchitis, bronchiolitis, and pneumonia in California.[447] Since then, it had been detected sporadically in the United States and elsewhere,[273] with small outbreaks identified. In the summer and fall of 2014, the largest recorded outbreak of acute respiratory illness due to EV-D68 occurred across the United States, with over 1,100 virologically confirmed cases from August through December, with the vast majority of cases occurring among children.[345] Since 2014, outbreaks of acute respiratory illness associated with EV-D68 have been identified globally.[203] Dyspnea, cough, and wheezing are some of the more prominent symptoms and patients with asthma were disproportionately affected. A high proportion of patients have been admitted to intensive care units and have required ventilator support.[345]

Herpangina and Hand-Foot-and-Mouth Disease

Herpangina is a febrile illness of relatively sudden onset with complaints of fever and sore throat. Characteristic lesions are found on the anterior tonsillar pillars, soft palate, uvula, and tonsils and on the posterior pharynx. The illness, which has a predilection for the young, is usually self-limited and disappears within a few days. At times, the disease is associated with more significant clinical abnormalities (e.g., meningitis). Hand-foot-and-mouth disease is an illness associated with vesicular lesions of the hands, feet, mouth, and, at times, buttocks.

A number of EVs have been identified as causes for herpangina, including CVA and CVB serotypes; echovirus types 6, 9, 11, 16, 17, 22, and 25[86]; and EV-A71. The main causes of hand-foot-and-mouth disease are CVA10 and CVA16 and EV-A71,[172] though CVA6 has recently emerged as a frequent cause, with cases also occurring in adults.[4,414] Most of the affected adults are parents or caregivers of young children. The pathogenesis of the lesions seen in herpangina is not clear; however, experimental infection of rhesus monkeys with CVA4 may provide a model system for the study of the pathogenesis of herpangina. In this system, ingestion of the virus by the oral route leads to multiplication in the lower gastrointestinal tract, followed by viremia, and then multiplication in the oropharynx.[460]

Neonate and Infant Disease

Neonates are at increased risk from enteroviral infections. This increased susceptibility is present in humans as well as experimental animals infected with varied EV.[88] Enteroviruses are among the most common sources of viral nosocomial infections in neonatal intensive care units (NICUs) and might account for as much as 15% of these infections.[92]

The increased risk of neonates to EV infection was apparent in the prevaccine era with respect to PV. Although the incidence of paralytic disease among neonates approached 40% in those born to mothers with poliomyelitis at the time of delivery, the overall incidence of neonatal poliomyelitis was an infrequent occurrence, perhaps related to the protective effect of maternal antibody.[528] Neonatal poliomyelitis generally had a shorter incubation period and a higher case fatality rate than found with disease later in life, demonstrating the increased susceptibility of immature hosts to EV infection. Infection of the mother early in gestation was associated with an increased risk of abortion, stillbirth, and prematurity.[88]

Nonpolio EV is a not infrequent cause of infection in neonates and infants. In a series from the CDC, EV isolates from patients less than 2 months of age included echoviruses (51%), CVB (45%), and CVA (4%).[353] Echovirus serotypes included

4, 9, 11, 17 to 20, 22 (now classified as HPeV1), and 31. A similar wide range of EV types was identified in a later review of CDC EV surveillance data for the period 1983–2003.[273] CVB1 to CVB4, E11, and E25 were significantly more common, whereas CVA16, E4, E9, E21, E30, and human parechovirus 1 (now termed PeV-A1) were less common among neonates than among persons aged ≥1 month.

The most frequent presentation in the neonate with nonpolio EV is asymptomatic infection.[241] Symptomatic cases most commonly manifest a self-contained febrile illness, at times associated with irritability and nonspecific signs of infection, making EV infection a leading cause of fever in the infant. A rash of variable character is seen in more than 30% of cases.[6] More serious infections can be seen, with the peak of symptoms correlating with viremia.[104] Nonpolio EVs are the most frequently identified cause of aseptic meningitis in infants less than a month of age and are believed responsible for more than a third of these cases.[456] An increased susceptibility of the neonatal CNS to CVB infection may be related to the virus' predilection for neonatal stem cells and the ability of the virus to damage these cells.[138,222] In a small series of patients with pneumonia in the first month of life, EVs were implicated in 15% of cases (6 of 40).[7] Usually, the mother has a history of fever or respiratory symptoms a week before the delivery, although mothers can be asymptomatic or have a more severe disease.

One of the serious infections caused by EV is a sepsis-like disease. In one series, EVs were implicated in 65% of infants less than 3 months of age admitted to the hospital for suspected sepsis.[105] In another series, evidence was seen of enteroviral genome in 80 of 345 infants less than 90 days of age admitted to a medical center with suspected sepsis.[63] A number of other studies have yielded similar results, emphasizing the importance of EV as a cause for a sepsis-like syndrome among neonates and infants.[104] In fact, EVs tend to be a more common cause of this syndrome than bacteria in the summer and fall.[63] There may be extensive multiorgan involvement in severely affected cases, especially ones that go on to a fatal outcome; the organs affected include the liver, lung, heart, pancreas, and brain.

The incidence and severity of EV infections among infants can be better appreciated by reviewing a study conducted in Nassau County, New York, from 1970 to 1979.[255] Of 153,250 live births, 77 infants younger than 3 months required hospitalization for CVB infection. These 77 cases were from a pool of 602 infants who tested positive for CVB, demonstrating the high frequency of CVB infection in infants. The attack rate might have been even higher than was found, because the positive samples from this study were from only a limited number of infants hospitalized in the community. A total of 24 mothers had evidence of a viral-like infection occurring within a period from 10 days before delivery to 5 days after delivery. The most common syndrome that was seen was aseptic meningitis. Some of the infections in the infants were very serious, as evidenced by the finding that eight children died from overwhelming CVB infection. All but one of these eight had evidence of myocarditis.

Severe EV disease in the young is associated with an early age of illness, prematurity, a more severe illness in the mother, multiorgan disease, low socioeconomic status, bottle-feeding, specific EV types, and an absence of neutralizing antibody to the pathogen.[6] The level of maternal neutralizing antibody appears to be important both for determining the risk of developing infection and for modulating disease severity.[8] Long-term sequelae following neonatal myocarditis or CNS infection appear infrequent.[6,435]

As discussed above, nonpolio enteroviral infection can affect the fetus, inducing clinical abnormalities and causing overt disease in the neonate. Reports exist of abortion and stillbirth associated with maternal EV infections, although these are infrequent. The relationship between maternal EV infection and congenital anomalies in the newborn remains unclear.

A number of routes exist by which EV can cause neonatal disease. Studies have found evidence of placentitis and viral infection in fetal tissues.[6] This would suggest that virus could be vertically transmitted from an infected mother to the fetus through the placenta, which forms the sole interface between the maternal and fetal compartments during pregnancy. No studies have investigated the ability of EV to infect placental tissue, but CVB can enter into primary human placental cells.[115] During delivery, virus could transmit to the neonate through feces or vaginal secretions. Infection can also occur from virus shed by other neonates or hospital staff in the nursery. In cases involving nursery outbreaks, implementation of infection controls (e.g., strict hand washing and the isolation of affected patients) has a role in prevention of new cases.

DIAGNOSIS

Differential and Presumptive Diagnosis

The process of diagnosing an EV infection or establishing that an EV infection produced a particular clinical syndrome can be complicated and challenging. This problem results from the biology and epidemiology of EV infections, as well as from limitations in current diagnostic methodologies. Although it is possible to demonstrate that a person is infected with an EV, this association does not necessarily prove likely disease causation. On the other hand, a presumptive diagnosis in certain epidemiologic and clinical situations can be possible with a high degree of certainty on clinical grounds alone.

Several related biologic properties complicate the diagnosis of EV-induced disease. The first is that most virus replication and infection typically occur in the respiratory and gastrointestinal tract. These infections are often asymptomatic, with few if any systemic clinical signs. Because these infections are extremely common, even random sampling of healthy individuals can demonstrate EV infections at substantial rates. For this reason, the simple recovery or detection of virus from certain nonsterile sites does not establish a firm linkage to disease, and it may be merely coincidental.

A second difficulty is that even when illness results from the EV infection, most of the signs and symptoms are relatively generic and usually lack specificity. The collection of appropriate clinical specimens for detection is critical to laboratory confirmation of EV infection. For example, the exclusive use of CNS specimens to diagnose meningitis and encephalitis limits the sensitivity for detection of infection. While it is possible to detect EV in the CSF from meningitis cases, it is uncommon to find virus in the CSF from cases of encephalitis wherein is seen a reasonable suspicion of EV as the cause; in other cases, the virus can be readily recovered from CSF, such as during the recent outbreaks of fatal EV71 encephalitis.[21] In general, however, the specimen with the highest sensitivity for establishing an acute infection is a stool specimen, regardless of clinical presentation,[346] followed by respiratory tract specimens. The difficulty with virus detection in some clinical conditions may be further compounded because virus shedding from the gastrointestinal and respiratory tracts may stop before the onset of symptoms, and, therefore, sensitivity for virus detection may be lower.

Sometimes, a presumptive diagnosis can be made on the basis of limited information because of the pronounced seasonality of EV infection in temperate latitudes and the tendency for EV to cause community outbreaks. For example, cases of aseptic meningitis occurring during the late summer and early autumn have a high probability of EV etiology. In this situation, a presumptive diagnosis of an EV infection could be made on the basis of signs and symptoms, exclusion of other nonviral pathogens, and detection in a specimen from some nonsterile site. Another example pertains to epidemic acute hemorrhagic conjunctivitis; in this case, the identification of an EV (either CVA24 variant or EV70) from a small number of patients precludes the need for further testing of specimens from other patients in that community with similar symptoms.

Laboratory Diagnosis

Molecular Detection

The application of molecular biology techniques to clinical virology has significantly changed approaches to EV diagnostics (see *Epidemiology*). Because of distinct advantages in speed, many of these procedures have supplanted traditional methods of detection and characterization such as virus isolation in cell culture. As with virus isolation and serotyping, the molecular methods attempt to detect the presence of EV in a specimen and, in some procedures, to further characterize the detected virus. The techniques can be grouped on the basis of their infrastructure and technical requirements and the types of specimens to which they are applicable. The most commonly used tests are based on the PCR, which is used primarily to detect EV genome in cell cultures, clinical specimens, and biopsy or autopsy tissues.[186,380,523] Additional procedures utilize genomic sequencing for the characterization of EV at the highest levels of specificity.

By far the most common use of PCR for EV diagnosis is the direct detection of virus in clinical specimens.[35,237,369,494] Numerous variations on the details of the procedures are found, but all methods that can generically detect EV have several common features. The most important property of these tests is that the primers are targeted to amplify the 5′-UTR of the virus genome. Several pan-EV real-time RT-PCR assays have been licensed for use in various countries, either as standalone assays or as part of a syndrome-specific multipathogen panel. The major advantage of the pan-EV PCR is that rapid detection of an EV is possible, even with very small amounts of clinical specimens such as spinal fluid. It is also possible to detect EVs that do not readily grow in cell culture. As with all PCR, the sensitivity of amplification of RNA from biologic specimens is extremely variable, depending on the nature of the specimen (e.g., stool).[474] Because of high-sequence conservation among enteroviruses and rhinoviruses in the 5′-UTR target sites, many "pan-EV" PCR assays cross-react with rhinoviruses,[182,380] though careful primer and probe selection can

minimize this effect.[256,319,369] Some commercial take advantage of the cross-reactivity to broaden the specificity of detection in respiratory samples, labeling the result "RV/EV-positive." A recent meta-analysis showed that empirical EV testing in febrile infants could reduce hospital costs and length of stay in the absence of a positive test for other causes of the illness (e.g., if blood cultures and other molecular tests are all negative).[505]

By changing the target for amplification, it is possible to characterize a particular EV using the PCR. Because the antigenic property of viruses that defines serotype is a property of the viral capsid proteins, certain sequences correspond to this conserved antigenic property within the capsid-coding region of the virus. Extensive studies of the capsid region of PV isolates have led to the design of primers that can selectively amplify isolates from a single serotype but not from other isolates of heterologous serotypes.[275] This is accomplished, despite the high rate of synonymous nucleotide substitutions, through the use of inosine in the primer synthesis. In an analogous manner, the ability of PV to uniquely bind to the CD155 is also an intrinsic property of the capsid proteins. The amino acids that are involved in receptor binding have been well characterized from studies of the three-dimensional structure of the virion. When primers are designed that correspond to these presumably PV-specific sequences, amplification is observed with all PV isolates but not with other EVs.[274] It has been possible to extend these principles to other EV receptor groups and serotypes and to provide tools for rapid serotype characterization of EV without the requirement for cell culture procedures.

A goal in virus identification is knowledge of the sequence of the viral genome. Encoded within this sequence are determinants for all the biologic properties that are attributable to a given virus. Therefore, the nucleic acid sequence information of a virus represents its ultimate characterization. All important information about a virus could potentially be obtained directly by PCR in conjunction with nucleic acid sequencing if all the molecular correlates of viral phenotypic determinants were understood. At present, however, the genetic location for many properties of the virus remains uncertain. Nevertheless, it is possible at present to use sequence information to assign an EV isolate to a particular serotype.[372,383–385,523] The molecular typing system is based on RT-PCR and nucleotide sequencing of all or a portion of the genomic region encoding VP1. The serotype of an unknown isolate is inferred by comparison of the VP1 sequence with a database containing VP1 sequences for the prototype and variant strains of all human EV serotypes. The following guidelines have been suggested:

"(i) a partial or complete VP1 nucleotide sequence identity of ≥75% (>85% amino acid identity) between a clinical EV isolate and serotype prototype strain may be used to establish the serotype of the isolate, on the provision that the second highest score is <70%; (ii) a best-match nucleotide sequence identity of <70% may indicate that the isolate represents an unknown (that is, new) serotype, and (iii) a sequence identity between 70% and 75% indicates that further characterization is required before the isolate can be identified firmly."[387]

Using these guidelines, strains of homologous serotypes can be easily discriminated from heterologous serotypes and new serotypes can be identified. This method can greatly reduce the time required to type an EV isolate and can be used to type isolates that are difficult or impossible to type using standard immunologic reagents. The technique is also useful to rapidly determine whether viruses isolated during an outbreak are epidemiologically related.

Virus Isolation

Many of the detailed procedures for the established laboratory diagnosis of EV infections using virus isolation have been described.[168] The traditional techniques for detecting and characterizing EV rely on the time-consuming and labor-intensive procedures of viral isolation in cell culture and neutralization by reference antisera. Isolation of EV from specimens using appropriate cultured cell lines is often possible within 2 or 3 days and remains a very sensitive method for detecting these viruses. The best specimens for isolation of virus are, in order of preference, stool specimens or rectal swabs, throat swabs or washings, and CSF. Throat swabs or washings and CSF are most likely to yield virus isolates if they are obtained early in the acute phase of the illness. For cases of acute hemorrhagic conjunctivitis, the best specimens are conjunctival swabs,[537] although occasionally virus can be isolated from tears.[538] Since the major pandemic in 1981, however, isolation of EV-D70 from patients with acute hemorrhagic conjunctivitis has been very difficult, and molecular methods provide the only sensitive method to detect this agent.[458]

The procedure for virus isolation involves inoculation of appropriate specimens onto susceptible cultured cells. No single cell line exists that is capable of growing all human enteroviruses. It is common practice to use several types of human and primate cells to increase the spectrum of viruses that can be detected.[87] Even with a variety of cells, however, several CVA serotypes fail to propagate in culture. The coxsackieviruses, including those that do not grow in cell culture, can be isolated and propagated in suckling mice.

As a consequence of current PV eradication activities and the importance of PV as a public health problem, specific diagnostic procedures have been developed to detect this virus. In general, PV grows well on a variety of primate and human cell culture lines, but it cannot be distinguished from other EVs solely on the basis of cytopathic effect. Polioviruses are unique in the use of CD155, which is distinct from receptors used by all other EVs to infect cells. This receptor has been transfected and expressed in a murine cell line that normally cannot be infected by most EV but is permissive to viral replication when the viral genome is present within the cell. One of these stably transfected murine cells, L20B, can grow PV and has been exploited selectively to isolate PV, even in the presence of other EVs.[211] When a specimen is inoculated onto these cells and a characteristic EV cytopathic effect is seen, the virus can be presumptively identified as a PV. A few strains of certain nonpolio EV serotypes are able to grow on the parent murine cells, however, and therefore growth on L20B cells is not a definitive identification of PV, and confirmatory testing is required.

Virus isolates may be typed by molecular methods as described for direct typing in clinical specimens, above. Attempting virus isolation may be useful in a case where typing is considered important (e.g., the index case in an outbreak or investigation of a nosocomial outbreak), the EV is of very low titer in the clinical specimen, and direct molecular typing is unsuccessful. For clinical management of routine cases, however, it is seldom critical to identify the specific nonpolio EV type. A high index of suspicion for an EV infection can be developed by reflecting on the clinical picture, the virus isolate's cytopathic effect and cell culture systems utilized, and knowledge of basic EV epidemiology.

Antibody Tests

Serologic diagnosis of EV infection can be made by comparing titers in acute and convalescent phase (*paired*) serum specimens. In general, however, EV serodiagnosis is more relevant to epidemiologic studies than to clinical diagnosis (see *Epidemiology*). The most basic serologic test is that of neutralization in cell culture. Many serologic studies rely on the detection of IgM antibody as evidence for recent EV infection, and this is now widely used as an alternative to the neutralization test. Several groups have developed an enzyme-linked immunosorbent assay (ELISA) for EV-specific IgM.[38,325] These tests have been found positive for nearly 90% of culture-confirmed CVB infections and can be performed rapidly. The ELISA has been successfully applied for epidemiologic investigations of outbreaks,[160] as well as for specific diagnostic use.[109]

In most cases, the IgM ELISA test is not serotype specific. Depending on the configuration and sensitivity of the test, from 10% to nearly 70% of serum samples show a heterotypic response caused by other EV infections. This heterotypic response has been exploited to measure broadly reactive antibody and the assay used to detect EV infection generically.[53,470] In attempting to characterize the exact nature of the response using different antigens, it is clear that the human immune response to EV infection includes antibodies that react with both serotype-specific epitopes and shared epitopes.[149] Despite this problem, which is inherently biologic, a fairly high concordance of results remains between assays of different configurations.[199] In summary, the IgM assays that are generally used in epidemiologic studies have very good sensitivity and appear to be very specific for EV infection; however, these assays detect heterotypic antibodies resulting from other EV infections and, therefore, cannot be considered strictly serotype specific.

PREVENTION AND CONTROL

Treatment

Although no currently available drug treatment for enteroviral infections is in clinical use, the effectiveness of a variety of drugs *in vitro*, as well as in animal models, has been documented. In addition, varied new directions for future therapeutic intervention are being pursued.

Pilot studies have been conducted administering intravenous immunoglobulin in neonates suspected of having enteroviral infection.[8] Pooled immunoglobulin delivered intravenously or via a shunt into the spinal fluid has also been used in patients who are agammaglobulinemic with chronic encephalitis and meningitis associated with nonpolio enteroviruses. Patients who are immunodeficient with persistent EV infections, including PV infections, represent a particular challenge to effective treatment. Although intravenous immunoglobulin may protect these patients from poliomyelitis and may appear to stabilize and improve some of the infections, the disease may progress; most of these infections, however, spontaneously cease. In some cases, efficacy may be limited by inadequate amounts of the relevant antibody in the immunoglobulin pool (e.g., if the infection involves an unusual and rare

EV serotype), as well as problems in the delivery of adequate levels of antibody to the infected cells. One report documented the failure to clear persistent PV excretion despite treatment with intravenous immunoglobulin, breast milk, and ribavirin (195a). Interestingly, a successful clearance of PV may apparently follow intercurrent diarrheal infections caused by other pathogens, perhaps because of damage to gut lymphoid tissue, which acts as a main site of PV replication.[272]

A number of specific antiviral compounds have been developed to target enteroviral proteins and steps in the virus' life cycle. The *WIN compounds* and related derivatives, which were originally shown to be effective against rhinovirus, have shown the most consistent results and have been those most studied mechanistically. These drugs bind a hydrophobic site near the surface of the virion called the *pocket*,[550] which lies in the floor of the *canyon* where the virion binds to the cellular receptor. By binding to the pocket, these compounds are believed to interfere with viral attachment and uncoating. Variations in activity of WIN compounds against different picornaviruses are presumably related to the particular fit of the drug into the pocket of a specific EV strain. Oral administration of WIN 54954 significantly decreased the number of upper respiratory infections following challenge with CVA21 (i.e., 3 of 27 patients in the treated group had an upper respiratory infection vs. 15 of 23 in the placebo group) with decreased associated symptoms and viral titers.[448] Adverse reactions, however, curtailed further investigations with this drug. Pleconaril or VP 63843 is a pocket-binding compound with a broad *in vitro* inhibitory activity against 95% of the 215 nonpolio EVs that were tested.[405] Significant activity was noted against some serotypes, such as echovirus 11. A randomized, double-blind study involving the administration of pleconaril following a challenge with CVA21 showed statistically significant decreases in viral shedding in nasal secretions, nasal mucus production, and total respiratory illness symptom scores in patients treated with pleconaril compared with subjects treated with placebo.[448] Another phase II trial of the same drug against enteroviral meningitis showed a statistically significant decrease in disease duration (9.5 days in the placebo group vs. 4.0 days in the controls).[436] A subsequent study, however, failed to have the statistical power to show efficacy in infants with enteroviral meningitis.[9] A problem with all of these antiviral compounds is that mutant viruses resistant to the drug can arise. In the case of resistance to rhinovirus, the mutant viruses tend to have bulky amino acid substitutions that sterically block entry of the drug into the pocket.[192] These mutant viruses may not be as significant a problem as expected, because drug-resistant CVB3 mutants that appeared in tissue culture following exposure to the WIN compounds tended to be attenuated when inoculated into mice.[173]

Enviroxime is an antiviral drug that targets nonstructural protein 3A, leading to a block in the synthesis of plus-strand viral RNA. Although this compound inhibits EV and rhinovirus *in vitro* infections, it is toxic and not effective in humans.[119] Resistance to enviroxime is determined by changes in the amino acid at position 30 in protein 3A.[191]

An antiviral strategy promoted recently involves the use of drug-sensitive dominantly inhibitory viruses, generated as a result of a targeted drug treatment, which interfere with growth of drug-resistant viruses.[102,476] Regions of the virus that can serve as targets for drugs that lead to the generation of these dominant defective viruses include (a) the capsid and polymerase-coding region, because of the proteins' oligomeric properties (i.e., there is interference during interactions with the respective wild-type protein); (b) cre and VPg (genome-linked virus protein), perhaps because their malfunction leads to inhibitory intermediates; and (c) 2A, perhaps because the uncleaved intramolecular cleavage of VP1-2A is inhibitory during assembly of the virus capsids. The 2A proteinase seemed to be an especially attractive target because of its inability to be rescued in *trans* and the dominant inhibition of the uncleaved product on virus growth.

Vaccines

Efforts have been initiated to develop a vaccine against EV71, and several approaches have been evaluated in animal models. Mice immunized with a DNA vaccine encoding VP1,[491,526] or with synthetic peptides encoding B-cell epitopes from vp1,[141] mount a neutralizing VP1-specific IgG response; passive transfer of vaccine-induced antibodies to neonatal mice conferred substantial protection against a normally lethal EV71 challenge.[142] A virus-like-particle (VLP) vaccine induced a strong and sustained neutralizing IgG response.[91] Finally, transgenic mice have been developed in which VP1 is expressed in the milk of nursing mothers; EV71-specific antibodies were induced in the suckling pups.[91] In both of the latter studies, the antibody responses protected neonatal mice against a normally lethal EV71 challenge.[83,91]

Poliovirus Vaccine and Eradication

The efforts to control PV over the last 60+ years benefitted from having more than one excellent vaccine, because both the inactivated (killed) vaccine of Salk administered by injection and the oral attenuated vaccine of Sabin were available. Both of these vaccines result in production of anti-PV antibody (Fig. 3.8) with subsequent protection from disease.[365,469] Although there has been a continuing advocacy for one or the other vaccine

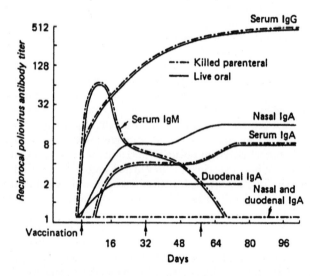

FIGURE 3.8 Serum and secretory antibody responses to oral administration of live attenuated polio vaccine and to intramuscular inoculation of killed PV vaccine. (From Ogra PL, Karzon DT. Formation and function of poliovirus antibody on different tissues. *Prog Med Virol* 1971;13:156–193, Ref.[393])

TABLE 3.8 Killed poliovirus vaccine: advantages and disadvantages

Advantages
   Safe because inactivation ensures no infectious virus exists
   Can be used in immunodeficient and immunosuppressed
      individuals
   Provides excellent systemic immunity

Disadvantages
   Requires intramuscular injection with repeated doses
   More expensive than live vaccine
   Potential hazards because of the use of wild seed virus in
      production
   Reduced intestinal immunity compared with natural infection

over the years, it is clear that each has advantages and disadvantages (Tables 3.8 and 3.9) and that appropriate circumstances exist for the use of each. As polio eradication efforts expanded in the developing world, it became evident that the question of the role of each of these vaccines is more complicated than originally thought. In the developed world, with the incidence of PV declining dramatically and VAPP the only significant source of disease associated with PV, many countries either never used OPV or switched to IPV. Like many other countries, the United States switched from OPV to the exclusive use of IPV in 2000 (with a routine schedule at 2 months, 4 months, 6–18 months, and 4–6 years of age). The main benefit from this change was the elimination of VAPP, and subsequent studies have shown that this was accomplished.[13]

In 1988, in part based on the rapid progress of eradication activities in the Americas, the World Health Assembly unanimously adopted a resolution calling for the global eradication of PV before the end of the 20th century (http://polioeradication.org/wp-content/uploads/2016/07/19880513_resolution-2.pdf). This resolution was reaffirmed in May of 1999, 2004, and 2011, and an acceleration of activities was urged with particular focus on the remaining endemic areas.

Four fundamental components constitute the strategy to eradicate PV.[227] First is the achievement and maintenance

TABLE 3.9 Live poliovirus vaccine: advantages and disadvantages

Advantages
   Confers strong systemic and intestinal immunity
   Relatively inexpensive
   Provides herd immunity because virus is excreted into the
      environment, expanding immunity
   Oral delivery
   Relatively safe

Disadvantages
   Can mutate to neurovirulent form, causing vaccine-associated
      paralytic poliomyelitis
   Contraindicated in immunodeficient and immunosuppressed
      individuals
   Requires monkeys for safety testing
   Can lead to circulating vaccine-derived polioviruses causing
      outbreaks of poliomyelitis

of high levels of routine immunization. With the accelerated activities resulting from the Expanded Program on Immunization of the WHO, routine coverage with three doses of OPV in children under 1 year of age reached nearly 90% of the world's children by 1990; however, maintenance of these levels has not been completely successful, and some erosion of routine immunization has occurred. Because of the inability of routine immunization to control PV circulation in many developing countries, the second element of the strategy is the use of National Immunization Days for the delivery of vaccine to all children under 5 years of age in a very short period of time, usually from one to a few days.[46] The mass immunization interferes with the spread of wild PV through a rapid increase in population immunity and abruptly decreases the *chains of transmission* in a country. This strategy was used in many early immunization efforts in the 1960s and was applied successfully in Cuba to achieve and maintain the elimination of PV from that country following three successive years of annual campaigns.[429] Multiple rounds in a given year are now routinely carried out for all endemic countries, and the National Immunization Days have grown in an extraordinary way as more countries have adopted this strategy. Some campaigns now represent the largest public health activities on record and often represent the largest multinational health events as well.

The third basic element of the strategy is the use of surveillance based on cases of AFP.[47] One of the major differences between the smallpox eradication program and the efforts to eradicate PV is the low rate of clinical disease following PV infection. Because less than 1% of infected susceptible individuals will develop paralytic illness, most infections are not clinically recognized. Following increased immunization, there are still fewer susceptible individuals who can be paralyzed, but immunity only partially prevents infection and therefore transmission can continue in partially immune populations with only a small number of cases evident. This creates a further challenge for finding the virus because of this complicated dynamic between immunity, disease, and surveillance.[249] Therefore, unlike smallpox, where almost all infections were symptomatic, PV is difficult to detect because most infections are sub-clinical. To improve the sensitivity of detecting PV infection and yet achieve a practical system, surveillance was developed around the unique clinical presentation of paralytic poliomyelitis. To avoid the requirement for extensive neurologic examinations, which are not feasible in many developing countries, the surveillance was simplified to include any case of AFP. This system reports many other diseases in addition to poliomyelitis, such as Guillain-Barré syndrome, transverse myelitis, and traumatic neuropathy. This loss of specificity, however, is compensated for by a gain in sensitivity, because most cases of true poliomyelitis are reported. The incidence of non–PV-induced flaccid paralysis is also used as an indicator of surveillance sensitivity (>2 case per 100,000 population under 15 years of age is considered an operational indicator of adequate quality), although it is not clear if the expected rate is the same in different countries or would be expected to be constant over time. Regardless, AFP surveillance has proved to be remarkably efficient for detection of wild PV circulation.

Once an AFP case is detected, the remaining part of surveillance is focused on detection of the virus. Two stool specimens are collected from all cases of AFP and tested in a global network of laboratories to attempt isolation of PV.[226]

The major advantages of this surveillance system are simplicity, practicality, and reasonable sensitivity for detection of PV. The major disadvantages are the requirements (a) to rapidly collect, transport, and test a large number of specimens from all areas of the world and (b) have high-quality laboratory testing. Despite these challenges, a global network of 146 laboratories was established and has been able to process more than 200,000 fecal specimens every year since 2011 and provide this information in a timely manner to the eradication program.[74]

The last element of the eradication strategy is the use of *mopping-up* activities.[112] This strategy focuses on an area or country where the previous three parts of the program have successfully reduced the number of PV cases to a small number and where surveillance has localized the remaining reservoirs of transmission. It is then possible to intensify immunization activities in those targeted communities that contain the remaining circulating virus, or the last *chains of transmission*. These intensified activities usually involve active searches in communities for children, including house-to-house or boat-to-boat immunization.[69] Teams visit all residences in the area and ensure that children are not missed for vaccination. With further reduction of PV circulation to only parts of a limited number of countries, further increase in vaccine coverage was achieved by more focused supplemental immunization activities (SIA). These immunization campaigns were focused on the remaining reservoirs of polio circulation within the endemic countries and conducted many times nearly year-round. At the late stages of the eradication program, the distinction between SIA and the original National Immunization Days has become blurred as greater flexibility of scope and timing has been introduced.

These four elements of PV eradication strategy have proven successful in most of the world. Because of this intensified effort, by the end of 2018, only two countries continued to report ongoing PV circulation. Since the program began, almost all countries are now free of indigenous PV circulation. This can be seen in Figure 3.9, where in 1988 PV was found on all

Polio Incidence: 1988

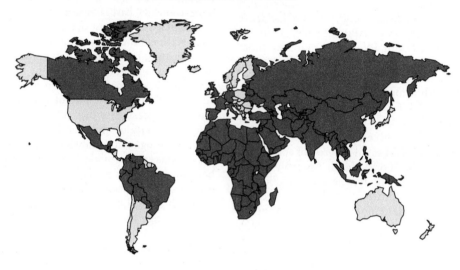

Polio Incidence: 2019

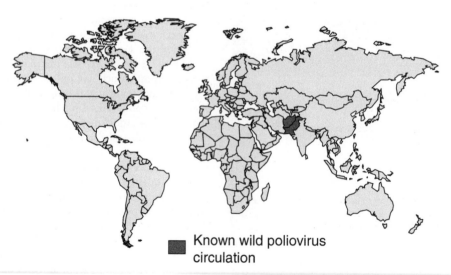

Known wild poliovirus circulation

FIGURE 3.9 Incidence of poliovirus in 1988 versus 2019.

the continents (except Australia), with estimates of more than 350,000 cases of PV each year. In 2011, the number of countries with PV was only 16, and by 2014, all of the Americas, Europe, Southeast Asia, and the Western Pacific Regions have been certified to be free of PV.[75] The only countries with endemic PV cases in 2018 were in South Asia (Pakistan and Afghanistan). The African Region reported its last case of wild PV in 2016. A weekly progress report on the global efforts to eradicate PV is provided on a Web site of the WHO.[524]

Numerous unknowns and potential obstacles remain to be faced in the eradication efforts. Because of the inherent insensitivity of detecting PV infection, it is important that surveillance quality be achieved and maintained for a period of time. Although the exact length of time required to be assured of success is not known in all circumstances, the minimal requirement for certification is 3 years. Previous experience indicates that if excellent surveillance is achieved and maintained, PV genotypes that have not been detected for a period of 1 year will not be detected ever again.[265] This has been true for more than three dozen genotypes that have been eliminated from circulation.

After wild virus circulation is interrupted, the accidental release of viruses from laboratories or vaccine-manufacturing facilities will represent a significant risk to the PV-free world. Therefore, it will be necessary to institute proper containment of the virus. A plan for these steps of containment has been drafted and will be implemented in phases as eradication proceeds. In the first pre-eradication phase, preparation for later phases is to be undertaken by conducting an inventory of all institutions and laboratories that have wild PV or potentially infectious materials. This survey for wild PV and potentially infectious materials has been completed in the polio-free regions of the world and has been completed in more than 100 countries, including the United States.[70] Wherever possible, use of vaccine strains of PV in the laboratory should be substituted for wild strains. In the second phase, after the last wild PV has been isolated anywhere in the world, all work with wild PV will be done at a higher biosafety level of containment (BSL-3/polio). Once all countries and regions have been certified as being free of circulating PV, and once all laboratories have properly contained, referred, or destroyed their PV stocks and potentially infectious materials, the Global Certification Commission will declare wild PV eradicated. The last phase of containment will occur sometime in the future when the decision is made to stop vaccination with OPV. At that time, all infectious PV will need to be in containment. The containment requirements for this last phase are being developed. In addition, the special containment needs associated with IPV production are being assessed. Of particular concern are the current use of wild strains and the associated risk of an accidental release of virus during vaccine production. One way to limit this danger that is under consideration and active development is to prepare the IPV from the live Sabin attenuated vaccine strains.[94]

Once eradication of wild PV is achieved, the only disease caused by PV in the world will be as a result of the use of live OPV. In most parts of the world that continue to use OPV, the disease burden caused by VAPP already exceeds that of wild PV and has for some time. In addition, the continued use of OPV also poses a risk for outbreaks from vaccine-derived polioviruses (VDPV). VDPV are derived from OPV, but differ from the OPV strains and from the frequent PV isolates seen soon after vaccination with OPV by having more than 1% nucleotide changes in the coding region for VP1. The demarcation of more than 1% is somewhat arbitrary, but is consistent with prolonged replication that may be associated with circulation of the virus. After observations of several recent outbreaks of VDPV, this definition has been modified for PV type 2 to be greater than 0.6% difference from the parent vaccine strain. Most OPV-like isolates and most PV excreted from patients with VAPP have less than 1% nucleotide change in the VP1 coding region and, therefore, are not classified as VDPV because the duration of infection is short and because random mutations do not accumulate and become genetically fixed as observed with VDPV and WPV.

VDPV fall into three groups: (a) circulating VDPV (cVDPV), (b) immunodeficiency-associated VDPV (iVDPV), and (c) ambiguous VDVP (aVDPV) in which the source of infection is unknown. Although recognized as a potential problem associated with OPV for more than 40 years, the occurrence of multiple outbreaks involving cVDPV in 26 different countries within the last 19 years has explicitly demonstrated this risk.[524] The first documented cVDPV outbreak of poliomyelitis occurred on the island of Hispaniola in 2000–2001, with 21 virologically confirmed cases in Haiti and the Dominican Republic and with many more apparent cases from which no specimens were collected.[269,270] Since this outbreak in Hispaniola, cVDPV outbreaks have occurred in numerous countries, including the large multiyear outbreak of type 2 cVDPV in Nigeria.[61] In addition, cVDPV have been recognized retrospectively in other countries, particularly Egypt, where the type 2 cVDPV virus was endemic for possibly 10 years.[535] Similar to wild PV, cVDPV often recombine with other species C enteroviruses during circulation, although nonrecombinant cVDPV have been observed. cVDPV circulate in regions that have inadequate vaccine coverage along with an absence of natural infection from circulating wild PV of the same serotype. The strains are of particular concern because they cause paralytic disease and have a capacity for sustained person-to-person transmission similar to wild PV of the same type.[131] The presence of cVDPV underscores the importance of maintaining excellent surveillance, the need to maintain high vaccine coverage, and the continued risk from suboptimal use of OPV, even in polio-free areas of the world.

Although not as great a concern as cVDPV, an issue that complicates PV eradication is the demonstrated excretion of iVDPV, in at least a few examples, for periods of more than a decade. The occurrence of iVDPV is rare, however, even in immunosuppressed patients. Although both iVDPV and cVDPV can occur in the absence of any recombination, recombination has only been observed in the case of iVDPV with other vaccine PV strains and not with other members of EV-C. This is presumably because of the absence of EV-C coinfections in the tissue supporting the chronic PV infection, in contrast to the frequent recombination observed between vaccine strains that occur in normal vaccinees. Interestingly, prolonged excretion with PV in immunodeficient individuals occurs with viruses derived from OPV and not with wild PV.[272] This may be because the greater neurovirulence of wild PV would be expected to lead to a uniformly fatal outcome in immunosuppressed individuals or because individuals with severe immunodeficiencies are likely to live in PV-free countries and, therefore, are only exposed to vaccine strains. Currently, no evidence indicates that patients with cell-mediated deficiencies are at increased risk for chronic PV infections. Prolonged excretion of PV has not been observed in studies undertaken specifically to look at human immunodeficiency virus–infected children and adults.[183,194]

Included in the VDPV group are ambiguous VDPV (aVDPV) in which the source of infection is unknown (e.g., VDPV isolates from environmental sources), no known immunodeficiency is found in the patient, or the isolate is associated with an AFP case, but without clear virologic or epidemiologic evidence of circulation.[62] For example, in more than 10,000 vaccine-related isolates studied in WHO Network laboratories in 2011, there were 67 cVDPV (from six recent outbreaks).[73,524]

Because of the risks evident from VAPP and VDPV, the WHO has concluded that continued use of OPV following wild PV eradication is incompatible with the ultimate goal of polio eradication. Therefore, sometime after the eradication of wild PV, all use of OPV for routine immunization will stop. This has significant implications for immunization policy decisions and raises two very important basic questions regarding the management of risks: What vaccination policies will be recommended for PV? How will future PV outbreaks or cases be controlled after OPV use has stopped? In the absence of any reported wild PV type 2 since 1999, the world has embarked on significant change to the routine vaccination recommendations with a focus on the withdrawal of type 2 containing OPV. The first step was the declaration of the eradication of indigenous wild PV type 2 in September 2015. The second step was the recommendation to introduce at least one dose of IPV into the routine program in all countries to provide continued type 2 immunity. The last step was the synchronized global switch in the more than 100 OPV-using countries from the trivalent OPV having all three types, to a bivalent OPV containing only types 1 and 3 in April 2016.[524] Despite the logistical and regulatory challenges, this effort was largely successful.[413]

One anticipated challenge that occurred after the switch was the detection of ongoing circulating VDPV type 2. To address the need to respond to these outbreaks, a stockpile of monovalent type 2 OPV was manufactured to be released only by authorization of the Director General of WHO. This control was needed to limit the exposure to the population of a live OPV strain that would have the potential risk of creating new circulating VDPV type 2 because of the outbreak response. Three years after the switch, the world is still struggling to complete this last step in the removal of all live type 2 PV from circulation in the world, one of the ultimate goals of eradication. These challenges with the removal of type 2 OPV will provide lessons for the final removal of the remaining type 1 and 3 OPV. This will provide the stage for future long-term polio vaccination policy.

Ideally, it should be possible to describe accurately all of the advantages and disadvantages of choices related to future vaccination policy. It is difficult, however, to estimate and quantitate risks for all populations associated with the cessation of OPV use because of inadequate knowledge about type-specific reversion of vaccine strains and viral genetic determinants for neurovirulence and transmissibility. It is also not clear what protective benefits are possible in the absence of high levels of routine IPV use. An attempt to use elements of decision analysis and disease modeling has been made to try to provide better information regarding risk assessments.[126,481]

Regardless of decisions made about immunization policies, future generations will have an increasing susceptibility to PV as immunization becomes the only source of immunity. For this reason, another key component of activities related to posteradication risk management is the establishment of a global stockpile of vaccine to respond to any outbreak in the future. In most developed countries in temperate climates, IPV has proved very effective in preventing outbreaks in the general population and may remain the vaccine of choice for small outbreaks in the countries. Much remains unknown about the potential for IPV to control PV circulation in developing countries because IPV induces a lower level of mucosal immunity than OPV.[155] Because OPV is the only vaccine that has ever been demonstrated to stop circulation of PV in developing countries, it will likely remain the vaccine of choice for the global stockpile. If an outbreak does occur, it is reasonable to expect that it will be caused by a single serotype in a specific place or time, prompting the maintenance of monovalent OPV strains in the stockpile. The use of monovalent OPV strains will eliminate the need to introduce undesirable additional strains into the population. Details remain, however, about the response plans and the use of the stockpile that need to be completed. In addition, issues remain about what should be done at the boundaries of the response population. It may be that the process of eliminating OPV may be as complicated and difficult as the process of eradicating the wild virus.

When the eradication program began, it was assumed that the vaccines available at the time were sufficient for the successful achievement of the goal. With the growing knowledge of the risks associated with OPV and the possible difficulties associated with either continuing or stopping its use in the future, hindsight indicates that the availability of additional options would be highly desirable. In the intervening years, many new approaches to vaccinology have been developed, raising the possibility of developing new PV vaccines (e.g., genetically engineered PV, noninfectious DNA, or immunogenic peptides). Despite the significant difficulties involving testing these new interventions, it seems appropriate to continue active investigations in this area.[196]

The world has endured the crippling effects of PV for millennia, yet the end of these particular viruses is approaching. It is possible that the next edition of this chapter will treat PV quite differently, possibly even as a historic footnote, rather than a major focus of public health activities.

PERSPECTIVES

For 25 to 50 years before the identification of acquired immunodeficiency syndrome, much of human virology was focused on PV. With the eradication of PV imminent, the picornavirology field is changing and will never be the same again. It is somewhat ironic to realize that, despite the incredible advances in our understanding of the molecular aspects of PV and the availability of extraordinarily powerful molecular tools for studying PV, the eradication of poliomyelitis will become a reality as a result of the use of the Salk and Sabin vaccines, vaccines that were generated empirically in the middle of the last century before the breakthroughs in our understanding of the molecular biology of PV.

But perhaps, it is unfair to belittle the achievements of modern techniques in the eradication of PV. Certainly, the tools of molecular biology were and will continue to be important in monitoring and tracking PV and identifying strains; it also may be that new technology and knowledge will make a better PV vaccine. Novel diagnostic methods developed to assist in surveillance of poliomyelitis are likely to aid in the identification of new enteroviruses, provide better and more accurate descriptions of the epidemiology of EV infections, and lead to new anti-EV drugs, nonpolio EV vaccines, and a better understanding of the relationship of EV to acute and chronic human disease.

What new directions will drive the field of picornavirology? Pressure exists to develop new antiviral treatments and vaccines. New antiviral approaches will take advantage of knowledge of virus receptors, structures of capsid and nonstructural proteins, and immunologic features of the disease. New vaccines will be pursued and developed. The ability of EV71 to mount large epidemics and to be a major cause of neurologic disease, especially AFP, is likely to have already generated special interest with respect to vaccine development. The many diseases that the coxsackieviruses cause also make this group of viruses of great interest from the point of view of vaccine development. In addition, investigations of coxsackieviral diseases may clarify the pathogenesis of virus-induced autoimmune diseases.

Despite the development of new treatments and vaccines, enteroviruses will still be very much with us, even after the eradication of PV.

REFERENCES

1. Abad FX, Pinto RM, Bosch A. Survival of enteric viruses on environmental fomites. *Appl Environ Microbiol* 1994;60(10):3704–3710.
2. Abad FX, Pinto RM, Bosch A. Disinfection of human enteric viruses on fomites. *FEMS Microbiol Lett* 1997;156(1):107–111.
3. Abed Y, et al. Development of a serological assay based on a synthetic peptide selected from the VP0 capsid protein for detection of human parechoviruses. *J Clin Microbiol* 2007;45(6):2037–2039.
4. Abedi GR, et al. Enterovirus and human parechovirus surveillance—United States, 2009–2013. *MMWR Morb Mortal Wkly Rep* 2015;64(34):940–943.
5. AbuBakar S, et al. Identification of enterovirus 71 isolates from an outbreak of hand, foot and mouth disease (HFMD) with fatal cases of encephalomyelitis in Malaysia. *Virus Res* 1999;61(1):1–9.
6. Abzug M. Perinatal enterovirus infections. In: Rotbart HA, ed. *Human Enterovirus Infections*. Washington: ASM Press; 1995:221–238.
7. Abzug MJ, et al. Viral pneumonia in the first month of life. *Pediatr Infect Dis J* 1990;9(12):881–885.
8. Abzug MJ, et al. Neonatal enterovirus infection: virology, serology, and effects of intravenous immune globulin. *Clin Infect Dis* 1995;20(5):1201–1206.
9. Abzug MJ, et al. Double blind placebo-controlled trial of pleconaril in infants with enterovirus meningitis. *Pediatr Infect Dis J* 2003;22(4):335–341.
10. Ackermann WW, Fujioka RS, Kurtz HB. Cationic modulation of the inactivation of poliovirus by heat. *Arch Environ Health* 1970;21(3):377–381.
11. Afif H, et al. Outbreak of poliomyelitis in Gizan, Saudi Arabia: cocirculation of wild type 1 polioviruses from three separate origins. *J Infect Dis* 1997;175(Suppl 1):S71–S75.
12. Alexander JP Jr, et al. Coxsackievirus B2 infection and aseptic meningitis: a focal outbreak among members of a high school football team. *J Infect Dis* 1993;167(5):1201–1205.
13. Alexander LN, et al. Vaccine policy changes and epidemiology of poliomyelitis in the United States. *JAMA* 2004;292(14):1696–1701.
14. Alexopoulou L, et al. Recognition of double-stranded RNA and activation of NF-kB by Toll-like receptor 3. *Nature* 2001;413(6857):732–738.
15. Aliabadi N, et al. Enterovirus D68 infection in children with acute flaccid myelitis, Colorado, USA, 2014. *Emerg Infect Dis* 2016;22(8):1387–1394.
16. Alirezaei M, et al. Pancreatic acinar cell-specific autophagy disruption reduces coxsackievirus replication and pathogenesis in vivo. *Cell Host Microbe* 2012;11(3):298–305.
17. Anderson DR, et al. Direct interactions of coxsackievirus B3 with immune cells in the splenic compartment of mice susceptible or resistant to myocarditis. *J Virol* 1996;70:4632–4645.
18. Andreoletti L, et al. Enteroviruses can persist with or without active viral replication in cardiac tissue of patients with end-stage ischemic or dilated cardiomyopathy. *J Infect Dis* 2000;182(4):1222–1227.
19. Andreoletti L, et al. Viral causes of human myocarditis. *Arch Cardiovasc Dis* 2009;102(6–7):559–568.
20. Anonymous. *Enterovirus Surveillance Report, 1970–1979*. Atlanta: Centers for Disease Control; 1981.
21. Anonymous. Deaths among children during an outbreak of hand, foot, and mouth disease—Taiwan, Republic of China, April–July 1998. *MMWR Morb Mortal Wkly Rep* 1998;47(30):629–632.
22. Archard LC, et al. The role of Coxsackie B viruses in the pathogenesis of myocarditis, dilated cardiomyopathy and inflammatory muscle disease. *Biochem Soc Symp* 1987;53:51–62.
23. Archard LC, et al. Characterization of Coxsackie B virus RNA in myocardium from patients with dilated cardiomyopathy by nucleotide sequencing of reverse transcription-nested polymerase chain reaction products. *Hum Pathol* 1998;29(6):578–584.
24. Arnesjo B, et al. Enterovirus infections in acute pancreatitis. *Scand J Gastroenterol* 1976;11(7):645–649.
25. Arola A, et al. Experimental myocarditis induced by two different coxsackievirus B3 variants: aspects of pathogenesis and comparison of diagnostic methods. *J Med Virol* 1995;47:251–259.
26. Asher DR, et al. Coxsackievirus and adenovirus receptor is essential for cardiomyocyte development. *Genesis* 2005;42(2):77–85.
27. Asturias EJ, et al. Poliovirus excretion in Guatemalan adults and children with HIV infection and children with cancer. *Biologicals* 2006;34(2):109–112.
28. Axelsson C, et al. Coxsackie B virus infections in women with miscarriage. *J Med Virol* 1993;39(4):282–285.
29. Aycock WL. The significance of the age distribution of poliomyelitis: evidence of transmission through contact. *Am J Hyg* 1928;8:35–54.
30. Baboonian C, Treasure T. Meta-analysis of the association of enteroviruses with human heart disease. *Heart* 1997;78(6):539–543.
31. Baboonian C, et al. Coxsackie B viruses and human heart disease. *Curr Top Microbiol Immunol* 1997;223:31–52.
32. Baggen J, et al. Enterovirus D68 receptor requirements unveiled by haploid genetics. *Proc Natl Acad Sci U S A* 2016;113(5):1399–1404.
33. Barral PM, et al. MDA-5 is cleaved in poliovirus-infected cells. *J Virol* 2007;81(8):3677–3684.
34. Basso NG, et al. Enterovirus isolation from foetal and placental tissues. *Acta Virol* 1990;34(1):49–57.
35. Beld M, et al. Highly sensitive assay for detection of enterovirus in clinical specimens by reverse transcription-PCR with an armored RNA internal control. *J Clin Microbiol* 2004;42(7):3059–3064.
36. Belkaya S, et al. Autosomal recessive cardiomyopathy presenting as acute myocarditis. *J Am Coll Cardiol* 2017;69(13):1653–1665.
37. Bell EJ, McCartney RA. A study of coxsackie B virus infections, 1972–1983. *J Hygiene* 1984;93(2):197–203.
38. Bell EJ, et al. Mu-antibody capture ELISA for the rapid diagnosis of enterovirus infections in patients with aseptic meningitis. *J Med Virol* 1986;19(3):213–217.
39. Bendig JWA, et al. Enterovirus sequences resembling coxsackievirus A2 detected in stool and spleen from a girl with fatal myocarditis. *J Med Virol* 2001;64:482–486.
40. Bendig JW, et al. Coxsackievirus B3 sequences in the blood of a neonate with congenital myocarditis, plus serological evidence of maternal infection. *J Med Virol* 2003;70(4):606–609.
41. Benschop KSM, et al. Human parechovirus infections in Dutch children and the association between serotype and disease severity. *Clin Infect Dis* 2006;42:204–210.
42. Bergelson JM, et al. Decay-accelerating factor (CD55), a glycosylphosphatidylinositol-anchored complement regulatory protein, is a receptor for several echoviruses. *Proc Natl Acad Sci U S A* 1994;91(13):6245–6248.
43. Berlin BS, Simon NM, Bovner RN. Myoglobinuria precipitated by viral infection. *JAMA* 1974;227(12):1414–1415.
44. Bersani I, et al. Neonatal acute liver failure due to enteroviruses: a 14 years single NICU experience. *J Matern Fetal Neonatal Med* 2019:1–5. doi:10.1080/14767058.2018.1555806.
45. Bird SW, et al. Nonlytic viral spread enhanced by autophagy components. *Proc Natl Acad Sci U S A* 2014;111(36):13081–13086.
46. Birmingham ME, et al. National immunization days: state of the art. *J Infect Dis* 1997;175(Suppl 1):S183–S188.
47. Birmingham ME, et al. Poliomyelitis surveillance: the compass for eradication. *J Infect Dis* 1997;175(Suppl 1):S146–S150.
48. Bodian D. Histopathologic basis of clinical findings in poliomyelitis. *Am J Med* 1949;6(5):563–578.
49. Bodian D. Viremia in experimental poliomyelitis II. Viremia and the mechanism of the provoking effect of injections or trauma. *Am J Hyg* 1954;60(3):358–370.
50. Bodian D. Some emerging concepts of poliomyelitis infection. *Science* 1955;122:105–108.
51. Bodian D, Morgan IM, Howe HA. Differentiation of types of poliomyelitis viruses. III. The grouping of fourteen strains into three basic immunological types. *Am J Hyg* 1949;49:234–245.
52. Boivin G, Abed Y, Boucher FD. Human parechovirus 3 and neonatal infections. *Emerg Infect Dis* 2005;11(1):103–105.
53. Boman J, Nilsson B, Juto P. Serum IgA, IgG, and IgM responses to different enteroviruses as measured by a coxsackie B5-based indirect ELISA. *J Med Virol* 1992;38(1):32–35.
54. Bothig B, Danes L, Dittmann S. Immunogenicity of oral poliomyelitis vaccine (OPV) against variants of wild poliovirus type 3. *Bull World Health Organ* 1990;68(5):597–600.
55. Bouin A, et al. Enterovirus persistence in cardiac cells of patients suffering from idiopathic dilated cardiomyopathy is linked to 5′ terminal genomic RNA-deleted viral populations with viral-encoded proteinase activities. *Circulation* 2019;139:2326–2338.
56. Bowles NE, et al. Detection of Coxsackie-B-virus-specific RNA sequences in myocardial biopsy samples from patients with myocarditis and dilated cardiomyopathy. *Lancet* 1986;1:1120–1123.
57. Brown BA, et al. Molecular epidemiology and evolution of enterovirus 71 strains isolated from 1970 to 1998. *J Virol* 1999;73(12):9969–9975.
58. Brown B, et al. Complete genomic sequencing shows that polioviruses and members of human enterovirus species C are closely related in the noncapsid coding region. *J Virol* 2003;77(16):8973–8984.
59. Buisman AM, et al. Preexisting poliovirus-specific IgA in the circulation correlates with protection against virus excretion in the elderly. *J Infect Dis* 2008;197(5):698–706.

60. Burnet FM. Poliomyelitis in the light of recent experimental work. *Health Bull (Melb)* 1945;(81–82):2173–2177.
61. Burns CC, et al. Multiple independent emergences of type 2 vaccine-derived polioviruses during a large outbreak in northern Nigeria. *J Virol* 2013;87(9):4907–4922.
62. Burns CC, et al. Vaccine-derived polioviruses. *J Infect Dis* 2014;210(Suppl 1):S283–S293.
63. Byington CL, et al. A polymerase chain reaction-based epidemiologic investigation of the incidence of nonpolio enteroviral infections in febrile and afebrile infants 90 days and younger. *Pediatrics* 1999;103(3):E27.
64. Caggana M, Chan P, Ramsingh A. Identification of a single amino acid residue in the capsid protein VP1 of coxsackievirus B4 that determines the virulent phenotype. *J Virol* 1993;67(8):4797–4803.
65. Carmona-Vicente N, et al. Phylogeny and prevalence of kobuviruses in dogs and cats in the UK. *Vet Microbiol* 2013;164(3–4):246–252.
66. Carson SD, et al. Endogenous low-level expression of the coxsackievirus and adenovirus receptor enables coxsackievirus B3 infection of RD cells. *J Gen Virol* 2007;88(Pt 11):3031–3038.
67. Carson SD, et al. Variation of coxsackievirus B3 capsid primary structure, ligands, and stability are selected in a coxsackievirus and adenovirus receptor-limited environment. *J Virol* 2011;85:3306–3314.
68. Cashman NR, et al. Late denervation in patients with antecedent paralytic poliomyelitis. *N Engl J Med* 1987;317(1):7–12.
69. Centers for Disease Control and Prevention. Final stages of poliomyelitis eradication—Western Pacific Region, 1997–1998. *JAMA* 1999;281(18):1690–1691.
70. Centers for Disease Control and Prevention. National laboratory inventory for global poliovirus containment—United States, November 2003. *MMWR Morb Mortal Wkly Rep* 2004;53(21):457–459.
71. Centers for Disease Control and Prevention. Outbreak of polio in adults—Namibia, 2006. *MMWR Morb Mortal Wkly Rep* 2006;55(44):1198–1201.
72. Centers for Disease Control and Prevention. Notes from the field: poliomyelitis outbreak—Republic of the Congo, September 2010—February 2011. *MMWR Morb Mortal Wkly Rep* 2011;60(10):312–313.
73. Centers for Disease Control and Prevention. Update on vaccine-derived polioviruses—worldwide, July 2009–March 2011. *MMWR Morb Mortal Wkly Rep* 2011;60(25):846–850.
74. Centers for Disease Control and Prevention. Tracking progress toward global polio eradication, 2010–2011. *MMWR Morb Mortal Wkly Rep* 2012;61:265–269.
75. Centers for Disease Control and Prevention. Progress toward interruption of wild poliovirus transmission—worldwide, January 2011–March 2012. *MMWR Morb Mortal Wkly Rep* 2012;61(19):353–357.
76. Cetta F, Michels VV. The autoimmune basis of dilated cardiomyopathy. *Ann Med* 1995;27(2):169–173.
77. Chambon M, Bailly JL, Peigue-Lafeuille H. Comparative sensitivity of the echovirus type 25 JV-4 prototype strain and two recent isolates to glutaraldehyde at low concentrations. *Appl Environ Microbiol* 1994;60(2):387–392.
78. Chapman NM, et al. Sites other than nucleotide 234 determine cardiovirulence in natural isolates of coxsackievirus B3. *J Med Virol* 1997;52(3):258–261.
79. Chapman NM, et al. 5′ terminal deletions in the genome of a coxsackievirus B2 strain occurred naturally in human heart. *Virology* 2008;375(2):480–491.
80. Charcot JM, Joffroy A. Cas de paralysie infantile spinale avec lesins des cornes anterieures de la substance grise de la moelle epiniere. *Arch Physiol Norm Pathol* 1870;3:134–152.
81. Chen SX, et al. Immunological status and pathology of coxsackie B viral myocarditis and dilated cardiomyopathy. *Chin Med J (Engl)* 1993;106:659–664.
82. Chen JW, et al. Cardiomyocyte-specific deletion of the coxsackievirus and adenovirus receptor results in hyperplasia of the embryonic left ventricle and abnormalities of sinuatrial valves. *Circ Res* 2006;98(7):923–930.
83. Chen HL, et al. Expression of VP1 protein in the milk of transgenic mice: a potential oral vaccine protects against enterovirus 71 infection. *Vaccine* 2008;26(23):2882–2889.
84. Chen YH, et al. Phosphatidylserine vesicles enable efficient en bloc transmission of enteroviruses. *Cell* 2015;160(4):619–630.
85. Chiou CC, et al. Coxsackievirus B1 infection in infants less than 2 months of age. *Am J Perinatol* 1998;15(3):155–159.
86. Chonmaitree T, Mann L. Respiratory infections. In: Rotbart HA, ed. *Human Enterovirus Infections*. Washington: ASM Press; 1995:255–270.
87. Chonmaitree T, et al. Comparison of cell cultures for rapid isolation of enteroviruses. *J Clin Microbiol* 1988;26(12):2576–2580.
88. Chow LH, Beisel KW, McManus BM. Enteroviral infection of mice with severe combined immunodeficiency. Evidence for direct viral pathogenesis of myocardial injury. *Lab Invest* 1992;66(1):24–31.
89. Christensen KK. Infection as a predominant cause of perinatal mortality. *Obstet Gynecol* 1982;59(4):499–508.
90. Chumakov M, et al. Enterovirus 71 isolated from cases of epidemic poliomyelitis-like disease in Bulgaria. *Arch Virol* 1979;60(3–4):329–340.
91. Chung YC, et al. Immunization with virus-like particles of enterovirus 71 elicits potent immune responses and protects mice against lethal challenge. *Vaccine* 2008;26(15):1855–1862.
92. Civardi E, et al. Viral outbreaks in neonatal intensive care units: what we do not know. *Am J Infect Control* 2013;41(10):854–856.
93. Clark CS, et al. Sewage worker's syndrome [letter]. *Lancet* 1977;1(8019):1009.
94. Cochi SL, Sutter RW, Aylward RB. Possible global strategies for stopping polio vaccination and how they could be harmonized. *Dev Biol (Basel)* 2001;105:153–158; discussion 159.
95. Codd MB, et al. Epidemiology of idiopathic dilated and hypertrophic cardiomyopathy. A population-based study in Olmsted County, Minnesota, 1975–1984. *Circulation* 1989;80(3):564–572.
96. Colbere-Garapin F, et al. An approach to understanding the mechanisms of poliovirus persistence in infected cells of neural or non-neural origin. *Clin Diagn Virol* 1998;9(2–3):107–113.
97. Conyn-Van Spaendonck MA, et al. Immunity to poliomyelitis in The Netherlands. *Am J Epidemiol* 2001;153(3):207–214.
98. Cooney MK, Hall CE, Fox JP. The Seattle virus watch. 3. Evaluation of isolation methods and summary of infections detected by virus isolations. *Am J Epidemiol* 1972;96(4):286–305.
99. Coyne CB, Bergelson JM. Virus-induced Abl and Fyn kinase signals permit coxsackievirus entry through epithelial tight junctions. *Cell* 2006;124(1):119–131.
100. Crainic R, et al. Natural variation of poliovirus neutralization epitopes. *Infect Immun* 1983;41(3):1217–1225.
101. Crotty S, et al. Poliovirus pathogenesis in a new poliovirus receptor transgenic mouse model: age-dependent paralysis and a mucosal route of infection. *J Gen Virol* 2002;83(Pt 7):1707–1720.
102. Crowder S, Kirkegaard K. Trans-dominant inhibition of RNA viral replication can slow growth of drug-resistant viruses. *Nat Genet* 2005;37(7):701–709.
103. D'Alessio DJ. A case–control study of group B coxsackievirus immunoglobulin M antibody prevalence and HLA-DR antigens in newly diagnosed cases of insulin-dependent diabetes mellitus. *Am J Epidemiol* 1992;135(12):1331–1338.
104. Dagan R, Menegus M. Nonpolio enteroviruses and the febrile infant. In: Rotbart HA, ed. *Human Enterovirus Infections*. Washington: ASM Press; 1995:239–254.
105. Dagan R, et al. Epidemiology and laboratory diagnosis of infection with viral and bacterial pathogens in infants hospitalized for suspected sepsis. *J Pediatr* 1989;115(3):351–356.
106. Dalakas MC. Enteroviruses and human neuromuscular diseases. In: Rotbart HA, ed. *Human Enterovirus Infections*. Washington: ASM Press; 1995:387–398.
107. Dales S, et al. Electron microscopic study of the formation of poliovirus. *Virology* 1965;26:379–389.
108. Dalldorf G, Sickles GM. An unidentified, filtrable agent isolated from the feces of children with paralysis. *Science* 1948;108:61–62.
109. Day C, Cumming H, Walker J. Enterovirus-specific IgM in the diagnosis of meningitis. *J Infect* 1989;19(3):219–228.
110. de Jong AS, et al. Functional analysis of picornavirus 2B proteins: effects on calcium homeostasis and intracellular protein trafficking. *J Virol* 2008;82(7):3782–3790.
111. de Leeuw N, et al. No evidence for persistent enterovirus infection in patients with end-stage idiopathic dilated cardiomyopathy. *J Infect Dis* 1998;178(1):256–259.
112. de Quadros CA, et al. Strategies for poliomyelitis eradication in developing countries. *Public Health Rev* 1993;21(1–2):65–81.
113. Dechkum N, et al. Coxsackie B virus infection and myopericarditis in Thailand, 1987–1989. *Southeast Asian J Trop Med Public Health* 1998;29(2):273–276.
114. Deibel R, Gross LL, Collins DN. Isolation of a new enterovirus (38506). *Proc Soc Exp Biol Med* 1975;148(1):203–207.
115. Delorme-Axford E, Sadovsky Y, Coyne CB. Lipid raft- and SRC family kinase-dependent entry of coxsackievirus B into human placental trophoblasts. *J Virol* 2013;87(15):8569–8581.
116. Deonarain R, et al. Protective role for interferon-beta in coxsackievirus B3 infection. *Circulation* 2004;110(23):3540–3543.
117. Dery P, Marks MI, Shapera R. Clinical manifestations of coxsackievirus infections in children. *Am J Dis Child* 1974;128(4):464–468.
118. Destombes J, et al. Persistent poliovirus infection in mouse motoneurons. *J Virol* 1997;71(2):1621–1628.
119. Diana GD, Pevear DC. Antipicornavirus drugs: current status. *Antivir Chem Chemother* 1997;8:401–408.
120. Dorner AA, et al. Coxsackievirus-adenovirus receptor (CAR) is essential for early embryonic cardiac development. *J Cell Sci* 2005;118(Pt 15):3509–3521.
121. Dorval BL, Chow M, Klibanov AM. Stabilization of poliovirus against heat inactivation. *Biochem Biophys Res Commun* 1989;159(3):1177–1183.
122. Douglas JD, Soike KF, Raynor J. The incidence of poliovirus in chimpanzees (Pan troglodytes). *Lab Anim Care* 1970;20(2):265–268.
123. Dowdle WR, Birmingham ME. The biologic principles of poliovirus eradication. *J Infect Dis* 1997;175(Suppl 1):S286–S292.
124. Drebot MA, Campbell JJ, Lee SH. A genotypic characterization of enteroviral antigenic variants isolated in eastern Canada. *Virus Res* 1999;59(2):131–140.
125. Drummond CG, et al. Enteroviruses infect human enteroids and induce antiviral signaling in a cell lineage-specific manner. *Proc Natl Acad Sci U S A* 2017;114(7):1672–1677.
126. Duintjer Tebbens RJ, et al. Uncertainty and sensitivity analyses of a decision analytic model for posteradication polio risk management. *Risk Anal* 2008;28:855–876.
127. Dunn JJ, et al. The stem loop II within the 5′ nontranslated region of clinical coxsackievirus B3 genomes determines cardiovirulence phenotype in a murine model. *J Infect Dis* 2003;187(10):1552–1561.
128. Enders JF, Weller TH, Robbins FC. Cultivation of the Lansing strain of poliomyelitis virus in cultures of various human embryonic tissues. *Science* 1949;109:85–87.
129. Esfandiarei M, McManus BM. Molecular biology and pathogenesis of viral myocarditis. *Annu Rev Pathol* 2008;3:127–155.
130. Essaidi-Laziosi M, et al. Propagation of respiratory viruses in human airway epithelia reveals persistent virus-specific signatures. *J Allergy Clin Immunol* 2018;141(6):2074–2084.
131. Estivariz CF, et al. A large vaccine-derived poliovirus outbreak on Madura Island—Indonesia, 2005. *J Infect Dis* 2008;197(3):347–354.
132. Estrin M, Smith C, Huber SA. Coxsackievirus B-3 myocarditis. T-cell autoimmunity to heart antigens is resistant to cyclosporin-A treatment. *Am J Pathol* 1986;125:244–251.
133. Evans DM, et al. Increased neurovirulence associated with a single nucleotide change in a noncoding region of the Sabin type 3 poliovaccine genome. *Nature* 1985;314:548–550.
134. Fairweather D, et al. IL-12 receptor $\beta 1$ and Toll-like receptor 4 increase IL-1β- and IL-18-associated myocarditis and coxsackievirus replication. *J Immunol* 2003;170(9):4731–4737.
135. Feachem R, Garelick H, Slade J. Enteroviruses in the environment. *Trop Dis Bull* 1981;78(3):185–230.
136. Feng Q, et al. Enterovirus 2Apro targets MDA5 and MAVS in infected cells. *J Virol* 2014;88(6):3369–3378.
137. Feuer R, et al. Cell cycle status affects coxsackievirus replication, persistence, and reactivation in vitro. *J Virol* 2002;76(9):4430–4440.
138. Feuer R, et al. Coxsackievirus B3 and the neonatal CNS: the roles of stem cells, developing neurons, and apoptosis in infection, viral dissemination, and disease. *Am J Pathol* 2003;163(4):1379–1393.

139. Feuer R, et al. Coxsackievirus replication and the cell cycle: a potential regulatory mechanism for viral persistence/latency. *Med Microbiol Immunol* 2004;193(2/3):83–90.
140. Flodstrom M, et al. Target cell defense prevents the development of diabetes after viral infection. *Nat Immunol* 2002;3(4):373–382.
141. Foo DG, et al. Identification of neutralizing linear epitopes from the VP1 capsid protein of Enterovirus 71 using synthetic peptides. *Virus Res* 2007;125(1):61–68.
142. Foo DG, et al. Passive protection against lethal enterovirus 71 infection in newborn mice by neutralizing antibodies elicited by a synthetic peptide. *Microbes Infect* 2007;9(11):1299–1306.
143. Foo DG, et al. Identification of human CD4 T-cell epitopes on the VP1 capsid protein of enterovirus 71. *Viral Immunol* 2008;21(2):215–224.
144. Fowlkes AL, et al. Enterovirus-associated encephalitis in the California encephalitis project, 1998–2005. *J Infect Dis* 2008;198(11):1685–1691.
145. Freistadt MS, Kaplan G, Racaniello VR. Heterogeneous expression of poliovirus receptor-related proteins in human cells and tissues. *Mol Cell Biol* 1990;10(11):5700–5706.
146. Frisancho-Kiss S, et al. Cutting edge: cross-regulation by TLR4 and T cell Ig mucin-3 determines sex differences in inflammatory heart disease. *J Immunol* 2007;178(11):6710–6714.
147. Frisk G, Diderholm H. Increased frequency of coxsackie B virus IgM in women with spontaneous abortion. *J Infect* 1992;24(2):141–145.
148. Frisk G, Lindberg MA, Diderholm H. Persistence of coxsackievirus B4 infection in rhabdomyosarcoma cells for 30 months. Brief report. *Arch Virol* 1999;144(11):2239–2245.
149. Frisk G, et al. Enterovirus IgM detection: specificity of mu-antibody-capture radioimmunoassays using virions and procapsids of Coxsackie B virus. *J Virol Methods* 1989; 24(1–2):191–202.
150. Fujii K, et al. Transgenic mouse model for the study of enterovirus 71 neuropathogenesis. *Proc Natl Acad Sci U S A* 2013;110(36):14753–14758.
151. Gauntt CJ, et al. Epitopes shared between coxsackievirus B3 (CVB3) and normal heart tissue contribute to CVB3-induced murine myocarditis. *Clin Immunol Immunopathol* 1993;68:129–134.
152. Gauntt CJ, et al. Molecular mimicry, anti-coxsackievirus B3 neutralizing monoclonal antibodies and myocarditis. *J Immunol* 1995;154:2983–2995.
153. Gelfand HM, et al. A continuing surveillance of enterovirus infections in healthy children in six United States cities. I. Viruses isolated during 1960 and 1961. *Am J Hyg* 1963;78:358–375.
154. George BP, Schneider EB, Venkatesan A. Encephalitis hospitalization rates and inpatient mortality in the United States, 2000–2010. *PLoS One* 2014;9(9):e104169.
155. Ghendon Y, Robertson SE. Interrupting the transmission of wild polioviruses with vaccines: immunological considerations. *Bull World Health Organ* 1994;72(6):973–983.
156. Girard S, et al. Poliovirus induces apoptosis in the mouse central nervous system. *J Virol* 1999;73(7):6066–6072.
157. Girard S, et al. Restriction of poliovirus RNA replication in persistently infected nerve cells. *J Gen Virol* 2002;83(Pt 5):1087–1093.
158. Gitlin L, et al. Essential role of mda-5 in type I IFN responses to polyriboinosinic:po lyribocytidylic acid and encephalomyocarditis picornavirus. *Proc Natl Acad Sci U S A* 2006;103(22):8459–8464.
159. Godeny EK, Gauntt CJ. In situ immune autoradiographic identification of cells in heart tissues of mice with coxsackievirus B3-induced myocarditis. *Am J Pathol* 1987;129:267–276.
160. Goldwater PN. Immunoglobulin M capture immunoassay in investigation of coxsackievirus B5 and B6 outbreaks in South Australia. *J Clin Microbiol* 1995;33(6):1628–1631.
161. Gomez RM, et al. Ultrastructural study of cell injury induced by coxsackievirus B3 in pancreatic and cardiac tissues. *Medicina (B Aires)* 1993;53:300–306.
162. Gondo K, et al. Echovirus type 9 epidemic in Kagoshima, southern Japan: seroepidemiology and clinical observation of aseptic meningitis. *Pediatr Infect Dis J* 1995;14(9):787–791.
163. Good CA, Wells A, Coyne CB. Type III interferon signaling restricts Enterovirus 71 infection of goblet cells. *Sci Adv* 2019;5:eaau4255.
164. Gorbea C, et al. A role for Toll-like receptor 3 variants in host susceptibility to enteroviral myocarditis and dilated cardiomyopathy. *J Biol Chem* 2010;285(30):23208–23223.
165. Gorgievski-Hrisoho M, et al. Detection by PCR of enteroviruses in cerebrospinal fluid during a summer outbreak of aseptic meningitis in Switzerland. *J Clin Microbiol* 1998;36(9):2408–2412.
166. Goubau D, et al. Antiviral immunity via RIG-I-mediated recognition of RNA bearing 5′-diphosphates. *Nature* 2014;514(7522):372–375.
167. Goyal SM, Gerba CP. Comparative adsorption of human enteroviruses, simian rotavirus, and selected bacteriophages to soils. *Appl Environ Microbiol* 1979;38(2):241–247.
168. Grandien M, Forsgren M, Ehrnst A. Enteroviruses and reoviruses. In: Lennette EH, Schmidt NJ, eds. *Diagnostic Procedures for Viral, Rickettsial, and Chlamydial Infections*. Washington: American Public Health Association; 1989:513–569.
169. Gravanis MB, Sternby NH. Incidence of myocarditis. A 10-year autopsy study from Malmo, Sweden. *Arch Pathol Lab Med* 1991;115(4):390–392.
170. Gregorio SB, Nakao JC, Beran GW. Human enteroviruses in animals and arthropods in the central Philippines. *Southeast Asian J Trop Med Public Health* 1972;3(1):45–51.
171. Grisariu S, et al. Enteroviral infection in patients treated with rituximab for non-Hodgkin lymphoma: a case series and review of the literature. *Hematol Oncol* 2017;35(4):591–598.
172. Grist NR, Bell EJ, Assaad F. Enteroviruses in human disease. *Prog Med Virol* 1978; 24:114–157.
173. Groarke JM, Pevear DC. Attenuated virulence of pleconaril-resistant coxsackievirus B3 variants. *J Infect Dis* 1999;179(6):1538–1541.
174. Gromeier M, Wimmer E. Mechanism of injury-provoked poliomyelitis. *J Virol* 1998; 72(6):5056–5060.
175. Guo R, et al. Preliminary studies on antigenic variation of poliovirus using neutralizing monoclonal antibodies. *J Gen Virol* 1987;68(Pt 4):989–994.
176. Haarmann CM, et al. Identification of serotype-specific and nonserotype-specific B-cell epitopes of coxsackie B virus using synthetic peptides. *Virology* 1994;200(2):381–389.
177. Halim SS, Collins DN, Ramsingh AI. A therapeutic HIV vaccine using coxsackie-HIV recombinants: a possible new strategy. *AIDS Res Hum Retroviruses* 2000;16(15): 1551–1558.
178. Halim S, Ramsingh AI. A point mutation in VP1 of coxsackievirus B4 alters antigenicity. *Virology* 2000;269(1):86–94.
179. Halim SS, et al. Immunogenicity of a foreign peptide expressed within a capsid protein of an attenuated coxsackievirus. *Vaccine* 2001;19(7–8):958–965.
180. Hall CE, Cooney MK, Fox JP. The Seattle virus watch program. I. Infection and illness experience of virus watch families during a communitywide epidemic of echovirus type 30 aseptic meningitis. *Am J Public Health Nations Health* 1970;60(8):1456–1465.
181. Haller AA, Stewart SR, Semler BL. Attenuation stem-loop lesions in the 5′ noncoding region of poliovirus RNA: neuronal cell-specific translation defects. *J Virol* 1996;70(3):1467–1474.
182. Halonen P, et al. Detection of enteroviruses and rhinoviruses in clinical specimens by PCR and liquid-phase hybridization. *J Clin Microbiol* 1995;33(3):648–653.
183. Halsey NA, et al. Search for poliovirus carriers in persons with primary immune deficiency diseases in the United States, Mexico and Brazil. *Bull World Health Organ* 2004;82:3–8.
184. Hartig PC, Webb SR. Coxsackievirus B4 heterogeneity: effect of passage on neutralization and mortality. *Acta Virol* 1986;30(6):475–486.
185. Harvala H, et al. Detection and genetic characterization of enteroviruses circulating among wild populations of chimpanzees in Cameroon; relationship with human and simian enteroviruses. *J Virol* 2011;85:4480–4486.
186. Harvala H, et al. Recommendations for enterovirus diagnostics and characterisation within and beyond Europe. *J Clin Virol* 2018;101:11–17.
187. Hashimoto I, Komatsu T. Myocardial changes after infection with Coxsackie virus B3 in nude mice. *Br J Exp Pathol* 1978;59(1):13–20.
188. Heck CF, Shumway SJ, Kaye MP. The registry of the International Society for Heart Transplantation: sixth official report—1989. *J Heart Transplant* 1989;8:271–276.
189. Heim A, et al. Synergistic interaction of interferon-beta and interferon-gamma in coxsackievirus B3-infected carrier cultures of human myocardial fibroblasts. *J Infect Dis* 1992;166:958–965.
190. Heine J. *Beobachtungen uber Lahmungszustande der untern Extermitaten und deren Behandlung*. Stuttgart: Kohler; 1840.
191. Heinz BA, Vance LM. Sequence determinants of 3A-mediated resistance to enviroxime in rhinoviruses and enteroviruses. *J Virol* 1996;70(7):4854–4857.
192. Heinz BA, et al. Genetic and molecular analyses of spontaneous mutants of human rhinovirus 14 that are resistant to an antiviral compound. *J Virol* 1989;63(6):2476–2485.
193. Henke A, et al. The role of CD8 + T lymphocytes in coxsackievirus B3-induced myocarditis. *J Virol* 1995;69(11):6720–6728.
194. Hennessey KA, et al. Poliovirus vaccine shedding among persons with HIV in Abidjan, Cote d'Ivoire. *J Infect Dis* 2005;192(12):2124–2128.
195. Herzum M, et al. Treatment of experimental murine Coxsackie B3 myocarditis. *Eur Heart J* 1991;12(Suppl D):200–202.
196. Heymann DL, Sutter RW, Aylward RB. A global call for new polio vaccines. *Nature* 2005;434(7034):699–700.
197. Hilfenhaus J, Nowak T. Inactivation of hepatitis A virus by pasteurization and elimination of picornaviruses during manufacture of factor VIII concentrate. *Vox Sang* 1994;67(Suppl 1):62–66.
198. Ho M, et al. An epidemic of enterovirus 71 infection in Taiwan. Taiwan Enterovirus Epidemic Working Group. *N Engl J Med* 1999;341(13):929–935.
199. Hodgson J, et al. Comparison of two immunoassay procedures for detecting enterovirus IgM. *J Med Virol* 1995;47(1):29–34.
200. Hofschneider PH, Klingel K, Kandolf R. Toward understanding the pathogenesis of enterovirus-induced cardiomyopathy: molecular and ultrastructural approaches. *J Struct Biol* 1990;104:32–37.
201. Hogle JM, Chow M, Filman DJ. Three-dimensional structure of poliovirus at 2.9 A resolution. *Science* 1985;229(4720):1358–1365.
202. Hogle JM, Filman DJ. The antigenic structure of poliovirus. *Philos Trans R Soc Lond B Biol Sci* 1989;323(1217):467–478.
203. Holm-Hansen CC, Midgley SE, Fischer TK. Global emergence of enterovirus D68: a systematic review. *Lancet Infect Dis* 2016;16(5):e64–e75.
204. Holtz LR, et al. Identification of a novel picornavirus related to cosaviruses in a child with acute diarrhea. *Virol J* 2008;5:159.
205. Holtz LR, et al. Klassevirus 1, a previously undescribed member of the family Picornaviridae, is globally widespread. *Virol J* 2009;6:86.
206. Honig EI, et al. An endemiological study of enteric virus infections: poliomyelitis, coxsackie, and orphan (ECHO) viruses isolated from normal children in two socioeconomic groups. *J Exp Med* 1956;103(2):247–262.
207. Hornung V, et al. 5′-Triphosphate RNA is the ligand for RIG-I. *Science* 2006;314(5801): 994–997.
208. Horstmann DM. Poliomyelitis: severity and type of disease in different age groups. *Ann N Y Acad Sci* 1955;61:956–967.
209. Horstmann DM. Enterovirus infections of the central nervous system. The present and future of poliomyelitis. *Med Clin North Am* 1967;51(3):681–692.
210. Horwitz MS, et al. Diabetes induced by Coxsackie virus: initiation by bystander damage and not molecular mimicry. *Nat Med* 1998;4(7):781–785.
211. Hovi T, Stenvik M. Selective isolation of poliovirus in recombinant murine cell line expressing the human poliovirus receptor gene. *J Clin Microbiol* 1994;32(5):1366–1368.
212. Huang CC, et al. Neurologic complications in children with enterovirus 71 infection. *N Engl J Med* 1999;341(13):936–942.
213. Huang SC, et al. Enterovirus 71-induced autophagy detected in vitro and in vivo promotes viral replication. *J Med Virol* 2009;81(7):1241–1252.
214. Huber SA. Autoimmunity in myocarditis: relevance of animal models. *Clin Immunol Immunopathol* 1997;83(2):93–102.
215. Huber SA. Autoimmunity in coxsackievirus B3 induced myocarditis. *Autoimmunity* 2006;39(1):55–61.
216. Huber SA, Born W, O'Brien R. Dual functions of murine gammadelta cells in inflammation and autoimmunity in coxsackievirus B3-induced myocarditis: role of Vgamma1+ and Vgamma4+ cells. *Microbes Infect* 2005;7(3):537–543.

217. Huber SA, Lodge PA. Coxsackievirus B-3 myocarditis in Balb/c mice. Evidence for autoimmunity to myocyte antigens. *Am J Pathol* 1984;116:21–29.
218. Huber SA, Lyden DC, Lodge PA. Immunopathogenesis of experimental Coxsackievirus induced myocarditis: role of autoimmunity. *Herz* 1985;10:1–7.
219. Huber SA, Moraska A, Cunningham M. Alterations in major histocompatibility complex association of myocarditis induced by coxsackievirus B3 mutants selected with monoclonal antibodies to group A streptococci. *Proc Natl Acad Sci U S A* 1994;91(12):5543–5547.
220. Huber S, Sartini D. T cells expressing the Vgamma1 T-cell receptor enhance virus-neutralizing antibody response during coxsackievirus B3 infection of BALB/c mice: differences in male and female mice. *Viral Immunol* 2005;18(4):730–739.
221. Huber S, Song WC, Sartini D. Decay-accelerating factor (CD55) promotes CD1d expression and Vgamma4+ T-cell activation in coxsackievirus B3-induced myocarditis. *Viral Immunol* 2006;19(2):156–166.
222. Hubner D, et al. Infection of iPSC lines with miscarriage-associated coxsackievirus and measles virus and teratogenic rubella virus as a model for viral impairment of early human embryogenesis. *ACS Infect Dis* 2017;3(12):886–897.
223. Hughes SA, Thaker HM, Racaniello VR. Transgenic mouse model for echovirus myocarditis and paralysis. *Proc Natl Acad Sci U S A* 2003;100(26):15906–15911.
224. Huhn MH, et al. IFN- g production dominates the early human natural killer cell response to coxsackievirus infection. *Cell Microbiol* 2008;10(2):426–436.
225. Huhn MH, et al. Melanoma differentiation-associated protein-5 (MDA-5) limits early viral replication but is not essential for the induction of type 1 interferons after coxsackievirus infection. *Virology* 2010;401(1):42–48.
226. Hull BP, Dowdle WR. Poliovirus surveillance: building the global Polio Laboratory Network. *J Infect Dis* 1997;175(Suppl 1):S113–S116.
227. Hull HF, et al. Paralytic poliomyelitis: seasoned strategies, disappearing disease. *Lancet* 1994;343(8909):1331–1337.
228. Huovilainen A, et al. Antigenic variation among 173 strains of type 3 poliovirus isolated in Finland during the 1984 to 1985 outbreak. *J Gen Virol* 1988;69(Pt 8):1941–1948.
229. Hurlbut HS. The recovery of poliomyelitis virus after parenteral introduction into cockroaches and houseflies. *J Infect Dis* 1950;86(1):103.
230. Hwang JH, et al. Coxsackievirus B infection is highly related with missed abortion in Korea. *Yonsei Med J* 2014;55(6):1562–1567.
231. Hyöty H, Hiltunen M, Lonnrot M. Enterovirus infections and insulin dependent diabetes mellitus—evidence for causality. *Clin Diagn Virol* 1998;9(2–3):77–84.
232. Hyypiä T, et al. Classification of enteroviruses based on molecular and biological properties. *J Gen Virol* 1997;78(Pt 1):1–11.
233. Ida-Hosonuma M, et al. Comparison of neuropathogenicity of poliovirus in two transgenic mouse strains expressing human poliovirus receptor with different distribution patterns. *J Gen Virol* 2002;83(Pt 5):1095–1105.
234. Ida-Hosonuma M, et al. The alpha/beta interferon response controls tissue tropism and pathogenicity of poliovirus. *J Virol* 2005;79(7):4460–4469.
235. Irvine DH, Irvine AB, Gardner PS. Outbreak of E.C.H.O. virus type 30 in a general practice. *Br Med J* 1967;4(582):774–776.
236. Ito M, et al. Isolation and identification of a novel human parechovirus. *J Gen Virol* 2004;85:391–398.
237. Iturriza-Gomara M, Megson B, Gray J. Molecular detection and characterization of human enteroviruses directly from clinical samples using RT-PCR and DNA sequencing. *J Med Virol* 2006;78(2):243–253.
238. Jackson WT, et al. Subversion of cellular autophagosomal machinery by RNA viruses. *PLoS Biol* 2005;3(5):e156.
239. Jankovic B, et al. Severe neonatal echovirus 17 infection during a nursery outbreak. *Pediatr Infect Dis J* 1999;18(4):393–394.
240. Jarasch N, et al. Influence of pan-caspase inhibitors on coxsackievirus B3-infected CD19 + B lymphocytes. *Apoptosis* 2007;12(9):1633–1643.
241. Jenista JA, Powell KR, Menegus MA. Epidemiology of neonatal enterovirus infection. *J Pediatr* 1984;104(5):685–690.
242. Johansson ME, et al. Intrauterine fetal death due to echovirus 11. *Scand J Infect Dis* 1992;24(3):381–385.
243. Johnson R. *Viral Infections of the Nervous System*. 2nd ed. Philadelphia: JB Lippincott-Raven; 1998.
244. Joki-Korpela P, Hyypia T. Diagnosis and epidemiology of echovirus 22 infections. *Clin Infect Dis* 1998;27(1):129–136.
245. Jones MJ, et al. Case reports Intrauterine echovirus type II infection. *Mayo Clin Proc* 1980;55(8):509–512.
246. Jubelt B, et al. Pathogenesis of human poliovirus infection in mice. I. Clinical and pathological studies. *J Neuropathol Exp Neurol* 1980;39(2):138–148.
247. Jubelt B, et al. Antibody titer to the poliovirus in blood and cerebrospinal fluid of patients with post-polio syndrome. *Ann N Y Acad Sci* 1995;753:201–207.
248. Juhela S, et al. Enterovirus infections and enterovirus specific T-cell responses in infancy. *J Med Virol* 1998;54(3):226–232.
249. Kalkowska DA, et al. Modeling undetected live poliovirus circulation after apparent interruption of transmission: implications for surveillance and vaccination. *BMC Infect Dis* 2015;15:66.
250. Kallewaard NL, et al. Tissue-specific deletion of the coxsackievirus and adenovirus receptor protects mice from virus-induced pancreatitis and myocarditis. *Cell Host Microbe* 2009;6(1):91–98.
251. Kanamitsu M, et al. Immunofluorescent study on the pathogenesis of oral infection of poliovirus in monkeys. *Jpn J Med Sci Biol* 1967;20(2):175–194.
252. Kandolf R. Molecular biology of viral heart disease. *Herz* 1993;18(4):238–244.
253. Kandolf R, Canu A, Hofschneider PH. Coxsackie B3 virus can replicate in cultured human foetal heart cells and is inhibited by interferon. *J Mol Cell Cardiol* 1985;17:167–181.
254. Kandolf R, et al. Mechanisms and consequences of enterovirus persistence in cardiac myocytes and cells of the immune system. *Virus Res* 1999;62(2):149–158.
255. Kaplan MH, et al. Group B coxsackievirus infections in infants younger than three months of age: a serious childhood illness. *Rev Infect Dis* 1983;5(6):1019–1032.
256. Kares S, et al. Real-time PCR for rapid diagnosis of entero- and rhinovirus infections using LightCycler. *J Clin Virol* 2004;29(2):99–104.
257. Kashimura T, et al. Spatiotemporal changes of coxsackievirus and adenovirus receptor in rat hearts during postnatal development and in cultured cardiomyocytes of neonatal rat. *Virchows Arch* 2004;444(3):283–292.
258. Kato H, et al. Differential roles of MDA5 and RIG-I helicases in the recognition of RNA viruses. *Nature* 2006;441(7089):101–105.
259. Kauder SE, Racaniello VR. Poliovirus tropism and attenuation are determined after internal ribosome entry. *J Clin Invest* 2004;113(12):1743–1753.
260. Kawamura N, et al. Determinants in the 5′ noncoding region of poliovirus Sabin 1 RNA that influence the attenuation phenotype. *J Virol* 1989;63(3):1302–1309.
261. Kaye SB, et al. Echovirus keratoconjunctivitis. *Am J Ophthalmol* 1998;125(2):187–190.
262. Kemball CC, Harkins S, Whitton JL. Enumeration and functional evaluation of virus-specific CD4+ and CD8+ T cells in lymphoid and peripheral sites of coxsackievirus B3 infection. *J Virol* 2008;82(9):4331–4342.
263. Kessler HH, et al. Rapid diagnosis of enterovirus infection by a new one-step reverse transcription-PCR assay. *J Clin Microbiol* 1997;35(4):976–977.
264. Kew OM, Nottay BK. Molecular epidemiology of polioviruses. *Rev Infect Dis* 1984;6(Suppl 2):S499–S504.
265. Kew O, Pallansch M. Breaking the last chains of poliovirus transmission: progress and challenges in global polio eradication. *Annu Rev Virol* 2018;5(1):427–451.
266. Kew OM, et al. Molecular epidemiology of wild poliovirus transmission. In: Kurstak E, et al., eds. *Virus Variability, Epidemiology, and Control*. New York: Plenum Medical Book Company; 1990:199–222.
267. Kew OM, et al. Molecular epidemiology of polioviruses. *Semin Virol* 1995;6:401–414.
268. Kew OM, et al. Prolonged replication of a type 1 vaccine-derived poliovirus in an immunodeficient patient. *J Clin Microbiol* 1998;36(10):2893–2899.
269. Kew OM, et al. Circulating vaccine-derived polioviruses: current state of knowledge. *Bull World Health Organ* 2004;82:16–23.
270. Kew OM, et al. Vaccine-derived polioviruses and the endgame strategy for global polio eradication. *Annu Rev Microbiol* 2005;59:587–635.
271. Khamrin P, Maneekarn N. Detection and genetic characterization of cosavirus in a pediatric patient with diarrhea. *Arch Virol* 2014;159(9):2485–2489.
272. Khetsuriani N, et al. Persistence of vaccine-derived polioviruses among immunodeficient persons with vaccine-associated paralytic poliomyelitis. *J Infect Dis* 2003;188:1845–1852.
273. Khetsuriani N, et al. Enterovirus surveillance—United States, 1970–2005. *MMWR Surveill Summ* 2006;55(SS-8):1–20.
274. Kilpatrick DR, et al. Group-specific identification of polioviruses by PCR using primers containing mixed-base or deoxyinosine residue at positions of codon degeneracy. *J Clin Microbiol* 1996;34(12):2990–2996.
275. Kilpatrick DR, et al. Serotype-specific identification of polioviruses by PCR using primers containing mixed-base or deoxyinosine residues at positions of codon degeneracy. *J Clin Microbiol* 1998;36(2):352–357.
276. Kim KS, et al. 5′-terminal deletions occur in coxsackievirus B3 during replication in murine hearts and cardiac myocyte cultures and correlate with encapsidation of negative-strand viral RNA. *J Virol* 2005;79(11):7024–7041.
277. Kitamura N, et al. Primary structure, gene organization and polypeptide expression of poliovirus RNA. *Nature* 1981;291(5816):547–553.
278. Klingel K, Kandolf R. The role of enterovirus replication in the development of acute and chronic heart muscle disease in different immunocompetent mouse strains. *Scand J Infect Dis Suppl* 1993;88:79–85.
279. Klingel K, et al. Pathogenesis of murine enterovirus myocarditis: virus dissemination and immune cell targets. *J Virol* 1996;70:8888–8895.
280. Knowles NJ, et al. Picornaviridae. In: King AMQ, et al., ed. *Virus Taxonomy: Classification and Nomenclature of Viruses: Ninth Report of the International Committee on Taxonomy of Viruses*. San Diego: Elsevier; 2011:855–880.
281. Koestner W, et al. Interferon-beta expression and type I interferon receptor signaling of hepatocytes prevent hepatic necrosis and virus dissemination in coxsackievirus B3-infected mice. *PLoS Pathog* 2018;14(8):e1007235.
282. Kogon A, et al. The virus watch program: a continuing surveillance of viral infections in metropolitan New York families VII. Observations on viral excretion, seroimmunity, intrafamilial spread and illness association in coxsackie and echovirus infections. *Am J Epidemiol* 1969;89(1):51–61.
283. Koide H, et al. Genomic detection of enteroviruses in the myocardium—studies on animal hearts with coxsackievirus B3 myocarditis and endomyocardial biopsies from patients with myocarditis and dilated cardiomyopathy. *Jpn Circ J* 1992;56(10):1081–1093.
284. Koike S, et al. Transgenic mice susceptible to poliovirus. *Proc Natl Acad Sci U S A* 1991;88(3):951–955.
285. Koike K, et al. Tumor necrosis factor-alpha stimulates prolactin release from anterior pituitary cells: a possible involvement of intracellular calcium mobilization. *Endocrinology* 1991;128(6):2785–2790.
286. Komatsu H, et al. Outbreak of severe neurologic involvement associated with Enterovirus 71 infection. *Pediatr Neurol* 1999;20(1):17–23.
287. Kono R. Apollo 11 disease or acute hemorrhagic conjunctivitis: a pandemic of a new enterovirus infection of the eyes. *Am J Epidemiol* 1975;101(5):383–390.
288. Konstantinidou A, et al. Transplacental infection of coxsackievirus B3 pathological findings in the fetus. *J Med Virol* 2007;79(6):754–757.
289. Kopecka H, Brown B, Pallansch M. Genotypic variation in coxsackievirus B5 isolates from three different outbreaks in the United States. *Virus Res* 1995;38(2–3):125–136.
290. Kramer M, et al. Echovirus infection causes rapid loss-of-function and cell death in human dendritic cells. *Cell Microbiol* 2007;9(6):1507–1518.
291. Kramer M, et al. Phagocytosis of picornavirus-infected cells induces an RNA-dependent antiviral state in human dendritic cells. *J Virol* 2008;82(6):2930–2937.
292. Kuss SK, Etheredge CA, Pfeiffer JK. Multiple host barriers restrict poliovirus trafficking in mice. *PLoS Pathog* 2008;4(6):e1000082.

293. Kuss SK, et al. Intestinal microbiota promote enteric virus replication and systemic pathogenesis. *Science* 2011;334(6053):249–252.
294. Labadie K, et al. Poliovirus mutants excreted by a chronically infected hypogammaglobulinemic patient establish persistent infections in human intestinal cells. *Virology* 2004;318(1):66–78.
295. Lafferty EI, et al. Unc93b1-dependent endosomal toll-like receptor signaling regulates inflammation and mortality during coxsackievirus B3 infection. *J Innate Immun* 2015;7(3):315–330.
296. Lancaster KZ, Pfeiffer JK. Limited trafficking of a neurotropic virus through inefficient retrograde axonal transport and the type I interferon response. *PLoS Pathog* 2010;6(3):e1000791.
297. Landsteiner K, Popper E. Mikroskopische Praparate von einem Menschlichen und zwei Affenruckenmarken. *Wien Klinische Wochenschrift* 1908;21:1830.
298. Lane JR, et al. LPS promotes CB3-induced myocarditis in resistant B10.A mice. *Cell Immunol* 1991;136(1):219–233.
299. Leake JP. Poliomyelitis following vaccination against this disease. *JAMA* 1935;105(26): 2152–2153.
300. Leff RL, et al. Viruses in idiopathic inflammatory myopathies: absence of candidate viral genomes in muscle. *Lancet* 1992;339(8803):1192–1195.
301. Lei X, et al. Cleavage of the adaptor protein TRIF by enterovirus 71 3C inhibits antiviral responses mediated by Toll-like receptor 3. *J Virol* 2011;85(17):8811–8818.
302. Leipner C, et al. Coxsackievirus B3-induced myocarditis in MHC class II-deficient mice. *J Hum Virol* 1999;2(2):102–114.
303. Leon-Monzon M, Dalakas MC. Absence of persistent infection with enteroviruses in muscles of patients with inflammatory myopathies. *Ann Neurol* 1992;32(2):219–222.
304. Leon-Monzon ME, Dalakas MC. Detection of poliovirus antibodies and poliovirus genome in patients with the post-polio syndrome. *Ann N Y Acad Sci* 1995;753:208–218.
305. Leparc-Goffart I, et al. Evidence of presence of poliovirus genomic sequences in cerebrospinal fluid from patients with postpolio syndrome. *J Clin Microbiol* 1996;34(8):2023–2026.
306. Li L, et al. A novel picornavirus associated with gastroenteritis. *J Virol* 2009;83(22): 12002–12006.
307. Li L, et al. Viruses in diarrhoeic dogs include novel kobuviruses and sapoviruses. *J Gen Virol* 2011;92(Pt 11):2534–2541.
308. Liljeqvist JA, et al. Failure to demonstrate enterovirus aetiology in Swedish patients with dilated cardiomyopathy. *J Med Virol* 1993;39(1):6–10.
309. Lim KH, Yin-Murphy M. An epidemic of conjunctivitis in Singapore in 1970. *Singapore Med J* 1971;12(5):247–249.
310. Lin YW, et al. Lymphocyte and antibody responses reduce enterovirus 71 lethality in mice by decreasing tissue viral loads. *J Virol* 2009;83(13):6477–6483.
311. Lin YW, et al. Human SCARB2 transgenic mice as an infectious animal model for enterovirus 71. *PLoS One* 2013;8(2):e57591.
312. Lind K, et al. Type III interferons are expressed by coxsackievirus-infected human primary hepatocytes and regulate hepatocyte permissiveness to infection. *Clin Exp Immunol* 2014;177(3):687–695.
313. Lipskaya G, et al. Geographical genotypes (geotypes) of poliovirus case isolates from the former Soviet Union: relatedness to other known poliovirus genotypes. *J Gen Virol* 1995;76(Pt 7):1687–1699.
314. Lisewski U, et al. The tight junction protein CAR regulates cardiac conduction and cell-cell communication. *J Exp Med* 2008;205(10):2369–2379.
315. Liu H-M, et al. Molecular evolution of a type 1 wild-vaccine poliovirus recombinant during widespread circulation in China. *J Virol* 2000;74:11153–11161.
316. Liu JY, et al. Hepatic damage caused by coxsackievirus B3 is dependent on age-related tissue tropisms associated with the coxsackievirus-adenovirus receptor. *Pathog Dis* 2013;68(2):52–60.
317. Lodge PA, et al. Coxsackievirus B-3 myocarditis. Acute and chronic forms of the disease caused by different immunopathogenic mechanisms. *Am J Pathol* 1987;128(3):455–463.
318. Loo YM, et al. Distinct RIG-I and MDA5 signaling by RNA viruses in innate immunity. *J Virol* 2008;82(1):335–345.
319. Lu X, et al. Real-time reverse transcription-PCR assay for comprehensive detection of human rhinoviruses. *J Clin Microbiol* 2008;46(2):533–539.
320. Lum LCS, et al. Fatal enterovirus 71 encephalomyelitis. *J Pediatr* 1998;133(6):795–798.
321. Ma JF, et al. Cell culture and PCR determination of poliovirus inactivation by disinfectants. *Appl Environ Microbiol* 1994;60(11):4203–4206.
322. Macadam AJ, et al. The 5′ noncoding region of the type 2 poliovirus vaccine strain contains determinants of attenuation and temperature sensitivity. *Virology* 1991;181(2):451–458.
323. Macadam AJ, et al. Genetic basis of attenuation of the Sabin type 2 vaccine strain of poliovirus in primates. *Virology* 1993;192(1):18–26.
324. Magnani JW, Dec GW. Myocarditis: current trends in diagnosis and treatment. *Circulation* 2006;113(6):876–890.
325. Magnius LO, et al. A solid-phase reverse immunosorbent test for the detection of enterovirus IgM. *J Virol Methods* 1988;20(1):73–82.
326. Mahfoud F, et al. Virus serology in patients with suspected myocarditis: utility or futility? *Eur Heart J* 2011;32:897–903.
327. Mahon BP, et al. Poliovirus-specific CD4 + Th1 clones with both cytotoxic and helper activity mediate protective humoral immunity against a lethal poliovirus infection in transgenic mice expressing the human poliovirus receptor. *J Exp Med* 1995;181(4):1285–1292.
328. Marchant D, et al. The impact of CVB3 infection on host cell biology. *Curr Top Microbiol Immunol* 2008;323:177–198.
329. Marroqui L, et al. Differential cell autonomous responses determine the outcome of coxsackievirus infections in murine pancreatic alpha and beta cells. *Elife* 2015;4:e06990.
330. Martin J, et al. Evolution of the Sabin strain of type 3 poliovirus in an immunodeficient patient during the entire 637-day period of virus excretion. *J Virol* 2000;74(7): 3001–3010.
331. Martino TA, et al. Enteroviral myocarditis and cardiomyopathy: a review of clinical and experimental studies. In: Rotbart HA, ed. *Human Enterovirus Infections*. Washington: ASM Press; 1995:291–351.
332. Matteucci D, et al. Group B coxsackieviruses readily establish persistent infections in human lymphoid cell lines. *J Virol* 1985;56(2):651–654.
333. McKay SL, et al. Increase in acute flaccid myelitis—United States, 2018. *MMWR Morb Mortal Wkly Rep* 2018;67(45):1273–1275.
334. McKinney RE Jr, Katz SL, Wilfert CM. Chronic enteroviral meningoencephalitis in agammaglobulinemic patients. *Rev Infect Dis* 1987;9(2):334–356.
335. Medin, O. 1891. Ueber eine Epidemie von spinaler Kinderlähmung. *Verhandl. d. 10. Internatl. med. Kongr.* 1890, 2, Abt. 6:37–47.
336. Melchers W, et al. The postpolio syndrome: no evidence for poliovirus persistence. *Ann Neurol* 1992;32(6):728–732.
337. Melnick JL. Enterovirus type 71 infections: a varied clinical pattern sometimes mimicking paralytic poliomyelitis. *Rev Infect Dis* 1984;6(Suppl 2):S387–S390.
338. Melnick JL. Current status of poliovirus infections. *Clin Microbiol Rev* 1996;9(3):293–300.
339. Melnick JL, Shaw EW, Curnen EC. A virus isolated from patients diagnosed as non-paralytic poliomyelitis or aseptic meningitis. *Proc Soc Exp Biol Med* 1949;71:344–349.
340. Mena I, et al. The role of B lymphocytes in coxsackievirus B3 infection. *Am J Pathol* 1999;155(4):1205–1215.
341. Mena I, et al. Coxsackievirus infection of the pancreas: evaluation of receptor expression, pathogenesis, and immunopathology. *Virology* 2000;271(2):276–288.
342. Mendelsohn CL, Wimmer E, Racaniello VR. Cellular receptor for poliovirus: molecular cloning, nucleotide sequence, and expression of a new member of the immunoglobulin superfamily. *Cell* 1989;56(5):855–865.
343. Mertens T, Pika U, Eggers HJ. Cross antigenicity among enteroviruses as revealed by immunoblot technique. *Virology* 1983;129(2):431–442.
344. Messacar K, et al. Encephalitis in US children. *Infect Dis Clin North Am* 2018;32(1): 145–162.
345. Midgley CM, et al. Severe respiratory illness associated with a nationwide outbreak of enterovirus D68 in the USA (2014): a descriptive epidemiological investigation. *Lancet Respir Med* 2015;3(11):879–887.
346. Mintz L, Drew WL. Relation of culture site to the recovery of nonpolio enteroviruses. *Am J Clin Pathol* 1980;74(3):324–326.
347. Misbah SA, et al. Chronic enteroviral meningoencephalitis in agammaglobulinemia: case report and literature review. *J Clin Immunol* 1992;12:266–270.
348. Modlin JF, et al. The humoral immune response to type 1 oral poliovirus vaccine in children previously immunized with enhanced potency inactivated poliovirus vaccine or live oral poliovirus vaccine. *Am J Dis Child* 1990;144(4):480–484.
349. Modlin JF, et al. Focal encephalitis with enterovirus infections. *Pediatrics* 1991;88(4):841–845.
350. Moore M. Enteroviral disease in the United States, 1970–1979. *J Infect Dis* 1982;146(1): 103–108.
351. Moore BE, Sagik BP, Sorber CA. Procedure for the recovery of airborne human enteric viruses during spray irrigation of treated wastewater. *Appl Environ Microbiol* 1979; 38(4):688–693.
352. Moore M, et al. Epidemiologic, clinical, and laboratory features of Coxsackie B1-B5 infections in the United States, 1970–79. *Public Health Rep* 1984;99(5):515–522.
353. Morens DM. Enteroviral disease in early infancy. *J Pediatr* 1978;92(3):374–377.
354. Morosky S, et al. The neonatal Fc receptor is a pan-echovirus receptor. *Proc Natl Acad Sci U S A* 2019;116(9):3758–3763.
355. Morrison ME, Racaniello VR. Molecular cloning and expression of a murine homolog of the human poliovirus receptor gene. *J Virol* 1992;66(5):2807–2813.
356. Muir P, et al. Evidence for persistent enterovirus infection of the central nervous system in patients with previous paralytic poliomyelitis. *Ann N Y Acad Sci* 1995;753:219–232.
357. Muir P, et al. Multicenter quality assessment of PCR methods for detection of enteroviruses. *J Clin Microbiol* 1999;37(5):1409–1414.
358. Mukherjee A, et al. The coxsackievirus B 3C protease cleaves MAVS and TRIF to attenuate host type I interferon and apoptotic signaling. *PLoS Pathog* 2011;7(3):e1001311.
359. Mulders MN, et al. Molecular epidemiology of wild poliovirus type 1 in Europe, the Middle East, and the Indian subcontinent. *J Infect Dis* 1995;171(6):1399–1405.
360. Nagata N, et al. A poliomyelitis model through mucosal infection in transgenic mice bearing human poliovirus receptor, TgPVR21. *Virology* 2004;321(1):87–100.
361. Nathanson N. The pathogenesis of poliomyelitis: what we don't know. *Adv Virus Res* 2008;71:1–50.
362. Nathanson N, Langmuir AD. Poliomyelitis following formaldehyde-inactivated poliovirus vaccination in the United States during the spring of 1955. *Am J Hyg* 1963;78:16–60.
363. Negishi H, et al. A critical link between Toll-like receptor 3 and type II interferon signaling pathways in antiviral innate immunity. *Proc Natl Acad Sci U S A* 2008;105(51):20446–20451.
364. Neu N, et al. Autoantibodies specific for the cardiac myosin isoform are found in mice susceptible to coxsackievirus B3-induced myocarditis. *J Immunol* 1987;138:2488–2492.
365. Neu N, et al. Cardiac myosin induces myocarditis in genetically predisposed mice. *J Immunol* 1987;139(11):3630–3636.
366. Nielsen JL, Berryman GK, Hankins GD. Intrauterine fetal death and the isolation of echovirus 27 from amniotic fluid. *J Infect Dis* 1988;158(2):501–502.
367. Nielsen AC, et al. Serious invasive Saffold virus infections in children, 2009. *Emerg Infect Dis* 2012;18(1):7–12.
368. Nielsen AC, et al. Gastroenteritis and the novel picornaviruses aichi virus, cosavirus, saffold virus, and salivirus in young children. *J Clin Virol* 2013;57(3):239–242.
369. Nijhuis M, et al. Rapid and sensitive routine detection of all members of the genus enterovirus in different clinical specimens by real-time PCR. *J Clin Microbiol* 2002;40(10):3666–3670.
370. Niklasson B, et al. A new picornavirus isolated from bank voles (*Clethrionomys glareolus*). *Virology* 1999;255(1):86–93.
371. Nishimura Y, et al. Human P-selectin glycoprotein ligand-1 is a functional receptor for enterovirus 71. *Nat Med* 2009;15(7):794–797.
372. Nix WA, Oberste MS, Pallansch MA. Sensitive, seminested PCR amplification of VP1 sequences for direct identification of all enterovirus serotypes from original clinical specimens. *J Clin Microbiol* 2006;44(8):2698–2704.

373. Nix WA, et al. Failure to detect enterovirus in the spinal cord of ALS patients using a sensitive RT-PCR method. *Neurology* 2004;62(8):1372–1377.
374. Nix WA, et al. Identification of enteroviruses in naturally infected captive primates. *J Clin Microbiol* 2008;46:2874–2878.
375. Noutsias M, et al. Human coxsackie-adenovirus receptor is colocalized with integrins alpha(v)beta(3) and alpha(v)beta(5) on the cardiomyocyte sarcolemma and upregulated in dilated cardiomyopathy: implications for cardiotropic viral infections. *Circulation* 2001;104(3):275–280.
376. O'Connell JB. The role of myocarditis in end-stage dilated cardiomyopathy. *Tex Heart Inst J* 1987;14:268–275.
377. Oberste MS, Maher K, Pallansch MA. Molecular phylogeny and proposed classification of the simian picornaviruses. *J Virol* 2002;76(3):1244–1251.
378. Oberste MS, Maher K, Pallansch MA. Evidence for frequent recombination within species human enterovirus B based on complete genomic sequences of all thirty-seven serotypes. *J Virol* 2004;78(2):855–867.
379. Oberste MS, Maher K, Pallansch MA. Complete genome sequences for nine simian enteroviruses. *J Gen Virol* 2007;88:3360–3372.
380. Oberste MS, Pallansch MA. Enterovirus molecular detection and typing. *Rev Med Microbiol* 2005;16:163–171.
381. Oberste MS, Penaranda S, Pallansch MA. RNA recombination plays a major role in genomic change during circulation of coxsackie B viruses. *J Virol* 2004;78(6):2948–2955.
382. Oberste MS, et al. Molecular epidemiology and genetic diversity of echovirus type 30 (E30): genotype correlates with temporal dynamics of E30 isolation. *J Clin Microbiol* 1999;37(12):3928–3933.
383. Oberste MS, et al. Typing of human enteroviruses by partial sequencing of VP1. *J Clin Microbiol* 1999;37(5):1288–1293.
384. Oberste MS, et al. Molecular evolution of the human enteroviruses: correlation of serotype with VP1 sequence and application to picornavirus classification. *J Virol* 1999;73(3):1941–1948.
385. Oberste MS, et al. Improved molecular identification of enteroviruses by RT-PCR and amplicon sequencing. *J Clin Virol* 2003;26(3):375–377.
386. Oberste MS, et al. Complete genome sequences of all members of the species Human enterovirus A. *J Gen Virol* 2004;85(Pt 6):1597–1607.
387. Oberste MS, et al. Molecular identification and characterization of two proposed new enterovirus serotypes, EV74 and EV75. *J Gen Virol* 2004;85(Pt 11):3205–3212.
388. Oberste MS, et al. Enteroviruses 76, 89, 90 and 91 represent a novel group within the species Human enterovirus A. *J Gen Virol* 2005;86(Pt 2):445–451.
389. Oberste MS, et al. Human encephalomyocarditis virus disease in Perú. *Emerg Infect Dis* 2009;15:640–646.
390. Oberste MS, et al. Naturally acquired picornavirus infections in nonhuman primates at the Dhaka Zoo. *J Virol* 2013;87:572–580.
391. Oberste MS, et al. Characterizing the picornavirus landscape among synanthropic nonhuman primates in Bangladesh, 2007–2008. *J Virol* 2013;87:558–571.
392. Ogilvie MM, Tearne CF. Spontaneous abortion after hand-foot-and-mouth disease caused by Coxsackie virus A16. *Br Med J* 1980;281(6254):1527–1528.
393. Ogra PL, Karzon DT. Formation and function of poliovirus antibody on different tissues. *Prog Med Virol* 1971;13:156–193.
394. Ohka S, et al. Retrograde transport of intact poliovirus through the axon via the fast transport system. *Virology* 1998;250(1):67–75.
395. Ohka S, et al. Receptor (CD155)-dependent endocytosis of poliovirus and retrograde axonal transport of the endosome. *J Virol* 2004;78(13):7186–7198.
396. Ohka S, et al. Receptor-dependent and -independent axonal retrograde transport of poliovirus in motor neurons. *J Virol* 2009;83(10):4995–5004.
397. Oostvogel PM, et al. Poliomyelitis outbreak in an unvaccinated community in The Netherlands, 1992–93. *Lancet* 1994;344(8923):665–670.
398. Otatume S, Addy P. Ecology of enteroviruses in tropics, I. Circulation of enteroviruses in healthy infants in tropical urban area. *Jpn J Microbiol* 1975;19(3):201–209.
399. Ozsvar Z, Deak J, Pap A. Possible role of Coxsackie-B virus infection in pancreatitis. *Int J Pancreatol* 1992;11(2):105–108.
400. Page GS, et al. Three-dimensional structure of poliovirus serotype 1 neutralizing determinants. *J Virol* 1988;62(5):1781–1794.
401. Paul JR. *A History of Poliomyelitis.* New Haven: Yale University Press; 1971.
402. Peigue-Lafeuille H, et al. Use of non-neutralizing monoclonal antibodies in an ELISA for intratypic differentiation of 28 echovirus type 25 clinical isolates. *J Virol Methods* 1992;36(1):91–99.
403. Pelletier I, Duncan G, Colbere-Garapin F. One amino acid change on the capsid surface of poliovirus sabin 1 allows the establishment of persistent infections in HEp-2c cell cultures. *Virology* 1998;241(1):1–13.
404. Pelletier I, et al. Molecular mechanisms of poliovirus persistence: key role of capsid determinants during the establishment phase. *Cell Mol Life Sci* 1998;54(12):1385–1402.
405. Pevear DC, et al. Activity of pleconaril against enteroviruses. *Antimicrob Agents Chemother* 1999;43(9):2109–2115.
406. Pezeshkpour GH, Dalakas MC. Pathology of spinal cord in post-poliomyelitis muscular atrophy. *Birth Defects Orig Artic Ser* 1987;23(4):229–236.
407. Pichlmair A, et al. RIG-I-mediated antiviral responses to single-stranded RNA bearing 5'-phosphates. *Science* 2006;314(5801):997–1001.
408. Pons-Salort M, et al. The seasonality of nonpolio enteroviruses in the United States: patterns and drivers. *Proc Natl Acad Sci U S A* 2018;115(12):3078–3083.
409. Pöyry T, et al. Relationships between simian and human enteroviruses. *J Gen Virol* 1999;80(3):635–638.
410. Prevots DR, et al. Outbreak of paralytic poliomyelitis in Albania, 1996: high attack rate among adults and apparent interruption of transmission following nationwide mass vaccination. *Clin Infect Dis* 1998;26(2):419–425.
411. Racaniello VR, Baltimore D. Molecular cloning of poliovirus cDNA and determination of the complete nucleotide sequence of the viral genome. *Proc Natl Acad Sci U S A* 1981;78(8):4887–4891.
412. Racaniello VR, Baltimore D. Cloned poliovirus complementary DNA is infectious in mammalian cells. *Science* 1981;214(4523):916–919.
413. Ramirez Gonzalez A, et al. Implementing the synchronized global switch from trivalent to bivalent oral polio vaccines-lessons learned from the global perspective. *J Infect Dis* 2017;216(Suppl_1):S183–S192.
414. Ramirez-Fort MK, et al. Coxsackievirus A6 associated hand, foot and mouth disease in adults: clinical presentation and review of the literature. *J Clin Virol* 2014;60(4):381–386.
415. Ramsingh AI. Coxsackieviruses and pancreatitis. *Front Biosci* 1997;2:e53–e62.
416. Ramsingh AI. CVB-induced pancreatitis and alterations in gene expression. *Curr Top Microbiol Immunol* 2008;323:241–258.
417. Ramsingh AI, Chapman N, Tracy S. Coxsackieviruses and diabetes. *Bioessays* 1997;19(9):793–800.
418. Ramsingh A, et al. Severity of disease induced by a pancreatropic Coxsackie B4 virus correlates with the H-2Kq locus of the major histocompatibility complex. *Virus Res* 1989;14(4):347–358.
419. Ren R, Racaniello VR. Poliovirus spreads from muscle to the central nervous system by neural pathways. *J Infect Dis* 1992;166(4):747–752.
420. Ren R, Racaniello VR. Human poliovirus receptor gene expression and poliovirus tissue tropism in transgenic mice. *J Virol* 1992;66(1):296–304.
421. Ren RB, et al. Transgenic mice expressing a human poliovirus receptor: a new model for poliomyelitis. *Cell* 1990;63(2):353–362.
422. Rewers M, Atkinson M. The possible role of enteroviruses in diabetes mellitus. In: Rotbart HA, ed. *Human Enterovirus Infections.* Washington: ASM Press; 1995:353–385.
423. Richer MJ, et al. Toll-like receptor 4-induced cytokine production circumvents protection conferred by TGF-beta in coxsackievirus-mediated autoimmune myocarditis. *Clin Immunol* 2006;121:339–349.
424. Richer MJ, et al. Toll-like receptor 3 signaling on macrophages is required for survival following coxsackievirus B4 infection. *PLoS One* 2009;4(1):e4127.
425. Rico-Hesse R, et al. Geographic distribution of wild poliovirus type 1 genotypes. *Virology* 1987;160(2):311–322.
426. Robbins FC, et al. Studies on the cultivation of poliomyelitis viruses in tissue culture. V. The direct isolation and serologic identification of virus strains in tissue culture from patients with nonparalytic and paralytic poliomyelitis. *Am J Hyg* 1951;54:286–293.
427. Robinson CM, Jesudhasan PR, Pfeiffer JK. Bacterial lipopolysaccharide binding enhances virion stability and promotes environmental fitness of an enteric virus. *Cell Host Microbe* 2014;15(1):36–46.
428. Robinson CM, Wang Y, Pfeiffer JK. Sex-dependent intestinal replication of an enteric virus. *J Virol* 2017;91(7).
429. Rodriguez Cruz R. Cuba: mass polio vaccination program, 1962–1982. *Rev Infect Dis* 1984;6(Suppl 2):S408–S412.
430. Roivainen M, et al. Several different enterovirus serotypes can be associated with prediabetic autoimmune episodes and onset of overt IDDM. Childhood Diabetes in Finland (DiMe) Study Group. *J Med Virol* 1998;56(1):74–78.
431. Rorabaugh ML, et al. Aseptic meningitis in infants younger than 2 years of age: acute illness and neurologic complications. *Pediatrics* 1993;92(2):206–211.
432. Rose NR, Herskowitz A, Neumann DA. Autoimmunity in myocarditis: models and mechanisms. *Clin Immunol Immunopathol* 1993;68:95–99.
433. Rose NR, Mackay IR. Molecular mimicry: a critical look at exemplary instances in human diseases. *Cell Mol Life Sci* 2000;57(4):542–551.
434. Ross ME, Hayashi K, Notkins AL. Virus-induced pancreatic disease: alterations in concentration of glucose and amylase in blood. *J Infect Dis* 1974;129(6):669–676.
435. Rotbart H. Meningitis and encephalitis. In: Rotbart H, ed. *Human Enterovirus Infections.* Washington: ASM Press; 1995:271–289.
436. Rotbart HA, O'Connell JF, McKinlay MA. Treatment of human enterovirus infections. *Antiviral Res* 1998;38(1):1–14.
437. Rotbart HA, et al. Enterovirus meningitis in adults. *Clin Infect Dis* 1998;27(4):896–898.
438. Rousset D, et al. Recombinant vaccine-derived poliovirus in Madagascar. *Emerg Infect Dis* 2003;9(7):885–887.
439. Rui Y, et al. Disruption of MDA5-mediated innate immune responses by the 3C proteins of coxsackievirus A16, coxsackievirus A6, and enterovirus D68. *J Virol* 2017;91(13).
440. Salazar-Grueso EF, et al. Immune responses in the post-polio syndrome [letter; comment]. *N Engl J Med* 1992;326(9):641; discussion 642.
441. Samuelson A, et al. Molecular basis for serological cross-reactivity between enteroviruses. *Clin Diagn Lab Immunol* 1994;1(3):336–341.
442. Sandelin K, Tuomioja M, Erkkila H. Echovirus type 7 isolated from conjunctival scrapings. *Scand J Infect Dis* 1977;9(2):71–73.
443. Santiana M, et al. Vesicle-cloaked virus clusters are optimal units for inter-organismal viral transmission. *Cell Host Microbe* 2018;24(2):208.e8–220.e8.
444. Sato S, et al. Persistence of replicating coxsackievirus B3 in the athymic murine heart is associated with development of myocarditic lesions. *J Gen Virol* 1994;75:2911–2924.
445. Satoh M, et al. Association between toll-like receptor 8 expression and adverse clinical outcomes in patients with enterovirus-associated dilated cardiomyopathy. *Am Heart J* 2007;154(3):581–588.
446. Sawyer LA, et al. An epidemic of acute hemorrhagic conjunctivitis in American Samoa caused by coxsackievirus A24 variant. *Am J Epidemiol* 1989;130(6):1187–1198.
447. Schieble JH, Fox VL, Lennette EH. A probable new human picornavirus associated with respiratory diseases. *Am J Epidemiol* 1967;85(2):297–310.
448. Schiff GM. Prophylactic efficacy of WIN 54954 in prevention of experimental human coxsackievirus A21 infection and illness. *Antiviral Res* 1992;17:92.
449. Schlegel A, et al. Cellular origin and ultrastructure of membranes induced during poliovirus infection. *J Virol* 1996;70(10):6576–6588.
450. Schoggins JW, et al. A diverse range of gene products are effectors of the type I interferon antiviral response. *Nature* 2011;472(7344):481–485.
451. Sejvar JJ, et al. Acute flaccid myelitis in the United States, August-December 2014: results of Nationwide surveillance. *Clin Infect Dis* 2016;63(6):737–745.

452. Seko Y, et al. Expression of perforin in infiltrating cells in murine hearts with acute myocarditis caused by coxsackievirus B3. *Circulation* 1991;84:788–795.
453. Seko Y, et al. Restricted usage of T cell receptor V alpha-V beta genes in infiltrating cells in the hearts of patients with acute myocarditis and dilated cardiomyopathy. *J Clin Investig* 1995;96(2):1035–1041.
454. Sharief MK, Hentges R, Ciardi M. Intrathecal immune response in patients with the post-polio syndrome. *N Engl J Med* 1991;325(11):749–755.
455. Sharp DG. Multiplicity reactivation of animal viruses. *Prog Med Virol* 1968;10:64–109.
456. Shattuck KE, Chonmaitree T. The changing spectrum of neonatal meningitis over a fifteen-year period. *Clin Pediatr (Phila)* 1992;31(3):130–136.
457. Shindarov LM, et al. Epidemiological, clinical, and pathomorphological characteristics of epidemic poliomyelitis-like disease caused by enterovirus 71. *J Hyg Epidemiol Microbiol Immunol* 1979;23(3):284–295.
458. Shulman LM, et al. Identification of a new strain of fastidious enterovirus 70 as the causative agent of an outbreak of hemorrhagic conjunctivitis. *J Clin Microbiol* 1997;35(8):2145–2149.
459. Sicinski P, et al. Poliovirus type 1 enters the human host through intestinal M cells. *Gastroenterology* 1990;98(1):56–58.
460. Simkova A, Petrovicova A. Experimental infection of rhesus monkeys with Coxsackie A 4 virus. *Acta Virol* 1972;16(3):250–257.
461. Simons J, Kutubuddin M, Chow M. Characterization of poliovirus-specific T lymphocytes in the peripheral blood of Sabin-vaccinated humans. *J Virol* 1993;67(3):1262–1268.
462. Slifka MK, et al. Using recombinant coxsackievirus B3 to evaluate the induction and protective efficacy of CD8 + T cells during picornavirus infection. *J Virol* 2001;75(5):2377–2387.
463. Smyth DJ, et al. A genome-wide association study of nonsynonymous SNPs identifies a type 1 diabetes locus in the interferon-induced helicase (IFIH1) region. *Nat Genet* 2006;38(6):617–619.
464. Sole MJ, Liu P. Viral myocarditis: a paradigm for understanding the pathogenesis and treatment of dilated cardiomyopathy. *J Am Coll Cardiol* 1993;22:99A–105A.
465. Solomon T, et al. Virology, epidemiology, pathogenesis, and control of enterovirus 71. *Lancet Infect Dis* 2010;10(11):778–790.
466. Staring J, et al. KREMEN1 is a host entry receptor for a major group of enteroviruses. *Cell Host Microbe* 2018;23(5):636.e5–643.e5.
467. Strikas RA, Anderson LJ, Parker RA. Temporal and geographic patterns of isolates of nonpolio enterovirus in the United States, 1970–1983. *J Infect Dis* 1986;153(2):346–351.
468. Suhy DA, Giddings TH Jr, Kirkegaard K. Remodeling the endoplasmic reticulum by poliovirus infection and by individual viral proteins: an autophagy-like origin for virus-induced vesicles. *J Virol* 2000;74(19):8953–8965.
469. Sutter RW, et al. Defining surrogate serologic tests with respect to predicting protective vaccine efficacy: poliovirus vaccination. In: Williams JC, et al., eds. *Combined Vaccines and Simultaneous Administration. Current Issues and Perspectives*. New York: New York Academy of Sciences;1995:289–299.
470. Swanink CM, et al. Coxsackievirus B1-based antibody-capture enzyme-linked immunosorbent assay for detection of immunoglobulin G (IgG), IgM, and IgA with broad specificity for enteroviruses. *J Clin Microbiol* 1993;31(12):3240–3246.
471. Takao S, et al. Seroepidemiological study of human Parechovirus 1. *Jpn J Infect Dis* 2001;54(2):85–87.
472. Tam PE, Messner RP. Molecular mechanisms of coxsackievirus persistence in chronic inflammatory myopathy: viral RNA persists through formation of a double-stranded complex without associated genomic mutations or evolution. *J Virol* 1999;73(12):10113–10121.
473. Tan CS, Cardosa MJ. High-titred neutralizing antibodies to human enterovirus 71 preferentially bind to the N-terminal portion of the capsid protein VP1. *Arch Virol* 2007;152(6):1069–1073.
474. Tanel RE, et al. Prospective comparison of culture vs genome detection for diagnosis of enteroviral meningitis in childhood. *Arch Pediatr Adolesc Med* 1996;150(9):919–924.
475. Tang TT, et al. Chronic myopathy associated with coxsackievirus type A9. A combined electron microscopical and viral isolation study. *N Engl J Med* 1975;292(12):608–611.
476. Tanner EJ, et al. Dominant drug targets suppress the emergence of antiviral resistance. *Elife* 2014;3.
477. Tassin M, et al. A case of congenital Echovirus 11 infection acquired early in pregnancy. *J Clin Virol* 2014;59(1):71–73.
478. Taylor MP, Kirkegaard K. Modification of cellular autophagy protein LC3 by poliovirus. *J Virol* 2007;81(22):12543–12553.
479. Taylor MP, Kirkegaard K. Potential subversion of autophagosomal pathway by picornaviruses. *Autophagy* 2008;4(3):286–289.
480. Taylor MP, et al. Role of microtubules in extracellular release of poliovirus. *J Virol* 2009;83(13):6599–6609.
481. Thompson KM, et al. The risks, costs, and benefits of future global policies for managing polioviruses. *Am J Public Health* 2008;98:1322–1330.
482. Too IH, et al. Enterovirus 71 infection of motor neuron-like NSC-34 cells undergoes a non-lytic exit pathway. *Sci Rep* 2016;6:36983.
483. Townsend TR, et al. Outbreak of coxsackie A1 gastroenteritis: a complication of bone-marrow transplantation. *Lancet* 1982;1(8276):820–823.
484. Tracy S, et al. Genetics of coxsackievirus B cardiovirulence and inflammatory heart muscle disease. *Trends Microbiol* 1996;4:175–179.
485. Trask JD. Poliomyelitis virus in human stools. *JAMA* 1938;111:6–11.
486. Triantafilou K, Triantafilou M. Coxsackievirus B4-induced cytokine production in pancreatic cells is mediated through toll-like receptor 4. *J Virol* 2004;78(20):11313–11320.
487. Triantafilou K, et al. Human cardiac inflammatory responses triggered by Coxsackie B viruses are mainly Toll-like receptor (TLR) 8-dependent. *Cell Microbiol* 2005;7(8):1117–1126.
488. Tsao KC, et al. Responses of IgM for enterovirus 71 infection. *J Med Virol* 2002;68(4):574–580.
489. Tu Z, et al. The cardiovirulent phenotype of coxsackievirus B3 is determined at a single site in the genomic 5′ nontranslated region. *J Virol* 1995;69:4607–4618.
490. Tucker SP, et al. Vectorial release of poliovirus from polarized human intestinal epithelial cells. *J Virol* 1993;67(7):4274–4282.
491. Tung WS, et al. DNA vaccine constructs against enterovirus 71 elicit immune response in mice. *Genet Vaccines Ther* 2007;5:6.
492. Uhlig J, Wiegers K, Dernick R. A new antigenic site of poliovirus recognized by an intertypic cross-neutralizing monoclonal antibody. *Virology* 1990;178(2):606–610.
493. Ursing B. Acute pancreatitis in coxsackie B infection. *Br Med J* 1973;3(879):524–525.
494. van Doornum GJ, et al. Development and implementation of real-time nucleic acid amplification for the detection of enterovirus infections in comparison to rapid culture of various clinical specimens. *J Med Virol* 2007;79(12):1868–1876.
495. Vekemans J, et al. T cell responses to vaccines in infants: defective IFN g production after oral polio vaccination. *Clin Exp Immunol* 2002;127(3):495–498.
496. Vella C, Brown CL, McCarthy DA. Coxsackievirus B4 infection of the mouse pancreas: acute and persistent infection. *J Gen Virol* 1992;73(6):1387–1394.
497. Vella C, Festenstein H. Coxsackievirus B4 infection of the mouse pancreas: the role of natural killer cells in the control of virus replication and resistance to infection. *J Gen Virol* 1992;73 (Pt 6):1379–1386.
498. Vella C, et al. Coxsackie virus B4 infection of the mouse pancreas: I. Detection of virus-specific RNA in the pancreas by in situ hybridisation. *J Med Virol* 1991;35(1):46–49.
499. Verboon-Maciolek MA, et al. Severe neonatal parechovirus infection and similarity with enterovirus infection. *Pediatr Infect Dis J* 2008;27(3):241–245.
500. Viskari HR, et al. Maternal first-trimester enterovirus infection and future risk of type 1 diabetes in the exposed fetus. *Diabetes* 2002;51(8):2568–2571.
501. Vuorinen T, et al. Coxsackievirus B3-induced acute pancreatitis: analysis of histopathological and viral parameters in a mouse model. *Br J Exp Pathol* 1989;70(4):395–403.
502. Wadia NH, et al. Polio-like motor paralysis associated with acute hemorrhagic conjunctivitis in an outbreak in 1981 in Bombay, India: clinical and serologic studies. *J Infect Dis* 1983;147(4):660–668.
503. Wagner DK, et al. Lymphocyte analysis in a patient with X-linked agammaglobulinemia and isolated growth hormone deficiency after development of echovirus dermatomyositis and meningoencephalitis. *Int Arch Allergy Appl Immunol* 1989;89(2–3):143–148.
504. Wahid R, Cannon MJ, Chow M. Virus-specific CD4 + and CD8 + cytotoxic T-cell responses and long-term T-cell memory in individuals vaccinated against polio. *J Virol* 2005;79(10):5988–5995.
505. Wallace SS, Lopez MA, Caviness AC. Impact of enterovirus testing on resource use in febrile young infants: a systematic review. *Hosp Pediatr* 2017;7(2):96–102.
506. Wang SM, et al. Clinical spectrum of enterovirus 71 infection in children in southern Taiwan, with an emphasis on neurological complications. *Clin Infect Dis* 1999;29(1):184–190.
507. Wang JP, et al. MDA5 and MAVS mediate type I IFN responses to Coxsackie B virus. *J Virol* 2010;84(1):254–260.
508. Wang B, et al. Enterovirus 71 protease 2Apro targets MAVS to inhibit anti-viral type I interferon responses. *PLoS Pathog* 2013;9(3):e1003231.
509. Ward C. Severe arrhythmias in Coxsackievirus B3 myopericarditis. *Arch Dis Child* 1978;53:174–176.
510. Wei W, et al. ICAM-5/telencephalin is a functional entry receptor for enterovirus D68. *Cell Host Microbe* 2016;20(5):631–641.
511. Weinzierl AO, et al. Effective chemokine secretion by dendritic cells and expansion of cross-presenting CD4–/CD8+ dendritic cells define a protective phenotype in the mouse model of coxsackievirus myocarditis. *J Virol* 2008;82(16):8149–8160.
512. Wells AI, Coyne CB. Type III interferons in antiviral defenses at barrier surfaces. *Trends Immunol* 2018;39(10):848–858.
513. Westrop GD, et al. Genetic basis of attenuation of the Sabin type 3 oral poliovirus vaccine. *J Virol* 1989;63(3):1338–1344.
514. Wickman I. *Beitrage zur Kenntnis der Heine-Medinschen Krankheit (Poliomyelitis acuta und verwandter Erkernkungen)*. Berlin: Karger; 1907.
515. Wilfert CM, et al. Persistent and fatal central-nervous-system ECHOvirus infections in patients with agammaglobulinemia. *N Engl J Med* 1977;296(26):1485–1489.
516. Winther B, et al. Histopathologic examination and enumeration of polymorphonuclear leukocytes in the nasal mucosa during experimental rhinovirus colds. *Acta Otolaryngol Suppl* 1984;413:19–24.
517. Winther B, et al. Viral-induced rhinitis. *Am J Rhinol* 1998;12(1):17–20.
518. Wolthers KC, et al. Human parechoviruses as an important viral cause of sepsislike illness and meningitis in young children. *Clin Infect Dis* 2008;47(3):358–363.
519. Wong CY, Woodruff JJ, Woodruff JF. Generation of cytotoxic T lymphocytes during coxsackievirus B-3 infection. III. Role of sex. *J Immunol* 1977;119(2):591–597.
520. Wong J, et al. Autophagosome supports coxsackievirus B3 replication in host cells. *J Virol* 2008;82(18):9143–9153.
521. Woodruff JF. Viral myocarditis. A review. *Am J Pathol* 1980;101(2):425–484.
522. Woodruff JF, Woodruff JJ. Involvement of T lymphocytes in the pathogenesis of coxsackie virus B3 heart disease. *J Immunol* 1974;113:1726–1734.
523. World Health Organization. *Enterovirus Surveillance Guidelines—Guidelines for Enterovirus Surveillance in Support of the Polio Eradication Initiative*. Copenhagen: World Health Organization Regional Office for Europe; 2015.
524. World Health Organization. Global Polio Eradication Initiative. 2019. Available at: http://www.polioeradication.org/
525. Wringe A, et al. Estimating the extent of vaccine-derived poliovirus infection. *PLoS One* 2008;3(10):e3433.
526. Wu X, Zhao T, Tian Y. [A bivalent VP1 gene vaccine against Coxsackie virus B1/B3]. *Zhonghua Yi Xue Za Zhi* 2001;81(8):480–484.
527. Wu B, et al. Structural basis for dsRNA recognition, filament formation, and antiviral signal activation by MDA5. *Cell* 2013;152(1–2):276–289.
528. Wyatt HV. Poliomyelitis in the fetus and the newborn. A comment on the new understanding of the pathogenesis. *Clin Pediatr* 1979;18(1):33–38.
529. Xiang Z, et al. Enterovirus 68 3C protease cleaves TRIF to attenuate antiviral responses mediated by Toll-like receptor 3. *J Virol* 2014;88(12):6650–6659.
530. Yagi S, Schnurr D, Lin J. Spectrum of monoclonal antibodies to coxsackievirus B-3 includes type- and group-specific antibodies. *J Clin Microbiol* 1992;30(9):2498–2501.

531. Yamashita T, et al. Complete nucleotide sequence and genetic organization of Aichi virus, a distinct member of the Picornaviridae associated with acute gastroenteritis in humans. *J Virol* 1998;72(10):8408–8412.

532. Yamayoshi S, et al. Scavenger receptor B2 is a cellular receptor for enterovirus 71. *Nat Med* 2009;15(7):798–801.

533. Yamayoshi S, et al. Functional comparison of SCARB2 and PSGL1 as receptors for enterovirus 71. *J Virol* 2013;87(6):3335–3347.

534. Yang WX, et al. Efficient delivery of circulating poliovirus to the central nervous system independently of poliovirus receptor. *Virology* 1997;229(2):421–428.

535. Yang CF, et al. Circulation of endemic type 2 vaccine-derived poliovirus in Egypt from 1983 to 1993. *J Virol* 2003;77(15):8366–8377.

536. Yang F, et al. Enterovirus 71 outbreak in the People's Republic of China in 2008. *J Clin Microbiol* 2009;47(7):2351–2352.

537. Yin-Murphy M. Acute hemorrhagic conjunctivitis. *Prog Med Virol* 1984;29:23–44.

538. Yin-Murphy M, et al. Early and rapid diagnosis of acute haemorrhagic conjunctivitis with tear specimens. *Bull World Health Organ* 1985;63(4):705–709.

539. Ylipaasto P, et al. Enterovirus infection in human pancreatic islet cells, islet tropism in vivo and receptor involvement in cultured islet beta cells. *Diabetologia* 2004;47(2):225–239.

540. Yoon JW, et al. Isolation of a virus from the pancreas of a child with diabetic ketoacidosis. *N Engl J Med* 1979;300(21):1173–1179.

541. Yoon JW, et al. Coxsackie virus B4 produces transient diabetes in nonhuman primates. *Diabetes* 1986;35(6):712–716.

542. Yoshihara Y, et al. An ICAM-related neuronal glycoprotein, telencephalin, with brain segment-specific expression. *Neuron* 1994;12(3):541–553.

543. Young DC, Sharp DG. Partial reactivation of chlorine-treated echovirus. *Appl Environ Microbiol* 1979;37(4):766–773.

544. Yousef GE, Isenberg DA, Mowbray JF. Detection of enterovirus specific RNA sequences in muscle biopsy specimens from patients with adult onset myositis. *Ann Rheum Dis* 1990;49(5):310–315.

545. Yu W, Tellier R, Wright JR Jr. Coxsackie virus A16 infection of placenta with massive perivillous fibrin deposition leading to intrauterine fetal demise at 36 weeks gestation. *Pediatr Dev Pathol* 2015;18(4):331–334.

546. Yu CK, et al. Neutralizing antibody provided protection against enterovirus type 71 lethal challenge in neonatal mice. *J Biomed Sci* 2000;7(6):523–528.

547. Zaoutis T, Klein JD. Enterovirus infections. *Pediatr Rev* 1998;19(6):183–191.

548. Zell R, et al. ICTV virus taxonomy profile: picornaviridae. *J Gen Virol* 2017;98(10):2421–2422.

549. Zhang S, Racaniello VR. Expression of the poliovirus receptor in intestinal epithelial cells is not sufficient to permit poliovirus replication in the mouse gut. *J Virol* 1997;71(7):4915–4920.

550. Zhang A, et al. Three-dimensional structure-activity relationships for antiviral agents that interact with picornavirus capsids. *Semin Virol* 1992;3(6):453–471.

551. Zhang G, et al. Molecular evolution of swine vesicular disease virus. *J Gen Virol* 1999;80(Pt 3):639–651.

552. Zheng DP, et al. Distribution of wild type 1 poliovirus genotypes in China. *J Infect Dis* 1993;168(6):1361–1367.

553. Zhu K, et al. TLR3 signaling in macrophages is indispensable for the protective immunity of invariant natural killer T cells against enterovirus 71 infection. *PLoS Pathog* 2015;11(1):e1004613.

554. Ziegler JB, Penny R. Fatal echo 30 virus infection and amyloidosis in X-linked hypogammaglobulinemia. *Clin Immunol Immunopathol* 1975;3(3):347–352.

555. Zoll J, Galama J, Melchers W. Intratypic genome variability of the coxsackievirus B1 2A protease region. *J Gen Virol* 1994;75(Pt 3):687–692.

Caliciviridae: The Viruses and Their Replication

Christiane E. Wobus • Kim Y. Green

The family *Caliciviridae* is composed of small (27–40 nm), nonenveloped, icosahedral viruses that possess a linear, positive-sense, single-stranded RNA (ssRNA) genome. The 11 genera of the family are *Norovirus, Sapovirus, Bavovirus, Lagovirus, Minovirus, Nacovirus, Nebovirus, Recovirus, Salovirus, Valovirus,* and *Vesivirus.*[625] The major human pathogens in the family are the noroviruses and sapoviruses, which cause acute

gastroenteritis. Important veterinary pathogens include vesiviruses such as feline calicivirus (FCV), which causes a respiratory disease in cats, and lagoviruses such as rabbit hemorrhagic disease virus (RHDV), which causes an often-fatal hemorrhagic disease in rabbits. This chapter provides a description of the family *Caliciviridae*, with major emphasis on the noroviruses because of their prominent role in sporadic and epidemic gastroenteritis.[5]

HISTORY

The establishment of a viral etiology for gastroenteritis in humans was a decades-long process that was hampered by the fastidious nature of many of these viruses for growth in cell culture.[255] Volunteer studies carried out in the 1940s and 1950s in the United States and Japan played a major role in establishing that filterable, nonbacterial infectious agents can cause enteric disease.[255] An important advance occurred in 1972 with the discovery of Norwalk virus (NV) by Kapikian et al.[256] Stool material from a rectal swab obtained from an ill individual involved in a gastroenteritis outbreak that had occurred at an elementary school in Norwalk, Ohio, in October 1968 was administered to adult volunteers as a bacteria-free filtrate and serially passaged to other volunteers, inducing acute gastroenteritis in certain individuals.[140,141] Virus particles (named Norwalk virus for the location of the original outbreak) were visualized in stool material from these volunteers by the technique of immune electron microscopy (IEM)[256] (Fig. 4.1). Hawaii virus (from a family outbreak of gastroenteritis that occurred in Honolulu in 1971) and Snow Mountain virus (from an outbreak in a Colorado resort camp in 1976) were subsequently discovered in 1977 and 1982, respectively, and shown to be antigenically distinct by IEM.[144,591] Norwalk virus would become the prototype strain for these and other "small round structured viruses," known now as the noroviruses.

In 1976, the teams of Madeley and Cosgrove[373] and Flewett and Davies[168] reported the presence of viruses in the stools of children that showed a striking morphologic similarity to previously characterized animal caliciviruses that were known to exhibit "classical" distinct cup-like depressions on the surface of the virion. Chiba et al.[110] described a "classical" calicivirus, associated with gastroenteritis, in infants and young children living in an infant home in Sapporo, Japan, in 1977.

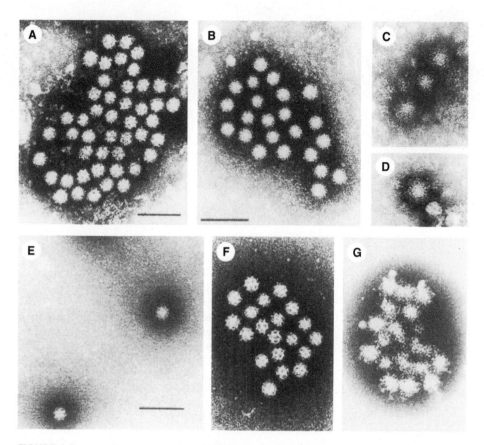

FIGURE 4.1 Norwalk virus (NV) (genus *Norovirus*) and Sapporo virus (genus *Sapovirus*) in stool material. A: NV particles in a stool filtrate visualized by immune electron microscopy (IEM). **B:** An aggregate observed after incubation of NV stool filtrate with a 1:5 dilution of volunteer's prechallenge serum. Particles have a light coating of antibody molecules. The amount of antibody present on this aggregate was given a rating of 1 to 2 to 2+, and the serum was given an overall rating of 1 to 2+ on a scale of 1 to 4. **C, D:** Three single particles (**C**) and one individual particle (**D**) observed after incubation of the NV stool filtrate with a 1:5 dilution of the same volunteer's postchallenge convalescent serum. Particles are heavily coated with antibody molecules. At high antibody levels (antibody excess), large aggregates may not be seen. The amount of antibody was given a rating of 4+, and the serum was given an overall rating of 4+ on a scale of 1 to 4. **E:** Sapporo virus particles in stool material visualized by direct electron microscopy (EM). The distinct, hollow cup-like structures are apparent. **F:** Sapporo virus particles after incubation with guinea pig hyperimmune serum. The amount of antibody was given a 1+ rating. **G:** An aggregate observed after incubation of Sapporo virus stool filtrate with guinea pig hyperimmune serum. The amount of antibody was given a rating of 4+ on a scale of 1 to 4. (**A–D** from Kapikian AZ, Wyatt RG, Dolin R, et al. Visualization by immune electron microscopy of a 27-nm particle associated with acute infectious nonbacterial gastroenteritis. *J Virol* 1972;10:1075–1081, with permission; **E–G** from Nakata S, Kogawa K, Numata K, et al. The epidemiology of human calicivirus/Sapporo/82/Japan. *Arch Virol* 1996;(Suppl 12):263–270, with permission.)

Another virus (later designated Sapporo/82/Japan) that exhibited classical calicivirus morphology was subsequently detected from this same infant home and characterized antigenically by IEM[422] (Fig. 4.1). The Sapporo virus would become the prototype strain for the "Sapporo-like viruses" or "classical caliciviruses," known now as the sapoviruses.

In the late 1980s, the stool filtrate derived from the Norwalk, Ohio, outbreak was fed to adults in volunteer studies to obtain adequate quantities of virus particles to characterize the viral genome.[242] This major advance by Jiang et al.[242] established the classification of NV as a member of the *Caliciviridae*. The complete RNA genome sequences of NV and the closely related Southampton virus were determined and found to be organized into three major open reading frames (ORF1,

ORF2, and ORF3) with a polyadenylated 3′ end[211,245,317,319] (see *Genome Structure and Organization*). The ORF1 was shown to encode a large polyprotein that was proteolytically processed into the mature nonstructural proteins.[345,348] The ORF2 encoded the major capsid protein, VP1, and ORF3 encoded a minor structural protein, VP2. The human noroviruses initially segregated into two major phylogenetic groups within what would become the genus *Norovirus* of the *Caliciviridae* that were designated as genogroups I (GI) and II (GII), with NV belonging to GI and the Hawaii and Snow Mountain viruses belonging to GII.[332,630] In addition, sequence analysis of the "classical caliciviruses" confirmed that they were distinct from the noroviruses, ultimately forming a separate genus, *Sapovirus*, within the *Caliciviridae*.[318,344,388,450]

CLASSIFICATION

Members of the virus family *Caliciviridae* have a virion protein, genome (VPg)-linked, positive-sense RNA genome that is polyadenylated and surrounded by a nonenveloped, icosahedral capsid of 27 to 40 nm in diameter. The capsid is constructed predominantly from a major structural protein, VP1, of approximately 60,000 Daltons (D). The 11 genera of Caliciviridae—*Norovirus, Sapovirus, Bavovirus, Lagovirus, Minovirus, Nacovirus, Nebovirus, Recovirus, Salovirus, Valovirus,* and *Vesivirus*—each represent a distinct phylogenetic clade in the family[625] (Fig. 4.2A). Within each genus, one or more species has been defined based primarily on genetic relatedness,

A Family: *Caliciviridae*

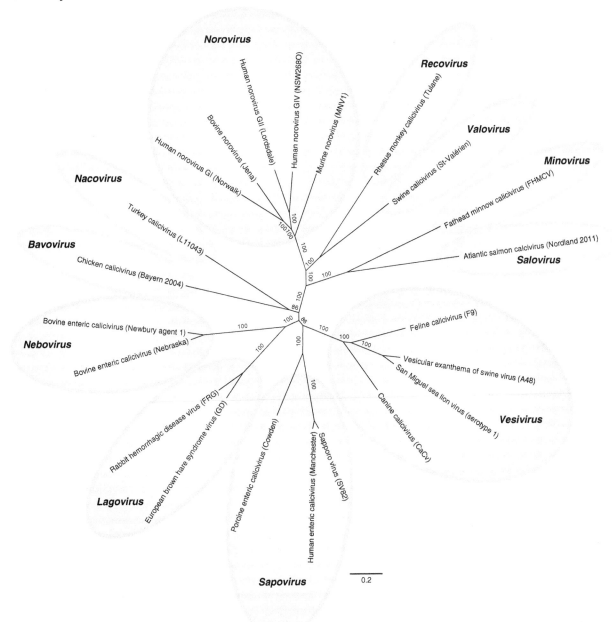

FIGURE 4.2 A: Phylogenetic relationships among representative members of the family *Caliciviridae*. The 11 established genera are *Norovirus, Sapovirus, Bavovirus, Lagovirus, Minovirus, Nacovirus, Nebovirus, Recovirus, Salovirus, Valovirus,* and *Vesivirus* according to the International Committee on Taxonomy of Viruses, with new genera recently approved shaded in *green*.[625] To generate this dendrogram, full-length genomic sequences were first aligned with the ClustalW algorithm in the MacVector, Inc. (Cary, NC) software package. Additional evolutionary analysis was conducted with the MEGA software package. Finally, phylogenetic relationships were inferred using the neighbor-joining method,[510] with the evolutionary distances computed by the Jukes-Cantor method.[249] The statistical support for tree nodes was evaluated by bootstrap analysis (1,000 replicates). The tree was drawn to scale, with branch lengths in the same units as those of the evolutionary distances used to infer the phylogenetic tree.

B Genus: *Norovirus*

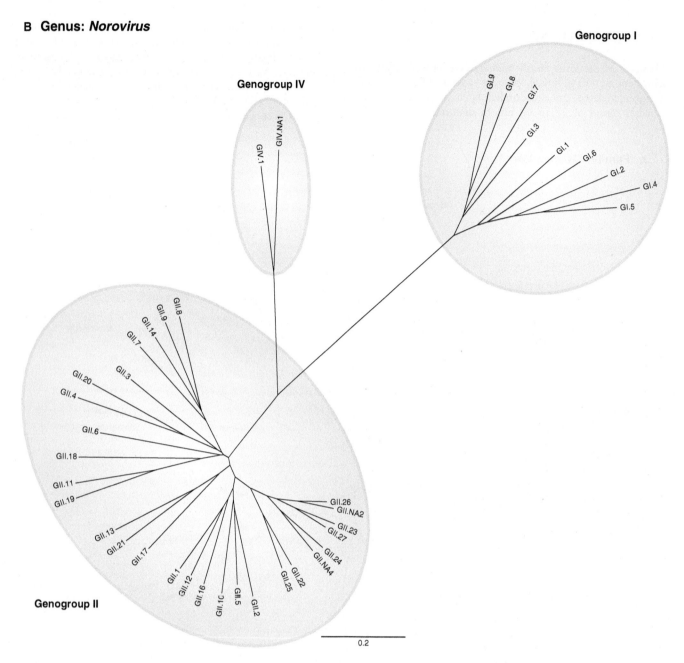

FIGURE 4.2 *(continued)* **B:** Phylogenetic relationships among the VP1 proteins from three representative genogroups (I, II, and IV) within the genus *Norovirus* that are characteristically associated with gastroenteritis in humans. This genotyping system is employed as an epidemiological tool to track the spread of genetically diverse noroviruses in susceptible populations (see Epidemiology and Table 4.5). (Analysis and figure from S.V. Sosnovtsev.)

and the current taxonomic structure of the *Caliciviridae* is shown in Table 4.1. Below the level of species in certain genera (*Norovirus* and *Sapovirus*), provisional genetic typing systems (consisting of genogroups subdivided into genetic clusters or genotypes) have proven useful in epidemiologic studies (see *Molecular Epidemiology*). The striking genetic diversity of noroviruses associated with human disease is illustrated in a phylogenetic analysis of strains representing different genotypes within GI, GII, and GIV (Fig. 4.2B).

VIRION STRUCTURE

Calicivirus virions exhibit $T = 3$ icosahedral symmetry. The capsid contains 90 dimers of the VP1 capsid protein that form a shell from which 90 arch-like capsomeres protrude at the local and strict twofold axes.[79,105,268,478,480,481,662] The dimers form two classes, A/B and C/C, with 60 A/B dimers located at the icosahedral quasi fivefold axis and 30 C/C dimers at the quasi twofold axis. The major capsid protein VP1 is organized into two major

TABLE 4.1   Taxonomic structure of the *Caliciviridae*

Genus	Species	Representative Strain[a]	GenBank Accession Number of Reference Genome
Bavovirus	*Bavaria virus*	Bavovirus/chicken/DE/2004/Bavaria V0021	HQ010042
Lagovirus	*Rabbit hemorrhagic disease virus*	Lagovirus/rabbit/DE1988/RHDV-FRG	M67473
	European brown hare syndrome virus	Lagovirus/hare/FR/1989/EBHSV-GD	Z69620
Minovirus	*Minovirus A*	Minovirus/fathead minnow/US/2012/FHMCV	KX371097
Nacovirus	*Nacovirus A*	Nacovirus/turkey/DE/2011/TC L11043	JQ347522
Norovirus	*Norwalk virus*	Norovirus/human/US/1968/Norwalk	M87661
Nebovirus	*Newbury 1 virus*	Nebovirus/bovine/UK/1976/Newbury-1	NC_007916
Recovirus	*Recovirus A*	Recovirus/rhesus macaque/US/2004/Tulane	EU391643
Salovirus	*Nordland virus*	Salovirus/salmon/NO/2011/Nordland	KJ577139
Sapovirus	*Sapporo virus*	Sapovirus/human/JP/1982/Sapporo	HM002617
Valovirus	*St. Valérien virus*	Valovirus/porcine/CA/2006/St. Valérien AB90	FJ355928
Vesivirus	*Vesicular exanthema of swine virus*	Vesivirus/porcine/US/1948/VESV-A48	AF181082
	Feline calicivirus	Vesivirus/feline/US/1958/FCV-F9	M86379

[a]The cryptogram is organized as follows: Genus/host of origin/country of origin/year of occurrence/strain name.

domains designated shell (S) and protruding (P) domain that are connected by a hinge region, as represented in a diagram of the NV VP1 (530 aa in length)[478] (Fig. 4.3). The N-terminal amino acids of VP1 form the N-terminal arm (NTA) that is found in the interior of the capsid and links the dimeric subunits (Fig. 4.3). The S domain is the most highly conserved region of the VP1 and forms a smooth inner shell that surrounds the RNA genome. The S domains of the A/B and C/C dimers adopt a "bent" versus "flat" conformation, respectively, to conform to the icosahedral $T = 3$ shape.[662] The P domains form the arch-like protrusions that emanate from the shell and contain the dimeric contacts. This domain is further subdivided into the P1 and the P2 subdomains. The P1 subdomains form the sides of the arch of the capsomeres and position the highly variable P2 subdomain at the top of the arch. These arches are arranged in such a way that 32 large hollows are formed at the icosahedral five- and threefold positions that appear as cup-like structures on the surface of caliciviruses (*calici* is derived from the Latin word *calyx*, or cup). Cryo-electron microscopy and computer image processing studies of representative caliciviruses show subtle variation in the capsid structures that are consistent with their differences in appearance by negative-stain EM that can range from a feathery appearance (many noroviruses, such as *Norwalk virus* in Fig. 4.1A) to the presence of sharply defined "cups" (many sapoviruses, such as Sapporo virus in Fig. 4.1E and the vesiviruses).[105,480] The exposure of the variable P2 domain on the surface is consistent with its role as the major antigenic site and in binding to cellular receptors and attachment factors.[83,276,351,429,478,528,575]

Structural comparisons of caliciviruses have shown major points of flexibility in the capsid protein. One region of flexibility is in the hinge between the S and P domains. As a result of this flexibility, the capsid protein in these viruses exhibits two distinct conformations, "closed" and "elevated." In the structures of NV, San Miguel sea lion virus (SMSV), and FCV, the capsid protein exhibits a "closed" conformation in which the P

domain interacts closely with the S domain,[105,457,479] whereas, in the structures of murine norovirus (MNV), RHDV, and Vietnam026 (human norovirus GII.10), the capsid protein exhibits an "elevated" conformation in which the P domain is rotated by about 40 to 53 degrees and significantly raised relative to the S domain[209,269,607] (Fig. 4.4). The biologic consequences or triggers for these movements are currently unknown. The other region of flexibility is within the P domain. X-ray crystallography of the MNV P domain captured a surface-exposed loop within the P domain in two conformations, "open" and "closed".[268] Engineered mutations that locked the loop into a closed conformation allowed the virus to escape neutralization by a potent neutralizing monoclonal antibody (A6.2) that had been mapped to this loop.[298] Molecular dynamics simulations suggest that escape from another neutralizing antibody (2D3) similarly affects the conformational relaxation of the MNV P domain even though the escape mutation is located distally from the antibody binding site at the top of the P domain.[299] The binding of bile acid has recently been shown to affect the conformation and stability of loop structures in the MNV P domain and enhance receptor binding.[275] Therefore, it is likely that capsid flexibility is an inherent feature of calicivirus virions and that this is critical during successful infection and pathogenesis.

Infectious virions also contain a minor capsid protein VP2 that associates with the S domain on the interior surface of the virion.[629] Roles for VP2 in viral entry (see below *Stages of Replication*) and assembly have been proposed.[115,629] Inside the virion, VP1 and VP2 interact via a highly conserved patch of residues in VP1 (IDPWI motif) that is located at the junction of the NTA and S domain. In particular, the first isoleucine residue of this motif (Ile-52 in NV) lies so that the two Ile-52 residues in a VP1 dimer are at the center of a negatively charged belt spanning the inner surface of the S dimers. Mutation of this residue ablates VP2 incorporation into particles. The VP1-interacting domain of VP2 was mapped to amino acids 108 to 152.[183] Computational analysis revealed that this region in VP2

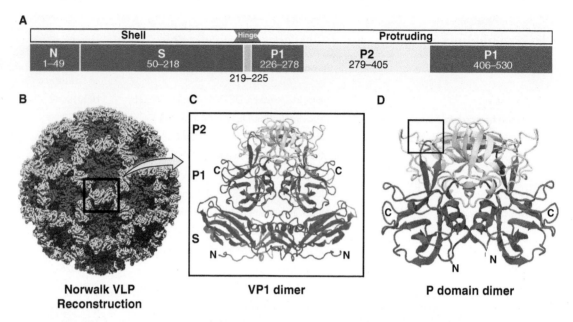

FIGURE 4.3 Organization of the norovirus major capsid protein, VP1. A: The Norwalk virus major capsid protein VP1 is 539 amino acids (aa) in length and is organized into two major parts, shell (S) and protruding (P), connected by a hinge (H) region. The aa borders of the defined domains are N-terminal (N) arm, 1 to 49; S, 50 to 218; hinge, 219 to 225; P1, 226 to 278 and 406 to 530; and P2, 279 to 405. **B:** (Adapted from Prasad BV, Hardy ME, Dokland T, et al. X-ray crystallographic structure of the Norwalk virus capsid. *Science* 1999;286:287–290.) Model of the *T* = 3 Norwalk virus whole capsid, determined at 3.4-Å resolution.[478] The capsid is composed of 90 dimers of VP1, with the S, P1, and P2 domains shown in *blue, red,* and *yellow,* respectively. The box highlights the arrangement of a VP1 dimer as it is displayed on the surface of the virion. **C:** Three-dimensional ribbon representation of a VP1 dimer derived from x-ray crystallography studies of Norwalk virus rVLPs at 3.4-Å, showing the presentation of the P2 domain at the top of an arch supported by two P1 domain "arms".[478] The S domain forms the internal scaffold of the virion that surrounds the RNA genome and positions the arch to the virion surface. The N-terminus (N) and C-terminus (C) of the VP1 are indicated. **D:** Three-dimensional ribbon representation of a P domain-only dimer, determined at 1.4-Å resolution.[112] The *box* highlights the location of an HBGA carbohydrate-binding site mapped within the P2 domain (see Fig. 4.11). (Images provided by B.V.V. Prasad.)

is hypervariable in GII.4 human norovirus strains, suggesting that VP1 and VP2 covary in virus evolution, such that when mutations in VP1 arise, VP2 adapts to the changed conformation.[95] Coevolution and strong selective pressure for a functional VP2[547] are consistent with VP1 and VP2 interactions that would be required to create a proposed VP2-constructed portal emanating from the capsid for the release of genomic RNA[115] (see below *Stages of Replication*) (Fig. 4.5).

Calicivirus VP1 proteins have the ability to self-assemble into virus-like particles (VLPs), a process that is efficient and does not require RNA or VP2.[244,328] However, coexpression of VP2 increases VLP stability and resistance to proteases.[51,335] This self-assembly feature has been especially useful in the study of the fastidious caliciviruses, because recombinant (r) VLPs have served as a surrogate for native virions[192,244,246] and are the basis for current vaccine development approaches (see *Vaccines*). Calicivirus VLPs self-assemble into two classes of particles. The *T* = 3 symmetry particles are made from 180 copies of rVP1 (~38 nm in diameter), while smaller VLPs (~23 nm in diameter) with *T* = 1 symmetry are composed of 60 copies of VP1.[38,79,640] In *T* = 3 particles, the NTA is involved in interlocking the S domains of VP1 capsomeres. Whether the NTA determines the switch between the two types of particles is unclear at present. The NTA was not visible in x-ray structural studies of *T* = 1 VLPs of FCV,[79] and N-terminal truncation mutants of NV VP1 did not result in smaller particles.[52]

In contrast, N-terminal truncations of the RHDV VP1 formed *T* = 1 VLPs.[38]

Knowledge of the capsid structure has also informed studies of capsid assembly. Capsid assembly is thought to occur in a series of successive steps that are highly dependent on solution pH, ionic strength, and VP1 concentration.[27,534] Based on the extensive dimer interfaces observed in the crystal structure of the recombinant NV capsid, a dimer of VP1, existing in equilibrium between "bent" and "flat" conformations, is proposed as the initial building block for the capsid assembly.[478] In support of VP1 dimers as the initial building block, norovirus VLPs disassemble into stable dimers of VP1, which can under the right conditions reassemble into particles.[27,534,602] Subsequent capsid assembly is proposed to involve association of pentamers of these dimers linked by an interstitial dimer, with the VP1 dimers adapting a bent or a flat conformation as required to form a closed icosahedral shell. Such a capsid assembly model predicts the coexistence of 10-mers (one pentamer of dimers) and 20-mers (association of two pentamers of dimers) as intermediates. Any pentamers of dimers were too transient to be detected by time-resolved small-angle x-ray scattering (SAXS) data in VLP assembly of a bovine norovirus VP1.[603] However, the data showed the existence of a stave-shaped intermediate with dimensions consistent with two pentamers of dimers connected by a single interstitial dimer (i.e., 11 dimers)[603] (Fig. 4.6). Formation of quasi 6-fold symmetry, as observed in the *T* = 3 structure, would be anticipated to be a

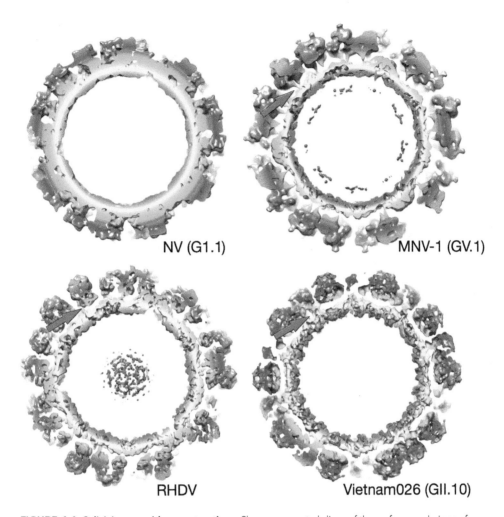

FIGURE 4.4 Calicivirus capsid reconstructions. Shown are central slices of the surface renderings of representative caliciviruses. The crystal structure of Norwalk virus (G1.1) was used to produce its corresponding image,[478] while the remaining three MNV-1,[269] RHDV,[268] and Vietnam026[209] were derived from their cryo-EM image reconstructions. The figures are colored according to radius with the *red hues* being the shortest radii and *purple* being the longest. The *pink arrows* indicate the region of flexibility between the S and P domain, where the P domain is "elevated" above the S domain. In contrast, the Norwalk virus P domain interacts closely with the S domain in a "closed" conformation. (Images provided by T. Smith.)

kinetically slow process that would occur only upon interlocking of intermediates into the final capsid (Fig. 4.6). Such contacts would require a switch in and neutralization of the negative charge of the NTA of VP1 around the quasi 6-fold axes. NTA charge neutralization is thought to be achieved by interaction with the internally located, positively charged VP2.[607,629] Consistent with this, VLPs produced by coexpression of VP2 and VP1 in contrast to VP1 alone are more stable and structurally homogenous.[51]

The inherent ability for calicivirus capsid self-assembly has facilitated genetic engineering and expression of modified and subviral forms of the capsid that have proven useful in several areas of research. For example, norovirus VLPs with a surface-exposed polyhistidine tag can be noncovalently modified to serve as nanocarriers,[296] while chimeric VLPs expressing foreign epitopes show utility as vaccine platforms.[124] The S domain alone has been engineered to provide a nanoparticle platform for peptide expression.[658] Engineering of the P domain via modifications of the C-terminus results in generation of subviral particles termed "P particles" or "small P particles." These

particles are assembled from 12 dimers of the P domain with $T = 1$ symmetry and have facilitated structure and function studies of the viral capsid.[572] Recombinantly expressed P domains from noroviruses, which form "P dimers," are recognized by antibodies and carbohydrates similarly to intact VLPs[574] and have been a critical tool in the field. In fact, most structural information on histoblood group antigen (HBGA) carbohydrate and antibody binding has originated from studies of recombinant P domain.[83,112,306,528,539,540,577,582]

GENOME STRUCTURE AND ORGANIZATION

Caliciviruses have a linear, single-stranded, positive-sense RNA genome (ranging from ~6.4 to 8.5 kb [kilobases] in length) (Fig. 4.7A). Genomes characteristically begin with a 5'-end terminal pGpU sequence that is covalently linked to a small protein, VPg. A short conserved region (CR) at the 5' end

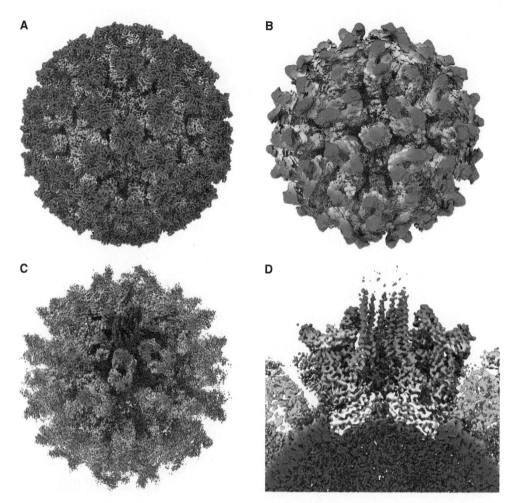

FIGURE 4.5 **A:** Structure of Feline calicivirus (FCV) strain F9, solved by cryogenic electron microscopy (cryo-EM) with imposition of icosahedral symmetry. **B:** Incubation of virus in the presence of a soluble fragment of feline junctional adhesion molecule A (fJAM-A) leads to binding of the receptor fragments to the outer face of the capsid P domains. Following receptor binding, the capsid undergoes conformational changes that break icosahedral symmetry—resulting in poorer resolution of the P domains and receptor. **C:** A low-symmetry reconstruction of the FCV-fJAM-A complex revealed the presence of a large portal-like assembly on the capsid surface, comprising 12 copies of the minor capsid protein VP2. The portal is located at a unique threefold symmetry axis (VP1, purple; fJAM-A, blue; VP2, orange). **D:** A close-up view of the portal-like assembly reveals an opening (indicated by *arrow*) in the capsid shell at the portal axis. (Images provided by D. Bhella and adapted from Conley MJ, McElwee M, Azmi L, et al. Calicivirus VP2 forms a portal-like assembly following receptor engagement. *Nature* 2019;565:377–381.)

is repeated internally in the genome near the beginning of a subgenomic-sized RNA transcript that is coterminal with the 3′ end of the genome.[218,319,404,410,426] The nonstructural proteins are encoded beginning near the 5′ end of the genome, and the structural proteins (VP1 and VP2) are encoded toward the 3′ end of the genome in the region corresponding to a subgenomic RNA. Calicivirus genomes are organized into two or more major ORFs, depending on the genus. Viruses in the genera *Norovirus*, *Recovirus*, and *Vesivirus* encode the VP1 structural protein in a separate ORF (ORF2), whereas those in *Bavovirus*, *Lagovirus*, *Minovirus*, *Nacovirus*, *Nebovirus*, *Salovirus*, *Sapovirus*, and *Valovirus* encode a VP1 that is contiguous with the large nonstructural polyprotein in ORF1 (Fig. 4.7B). All caliciviruses have a relatively small ORF near the 3′ end that encodes the minor structural protein, VP2. The VP2 is variable in size (12,000–30,000 D) and sequence identity among

the caliciviruses.[85,524] MNV genomes analyzed thus far also contain a unique conserved ORF (ORF4)[586] overlapping with and beginning near the 5′ end of ORF2. ORF4 encodes a protein of 23,800 D (designated VF1) that has been implicated in modulation of the host immune response.[397,674] Some sapoviruses have a predicted ORF3 overlapping the capsid encoding region in ORF1, but a protein product has not been verified.[164,523]

Reverse genetics systems based on full-length infectious cDNA clones (and positive-sense RNA transcripts derived from these clones) have been developed for a number of caliciviruses, including FCV and Hom-1 (*Vesivirus*),[545,551,595] porcine enteric calicivirus (PEC) (*Sapovirus*),[99] Tulane virus (*Recovirus*),[636] RHDV (*Lagovirus*),[347] MNV (*Norovirus*),[17,103,512,632,664] and human norovirus (*Norovirus*).[20,267,453] A replicon-bearing continuous cell line derived from the NV genome was also developed[100] and has provided a useful platform for evaluating

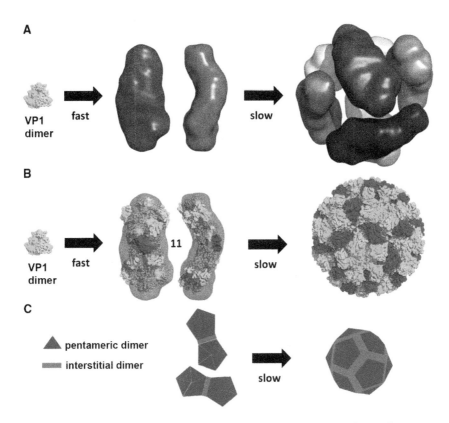

FIGURE 4.6 Norovirus capsid assembly model. All assemblies in A and B are drawn to the same scale. **A:** Small-angle x-ray scattering reconstruction shows that the VP1 dimer (*left*) of the capsid protein of a norovirus forms 10- or 11-dimer stave-like intermediates (*middle*) when assembling into the capsid. The intermediates are proposed to interlock to form the capsid (*right*).[603] **B:** A possible model for the intermediate consisting of 11 dimers is shown. VP1 dimers (*left*) assemble into two pentamers of VP1 dimers that are linked via an interstitial dimer (*middle, pink*), which self-assemble into the *T* = 3 capsid (90 dimers, *right*). The model is based on pieces of the NV capsid atomic structure.[478] In this scheme, the quasi sixfold axes are completed only at the final stage and imply neutralization of negative charges in the NTA,[607] a process that may be assisted by the positively charged VP2 (not shown). **C:** Cartoon of the 11-dimer intermediate structures (*left*) and a self-assembled capsid (*right*). (Images provided by S. Bressanelli; adapted from Tresset G, Le Coeur C, Bryche JF, et al. Norovirus capsid proteins self-assemble through biphasic kinetics via long-lived stave-like intermediates. (*J Am Chem Soc* 2013;135:15373–15381.)

inhibitors of human norovirus replication. Transposon insertional mutagenesis scanning of the FCV[2] and MNV[590] genomes has been applied to genetic engineering of inserted (albeit unstable over multiple passages) foreign sequences.

Viral Proteins

Structural Proteins

Three proteins are found in mature calicivirus virions: VP1, VP2, and VPg.[546] The VP1 (~60,000 D), which is the major structural protein of the virus, is present in 180 copies (90 dimers) per virion.[478] The predominance of VP1 in the formation of the viral capsid structure (see *Virion Structure*) is consistent with its critical role in determining the antigenic phenotype of the virus and its interactions with host cells.

The VP2 (12,000–29,000 D) is considered a minor structural protein because it is less abundant in virion particles.[182,183,546] Evidence for a direct interaction between the VP1 and VP2 capsid proteins has been reported for both NV[95,182,183] and FCV[134,253] (See *Virion Structure*). Recent structural studies

of FCV have shown that VP2 forms a portal at a specialized vertex of the capsid for the release of genomic RNA from the endosome[115] (See *Virion Structure*). Consistent with a role in the initiation of infection, the ablation of VP2 expression in an infectious FCV complementary DNA (cDNA) clone by the introduction of a stop codon in its reading frame did not abolish RNA replication; however, infectious virions could not be recovered without an intact VP2.[547]

The VPg is covalently linked to the genomic and subgenomic RNA in infected cells[148,219] and is a minor component in virions at an estimated one or two copies per particle.[518,546] Although the VPg is present in virions, it likely functions primarily as a nonstructural protein during replication (see *Nonstructural Proteins*).

Nonstructural Proteins

Caliciviruses derive their mature nonstructural proteins (designated here as NS1 through NS7) by proteolytic cleavage of a large polyprotein encoded in ORF1 (Fig. 4.7C).[544] The length

A Genome Organization

B Reading Frame Usage

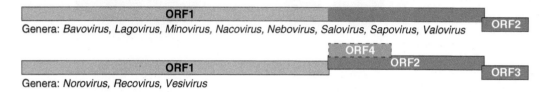

C Gene Order and Cleavage Sites

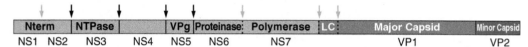

FIGURE 4.7 Comparative features of calicivirus genomes. A: The positive-sense RNA genome is covalently linked to a VPg protein at the 5′ end and polyadenylated at the 3′ end. Nonstructural proteins are encoded beginning from the 5′ end of the genome, and the structural proteins are encoded toward the 3′ end. A conserved region (CR) of nucleotide sequence is shared between the 5′ end of the viral genome and the 5′ end of an abundant subgenomic RNA species produced during replication that serves as a template for translation of the viral structural proteins. **B:** Calicivirus genome organization. Calicivirus genomes are organized so that the major capsid protein coding sequence is either in frame or not with the upstream nonstructural protein sequence. The genera of the *Caliciviridae* associated with each type of organization are indicated. A unique ORF4 has been identified in MNV, comprising genogroup (V) of the genus *Norovirus*. **C:** A large polyprotein (encoded in ORF1) is translated from the viral RNA genome, and it is processed into precursors and final products by a virus-encoded protease. The proteolytic processing strategy varies among the caliciviruses, but all viruses encode domains for at least seven protein functions indicated here as nonstructural (NS) proteins NS1 through NS7.[548] An extra cleavage site is present in the ORF1 of most caliciviruses in which the capsid protein sequence is in frame with the nonstructural polyprotein encoded in ORF1. Cleavage at this site is thought to release the VP1 from the polyprotein so that the RNA-dependent RNA polymerase (NS7) can adopt an active conformation early in the replicative cycle. A cleavage site unique to the vesiviruses is present to release the leader of the capsid protein (LC), from a capsid precursor encoded in ORF2.[552] Mapped cleavage sites conserved and utilized among all calicivirus genera are indicated with a *dark arrow*; cleavage sites that vary in utilization among the family are indicated with a *light arrow* (see text).

of the uncleaved polyprotein precursor is approximately 200,000 D (excluding in-frame VP1 capsid protein sequences). This large precursor has never been observed, most likely because proteolytic processing is rapid and cotranslational.[345,348,553] The proteolytic cleavages are mediated by a virus-encoded cysteine proteinase (NS6[Pro]).[66] The location of the cleavage sites in the ORF1 polyprotein that define the borders of the final nonstructural protein cleavage products has been determined for calicivirus strains representing the genera *Norovirus*,[48,345,348,548] *Vesivirus*,[549] *Lagovirus*,[302,650] and *Sapovirus*.[451] Some variation is seen among the proteolytic processing strategies, but the overall gene order of the calicivirus nonstructural proteins is conserved. The lagoviruses, represented by RHDV, have the highest number (six) of mapped cleavage sites. The polyprotein of RHDV is cleaved at these six sites to release seven final products (designated as NS1 through NS7 in Fig. 4.7C and Table 4.2). Five cleavage sites for the norovirus ORF1 polyprotein (represented by Southampton virus) have been mapped that release six mature products.[345,348] The noroviruses differ from the lagoviruses in that a protease cleavage site has not been directly mapped in the extreme N-terminal protein, although evidence suggests that additional processing (or modification) of the protein can occur in cells.[525,548] For example, at least 10 protease-containing precursors were identified in

MNV-infected cells, whose activity is temporally and spatially regulated.[152] The vesivirus cleavage map (represented by FCV) contains five mapped cleavage sites to release six mature nonstructural proteins, and each cleavage event is essential in the virus replication cycle.[549] The vesiviruses show yet another variation in processing, in that no evidence exists for efficient viral protease–mediated cleavage between the protease (Pro) and polymerase (Pol) proteins, even in virus-infected cells.[385,549,553] In addition, vesiviruses bear a unique cleavage site in the capsid protein precursor protein that is processed by NS6[Pro] to release the leader of the capsid (LC) from the major capsid protein, VP1[552,598] (Fig. 4.7C). The predicted nonstructural protein cleavage map of human sapovirus strain, Mc10, shows an overall similarity with that of the vesiviruses.[451] Sapoviruses (and several other caliciviruses in which the capsid region is in frame with the nonstructural polyprotein) bear an additional protease cleavage site in the ORF1 polyprotein between the polymerase and capsid coding regions. A number of stable precursor proteins have been described also for the caliciviruses, and it is likely that these proteins have unique functions in replication beyond those of the fully processed mature forms.[544]

The calicivirus dipeptide cleavage recognition sites are consistent with those described for the picornavirus 3C cysteine proteinase.[212] The calicivirus cleavage sites identified thus far

TABLE 4.2   Calicivirus nonstructural proteins

Calicivirus Nonstructural Protein (NS)	Common Designations	Reported Properties (Virus[b])	References
NS1	p5.6, p16	Cleavage and release essential for replication (FCV)	549
		Cytoplasmic and nuclear localization (RHDV)	612
NS1/2 or NS2[a]	N-term, p48	Binding partner with host cell VAP-A (HNV)	159
		FFAT mimic motif interacts with VAP-A (MNV)	394
		Golgi colocalization and disassembly (HNV)	167
		C-terminal hydrophobic region (HNV)	159,167
		Smooth ER membrane proliferation (HNV)	136
		Proximal association with lipid droplets (MNV)	136
		Predicted hydrolase domain (HNV)	136
		Determinant of colon tropism and persistence in mice (MNV)	67,440
		Bears caspase cleavage sites (MNV)	548
		Inherent structural disorder and multimerization (MNV)	33
NS3	NTPase, p39	NTP binding, hydrolysis of NTP (RHDV, HNV)	381,471
		ATP-dependent RNA helicase activity (HNV)	334
		Induction of membrane rearrangements (HNV)	136,661
		RNA chaperone–like activity (MNV, HNV)	205,334
		Lipid and microtubule associated (MNV, HNV)	120
		Suppresses IRF3 activation (FCV)	663
NS4	"3A-like," p20, p22	Forms stable precursor with VPg: proposed VPg anchor (FCV)	549
		Inhibits actin cytoskeleton remodeling (HNV)	222
		ER/Golgi trafficking antagonist (HNV)	529
		Induction of single-, double-, and multimembraned structures (HNV)	136
NS5	VPg	Present in virions, covalently linked to RNA (VESV, FCV)	80,219
		Sequence homology with eIF1A (HNV, FCV)	553
		Binding partner with eIF3 (HNV)	128
		VPg-linked translation requires eIF4a unwinding activity (FCV, MNV, PSV)	102,228
		Binding partner and translation function with eIF4E (FCV, PSV)	188,227
		Binding partner with eIF4G (MNV)	113
		Nucleotidylated by RdRP at conserved tyrosine (RHDV, HNV)	47,372
		Conserved tyrosine essential for replication of virus (FCV, NV)	406,560
		Functions in protein-primed RNA synthesis (NV)	503
		Linked to cellular trans-Golgi network protein 2 RNA in cells (NV)	560
		Compact helical core domains with flexible N and C termini (FCV, MNV)	327
NS6	Proteinase (Pro)	Proteinase activity, cysteine in active site (HNV, FCV, RHDV, SV)	66,348,448,553
		Mediates cleavage of ORF1 polyprotein (HNV, FCV, HSV, RHDV)	348,449,553,649
		Mediates cleavage of capsid precursor protein, PreVP1 (FCV)	553
		Cleaves cellular proteins (FCV, HNV)	153,315,647
		Structural analysis shows chymotrypsin-like folding (NV)	421
		RNA-binding activity	627

(continued)

TABLE 4.2 Calicivirus nonstructural proteins *(Continued)*

Calicivirus Nonstructural Protein (NS)	Common Designations	Reported Properties (Virus[b])	References
NS7	Polymerase (Pol), RdRP	Contains RdRP motif hYGDDhhY/V (FCV, HNV, RHDV, HSV)	242,388,403,424
		In vitro activity is primer-independent (RHDV, HNV, FCV)	46,170,618,637
		Protein (VPg)-primed RNA polymerase activity (HNV)	503
		Transcription activity on negative-strand template (RHDV)	410
		Enzymatically active as ProPol (NS6-7) precursor form (FCV, HNV)	46,637
		Active as a homodimer (HNV)	226
		Interacts with VPg (FCV, MNV)	253,325
		Structural analysis reveals carboxy terminus in active site cleft (HNV, HSV)	171,436
		Phosphorylated by signaling kinase Akt (HNV)	149

[a]The predominant form of the N-terminal ORF1 protein in noroviruses consists of an NS1/NS2 precursor that is not cleaved by the virus-encoded proteinase. In this table, the known properties of the norovirus NS1/NS2 protein are listed under NS2.
[b]Virus abbreviations: FCV, Feline calicivirus, and VESV, vesicular exanthema of swine virus, in genus *Vesivirus*; RHDV, rabbit hemorrhagic disease virus, in genus *Lagovirus*; HNV, human norovirus, and MNV, murine norovirus, in genus *Norovirus*; HSV, human sapovirus, and PSV, porcine sapovirus, in genus *Sapovirus*.

have either a negatively charged glutamic acid (E) or polar glutamine (Q) in the first position (designated P1). More variation exists within the second position of the dipeptide cleavage site (designated P1'). Studies of the calicivirus proteinase substrate specificity have shown some tolerance in the P1' position at certain cleavage sites.[212,552,649] The conformation of the protein surrounding the dipeptide recognition site is also important for efficient cleavage by the proteinase.[212,553]

The availability of proteolytic cleavage maps for the calicivirus nonstructural polyproteins has enabled studies that elucidate the functions and structures of individual proteins. Biochemical studies first confirmed enzymatic activities in calicivirus proteins corresponding to an NTPase (NTPase or NS3[NTPase]),[381] a chymotrypsin-like cysteine proteinase (Pro or NS6[Pro]),[66] and an RNA-dependent RNA polymerase (Pol or NS7[Pol]).[618] The three-dimensional structures for the latter two enzymes have

been reported. The norovirus Pro shares structural similarities with classical chymotrypsin-like serine proteases.[166,235,419,421,543,669] A cleft containing the active site catalytic residues (His 30, Glu 54, and Cys 139 for Norwalk virus) involved in substrate cleavage is located between the N-terminal β-barrel and the C-terminal twisted β-sheet domains. Substrate-binding pockets are shown to undergo slight conformational changes in response to sequence variations in the polyprotein cleavage sites.[417] Comparison of a recently determined structure of catalytically active GII.4 norovirus protease with that of the GI.1 Norwalk virus shows a similar overall organization, but with noticeable conformational changes in the substrate-binding pockets and also in the three catalytic residues, which are arranged in a slightly different conformation (Fig. 4.8).[626,669] Furthermore, an Arg residue (R122) is located within the active cleft that is observed to make a cation-pi interaction with the catalytic His residue (Fig. 4.8, inset), thereby affecting GII.4

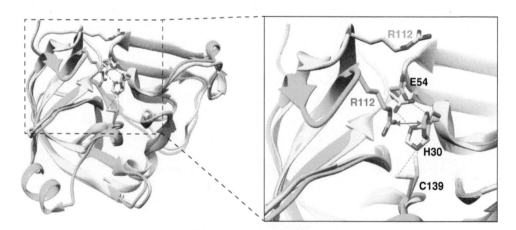

FIGURE 4.8 Comparison of GI and GII norovirus protease active sites. Structural overlay of GII.4 HOV (*cyan*; PDB: 6NIR) and GI.1 Norwalk virus (*yellow*; PDB: 2FYQ) proteases. The **inset** shows the structural changes of bII-cII loop between HOV and NV proteases. Active site residues H30, E54, and C139 and the S2 substrate–binding pocket residues R112 are shown as stick models with nitrogen and oxygen atoms colored in *blue* and *red*, respectively. The cation-π interaction between R112 and H30 in HOV protease is indicated by a *red double arrow*. (Images provided by L. Hu and B.V.V. Prasad; adapted from Viskovska MA, Zhao B, Shanker S, et al. GII.4 norovirus protease shows pH-sensitive proteolysis with a unique ARG-HIS pairing in the catalytic site. *J Virol* 2019;93(6). doi:10.1128/JVI.01479-18; Zeitler CE, Estes MK, Venkataram Prasad BV. X-ray crystallographic structure of the Norwalk virus protease at 1.5-Å resolution. *J Virol* 2006;80:5050–5058.)

Norovirus RNA-Dependent RNA Polymerase

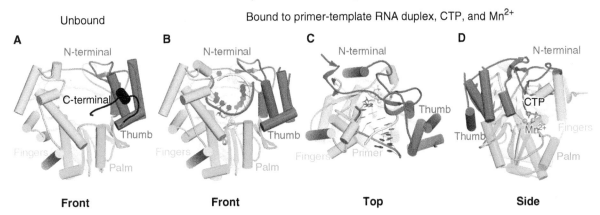

FIGURE 4.9 **Structure of the norovirus RNA–dependent RNA polymerase. A:** The norovirus RNA–dependent RNA polymerase adopts the classic "right-hand" structure characteristic of polynucleotide polymerases as shown in this stick model. The fingers (*blue*) and palm (*green*) domains form a rigid unit, while the thumb (*red*) domain is flexible and can assume either a "closed" or "open" conformation. An N-terminal domain bridges the fingers and thumb domains. When the polymerase is unbound to template, the C-terminal end of the protein appears to lie within the active site cleft.[436] **B–D:** The front, top, and side views, respectively, of the Norwalk RNA polymerase bound to a primer-RNA duplex, CTP, and metal divalent cation, Mn[2+]. (Images provided by K. Ng; adapted from Ng KK, Cherney MM, Vazquez AL, et al. Crystal structures of active and inactive conformations of a caliciviral RNA-dependent RNA polymerase. *J Biol Chem* 2002;277:1381–1387; Ng KK, Pendas-Franco N, Rojo J, et al. Crystal structure of norwalk virus polymerase reveals the carboxyl terminus in the active site cleft. *J Biol Chem* 2004;279:16638–16645; Zamyatkin DF, Parra F, Alonso JM, et al. Structural insights into mechanisms of catalysis and inhibition in Norwalk virus polymerase. *J Biol Chem* 2008;283:7705–7712. Ref.[435])

protease sensitivity to pH. Such differences might be important in the design of norovirus protease inhibitors among diverse strains. The norovirus RNA-dependent RNA polymerase has a classical "right-hand" (finger, thumb, and palm) organization,[436,668] with the C-terminus of the protein positioned in the active site cleft (Fig. 4.9A). Modeling of the interaction of Pol with an RNA template in the presence of manganese and CTP shows that the initiation of RNA synthesis occurs within the active site cleft (Fig. 4.9B–D). Binding of the primer/template RNA duplex displaces the C-terminal tail away from the active site, allowing the central helix of the thumb domain to position itself for interaction with the primer strand and minor groove of the primer–template duplex.[668] Two divalent metal ions (likely Mg[2+] in cells) help mediate catalysis by forming coordination bonds with three highly conserved aspartic acid residues and the nucleoside triphosphate (NTP). After nucleotidyl transfer has occurred, the pyrophosphate is released from the enzyme. The primer–template duplex is predicted to translocate in a manner that places the newly incorporated nucleotide into the same position as that of the 3' end of the primer strand immediately prior to nucleotidyl transfer. This translocation process provides the space needed to form the binding site for the next incoming nucleoside triphosphate.

Structure and function studies of the mapped calicivirus nonstructural proteins encoded in ORF1 are summarized in Table 4.2. The activities of replicative enzymes NS3 (NTPase), NS6 (proteinase), and NS7 (polymerase) are established, and knowledge of their structure has informed investigations of targeted inhibitors. The NS5 (VPg), required for the infectivity of genomic RNA, is multifunctional, playing a role in both translation and RNA replication. The remaining proteins (NS1, NS2, and NS4) have all been associated, in some capacity, with intracellular membrane interactions. These interactions are likely important in forming a scaffold for the assembly of viral replication complexes in the cell,[136,239,588] and elucidation of their effects on host cell pathways may also inform the design of therapeutic interventions.

STAGES OF REPLICATION

Replication Strategy

The calicivirus replication strategy shares many features with those of other positive-strand RNA viruses (Fig. 4.10).[588] Caliciviruses attach and enter the cell, the RNA genome is released, and translation of the VPg-linked genome occurs via the host cell machinery. Certain newly translated viral proteins interact with the host cell to establish defined sites of virus replication (characteristically involving reorganized intracellular membranes), while other proteins function as replicative enzymes. Newly synthesized positive-strand RNA genomes are covalently linked to VPg and packaged into virions that are released from cells via lytic and nonlytic mechanisms. The replication cycle of a calicivirus is rapid: new viral progeny can be detected within hours after infection.

Mechanism of Attachment

Many caliciviruses interact with host cell surface glycans that serve as attachment factors to facilitate infection (Fig. 4.11). The specificity of these interactions plays an important role in the determination of host range and tissue tropism, and there is considerable diversity among calicivirus strains in their glycan binding profiles (Table 4.3). Human and bovine noroviruses bind to various HBGA carbohydrate moieties, heparan sulfate proteoglycans, and sialylated glycans.[10,382,571,579,635,666] MNVs recognize sialic acids on glycolipids and N- and/or O-linked glycoproteins.[580,581] Glycan interactions have been described for lagoviruses,[443,444,484] recoviruses,[576] sapoviruses,[280,670] and vesiviruses.[310,558] Structure and function studies have verified a number of these interactions and defined the location of glycan binding sites on calicivirus capsids[83,112,305,376] (Fig. 4.12). Additional binding ligands for noroviruses have been noted (such as bacterial HBGA-like moieties), but their role in the initiation of infection is not known.[10]

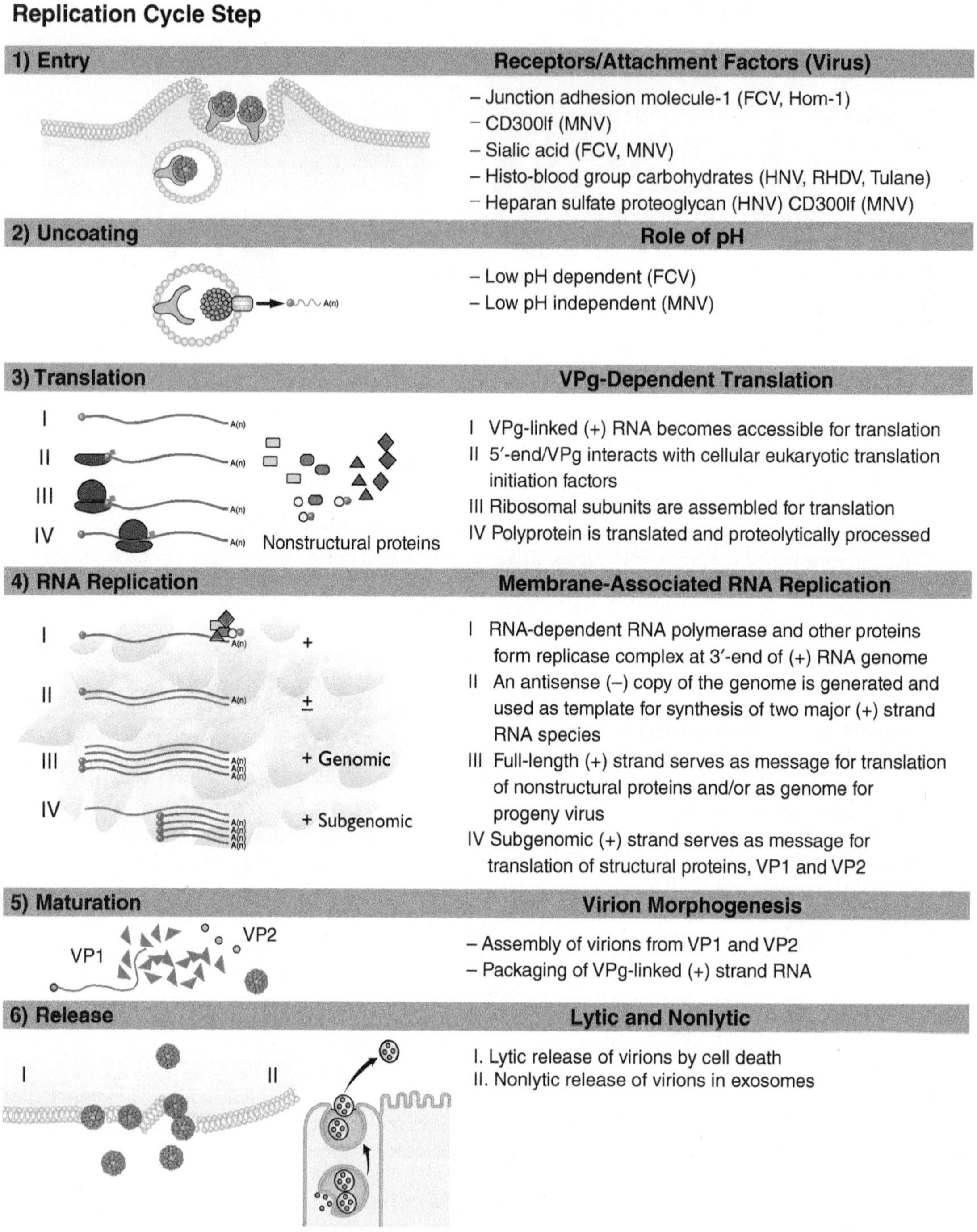

Replication Cycle Step

1) Entry

Receptors/Attachment Factors (Virus)

– Junction adhesion molecule-1 (FCV, Hom-1)
– CD300lf (MNV)
– Sialic acid (FCV, MNV)
– Histo-blood group carbohydrates (HNV, RHDV, Tulane)
– Heparan sulfate proteoglycan (HNV) CD300lf (MNV)

2) Uncoating

Role of pH

– Low pH dependent (FCV)
– Low pH independent (MNV)

3) Translation

Nonstructural proteins

VPg-Dependent Translation

I   VPg-linked (+) RNA becomes accessible for translation
II 5′-end/VPg interacts with cellular eukaryotic translation initiation factors
III Ribosomal subunits are assembled for translation
IV Polyprotein is translated and proteolytically processed

4) RNA Replication

+
±
+ Genomic
+ Subgenomic

Membrane-Associated RNA Replication

I   RNA-dependent RNA polymerase and other proteins form replicase complex at 3′-end of (+) RNA genome
II An antisense (–) copy of the genome is generated and used as template for synthesis of two major (+) strand RNA species
III Full-length (+) strand serves as message for translation of nonstructural proteins and/or as genome for progeny virus
IV Subgenomic (+) strand serves as message for translation of structural proteins, VP1 and VP2

5) Maturation

VP1   VP2

Virion Morphogenesis

– Assembly of virions from VP1 and VP2
– Packaging of VPg-linked (+) strand RNA

6) Release

I   II

Lytic and Nonlytic

I. Lytic release of virions by cell death
II. Nonlytic release of virions in exosomes

FIGURE 4.10 Schematic diagram of the proposed replication strategy of the caliciviruses. Consistent with other positive-strand RNA viruses, the replication cycle of a calicivirus involves the following stages: (1) entry, (2) uncoating, (3) translation, (4) RNA replication, (5) maturation, and (6) release, as reviewed in the text.

Following the interaction with carbohydrate attachment factors, caliciviruses interact with a proteinaceous entry receptor. The identity of the first experimentally verified cellular receptor was for FCV, the junction adhesion molecule-1 (JAM-1, also called JAM-A), an immunoglobulin-like cellular membrane protein.[374] A homologous protein, human JAM-1 (JAM-A), also serves as the receptor for Hom-1 vesivirus.[551] FCV interacts with feline (f) JAM-1 through binding of the P2 domain of the capsid to the distal membrane domain (D1)

of fJAM-1 and triggers irreversible conformational changes in the virus capsid.[53] Mutational analysis has confirmed two residues in the viral capsid that bind to the receptor.[364] The second verified proteinaceous receptor for caliciviruses is the MNV entry receptor CD300lf (also named CLM-1, CMRF35, MAIR-V, LMIR3). It was independently identified by two groups through an unbiased CRISPR/Cas9 screen in BV2 (murine microglial cells) or RAW 264.7 cells (murine macrophages) using multiple MNV strains.[201,454] CD300lf is a

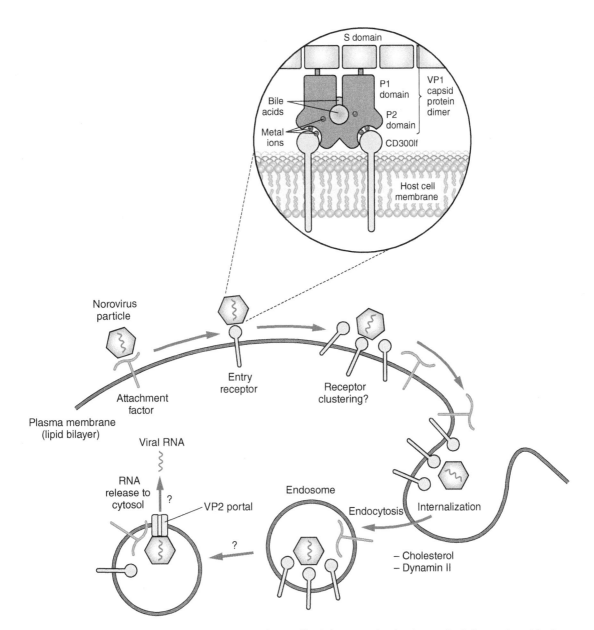

FIGURE 4.11 Schematics of calicivirus entry into host cells. Caliciviruses bind to host cells via interaction with glycans, which serve as attachment factors. This is followed by engagement with a proteinaceous entry receptor. These receptor interactions likely trigger receptor clustering and initiate internalization of virus particles by the endocytic pathway. The uptake pathway differs among caliciviruses. Murine norovirus uptake is pH independent[469] but dependent on cholesterol and dynamin II[180,468] and via a nonclathrin and noncaveolin pathway. *Feline calicivirus* entry is pH dependent and via clathrin-mediated endocytosis.[557] Porcine sapovirus entry requires dynamin II, cholesterol, and actin to enter via clathrin-mediated endocytosis.[542] Escape from the endosome may then be mediated by the minor capsid VP2, which forms a portal across the endosomal membrane in FCV infection.[115] **Inset:** In the case of murine norovirus, interaction with the proteinaceous receptor CD300lf[455] occurs in place of the natural lipid ligands with CD300lf and is facilitated by cofactors bile acids and cations.[429]

cell surface-expressed, immunoglobulin (Ig)-like domain-containing, lipid-binding protein (e.g., ceramide, phosphatidylcholine, phosphatidylserine). MNV binding and infection are blocked by incubation with an anti-CD300lf antibody, soluble CD300lf ectodomain, or deletion of the gene. Expression of murine CD300lf or the related molecule CD300ld (which have highly homologous ectodomains), but not human CD300f, makes cells susceptible to MNV infection, includ-

ing non-murine cells. CD300lf is the primary receptor *in vivo* since CD300lf-deficient mice are resistant to MNV infection as indicated by the absence of fecal shedding.[454] Thus, receptor availability is a major determinant of species specificity and tissue tropism. Mutational and structural analysis identified residues in the CC' and CDR3 loops of CD300lf and the capsid P2 domain that mediate the interaction.[201,276,429,454] Virus binding to the receptor occurs in the same location as

TABLE 4.3   Glycans associated with binding to calicivirus capsids

Glycan Moiety	Virus	References
Histoblood group antigens (HBGA)	Human norovirus GI and GII (H type 1, H type 2, H type 3)	83,112,230,343,382,507
	Canine norovirus (α1,2-fucose-containing H and A antigens)	81
	Simian recovirus (*Tulane*) (B types 1-4 and A type 3/4)	163,670
	Bat calicivirus (H type 1)	295
	Rabbit hemorrhagic disease virus (H type 2)	444,505
	European brown hare syndrome virus (H type 2)	353
	Bovine nebovirus (H type 2)	111
Lewis antigens	Human norovirus GI and GII (LeA, LeB, LeX, and LeY)	204,231,314,343,375,505,533,541,666
	Human norovirus GII (sLeX)	507
Alpha gal (Galactose-*alpha*-1,3-galactose)	Bovine norovirus (α-gal epitope)	666
Heparan sulfate proteoglycan	Human norovirus GII	571
Sialic acids	Human norovirus (α2,6-linked and α2,3-linked)	206,635
	Bovine norovirus	392
	Murine norovirus (α2,6-linked and α2,3-linked)	580,581
	Bat norovirus (α2,6-linked)	295
	Porcine sapovirus (α2,6-linked and α2,3-linked)	280
	Simian recovirus (*Tulane*) (α2,3-linked)	576
	Bat calicivirus (α2,6-linked)	295
	Feline calicivirus (α2,6-linked)	558
Milk oligosaccharides	Human norovirus	207,243,522
Plant cell wall carbohydrates	Human norovirus	158
Bacterial HBGA-like glycans	Human norovirus	407
Bivalve mollusks HBGA-like glycans	Human norovirus	321,597

lipid binding, making this interaction an example of viral mimicry of a natural ligand.[429] Furthermore, the receptor binding site on the viral capsid overlaps with the epitopes of two neutralizing antibodies (named A6.2, 2D3), suggesting inhibition of receptor binding as one mechanism of neutralization.[276,429] The binding affinity between one CD300lf molecule and one viral capsid protein is low (KD ~ 25 μM) in biochemical assays,[429] indicating other factors strengthen the interaction. Structural and functional analysis identified divalent cations and bile acids (especially GCDCA) as cofactors that enhance binding and infection[275,429] (Fig. 4.11, inset). The binding sites for two bile acid molecules and three cations in each capsid protein are distant from the CD300lf binding site, and none of these interactions induced structural rearrangements in the MNV P domain visible by crystallography.[429] Clustering of CD300lf molecules to increase avidity is another proposed factor that likely strengthens the interaction between the virion and the receptor (Fig. 4.11). Other proteins that facilitate calicivirus entry have also been identified. Specifically, the tight junction protein occludin was

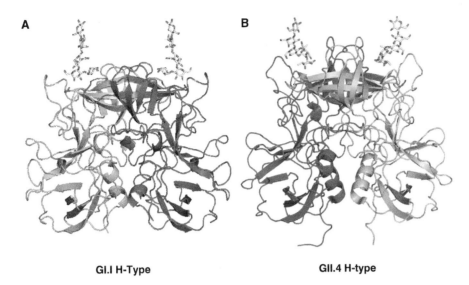

A **B**

GI.I H-Type   GII.4 H-type

FIGURE 4.12 Interaction of representative norovirus VP1 dimers with H carbohydrates from histoblood group antigens. For both GI.1 and GII.4 noroviruses, HBGA carbohydrates interact with the distal surface of the capsid, but differences in these interactions have been noted. **A:** The Norwalk virus (GI.1) carbohydrate-binding site contains residues that project from a well-structured antiparallel β-sheet near the P domain dimeric interface and favors a precise and limited recognition of a terminal Gal-Fuc or Gal-acetamido combination. **B:** In contrast, the VA387 (GII.4) binding site is formed by residues located in two surface-exposed loops near the P domain dimeric interface that broadly recognize a terminal fucosyl moiety. (Images provided by B.V.V. Prasad with data adapted from Cao S, Lou Z, Tan M, et al. Structural basis for the recognition of blood group trisaccharides by norovirus. *J Virol* 2007;81:5949–5957; Choi JM, Hutson AM, Estes MK, et al. Atomic resolution structural characterization of recognition of histo-blood group antigens by Norwalk virus. *Proc Natl Acad Sci U S A* 2008;105:9175–9180.)

shown to directly bind to porcine sapovirus and to function as a coreceptor, while claudin 1 did not directly bind to the virus but facilitated infection and was thus proposed to serve as an entry factor.[6] In addition to CD300lf, MNV-1 also binds to the extracellular domains of murine CD36, CD98 heavy chain (CD98), and transferrin receptor 1 TfRc, which promoted binding to dendritic cells (CD36) or murine macrophages (CD98 and TfRc) in a cell-type–specific manner.[70]

Mechanism of Entry and Intracellular Trafficking

Following engagement with viral receptors, clustering of receptors in membrane domains may contribute to virion internalization (Fig. 4.11). Consistent with receptor clustering are the following data: (a) Engagement of HBGAs on glycolipids by human norovirus VLPs results in invaginations in unilamellar vesicles and VLP clustering,[463,508] (b) MNV entry is dependent on cholesterol,[180,468] virion binding leads to the aggregation of detergent-resistant membrane domains,[29] and (c) inhibition of synthesis of sphingolipid and ceramide, molecules required for membrane fluidity and dynamics, is critical for CD300lf cell surface arrangement and MNV infection.[455] Endocytic uptake of MNV further requires dynamin II, but not clathrin, caveolin, or low pH[180,468,469] (Fig. 4.11). FCV, on the other hand, requires low pH and is endocytosed via a clathrin-mediated uptake pathway.[309,557] Its internalization was proposed to be initiated following binding to fJAM-1 and disruption of the fJAM-1 homodimer.[115] In the case of porcine sapovirus, virions are internalized by clathrin- and cholesterol-mediated endocytosis that requires dynamin II and actin rearrangement and traffic to late endosomes via early endosomes in complex with the coreceptor occludin.[6,542]

Uncoating

The uncoating events that allow the calicivirus positive-sense RNA genome to become accessible to the cellular translational machinery have not been defined in detail. However, similar to other viruses, receptor engagement, low pH, and/or ion flux in endosomes may all serve as triggers for RNA release into the cytosol (Fig. 4.11). Uncoating is a rapid process: MNV genome was released within 1 hour after infection[468] but independent of pH.[469] Consistent with a pH-independent trigger, norovirus (NV) VLPs are stable under acidic conditions, but disassociation occurs under alkaline conditions.[534] In FCV, binding to the cellular receptor induces a conformational change in the capsid,[53] which ultimately leads to the formation of a portal vertex at a unique 3-fold axis.[115] A dodecameric assembly of VP2 protrudes from this vertex to form a channel through which viral RNA is released from the endosome into the cytosol[115] (Fig. 4.11). Intriguingly, no significant structural rearrangements are observed upon CD300lf binding to the MNV P domain.[429] However, no structural information of the full-length VP1 capsid protein or virions during receptor binding is currently available.

Translation

Calicivirus genomic RNA in virions requires the presence of the covalently linked VPg protein in order to establish an infection after release (or transfection) into cells.[80] The initiation of translation of the incoming positive-strand genome is likely mediated through interactions of the VPg protein with the cellular translation machinery.[102,128,188] Direct interactions of host cell proteins with viral RNA may also mediate translation efficiency.[198,199,220,259] Calicivirus replication is associated with an inhibition of host cell translation, and the viral proteinase

TABLE 4.4   Pathogenesis and disease manifestations of representative calicivirus strains

Calicivirus Strain	Genus	Host	Site of Replication[a]	Clinical Disease[b]
Norwalk virus	*Norovirus*	Human	Enteric	Gastroenteritis
Jena virus	*Norovirus*	Cattle	Enteric	Gastroenteritis
Murine norovirus (MNV-1-like)	*Norovirus*	Mouse	Distal SI, lymphoid	Acute systemic but limited disease[c]
Murine norovirus (CR6-like)	*Norovirus*	Mouse	Colon (tuft cells)	Persistent, asymptomatic
Pistoia virus	*Norovirus*	Lion	Enteric	Hemorrhagic enteritis
Canine norovirus	*Norovirus*	Dog	Enteric	Gastroenteritis
Porcine norovirus CH6	*Norovirus*	Pig	Enteric	Gastroenteritis
Sapporo virus	*Sapovirus*	Human	Enteric	Gastroenteritis
Porcine enteric calicivirus (Cowden)	*Sapovirus*	Pig	Enteric	Gastroenteritis
Mink enteric calicivirus	*Sapovirus*	Mink	Enteric	Gastroenteritis
Rabbit hemorrhagic disease virus	*Lagovirus*	Rabbit	Liver, systemic	Organ dysfunction, pulmonary hemorrhage[e]
Rabbit calicivirus	*Lagovirus*	Rabbit	Liver	Asymptomatic
European brown hare syndrome virus	*Lagovirus*	Hare	Liver, systemic	Organ dysfunction, pulmonary hemorrhage[e]
Bovine enteric calicivirus (Newbury-1 virus)	*Nebovirus*	Cattle	Enteric	Gastroenteritis
Bovine enteric calicivirus (Nebraska virus)	*Nebovirus*	Cattle	Enteric	Gastroenteritis
Feline calicivirus	*Vesivirus*	Cat	Mouth, upper respiratory	Stomatitis, pneumonia
Feline calicivirus-VS	*Vesivirus*	Cat	Systemic	Fulminant organ dysfunction[f]
San Miguel sea lion virus (SMSV)	*Vesivirus*	Sea lion	Mucosal, systemic	Skin (flipper) lesions, pneumonia
Canine calicivirus (No. 48)	*Vesivirus*	Dog	Enteric	Gastroenteritis
Vesivirus isolate 2117	*Vesivirus*	Unknown	Unknown	Unknown[g]
Hom-1 (SMSV to human)	*Vesivirus*	Human	Mucosal	Skin lesions
Tulane virus	*Recovirus*	Monkey	Enteric	Gastroenteritis
St. Valérien virus (AB90)	*Valovirus*	Pig	Enteric	Not established
Bayern virus	*Bavovirus*	Chicken	Enteric	Not established

[a]Site of replication is based on observed pathological effects in tissue and, in some cases, confirmed by immunohistochemistry. For many caliciviruses, the primary site of replication in the host has not been fully established. In general, infection outcome in the family *Caliciviridae* can range from asymptomatic (subclinical) to lethal.

[b]The characteristic clinical disease associated with each representative calicivirus strain is shown. St. Valérien virus[316] and Bayern virus[654] were detected in screening surveys of nonselected stool specimens: the clinical disease outcome has not been established. *Norwalk virus*, representative of the human noroviruses associated with acute gastroenteritis, is generally associated with self-limiting vomiting and diarrhea of 24- to 48-hour duration. However, the illness can be severe and life-threatening in certain individuals (see text).

[c]Most variants of the MNV-1 strain of murine norovirus are lethal only in certain mice that lack an innate immune system, but evidence exists for varying pathogenicity among MNV strains and variants.[265,586]

[d]Sapporo virus, representative of the human sapoviruses associated with acute gastroenteritis, has most often been associated with self-limiting gastroenteritis in younger age groups, as opposed to norovirus, which occurs in all age groups.[109]

[e]Rabbit hemorrhagic disease virus was first recognized as a highly lethal disease in rabbits, but there are a wide range of disease manifestations in lagomorphs.[323]

[f]Feline calicivirus strains have emerged in recent years designated as "virulent systemic" (VS) that are associated with high morbidity and mortality in cats. In addition, the virus can cause a persistent, asymptomatic infection in cats.[485]

[g]Vesivirus 2117 was discovered as a contaminant in cultured Chinese hamster ovary cells.[447]

(NS6^{Pro}) has been shown to cleave certain cellular proteins involved in translation, which may, in part, give the viral RNA a competitive advantage.[315] The ORF1 of the virus is translated first to produce a large polyprotein, which is processed rapidly into precursors and products by NS6^{Pro} at several essential cleavage sites.[549] Certain of these nonstructural proteins and their precursors function to set up replication sites within the host cell,[30,136,239] while others (such as the RNA-dependent RNA polymerase, NS7^{Pol}) play a direct role in replication of the viral RNA (Table 4.2).

An abundant VPg-linked subgenomic positive-strand RNA serves as a bicistronic message for translation of the structural proteins, VP1 and VP2.[218,426] Regulation of translation of VP2 from the subgenomic RNA (translated at ~20% of the levels of VP1) was mapped to an upstream RNA sequence element in the 3′-end VP1 coding region of approximately 70 nucleotides designated as the termination upstream ribosomal binding site (TURBS).[200,401,402,638] The TURBS site contains two motifs, one of which mediates base pairing between the viral subgenomic messenger RNA and the cellular 18S ribosomal subunit.[402] This interaction may function as a "tether," positioning the ribosome for immediate reinitiation of translation following termination of translation of the VP1 gene.[367] Translation of the VF1 protein, encoded in an alternative ORF[4] within the VP1 coding region of the MNV genome, likely occurs through a leaky scanning mechanism.[397]

Replication of Genomic Nucleic Acid

As with all other positive-strand RNA viruses, the replication of calicivirus RNA is associated with host cell membranes.[30,136,193,239] A marked rearrangement of intracellular membranes occurs, and evidence exists for the initiation of RNA replication in a perinuclear site that contains membranes associated with endoplasmic reticulum, trans-Golgi network, and endosomal membrane markers.[30,136,239] This early replication complex is localized proximal to the microtubule-organizing center in MNV-infected cells, with VP1 associated with the redistribution of acetylated tubulin to the complex.[238] The initiation of synthesis of an antisense (negative) strand RNA from the genomic RNA template occurs beginning at the 3′ end of the genomic positive-strand RNA, and interactions with a number of cellular proteins with viral RNA have been identified that could play a role in RNA transcription and replication.[199,355,516] The negative-strand RNA, in turn, serves as a template for transcription of two major positive-strand RNA species corresponding to the full-length genome (genomic RNA) and the approximately one-third of the genome toward the 3′ end (subgenomic RNA).[426]

The calicivirus RNA genome bears conserved regions of secondary structure,[368,476,536] and functional RNA regulatory elements have been mapped both internally and near the ends of the genome.[8,31] Transcription from the start site for the subgenomic RNA species on the negative-strand template (nt 5,296 of RHDV) was found to require an upstream sequence of 50 nt for full polymerase activity in *in vitro* studies,[410] consistent with its role in the formation of a subgenomic promoter. The corresponding region of MNV was mapped also as bearing a promoter for subgenomic RNA synthesis from the negative-strand template[336,665]

Assembly

A two-stage process has been proposed for the maturation of calicivirus (FCV) particles.[301] The first stage involves the rapid aggregation and assembly of capsid precursor proteins into 5S subunits that then pass through several intermediate forms (with varying stability) to form stable 15S subunits. The second stage involves the association of 15S subunits with newly synthesized RNA genomes to form infectious particles (that sediment at 170S). Protein–protein interactions have been detected between the FCV VPg (covalently linked to the RNA genome) and the capsid precursor as well as between the RNA-dependent RNA polymerase NS7[Pol] and the capsid precursor, suggesting that these interactions may be related to packaging of the newly synthesized RNA into the viral capsid.[253] In addition, successful assembly of the infectious FCV virions was linked to an efficient expression of the virus minor capsid protein, VP2.[547]

The VPg-linked genomic and subgenomic positive-strand RNA species are found in FCV and RHDV particles of distinct densities, indicating that they are not packaged together in the same virion.[404,425] The incorporation of subgenomic RNA into the lower density (LD) particles suggests that a packaging signal is located within the 3′ terminal 2,400 nucleotides of the genome. It has been suggested that LD particles (which would not be infectious) may be associated with FCV strains of higher virulence, but their function, if any, in the virus life cycle is unknown.[425] The existence of defective interfering (DI) particles has been suggested, but not confirmed experimentally for caliciviruses.[486]

Release

Virus progeny can be detected in cell culture medium within hours of infection, prior to visible cytopathic effect and cell lysis. One mechanism for this early nonlytic release may involve the egress of viruses within exosomal vesicles, utilizing intracellular membrane trafficking pathways.[515] Eventually, calicivirus-infected cells undergo cell death and lysis, and it is presumed that the majority of progeny viruses are released during this process. The triggering of apoptosis has been associated with calicivirus infection both *in vitro*[12,64,172,423,550] and *in vivo*,[104,270,413,418,490,604] and apoptotic changes in cellular membranes may be one of the death mechanisms by which cells lyse and release viral particles.

PATHOGENESIS AND PATHOLOGY

Caliciviruses cause a broad range of diseases in many different animal hosts (Table 4.4). This section will focus on the noroviruses, but there are important common themes in pathogenesis shared by all caliciviruses. Illnesses range from mild to life threatening, and evidence exists for the emergence of calicivirus strains with increased virulence. Asymptomatic infections occur in susceptible populations,[360,474] and shedding of virus can occur days to weeks after resolution of acute symptoms.[25,177,288,499] Caliciviruses can establish a chronic carrier state in a number of hosts, with varying proposed mechanisms of persistence.[121,191,617]

Adult volunteer studies have been successful in defining important features of human norovirus gastroenteritis, pathogenesis, and immunity.[255] Presently, there is no animal model that directly recapitulates the full range of disease symptoms observed in humans (see *Clinical Features*),[651] but animals in which evidence for infection has been reported following challenge with human noroviruses include gnotobiotic piglets[104] and calves,[554] monkeys[498,561] and chimpanzees,[63,657] and immunocompromised mice.[578] In addition, much information about norovirus biology has been learned from MNV infection of mice as detailed below.[263]

Entry into the Host

Noroviruses enter the body predominantly via the oral route. Studies in human volunteers demonstrated that the Norwalk, Hawaii, Montgomery County, and Snow Mountain viruses induced gastroenteritis when administered orally.[140,141,247,331,411,555,656] Virions are acid stable, consistent with an ability to survive passage through the stomach. Indirect evidence from epidemiologic studies suggests that human noroviruses can enter also via aerosols, such as those generated by the explosive vomiting that often occurs during illness.[86,90,289,383,384,464] During experimental infection, MNV is also infectious via intranasal and intracerebral routes during experimental infection,[265] while human noroviruses establish an enteric infection in gnotobiotic piglets[104] and chimpanzees[63] when administered by the intravenous route.

The mechanism by which caliciviruses enter the host following exposure by various routes remains ill-defined. Studies with MNV have demonstrated a critical role for microfold (M) cells as the portal of entry into the host intestine.[264] M cells are specialized intestinal epithelial cells primarily located in follicle-associated epithelium overlaying mucosa-associated lymphoid tissues. These cells transcytose particulate antigen from the lumen into the host interior. Mice deficient in Peyer patches (small intestinal lymphoid follicles) and associated M cells are resistant to oral infection with at least two MNV strains (MNV-1 and MNV.CR3).[297] Furthermore, antibody depletion of M cells via successive rounds of anti-RANKL antibody administration in Balb/c mice significantly reduced MNV infectious titers in multiple intestinal sites and in fecal shedding.[187] The ability of MNV to be transcytosed across an intestinal epithelial monolayer via M cells was also recapitulated in cell culture.[186] No infection of M cells was observed either *in vitro* or *in vivo*, consistent with the absence of expression of the MNV receptor CD300lf in this cell type. Thus, M cells are not an MNV target cell but instead mediate viral transport across the epithelial monolayer for subsequent infection of target cells. Whether M cells play a similar role during infection with other noroviruses or caliciviruses in general is unknown.

Site of Primary Replication

The tissue site of primary replication has been established for MNV. Depending on the virus strain, infection initiates in Peyer patches of the distal small intestine (MNV-1 strain), or in the cecum (MNV.CR3 strain), following M cell transcytosis.[187,190] For other noroviruses, there is evidence for primary replication in the upper intestinal tract. Consistent with this, human intestinal enteroids derived from the small intestine (jejunum, duodenum, ileum) but not the large intestine (colon) support human norovirus infection *in vitro*.[118,160] Further support comes from *in vivo* analysis. Jejunal biopsies of volunteers who develop gastrointestinal illness following oral administration of Norwalk or Hawaii virus exhibit histopathologic lesions.[4,142,520,521] Histologic lesions are not observed in the gastric fundus, antrum, or rectal mucosa of volunteers with NV-induced illness.[644] During acute infection, a broadening and blunting of the villi of the proximal small intestine and infiltration of mononuclear cells occur. Characteristic jejunal lesions have also been observed in volunteers who were fed NV or Hawaii virus but who did not become ill.[398,520,521] Cellular infiltrates and villus blunting are also observed in pediatric patients infected with human norovirus[413] and in duodenal biopsies from immunocompetent individuals with acute norovirus gastroenteritis.[604] For large animal caliciviruses, blunting and atrophy of the villi is observed in the small intestines of pigs infected with PEC, a sapovirus,[169] and in newborn calves infected with Jena virus, a bovine norovirus.[458]

Cell and Tissue Tropism

MNV has an established dual target cell tropism of immune cells and tuft cells, a specialized intestinal epithelial cell type.[652]

Cellular tropism is determined by expression of the viral receptor CD300lf on cells,[454] but genetic differences among MNV strains may influence *in vivo* tropism. Consistent with this, CD300lf-expressing immune cells in gastrointestinal lymphoid tissues have been established as the primary target cells for many MNV strains (such as MNV-1) during acute infection.[190] Certain other MNV strains (such as CR6) have been detected in rare CD300lf-expressing tuft cells[645] during persistent infection. It is not yet clear whether these strains also infect tuft cells during the initial infection to establish the persistent reservoir. MNV also infects inflammatory monocytes and neutrophils, which can promote dissemination of the virus under certain conditions.[617] The *in vivo* tropism for immune cells is largely recapitulated *in vitro*, whereby MNV infects macrophages, dendritic cells, and T and B cells in culture.[190,248,653]

The cellular tropisms of other noroviruses will not be clarified until their entry receptors are identified. To date, immunofluorescence studies of intestinal biopsies from immunocompromised patients detected norovirus capsid antigen-positive cells in enterocytes at the villus tips and cells positive for CD3, CD68, or DC-SIGN, which are markers for T cells, macrophages, and dendritic cells, respectively.[260] In this same study, co-localization of capsid and nonstructural protein expression was observed only in enterocytes, leading the authors to conclude that epithelial cells could support viral replication.[260] A non-epithelial tropism is consistent with a previous study in humans, in which Sakai virus (a GII norovirus) was shown to bind to cells within the lamina propria and Brunner glands of human duodenum but not the epithelium.[94] However, in another binding study, NV virus VLPs bound to the surface of epithelial cells in human biopsies, but not lamina propria.[382] Chimpanzees infected with NV displayed NV capsid antigen-positive cells within the lamina propria of the upper small intestine.[63] GII.4 human norovirus antigen was detected in macrophages in immunocompromised mice[578] and in enterocytes in the duodenum and jejunum of gnotobiotic piglets.[104] Lastly, macrophages, dendritic cells, and lymphocytes were positive for GII human norovirus capsid protein in miniature piglets.[527] Taken together, these data implicate the involvement of epithelial and non-epithelial cell types during human norovirus infection. However, binding of virus or VLPs to tissue or the presence of capsid antigen in cells may not necessarily reflect active replication. Thus, it will be critical in the future to confirm these findings with additional evidence such as the detection of negative-sense RNA as was demonstrated with MNV.[190]

Two newly developed *in vitro* culture systems support a possible dual-tropic nature of human noroviruses. Some GII human noroviruses infect established human B-cell lines in culture.[248] Infection is dependent on the viral attachment factor HBGA, in synthetic form or expressed by commensal bacteria. In a second cell culture model, multiple human norovirus strains were shown to replicate in human intestinal organoids derived from the small intestine.[160] Only differentiated cultures enriched in mature enterocytes (i.e., absorptive columnar intestinal epithelial cells) supported infection. Bile enhanced or was required for viral replication in a virus genotype-dependent manner. This culture system also recapitulated the dependence of some genotypes on HBGAs. However, in contrast to the B-cell system, HBGAs were expressed on the surface of the intestinal epithelial cells.

While noroviruses infect many different mammals, bovine norovirus is the only other norovirus whose cellular tropism has been investigated to date. Following Jena virus infection of calves, intestinal epithelial cells stained positive for capsid antigens in the cytoplasm, while macrophage-like cells in the lamina propria and Peyer patch domes contained capsid antigen-positive granular deposits.[458] Whether the latter represent phagocytosed infected epithelial cells as proposed by the authors or bona fide infected cells remains to be determined. To date, no cell culture system has been described for bovine noroviruses to verify the cellular tropism.

Taken together, the long-held assumption that noroviruses exclusively infect intestinal epithelial cells has changed over the past decade. Recent data support a more complex tropism and interplay of intestinal epithelial and nonepithelial cells during norovirus pathogenesis. Additional studies in humans with fully functioning immune systems and with norovirus strains from different genogroups as well as different mammalian hosts are required to reveal the complete extent of the cell and tissue tropism for viruses across the family.

Spread in the Host

Following virus replication at the initial site of infection, noroviruses can spread inside the host beyond the initial site of replication in the intestine. In the case of MNV, the extent of extraintestinal spread is strain dependent. The acutely replicating strain MNV-1 (isolates CW3 or CW1) and the persistently replicating strain MNV.CR3 can spread to mesenteric lymph nodes and the spleen but less frequently to the liver or lung.[418,580] Other persistent strains (e.g., MNV.CR6, MNV-3) typically do not spread beyond the mesenteric lymph nodes.[252,437] Spread to secondary lymphoid tissues is mediated by CD11c-positive dendritic cells, since MNV.CR3 is unable to spread to the mesenteric lymph nodes or spleen when these cells are depleted from mice.[150] In the case of MNV-1, systemic spread was mediated by recruitment of susceptible monocytes and neutrophils following virus-triggered inflammation.[617]

Human norovirus RNA has not been detected in the sera of immunocompetent infected adult volunteers.[432] However, there are reports of the detection of norovirus RNA in various clinical specimens, suggesting that under certain conditions, the virus might spread beyond the initial site of infection in the intestine. Viral RNA has been detected in the serum and cerebrospinal fluid of a 23-month-old patient with encephalopathy.[241] Norovirus has also been associated with cases of benign convulsions with mild gastroenteritis[277] and more severe outcomes of encephalitis/encephalopathy, particularly in very young children.[531] However, only stool samples were tested for viral RNA, and/or viral RNA was undetectable in the cerebrospinal fluid. Additional studies have also detected human norovirus RNA in the serum of some patients, suggesting viremia occurs under some circumstances, such as in the context of very young patient age, increased disease severity, and/or high viral loads during acute norovirus gastroenteritis.[233,494,567]

Immune Response

Immunity to noroviruses in humans is poorly understood. Human norovirus infections can be symptomatic or asymptomatic, with up to one-third of individuals being asymptomatically infected.[431] Resistance to norovirus illness involves a complex interplay between host genetics (see *Mechanisms of Attachment*), immune status, and exposure to evolving norovirus strains. Studies in the MNV mouse model have demonstrated that innate immune responses control the extent of norovirus infection, while adaptive immune responses are critical in clearing infection.

Innate Immunity

The innate immune response is of critical importance in limiting norovirus infection and initiating memory-generating adaptive responses. Human norovirus replication is inhibited by exogenous type I, II, or III interferon (IFN) treatment *in vitro* and *in vivo*.[100,127,250,482] A screen of known interferon-stimulated genes (ISGs) in NV replicon-containing cells identified IRF1, RIG-I, and MDA5 as potent anti-norovirus effectors, while RTP4 and HPSE had moderate antiviral activity.[127] Paradoxically, no IFN-β responses or ISGs are induced during human norovirus RNA replication (GI.1 and GII.3) following transfection or addition of VLPs in transformed cells.[127,482] However, no data are yet available regarding innate antiviral responses during human norovirus infection in primary cells. Innate immune responses are also critically important in the control of MNV infections.[35] Indeed, MNV-1 causes a disseminated, lethal infection in certain mouse strains deficient in components of the innate immune system (i.e., STAT1, IFNAR/IFNAGR double knockout, or IRF3/5/7 triple knockout)[265,320] and replicates to higher titers in mice deficient in pattern recognition receptors (specifically MDA5, TLR3, and NLRP6) or interferon signal transduction components (IRF1, IRF3, IRF7).[379,585,631] Similarly, HOIL-1 (heme-oxidized IRP2 ubiquitin ligase-1), a component of LUBAC (linear ubiquitin chain assembly complex), which mediates type I and III IFN induction via MDA5 and IRF3, also reduces viral infection.[371] For the persistent MNV.CR6 strain, mice with the aforementioned defects display higher viral loads and increased fecal shedding (i.e., IFNLR1 −/−, STAT1−/−) or systemic infection (i.e., IFNAR−/−). In most cases, increased viral replication is also seen *in vitro* in bone marrow–derived macrophages and dendritic cells lacking these molecules, confirming the essential role of IFN signaling for control of MNV infection at the cellular and host level. One of the ISGs that has been further investigated during infection is ISG15. It limits MNV infection early in the viral life cycle during entry or uncoating.[500] Taken together, a picture emerges whereby type I IFNs control systemic MNV infection in myeloid cells, while type III IFNs control persistent infection in tuft cells. Opposing these multiple host defense mechanisms is the viral protein VF1 (virulence factor 1), which delays the IFN response via an unknown mechanism.[397] Other mediators of the intrinsic host response also exhibit anti-MNV activity. Specifically, autophagy-related gene proteins (i.e., Atg5, Atg7, Atg12, Atg16L1) mark viral replication complexes and recruit interferon-inducible GTPases to block viral replication in an IFN-dependent manner.[54] In addition, a recent genome-wide CRISPR activation screen in HeLa cells expressing the MNV receptor CD300lf identified a number of genes with anti-MNV activity that functioned not only in IFN signaling and cytokine responses but also in genes involved in RNA polymerase expression and embryogenesis.[454] Transcriptomic analysis showed that innate immune pathways are major response pathways of cells to MNV infection.[154,330]

Other caliciviruses have also been shown to be sensitive to various types of interferon *in vitro*, and infections are limited by ISGs.[98,100,101,283,346,408,663]

Adaptive Immunity

Information about human norovirus immunity comes largely from human volunteer studies and vaccine trials, and identifying determinants of protective immunity is still an area of active investigation. Early volunteer studies in adults established that protection from reinfection is relatively short, ranging from 2 months to 2 years, in susceptible individuals.[247,462,492] Investigations of natural human norovirus infections in children indicated protection of up to 3 years.[58] In contrast, a mathematical model estimated the duration of human norovirus immunity to be slightly longer, ranging from 4 to 9 years.[537] Protective immunity induced by a single MNV infection waned after a few months.[674]

The discovery that NV and other human noroviruses utilize HBGAs as attachment factors has led to the development of assays to measure HBGA carbohydrate–blocking activity (or "blockade") of serum antibodies.[350] Since antibodies that block binding of norovirus VLPs to HBGA glycans correlate with protection from illness in adult volunteers, HBGA-blocking assays have been used as surrogate tests for neutralization in the absence of traditional cell culture-based virus neutralization assays.[339,492] Application of this technique in the first efficacy study of norovirus vaccines in adult volunteers showed a correlation between levels of prechallenge HBGA-blocking titers and protection from illness.[22] A hemagglutination-inhibition assay (HAI) was another surrogate assay used to analyze serum antibodies and was shown also to correlate with protection from illness in volunteers challenged with NV.[125,237] Studies in adult volunteers further demonstrated that higher titer prechallenge or postchallenge serum antibodies that blocked norovirus binding to HBGA glycans correlated with protection from gastroenteritis.[22,492] In addition, development of a rapid mucosal IgA response (indicating prior exposure to NV or a related norovirus) was also associated with resistance to illness following challenge with NV.[341] In another NV challenge study, NV-specific salivary IgA and NV-specific memory IgG cells were identified as correlates of protection from gastroenteritis, while prechallenge levels of NV-specific fecal IgA correlated with reduced viral loads.[489] In the case of a GII.4 volunteer study, higher prechallenge levels of serum IgA antibodies were also associated with less illness and a lower frequency of infection.[23]

The anti–norovirus antibody responses following primary infections in children are not only short-lived but also of low avidity.[442] Primary infections in children generate blocking antibodies that provide homotypic protection, while heterotypic protection develops over time and with additional infections.[59,378] Studies indicate that during the first year of life, a child may have one to three norovirus infections.[60,362,509] Higher avidity antibodies were detected in older children following repeat infections and protection correlated with the ability to block HBGA binding.[442] Timing of the first norovirus infection appears to be determined by the quality of the maternal antibodies. In a study following two children from birth to age 8, higher titer, greater avidity, and increased HBGA-blocking ability of maternal antibodies correlated with longer protection and a later time point in life of the first infection.[58]

The antibody responses that develop to human noroviruses can be strain, genotype, genogroup, or intergenogroup specific. Strain-specific or genotype-specific epitopes are often located in the hypervariable VP1 P2 domain,[84,176] while more broadly reactive epitopes are commonly found in the more conserved VP1 S and P1 domains.[123,460] Similarly, antibodies to MNV directed against the P domain are strain or genotype specific, while the S domain antibody was broadly cross-reactive and even recognized human norovirus VLPs.[300] However, only antibodies directed to the MNV P domain had neutralizing activity.[269,300]

An *in vitro* culture system for human norovirus has enabled analysis of true neutralizing activities.[160] Characterization of a panel of pandemic GII.4 Sydney reactive human monoclonal IgG and IgA antibodies identified three major antigenic epitopes in the P domain, and most showed neutralization capabilities in the two surrogate neutralization assays: of those tested, all inhibited norovirus replication in human intestinal enteroid monolayers.[13] The majority of tested mAbs had lower neutralization titers than blockade or HAI titers, indicating that the true neutralization assay is more sensitive than either surrogate assay and thus that additional factors beyond glycan interaction contribute to virus neutralization.

In addition to B-cell responses, human norovirus infection also leads to Th1-skewed immunity with some Th2 involvement. When cell-mediated immune responses were studied in volunteers following oral immunization with NV rVLPs, an increase in IFN-γ in the absence of IL-4 production was detected, consistent with a dominant Th-1 pattern of cytokine production.[566] Serum sample analysis from two human norovirus challenge studies with NV demonstrated a rise in Th1 (IFN-γ, IL-2, IL12p70, TNF-α) and Th2 cytokines (IL-6, IL-10) as well as IL-8 and MCP-1 in infected versus uninfected volunteers.[434] Cytokines peaked at day 2 postchallenge. In a study of 15 volunteers infected with Snow Mountain virus (GII.2), significant increases in serum IFN-γ, IL-2 (Th1 cytokines), and IL-5 (a Th2 cytokine), but not IL-6 or IL-10, were detected on day 2 after challenge.[340] Depletion of CD4+ cells prior to stimulation of peripheral blood mononuclear cells with norovirus antigen led to a decrease in IFN-γ, implicating these T cells as the major source of this cytokine.[340] The Th1 cytokines IFN-γ and TNF-α, but also the Th2 cytokine IL-6, were secreted following stimulation of PBMCs with GII.4 VLPs.[477] IFN-γ is also secreted following VLP stimulation of PBMCs from eight healthy human donors previously infected by human norovirus.[377] This study also identified a peptide in the VP1 S domain from two donors as a CD8+ T-cell epitope. Evidence for cross-reactive T-cell epitopes shared among different norovirus genogroups and genotypes was found in mice immunized with human and MNVs VLPs.[349]

The combined action of T and B cells is critical to clear human norovirus infection since the lack of functional T- and B-cell responses in immunocompromised patients results in chronic norovirus infection.[91,191] Immune reconstitution following gene therapy and improvement of T-cell levels have both been associated with clearance of chronic human norovirus infection.[130,648]

A similar picture has emerged from studies of the MNV model. Mice lacking T cells and/or B cells (i.e., Rag1−/−, μMT−/−, Ighm−/−) or their function are persistently infected by the acute strain MNV-1, while transfer of antibody, splenocytes, or T cells reduced persistent viral loads and could clear infection.[88,89,265,673] In contrast, persistent MNV strains (e.g., MNV.CR6) elicited fewer virus-specific T cells and generated less effective T-cell responses compared to acute MNV-1 infection.[599] While the MNV.CR6-specific CD8+ T cells were functional, they were unable to detect viral replication in intestinal epithelial tuft cells, an immune-privileged site, enabling persistence[600] (see *Persistence*).

Taken together, individual human volunteer studies have identified several antibody-based correlates of protection from illness or infection.[488] Work in the mouse model has also indicated a role for cell-mediated and innate immunity in protection. Future studies with larger cohorts will be needed to identify the best predictor of protection while simultaneously increasing our knowledge of human norovirus immunity.

Release from Host and Transmission

Noroviruses are released from the enteric tract of the host in feces and have been detected also in vomitus.[194,195,274,396] Viral RNA can be detected in feces before the onset of symptoms and shedding in stool can last several days to weeks in immunocompetent individuals[25,179,189,197,452] and even longer in immunocompromised patients.[21,191] Studies of the natural history of norovirus in a community found that 26% of the examined 99 patients shed virus (detected by RT-PCR) up to 3 weeks after the onset of illness, with the highest rate (38%) of prolonged shedding in children younger than 1 year of age.[499] This observation indicates that infected individuals recovering from norovirus illness can continue to shed virus beyond the symptomatic period, a finding that has implications in the management of outbreaks.[445] In addition, a time-course study comparing shedding of 102 asymptomatic and symptomatic individuals detected no difference in the duration of shedding (average 8–60 days) and peak amounts of virus shed.[584] Norovirus RNA has been detected in washings from the mouths of individuals who experienced norovirus infection for several days after symptoms subsided, suggesting that oral-to-oral transmission of norovirus might occur.[287] The detection of norovirus RNA in the sera of children with gastroenteritis has been reported, but it is not known whether this RNA corresponds to that of circulating infectious virus (viremia) or noninfectious (inactivated) virus present in circulating immune cells.[567]

Noroviruses are spread by several modes of transmission. The predominant modes of transmission for the noroviruses are person-to-person contact and food- or waterborne spread.[313] Contamination of surfaces and objects by infected individuals can lead to inadvertent exposure.[357] Several epidemiological investigations have also linked exposure to noroviruses in air or in aerosolized vomitus with infection.[65,87,286,289] However, in infected volunteers, norovirus RNA in vomitus is less frequent and detected at lower amounts than in stool samples.[26]

The explosive nature of some norovirus outbreaks, in which a large number of persons become ill within 24 to 48 hours, indicates that infection is often acquired from a common source. This was suggested in the original NV outbreak, but a common-source exposure could not be identified.[3] Later, a review of 38 human norovirus-associated outbreaks suggested that a common source of infection was likely in 31 (82%).[257] The vehicle of transmission was water in 13 instances and food

in 4 others. Secondary transmission was observed in most outbreaks, with attack rates ranging from 4% to 32% and being highest in children under 10 years of age. The median duration of the 38 outbreaks was 7 days (ranging from 1 day to 3 months). The number of individuals who became ill ranged from 2 to 2,000, with the attack rate being higher in common-source outbreaks (median 60%, range 23%–93%) than in primary person-to-person outbreaks (median 39%, range 31%–42%).[258] A similar attack rate from children with norovirus diarrhea (33%) was observed in a household transmission study, while the attack rates of asymptomatic controls were lower (18%).[178] The efficient transmission of human caliciviruses by contaminated food and water vehicles has raised concerns about public safety in a global market economy.[491]

The infectious dose for noroviruses is low, with an estimated median infectious dose of 18–1,015 genome equivalents.[583] Another human volunteer challenge study determined the 50% human infectious dose for NV at approximately 1,230 genome equivalents for blood group O and A individuals and approximately 2,800 for all secretor-positive individuals.[26] Exposure to higher levels of virus likely increases the risk of illness.[363] In a study that examined norovirus fecal load, higher numbers (>100-fold) of norovirus genome copies were detected in individuals shedding GII (median, 3.0×10^8 genome copies per gram feces) strains compared to GI (median, 8.4×10^5 genome copies per gram feces).[96] It was proposed that the higher levels of GII shedding might account for a higher transmissibility of these viruses through the fecal–oral route.[96] However, high levels of GI shedding have also been reported: the median peak of GI NV shed in the stool of 16 volunteers was 9.5×10^{10} genome copies per gram feces.[25]

Noroviruses are remarkably stable. Norwalk virus retains infectivity for volunteers following (a) exposure of the stool filtrate to pH 2.7 for 3 hours at room temperature, (b) treatment with 20% ether at 4°C for 18 hours, or (c) incubation at 60°C for 30 minutes.[141] Norwalk virions remain infectious when stored in groundwater at room temperature in the dark for as long as 61 days, and RNA could be detected in such samples after storage at room temperature for 3 years.[526] Using the new human intestinal organoid culture system, GII.4 noroviruses in human stool samples have for the first time been tested directly for their inactivation patterns.[118] Virions were not completely inactivated by 5-minute incubation in 70% ethanol or 70% isopropanol, although some reduction in viral infectivity was observed. However, infectivity was effectively destroyed by 1 minute in greater than 50 ppm chlorine, while viral RNA was only destroyed at concentrations of greater than 600 ppm. This demonstrates that previous human norovirus inactivation studies using measurements of RNA integrity should be re-evaluated using the more sensitive infectivity–based culture systems.

Although norovirus virions are highly stable and are shed at high levels, the viral RNA-dependent RNA polymerase introduces many mutations, the majority of which are expected to be lethal.[513] Furthermore, the host's gastrointestinal tract is large (i.e., the human intestine is the size of half a badminton court)[217] and covered with host mucins that can inhibit norovirus VLP binding to HBGAs and Caco-2 cells.[596] Thus, how noroviruses maintain their high infectivity and achieve high recombination rates (which requires coinfection of cells with at least two virions) was puzzling. A recent study has provided evidence of multiple murine and human norovirus particles packaged into membrane-cloaked vesicles in the stool of infected hosts.[515] Studies in the rotavirus mouse model demonstrated that these virion-containing vesicles improve viral infection. Previous studies have also demonstrated that multiple norovirus virions bind to various bacterial species.[11] In the case of poliovirus, this concentration of virions on intestinal bacteria facilitated coinfection and recombination.[156] These data suggest that aggregation of virus particles via vesicles or bacteria likely increases norovirus coinfection rates and complementation via recombination, which results in increased infectivity and viral shedding.[405]

Virulence

Virulence determinants are being defined mechanistically for MNV but have not been well defined for the human noroviruses. Studies with MNV have identified determinants that fall into three general groups: host determinants (see *Immune Response*), virus determinants, and the microbiota[35] (see below).

Viral Determinants

The ability to genetically manipulate MNV has resulted in the identification of various roles in pathogenesis for multiple viral proteins. The viral proteins NS1/2, virulence factor 1 (VF1) encoded by ORF4, and both the major and minor capsid proteins VP1 and VP2 are known to play critical role during pathogenesis. The nonstructural protein NS1/2 (N-term) determines colonic tropism and viral persistence[440] (see *Persistence*). VF1 antagonizes the antiviral innate immune response, and thus VF1-deletion viruses are attenuated *in vivo*.[397] VF1 may also play a role in the induction of protective immunity via regulation of cytokine induction.[674] VP1 is linked to virulence. Specifically, a single amino acid (residue 296) in the variable P2 domain of VP1, which arises during tissue culture passage and persistent infection, contributes to virulence of MNV.[32,556,653,675] Viruses with a lysine at this position are more virulent and cause increased lethality in mice, while those with a glutamic acid are attenuated. However, the importance of this residue differs depending on mouse background, and additional virulence determinants are present in the VP1 P domain that contribute to viral replication, histopathology, and lethality in STAT1-deficient mice.[556] Although not sufficient, the S domain may also contribute to virulence.[556] Additional residues in the VP1 P1 and P2 domains contribute to *in vitro* B-cell (but not macrophage) growth and replication *in vivo*.[675] Lastly, studies of viruses from the same cluster revealed that VP2 controls antigen presentation in B cells and macrophages *in vitro* and induction of protective immunity *in vivo*.[673,674] Specifically, VP2 of the MNV-3 strain, which induced higher systemic and mucosal antibody responses compared to MNV-1, induced upregulation of antigen presentation in macrophages and enhanced protective immunity.[674] In contrast, VP2 of MNV-1 (but not MNV-3) induced upregulation of antigen presentation molecules on B cells, which contributed to the control of acute MNV-1 infection.[673] These striking cell-type and virus-strain–specific differences observed with MNV suggest that similar phenomena likely exist for human noroviruses and animal caliciviruses. Indeed, virus strain–specific differences in clinical outcome, ranging from asymptomatic infection to life-threatening diarrhea, are observed[234] (Table 4.4).

Norovirus–Microbiota Interactions

Noroviruses encounter members of the microbiota (a collection of bacteria, viruses, fungi, and other microorganisms) during intestinal infection. Human noroviruses, for example, bind to selected pathogenic and nonpathogenic bacterial species.[11,407] Binding was mediated by HBGA-like molecules on the bacteria.[407] It remains unclear whether interactions can be mediated by other factors or whether other noroviruses can similarly bind to bacteria. The microbiota influences viral pathogenesis by direct and indirect mechanisms.[261] Direct effects of bacterial binding to human noroviruses described to date are (a) increased heat stability[333] and (b) enhanced attachment and infection of human BJAB B cells by human norovirus.[248] Indirect mechanisms are those whereby the microbiota induces host cell responses that affect viral pathogenesis via innate or adaptive immunity. Interestingly, MNV can replace the beneficial effects of the microbiota via type I IFN signaling in the absence of commensal bacteria.[272] Studies in the MNV system have revealed multiple reciprocal interactions between the host, the virus, and the microbiome. In IL10- or ATG16L1-deficient mice (i.e., models for inflammatory bowel disease), MNV infection causes intestinal inflammation in the presence of the microbiota.[44,82] MNV can also exacerbate intestinal inflammation and lethality during bacterial superinfection by enhancing host responses.[282] Commensal bacteria are critical for the establishment of persistent MNV infection in a mechanism dependent on intact IFN-λ responses.[34] In the case of acute MNV infection, commensal bacteria and host secretory immunoglobulins are needed for a homeostatic environment conducive to infection, as the lack of secretory immunoglobulins or commensal bacteria leads to reduced infection.[610] Commensal bacteria also suppress the maintenance of an antiviral antibody response. For human noroviruses, a link between the abundance of specific bacterial species, host genetics, and antinorovirus IgA antibodies is observed.[501] Another member of the microbiota, helminths, also has immunomodulatory functions. Colonization of the host by helminths resulted in immune skewing that resulted in reduced antiviral immunity to MNV infection and thus elevated viral loads.[456,645] While these examples speak to the ability of the host and the microbiota to influence norovirus pathogenesis, norovirus infections under some circumstances may also influence the bacterial communities in the intestine. A subset (~20%) of human norovirus–infected patients exhibited bacterial dysbiosis characterized by increased *Proteobacteria*.[428] Bacterial communities remained mostly unaltered during infection of mice with multiple MNV strains under standard housing conditions.[427] However, dramatic alterations in the intestinal bacteria were observed under malnutrition conditions in mice.[221] Therefore, a complex network of interactions occurs between the host, the microbiota, and noroviruses.

Persistence

Human noroviruses have been associated with prolonged infections in immunocompromised patients, including those with primary immunodeficiencies and transplant patients.[470] For example, nine adult patients receiving kidney allografts and undergoing immunosuppression were shown to shed norovirus for periods ranging from 97 to 898 days.[519] Another study described a chronic norovirus infection lasting at least 6 years in an immunocompromised patient with X-linked syndrome.[138] Chronic norovirus shedders can contribute to nosocomial transmissions[562] and were proposed to be a source of emergent norovirus infections.[262] However, the full contribution of chronic norovirus infections to disease burden remains unclear.

The ability of noroviruses to persist in infected hosts is well established for MNV, and differences in pathogenicity have been documented among MNV strains. While MNV-1 (isolated following a series of intracranial injections in RAG/STAT1-deficient animals)[265] causes an acute and rapidly cleared infection in immunocompetent animals, certain other MNV strains (characteristically isolated from feces) can establish persistent infection in the intestine with shedding for at least 35 days.[439,586] Studies using MNV have demonstrated that persistence occurs in the face of a robust cytotoxic T-cell response[600] but the infection can be cleared by the action of the innate immune response, specifically IFN-λ.[34,437,563] Genetic studies with the acute MNV-1.CW3 and persistent MNV.CR6 strains revealed a unique role for IFN-λ in the intestinal epithelium in concert with the viral NS1/2 protein in establishment of persistence. NS1/2, and in particular a single amino acid residue (glutamic acid at position 94), is necessary and sufficient for replication in the large intestine and persistence.[440] The reservoir of persistent norovirus infection is in intestinal epithelial cells, specifically tuft cells.[326,645] The ability of MNV.CR6 to persist in these specialized intestinal epithelial cells is dependent on the NS1 protein, which antagonizes IFN-λ–mediated antiviral immunity.[326] Hence, chimeric MNV-1 carrying the MNV.CR6 NS1 gene or MNV-1 infection of mice lacking the IFN-λ receptor similarly leads to persistence. In addition, the viral capsid protein VP1 further contributes to persistence in a dose-dependent manner since high infectious doses of MNV-1.CW3 only established persistent infection when carrying both the mutation in NS1 (E94) and VP1 of MNV.CR6.[437] When MNV-1.CW3 was carrying its own VP1, however, high doses elicited strong stimulation of type I and III IFN responses in Peyer patches and mesenteric lymph nodes, leading to eventual clearance.[437] Interestingly, depletion of the intestinal microbiota via antibiotics also prevented the establishment of persistent MNV.CR6 infection.[34] The phenotype did not occur in IFNLR-deficient animals, further pointing to the importance of IFN-λ during persistent norovirus infection in the intestine. On the other hand, type I IFNs only play a role during systemic infection, and deletion of IFNAR on CD11c-positive myeloid cells permits persistence of MNV-1.[438] Furthermore, adaptive immunity does not regulate intestinal persistence, although it is required for clearing systemic infections.[88] Taken together, MNV persistence is controlled by a combination of viral (NS1, VP1, and maybe others) and host factors (in particular, IFN-λ) and further modulated by the microbiota.

EPIDEMIOLOGY

Age

Noroviruses have been associated with infection and disease in all age groups.[202] Age is a risk factor for severe disease, with infants and young children (<5 years old)[213,473] and older adults (>65 years old)[342] at highest risk. A review of pediatric cases in over 5,000 infants and young children in 23 countries found that approximately 70% of noroviruses illnesses occurred

between 6 and 23 months of age, with less than 15% occurring in the first 6 months of life.[532] Norovirus infection has also been detected in neonates[400,609] and preterm infants,[18] with varying clinical manifestations.

Morbidity and Mortality

Although precise data on morbidity and mortality are not available,[9] recent estimates confirm their predominant role in diarrheal disease. Global estimates of norovirus illness have projected nearly 700 million cases and 218,800 deaths annually.[5,43] In the surveillance period following efficacious rotavirus vaccination in pediatric populations, norovirus has emerged as the single most important cause of life-threatening gastroenteritis in infants and young children.[74,303,466] In a review of 39 published studies that surveyed severe gastroenteritis in individuals older than 65 years of age, norovirus was responsible for an approximate 10% to 20% of hospitalizations and 10% to 15% of all-cause gastroenteritis deaths.[342]

Morbidity is reflected in the number of hospitalizations due to norovirus disease. In the United States, an estimated 71,000 hospitalizations were associated with norovirus gastroenteritis each year, at a cost of $493 million per year, and an estimated 570 to 800 deaths.[202,358] In Germany, an estimated 53,000 to 90,000 hospitalizations per year were attributed to norovirus gastroenteritis with an annual cost of €31 to 43 million.[308] An estimated 4,000 to 11,000 hospitalizations per year were associated with norovirus in Canada.[415] Of patients hospitalized in Canada from 2001 to 2004, noroviruses were responsible for a mean hospitalization incidence rate of 1.6 cases per 100,000, and the average age of hospitalized patients was 59 years old.[506] Over this 4-year period, 43 deaths were attributed to noroviruses, making it a leading cause of mortality among the enteric pathogens studied.[506] In England, noroviruses were the second largest cause of hospitalization due to gastroenteritis (after *Campylobacter*)[511] and have likely been underestimated.[622] This results in an estimated 0.3 to 1.2 years of healthy life lost per thousand cases of norovirus.[214] Noroviruses are also an important cause of illness in China, detected in 29% of adults and the elderly and 22% in children 6 to 35 months old with acute gastroenteritis.[672] An estimated 171,000 hospitalizations per year in Japan were modeled from a review of medical insurance claims.[97] In Lebanon, noroviruses were detected in 11.2% of stool samples from children less than 5 years old presenting with acute gastroenteritis to six large hospitals over a 2-year period[399] and in 27% of children hospitalized for gastroenteritis in Spain.[185]

Noroviruses have been associated with increased morbidity and mortality in patients with an underlying illness such as cardiovascular disease or who are immunosuppressed or receiving cancer chemotherapy.[62,191,390] In a review of hospitalization and emergency room visits in the United States from July 2002 to December 2013, over 51% of the norovirus illnesses occurred in 37% of patients with a chronic medical condition who were hospitalized for gastroenteritis.[623]

Origin and Spread of Epidemics

Noroviruses are the single most important cause of nonbacterial gastroenteritis outbreaks. In an analysis of 233 nonbacterial gastroenteritis outbreaks reported to the Centers for Disease Control and Prevention (CDC) between July 1997 and June 2000, 217 (93%) were associated with noroviruses.[162] In a larger survey of 3,714 nonbacterial gastroenteritis outbreaks that occurred in Europe between 1995 and 2000, 85% were associated with norovirus.[359] A review of 666 norovirus outbreak reports from multiple countries linked 362 (54%) of these to foodborne illness, 174 (26%) to person-to-person transmission, 70 (11%) to water contamination, and 60 (9%) to environmental exposure.[389] Noroviruses are estimated to cause as many as 47% to 96% of acute gastroenteritis outbreaks in pediatric populations and 5% to 36% of sporadic cases.[157]

Norovirus outbreaks characteristically occur in settings that facilitate rapid person-to-person spread or single-source exposure to contaminated food, water, or surfaces. These settings include hospitals, long-term care facilities, camps (recreational and evacuee), recreational areas, schools, universities, daycare centers, cruise ships, stadiums, retirement centers, restaurants, social events with catered meals, families, the military, prisons, and community events. Outbreaks can vary in size, involving small family groups to hundreds of individuals.[240,660] Outbreaks can be prolonged, with recurring sharp peaks, and the modes of transmission can vary within an outbreak.[7,129] While norovirus infection occurs year-round, a seasonal pattern of occurrence (typically peaking in cooler months of the year) has been described that varies according to the climate of the region.[92,416,502] Food service and cooler months were risk factors for higher attack rates within outbreaks.[389]

Noroviruses are the leading cause of foodborne illness in the United States (followed by *Salmonella* (nontyphoidal), *Clostridium perfringens*, *Campylobacter* spp., and *Staphylococcus aureus*), accounting for approximately 26% of all reported outbreaks.[517] An analysis of 8,271 foodborne outbreaks reported to the CDC (1991–2000) showed that norovirus outbreaks were often larger than bacterial outbreaks (median persons affected: 25 vs. 15), with 10% of the affected individuals seeking medical care and 1% being hospitalized.[643] In a study of waterborne outbreaks in Finland, 18 (64%) of 28 outbreaks evaluated were associated with norovirus.[391] Bivalve mollusks (such as oysters and mussels) are an important cause of foodborne norovirus outbreaks.[291,356,370,395,414,639] In fact, a recent review of foodborne norovirus outbreaks identified shellfish and seafood as the most common foods implicated, followed by lettuce and raspberries.[210]

Noroviruses have been documented as important agents of gastroenteritis in military populations in different areas of the world.[19,68,225,354,393,495,593,633] Norovirus illness can be severe in troops who may already be physically stressed.[132] Large-scale outbreaks of gastroenteritis have been attributed to noroviruses on ships such as aircraft carriers on which hundreds of crew members became ill.[61,117,459,530]

Although the majority of traveler's diarrhea has been attributed to enterotoxigenic *Escherichia coli*,[55] prevalence rates ranging from 10% to 65% have been associated with norovirus.[538] The global distribution of diverse norovirus strains and limited use of diagnostic confirmation suggest that norovirus illnesses have been underestimated in traveler's diarrhea.[37,538] Norovirus transmission during airplane travel[290,592] in addition to that on recreational cruise ships[620,642] illustrates the potential ease with which strains can be spread globally.

Prevalence and Seroepidemiology

Norovirus has been estimated to cause a fifth of all acute gastroenteritis illnesses, consistent with its widespread distribution in the human population.[5] In a review of studies that incorporated norovirus diagnostic confirmation in approximately 190,000 patients, the overall prevalence of norovirus in individuals with acute gastroenteritis was 18%.[5] Norovirus prevalence rates in this report were 24%, 20%, and 17% in cases of acute gastroenteritis in the community, outpatient, and inpatient settings, respectively.[5] The prevalence of norovirus in pediatric populations has been evaluated in a birth cohort of 1,457 children in a multinational study (MAL-ED).[504] Approximately 89% of children had evidence of a norovirus infection by 2 years of age, and 22.7% of the diarrheal stools were norovirus positive.[504] The prevalence of antibody to the GII viruses appears to be greater than that of the GI viruses in most studies, likely reflecting the predominance of circulating GII strains.[504,615] In Finnish infants and children, aged 0 to 14 years, the antibody prevalence against GII.4 noroviruses reached 91.2% in children above 5 years of age.[442]

The incidence of norovirus gastroenteritis has been estimated in several community-based studies. In the United States, an enhanced surveillance study of acute gastroenteritis (that included pathogen identification with diagnostic assays) in a single state (Georgia) estimated that norovirus was the predominant cause of acute gastroenteritis, accounting for 6,500 (16%) and 640 (12%) per 100,000 person-years of community and outpatient acute gastroenteritis episodes, respectively.[203] In the Netherlands, 18% of the community cases of gastroenteritis over a single winter season and at least 5% of gastroenteritis cases that resulted in a visit to a physician were associated with norovirus infection.[304] Furthermore, a 1-year prospective population-based cohort study showed that noroviruses were the single most important cause of gastroenteritis overall in nearly all age groups in the Netherlands.[131] In Germany, the incidence of norovirus gastroenteritis in the community requiring medical attention was reported as 626 cases/100,000 person-years, making it the predominant known cause of acute gastroenteritis in that country.[266] In England, the community incidence of norovirus gastroenteritis was 4.5 cases/100 person-years, corresponding to approximately 2 million episodes per year.[474] In a community cohort study in the United Kingdom over a 1-year period (2007–2008), noroviruses were the most common organism detected, with incidence rates of 47 community cases per 1,000 person-years.[568] In China, the incidence was estimated to be 15.6/100 children/year among children less than 5 years of age.[672]

Genetic Diversity of Virus

Molecular epidemiologic studies have demonstrated a marked genetic diversity among circulating noroviruses.[613] Genetic typing of circulating strains has proven to be a useful tool in elucidating the source and spread of outbreaks,[312,621] and regional data sharing networks have been established in several areas of the world.[613] A dual genotyping system that identifies both the VP1 and NS7[Pol] has been developed to track the emergence of recombinant strains in the population.[311] The VP1 system is defined by the amino acid sequence identities of complete VP1 capsid proteins, which presumably would correlate with the antigenic specificity.[107,311,671] Classification of the VP1 shows the division of the genus *Norovirus* into 10 major phylogenetic genogroups, designated GI through GX, with two additional "nonassigned" (NA) genogroups pending (Table 4.5). Genogroups I, II, and III are further subdivided into 9, 26,

TABLE 4.5 Norovirus genogroups and genotypes as determined by VP1 relatedness

Reference Virus	Genogroup	Genetic Cluster	GenBank Accession Number
GI/Hu/US/1968/GI.1/Norwalk	I	1	M87661
GI/Hu/GB/1991/GI.2/Southampton	I	2	L07418
GI/Hu/SA/1990/GI.3/DesertShield395	I	3	U04469
GI/Hu/JP/1987/GI.4/Chiba407	I	4	AB022679
GI/Hu/GB/1989/GI.5/Musgrove	I	5	AJ277614
GI/Hu/DE/1997/GI.6/BS5(Hesse)	I	6	AF093797
GI/Hu/GB/1994/GI.7/Winchester	I	7	AJ277609
GI/Hu/US/2001/GI.8/Boxer	I	8	AF538679
GI/Hu/CA/2004/GI.9/Vancouver730	I	9	HQ637267
GII/Hu/US/1971/GII.1/Hawaii	II	1	U07611
GII/Hu/GB/1994/GII.2/Melksham	II	2	X81879
GII/Hu/CA/1991/GII.3/Toronto	II	3	U02030
GII/Hu/GB/1993/GII.4/Bristol	II	4	X76716
GII/Hu/GB/1990/GII.5/Hillingdon	II	5	AJ277607
GII/Hu/GB/1990/GII.6/Seacroft	II	6	AJ277620
GII/Hu/GB/1990/GII.7/Leeds	II	7	AJ277608
GII/Hu/NL/1998/GII.8/Amsterdam	II	8	AF195848
GII/Hu/US/1997/GII.9/VA97207	II	9	AY038599
GII/Hu/DE/2000/GII.10/Erfurt546	II	10	AF427118
GII/Po/JP/1997/GII.11/Sw918	II	11	AB074893
GII/Hu/GB/1990/GII.12/Wortley	II	12	AJ277618
GII/Hu/US/1998/GII.13/Fayetteville	II	13	AY113106
GII/Hu/US/1999/GII.14/M7	II	14	AY130761
GII/Hu/US/1999/GII.16/Tiffin	II	16	AY502010
GII/Hu/US/2002/GII.17/CS-E1	II	17	AY502009
GII/Po/US/2003/GII.18/OH-QW101	II	18	AY823304
GII/Po/US/2003/GII.19/OH-QW170	II	19	AY823306
GII/Hu/DE/2002/GII.20/Luckenwalde591	II	20	EU424333
GII/Hu/IQ/2002/GII.21/IF1998	II	21	AY675554
GII/Hu/JP/2003/GII.22/Yuri	II	22	AB083780
GII/Hu/PE/2010/GII.23/Loreto1847	II	23	KT290889
GII/Hu/PE/2013/GII.24/Loreto1972	II	24	KY225989
GII/Hu/CN/2007/GII.25/Beijing53931	II	25	GQ856469
GII/Hu/NI/2005/GII.26/Leon4509	II	26	KU306738
GII/Hu/PE/2012/GII.NA1/Loreto0959	II	27	MG495077
GII/Hu/PE/2013/GII.NA2/Loreto1257	II	NA2	MG495079
GII/Hu/PE/2008/GII.NA4/PNV06929	II	NA4	MG706448
GIII/Bo/DE/1980/GIII.1/Jena	III	1	AJ011099
GIII/Bo/GB/1976/GIII.2/Newbury	III	2	AF097917
GIII/Ov/NZ/2007/GIII.3/Norsewood30	III	3	EU193658
GIV/Hu/NL/1998/GIV.1/Alphatron	IV	1	AF195847
GIV/Ca/IT/2006/GIV.2/Pistoia	IV	2	EF450827
GIV/Hu/US/2016/GIV.NA1/WI7002	IV	NA1	KX907728
GV/Mu/US/2002/GV.1/MNV-1	V	1	AY228235
GV/Rn/HK/2011/GV.2/HKU-CT2	V	2	JX486101
GVI/Ca/IT/2007/GVI.1/Bari91	VI	1	FJ875027
GVI/Ca/PT/2007/GVI.2/Viseu	VI	2	GQ443611

Genotypes are defined based on the complete VP1 sequence.[107]

and 2 genotypes, respectively. To facilitate global tracking of emerging norovirus strains, online genotyping tools are available that can identify the VP1 and Pol genotype when interrogated with full or partial genomic sequences.[312]

Large-scale molecular epidemiologic studies have given insight into the role of norovirus genotypes, variants, and recombinants.[613] The GII noroviruses, particularly those of the GII.4 cluster, are the predominant viruses detected, and this distribution reflects the epidemiologic pattern observed in most other parts of the world.[613] Major shifts in the predominant circulating GII.4 variant can occur.[77,174,338,535] Different norovirus genotypes, such as GII.17, can emerge and displace the predominant GII.4 variant in a population for a period of time, but it is not clear whether such displacements are permanent.[232] Sequence analysis of the GII.4 noroviruses that emerged on a global level in the early 2000s identified the presence of an amino acid insertion in the VP1 P2 domain, suggesting a possible change in the antigenic or receptor recognition phenotype.[135] Further evolution in the GII.4 cluster was described,[77] and several studies have examined the possibly unique propensity of this genotype to undergo genetic (and antigenic) drift.[337,461] Genetic variation has been detected in other regions of the genome such as the emergence of the "GGIIb-pol" polymerase type that was found in norovirus strains in combination with several different VP1 genotypes.[493] Additional reports of unique polymerase sequences have led to the conclusion that recombination is a driving mechanism of norovirus evolution.[76,181,366] There is epidemiological evidence that disease with GII.4 may be more severe.[78,133,234] Epidemiological data indicate a higher association of GI noroviruses with environmental outbreaks (such as waterborne and shellfish) as compared to GII, which was more prevalent in health care settings and in outbreaks occurring in cooler months.[389]

Evidence for mixed norovirus infections within the same individual or within the same outbreak has been reported in many epidemiologic studies.[667] In addition, a marked genotypic diversity among norovirus strains has been documented in pediatric patients.[173,208,292,386,677] The presence of diverse norovirus sequences in shellfish and environmental samples is common,[616] suggesting another potential source for mixed infection. Such diverse and mixed infections likely enable recombination between norovirus RNA genomes, a possibility suggested from sequence analyses of naturally occurring noroviruses in several species.[76] Immunocompromised individuals with chronic norovirus infection can be superinfected with a different norovirus and sustain a prolonged mixed infection.[73] Viral RNA populations are genetically heterogenous, especially during chronic infection, which further drives evolution of new strains.[75,619] Infection of feline kidney cells with two distinct recombinant FCV strains bearing different fluorescent markers has demonstrated that coinfection of the same cell can readily occur, further supporting the potential for recombination of RNA genomes during replication.[2]

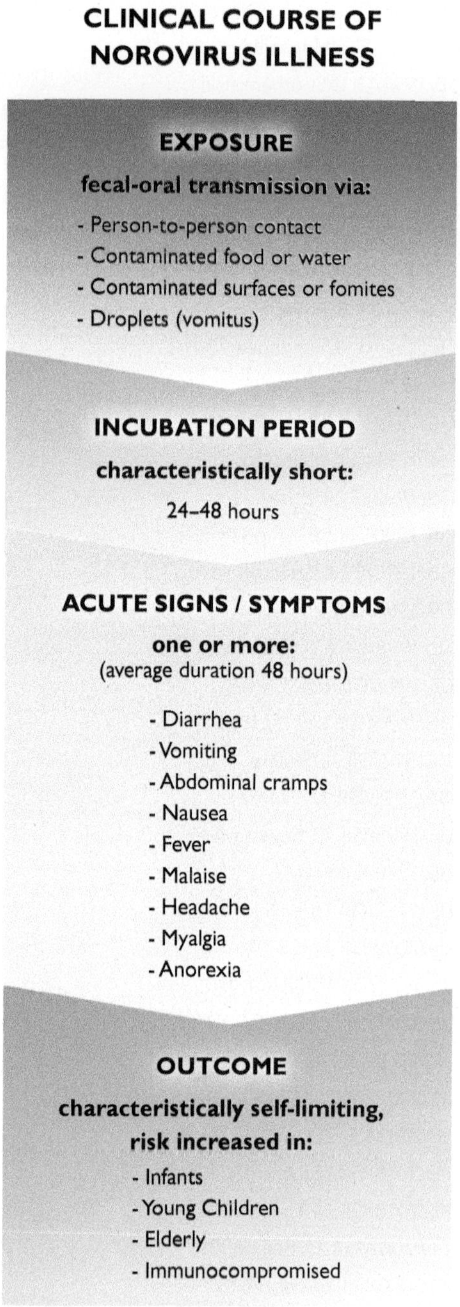

CLINICAL FEATURES

Viral gastroenteritis is generally considered to be mild and self-limiting, although the illness can be incapacitating during the symptomatic phase that usually lasts 24 to 48 hours[496] (Fig. 4.13). Illness induced by the noroviruses can be sufficiently

CLINICAL COURSE OF NOROVIRUS ILLNESS

EXPOSURE

fecal-oral transmission via:

- Person-to-person contact
- Contaminated food or water
- Contaminated surfaces or fomites
- Droplets (vomitus)

INCUBATION PERIOD

characteristically short:

24–48 hours

ACUTE SIGNS / SYMPTOMS

one or more:
(average duration 48 hours)

- Diarrhea
- Vomiting
- Abdominal cramps
- Nausea
- Fever
- Malaise
- Headache
- Myalgia
- Anorexia

OUTCOME

characteristically self-limiting, risk increased in:

- Infants
- Young Children
- Elderly
- Immunocompromised

FIGURE 4.13 Clinical course of norovirus gastroenteritis. Norovirus disease is characterized by a short incubation period and acute onset. Symptoms and signs vary, but vomiting and diarrhea are common manifestations of disease. In otherwise healthy individuals, illness is characteristically self-limiting without serious sequelae. Risk factors for severe disease include young and old age, a compromised immune system, or a debilitating underlying illness or condition.

severe to require medical intervention, with an increased risk for life-threatening dehydration at both ends of the age spectra (See *Morbidity and Mortality*). Immunocompromised patients with norovirus infection are at increased risk for morbidity and mortality, and an increasing number of reports have linked norovirus to chronic gastroenteritis in patients undergoing transplantation or chemotherapy[191] (see *Treatment*).

Based on volunteer studies with human NV, the incubation period is short, ranging from 10 to 51 hours, with a mean of 24 hours.[25,56,140,141,555,656] This brief incubation period is consistent with the pattern of illness in outbreak investigations.[324] The incubation period recorded in 22 naturally occurring outbreaks of NV gastroenteritis was between 24 and 48 hours in 20 of the outbreaks, and the range was from 4 to 77 hours.[258] The incubation period of experimentally induced Snow Mountain virus illness ranged from 19 to 41 hours, with a mean of 27 hours.[144] Acute illness usually lasts about 24 to 48 hours.

A transient malabsorption of fat, D-xylose, and lactose is observed during experimentally induced NV illness.[56,520] Levels of small intestinal brush-border enzymes (trehalase and alkaline phosphatase) were significantly decreased when compared with baseline and convalescent-phase values, whereas adenylate cyclase activity in the jejunum was not elevated following NV or Hawaii virus-induced illness.[4,331] Gastric secretion of hydrochloric acid, pepsin, and intrinsic factor did not appear to be altered during NV illness.[398] Elevation of serum transaminase levels was reported in four pediatric patients at approximately 2 weeks following acute illness.[606]

Of 16 volunteers who developed illness following Norwalk or Hawaii virus infection, 14 developed transient lymphopenia.[143] This was attributed to a redistribution of circulating lymphocytes to the site of viral infection in the small intestine. The lymphocytes remaining in the circulation responded normally or exhibited an exaggerated response to mitogenic stimuli.

A marked delay in gastric emptying was observed in infected volunteers who became ill and developed the typical jejunal mucosal lesion.[398] It has been proposed that abnormal gastric motor function is responsible for the nausea and vomiting associated with these viral agents[398]; however, the mechanisms of illness are not clear. An analysis of epithelial barrier and secretion function in norovirus-positive human duodenal biopsy tissue showed that tight junction proteins occludin, claudin-4, and claudin-5 were reduced and anion secretion was stimulated.[604] In addition, a comparison of asymptomatic and symptomatically infected human volunteers identified increased serum cytokines in symptomatic patients only, while viral RNA levels and shedding were similar.[433] Thus, norovirus diarrhea could result from one or more of the following mechanisms: loss of epithelial barrier integrity, secretory pathway dysfunction, and immune system hyperactivation.

Clinical manifestations observed in 31 volunteers experimentally infected with noroviruses who became ill included the following: fever above 99.4°F (45%), diarrhea (81%), vomiting (65%), abdominal discomfort (68%), anorexia (90%), headache (81%), and myalgias (58%).[656] The illnesses were characteristically mild and usually lasted 24 to 48 hours; however, one volunteer was given parenteral fluid because he vomited 20 times within a 24-hour period. The number of clinical signs and symptoms can vary among volunteers receiving the same inoculum.[140] Illnesses induced by the Hawaii, Montgomery County, and Snow Mountain viruses in volunteers cannot be distinguished clinically from those caused by NV.[144,656] Subclinical infections with Norwalk or Hawaii virus have been observed under experimental as well as natural conditions.

Clinical manifestations observed in 38 outbreaks associated with NV included the following (expressed as the median percentage of patients): nausea (79%), vomiting (69%), diarrhea (66%), abdominal cramps (30%), headache (22%), fever (subjective) (37%), chills (32%), myalgias (26%), and sore throat (18%).[258] Bloody stools were not reported. Vomiting occurred more frequently than diarrhea in children, whereas in adults, the reverse was observed. The duration of illness in 28 outbreaks ranged from 2 hours to several days, with a mean or median of between 12 and 60 hours in 26 of the 28 outbreaks. In 6 outbreaks, illness lasted more than 3 days in up to 15% of the affected individuals. The attack rates did not differ significantly with age or sex in 6 outbreaks in which this was analyzed.[258]

A 2-year study in children (≤5 years of age) compared the severity of acute diarrheal episodes caused by noroviruses with rotaviruses in hospital emergency and outpatient settings; most cases for both viruses ranged from moderate to severe, although illness was overall less severe for norovirus-infected individuals.[446] The clinical course of norovirus illness in preterm infants has been reported to include a distended abdomen and symptoms such as apnea or a sepsis-like appearance: vomiting was not a predominant symptom in these patients.[18,467] Noroviruses have been reported as associated with the following rare conditions or sequelae[496]: convulsions,[1,93] seizures,[42,106,229,279] encephalitis/encephalopathy,[241,284,531] intestinal perforation,[465,611,641] transient liver dysfunction,[420] and necrotizing enterocolitis.[559] Noroviruses have been associated with enteropathy in certain immunocompromised patients.[215,655] However, its role in inflammatory bowel disease remains unclear with studies ranging from no effect to exacerbation of disease.[28,273,470]

The determinants of susceptibility and resistance to norovirus disease are clearly complex (See *Immunity*). Expression of HBGAs ABH and Lewis carbohydrate antigens in the intestinal epithelium is considered a genetic susceptibility factor for human norovirus infection.[254,594] These glycans can serve as norovirus attachment factors (see *Mechanisms of Attachment*, Table 4.3), and their synthesis is controlled by enzymes that are products of alleles at the ABO, FUT2, and FUT3 loci. Individuals with two mutated FUT2 alleles, who are therefore devoid of H-type antigens on their gut and other mucosal epithelial cells, are called nonsecretors. Human volunteer studies previously identified that the secretor status of an individual were a major correlate in susceptibility to infection with NV.[341] On oral challenge with NV, only secretor individuals with H-type 1 antigens were susceptible to infection, whereas nonsecretors were resistant. This was confirmed in a retrospective analysis of volunteers.[236] However, variation exists among the noroviruses in their recognition of host cell carbohydrates.[322] For example, infection in volunteers challenged with GII Snow Mountain virus (unlike those challenged with NV) showed no correlation between ABH secretor status and susceptibility.[340]

DIAGNOSIS

Differential

An analysis of the common features of 38 NV outbreaks indicates that a provisional diagnosis of illness by the noroviruses can be made during an outbreak if the following criteria are met: (a) bacterial or parasitic pathogens are not detected, (b) vomiting occurs in more than 50% of cases, (c) the mean or median duration of illness ranges from 12 to 60 hours, and (d) the incubation period is 24 to 48 hours.[257] These so-called Kaplan criteria were found to be highly (99%) specific and moderately (68%) sensitive for the provisional diagnosis of a norovirus outbreak when re-evaluated with samples confirmed as norovirus positive.[608] Suspected foodborne illness presents as abdominal cramps, diarrhea (more common in adults), fever, headache, nausea, and vomiting (more common in children).[564]

Differential diagnosis of sporadic norovirus illness in individual patients is difficult, due to shared clinical features with a wide range of enteric pathogens and disease syndromes (see *Clinical Features*). Laboratory diagnosis is required to confirm etiology, but empiric treatment of symptoms should not be delayed due to the rapid progression of dehydration.[564]

Laboratory

Reverse Transcriptase Polymerase Chain Reaction

Currently, RT-PCR is the most widely used technique for detection of noroviruses.[624] With this method, noroviruses can be detected in clinical specimens (feces is preferred because it contains highest quantity of virus) and contaminated food, water, or fomites. The application of real-time quantitative (q) RT-PCR has gained widespread use because it allows rapid detection as well as comparison of viral RNA levels.[251,472,605] The choice of primers is important, because considerable genetic diversity exists among circulating strains.[624,659,676] The application of RT-PCR to amplify partial or complete genomes, coupled with sequence analysis of the amplicons, has been used extensively to detect and characterize noroviruses in various outbreaks.[72,119,461,614] Norovirus identification is included in multiplex PCR–based assays (several commercially available) that detect a wide array of enteric pathogens, and these are an important advance in managing and treating infectious gastroenteritis.[49,108] The association of norovirus with an outbreak requires a limited number of specimens.[147]

Immunoassays

Immunoassays for the detection of noroviruses in clinical specimens are commercially available.[646] These assays characteristically utilize hyperimmune sera and monoclonal antibodies generated against recombinant norovirus antigens. Point of care assays that quickly identify norovirus antigen in stool are in development that can distinguish between viral and bacterial gastroenteritis in a clinical setting, and informing the use of antibiotics.[137,369,587]

Immunoassays that use recombinant proteins (such as rVLPs) as antigen to detect serological responses are specific, sensitive, and efficient for detecting infection with the human caliciviruses and have been used in several large-scale seroepidemiologic studies (see *Prevalence and Seroepidemiology*). The Norwalk rVLP ELISA has been shown to detect broadly reactive antibody responses in volunteers given NV, Hawaii virus, or Snow Mountain virus, although the maximal response was observed in volunteers challenged with the NV.[189,192,409,601] Thus, it is difficult to identify conclusively the antigenic type of an infecting norovirus strain by serologic analysis because of shared cross-reactive antigens.[45,441] The demonstration of an antibody response in 50% or more of the individuals involved (or examined) in an outbreak to a calicivirus antigen is strong evidence linking the virus with the outbreak.[258] Newer approaches to detect antibodies include noninvasive assays that utilize saliva to measure norovirus-specific IgA.[24,475,570]

PREVENTION AND CONTROL

Treatment

Noroviruses characteristically induce a mild, self-limited gastroenteritis that normally resolves without complications.[56,139–141,247,555,656] As noted, hospitalization for severe dehydration, although rare, can occur with norovirus gastroenteritis. Oral fluid and electrolyte replacement therapy is usually sufficient to replace fluid loss.[14,15,122] Oral rehydration therapy should not be administered to patients with depressed consciousness because of the possibility of fluid aspiration. Parenteral administration of fluids may be necessary, however, if severe vomiting or diarrhea occurs.

Oral administration of bismuth subsalicylate after onset of symptoms significantly reduced the severity and duration of abdominal cramps during experimentally induced norovirus illness in adults.[555] In addition, the median duration of gastrointestinal symptoms was reduced from 20 to 14 hours. The number, weight, and water content of stools, as well as the extent of virus excretion, were not significantly affected by treatment. The use of various medications for symptomatic treatment of acute diarrhea in infants and young children (aged 1 month to 5 years) was reviewed: bismuth subsalicylate, loperamide, anticholinergic agents, adsorbents, or *Lactobacillus*-containing compounds were not recommended by the American Academy of Pediatrics, and, in addition, the use of opiates as well as opiate and atropine combination drugs was contraindicated.[14,15]

A need for norovirus-targeted therapy has been recognized in the management of immunocompromised patients with chronic norovirus infection.[271] Treatment protocols implemented for other pathogens have been evaluated in a small number of individuals with norovirus disease, with varying success.[430] Improvement in chronic norovirus diarrhea has been reported in immunocompromised patients following reduction in immunosuppressive therapy (IST) drugs; however, careful monitoring of these patients is required.[62] The effect of exclusion diets, enteral and intravenous immunoglobulins, breast milk, immunosuppressants, ribavirin, and nitazoxanide has also been examined in this patient population with differing efficacies.[71]

Efforts are in progress to develop antiviral drugs to target specific stages of the norovirus life cycle, but their safety and clinical efficacy have not been established.[589] The selection of drug-resistant viruses during treatment will be a continuing challenge,[293] and it is likely that a combined therapy approach will be needed.[16] Improvements in tools for high-throughput drug screening,[483,634] structure-guided drug development,[126,165] and innovative inhibitors[145] are in development. Ideally, drugs or host immune modulators (such as IFN-lambda or TLR agonists) will be identified that would protect against diverse norovirus genotypes.[155,437,497]

Vaccines

Recognition of the disease burden and economic impact of noroviruses has informed research to develop a vaccine.[361,487] As noted earlier, improved surveillance in concert with diagnostic confirmation has allowed more accurate assessment of morbidity and mortality (see *Morbidity and Mortality*). Globally, norovirus incurs billions of dollars each year in direct health care system costs ($4.2 billion US) and even more in indirect societal costs ($60.3 billion US).[43] A vaccine would be of special importance to infants and young children, health care workers, food handlers, college students, military personnel, nursing home residents, and individuals in various institutional settings. Although norovirus gastroenteritis tends to be a mild illness, a reduction in diarrheal episodes may be especially important in the debilitated, malnourished infant, because it has been suggested that repeated diarrheal episodes may be a precipitating factor in the development of malnutrition through sequential damage to the intestinal mucosa.[387,504] The impact of norovirus infection on normal gastrointestinal microbiota or underlying disease conditions when elucidated may provide additional avenues to support norovirus immunoprophylaxis (see *Norovirus-Microbiota Interactions*).

A vaccine for the control of norovirus gastroenteritis is not yet available, but a number of vaccine candidates are in development.[116,294,365] Various routes of administration, formulations, and expression systems for rVLPs (or subunit forms) are under investigation.[36,40,63,151,161,196,224,278,514,565,566,569,573] Two-phase I/II trials have shown that norovirus rVLPs are safe and provide some protection against illness at the doses, routes, and adjuvants tested. In the first trial, NV (GI.1) rVLPs were administered by an intranasal route followed by oral challenge with infectious NV.[22] The second trial evaluated a bivalent formulation comprised of NV(GI.1) and a GII.4 consensus rVLP administered by intramuscular injection, followed by challenge with infectious GII.4 norovirus.[50] Although both trials showed some evidence for protective immunity, larger placebo-controlled phase III trials will be needed to establish the efficacy of these vaccines. A phase I trial of an adenovirus-vectored norovirus vaccine administered orally in tablet form was also recently completed with promising results and will likely progress further in clinical trials.[281] Because noroviruses are antigenically diverse, additional work will be needed to determine the number of antigenic components required to provide protection against a broad range of norovirus antigenic types and variants.

Infection Control

Specific methods are not available for the prevention of norovirus infection and illness. Outbreak management generally focuses on containment by the prevention of spread to other areas by ill or exposed individuals, frequent handwashing, and effective environmental decontamination.[39] Shedding can occur beyond the resolution of symptoms as well as in the prodromal stage of infection,[184] presenting challenges to infection control.

The noroviruses are generally resistant to detergent or ethanol-based cleaning of environmental surfaces and fomites and require additional chemical disinfection.[41,146] Reliance on the use of alcohol-based hand sanitizers over handwashing has been reported to actually increase the risk of norovirus transmission and infection in patient care settings.[57,628] Effective disinfectants have been reported to include hypochlorite at 5,000 ppm (domestic bleach is ~5% sodium hypochlorite and can be used as a 10% solution), hydrogen peroxide–based cleaners, and phenolic-based cleaners.[41] Inactivation has been difficult to evaluate in the absence of *in vitro* infectivity assays, and surrogates for human noroviruses have been employed, with variable success.[114] However, recent advances should facilitate this analysis.[380] The poor disinfecting properties of alcohols and the efficacious properties of chlorine against human norovirus have recently been verified in an *in vitro* infectivity assay in human enteroids.[118]

Special care must be given to the hygienic processing of food in view of the frequent occurrence of foodborne outbreaks.[69] Depuration of oysters does not adequately clear tissues of NV,[216] and recent studies have shown that certain norovirus genotypes (such as GI) bind more avidly to HBGA-like glycans in oyster tissues.[321,370] Leafy greens such as lettuce may also bear HBGA-like ligands that bind norovirus.[175] Precaution must be taken to prevent contamination of oyster beds and farm fields with feces, vomitus, or sewage treatment plant effluent. Measures that increase the purity of drinking water or swimming pool water should also decrease the frequency of outbreaks.[352] Various technological processes are under development to inactivate noroviruses in agricultural food products and shellfish prior to market.[223,285,307,329,412,491]

PERSPECTIVE

The past few years have seen remarkable progress in the calicivirus field, but in particular, major advances were made in our understanding of noroviruses. Chiefly among them was the discovery of two human norovirus culture systems, human intestinal enteroid cultures and transformed human B-cell lines (e.g., BJAB). Admittedly, improvements need to be made in several aspects of both systems to realize the full potential of these culture models. Nevertheless, since this lack of a cell culture model has been hampering progress in the field for decades, these initial steps are vital to spur the many new discoveries in the future that will undoubtedly follow. Furthermore, the MNV model with its many tools continues to reveal fascinating new biology about these viruses. Among them was the discovery of the first norovirus proteinaceous receptor CD300lf, an Ig-like lipid-binding protein, whose presence regulates the cellular tropism of MNVs. Study with MNV also uncovered for the first time that tuft cells, specialized chemosensory cells in the intestinal epithelium, are infected by a virus and that these cells can provide an immuno-privileged location for long-term viral persistence in the intestine. Studies with both human and MNVs also demonstrated an intricate interplay of these enteric viruses with the microbiota. Thus, in addition to host factors, viral biology and pathogenesis are also impacted by members of other kingdoms of life, highlighting the need to broaden our reductionist approaches, if we want to fully understand these emerging viruses. Advances in genomic technologies continue to uncover additional genetic diversity in the calicivirus family, leading to the recent description of six new calicivirus genera. Individual members of these genera hold the potential for additional animal and cell culture models to increase the versatility of existing tools and models in the field. Combining the enormous technical advances being made in other scientific fields with the calicivirus knowledge and tools from the past decades promises additional scientific breakthroughs in the field as well as effective ways to treat and prevent their infections in the near future.

REFERENCES

1. Abe T, Kobayashi M, Araki K, et al. Infantile convulsions with mild gastroenteritis. *Brain Dev* 2000;22:301–306.
2. Abente EJ, Sosnovtsev SV, Bok K, et al. Visualization of feline calicivirus replication in real-time with recombinant viruses engineered to express fluorescent reporter proteins. *Virology* 2010;400:18–31.
3. Adler JL, Zickl R. Winter vomiting disease. *J Infect Dis* 1969;119:668–673.

4. Agus SG, Dolin R, Wyatt RG, et al. Acute infectious nonbacterial gastroenteritis: intestinal histopathology. Histologic and enzymatic alterations during illness produced by the Norwalk agent in man. *Ann Intern Med* 1973;79:18–25.
5. Ahmed SM, Hall AJ, Robinson AE, et al. Global prevalence of norovirus in cases of gastroenteritis: a systematic review and meta-analysis. *Lancet Infect Dis* 2014;14:725–730.
6. Alfajaro MM, Cho EH, Kim DS, et al. Early porcine sapovirus infection disrupts tight junctions and uses occludin as a coreceptor. *J Virol* 2019;93:e01773–18.
7. Alfano-Sobsey E, Sweat D, Hall A, et al. Norovirus outbreak associated with undercooked oysters and secondary household transmission. *Epidemiol Infect* 2012;140:276–282.
8. Alhatlani B, Vashist S, Goodfellow I. Functions of the 5' and 3' ends of calicivirus genomes. *Virus Res* 2015;206:134–143.
9. Allen DJ, Harris JP. Methods for ascertaining norovirus disease burdens. *Hum Vaccin Immunother* 2017;13:2630–2636.
10. Almand EA, Moore MD, Jaykus LA. Norovirus binding to ligands beyond histo-blood group antigens. *Front Microbiol* 2017;8:2549.
11. Almand EA, Moore MD, Outlaw J, et al. Human norovirus binding to select bacteria representative of the human gut microbiota. *PLoS One* 2017;12:e0173124.
12. Al-Molawi N, Beardmore VA, Carter MJ, et al. Caspase-mediated cleavage of the feline calicivirus capsid protein. *J Gen Virol* 2003;84:1237–1244.
13. Alvarado G, Ettayebi K, Atmar RL, et al Human monoclonal antibodies that neutralize pandemic GII.4 noroviruses. *Gastroenterology* 2018;155:1898–1907.
14. Anonymous. Practice parameter: the management of acute gastroenteritis in young children. American Academy of Pediatrics, Provisional Committee on Quality Improvement, Subcommittee on Acute Gastroenteritis [see comments]. *Pediatrics* 1996;97:424–435.
15. Anonymous. Updated norovirus outbreak management and disease prevention guidelines. *MMWR Recomm Rep* 2011;60:1–18.
16. Arias A, Emmott E, Vashist S, et al. Progress towards the prevention and treatment of norovirus infections. *Future Microbiol* 2013;8:1475–1487.
17. Arias A, Urena L, Thorne L, et al. Reverse genetics mediated recovery of infectious murine norovirus. *J Vis Exp* 2012;(64):4145.
18. Armbrust S, Kramer A, Olbertz D, et al. Norovirus infections in preterm infants: wide variety of clinical courses. *BMC Res Notes* 2009;2:96.
19. Armed Forces Health Surveillance Branch. Surveillance snapshot: norovirus outbreaks among military forces, 2008–2016. *MSMR* 2017;24:30–31.
20. Asanaka M, Atmar RL, Ruvolo V, et al. Replication and packaging of Norwalk virus RNA in cultured mammalian cells. *Proc Natl Acad Sci U S A* 2005;102:10327–10332.
21. Atmar J, Mullen E. Norovirus in immunocompromised patients. *Oncol Nurs Forum* 2013;40:434–436.
22. Atmar RL, Bernstein DI, Harro CD, et al. Norovirus vaccine against experimental human Norwalk Virus illness. *N Engl J Med* 2011;365:2178–2187.
23. Atmar RL, Bernstein DI, Lyon GM, et al. Serological correlates of protection against a GII.4 Norovirus. *Clin Vaccine Immunol* 2015;22:923–929.
24. Atmar RL, Cramer JP, Baehner F, et al. An exploratory study of the salivary IgA responses to one dose of a Norovirus VLP candidate vaccine in healthy adults. *J Infect Dis* 2019;219(3):410–414.
25. Atmar RL, Opekun AR, Gilger MA, et al. Norwalk virus shedding after experimental human infection. *Emerg Infect Dis* 2008;14:1553–1557.
26. Atmar RL, Opekun AR, Gilger MA, et al. Determination of the 50% human infectious dose for Norwalk virus. *J Infect Dis* 2014;209:1016–1022.
27. Ausar SF, Foubert TR, Hudson MH, et al. Conformational stability and disassembly of Norwalk virus-like particles. Effect of pH and temperature. *J Biol Chem* 2006;281:19478–19488.
28. Axelrad JE, Joelson A, Green PHR, et al. Enteric infections are common in patients with flares of inflammatory bowel disease. *Am J Gastroenterol* 2018;113:1530–1539.
29. Aybeke EN, Belliot G, Lemaire-Ewing S, et al. HS-AFM and SERS analysis of murine norovirus infection: involvement of the lipid rafts. *Small* 2017;13:1600918.
30. Bailey D, Kaiser WJ, Hollinshead M, et al. Feline calicivirus p32, p39 and p30 proteins localize to the endoplasmic reticulum to initiate replication complex formation. *J Gen Virol* 2010;91:739–749.
31. Bailey D, Karakasiliotis I, Vashist S, et al. Functional analysis of RNA structures present at the 3' extremity of the murine norovirus genome: the variable polypyrimidine tract plays a role in viral virulence. *J Virol* 2010;84:2859–2870.
32. Bailey D, Thackray LB, Goodfellow IG. A single amino acid substitution in the murine norovirus capsid protein is sufficient for attenuation in vivo. *J Virol* 2008;82:7725–7728.
33. Baker ES, Luckner SR, Krause KL, et al. Inherent structural disorder and dimerisation of murine norovirus NS1-2 protein. *PLoS One* 2012;7:e30534.
34. Baldridge MT, Nice TJ, McCune BT, et al. Commensal microbes and interferon-lambda determine persistence of enteric murine norovirus infection. *Science* 2015;347:266–269.
35. Baldridge MT, Turula H, Wobus CE. Norovirus regulation by host and microbe. *Trends Mol Med* 2016;22:1047–1059.
36. Ball JM, Graham DY, Opekun AR, et al. Recombinant Norwalk virus-like particles given orally to volunteers: phase I study [see comments]. *Gastroenterology* 1999;117:40–48.
37. Ballard SB, Saito M, Mirelman AJ, et al. Tropical and travel-associated norovirus: current concepts. *Curr Opin Infect Dis* 2015;28:408–416.
38. Barcena J, Verdaguer N, Roca R, et al. The coat protein of rabbit hemorrhagic disease virus contains a molecular switch at the N-terminal region facing the inner surface of the capsid. *Virology* 2004;322:118–134.
39. Barclay L, Park GW, Vega E, et al. Infection control for norovirus. *Clin Microbiol Infect* 2014;20:731–740.
40. Baric RS, Yount B, Lindesmith L, et al. Expression and self-assembly of norwalk virus capsid protein from venezuelan equine encephalitis virus replicons. *J Virol* 2002;76:3023–3030.
41. Barker J, Vipond IB, Bloomfield SF. Effects of cleaning and disinfection in reducing the spread of Norovirus contamination via environmental surfaces. *J Hosp Infect* 2004;58:42–49.
42. Bartolini L, Mardari R, Toldo I, et al. Norovirus gastroenteritis and seizures: an atypical case with neuroradiological abnormalities. *Neuropediatrics* 2011;42:167–169.
43. Bartsch SM, Lopman BA, Ozawa S, et al. Global economic burden of norovirus gastroenteritis. *PLoS One* 2016;11:e0151219.
44. Basic M, Keubler LM, Buettner M, et al. Norovirus triggered microbiota-driven mucosal inflammation in interleukin 10-deficient mice. *Inflamm Bowel Dis* 2014;20:431–443.
45. Belliot G, Noel JS, Li J-F, et al. Characterization of three new genetically distinct "Norwalk-like viruses" expressed by using the baculovirus system. *J Clin Microbiol* 2001;39(12):4288–4295.
46. Belliot G, Sosnovtsev SV, Chang KO, et al. Norovirus proteinase-polymerase and polymerase are both active forms of RNA-dependent RNA polymerase. *J Virol* 2005;79:2393–2403.
47. Belliot G, Sosnovtsev SV, Chang KO, et al. Nucleotidylylation of the VPg protein of a human norovirus by its proteinase-polymerase precursor protein. *Virology* 2008;374:33–49.
48. Belliot G, Sosnovtsev SV, Mitra T, et al. In vitro proteolytic processing of the MD145 norovirus ORF1 nonstructural polyprotein yields stable precursors and products similar to those detected in calicivirus-infected cells. *J Virol* 2003;77:10957–10974.
49. Bennett S, Gunson RN. The development of a multiplex real-time RT-PCR for the detection of adenovirus, astrovirus, rotavirus and sapovirus from stool samples. *J Virol Methods* 2017;242:30–34.
50. *Bernstein DI, Atmar RL, Lyon GM, et al. Norovirus vaccine against experimental human GII.4 virus illness: a challenge study in healthy adults. J Infect Dis 2015;211:870–878.*
51. Bertolotti-Ciarlet A, Crawford SE, Hutson AM, et al. The 3' end of Norwalk virus mRNA contains determinants that regulate the expression and stability of the viral capsid protein VP1: a novel function for the VP2 protein. *J Virol* 2003;77:11603–11615.
52. Bertolotti-Ciarlet A, White LJ, Chen R, et al. Structural requirements for the assembly of Norwalk virus-like particles. *J Virol* 2002;76:4044–4055.
53. Bhella D, Gatherer D, Chaudhry Y, et al. Structural insights into calicivirus attachment and uncoating. *J Virol* 2008;82:8051–8058.
54. Biering SB, Choi J, Halstrom RA, et al. Viral replication complexes are targeted by LC3-guided interferon-inducible GTPases. *Cell Host Microbe* 2017;22:74.e7–85.e7.
55. Black RE. Epidemiology of travelers' diarrhea and relative importance of various pathogens. *Rev Infect Dis* 1990;12(Suppl 1):S73–S79.
56. Blacklow NR, Dolin R, Fedson DS, et al. Acute infectious nonbacterial gastroenteritis: etiology and pathogenesis. A combined clinical staff conference at the Clinical Center of the National Institutes of Health. *Ann Intern Med* 1972;76:993–1008.
57. Blaney DD, Daly ER, Kirkland KB, et al. Use of alcohol-based hand sanitizers as a risk factor for norovirus outbreaks in long-term care facilities in northern New England: December 2006 to March 2007. *Am J Infect Control* 2011;39:296–301.
58. Blazevic V, Malm M, Honkanen H, et al. Development and maturation of norovirus antibodies in childhood. *Microbes Infect* 2016;18:263–269.
59. Blazevic V, Malm M, Vesikari T. Induction of homologous and cross-reactive GII.4-specific blocking antibodies in children after GII.4 New Orleans norovirus infection. *J Med Virol* 2015;87(10):1656–1661.
60. Blazevic V, Malm M, Salminen M, et al. Multiple consecutive norovirus infections in the first 2 years of life. *Eur J Pediatr* 2015;174:1679–1683.
61. Bohnker BK, Thornton S. Explosive outbreaks of gastroenteritis in the shipboard environment attributed to Norovirus. *Mil Med* 2003;168:iv.
62. Bok K, Green KY. Norovirus gastroenteritis in immunocompromised patients. *N Engl J Med* 2012;367:2126–2132.
63. Bok K, Parra GI, Mitra T, et al. Chimpanzees as an animal model for human norovirus infection and vaccine development. *Proc Natl Acad Sci U S A* 2011;108:325–330.
64. Bok K, Prikhodko VG, Green KY, et al. Apoptosis in murine norovirus-infected RAW264.7 cells is associated with downregulation of survivin. *J Virol* 2009;83:3647–3656.
65. Bonifait L, Charlebois R, Vimont A, et al. Detection and quantification of airborne norovirus during outbreaks in healthcare facilities. *Clin Infect Dis* 2015;61(3):299–304.
66. Boniotti B, Wirblich C, Sibilia M, et al. Identification and characterization of a 3C-like protease from rabbit hemorrhagic disease virus, a calicivirus. *J Virol* 1994;68:6487–6495.
67. Borin BN, Tang W, Nice TJ, et al. Murine norovirus protein NS1/2 aspartate to glutamate mutation, sufficient for persistence, reorients side chain of surface exposed tryptophan within a novel structured domain. *Proteins* 2014;82(7):1200–1209.
68. Bourgeois AL, Gardiner CH, Thornton SA, et al. Etiology of acute diarrhea among United States military personnel deployed to South America and west Africa. *Am J Trop Med Hyg* 1993;48:243–248.
69. Bouwknegt M, Verhaelen K, Rzezutka A, et al. Quantitative farm-to-fork risk assessment model for norovirus and hepatitis A virus in European leafy green vegetable and berry fruit supply chains. *Int J Food Microbiol* 2015;198:50–58.
70. Bragazzi Cunha J, Wobus CE. Select membrane proteins modulate MNV-1 infection of macrophages and dendritic cells in a cell type-specific manner. *Virus Res* 2016;222:64–70.
71. Brown LK, Clark I, Brown JR, et al. Norovirus infection in primary immune deficiency. *Rev Med Virol* 2017;27(3):e1926.
72. Brown JR, Roy S, Shah D, et al. Norovirus transmission dynamics in a paediatric hospital using full genome sequences. *Clin Infect Dis* 2019;68(2):222–228.
73. Brown JR, Roy S, Tutill H, et al. Super-infections and relapses occur in chronic norovirus infections. *J Clin Virol* 2017;96:44–48.
74. Bucardo F, Lindgren PE, Svensson L, et al. Low prevalence of rotavirus and high prevalence of norovirus in hospital and community wastewater after introduction of rotavirus vaccine in Nicaragua. *PLoS One* 2011;6:e25962.
75. Bull RA, Eden JS, Luciani F, et al. Contribution of intra- and interhost dynamics to norovirus evolution. *J Virol* 2012;86:3219–3229.
76. Bull RA, Hansman GS, Clancy LE, et al. Norovirus recombination in ORF1/ORF2 overlap. *Emerg Infect Dis* 2005;11:1079–1085.
77. Bull RA, Tu ET, McIver CJ, et al. Emergence of a new norovirus genotype II.4 variant associated with global outbreaks of gastroenteritis. *J Clin Microbiol* 2006;44:327–333.

78. Burke RM, Shah MP, Wikswo ME, et al. The norovirus epidemiologic triad: predictors of severe outcomes in US norovirus outbreaks, 2009–2016. *J Infect Dis* 2019;219(9): 1364–1372.

79. Burmeister WP, Buisson M, Estrozi LF, et al. Structure determination of feline calicivirus virus-like particles in the context of a pseudo-octahedral arrangement. *PLoS One* 2015;10:e0119289.

80. Burroughs JN, Brown F. Presence of a covalently linked protein on calicivirus RNA. *J Gen Virol* 1978;41:443–446.

81. Caddy S, Breiman A, Le Pendu J, et al. Genogroup IV and VI canine noroviruses interact with histo-blood group antigens. *J Virol* 2014;88:10377–10391.

82. Cadwell K, Patel KK, Maloney NS, et al. Virus-plus-susceptibility gene interaction determines Crohn's disease gene Atg16L1 phenotypes in intestine. *Cell* 2010;141:1135–1145.

83. Cao S, Lou Z, Tan M, et al. Structural basis for the recognition of blood group trisaccharides by norovirus. *J Virol* 2007;81:5949–5957.

84. Carmona-Vicente N, Vila-Vicent S, Allen D, et al. Characterization of a novel conformational GII.4 norovirus epitope: implications for norovirus-host interactions. *J Virol* 2016;90:7703–7714.

85. Cauchi MR, Doultree JC, Marshall JA, et al. Molecular characterization of Camberwell virus and sequence variation in ORF3 of small round-structured (Norwalk-like) viruses. *J Med Virol* 1996;49:70–76.

86. Caul EO. Small round structured viruses: airborne transmission and hospital control [see comments]. *Lancet* 1994;343:1240–1242.

87. Caul EO. Hyperemesis hiemis—a sick hazard. *J Hosp Infect* 1995;30(Suppl):498–502.

88. Chachu KA, LoBue AD, Strong DW, et al. Immune mechanisms responsible for vaccination against and clearance of mucosal and lymphatic norovirus infection. *PLoS Pathog* 2008;4:e1000236.

89. Chachu KA, Strong DW, LoBue AD, et al. Antibody is critical for the clearance of murine norovirus infection. *J Virol* 2008;82:6610–6617.

90. Chadwick PR, McCann R. Transmission of a small round structured virus by vomiting during a hospital outbreak of gastroenteritis. *J Hosp Infect* 1994;26:251–259.

91. Chagla Z, Quirt J, Woodward K, et al. Chronic norovirus infection in a transplant patient successfully treated with enterally administered immune globulin. *J Clin Virol* 2013;58:306–308.

92. Chan MC, Kwok K, Zhang LY, et al. Bimodal seasonality and alternating predominance of norovirus GII.4 and non-GII.4, Hong Kong, China, 2014–2017. *Emerg Infect Dis* 2018;24:767–769.

93. Chan CM, Chan CW, Ma CK, et al. Norovirus as cause of benign convulsion associated with gastro-enteritis. *J Paediatr Child Health* 2011;47:373–377.

94. Chan MC, Ho WS, Sung JJ. In vitro whole-virus binding of a norovirus genogroup II genotype 4 strain to cells of the lamina propria and Brunner's glands in the human duodenum. *J Virol* 2011;85:8427–8430.

95. Chan MC, Lee N, Ho WS, et al. Covariation of major and minor viral capsid proteins in norovirus genogroup II genotype 4 strains. *J Virol* 2012;86:1227–1232.

96. Chan MC, Sung JJ, Lam RK, et al. Fecal viral load and norovirus-associated gastroenteritis. *Emerg Infect Dis* 2006;12:1278–1280.

97. Chang CH, Sakaguchi M, Weil J, et al. The incidence of medically-attended norovirus gastro-enteritis in Japan: modelling using a medical care insurance claims database. *PLoS One* 2018;13:e0195164.

98. Chang KO, Sosnovtsev SV, Belliot G, et al. Bile acids are essential for porcine enteric calicivirus replication in association with down-regulation of signal transducer and activator of transcription 1. *Proc Natl Acad Sci U S A* 2004;101:8733–8738.

99. Chang KO, Sosnovtsev SS, Belliot G, et al. Reverse genetics system for porcine enteric calicivirus, a prototype sapovirus in the Caliciviridae. *J Virol* 2005;79:1409–1416.

100. Chang KO, Sosnovtsev SV, Belliot G, et al. Stable expression of a Norwalk virus RNA replicon in a human hepatoma cell line. *Virology* 2006;353:463–473.

101. Changotra H, Jia Y, Moore TN, et al. Type I and type II interferons inhibit the translation of murine norovirus proteins. *J Virol* 2009;83:5683–5692.

102. Chaudhry Y, Nayak A, Bordeleau ME, et al. Caliciviruses differ in their functional requirements for eIF4F components. *J Biol Chem* 2006;281:25315–25325.

103. Chaudhry Y, Skinner MA, Goodfellow IG. Recovery of genetically defined murine norovirus in tissue culture by using a fowlpox virus expressing T7 RNA polymerase. *J Gen Virol* 2007;88:2091–2100.

104. Cheetham S, Souza M, Meulia T, et al. Pathogenesis of a genogroup II human norovirus in gnotobiotic pigs. *J Virol* 2006;80:10372–10381.

105. Chen R, Neill JD, Noel JS, et al. Inter- and intragenus structural variations in caliciviruses and their functional implications. *J Virol* 2004;78:6469–6479.

106. Chen SY, Tsai CN, Lai MW, et al. Norovirus infection as a cause of diarrhea-associated benign infantile seizures. *Clin Infect Dis* 2009;48:849–855.

107. Chhabra P, de Graaf M, Parra GI, et al. Updated classification of norovirus genogroups and genotypes. *J Gen Virol* 2019;100:1393–1406.

108. Chhabra P, Gregoricus N, Weinberg GA, et al. Comparison of three multiplex gastrointestinal platforms for the detection of gastroenteritis viruses. *J Clin Virol* 2017;95:66–71.

109. Chiba S, Nakata S, Numata-Kinoshita K, et al. Sapporo virus: history and recent findings. *J Infect Dis* 2000;181:S303–S308.

110. Chiba S, Sakuma Y, Kogasaka R, et al. An outbreak of gastroenteritis associated with calicivirus in an infant home. *J Med Virol* 1979;4:249–254.

111. Cho EH, Soliman M, Alfajaro MM, et al. Bovine nebovirus interacts with a wide spectrum of histo-blood group antigens. *J Virol* 2018;92:e02160–17.

112. Choi JM, Hutson AM, Estes MK, et al. Atomic resolution structural characterization of recognition of histo-blood group antigens by Norwalk virus. *Proc Natl Acad Sci U S A* 2008;105:9175–9180.

113. Chung L, Bailey D, Leen EN, et al. Norovirus translation requires an interaction between the C Terminus of the genome-linked viral protein VPg and eukaryotic translation initiation factor 4G. *J Biol Chem* 2014;289:21738–21750.

114. Clayton JS, Bolinger HK, Jaykus LA. Disinfectant testing against human norovirus surrogates-what infection preventionists need to know. *Infect Control Hosp Epidemiol* 2018;39:1388–1389.

115. Conley MJ, McElwee M, Azmi L, et al. Calicivirus VP2 forms a portal-like assembly following receptor engagement. *Nature* 2019;565:377–381.

116. Cortes-Penfield NW, Ramani S, Estes MK, et al. Prospects and challenges in the development of a norovirus vaccine. *Clin Ther* 2017;39:1537–1549.

117. Corwin AL, Soderquist R, Edwards M, et al. Shipboard impact of a probable Norwalk virus outbreak from coastal Japan. *Am J Trop Med Hyg* 1999;61:898–903.

118. Costantini V, Morantz EK, Browne H, et al. Human norovirus replication in human intestinal enteroids as model to evaluate virus inactivation. *Emerg Infect Dis* 2018;24:1453–1464.

119. Cotten M, Koopmans M. Next-generation sequencing and norovirus. *Future Virol* 2016;11:719–722.

120. Cotton BT, Hyde JL, Sarvestani ST, et al. The norovirus NS3 protein is a dynamic lipid- and microtubule-associated protein involved in viral RNA replication. *J Virol* 2017;91:e02138–16.

121. Coyne KP, Gaskell RM, Dawson S, et al. Evolutionary mechanisms of persistence and diversification of a calicivirus within endemically infected natural host populations. *J Virol* 2007;81:1961–1971.

122. Crane JK, Guerrant RL. *Acute Watery Diarrhea*. New York: Raven Press Ltd.; 1995.

123. Crawford SE, Ajami N, Parker TD, et al. Mapping broadly reactive norovirus genogroup I and II monoclonal antibodies. *Clin Vaccine Immunol* 2015;22:168–177.

124. Crisci E, Fraile L, Moreno N, et al. Chimeric calicivirus-like particles elicit specific immune responses in pigs. *Vaccine* 2012;30:2427–2439.

125. Czako R, Atmar RL, Opekun AR, et al. Serum hemagglutination inhibition activity correlates with protection from gastroenteritis in persons infected with Norwalk virus. *Clin Vaccine Immunol* 2012;19:284–287.

126. Damalanka VC, Kim Y, Galasiti Kankanamalage AC, et al. Structure-guided design, synthesis and evaluation of oxazolidinone-based inhibitors of norovirus 3CL protease. *Eur J Med Chem* 2018;143:881–890.

127. Dang W, Xu L, Yin Y, et al. IRF-1, RIG-I and MDA5 display potent antiviral activities against norovirus coordinately induced by different types of interferons. *Antiviral Res* 2018;155:48–59.

128. Daughenbaugh KF, Fraser CS, Hershey JW, et al. The genome-linked protein VPg of the Norwalk virus binds eIF3, suggesting its role in translation initiation complex recruitment. *EMBO J* 2003;22:2852–2859.

129. de Laval F, Nivoix P, Pommier de Santi V, et al. Severe norovirus outbreak among soldiers in the field: foodborne followed by person-to-person transmission. *Clin Infect Dis* 2011;53:399–400.

130. De Ravin SS, Wu X, Moir S, et al. Lentiviral hematopoietic stem cell gene therapy for X-linked severe combined immunodeficiency. *Sci Transl Med* 2016;8:335ra57.

131. de Wit MA, Koopmans MP, Kortbeek LM, et al. Sensor, a population-based cohort study on gastroenteritis in the Netherlands: incidence and etiology. *Am J Epidemiol* 2001;154:666–674.

132. Delacour H, Dubrous P, Koeck JL. Noroviruses: a challenge for military forces. *J R Army Med Corps* 2010;156:251–254.

133. Desai R, Hembree CD, Handel A, et al. Severe outcomes are associated with genogroup 2 genotype 4 norovirus outbreaks: a systematic literature review. *Clin Infect Dis* 2012;55:189–193.

134. Di Martino B, Marsilio F. Feline calicivirus VP2 is involved in the self-assembly of the capsid protein into virus-like particles. *Res Vet Sci* 2010;89:279–281.

135. Dingle KE. Mutation in a Lordsdale norovirus epidemic strain as a potential indicator of transmission routes. *J Clin Microbiol* 2004;42:3950–3957.

136. Doerflinger SY, Cortese M, Romero-Brey I, et al. Membrane alterations induced by nonstructural proteins of human norovirus. *PLoS Pathog* 2017;13:e1006705.

137. Doerflinger SY, Tabatabai J, Schnitzler P, et al. Development of a nanobody-based lateral flow immunoassay for detection of human norovirus. *mSphere* 2016;1:e00219–16.

138. Doerflinger SY, Weichert S, Koromyslova A, et al. Human norovirus evolution in a chronically infected host. *mSphere* 2017;2:e00352–16.

139. Dolin R. *Norwalk-Like Agents of Gastroenteritis*. New York: John Wiley & Sons; 1979.

140. Dolin R, Blacklow NR, DuPont H, et al. Transmission of acute infectious nonbacterial gastroenteritis to volunteers by oral administration of stool filtrates. *J Infect Dis* 1971;123:307–312.

141. Dolin R, Blacklow NR, DuPont H, et al. Biological properties of Norwalk agent of acute infectious nonbacterial gastroenteritis. *Proc Soc Exp Biol Med* 1972;140:578–583.

142. Dolin R, Levy AG, Wyatt RG, et al. Viral gastroenteritis induced by the Hawaii agent. Jejunal histopathology and serologic response. *Am J Med* 1975;59:761–768.

143. Dolin R, Reichman RC, Fauci AS. Lymphocyte populations in acute viral gastroenteritis. *Infect Immun* 1976;14:422–428.

144. Dolin R, Reichman RC, Roessner KD, et al. Detection by immune electron microscopy of the Snow Mountain agent of acute viral gastroenteritis. *J Infect Dis* 1982;146:184–189.

145. Dong X, Moyer MM, Yang F, et al. Carbon dots' antiviral functions against noroviruses. *Sci Rep* 2017;7:519.

146. Duizer E, Bijkerk P, Rockx B, et al. Inactivation of caliciviruses. *Appl Environ Microbiol* 2004;70:4538–4543.

147. Duizer E, Pielaat A, Vennema H, et al. Probabilities in norovirus outbreak diagnosis. *J Clin Virol* 2007;40:38–42.

148. Dunham DM, Jiang X, Berke T, et al. Genomic mapping of a calicivirus VPg. *Arch Virol* 1998;143:2421–2430.

149. Eden JS, Sharpe LJ, White PA, et al. Norovirus RNA-dependent RNA polymerase is phosphorylated by an important survival kinase, Akt. *J Virol* 2011;85:10894–10898.

150. Elftman MD, Gonzalez-Hernandez MB, Kamada N, et al. Multiple effects of dendritic cell depletion on murine norovirus infection. *J Gen Virol* 2013;94:1761–1768.

151. El-Kamary SS, Pasetti MF, Mendelman PM, et al. Adjuvanted intranasal Norwalk virus-like particle vaccine elicits antibodies and antibody-secreting cells that express homing receptors for mucosal and peripheral lymphoid tissues. *J Infect Dis* 2010;202: 1649–1658.

152. Emmott E, de Rougemont A, Hosmillo M, et al. Polyprotein processing and intermolecular interactions within the viral replication complex spatially and temporally control norovirus protease activity. *J Biol Chem* 2019;294(11):4259–4271.

153. Emmott E, Sorgeloos F, Caddy SL, et al. Norovirus-mediated modification of the translational landscape via virus and host-induced cleavage of translation initiation factors. *Mol Cell Proteomics* 2017;16(4 Suppl 1):S215–S229.

154. Enosi Tuipulotu D, Netzler NE, Lun JH, et al. RNA sequencing of murine norovirus-infected cells reveals transcriptional alteration of genes important to viral recognition and antigen presentation. *Front Immunol* 2017;8:959.

155. Enosi Tuipulotu D, Netzler NE, Lun JH, et al. TLR7 agonists display potent antiviral effects against norovirus infection via innate stimulation. *Antimicrob Agents Chemother* 2018;62:e02417–17.

156. Erickson AK, Jesudhasan PR, Mayer MJ, et al. Bacteria facilitate enteric virus co-infection of mammalian cells and promote genetic recombination. *Cell Host Microbe* 2018;23:77.e5–88.e5.

157. Esposito S, Ascolese B, Senatore L, et al. Pediatric norovirus infection. *Eur J Clin Microbiol Infect Dis* 2014;33:285–290.

158. Esseili MA, Wang Q, Saif LJ. Binding of human GII.4 norovirus virus-like particles to carbohydrates of romaine lettuce leaf cell wall materials. *Appl Environ Microbiol* 2012;78:786–794.

159. Ettayebi K, Hardy ME. Norwalk virus nonstructural protein p48 forms a complex with the SNARE regulator VAP-A and prevents cell surface expression of vesicular stomatitis virus G protein. *J Virol* 2003;77:11790–11797.

160. Ettayebi K, Crawford SE, Murakami K, et al. Replication of human noroviruses in stem cell-derived human enteroids. *Science* 2016;353:1387–1393.

161. Fang H, Tan M, Xia M, et al. Norovirus P particle efficiently elicits innate, humoral and cellular immunity. *PLoS One* 2013;8:e63269.

162. Fankhauser RL, Monroe SS, Noel JS, et al. Epidemiologic and molecular trends of "Norwalk-like viruses" associated with outbreaks of gastroenteritis in the United States. *J Infect Dis* 2002;186:1–7.

163. Farkas T, Cross RW, Hargitt E III, et al. Genetic diversity and histo-blood group antigen interactions of rhesus enteric caliciviruses. *J Virol* 2010;84:8617–8625.

164. Farkas T, Zhong WM, Jing Y, et al. Genetic diversity among sapoviruses. *Arch Virol* 2004;149:1309–1323.

165. Ferla S, Netzler NE, Ferla S, et al. In silico screening for human norovirus antivirals reveals a novel non-nucleoside inhibitor of the viral polymerase. *Sci Rep* 2018;8:4129.

166. Fernandes H, Leen EN, Cromwell H Jr, et al. Structure determination of Murine Norovirus NS6 proteases with C-terminal extensions designed to probe protease-substrate interactions. *PeerJ* 2015;3:e798.

167. Fernandez-Vega V, Sosnovtsev SV, Belliot G, et al. Norwalk virus N-terminal nonstructural protein is associated with disassembly of the Golgi complex in transfected cells. *J Virol* 2004;78:4827–4837.

168. Flewett TH, Davies H. Letter: caliciviruses in man. *Lancet* 1976;1:311.

169. Flynn WT, Saif LJ, Moorhead PD. Pathogenesis of porcine enteric calicivirus-like virus in four-day-old gnotobiotic pigs. *Am J Vet Res* 1988;49:819–825.

170. Fukushi S, Kojima S, Takai R, et al. Poly(A)- and primer-independent RNA polymerase of Norovirus. *J Virol* 2004;78:3889–3896.

171. Fullerton SW, Blaschke M, Coutard B, et al. Structural and functional characterization of sapovirus RNA-dependent RNA polymerase. *J Virol* 2007;81:1858–1871.

172. Furman LM, Maaty WS, Petersen LK, et al. Cysteine protease activation and apoptosis in Murine norovirus infection. *Virol J* 2009;6:139.

173. Gallimore CI, Cubitt DW, Richards AF, et al. Diversity of enteric viruses detected in patients with gastroenteritis in a tertiary referral paediatric hospital. *J Med Virol* 2004;73:443–449.

174. Gallimore CI, Iturriza-Gomara M, Xerry J, et al. Inter-seasonal diversity of norovirus genotypes: emergence and selection of virus variants. *Arch Virol* 2007;152:1295–1303.

175. Gao X, Esseili MA, Lu Z, et al. Recognition of histo-blood group antigen-like carbohydrates in lettuce by human GII.4 norovirus. *Appl Environ Microbiol* 2016;82:2966–2974.

176. Garaicoechea L, Aguilar A, Parra GI, et al. Llama nanoantibodies with therapeutic potential against human norovirus diarrhea. *PLoS One* 2015;10:e0133665.

177. Garcia C, DuPont HL, Long KZ, et al. Asymptomatic norovirus infection in Mexican children. *J Clin Microbiol* 2006;44:2997–3000.

178. Gastanaduy PA, Vicuna Y, Salazar F, et al. Transmission of norovirus within households in Quininde, Ecuador. *Pediatr Infect Dis J* 2015;34:1031–1033.

179. Gaulin C, Frigon M, Poirier D, et al. Transmission of calicivirus by a foodhandler in the pre-symptomatic phase of illness [In process citation]. *Epidemiol Infect* 1999;123:475–478.

180. Gerondopoulos A, Jackson T, Monaghan P, et al. Murine norovirus-1 cell entry is mediated through a non-clathrin-, non-caveolae-, dynamin- and cholesterol-dependent pathway. *J Gen Virol* 2010;91:1428–1438.

181. Giammanco GM, Rotolo V, Medici MC, et al. Recombinant norovirus GII.g/GII.12 gastroenteritis in children. *Infect Genet Evol* 2012;12:169–174.

182. Glass PJ, White LJ, Ball JM, et al. Norwalk virus open reading frame 3 encodes a minor structural protein. *J Virol* 2000;74:6581–6591.

183. Glass PJ, Zeng CQ, Estes MK. Two nonoverlapping domains on the Norwalk virus open reading frame 3 (ORF3) protein are involved in the formation of the phosphorylated 35K protein and in ORF3-capsid protein interactions. *J Virol* 2003;77:3569–3577.

184. Goller JL, Dimitriadis A, Tan A, et al. Long-term features of norovirus gastroenteritis in the elderly. *J Hosp Infect* 2004;58:286–291.

185. Gonzalez-Galan V, Sanchez-Fauqier A, Obando I, et al. High prevalence of community-acquired norovirus gastroenteritis among hospitalized children: a prospective study. *Clin Microbiol Infect* 2011;17:1895–1899.

186. Gonzalez-Hernandez MB, Liu T, Blanco LP, et al. Murine norovirus transcytosis across an in vitro polarized murine intestinal epithelial monolayer is mediated by M-like cells. *J Virol* 2013;87:12685–12693.

187. Gonzalez-Hernandez MB, Liu T, Payne HC, et al. Efficient norovirus and reovirus replication in the mouse intestine requires microfold (M) cells. *J Virol* 2014;88:6934–6943.

188. Goodfellow I, Chaudhry Y, Gioldasi I, et al. Calicivirus translation initiation requires an interaction between VPg and eIF 4 E. *EMBO Rep* 2005;6:968–972.

189. Graham DY, Jiang X, Tanaka T, et al. Norwalk virus infection of volunteers: new insights based on improved assays. *J Infect Dis* 1994;170:34–43.

190. Grau KR, Roth AN, Zhu S, et al. The major targets of acute norovirus infection are immune cells in the gut-associated lymphoid tissue. *Nat Microbiol* 2017;2:1586–1591.

191. Green KY. Norovirus infection in immunocompromised hosts. *Clin Microbiol Infect* 2014;20:717–723.

192. Green KY, Lew JF, Jiang X, et al. Comparison of the reactivities of baculovirus-expressed recombinant Norwalk virus capsid antigen with those of the native Norwalk virus antigen in serologic assays and some epidemiologic observations. *J Clin Microbiol* 1993;31:2185–2191.

193. Green KY, Mory A, Fogg MH, et al. Isolation of enzymatically active replication complexes from feline calicivirus-infected cells. *J Virol* 2002;76:8582–8595.

194. Green J, Wright PA, Gallimore CI, et al. The role of environmental contamination with small round structured viruses in a hospital outbreak investigated by reverse-transcriptase polymerase chain reaction assay. *J Hosp Infect* 1998;39:39–45.

195. Greenberg HB, Wyatt RG, Kapikian AZ. Norwalk virus in vomitus [letter]. *Lancet* 1979;1:55.

196. Guo L, Wang J, Zhou H, et al. Intranasal administration of a recombinant adenovirus expressing the norovirus capsid protein stimulates specific humoral, mucosal, and cellular immune responses in mice. *Vaccine* 2008;26:460–468.

197. Gustavsson L, Norden R, Westin J, et al. Slow clearance of norovirus following infection with emerging variants of genotype GII.4 strains. *J Clin Microbiol* 2017;55(5):1533–1539. doi: 10.1128/JCM.00061-17.

198. Gutierrez-Escolano AL, Brito ZU, del Angel RM, et al. Interaction of cellular proteins with the 5' end of Norwalk virus genomic RNA. *J Virol* 2000;74:8558–8562.

199. Gutierrez-Escolano AL, Vazquez-Ochoa M, Escobar-Herrera J, et al. La, PTB, and PAB proteins bind to the 3(') untranslated region of Norwalk virus genomic RNA. *Biochem Biophys Res Commun* 2003;311:759–766.

200. Habeta M, Luttermann C, Meyers G. Feline calicivirus can tolerate gross changes of its minor capsid protein expression levels induced by changing translation reinitiation frequency or use of a separate VP2-coding mRNA. *PLoS One* 2014;9:e102254.

201. Haga K, Fujimoto A, Takai-Todaka R, et al. Functional receptor molecules CD300lf and CD300ldwithin the CD300 family enable murine noroviruses to infect cells. *Proc Natl Acad Sci U S A* 2016;113(41):E6248–E6255.

202. Hall AJ, Lopman BA, Payne DC, et al. Norovirus disease in the United States. *Emerg Infect Dis* 2013;19:1198–1205.

203. Hall AJ, Rosenthal M, Gregoricus N, et al. Incidence of acute gastroenteritis and role of norovirus, Georgia, USA, 2004-2005. *Emerg Infect Dis* 2011;17:1381–1388.

204. Han L, Kitov PI, Kitova EN, et al. Affinities of recombinant norovirus P dimers for human blood group antigens. *Glycobiology* 2013;23:276–285.

205. Han KR, Lee JH, Kotiguda GG, et al. Nucleotide triphosphatase and RNA chaperone activities of murine norovirus NS3. *J Gen Virol* 2018;99:1482–1493.

206. Han L, Tan M, Xia M, et al. Gangliosides are ligands for human noroviruses. *J Am Chem Soc* 2014;136:12631–12637.

207. Hanisch FG, Hansman GS, Morozov V, et al. Avidity of alpha-fucose on human milk oligosaccharides and blood group-unrelated oligo/poly-fucoses is essential for potent norovirus binding targets. *J Biol Chem* 2018;293(30):11955–11965.

208. Hansman GS, Katayama K, Maneekarn N, et al. Genetic diversity of norovirus and sapovirus in hospitalized infants with sporadic cases of acute gastroenteritis in Chiang Mai, Thailand. *J Clin Microbiol* 2004;42:1305–1307.

209. Hansman GS, Taylor DW, McLellan JS, et al. Structural basis for broad detection of genogroup II noroviruses by a monoclonal antibody that binds to a site occluded in the viral particle. *J Virol* 2012;86:3635–3646.

210. Hardstaff JL, Clough HE, Lutje V, et al. Foodborne and food-handler norovirus outbreaks: a systematic review. *Foodborne Pathog Dis* 2018;15:589–597.

211. Hardy ME, Estes MK. Completion of the Norwalk virus genome sequence. *Virus Genes* 1996;12:287–290.

212. Hardy M, Crone T, Brower J, et al. Substrate specificity of the Norwalk virus 3C-like proteinase. *Virus Res* 2002;89:29.

213. Harris JP, Iturriza-Gomara M, Allen DJ, et al. Norovirus strain types found within the second infectious intestinal diseases (IID2) study an analysis of norovirus circulating in the community. *BMC Infect Dis* 2019;19:87.

214. Harris JP, Iturriza-Gomara M, O'Brien SJ. Estimating disability-adjusted life years (DALYs) in community cases of norovirus in England. *Viruses* 2019;11.

215. Hartono S, Bhagia A, Joshi AY. No! When the immunologist becomes a virologist: Norovirus—an emerging infection in immune deficiency diseases. *Curr Opin Allergy Clin Immunol* 2016;16:557–564.

216. Hassard F, Sharp JH, Taft H, et al. Critical review on the public health impact of norovirus contamination in shellfish and the environment: a UK perspective. *Food Environ Virol* 2017;9(2):123–141.

217. Helander HF, Fandriks L. Surface area of the digestive tract—revisited. *Scand J Gastroenterol* 2014;49:681–689.

218. Herbert TP, Brierley I, Brown TD. Detection of the ORF3 polypeptide of feline calicivirus in infected cells and evidence for its expression from a single, functionally bicistronic, subgenomic mRNA. *J Gen Virol* 1996;77:123–127.

219. Herbert TP, Brierley I, Brown TD. Identification of a protein linked to the genomic and subgenomic mRNAs of feline calicivirus and its role in translation. *J Gen Virol* 1997;78:1033–1040.

220. Hernandez BA, Sandoval-Jaime C, Sosnovtsev SV, et al. Nucleolin promotes in vitro translation of feline calicivirus genomic RNA. *Virology* 2016;489:51–62.

221. Hickman D, Jones MK, Zhu S, et al. The effect of malnutrition on norovirus infection. *MBio* 2014;5:e01032-13.

222. Hillenbrand B, Gunzel D, Richter JF, et al. Norovirus non-structural protein p20 leads to impaired restitution of epithelial defects by inhibition of actin cytoskeleton remodelling. *Scand J Gastroenterol* 2010;45:1307–1319.

223. Hirneisen KA, Markland SM, Kniel KE. Ozone inactivation of norovirus surrogates on fresh produce. *J Food Prot* 2011;74:836–839.

224. Hjelm BE, Kilbourne J, Herbst-Kralovetz MM. TLR7 and 9 agonists are highly effective mucosal adjuvants for norovirus virus-like particle vaccines. *Hum Vaccin Immunother* 2013;10(2):410–416.
225. Ho ZJ, Vithia G, Ng CG, et al. Emergence of norovirus GI.2 outbreaks in military camps in Singapore. *Int J Infect Dis* 2015;31:23–30.
226. Hogbom M, Jager K, Robel I, et al. The active form of the norovirus RNA-dependent RNA polymerase is a homodimer with cooperative activity. *J Gen Virol* 2009;90:281–291.
227. Hosmillo M, Chaudhry Y, Kim DS, et al. Sapovirus translation requires an interaction between VPg and the cap binding protein eIF4E. *J Virol* 2014;88:12213–12221.
228. Hosmillo M, Sweeney TR, Chaudhry Y, et al. The RNA helicase eIF4A is required for sapovirus translation. *J Virol* 2016;90:5200–5204.
229. Hu MH, Lin KL, Wu CT, et al. Clinical characteristics and risk factors for seizures associated with norovirus gastroenteritis in childhood. *J Child Neurol* 2017;32:810–814.
230. Huang P, Farkas T, Marionneau S, et al. Noroviruses bind to human ABO, Lewis, and secretor histo-blood group antigens: identification of 4 distinct strain-specific patterns. *J Infect Dis* 2003;188:19–31.
231. Huang P, Farkas T, Zhong W, et al. Norovirus and histo-blood group antigens: demonstration of a wide spectrum of strain specificities and classification of two major binding groups among multiple binding patterns. *J Virol* 2005;79:6714–6722.
232. Huang XY, Su J, Lu QC, et al. A large outbreak of acute gastroenteritis caused by the human norovirus GII.17 strain at a university in Henan Province, China. *Infect Dis Poverty* 2017;6:6.
233. Huhti L, Hemming-Harlo M, Vesikari T. Norovirus detection from sera of young children with acute norovirus gastroenteritis. *J Clin Virol* 2016;79:6–9.
234. Huhti L, Szakal ED, Puustinen L, et al. Norovirus GII-4 causes a more severe gastroenteritis than other noroviruses in young children. *J Infect Dis* 2011;203:1442–1444.
235. Hussey RJ, Coates L, Gill RS, et al. Crystallization and preliminary X-ray diffraction analysis of the protease from Southampton norovirus complexed with a Michael acceptor inhibitor. *Acta Crystallogr Sect F Struct Biol Cryst Commun* 2010;66:1544–1548.
236. Hutson AM, Airaud F, Lependu J, et al. Norwalk virus infection associates with secretor status genotyped from sera. *J Med Virol* 2005;77:116–120.
237. Hutson AM, Atmar RL, Marcus DM, et al. Norwalk virus-like particle hemagglutination by binding to h histo-blood group antigens. *J Virol* 2003;77:405–415.
238. Hyde JL, Gillespie LK, Mackenzie JM. Mouse norovirus 1 utilizes the cytoskeleton network to establish localization of the replication complex proximal to the microtubule organizing center. *J Virol* 2012;86:4110–4122.
239. Hyde JL, Sosnovtsev SV, Green KY, et al. Mouse norovirus replication is associated with virus-induced vesicle clusters originating from membranes derived from the secretory pathway. *J Virol* 2009;83:9709–9719.
240. Inouye S, Yamashita K, Yamadera S, et al. Surveillance of viral gastroenteritis in Japan: pediatric cases and outbreak incidents. *J Infect Dis* 2000;181:S270–S274.
241. Ito S, Takeshita S, Nezu A, et al. Norovirus-associated encephalopathy. *Pediatr Infect Dis J* 2006;25:651–652.
242. Jiang X, Graham DY, Wang K, et al. Norwalk virus genome cloning and characterization. *Science* 1990;250:1580–1583.
243. Jiang X, Huang P, Zhong W, et al. Human milk contains elements that block binding of noroviruses to histo-blood group antigens in saliva. *Adv Exp Med Biol* 2004;554:447–450.
244. Jiang X, Wang M, Graham DY, et al. Expression, self-assembly, and antigenicity of the Norwalk virus capsid protein. *J Virol* 1992;66:6527–6532.
245. Jiang X, Wang M, Wang K, et al. Sequence and genomic organization of Norwalk virus. *Virology* 1993;195:51–61.
246. Jiang X, Wilton N, Zhong WM, et al. Diagnosis of human caliciviruses by use of enzyme immunoassays. *J Infect Dis* 2000;181:S349–S359.
247. Johnson PC, Mathewson JJ, DuPont HL, et al. Multiple-challenge study of host susceptibility to Norwalk gastroenteritis in US adults. *J Infect Dis* 1990;161:18–21.
248. Jones MK, Watanabe M, Zhu S, et al. Enteric bacteria promote human and mouse norovirus infection of B cells. *Science* 2014;346:755–759.
249. Jukes TH. Recent advances in studies of evolutionary relationships between proteins and nucleic acids. *Space Life Sci* 1969;1:469–490.
250. Jung K, Wang Q, Kim Y, et al. The effects of simvastatin or interferon-alpha on infectivity of human norovirus using a gnotobiotic pig model for the study of antivirals. *PLoS One* 2012;7:e41619.
251. Kageyama T, Kojima S, Shinohara M, et al. Broadly reactive and highly sensitive assay for Norwalk-like viruses based on real-time quantitative reverse transcription-PCR. *J Clin Microbiol* 2003;41:1548–1557.
252. Kahan SM, Liu G, Reinhard MK, et al. Comparative murine norovirus studies reveal a lack of correlation between intestinal virus titers and enteric pathology. *Virology* 2011;421:202–210.
253. Kaiser WJ, Chaudhry Y, Sosnovtsev SV, et al. Analysis of protein-protein interactions in the feline calicivirus replication complex. *J Gen Virol* 2006;87:363–368.
254. Kambhampati A, Payne DC, Costantini V, et al. Host genetic susceptibility to enteric viruses: a systematic review and metaanalysis. *Clin Infect Dis* 2016;62:11–18.
255. Kapikian AZ. The discovery of the 27-nm Norwalk virus: An historic perspective. *J Infect Dis* 2000;181:S295–S302.
256. Kapikian AZ, Wyatt RG, Dolin R, et al. Visualization by immune electron microscopy of a 27-nm particle associated with acute infectious nonbacterial gastroenteritis. *J Virol* 1972;10:1075–1081.
257. Kaplan JE, Feldman R, Campbell DS, et al. The frequency of a Norwalk-like pattern of illness in outbreaks of acute gastroenteritis. *Am J Public Health* 1982;72:1329–1332.
258. Kaplan JE, Gary GW, Baron RC, et al. Epidemiology of Norwalk gastroenteritis and the role of Norwalk virus in outbreaks of acute nonbacterial gastroenteritis. *Ann Intern Med* 1982;96:756–761.
259. Karakasiliotis I, Vashist S, Bailey D, et al. Polypyrimidine tract binding protein functions as a negative regulator of feline calicivirus translation. *PLoS One* 2010;5:e9562.
260. Karandikar UC, Crawford SE, Ajami NJ, et al. Detection of human norovirus in intestinal biopsies from immunocompromised transplant patients. *J Gen Virol* 2016;97:2291–2300.
261. Karst SM. The influence of commensal bacteria on infection with enteric viruses. *Nat Rev Microbiol* 2016;14:197–204.
262. Karst SM, Baric RS. What is the reservoir of emergent human norovirus strains? *J Virol* 2015;89(11):5756–5759.
263. Karst SM, Wobus CE. Viruses in rodent colonies: lessons learned from murine noroviruses. *Annu Rev Virol* 2015;2:525–548.
264. Karst SM, Wobus CE. A working model of how noroviruses infect the intestine. *PLoS Pathog* 2015;11:e1004626.
265. Karst SM, Wobus CE, Lay M, et al. STAT1-dependent innate immunity to a Norwalk-like virus. *Science* 2003;299:1575–1578.
266. Karsten C, Baumgarte S, Friedrich AW, et al. Incidence and risk factors for community-acquired acute gastroenteritis in north-west Germany in 2004. *Eur J Clin Microbiol Infect Dis* 2009;28:935–943.
267. Katayama K, Murakami K, Sharp TM, et al. Plasmid-based human norovirus reverse genetics system produces reporter-tagged progeny virus containing infectious genomic RNA. *Proc Natl Acad Sci U S A* 2014;111:E4043–E4052.
268. Katpally U, Voss NR, Cavazza T, et al. High-resolution cryo-electron microscopy structures of murine norovirus 1 and rabbit hemorrhagic disease virus reveal marked flexibility in the receptor binding domains. *J Virol* 2010;84:5836–5841.
269. Katpally U, Wobus CE, Dryden K, et al. Structure of antibody-neutralized murine norovirus and unexpected differences from viruslike particles. *J Virol* 2008;82:2079–2088.
270. Kaufman SS, Chatterjee NK, Fuschino ME, et al. Characteristics of human calicivirus enteritis in intestinal transplant recipients. *J Pediatr Gastroenterol Nutr* 2005;40:328–333.
271. Kaufman SS, Green KY, Korba BE. Treatment of norovirus infections: moving antivirals from the bench to the bedside. *Antiviral Res* 2014;105:80–91.
272. Kernbauer E, Ding Y, Cadwell K. An enteric virus can replace the beneficial function of commensal bacteria. *Nature* 2014;516:94–98.
273. Khan RR, Lawson AD, Minnich LL, et al Gastrointestinal norovirus infection associated with exacerbation of inflammatory bowel disease. *J Pediatr Gastroenterol Nutr* 2009;48:328–333.
274. Kilgore PE, Belay ED, Hamlin DM, et al. A university outbreak of gastroenteritis due to a small round- structured virus. Application of molecular diagnostics to identify the etiologic agent and patterns of transmission. *J Infect Dis* 1996;173:787–793.
275. Kilic T, Koromyslova A, Hansman GS. Structural basis for human norovirus capsid binding to bile acids. *J Virol* 2019;93:e01581–18.
276. Kilic T, Koromyslova A, Malak V, et al. Atomic structure of the murine norovirus protruding domain and soluble CD300lf receptor complex. *J Virol* 2018;92.
277. Kim GH, Byeon JH, Lee DY, et al. Norovirus in benign convulsions with mild gastroenteritis. *Ital J Pediatr* 2016;42:94.
278. Kim SH, Chen S, Jiang X, et al. Newcastle disease virus vector producing human norovirus-like particles induces serum, cellular, and mucosal immune responses in mice. *J Virol* 2014;88:9718–9727.
279. Kim BR, Choi GE, Kim YO, et al. Incidence and characteristics of norovirus-associated benign convulsions with mild gastroenteritis, in comparison with rotavirus ones. *Brain Dev* 2018;40(8):699–706.
280. Kim DS, Hosmillo M, Alfajaro MM, et al. Both alpha2,3- and alpha2,6-linked sialic acids on o-linked glycoproteins act as functional receptors for porcine sapovirus. *PLoS Pathog* 2014;10:e1004172.
281. Kim L, Liebowitz D, Lin K, et al. Safety and immunogenicity of an oral tablet norovirus vaccine, a phase I randomized, placebo-controlled trial. *JCI Insight* 2018;3.
282. Kim YG, Park JH, Reimer T, et al. Viral infection augments Nod1/2 signaling to potentiate lethality associated with secondary bacterial infections. *Cell Host Microbe* 2011;9:496–507.
283. Kim Y, Thapa M, Hua DH, et al. Biodegradable nanogels for oral delivery of interferon for norovirus infection. *Antiviral Res* 2011;89:165–173.
284. Kimura E, Goto H, Migita A, et al. An adult norovirus-related encephalitis/encephalopathy with mild clinical manifestation. *BMJ Case Rep* 2010;2010.
285. Kingsley DH, Holliman DR, Calci KR, et al. Inactivation of a norovirus by high-pressure processing. *Appl Environ Microbiol* 2007;73:581–585.
286. Kirby A, Ashton L, Hart IJ. Detection of norovirus infection in the hospital setting using vomit samples. *J Clin Virol* 2011;51:86–87.
287. Kirby A, Dove W, Ashton L, et al. Detection of norovirus in mouthwash samples from patients with acute gastroenteritis. *J Clin Virol* 2010;48:285–287.
288. Kirby AE, Shi J, Montes J, et al. Disease course and viral shedding in experimental Norwalk virus and Snow Mountain virus infection. *J Med Virol* 2014;86:2055–2064.
289. Kirby AE, Streby A, Moe CL. Vomiting as a symptom and transmission risk in norovirus illness: evidence from human challenge studies. *PLoS One* 2016;11:e0143759.
290. Kirking HL, Cortes J, Burrer S, et al. Likely transmission of norovirus on an airplane, October 2008. *Clin Infect Dis* 2010;50:1216–1221.
291. Kirkland KB, Meriwether RA, Leiss JK, et al. Steaming oysters does not prevent Norwalk-like gastroenteritis. *Public Health Rep* 1996;111:527–530.
292. Kirkwood CD, Clark R, Bogdanovic-Sakran N, et al. A 5-year study of the prevalence and genetic diversity of human caliciviruses associated with sporadic cases of acute gastroenteritis in young children admitted to hospital in Melbourne, Australia (1998–2002). *J Med Virol* 2005;77:96–101.
293. Kitano M, Hosmillo M, Emmott E, et al. Selection and characterization of rupintrivir-resistant Norwalk virus replicon cells in vitro. *Antimicrob Agents Chemother* 2018;62:e00201–18.
294. Kocher J, Yuan L. Norovirus vaccines and potential antinorovirus drugs: recent advances and future perspectives. *Future Virol* 2015;10:899–913.
295. Kocher JF, Lindesmith LC, Debbink K, et al. Bat caliciviruses and human noroviruses are antigenically similar and have overlapping histo-blood group antigen binding profiles. *MBio* 2018:9;e00869–18.
296. Koho T, Ihalainen TO, Stark M, et al. His-tagged norovirus-like particles: a versatile platform for cellular delivery and surface display. *Eur J Pharm Biopharm* 2015;96:22–31.
297. Kolawole AO, Gonzalez-Hernandez MB, Turula H, et al. Oral norovirus infection is blocked in mice lacking Peyer's patches and mature M cells. *J Virol* 2016;90: 1499–1506.

298. Kolawole AO, Li M, Xia C, et al. Flexibility in surface-exposed loops in a virus capsid mediates escape from antibody neutralization. *J Virol* 2014;88:4543–4557.
299. Kolawole AO, Smith HQ, Svoboda SA, et al. Norovirus escape from broadly neutralizing antibodies is limited to allostery-like mechanisms. *mSphere* 2017;2:e00334–17.
300. Kolawole AO, Xia C, Li M, et al. Newly isolated mAbs broaden the neutralizing epitope in murine norovirus. *J Gen Virol* 2014;95:1958–1968.
301. Komolafe OO, Jarrett O. A possible maturation pathway of calicivirus particles. *Microbios* 1986;46:103–111.
302. Konig M, Thiel HJ, Meyers G. Detection of viral proteins after infection of cultured hepatocytes with rabbit hemorrhagic disease virus. *J Virol* 1998;72:4492–4497.
303. Koo HL, Neill FH, Estes MK, et al. Noroviruses: the most common pediatric viral enteric pathogen at a large university hospital after introduction of rotavirus vaccination. *J Pediatric Infect Dis Soc* 2013;2:57–60.
304. Koopmans M, Vinje J, de Wit M, et al. Molecular epidemiology of human enteric caliciviruses in The Netherlands. *J Infect Dis* 2000;181:S262–S269.
305. Koromyslova AD, Leuthold MM, Bowler MW, et al. The sweet quartet: binding of fucose to the norovirus capsid. *Virology* 2015;483:203–208.
306. Koromyslova AD, Morozov VA, Hefele L, et al. Human norovirus neutralized by a monoclonal antibody targeting the HBGA pocket. *J Virol* 2019;93:e02174–18.
307. Kovac K, Diez-Valcarce M, Raspor P, et al. Effect of high hydrostatic pressure processing on norovirus infectivity and genome stability in strawberry puree and mineral water. *Int J Food Microbiol* 2012;152:35–39.
308. Kowalzik F, Binder H, Zoller D, et al. Norovirus gastroenteritis among hospitalized patients, Germany, 2007-2012. *Emerg Infect Dis* 2018;24:2021–2028.
309. Kreutz LC, Seal BS. The pathway of feline calicivirus entry. *Virus Res* 1995;35:63–70.
310. Kreutz LC, Seal BS, Mengeling WL. Early interaction of feline calicivirus with cells in culture. *Arch Virol* 1994;136:19–34.
311. Kroneman A, Vega E, Vennema H, et al. Proposal for a unified norovirus nomenclature and genotyping. *Arch Virol* 2013;158:2059–2068.
312. Kroneman A, Vennema H, Deforche K, et al. An automated genotyping tool for enteroviruses and noroviruses. *J Clin Virol* 2011;51:121–125.
313. Kroneman A, Verhoef L, Harris J, et al. Analysis of integrated virological and epidemiological reports of norovirus outbreaks collected within the Foodborne Viruses in Europe network from 1 July 2001 to 30 June 2006. *J Clin Microbiol* 2008;46:2959–2965.
314. Kubota T, Kumagai A, Ito H, et al. Structural basis for the recognition of Lewis antigens by genogroup I norovirus. *J Virol* 2012;86:11138–11150.
315. Kuyumcu-Martinez M, Belliot G, Sosnovtsev SV, et al. Calicivirus 3C-like proteinase inhibits cellular translation by cleavage of poly(A)-binding protein. *J Virol* 2004;78:8172–8182.
316. L'Homme Y, Sansregret R, Plante-Fortier E, et al. Genetic diversity of porcine Norovirus and Sapovirus: Canada, 2005–2007. *Arch Virol* 2009;154:581–593.
317. Lambden PR, Caul EO, Ashley CR, et al. Sequence and genome organization of a human small round-structured (Norwalk-like) virus. *Science* 1993;259:516–519.
318. Lambden PR, Caul EO, Ashley CR, et al. Human enteric caliciviruses are genetically distinct from small round structured viruses [letter]. *Lancet* 1994;343:666–667.
319. Lambden PR, Liu B, Clarke IN. A conserved sequence motif at the 5' terminus of the Southampton virus genome is characteristic of the Caliciviridae. *Virus Genes* 1995;10:149–152.
320. Lazear HM, Lancaster A, Wilkins C, et al. IRF-3, IRF-5, and IRF-7 coordinately regulate the type I IFN response in myeloid dendritic cells downstream of MAVS signaling. *PLoS Pathog* 2013;9:e1003118.
321. Le Guyader F, Loisy F, Atmar RL, et al. Norwalk virus-specific binding to oyster digestive tissues. *Emerg Infect Dis* 2006;12:931–936.
322. Le Pendu J. Histo-blood group antigen and human milk oligosaccharides: genetic polymorphism and risk of infectious diseases. *Adv Exp Med Biol* 2004;554:135–143.
323. Le Pendu J, Abrantes J, Bertagnoli S, et al. Proposal for a unified classification system and nomenclature of lagoviruses. *J Gen Virol* 2017;98:1658–1666.
324. Lee RM, Lessler J, Lee RA, et al. Incubation periods of viral gastroenteritis: a systematic review. *BMC Infect Dis* 2013;13:446.
325. Lee JH, Park BS, Han KR, et al. Insight into the interaction between RNA polymerase and VPg for murine norovirus replication. *Front Microbiol* 2018;9:1466.
326. Lee S, Wilen CB, Orvedahl A, et al. Norovirus cell tropism is determined by combinatorial action of a viral non-structural protein and host cytokine. *Cell Host Microbe* 2017;22:449. e4–459.e4.
327. Leen EN, Kwok KY, Birtley JR, et al. Structures of the compact helical core domains of feline calicivirus and murine norovirus VPg proteins. *J Virol* 2013;87:5318–5330.
328. Leite JP, Ando T, Noel JS, et al. Characterization of Toronto virus capsid protein expressed in baculovirus. *Arch Virol* 1996;141:865–875.
329. Leon JS, Kingsley DH, Montes JS, et al. Randomized, double-blinded clinical trial for human norovirus inactivation in oysters by high hydrostatic pressure processing. *Appl Environ Microbiol* 2011;77:5476–5482.
330. Levenson EA, Martens C, Kanakabandi K, et al. Comparative transcriptomic response of primary and immortalized macrophages to murine norovirus infection. *J Immunol* 2018;200:4157–4169.
331. Levy AG, Widerlite L, Schwartz CJ, et al. Jejunal adenylate cyclase activity in human subjects during viral gastroenteritis. *Gastroenterology* 1976;70:321–325.
332. Lew JF, Kapikian AZ, Valdesuso J, et al. Molecular characterization of Hawaii virus and other Norwalk-like viruses: evidence for genetic polymorphism among human caliciviruses. *J Infect Dis* 1994;170:535–542.
333. Li D, Breiman A, le Pendu J, et al. Binding to histo-blood group antigen-expressing bacteria protects human norovirus from acute heat stress. *Front Microbiol* 2015;6:659.
334. Li TF, Hosmillo M, Schwanke H, et al. Human norovirus NS3 has RNA helicase and chaperoning activities. *J Virol* 2018;92:e01606–17.
335. Lin Y, Fengling L, Lianzhu W, et al. Function of VP2 protein in the stability of the secondary structure of virus-like particles of genogroup II norovirus at different pH levels: function of VP2 protein in the stability of NoV VLPs. *J Microbiol* 2014;52:970–975.
336. Lin X, Thorne L, Jin Z, et al. Subgenomic promoter recognition by the norovirus RNA-dependent RNA polymerases. *Nucleic Acids Res* 2015;43:446–460.
337. Lindesmith LC, Brewer-Jensen PD, Mallory ML, et al. Human norovirus epitope D plasticity allows escape from antibody immunity without loss of capacity for binding cellular ligands. *J Virol* 2019;93.
338. Lindesmith LC, Donaldson EF, Baric RS. Norovirus GII.4 strain antigenic variation. *J Virol* 2011;85:231–242.
339. Lindesmith LC, Mallory ML, Debbink K, et al. Conformational occlusion of blockade antibody epitopes, a novel mechanism of GII.4 human norovirus immune evasion. *mSphere* 2018;3:e00518–17.
340. Lindesmith L, Moe C, Lependu J, et al. Cellular and humoral immunity following Snow Mountain virus challenge. *J Virol* 2005;79:2900–2909.
341. Lindesmith L, Moe C, Marionneau S, et al. Human susceptibility and resistance to Norwalk virus infection. *Nat Med* 2003;9:548–553.
342. Lindsay L, Wolter J, De Coster I, et al. A decade of norovirus disease risk among older adults in upper-middle and high income countries: a systematic review. *BMC Infect Dis* 2015;15:425.
343. Liu W, Chen Y, Jiang X, et al. A unique human norovirus lineage with a distinct HBGA binding interface. *PLoS Pathog* 2015;11:e1005025.
344. Liu BL, Clarke IN, Caul EO, et al. Human enteric caliciviruses have a unique genome structure and are distinct from the Norwalk-like viruses. *Arch Virol* 1995;140: 1345–1356.
345. Liu B, Clarke IN, Lambden PR. Polyprotein processing in Southampton virus: identification of 3C-like protease cleavage sites by in vitro mutagenesis. *J Virol* 1996;70:2605–2610.
346. Liu Y, Liu X, Kang H, et al. Identification of feline interferon regulatory factor 1 as an efficient antiviral factor against the replication of feline calicivirus and other feline viruses. *Biomed Res Int* 2018;2018:2739830.
347. Liu G, Ni Z, Yun T, et al. A DNA-launched reverse genetics system for rabbit hemorrhagic disease virus reveals that the VP2 protein is not essential for virus infectivity. *J Gen Virol* 2008;89:3080–3085.
348. Liu BL, Viljoen GJ, Clarke IN, et al. Identification of further proteolytic cleavage sites in the Southampton calicivirus polyprotein by expression of the viral protease in *E. coli*. *J Gen Virol* 1999;80:291–296.
349. LoBue AD, Lindesmith LC, Baric RS. Identification of cross-reactive norovirus CD4+ T cell epitopes. *J Virol* 2010;84:8530–8538.
350. LoBue AD, Lindesmith L, Yount B, et al. Multivalent norovirus vaccines induce strong mucosal and systemic blocking antibodies against multiple strains. *Vaccine* 2006;24:5220–5234.
351. Lochridge VP, Hardy ME. A single-amino-acid substitution in the P2 domain of VP1 of murine norovirus is sufficient for escape from antibody neutralization. *J Virol* 2007;81:12316–12322.
352. Lodder WJ, Vinje J, van De Heide R, et al. Molecular detection of Norwalk-like caliciviruses in sewage. *Appl Environ Microbiol* 1999;65:5624–5627.
353. Lopes AM, Breiman A, Lora M, et al. Host specific glycans are correlated with susceptibility to infection by lagoviruses, but not with their virulence. *J Virol* 2018;92:e01759–17.
354. Lopes-Joao A, Mesquita JR, de Sousa R, et al. Country-wide surveillance of norovirus outbreaks in the Portuguese Army, 2015-2017. *J R Army Med Corps* 2018;164:419–422.
355. Lopez-Manriquez E, Vashist S, Urena L, et al. Norovirus genome circularization and efficient replication are facilitated by binding of PCBP2 and hnRNP A1. *J Virol* 2013;87:11371–11387.
356. Lopman BA, Adak GK, Reacher MH, et al. Two epidemiologic patterns of norovirus outbreaks: surveillance in England and wales, 1992-2000. *Emerg Infect Dis* 2003;9:71–77.
357. Lopman B, Gastanaduy P, Park GW, et al. Environmental transmission of norovirus gastroenteritis. *Curr Opin Virol* 2012;2:96–102.
358. Lopman BA, Hall AJ, Curns AT, et al. Increasing rates of gastroenteritis hospital discharges in US adults and the contribution of norovirus, 1996-2007. *Clin Infect Dis* 2011;52:466–474.
359. Lopman BA, Reacher MH, Van Duijnhoven Y, et al. Viral gastroenteritis outbreaks in Europe, 1995–2000. *Emerg Infect Dis* 2003;9:90–96.
360. Lopman B, Simmons K, Gambhir M, et al. Epidemiologic implications of asymptomatic reinfection: a mathematical modeling study of norovirus. *Am J Epidemiol* 2014;179:507–512.
361. Lopman BA, Steele D, Kirkwood CD, et al. The vast and varied global burden of norovirus: prospects for prevention and control. *PLoS Med* 2016;13:e1001999.
362. Lopman BA, Trivedi T, Vicuna Y, et al. Norovirus infection and disease in an ecuadorian birth cohort: association of certain norovirus genotypes with host FUT2 secretor status. *J Infect Dis* 2015;211(11):1813–1821.
363. Lowther JA, Gustar NE, Hartnell RE, et al. Comparison of norovirus RNA levels in outbreak-related oysters with background environmental levels. *J Food Prot* 2012;75:389–393.
364. Lu Z, Ledgerwood ED, Hinchman MM, et al. Conserved surface residues on the feline calicivirus capsid are essential for interaction with its receptor feline junctional adhesion molecule A (fJAM-A). *J Virol* 2018;:e00035–18.
365. Lucero Y, Vidal R, O'Ryan GM. Norovirus vaccines under development. *Vaccine* 2018;36:5435–5441.
366. Ludwig-Begall LF, Mauroy A, Thiry E. Norovirus recombinants: recurrent in the field, recalcitrant in the lab—a scoping review of recombination and recombinant types of noroviruses. *J Gen Virol* 2018;99:970–988.
367. Luttermann C, Meyers G. A bipartite sequence motif induces translation reinitiation in feline calicivirus RNA. *J Biol Chem* 2007;282:7056–7065.
368. Luttermann C, Meyers G. The importance of inter- and intramolecular base pairing for translation reinitiation on a eukaryotic bicistronic mRNA. *Genes Dev* 2009;23:331–344.
369. Ma D, Shen L, Wu K, et al. Low-cost detection of norovirus using paper-based cell-free systems and synbody-based viral enrichment. *Synth Biol (Oxf)* 2018;3:ysy018.
370. Maalouf H, Schaeffer J, Parnaudeau S, et al. Strain-dependent norovirus bioaccumulation in oysters. *Appl Environ Microbiol* 2011;77:3189–3196.

371. MacDuff DA, Baldridge MT, Qaqish AM, et al. HOIL1 is essential for the induction of type I and III interferons by MDA5 and regulates persistent murine norovirus infection. *J Virol* 2018;92:e01368–18.
372. Machin A, Martin Alonso JM, Parra F. Identification of the amino acid residue involved in rabbit hemorrhagic disease virus VPg uridylylation. *J Biol Chem* 2001;276:27787–27792.
373. Madeley CR, Cosgrove BP. Letter: Caliciviruses in man. *Lancet* 1976;1:199–200.
374. Makino A, Shimojima M, Miyazawa T, et al. Junctional adhesion molecule 1 is a functional receptor for feline calicivirus. *J Virol* 2006;80:4482–4490.
375. Mallagaray A, Lockhauserbaumer J, Hansman G, et al. Attachment of norovirus to histo blood group antigens: a cooperative multistep process. *Angew Chem Int Ed Engl* 2015;54:12014–12019.
376. Mallagaray A, Rademacher C, Parra F, et al. Saturation transfer difference nuclear magnetic resonance titrations reveal complex multistep-binding of l-fucose to norovirus particles. *Glycobiology* 2017;27:80–86.
377. Malm M, Tamminen K, Vesikari T, et al. Norovirus-specific memory T cell responses in adult human donors. *Front Microbiol* 2016;7:1570.
378. Malm M, Uusi-Kerttula H, Vesikari T, et al. High serum levels of norovirus genotype-specific blocking antibodies correlate with protection from infection in children. *J Infect Dis* 2014;210:1755–1762.
379. Maloney NS, Thackray LB, Goel G, et al. Essential cell-autonomous role for interferon (IFN) regulatory factor 1 in IFN-gamma-mediated inhibition of norovirus replication in macrophages. *J Virol* 2012;86:12655–12664.
380. Manuel CS, Moore MD, Jaykus LA. Predicting human norovirus infectivity—recent advances and continued challenges. *Food Microbiol* 2018;76:337–345.
381. Marin MS, Casais R, Alonso Martin JM, et al. ATP binding and ATPase activities associated with recombinant rabbit hemorrhagic disease virus 2C-like polypeptide. *J Virol* 2000;74:10846–10851.
382. Marionneau S, Ruvoen N, Le Moullac-Vaidye B, et al. Norwalk virus binds to histo-blood group antigens present on gastroduodenal epithelial cells of secretor individuals. *Gastroenterology* 2002;122:1967–1977.
383. Marks PJ, Vipond IB, Carlisle D, et al. Evidence for airborne transmission of Norwalk-like virus (NLV) in a hotel restaurant. *Epidemiol Infect* 2000;124:481–487.
384. Marks PJ, Vipond IB, Regan FM, et al. A school outbreak of Norwalk-like virus: evidence for airborne transmission. *Epidemiol Infect* 2003;131:727–736.
385. Martin-Alonso JM, Skilling DE, Gonzalez-Molleda L, et al. Isolation and characterization of a new Vesivirus from rabbits. *Virology* 2005;337:373–383.
386. Martinez N, Espul C, Cuello H, et al. Sequence diversity of human caliciviruses recovered from children with diarrhea in Mendoza, Argentina, 1995–1998. *J Med Virol* 2002;67:289–298.
387. Mata LJ, Urrutia JJ, Gordon JE. Diseases and disabilities. In: Mata LJ, ed. *The Children of Santa Maria Cauque: A Prospective Field Study of Health and Growth*. Cambridge, MA: MIT Press; 1978:254–292.
388. Matson DO, Zhong WM, Nakata S, et al. Molecular characterization of a human calicivirus with sequence relationships closer to animal caliciviruses than other known human caliciviruses. *J Med Virol* 1995;45:215–222.
389. Matthews JE, Dickey BW, Miller RD, et al. The epidemiology of published norovirus outbreaks: a review of risk factors associated with attack rate and genogroup. *Epidemiol Infect* 2012;140:1161–1172.
390. Mattner F, Sohr D, Heim A, et al. Risk groups for clinical complications of norovirus infections: an outbreak investigation. *Clin Microbiol Infect* 2006;12:69–74.
391. Maunula L, Miettinen IT, von Bonsdorff CH. Norovirus outbreaks from drinking water. *Emerg Infect Dis* 2005;11:1716–1721.
392. Mauroy A, Gillet L, Mathijs E, et al. Alternative attachment factors and internalization pathways for GIII.2 bovine noroviruses. *J Gen Virol* 2011;92:1398–1409.
393. McCarthy M, Estes MK, Hyams KC. Norwalk-like virus infection in military forces: Epidemic potential, sporadic disease, and the future direction of prevention and control efforts. *J Infect Dis* 2000;181:S387–S391.
394. McCune BT, Tang W, Lu J, et al. Noroviruses co-opt the function of host proteins VAPA and VAPB for replication via a phenylalanine-phenylalanine-acidic-tract-motif mimic in nonstructural viral protein NS1/2. *MBio* 2017;8:e00668–17.
395. McDonnell S, Kirkland KB, Hlady WG, et al. Failure of cooking to prevent shellfish-associated viral gastroenteritis. *Arch Intern Med* 1997;157:111–116.
396. McEvoy M, Blake W, Brown D, et al. An outbreak of viral gastroenteritis on a cruise ship. *Commun Dis Rep CDR Rev* 1996;6:R188–R192.
397. McFadden N, Bailey D, Carrara G, et al. Norovirus regulation of the innate immune response and apoptosis occurs via the product of the alternative open reading frame 4. *PLoS Pathog* 2011;7:e1002413.
398. Meeroff JC, Schreiber DS, Trier JS, et al. Abnormal gastric motor function in viral gastroenteritis. *Ann Intern Med* 1980;92:370–373.
399. Melhem NM, Zaraket H, Kreidieh K, et al. Clinical and epidemiological characteristics of norovirus gastroenteritis among hospitalized children in Lebanon. *World J Gastroenterol* 2016;22:10557–10565.
400. Menon VK, George S, Ramani S, et al. Genogroup IIb norovirus infections and association with enteric symptoms in a neonatal nursery in southern India. *J Clin Microbiol* 2010;48:3212–3215.
401. Meyers G. Translation of the minor capsid protein of a calicivirus is initiated by a novel termination-dependent reinitiation mechanism. *J Biol Chem* 2003;278(36):34051–34060.
402. Meyers G. Characterization of the sequence element directing translation reinitiation in RNA of the calicivirus rabbit hemorrhagic disease virus. *J Virol* 2007;81:9623–9632.
403. Meyers G, Wirblich C, Thiel H-J. Rabbit hemorrhagic disease virus—molecular cloning and nucleotide sequencing of a calicivirus genome. *Virology* 1991;184:664–676.
404. Meyers G, Wirblich C, Thiel HJ. Genomic and subgenomic RNAs of rabbit hemorrhagic disease virus are both protein-linked and packaged into particles. *Virology* 1991;184:677–686.
405. Mirabelli C, Wobus CE. All aboard! Enteric viruses travel together. *Cell Host Microbe* 2018;24:183–185.
406. Mitra T, Sosnovtsev SV, Green KY. Mutagenesis of tyrosine 24 in the VPg protein is lethal for feline calicivirus. *J Virol* 2004;78:4931–4935.
407. Miura T, Sano D, Suenaga A, et al. Histo-blood group antigen-like substances of human enteric bacteria as specific adsorbents for human noroviruses. *J Virol* 2013;87:9441–9451.
408. Mochizuki M, Nakatani H, Yoshida M. Inhibitory effects of recombinant feline interferon on the replication of feline enteropathogenic viruses in vitro. *Vet Microbiol* 1994;39:145–152.
409. Monroe SS, Stine SE, Jiang X, et al. Detection of antibody to recombinant Norwalk virus antigen in specimens from outbreaks of gastroenteritis. *J Clin Microbiol* 1993;31:2866–2872.
410. Morales M, Barcena J, Ramirez MA, et al. Synthesis in vitro of rabbit hemorrhagic disease virus subgenomic RNA by internal initiation on (-)sense genomic RNA: mapping of a subgenomic promoter. *J Biol Chem* 2004;279:17013–17018.
411. Morens DM, Zweighaft RM, Vernon TM, et al. A waterborne outbreak of gastroenteritis with secondary person-to- person spread. Association with a viral agent. *Lancet* 1979;1:964–966.
412. Mormann S, Heissenberg C, Pfannebecker J, et al. Tenacity of human norovirus and the surrogates feline calicivirus and murine norovirus during long-term storage on common nonporous food contact surfaces. *J Food Prot* 2015;78:224–229.
413. Morotti RA, Kaufman SS, Fishbein TM, et al. Calicivirus infection in pediatric small intestine transplant recipients: pathological considerations. *Hum Pathol* 2004;35:1236–1240.
414. Morse DL, Guzewich JJ, Hanrahan JP, et al. Widespread outbreaks of clam- and oyster-associated gastroenteritis. Role of Norwalk virus. *N Engl J Med* 1986;314:678–681.
415. Morton VK, Thomas MK, Mc ES. Estimated hospitalizations attributed to norovirus and rotavirus infection in Canada, 2006–2010. *Epidemiol Infect* 2015;143(16):3528–3537.
416. Mounts AW, Ando T, Koopmans M, et al. Cold weather seasonality of gastroenteritis associated with Norwalk-like viruses. *J Infect Dis* 2000;181(Suppl 2):S284–S287.
417. Muhaxhiri Z, Deng L, Shanker S, et al. Structural basis of substrate specificity and protease inhibition in Norwalk virus. *J Virol* 2013;87:4281–4292.
418. Mumphrey SM, Changotra H, Moore TN, et al. Murine norovirus 1 infection is associated with histopathological changes in immunocompetent hosts, but clinical disease is prevented by STAT1-dependent interferon responses. *J Virol* 2007;81:3251–3263.
419. Muzzarelli KM, Kuiper BD, Spellmon N, et al. Structural and antiviral studies of the human norovirus GII.4 protease. *Biochemistry* 2019;58(7):900–907.
420. Nakajima H, Watanabe T, Miyazaki T, et al. Acute liver dysfunction in the course of norovirus gastroenteritis. *Case Rep Gastroenterol* 2012;6:69–73.
421. Nakamura K, Someya Y, Kumasaka T, et al. A norovirus protease structure provides insights into active and substrate binding site integrity. *J Virol* 2005;79:13685–13693.
422. Nakata S, Kogawa K, Numata K, et al. The epidemiology of human calicivirus/Sapporo/82/Japan. *Arch Virol* 1996;(Suppl 12):263–270.
423. Natoni A, Kass GE, Carter MJ, et al. The mitochondrial pathway of apoptosis is triggered during feline calicivirus infection. *J Gen Virol* 2006;87:357–361.
424. Neill JD. Nucleotide sequence of a region of the feline calicivirus genome which encodes picornavirus-like RNA-dependent RNA polymerase, cysteine protease and 2C polypeptides. *Virus Res* 1990;17:145–160.
425. Neill JD. The subgenomic RNA of feline calicivirus is packaged into viral particles during infection. *Virus Res* 2002;87:89–93.
426. Neill JD, Mengeling WL. Further characterization of the virus-specific RNAs in feline calicivirus infected cells. *Virus Res* 1988;11:59–72.
427. Nelson AM, Elftman MD, Pinto AK, et al. Murine norovirus infection does not cause major disruptions in the murine intestinal microbiota. *Microbiome* 2013;1:7.
428. Nelson AM, Walk ST, Taube S, et al. Disruption of the human gut microbiota following Norovirus infection. *PLoS One* 2012;7:e48224.
429. Nelson CA, Wilen CB, Dai YN, et al. Structural basis for murine norovirus engagement of bile acids and the CD300lf receptor. *Proc Natl Acad Sci U S A* 2018;115:E9201–E9210.
430. Netzler NE, Enosi Tuipulotu D, White PA. Norovirus antivirals: where are we now? *Med Res Rev* 2019;39(3):860–886.
431. Newman KL, Leon JS. Norovirus immunology: of mice and mechanisms. *Eur J Immunol* 2015;45(10):2742–2757.
432. Newman KL, Marsh Z, Kirby AE, et al. Immunocompetent adults from human norovirus challenge studies do not exhibit norovirus viremia. *J Virol* 2015;89:6968–6969.
433. Newman KL, Moe CL, Kirby AE, et al. Norovirus in symptomatic and asymptomatic individuals: cytokines and viral shedding. *Clin Exp Immunol* 2016;184:347–357.
434. Newman KL, Moe CL, Kirby AE, et al. Human norovirus infection and the acute serum cytokine response. *Clin Exp Immunol* 2015;182(2):195–203.
435. Ng KK, Cherney MM, Vazquez AL, et al. Crystal structures of active and inactive conformations of a caliciviral RNA-dependent RNA polymerase. *J Biol Chem* 2002;277:1381–1387.
436. Ng KK, Pendas-Franco N, Rojo J, et al. Crystal structure of norwalk virus polymerase reveals the carboxyl terminus in the active site cleft. *J Biol Chem* 2004;279:16638–16645.
437. Nice TJ, Baldridge MT, McCune BT, et al. Interferon-lambda cures persistent murine norovirus infection in the absence of adaptive immunity. *Science* 2015;347:269–273.
438. Nice TJ, Osborne LC, Tomov VT, et al. Type I interferon receptor deficiency in dendritic cells facilitates systemic murine norovirus persistence despite enhanced adaptive immunity. *PLoS Pathog* 2016;12:e1005684.
439. Nice TJ, Robinson BA, Van Winkle JA. The role of interferon in persistent viral infection: insights from murine norovirus. *Trends Microbiol* 2018;26:510–524.
440. Nice TJ, Strong DW, McCune BT, et al. A single-amino-acid change in murine norovirus NS1/2 is sufficient for colonic tropism and persistence. *J Virol* 2013;87:327–334.
441. Noel JS, Ando T, Leite JP, et al. Correlation of patient immune responses with genetically characterized small round-structured viruses involved in outbreaks of nonbacterial acute gastroenteritis in the United States, 1990 to 1995. *J Med Virol* 1997;53:372–383.
442. Nurminen K, Blazevic V, Huhti L, et al. Prevalence of norovirus GII-4 antibodies in Finnish children. *J Med Virol* 2011;83:525–531.

443. Nystrom K, Abrantes J, Lopes AM, et al. Neofunctionalization of the Sec1 alpha1,2fucosyltransferase paralogue in leporids contributes to glycan polymorphism and resistance to rabbit hemorrhagic disease virus. *PLoS Pathog* 2015;11:e1004759.

444. Nystrom K, Le Gall-Recule G, Grassi P, et al. Histo-blood group antigens act as attachment factors of rabbit hemorrhagic disease virus infection in a virus strain-dependent manner. *PLoS Pathog* 2011;7:e1002188.

445. O'Brien SJ, Sanderson RA, Rushton SP. Control of norovirus infection. *Curr Opin Gastroenterol* 2019;35:14–19.

446. O'Ryan ML, Lucero Y, Prado V, et al. Symptomatic and asymptomatic rotavirus and norovirus infections during infancy in a Chilean birth cohort. *Pediatr Infect Dis J* 2009;28:879–884.

447. Oehmig A, Buttner M, Weiland F, et al. Identification of a calicivirus isolate of unknown origin. *J Gen Virol* 2003;84:2837–2845.

448. Oka T, Katayama K, Ogawa S, et al. Cleavage activity of the sapovirus 3C-like protease in Escherichia coli. *Arch Virol* 2005;150:2539–2548.

449. Oka T, Katayama K, Ogawa S, et al. Proteolytic processing of sapovirus ORF1 polyprotein. *J Virol* 2005;79:7283–7290.

450. Oka T, Wang Q, Katayama K, et al. Comprehensive review of human sapoviruses. *Clin Microbiol Rev* 2015;28:32–53.

451. Oka T, Yamamoto M, Katayama K, et al. Identification of the cleavage sites of sapovirus open reading frame 1 polyprotein. *J Gen Virol* 2006;87:3329–3338.

452. Okhuysen PC, Jiang X, Ye L, et al. Viral shedding and fecal IgA response after Norwalk virus infection. *J Infect Dis* 1995;171:566–569.

453. Oliveira LM, Blawid R, Orilio AF, et al. Development of an infectious clone and replicon system of norovirus GII.4. *J Virol Methods* 2018;258:49–53.

454. Orchard RC, Wilen CB, Doench JG, et al. Discovery of a proteinaceous cellular receptor for a norovirus. *Science* 2016;353:933–936.

455. Orchard RC, Wilen CB, Virgin HW. Sphingolipid biosynthesis induces a conformational change in the murine norovirus receptor and facilitates viral infection. *Nat Microbiol* 2018;3:1109–1114.

456. Osborne LC, Monticelli LA, Nice TJ, et al. Coinfection. Virus-helminth coinfection reveals a microbiota-independent mechanism of immunomodulation. *Science* 2014;345:578–582.

457. Ossiboff RJ, Zhou Y, Lightfoot PJ, et al. Conformational changes in the capsid of a calicivirus upon interaction with its functional receptor. *J Virol* 2010;84:5550–5564.

458. Otto PH, Clarke IN, Lambden PR, et al. Infection of calves with bovine norovirus GIII.1 strain Jena virus: an experimental model to study the pathogenesis of norovirus infection. *J Virol* 2011;85:12013–12021.

459. Oyofo BA, Soderquist R, Lesmana M, et al. Norwalk-like virus and bacterial pathogens associated with cases of gastroenteritis onboard a US Navy ship. *Am J Trop Med Hyg* 1999;61:904–908.

460. Parra GI, Azure J, Fischer R, et al. Identification of a broadly cross-reactive epitope in the inner shell of the norovirus capsid. *PLoS One* 2013;8:e67592.

461. Parra GI, Squires RB, Karangwa CK, et al. Static and evolving norovirus genotypes: implications for epidemiology and immunity. *PLoS Pathog* 2017;13:e1006136.

462. Parrino TA, Schreiber DS, Trier JS, et al. Clinical immunity in acute gastroenteritis caused by Norwalk agent. *N Engl J Med* 1977;297:86–89.

463. Parveen N, Rimkute I, Block S, et al. Membrane deformation induces clustering of norovirus bound to glycosphingolipids in a supported cell-membrane mimic. *J Phys Chem Lett* 2018;9:2278–2284.

464. Patterson W, Haswell P, Fryers PT, et al. Outbreak of small round structured virus gastroenteritis arose after kitchen assistant vomited. *Commun Dis Rep CDR Rev* 1997;7:R101–R103.

465. Pawa N, Vanezis AP, Tutton MG. Spontaneous bowel perforation due to norovirus: a case report. *Cases J* 2009;2:9101.

466. Payne DC, Vinje J, Szilagyi PG, et al. Norovirus and medically attended gastroenteritis in U.S. children. *N Engl J Med* 2013;368:1121–1130.

467. Pelizzo G, Nakib G, Goruppi I, et al. Isolated colon ischemia with norovirus infection in preterm babies: a case series. *J Med Case Rep* 2013;7:108.

468. Perry JW, Wobus CE. Endocytosis of murine norovirus 1 into murine macrophages is dependent on dynamin II and cholesterol. *J Virol* 2010;84:6163–6176.

469. Perry JW, Taube S, Wobus CE. Murine norovirus-1 entry into permissive macrophages and dendritic cells is pH-independent. *Virus Res* 2009;143:125–129.

470. Petrignani M, Verhoef L, de Graaf M, et al. Chronic sequelae and severe complications of norovirus infection: a systematic review of literature. *J Clin Virol* 2018;105:1–10.

471. Pfister T, Wimmer E. Polypeptide p41 of a Norwalk-like virus is a nucleic acid-independent nucleoside triphosphatase. *J Virol* 2001;75:1611–1619.

472. Phillips G, Lopman B, Tam CC, et al. Diagnosing norovirus-associated infectious intestinal disease using viral load. *BMC Infect Dis* 2009;9:63.

473. Phillips G, Tam CC, Conti S, et al. Community incidence of norovirus-associated infectious intestinal disease in England: improved estimates using viral load for norovirus diagnosis. *Am J Epidemiol* 2010;171:1014–1022.

474. Phillips G, Tam CC, Rodrigues LC, et al. Prevalence and characteristics of asymptomatic norovirus infection in the community in England. *Epidemiol Infect* 2010;138:1454–1458.

475. Pisanic N, Ballard SB, Colquechagua FD, et al. Minimally invasive saliva testing to monitor norovirus infection in community settings. *J Infect Dis* 2019;219(8):1234–1242.

476. Pletneva MA, Sosnovtsev SV, Green KY. The genome of Hawaii virus and its relationship with other members of the Caliciviridae. *Virus Genes* 2001;23:5–16.

477. Ponterio E, Petrizzo A, Di Bartolo I, et al. Pattern of activation of human antigen presenting cells by genotype GII.4 norovirus virus-like particles. *J Transl Med* 2013;11:127.

478. Prasad BV, Hardy ME, Dokland T, et al. X-ray crystallographic structure of the Norwalk virus capsid. *Science* 1999;286:287–290.

479. Prasad BV, Hardy ME, Jiang X, et al. Structure of Norwalk virus. *Arch Virol* 1996;(Suppl 12):237–242.

480. Prasad BV, Matson DO, Smith AW. Three-dimensional structure of calicivirus. *J Mol Biol* 1994;240:256–264.

481. Prasad BV, Rothnagel R, Jiang X, et al. Three-dimensional structure of baculovirus-expressed Norwalk virus capsids. *J Virol* 1994;68:5117–5125.

482. Qu L, Murakami K, Broughman JR, et al. Replication of human norovirus RNA in mammalian cells reveals lack of interferon response. *J Virol* 2016;90:8906–8923.

483. Qu L, Vongpunsawad S, Atmar RL, et al. Development of a Gaussia luciferase-based human norovirus protease reporter system: cell type-specific profile of Norwalk virus protease precursors and evaluation of inhibitors. *J Virol* 2014;88:10312–10326.

484. Rademacher C, Krishna NR, Palcic M, et al. NMR experiments reveal the molecular basis of receptor recognition by a calicivirus. *J Am Chem Soc* 2008;130:3669–3675.

485. Radford AD, Addie D, Belak S, et al. Feline calicivirus infection. ABCD guidelines on prevention and management. *J Feline Med Surg* 2009;11:556–564.

486. Radford AD, Turner PC, Bennett M, et al. Quasispecies evolution of a hypervariable region of the feline calicivirus capsid gene in cell culture and in persistently infected cats. *J Gen Virol* 1998;79:1–10.

487. Ramani S, Atmar RL, Estes MK. Epidemiology of human noroviruses and updates on vaccine development. *Curr Opin Gastroenterol* 2014;30:25–33.

488. Ramani S, Estes MK, Atmar RL. Correlates of protection against norovirus infection and disease-where are we now, where do we go? *PLoS Pathog* 2016;12:e1005334.

489. Ramani S, Neill FH, Opekun AR, et al. Mucosal and cellular immune responses to norwalk virus. *J Infect Dis* 2015;212:397–405.

490. Ramiro-Ibanez F, Martin-Alonso JM, Garcia Palencia P, et al. Macrophage tropism of rabbit hemorrhagic disease virus is associated with vascular pathology. *Virus Res* 1999;60:21–28.

491. Randazzo W, D'Souza DH, Sanchez G. Norovirus: the burden of the unknown. *Adv Food Nutr Res* 2018;86:13–53.

492. Reeck A, Kavanagh O, Estes MK, et al. Serological correlate of protection against norovirus-induced gastroenteritis. *J Infect Dis* 2010;202:1212–1218.

493. Reuter G, Krisztalovics K, Vennema H, et al. Evidence of the etiological predominance of norovirus in gastroenteritis outbreaks—emerging new-variant and recombinant noroviruses in Hungary. *J Med Virol* 2005;76:598–607.

494. Reymao TKA, Fumian TM, Justino MCA, et al. Norovirus RNA in serum associated with increased fecal viral load in children: detection, quantification and molecular analysis. *PLoS One* 2018;13:e0199763.

495. Rha B, Lopman BA, Alcala AN, et al. Incidence of norovirus-associated medical encounters among active duty United States military personnel and their dependents. *PLoS One* 2016;11:e0148505.

496. Robilotti E, Deresinski S, Pinsky BA. Norovirus. *Clin Microbiol Rev* 2015;28:134–164.

497. Rocha-Pereira J, Nascimento MS, Ma Q, et al. The enterovirus protease inhibitor rupintrivir exerts cross-genotypic anti-norovirus activity and clears cells from the norovirus replicon. *Antimicrob Agents Chemother* 2014;58:4675–4681.

498. Rockx BH, Bogers WM, Heeney JL, et al. Experimental norovirus infections in non-human primates. *J Med Virol* 2005;75:313–320.

499. Rockx B, De Wit M, Vennema H, et al. Natural history of human calicivirus infection: a prospective cohort study. *Clin Infect Dis* 2002;35:246–253.

500. Rodriguez MR, Monte K, Thackray LB, et al. ISG15 functions as an interferon-mediated antiviral effector early in the murine norovirus life cycle. *J Virol* 2014;88:9277–9286.

501. Rodriguez-Diaz J, Garcia-Mantrana I, Vila-Vicent S, et al. Relevance of secretor status genotype and microbiota composition in susceptibility to rotavirus and norovirus infections in humans. *Sci Rep* 2017;7:45559.

502. Rohayem J. Norovirus seasonality and the potential impact of climate change. *Clin Microbiol Infect* 2009;15:524–527.

503. Rohayem J, Robel I, Jager K, et al. Protein-primed and de novo initiation of RNA synthesis by norovirus 3Dpol. *J Virol* 2006;80:7060–7069.

504. Rouhani S, Penataro Yori P, Paredes Olortegui M, et al. Norovirus infection and acquired immunity in 8 countries: results from the MAL-ED study. *Clin Infect Dis* 2016;62:1210–1217.

505. Ruvoen-Clouet N, Ganiere JP, Andre-Fontaine G, et al. Binding of rabbit hemorrhagic disease virus to antigens of the ABH histo-blood group family. *J Virol* 2000;74:11950–11954.

506. Ruzante JM, Majowicz SE, Fazil A, et al. Hospitalization and deaths for select enteric illnesses and associated sequelae in Canada, 2001–2004. *Epidemiol Infect* 2011;139:937–945.

507. Rydell GE, Nilsson J, Rodriguez-Diaz J, et al. Human noroviruses recognize sialyl Lewis x neoglycoprotein. *Glycobiology* 2009;19:309–320.

508. Rydell GE, Svensson L, Larson G, et al. Human GII.4 norovirus VLP induces membrane invaginations on giant unilamellar vesicles containing secretor gene dependent alpha1,2-fucosylated glycosphingolipids. *Biochim Biophys Acta* 2013;1828:1840–1845.

509. Saito M, Goel-Apaza S, Espetia S, et al. Multiple norovirus infections in a birth cohort in a Peruvian Periurban community. *Clin Infect Dis* 2014;58:483–491.

510. Saitou N, Nei M. The neighbor-joining method: a new method for reconstructing phylogenetic trees. *Mol Biol Evol* 1987;4:406–425.

511. Sandmann FG, Shallcross L, Adams N, et al. Estimating the hospital burden of norovirus-associated gastroenteritis in England and its opportunity costs for non-admitted patients. *Clin Infect Dis* 2018;67(5):693–700.

512. Sandoval-Jaime C, Green KY, Sosnovtsev SV. Recovery of murine norovirus and feline calicivirus from plasmids encoding EMCV IRES in stable cell lines expressing T7 polymerase. *J Virol Methods* 2015;217:1–7.

513. Sanjuan R, Moya A, Elena SF. The distribution of fitness effects caused by single-nucleotide substitutions in an RNA virus. *Proc Natl Acad Sci U S A* 2004;101:8396–8401.

514. Santi L, Batchelor L, Huang Z, et al. An efficient plant viral expression system generating orally immunogenic Norwalk virus-like particles. *Vaccine* 2008;26:1846–1854.

515. Santiana M, Ghosh S, Ho BA, et al. Vesicle-cloaked virus clusters are optimal units for inter-organismal viral transmission. *Cell Host Microbe* 2018;24:208.e8–220.e8.

516. Santos-Valencia JC, Cancio-Lonches C, Trujillo-Uscanga A, et al. Annexin A2 associates to feline calicivirus RNA in the replication complexes from infected cells and participates in an efficient viral replication. *Virus Res* 2018;261:1–8.

517. Scallan E, Hoekstra RM, Angulo FJ, et al. Foodborne illness acquired in the United States—major pathogens. *Emerg Infect Dis* 2011;17:7–15.

518. Schaffer FL, Ehresmann DW, Fretz MK, et al. A protein, VPg, covalently linked to 36S calicivirus RNA. *J Gen Virol* 1980;47:215–220.
519. Schorn R, Hohne M, Meerbach A, et al. Chronic norovirus infection after kidney transplantation: molecular evidence for immune-driven viral evolution. *Clin Infect Dis* 2010;51:307–314.
520. Schreiber DS, Blacklow NR, Trier JS. The mucosal lesion of the proximal small intestine in acute infectious nonbacterial gastroenteritis. *N Engl J Med* 1973;288:1318–1323.
521. Schreiber DS, Blacklow NR, Trier JS. The small intestinal lesion induced by Hawaii agent acute infectious nonbacterial gastroenteritis. *J Infect Dis* 1974;129:705–708.
522. Schroten H, Hanisch FG, Hansman GS. Human norovirus interactions with histo-blood group antigens and human milk oligosaccharides. *J Virol* 2016;90:5855–5859.
523. Schuffenecker I, Ando T, Thouvenot D, et al. Genetic classification of "Sapporo-like viruses". *Arch Virol* 2001;146:2115–2132.
524. Seah EL, Gunesekere IC, Marshall JA, et al. Variation in ORF3 of genogroup 2 Norwalk-like viruses. *Arch Virol* 1999;144:1007–1014.
525. Seah EL, Marshall JA, Wright PJ. Trans activity of the norovirus Camberwell proteinase and cleavage of the N-terminal protein encoded by ORF1. *J Virol* 2003;77:7150–7155.
526. Seitz SR, Leon JS, Schwab KJ, et al. Norovirus infectivity in humans and persistence in water. *Appl Environ Microbiol* 2011;77:6884–6888.
527. Seo DJ, Jung D, Jung S, et al. Experimental miniature piglet model for the infection of human norovirus GII. *J Med Virol* 2018;90:655–662.
528. Shanker S, Czako R, Sapparapu G, et al. Structural basis for norovirus neutralization by an HBGA blocking human IgA antibody. *Proc Natl Acad Sci U S A* 2016;113:E5830–E5837.
529. Sharp TM, Guix S, Katayama K, et al. Inhibition of cellular protein secretion by norwalk virus nonstructural protein p22 requires a mimic of an endoplasmic reticulum export signal. *PLoS One* 2010;5:e13130.
530. Sharp TW, Hyams KC, Watts D, et al. Epidemiology of Norwalk virus during an outbreak of acute gastroenteritis aboard a US aircraft carrier. *J Med Virol* 1995;45:61–67.
531. Shima T, Okumura A, Kurahashi H, et al. A nationwide survey of norovirus-associated encephalitis/encephalopathy in Japan. *Brain Dev* 2019;41:263–270.
532. Shioda K, Kambhampati A, Hall AJ, et al. Global age distribution of pediatric norovirus cases. *Vaccine* 2015;33:4065–4068.
533. Shirato H, Ogawa S, Ito H, et al. Noroviruses distinguish between type 1 and type 2 histo-blood group antigens for binding. *J Virol* 2008;82:10756–10767.
534. Shoemaker GK, van Duijn E, Crawford SE, et al. Norwalk virus assembly and stability monitored by mass spectrometry. *Mol Cell Proteomics* 2010;9:1742–1751.
535. Siebenga JJ, Vennema H, Renckens B, et al. Epochal evolution of GGII.4 norovirus capsid proteins from 1995 to 2006. *J Virol* 2007;81:9932–9941.
536. Simmonds P, Karakasiliotis I, Bailey D, et al. Bioinformatic and functional analysis of RNA secondary structure elements among different genera of human and animal caliciviruses. *Nucleic Acids Res* 2008;36:2530–2546.
537. Simmons K, Gambhir M, Leon J, et al. Duration of immunity to norovirus gastroenteritis. *Emerg Infect Dis* 2013;19:1260–1267.
538. Simons MP, Pike BL, Hulseberg CE, et al. Norovirus: new developments and implications for travelers' diarrhea. *Trop Dis Travel Med Vaccines* 2016;2:1.
539. Singh BK, Glatt S, Ferrer JL, et al. Structural analysis of a feline norovirus protruding domain. *Virology* 2015;474:181–185.
540. Singh BK, Koromyslova A, Hansman GS. Structural analysis of bovine norovirus protruding domain. *Virology* 2016;487:296–301.
541. Singh BK, Leuthold MM, Hansman GS. Human noroviruses' fondness for histo-blood group antigens. *J Virol* 2015;89:2024–2040.
542. Soliman M, Kim DS, Kim C, et al. Porcine sapovirus Cowden strain enters LLC-PK cells via clathrin- and cholesterol-dependent endocytosis with the requirement of dynamin II. *Vet Res* 2018;49:92.
543. Someya Y. From head to toe of the norovirus 3C-like protease. *Biomol Concepts* 2012;3:41–56.
544. Sosnovtsev SV. Proteolytic cleavage and viral proteins. In: Hansman GS, Jiang X, Green KY, eds. *Caliciviruses: Molecular and Cellular Virology*. Norfolk, UK: Caister Academic Press; 2010:65–94.
545. Sosnovtsev S, Green KY. RNA transcripts derived from a cloned full-length copy of the feline calicivirus genome do not require VPg for infectivity. *Virology* 1995;210:383–390.
546. Sosnovtsev SV, Green KY. Identification and genomic mapping of the ORF3 and VPg proteins in feline calicivirus virions. *Virology* 2000;277:193–203.
547. Sosnovtsev SV, Belliot G, Chang KO, et al. Feline calicivirus VP2 is essential for the production of infectious virions. *J Virol* 2005;79:4012–4024.
548. Sosnovtsev SV, Belliot G, Chang KO, et al. Cleavage map and proteolytic processing of the murine norovirus nonstructural polyprotein in infected cells. *J Virol* 2006;80:7816–7831.
549. Sosnovtsev SV, Garfield M, Green KY. Processing map and essential cleavage sites of the nonstructural polyprotein encoded by ORF1 of the feline calicivirus genome. *J Virol* 2002;76:7060–7072.
550. Sosnovtsev SV, Prikhod'ko EA, Belliot G, et al. Feline calicivirus replication induces apoptosis in cultured cells. *Virus Res* 2003;94:1–10.
551. Sosnovtsev SV, Sandoval-Jaime C, Parra GI, et al. Identification of human junctional adhesion molecule 1 as a functional receptor for the Hom-1 calicivirus on human cells. *MBio* 2017;8:e00031–17.
552. Sosnovtsev SV, Sosnovtseva SA, Green KY. Cleavage of the feline calicivirus capsid precursor is mediated by a virus-encoded proteinase. *J Virol* 1998;72:3051–3059.
553. Sosnovtseva SA, Sosnovtsev SV, Green KY. Mapping of the feline calicivirus proteinase responsible for autocatalytic processing of the nonstructural polyprotein and identification of a stable proteinase-polymerase precursor protein. *J Virol* 1999;73:6626–6633.
554. Souza M, Azevedo MS, Jung K, et al. Pathogenesis and immune responses in gnotobiotic calves after infection with the genogroup II.4-HS66 strain of human norovirus. *J Virol* 2008;82:1777–1786.
555. Steinhoff MC, Douglas RG Jr, Greenberg HB, et al. Bismuth subsalicylate therapy of viral gastroenteritis. *Gastroenterology* 1980;78:1495–1499.
556. Strong DW, Thackray LB, Smith TJ, et al. Protruding domain of capsid protein is necessary and sufficient to determine murine norovirus replication and pathogenesis in vivo. *J Virol* 2012;86:2950–2958.
557. Stuart AD, Brown TD. Entry of feline calicivirus is dependent on clathrin-mediated endocytosis and acidification in endosomes. *J Virol* 2006;80:7500–7509.
558. Stuart AD, Brown TD. Alpha2,6-linked sialic acid acts as a receptor for Feline calicivirus. *J Gen Virol* 2007;88:177–186.
559. Stuart RL, Tan K, Mahar JE, et al. An outbreak of necrotizing enterocolitis associated with norovirus genotype GII.3. *Pediatr Infect Dis J* 2010;29:644–647.
560. Subba-Reddy CV, Goodfellow I, Kao CC. VPg-primed RNA synthesis of norovirus RNA-dependent RNA polymerases by using a novel cell-based assay. *J Virol* 2011;85:13027–13037.
561. Subekti DS, Tjaniadi P, Lesmana M, et al. Experimental infection of Macaca nemestrina with a Toronto Norwalk-like virus of epidemic viral gastroenteritis. *J Med Virol* 2002;66:400–406.
562. Sukhrie FH, Siebenga JJ, Beersma MF, et al. Chronic shedders as reservoir for nosocomial transmission of norovirus. *J Clin Microbiol* 2010;48:4303–4305.
563. Swamy M, Abeler-Dorner L, Chettle J, et al. Intestinal intraepithelial lymphocyte activation promotes innate antiviral resistance. *Nat Commun* 2015;6:7090.
564. Switaj TL, Winter KJ, Christensen SR. Diagnosis and management of foodborne illness. *Am Fam Physician* 2015;92:358–365.
565. Tacket CO. Plant-derived vaccines against diarrheal diseases. *Vaccine* 2005;23:1866–1869.
566. Tacket CO, Sztein MB, Losonsky GA, et al. Humoral, mucosal, and cellular immune responses to oral Norwalk virus-like particles in volunteers. *Clin Immunol* 2003;108:241–247.
567. Takanashi S, Hashira S, Matsunaga T, et al. Detection, genetic characterization, and quantification of norovirus RNA from sera of children with gastroenteritis. *J Clin Virol* 2009;44:161–163.
568. Tam CC, Rodrigues LC, Viviani L, et al. Longitudinal study of infectious intestinal disease in the UK (IID2 study): incidence in the community and presenting to general practice. *Gut* 2012;61:69–77.
569. Tamminen K, Lappalainen S, Huhti L, et al. Trivalent combination vaccine induces broad heterologous immune responses to norovirus and rotavirus in mice. *PLoS One* 2013;8:e70409.
570. Tamminen K, Malm M, Vesikari T, et al. Norovirus-specific mucosal antibodies correlate to systemic antibodies and block norovirus virus-like particles binding to histo-blood group antigens. *Clin Immunol* 2018;197:110–117.
571. Tamura M, Natori K, Kobayashi M, et al. Genogroup II noroviruses efficiently bind to heparan sulfate proteoglycan associated with the cellular membrane. *J Virol* 2004;78:3817–3826.
572. Tan M, Jiang X. The p domain of norovirus capsid protein forms a subviral particle that binds to histo-blood group antigen receptors. *J Virol* 2005;79:14017–14030.
573. Tan M, Jiang X. Norovirus P particle: a subviral nanoparticle for vaccine development against norovirus, rotavirus and influenza virus. *Nanomedicine (Lond)* 2012;7:889–897.
574. Tan M, Hegde RS, Jiang X. The P domain of norovirus capsid protein forms dimer and binds to histo-blood group antigen receptors. *J Virol* 2004;78:6233–6242.
575. Tan M, Huang P, Meller J, et al. Mutations within the P2 domain of norovirus capsid affect binding to human histo-blood group antigens: evidence for a binding pocket. *J Virol* 2003;77:12562–12571.
576. Tan M, Wei C, Huang P, et al. Tulane virus recognizes sialic acids as cellular receptors. *Sci Rep* 2015;5:11784.
577. Tan M, Xia M, Cao S, et al. Elucidation of strain-specific interaction of a GII-4 norovirus with HBGA receptors by site-directed mutagenesis study. *Virology* 2008;379:324–334.
578. Taube S, Kolawole AO, Hohne M, et al. A mouse model for human norovirus. *MBio* 2013;4:e00450–13.
579. Taube S, Mallagaray A, Peters T. Norovirus, glycans and attachment. *Curr Opin Virol* 2018;31:33–42.
580. Taube S, Perry JW, McGreevy E, et al. Murine noroviruses bind glycolipid and glycoprotein attachment receptors in a strain-dependent manner. *J Virol* 2012;86:5584–5593.
581. Taube S, Perry JW, Yetming K, et al. Ganglioside-linked terminal sialic acid moieties on murine macrophages function as attachment receptors for murine noroviruses. *J Virol* 2009;83:4092–4101.
582. Taube S, Rubin JR, Katpally U, et al. High-resolution x-ray structure and functional analysis of the murine norovirus 1 capsid protein protruding domain. *J Virol* 2010;84:5695–5705.
583. Teunis PF, Moe CL, Liu P, et al. Norwalk virus: how infectious is it? *J Med Virol* 2008;80:1468–1476.
584. Teunis PF, Sukhrie FH, Vennema H, et al. Shedding of norovirus in symptomatic and asymptomatic infections. *Epidemiol Infect* 2015;143:1710–1717.
585. Thackray LB, Duan E, Lazear HM, et al. Critical role for interferon regulatory factor 3 (IRF-3) and IRF-7 in type I interferon-mediated control of murine norovirus replication. *J Virol* 2012;86:13515–13523.
586. Thackray LB, Wobus CE, Chachu KA, et al. Murine noroviruses comprising a single genogroup exhibit biological diversity despite limited sequence divergence. *J Virol* 2007;81:10460–10473.
587. Thongprachum A, Khamrin P, Tran DN, et al. Evaluation and comparison of the efficiency of immunochromatography methods for norovirus detection. *Clin Lab* 2012;58:489–493.
588. Thorne LG, Goodfellow IG. Norovirus gene expression and replication. *J Gen Virol* 2014;95:278–291.
589. Thorne L, Arias A, Goodfellow I. Advances toward a norovirus antiviral: from classical inhibitors to lethal mutagenesis. *J Infect Dis* 2016;213(Suppl 1):S27–S31.
590. Thorne L, Bailey D, Goodfellow I. High-resolution functional profiling of the norovirus genome. *J Virol* 2012;86:11441–11456.
591. Thornhill TS, Wyatt RG, Kalica AR, et al. Detection by immune electron microscopy of 26- to 27-nm viruslike particles associated with two family outbreaks of gastroenteritis. *J Infect Dis* 1977;135:20–27.
592. Thornley CN, Emslie NA, Sprott TW, et al. Recurring norovirus transmission on an airplane. *Clin Infect Dis* 2011;53:515–520.
593. Thornton SA, Sherman SS, Farkas T, et al. Gastroenteritis in US Marines during Operation Iraqi Freedom. *Clin Infect Dis* 2005;40:519–525.

594. Thorven M, Grahn A, Hedlund KO, et al. A homozygous nonsense mutation (428G->A) in the human secretor (FUT2) gene provides resistance to symptomatic norovirus (GGII) infections. *J Virol* 2005;79:15351–15355.

595. Thumfart JO, Meyers G. Feline calicivirus: recovery of wild-type and recombinant viruses after transfection of cRNA or cDNA constructs. *J Virol* 2002;76:6398–6407.

596. Tian P, Brandl M, Mandrell R. Porcine gastric mucin binds to recombinant norovirus particles and competitively inhibits their binding to histo-blood group antigens and Caco-2 cells. *Lett Appl Microbiol* 2005;41:315–320.

597. Tian P, Engelbrektson AL, Jiang X, et al. Norovirus recognizes histo-blood group antigens on gastrointestinal cells of clams, mussels, and oysters: a possible mechanism of bioaccumulation. *J Food Prot* 2007;70:2140–2147.

598. Tohya Y, Shinchi H, Matsuura Y, et al. Analysis of the N-terminal polypeptide of the capsid precursor protein and the ORF3 product of feline calicivirus [In process citation]. *J Vet Med Sci* 1999;61:1043–1047.

599. Tomov VT, Osborne LC, Dolfi DV, et al. Persistent enteric murine norovirus infection is associated with functionally suboptimal virus-specific CD8 T cell responses. *J Virol* 2013;87:7015–7031.

600. Tomov VT, Palko O, Lau CW, et al. Differentiation and protective capacity of virus-specific CD8+ T cells suggest murine norovirus persistence in an immune-privileged enteric niche. *Immunity* 2017;47:723.e5–738.e5.

601. Treanor JJ, Jiang X, Madore HP, et al. Subclass-specific serum antibody responses to recombinant Norwalk virus capsid antigen (rNV) in adults infected with Norwalk, Snow Mountain, or Hawaii virus. *J Clin Microbiol* 1993;31:1630–1634.

602. Tresset G, Decouche V, Bryche JF, et al. Unusual self-assembly properties of Norovirus Newbury2 virus-like particles. *Arch Biochem Biophys* 2013;537:144–152.

603. Tresset G, Le Coeur C, Bryche JF, et al. Norovirus capsid proteins self-assemble through biphasic kinetics via long-lived stave-like intermediates. *J Am Chem Soc* 2013;135:15373–15381.

604. Troeger H, Loddenkemper C, Schneider T, et al. Structural and functional changes of the duodenum in human norovirus infection. *Gut* 2009;58:1070–1077.

605. Trujillo AA, McCaustland KA, Zheng DP, et al. Use of TaqMan real-time reverse transcription-PCR for rapid detection, quantification, and typing of norovirus. *J Clin Microbiol* 2006;44:1405–1412.

606. Tsuge M, Goto S, Kato F, et al. Elevation of serum transaminases with norovirus infection. *Clin Pediatr (Phila)* 2010;49:574–578.

607. Tubiana T, Boulard Y, Bressanelli S. Dynamics and asymmetry in the dimer of the norovirus major capsid protein. *PLoS One* 2017;12:e0182056.

608. Turcios RM, Widdowson MA, Sulka AC, et al. Reevaluation of epidemiological criteria for identifying outbreaks of acute gastroenteritis due to norovirus: United States, 1998–2000. *Clin Infect Dis* 2006;42:964–969.

609. Turcios-Ruiz RM, Axelrod P, St John K, et al. Outbreak of necrotizing enterocolitis caused by norovirus in a neonatal intensive care unit. *J Pediatr* 2008;153:339–344.

610. Turula H, Bragazzi Cunha J, Mainou BA, et al. Natural secretory immunoglobulins promote enteric viral infections. *J Virol* 2018;92:e00826–18.

611. Ueda N. Gastroduodenal perforation and ulcer associated with rotavirus and norovirus infections in Japanese children: a case report and comprehensive literature review. *Open Forum Infect Dis* 2016;3:ofw026.

612. Urakova N, Frese M, Hall RN, et al. Expression and partial characterisation of rabbit haemorrhagic disease virus non-structural proteins. *Virology* 2015;484:69–79.

613. van Beek J, de Graaf M, Al-Hello H, et al. Analysis of norovirus molecular surveillance data collected through the NoroNet network, 2005–2016. *Lancet Infect Dis* 2017;18:545–553.

614. van Beek J, de Graaf M, Smits S, et al. Whole-genome next-generation sequencing to study within-host evolution of norovirus (NoV) among immunocompromised patients with chronic NoV infection. *J Infect Dis* 2017;216:1513–1524.

615. van Beek J, de Graaf M, Xia M, et al. Comparison of norovirus genogroup I, II and IV seroprevalence among children in the Netherlands, 1963, 1983 and 2006. *J Gen Virol* 2016;97:2255–2264.

616. van den Berg H, Lodder W, van der Poel W, et al. Genetic diversity of noroviruses in raw and treated sewage water. *Res Microbiol* 2005;156:532–540.

617. Van Winkle JA, Robinson BA, Peters AM, et al. Persistence of systemic murine norovirus is maintained by inflammatory recruitment of susceptible myeloid cells. *Cell Host Microbe* 2018;24(5):665.e4–676.e4.

618. Vazquez AL, Martin Alonso JM, Casais R, et al. Expression of enzymatically active rabbit hemorrhagic disease virus RNA-dependent RNA polymerase in *Escherichia coli*. *J Virol* 1998;72:2999–3004.

619. Vega E, Donaldson E, Huynh J, et al. RNA populations in immunocompromised patients as reservoirs for novel norovirus variants. *J Virol* 2014;88:14184–14196.

620. Verhoef L, Depoortere E, Boxman I, et al. Emergence of new norovirus variants on spring cruise ships and prediction of winter epidemics. *Emerg Infect Dis* 2008;14:238–243.

621. Verhoef L, Williams KP, Kroneman A, et al. Selection of a phylogenetically informative region of the norovirus genome for outbreak linkage. *Virus Genes* 2012;44:8–18.

622. Verstraeten T, Cattaert T, Harris J, et al. Estimating the burden of medically attended norovirus gastroenteritis: modeling linked primary care and hospitalization datasets. *J Infect Dis* 2017;216:957–965.

623. Verstraeten T, Jiang B, Weil JG, et al. Modelling estimates of norovirus disease in patients with chronic medical conditions. *PLoS One* 2016;11:e0158822.

624. Vinje J. Advances in laboratory methods for detection and typing of norovirus. *J Clin Microbiol* 2015;53:373–381.

625. Vinje J, Estes MK, Esteves P, et al. ICTV virus taxonomy profile: Caliciviridae. *J Gen Virol* 2019.

626. Viskovska MA, Zhao B, Shanker S, et al. GII.4 norovirus protease shows pH-sensitive proteolysis with a unique ARG-HIS pairing in the catalytic site. *J Virol* 2019;93(6).

627. Viswanathan P, May J, Uhm S, et al. RNA binding by human Norovirus 3C-like proteases inhibits protease activity. *Virology* 2013;438:20–27.

628. Vogel L. Hand sanitizers may increase norovirus risk. *CMAJ* 2011;183:E799–E800.

629. Vongpunsawad S, Venkataram Prasad BV, Estes MK. Norwalk virus minor capsid protein VP2 associates within the VP1 shell domain. *J Virol* 2013;87:4818–4825.

630. Wang J, Jiang X, Madore HP, et al. Sequence diversity of small, round-structured viruses in the Norwalk virus group. *J Virol* 1994;68:5982–5990.

631. Wang P, Zhu S, Yang L, et al. Nlrp6 regulates intestinal antiviral innate immunity. *Science* 2015;350:826–830.

632. Ward VK, McCormick CJ, Clarke IN, et al. Recovery of infectious murine norovirus using pol II-driven expression of full-length cDNA. *Proc Natl Acad Sci U S A* 2007;104:11050–11055.

633. Watier-Grillot S, Boni M, Tong C, et al. Challenging investigation of a norovirus foodborne disease outbreak during a military deployment in Central African Republic. *Food Environ Virol* 2017;9:498–501.

634. Weerasekara S, Prior AM, Hua DH. Current tools for norovirus drug discovery. *Expert Opin Drug Discov* 2016;11:529–541.

635. Wegener H, Mallagaray A, Schone T, et al. Human norovirus GII.4(MI001) P dimer binds fucosylated and sialylated carbohydrates. *Glycobiology* 2017;27:1027–1037.

636. Wei C, Farkas T, Sestak K, et al. Recovery of infectious virus by transfection of in vitro-generated RNA from tulane calicivirus cDNA. *J Virol* 2008;82:11429–11436.

637. Wei L, Huhn JS, Mory A, et al. Proteinase-polymerase precursor as the active form of feline calicivirus RNA-dependent RNA polymerase. *J Virol* 2001;75:1211–1219.

638. Wennesz R, Luttermann C, Kreher F, et al. Structure-function relationship in the 'termination upstream ribosomal binding site' of the calicivirus rabbit hemorrhagic disease virus. *Nucleic Acids Res.* 2019;47(4):1920–1934.

639. Westrell T, Dusch V, Ethelberg S, et al. Norovirus outbreaks linked to oyster consumption in the United Kingdom, Norway, France, Sweden and Denmark, 2010. *Euro Surveill* 2010;15(12).

640. White LJ, Hardy ME, Estes MK. Biochemical characterization of a smaller form of recombinant Norwalk virus capsids assembled in insect cells. *J Virol* 1997;71:8066–8072.

641. Wi SW, Lee SJ, Kang EK, et al. Ileal perforation with norovirus gastroenteritis in a 3-month-old infant. *Pediatr Gastroenterol Hepatol Nutr* 2017;20:130–133.

642. Widdowson MA, Cramer EH, Hadley L, et al. Outbreaks of acute gastroenteritis on cruise ships and on land: identification of a predominant circulating strain of norovirus—United States, 2002. *J Infect Dis* 2004;190:27–36.

643. Widdowson MA, Sulka A, Bulens SN, et al. Norovirus and foodborne disease, United States, 1991–2000. *Emerg Infect Dis* 2005;11:95–102.

644. Widerlite L, Trier JS, Blacklow NR, et al. Structure of the gastric mucosa in acute infectious bacterial gastroenteritis. *Gastroenterology* 1975;68:425–430.

645. Wilen CB, Lee S, Hsieh LL, et al. Tropism for tuft cells determines immune promotion of norovirus pathogenesis. *Science* 2018;360:204–208.

646. Wilhelmi de Cal I, Revilla A, del Alamo JM, et al. Evaluation of two commercial enzyme immunoassays for the detection of norovirus in faecal samples from hospitalised children with sporadic acute gastroenteritis. *Clin Microbiol Infect* 2007;13:341–343.

647. Willcocks MM, Carter MJ, Roberts LO. Cleavage of eukaryotic initiation factor eIF4G and inhibition of host-cell protein synthesis during feline calicivirus infection. *J Gen Virol* 2004;85:1125–1130.

648. Wingfield T, Gallimore CI, Xerry J, et al. Chronic norovirus infection in an HIV-positive patient with persistent diarrhoea: a novel cause. *J Clin Virol* 2010;49:219–222.

649. Wirblich C, Sibilia M, Boniotti MB, et al. 3C-like protease of rabbit hemorrhagic disease virus: identification of cleavage sites in the ORF1 polyprotein and analysis of cleavage specificity. *J Virol* 1995;69:7159–7168.

650. Wirblich C, Thiel HJ, Meyers G. Genetic map of the calicivirus rabbit hemorrhagic disease virus as deduced from in vitro translation studies. *J Virol* 1996;70:7974–7983.

651. Wobus CE, Cunha JB, Elftman MD, et al. Animal models of norovirus infection. In Svensson, L., Desselberger, U., Greenberg, H.B., Estes, M.K, eds. *Viral Gastroenteritis: Molecular Epidemiology and Pathogenesis*. Elsevier;2016:397–422.

652. Wobus CE. The dual tropism of noroviruses. *J Virol* 2018;92:e01010–17.

653. Wobus CE, Karst SM, Thackray LB, et al. Replication of Norovirus in cell culture reveals a tropism for dendritic cells and macrophages. *PLoS Biol* 2004;2:e432.

654. Wolf S, Reetz J, Otto P. Genetic characterization of a novel calicivirus from a chicken. *Arch Virol* 2011;156:1143–1150.

655. Woodward J, Gkrania-Klotsas E, Kumararatne D. Chronic norovirus infection and common variable immunodeficiency. *Clin Exp Immunol* 2017;188:363–370.

656. Wyatt RG, Dolin R, Blacklow NR, et al. Comparison of three agents of acute infectious nonbacterial gastroenteritis by cross-challenge in volunteers. *J Infect Dis* 1974;129:709–714.

657. Wyatt RG, Greenberg HB, Dalgard DW, et al. Experimental infection of chimpanzees with the Norwalk agent of epidemic viral gastroenteritis. *J Med Virol* 1978;2:89–96.

658. Xia M, Huang P, Sun C, et al. Bioengineered norovirus S60 nanoparticles as a multifunctional vaccine platform. *ACS Nano* 2018;12(11):10665–10682.

659. Yang S, Li M, Cheng J, et al. Diagnostic determination of Norovirus infection as one of the major causes of infectious diarrhea in HIV patients using a multiplex polymerase chain reaction assay. *Int J STD AIDS* 2019;30(6):550–556.

660. Yee EL, Palacio H, Atmar RL, et al. Widespread outbreak of norovirus gastroenteritis among evacuees of Hurricane Katrina residing in a large "megashelter" in Houston, Texas: lessons learned for prevention. *Clin Infect Dis* 2007;44:1032–1039.

661. Yen JB, Wei LH, Chen LW, et al. Subcellular localization and functional characterization of GII.4 norovirus-encoded NTPase. *J Virol* 2018;92:e01824–17.

662. Yu G, Zhang D, Guo F, et al. Cryo-EM structure of a novel calicivirus, Tulane virus. *PLoS One* 2013;8:e59817.

663. Yumiketa Y, Narita T, Inoue Y, et al. Nonstructural protein p39 of feline calicivirus suppresses host innate immune response by preventing IRF-3 activation. *Vet Microbiol* 2016;185:62–67.

664. Yunus MA, Chung LM, Chaudhry Y, et al. Development of an optimized RNA-based murine norovirus reverse genetics system. *J Virol Methods* 2010;169:112–118.

665. Yunus MA, Lin X, Bailey D, et al. The murine norovirus core subgenomic RNA promoter consists of a stable stem-loop that can direct accurate initiation of RNA synthesis. *J Virol* 2015;89:1218–1229.

666. Zakhour M, Ruvoen-Clouet N, Charpilienne A, et al. The alphaGal epitope of the histo-blood group antigen family is a ligand for bovine norovirus Newbury2 expected to prevent cross-species transmission. *PLoS Pathog* 2009;5:e1000504.

667. Zambruni M, Luna G, Silva M, et al. High prevalence and increased severity of norovirus mixed infections among children 12-24 months of age living in the suburban areas of Lima, Peru. *J Pediatric Infect Dis Soc* 2016;5:337–341.

668. Zamyatkin DF, Parra F, Alonso JM, et al. Structural insights into mechanisms of catalysis and inhibition in Norwalk virus polymerase. *J Biol Chem* 2008;283:7705–7712.

669. Zeitler CE, Estes MK, Venkataram Prasad BV. X-ray crystallographic structure of the Norwalk virus protease at 1.5-A resolution. *J Virol* 2006;80:5050–5058.

670. Zhang D, Huang P, Zou L, et al. Tulane virus recognizes the A type 3 and B histo-blood group antigens. *J Virol* 2015;89:1419–1427.

671. Zheng DP, Ando T, Fankhauser RL, et al. Norovirus classification and proposed strain nomenclature. *Virology* 2006;346:312–323.

672. Zhou HL, Zhen SS, Wang JX, et al. Burden of acute gastroenteritis caused by norovirus in China: a systematic review. *J Infect* 2017;75:216–224.

673. Zhu S, Jones MK, Hickman D, et al. Norovirus antagonism of B-cell antigen presentation results in impaired control of acute infection. *Mucosal Immunol* 2016;9:1559–1570.

674. Zhu S, Regev D, Watanabe M, et al. Identification of immune and viral correlates of norovirus protective immunity through comparative study of intra-cluster norovirus strains. *PLoS Pathog* 2013;9:e1003592.

675. Zhu S, Watanabe M, Kirkpatrick E, et al. Regulation of norovirus virulence by the VP1 protruding domain correlates with B cell infection efficiency. *J Virol* 2015;90:2858–2867.

676. Zhuo R, Cho J, Qiu Y, et al. High genetic variability of norovirus leads to diagnostic test challenges. *J Clin Virol* 2017;96:94–98.

677. Zintz C, Bok K, Parada E, et al. Prevalence and genetic characterization of caliciviruses among children hospitalized for acute gastroenteritis in the United States. *Infect Genet Evol* 2005;5:281–290.

Togaviridae: The Viruses and Their Replication

Richard J. Kuhn

The *Togaviridae* are simple enveloped plus-strand RNA viruses that are spherical in appearance and contribute significantly to human disease. Although they were originally classified together with several groups of viruses predominantly transmitted by insects, more recent analyses have defined them into a distinct family with two genera: the alphaviruses and the rubiviruses.[165] The alphavirus genus is by far the larger of the two with about 31 recognized members, while the *Rubivirus* genus is composed of a single member, rubella virus. Virus classification into each group is determined by genome organization and nucleotide homologies. The alphaviruses are responsible for a variety of human and animal diseases, involving encephalitis, arthritis, fever, rash, and arthralgia, and are transmitted primarily by arthropod vectors. Viruses such as chikungunya (CHIKV) and Venezuelan equine encephalitis virus (VEEV) have been responsible for recent human outbreaks and have raised awareness of the significance and potential threat of alphaviruses to human health. Rubella virus is a common childhood illness for which an effective vaccine is available. However, in the absence of immunity, the virus can induce severe congenital defects in the fetus of infected women.

Sindbis virus (SINV), the type member of the alphavirus genus, has been extensively studied in large part due to its facile growth in cell culture and its ability to cause mild or inapparent illness in humans. The virus has an 11.7-kb RNA genome that is capped at its 5′ end and contains a poly (A) tract at its 3′ terminus.[255] Virions have a spherical icosahedral arrangement of proteins that has facilitated their structural analysis. The detailed knowledge of the viral life cycle, which is the focus of this chapter, has been exploited for the development of alphavirus gene expression vectors. Many members of this virus group have been studied for their role in pathogenesis. Rubella virus, as expected from its classification, shares a number of properties with the alphaviruses, yet has several important distinctions that are highlighted throughout the chapter.

CLASSIFICATION OF VIRUSES WITHIN THE *TOGAVIRIDAE* FAMILY

Viruses transmitted by arthropods have been referred to as arboviruses. It was originally observed by electron microscopy that many arboviruses had a similar morphological appearance that resembled a Roman cloak (in Latin, *toga*), hence the name togaviruses. Originally, the family *Togaviridae* consisted of Group A (alphaviruses) and Group B (flaviviruses); however, the genera rubiviruses and pestiviruses were later added based on their similar physical properties but despite their lack of arthropod transmission. With the development of sequencing, it became apparent that the original joint classification for these viruses was in error. The togaviruses have nonstructural or replication proteins encoded at the 5′ end of their genome RNA, while the 3′ end encoded the proteins that constitute the virus particle or virion. In the togaviruses, these structural proteins are translated from a subgenomic mRNA that derives from, and is coterminal with, the 3′ end of the genome.[215,255]

The larger of the two genera within togaviruses, the alphaviruses, has been classified into several antigenically related complexes.[207] Most phylogenetic analyses support this classification, but several recent additions add complexity to the organization. The alphaviruses have a worldwide geographic distribution, including the continent of Antarctica. The alphaviruses have classically been described as either Old World or New World viruses, depending on their distribution, and it is likely that several transoceanic exchanges have occurred.[207] Most alphaviruses are transmitted by arthropod vectors that probably control their geographic dispersal. However, the identification of the salmonid viruses, salmon pancreas disease virus, and sleeping disease virus (infecting rainbow trout) presents examples of alphaviruses for which arthropod transmission is unlikely.[299] These salmonid viruses appear to have diverged from the Old World to New World lineages early in alphavirus evolution, with no present-day close relatives. Another identified alphavirus, southern elephant seal virus, has been isolated from the louse *Lepidophthirus macrorhini*.[148] This isolation demonstrates not only that alphaviruses can be transmitted by lice but also that they can infect marine mammals, and a recent report suggests a marine origin for the alphaviruses.[50] However, the recent isolation of insect-specific alphaviruses such as Eilat virus, which are unable to replicate in vertebrate cells, suggests a potentially ancestral alphavirus.[182]

Although the alphaviruses and rubella virus have been classified within the same family, the evolutionary relationship between them is obscure.[52] They have a similar genome organization, and their virions share physical similarities, yet their replication and assembly strategies are sufficiently diverse to question whether they arose from a direct ancestor.

VIRION STRUCTURE

Structure of Mature Virion

The structure of the alphavirus virion has been extensively studied, and numerous high-resolution structural studies now provide an atomic view of the virion. Although a variety of biophysical methods were used to elaborate the alphavirus structure, work

that has advanced the field the most has come from cryoelectron microscopy (cryo-EM) and image reconstruction techniques.[27,28,89,90,277,278] The virion is 70 nm in diameter, with a molecular mass of 52×10^6 Da and a density of 1.22 g per cc. It is composed of repeating units of the E1 and E2 transmembrane glycoproteins, the capsid protein (C, sometimes referred to as the nucleocapsid protein), a host-derived lipid bilayer, and a single molecule of genome RNA. The protein components of the virion are arranged as a T = 4 icosahedral lattice, with 240 copies of each subunit.[28,198,201] These subunits interact with one another to form a rigid structure across the membrane in a one-to-one relationship between glycoproteins E2 and C. Smaller amounts of another membrane-associated protein, 6K, are also found in the virus particle.[64,157] It has been discovered that another small protein, the TransFrame (TF) protein, is found in substoichiometric amounts in the virion.[46] The lipid bilayer is derived from the host plasma membrane and is enriched in cholesterol and sphingolipid, molecules that are required for entry and budding.[110] Inside the bilayer, the C surrounds the genome RNA and forms an icosahedral shell. Thus, the alphaviruses are composed of multiple organized shells of molecules that effectively protect and deliver the viral RNA to susceptible host cells.

Cryo-EM has been extensively used to study the structure of alphaviruses, including SINV,[198] Semliki Forest virus (SFV),[273] Ross River virus (RRV),[28] VEEV,[196,308] Western equine encephalitis virus (WEEV),[238] Eastern equine encephalitis virus (EEEV),[91] Aura virus,[306] CHIKV,[260] and Barmah Forest virus (BFV).[120] The most recent studies with SINV are the most advanced, with a resolution of 3.5 Å reported for these viruses.[27] The surface view of the virion, seen in Figure 5.1 for

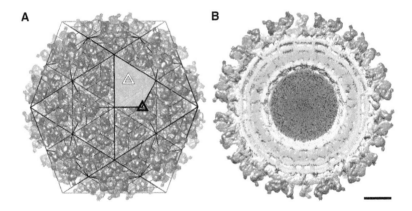

FIGURE 5.1 Structure of an alphavirus determined using cryo-EM. **A:** Surface-shaded view of Sindbis virus as determined by cryo-EM at 7.0 Å. The trimeric petal-shaped spikes are visible, with *solid triangles* representing the threefold axes and *white triangles* representing quasi-threefold axes. One of the asymmetric units is highlighted by *green shading*. **B:** The same view as shown in **(A)** but with the front half of the reconstructed structure removed. The outer layer containing spikes is shown in *blue*, while the underlying skirt density is in *magenta*. Crossing the lipid bilayer (*cyan*) reveals the ordered capsid protein (*green*; residues 114–264), a disordered region containing a mix of protein and RNA (*yellow*), and a region containing the remainder of the RNA genome (*red*). The transmembrane densities of E1 and E2 are seen spanning the outer and inner leaflets of the lipid bilayer (*cyan*). (Reprinted from Tang J, Jose J, Chipman P, et al. Molecular links between the E2 envelope glycoprotein and nucleocapsid core in Sindbis virus. *J Mol Biol* 2011;414(3):442–459, copyright 2011 with permission from Elsevier.)

SINV, reveals a spherical particle with spike protrusions rising 100 Å from the lipid membrane surface. The icosahedral nature of the particle results in an ordered distribution of the petal-like spikes. The asymmetric unit, which is shaded in green in Figure 5.1A, contains four E1–E2 heterodimers. Each spike consists of three heterodimers of E1 and E2 glycoproteins. A total of 80 spikes reside on icosahedral threefold (solid black triangle in Fig. 5.1A) and quasi-threefold axes (open white triangle in Fig. 5.1A). Earlier biochemical studies established the nature of the heterodimer, and this relationship has been confirmed by cryo-EM reconstructions[312] and by x-ray crystallography.[142,279] Although the protein lattice occupies a substantial surface area, small openings are present in the virion that reveals the underlying lipid bilayer. These openings are most pronounced at the twofold axes but can also be found at the fivefold axes and around the base of each spike.

The transmembrane components of the two glycoproteins are clearly seen in the cryo-EM reconstructions (Fig. 5.1B). The shape of density demonstrates that each transmembrane segment traverses the bilayer as a helix, although the E1 transmembrane domain is better represented by two alpha helices separated by a two–amino acid kink.[308] The E1 glycoprotein has 5 amino acid residues that penetrate across to the inner side of the membrane (cdE1), while E2 has 33 amino acids (cdE2) that interact with the nucleocapsid core.[146,149,262,308] This interaction is observed in cryo-EM reconstructions and demonstrates that each E2 molecule makes specific contacts with each capsid protein. The nucleocapsid core has a T = 4 arrangement of capsid protein, with the C-terminal protease domain forming pentameric and hexameric projections that appear as capsomeres on the surface of nucleocapsid cores (shown in green in Fig. 5.1B). The genome RNA does not appear to assume regular symmetry within the nucleocapsid core and is not ordered in the reconstructions (red in Fig. 5.1B).

Structure of Immature Virion

The structure of the immature virus containing an uncleaved precursor to E2, called PE2 or p62, has also been solved using cryo-EM.[45,200] Mutant versions of both SINV and SFV were used for independent structure determinations resulting in

similar structures. The extra density corresponding to the small protein E3 was found predominantly between the petals of the spike resulting in a dual-lobed petal. At a resolution of 25 Å, no apparent differences were found in the skirt or other regions of the spike and suggest that following cleavage of PE2 and release of E3, no significant conformational changes occur in the virus structure. These results have been further validated by a 6.8 Å cryo-EM structure of an immature CHIKV virus-like particle.[304] Slight differences were observed in the transmembrane helices and the radius of the spikes when compared with mature particles. The immature form of the virus has been proposed to stabilize the fusion protein as it transits the mildly acidic environment of the Golgi.[152,154,281] At some point in the transit of the particle post-Golgi, the pE2 precursor protein is cleaved by furin; however, the processed E3 remains bound to the particle.[269]

The Structural Proteins of the Virion

The proteins that constitute the alphavirus virion are synthesized as a polyprotein from a subgenomic RNA and are shown in Figure 5.2. The structures of the three major virion proteins have been determined by x-ray crystallography to high resolution. The capsid protein functions to encapsidate the genome RNA and forms a T = 4 icosahedron prior to release from the cell. The 264–amino acid capsid protein of SINV was crystallized, although the N-terminal 105 residues have been absent in the final structures.[30] It was suggested that the highly basic N-terminal domain was susceptible to proteases and degraded during crystal growth. A similar observation was made for the SFV capsid protein.[29] The C-terminal residues 114 to 264 of the SINV capsid protein form a chymotrypsin-like fold with the ultimate residue tryptophan 264 bound in the active site protease pocket. The fold contains two Greek key β–barrel domains that bring the catalytic triad of Ser215, His141, and Asp163 into juxtaposition for activity.[83] This structure substantiated biochemical and genetic data that proposed that the capsid protein had an autocatalytic serine protease activity.[10,84,166] The atomic structure of the capsid protein was used to generate a "pseudoatomic" resolution structure of the alphavirus nucleocapsid core (Fig. 5.3C) by fitting its coordinates

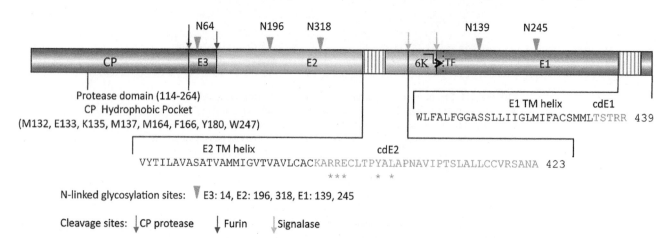

N-linked glycosylation sites: ▼ E3: 14, E2: 196, 318, E1: 139, 245

Cleavage sites: ↓CP protease ↓ Furin ↓ Signalase

FIGURE 5.2 A schematic of the Sindbis virus structural polyprotein. The individual proteins are color-coded with protease cleavage sites indicated by an *arrow.* N-linked glycosylation sites are shown by *green arrowheads.* The amino acids that constitute the transmembrane and cytoplasmic domains of both E1 and E2 are shown. *Asterisks* indicate residues of cdE2 that interact with the capsid protein. The TF protein is identified by the *bent arrow* followed by the *dotted line* crossing E1.

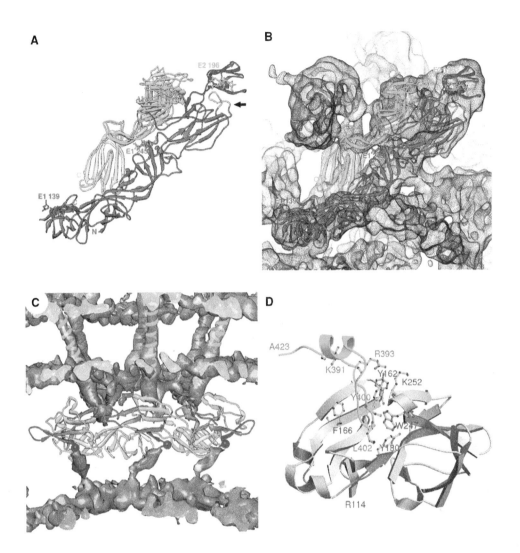

FIGURE 5.3 Pseudoatomic representation of the Sindbis virus structural proteins based on the 7.0 Å cryo-EM reconstruction. A: The structure of E1 and E2 of Sindbis virus. E1 is shown in *red*. The A and C domains of E2 are shown in two colors with one representing the structure from the crystal structure (*cyan*) and the one obtained by fitting the crystal structure into the cryo-EM map (*green*). The B domain of E2 (*blue*) is a homology-modeled structure derived from the chikungunya crystal structure. The *arrow* points to the E1 fusion peptide (*yellow*). **B:** Same as in **(A)** but fitted into the cryo-EM density (*gray mesh*). **C:** Cross section of the fitted cryo-EM structure showing the transmembrane helices of E1 (*red*) and E2 (*green*) and the underlying N-terminal protease domain of the capsid protein (residues 114–264). Below capsid residue 114 (*blue ball*), the remaining N-terminal residues of the capsid are not identified but must interact with the underlying genome RNA. Additional EM density is shown in *gray*. **D:** Interactions between the capsid protein and the cdE2. The residues that constitute cdE2 (amino acids 391–423) were modeled based on the cryo-EM density and are shown as they interact with the hydrophobic pocket of the capsid protein. Residues of the capsid that have been shown as important in this interaction, F166, Y180, and W247, are highlighted. (Reprinted from Tang J, Jose J, Chipman P, et al. Molecular links between the E2 envelope glycoprotein and nucleocapsid core in Sindbis virus. *J Mol Biol* 2011;414(3):442–459, copyright 2011 with permission from Elsevier.)

into the cryo-EM density.[166,177,222] This was accomplished and suggested that the missing residues of the N-terminus would point inward from the core surface and interact with the negatively charged viral RNA. The recent 4.4 Å cryo-EM structure of EEEV provides support for the earlier fitted structures and provides additional insight into the position of the N-terminal residues 82 to 112 (Fig. 5.4) that were implicated in genome RNA binding.[91]

The E1 protein functions as a class II fusion machine to promote the joining of viral and cellular membranes under conditions of low pH. The structure of the prefusion form of the E1 molecule from SFV was solved using x-ray crystallography.[137,297] The structure of the E1 ectodomain (residues 1–383) is shown in Figure 5.3A and B and contains three β–barrel domains. Domain I, the so-called central domain, links domains II and III. The extended domain II contains at

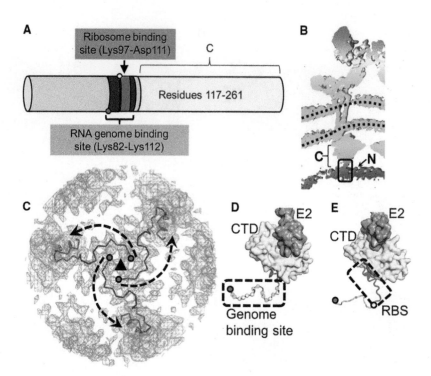

FIGURE 5.4 Structure/topology of the alphavirus capsid protein. A: Schematic representation of the EEEV capsid protein with the N-terminal disordered domain (residues 1–81) shown in *gray* and the C-terminal serine protease domain (residues 117–261) shown in *yellow*. The putative RNA genome–binding and ribosome-binding sites (residues 82–112) are shown between the N and C domains. **B:** Cross-sectional density of the 4.4 Å EEEV reconstruction showing a set of E1–E2–C proteins radially colored with the outer tip of E2 shown in *red* and the inner capsid/RNA genome shown in *blue*. The *dashed lines* represent the inner and outer lipid bilayer head groups. **C:** The genome RNA-binding sequence is shown by the *brown* chain with residue 82 represented by the *red circle* at the radius of the capsid. **D:** A surface-shaded representation of the C-terminal domain of the capsid is shown in *yellow* with the E2 glycoprotein bound in the hydrophobic pocket of the capsid. On the other side (facing RNA genome) of the capsid C-terminal domain are the residues (82–112) of the RNA-binding site. **E:** As in **(D)**, except the ribosome-binding site is highlighted (residues 97–111), and residue Lys97 is shown with a *yellow circle*. (Reprinted from Hasan SS, Sun C, Kim AS, et al. Cryo-EM structures of eastern equine encephalitis virus reveal mechanisms of virus disassembly and antibody neutralization. *Cell Rep* 2018;25(11):3136.e5–3147.e5, copyright 2018 with permission from Cell Press.)

its distal end the fusion peptide, a short loop of hydrophobic amino acids that promotes insertion of the protein into the target membrane. Domain III has an Ig-like fold and connects at its C-terminus with the transmembrane domain of the protein.

The structure of E1 is remarkably similar to the flavivirus E protein.[214,259] Unlike the alphaviruses, the flavivirus E protein functions both in receptor attachment and in membrane fusion. In the alphaviruses, these two activities are carried out by proteins E2 and E1, respectively. In the flaviviruses, the E protein is oriented roughly parallel to the lipid membrane, and it was anticipated that E1 might assume a similar orientation in the alphavirus virion.[123] This was essentially verified once the E1 atomic structure was fitted into the cryo-EM density. This fitting was accomplished for both SFV and SINV and recently for CHIKV.[137,142,206,279] Furthermore, for SINV, the two sites of E1 glycosylation were mapped onto the cryo-EM structure,

and these sites at Asn139 and Asn245 were used as positional markers to fix the position of E1 in the virion.[206] E1 lies at an angle of approximately 50 degrees relative to the surface of the membrane (Fig. 5.3B), and it forms an icosahedral lattice constituting the region that has been referred to as the skirt.[137,206] The crystallographic E1 dimer, which is a back-to-back dimer as opposed to a face-to-face dimer seen in the flaviviruses, is essentially preserved in the arrangement of E1 in the virion. The interface residues that make contact in the crystallographic dimer are presumably those that are important for forming the icosahedral lattice in the virion.

Although E1 constitutes the skirt region of the alphavirus surface, the majority of the protruding spike is composed of the E2 molecule. E2 constitutes the petals that make up the spike and covers the distal end of the E1 molecule that points outward. E2 serves to engage cell surface receptor molecules required for entry of the virion into the cell. The crystal structure of E2 together with both E1 and E3 for CHIKV was solved and reveals a three-immunoglobulin domain protein.[279] Domain B is located at the outermost point of the spike and contains the residues that have been implicated in receptor binding and as well as those involved in binding neutralizing antibodies. Domain B exhibits mobility in the context of the spike and was absent from the intact SINV E1–E2 trimer structure done at low pH. At the other end of the protein, located closest to the viral membrane is the C-terminal domain C. The N-terminal domain A (residues 1–132 in SINV) is the central bridge of E2, and connections are made to the B domain by the β−ribbon connector. The β−ribbon connector is flanked by a pair of well-conserved histidine residues, with E2 residue His170 shown to function as an acid switch to release the connector and B domain under acidic conditions. While E3 does not directly contact E1, its contact with the β−ribbon connector holds it in place to prevent movement of the B domain while the virus exits the cell in an immature state. The furin cleavage of the p62 to release E3, therefore, releases the clamp holding the B domain and activating the complex for pH-triggered fusion. E1 and E2 have extensive contacts with each other promoting the spike architecture (Fig. 5.3A, B). A recent high-resolution 3.5 Å cryo-EM reconstruction of SINV revealed the existence of a hydrophobic pocket that was occupied by a 20-Å-long linear molecule.[27] This pocket, similar to one seen in a lower-resolution structure of VEEV,[308] lies above the lipid membrane and is bound by conserved amino acids (Fig. 5.5). It has been hypothesized that this pocket stabilizes

the glycoprotein interactions, and when exposed to low pH, several conserved histidines may be protonated and cause the release of this "pocket factor" facilitating the resulting low pH-induced conformational changes.

In addition to the three major structural proteins identified by cryo-EM in the virion, two small transmembrane proteins are present in substoichiometric amounts and can be identified using purified virus and mass spectrometry. The existence of the 6K protein in the virion has been well established, but more recently the TF protein (~8 kDa) has also been found within SFV particles.[46] Given the low abundance and presumably random distribution of these small transmembrane proteins, they have not been detected using high-resolution cryo-EM, and their membrane architecture has to date prevented x-ray crystal structures. Whether the TF and 6K proteins exist as oligomers is also unknown.

GENOME STRUCTURE AND ORGANIZATION

The *Togavirus* genome resides on a positive strand RNA that contains a 5′ terminal 7-methylguanosine and a 3′ terminus that is polyadenylated (Fig. 5.6). The alphavirus genome, represented in Figure 5.6 by the type virus SINV, is approximately 11.7 kb in length, while rubella virus is nearly 2 kb shorter at 9.8 kb.[38,255] The genomes segregate their replication and virion proteins coding regions into two segments with the replication region mapping to the 5′ two-thirds and the structural region mapping to the 3′ one-third. Limited nucleotide homology exists between genomes in the two genera, although there are several sequences in both translated and nontranslated regions (NTRs) that do have homology; however, most evidence suggests that their replication and assembly strategies are quite different.[38] The nonstructural or replication proteins are translated from the genome RNA, whereas the structural or virion proteins are translated from a subgenomic mRNA.[190] In SINV, the 5′ NTR is 59 nucleotides, about average for the alphaviruses, while the 3′ NTR is also close to the average in length at 322 nucleotides.

Using comparative genome analyses and functional genetic studies of defective interfering (DI) particles and viruses, four conserved regions (conserved sequence element [CSE]) of the alphavirus genome were identified as cis-acting elements important for replication.[141] Two conserved regions are found near the 5′ end of the genome, one is found in the junction region between nonstructural and structural genes, and one is found at the 3′ end immediately preceding the poly (A). Three presumably similar functioning CSEs can also be found in the rubella genome.[38] In the alphaviruses, each CSE has been shown to interact in a host-dependent manner, suggesting that host factors may play a role in their function.[43,122,185,186] It has been shown that a U-rich region in the 3′ NTR of SINV contains elements responsible for viral RNA stability and that the cellular HuR protein binds this region decreasing the rate of cell-mediated decay of the genome RNA.[250] In addition, studies have shown that host proteins bind to the 3′ end of the minus-strand RNA of SINV, and in one case, the protein was identified as the mosquito homolog to the La protein.[193–195]

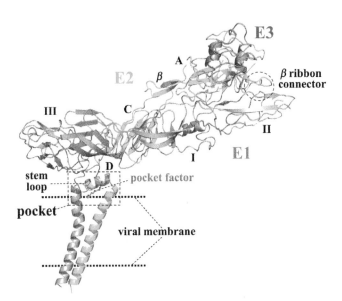

FIGURE 5.5 The C-α backbone of the 3.5 Å cryo-EM structure of SINV showing E1/E2/E3 glycoproteins. The atomic model of the glycoproteins was built directly from the cryo-EM density. The *dashed box* shows the location of the hydrophobic pocket that is occupied by an extended lipid molecule (*red*). It is suggested that the collapse of the pocket upon acidification results in ejection of the pocket factor and the ability of the glycoproteins to undergo movement necessary for fusion. (Reprinted from Chen L, Wang M, Zhu D, et al. Implication for alphavirus host-cell entry and assembly indicated by a 3.5 Å resolution cryo-EM structure. *Nat Commun* 2018;9(1):5326, copyright 2018 with permission from Springer Nature.)

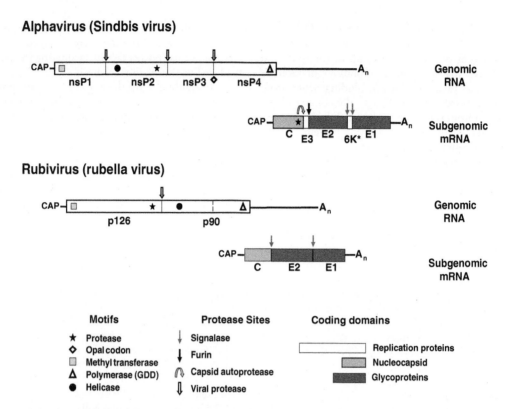

FIGURE 5.6 The genomes of SINV and rubella virus. Nontranslated regions are shown by the *solid line*, and translated regions are shown in *boxes*. *Open boxes* indicate replication proteins and *shaded boxes* represent structural or virion proteins. Motifs and cleavage sites are indicated according to the scheme. The subgenomic mRNAs are not shown to scale with the genomic RNAs.

ALPHAVIRUS REPLICATION

Mechanism of Attachment and Receptors

Alphaviruses display an extremely broad host range, both in terms of susceptible animal species and in terms of cells in culture. This broad host range has prompted speculation as to the nature of the receptor with two hypotheses proposed to explain this phenomenon.[256] In the first, the virus E2 glycoprotein contains multiple receptor-binding sites so distinct cellular receptors can bind the viral surface protein. The second hypothesis proposes that the virus uses a ubiquitous receptor that is highly conserved across species, including both mammals and mosquitoes. Data exist to support each model, and it is likely that a combination of the two is the true strategy for alphavirus attachment to the cell.

The variety of molecules that have been implicated for SINV argues for multiple distinct receptor-binding sites on E2.[256] The use of the laminin receptor with its high conservation across species suggests that it might serve as a receptor in multiple cell types and multiple host species.[285] However, the picture remains obscure for SINV because laminin receptor functions in baby hamster kidney cells but not in chicken embryo fibroblasts, where a 63-kDa protein has been implicated.[288] In mouse neuroblastoma cells, proteins of 74 and 110 kDa have been reported as possible SINV cellular receptors.[288] DC-SIGN and L-SIGN, C-type lectins that bind mannose-enriched carbohydrates, have also been implicated as receptors of alphaviruses that have been produced in mosquito cells.[116]

Studies using a genome-wide RNAi screen in Drosophila cells identified the natural resistance-associated macrophage protein (NRAMP) as a cellular receptor functioning to permit SINV infection.[220] Likewise, NRAMP2, the vertebrate homolog, is allowed for SINV, but not RRV, entry into mammalian cells. This finding raises the possibility that a family of related conserved multipass membrane proteins may serve as receptors for other alphaviruses. However, it has recently been shown using a genome-wide CRISPR–Cas9 screen for host factors involved in CHIKV infection that a membrane adhesion protein, Mxra8, functions as a cellular receptor for CHIKV, RRV, and other related arthritogenic alphaviruses.[309] The virus did bind to Mxra8, and antibodies against the protein were able to block CHIKV infection validating this protein as an authentic alphavirus receptor. A cryo-EM structure of CHIKV bound to Mxra8 reveals the binding of the receptor into a cleft formed by neighboring E1–E2 heterodimers within a spike and engaging a neighboring spike.

Natural isolates of EEEV utilize cell surface heparan sulfate as an attachment receptor.[65] This use of heparan sulfate may direct tropism of EEEV and promote enhanced neurovirulence. In contrast, passage of several other alphaviruses in culture leads to the accumulation of adaptive mutations, some of which introduce basic amino acids in their E2 glycoprotein.[19,21,22,117] This increase of positively charged amino acids in E2 leads to high-efficiency attachment to cells through heparan sulfate molecules. The importance of this interaction was demonstrated genetically by the generation of a Chinese hamster ovary cell line using retroviral insertional mutagenesis that was deficient in the expression of heparan sulfate and chondroitin sulfate.[104] These cells were resistant to SINV infection and defective in binding virus. The substitution of a single residue on the E2 glycoprotein of RRV was sufficient to permit heparan sulfate binding, and this attachment was mapped using cryo-EM to the distal tip of the spike.[94,307] The binding of heparan sulfate does not result in conformational changes in the virion, nor does it enhance the fusion process.[247,307] Therefore, it likely serves simply as a mechanism to attach the particle to the cell surface so an efficient interaction with the entry receptor can occur. In contrast to what is observed in cell culture with SINV, infection of mice results in the development of large-plaque viral mutants with a reduced affinity for heparan sulfate and a greater viremia.[22] However, given these diverse observations, the utilization of heparan sulfate and its role in

pathogenesis among the different alphaviruses requires further investigation. This model in which viruses first use a low affinity ubiquitous cell surface molecule to attach to the cell so that a more limited two-dimensional search for the entry receptor is likely employed by many of the alphaviruses.

Mechanisms of Entry, Membrane Fusion, and Uncoating

Following attachment to cells and engagement with an entry receptor, alphaviruses proceed via the endocytic pathway to gain access to the cell interior (Fig. 5.7).[36,95,162] Structural and biochemical experiments demonstrate that binding of RRV to heparan sulfate does not induce conformational changes in the virion.[307] However, other receptors may induce conformational changes in the particle that might mediate entry such as the reduction of disulfide bonds to disrupt protein–protein

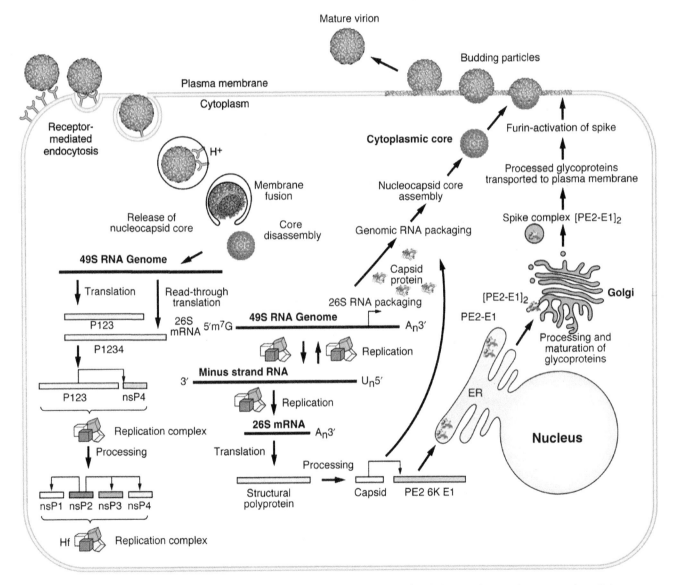

FIGURE 5.7 Life cycle of an alphavirus. The start of the life cycle is shown on the *left* with the attachment of a virion to the cellular receptor. Following fusion of the viral envelope, disassembly of the core, and release of the genome RNA, replication proteins are translated and processed (*bottom left*). These proteins enable the replication of the input genome RNA (*bottom center*) and translation of the subgenomic mRNA into structural proteins. Cytoplasmic assembly of genome RNA and capsid produces the nucleocapsid core that associates with processed glycoproteins (*right*) at the plasma membrane resulting in budding. Scale varies.

interactions.[1,11,199,230] Despite these suggestions that disulfide exchange may play a role in alphavirus entry, the use of thiol-blocking reagents failed to show a significant inhibition of infection.[75] However, it is clear that the attachment of SINV to cells results in the exposure of new epitopes defined by monoclonal antibodies and suggests that protein rearrangements occur following receptor engagement.[47,170] Similar observations have been made using purified virus and treatment with heat, pH, and reducing agents.[169] In addition, the recent observations on the role of virion and protein dynamics in the flavivirus life cycle suggest that other structurally related viruses might employ particle dynamics to sense their environment as they search for an entry receptor.[121] In addition to the role of thiol exchange reactions that have been proposed to play a role in alphavirus entry, there has even been a suggestion that cell penetration may occur at the cell surface in the absence of fusion by conformational rearrangements in the envelope glycoproteins.[1,199] However, it has been fairly well established that membrane fusion triggered by an exposure to acidic conditions is the gateway for the release of genome RNA into the cytoplasm (Fig. 5.8). Finally, a virus receptor may not need to induce a conformational change in the virion to function as a receptor and for the particle to gain entry.

Receptor-bound viruses undergo endocytosis into coated vesicles using a clathrin-dependent pathway. This pathway was demonstrated by DeTulleo and Kirchhausen using dominant-negative mutants of dynamin to block the formation of clathrin-coated pits and prevent entry of SFV and SINV.[36] The vesicles are subsequently acidified, providing the trigger for fusion between viral and cellular membranes. Acid-induced fusion is supported by numerous studies but most convincingly by the use of lysosomotropic weak bases that raise the pH of endocytic vesicles and prevent entry of alphaviruses.[75,96] Although it has been argued that viral RNA replication might also be affected by the acidification, pseudotyped viruses containing

alphavirus envelope proteins are also inhibited in entry by this treatment.[41,97,237] Entry is aided by several host proteins in the endosomal pathway, with TSPAN9 being one that functions in the early endosome to make it more permissive for membrane fusion.[252]

The role of the alphavirus E1 and E2 glycoproteins in the entry process has been firmly established (Figs. 5.8 and 5.9). In the presence of acidic pH, the E1–E2 heterodimer is destabilized and the two proteins dissociate.[281,283] The dissociation of the proteins results in the exposure of the fusion peptide that is found on the distal tip of E1.[4,72,85,137] The fusion peptide of E1 inserts into the target membrane in a cholesterol-dependent manner followed by the trimerization of E1.[4,72,85,137] A large conformational change in E1 results in domain III and the stem anchor region of the protein packing against domain II, resulting in the viral and target membranes being brought into close opposition (Fig. 5.8).[74] A set of E1 trimers, possibly resembling what has been seen in liposomes, results in membrane deformation and promotes membrane mixing.[72] Finally, a fusion pore will form as the two membranes complete the process, and the nucleocapsid core will be released into the cytoplasm (Fig. 5.9).

Lescar et al.[137] recognized that the structural features of the alphavirus E1 and flavivirus E proteins were distinct from the structures of other previously identified fusion proteins, such as HA from influenza, and proposed that they represented a novel class of fusion machines. They termed these class II membrane fusion proteins and elaborated several distinguishing features that separated the two classes. Class II fusion proteins are predominantly composed of β-strands, contain an internal fusion peptide, and have a companion protein that stabilized the structure; this companion protein forms an activated metastable structure following proteolytic processing of a precursor protein. In the alphaviruses, PE2 is proteolytically activated by cleavage to generate E3 and E2, with E2 and E1 forming

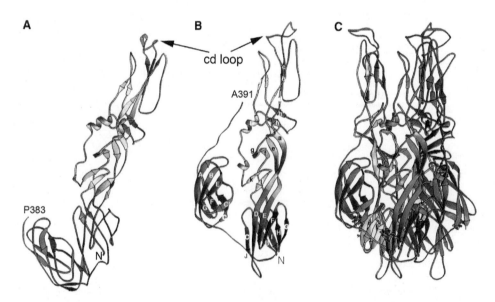

FIGURE 5.8 Postfusion structure of the Semliki Forest virus E1 protein. Panels A and **B** represent the neutral and low pH forms of the soluble E1 ectodomain lacking amino acid residues 392 to 438, respectively. The orientation of the protein presents the fusion loop (cd loop) toward the target membrane (*top*). This rearrangement would occur after E1 has undergone trimerization as shown in **panel C**. (This figure was modified using an image kindly provided courtesy of Dr. Felix Rey.[137])

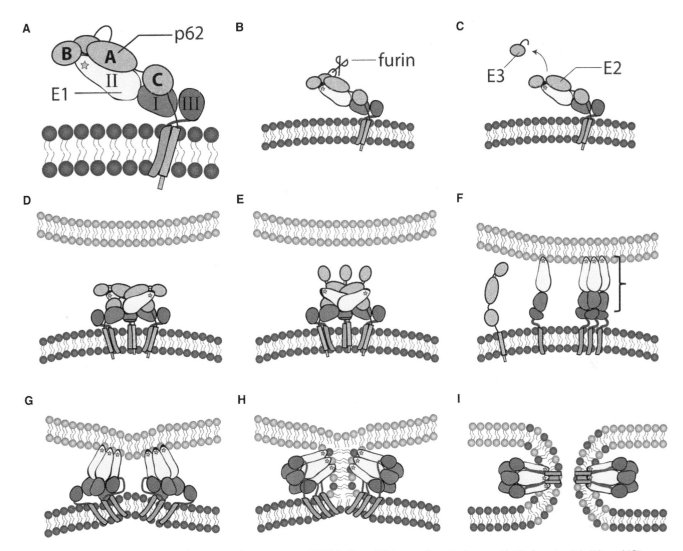

FIGURE 5.9 Model of alphavirus fusion. A: The immature p62/E1 (p62 = pE2) heterodimer is shown with E2 domains **(A)**, **(B)**, and **(C)** shown in *gray*, E3 in *pink*, and E1 domains I, II, and III in *red, yellow,* and *blue*, respectively, covering the E1 fusion peptide (*star*). **B:** Cleavage of p62 by host furin, although it remains bound protecting E1 in the low pH of the trans-Golgi. **C:** E3 may be released depending on pH conditions as the virus is secreted from the cell. **D:** The mature form of the E2/E1 trimer of heterodimers. **E:** At low pH, domain B of E2 rearranges to expose the E1 fusion loop. **F:** Low pH releases E2 from the heterodimer, and E1 inserts into the target membrane. **G:** Fold-back process by which domain III and the stem region move toward the fusion loop. **H:** Folding of domain III and the stem region against domain II of the trimer pulls the transmembrane domains toward one another distorting the viral membrane and initiating hemifusion of viral and target membranes. **I:** Close opposition of the fusion peptides and transmembrane domains resolve into the fusion pore. (This figure was kindly provided courtesy of Margaret K from *Nature*: Felix AR. Virus membrane-fusion proteins: more than one way to make a hairpin. *Nat Rev Microbiol* 2006;4(1):67–76. Copyright © 2006 Springer Nature.)

a stable heterodimer.[152,153] Mutagenesis experiments have provided insight into the fusion process and the residues that play regulatory and supporting roles in this process. As predicted, a pH-sensitive histidine residue in E1 (SFV H3) appears to regulate the low pH-dependent folding of E1 that is required for fusion.[212] Several other well-conserved histidines in E1 were evaluated and found unable to influence the activity. Kielian and colleagues also found that a salt bridge is formed within domain II of the E1 trimer core, which appears critical for stabilizing the homotrimer fusion intermediate.[150] These have been supported by computational analyses of the envelope proteins undergoing a low pH transition.[305]

Biochemical experiments with SFV have defined the requirements and steps in the alphavirus fusion process. Kielian et al. demonstrated a strict dependence on cholesterol for fusion.[111,156,205] This requirement has been narrowed down to the sterol 3β hydroxyl group in cholesterol.[31,174,280,301] A mutant was isolated (named *srf-3* for sterol requirement in function) that was cholesterol independent and had an amino acid substitution of a proline to serine at E1 residue 226. This mutation did not affect fusion with normal membranes but significantly enhanced fusion to cholesterol-free membranes.[25,271] In mosquito cells, the *srf-3* mutant grew better than wild-type virus.[5] The importance of this region of E1, which lies in the ij loop, for alphavirus fusion was further demonstrated by mutation of a conserved histidine at position 230 to alanine with the resulting virus particles being noninfectious but capable of proceeding through E1 homotrimer formation under low pH conditions and suggesting a late step in fusion.[24] However, the exact role of cholesterol to promote fusion is not known. The structure of the postfusion form of E1 has been determined using x-ray crystallography.[72–74] This was accomplished using a soluble form of the E1 ectodomain known as E1* following exposure to low pH in the presence of liposomes and solubilization with detergents. The structure of this homotrimer reveals the movement of domain III by 37 Å toward the fusion peptide and target membrane (Fig. 5.8)[74] and is similar to changes that are induced by class I fusion protein activation.[112] Importantly, the addition of exogenous domain III can inhibit fusion by binding to E1 and preventing fold-back of the endogenous domain III.[145] A complete picture of the virion during the fusion process is not available, despite several attempts using cryo-EM to examine these steps.[45,62,81,199]

Following the fusion of the viral and cellular membranes, the nucleocapsid core is released into the cytoplasm. The stability of that core is not known, but uncoating has been suggested to require the interaction of the core with ribosomes. This is based on several reports that suggest that ribosomal RNA competes for a site on the capsid protein and that displacement of this site results in disassembly.[243,244,295] This site has been identified in SINV capsid protein between residues 94 and 105 and coincides with a predicted site for genome RNA binding.[298] It has also been suggested that the core might be primed for uncoating by exposure to low pH, which causes the core to become unstable.[293,296] This exposure to low pH could occur in the endosome because both E1 and 6K have been proposed to have ion channel properties.[155,167,294] However, studies using preformed cores microinjected into naïve cells demonstrated that these cores do uncoat presumably devoid of conditions of low pH.[248] Whether these cores interact with ribosomes to promote disassembly and release of genome RNA remains to be shown.

Translation and the Role of Viral-Encoded Replication Proteins

The genome RNA serves as a messenger RNA for the synthesis of the nonstructural or replication proteins (Fig. 5.6). These are produced by two polyproteins that originate translation at nucleotide 60 in SINV.[258] The smaller but more abundant polyprotein P123 terminates translation at an opal codon following 1897 amino acids. Readthrough of the opal codon occurs with a low frequency (~10%–20%) and results in the production of the larger P1234 polyprotein. Not all alphaviruses have a termination codon to control the production of the two polyproteins, but mutagenesis of the opal codon in SINV adversely affects replication.[144] Processing of the polyproteins occurs through the action of a virus-encoded protease located within the nonstructural protein 2 (nsP2).[37,87,88] The processing of the polyprotein to generate precursor and end product nsPs is believed to regulate the synthesis of viral RNAs.[34,136,240] Translation of the structural polyprotein proceeds through a subgenomic mRNA that is initiated near the coding region for the C-terminus of P1234. The subgenomic mRNA is 3′ coterminal with the genome RNA and is produced later in the infection.[258]

Initial studies of the replication proteins used temperature-sensitive mutants that were conditional lethal for viral replication. These studies established complementation groups and identified specific functions of the replication proteins.[254] Four complementation groups were identified, and these correlated with the four nsPs. Once sequence information was available, motifs were identified that verified function and permitted phylogenetic relationships between other virus families to be established. This resulted in the suggestion of an alphavirus-like superfamily that contained RNA virus members from several plant families and argued for an evolutionary relationship between them.[3,257]

The nsPs are multifunctional proteins with some of their activities shown in Table 5.1. However, it is likely that additional unknown activities exist. Guanine-7-methyltransferase and guanylyltransferase activities necessary for mRNA and genome RNA capping have been shown to reside within nsP1.[126,171,172] This capping activity is distinct from cellular capping enzymes in substrate preference.[6] Several genetic studies have confirmed the identity of amino acids critical for the methyltransferase function, but the domain required for guanylyltransferase activity has not be identified and may flank the conserved methyltransferase domain.[8,221] A ts mutant that mapped to Ala348 of nsP1 in SINV demonstrated a role of the protein in minus-strand RNA synthesis.[82] A defect in

TABLE 5.1   Translation products of alphaviruses (sindbis virus)

Protein	Size (aa)	Function
Nonstructural proteins		
nsP1	540	Methyltransferase and guanylyltransferase; anchors replicase complex to membranes
nsP2	807	NTPase, helicase, RNA triphosphatase, protease responsible for processing of nonstructural polyprotein
nsP3	556	Phosphoprotein important for initiation of RNA synthesis; contains macro domain and SH3-binding regions with ADP-ribosyl–binding/hydrolase activities, zinc-binding oligomerization domain
nsP4	610	RNA-dependent RNA polymerase (RdRp), terminal transferase
Structural proteins		
Capsid	264	Encapsidates genomic RNA to form nucleocapsid core; carboxyl domain is an autocatalytic serine protease
E3	64	N-terminal domain is uncleaved leader peptide for E2; E3+E2 = pE2
E2	423	Presents the major neutralizing epitopes and is responsible for receptor binding
6K	55	Leader peptide for E1, enhances particle release, putative ion channel
TF	70	TransFrame protein, putative ion channel, enhances particle infectivity, expression prevents synthesis of E1
E1	439	Responsible for membrane fusion activity

minus-strand synthesis has also been seen with mutations in nsP4, and some of these have been complemented with changes in nsP1 at residues 349 and 374, suggesting sites for nsP1 and nsP4 interaction.[42] nsP1 is the only alphavirus nonstructural protein that has been shown to be membrane associated.[127,202] The membrane association has been suggested to occur by a palmitoylated cysteine at residue 420 (in SINV).[7,126] Mutations that disrupt palmitoylation did not alter the distribution of replication complexes and show only modest reductions in growth. However, nsP1 can still bind to membranes through a patch of positively charged and hydrophobic amino acids between residues 245 and 264.[9] Nuclear magnetic resonance spectroscopy of a corresponding peptide suggests that this sequence can form an amphipathic α-helix that can interact with liposomes.[128] This membrane anchoring of the replication complex associated with nsP1 is probably required for efficient replicase activity.

The largest of the replication proteins is nsP2, with a length of about 800 amino acids. The N-terminal half of the protein has helicase, nucleoside triphosphatase, and RNA triphosphatase activities,[76,77,217] while the C-terminal half contains a novel cysteine protease domain and a nonfunctional methyltransferase domain.[253,272] The structure for the C-terminal two domains of the VEEV nsP2 was solved by Watowich and colleagues using x-ray crystallography (Fig. 5.10).[228] The structure shows that the active site of the protease is positioned close to the inter-face between the two domains. Although related to proteases papain and cathepsin X, the fold of the nsP2 protease domain appears to be unique and a new form of cysteine protease structure. Although having a similar tertiary structure with known methyltransferases such as FtsJ, the SAM substrate binding site is very different in backbone alignment and sequence, arguing against any methyltransferase activity. However, by mapping several previously identified *ts* mutants affected in RNA synthesis onto the C-terminal domain, it was suggested that the domain functions as an RNA-binding scaffold that regulates protease activity and RNA synthesis.[227,228] The structure of the N-terminal helicase domain from CHIKV has been solved by Law and colleagues and reveals a unique fold for its N-terminal region followed by a superfamily 1 RNA helicase domain.[131]

The nsP2 protein has a nuclear localization sequence that results in 50% of the protein reaching the nucleus,[216,217] and it has been reported that nsP2 of VEEV undergoes both nuclear import as well as export.[175] Abrogation of the signal results in a slightly defective virus, but at least in SFV, the mutant has lost neuropathogenesis, arguing for a role of nsP2 in host interactions.[216] Studies have identified a role for nsP2 from the Old World alphaviruses in the induction of cytopathic effects and the establishment of persistent infections, and this is discussed later in the chapter.[39,54] Experiments have also provided a link between nsP2 and the host response, resulting in shutoff of minus-strand RNA synthesis.[66,233] Genetic studies identified conditional lethal mutations demonstrating RNA-defective phenotypes that implicated nsP2 in the regulation of minus-strand synthesis and in the initiation of subgenomic RNA synthesis.[82] Furthermore, the role of the protease activity to regulate the temporal control of RNA synthesis has been well established and is described later.[34,136]

The function of the nsP3 protein remains obscure, although genetic analyses indicate that it plays a role in RNA synthesis and neurovirulence.[2,130,267,287] The protein is highly conserved among alphaviruses at its N-terminus, while the C-terminal 200 amino acids are rich in serine and threonine residues. The protein is phosphorylated on serines and threonine, although this modification is not required for replication and its function in the virus life cycle is not known.[129,130,143,203,274,275] The protein has a weak affinity for membranes and will associate with them when expressed in the absence of the other nsPs.[274] A crystal structure of both the CHIKV and VEEV N-terminal 160 residues of nsP3 confirmed previous suggestions that this region contains a macro domain (the VEEV structure is shown in Fig. 5.11).[158,239] These domains function as ADP-ribose binding modules and have also been shown capable of single-strand RNA binding.[2] The exact function(s) of the macro domain awaits additional studies. While the C-terminal end of nsP3 is not well conserved, a proline-rich sequence found in most alphaviruses was identified as a target site for Src-homology 3 domain containing proteins amphiphysin-1 and amphiphysin-2.[183] Disruption of the binding sequence by mutation or reduction of amphiphysin-2 by RNAi reduced replication in both SINV and SFV. It is unclear how this interaction influences RNA replication; however, the amphiphysins have been implicated as membrane-binding proteins, endocytosis, and membrane trafficking, and the virus may usurp these functions to facilitate RNA synthesis. Furthermore, the C-terminus of nsP3 has been shown to bind to FXR and G3BP that help facilitate formation of viral replication complexes.[115]

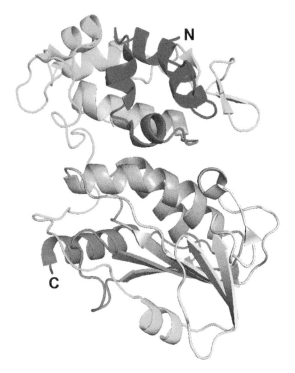

FIGURE 5.10 Structure of the Venezuelan equine encephalitis virus nsP2 protease. A ribbon diagram showing the protease colored from *blue* (N-terminus) through *red* (C-terminus) representing residues N468 to S787. The catalytic dyad residues, C477 and H546, are found in the N-terminal protease domain (*top*), while the methyltransferase-like domain (*bottom*) constitutes the C-terminal domain. (This figure was generated in PyMol using the PDB coordinates 2HWK from Russo and colleagues[228] and was kindly provided courtesy of Dr. Joyce Jose.)

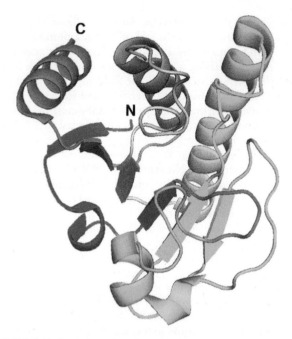

FIGURE 5.11 Structure of the Venezuelan equine encephalitis virus nsP3 macro domain. A ribbon diagram showing the nsP3 macro domain colored from *blue* (N-terminus) through *red* (C-terminus) representing residues A1 to E160. The structure consists of a six-stranded β-sheet ringed by three α-helices. (This figure was generated in PyMol using the PDB coordinates 3GQE from Malet and colleagues[76] and was kindly provided courtesy of Dr. Joyce Jose.)

The core of the virus replication complex is the RNA-dependent RNA polymerase (RdRp) that maps to nsP4.[82,119] Interestingly, because of the opal codon in SINV, synthesis of P123 is significantly greater than the level of P1234, and thus, nsP4 levels are lower than that of the other nsPs. Furthermore, modifications that increase the synthesis of nsP4, such as the removal of the opal termination codon, result in reduced virus replication.[144] The majority of the protein from the C-terminus constitutes the RdRp domain based on homology with other polymerases and predicted secondary structures.[107] A short region exists at the N-terminus that lacks a counterpart in other viral polymerases, and it has been suggested that it might be a binding domain for the other nsPs. The N-terminus of nsP4 also contains a conserved tyrosine residue, and this serves to make the protein unstable in infected cells.[35,241] de Groot et al.[35] examined the degradation of nsP4 and showed that it was degraded by the N-end rule pathway. It has been suggested that free nsP4 is rapidly degraded, whereas nsP4 that is a component of replicase complexes is protected and relatively stable. Thus, it was not a surprise that attempts to express the full-length nsP4 in heterologous systems were initially unsuccessful. However, expression of nsP4 lacking the first 97 amino acids was successful, and this truncated nsP4 displayed a terminal adenylyltransferase activity.[266] This terminal transferase activity was suggested to play a role in the maintenance of the poly (A) tract at the 3′ end of positive strand RNAs. The nsP4 protein was subsequently expressed as an N-terminal SUMO fusion protein that was cleaved after purification, and nsP4 was shown to possess *de novo* minus-strand synthesis activity that was dependent on the correct 3′ end of positive strand template.[223] Proteomic studies have been used to identify host

proteins that might interact with nsP4 during virus infection.[32] In this study, the authors demonstrated a total of 29 host proteins were associated with nsP4 in a temporally regulated pattern. Among the proteins identified, two proteins known as GTPase-activating protein SH3-domain–binding proteins 1 and 2 (G3BP1 and G3BP2) were also shown to interact with nsP2 and nsP3.[32] However, the role of these proteins is unclear, and they may function to reduce the pool of RNAs available for translation by recruiting the viral RNA to the stress granule pathway.

Transcription and Replication of Genomic Nucleic Acid

Alphavirus-infected cells produce three species of RNAs: genome plus-strand RNA, complementary minus-strand RNA, and subgenomic mRNA. The synthesis of these three species is tightly regulated by the availability of specific nsPs (Fig. 5.12).[34,134,136] Replication is initiated on the cytoplasmic surface of endosomes and lysosomes on structures termed cytopathic vacuoles.[61] All four nsPs can be found associated with each other and within these vacuoles.[125] In elegant studies by DeGroot et al.,[34] it was shown that proteolytic site selection controlled the processing of the nsPs and determined the components of the replicase complex. This was accomplished by assessing cleavage site preferences and determining which enzymes (nsP2 or its precursors) could affect processing. Additional studies by the Sawicki laboratory using temperature-sensitive mutants established the biochemical nature of the replicase complex.[15,232,234] In complementary work, the Rice laboratory carried out *in vivo* replication studies using nsPs expressed in a vaccinia vector to discern the functional complexes.[134–136] Despite earlier problems, they were successful in developing a system for template-dependent initiation of SINV.[133]

RNA replication begins with the initiation of minus-strand synthesis. This event requires the 3′ CSE and host proteins/factors.[56,70,122] *In vitro* studies using polymerase extracts suggest the poly (A) tract may not serve as template for the initiation of minus-strand synthesis, although the details of this initiation event are not known.[86] Minus-strand synthesis requires P123 or P23 and nsP4, but a cleavage-defective P1234 is not functional.[134–136] Similarly, in the vaccinia system, expression of the individual nsPs was not sufficient for complex formation and minus-strand synthesis. As minus-strand synthesis continues, nsPs continue to be translated, and concentrations of the protease precursors increase. Cleavage at the nsP1–nsP2 and nsP2–nsP3 junctions results in the switch over to plus-strand synthesis presumably by a change in the conformation and composition of the replicase complex (Fig. 5.12). Synthesis of minus strands by the replicase requires continuous protein synthesis, and it has been suggested that nsP2 engages the host response by using the RNase L–dependent pathway to inhibit host cell translation.[79,233] As with most plus-strand RNA viruses, synthesis is asymmetric with minus-strand synthesis about 2% to 5% the level of plus-strand genome RNA.[286]

Although the viral protein composition of the minus and plus-strand replicases is known, the role of host proteins in the complex is not. From studies with the CSEs, host cell–dependent effects were observed, and several host proteins were shown to bind to the conserved RNA elements.[56,193–195] Furthermore, Fayzulin and Frolov[43] showed that although the 51 nt CSE is dispensable in mammalian cells, in mosquito cells mutations

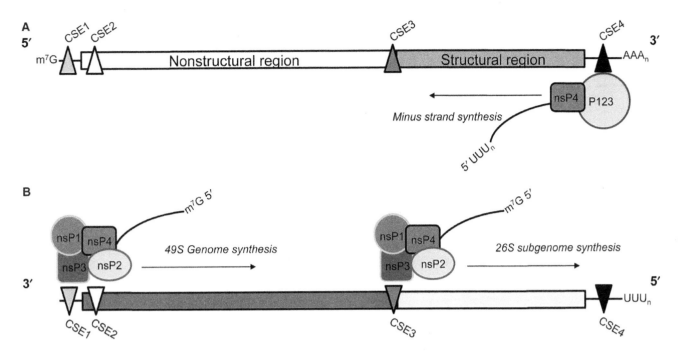

FIGURE 5.12 The conserved sequence elements (CSE) and nonstructural proteins involved in alphavirus genome replication.
A: A schematic of minus-strand synthesis from a plus-strand template. A protein complex composed of P123 and nsP4, and presumably host proteins (not shown) initiate synthesis of the minus strand from the 3' end of the genome. CSE4, a 19nt element, is found just upstream of the poly **(A)** tract. CSE4 is thought to act as a promoter for minus-strand synthesis, perhaps via a cyclization event with CSE2, a 51nt element located within the nsP1 coding region (not shown). **B:** A schematic of full-length 49S genomic and 26S subgenomic RNA syntheses from a minus-strand template. An accumulation of P123 allows processing of P123 polyproteins in *trans* into the individual nonstructural proteins. Presumably, the altered conformation of the replicase complex shifts template preference to the minus strand. CSE1, composed of the first 44nt of the 5' genome, act as a promoter for synthesis of full-length 49S genomic RNA from a minus-strand template, perhaps in conjunction with CSE2. Fully processed replicase complexes also associate on the CSE3 element, which spans the 3' end of the nsP4 coding sequence and the junction region between the nonstructural and structural genes. These CSE3-associated replicase complexes efficiently transcribe the 26S subgenomic message. Note that a replicase complex composed of nsP1, P23, and nsp4 may also be capable of plus-strand synthesis (not shown). (This figure was kindly provided courtesy of Jonathan Snyder.)

have a deleterious effect. Interestingly, adaptive mutations occur in the 5' NTR, as well as in nsP2 and nsP3, suggesting their involvement in CSE function. Frolov et al.,[56] using chimeric templates and trans-competition experiments, showed that the 5' NTR is a component of the promoter for not only plus-strand synthesis but also minus-strand synthesis. From these data, they proposed a model for the initiation of minus-strand RNA synthesis that requires the 5' and 3' ends of the genome RNA to be brought together. This would be accomplished using components of the host translational machinery, which is involved in cap and poly (A) binding. Despite the attractiveness of the model, the lack of a purified reconstituted system for RNA synthesis has hampered progress in understanding alphavirus RNA replication.

The synthesis of the subgenomic mRNA is controlled by a minimal promoter element that spans from −19 to +5 relative to the start of mRNA synthesis. A larger fragment from −98 to +14 provides three- to sixfold more activity and constitutes the fully active promoter. As with the 5' and 3' CSEs, the subgenomic promoter appears to interact with host factors as mutations in the promoter have differential effects, depending on replication in vertebrate versus invertebrate hosts.[98,99,300] This promoter has been extensively employed in gene expression and replicon studies using alphaviruses, including the use of multiple tandem promoters.[20,57,59]

Perhaps the most informative studies on alphavirus replication in recent years have emerged using advanced imaging techniques.[55,106,163,164,311] These approaches have shed light on the spatial and temporal assembly of replication complexes. Most intriguing is the observation that membrane-derived structures competent for RNA synthesis appear to form initially at the plasma membrane (Fig. 5.13). Studies from both SFV and SINV demonstrate the membrane invaginations referred to as spherules first accumulate on the plasma membrane and are later internalized using the actin–myosin network.[60] These structures appear to contain all of the nonstructural proteins as well as double-stranded RNA but are devoid of any structural proteins. Structures known as cytopathic vacuoles type 1 and type 2 (CPV1 and CPV2) were previously described to contain the replication proteins and viral glycoproteins, respectively. The role of CPV2 appears to guide the glycoproteins to the site of budding; however, the role of CPV1 for RNA synthesis is not as clear. CPV1 structures form later in RNA replication, probably as a result of spherule recruitment from the plasma membrane, but it has been suggested that they may not be the major site for viral RNA synthesis at least in mammalian cells.[60]

Assembly of Nucleocapsid Core, Glycoprotein Synthesis, and Processing
The subgenomic RNA, which is made at approximately three times the level of the genomic RNA, is translated to produce

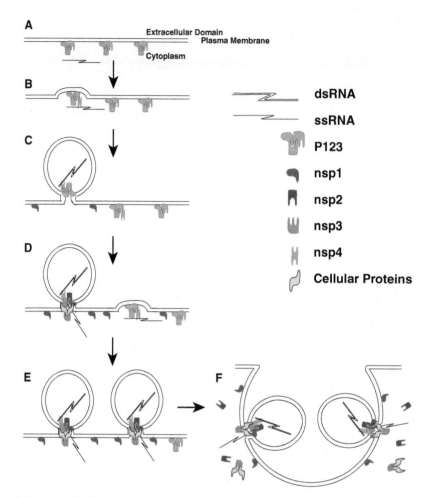

FIGURE 5.13 Assembly of alphavirus replication complexes. A: Replication complexes consisting of P123 and genome RNA are found at the plasma membrane; **(B)** with the addition of nsP4, the RdRp, synthesis of dsRNA occurs **(C)** along with the formation of membrane spherules. Upon processing of P123 **(D)**, replication complexes switch to the synthesis of genomic and subgenomic RNA. As replication continues **(E and F)**, free nsP1, nsP2, and nsP3 are found, with the latter protein associating with specific host proteins and nsP1 remaining membrane associated. At latter stages, multiple spherules coalesce into CPV1 within the cytoplasm. (This figure was adapted by Thomas Edwards and R.J.K. with permission from Drs. Elena Frolova and Ilya Frolov. From Frolova EI, Gorchakov R, Pereboeva L, Atasheva S, Frolov I. Functional Sindbis virus replicative complexes are formed at the plasma membrane. *J Virol* 2010;84(22):11679–11695. doi: 10.1128/JVI.01441-10. Reprinted with permission from American Society for Microbiology.)

the structural or virion proteins.[213] The order of translation is capsid-PE2(E3+E2)-6K-E1 (Fig. 5.6). Translation of the structural polyprotein is enhanced due to the presence of a hairpin secondary structure in the subgenomic mRNA between residues 77 and 139.[59] The polyprotein is processed by host and viral proteases to generate the authentic structural proteins that will end up in the virion, and the membrane topology of the glycoproteins is shown in Figure 5.12. The capsid protein is translated first and is released by proteolysis immediately after the ribosome clears the junction between it and PE2. The capsid functions as an autoprotease, and sequence and mutational analyses suggested that the C-terminal domain of the capsid contained a serine-like protease.[10,83] This hypothesis was confirmed by the x-ray crystal structure of the C-terminal domain from SINV.[30] The protein has a chymotrypsin-like fold, with His141, Asp163, and Ser215 forming the catalytic triad. Interestingly, the C-terminal residue, Trp264, remains in the active site pocket and presumably prevents transcleavage by the protease. With

the self-cleavage of the capsid protein, the new N-terminus of the polyprotein now contains a signal sequence for translocation of the PE2 sequence across the ER membrane.[67] Additional signal sequences are present at the C-terminus of E2, permitting translocation of 6K, and at the C-terminus of 6K, permitting translocation of E1 (Fig. 5.14). The expression of TF protein, which contains the first 43 amino acids of 6K, contains a stop codon that prevents the synthesis of E1. Proteins E1, E2, 6K, and TF are transmembrane proteins, while E3 is released from most alphavirus particles following cleavage of its PE2 precursor.[92,208,209,226] SFV retains the cleaved E3 with the virion; however, it is unclear whether it has a postcleavage function.[312]

Following autoproteolysis, the capsid protein transiently associates with the ribosome, and assembly into a core particle appears to be both rapid and efficient, with no observed intermediates.[249,270] A specific "packaging sequence" has been identified in the genome RNA in SINV that promotes encapsidation of RNA into the assembling core.[290] In SINV, this

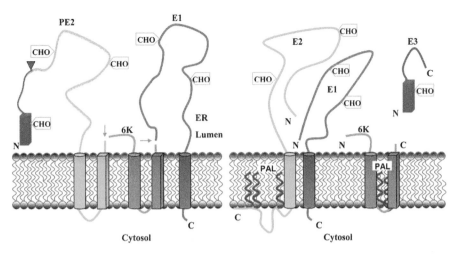

FIGURE 5.14 Schematic model for the configuration of the E1 and E2 glycoproteins in the membrane. Left: Configuration of the glycoproteins after signalase cleavage of 6K and E1 but before cleavage of PE2. **Right:** Configuration of glycoproteins after the maturation cleavage of PE2 into E3 and E2. Note the *dark red jagged lines* on the cytoplasmic side of E2 and 6K that represent palmitoylation sites (PAL). Glycosylation sites are indicated by CHO. Signal sequences are indicated as colored rectangular blocks. Stop-transfer sequences are indicated as colored cylinders. The shape of the polypeptides does not imply their native configuration. (This figure was kindly provided courtesy of Dr. Joyce Jose.)

sequence has been identified as nucleotides 945 to 1,076, and attempts to identify the nature of the recognition element have met with limited success. However, there is conservation of structural and functional components of packaging signal across diverse alphaviruses.[114] The packaging sequence on the genome RNA is recognized by residues 81 to 113 in the capsid protein.[69,289] A deletion of residues 97 to 106 results in a failure to efficiently package genome RNA, although cores still form with heterologous RNA incorporated.[191] Although most alphaviruses package their genomes with high efficiency, Aura virus has been described as an alphavirus that packages its subgenomic mRNA as well.[224,225] The development of alphaviruses as gene expression vectors has prompted much investigation into the packaging requirements, and in VEEV, packaging has been shown to require expression of nsP123, although the mechanism and the generality of this requirement have not been shown.[276]

Although *in vitro* systems for core assembly have been described, the stepwise assembly process has not been clearly elaborated.[263–265,291,292] The capsid protein requires the addition of nucleic acid to initiate the assembly process, and in the presence of full-length wild-type protein, assembly proceeds rapidly. Using a truncated capsid protein, the initial step appears to involve a protein dimer complexed with RNA.[263–265] Cores are found in the cytoplasm and attached to membranes, probably through their interaction with E2. Cytoplasmic cores have a well-defined size and T = 4 icosahedral symmetry, similar to *in vitro* assembled cores, but not identical to the well-ordered T = 4 symmetry in cores found within virus particles.[176,197] However, the symmetry of the core does not necessarily dictate the symmetry of the virion, and it is likely that the icosahedral architecture of the glycoprotein scaffold is the driving force behind the strict T = 4 organization of alphavirus.[197] This is supported by the observation from Forsell et al.,[51] who produced a SFV capsid protein with a deletion in residues 40 to

118. This mutant was unable to assemble cores, but virus particles were produced that had the expected T = 4 symmetry.

In parallel with the formation of the nucleocapsid in the cytoplasm, the envelope proteins that were translocated into the ER are processed and undergo posttranslational modifications. High mannose chains are added to all potential N-linked glycosylation sites, and the oligosaccharide chains are trimmed depending on the availability of the site.[236] Palmitoylation occurs at several sites in E2 and 6K/TF.[18,64] In a set of elegant studies, Brown et al. showed that E1 and PE2 undergo a complex series of folding intermediates.[23,118,178,179] These intermediates require chaperones and disulfide bond formation and exchange. The E1 and E2 glycoproteins form a heterodimer in the ER, but it is not known whether higher-order oligomerization takes place here.[312] Oligomerization of PE2 and E1 is also a requirement for the transport of the glycoproteins, but the presence of the CP is not required.[68,154] It has been shown that PE2 oligomerizes with a partially folded intermediate of E1 and that this oligomerization is sufficient for the proteins to exit the ER. After the heterodimer reaches the trans-Golgi network, but prior to arrival at the plasma membrane, PE2 is cleaved by furin.[33] This cleavage is required for virion entry and fusion activation in new cells, although revertants can be readily isolated that suppress the requirement for cleavage.[93,209] The E3 protein can be retained on the virion postrelease depending upon the pH of the media.[245]

Virion Budding

The final stage of the virus life cycle is the effective interaction between the capsid protein and the glycoproteins to promote virus budding. Thin-section electron microscopy of infected cells has shown a clustering of nucleocapsid cores at the plasma membrane at sites of budding, but it is likely that the interaction occurs earlier, perhaps in the vicinity of CPV2.[251] All evidence suggests that a proper interaction between the cores and glycoprotein spikes is required for budding.[106,164] When the glycoproteins have been expressed in the absence of the capsid protein, virus-like particles have not been observed. In SFV, virions have been shown to bud from specific sites in polarized cells,[219] and virus has been reported to bud intracellularly in insect cells.[173] There also appears to be a requirement for cholesterol in the membrane to support budding,[156,161] and host cell lipid metabolism has also been implicated.[184] Several systems have been reported that show the exogenously produced capsid cores can be introduced into naïve cells expressing the viral glycoproteins and particles can be released, suggesting that RNA synthesis is not required for budding.[248]

The interaction between the capsid protein and the envelope glycoproteins has been extensively investigated with most of the available data coming from molecular genetic and structural studies.[262] X-ray crystallography of the capsid protein identified a hydrophobic pocket that was occupied by the amino terminal arm of a neighboring capsid protein. The nature of the arm residues bound in the hydrophobic pocket suggested that a tyr-ala-leu motif found in the cytoplasmic domain of the E2 glycoprotein might function in a similar manner and bind into the capsid protein pocket.[132,246] Residues of the E2 cytoplasmic domain were shown to be important for the interaction with the tyrosine found in the hydrophobic pocket of the capsid protein, which is conserved in the alphaviruses.[105,192,261,262,310] E2 peptides have also been used to inhibit budding, suggesting residues involved in process and similar peptides were shown to bind to capsids.[168] In addition, cryo-EM studies have shown that the cytoplasmic domain of E2 clearly extends down into the core to the site of the hydrophobic pocket.[27,262] As was mentioned previously, deletions that disrupt the accumulation of nucleocapsid cores do not prevent budding because lateral interaction between the glycoproteins appear to be the driving force as long as capsid interactions do occur.[27]

The 6K protein, which has been estimated at 5 to 10 molecules per virion, has been implicated in the budding process and in the formation of virions.[63,64] Removal of 6K from the genome of SFV did not influence the formation of the E1–E2 heterodimer or its transport to the cell surface, but it did reduce budding.[63,64] Other studies have shown that mutations in 6K can influence glycoprotein trafficking and virion assembly.[231] E2 and 6K appear to interact as mutations in 6K can be suppressed by mutations in E2, and chimeric viruses containing a SINV glycoprotein and a RRV 6K are highly defective for virus formation.[303] Recently, it has been shown that a frame shift occurs at a low frequency during translation of the region encoding 6K resulting in the production of the TF protein shown in Figure 5.15. The TF protein shares 47 amino acids with 6K and contains the transmembrane domain that has been implicated in channel formation. The remaining 23 residues are unique to TF, and end in a termination codon with no E1 is produced from this polyprotein. Preliminary data suggest that TF also has a role in virus replication and is incorporated into the virion, but whether its function(s) overlaps with 6K is not yet known.

Effects on the Host Cell

Alphaviruses have a wide host range and must interact with a variety of cellular receptors, either ubiquitous or unrelated molecules. Because the nature of these receptors is largely unknown, equally unknown is the signaling that such molecules might

engage in following virion attachment and early steps in entry. Clearly, the response of most vertebrate cells to viral infection is distinct from the response of invertebrate cells. However, in both cases, there appears to be a balance between the needs of the virus to effectively propagate and the needs of the host to control virus infection and dissemination. Host macromolecular synthesis is inhibited in vertebrate cells shortly after infection. Host protein synthesis is shut off at 3 hours after infection, although virus protein translation continues unabated. This has been an intensive area of investigation, and four mechanisms for shutoff have been proposed: (a) an altered intracellular environment such as K+ concentration that would favor viral translation, (b) direct competition for translational machinery, (c) inhibition of cellular translation by the capsid protein, and (d) inhibition of translation by one of the nonstructural proteins. The development and use of replicon systems that contain only the cis-acting replication signals and the coding region for

A

SINV	CUGCCUGCC<u>UUUUUUA</u>GUGGUUGCC	(10022)
WEEV	CUGCAUGCCUUUUUUAUUGGUUGCA	(9821)
EEEV	UGGGCCGGCUUUUUUACUUGUCUGC	(9955)
CHIKV	AACGUUGGCUUUUUUAGCCGUAAUG	(9951)
RRV	GCCAUUUUCUUUUUUAGUGUUACUG	(9973)
SFV	GAGCCUUUCUUUUUUAGUGCUACUG	(9825)

B

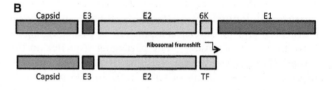

C

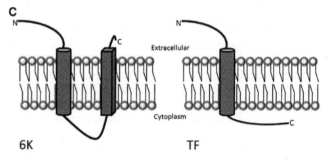

6K   TF

FIGURE 5.15 Ribosomal frame shifting during translation of the 26S subgenomic RNA yields a newly described protein, TF. A: Sequence alignment of various alphaviruses demonstrates the conservation of a putative slippery site motif within the 6K gene (underlined for SINV). The coordinate of the first nucleotide of the slippery site is indicated in parentheses for each virus. **B:** The typical protein products obtained from normal translation of the 26S subgenomic RNA (*top*) and the protein products obtained in the case of a frame shift event (*bottom*). Note that the amino terminal region of the 6K and TF proteins shares the same sequence. **C:** A model of the putative membrane topology of the mature 6K and TF proteins. The N- and C-termini are denoted. 6K (*left*) contains both a transmembrane anchor (*cylindrical*) and a membrane spanning region that acts as the signal sequence for E1 (*rectangular*). TF contains only the transmembrane anchor (*cylindrical*); the frameshift event prevents production of the E1 signal sequence. (This figure was kindly provided courtesy of Jonathan Snyder.)

replication proteins suggested that the structural proteins were not responsible for translational shutoff.[58] Furthermore, studies investigating the establishment of persistence identified changes in SINV nsP2, at Pro726 to serine, which reduced cytopathic effects of the virus.[54] A variety of studies suggest that alphavirus infection promotes the double-stranded RNA-activated protein kinase (PKR)–dependent and PKR-independent pathways to reduce host cell translation.[229] Mutations in nsP2 suggest that the shutoff of host cell transcription and translation are distinct events and strongly influence the decreased production of a α/β interferon.[78] However, the role of nsP2 in host cell shutoff appears to function only in the Old World alphaviruses. It has been shown that in VEEV and other New World alphaviruses that a region of the capsid protein encompassing residues 33 to 68 and not nsP2 is responsible for transcriptional shutoff and cytopathogenicity.[66] This region of the VEEV capsid protein has also been shown to be responsible for nuclear trafficking of the protein to the nucleus.[12,13,113]

Most infections by alphaviruses of vertebrate cells in culture lead to the induction of apoptosis.[139] Apoptosis of infected neurons is a major determinant of neurovirulence, as demonstrated for SINV.[138] In contrast, mosquito cells can undergo a variety of effects from persistent infections to cell death caused by necrosis.[108] It has also been possible to establish persistent infection of vertebrate cells using DI particles, followed by genetic changes to the helper virus in nsP2.[39] An alternative method was used by selecting for replicons that were noncytopathic to BHK cells, and again, amino acid substitutions were detected in the coding region for nsP2,[54] suggesting a major role for this protein in modulating the virus–host interaction.

A number of antiviral proteins produced in infected cells have been described for the alphaviruses. A small hydrophobic peptide of 3,200 Da was shown to be produced in persistently infected mosquito cells, and this peptide could activate an antiviral state. This peptide induced the synthesis of a 55-kDa protein and inhibited the replication of alphavirus RNA. The rat zinc-finger antiviral protein (ZAP), originally identified as a retrovirus resistance protein, was shown to inhibit multiple alphaviruses.[17] This protein inhibited viral translation by binding to viral mRNA, although its exact mechanism of action is not known.[80] It is likely that many additional proteins, such as interferon-stimulated genes, will demonstrate direct antiviral activity and might be exploited to control alphavirus infection.

Defective Interfering Genomes and Replicon Systems

Defective interfering genomes replicate and are packaged in the presence of helper virus and retain all cis-acting sequences necessary for RNA replication. Several alphavirus DI genomes have been molecularly characterized, and all retain the 3′ CSE that was previously described. The 5′ end of the DI genomes was found to be more heterogenous, with the 5′ CSE, cellular tRNA sequences, or the 5′ 142 nucleotides from the subgenomic mRNA located at the 5′ end of the DI RNA. The study of DI genomes provided a powerful genetic tool to identify the location and function of required cis-acting sequence elements.[141] The development of DI genomes for genetic purposes gave way to the construction of replicons, which supported RNA replication but were incapable of infection of new cells because they lacked the structural proteins.[140,302] The structural proteins could be supplied by additional helper RNAs so that the replicons could be packaged and used to efficiently infect target cells.[20]

The alphavirus replicon has become a standard gene expression system. The system has proven useful for examining protein expression in heterogenous systems and the development of vaccines.[235] SINV, SFV, and VEEV replicons have been widely used and can allow for targeting to specific cells.[147] By introducing a mutation in nsP2 that renders the replicon noncytopathic, continuous replication in the absence of cell death can occur for SINV. For VEEV, mutations in the 5′ NTR and nsP3 were also required for persistent infection by the replicon.[204] Multiple subgenomic promoters can be employed for the expression of several proteins of interest in a regulated fashion. To further reduce the chance of recombination between replicon and helper RNAs to generate an infectious genome, tricomponent replicon systems have been developed that can produce at least 1,000 packaged replicons per cell.[44]

RUBIVIRUS REPLICATION

Virion Structure and Entry

Although once considered a close cousin of the alphaviruses, molecular analyses of rubella virus have revealed significant differences.[52] Whereas rubella virions are similar to alphaviruses in protein composition and morphology, the particles have yet to yield to high-resolution structural analysis, and it is unlikely that the particles share the property of icosahedral symmetry with the alphaviruses. The rubella virion is composed of three structural proteins that share the same name as alphaviruses yet differ in amino acid sequence.[38] The virions are pleomorphic in shape and are around 60 to 70 nm in diameter.[16,159] The two type I envelope glycoproteins, E1 and E2, form heterodimers and have 13 and 7 amino acids on their inner cytoplasmic face. All three structural proteins are membrane associated with the C-terminus of the capsid containing the signal sequence for E2.[188–190] The structural proteins are cleaved by signal peptidase, with the signal sequence for E1 present at the C-terminus of E2.[100,101] The capsid protein is a phosphoprotein of 293 or 300 amino acids, depending on which AUG codon is used to initiate the polyprotein.[53]

Rubella virus is restricted to growth in humans and is not transmitted by insects, as are the alphaviruses. However, the virus can replicate in a wide range of mammalian cell types and can infect experimental animals producing subclinical results. Thus, like alphaviruses, a ubiquitous cellular receptor may function in entry, although none has yet been identified. The virus also appears to enter through a receptor-mediated endocytosis pathway with membrane fusion promoted by an acidified endosome,[109] and a class II fusion mechanism is expected.

Transcription, Translation, and Genome Replication

The placement of rubella virus in the family *Togaviridae* implies a common genome structure and replication strategy. Complete nucleotide sequences are available for several strains of rubella virus.[52,210] The 9,762 nucleotide genome RNA contains a 5′ terminal 7-methylguanosine and a 3′ terminus that is polyadenylated.[190,284] The genomes of rubiviruses and alphaviruses are compared in Figure 5.6. The replication proteins P150 and P90 are encoded by the genome RNA, whereas the structural proteins are derived from the subgenomic mRNA. Although there is no amino acid sequence homology among the structural proteins, limited homologies do exist within the replication proteins. The construction of a rubella virus cDNA clone from which infectious RNA could be generated permitted molecular genetic studies on the virus that were, up until then, quite limited.[211,284]

Three species of RNA are synthesized in infected cells: complementary minus-strand RNA, genome RNA, and subgenomic mRNA. On infection, the genome RNA is translated into a 200-kDa polyprotein that is cleaved by a virus-encoded protease.[49] Unlike its alphavirus counterpart, the rubella enzyme is a metalloprotease that contains zinc-binding domains, and it cleaves P200 *in trans*. Virus replication complexes can be found in association with cellular membranes. Virus-specific vacuoles have been identified and colocalize with lysosomal markers, similar to those found for alphaviruses.[124] There is a close association between these replication complexes, identified with antibodies to P150, and ER and Golgi membranes, presumably to facilitate translation and packaging of genome RNAs.[218]

Attempts to identify cellular proteins that might participate in RNA replication have focused on proteins that bind to the 5′ and 3′ NTRs. A 5′ stem-loop structure predicted to form on the plus-strand RNA was shown to bind to the La autoantigen. Several cellular proteins were shown to bind to the 3′ NTR.[180,181] One of these proteins was identified as calreticulin, although decreased binding of calreticulin did not correlate with reduced virus replication.[242] The nonstructural protein P90 has been shown to bind to the retinoblastoma protein Rb through an Rb-binding motif.[14] Mutation of this motif reduces virus replication, but it is unclear whether the defect is related to a reduction in binding.[48]

The capsid protein has also been implicated in RNA replication. It has been shown to complement a replication defect resulting from a deletion of 169 amino acids from P150.[268] Exactly how this might function is not known, but the amino terminal 88 residues of the capsid were sufficient for complementation, and these might function by binding to RNA. In addition, the capsid protein has been shown to influence the replication of rubella replicons,[26] although once again the mechanism is not known. The capsid protein has also been shown to bind to mitochondrial matrix protein p32 and the proapoptotic protein Bax.[103] The function of capsid in binding these proteins is to prevent apoptosis and enhance RNA replication.

Virus Assembly

A packaging signal has been located between nucleotides 347 and 375 of the genome RNA, and it interacts with capsid residues 28 to 56. Phosphorylation of the capsid protein occurs and has been suggested to act as a regulatory mechanism to prevent binding of nonviral RNAs to the capsid.[151] With the retention of the capsid protein signal sequence at its C-terminus, the capsid remains associated with the ER membrane. This association may be important for ensuring close connectivity with the envelope glycoproteins through their transmembrane domains. Glycoproteins E1 and E2 are believed to have functions similar to their alphavirus counterparts, although rubella virions bud into the Golgi.[102] Indeed the crystal structure of rubella E1 protein revealed it to be a class II fusion protein with a metal binding site not seen in the alphavirus or flavivirus fusion proteins.[40]

Virions undergo a maturation step after Golgi budding that may release the capsid signal sequence because morphological changes occur in the core of the virion.[218] The structure of the mature rubella virions using electron tomography revealed a helical particle that lacks the icosahedral symmetry present in the alphaviruses.[160]

PERSPECTIVES

Our knowledge of togaviruses has grown dramatically thanks in large part to the ability to genetically manipulate these relatively "simple" plus-strand RNA viruses. Insights into alphaviruses have been obtained more quickly than for rubella virus due to their greater replication efficiency in cultured cells and their well-organized virions. Structural studies of the alphaviruses have progressed rapidly leveraging the icosahedral nature of the virus particles and the ability to obtain large quantities of homogeneous preparations. The ability to express capsid proteins in heterologous systems has facilitated both structural and biochemical studies of capsid structure and its assembly pathway. The structure determinations of the native and postfusion forms of the E1 protein have provided exceptional insights into the entry process and the structure of the virion. The atomic structure of the E1 and E2 heterodimer in both a low pH and neutral form has provided insight into the sequential entry process employed by these viruses. Structures of the replication proteins are coming slowly but beginning to provide greater insight into the replication process.

Significant gaps still persist in understanding the replication process of the togaviruses. The ability to reconstitute purified and functional replication complexes will be an important milestone to decipher RNA replication. In contrast, significant progress has been made in understanding the cellular response to viral infection and the recruitment of cellular proteins to promote or inhibit the virus replication complex. Systems-level studies to evaluate the total cellular environment altered in virus infection are beginning to yield a comprehensive picture of how the virus perturbs and subjugates the cell. The use of advanced and real-time optical imaging as well as electron tomography promises to provide a temporal and spatial view of virus infection. However, most studies continue to rely on standard cell culture systems, and it will be important to verify what occurs in more natural target cells such as neurons.

With the growing knowledge of togaviruses, their utility in gene expression and gene therapy continues to be exploited and expanded. Future directions that will further benefit this system will be in understanding the nature of the cellular receptors and the structure of the E2 protein that is involved in binding these receptors. With this knowledge, newly designed alphavirus vectors will be engineered to specifically and efficiently target the replicon to cells and tissues of interest.

REFERENCES

1. Abell BA, Brown DT. Sindbis virus membrane fusion is mediated by reduction of glycoprotein disulfide bridges at the cell surface. *J Virol* 1993;67(9):5496–5501.
2. Abraham R, Hauer D, McPherson RL, et al. ADP-ribosyl-binding and hydrolase activities of the alphavirus nsP3 macrodomain are critical for initiation of virus replication. *Proc Natl Acad Sci U S A* 2018;115(44):E10457–E10466.
3. Ahlquist P, Strauss EG, Rice CM, et al. Sindbis virus proteins nsP1 and nsP2 contain homology to nonstructural proteins from several RNA plant viruses. *J Virol* 1985;53:536–542.
4. Ahn A, Klimjack MR, Chatterjee PK, et al. An epitope of the Semliki Forest virus fusion protein exposed during virus-membrane fusion. *J Virol* 1999;73(12):10029–10039.

5. Ahn A, Schoepp RJ, Sternberg D, et al. Growth and stability of a cholesterol-independent Semliki Forest virus mutant in mosquitoes. *Virology* 1999;262(2):452–456.

6. Ahola T, Kaariainen L. Reaction in alphavirus mRNA capping: formation of a covalent complex of nonstructural protein nsP1 with 7-methyl-GMP. *Proc Natl Acad Sci* 1995;92(2):507–511.

7. Ahola T, Kujala P, Tuittila M, et al. Effects of palmitoylation of replicase protein nsP1 on alphavirus infection. *J Virol* 2000;74:6725–6733.

8. Ahola T, Laakkonen P, Vihinen H, et al. Critical residues of Semliki Forest virus RNA capping enzyme involved in methyltransferase and guanylyltransferase-like activities. *J Virol* 1997;71(1):392–397.

9. Ahola T, Lampio A, Auvinen P, et al. Semliki Forest virus mRNA capping enzyme requires association with anionic membrane phospholipids for activity. *EMBO J* 1999;18(11):3164–3172.

10. Aliperti G, Schlesinger MJ. Evidence for an autoprotease activity of Sindbis virus capsid protein. *Virology* 1978;90:366–369.

11. Anthony RP, Pardes AM, Brown DT. Disulfide bonds are essential for the stability of the Sindbis virus envelope. *Virology* 1993;190:330–336.

12. Atasheva S, Fish A, Fornerod M, et al. Venezuelan equine Encephalitis virus capsid protein forms a tetrameric complex with CRM1 and importin alpha/beta that obstructs nuclear pore complex function. *J Virol* 2010;84(9):4158–4171.

13. Atasheva S, Garmashova N, Frolov I, et al. Venezuelan equine encephalitis virus capsid protein inhibits nuclear import in Mammalian but not in mosquito cells. *J Virol* 2008;82(8):4028–4041.

14. Atreya CD, Lee NS, Forng RY, et al. The rubella virus putative replicase interacts with the retinoblastoma tumor suppressor protein. *Virus Genes* 1998;16(2):177–183.

15. Barton DJ, Sawicki SG, Sawicki DL. Demonstration *in vitro* of temperature-sensitive elongation of RNA in Sindbis virus mutant *ts6*. *J Virol* 1988;62:3597–3602.

16. Battisti AJ, Yoder JD, Plevka P, et al. Cryo-electron tomography of rubella virus. *J Virol* 2012;86:11078–11085.

17. Bick MJ, Carroll JW, Gao G, et al. Expression of the zinc-finger antiviral protein inhibits alphavirus replication. *J Virol* 2003;77(21):11555–11562.

18. Bonatti S, Migliaccio G, Simons K. Palmitoylation of viral membrane glycoproteins takes place after exit from the endoplasmic reticulum. *J Biol Chem* 1989;264(21):12590–12595.

19. Brault AC, Powers AM, Holmes EC, et al. Positively charged amino acid substitutions in the E2 envelope glycoprotein are associated with the emergence of Venezuelan equine encephalitis virus. *J Virol* 2002;76(4):1718–1730.

20. Bredenbeek PJ, Frolov I, Rice CM, et al. Sindbis virus expression vectors: packaging of RNA replicons by using defective helper RNAs. *J Virol* 1993;67(11):6439–6446.

21. Byrnes AP, Griffin DE. Binding of Sindbis virus to cell surface heparan sulfate. *J Virol* 1998;72(9):7349–7356.

22. Byrnes AP, Griffin DE. Large-plaque mutants of Sindbis virus show reduced binding to heparan sulfate, heightened viremia, and slower clearance from the circulation. *J Virol* 2000;74(2):644–651.

23. Carleton M, Brown DT. Disulfide bridge-mediated folding of Sindbis virus glycoproteins. *J Virol* 1996;70(8):5541–5547.

24. Chanel-Vos C, Kielian M. A conserved histidine in the ij loop of the Semliki Forest virus E1 protein plays an important role in membrane fusion. *J Virol* 2004;78(24):13543–13552.

25. Chatterjee PK, Vashishtha M, Kielian M. Biochemical consequences of a mutation that controls the cholesterol dependence of Semliki Forest virus fusion. *J Virol* 2000;74(4):1623–1631.

26. Chen MH, Icenogle JP. Rubella virus capsid protein modulates viral genome replication and virus infectivity. *J Virol* 2004;78:4314–4322.

27. Chen L, Wang M, Zhu D, et al. Implication for alphavirus host-cell entry and assembly indicated by a 3.5Å resolution cryo-EM structure. *Nat Commun* 2018;9(1):5326.

28. Cheng RH, Kuhn RJ, Olson NH, et al. Nucleocapsid and glycoprotein organization in an enveloped virus. *Cell* 1995;80(4):621–630.

29. Choi HK, Lu G, Lee S, et al. Structure of Semliki Forest virus core protein. *Proteins* 1997;27:345–359.

30. Choi HK, Tong L, Minor W, et al. Structure of Sindbis virus core protein reveals a chymotrypsin-like serine proteinase and the organization of the virion. *Nature* 1991;354:37–43.

31. Corver J, Moesby L, Erukulla RK, et al. Sphingolipid-dependent fusion of Semliki Forest virus with cholesterol-containing liposomes requires both the 3-hydroxyl group and the double bond of the sphingolipid backbone. *J Virol* 1995;69(5):3220–3223.

32. Cristea IM, Carroll JW, Rout MP, et al. Tracking and elucidating alphavirus-host protein interactions. *J Biol Chem* 2006;281(40):30269–30278.

33. de Curtis I, Simons K. Dissection of Semliki Forest virus glycoprotein delivery from the trans-Golgi network to the cell surface in permeabilized BHK cells. *Proc Natl Acad Sci U S A* 1988;85(21):8052–8056.

34. de Groot RJ, Hardy RH, Shirako Y, et al. Cleavage-site preferences of Sindbis virus polyproteins containing the nonstructural proteinase: evidence for temporal regulation of polyprotein processing in vivo. *EMBO J* 1990;9:2631–2638.

35. de Groot RJ, Rümenapf T, Kuhn RJ, et al. Sindbis virus RNA polymerase is degraded by the N-end rule pathway. *Proc Natl Acad Sci U S A* 1991;88:8967–8971.

36. DeTulleo L, Kirchhausen T. The clathrin endocytic pathway in viral infection. *EMBO J* 1998;17(16):4585–4593.

37. Ding M, Schlesinger MJ. Evidence that Sindbis virus nsP2 is an autoprotease which processes the virus nonstructural polyprotein. *Virology* 1989;171:280–284.

38. Dominguez G, Wang C-Y, Frey TK. Sequence of the genome RNA of rubella virus: Evidence for genetic rearrangement during togavirus evolution. *Virology* 1990;177:225–238.

39. Dryga SA, Dryga OA, Schlesinger S. Identification of mutations in a Sindbis virus variant able to establish persistent infection in BHK cells: the importance of a mutation in the nsP2 gene. *Virology* 1997;228:74–83.

40. DuBois RM, Vaney MC, Tortorici MA, et al. Functional and evolutionary insight from the crystal structure of rubella virus protein E1. *Nature* 2013;493(7433):552–556.

41. Edwards J, Brown DT. Sindbis virus infection of a Chinese hamster ovary cell mutant defective in the acidification of endosomes. *Virology* 1991;182:28–33.

42. Fata CL, Sawicki G, Sawicki DL. Modification of Asn374 of nsP1 suppresses a Sindbis virus nsP4 minus-strand polymerase mutant. *J Virol* 2002;76:8641–8649.

43. Fayzulin R, Frolov I. Changes of the secondary structure of the 5′ end of the sindbis virus genome inhibit virus growth in mosquito cells and lead to accumulation of adaptive mutations. *J Virol* 2004;78:4953–4964.

44. Fayzulin R, Gorchakov R, Petrakova O, et al. Sindbis virus with a tricomponent genome. *J Virol* 2005;79(1):637–643.

45. Ferlenghi I, Gowen B, de Haas F, et al. The first step: activation of the Semliki Forest virus spike protein precursor causes a localized conformational change in the trimeric spike. *J Mol Biol* 1998;283:71–81.

46. Firth AE, Chung BY, Fleeton MN, et al. Discovery of frameshifting in Alphavirus 6K resolves a 20-year enigma. *Virol J* 2008;5:108.

47. Flynn DC, Meyer WJ, MacKenzie JM, et al. A conformational change in Sindbis glycoprotein E1 and E2 is detected at the plasma membrane as a consequence of early virus-cell interaction. *J Virol* 1990;64:3643–3653.

48. Forng RY, Atreya CD. Mutations in the retinoblastoma protein-binding LXCXE motif of rubella virus putative replicase affect virus replication. *J Gen Virol* 1999;80(Pt 2):327–332.

49. Forng RY, Frey TK. Identification of the rubella virus nonstructural proteins. *Virology* 1995;206(2):843–853.

50. Forrester NL, Palacios G, Tesh RB, et al. Genome-scale phylogeny of the alphavirus genus suggests a marine origin. *J Virol* 2012;86(5):2729–2738.

51. Forsell K, Xing L, Kozlovska T, et al. Membrane proteins organize a symmetrical virus. *EMBO J* 2000;19:5081–5091.

52. Frey TK. Molecular biology of rubella virus. *Adv Virus Res* 1994;44:69–160.

53. Frey TK, Marr LD. Sequence of the region coding for virion proteins C and E2 and the carboxy terminus of the nonstructural proteins of rubella virus: comparison with alphaviruses. *Gene* 1988;62(1):85–99.

54. Frolov I, Agapov E, Hoffman TA Jr, et al. Selection of RNA replicons capable of persistent noncytopathic replication in mammalian cells. *J Virol* 1999;73(5):3854–3865.

55. Frolov I, Akhrymuk M, Akhrymuk I, et al. Early events in alphavirus replication determine the outcome of infection. *J Virol* 2012;86(9):5055–5066.

56. Frolov I, Hardy R, Rice CM. Cis-acting RNA elements at the 5′ end of Sindbis virus genome RNA regulate minus- and plus-strand RNA synthesis. *RNA* 2001;7(11):1638–1651.

57. Frolov I, Hoffman TA, Pragai BM, et al. Alphavirus-based expression vectors: strategies and applications. *Proc Natl Acad Sci U S A* 1996;93(21):11371–11377.

58. Frolov I, Schlesinger S. Comparison of the effects of Sindbis virus and Sindbis virus replicons on host cell protein synthesis and cytopathogenicity in BHK cells. *J Virol* 1994;68(3):1721–1727.

59. Frolov I, Schlesinger S. Translation of Sindbis virus mRNA: analysis of sequences downstream of the initiating AUG codon that enhance translation. *J Virol* 1996;70:1182–1190.

60. Frolova EI, Gorchakov R, Pereboeva L, et al. Functional Sindbis virus replicative complexes are formed at the plasma membrane. *J Virol* 2010;84(22):11679–11695.

61. Froshauer S, Kartenbeck J, Helenius A. Alphavirus RNA replicase is located on the cytoplasmic surface of endosomes and lysosomes. *J Cell Biol* 1988;107(6):2075–2086.

62. Fuller SD, Berriman JA, Butcher SJ, et al. Low pH induces swiveling of the glycoprotein heterodimers in the Semliki Forest virus spike complex. *Cell* 1995;81(5):715–725.

63. Gaedigk-Nitschko K, Ding M, Schlesinger MJ. Site-directed mutations in the Sindbis virus 6K protein reveal sites for fatty acylation and the underacylated protein affects virus release and virion structure. *Virology* 1990;175:282–291.

64. Gaedigk-Nitschko K, Schlesinger MJ. The Sindbis virus 6K protein can be detected in virions and is acylated with fatty acids. *Virology* 1990;175(1):274–281.

65. Gardner CL, Ebel GD, Ryman KD, et al. Heparan sulfate binding by natural eastern equine encephalitis viruses promotes neurovirulence. *Proc Natl Acad Sci U S A* 2011;108(38):16026–16031.

66. Garmashova N, Atasheva S, Kang W, et al. Analysis of Venezuelan equine encephalitis virus capsid protein function in the inhibition of cellular transcription. *J Virol* 2007;81(24):13552–13565.

67. Garoff H, Huylebroeck D, Robinson A, et al. The signal sequence of the p62 protein of Semliki Forest virus is involved in initiation but not in completing chain translocation. *J Cell Biol* 1990;111(3):867–876.

68. Garoff H, Kondor-Koch C, Petterson R, et al. Expression of Semliki Forest virus proteins from cloned complementary DNA. II. The membrane-spanning glycoprotein E2 is transported to the cell surface without its normal cytoplasmic domain. *J Cell Biol* 1983;97:652.

69. Geigenmüller-Gnirke U, Nitschko H, Schlesinger S. Deletion analysis of the capsid protein of Sindbis virus: Identification of the RNA binding region. *J Virol* 1993;67:1620–1626.

70. George J, Raju R. Alphavirus RNA genome repair and evolution: molecular characterization of infectious Sindbis virus isolates lacking a known conserved motif at the 3′ end of the genome. *J Virol* 2000;74:9776–9785.

71. Gibbons DL, Ahn A, Chatterjee PK, et al. Formation and characterization of the trimeric form of the fusion protein of Semliki Forest virus. *J Virol* 2000;74(17):7772–7719.

72. Gibbons DL, Erk I, Reilly B, et al. Visualization of the target-membrane-inserted fusion protein of Semliki Forest virus by combined electron microscopy and crystallography. *Cell* 2003;114:573–583.

73. Gibbons DL, Reilly B, Ahn A, et al. Purification and crystallization reveal two types of interactions of the fusion protein homotrimer of Semliki Forest virus. *J Virol* 2004;78(7):3514–3523.

74. Gibbons DL, Vaney M-C, Roussel A, et al. Conformational change and protein-protein interactions of the fusion protein of Semliki Forest virus. *Nature* 2004;427:322–325.

75. Glomb-Reinmund S, Kielian M. The role of low pH and disulfide shuffling in the entry and fusion of Semliki Forest virus and Sindbis virus. *Virology* 1998;248(2):372–381.

76. Gomez de Cedron M, Ehsani N, Mikkola ML, et al. RNA helicase activity of Semliki Forest virus replicase protein NSP2. *FEBS Lett* 1999;448(1):19–22.

77. Gorbalenya AE, Koonin EV, Donchenko AP, et al. A novel superfamily of nucleoside triphosphate-binding motif containing proteins which are probably involved in duplex unwinding in DNA and RNA replication and recombination. *FEBS Lett* 1988;235:16–24.

78. Gorchakov R, Frolova E, Frolov I. Inhibition of transcription and translation in Sindbis virus-infected cells. *J Virol* 2005;79:9397–9409.
79. Gorchakov R, Frolova E, Sawicki S, et al. A new role for ns polyprotein cleavage in Sindbis virus replication. *J Virol* 2008;82(13):6218–6231.
80. Guo X, Carroll JW, Macdonald MR, et al. The zinc finger antiviral protein directly binds to specific viral mRNAs through the CCCH zinc finger motifs. *J Virol* 2004;78(23):12781–12787.
81. Haag L, Garoff H, Xing L, et al. Acid-induced movements in the glycoprotein shell of an alphavirus turn the spikes into membrane fusion mode. *EMBO J* 2002;21(17):4402–4410.
82. Hahn YS, Grakoui A, Rice CM, et al. Mapping of RNA- temperature-sensitive mutants of Sindbis virus: complementation group F mutants have lesions in nsP4. *J Virol* 1989;63:1194–1202.
83. Hahn CS, Strauss JH. Site-directed mutagenesis of the proposed catalytic amino acids of the Sindbis virus capsid protein autoprotease. *J Virol* 1990;64:3069–3073.
84. Hahn CS, Strauss EG, Strauss JH. Sequence analysis of three Sindbis virus mutants temperature-sensitive in the capsid autoprotease. *Proc Natl Acad Sci U S A* 1985;82:4648–4652.
85. Hammar L, Markarian S, Haag L, et al. Prefusion rearrangements resulting in fusion Peptide exposure in Semliki Forest virus. *J Biol Chem* 2003;278(9):7189–7198.
86. Hardy RW. The role of the 3′ terminus of the sindbis virus genome in minus-strand initiation site selection. *Virology* 2006;345:520–531.
87. Hardy WR, Strauss JH. Processing of the nonstructural polyproteins of Sindbis virus: study of the kinetics in vivo using monospecific antibodies. *J Virol* 1988;62:998–1007.
88. Hardy WR, Strauss JH. Processing the nonstructural proteins of Sindbis virus: nonstructural proteinase is in the C-terminal half of nsP2 and functions both in *cis* and *trans*. *J Virol* 1989;63:4653–4664.
89. Harrison SC, David A, Jumblatt J, et al. Lipid and protein organization in Sindbis virus. *J Mol Biol* 1971;60:532.
90. Harrison SC, Strong RK, Schlesinger S, et al. Crystallization of Sindbis virus and its nucleocapsid. *J Mol Biol* 1992;226:277–280.
91. Hasan SS, Sun C, Kim AS, et al. Cryo-EM structures of eastern equine encephalitis virus reveal mechanisms of virus disassembly and antibody neutralization. *Cell Rep* 2018;25(11):3136.e5–3147.e5.
92. Heidner HW, Knott TA, Johnston RE. Differential processing of sindbis virus glycoprotein PE2 in cultured vertebrate and arthropod cells. *J Virol* 1996;70(3):2069–2073.
93. Heidner HW, McKnight KL, Davis NL, et al. Lethality of PE2 incorporation into Sindbis virus can be suppressed by second-site mutations in E3 and E2. *J Virol* 1994;68(4):2683–2692.
94. Heil ML, Albee A, Strauss JH, et al. An amino acid substitution in the coding region of the E2 glycoprotein adapts Ross River Virus to utilize heparan sulfate as an attachment moiety. *J Virol* 2001;7:6303–6309.
95. Helenius A, Kartenbeck J, Simons K, et al. On the entry of Semliki Forest virus into BHK-21 cells. *J Cell Biol* 1980;84:404–420.
96. Helenius A, Marsh M, White J. Inhibition of Semliki Forest virus penetration by lysosomotropic weak bases. *J Gen Virol* 1982;58:47–61.
97. Hernandez R, Luo TC, Brown DT. Exposure to low pH is not required for penetration of mosquito cells by Sindbis virus. *J Virol* 2001;75(4):2010–2013.
98. Hertz JM, Huang HV. Host-dependent evolution of the Sindbis virus promoter for subgenomic mRNA synthesis. *J Virol* 1995;69(12):7775–7781.
99. Hertz JM, Huang HV. Evolution of the Sindbis virus subgenomic mRNA promoter in cultured cells. *J Virol* 1995;69(12):7768–7774.
100. Hobman TC, Gillam S. *In vitro* and *in vivo* expression of rubella virus glycoprotein E2: the signal peptide is contained in the C-terminal region of capsid protein. *Virology* 1989;173:241–250.
101. Hobman TC, Lundstrom ML, Mauracher CA, et al. Assembly of rubella virus structural proteins into virus-like particles in transfected cells. *Virology* 1994;202(2):574–585.
102. Hobman TC, Woodward L, Farquhar MG. Targeting of a heterodimeric membrane protein complex to the Golgi: rubella virus E2 glycoprotein contains a transmembrane Golgi retention signal. *Mol Biol Cell* 1995;6(1):7–20.
103. Ilkow CS, Goping IS, Hobman TC. The rubella virus capsid is an anti-apoptotic protein that attenuates the pore-forming ability of Bax. *PLoS Pathog* 2011;7:e1001291.
104. Jan JT, Byrnes AP, Griffin DE. Characterization of a Chinese hamster ovary cell line developed by retroviral insertional mutagenesis that is resistant to Sindbis virus infection. *J Virol* 1999;73(6):4919–4924.
105. Jose J, Przybyla L, Edwards TJ, et al. Interactions of the cytoplasmic domain of Sindbis virus E2 with nucleocapsid cores promote alphavirus budding. *J Virol* 2012;86(5):2585–2599.
106. Jose J, Taylor AB, Kuhn RJ. Spatial and temporal analysis of alphavirus replication and assembly in mammalian and mosquito cells. *MBio* 2017;8(1):2294–2316.
107. Kamer G, Argos P. Primary structural comparison of RNA-dependent polymerases from plant, animal and bacterial viruses. *Nucleic Acids Res* 1984;12:7269–7282.
108. Karpf AR, Blake JM, Brown DT. Characterization of the infection of Aedes albopictus cell clones by Sindbis virus. *Virus Res* 1997;50(1):1–13.
109. Katow S, Sugiura A. Low pH-induced conformational change of rubella virus envelope proteins. *J Gen Virol* 1988;69(Pt 11):2797–2807.
110. Kielian M, Chatterjee PK, Gibbons DL, et al. Specific roles for lipids in virus fusion and exit. Examples from the alphaviruses. *Subcell Biochem* 2000;34:409–455.
111. Kielian MC, Helenius A. Role of cholesterol in fusion of Semliki Forest virus with membranes. *J Virol* 1984;52:281–283.
112. Kielian M, Rey FA. Virus membrane-fusion proteins: more than one way to make a hairpin. *Nat Rev Microbiol* 2006;4:67–76.
113. Kim DY, Atasheva S, Frolova EI, et al. Venezuelan equine encephalitis virus nsP2 protein regulates packaging of the viral genome into infectious virions. *J Virol* 2013;87(8):4202–4213.
114. Kim DY, Firth AE, Atasheva S, et al. Conservation of a packaging signal and the viral genome RNA packaging mechanism in alphavirus evolution. *J Virol* 2011;85(16):8022–8036.
115. Kim DY, Reynaud JM, Rasalouskaya A, et al. New world and old world alphaviruses have evolved to exploit different components of stress granules, FXR and G3BP proteins, for assembly of viral replication complexes. *PLoS Pathog* 2016;12(8):e1005810.
116. Klimstra WB, Nangle EM, Smith MS, et al. DC-SIGN and L-SIGN can act as attachment receptors for alphaviruses and distinguish between mosquito cell- and mammalian cell-derived viruses. *J Virol* 2003;77(22):12022–12032.
117. Klimstra WB, Ryman KD, Johnston RE. Adaptation of Sindbis virus to BHK cells selects for use of heparan sulfate as an attachment receptor. *J Virol* 1998;72(9):7357–7366.
118. Knipfer KW, Brown DT. Intracellular transport and processing of Sindbis virus glycoproteins. *Virology* 1989;170(1):117–122.
119. Koonin EV, Dolja VV. Evolution and taxonomy of positive-strand RNA viruses: implications of comparative analysis of amino acid sequences. *Crit Rev Biochem Mol Biol* 1993;28:375–430.
120. Kostyuchenko VA, Jakana J, Liu X, et al. The structure of Barmah Forest virus as revealed by cryo-electron microscopy at a 6-angstrom resolution has detailed transmembrane protein architecture and interactions. *J Virol* 2011;85(18):9327–9333.
121. Kuhn RJ, Dowd KA, Beth Post C, et al. Shake, rattle, and roll: impact of the dynamics of flavivirus particles on their interactions with the host. *Virology* 2015;479–480:508–517.
122. Kuhn RJ, Hong Z, Strauss JH. Mutagenesis of the 3′ nontranslated region of Sindbis virus RNA. *J Virol* 1990;64:1465–1476.
123. Kuhn RJ, Zhang W, Rossmann MG, et al. Structure of dengue virus: implications for flavivirus organization, maturation, and fusion. *Cell* 2002;108(5):717–725.
124. Kujala P, Ahola T, Ehsani N, et al. Intracellular distribution of rubella virus nonstructural protein P150. *J Virol* 1999;73(9):7805–7811.
125. Kujala P, Ikaheimonen A, Ehsani N, et al. Biogenesis of the Semliki Forest virus RNA replication complex. *J Virol* 2001;75(8):3873–3884.
126. Laakkonen P, Ahola T, Kaariainen L. The effects of palmitoylation on membrane association of Semliki forest virus RNA capping enzyme. *J Biol Chem* 1996;271(45):28567–28571.
127. Laakkonen P, Hyvonen M, Peranen J, et al. Expression of Semliki Forest virus nsP1-specific methyltransferase in insect cells and in Escherichia coli. *J Virol* 1994;68(11):7418–7425.
128. Lampio A, Kilpelainen I, Pesonen S, et al. Membrane binding mechanism of an RNA virus-capping enzyme. *J Biol Chem* 2000;275(48):37853–37859.
129. Lastarza MW, Grakoui A, Rice CM. Deletion and duplication mutations in the C-terminal nonconserved region of Sindbis virus nsP3: effects on phosphorylation and on virus replication in vertebrate and invertebrate cells. *Virology* 1994;202(1):224–232.
130. LaStarza MW, Lemm JA, Rice CM. Genetic analysis of the nsP3 region of Sindbis virus: evidence for roles in minus-strand and subgenomic RNA synthesis. *J Virol* 1994;68(9):5781–5791.
131. Law YS, Utt A, Tan YB, et al. Structural insights into RNA recognition by the Chikungunya virus nsP2 helicase. *Proc Natl Acad Sci U S A* 2019;116(19):9558–9567.
132. Lee S, Owen KE, Choi H-K, et al. Identification of a protein binding site on the surface of the alphavirus nucleocapsid and its implication in virus assembly. *Structure* 1996;4:531–541.
133. Lemm JA, Bergqvist A, Read CM, et al. Template-dependent initiation of Sindbis virus RNA replication in vitro. *J Virol* 1998;72(8):6546–6553.
134. Lemm JA, Rice CM. Roles of nonstructural polyproteins and cleavage products in regulating Sindbis virus RNA replication and transcription. *J Virol* 1993;67(4):1916–1926.
135. Lemm JA, Rice CM. Assembly of functional Sindbis virus RNA replication complexes: requirement for coexpression of P123 and P34. *J Virol* 1993;67(4):1905–1915.
136. Lemm JA, Rumenapf T, Strauss EG, et al. Polypeptide requirements for assembly of functional Sindbis virus replication complexes: a model for the temporal regulation of minus- and plus-strand RNA synthesis. *EMBO J* 1994;13(12):2925–2934.
137. Lescar J, Roussel A, Wein MW, et al. The fusion glycoprotein shell of Semliki Forest virus: an icosahedral assembly primed for fusogenic activation at endosomal pH. *Cell* 2001;105:137–148.
138. Levine B, Goldman JE, Jiang HH, et al. Bcl-2 protects mice against fatal alphavirus encephalitis. *Proc Natl Acad Sci U S A* 1996;93(10):4810–4815.
139. Levine B, Huang Q, Isaacs JT, et al. Conversion of lytic to persistent alphavirus infection by the bcl-2 cellular oncogene. *Nature* 1993;361(6414):739–742.
140. Levis R, Huang H, Schlesinger S. Engineered defective interfering RNAs of Sindbis virus express bacterial chloramphenicol acetyltransferase in avian cells. *Proc Natl Acad Sci U S A* 1987;84(14):4811–4815.
141. Levis R, Weiss BG, Tsiang M, et al. Deletion mapping of Sindbis virus DI RNAs derived from cDNAs defines the sequences essential for replication and packaging. *Cell* 1986;44:137–145.
142. Li L, Jose J, Xiang Y, et al. Structural changes of envelope proteins during alphavirus fusion. *Nature* 2010;468:705–708.
143. Li G, LaStarza MW, Hardy WR, et al. Phosphorylation of Sindbis virus nsP3 *in vivo* and *in vitro*. *Virology* 1990;179:416–427.
144. Li G, Rice CM. Mutagenesis of the in-frame opal termination codon preceding nsP4 of Sindbis virus: studies of translational readthrough and its effect on virus replication. *J Virol* 1989;63:1326–1337.
145. Liao M, Kielian M. Domain III from class II fusion proteins functions as a dominant-negative inhibitor of virus membrane fusion. *J Cell Biol* 2005;171(1):111–120.
146. Liljeström P, Garoff H. Internally located cleavable signal sequences direct the formation of Semliki Forest virus membrane proteins from a polyprotein precursor. *J Virol* 1991;65:147–154.
147. Liljeström P, Garoff H. A new generation of animal cell expression vectors based on the Semliki Forest virus replicon. *Biotechnology* 1991;9:1356–1361.
148. Linn ML, Gardner J, Warrilow D, et al. Arbovirus of marine mammals: a new alphavirus isolated from the elephant seal louse, Lepidophthirus macrorhini. *J Virol* 2001;75(9):4103–4109.
149. Liu N, Brown DT. Transient translocation of the cytoplasmic (Endo) domain of a type I membrane glycoprotein into cellular membranes. *J Cell Biol* 1993;120:877–883.
150. Liu CY, Kielian M. E1 mutants identify a critical region in the trimer interface of the Semliki forest virus fusion protein. *J Virol* 2009;83(21):11298–11306.
151. Liu Z, Yang D, Qiu Z, et al. Identification of domains in rubella virus genomic RNA and capsid protein necessary for specific interaction. *J Virol* 1996;70(4):2184–2190.
152. Lobigs M, Garoff H. Fusion function of the Semliki Forest virus spike is activated by proteolytic cleavage of the envelope glycoprotein precursor p62. *J Virol* 1990;64(3):1233–1240.

153. Lobigs M, Wahlberg JM, Garoff H. Spike protein oligomerization control of Semliki Forest virus fusion. *J Virol* 1990;64(10):5214–5218.

154. Lobigs M, Zhao HX, Garoff H. Function of Semliki Forest virus E3 peptide in virus assembly: replacement of E3 with an artificial signal peptide abolishes spike heterodimerization and surface expression of E1. *J Virol* 1990;64(9):4346–4355.

155. Loewy A, Smyth J, von Bonsdorff CH, et al. The 6-kilodalton membrane protein of Semliki Forest virus is involved in the budding process. *J Virol* 1995;69(1):469–475.

156. Lu YE, Cassese T, Kielian M. The cholesterol requirement for sindbis virus entry and exit and characterization of a spike protein region involved in cholesterol dependence. *J Virol* 1999;73(5):4272–4278.

157. Lusa S, Garoff H, Liljestrom P. Fate of the 6K membrane protein of Semliki Forest virus during virus assembly. *Virology* 1991;185(2):843–846.

158. Malet H, Egloff MP, Selisko B, et al. Crystal structure of the RNA polymerase domain of the West Nile virus non-structural protein 5. *J Biol Chem* 2007;282(14):10678–10689.

159. Mangala Prasad V, Fokine A, Battisti AJ, et al. Rubella virus capsid protein structure and its role in virus assembly and infection. *Proc Natl Acad Sci U S A* 2013;110:20105–20110.

160. Mangala Prasad V, Klose T, Rossmann MG. Assembly, maturation and three-dimensional helical structure of the teratogenic rubella virus. *PLoS Pathog* 2017;13(6):e1006377.

161. Marquardt MT, Phalen T, Kielian M. Cholesterol is required in the exit pathway of Semliki Forest virus. *J Cell Biol* 1993;123(1):57–65.

162. Marsh M, Bolzau E, Helenius A. Penetration of Semliki Forest virus from acidic prelysosomal vacuoles. *Cell* 1983;32:931–940.

163. Martinez MG, Kielian M. Intercellular extensions are induced by the alphavirus structural proteins and mediate virus transmission. *PLoS Pathog* 2016;12(12):e1006061.

164. Martinez MG, Snapp EL, Perumal GS, et al. Imaging the alphavirus exit pathway. *J Virol* 2014;88(12):6922–6933.

165. Matthews REF. Classification and nomenclature of viruses. *Intervirology* 1982;17:1–199.

166. Melancon P, Garoff H. Processing of the Semliki Forest virus structural polyprotein: role of the capsid protease. *J Virol* 1987;61:1301–1309.

167. Melton JV, Ewart GD, Weir RC, et al. Alphavirus 6K proteins form ion channels. *J Biol Chem* 2002;277:46923–46931.

168. Metsikkö K, Garoff H. Oligomers of the cytoplasmic domain of the p62/E2 membrane protein of Semliki Forest virus bind to the nucleocapsid in vitro. *J Virol* 1990;64:4678–4683.

169. Meyer WJ, Gidwitz S, Ayers VK, et al. Conformational alteration of Sindbis virion glycoproteins induced by heat, reducing agents, or low pH. *J Virol* 1992;66(6):3504–3513.

170. Meyer WJ, Johnston RE. Structural rearrangement of infecting Sindbis virions at the cell surface: mapping of newly accessible epitopes. *J Virol* 1993;67:5117–5125.

171. Mi S, Durbin R, Huang HV, et al. Association of the Sindbis virus RNA methyltransferase activity with the nonstructural protein nsP1. *Virology* 1989;170:385–391.

172. Mi S, Stollar V. Expression of Sindbis virus nsP1 and methyltransferase activity in Escherichia coli. *Virology* 1991;184(1):423–427.

173. Miller ML, Brown DT. Morphogenesis of Sindbis virus in three subclones of Aedes albopictus (mosquito) cells. *J Virol* 1992;66(7):4180–4190.

174. Moesby L, Corver J, Erukulla RK, et al. Sphingolipids activate membrane fusion of Semliki Forest virus in a stereospecific manner. *Biochemistry* 1995;34(33):10319–10324.

175. Montgomery SA, Johnston RE. Nuclear import and export of Venezuelan equine encephalitis virus nonstructural protein 2. *J Virol* 2007;81(19):10268–10279.

176. Mukhopadhyay S, Chipman PR, Hong EM, et al. In vitro-assembled alphavirus core-like particles maintain a structure similar to that of nucleocapsid cores in mature virus. *J Virol* 2002;76(21):11128–11132.

177. Mukhopadhyay S, Zhang W, Gabler S, et al. Mapping the structure and function of the E1 and E2 glycoproteins in alphaviruses. *Structure* 2006;14:63–73.

178. Mulvey M, Brown DT. Formation and rearrangement of disulfide bonds during maturation of the Sindbis virus E1 glycoprotein. *J Virol* 1994;68(2):805–812.

179. Mulvey M, Brown DT. Assembly of the Sindbis virus spike protein complex. *Virology* 1996;219(1):125–132.

180. Nakhasi HL, Cao X-Q, Rouault TA, et al. Specific binding of host cell proteins to the 3′-terminal stem-loop structure of rubella virus negative-strand RNA. *J Virol* 1991;65(11):5961–5967.

181. Nakhasi HL, Rouault TA, Haile DJ, et al. Specific high-affinity binding of host cell proteins to the 3′ region of rubella virus RNA. *New Biol* 1990;2:255–264.

182. Nasar F, Palacios G, Gorchakov RV, et al. Eilat virus, a unique alphavirus with host range restricted to insects by RNA replication. *Proc Natl Acad Sci U S A* 2012;109(36):14622–14627.

183. Neuvonen M, Kazlauskas A, Martikainen M, et al. SH3 domain-mediated recruitment of host cell amphiphysins by alphavirus nsP3 promotes viral RNA replication. *PLoS Pathog* 2011;7(11):e1002383.

184. Ng CG, Coppens I, Govindarajan D, et al. Effect of host cell lipid metabolism on alphavirus replication, virion morphogenesis, and infectivity. *Proc Natl Acad Sci U S A* 2008;105(42):16326–16331.

185. Niesters HGM, Strauss JH. Mutagenesis of the conserved 51-nucleotide region of Sindbis virus. *J Virol* 1990;64:1639–1647.

186. Niesters HGM, Strauss JH. Defined mutations in the 5′ nontranslated sequence of Sindbis virus RNA. *J Virol* 1990;64:4162–4168.

187. Nieva JL, Bron R, Corver J, et al. Membrane fusion of Semliki Forest virus requires sphingolipids in the target membrane. *EMBO J* 1994;13(12):2797–2804.

188. Oker-Blom C. The gene order for Rubella virus structural proteins is NH2-C-E2-E1-COOH. *J Virol* 1984;51:354–358.

189. Oker-Blom C, Kalkkinen N, Kääriäinen L, et al. Rubella virus contains one capsid protein and three envelope glycoproteins, E1, E2a, and E2b. *J Virol* 1983;46:964–973.

190. Oker-Blom C, Ulmanen I, Kääriäinen L, et al. Rubella virus 40S genome RNA specifies a 24S subgenomic mRNA that codes for a precursor to structural proteins. *J Virol* 1984;49:403–408.

191. Owen KE, Kuhn RJ. Identification of a region in the Sindbis virus nucleocapsid protein that is involved in specificity of RNA encapsidation. *J Virol* 1996;70:2757–2763.

192. Owen KE, Kuhn RJ. Alphavirus budding is dependent on the interaction between the nucleocapsid and hydrophobic amino acids on the cytoplasmic domain of the E2 envelope glycoprotein. *Virology* 1997;230(2):187–196.

193. Pardigon N, Lenches E, Strauss JH. Multiple binding sites for cellular proteins in the 3′ end of Sindbis alphavirus minus-sense RNA. *J Virol* 1993;67:5003–5011.

194. Pardigon N, Strauss JH. Cellular proteins bind to the 3′ end of Sindbis virus minus strand RNA. *J Virol* 1992;66(2):1007–1015.

195. Pardigon N, Strauss JH. Mosquito homolog of the La autoantigen binds to Sindbis virus RNA. *J Virol* 1996;70(2):1173–1181.

196. Paredes A, Alwell-Warda K, Weaver SC, et al. Venezuelan equine encephalomyelitis virus structure and its divergence from old world alphaviruses. *J Virol* 2001;75(19):9532–9537.

197. Paredes A, Alwell-Warda K, Weaver SC, et al. Structure of isolated nucleocapsids from venezuelan equine encephalitis virus and implications for assembly and disassembly of enveloped virus. *J Virol* 2003;77(1):659–664.

198. Paredes AM, Brown DT, Rothnagel R, et al. Three-dimensional structure of a membrane-containing virus. *Proc Natl Acad Sci U S A* 1993;90:9095–9099.

199. Paredes AM, Ferreira D, Horton M, et al. Conformational changes in Sindbis virions resulting from exposure to low pH and interactions with cells suggest that cell penetration may occur at the cell surface in the absence of membrane fusion. *Virology* 2004;324:373–386.

200. Paredes AM, Heidner H, Thuman-Commike P, et al. Structural localization of the E3 glycoprotein in attenuated Sindbis virus mutants. *J Virol* 1998;72(2):1534–1541.

201. Paredes AM, Simon ML, Brown DT. The mass of the Sindbis virus nucleocapsid suggests it has T = 4 icosahedral symmetry. *Virology* 1993;187:329–332.

202. Peranen J, Laakkonen P, Hyvonen M, et al. The alphavirus replicase protein nsP1 is membrane-associated and has affinity to endocytic organelles. *Virology* 1995;208(2):610–620.

203. Peränen J, Takkinen K, Kalkkinen N, et al. Semliki Forest virus-specific non-structural protein nsP3 is a phosphoprotein. *J Gen Virol* 1988;69:2165–2178.

204. Petrakova O, Volkova E, Gorchakov R, et al. Noncytopathic replication of Venezuelan equine encephalitis virus and eastern equine encephalitis virus replicons in Mammalian cells. *J Virol* 2005;79(12):7597–7608.

205. Phalen T, Kielian M. Cholesterol is required for infection by Semliki Forest virus. *J Cell Biol* 1991;112(4):615–623.

206. Pletnev SV, Zhang W, Mukhopadhyay S, et al. Locations of carbohydrate sites on alphavirus glycoproteins show that E1 forms an icosahedral scaffold. *Cell* 2001;105:127–136.

207. Powers AM, Brault AC, Shirako Y, et al. Evolutionary relationships and systematics of the alphaviruses. *J Virol* 2001;75(21):10118–10131.

208. Presley JF, Brown DT. The proteolytic cleavage of PE2 to envelope glycoprotein E2 is not strictly required for the maturation of Sindbis virus. *J Virol* 1989;63(5):1975–1980.

209. Presley JF, Polo JM, Johnston RE, et al. Proteolytic processing of the Sindbis virus membrane protein precursor PE2 is nonessential for growth in vertebrate cells but is required for efficient growth in invertebrate cells. *J Virol* 1991;65:1905–1909.

210. Pugachev KV, Abernathy ES, Frey TK. Genomic sequence of the RA27/3 vaccine strain of rubella virus. *Arch Virol* 1997;142(6):1165–1180.

211. Pugachev KV, Abernathy ES, Frey TK. Improvement of the specific infectivity of the rubella virus (RUB) infectious clone: determinants of cytopathogenicity induced by RUB map to the nonstructural proteins. *J Virol* 1997;71(1):562–568.

212. Qin ZL, Zheng Y, Kielian M. Role of conserved histidine residues in the low-pH dependence of the Semliki Forest virus fusion protein. *J Virol* 2009;83(9):4670–4677.

213. Raju R, Huang HV. Analysis of Sindbis virus promoter recognition in vivo, using novel vectors with two subgenomic mRNA promoters. *J Virol* 1991;65:2501–2510.

214. Rey FA, Heinz FX, Mandl C, et al. The envelope glycoprotein from tick-borne encephalitis virus at 2 Å resolution. *Nature* 1995;375:291–298.

215. Rice CM, Strauss JH. Nucleotide sequence of the 26S mRNA of Sindbis virus and deduced sequence of the encoded virus structural proteins. *Proc Natl Acad Sci U S A* 1981;78:2062–2066.

216. Rikkonen M. Functional significance of the nuclear-targeting and NTP-binding motifs of Semliki Forest virus nonstructural protein nsP2. *Virology* 1996;218:352–361.

217. Rikkonen M, Peranen J, Kaariainen L. Nuclear and nucleolar targeting signals of Semliki Forest virus nonstructural protein nsP2. *Virology* 1992;189:462–473.

218. Risco C, Carrascosa JL, Frey TK. Structural maturation of rubella virus in the Golgi complex. *Virology* 2003;312(2):261–269.

219. Roman LM, Garoff H. Alteration of the cytoplasmic domain of the membrane-spanning glycoprotein p62 of Semliki Forest virus does not affect its polar distribution in established lines of Madin-Darby canine kidney cells. *J Cell Biol* 1986;103(6 Pt 2):2607–2618.

220. Rose PP, Hanna SL, Spiridigliozzi A, et al. Natural resistance-associated macrophage protein is a cellular receptor for sindbis virus in both insect and mammalian hosts. *Cell Host Microbe* 2011;10(2):97–104.

221. Rosenblum CI, Scheidel LM, Stollar V. Mutations in the nsP1 coding sequence of Sindbis virus which restrict viral replication in secondary cultures of chick embryo fibroblasts prepared from aged primary cultures. *Virology* 1994;198:100–108.

222. Roussel A, Lescar J, Vaney M-C, et al. Structure and interactions at the viral surface of the envelope protein E1 of Semliki Forest virus. *Structure* 2006;14:75–86.

223. Rubach JK, Wasik BR, Rupp JC, et al. Characterization of purified Sindbis virus nsP4 RNA-dependent RNA polymerase activity in vitro. *Virology* 2009;384(1):201–208.

224. Rümenapf T, Brown DT, Strauss EG, et al. Aura alphavirus subgenomic RNA is packaged into virions of two sizes. *J Virol* 1995;69:1741–1746.

225. Rümenapf T, Strauss EG, Strauss JH. Subgenomic mRNA of Aura alphavirus is packaged into virions. *J Virol* 1994;68:56–62.

226. Russell DL, Dalrymple JM, Johnston RE. Sindbis virus mutations which coordinately affect glycoprotein processing, penetration and virulence in mice. *J Virol* 1989;63:1619–1629.

227. Russo AT, Malmstrom RD, White MA, et al. Structural basis for substrate specificity of alphavirus nsP2 proteases. *J Mol Graph Model* 2010;29(1):46–53.

228. Russo AT, White MA, Watowich SJ. The crystal structure of the Venezuelan equine encephalitis alphavirus nsP2 protease. *Structure* 2006;14(9):1449–1458.

229. Ryman KD, Meier KC, Nangle EM, et al. Sindbis Virus translation is inhibited by a PKR/RNase L-independent effector induced by alpha/beta interferon priming of dendritic cells. *J Virol* 2005;79:1487–1499.

230. Sanders DA. Sulfhydryl involvement in fusion mechanisms. In: Hilderson H, Fuller S, eds. *Fusion of Biological Membranes and Related Problems.* New York: Kluwer Academic/Plenum Publishers; 2000:483–514.

231. Sanz MA, Carrasco L. Sindbis virus variant with a deletion in the 6K gene shows defects in glycoprotein processing and trafficking: lack of complementation by a wild-type 6K gene in trans. *J Virol* 2001;75(16):7778–7784.

232. Sawicki D, Barkhimer DB, Sawicki SG, et al. Temperature sensitive shut-off of alphavirus minus strand RNA synthesis maps to a nonstructural protein, nsP4. *Virology* 1990;174(1):43–52.

233. Sawicki DL, Perri S, Polo JM, et al. Role for nsP2 proteins in the cessation of alphavirus minus-strand synthesis by host cells. *J Virol* 2006;80:360–371.

234. Sawicki SG, Sawicki DL, Kääriäinen L, et al. A Sindbis virus mutant temperature-sensitive in the regulation of minus-strand RNA synthesis. *Virology* 1981;115:161–172.

235. Schlesinger S. Alphavirus expression vectors. *Adv Virus Res* 2000;55:565–577.

236. Sefton BM. Immediate glycosylation of Sindbis virus membrane proteins. *Cell* 1977;10:659–668.

237. Sharkey CM, North CL, Kuhn RJ, et al. Ross River virus glycoprotein-pseudotyped retroviruses and stable cell lines for their production. *J Virol* 2001;75(6):2653–2659.

238. Sherman MB, Weaver SC. The structure of the recombinant alphavirus, western equine encephalitis virus, revealed by cryoelectron microscopy. *J Virol* 2010;84:9775–9782.

239. Shin G, Yost SA, Miller MT, et al. Structural and functional insights into alphavirus polyprotein processing and pathogenesis. *Proc Natl Acad Sci U S A* 2012;109(41):16534–16539.

240. Shirako Y, Strauss JH. Regulation of Sindbis virus RNA replication: uncleaved P123 and nsP4 function in minus-strand RNA synthesis, whereas cleaved products from P123 are required for efficient plus-strand RNA synthesis. *J Virol* 1994;68:1874–1885.

241. Shirako Y, Strauss EG, Strauss JH. Suppressor mutations that allow sindbis virus RNA polymerase to function with nonaromatic amino acids at the N-terminus: evidence for interaction between nsP1 and nsP4 in minus-strand RNA synthesis. *Virology* 2000;276:148–160.

242. Singh NK, Atreya CD, Nakhasi HL. Identification of calreticulin as a rubella virus RNA binding protein. *Proc Natl Acad Sci U S A* 1994;91(26):12770–12774.

243. Singh I, Helenius A. Role of ribosomes in Semliki Forest virus nucleocapsid uncoating. *J Virol* 1992;66:7049–7058.

244. Singh IR, Suomalainen M, Varadarajan S, et al. Multiple mechanisms for the inhibition of entry and uncoating of superinfecting Semliki Forest virus. *Virology* 1997;231(1):59–71.

245. Sjoberg M, Lindqvist B, Garoff H. Activation of the alphavirus spike protein is suppressed by bound E3. *J Virol* 2011;85(11):5644–5650.

246. Skoging U, Vihinen M, Nilsson L, et al. Aromatic interactions define the binding of the alphavirus spike to its nucleocapsid. *Structure* 1996;4(5):519–529.

247. Smit JM, Waarts B-L, Kimata K, et al. Adaptation of alphaviruses to heparan sulfate: interaction of Sindbis and Semliki Forest virus with liposomes containing lipid-conjugated heparin. *J Virol* 2002;76:10128–10137.

248. Snyder JE, Azizgolshani O, Wu B, et al. Rescue of infectious particles from preassembled alphavirus nucleocapsid cores. *J Virol* 2011;85(12):5773–5781.

249. Söderlund H, Ulmanen I. Transient association of Semliki Forest virus capsid protein with ribosomes. *J Virol* 1977;24:907–909.

250. Sokoloski KJ, Dickson AM, Chaskey EL, et al. Sindbis virus usurps the cellular HuR protein to stabilize its transcripts and promote productive infections in mammalian and mosquito cells. *Cell Host Microbe* 2010;8(2):196–207.

251. Soonsawad P, Xing L, Milla E, et al. Structural evidence of glycoprotein assembly in cellular membrane compartments prior to Alphavirus budding. *J Virol* 2010;84(21):11145–11151.

252. Stiles KM, Kielian M. Role of TSPAN9 in alphavirus entry and early endosomes. *J Virol* 2016;90(9):4289–4297.

253. Strauss EG, De Groot RJ, Levinson R, et al. Identification of the active site residues in the nsP2 proteinase of Sindbis virus. *Virology* 1992;191(2):932–940.

254. Strauss EG, Lenches EM, Strauss JH. Mutants of Sindbis Virus. I. Isolation and partial characterization of 89 new temperature-sensitive mutants. *Virology* 1976;74:154–168.

255. Strauss EG, Rice CM, Strauss JH. Complete nucleotide sequence of the genomic RNA of Sindbis virus. *Virology* 1984;133:92–110.

256. Strauss JH, Rümenapf T, Weir RC, et al. Cellular receptors for alphaviruses. In: Wimmer E, ed. *Cellular Receptors for Animal Viruses.* Cold Spring Harbor: Cold Spring Harbor Press; 1994:141–163.

257. Strauss JH, Strauss EG. Evolution of RNA viruses. *Ann Rev Microbiol* 1988;42:657–683.

258. Strauss JH, Strauss EG. The alphaviruses: gene expression, replication, and evolution. *Microbiol Rev* 1994;58(3):491–562.

259. Strauss JH, Strauss EG. Virus evolution: how does an enveloped virus make a regular structure? *Cell* 2001;105:5–8.

260. Sun S, Xiang Y, Akahata W, et al. Structural analyses at pseudo atomic resolution of Chikungunya virus and antibodies show mechanisms of neutralization. *Elife* 2013;2:e00435.

261. Suomalainen M, Liljestrom P, Garoff H. Spike protein-nucleocapsid interactions drive the budding of alphaviruses. *J Virol* 1992;66(8):4737–4747.

262. Tang J, Jose J, Chipman P, et al. Molecular links between the E2 envelope glycoprotein and nucleocapsid core in Sindbis virus. *J Mol Biol* 2011;414(3):442–459.

263. Tellinghuisen TL, Hamburger AE, Fisher BR, et al. In vitro assembly of alphavirus cores by using nucleocapsid protein expressed in Escherichia coli. *J Virol* 1999;73(7):5309–5319.

264. Tellinghuisen TL, Kuhn RJ. Nucleic acid-dependent cross-linking of the nucleocapsid protein of Sindbis virus. *J Virol* 2000;74(9):4302–4309.

265. Tellinghuisen TL, Perera R, Kuhn RJ. In vitro assembly of Sindbis virus core-like particles from cross-linked dimers of truncated and mutant capsid proteins. *J Virol* 2001;75(6):2810–2817.

266. Tomar S, Hardy RW, Smith JL, et al. Catalytic core of alphavirus nonstructural protein nsP4 possesses terminal adenylyltransferase activity. *J Virol* 2006;80:9962–9969.

267. Tuittila M, Hinkkanen AE. Amino acid mutations in the replicase protein nsP3 of Semliki Forest virus cumulatively affect neurovirulence. *J Gen Virol* 2003;84:1525–1533.

268. Tzeng WP, Frey TK. Complementation of a deletion in the rubella virus p150 nonstructural protein by the viral capsid protein. *J Virol* 2003;77(17):9502–9510.

269. Uchime O, Fields W, Kielian M. The role of E3 in pH protection during alphavirus assembly and exit. *J Virol* 2013;87(18):10255–10262.

270. Ulmanen I, Soderlund H, Kaariainen L. Semliki Forest virus capsid protein associates with the 60S ribosomal subunit in infected cells. *J Virol* 1976;20:203–210.

271. Vashishtha M, Phalen T, Marquardt MT, et al. A single point mutation controls the cholesterol dependence of Semliki Forest virus entry and exit. *J Cell Biol* 1998;140(1):91–99.

272. Vasiljeva L, Valmu L, Kaariainen L, et al. Site-specific protease activity of the carboxyl-terminal domain of Semliki Forest virus replicase protein nsP2. *J Biol Chem* 2001;276(33):30786–30793.

273. Venien-Bryan C, Fuller SD. The organization of the spike complex of Semliki Forest virus. *J Mol Biol* 1994;236(2):572–583.

274. Vihinen H, Ahola T, Tuittila M, et al. Elimination of phosphorylation sites of Semliki Forest virus replicase protein nsP3. *J Biol Chem* 2001;276(8):5745–5752.

275. Vihinen H, Saarinen J. Phosphorylation site analysis of Semliki Forest virus nonstructural protein 3. *J Biol Chem* 2000;275:27775–27783.

276. Volkova E, Gorchakov R, Frolov G. The efficient packaging of Venezuelan equine encephalitis virus-specific RNAs into viral particles is determined by nsP1-3 synthesis. *Virology* 2006;344:315–327.

277. von Bonsdorff CH, Harrison SC. Sindbis virus glycoproteins form a regular icosahedral surface lattice. *J Virol* 1975;16:141–145.

278. von Bonsdorff CH, Harrison SC. Hexagonal glycoprotein arrays from Sindbis virus membranes. *J Virol* 1978;28:578–583.

279. Voss JE, Vaney MC, Duquerroy S, et al. Glycoprotein organization of Chikungunya virus particles revealed by X-ray crystallography. *Nature* 2010;468(7324):709–712.

280. Waarts B-L, Bittman R, Wilschut J. Sphingolipid and cholesterol dependence of alphavirus membrane fusion. *J Biol Chem* 2002;277:38141–38147.

281. Wahlberg JM, Boere WA, Garoff H. The heterodimeric association between the membrane proteins of Semliki Forest virus changes its sensitivity to low pH during virus maturation. *J Virol* 1989;63(12):4991–4997.

282. Wahlberg JM, Bron R, Wilschut J, et al. Membrane fusion of Semliki Forest virus involves homotrimers of the fusion protein. *J Virol* 1992;66(12):7309–7318.

283. Wahlberg JM, Garoff H. Membrane fusion process of Semliki Forest virus I: low pH-induced rearrangement in spike glycoprotein quaternary structure precedes virus penetration into cells. *J Cell Biol* 1992;116:339–348.

284. Wang CY, Dominguez G, Frey TK. Construction of rubella virus genome-length cDNA clones and synthesis of infectious RNA transcripts. *J Virol* 1994;68(6):3550–3557.

285. Wang KS, Kuhn RJ, Strauss EG, et al. High-affinity laminin receptor is a receptor for Sindbis virus in mammalian cells. *J Virol* 1992;66(8):4992–5001.

286. Wang YF, Sawicki SG, Sawicki DL. Sindbis virus nsP1 functions in negative-strand RNA synthesis. *J Virol* 1991;65(2):985–988.

287. Wang Y-F, Sawicki SG, Sawicki D. Alphavirus nsP3 functions to form replication complexes transcribing negative-strand RNA. *J Virol* 1994;68:6466–6475.

288. Wang K-S, Schmaljohn AL, Kuhn RJ, et al. Antiidiotypic antibodies as probes for the Sindbis virus receptor. *Virology* 1991;181:694–702.

289. Weiss B, Geigenmüller-Gnirke U, Schlesinger S. Interactions between Sindbis virus RNAs and a 68 amino acid derivative of the viral capsid protein further defines the capsid binding site. *Nucleic Acids Res* 1994;22:780–786.

290. Weiss B, Nitschko H, Ghattas I, et al. Evidence for specificity in the encapsidation of Sindbis virus RNAs. *J Virol* 1989;63:5310–5318.

291. Wengler G. The mode of assembly of alphavirus cores implies a mechanism for the disassembly of the cores in the early stages of infection. *Arch Virol* 1987;94:1–14.

292. Wengler G, Boege U, Wengler G, et al. The core protein of the alphavirus Sindbis virus assembles into core-like nucleoproteins with the viral genome RNA and with other single-stranded nucleic acids in vitro. *Virology* 1982;118:401–410.

293. Wengler G, Gros C, Wengler G. Analyses of the role of structural changes in the regulation of uncoating and assembly of alphavirus cores. *Virology* 1996;222:123–132.

294. Wengler G, Koschinski A, Wengler G, et al. Entry of alphaviruses at the plasma membrane converts the viral surface proteins into an ion-permeable pore that can be detected by electrophysiological analyses of whole-cell membrane currents. *J Gen Virol* 2003;84:173–181.

295. Wengler G, Wengler G. Identification of a transfer of viral core protein to cellular ribosomes during the early stages of alphavirus infection. *Virology* 1984;134:435.

296. Wengler G, Wengler G. In vitro analysis of factors involved in the disassembly of Sindbis virus cores by 60S ribosomal subunits identifies a possible role of low pH. *J Gen Virol* 2002;83:2417–2426.

297. Wengler G, Wengler G, Rey FA. The isolation of the ectodomain of the alphavirus E1 protein as a soluble hemagglutinin and its crystallization. *Virology* 1999;257:472–482.

298. Wengler G, Würkner D, Wengler G. Identification of a sequence element in the alphavirus core protein which mediates interaction of cores with ribosomes and the disassembly of cores. *Virology* 1992;191:880–888.

299. Weston JH, Welsh MD, McLoughlin MF, et al. Salmon pancreas disease virus, an alphavirus infecting farmed Atlantic salmon, Salmo salar L. *Virology* 1999;256(2):188–195.

300. Wielgosz MM, Raju R, Huang HV. Sequence requirements for Sindbis virus subgenomic mRNA promoter function in cultured cells. *J Virol* 2001;75(8):3509–3519.

301. Wilschut J, Corver J, Nieva JL, et al. Fusion of Semliki Forest virus with cholesterol-containing liposomes at low pH: a specific requirement for sphingolipids. *Mol Membr Biol* 1995;12(1):143–149.

302. Xiong C, Levis R, Shen P, et al. Sindbis virus: an efficient, broad host range vector for gene expression in animal cells. *Science* 1989;243:1188–1191.

303. Yao JS, Strauss EG, Strauss JH. Interactions between PE2, E1, and 6K required for assembly of alphaviruses studied with chimeric viruses. *J Virol* 1996;70(11):7910–7920.

304. Yap ML, Klose T, Urakami A, et al. Structural studies of Chikungunya virus maturation. *Proc Natl Acad Sci U S A* 2017;114(52):13703–13707.

305. Zeng X, Mukhopadhyay S, Brooks CL III. Residue-level resolution of alphavirus envelope protein interactions in pH-dependent fusion. *Proc Natl Acad Sci U S A* 2015;112(7):2034–2039.

306. Zhang W, Fisher BR, Olson NH, et al. Aura virus structure suggests that the T = 4 organization is a fundamental property of viral structural proteins. *J Virol* 2002;76(14):7239–7246.

307. Zhang W, Heil ML, Kuhn RJ, et al. Heparin binding sites on Ross River Virus revealed by electron cryo-microscopy. *Virology* 2005;332:511–518.

308. Zhang R, Hryc CF, Cong Y, et al. 4.4 Å cryo-EM structure of an enveloped alphavirus Venezuelan equine encephalitis virus. *EMBO J* 2011;30(18):3854–3863.

309. Zhang R, Kim AS, Fox JM, et al. Mxra8 is a receptor for multiple arthritogenic alphaviruses. *Nature* 2018;557(7706):570–574.

310. Zhao H, Lindqvist B, Garoff H, et al. A tyrosine-based motif in the cytoplasmic domain of the alphavirus envelope protein is essential for budding. *EMBO J* 1994;13:4204–4211.

311. Zheng Y, Kielian M. Imaging of the alphavirus capsid protein during virus replication. *J Virol* 2013;87(17):9579–9589.

312. Ziemiecki A, Garoff H. Subunit composition of the membrane glycoprotein complex of Semliki Forest virus. *J Mol Biol* 1978;122:259–269.

Alphaviruses

Diane E. Griffin • Scott C. Weaver

The genus *Alphavirus* in the family *Togaviridae* includes 31 species that can be classified antigenically or genetically into at least 8 complexes (Table 6.1). Alphaviruses are geographically restricted in their distributions and have been found on all continents and on many islands, as well as in marine mammals. In nature, most alphaviruses are zoonotic arthropod-borne (arbo) viruses that cycle between invertebrate insect vectors and vertebrate hosts. For most alphaviruses, the vectors are mosquitoes, but other hematophagous arthropods, such as lice or mites, are vectors for a few. The vertebrate hosts are mostly wild mammals or birds, and birds, but fish are hosts for some aquatic alphaviruses. In general, the pathogenic alphaviruses are divided into the viruses that cause human disease characterized by rash and arthritis, primarily found originally in the Old World (OW), and viruses that cause encephalitis, primarily found in the New World (NW). For many alphaviruses, no human or veterinary disease has been recognized. Larger mammals, such as humans and horses, that tend to develop severe or fatal disease are often dead-end hosts unimportant to the enzootic/endemic virus transmission cycles, but can be important for sustaining epidemics.

HISTORY

Records of diseases almost certainly due to alphaviruses date to the 18th and 19th centuries when epidemics of fatal encephalitis in horses in the northeastern United States (USA) and outbreaks of arthritis in Southeast Asia were recognized and recorded. The first clear report of epidemic encephalitis comes from the summer of 1831 when 75 horses died in Massachusetts.[372] Over the next 100 years, several local outbreaks of encephalitis in horses were noted along the Atlantic seaboard of the United States and in the pampas regions of South America.[838] However, the first alphavirus to be cultured was western equine encephalitis virus (WEEV). This virus was isolated in 1930 from the central nervous system (CNS) tissues of two horses involved in an epidemic of equine encephalitis in the San Joaquin Valley of California.[639] The eastern equine encephalitis virus (EEEV) was isolated from the brains of affected horses in New Jersey and Virginia in 1933.[106] Both diseases occurred in summertime epidemics, suggesting an arthropod vector, and in 1933, Kelser showed WEEV transmission by mosquitoes.[478] In 1936, an epizootic of equine encephalitis occurred in the Guajira region of Venezuela, and the virus isolated was not neutralized by antisera against EEEV or WEEV and was designated Venezuelan equine encephalitis virus (VEEV).[512]

TABLE 6.1   Alphaviruses, abbreviations, biologic features, and association with disease

Virus (Abbreviation)[a]	Antigenic Complex	Principal Vertebrate Reservoir Host	Geographic Distribution	Human Disease	Animal Disease
Aura virus (AURAV)	WEE	Unknown	S. America		
Barmah Forest virus (BFV)	BF	Birds	Australia	Fever, arthritis, rash	
Bebaru virus (BEBV)	SF	Unknown	Asia		
Cabassou virus (CABV)	VEE	Unknown	French Guiana		
Chikungunya virus (CHIKV)	SF	Primates	Africa, SE Asia, Philippines, Indonesia	Fever, arthritis, rash	
Eastern equine encephalitis virus (EEEV)	EEE	Birds, possibly reptiles	S. Amer., Caribbean	Fever, encephalitis	Horse, pheasant, emu, pigeon, turkey
Eilat virus (EILV)	None described	None	Israel, S. America	None (replication defective)	None (replication defective)
Everglades virus (EVEV)	VEE	Mammals	Florida	Fever, encephalitis	
Fort Morgan virus (FMV)	WEE	Birds	Colorado		
Getah virus (GETV)	SF	Mammals	Asia	Fever	Horse
Highlands J virus (HJV)	WEE	Birds	N. America		Horse, turkey, emu, pheasant, duck, crane
Madariaga virus (MADV)	EEE	S. America, Caribbean	S. America	Fever, encephalitis	Horse
Mayaro virus (MAYV)	SF	Mammals	S. America	Fever, arthritis, rash	
Middelburg virus (MIDV)	MID	Unknown	Africa		
Mosso das Pedras virus /78V3531 (MDPV)	VEE	Mammals	S. Amer.		
Mucambo virus (MUCV)	VEE	Mammals	S. Amer., Caribbean		
Ndumu virus (NDUV)	NDU	Unknown	Africa		
O'nyong-nyong virus (ONNV)	SF	Unknown	East Africa	Fever, arthritis, rash	
Pixuna virus (PIXV)	VEE	Mammals	Brazil		
Rio Negro virus/AG80 (RNV)	VEE	Mammals	Argentina		
Ross River virus (RRV)	SF	Mammals	Australia, S. Pacific	Fever, arthritis, rash	
Salmonid alphavirus (SAV)	None described	Fish	North Atlantic		Trout, salmon
Semliki Forest virus (SFV)	SF	Unknown	Africa	Fever, encephalitis	Horse
Sindbis virus (SINV)	WEE	Birds	Australia, Africa, N. Europe, Middle East	Fever, arthritis, rash	
Southern elephant seal virus (SESV)	None described	Seals	Antarctica		
Tonate virus (TONV)	VEE	Birds	S. Amer.	Fever, encephalitis	
Trocara virus (TROV)	WEE	Unknown	S. Amer.		
Una virus (UNAV)	SF	Unknown	S. Amer., Trinidad		Horse
Venezuelan equine encephalitis virus (VEEV)	VEE	Mammals	S. Amer., N. Amer.	Fever, encephalitis	Horse
Western equine encephalitis virus (WEEV)	WEE	Birds, mammals	N. Amer., S. Amer.	Fever, encephalitis	Horse, emu
Whataroa virus (WHATV)	WEE	Birds	New Zealand, Australia		

[a]All are also considered species by the International Committee on Taxonomy of Viruses.

Summertime epidemics of polyarthritis were recognized in Australia and New Guinea in 1928,[220,698] and subsequent outbreaks of polyarthritis were reported in Northern Europe, Africa, and Southeast Asia.[895] It is likely, of course, that the alphavirus-induced arthritic diseases are much older than these dates but were not clearly described or differentiated from more prevalent infections in these regions, such as dengue. This is considered to be particularly true of outbreaks of chikungunya virus (CHIKV) infection that have occurred in India and Southeast Asia over the last 200 years[141,971] and probably also in the Americas.[370] Viruses associated with epidemic polyarthritis were eventually isolated, both from mosquitoes collected in the areas of human disease and later from humans. The first of these viruses was isolated in 1952 from a pool of *Culex* spp. mosquitoes collected near Sindbis, Egypt.[963] However, it was many years before Sindbis virus (SINV) was linked to human disease.[604]

The first clear association of an alphavirus with arthritic disease came in 1953 when CHIKV was isolated in present-day Tanzania from the blood of people with severe arthritis.[820] During the next several years, a number of viruses causing arthritis, often accompanied by a rash, were isolated in Africa, Australia, and South America.[156,654,1083] These viruses were added to the growing list of arboviruses, defined by the World Health Organization in 1967 as "viruses which are maintained in nature principally, or to an important extent, through biological transmission between susceptible vertebrate hosts by haematophagous arthropods; they multiply and produce viremia in the vertebrates, multiply in the tissues of arthropods, and are passed on to new vertebrates by the bites of arthropods after a period of extrinsic incubation."

In 1954, arboviruses were divided by Casals and Brown into three serologic groups A, B, and C, based on cross-reactivity in hemagglutination inhibition (HI) and complement fixation (CF) tests. EEE, WEE, and VEE viruses constituted the group A arboviruses. A second cross-reacting set, including dengue, St. Louis encephalitis, and yellow fever viruses, constituted the group B arboviruses, and the nonreactive viruses were designated group C. As viruses became classified on the fundamental properties of the virion and the genome, the group A viruses became the *Alphavirus* genus within the *Togaviridae* family of enveloped RNA viruses.

INFECTIOUS AGENTS

Alphaviruses are enveloped plus-strand RNA viruses with icosahedral symmetry (Fig. 6.1). The virions are *ca.* 70 nm in diameter and sensitive to ether and detergent. Cryoelectron microscopy structures are available for many.[508,606,890,1106,1107,1109] The RNA is contained within a capsid formed by a single protein arranged as an icosahedron with T = 4 symmetry. The nucleocapsid is enclosed in a lipid envelope derived from the host cell plasma membrane that contains the viral-encoded glycoproteins, E1 and E2. These proteins form heterodimers that are grouped as trimers to form 80 knobs on the virion surface. Glycoproteins are arranged such that 240 copies of each cytoplasmic E2 tail interact with 240 copies of capsid protein.[169]

The 42-49S genome is composed of a single-strand, nonsegmented, capped, and polyadenylated message-sense RNA that is infectious. Complete genomic sequences are available for representatives of all currently known alphavirus species. The genomes are 11 to 12 kb in size and have two open reading frames organized with the nonstructural proteins (nsPs) at the 5′ end and the structural proteins at the 3′ end. The nsPs are translated as a polyprotein from genomic RNA, and the structural proteins are translated as a polyprotein from a subgenomic RNA.[943] Four nsPs are sequentially processed to replicate the viral genomic RNA and produce the subgenomic RNA

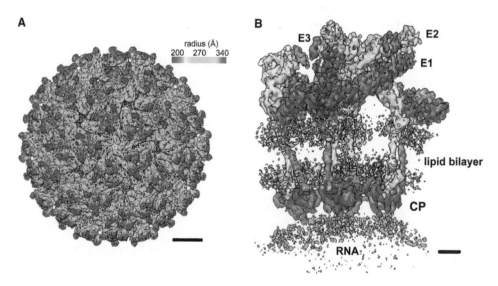

FIGURE 6.1 Three-dimensional reconstruction of the VEEV virion. A: Radially colored 3D reconstruction of VEEV showing the E1 basal triangle (*green*) and E2 central protrusion (*blue*) for each spike. Scale bar: 10 nm. **B:** One asymmetric unit of the virus containing four unique copies of E1 (*magenta*), E2 (*cyan*), E3 (*orange*), and capsid (CP, *blue*). The cryo-EM densities for the viral membrane (*yellow*) and genomic RNA (*green*) are also displayed at slightly lower isosurface threshold. (Courtesy of Wah Chiu and reproduced with permission from Zhang R, Hryc CF, Cong Y, et al. 4.4 Å cryo-EM structure of an enveloped alphavirus Venezuelan equine encephalitis virus. *EMBO J* 2011;30(18):3854–3863.)

(covered in chapter on Togaviruses). nsP1 has methyl- and guanylyl transferase capping activities, anchors the replication complex to membranes, and initiates minus-strand synthesis.[21,22,525,1042] nsP2 has N-terminal helicase, NTPase and RNA triphosphatase, and C-terminal protease activities.[323,472,633,808,1022] nsP3 is a phosphoprotein that interacts with viral and cellular proteins to regulate replication and is a major determinant of cell-type–specific replication, host range, and virulence.[328,533,741,780] The N-terminal macrodomain is highly conserved in alphaviruses and binds and removes ADP-ribose from proteins,[326,627] while the intrinsically disordered hypervariable domain provides a hub for at least three different host protein families.[332] nsP4 is the RNA-dependent RNA polymerase.[856]

Five potential structural proteins (C, E3, E2, 6K, and E1) are encoded in the subgenomic RNA, and an additional transframe protein (TF) is produced by -1 ribosomal frameshifting within the 6K coding region extending into E1.[177,265,779] The N-terminal portion of C is basic and binds the viral genomic RNA, while the more conserved C-terminal portion proteolytically cleaves C from the nascent chain, interacts with other copies of C to form the nucleocapsid, and binds the cytoplasmic tail of E2 for virion assembly and budding.[587,612,722,921,926,959,1107,1110]

E3 is a small cysteine-rich glycoprotein that serves as a signal sequence for pE2 (the E2 precursor composed of E3 and E2), mediates proper folding of E2, and is necessary for pE2 to heterodimerize with E1 for transport to the cell surface.[572,734] As part of the pE2-E1 heterodimer, E3 prevents premature activation of E1 in the secretory pathway.[443,1013,1035] E3 is cleaved from E2 by furin in the trans-Golgi, remains associated with the spike under acidic conditions, and needs to be shed when virions bud from the cell surface for particles to be infectious.[910,1105]

The E2 glycoprotein is a transmembrane protein that has two or three N-linked carbohydrates and contains the most important epitopes for neutralizing antibody. E2 is organized into three immunoglobulin ectodomains (A, B, and C) and a subdomain (D) (Fig. 6.2). Domain A (residues 1–132) is at the center and top of the heterotrimer and has receptor and neutralizing antibody–binding sites. Domain B is at the spike tip and probably interacts with cellular receptors, and C is toward the viral membrane.[558,1018,1032] Subdomain D connects C with the transmembrane helix.[168,1107] The intracytoplasmic portion

interacts with the capsid and has a second stretch of hydrophobic amino acids and myristoylation sites that tether it to the inner surface of the membrane.

The E1 protein has one or two N-linked carbohydrates, a short (one or two residues) intracytoplasmic tail, and a positionally conserved internal hydrophobic stretch of amino acids in the N-terminal portion that serves as the fusion peptide for virion entry into the cell. E1 is organized into three β-sheet–rich domains (I, II, and III) similar to the flavivirus E protein with the internal fusion loop at the tip of domain II[311] (Fig. 6.2). 6K is the signal peptide for E1, is cleaved from E1 and E2 by signalase, and has characteristics of a viroporin. TF has the same N-terminus as 6K, is palmitoylated, is important for virus virulence, and regulates virus budding with small amounts incorporated into virions.[265,779,922]

Propagation and Assay in Tissue Culture

Initial isolations of alphaviruses were accomplished by intracerebral inoculation into suckling mice, a host very susceptible to infection with most alphaviruses. Many alphaviruses can also be isolated and propagated efficiently in primary chicken embryo fibroblasts (CEF) and in a wide variety of continuous mammalian cell lines such as human epithelial (HeLa, MRC5) cells, baby hamster kidney (BHK) cells, monkey kidney (Vero) cells, and mouse fibroblast and neuroblastoma cells (Fig. 6.3).

Most alphaviruses will form plaques on susceptible mammalian or avian cells under an agar overlay. Mosquito cell lines also support replication, but often without overt cytopathic effect (CPE).[777,939] The first plaque assay of an animal virus was performed using WEEV on CEF cells,[231] and plaque assay remains a convenient and sensitive way to quantify infectious virus. Plaque size has been used to differentiate strains and is determined by the type of overlay used, by relative virus binding to negatively charged sulfated polysaccharides present in the overlay, and by replication efficiency.[111,125,954] Plaque size is sometimes, but not always, associated with virulence differences among virus strains.[1039]

Biological Characteristics

Hemagglutination

Alphaviruses can hemagglutinate avian (e.g., goose, chicken) erythrocytes,[839] and hemagglutination has been used as a method for quantifying virus and HI for measuring antiviral antibody. Hemagglutination requires prior exposure of the virus to acidic pH, is dependent primarily on the E1 glycoprotein, and reflects binding of the fusion domain of the E1 glycoprotein to lipids in the erythrocyte membrane.[159,1016,1069] E2 also participates in hemagglutination because some monoclonal antibodies (mAbs) specific for E2 also have HI activity.[90,785] The HI test is not currently in common use but has been helpful for determining antigenic relationships among alphaviruses and in screening diverse animal sera for antibodies where its cross-reactivity can be advantageous.[137]

Cellular Receptors

Binding of virus to the cell surface and entry into the cell is a multistep process that is dependent on virus glycoproteins E1 and E2, cell-surface molecules, low pH in the endosome, and fusion of membrane lipids. Variations in any of these components will affect the efficiency of infection and the likelihood

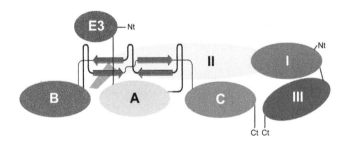

FIGURE 6.2 Domain structure of the glycoprotein spike. Schematic diagram of the E1pE2 heterodimer drawn "untwisted" to show the domains positioned with respect to one another and their connectivity. Domains of E1 (I, red; II, yellow; III, blue; fusion loop, orange) and pE2 (A, cyan; B, dark green; C, pink; E3, gray) are shown. Ct, C-terminus. (Courtesy of Felix Rey and reproduced with permission from Voss JE, Vaney MC, Duquerroy S, et al. Glycoprotein organization of Chikungunya virus particles revealed by X-ray crystallography. *Nature* 2010;468(7324):709–712.)

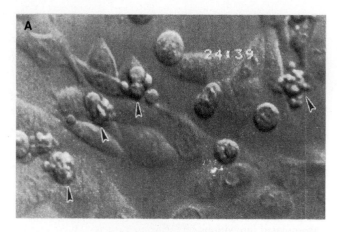

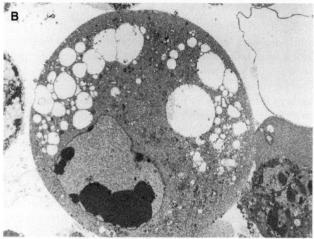

FIGURE 6.3 Effects of Sindbis virus infection on vertebrate cells.
A: Cytopathic effects (CPE) of rounding, shrinkage, and cytoplasmic blebbing in BHK cells infected at a low multiplicity (arrowheads).
B: Electron micrograph of an infected BHK cell showing chromosomal condensation and cytopathic vacuoles.

that any particular cell will become infected. Virus-specific attachment to cells is primarily a function of the E2 glycoprotein. The important role for E2 in initiating virus–cell interaction is evidenced by the ability of anti-E2 mAbs to inhibit binding to cells,[125] of anti-idiotypic antibodies to E2-specific mAbs to recognize putative virus receptors on cells,[1043] and of amino acid changes in E2 to alter virus binding to cells of different types.[230,539]

Identification of specific alphavirus receptors has been difficult and complicated by experimental use of virus strains that are adapted to replicate in tissue culture.[500] Because each alphavirus infects a wide range of hosts, often including birds, mammals, and insects, they must use either an evolutionarily well-conserved cell-surface molecule or multiple molecules as receptors. Specificity in infection is generally maximal for oral infection of even closely related mosquitoes, suggesting a role for processes beyond binding to proteins on the apical surface of midgut cells. None of the alphavirus receptors identified to date appears to be used exclusively, suggesting the possibility of several receptors. Alternatively, alphaviruses may use attachment molecule–receptor–coreceptor combinations to achieve wide host range and the specific tropisms observed *in vivo*.

The first alphavirus receptor to be identified was the major histocompatibility complex (MHC) class I molecule receptor for Semliki Forest virus (SFV) on mouse and human cells.[391] However, cells lacking MHC molecules can still be infected with SFV.[710] The high-affinity laminin receptor is a receptor for SINV on BHK cells and a potential receptor for SINV and VEEV on C6/36 mosquito cells.[581,1040] Again, this molecule appears to account for only a portion of the total virus interaction with the cells studied and does not contribute to SINV binding to avian cells.[1040] Ross River virus (RRV) uses the $\alpha_1\beta_1$-integrin on HeLa cells for binding.[523] SINV and VEEV can use natural resistance–associated macrophage protein (NRAMP) for binding to insect and mammalian cells,[816] and adhesion molecule Mxra8 improves binding of CHIKV, o'nyong-nyong virus (ONNV), RRV, and Mayaro virus (MAYV) to mouse fibroblasts.[1108] The type of cell in which the virus is grown can also influence initial virus–receptor interactions. For instance, SINV grown in mosquito cells is enriched in high-mannose carbohydrates that bind the C-type lectins DC-SIGN and L-SIGN on the surface of dendritic cells (DCs).[499]

Heparan sulfate (HS), a ubiquitously expressed glycosaminoglycan, is an important initial binding molecule for many alphaviruses. Interaction with HS, a highly sulfated, negatively charged molecule, probably explains the effects of ionic strength and charge on the attachment of virus to cells.[610,752] Use of HS is selected by virus passage in vertebrate cells. However, wild-type strains of EEEV bind HS, so this property is not exclusively determined by passage in tissue culture.[298] For these viruses, addition of heparin or lactoferrin, treatment of cells with heparinase, or use of cells deficient in HS decreases binding to cells and plaque formation. The heparin-binding domain of the E2 glycoprotein is on domain A and overlaps a neutralizing epitope (Fig. 6.2). Changes toward more positively charged amino acids in the region around E2-70 increase the efficiency of attachment to cells in tissue culture.[79,126,500]

Entry requires interaction with the cell membrane followed by a conformational change in the trimer of E1–E2 heterodimers.[389,505,897,912,1075] This conformational change is generally induced by low pH in the endosome, but entry may also occur at the plasma membrane.[930,1017] At neutral pH, the E1 fusion peptide is protected in the virion heterotrimer by domain B of E2 and this association is stabilized by E3.[558,1032] When exposed to acidic pH, E1 dissociates from E2 and forms stable E1 homotrimers in the presence of cholesterol-containing membranes.[140,1102] During this conformational change, the fusion peptide is exposed and inserted into the outer leaflet of the endosomal membrane lipid bilayer.[108,311] E1 folds back to bring the viral and endosomal membranes together, promoting fusion. Efficient fusion with the cell membrane to initiate infection is dependent on cellular factors including presence of a membrane potential, cholesterol, sphingolipid, and tetraspanin TSPAN9.[390,694,718]

Effects on Vertebrate Cells

Alphaviruses replicate rapidly in most vertebrate cell lines with the release of progeny virus typically within 4 to 6 hours after infection. At the time of virus entry, there is an increase in permeability perhaps due to pore formation by the E1, 6K, and/or TF proteins.[602,1067,1068] Insertion of newly synthesized glycoproteins into the plasma membrane for virion budding renders infected cells capable of ATP-dependent polykaryocyte formation upon exposure to acid pH.[479] Infection causes extensive

CPE in a variety of cell lines characterized by cell rounding, shrinkage, and cytoplasmic blebbing (Fig. 6.3A) with the death of infected cells within 24 to 48 hours.[552,777] Alphavirus-induced CPE has been linked to shutoff of host cell transcription and translation, endoplasmic reticulum (ER) stress, the unfolded protein response, and induction of apoptosis.[28,56,303,316,433,552,700] The ability of alphaviruses to induce cell death, combined with the ability to express heterologous genes, has led to their development as potential oncolytic agents.[421,776,830,994]

Shutoff of host cell functions by OW viruses (e.g., SINV, SFV, CHIKV) differs from that of NW viruses (e.g., VEEV, EEEV).[304] Transcription of cellular mRNAs including antiviral response genes is inhibited by nsP2 from OW viruses and by capsid from NW viruses.[18,42,302,303,320] nsP2 of OW viruses translocates to the nucleus[740] and induces degradation of RPB1, the catalytic subunit of RNA polymerase II to shut off cellular transcription.[24] Mutations at nsP2 P726 that impair this function result in viruses that replicate less well and are less cytopathic.[23,290] Capsid of NW viruses inhibits nuclear import by forming a complex with the nuclear export receptor CRM1 and the nuclear import receptor importin-α/β.[41]

Several factors probably contribute in cell type–specific ways to shut off host cell translation.[144] One important factor is activation of RNA-dependent protein kinase (PKR) by interaction with double-stranded RNA (dsRNA) or capsid that results in phosphorylation of eIF2α, which inhibits translation of genomic viral RNA for the nonstructural polyprotein and host mRNAs without affecting translation of viral 26S subgenomic RNA for the structural proteins.[18,255,1026] In many alphaviruses, escape from eIF2α phosphorylation for subgenomic RNA translation is due to the presence of a hairpin loop structure downstream of the initiation codon that allows the 40S ribosome to initiate translation in the absence of eIF2 and eIF4.[144,222,647,850,911,1025]

The apoptotic process in virus-infected cell lines is associated with blebbing of the plasma membrane, condensation of nuclear chromatin, and formation of apoptotic bodies (Fig. 6.3B). Viral proteins are concentrated in the surface blebs from which budding continues to occur.[511,817] This process does not hamper, and may enhance, virus replication because inhibition of apoptosis usually decreases virus yield.[548,561,860]

The mechanism(s) by which alphaviruses induce apoptosis can involve both intrinsic and extrinsic pathways and likely differs with virus and type of target cell.[458,510] Apoptosis of cultured cells can be initiated at the endosomal membrane during SINV fusion resulting in activation of membrane-bound sphingomyelinases that release ceramide, an efficient inducer of cellular apoptosis.[444,445,449] SFV-induced apoptosis requires accumulation of viral RNA and is independent of p53.[317,956,1015] Cellular caspases are activated with cleavage of caspase-3 substrates and fragmentation of chromosomal DNA.[1011] Other events in alphavirus-induced cell death often include early activation of poly(ADP-ribose) polymerase-1,[684,730] activation of proapoptotic Bcl-2 family member proteins Bad or Bak,[657] loss of mitochondrial membrane integrity, and release of cytochrome c.[66,1015]

Apoptotic death is accelerated by glycoprotein-induced ER stress,[66] sphingomyelinase deficiency,[692] low levels of extracellular Ca++,[1011] expression of Bax,[700] and activation of Bid.[1015] Alphavirus-induced apoptosis can be slowed or prevented by expression of ceramidase,[444] altered Ras signaling,[448,502] expression of p21WAF1/CIP1,[418] expression of Bcl-2 family member and interacting proteins,[337,552,555,561,657,672,700,860,1012,1015] expression of the ER stress protective protein Parkin,[700] mutation of nsP2,[303,700] phosphorylation of protein kinase C-delta (PKCδ),[1115] inhibition of constitutive expression of NF-κB,[564] and caspase inhibition.[686,852,1015] Apoptotic cell death is delayed by the cell type–specific induction of autophagy.[458,486,511]

Autophagy serves for lysosomal degradation of damaged cellular organelles and also for defense against intracellular pathogens.[207,553] Autophagy can be activated by viral stimulation of cellular pattern recognition receptors or cytokines such as IFNγ and can serve to deliver viral nucleic acids to endosomal toll-like receptors (TLRs) to amplify innate responses.[950] Autophagy delays neuronal cell death and facilitates SINV clearance through a selective process by which the adaptor protein p62, along with other selective factors in the autophagy pathway, targets nucleocapsids for delivery to autophagosomes.[541,719,720,951] CHIKV-induced autophagy promotes virus replication in HEK293 cells and mouse embryo fibroblasts (MEFs).[458,511]

Alphavirus-induced vertebrate cell death can also occur by caspase-independent, nonapoptotic mechanisms. Alphaviruses efficiently shut down protein, rRNA, and mRNA synthesis in infected cells,[303,327,621,675] deplete nicotinamide adenine dinucleotide (NAD) and energy stores,[240,1011] and induce dysfunction of Na+K+ATPase causing loss of membrane potential and changes in intracellular cation concentrations.[67,1014] Genome replication without structural protein synthesis can also induce cell death.[1015] For Old World viruses, expression of nsP2 alone is cytotoxic, and this property can be separated from its protease activity and the effects of nsP2 on host transcription.[226,287,303,304,327,617,742,956]

Although immature neurons die by apoptosis, mature neurons are more resistant to apoptotic cell death.[316,379] This resistance is due to an intrinsic ability to suppress virus replication.[153,871,1027] Mature motor neurons, infected by virulent strains of virus, die by a necrotic process and are not protected from death by Bcl-2 family proteins.[379,483] Autophagic clearance of viral proteins may promote neuronal survival.[719]

Persistent infection can occasionally be established in mammalian cell cultures. Mouse fibroblasts producing interferon (IFN), or BHK cells with a high concentration of defective interfering particles, can establish SINV-persistent infection.[427,1064] Infection with SINV or SINV replicons (incomplete genomes that retain replicative ability) that have mutations in the C-terminal methyltransferase-like domain of nsP2 results in reduced viral RNA synthesis, decreased CPE, and persistent infection in some vertebrate cell lines.[11,226,287,288,617,742] Persistent infection can also be established if the cell infected is resistant to virus-induced apoptosis.[117,552,1010,1027]

Effects on Invertebrate Cells

Studies of alphavirus infection of cell lines derived from *Aedes albopictus* (e.g., C6/36, U4.4) and *Aedes aegypti* (e.g., Aag2) mosquito larvae demonstrate fundamental differences in alphavirus replication between vertebrate and invertebrate cells. The time course of virus replication is similar, but there is only a modest effect on host gene expression,[278,853] and persistent noncytopathic infection, or death by a nonapoptotic process,[473] is more common than in vertebrate cells. Infection of mosquito cells does not lead to host cell transcriptional and translational shutoff as seen in vertebrate cells, and this is probably the main factor permitting persistent infection of mosquitoes *in vivo* as well as mosquito cells *in vitro*.[327] Interaction of the nsP3 hypervariable C-terminal domain with SH3-containing domain proteins is particularly important for replication.[636] In culture, virion maturation is often observed within vesicular structures with virion release by exocytosis rather than at the plasma membrane,[640,941] while in polarized cells of the mosquito midgut digestive and salivary gland acinar cells, in vivo maturation generally occurs via budding from the plasma membrane, often in a directed manner.[224,1059]

Virions produced by mosquito cells are relatively deficient in cholesterol (mosquitoes are auxotrophs for cholesterol, which is derived in the adult stage from blood feeding) compared to virions produced by vertebrate cells and have detectable differences in structure and glycosylation of the envelope proteins that can affect infection.[366,386,417,689,931] Recent studies have shown that several alphaviruses produced by mosquito cells are denser than some populations from vertebrate cells, and contain components of the small subunit of the host cell ribosome. These "heavy" virions are more infectious for vertebrate cells than their less dense counterparts from vertebrate cells. However, the "light" particles are more infectious for mosquitoes and induce a stronger innate response in the vector.[600]

The uncloned lines derived from *Ae. albopictus* larvae contain many types of cells with properties representative of different mosquito tissues. Lytic infection occurs in some clones that support high levels of virus replication,[640,984] while persistent infection is associated with a short period of relatively high virus replication followed by a decrease in virus production and in the numbers of cells in the culture that are producing virus.[200,668,669] The decrease in virus production is not associated with activation of the signal transducer and activator of transcription (STAT), immune deficiency (IMD), or toll insect innate response pathways but is associated with decreased processing of the nonstructural polyprotein and expression of the protease inhibitor TEPII.[278,668] However, in *Ae. aegypti* infection, SINV up-regulation of the IMD pathway is dependent on the mosquito microbiome.[62] Transcriptional analysis of persistently infected cells shows an increase in mRNAs associated with vesicle formation and the Notch signaling pathway.[668] Lytic infection can also be induced by viruses engineered to express death-inducing insect proteins such as reaper or Michelob_x.[1038] Insect-specific viruses present in U4.4 cells (and lines from other mosquito species), but not in C6/36 *Ae. albopictus*–derived cell lines, may also affect infection with alphaviruses.[1063] Studies expressing the proapoptotic gene reaper from a SINV vector suggest that apoptosis is also important for controlling alphavirus infection of mosquitoes.[716]

RNAi is an important insect defense mechanism, and modulation of viral replication in mosquito cells is due in large part to the RNAi pathway. SFV infection of U4.4 or Aag2 cells leads to production of viral RNAs derived from replicative dsRNA that are unevenly distributed across the genome and variable in efficiency for mediating antiviral RNAi.[909] This RNAi signal can spread from cell-to-cell and inhibit replication.[46] The RNAi pathway is defective in C6/36 cells,[97] but the IMD, and not the toll innate response pathway, can suppress SINV replication in these cells.[52] The small interfering RNA (siRNA) pathway is regarded as the principal antialphaviral pathway, and CHIKV nsP2 and nsP3 appear to exhibit RNAi suppressor activity.[615] Knockdown of virus-specific PIWI-interacting RNA (piRNA) pathway components in *Ae. aegypti* cells to reduce CHIKV-

specific RNAs does not affect CHIKV replication, suggesting that this pathway is not critical to modulating viral replication. However, knockdown of the helicase Spindle-E (SpnE), essential to the piRNA pathway in *Drosophila melanogaster*, increases CHIKV and SFV replication in *Ae. aegypti cells* independent of the siRNA and piRNA pathways. This suggests a small RNA-independent antiviral function for SpnE.[1021] In addition, *Ae. aegypti* microRNAs appear to modulate CHIKV infection of mosquito cells.[227]

Superinfection Exclusion

Vertebrate and invertebrate cells infected with one alphavirus often cannot be productively infected with the same, or a closely related, alphavirus at a later time. Exclusion is established after translation of the nsP genes of the first virus to enter. The superinfecting genome can be translated, but not replicated[940] possibly due to the presence of the transacting nsP2 protease that prematurely cleaves the replicase polyprotein required for minus-strand synthesis.[474] Experimental coinfection of *Ae. aegypti* by CHIKV and the often cocirculating dengue-2 and Zika flaviviruses does not appear to be less efficient than single-virus infection.[824]

Antigenic Composition

All alphaviruses are related and share common antigenic sites, as revealed by HI and CF tests with polyclonal immune sera[137] and by cytotoxic T-cell lysis of infected cells.[568,670] Antigenic cross-reactivities may confer some cross protection and interfere with sequential alphavirus immunizations.[136,218,344,568,619] These cross-reactivities formed the basis for the original classification into the group A arboviruses (later the alphaviruses) and continue to be a valuable means for initial identification and classification of alphaviruses.[137] Closely related viruses within a serogroup form a complex. Seven broad antigenic complexes have been identified within the alphavirus serogroup: Barmah Forest (BF), EEE, Middelburg (MID), Ndumu (NDU), SF, VEE, and WEE.[524,767,990] However, several more recently discovered alphaviruses have not been extensively characterized antigenically, so their classification into new complexes is based on extrapolation from sequences alone; examples include Trocara,[990] Eilat,[685] and Tai Forest[398] (Table 6.1). The BF, EEE, MID, and NDU complexes each contain only a single virus, while the SF, VEE, and WEE complexes include several viruses. Viruses within each complex can be subtyped using reactivity with mAbs, kinetic HI, or neutralization assays.[128]

Antibodies to E1 are more likely to cross-react with other alphaviruses than are antibodies to E2.[90,424,1094] This is consistent with the documented greater sequence conservation in the E1 protein. Competitive binding assays using mAbs have identified approximately seven epitopes on the E1 glycoproteins of SINV, SFV, WEEV, and VEEV.[90,424,632,814,867] Most E1 epitopes are not exposed on the virion surface but are present on the surface of infected cells or on acid-exposed virions.[19,399,632,867] These transitional epitopes map to domain III in a region buried at the spike interfaces (Fig. 6.4).[1032] The *in vitro* biologic activities of antibodies to E1 include HI, neutralization of virus infectivity, and inhibition of fusion.[19,90,424,867] Neutralizing epitopes map to domains I, II, and III.[558]

Antibodies to E2 are usually alphavirus specific, but can be cross-reactive and block multiple steps in the replication cycle including both entry and egress through cross-linking of

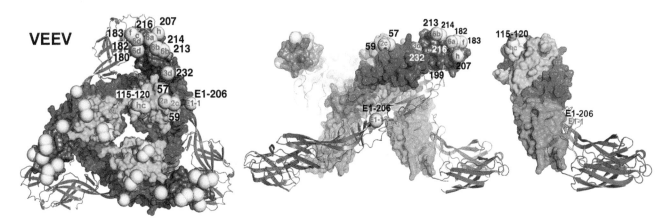

FIGURE 6.4 Neutralization escape mutations and positions affecting host range and tissue tropism mapped on the VEEV spike. Neutralizing antibody escape mutations displayed as yellow spheres on the spike with epitope written in the spheres. E1 is shown in ribbons and E2 in surface rendering using the colors defined in Figure 6.2. The **left panel** shows a top-down view of the spike, the **middle panel** shows the spike from the side, and the **right panel** shows the far right dimer from the middle panel. (Courtesy of Felix Rey and reproduced with permission from Voss JE, Vaney MC, Duquerroy S, et al. Glycoprotein organization of Chikungunya virus particles revealed by X-ray crystallography. *Nature* 2010;468(7324):709–712.).

neighboring spikes.[276] Competitive binding assays using mAbs identify 4 to 5 epitopes on the E2 glycoproteins of SINV, SFV, RRV, and VEEV.[90,482,632,714,814] *In vitro* biologic activities of antibodies to E2 include HI, neutralization of virus infectivity, and blocking of virus binding to the cell surface.[814] Many anti-E2 mAbs have both neutralizing and HI activities suggesting that these functions overlap. Neutralization-escape mutants, naturally occurring variants, λgt11 expression libraries, site-directed mutagenesis of cDNAs, and recombinant viruses have been used to identify amino acids contributing to the various epitopes on E2 and have identified two major neutralizing sites[868,935,1044] that have been mapped onto domain B of the crystal structure of the E1–E2 heterodimer and trimerized spike[558,1032] (Fig. 6.4). This is an exposed hydrophilic region that often includes an N-linked carbohydrate. There are linear, as well as conformational, determinants in this region because these mAbs frequently react in Western blots and recognize λ-fusion proteins, and antibodies to peptides from this region are protective against challenge.[1044]

The second neutralizing epitope on E2 appears to be primarily conformational and is in domain A (Fig. 6.4). This region is responsible for binding to HS and is obscured if pE2 is not cleaved.[1032] Visualization by cryoelectron microscopy of the binding of HS and mAbs to this epitope on SINV and RRV identifies the domain A knob on the glycoprotein spike.[913,1106]

Monoclonal antibodies against EEEV that bind to E2 domains A or B can protect mice and nonhuman primates when administered passively.[107,196,488,916,1050] One CHIKV mAb that bridges domains A and B prevents entry by interfering with movement of the B domain away from the E1 fusion loop.[576] Other mAbs bind a footprint that spans different domains on adjacent E2 proteins[447] or bind the E2 proteins in the plasma membrane to prevent budding by inducing coalescence leaving nucleocapsids accumulating in the cytosol to activate Fc receptors.[446]

Evolution and Phylogeny

Alphaviruses, which replicate in arthropods, birds, reptiles, fish, and mammals, derive from a single unknown protoalphavirus within the alphavirus superfamily of viruses. Viruses in this superfamily, including many RNA plant viruses, have a similar genetic organization and replicase proteins with homologous conserved motifs, but diverse coat proteins.[507] Amino acids important in secondary structure (e.g., cysteines and those close to one another in adjacent β-sheets and α-helices) have been conserved for the glycoproteins E1, E2, and E3, consistent with a similar conserved three-dimensional structure of the virion.[270] Highly conserved regions in the nsP1 and nsP4 genes have allowed for the development of primers to detect a broad range of alphaviruses by RT-PCR.[247,314,357] The most variable regions of the open reading frames are in the C-terminus of nsP3 (hypervariable domain) and the N-terminus of C.[270] Sequence information from the entire genome generally groups the viruses similarly to that derived by antigenic analysis (Fig. 6.5) and has detected at least one ancient recombination event.[368] Criteria for species demarcation of alphaviruses combine genetic, ecological, and antigenic information. Species generally have distinct transmission cycles and differ by more than 23% at the nucleotide level and 10% in amino acid sequence when E1 genes are compared.

The origin of the alphaviruses is unclear. Partial genome sequencing has suggested origins both in the Americas and in the Old World.[333,535,767,1054] Recently, comparison of whole genome sequences from all known alphaviruses has suggested an origin from an ancestor of the louse-borne aquatic alphaviruses[270] (Fig. 6.5). However, the discovery of geographically diverse "insect-specific" alphaviruses,[398,685,986] which infect mosquitoes but are fundamentally defective for replication in vertebrates, suggests that they may represent the ancestral alphaviruses. All of these scenarios require repeated movement across the globe to explain the current virus distributions.

Like other RNA viruses, alphaviruses undergo genetic change primarily by accumulation of point mutations in the genomic RNA, but deletions and duplications also occur, especially in the C-terminal hypervariable domain of the nsP3 gene and the highly variable 3′-untranslated region (UTR).[3,167,268] Mutation occurs at a rate that is slower (1–7 × 10^{-4} substitutions/nucleotide/year) than is estimated for some other RNA viruses,[120,179] presumably because "tradeoff" fitness must be maintained in both insect vectors and vertebrate hosts.[183] Recombination between

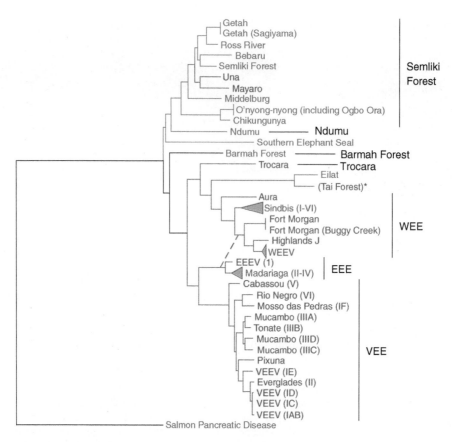

FIGURE 6.5 Unrooted phylogenetic tree of all alphavirus species generated from a conserved region of envelope protein gene nucleotide sequences (2184 nt) using the GTR+I+G substitution model and maximum likelihood method. *Red color* indicates location in the Old World; *green* indicates New World. Parentheses indicate major subtypes; *asterisks* indicates unclassified virus. *Black lines and labels* indicate alphavirus complexes based on antigenic and/or genetic similarities. Abbreviations: EEE, eastern equine encephalitis; VEE, Venezuelan equine encephalitis; WEE, western equine encephalitis. (Courtesy of Rubing Chen.)

alphaviruses can be demonstrated *in vitro*, but is infrequent and usually puts the chimeric virus at a replicative disadvantage.[120,179] However, successful recombination has occurred at least occasionally in nature as evidence by the fact that WEEV is the result of an ancient recombination between EEE- and SIN-like viruses (Fig. 6.5) at the junction of E3 and capsid.[27,270,368,513]

Alphaviruses replicate in and are transmitted horizontally by a wide range of invertebrate, primarily mosquito, species. However, each virus usually has a principal or preferred vector for the enzootic cycle. Most alphaviruses can infect a variety of vertebrates, but have birds, mammals, or fish as their primary amplifying and reservoir hosts (Table 6.1). The specific invertebrate vector and vertebrate host used by an alphavirus typically contribute significantly to determining the enzootic geographic distribution of that virus. Experiments modeling evolution *in vitro* show that fewer mutations accumulate if replication alternates between vertebrate and invertebrate cells, but diversity, fitness, and adaptability are greater with serial passage in a single host system.[185,186,189,343,1049] Experiments employing *in vivo* passage show that serial passage in mosquitoes increases mosquito infection efficiency and passage in vertebrates produces higher viremias in vertebrates, but alternately passaged viruses do not change fitness.[185]

It is hypothesized that host mobility influences alphavirus genetic diversity and evolution in a given geographic region.[179,1053] Viruses using avian enzootic hosts (e.g., EEEV, WEEV, SINV) extend over wide geographic regions and evolve as a few highly conserved genotypes, while viruses using mammalian enzootic hosts with a more limited range of dispersal (e.g., RRV, enzootic VEEV, enzootic CHIKV) evolve within multiple geographically restricted genotypes.[166,599,842] However, human-amplified lineages of CHIKV and equine-amplified strains of VEEV have the opportunity to spread even more rapidly and extensively than do avian-amplified alphaviruses.[1048]

Some strains of alphaviruses associated with epidemics or epizootics are antigenically and biologically distinguishable from enzootic strains. Phylogenetic evidence indicates that, at least for VEEV and some strains of WEEV, the virulent epizootic strains evolve by mutation from avirulent viruses being maintained in the enzootic cycle.[31,82,770,806] For CHIKV, several human-amplified lineages have been evolving independent of the enzootic, African lineages for several years to many decades.[1050]

PATHOGENESIS AND PATHOLOGY IN VERTEBRATES

Excellent and well-studied model systems exist for several alphaviruses, and much of our detailed knowledge about alphavirus pathogenesis comes from investigations in mice. Information from these models will be combined where appropriate with information from studies of humans with alphavirus-induced disease to deduce the pathogenesis of infection. Specifics will be covered in sections on the individual viruses.

Entry

The primary mode of alphavirus transmission to vertebrates is through the bite of an infected insect, most often a mosquito. Mosquitoes salivate during feeding and deposit virus-infected saliva mainly extravascularly.[1006] Saliva virus titers are highest early after the mosquito is infected and sometimes decline, along with transmission rates, after 1 to 2 weeks, but mosquitoes remain infected for life.[642,1023] The high-mannose glycans on virus from mosquitoes inhibit induction of IFN by myeloid DCs,[885] and proteins in saliva further facilitate transmission by skewing the host cellular immune response toward Th2 cytokines.[977]

Sites of Primary Replication

The initial sites of virus replication vary with the virus and host. Mice have received the most extensive study. After subcutaneous inoculation, viruses may infect skeletal muscle or fibroblasts at the local site (e.g., EEEV, WEEV, SFV, RRV, SINV, and Getah virus) or be taken up by and infect Langerhans cells in the skin (e.g., VEEV)[354,404,571,671] (Fig. 6.6). Langerhans cells and DCs transport virus to lymph nodes draining the site of inoculation that also may become infected.[298,596] *In vitro*, human DCs are susceptible to infection with VEEV, but not to infection with CHIKV or EEEV,[296,699,865,929] so the importance of DC infection after mosquito inoculation is likely to differ with the infecting virus.

Spread

Alphaviruses induce a substantial plasma viremia in their amplifying hosts and in hosts susceptible to disease (Fig. 6.7). The ability to mount and sustain a viremia is dependent on the continued efficient production of virus, delivery of virus into the vascular system, and slow clearance from the blood. Animal studies have shown that small-plaque viruses are generally less virulent because they are cleared more rapidly from the circulation than are large-plaque viruses.[436,440,763] This phenomenon is related to the ability of small-plaque viruses to bind HS and thus to be rapidly removed from the circulation by the highly sulfated glycosaminoglycans in the liver.[126] An exception is VEEV, where naturally small-plaque variants produce higher viremia titers in equids, allowing for epizootic amplification.[102] Ability to invade target organs is dependent in part on the duration and height of the viremia, but also on other characteristics of the virus important for tissue invasion.[593]

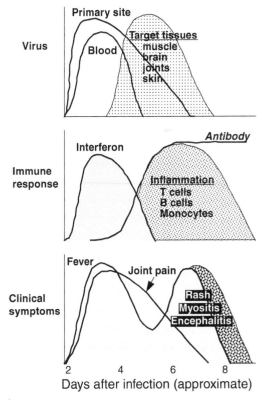

FIGURE 6.7 Schematic diagram of the pathogenesis of alphavirus-induced disease. Viremia may be accompanied by production of interferon and other proinflammatory cytokines and fever. Virus then spreads through the blood to other target tissues. As the immune response is induced, the viremia is terminated, but fever is renewed with appearance of a mononuclear inflammatory response in the infected tissue. In infections that lead to rash and arthritis, joint pain usually appears early after infection and prior to the appearance of the rash.

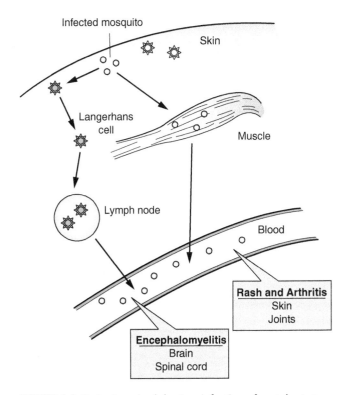

FIGURE 6.6 Basic steps in alphavirus infection of vertebrates. Virus is delivered extravascularly by an infected mosquito and infects local muscle cells or Langerhans cells in the skin. Langerhans cells can carry virus to local lymph nodes where further replication may occur. Virus is delivered to the blood and spreads to target tissues such as skin, joints, and the central nervous system, in addition to distant muscle and lymphatic tissue.

Cell and Tissue Tropism

Viruses that replicate initially in skeletal muscle and lymph nodes near the site of inoculation often spread through the bloodstream to more distant skeletal muscles and other lymphatic tissues. In addition, cardiac myocytes, osteoblasts, brain and spinal cord neurons, and brown fat cells are secondary sites of replication for many alphaviruses in mice (Fig. 6.6).[12,571,652,673] RRV and Getah virus cause polymyositis[404,878]; EEEV, WEEV, SFV, and SINV cause encephalitis[57,298,432,571,1030]; RRV and CHIKV cause arthritis[294,661,1111]; and VEEV causes lymphoid depletion and encephalitis.[319,441,1036]

In humans, the skin is a target for alphaviruses that cause a rash,[284,412,520,604] the joints for alphaviruses that cause arthritis,[283,407,661] muscle for alphaviruses that cause myalgia,[723] and the nervous system for alphaviruses that cause encephalitis.[301,901] RRV and SINV have been recovered from skin biopsies.[519,520,604] RRV replicates in skin basal epidermal and eccrine duct epithelial cells.[284] Human synovial cells support RRV infection in vitro[459] and RRV RNA is detected in synovial biopsy specimens.[923] Joint fluid taken from humans with acute arthritis has not yielded infectious virus, but viral antigen and RNA can be detected in fibroblasts and macrophages and these cells support RRV and CHIKV replication in vitro.[407,459,526]

The mechanism by which encephalitic alphaviruses enter the CNS is not entirely clear. Neuroinvasiveness is a component of virulence that varies between viruses, virus strains, and route of inoculation.[229] Murine studies have shown infection or transport by cerebrovascular endothelial cells,[485,737,924] choroid plexus epithelial cells,[571] olfactory neurons,[127,162,749,823,975,1029] and peripheral nerves.[188] Once within the CNS, virus can spread from cell to cell or through the cerebrospinal fluid (CSF).[431,711,975] For most encephalitic alphaviruses, the targeted cell within the CNS is the neuron[432,571,711] where cellular protein synthesis is suppressed[985] and damage can be severe and irreversible. In mice that recover from neuronal infection, infectious virus is cleared, but viral RNA persists.[278,549,638,1008] SFV, RRV, and VEEV can also cause persistent infection of microglial and oligodendroglial cells leading to demyelination.[122,196,279,878]

Immune Responses

Innate Responses

Early responses to alphavirus infection include production of cytokines and chemokines and activation of natural killer (NK) cells.[338] Type I (α/β) IFN is induced in vivo by many, but not all, alphavirus infections of experimental animals[298,313,439,889,991] and humans[407,832,865,1045] (Fig. 6.7). The amount of IFN produced by infected tissues is usually linked to the level of virus replication, and IFN production continues if virus is not cleared.[118,277,363,407,439,865] IFN rapidly appears in serum, and levels are diminished by splenectomy or failure to replicate in hematopoietic cells, suggesting that lymphoid tissue is one important source.[298,439,504,506]

Different cell systems have been used to determine the mechanisms by which alphaviruses induce and control synthesis of IFN in response to infection. Viruses vary in their ability to induce IFN production by different types of cells,[763,865,889] and the cellular sources of IFN probably differ with time after infection. In tissue culture cell lines, IFN production, shutoff of host protein synthesis, and CPE are controlled by nsP2 (SINV, SFV) or C (VEEV, EEEV).[18,104,288,303,304] In these cells, shutoff of host gene expression suppresses antiviral responses.[18,104,304,1096]

Alphaviruses can also interfere with IFN signaling by decreasing JAK activation and STAT phosphorylation and nuclear translocation.[289,904,905]

The primary source of early IFN in vivo may be plasmacytoid DCs for some alphaviruses,[898] but not for others.[865] SFV induction of IFN by myeloid DCs requires fusion and IFN regulatory factor (IRF)-3, but not replication, and is independent of MyD88.[403] For SINV and RRV, N-linked glycans on E2 are important determinants of IFN production by DCs.[886]

In cells other than DCs, induction of IFN and IFN-stimulated genes (ISGs) requires viral entry and RNA synthesis.[74,1078] Data from ts mutants suggest that formation of dsRNA is the necessary step in replication for IFN induction. NsP1/nsP2 cleavage affects IRF3 activation and IFN induction by SINV without affecting shutoff of host transcription or translation.[194] Viruses with mutations in the protease domain of nsP2, which cannot process the nonstructural polyprotein to initiate plus-strand RNA synthesis, do not induce IFN.[367,609] In infected or transfected fibroblasts and epithelial cells, dsRNA and higher-ordered RNA structures convert host cell RNA into 5′-ppp dsRNA to activate MDA5 and PKR, important intracellular sensors of alphavirus infection,[65,696] and stimulate phosphorylation of IRF3[751,872] and formation of the IRF3/CBP/p300 transcriptional activation complex for induction of immediate early IFNs.[74] This process is independent of mTOR pathway activation.[211] Virulent strains of EEEV do not induce IFN after fibroblast infection, while attenuated strains do, potentially associated with differences in binding to HS.[300]

Production of IFN often follows the initial release of virus from infected cells by 2 to 3 hours[406] and for some but not all alphavirus strains is regulated by whether host protein synthesis is shut off before IFN can be synthesized.[104,119,1078] The ability of CHIKV to induce IFN mRNA and protein is cell type dependent.[865] Primary human monocytes infected by CHIKV produce IFN-α, IL-6, and IL-12.[396] Replication in primary human fibroblasts is controlled by TLR signaling with production of IFN-β mRNA, but no protein because the mRNA is not translated.[397,1078]

IFN is an important part of the host response to alphavirus infection and virus replication is generally sensitive to its effects.[16,191,208,439,545,659,835,885,929,1103] Mutations associated with altered sensitivity to antiviral activities of IFN have been mapped to the 5′ UTR, nsP1, and nsP2,[288,455,819,933,1079] and this variation in sensitivity may or may not correlate with virulence.[32,91,210,425,933,1096]

Animals can be protected from lethal infection if treated with type I IFN or IFN-inducers before or soon after infection.[16,439,461,584,772,879] Animals unable to respond to IFN due to deletions of the α-chain of the IFN receptor or crucial IFN signaling molecules develop more severe disease than wild-type mice.[16,124,191,193,258,277,346,825,834,865,870,884,933,1079] Furthermore, absence of an IFN response allows virus replication in cells previously resistant to infection.[277,833,834,995] IFN appears to primarily limit virus replication early while the adaptive immune response is being induced (Fig. 6.7). Roles for several ISGs have been identified with effects on entry, genome translation, replication complex formation, structural protein synthesis, and morphogenesis.[84,275,970]

Antiviral proteins PKR and RNase L have a limited role in the IFN-induced antiviral response in vitro and in vivo.[836] However, activation of PKR improves the stability of IFN mRNA,[65,872] and RNase L–deficient fibroblasts fail to shut off minus-strand RNA synthesis or form stable replication complexes and establish persistent infection suggesting a role for RNase L in regulating viral RNA synthesis.[857] Several IFN-induced proteins have been demonstrated, often through overexpression studies, to inhibit alphavirus replication *in vitro*, and through studies of transgenic or knockout mice *in vivo*. Transgenic expression of MxA, a large cytoplasmic GTPase, in IFN-α/β receptor-deficient mice results in decreased SFV replication by preventing accumulation of genomic and subgenomic RNA and provides some protection against fatal disease.[387,531] Zinc finger antiviral protein (ZAP/PARP13) is an RNA-binding protein that blocks translation of incoming viral genomic RNA[84,358] by binding to specific viral mRNA sequences, interaction with the host DEAD box helicase p72, and degradation by the RNA-processing exosome.[84,165,359,481,536,597,1103] Viperin (Rsad2) is a conserved multifunctional protein that can bind Fe-S clusters and associates with the cytosolic face of the ER and lipid droplets to inhibit the replication of many viruses.[388,883,967,1103] The large form of 2′-5′-oligoadenylate synthetase (OAS3) is associated with ribosomes and blocks early stages of replication independent of RNase L.[105] Tetherin (Bst2) is a transmembrane protein that blocks alphavirus release from the plasma membrane.[455,717] Tetherin-deficient mice have increased viral loads and decreased inflammatory responses suggesting an additional regulatory role for this ISG.[603] ISG15 is an ubiquitin-like molecule that exerts its antiviral effect by conjugating proteins, and ISG15-deficient mice have increased mortality with increased levels of proinflammatory cytokines.[310,544,545,1070] ISG20 is a nuclear DEDD family 3′-5′ exonuclease that inhibits alphavirus replication by increasing expression of antiviral ISGs such as IFN-induced protein with tetratricopeptide repeats (IFITs).[1065,1103] IFIT1 (ISG56) is a cytoplasmic protein that inhibits translation by binding 5′-ppp or incompletely capped (cap 0) viral RNAs and components of the eIF3 translation initiation complex.[7,260,517,750] IFIT1-deficient mice have increased susceptibility to infection, but virulent alphaviruses with a secondary structural motif in the 5′ UTR escape IFIT1 binding and function.[425,802] IFN-induced transmembrane protein (IFITM)-3 is present in early endosomes and blocks pH-dependent virus fusion required for entry, and deficiency leads to increased viral load in tissues.[759,1072]

IFN may also contribute to alphavirus-induced disease. Fever during the viremic phase of infection, as is seen with CHIKV and RRV, is probably a response to the IFN induced early after infection (Fig. 6.7). It has been postulated that the rapidly fatal disease induced by alphaviruses in newborn mice may be due to the production of large amounts of IFN and proinflammatory cytokines.[991] Acute phase responses induced by alphaviruses prior to the virus-specific adaptive immune response often reflect the extent of virus replication and include up-regulation of TLR expression and increased production of tumor necrosis factor (TNF), interleukin (IL)-1 and IL-6, as well as IFN-α/β.[345,623,865,991,1071] Adult mice deficient in IL-1β have reduced mortality after CNS infection with a neurovirulent strain of SINV, suggesting that cytokine production may also contribute to disease.[560]

Virus-Specific Adaptive Responses

Both cellular and humoral immune responses are induced by infection[275] (Fig. 6.7). In experimentally infected adult mice, antiviral IgM is usually detected in serum within 3 to 4 days after infection.[347,585,725,878] The cellular immune response, manifested by the presence of virus-reactive lymphocytes in draining lymph nodes and blood and the infiltration of mononuclear cells into infected tissues, also appears within 3 to 4 days after infection.[350,620] These responses appear later (7–10 days after infection) in neonatal mice.[889] Both play a role in recovery from infection and protection against reinfection.

Humoral immunity

Virus-specific IgM antibody is detectable very early in human disease, which often provides a means for rapid diagnosis of infection when it is short-lived or when seroconversion is detected, but it can also persist for many months after recovery.[92,129,133,142,148,355,407,519,605,695] Appearance of antibody correlates with cessation of viremia (Fig. 6.7). Virus-specific IgA also appears early in infection, but declines rapidly.[147] IgG antibody is present in serum after 7 to 14 days and is maintained at relatively high levels for years.[131,220] Many lines of evidence support the hypothesis that recovery from alphavirus infection is dependent in large part on the antibody response and that either IgM or IgG is sufficient.[118,351,585,697,761] Rapidity of antibody synthesis within the CNS is predictive of outcome from encephalitis in both mice and humans. Those without evidence of early antibody synthesis are most likely to die.[70,129] Antibody in the periphery can neutralize virus infectivity and promote virus clearance by the reticuloendothelial system in conjunction with complement.

The most extensive experimental studies to define the relevant antibody specificities and the mechanisms of antibody-mediated recovery and protection have been done using VEEV, SFV, CHIKV, and SINV infection of mice. Passive transfer of antibody before or after infection is protective. Both neutralizing and nonneutralizing mAbs against multiple epitopes on the E1, E2, and E3 glycoproteins can protect against alphavirus challenge and promote recovery.[88,89,107,356,424,488,613,632,732,934,1094]

Treatment of immune-deficient mice persistently infected with SINV or SFV with antiviral antibody clears infectious virus from the CNS without causing neurologic damage.[29,551] Similarly, antibody clears CHIKV from the joints of infected mice.[382,383,761] E2-specific mAbs can down-regulate intracellular virus replication *in vivo* and *in vitro* by a nonlytic mechanism.[551,1010] Antibody against an N-terminal peptide of VEEV E2 that is not neutralizing can limit virus replication *in vivo*,[423] and a nonneutralizing mAb to SFV E2 can limit virus replication *in vitro*.[89] Anti-E3 mAbs inhibit production of VEEV.[732] Anti-E1 mAbs may also be able to alter intracellular virus replication.[158]

In vitro studies show that the process by which antibody alters intracellular virus replication requires bivalent antibody, but does not require the Fc portion of the MAb, complement, or other cells.[551,1010] However, the effects of antibody are amplified by treatment of infected cells with IFN-α.[208] Soon after antibody binding, virion budding from the plasma membrane is inhibited.[209] *In vivo* studies also show that IFN and antibody act synergistically to promote recovery and that germ-line IgM as well as IgG is effective, but the mechanisms by which these systems interact have not been identified.[124,190,697]

Clearance of infectious virus is rapid, while the decline in viral RNA occurs more slowly.[549,551,638] After recovery from encephalitis or arthritis, viral RNA often remains detectable in murine tissues for life. Therefore, one consequence of a nonlytic mechanism for clearance of virus from tissue is that the virus genome is not completely eliminated if the originally infected cells survive.[549,551,1008] This leads to a need for long-term control of virus replication that is accomplished in part by infiltration and maintenance of antibody-producing B cells in the CNS.[348,637,638,1008]

Antibody also is important for protection from infection.[656] Inactivated or replication-defective vaccines protect against EEEV, VEEV, and WEEV.[245,781,783] Delivered before or shortly after infection, passive transfer of antibody can protect from acute disease, but may predispose to late disease.[351,490,877]

Cellular immunity

Alphavirus infection induces virus-specific lymphoproliferative, cytokine, and cytotoxic T-cell responses.[2,350] After epidermal virus inoculation, Langerhans cells increase expression of MHC class II antigens and accessory and costimulatory molecules that enhance activation of naïve T cells.[453] The mononuclear inflammatory process in response to alphavirus infection is immunologically specific and includes infiltration of NK cells, CD4+ and CD8+ T lymphocytes, B cells, and macrophages.[428,620,638,646,658] Relative proportions of these mononuclear cells vary with the time after infection.[428,638,646] T cells play a role in virus clearance and in protection from challenge.[242,1100] Cytokines and chemokines increased in plasma during acute disease include IL-4, IL-6, IL-10, IL-12, IL-13, IFNγ, CCL2, and CXCL10.[407,1045] Mice lacking the ability to produce antibody can clear infectious virus from some populations of neurons through production of IFNγ,[85,109] and IFNγ downregulates SINV replication in mature neurons *in vitro* through a JAK-/STAT-dependent mechanism.[116,117] Viral RNA levels in the CNS of SINV-infected mice decrease more rapidly when CD8+ T cells are present.[489] In animals infected with virulent strains of virus, cellular immune responses contribute to tissue damage and fatal disease and can be modulated by regulatory T cells.[340,490,514–516,542,608,683,822] Humans with persistent symptoms have prolonged elevations of IFN, cytokines, and chemokines indicating ongoing immune activation.[175,407,866]

Pathological Changes

Encephalomyelitis

Pathological changes in the CNS of humans with fatal neurologic disease and mice with experimentally induced encephalomyelitis begin with perivascular infiltration of mononuclear and polymorphonuclear inflammatory cells.[620,646,703] Adhesion molecules (e.g., ICAM-1, VCAM-1) are up-regulated on endothelial cells, and integrins LFA-1 and VLA-4 are important mediators of mononuclear cell entry.[429,915,925] This phase of infection may include extravasation of red blood cells and endothelial cell swelling and hyperplasia.[703] Lymphocytes and monocytes move from the perivascular regions to areas of the parenchyma with virus-infected neurons. This inflammatory process is accompanied by gliosis and evidence of inflammatory and glial cell apoptosis.[301]

Neonatal mice and human infants may die with widespread virus-induced neuronal cell death before the inflammatory process, a manifestation of the cellular immune response, can be initiated.[674] Immature neurons die by an apoptotic process,[556] while death of mature neurons may be characterized by cytoplasmic swelling, vacuolation, membrane breakdown, and cellular degeneration suggesting necrosis.[301,379,674] Demyelination has been described as a consequence of EEEV

and WEEV infection in humans[68,702,703] and of WEEV, RRV, and SFV infection of mice, probably as a result of infection of oligodendrocytes.[122,648,880]

Reticuloendothelial Infection

The pathology of VEE in horses includes cellular depletion of bone marrow, spleen, and lymph node tissue and pancreatic necrosis.[496] Small mammals also develop widespread infection of reticuloendothelial system tissues and may develop fatal ileal necrosis.[51,331,1036]

Arthritis

In CHIKV- and RRV-induced arthritis, there is hyperplasia of the synovial lining, vascular proliferation, and mononuclear cell infiltration.[407,923] Synovial fluid contains increased protein, CD4+ T lymphocytes, activated NK cells and macrophages, and increased levels of monocyte chemotactic protein (MCP)-1/CCL2, IL-6, and IL-8.[182,283,407] Evidence of persistent human infection as a cause of chronic arthritis includes the presence of RRV RNA 5 weeks after onset of symptoms[923] and CHIKV antigen and RNA in synovial macrophages 18 months after acute disease.[407]

Rash

Skin biopsies taken from patients with RRV-induced rash show perivascular infiltration of lymphocytes (primarily CD8+ T cells) and monocytes without evidence of immune complex deposition.[284]

Release and Transmission

A common feature of alphaviruses is their transmission by insects and maintenance in a natural cycle of replication in vertebrate and invertebrate hosts. Arthropod vectors become infected by feeding on a viremic host, are able to transmit the virus 2 to 10 days later (extrinsic incubation), and remain persistently infected. Maintenance of this cycle requires an amplifying host that develops a viremia of sufficient magnitude to infect feeding mosquitoes. For many alphaviruses, humans and horses are dead-end hosts unable to infect mosquitoes efficiently due to insufficient viremia. However, human–mosquito–human transmission has been important in epidemics of RRV-, ONNV-, and CHIKV-induced polyarthritis,[586,845,973] and equid–mosquito–equid transmission is important in epizootics of VEE.[810,948]

Other modes of transmission are occasionally important. Horses infected with VEEV may shed virus in nasal, eye, and mouth secretions as well as in urine and milk resulting in the potential for respiratory and oral route.[151,496] CHIKV can also be transmitted through oral secretions from animals with hemorrhagic manifestations[299] and during childbirth.[1052] Aerosol transmission of VEEV, CHIKV, and MAYV has occurred in laboratory settings,[151,464,543,971,981] and aerosolized VEEV has been developed as an agent of biological warfare.[896] EEEV persists in the feather follicles of infected pheasants, and transmission among penned pheasants can occur through feather picking and cannibalism.[854] Person-to-person transmission has not been reported.[543,810]

Veterinary Correlates and Animal Models

WEEV, EEEV, and VEEV, the first alphaviruses to be cultured, came to the attention of virologists because they caused fatal disease in horses and these viruses remain important equine pathogens.[106,219,639] EEEV and WEEV cause encephalitis in horses, while VEEV causes severe respiratory disease associated with leukopenia; encephalitis occurs with some epizootic strains. Getah virus causes an urticarial rash and hind leg edema in horses.[690] WEEV, EEEV, and Highlands J virus (HJV) cause disease in domesticated birds such as chickens, pigeons, pheasants, turkeys, and emus,[54,203,263,273,583,1009] and EEEV causes fatal disease in swine.[243] The alphaviruses associated with arthritis in humans have not been recognized as important causes of disease in animals or birds.

Good small animal models have been developed for many alphaviruses. In mice, alphaviruses generally infect lymphatic tissue, muscle, brown fat, brain, and spinal cord, but the extent and relative importance of infection at these sites differ among these viruses. For instance, RRV and Getah virus cause primarily myositis, VEEV causes reticuloendothelial infection, and WEEV and EEEV cause encephalitis with neurons as the main target cells.[12,643,673] In mice infected with relatively avirulent strains of SFV, RRV, and VEEV, the acute encephalitic phase is accompanied by infection of oligodendroglial cells and demyelination.[122,880] For all alphaviruses, fatal disease in immunocompetent mice is usually associated with CNS infection even if encephalitis is not a manifestation of the human infection. For instance, SINV and SFV infections of mice are studied as models for acute viral encephalitis although these viruses usually cause fever, arthritis, or rash, and rarely CNS disease, in humans.[10,431,598,614,1007] Specifics of these animal model systems are discussed with the individual viruses.

Virulence

Virulence is a measure of the ability of the virus to cause fatal or severe disease. For most alphaviruses, this usually reflects the severity of neurologic disease, but disease in other organs can also reflect viral virulence. Outcome is influenced by characteristics of both the host and the virus. An early virus determinant of virulence is induction of IFN and susceptibility to IFN-mediated inhibition of replication. Viruses that induce IFN and are susceptible to IFN are generally attenuated.[16,119,194,288,300,905,933,1079] Most alphaviruses show an age-dependent susceptibility to disease.[12,98,363,673,711,878] Resistance increases with maturation and is associated with decreased virus replication in tissues at the site of virus inoculation and in target tissues (e.g., brain) and not with changes in induction of IFN or the ability of infected mice to mount a virus-specific immune response[347,354,673] although older mice increase ISG12 while young mice do not.[528] Avirulent alphavirus strains may replicate poorly even in newborn animals, while virulent strains can usually replicate well and cause disease in adult as well as newborn animals. The ability of a virus strain to cause fatal disease or a particular complication of infection is also often dependent on the genetic background of the host,[225,514,936,975,1001] but the genetic determinants of susceptibility are just beginning to be identified.[514,976]

For encephalitic alphaviruses, another viral determinant of virulence is their ability to enter the CNS efficiently (neuroinvasiveness). Many alphavirus strains can cause fatal disease after intracerebral or intranasal inoculation, but not after subcutaneous or intraperitoneal inoculation, while others cause fatal disease after peripheral inoculation as well. The duration of viremia often correlates with virulence with virulent strains having slower clearance and sustaining longer viremias than avirulent strains.[437,438,440] Peripheral replication, viremia, neuroinvasiveness, and neurotropism (ability to replicate in CNS cells) all contribute to virulence.

The viral determinants of virulence have been most extensively studied in murine models for SINV, SFV, RRV, CHIKV, and VEEV infections. Viruses with altered virulence have been selected after chemical mutagenesis,[64,113] by passage in tissue culture,[75,202,484,554,964] by passage in mice,[351,629,964] by isolation of mAb escape mutants[1034] or plaque variants,[436] and by manipulation of cDNA virus clones. Nucleotide and amino acid changes affecting virulence have been mapped to the 5′ UTR, nsP1, nsP2, nsP3, E1, and E2, particularly the receptor-binding regions of the A and B domains[1032] (Fig. 6.4). Specifics are covered in the sections dealing with each of these viruses.

Persistence

There is substantial evidence that alphaviruses can persist after appearance of an immune response and clearance of infectious virus from the circulation and from tissue.[550] An active inflammatory process is present in CNS tissue from human cases of progressive WEEV months to years after resolution of acute encephalitis.[701,703] Viral RNA and proteins can be detected in the nervous system long after recovery of mice from SINV- or SFV-induced encephalitis and in the joints of humans and mice with CHIKV- and RRV-induced arthritis.[225,353,383,407,485,550,638,923,1008] It is postulated that this persistence of RNA is due to failure of the virus or the immune system to eliminate infected cells. Interestingly, passive antibody protection predisposes to transmission persistent infection and the late onset of progressive disease.[490,877]

Congenital Infection

Alphaviruses can be transmitted transplacentally. This has been documented in mice for RRV, SFV, VEEV, and Getah virus[1,38,641,932] and in humans for RRV, WEEV, VEEV, and CHIKV.[5,285,467,891,988] In mice, the virus infects the placenta where it is able to persist and spread to the fetus despite the development of maternal antibody. The outcome of fetal infection is dependent on the timing of infection relative to transfer of maternal antiviral IgG to the fetus. Fetuses are protected if transfer occurs prior to infection, but transfer of antibody after fetal infection does not mediate recovery.[641] In monkeys, congenital infection with VEEV induces malformations of the brain and eye.[575] In humans, no abnormalities were observed in infants infected with RRV at 11 to 19 weeks' gestation; however, earlier infection may lead to fetal death.[5] Epidemics of VEE are associated with increases in spontaneous abortion.[810,1057] No effect on pregnancy outcome was identified during the CHIKV outbreak on Réunion Island,[285] although perinatal infection rates have approached 50% in Latin America.[988]

PATHOGENESIS AND PATHOLOGY IN MOSQUITOES

The ability of alphaviruses to infect mosquitoes efficiently with dissemination to and replication in the salivary glands is essential for maintaining the natural cycle of transmission. Not all mosquitoes taking a blood meal from a viremic host will become infected, and not all infected mosquitoes develop disseminated infections required for transmission. Many alphaviruses preferentially infect a narrow range of mosquito species, and this host specificity plays an important role in determining the geographic distribution of the virus. Even within a species, strains of mosquitoes may vary in susceptibility to infection. *Ae. albopictus* collected from different geographic regions show differences in susceptibility to infection with CHIKV and in the amount of virus produced after infection.[972] Field and laboratory populations of *Culex tarsalis* differ in susceptibility to WEEV.[413] These differences may reflect geographic genetic variation or differences in the microbiome composition, which can affect innate immune activity and responses as well as susceptibility and transmission. Strains of virus also differ in their abilities to infect mosquitoes, and laboratory-adapted strains may establish infection relatively inefficiently.[676,875,876,1019,1023]

The extrinsic incubation period, or time between taking an infected blood meal and ability to transmit infection, is dependent on the rapidity of virus replication and dissemination to the salivary glands. This period is relatively short (2–7 days) for alphaviruses compared to other arboviruses.[228,875]

Entry and Sites of Primary Replication

Posterior midgut epithelial cells are the initial sites of infection,[100,677,753,873,1059] and infection is facilitated when virus in the serum is concentrated next to these cells as the blood meal clots (Fig. 6.8).[1061] Susceptibility of mosquitoes to alphavirus infection is determined in large part by the ability of the virus to infect midgut epithelial cells.[413,487,875] Changes both in the virus and vector can affect this interaction.[1090] WEEV rapidly fuses with microvillar membrane preparations from *Cx. tarsalis* mosquitoes, and both WEEV and CHIKV bind better to membranes from susceptible mosquitoes than to membranes from refractory mosquitoes[413,666] consistent with a role for viral

structural proteins as determinants of vector specificity, midgut infection, and dissemination.[753,1000,1020,1023] Natural mutations in both the E2 and E1 proteins of CHIKV increase initial infection of *Ae. albopictus* midgut cells to permit more efficient transmission by this invasive species.[998,999] nsP3, a determinant of vector transmission by ONNV, the only alphavirus transmitted by *Anopheles* mosquitoes, is sufficient to confer CHIKV infection competence for these mosquitoes.[676,858]

Receptors for mosquito infection by alphaviruses remain enigmatic. The high-affinity laminin receptor A can serve as a receptor for VEEV and SINV on the surface of C6/36 larval *Ae. albopictus* cells,[581,1040] and proteins of 60 and 38 kDa have been identified as putative receptors for CHIKV on brush-border membranes from *Ae. aegypti.*[666] However, the roles of these proteins remain unclear because their distribution does not explain alphavirus–vector specificity. The recently identified cell adhesion molecule Mxra8, which serves as a receptor for arthritogenic, but not encephalitic alphavirus infection of vertebrate cells, does not appear to have a mosquito ortholog.[1108]

Host cell membrane cholesterol levels affect the efficiency of alphavirus entry.[579] Mosquitoes, like other insects, do not synthesize cholesterol and obtain sterols needed for reproduction and development from dietary blood. Cholesterol-independent mutants of SFV replicate better than parental SFV in cholesterol-depleted C6/36 cells and in adult *Ae. albopictus* mosquitoes.[20]

Replication in midgut epithelial cells is regulated by the RNAi innate antiviral response that is triggered by virus-derived dsRNA and siRNAs.[138,476,487,678] RNAi affects infection rate of the midgut, intensity of infection, and virus dissemination to secondary tissues and is probably an important determinant of vector competence, which depends on modulating virus replication to allow the vector to survive for transmission.[476,487] In addition to small RNAs, CHIKV-infected mosquitoes generate a viral-derived DNA (vDNA) that is essential for viral tolerance and survival.[321]

Spread

For the mosquito to become capable of transmission after a viremic blood meal, virus must disseminate from the midgut into the hemocoel to reach the salivary glands via the hemolymph.[875] Virus buds primarily from the basolateral surface of the infected midgut epithelial cells and accumulates next to the basal lamina,[875] a layered structure composed of mucopolysaccharide that acts as a barrier to hemocoel entry. Dissemination of SINV from the midgut of *Ae. aegypti* mosquitoes is dependent on expression of endosomal proteins UNC93A and synaptic vesicle-2.[139] Replication of ONNV in *Anopheles gambiae* is controlled by expression of heat shock protein cognate 70B.[902,903] Although the basal lamina surrounding the midgut appears to be a major barrier to dissemination, it is degraded by matrix metalloproteinases during blood meal digestion, probably providing an opportunity for virus escape into the hemocoel.[223] Infected midgut epithelial cells can degenerate and slough into the lumen 36 to 48 hours after infection, and this process may facilitate penetration of the virus into the hemocoel.[875,1060]

Infection of salivary gland acinar cells requires that the virus again traverse a basal lamina, a process that may depend on hemolymph titer and replication in adjacent organs such as the fat body, an important site for virus amplification.[1047,1059]

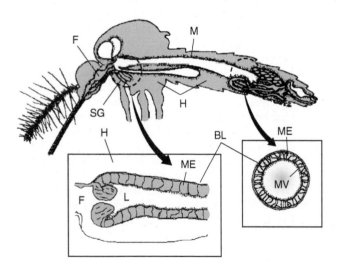

FIGURE 6.8 Diagram of mosquito internal anatomy showing the essential sites for alphavirus infection. BL, basal lamina; L, lumen; F, foregut; M, midgut; ME, midgut epithelium; MV, microvilli or brush border; SG, salivary gland. (Adapted from Weaver SC, Scott TW, Lorenz LH, Lerdthusnee K, Romoser WS. Togavirus-associated pathologic changes in the midgut of a natural mosquito vector. *J Virol* 1988;62(6):2083–2090.)

Other organs may or may not become infected. In addition to the midgut, EEEV infects the fat body, muscle, and salivary glands without involving the nervous system or the ovarioles,[873,1059] while VEEV infects the nervous system[1047] and SINV infects respiratory tissue.[96]

Once salivary gland infection is established, virus matures by budding into apical cavities or randomly into vesicles, basolaterally and apically. This process may be associated with cytopathic changes in the salivary glands.[642] The rapidity of virus replication and dissemination to the salivary glands is dependent on the ambient temperature and can be as short as 2 to 3 days for EEEV[875] or CHIKV.[228] Higher temperatures may accelerate the alphavirus transmission cycle in warm months,[795,1003] although WEEV transmission by *Cx. tarsalis* can decrease with temperatures greater than 30°C.[796] In general, virus content of an individual mosquito reaches a peak within 4 to 7 days after infection.[642,875] Some tissues (e.g., fat body) produce large amounts of virus, while others (e.g., head ganglia) produce small amounts and others (e.g., ovarioles and malpighian tubules) remain virus-negative.[640]

Vector competence for alphaviruses is also dependent on the microbiome[34,62] and the introduction of endosymbiotic *Wolbachia* bacteria into *Ae. aegypti* and *Ae. albopictus* decreases vector competence for CHIKV[25,655,667]; conversely, CHIKV infection alters the microbiome diversity in *Ae. albopictus*.[1114] In a *Drosophila* cell culture model, a comparable effect of *Wolbachia* on SFV infection involves early inhibition of viral genome replication without a role for the bacterial transcriptional response of the insect cell small RNA pathways.[778]

For transovarial transmission to occur, virus must be able to infect oocytes early in development. Failure to infect ovarioles precludes efficient transovarial transmission of most alphaviruses.[96,213,873,1047] However, the presence of RRV and CHIKV in field-caught male mosquitoes suggests that vertical transmission can occur.[565,784,978] Eggs can also be infected after they have been fertilized. Low levels of vertical transmission have been documented in the laboratory for RRV in *Aedes vigilax*, for SINV in *Aedes australis*, and for CHIKV in *Ae. aegypti* and *Ae. albopictus*,[174,616,721] and venereal transmission of the latter has also been reported.[616] Vertical transmission in nature has been reported for RRV, SINV, and WEEV.[213,291,565] However, reports of the persistence of CHIKV RNA without the presence of infectious virus after putative vertical transmission underscore the need to perform infectious assays rather than relying on RT-PCR alone.[1088]

Pathology, Persistence, and Host Response

Although generally considered to be benign for the invertebrate vector, alphavirus infection may generate CPEs in the vector midgut and can reduce survival and reproductive capacity.[874,875] The IMD pathway of innate immunity can be activated by infection to decrease virus replication.[52] Suppression of the RNAi response increases virus replication and mosquito mortality after infection.[180,476] Mosquitoes generally remain infected and infectious for life,[642,875] although WEEV transmission efficiency decreases with time after peaking about 7 to 10 days after oral infection.[796] In the fat body and salivary glands, EEEV infection is persistent, although titers decline after the acute phase of infection, decreasing efficiency of transmission.[873,1059]

ALPHAVIRUSES ASSOCIATED PRIMARILY WITH ENCEPHALITIS

Eastern Equine Encephalitis

EEE was first recognized as a disease of horses in the northeastern United States. In the summer of 1831, more than 75 horses died in 3 coastal counties of Massachusetts.[372] Between 1845 and 1912, epizootics were recorded on Long Island, in North Carolina, New Jersey, Florida, Maryland, and Virginia.[372,875] The virus responsible for EEE was first isolated in 1933 from the brains of affected horses in New Jersey and Virginia during a widespread outbreak that also involved coastal areas of Delaware and Maryland.[106] A South American virus originally considered a subtype of EEEV, but recently reclassified to the species *Madariaga virus* (MADV), was first isolated in 1936 from a horse in Argentina.[838] Although human EEE was suspected earlier, it was not demonstrated until 1938 when an outbreak in the northeastern United States resulted in 30 cases of fatal encephalitis in children living in the same areas as equine cases. At that time, EEEV was isolated from the CNS of humans, as well as from pigeons and pheasants.[273,1062]

Based on seasonality, location of cases near salt-marsh areas, lack of evidence of transmission from horse-to-horse through contact, short period of equine viremia, and geographic distribution of cases, it was postulated that insects transmitted infection and that birds were likely to be the reservoir hosts.[966] The first arthropod isolates were actually from chicken mites and lice that can transmit infection only inefficiently.[234,875] Transmission of EEEV by *Aedes sollicitans* in the laboratory was accomplished in 1934,[635] and subsequently multiple *Aedes* species were shown to be competent vectors. However, recovery of EEEV from naturally infected mosquitoes did not occur until 1949 with isolates from *Mansonia perturbans* in Georgia[415] and *Culiseta melanura* in Louisiana.[157] Subsequent work showing the competence of *Cs. melanura* and a consistent association between infected birds and the isolation of virus from this vector has led to the current understanding that *Cs. melanura* is the primary enzootic vector for North American EEEV (NA-EEEV) strains.[35,197,538,875] However, in some Gulf Coast regions, *Culex* mosquitoes are considered the primary enzootic vectors.[195]

Epidemiology

NA-EEEV causes localized outbreaks of equine, pheasant, and human encephalitis in the summer. NA-EEEV is enzootic in North America from Maine southward along the Atlantic seaboard and Gulf Coast to Texas, in the Caribbean, and in Central America[312] (Fig. 6.9). Inland foci exist in the Great Lakes region and have extended to South Dakota and Quebec.[170,567] In the northeastern United States, the primary enzootic cycle is maintained in shaded swamps where the vector is the ornithophilic mosquito *Cs. melanura*[35,875] (Fig. 6.10). Modeling suggests that in Florida, transmission is associated with tree plantations and cardinal abundance.[251,477] In most locations, birds are the primary reservoir host and many species are susceptible to infection.[495] The amplifying species for NA-EEEV are wading birds, migratory passerine songbirds, and starlings.[197,250,503,625] Young birds are probably important

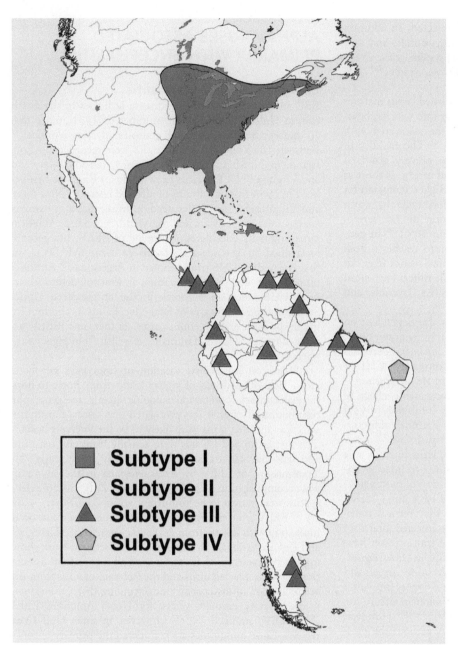

FIGURE 6.9 Geographic distribution of EEEV. The map shows the locations for isolation of NA-EEEV (subtype I) and the three SA-EEEV lineages (subtypes I, II, and III; now Madariaga virus) (From Weaver SC, Powers AM, Brault AC, Barrett AD. Molecular epidemiological studies of veterinary arboviral encephalitides. *Vet J* 1999;157(2):123–138.)

for virus amplification because they are more susceptible to infection, have a prolonged viremia, and are less defensive toward mosquitoes.[197] In addition to occasional mammalian blood feeding by *Cs. melanura*,[650] multiple mosquito species, such as *Coquillettidia perturbans*, Ae. (*Ochlerotatus*) *canadensis*, and various *Aedes* species, may serve as bridge vectors for transmission to susceptible mammals.[35,195,645,875] In temperate areas, the virus is probably periodically reintroduced from subtropical areas of year-round transmission by migratory viremic birds or wind-borne infected mosquitoes.[881,1056,1077,1099] Reptiles and amphibians with viremias that are prolonged and persist through hibernation may maintain the virus focally.[86,195,335,1076] There is no convincing evidence for overwintering in mosquitoes and ovarioles are not involved after experimental EEEV infection of *Cs. melanura*.[873]

MADV, originally comprising three antigenic South American subtypes of EEEV (SA-EEEV), is enzootic in Central and South America including the Amazon Basin (Fig. 6.9).[155] In South and Central America, the enzootic cycle is maintained in moist forests where *Culex* (*Melanoconion*) spp. appear to be the primary vectors.[875,1005] Forest-dwelling rodents, bats, and marsupials are frequently infected and may provide a reservoir, but these transmission cycles are not well characterized.[36,875]

Morbidity and mortality

EEEV is the most virulent of the encephalitic alphaviruses with a high mortality due to encephalitis. Most cases are associated with exposure to wooded areas adjacent to swamps and marshes[128] with more cases in males than females.[259,567] Children under 10 years of age are most

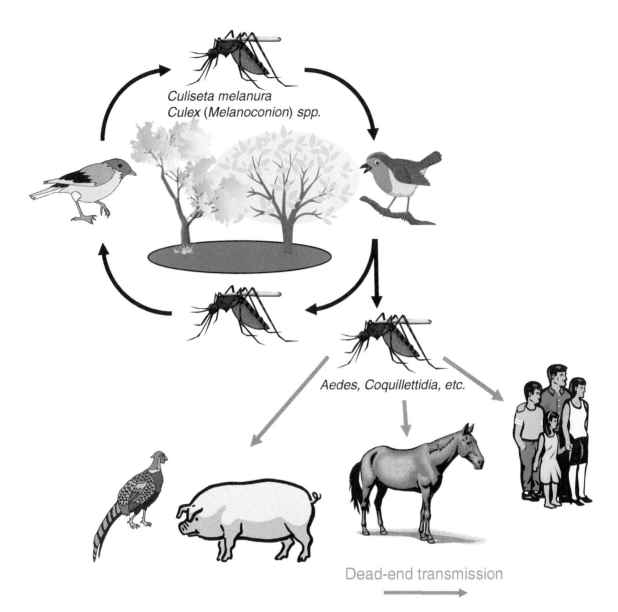

FIGURE 6.10 Enzootic transmission cycle of EEEV in North America. This is an example of an alphavirus that uses a species of mosquito with different host preferences to bridge from the enzootic avian-ornithophilic mosquito (*Culiseta melanura*) cycle to infect mammals such as humans and horses. In Alabama, *Culex* (*Melanoconion*) spp. mosquitoes with broader host feeding patterns serve as enzootic EEEV vector, as they do for the closely related Madariaga virus in Central and South America, where rodents may also serve as enzootic hosts in addition to birds. Similar mechanisms are operative in transmission of Sindbis virus to humans.

susceptible[259] with 1 in 8 infections resulting in encephalitis compared to 1 in 23 for adults.[322] The case-fatality rate was 60% to 70% in earlier studies and 30% to 50% in more recent studies, with the highest rates in children and the elderly[246,680,660,682,683] Most strains of MADV appear to be much less virulent, but lineage III viruses can cause fever and encephalitis.[17,87,146,155,217,837]

Origin and spread of epidemics
In the northern part of the North American range, human and equine cases of EEE occur between July and October, while in the southern region, cases can occur throughout the year.[775] In the Caribbean, outbreaks appear to be linked to virus introduction by southbound migratory songbirds.[875] In North America,

human and equine cases usually occur near hardwood freshwater swamps maintaining enzootic transmission among passerine birds. Outbreaks are initiated when the virus spreads from the enzootic cycle involving ornithophilic mosquitoes into mosquito populations that feed on a wider variety of hosts (Fig. 6.10). Multiple species of mosquitoes with catholic feeding habits have been implicated as potential bridge vectors in different regions.[35,195,645,712,851,875]

Cases of equine encephalitis are usually the first indication of an outbreak. In the absence of equid immunization, epizootics appear approximately every 5 to 10 years and are associated with heavy rainfall and warmer water temperatures that increase the populations of enzootic and epizootic mosquito vectors.[547] Many epidemics have occurred in Massachusetts and surrounding states,[259,567] but the largest recorded outbreak

Eastern Equine Encephalitis: US

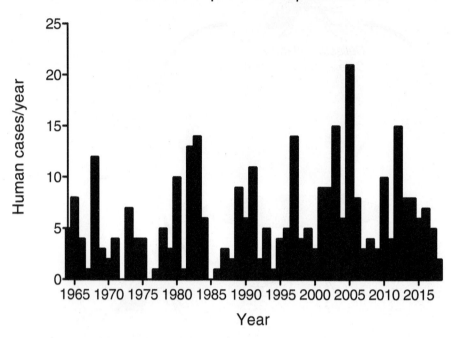

FIGURE 6.11 Numbers of human cases of eastern equine encephalitis reported annually in the United States since 1964. Based on data from the Centers for Disease Control and Prevention.

occurred in 1947 in Louisiana and Texas with 14,344 cases of equine encephalitis and 11,722 horse deaths. The virus is widespread, but since 1955, only an average of 8 cases of EEE have been diagnosed in humans each year[567] (Fig. 6.11). Recently, outbreaks and enzootic EEEV activity have been detected as far north as Vermont, Maine, and Nova Scotia, suggesting a northward expansion.[78,567,580,859] As of late October, 2019, more than 30 human EEE cases were reported in the United States, the most in over 50 years (https://www.cdc.gov/easternequine-encephalitis/index.html).

Molecular epidemiology

Antigenic differences between EEEV and MADV (formerly SA-EEEV) have long been recognized,[150] and the viruses can be distinguished by reactivity with mAbs to the E1 glycoprotein,[815] as well as by neutralization assays.[101] Based on their sequence divergence as well as ecologic and pathogenesis differences, the three SA-EEEV lineages were recently classified as a different alphavirus species, MADV.[37] Sequence comparisons indicate that EEEV/MADV has evolved independently in North and South America for thousands of years or longer reaching 23% to 24% nucleotide and 9% to 11% amino acid sequence divergence.[37] There is one lineage of EEEV and three lineages of MADV: on the coasts of South and Central America (originally EEEV lineage II), in the Amazon Basin (lineage III), and in Brazil (lineage IV)[101,1056] (Fig. 6.9). Isolates of EEEV are highly conserved, differing over a large geographic range and nearly 100 years by less than 3% in nucleotide sequence consistent with birds as highly mobile vertebrate reservoir hosts. The calculated annual nucleotide substitution rates are 2.1×10^{-4} for MADV and 2.7×10^{4} for EEEV.[101,1056] EEEV enzootic in Florida appears to be the source of frequent introductions

into the northeastern United States.[957] The two main lineages of MADV (II and III) exhibit 17% to 21% nucleotide divergence and 3% to 5% amino acid divergence and are evolving at a slower rate (1.2×10^{-4} substitutions/nt/year).[37] MADV lineages appear to be evolving locally, consistent with small mammals as the reservoir hosts.[37,1053,1056] The recent detection of MADV in Haiti suggests a possible expansion in its geographic range.[87]

Clinical Disease and Pathology

Illness caused by infection with EEEV may consist of 1 to 2 weeks of fever, chills, malaise, and myalgias followed by recovery. In cases of encephalitis, these prodromal symptoms are followed by the fulminant onset of increased headache, vomiting, restlessness, irritability, seizures, obtundation, and coma.[206,254,259,901] Meningismus is frequent, and focal signs including cranial nerve palsies and hemipareses are not uncommon.[206,775] Hyponatremia due to inappropriate secretion of antidiuretic hormone is a common complication, and edema of the face and extremities has been noted.[206,254] Death typically occurs 2 to 10 days after onset of encephalitis.

CSF examination shows increased pressure and white cell counts ranging from 10 to 2,000/μL. Polymorphonuclear leukocytes are often abundant early in disease with a shift to mononuclear cells over the first few days of illness.[206,900] The presence of red blood cells or xanthochromia is not uncommon.[775] CSF protein levels are increased, while glucose is low to normal.[254,775] EEG findings are relatively nonspecific, usually showing slowing.[206] CT scans may be normal or show only edema.[206,775] Magnetic resonance imaging (MRI) scans are more often abnormal with focal lesions most commonly observed in the thalamus, basal ganglia, and brainstem.[206]

Poor outcome is predicted by high CSF white cell count or severe hyponatremia, but not by the size of the radiographic lesions.[206] Recovery is more likely in individuals who have a long (5–7 days) prodrome and do not develop coma.[775,900] Sequelae, including paralysis, seizures, and cognitive deficits, are common, with 35% to 80% of survivors, particularly children, having significant long-term neurological impairment.[206,254,259]

Histopathology on fatal cases demonstrates a diffuse meningoencephalitis with edema, widespread neuronal destruction, perivascular cuffing with polymorphonuclear as well as mononuclear leukocytes, and vasculitis with vessel occlusion in the cortex, basal ganglia, and brainstem. The spinal cord is frequently spared.[254,274,937] Virus antigen is localized to neurons and neuronal death is marked by cytoplasmic swelling and nuclear pyknosis.[301,901] Apoptotic glial and inflammatory cells are frequently found in the regions of affected neurons.[254,301]

Veterinary Correlates, Host Range, and Animal Models

EEEV is an important cause of disease in horses, pheasants, emus, and turkeys and can also cause encephalitis in penguins, sheep, deer, dogs, seals, and pigs.[69,203,273,360,583,618,854,962] Horses develop signs of depression, progressive incoordination, seizures, and prostration. The case-fatality rate is 80% to 90%. Most survivors are left with neurologic sequelae.[875] Birds vary in their susceptibility, with some species developing disease, while many others show no morbidity or mortality despite a prolonged viremia.[495,583] Chickens, turkeys, emus, and whooping cranes often develop fatal viscerotropic disease with multifocal necrosis in the heart, kidney, and pancreas and lymphoid depletion in the thymus, spleen, and bursa.[203,360,1009] Pheasants develop encephalitis with 50% to 70% mortality, while penguins develop nonfatal encephalitis.[583,854]

Laboratory studies of macaques, marmosets, mice, guinea pigs, and hamsters generally confirm the neurovirulence of EEEV for mammals.[106,274,571,725,823,937,1030,1095] Peripheral replication is in fibroblasts, skeletal muscle, and osteoblasts, while macrophages are resistant to infection due to restriction by hematopoietic cell–specific miRNA 142-3p.[992,1030] Macaques and marmosets develop encephalitis, while New World *Aotus* owl monkeys develop viremia without evidence of disease.[248] EEEV can initiate CNS infection in experimental animals by infecting choroid plexus epithelial cells or olfactory neurons.[571,937] Young mice show extensive neuronal damage and rapid death.[1030] Older mice are more resistant to peripheral inoculation, but can develop fatal disease and after intracerebral inoculation develop seizures and die rapidly.[298,571] Guinea pigs develop encephalitis after aerosol exposure to EEEV with neuronal death, inflammation, and vasculitis.[823] Hamsters develop a biphasic fatal illness with hepatitis and lymphatic organ infection followed by encephalitis characterized by extensive vasculitis and microhemorrhages.[725]

Virulence

EEEV is generally more virulent than MADV in humans and most experimental animals.[16,155,875] Construction of chimeric viruses and testing in mice indicate that both structural and nonstructural proteins contribute to virulence.[13] Viruses with a temperature-sensitive, small-plaque phenotype and decreased virulence for mice and hamsters have been selected after chemical mutagenesis.[113] One determinant of the neurovirulence of

EEEV is the ability to bind HS. Increased E2 HS binding and miR2142-3p are associated with decreased tropism for lymphoid tissue and production of little IFN leading to increased likelihood of virus spread to the CNS.[297,298,992,993]

Diagnosis, Treatment, and Prevention

Diagnosis is based on virus isolation, detection of RNA, or serology (IgM or seroconversion for IgG). Virus can be isolated from CSF, blood, or CNS tissue by inoculation into newborn mice or a variety of tissue culture cells. Detection and identification of virus in field and clinical samples can also be accomplished through various nucleic acid amplification assays.[529] Antibody is usually measured by enzyme immunoassay (EIA) with detection of IgM in serum and CSF particularly useful.[129,130] Although specific therapies are in development for EEE,[456] currently treatment is supportive.[790]

Infection in mosquito populations can be monitored by virus isolation, by nucleic acid amplification, or by seroconversion of sentinel pheasants or chickens. This information can be used to guide insecticide spraying to reduce adult and larval mosquito populations and prevent human cases. A formalin-inactivated vaccine (EEEV PE-6) is available for horses and emus and for investigational use in humans to protect laboratory workers. This vaccine does not induce significant neutralizing or anti-E2 antibody to MADV.[944] Experimental vaccines include replicon particles and chimeric viruses and rationally attenuated viruses.[246,729,786,823]

Western Equine Encephalitis

Epizootics of viral encephalitis in horses were described in 1908 in Argentina, and in 1912, 25,000 horses were estimated to have died in the central plains of the United States.[838] In the summer of 1930, a similar epizootic occurred in the San Joaquin Valley of California causing an estimated 6,000 cases of equine encephalitis. During this outbreak, WEEV was isolated from the brains of two affected horses by intraocular inoculation of another horse, and this virus was subsequently used to infect other animals.[639] WEEV was suspected at that time to be a cause of human disease, and in 1938, WEEV was recovered from the brain of a child with fatal encephalitis.[415]

Mosquitoes were implicated in WEEV transmission when it was demonstrated that horses developed a viremia[414] and that experimentally infected *Ae. aegypti* mosquitoes were capable of transmitting the virus to horses.[478] However, it was not until the summer of 1941 during a widespread epidemic in the northern plains of the United States and Canada that the virus was isolated from naturally infected *Cx. tarsalis* mosquitoes.[371] Subsequently, WEEV was isolated from *Cx. tarsalis* in other epizootic sites and recognized to be the principal vector.

Other New-World WEEV Complex Viruses

The WEE complex in the New World includes three viruses in addition to WEEV: HJV, Fort Morgan virus (FMV, including the subtype Buggy Creek), and Aura virus.[132] These viruses have different ecological niches and vary in virulence. Only WEEV is recognized to cause human disease.[128] Viruses in the WEE complex found in the Old World (e.g., SINV and Whataroa virus) are discussed in the section on SINV. WEEV, HJV, and FMV all belong to the lineage that diverged since recombination between a SIN-like virus and an EEE-like virus.[368] Aura virus is a "prerecombinant" virus (Fig. 6.5).

Highlands J virus

WEEV-like viruses were first isolated in the eastern part of the United States in 1952, and in 1960, the prototype HJV was isolated from a blue jay in Florida.[393] HJV is enzootic on the U.S. East Coast and is maintained in a cycle similar to that of EEEV with *Cs. melanura* the primary vector and migrating birds the primary reservoir. All alphaviruses in the WEEV complex isolated in the eastern United States are strains of HJV.[385] Rates of divergence of WEEV and HJV of 0.1% to 0.2% per year have been estimated.[179] HJV can occasionally cause encephalitis in horses[469] and is a recognized pathogen for a variety of avian species including turkeys, pheasants, partridges, ducks, emus, hawks, and whooping cranes.[26,263,360,1056]

Fort Morgan, Buggy Creek, and Stone Lakes viruses

FMV and its close relatives Buggy Creek virus (BCRV) and Stone Lakes virus have been isolated from cliff swallows, sparrows, and swallow nest bugs.[99,384,411] These viruses are found primarily in the western regions of North America[724,745] and are transmitted to swallows and sparrows that parasitize swallow nests by cimicid swallow nest bugs (*Oeciacus vicarius*).[110,112,135,708] These viruses cause encephalitis in nestling house sparrows, but are not recognized as pathogens for humans.[707]

Aura virus

Aura virus was isolated in 1959 in Brazil from *Culex* (*Melanoconion*) spp. collected near the Aura River and later from *Aedes serratus* in Brazil and Argentina.[154] This virus may be related to the New World "SIN-like" virus that recombined with EEEV to produce WEEV and related postrecombinant viruses.[27,829] It is relatively nonpathogenic for mice and has not been linked to human disease.

Epidemiology

WEEV is widely distributed in the western plains and valleys of the United States and Canada and in South America. In North America, WEEV is maintained in an endemic cycle involving domestic and passerine birds (particularly finches and sparrows) and *Cx. tarsalis*, a mosquito well-adapted to irrigated agricultural areas.[128] Occasional isolations have been made from *Aedes melanimon* and *Aedes dorsalis*, also competent vectors. There is evidence for a secondary transmission cycle involving *Aedes melanimon* and the blacktail jackrabbit[128,374] in addition to the *Cx. tarsalis*–avian cycle. Increased transmission is associated with greater abundance of *Cx. tarsalis*.[61] Serosurveys and virus isolations provide evidence of natural infection in chickens, pheasants, rodents, rabbits, ungulates, tortoises, and snakes. In some areas of South America, most mosquitoes from which WEEV has been isolated feed primarily on mammals, and antibodies are common in small mammals including rats and rabbits, while in other areas antibodies are found primarily in birds.[894,1056] A survey of horses in the Pantanal region of Brazil found 36% seropositivity for WEEV.[738] Interseasonal persistence can occur in saltwater marshes perhaps by overwintering in adults.[793,794]

Morbidity and mortality

WEEV in the western United States has caused epidemics of encephalitis in humans, horses, and emus, but the case-fatality rate of 3% for humans, 20% to 40% for horses, and 10% for emus is lower than for NA-EEEV. In older children and adults,

males are two to three times more likely to develop disease than females.[578] The estimated case-to-infection ratio is 1:58 in children under 5 years and 1:1,150 in adults.[128] Clinically apparent disease is most common in the very young and those over 50.[578] Severe disease, seizures, fatal encephalitis, and significant sequelae are more likely to occur in infants and in young children.[235,501] The case-fatality rate rises to 8% in those over 50.[578] Accidental infections involving aerosolized virus in the laboratory have been reported and WEEV is regarded as a potential bioterrorist threat.[896] The rare occurrence of significant human disease during equine outbreaks of WEE in South America may be related to the feeding habits of the vector or to a lower virulence of South American strains for humans and horses.[205,838]

Origin and spread of epidemics

During the 20th century, large, often widespread, epidemics of equine encephalitis occurred from mid-June to late September in North America with significant spillover into the human population. These outbreaks correlated with regional increases in the population densities of *Cx. tarsalis*.[715] Major epizootics occurred every 2 to 3 years in the United States from 1931 to 1952. In 1941, more than 3,400 human WEE cases were reported in the plains of the western United States and Canada with attack rates of up to 167 cases/100,000 population.[128] During the 1952 epidemic in California's Central Valley, attack rates were 36 cases/100,000 humans and 1,120/100,000 equids.[128] Seroprevalence in humans was 34% in rural areas of California endemic for WEEV in 1960[286] but only 1.3% to 2.6% in similar areas in 1993 to 1995.[791] Beginning in the late 20th century, human cases of WEE steadily declined with the last detected in North America in 1998[77] (Fig. 6.12) and in South America in 2009.[205] This decline does not appear to be due to a decrease in virus virulence or a change in vector competence,[269,792,1104] but WEEV population declines and genetic drift could provide a partial explanation.[77,664] However, recent reverse genetic studies indicate no loss in fitness, suggesting ecologic changes as the explanation for the decline in WEEV circulation.

In South America, both epizootic (equine-virulent) and enzootic (not associated with disease) strains circulate.[82] Sequence analysis of the viruses found at the initial focus of the 1982 WEE epizootic in Argentina suggested that the enzootic virus was the source of a virulent variant, which emerged by mutation or selection to cause the epizootic. An epizootic vector in South America is *Aedes albifasciatus* and rabbits may serve as an amplifying host.[1056]

Molecular epidemiology

WEEV has three major lineages: one was isolated during the 1982 to 1983 epizootic in Argentina, a second has been sampled in Brazil and Argentina, and a third is widely distributed in the western half of North America.[77,1054,1056] Within California, separately evolving lineages have been identified in the Central Valley and the southern part of the state.[509]

Clinical Features and Pathology

WEEV causes encephalitis with signs and symptoms similar to those of EEE. Transmission can occur by aerosols as well as by mosquitoes.[787] There is a 3- to 5-day prodrome of fever and headache that may progress to restlessness, tremor, irritability, nuchal rigidity, photophobia, altered mental status,

Western Equine Encephalitis: US

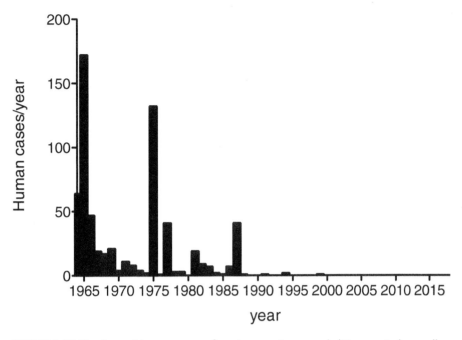

FIGURE 6.12 Numbers of human cases of western equine encephalitis reported annually in the United States since 1964. Based on data from the Centers for Disease Control and Prevention.

and paralysis.[264,501,628] Infants develop rigidity, seizures, and a bulging fontanel.[264,628] Transplacental transmission results in perinatal infection manifesting within the first week of life as fever, failure to feed, and seizures.[628,891] CSF pleocytosis is typical with 100 to 1,500 cells/μL. Neutrophils are present early in disease and mononuclear cells later.[628] In infants less than 1 year of age, approximately 60% of survivors have brain damage, and in some, the disease is progressive.[628,701] Common problems are cognitive deficits associated with quadriplegia, spasticity, recurring seizures, cortical atrophy, ventricular dilation, and intracranial calcification.[235,264,702,927] In older individuals, recovery is typically rapid with remission of signs and symptoms within 5 to 10 days, and sequelae are less common (5%).[264] Increased susceptibility of the very young compared to adults is likely related to the maturation-dependent ability of neurons to respond to IFN and limit virus replication.[153]

Pathology of acute cases of WEE shows leptomeningitis and perivascular cuffing with neutrophils in the earliest cases and lymphocytes, plasma cells, and macrophages at later times. In areas of neuronal degeneration, there is inflammation accompanied by endothelial hyperplasia, petechial hemorrhages, and glial nodules. Lesions are found primarily in the basal ganglia, brainstem, cerebellum, cerebral cortex, and spinal cord with areas of focal necrosis and demyelination in the subcortical white matter and basal ganglia.[264,702,703]

Occasionally in infants and children, there is pathologic evidence of progressive disease consistent with persistent infection.[628,702,703] Individuals surviving months to years after onset of encephalitis (often with progressive disease) may have cystic lesions, gliosis, and demyelination with areas of active mononuclear inflammation.[702,703]

Veterinary Correlates, Host Range, and Animal Models

WEE was first recognized as a neurologic disease of equids characterized by fever, incoordination, drowsiness, and anorexia leading to prostration, coma, and death in approximately 40% of the affected animals.[219] Emus also develop symptomatic, often fatal, disease characterized by ataxia, paralysis, and tremors.[54] As a part of its enzootic cycle, WEEV infects sparrows, finches, blackbirds, mourning doves, pheasants, cowbirds, swallows, and chickens. The virus can cause fatal disease in sparrows, while chickens, which are often used as sentinels, develop inapparent infection.[797]

Experimentally infected newborn mice die within 48 hours after infection with involvement of skeletal muscle, cartilage, and bone marrow. In weanling mice, brain, heart, lung, and brown fat appear to be the primary target tissues.[12] After intracerebral inoculation, there is infection of the choroid plexus and ependyma with spread to neurons and glial cells in the brain, cerebellum, and brainstem and to motor neurons in the spinal cord.[571] After intranasal inoculation, olfactory neurons are infected with subsequent neuronal spread.[749] After peripheral inoculation, WEEV replicates in skeletal and cardiac muscle cells, causes a necrotizing myocarditis, and occasionally spreads to the CNS.[571,652] Virus is first detected in the cerebral circumventricular organs followed by centripetal spread via the neuronal axis.[748] Hamsters are more susceptible to WEEV-induced disease than mice with high mortality due to encephalitis after intranasal or intraperitoneal inoculation.[461] Neurons are infected and neuropathological changes include perivascular inflammation, microcavitation, and astrocytic hypertrophy.[1112] Cynomolgus and rhesus macaques are susceptible to intranasal and aerosol, as well as intracerebral, infection and develop dose-dependent signs of encephalitis with fever, tremors, and altered consciousness. Pathology shows encephalitis with infection of neurons accompanied by mononuclear inflammation.[787,1095]

Virulence

Variants of WEEV with decreased pathogenicity for mice and hamsters (e.g., B628 clone 15) have been selected by passage on CEF cells.[1112] Large-plaque strains tend to be more virulent than small-plaque strains.[436] Epizootic strains appear to be optimized for viremia and neuroinvasiveness and are generally more virulent for mice and guinea pigs than are enzootic strains.[82,83,375] North American isolates vary substantially in their virulence for mice, but are generally more virulent than South American strains.[269,573,680] Differences in mouse virulence are determined in part by E2 sequence changes.[664]

Diagnosis, Treatment, and Prevention

Diagnosis can be made by detection of WEEV-specific IgM in serum, by IgG seroconversion, or by isolation of virus in mice or cultured cells or by nucleic acid amplification.[129,529] Small molecule screening has identified lead compounds that inhibit WEEV replication and are partially protective in mice.[463,739] An inactivated vaccine is available for horses and as an experimental preparation for laboratory workers.[783] Preclinical studies of approaches to protection include activation of innate immunity,[574] DNA virus vectors expressing IFN or viral proteins, and chimeric alphaviruses.[43,60,305,679,786,953,1092,1093]

Venezuelan Equine Encephalitis

Equine disease was recognized in South America in the 1920s, and a virus (VEEV) was isolated from the brains of encephalitic horses in 1936 during an outbreak of equine encephalitis that may have spread from the central river valleys of Colombia into the Guajira region of Venezuela. This virus was antigenically distinct from the viruses causing equine encephalitis in the eastern and western portions of North America (EEEV and WEEV) and became the third encephalitic alphavirus identified in the Americas.[73,512] Between 1943 and 1980, many VEEV-related viruses, including the prototypic Trinidad donkey (TrD) strain,[782] were isolated in South America, Central America, and southern regions of the United States.[14] The first reported human cases of VEE were in laboratory workers,[151,543] and subsequently human disease was documented in the general population during equine outbreaks and virus was isolated from ill humans.[782,848,1051]

Studies in Central America during this period indicated an enzootic cycle involving *Culex (Melanoconion)* spp. mosquitoes and rodents,[292] and human cases in Colombia in the absence of equine disease also reflected enzootic circulation and spillover.[848] In 1969, an epizootic/epidemic of VEE appeared and spread from Peru or Ecuador and through Central America and into Texas causing human disease and a high mortality in horses.[14] Virus isolations during the epizootic were primarily from *Psorophora confinnis* and *Ae. sollicitans* and Ae. taeniorhynchus mosquitoes and from horses suggesting that the epizootic and enzootic transmission cycles differed.[494,948] The latest major epizootic/epidemic in 1995 involved northern Venezuela and Colombia with an estimated 100,000 human cases.[1057]

Other VEEV Complex Viruses

Using a short-incubation (kinetic) HI test, isolates of viruses related to VEEV were originally classified into subtypes I to IV: VEE (I), Everglades (EVE, II), Mucambo (MUC, III), and Pixuna (PIX, IV).[1098] When Cabassou (CAB) and AG80-663 (Rio Negro, RN) viruses were isolated and shown to be within the VEE antigenic complex, they became subtypes V and VI.[134,218] The VEE subtype I viruses were further subdivided serologically into IAB, IC, ID, IE, and IF (Mosso das Pedras)[134,1051,1098] and the MUC subtype III viruses into IIIA, IIIB (Tonate/Bijou Bridge), IIIC, and IIID.[493,1051] Analysis of the phylogenetic relationships of the VEE complex viruses gained from sequencing led to a recognition of eight distinct species, with the species VEEV now comprising only subtypes IAB, IC, ID, and IE (Table 6.1)[492,631,770] (Fig. 6.13).

1. *Everglades*—EEEV (*subtype II*) was first recognized in southern Florida in the 1960s in persons living near Everglades National Park. Transmission is widespread in Florida with *Cx. (Melanoconion) cedecei* as the primary vector and cotton rats (*Sigmodon hispidus*) the main vertebrate reservoir.[184,1058] Disease in humans is usually mild.[239]

2. *Mucambo*—MUCV (subtype IIIA) was first isolated (strain BeAn 8) from a Brazilian monkey in 1954.[155] Three clades have been identified with temporally defined clades 1 and 2 from Trinidad and clade 3 from Brazil.[48,50] The virus causes fatal disease in newborn and adult mice after intracerebral, but not peripheral, inoculation. Experimentally inoculated guinea pigs and horses survive infection.[893] More recently, genetically distinct subtype IIIC[862] and IIID[15] VEE complex virus strains, now formally part of the species MUCV, have been identified in eastern Peru. All appear to be maintained in enzootic, sylvatic transmission cycles with direct spillover human infections documented only for IIIA and IIID.

3. *Tonate*—TONV (subtype IIIB) was first isolated in 1973 from a bird (*Psarocolius decumanus*) captured in French Guiana[218] and subsequently from *Cx. (Melanoconion) portesi*.[728] The close relative TONV (strain Bijou Bridge) has also been recovered from cliff swallow bugs and birds in North America.[653] Human seropositivity is 11.9% in French Guiana with the highest rates in savannah areas.[955] Infection is most often associated with a mild dengue-like illness, but fatal encephalitis has also been reported in a young child.[410]

4. *Pixuna*—PIXV (subtype IV) was first isolated (BeAr 35645) from *Anopheles (Stethomyia) nimbus* mosquitoes in Belém, Brazil, in 1961[893] and has also been identified in Argentina.[754,756] There is no evidence that it causes disease in humans or equids.

5. *Cabassou*—CABV (subtype V) was first isolated (strain CaAr508) from mosquitoes in French Guiana in 1974.[218] CABV is not neurovirulent for adult mice or guinea pigs.

6. *Rio Negro*—RNV (subtype VI) was first isolated (strain AG80-663) from *Cx. (Melanoconion) delpontei* near the Rio Negro in Argentina in 1980.[134] RNV circulates in neotropical regions of Argentina[644,754,756] where it has caused outbreaks of acute febrile illness.[187] Suckling mice die within 2 to 3 days, but adult mice and guinea pigs survive infection.[1340]

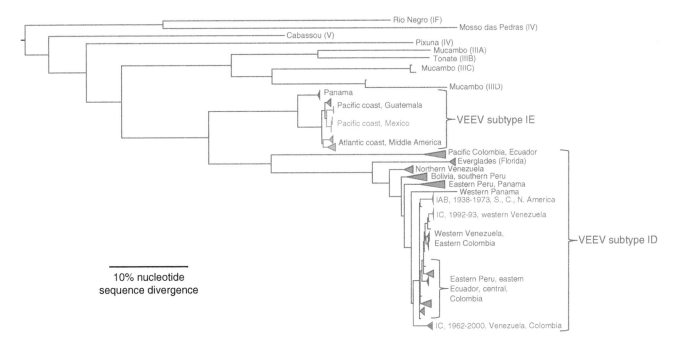

10% nucleotide sequence divergence

FIGURE 6.13 VEEV phylogenetic tree showing relationships of epizootic (colored *red* and *orange*) and enzootic/endemic strains (colored *green*). Strains are abbreviated with country followed by year of collection. The tree was generated using 817 nt sequences from the PE2 envelope glycoprotein gene using maximum likelihood methods. Courtesy of Naomi Forrester.

Epidemiology

Enzootic VEE complex viruses are involved in perennially active transmission cycles in subtropical and tropical areas of the Americas (e.g., EVE in Florida; VEE ID and IE in Central America; IF Mosso das Pedras, MUCV (IIIA, C, D), PIXV, CABV, and RNV in South America). In enzootic areas, mosquito isolates are primarily from *Culex* (*Melanoconion*) spp. mosquitoes that live in tropical and subtropical swamps and forests throughout the Americas, with larval habitats often associated with aquatic plants and which typically blood-feed at dawn, dusk, and nighttime on a wide variety of rodents, birds, and other vertebrates.[14,262,292,339] Wild birds are susceptible to infection, but mammals, such as cotton rats, spiny rats, other rodents, and sometimes bats, are the most likely reservoir hosts of all but TONV, as determined by virus isolation, levels of viremia, serology and resistance to disease.[63,143,252,339,361,1051] Although enzootic circulation is typically associated with sylvatic habitats, it also occurs in periurban regions with large numbers of human spillover infections.[14]

Morbidity and mortality

Clinically evident, including fatal, human infection can occur with most, if not all, enzootic, as well as epizootic, VEE complex viruses.[14,239,410,955,1051] Humans living in areas of enzootic transmission have a high prevalence of antibody due to infection associated mostly with undiagnosed mild febrile illnesses, often assumed in the absence of laboratory diagnostics to be dengue.[14,252,339,755,863,955] During epizootics, human attack rates vary widely, but recent epidemic estimates approach 30%.[810] In some outbreaks, most infections are asymptomatic with the apparent-to-inapparent infection ratio estimates as low as 1:11[95,239]; however, attack rates up to 30% during 1995 suggest a much higher rate of symptomatic infection.[810] All ages and both sexes are equally susceptible to infection, but disease manifestations vary with age.[810] Individuals under the age of 15 are more likely to develop fulminant disease with reticuloendothelial infection, lymphoid depletion, and encephalitis. In older children and young adults, a relatively benign influenza-like illness is most common.[239] Individuals over 50 are prone to develop encephalitis, but most recover.[239] The incidence of encephalitis in clinically ill humans is generally less than 5% and the mortality less than 1%.[810] Essentially all deaths occur in children.

Origin and spread of epidemics

Since the 1920s, VEE epizootics/epidemics have occurred at approximately 10- to 20-year intervals in cattle ranching areas of Venezuela, Colombia, Peru, and Ecuador when heavy rainfall leads to increased populations of epizootic mosquito vectors and when herd immunity decreases with equine population turnover.[810] Formalinized vaccines containing residual live virus were probably responsible for initiating all IAB outbreaks since the 1940s, including ones in South and Central America/Texas between 1969 and 1972[494] and another in Peru in 1973.[770,1055] VEE complex viruses causing epizootics are members of subtypes IAB, IC, or IE, while enzootic viruses include ID, IE, and all other subtypes/species. During 1995, a major IC outbreak occurred in coastal areas of Venezuela and Colombia causing disease in 75,000 to 100,000 people. This region had experienced a similar outbreak in 1962 to 1964. Subtype ID VEEV strains obtained from mosquitoes and sentinel animals in western Venezuela and eastern Colombia when there was no epidemic activity have sequences that are closely related to the predicted epizootic IAB and IC progenitors, indicating that epizootic strains are not maintained in a separate cycle, but rather evolve by mutation from enzootic ID strains[770,806,1057] (Figs. 6.13 and 6.14). Epizootic potential is correlated with positive charge mutations in E2 that increase the level of viremia

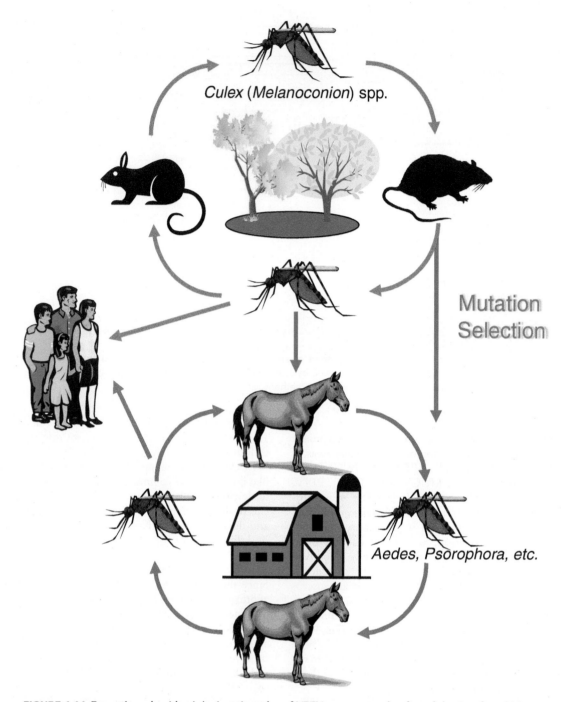

Culex (Melanoconion) spp.

Mutation
Selection

Aedes, Psorophora, etc.

FIGURE 6.14 Enzootic and epidemic/epizootic cycles of VEEV as an example of an alphavirus for which epizootic strains arise by mutation and selection for equine viremia or epizootic vector transmission from the enzootic virus.

in equids and may also increase infectivity for the mosquito vector *Aedes* (*Ochlerotatus*) *taeniorhynchus,*[31,103,342] and one of these mutations was shown using reverse genetics to transform a subtype ID enzootic strain to an equine amplification-competent, subtype IC phenotype.[31] During epizootics, horses are an important amplifying species, and susceptible equids provide a means for virus amplification and spread.[948]

Detailed phylogenetic studies have delineated six major lineages of enzootic VEEV including five subtype ID strains and the subtype IE lineage (Fig. 6.13). All epizootic strains from major outbreaks fall into a clade nested within one of

these lineages.[1051] Enzootic IE viruses were the source of epizootic IE strains in two recent equine epizootics in Mexico.[705] Interestingly, these epizootic IE strains cause encephalitis in horses with little viremia.[324,840] A substitution in E2 that appeared prior to outbreaks along the Pacific Coast of Mexico appears to have adapted the local enzootic IE strains for more efficient transmission by *Ae. taeniorhynchus.*

During outbreaks, VEEV has been isolated from several species of mosquitoes. Those most incriminated as VEEV vectors include *Ae.* (*Ochlerotatus*) *sollicitans*, *Ae. taeniorhynchus*, *Psorophora columbiae*, and *Psorophora confinnis.*[948,1051]

After an epizootic, IC viruses may persist in a natural cycle and serve as a source for subsequent smaller outbreaks.[687]

Molecular epidemiology

Sequence analysis of the VEE complex viruses shows the greatest divergence for the E2 glycoprotein and the C-terminal region of nsP3.[271,631,770] At least five enzootic subtype ID lineages have been identified: Colombia and coastal Ecuador; Panama/Peru; Colombia, western Venezuela, and northern Peru; north central Venezuela; and Peru/Bolivia (Fig. 6.13). All epizootic IAB and IC strains are related to ID strains from Colombia, Venezuela, and Peru.[770,1051] Three distinct geographically separate IE lineages have also been recognized: northwestern Panama, Pacific Coast (Mexico and Guatemala), and Gulf/Caribbean Coast (Mexico and Belize).[706]

Clinical Features and Pathology

Infection with enzootic, as well as epizootic, strains of VEEV can cause significant human disease with the most common signs and symptoms being fever, headache, tremors, prostration, nausea, and vomiting that last 3 to 4 days.[14] Accidental laboratory aerosol infections of young adults with epizootic strains of VEEV caused a febrile illness with the abrupt onset of chills, headache, myalgia, somnolence, vomiting, diarrhea, and pharyngitis 2 to 5 days after exposure without evidence of encephalitis.[151,239,543] Natural epidemic human infection was first described in 1952 in Colombia and subsequently in Venezuela during the 1962 to 1964 outbreak that resulted in 32,000 human cases and 190 deaths.[239,452] The 1995 outbreak in Colombia caused an estimated 75,000-100,000 human cases, 3,000 with neurologic complications and 300 deaths.[810,1057] The case-fatality rate is 0.7% to 1%. Neurologic disease tends to appear 4 to 10 days after onset of illness with headache and vomiting the most common initial symptoms. Specific neurologic signs include focal or generalized seizures, paresis, behavioral changes, and stupor or coma.[810,1057] Children recovering from encephalitis may be left with neurological deficits, particularly seizure disorders.[546] Fetal abnormalities, spontaneous abortions, and stillbirths may occur with infection during pregnancy.[810,1057]

Laboratory studies often show lymphopenia. Pathology on fatal cases has shown myocarditis, focal centrilobular hepatic necrosis and inflammation, generalized lymphoid depletion, cerebral edema, and vasculitis.[452] Congenitally infected infants show severe neurologic damage with widespread necrosis, hemorrhage, and hypoplasia resulting, in the most severe cases, in hydranencephaly.[1066]

Veterinary Correlates, Host Range, and Animal Models

Enzootic strains of the VEE complex can infect horses, but these infections are typically asymptomatic or cause short-term fever, low-level viremia, and little clinical illness and may immunize horses against infection with epizootic strains (IAB, IC, and IE).[392,1051] Equine disease induced by epizootic strains is characterized by fever, depression, and diarrhea leading to death 6 to 8 days after infection. Viremia persists until death with titers up to 10^8 infectious units/mL blood. Virus can also be recovered from eye washings, nasal washings, and urine. Leukopenia coincides with the viremia and is progressive in fatal cases. In animals that recover, antibody appears approximately 7 days after infection.[496] Pathology on fatal cases shows

pancreatic necrosis and cellular depletion in the bone marrow, lymph nodes, and spleen. The brains of horses with signs of neurologic disease show swollen cerebrovascular endothelial cells, edema, extravasation of blood, and leukocytic infiltration into the perivenular spaces.[319,496]

Infection of macaques by aerosol or subcutaneous inoculation with enzootic and epizootic strains of virus elicits a biphasic febrile response—the first phase is coincident with the viremia and the second phase with termination of viremia, that is, the appearance of the immune response[319,651,789] (Fig. 6.7). Leukopenia is common. Symptom signs are usually mild, consisting of anorexia, loose stools, irritability, and occasionally loss of balance, tremor, or myoclonus.[651,937] Examination of tissues shows lymphocyte depletion early, mild hepatitis, myocarditis, and encephalitis. Lesions in the brain are found primarily in the olfactory cortex and basal ganglia and consist of lymphocytic perivascular cuffing and glial nodules.[319]

Experimental infection of small laboratory animals with VEEV produces a variety of disease patterns. After subcutaneous inoculation of guinea pigs, rabbits, or hamsters with virulent strains of VEEV, there is a viremia. Virus replicates in the bone marrow, lymph nodes, spleen, and brain with rapid destruction of myeloid and lymphoid cells in lymph nodes, spleen, thymus, intestinal and conjunctival lymphoid tissue, liver, and bone marrow, damage to the intestinal wall and pancreas, cerebral hemorrhage, and neuronal cell death.[319,441,1036] Death occurs 2 to 4 days after infection and may be associated with ileal necrosis, bacteremia, and endotoxemia.[331] EVEV, MUCV, and PIXV are progressively less virulent.[441]

In addition to myeloid and lymphoid necrosis, susceptible strains of mice develop encephalomyelitis leading to death in 6 to 9 days after infection with the TC-83 vaccine strain, as well as wild-type strains of VEEV.[319,462,582] After subcutaneous inoculation, virus replicates first in DCs or Langerhans cells that migrate to the draining lymph node where virus is amplified[596] (Fig. 6.6). Virus enters the CNS by the olfactory route after respiratory or peripheral inoculation, although cerebral infection can also follow hematogenous seeding of the circumventricular organs.[748] Initial infection is of olfactory epithelium with spread to olfactory neurons and then caudally to all regions of the brain, causing encephalitis and neuronal apoptosis.[162,433,936,937,1029] Virus also infects the pancreas, liver, and teeth. Fatal disease has an immunopathological component dependent on the strain of mouse infected.[161,937] There can also be transplacental transmission of infection.[932]

Virulence

Comparative studies of the virulent TrD and avirulent TC-83 strains of the IAB serotype and construction of recombinant viruses have led to identification of the 5' UTR (nt 3) and the E2 glycoprotein (residue 120) as important determinants of VEEV virulence for mice.[202,491] Attenuated viruses infect DCs less efficiently and replicate less well in lymphoid tissue and in the CNS than virulent viruses.[596,936] Virulence for guinea pigs is determined by both envelope and nonenvelope genes.[341,766] Determinants of equine virulence are different from determinants of murine virulence, but also lie largely within the E2 glycoprotein.[102,342,770] Changes most frequently associated with acquisition of equine virulence for ID strains are replacement of uncharged residues with Arg at positions 193 and 213 of

E2.[31,1037] Acquisition of surface charge changes in E2 is also associated with emergence of epizootic IE strains.[102]

Diagnosis, Treatment, and Prevention

Diagnosis can be made by virus isolation from blood or pharynx[151,543,1057] or by documenting the presence of anti-VEEV IgM or a rise in IgG antibody. HI, CF, neutralization, or EIA tests can be used for serologic diagnosis and nucleic acid amplification for detection of viral RNA. Antibody responses to enzootic versus epizootic strains can be differentiated with an epitope-blocking EIA.[1041]

Treatment is generally supportive, but passive transfer of antibody can protect mice before or up to 24 hours after challenge.[325,420,422] The D-(−) enantiomer of carbodine, an inhibitor of cellular cytidine triphosphate synthetase, and antisense morpholino oligomers suppress VEEV replication *in vitro* and improve the outcome of infected mice.[460,726]

The earliest vaccines developed for horses and laboratory workers were formalin-inactivated preparations.[781,783] These vaccines had repeated problems with residual live virus producing disease and initiating equine-amplified outbreaks and with poor immunogenicity and are no longer in use.[494,770,1055] A live attenuated vaccine (TC-83), developed by serial passage of the virulent TrD strain in guinea pig heart tissue culture cells,[75] is protective for horses and laboratory workers, but 15% to 30% of recipients develop fever and pharyngeal viral shedding.[758] Therefore, a formalin-inactivated TC-83 vaccine (C-84) was produced.[237] Both the live and inactivated vaccines are immunogenic, but live TC-83 provides better protection against aerosol challenge in hamsters than C-84 and is therefore preferred despite the reactogenicity.[442] To produce a more optimal vaccine, several experimental DNA, inactivated, live attenuated, chimeric, and replicon particle vaccines are at various stages of development.[160,232,233,246,611,727,786,788,821]

A number of measures are effective in controlling outbreaks. These include immunizing equids, limiting equine movements from regions of infection, applying larvacides to mosquito-breeding sites, and spraying insecticides to control adult mosquitoes.[810,948,1051] Protection of human populations relies primarily on personal protection from mosquito bites.

ALPHAVIRUSES ASSOCIATED PRIMARILY WITH RASH AND POLYARTHRITIS

Chikungunya

An outbreak of a crippling arthritic disease of sudden onset was first recorded in the Newala District of Tanzania in 1952.[812] Retrospective case reviews have suggested that CHIKV epidemics in Africa, Asia, and the Americas occurred as early as 1779, but were confused with dengue.[141,370] Because of the severe arthritic symptoms, the disease was given the name of "chikungunya" meaning "to walk bent over" in the Kimakonde language of Mozambique.[407,812] The virus, isolated in 1953 from serum and from *Aedes* spp. and *Culex* spp. mosquitoes, was related to the group A arboviruses (Fig. 6.5).[820] Subsequent epidemics were recognized in the Transvaal of South Africa, Zambia, India, Southeast Asia, and the Philippines. From 2004 to 2007, a large epidemic affected islands in the Indian Ocean

and India with spread to SE Asia and Europe,[769,801] and in 2013 and 2014, CHIKV was introduced into the Caribbean and Central and South America.[1050,1052]

Epidemiology

CHIKV causes epidemics of rash and arthritis in India, Southeast Asia, Indonesia, the Philippines, most of sub-Saharan Africa, and Indian Ocean islands with recent extension into southern Europe and the Americas[336,532,803,971] (Fig. 6.15). In Africa, the virus is maintained in cycles similar to that of yellow fever virus. There is a rural cycle involving *Aedes africanus*, *Aedes furcifer*, nonhuman primates, and other mammals and an urban cycle involving *Ae. aegypti* or *Ae. albopictus* and humans.[171,214,996] In rural areas, the disease is endemic with small numbers of cases occurring most years.[214] In urban areas, outbreaks are sporadic and explosive with infection of a large proportion of the susceptible population within a few weeks.[309,736,801,812,813] In Asia, there is no evidence for a sylvatic cycle; rather, urban transmission is by *Ae. aegypti* and suburban rural transmission is by *Ae. albopictus* in a human–mosquito–human cycle.[405,693,768] Laboratory-acquired infections have also been reported.[981]

Morbidity and mortality

All ages and both sexes are susceptible and disease is usually self-limiting and rarely life threatening. However, approximately 0.3% of cases are atypical or severe with nephritis, hepatitis, meningoencephalitis, thrombocytopenia, or encephalopathy, and the case-fatality rate has been estimated at 1 in 1,000 with most of the deaths either in neonates infected peripartum, adults with underlying conditions, or the elderly.[152,236,801,811] The epidemic on Réunion Island affected almost 40% of the population (estimated 300,000 cases) and led to an excess of 254 deaths.[309,395,800] Infants infected at birth are susceptible to CNS complications including cerebral edema and hemorrhage resulting in long-term disabilities.[307,988] Musculoskeletal symptoms are recurrent or persistent in approximately 40% of adults and more likely to affect females than males.[928,1086]

Origin and spread of epidemics

CHIKV is believed to have originated in sylvatic, enzootic African transmission cycles involving nonhuman primates and arboreal *Aedes* spp. vectors. However, this cycle was identified after the first epidemics were recognized in the 1950s in Africa and Asia (although outbreaks probably occurred for the past few centuries in both Asia and the Americas following the spread of both CHIKV and *Ae. aegypti* mosquitoes from Africa).[370,1050] After an epidemic, the disease usually disappears from an affected region for years, probably due to herd immunity. An unprecedented series of epidemics began in Kenya in 2004 with spread to Comoros, Réunion Island, the Seychelles, Mauritius, and Mayotte in 2005. This epidemic strain, called the Indian Ocean Lineage (IOL), was derived from one of the two main African enzootic genotypes called the East/Central/South African (ECSA) lineage[470,869] (Fig. 6.16). The same IOL strain subsequently spread from Africa to the Indian subcontinent and then to Southeast Asia with smaller outbreaks in France and Italy following imported cases.[395,733] Some IOL strains increased their ability to be transmitted by *Ae. albopictus*, not previously implicated in CHIKV transmission, through a series of mutations in the envelope glycoprotein genes.[405,997,1023] Because susceptible urban vectors are widely distributed,

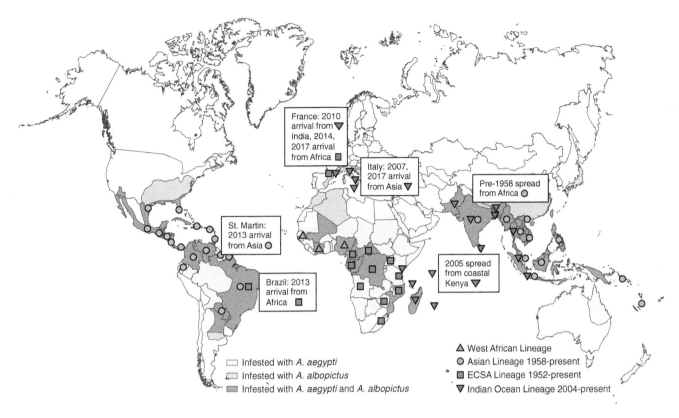

FIGURE 6.15 Time course of worldwide spread and current geographic distribution of lineages of chikungunya virus along with the distribution of the relevant *Aedes aegypti* and *Ae. albopictus* mosquito vectors. Adapted from reference 805, with permission.

travelers provide a source of CHIKV introduction into many other geographic regions.[395,733,799] There is some evidence that virus can be maintained within mosquito populations by low rates of transovarial or venereal transmission.[616,784,978]

Molecular epidemiology

CHIKV is a member of the SFV complex evolved from an enzootic ancestor in Africa, and the first permanently endemic (human-amplified and *Ae. aegypti*–transmitted) virus was probably introduced into Asia about a century ago.[1031] Two distinct enzootic lineages exist, transmitted in sylvatic locations among nonhuman primates by arboreal *Aedes* mosquitoes: West African and ECSA[768,769,869] (Fig. 6.16). All extant endemic/epidemic strains analyzed were derived from the latter.[166,373,470,869,1031] Of the two endemic/epidemic lineages, only the IOL has adapted for more efficient transmission by *Ae. albopictus*. The Asian lineage, which was introduced into the Americas in 2013, is constrained by an epistatic interaction between threonine at E1-98 and the adaptive E1-226 alanine-to-valine substitution.[996] The second lineage to reach the Americas, from Angola into Brazil in 2014, is constrained in the same manner by a different epistatic interaction at E2-211, where a threonine residue is required for the effect of E1-226 to be realized,[1000] while isoleucine found in the Brazilian ECSA strain does not allow penetrance of the 226 substitution. Another constraint on this adaptation is the geographic source of *Ae. albopictus*; unlike other populations tested, this species derived from the Democratic Republic of the Congo is not more susceptible to the E1-226V mutant.[1024]

After identification of the E1-A226 mutation, additional *Ae. albopictus*–adaptive mutations were identified in E2, all involving glutamine or glutamic acid substitutions of various amino acids.[998] Structural mapping of these mutations combined with their common derived amino acids allowed for additional *Ae. albopictus*–adaptive mutations, never observed in nature, to be predicted and confirmed experimentally. These results suggested that CHIKV has additional potential for adaptation to this invasive vector species. In addition to having two major epidemic vectors, IOL strains also appear to be more virulent than those of the Asian lineage.[306,1097]

Clinical Features and Pathology

The disease is of sudden onset with an incubation period estimated at 3 to 12 days.[812] No prodrome is recognized and most infections result in disease with children more likely than adults to have mild symptoms.[142,330,809,907,908] Fever rises rapidly to 103°F to 104°F and may be accompanied by a rigor. The onset of fever corresponds to the period of viremia and may be related to the ability of this virus to induce large amounts of type I IFN, IFN pathway genes, and proinflammatory cytokines[175,267,967,968,1045] (Fig. 6.7). Disease severity and levels of neutralizing antibody are associated with TLR3 polymorphisms.[397] Monocytes are infected and are a source of IFN.[396,967] Virus titers in blood can reach greater than 10^6 PFU/ml and virus load correlates with disease severity and IFN production.[142,175,407,865] Joint pain appears suddenly and can be incapacitating and chronic. Essentially any joint can be involved and pain may be accompanied by swelling and paresthesias.[92,480,691] Headache, conjunctivitis, and gastrointestinal symptoms are common, and in 80%, a maculopapular rash appears 4 to 8 days after the initial illness. The rash may be associated with a second rise in fever (Fig. 6.7), lasts approximately 2 days, and is described as "irritating" or "itchy."[93,812] Meningoencephalitis associated with

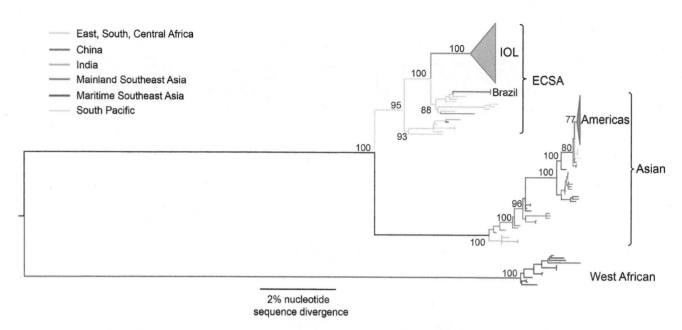

FIGURE 6.16 CHIKV phylogenetic tree derived from nucleotide sequences encoding the two ORFs using Bayesian methods. The major enzootic lineages (West African and East/Central/South African) are shown as well as the two endemic/epidemic lineages that involve human–mosquito transmission cycles in urban settings: Asian and Indian Ocean Lineage (IOL). Endemic/epidemic strains circulating in the Americas from Asian and ECSA lineages are shown in *red*, and legend indicates the geographic locations of other strains. All posterior probability values were 1.0. (Courtesy of Rubing Chen.)

CNS infection can result in death or permanent disability and is more common with CHIKV than with other alphaviruses causing primarily rash and arthritis.[152,308,630,811,844] In addition, atypical cases with severe disease and increased mortality can develop hepatitis, myocarditis, bullous dermatosis, myelopathy, pneumonia, and diabetes.[176,178,236,416,958,987] Fibroblasts in the skin and joints and satellite cells in the muscle are targets for infection.[191,723] Leukopenia and thrombocytopenia are frequent.[93,175,407,1086]

There are multiple indications of virus persistence after resolution of acute infection. Episodes of joint pain and myalgia and detection of viral RNA and sometimes antigen often continue for many months to years after the original illness.[58,92,204,241,407,820,866,928] Chronic pain is more likely in females and those over 60 years of age with a high viral load during the acute illness.[407,1086] Synovial tissue harbors persistently infected perivascular macrophages, fibroblast hyperplasia, activated NK cells, and CD4+ T cells, but few CD8+ T cells.[407] Cytokines are increased during acute infection, and persistent arthralgia is associated with elevated plasma levels of IL-6 and granulocyte–macrophage colony-stimulating factor.[173,175,691] Joint x-rays are usually normal or show soft tissue swelling without evidence of bone or joint damage, although bone erosion has been reported.[480,605,607] Osteoblasts can be infected and express osteoclast-activating factors such as IL-6 and RANKL.[704] In India, but not Africa, inguinal lymphadenopathy and red swollen ears are also observed as part of the clinical picture.[142]

Animal Models, Host Range, and Virulence

Mice and nonhuman primates can be infected with CHIKV.[365] In wild-type mice, disease severity is age-dependent.[191] Neonatal mice develop fatal disease.[212,681] One- to two-week-old mice survive infection, but develop weight loss, difficulty walking, myositis, foot swelling, tenosynovitis, and vasculitis with virus replication in multiple organs, including the CNS.[280,661,1111]

Local inoculation of adult mice causes biphasic foot swelling associated with macrophage and CD4+ T-cell infiltration and production of inflammatory cytokines, particularly TNF, IFNγ, and MCP-1.[275,294,827,969] Virulence is associated with changes in the 3′ UTR, nsP3, and E2.[8,39,329,381,627]

Fibroblasts and macrophages are target cells for CHIKV infection in the periphery, recruited to sites of virus replication and a major source of IFN-α/β.[294,827,865] In the CNS, neurons and astrocytes are target cells with up-regulation of multiple innate response genes.[199,280,681,772] Adult IFN-α/β receptor (IFNAR)-, IRF3-/IRF7-, and STAT1-deficient mice develop fatal disease with replication in macrophages, liver, muscle, joint, and skin fibroblasts; occasional dissemination to the choroid plexus, leptomeninges, and ependyma of the CNS; and features of hemorrhagic shock.[191,295,299,825,864,865] Viperin (Rsad2)-deficient and TLR3-deficient mice survive but have higher viremias, wider virus dissemination, and more joint inflammation than WT mice.[397,967] Infection of pregnant mice does not result in fetal infection.[193]

The adaptive immune response mediates much of the inflammation and is required for clearance of infectious virus.[275] Virus clearance is associated with production of antibody to the E1 and E2 surface glycoproteins.[382,468,585] Antibody-deficient mice develop persistent infection even after infection with an attenuated virus strain.[382] Higher viral loads in TLR3-deficient mice are associated with decreased production of neutralizing antibody to a linear B-cell epitope in E2.[397] Viral RNA persists in joint-associated tissues for months after infection.[382,383]

Adult cynomolgus macaques infected intravenously, subcutaneously, or intradermally develop a dose-dependent viremia, fever, rash, gingival bleeding, liver enzyme elevation, arthritis, and meningoencephalitis with astrocyte activation.[299,426,526] IFN-α/β production correlates with the viremia. Pathology shows persistent mononuclear cell infiltration into lymphatic tissue, joints, muscle, and liver associated with prolonged presence of CHIKV RNA in macrophages at these sites.[526] Pregnant rhesus macaques infected with enzootic West African and epidemic Indian strains of CHIKV develop viremia, rash, joint swelling, leukopenia, and cytokine increases after infection, but fetuses did not become infected providing further evidence that transplacental transmission is infrequent.[163]

Diagnosis, Treatment, and Prevention

The primary differential diagnoses for CHIK fever are dengue and Zika and, in Africa, ONN fevers. Dengue and Zika overlap the CHIK geographic distribution extensively, but are characterized more by myalgia than arthralgia.[480] ONN is clinically similar, but has geographic overlap only in Africa (Fig. 6.17).[142] Routine laboratory parameters are variable and not particularly helpful in the diagnosis.[769] CHIKV can be isolated from plasma or detected by nucleic acid amplification during the initial fever.[355,451,735,820,965] Detection of IgM antibody provides a means of early diagnosis and can persist for months, particularly in those with persistent symptoms.[92,130,355] In some locations, slight cross-reactions in EIA with other SF complex alphaviruses such as RRV or MAYV must be ruled out.[244]

Treatment is generally symptomatic with anti-inflammatory agents, and in mice, inhibition of IL-1β signaling decreases bone loss and inhibition of MCP-1 synthesis decreases muscle and joint inflammation.[827,1087] Passive transfer of immunoglobulin containing antibody to CHIKV can protect neonatal wild-type mice and IFNAR-/- mice from fatal infection.[192] IFN-α is protective in mice if given prior to infection and activity in peripheral joints is promoted at warm ambient temperatures.[294,774]

A live attenuated vaccine has been developed by passage of a CHIKV isolate from Thailand in MRC-5 cells.[238,554] This vaccine (strain 181/clone 25) induces long-term production of neutralizing antibody and can be used to protect laboratory workers from infection.[619,769] A formalin-inactivated vaccine can elicit protective immune responses in mice.[294,979] Additional approaches to vaccination include DNA, chimeric and rationally attenuated engineered viruses, and virus-like particles with a measles virus–vectored vaccine recently shown to be safe and immunogenic in a phase 2 human trial.[245,798,805]

O'nyong-Nyong

In 1959, an outbreak of a new disease, originally mistaken for dengue, was reported from northwestern Uganda,[364,895] and it is likely that a similar epidemic occurred in the same region in 1904 to 1906.[895] The name o'nyong-nyong originated from one of the first tribes to be affected, the Acholi, and refers to the painful joints characteristic of the disease.[364] During the 1959 outbreak, ONNV was isolated from the serum of a patient with acute arthritis[1083] and from anopheline mosquitoes.[1084] ONNV is a member of the SF complex and antigenically most closely related to CHIKV from which it is estimated to have diverged at least thousands of years ago.[768,1083] The virus reemerged in southern Uganda in 1996 to 1997 suggesting a 30- to 50-year epidemic cycle.[530] In 1967, Igbo-Ora, now recognized to be a strain of ONNV,[530,768] was isolated from humans in western Nigeria.[654]

Epidemiology

ONNV causes sporadic, widespread outbreaks of fever, rash, and arthritis with high attack rates like CHIKV. The first epidemic recognized originated in northwestern Uganda in 1959 and spread south and east to Kenya, Tanzania, Zaire, Malawi, Mozambique, and Zambia to affect greater than 2 million people.[1085] Another major outbreak occurred in southern Uganda in 1996.[845] More recent evidence of widespread ONNV infection has been documented in West, Central, and East Africa.[80,518,527,557,762,804,960]

The presumed enzootic vector and vertebrate reservoir host for ONNV are unknown. Interepidemic seroconversions and mosquito isolations suggest continuous sporadic transmission in East Africa, and it is possible that humans or nonhuman primates are the primary reservoir.[530] During outbreaks, ONNV is transmitted principally by *Anopheles funestus* and *An. gambiae* mosquitoes and is the only alphavirus known to be transmitted by anopheline mosquitoes.[595,1084] Human–mosquito–human transmission occurs during epidemics, and spread from one region to another occurs through the movement of infected humans.[845] The most recent outbreak began near swamps and lakes in the rural Rakai district of south central Uganda in 1996. Serosurveys showed infection rates of 45% to 96% in areas of epidemic transmission with the ratio of apparent-to-inapparent infection ranging from 1:4 to 1:24.[557,654,845] All ages and both sexes are equally susceptible.[497] Among domestic animals in the same region, cattle have the highest seroprevalence (40%),[709] but few animals have been studied, so the putative enzootic reservoir is not known.

Clinical Features

The onset of fever is sudden and often accompanied by a rigor. The characteristic syndrome includes joint pains, rash, lymphadenitis, and conjunctivitis. Fever is typically moderate (100°F–101°F) and lasts approximately 5 days. Joint pain most often occurs in the knees, but ankles, elbows, wrists, and fingers can also be affected. The pain usually lasts 6 to 7 days and is severe enough to be immobilizing in 80% to 90% of patients and can persist for up to 3 months. The generalized morbilliform maculopapular rash erupts 4 to 7 days after the onset of symptoms and is similar to that of CHIK. It begins on the face and extends to the trunk and extremities occasionally affecting

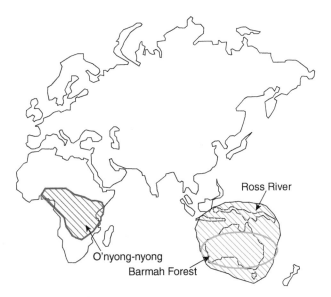

FIGURE 6.17 Geographic distributions of several alphaviruses that cause epidemic polyarthritis and rash: O'nyong-nyong, Barmah Forest, and Ross River viruses.

the palms. Cervical lymphadenopathy distinguishes the disease from CHIK, occurs in approximately half of the patients, and most frequently involves posterior cervical lymph nodes. Leukopenia is common. Fatalities have not been described, but morbidity is substantial.[497,557,654,895]

Diagnosis

The disease is often clinically confused with malaria, measles, dengue, and rubella,[762,895] but also resembles CHIK. Virus can be isolated, or nucleic acid amplified, from blood early in the illness.[80,762,1085] Diagnostic serology includes a positive IgM EIA and neutralizing antibody to ONNV that is more than twofold greater than that to CHIKV.[845] IgM persists for about 60 days after infection.[497]

Ross River

Epidemics of polyarthritis in Australia probably date from at least 1886, but were first clearly described in towns on the Murrumbidgee River in New South Wales in 1928 and then in troops stationed in the Northern Territory and Queensland during World War II.[378,435,598] Serological studies suggested an alphavirus as the causative agent and RRV (strain T48) was first isolated from *Ae. vigilax* mosquitoes trapped near the Ross River in Queensland in 1959.[378,598] The first human isolate was made in 1971 from the blood of a child with fever.[221] In 1979, RRV spread from Australia to Fiji, Samoa, and the Cook Islands causing an explosive outbreak of tens of thousands of cases of polyarthritis on these Pacific Islands.[378] Virus was first isolated from the serum of patients with polyarthritis during this epidemic.

Epidemiology

RRV is endemic throughout the coastal regions of much of northern and central Australia and epidemic in the rest of Australia, Papua New Guinea, and the Solomon Islands.[818,973] In general, the Wallace and Weber hypothetical lines in the Indo–Australian archipelago that separate the fauna of the Oriental and Australian regions appear also to have separated the geographic distributions of CHIKV and RRV[598] (Fig. 6.17). RRV is the most common mosquito-borne pathogen in Australia with approximately 5,000 cases reported each year, an annual incidence of 14 to 50/100,000 population, and 10-year seroconversion rates of 24% in some areas.[831] Cases are most common in the north and occur primarily in late summer and early autumn with some evidence of an increasing incidence.[378,598,831] Two salt marsh–breeding mosquitoes *Aedes camptorhynchus* and *Ae. vigilax* are probably the major vectors in coastal regions of Australia.[831] In inland areas, the freshwater-breeding mosquito *Culex annulirostris* is the major vector, and in urban areas, *Aedes notoscriptus* appears to be involved in transmission.[831] Both urban and rural cycles of transmission occur. A wide variety of mammals, primarily macropods such as kangaroos and wallabies and potentially pteropid bats, appear to serve as vertebrate hosts for the enzootic cycle, although placental mammals and birds have not been studied adequately to rule them out as reservoirs.[149,181,378,764,831,938] In urban areas, horses and brushtail opossums are likely involved in transmission.[475]

Morbidity and mortality

Infection rates can be as high as 1:30 during outbreaks.[598] Estimates of apparent-to-inapparent infections range from 1:3 to 1:1.[378,739] Seroprevalence and disease incidence are similar in males and females. Clinically apparent infections are rare in children and the highest incidence of disease is in the 25- to 40-year age group.[378,434]

Origin and spread of epidemics

In Australia, a wide variety of mosquito species is believed to be involved in RRV transmission.[181] Outbreaks are seasonal and have been associated with prolonged inundation of salt marshes due to increased tidal heights or heavy rains during the summer[419,435,598,982,1082] and with a loss of herd immunity in reservoir populations.[149] In arid regions, outbreaks often occur within 2 or 3 weeks of heavy rains suggesting that RRV survives in desiccation-resistant mosquito eggs with vertical transmission.[565] This is further suggested by isolation of RRV from field-caught immature and male *Ae. vigilax* and *Aedes tremulus* mosquitoes.[565]

Epidemic polyarthritis, initiated by a viremic traveler from Australia to Fiji, spread to several South Pacific Islands between 1979 and 1980 in explosive outbreaks similar to urban CHIK with a man–mosquito–man transmission cycle and *Aedes polynesiensis* as the vector.[818,973] Human viremias of greater than 10^6 mosquito ID$_{50}$/mL have been documented.[973] Cases in travelers suggest that RRV has been reintroduced to Fiji,[498] and serosurveys in American Samoa and French Polynesia indicate ongoing silent circulation.[47,534]

Molecular epidemiology

Strains of RRV originally isolated from the northeastern (Queensland), southeastern (New South Wales), and western regions of Australia are antigenically and genetically distinguishable.[454,842,1089] However, the northeastern lineage has not been recovered since 1977 and, along with the western lineage, has been replaced by the southeastern lineage.[3,454] This replacement accompanied the appearance of a duplication in the C-terminal hypervariable domain of nsP3 first identified in a strain recovered in 1979 from a patient in Fiji.[3,4] The data suggest genetic divergence and independent evolution of RRV within geographically isolated enzootic foci consistent with mammals as a vertebrate reservoir.[842] However, overall diversity is low, perhaps due to purifying selection.[454] Sequencing of intrahost populations of RRV reveals substantial diversity and evidence of mixed infections.[569]

Clinical Features and Pathology

RRV infection most often induces fever, arthralgia, and rash (Fig. 6.7), but not all patients develop all three signs/symptoms.[380,971] Usually, the illness has a sudden onset after a 7- to 9-day incubation period. Fever is the initial symptom, is low grade, and is typically followed by the onset of pain, swelling, and tenderness in multiple joints. Joint involvement is usually symmetrical and both small and large joints can be affected. Characteristically, the rash appears on the 3rd or 4th day of illness; is maculopapular, nonpruritic, and present on the face, trunk, and extremities with occasional involvement of the palms and soles; and generally lasts 3 to 4 days. Frequent accompanying signs and symptoms include lymphadenopathy, lethargy, headache, myalgias, and photophobia. The average period of incapacity is 6 weeks and symptoms gradually resolve in most affected individuals over 3 to 6 months.[282,376,380,570]

Examination of synovial fluid shows increased protein, CD4$^+$ T lymphocytes, monocytes, and activated macrophages and increased levels of RANKL, TRAP56, TNF, IFNγ, and MCP-1.[164,182,283,563] Cell counts are moderately increased, ranging from 1,500 to 15,000 cells/mm[283]and RRV RNA is present.[923] RRV replicates in osteoblasts and can cause persistent infection of synovial macrophages *in vitro*,[1046] and it is postulated that infection of these cells leads to cytokine production and inflammatory arthritis *in vivo*.[949] For instance, osteoblast infection induces inflammatory cytokine production and increases RANKL relative to its decoy receptor osteoprotegerin favoring osteoclast formation.[164] Serum levels of complement pathway protein long pentraxin 3 are increased.[267]

The skin lesions show mononuclear perivascular inflammation without evidence of immune complex deposition. Most of the infiltrating cells are CD8+ T lymphocytes. RRV antigen is present in the basal epidermal and eccrine duct epithelial cells.[284]

Animal Models and Host Range

Despite its extensive host range, RRV induces clinically evident disease only in humans, mice, and horses.[55,964] The prototype T48 strain has been extensively passaged in mice and virulence is age-dependent.[643,673] In newborn mice, T48 infects cardiac muscle causing myocardial necrosis and death 3 to 4 days after infection.[673,880] One-week-old mice survive and infection of the CNS leads to demyelination and destruction of the internal granule cell layer of the cerebellum.[880] In 2- to 3-week-old mice, RRV causes myositis, arthritis, and weakness with virus replication in muscle, perichondrium, periosteum, bone, and skin.[164,663] Macrophages are prominent components of the disease-inducing inflammatory and virus control processes.[369,563,570,828] Soluble mediators that contribute to disease pathogenesis include complement, pentraxin 3, TNF, IFN-α/β, IFNγ, IL-6, MCP-1, and macrophage inhibitory factor (MIF).[164,369,401,562,563,660,662] Treatment with antibody to IL-6 decreases bone loss.[164] CD8+ T cells contribute to virus clearance from muscle, but not joint tissue,[121,563] and mice deficient in TLR7 signaling have more severe disease, inadequate production of neutralizing antibody, and poor virus clearance.[688] Mice deficient in pentraxin 3 have decreased inflammation and virus replication with improved outcome.[267] Adult mice develop an asymptomatic viremia that persists for 5 to 9 days.[887] In pregnant mice, virus can replicate in the placenta and spread to the fetus.[641]

The less virulent NB5092 strain induces severe myositis and muscle cell death in newborn mice after subcutaneous inoculation.[673] Mice become stiff and unable to move and then gradually regenerate muscle and recover function after virus is cleared.[673] CNS disease is minimal with patchy infection of ependymal cells and ependymitis leading to hydrocephalus. Neurons are only occasionally infected.[643] Brown fat is another important site of virus replication.[673] By 1 week of age, mice no longer develop signs of disease.[673]

Virulence

To identify determinants of virulence for mice, virulent T48 has been compared to the less virulent NB5092 and DC5692 strains with different passage histories.[253,293] Virulence has been associated primarily with amino acid differences in nsP1 and E2.[465,466,484,629,964,1033,1034] Changes in nsP1 affect disease without affecting virus replication, while changes in E2 usually affect replication. Induction and susceptibility to IFN also influence

disease development.[369,562] Of unproven but possible significance is the fact that the epidemic strain of RRV in the Pacific differed from the parent Australian strain by a change from Thr to Ala at E2-219 and a duplication in nsP3.[3,120]

Diagnosis, Treatment, and Prevention

Diagnosis is aided by geographic location and travel history. The differential diagnosis includes rubella, other alphavirus-induced arthritides, and Henoch-Schonlein syndrome.[282] Virus can be recovered from blood early in disease,[818,1092] but most diagnoses are made using serology. The IgM capture EIA is sensitive, but can remain positive for 1 to 2 years after the onset of disease.[148] Neutralization assays can distinguish between viruses in the SF complex.[394]

In mice, treatment with drugs to block NF-κB, MCP-1 synthesis, or IL-1β signaling can decrease inflammation and tissue damage.[563,826,1087] In contrast, treatment to block TNF enhances virus replication, inflammation, and tissue damage.[1101]

Vector control and personal protection against mosquito bites remain the primary means of prevention.[377,980] An aluminum hydroxide–adjuvanted inactivated whole-virus vaccine that protects mice from infection and disease induces neutralizing antibody in humans at levels predicted to be protective and is in phase 3 clinical development.[6,409,1091]

Sindbis

The prototype strain of SINV, AR339, was initially isolated from *Culex univittatus* mosquitoes collected near Sindbis, Egypt, in 1952.[963] Humans living in the Nile Delta at that time had a seroprevalence of 27%, but no disease was associated with infection.[963] Over the next 25 years, SINV was isolated in Europe, the Middle East, Africa, India, Asia, Australia, and the Philippines from a variety of mosquito and vertebrate species. SINV was first isolated from the blood of febrile humans in Uganda in 1961 and recognized as a cause of rash and arthritis in South Africa in 1963.[604]

Epidemiology

SINV is the most widely distributed of the alphaviruses causing arthritis in man, but is not recognized as a cause of disease in much of its range (Fig. 6.18). The primary sites of recognized SINV-mediated human disease are in Northern Europe (Ockelbo fever in Sweden, Pogosta fever in Finland, and Karelian fever in Russia)[249] and South Africa[467] (Fig. 6.18). In the many other regions where the virus exists, human infection occurs, but results only in subclinical disease, fever, or mild arthralgias. The basic maintenance cycle of SINV is between *Culex* spp. or *Culiseta* spp. mosquitoes and wild birds.[598] In Sweden, the enzootic cycle involves *Culex torrentium*, *Culiseta morsitans*, and passerine birds.[281,402,589,591] In Finland, grouse are an important vertebrate host.[521]

Morbidity and mortality

The age-adjusted prevalence for SINV is 2% to 8% in endemic regions of Northern Europe and 0.1% to 0.2% in neighboring nonendemic areas. Risk is highest between the 60th and 64th parallels and is associated with spending time in the woods or marshland and exposure to mosquito bites.[114,249,521,588,846] The ratio of symptomatic to asymptomatic cases is 1:17 with 45- to 65-year-old females most likely to develop disease.[114]

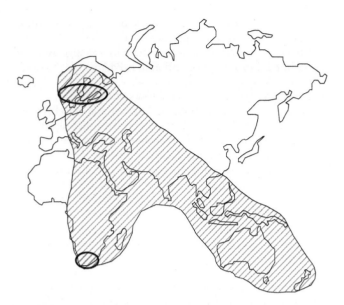

FIGURE 6.18 Geographic distribution of Sindbis virus. Northern Europe and South Africa, regions with significant outbreaks of arthritis and rash disease in humans, are designated in *blue*.

Origin and spread of epidemics

Spread of SINV from its enzootic cycle between passerine birds and ornithophilic mosquitoes to humans involves bridge vectors with less specialized feeding habits[1004] (Fig. 6.10). In Northern Europe, the primary bridge vector is *Aedes cinereus* and availability of this species may determine the frequency of human infection. Cases begin to appear in late July and continue into the fall. Large outbreaks occur approximately every 7 years, perhaps in association with fluctuating grouse populations.[588,846] During a 2013 Swedish outbreak, *Cs. morsitans* was naturally infected and the SINV strain detected was closely related to recent Finnish SINV isolates.[76] Vertical transmission in mosquitoes can occur.[213] Detection of SINV in mosquito larvae of three species (*Aedes* [*Ochlerotatus*] *communis*, *Aedes* [*Ochlerotatus*] *punctor*, and *Aedes* [*Ochlerotatus*] *diantaeus*) in Sweden also indicates natural transovarial transmission as a maintenance mechanism. In South Africa, cases appear annually, mainly during late summer and early autumn in the central plateau region.[942]

Molecular epidemiology

Antigenic and genetic analyses of strains from different locations indicate the presence of five geographically distributed distinct genotypes: Africa and Europe (I), Australia (II), East Asia (III), Azerbaijan and China (IV), and New Zealand (V, Whataroa).[590,591,841,843,899] Strains isolated in Northern Europe and South Africa, where most SINV-induced disease occurs, are more closely related to each other than to strains isolated in south and central Europe and the Middle East where disease is rare.[457,892] Israeli SINV strains together with those from Saudi Arabia comprise a Middle Eastern clade within genotype I.[53] Patterns of SINV clade distributions are consistent with a major role for migratory birds in dispersal.[590,843]

Clinical Features

The primary clinical manifestations are itching rash, arthritis, fever, and muscle pain.[10,249,519,1007] The rash is distributed diffusely over the trunk and limbs and can affect the palms and soles. Skin lesions have a macular base with central vesicle formation and a pale halo and are occasionally hemorrhagic.[249,604] Joint pain preferentially affects large joints and may be severe enough to be immobilizing. Macrophages infected with SINV become activated; release MIF, TNF, IL-1β, and IL-6; and express matrix metalloproteinases.[40] Most patients recover within 14 days, but joint pain and muscle stiffness may persist for months to years.[249,362,519,847,1007] In Australia, SINV-induced arthritis and rash are milder and less frequent than RRV-induced disease or SINV-induced disease in Northern Europe and Africa.[598]

Animal Models and Host Range

SINV can infect a wide variety of vertebrates and has been extensively studied in mice as a model for acute encephalomyelitis. In mice, there is an age-dependent susceptibility to fatal encephalitis.[450] In young mice, virus replicates to high titer and spreads rapidly, causing death in 3 to 5 days. In older mice, virus replication is more restricted and mice often recover. After peripheral inoculation, virus replicates in muscle, produces a viremia, and then spreads to the brain and spinal cord where the primary target cells are neurons.[431] The ability of SINV to spread to the CNS and cause fatal disease is dependent on the strain of virus and the genetic background of the mouse.[432,592,593,889,975,1001] C57BL/6 mice are most susceptible to fatal encephalomyelitis after infection with neurovirulent strains, and this is determined in part by a gene on chromosome 2.[975,976,1001] Neuronal death requires host contributions such as glutamate excitotoxicity and T-cell–mediated immunopathology.[198,340,514,515,608,683,822] Mice with deficiencies of IFN signaling, IRF7, or acid sphingomyelinase have increased susceptibility to fatal encephalitis.[124,692,870]

In nonfatal encephalitis, a SINV-specific perivascular mononuclear inflammatory response consisting of T cells and monocytes appears in the CNS within 3 to 4 days after infection followed by entry of antibody-secreting B cells.[638,646] Spread of infection is limited initially by IFN-α/β,[124] and infectious virus is cleared within 7 to 8 days after infection primarily through the effects of antiviral IgM antibody and IFNγ.[85,116,117,352,551,697] Viral RNA persists in the CNS after clearance of infectious virus, and reactivation of infection appears to be prevented by continued presence of T lymphocytes and antibody-secreting B cells within the CNS.[353,550,638,1008]

Virulence

Strains of SINV differing in virulence have been derived from independent isolates from Egypt (AR339), South Africa (SR86), and Israel (SV-Peleg). Variants of AR339 and SV-Peleg differing in virulence have been derived by passage in mice and in tissue culture.[351,592] Virulence is determined primarily by the 5′ UTR, nsP3, and the E2 glycoprotein, but is also influenced by changes in E1, capsid, and the other nsPs.[201,594,624,627,731,926,952] Changes from A to G in nucleotide 5 or 8 in the 5′ UTR decrease recognition by IFIT1 and increase neurovirulence.[229,425,624] The N-terminal nsP3 macrodomain affects efficiency of replication in neurons.[731] Amino acid changes in the E2 glycoprotein alter efficiency of virus entry into the CNS and can enhance neuronal infection.[71,201,539,1002] Neuroinvasion is affected by changes at residues 55 and 190 of E2.[229] A Gln to His change at E2-55 increases efficiency of infection of neurons and is a major determinant of increased virulence in older mice.[539,1002]

Diagnosis, Treatment, and Prevention

The major differential is with other causes of acute rash and arthritis, such as parvovirus B19 and rubella. SINV can be recovered from skin lesions and from blood,[519,520,604] but the diagnosis is most often made by serology. SINV-specific IgM increases during the acute phase of the disease and then tends to decrease slowly for 3 to 4 years independent of persistent symptoms.[695]

Mice can be protected from fatal encephalitis by treatment with drugs that inhibit inflammation and glutamate excitotoxicity.[340,430,608,773] Mice can also be passively protected with antibody, but develop progressive destruction of infected regions of the brain.[490]

Barmah Forest

Barmah Forest virus (BFV) was first isolated in 1974 from *Cx. annulirostris* mosquitoes collected in the BF in the Murray River Valley region of southeastern Australia and soon thereafter in southwest Queensland.[33] It is the only recognized member of the BFV complex and has a unique E2 protein without N-linked glycosylation.[94,508,540] Human disease was first reported in 1986 with an epidemic of polyarthritis in New South Wales,[94] and BFV was first isolated from the blood of a patient in 1988.[747] The geographic range of BFV is expanding although problems with serologic diagnosis have been identified.[522,983] In 1989, BFV, previously restricted to eastern portions of Australia, was isolated in Western Australia with subsequent outbreaks of human disease.[566]

The vertebrate reservoir host is unknown, but serosurveys suggest that horses and marsupials, particularly brushtail possums, may play a role.[475,566] On the other hand, sequence analysis shows a high degree of sequence identity over the geographic distribution consistent with an avian vertebrate host.[760] Newborn mice are susceptible to experimental infection with virus replication in muscle and brain, but disease is less severe than that induced by RRV.[400] The main mosquito vectors are not well established, but appear to include *Cx. annulirostris*, *Ae. vigilax*, *Ae. notoscriptus*, and *Ae. camptorhynchus*.[434,566] Transmission in coastal areas is influenced by temperature, tides, and socioeconomic factors.[682]

Disease is most common in the 30- to 50-year age group with males and females equally affected.[72] The most common clinical features are fever, lethargy, polyarthritis, and myalgia accompanied by a vesicular rash.[33,72,747] Diagnosis may not be made because the illness is frequently mild and overlaps the clinical spectrum and geographic distribution of RRV and SINV infections (Figs. 6.17 and 6.18). Rash is more prominent in BFV, while arthritis is more prominent in RRV[266] and the serology is distinct.[747] In over half of infected individuals, recovery takes several weeks, with lethargy the most prominent persisting symptom.[72]

Mayaro and Una

MAYV was first isolated in 1954 from febrile forest workers in Trinidad and then from several individuals with fever and frontal headache in the Guamá River area of Brazil.[30,156] The virus is widely distributed in South America,[272,665,974] and evidence of human infection has been obtained in Haiti[537] and Panama[145] suggesting recent spread. Human cases are sporadic and occur primarily in persons with recent contact with humid tropical forests.[989] There are three distinct genotypes. Genotype

D contains isolates from Trinidad and north central South America, genotype L contains isolates from Brazil, and genotype N is represented by a single isolate from eastern Peru.[49,765] The principal mosquito vectors are in the forest-dwelling genus *Haemagogus* and the vertebrate hosts are mammals, mainly nonhuman primates. Airborne transmission to laboratory personnel has also occurred.[464] However, experimentally, MAYV can be transmitted by *Ae. aegypti* and *Ae. albopictus*,[577,914,1080] and human viremia levels suggest the possibility of urban, human-amplified transmission like that exhibited by CHIKV.[577] Recent studies also demonstrate laboratory vector competence by *Anopheles* mosquitoes.[115]

Signs and symptoms of MAYV infection, which, like CHIKV, is usually symptomatic, include fever, headache, arthralgia, myalgia, vomiting, diarrhea, and rash that last 3 to 5 days.[665] The diagnosis can be made by isolation of virus from blood or by serology using an IgM capture EIA or neutralization assay.[130,394]

Una virus is closely related to MAYV and was first isolated from *Psorophora ferox* mosquitoes in the Amazonian region of Brazil in 1959.[154] It is widely distributed in Central and South America.[154,215,216] Vertebrate hosts include nonhuman primates.[215] Una virus is pathogenic for mice, but is not recognized to cause human disease.

OTHER ALPHAVIRUSES

Semliki Forest

SFV was first isolated in 1942 from *Aedes abnormalis* collected in the Semliki Forest (SF) of western Uganda.[917] It is widely distributed in Africa with mosquito (e.g., *Ae. africanus*, *Ae. argenteopunctatus*) isolates documented from Mozambique, Nigeria, and the Central African Republic.[601,614,622] Although SFV is one of the most extensively studied of the alphaviruses and serosurveys indicate that human infection is relatively common,[614,917] it has been linked to human disease on only two occasions. In the first case, reported in 1979, a 26-year-old laboratory worker in Germany with a 1-year history of "purulent bronchitis" working with the Osterrieth strain of SFV developed fever and headache followed by seizures, coma, and death from encephalitis. SFV was isolated from the CSF and from the brain. No antiviral antibody was detectable at the time the CNS symptoms began, but was detected at the time of death 1 week later.[1081] The history of chronic pulmonary infections and failure to rapidly produce antiviral antibody suggest that this individual had an immunodeficiency disorder involving antibody production. In 1987, SFV was isolated from serum samples of individuals in the Central African Republic with fever, persistent headache, myalgias, and arthralgias.[614]

Animal Models

SFV can cause encephalitis in horses, mice, rats, hamsters, rabbits, and guinea pigs.[45,98,917,1113] Severity and type of disease are dependent on the age of the animal at the time of infection, on the route of inoculation, and on the virulence of the strain of SFV used for infection.[98,354] Mice have been most extensively studied and the strain of inbred mouse infected can also influence outcome.[946]

In newborn and suckling mice, inoculated peripherally virulent and avirulent strains of SFV replicate rapidly and extensively in the muscle, elicit a high-titered viremia, spread to the CNS, and cause death within 2 to 4 days.[256,354,671] Evidence suggests that SFV enters the brain across cerebrovascular endothelial cells.[256,485,924] Once within the CNS, the virus replicates primarily in neurons and spreads rapidly along neural pathways producing neuronal cell death.[711]

In weanling (3–5 weeks old) mice, SFV replicates rapidly, but reaches lower peak titers in muscle, blood, and brain than in younger animals.[354] Virus enters perivascular regions of the brain and initiates foci of infection within the CNS. After intranasal inoculation, virus infects olfactory neurons and then spreads within the CNS.[711] The primary target cells in the brain are neurons that control virus replication more effectively than oligodendrocytes.[45,256,279,485] A mononuclear inflammatory response consisting of T lymphocytes, B lymphocytes, and monocytes is apparent 3 to 4 days after infection, peaks at 2 to 3 weeks, and is mostly resolved by 6 weeks.[658]

Mice infected with virulent strains can be passively protected from fatal encephalitis with immune serum, but then develop a delayed disease associated with persistent infection, inflammation, and neuronal degeneration.[877] Mice that survive infection develop demyelination, accompanied by mild paralysis, 2 to 4 weeks after infection.[172,947] Clearance of infectious virus is complete 7 to 10 days after infection and this clearance is mediated by antibody.[256] Viral RNA and protein persist for months.[225,485] Focal areas of demyelination are found 14 to 21 days after SFV infection and are characterized initially by swelling and vacuolation of oligodendrocytes and loss of myelin sheaths followed by remyelination.[122] Demyelination is macrophage-mediated and appears to be the result of oligodendrocyte infection, the immune response to infection, and induction of an autoimmune response to myelin.[257,648,945] SJL mice have more prolonged inflammatory responses and demyelination after infection compared with other strains of mice.[225,918]

SFV infection of the CNS can also increase the susceptibility of mice to induction of experimental autoimmune encephalomyelitis[649] apparently by damaging the blood–brain barrier, increasing adhesion molecule expression on endothelial cells, and facilitating entry of autoimmune T lymphocytes into the CNS.[924,925]

Virulence

Isolates from mosquitoes collected in 1942 in Bwamba, Uganda,[917] in 1948 in Kumba, Nigeria,[601] and in 1959 in Namacurra, Mozambique,[622] have given rise to a variety of laboratory strains of SFV with differing levels of virulence. The most commonly studied are virulent strains V12, V13, and L10 (Uganda strain independently passaged in mice in Bethesda [V] and London [L]) and avirulent strain A7 (Mozambique strain AR2066 passaged in mice) and its less virulent derivative A7-74.[98] In addition, avirulent strains of L10 have been derived by chemical mutagenesis (e.g., m9).[64] Virulent and avirulent strains differ in their ability to invade and replicate in the CNS of weanling mice and rats after peripheral inoculation, but all strains cause fatal disease in newborn or suckling mice.[45,256,354,671] In 3- to 4-week-old mice, avirulent SFV is restricted in replication and spread in the CNS compared to virulent strains of virus and compared to avirulent strains in younger mice.[713] This difference in replication is associated with decreased budding of infectious virus and is independent of the host immune response.[256] Mature neurons and pancreatic and myocardial cells can be made more susceptible to avirulent

virus by treatment with aurothiolate compounds that induce intracellular membrane proliferation.[256,861] In general, reduced virulence correlates with reduced replication in neurons.[57]

In vitro studies of the differences between virulent and avirulent strains of SFV have shown differential replication in neuronal cells[44] and differences in susceptibility to IFN.[210] Efforts to identify specific nucleotide and amino acid changes important for virulence have utilized comparative sequence analysis and an infectious SFV cDNA clone pSP6-SFV4 derived from the prototype virulent L10 strain. Construction of SFV4/A7 chimeric viruses has shown that determinants of virulence reside in both the structural and nonstructural regions of the genome[961] with changes in E2, nsP2, and nsP3 identified as particularly important.[256,261,315,318,807,849,855]

Other SFV-Related Viruses

The SFV complex includes eight viruses and has representatives in both the Old World (BEBV, CHIKV, GETV, ONNV, RRV, and SFV) and the New World (MAYV and Una virus) (Table 6.1; Fig. 6.5). Southern elephant seal (SES) virus is phylogenetically, but not antigenically, related to SFV. Human disease, when present, is generally characterized by fever that may be accompanied by arthritis and rash. CHIKV, ONNV, RRV, and SFV have been discussed previously.

Getah

Getah virus was first isolated from *Culex* spp. mosquitoes collected in Malaysia in 1955 and causes myositis when inoculated into mice.[404] It is maintained in a cycle similar to Japanese encephalitis virus with transmission by *Culex tritaeniorhynchus* and amplification in domestic pigs.[906] Getah virus is widespread and ranges from Eurasia to Southeast and Far East Asia, Pacific Islands, and Australasia. Disease in humans is limited to fever,[559] but it causes abortion in pigs and is an important pathogen of horses.[59,690,882] The equine disease is characterized by fever, an urticarial rash, and hind leg edema, but is not life-threatening.[882]

Southern Elephant Seal

SES virus was isolated from lice residing on Southern elephant seals on Macquarie Island, Australia. It is phylogenetically related to SFV, but does not cross-react serologically. No disease has been recognized in infected seals and it is not known whether lice are responsible for transmission.[524]

Salmonid Alphaviruses

Salmonid alphaviruses (SAV), formally multiple subtypes of the species salmon pancreatic disease virus (SPDV), cause sleeping disease in rainbow trout and pancreas disease in farmed Atlantic salmon.[408,1028,1073,1074] SPDV has unusually large E1 and E2 structural glycoproteins and relatively low (30%–34%) homology to other alphaviruses.[1028,1074] Six subtypes have been identified that likely evolved from a wild reservoir.[471,919] Subtypes 1, 4, and 5 are closely related and have been isolated from farms in Britain with pancreas disease. Subtype 3 causes disease on salmon farms in Norway and subtype 2 causes sleeping disease in Europe. Subtype 6 is represented by a single isolate from Ireland. SPDV causes significant disease on fish farms characterized by abnormal swimming behavior and lack of appetite. SPDV replicates in muscle satellite stem cells with frequent generation of deletion mutants and E2 is a determinant of virulence.[81,634,744] Histopathology shows degeneration of the pancreas and of cardiac and skeletal muscles.[626] SPDV is shed in feces and mucus and can be horizontally transmitted.[334] Sea lice can be infected, but their role in transmission is unclear.[743] Subtype 5 SAV RNA sequences have been detected in wild marine fish further suggesting that marine reservoirs exist.[920]

DIAGNOSIS

The differential diagnosis of alphavirus-induced diseases often includes more than one alphavirus in addition to other mosquito-borne febrile viral diseases such as dengue and Zika and West Nile fevers, other rash diseases such as rubella and parvovirus B19, and other causes of encephalitis. IgM capture EIAs can be used for diagnosis early in disease.[129,130,133] The IgM response is relatively specific for each antigenic complex and is useful even at later times, because IgM persists for at least 2 to 3 weeks after onset of disease.[130] In regions where two or more viruses in a given antigenic complex occur, virus-specific IgM EIAs or neutralization assays may be required to rule out cross-reactions. Virus isolation remains useful, but nucleic acid amplification tests have simplified virus identification in clinical samples.[771] RT-PCR primers have been designed that can amplify the conserved region of all alphaviruses,[247,357,746] as well as alphavirus-specific regions,[529] and are useful for rapid diagnosis.

PREVENTION AND CONTROL

Treatment

There is currently no available specific antiviral treatment for any alphavirus-induced disease, although compound screening and molecular docking studies have identified many potential antiviral therapies for evaluation in animals along with therapeutic monoclonal antibodies, IFN, and immune system activators.[9,123,570] Several neuroprotective drugs can protect mice from fatal encephalomyelitis and supportive treatment can be lifesaving.[349] Symptomatic treatment for arthritis with anti-inflammatory drugs and immune modulators can be beneficial.[570]

Vaccines

Formalin-inactivated vaccines against EEE, WEE, and VEE are available for horses and against EEE for birds. Experimental inactivated vaccines against EEE, WEE, and VEE are also available for laboratory workers exposed to these agents with yearly booster doses required for EEE and WEE.[237] PE-6, the investigational inactivated EEE vaccine for humans, induces good immunoreactivity against the NA-EEEV, but not MADV.[944] Because formalin inactivation of TrD for VEE vaccination was sometimes incomplete, other virus strains and methods of inactivation have been evaluated.[888] An inactivated RRV vaccine was safe and immunogenic in a phase 3 human trial.[1091] Live attenuated vaccines for VEEV (TC-83) and CHIKV (181/25) have been tested in clinical trials,[554,888] but substantial side effects are common with both. Alternative approaches at various stages of preclinical development for prevention of CHIKV, VEEV, and RRV infection include monoclonal antibodies and DNA, subunit, replicon, virus-like particle, and virus-vectored vaccines.[245,570,888] In both horses and humans, prior vaccination against one alphavirus can interfere with development of neutralizing antibody to subsequent alphavirus vaccines.[136,619,757]

Other

Prevention of infection with most alphaviruses relies primarily on efforts to control mosquito populations with insecticides and elimination of aquatic larval habitats. A variety of means can be used for assessing the need for mosquito abatement. These include monitoring mosquito population densities, seroconversion of sentinel animals, and presence of virus in populations of mosquitoes capable of transmitting virus to humans or domestic animals. Individual use of protective measures, such as mosquito repellents and protective clothing, is important. New methods directed against *Ae. aegypti*, including population reductions based on release of *Wolbachia*-infected or transgenic males to effectively sterilize wild females, or the introduction of *Wolbachia* that interfere with CHIKV transmission, are in widespread trials.[1050]

PERSPECTIVE

The ability to construct full-length cDNA alphavirus clones that can be transcribed into infectious RNA has advanced understanding of the functions of various genes and their importance for replication and virulence in the multiple hosts necessary for maintenance of these viruses in their natural cycles. An understanding of the three-dimensional structures of proteins in the virion has greatly aided interpretation of much of the sequence and virulence data previously acquired. Further sequence information on virulent and avirulent strains, functional and structural analysis of the nonstructural proteins and polyproteins, and assessment of cell-type–specific virus interactions is likely to provide the next level of understanding of virus–host relationships.

In addition, there is a need for improved approaches to prevention and treatment. There is a particular need for understanding the components of the immune response necessary for noncytolytic virus clearance, protection from reinfection, immunomodulation of disease, mechanisms of chronic arthralgia, and importance of persistent viral RNA in tissues. New and improved vaccines are needed for protection during outbreaks and for laboratory workers. In addition, there is a need for effective antialphaviral drugs, and an understanding of the structure of viral proteins may offer new approaches to therapeutics. These areas have implications for biological defense purposes because many alphaviruses can be transmitted by aerosol and VEEV, EEEV, and WEEV are considered potential agents of biowarfare.[9] Finally, improved, inexpensive, point of care diagnostics are needed so that alphaviruses such as CHIKV, MAYV, and VEEV are not misdiagnosed as dengue and other common infections. This could lead to major improvements in surveillance and control measures, as well as identification of endemic locations suitable for clinical efficacy testing of vaccines and therapeutics.[805]

REFERENCES

1. Aaskov JG, Davies CE, Tucker M, et al. Effect on mice of infection during pregnancy with three Australian arboviruses. *Am J Trop Med Hyg* 1981;30(1):198–203.
2. Aaskov JG, Fraser JR, Dalglish DA. Specific and non-specific immunological changes in epidemic polyarthritis patients. *Aust J Exp Biol Med Sci* 1981;59(Pt 5):599–608.
3. Aaskov J, Jones A, Choi W, et al. Lineage replacement accompanying duplication and rapid fixation of an RNA element in the nsP3 gene in a species of alphavirus. *Virology* 2011;410(2):353–359.

4. Aaskov JG, Mataika JU, Lawrence GW, et al. An epidemic of Ross River virus infection in Fiji, 1979. *Am J Trop Med Hyg* 1981;30(5):1053–1059.

5. Aaskov JG, Nair K, Lawrence GW, et al. Evidence for transplacental transmission of Ross River virus in humans. *Med J Aust* 1981;2(1):20–21.

6. Aaskov J, Williams L, Yu S. A candidate Ross River virus vaccine: preclinical evaluation. *Vaccine* 1997;15(12–13):1396–1404.

7. Abbas YM, Pichlmair A, Gorna MW, et al. Structural basis for viral 5'-PPP-RNA recognition by human IFIT proteins. *Nature* 2013;494(7435):60–64.

8. Abraham R, Hauer D, McPherson RL, et al. ADP-ribosyl-binding and hydrolase activities of the alphavirus nsP3 macrodomain are critical for initiation of virus replication. *Proc Natl Acad Sci U S A* 2018;115(44):E10457–E10466.

9. Abu Bakar F, Ng LFP. Nonstructural proteins of alphavirus-potential targets for drug development. *Viruses* 2018;10(2).

10. Adouchief S, Smura T, Sane J, et al. Sindbis virus as a human pathogen-epidemiology, clinical picture and pathogenesis. *Rev Med Virol* 2016;26(4):221–241.

11. Agapov EV, Frolov I, Lindenbach BD, et al. Noncytopathic Sindbis virus RNA vectors for heterologous gene expression. *Proc Natl Acad Sci U S A* 1998;95(22):12989–12994.

12. Aguilar MJ. Pathological changes in brain and other target organs of infant and weanling mice after infection with non-neuroadapted Western equine encephalitis virus. *Infect Immun* 1970;2(5):533–542.

13. Aguilar PV, Adams AP, Wang E, et al. Structural and nonstructural protein genome regions of eastern equine encephalitis virus are determinants of interferon sensitivity and murine virulence. *J Virol* 2008;82(10):4920–4930.

14. Aguilar PV, Estrada-Franco JG, Navarro-Lopez R, et al. Endemic Venezuelan equine encephalitis in the Americas: hidden under the dengue umbrella. *Future Virol* 2011;6(6):721–740.

15. Aguilar PV, Greene IP, Coffey LL, et al. Endemic Venezuelan equine encephalitis in northern Peru. *Emerg Infect Dis* 2004;10(5):880–888.

16. Aguilar PV, Paessler S, Carrara AS, et al. Variation in interferon sensitivity and induction among strains of eastern equine encephalitis virus. *J Virol* 2005;79(17):11300–11310.

17. Aguilar PV, Robich RM, Turell MJ, et al. Endemic eastern equine encephalitis in the Amazon region of Peru. *Am J Trop Med Hyg* 2007;76(2):293–298.

18. Aguilar PV, Weaver SC, Basler CF. Capsid protein of eastern equine encephalitis virus inhibits host cell gene expression. *J Virol* 2007;81(8):3866–3876.

19. Ahn A, Klimjack MR, Chatterjee PK, et al. An epitope of the Semliki Forest virus fusion protein exposed during virus-membrane fusion. *J Virol* 1999;73(12):10029–10039.

20. Ahn A, Schoepp RJ, Sternberg D, et al. Growth and stability of a cholesterol-independent Semliki Forest virus mutant in mosquitoes. *Virology* 1999;262(2):452–456.

21. Ahola T, Kaariainen L. Reaction in alphavirus mRNA capping: formation of a covalent complex of nonstructural protein nsP1 with 7-methyl-GMP. *Proc Natl Acad Sci U S A* 1995;92(2):507–511.

22. Ahola T, Lampio A, Auvinen P, et al. Semliki Forest virus mRNA capping enzyme requires association with anionic membrane phospholipids for activity. *EMBO J* 1999;18(11):3164–3172.

23. Akhrymuk I, Frolov I, Frolova EI. Sindbis virus infection causes cell death by nsP2-induced transcriptional shutoff or by nsP3-dependent translational shutoff. *J Virol* 2018;92(23).

24. Akhrymuk I, Kulemzin SV, Frolova EI. Evasion of the innate immune response: the Old World alphavirus nsP2 protein induces rapid degradation of Rpb1, a catalytic subunit of RNA polymerase II. *J Virol* 2012;86(13):7180–7191.

25. Aliota MT, Walker EC, Uribe Yepes A, et al. The wMel strain of Wolbachia reduces transmission of chikungunya virus in *Aedes aegypti*. *PLoS Negl Trop Dis* 2016;10(4):e0004677.

26. Allison AB, Stallknecht DE. Genomic sequencing of Highlands J virus: a comparison to western and eastern equine encephalitis viruses. *Virus Res* 2009;145(2):334–340.

27. Allison AB, Stallknecht DE, Holmes EC. Evolutionary genetics and vector adaptation of recombinant viruses of the western equine encephalitis antigenic complex provides new insights into alphavirus diversity and host switching. *Virology* 2015;474:154–162.

28. Allsopp TE, Scallan MF, Williams A, et al. Virus infection induces neuronal apoptosis: a comparison with trophic factor withdrawal. *Cell Death Differ* 1998;5(1):50–59.

29. Amor S, Scallan MF, Morris MM, et al. Role of immune responses in protection and pathogenesis during Semliki Forest virus encephalitis. *J Gen Virol* 1996;77(Pt 2):281–291.

30. Anderson CR, Downs WG, Wattley GH, et al. Mayaro virus: a new human disease agent. II. Isolation from blood of patients in Trinidad, B.W.I. *Am J Trop Med Hyg* 1957;6(6):1012–1016.

31. Anishchenko M, Bowen RA, Paessler S, et al. Venezuelan encephalitis emergence mediated by a phylogenetically predicted viral mutation. *Proc Natl Acad Sci U S A* 2006;103(13):4994–4999.

32. Anishchenko M, Paessler S, Greene IP, et al. Generation and characterization of closely related epizootic and enzootic infectious cDNA clones for studying interferon sensitivity and emergence mechanisms of Venezuelan equine encephalitis virus. *J Virol* 2004;78(1):1–8.

33. Anonymous. Barmah Forest virus. *Lancet* 1991;337:948–949.

34. Apte-Deshpande AD, Paingankar MS, Gokhale MD, et al. Serratia odorifera mediated enhancement in susceptibility of *Aedes aegypti* for chikungunya virus. *Indian J Med Res* 2014;139(5):762–768.

35. Armstrong PM, Andreadis TG. Eastern equine encephalitis virus in mosquitoes and their role as bridge vectors. *Emerg Infect Dis* 2010;16(12):1869–1874.

36. Arrigo NC, Adams AP, Watts DM, et al. Cotton rats and house sparrows as hosts for North and South American strains of eastern equine encephalitis virus. *Emerg Infect Dis* 2010;16(9):1373–1380.

37. Arrigo NC, Adams AP, Weaver SC. Evolutionary patterns of eastern equine encephalitis virus in North versus South America suggest ecological differences and taxonomic revision. *J Virol* 2010;84(2):1014–1025.

38. Asai T, Shibata I, Uruno K. Susceptibility of pregnant hamster, guinea pig, and rabbit to the transplacental infection of Getah virus. *J Vet Med Sci* 1991;53(6):1109–1111.

39. Ashbrook AW, Burrack KS, Silva LA, et al. Residue 82 of the Chikungunya virus E2 attachment protein modulates viral dissemination and arthritis in mice. *J Virol* 2014;88(21):12180–12192.

40. Assuncao-Miranda I, Bozza MT, Da Poian AT. Pro-inflammatory response resulting from sindbis virus infection of human macrophages: implications for the pathogenesis of viral arthritis. *J Med Virol* 2010;82(1):164–174.

41. Atasheva S, Fish A, Fornerod M, et al. Venezuelan equine encephalitis virus capsid protein forms a tetrameric complex with CRM1 and importin alpha/beta that obstructs nuclear pore complex function. *J Virol* 2010;84(9):4158–4171.

42. Atasheva S, Krendelchtchikova V, Liopo A, et al. Interplay of acute and persistent infections caused by Venezuelan equine encephalitis virus encoding mutated capsid protein. *J Virol* 2010;84(19):10004–10015.

43. Atasheva S, Wang E, Adams AP, et al. Chimeric alphavirus vaccine candidates protect mice from intranasal challenge with western equine encephalitis virus. *Vaccine* 2009;27(32):4309–4319.

44. Atkins GJ. The avirulent A7 Strain of Semliki Forest virus has reduced cytopathogenicity for neuroblastoma cells compared to the virulent L10 strain. *J Gen Virol* 1983;64(Pt 6):1401–1404.

45. Atkins GJ, Sheahan BJ, Mooney DA. Pathogenicity of Semliki Forest virus for the rat central nervous system and primary rat neural cell cultures: possible implications for the pathogenesis of multiple sclerosis. *Neuropathol Appl Neurobiol* 1990;16(1):57–68.

46. Attarzadeh-Yazdi G, Fragkoudis R, Chi Y, et al. Cell-to-cell spread of the RNA interference response suppresses Semliki Forest virus (SFV) infection of mosquito cell cultures and cannot be antagonized by SFV. *J Virol* 2009;83(11):5735–5748.

47. Aubry M, Finke J, Teissier A, et al. Silent circulation of Ross River Virus in French Polynesia. *Int J Infect Dis* 2015;37:19–24.

48. Auguste AJ, Adams AP, Arrigo NC, et al. Isolation and characterization of sylvatic mosquito-borne viruses in Trinidad: enzootic transmission and a new potential vector of Mucambo virus. *Am J Trop Med Hyg* 2010;83(6):1262–1265.

49. Auguste AJ, Liria J, Forrester NL, et al. Evolutionary and ecological characterization of Mayaro virus strains isolated during an outbreak, Venezuela, 2010. *Emerg Infect Dis* 2015;21(10):1742–1750.

50. Auguste AJ, Volk SM, Arrigo NC, et al. Isolation and phylogenetic analysis of Mucambo virus (Venezuelan equine encephalitis complex subtype IIIA) in Trinidad. *Virology* 2009;392(1):123–130.

51. Austin FJ, Scherer WF. Studies of viral virulence. I. Growth and histopathology of virulent and attenuated strains of Venezuelan encephalitis virus in hamsters. *Am J Pathol* 1971;62(2):195–210.

52. Avadhanula V, Weasner BP, Hardy GG, et al. A novel system for the launch of alphavirus RNA synthesis reveals a role for the Imd pathway in arthropod antiviral response. *PLoS Pathog* 2009;5(9):e1000582.

53. Avizov N, Zuckerman N, Orshan L, et al. High endemicity and distinct phylogenetic characteristics of Sindbis Virus in Israel. *J Infect Dis* 2018;218(9):1500–1506.

54. Ayers JR, Lester TL, Angulo AB. An epizootic attributable to western equine encephalitis virus infection in emus in Texas. *J Am Vet Med Assoc* 1994;205(4):600–601.

55. Azuolas JK, Wishart E, Bibby S, et al. Isolation of Ross River virus from mosquitoes and from horses with signs of musculo-skeletal disease. *Aust Vet J* 2003;81(6):344–347.

56. Baer A, Lundberg L, Swales D, et al. Venezuelan equine encephalitis virus induces apoptosis through the unfolded protein response activation of EGR1. *J Virol* 2016;90(7):3558–3572.

57. Balluz IM, Glasgow GM, Killen HM, et al. Virulent and avirulent strains of Semliki Forest virus show similar cell tropism for the murine central nervous system but differ in the severity and rate of induction of cytolytic damage. *Neuropathol Appl Neurobiol* 1993;19(3):233–239.

58. Bandeira AC, Campos GS, Rocha VF, et al. Prolonged shedding of Chikungunya virus in semen and urine: a new perspective for diagnosis and implications for transmission. *IDCases* 2016;6:100–103.

59. Bannai H, Nemoto M, Niwa H, et al. Geospatial and temporal associations of Getah virus circulation among pigs and horses around the perimeter of outbreaks in Japanese racehorses in 2014 and 2015. *BMC Vet Res* 2017;13(1):187.

60. Barabe ND, Rayner GA, Christopher ME, et al. Single-dose, fast-acting vaccine candidate against western equine encephalitis virus completely protects mice from intranasal challenge with different strains of the virus. *Vaccine* 2007;25(33):6271–6276.

61. Barker CM, Johnson WO, Eldridge BF, et al. Temporal connections between *Culex tarsalis* abundance and transmission of western equine encephalomyelitis virus in California. *Am J Trop Med Hyg* 2010;82(6):1185–1193.

62. Barletta AB, Nascimento-Silva MC, Talyuli OA, et al. Microbiota activates IMD pathway and limits Sindbis infection in *Aedes aegypti*. *Parasit Vectors* 2017;10(1):103.

63. Barrera R, Ferro C, Navarro JC, et al. Contrasting sylvatic foci of Venezuelan equine encephalitis virus in northern South America. *Am J Trop Med Hyg* 2002;67(3):324–334.

64. Barrett PN, Sheahan BJ, Atkins GJ. Isolation and preliminary characterization of Semliki Forest virus mutants with altered virulence. *J Gen Virol* 1980;49(1):141–147.

65. Barry G, Breakwell L, Fragkoudis R, et al. PKR acts early in infection to suppress Semliki Forest virus production and strongly enhances the type I interferon response. *J Gen Virol* 2009;90(Pt 6):1382–1391.

66. Barry G, Fragkoudis R, Ferguson MC, et al. Semliki forest virus-induced endoplasmic reticulum stress accelerates apoptotic death of mammalian cells. *J Virol* 2010;84(14):7369–7377.

67. Bashford CL, Alder GM, Gray MA, et al. Oxonol dyes as monitors of membrane potential: the effect of viruses and toxins on the plasma membrane potential of animal cells in monolayer culture and in suspension. *J Cell Physiol* 1985;123(3):326–336.

68. Bastian FO, Wende RD, Singer DB, et al. Eastern equine encephalomyelitis. Histopathologic and ultrastructural changes with isolation of the virus in a human case. *Am J Clin Pathol* 1975;64(1):10–13.

69. Bauer RW, Gill MS, Poston RP, et al. Naturally occurring eastern equine encephalitis in a Hampshire weather. *J Vet Diagn Invest* 2005;17(3):281–285.

70. Baxter VK, Troisi EM, Pate NM, et al. Death and gastrointestinal bleeding complicate encephalomyelitis in mice with delayed appearance of CNS IgM after intranasal alphavirus infection. *J Gen Virol* 2018.

71. Bear JS, Byrnes AP, Griffin DE. Heparin-binding and patterns of virulence for two recombinant strains of Sindbis virus. *Virology* 2006;347(1):183–190.

72. Beard JR, Trent M, Sam GA, et al. Self-reported morbidity of Barmah Forest virus infection on the north coast of New South Wales. *Med J Aust* 1997;167(10):525–528.
73. Beck CE, Wyckoff RW. Venezuelan equine encephalomyelitis. *Science* 1938;88(2292):530.
74. Behr M, Schieferdecker K, Buhr P, et al. Interferon-stimulated response element (ISRE)-binding protein complex DRAF1 is activated in Sindbis virus (HR)-infected cells. *J Interferon Cytokine Res* 2001;21(11):981–990.
75. Berge TO, Tigertt WD, Banks IS. Attenuation of Venezuelan equine encephalomyelitis virus by in vitro cultivation in guinea-pig heart cells. *Am J Hyg* 1961;73(2):209–218.
76. Bergqvist J, Forsman O, Larsson P, et al. Detection and isolation of Sindbis virus from mosquitoes captured during an outbreak in Sweden, 2013. *Vector Borne Zoonotic Dis* 2015;15(2):133–140.
77. Bergren NA, Auguste AJ, Forrester NL, et al. Western equine encephalitis virus: evolutionary analysis of a declining alphavirus based on complete genome sequences. *J Virol* 2014;88(16):9260–9267.
78. Bergren NA, Haller SH, Rossi SL, et al. "Submergence" of western equine encephalitis virus: evidence of positive selection argues against genetic drift and fitness reductions. *PLoS Pathog* 2019:in press.
79. Berl E, Eisen RJ, MacMillan K, et al. Serological evidence for eastern equine encephalitis virus activity in white-tailed deer, Odocoileus virginianus, in Vermont, 2010. *Am J Trop Med Hyg* 2013;88(1):103–107.
80. Bernard KA, Klimstra WB, Johnston RE. Mutations in the E2 glycoprotein of Venezuelan equine encephalitis virus confer heparan sulfate interaction, low morbidity, and rapid clearance from blood of mice. *Virology* 2000;276(1):93–103.
81. Bessaud M, Peyrefitte CN, Pastorino BA, et al. O'nyong-nyong Virus, Chad. *Emerg Infect Dis* 2006;12(8):1248–1250.
82. Biacchesi S, Jouvion G, Merour E, et al. Rainbow trout (Oncorhynchus mykiss) muscle satellite cells are targets of salmonid alphavirus infection. *Vet Res* 2016;47:9.
83. Bianchi TI, Aviles G, Monath TP, et al. Western equine encephalomyelitis: virulence markers and their epidemiologic significance. *Am J Trop Med Hyg* 1993;49(3):322–328.
84. Bianchi TI, Aviles G, Sabattini MS. Biological characteristics of an enzootic subtype of western equine encephalomyelitis virus from Argentina. *Acta Virol* 1997;41(1):13–20.
85. Bick MJ, Carroll JW, Gao G, et al. Expression of the zinc-finger antiviral protein inhibits alphavirus replication. *J Virol* 2003;77(21):11555–11562.
86. Binder GK, Griffin DE. Interferon-gamma-mediated site-specific clearance of alphavirus from CNS neurons. *Science* 2001;293(5528):303–306.
87. Bingham AM, Graham SP, Burkett-Cadena ND, et al. Detection of eastern equine encephalomyelitis virus RNA in North American snakes. *Am J Trop Med Hyg* 2012;87(6):1140–1144.
88. Blohm GM, Lednicky JA, White SK, et al. Madariaga virus: identification of a lineage III strain in a venezuelan child with acute undifferentiated febrile illness, in the setting of a possible equine epizootic. *Clin Infect Dis* 2018;67(4):619–621.
89. Boere WA, Benaissa-Trouw BJ, Harmsen M, et al. Neutralizing and non-neutralizing monoclonal antibodies to the E2 glycoprotein of Semliki Forest virus can protect mice from lethal encephalitis. *J Gen Virol* 1983;64(Pt 6):1405–1408.
90. Boere WA, Benaissa-Trouw BJ, Harmsen T, et al. Mechanisms of monoclonal antibody-mediated protection against virulent Semliki Forest virus. *J Virol* 1985;54(2):546–551.
91. Boere WA, Harmsen T, Vinje J, et al. Identification of distinct antigenic determinants on Semliki Forest virus by using monoclonal antibodies with different antiviral activities. *J Virol* 1984;52(2):575–582.
92. Bordi L, Meschi S, Selleri M, et al. Chikungunya virus isolates with/without A226V mutation show different sensitivity to IFN-a, but similar replication kinetics in non human primate cells. *New Microbiol* 2011;34(1):87–91.
93. Borgherini G, Poubeau P, Jossaume A, et al. Persistent arthralgia associated with chikungunya virus: a study of 88 adult patients on reunion island. *Clin Infect Dis* 2008;47(4):469–475.
94. Borgherini G, Poubeau P, Staikowsky F, et al. Outbreak of chikungunya on Reunion Island: early clinical and laboratory features in 157 adult patients. *Clin Infect Dis* 2007;44(11):1401–1407.
95. Boughton CR, Hawkes RA, Naim HM. Illness caused by a Barmah Forest-like virus in New South Wales. *Med J Aust* 1988;148(3):146–147.
96. Bowen GS, Calisher CH. Virological and serological studies of Venezuelan equine encephalomyelitis in humans. *J Clin Microbiol* 1976;4(1):22–27.
97. Bowers DF, Abell BA, Brown DT. Replication and tissue tropism of the alphavirus Sindbis in the mosquito *Aedes albopictus*. *Virology* 1995;212(1):1–12.
98. Brackney DE, Scott JC, Sagawa F, et al. C6/36 *Aedes albopictus* cells have a dysfunctional antiviral RNA interference response. *PLoS Negl Trop Dis* 2010;4(10):e856.
99. Bradish CJ, Allner K, Maber HB. The virulence of original and derived strains of Semliki forest virus for mice, guinea-pigs and rabbits. *J Gen Virol* 1971;12(2):141–160.
100. Brault AC, Armijos MV, Wheeler S, et al. Stone Lakes virus (family Togaviridae, genus Alphavirus), a variant of Fort Morgan virus isolated from swallow bugs (Hemiptera: Cimicidae) west of the Continental Divide. *J Med Entomol* 2009;46(5):1203–1209.
101. Brault AC, Foy BD, Myles KM, et al. Infection patterns of o'nyong nyong virus in the malaria-transmitting mosquito, *Anopheles gambiae*. *Insect Mol Biol* 2004;13(6):625–635.
102. Brault AC, Powers AM, Chavez CL, et al. Genetic and antigenic diversity among eastern equine encephalitis viruses from North, Central, and South America. *Am J Trop Med Hyg* 1999;61(4):579–586.
103. Brault AC, Powers AM, Holmes EC, et al. Positively charged amino acid substitutions in the e2 envelope glycoprotein are associated with the emergence of venezuelan equine encephalitis virus. *J Virol* 2002;76(4):1718–1730.
104. Brault AC, Powers AM, Ortiz D, et al. Venezuelan equine encephalitis emergence: enhanced vector infection from a single amino acid substitution in the envelope glycoprotein. *Proc Natl Acad Sci U S A* 2004;101(31):11344–11349.
105. Breakwell L, Dosenovic P, Karlsson Hedestam GB, et al. Semliki Forest virus nonstructural protein 2 is involved in suppression of the type I interferon response. *J Virol* 2007;81(16):8677–8684.
106. Brehin AC, Casademont I, Frenkiel MP, et al. The large form of human 2',5'-Oligoadenylate Synthetase (OAS3) exerts antiviral effect against Chikungunya virus. *Virology* 2009;384(1):216–222.
107. Broeck CT, Merrill MH. A serological difference between eastern and western equine encephalomyelitis virus. *Exp Biol Med* 1933;31(2):217–220.
108. Broeckel R, Fox JM, Haese N, et al. Therapeutic administration of a recombinant human monoclonal antibody reduces the severity of chikungunya virus disease in rhesus macaques. *PLoS Negl Trop Dis* 2017;11(6):e0005637.
109. Bron R, Wahlberg JM, Garoff H, et al. Membrane fusion of Semliki Forest virus in a model system: correlation between fusion kinetics and structural changes in the envelope glycoprotein. *EMBO J* 1993;12(2):693–701.
110. Brooke CB, Deming DJ, Whitmore AC, et al. T cells facilitate recovery from Venezuelan equine encephalitis virus-induced encephalomyelitis in the absence of antibody. *J Virol* 2010;84(9):4556–4568.
111. Brown CR, Moore AT, Young GR, et al. Persistence of Buggy Creek virus (Togaviridae, Alphavirus) for two years in unfed swallow bugs (Hemiptera: Cimicidae: *Oeciacus vicarius*). *J Med Entomol* 2010;47(3):436–441.
112. Brown LN, Packer RA. Some factors affecting plaque size of western equine encephalomyelitis virus. *Am J Vet Res* 1964;25:487–493.
113. Brown CR, Strickler SA, Moore AT, et al. Winter ecology of Buggy Creek virus (Togaviridae, Alphavirus) in the Central Great Plains. *Vector Borne Zoonotic Dis* 2010;10(4):355–363.
114. Brown A, Vosdingh R, Zebovitz E. Attenuation and immunogenicity of ts mutants of Eastern encephalitis virus for mice. *J Gen Virol* 1975;27(1):111–116.
115. Brummer-Korvenkontio M, Vapalahti O, Kuusisto P, et al. Epidemiology of Sindbis virus infections in Finland 1981-96: possible factors explaining a peculiar disease pattern. *Epidemiol Infect* 2002;129(2):335–345.
116. Brustolin M, Pujhari S, Henderson CA, et al. Anopheles mosquitoes may drive invasion and transmission of Mayaro virus across geographically diverse regions. *PLoS Negl Trop Dis* 2018;12(11):e0006895.
117. Burdeinick-Kerr R, Govindarajan D, Griffin DE. Noncytolytic clearance of sindbis virus infection from neurons by gamma interferon is dependent on Jak/STAT signaling. *J Virol* 2009;83(8):3429–3435.
118. Burdeinick-Kerr R, Griffin DE. Gamma interferon-dependent, noncytolytic clearance of sindbis virus infection from neurons in vitro. *J Virol* 2005;79(9):5374–5385.
119. Burdeinick-Kerr R, Wind J, Griffin DE. Synergistic roles of antibody and interferon in noncytolytic clearance of Sindbis virus from different regions of the central nervous system. *J Virol* 2007;81(11):5628–5636.
120. Burke CW, Gardner CL, Steffan JJ, et al. Characteristics of alpha/beta interferon induction after infection of murine fibroblasts with wild-type and mutant alphaviruses. *Virology* 2009;395(1):121–132.
121. Burness AT, Pardoe I, Faragher SG, et al. Genetic stability of Ross River virus during epidemic spread in nonimmune humans. *Virology* 1988;167(2):639–643.
122. Burrack KS, Montgomery SA, Homann D, et al. CD8+ T cells control Ross River virus infection in musculoskeletal tissues of infected mice. *J Immunol* 2015;194(2):678–689.
123. Butt AM, Tutton MG, Kirvell SL, et al. Morphology of oligodendrocytes during demyelination in optic nerves of mice infected with Semliki Forest virus. *Neuropathol Appl Neurobiol* 1996;22(6):540–547.
124. Byler KG, Collins JT, Ogungbe IV, et al. Alphavirus protease inhibitors from natural sources: a homology modeling and molecular docking investigation. *Comput Biol Chem* 2016;64:163–184.
125. Byrnes AP, Durbin JE, Griffin DE. Control of Sindbis virus infection by antibody in interferon-deficient mice. *J Virol* 2000;74(8):3905–3908.
126. Byrnes AP, Griffin DE. Binding of Sindbis virus to cell surface heparan sulfate. *J Virol* 1998;72(9):7349–7356.
127. Byrnes AP, Griffin DE. Large-plaque mutants of Sindbis virus show reduced binding to heparan sulfate, heightened viremia, and slower clearance from the circulation. *J Virol* 2000;74(2):644–651.
128. Cain MD, Salimi H, Gong Y, et al. Virus entry and replication in the brain precedes blood-brain barrier disruption during intranasal alphavirus infection. *J Neuroimmunol* 2017;308:118–130.
129. Calisher CH. Medically important arboviruses of the United States and Canada. *Clin Microbiol Rev* 1994;7(1):89–116.
130. Calisher CH, Berardi VP, Muth DJ, et al. Specificity of immunoglobulin M and G antibody responses in humans infected with eastern and western equine encephalitis viruses: application to rapid serodiagnosis. *J Clin Microbiol* 1986;23(2):369–372.
131. Calisher CH, el-Kafrawi AO, Al-Deen Mahmud MI, et al. Complex-specific immunoglobulin M antibody patterns in humans infected with alphaviruses. *J Clin Microbiol* 1986;23(1):155–159.
132. Calisher CH, Emerson JK, Muth DJ, et al. Serodiagnosis of western equine encephalitis virus infections: relationships of antibody titer and test to observed onset of clinical illness. *J Am Vet Med Assoc* 1983;183(4):438–440.
133. Calisher CH, Karabatsos N, Lazuick JS, et al. Reevaluation of the western equine encephalitis antigenic complex of alphaviruses (family Togaviridae) as determined by neutralization tests. *Am J Trop Med Hyg* 1988;38(2):447–452.
134. Calisher CH, Meurman O, Brummer-Korvenkontio M, et al. Sensitive enzyme immunoassay for detecting immunoglobulin M antibodies to Sindbis virus and further evidence that Pogosta disease is caused by a western equine encephalitis complex virus. *J Clin Microbiol* 1985;22(4):566–571.
135. Calisher CH, Monath TP, Mitchell CJ, et al. Arbovirus investigations in Argentina, 1977-1980. III. Identification and characterization of viruses isolated, including new subtypes of western and Venezuelan equine encephalitis viruses and four new bunyaviruses (Las Maloyas, Resistencia, Barranqueras, and Antequera). *Am J Trop Med Hyg* 1985;34(5):956–965.
136. Calisher CH, Monath TP, Muth DJ, et al. Characterization of Fort Morgan virus, an alphavirus of the western equine encephalitis virus complex in an unusual ecosystem. *Am J Trop Med Hyg* 1980;29(6):1428–1440.
137. Calisher CH, Sasso DR, Sather GE. Possible evidence for interference with Venezuelan equine encephalitis virus vaccination of equines by pre-existing antibody to Eastern or Western Equine encephalitis virus, or both. *Appl Microbiol* 1973;26(4):485–488.

138. Calisher CH, Shope RE, Brandt W, et al. Proposed antigenic classification of registered arboviruses I. Togaviridae, Alphavirus. *Intervirology* 1980;14(5–6):229–232.
139. Campbell CL, Keene KM, Brackney DE, et al. *Aedes aegypti* uses RNA interference in defense against Sindbis virus infection. *BMC Microbiol* 2008;8:47.
140. Campbell CL, Lehmann CJ, Gill SS, et al. A role for endosomal proteins in alphavirus dissemination in mosquitoes. *Insect Mol Biol* 2011;20(4):429–436.
141. Cao S, Zhang W. Characterization of an early-stage fusion intermediate of Sindbis virus using cryoelectron microscopy. *Proc Natl Acad Sci U S A* 2013;110(33):13362–13367.
142. Carey DE. Chikungunya and dengue: a case of mistaken identity? *J Hist Med Allied Sci* 1971;26(3):243–262.
143. Carey DE, Myers RM, DeRanitz CM, et al. The 1964 chikungunya epidemic at Vellore, South India, including observations on concurrent dengue. *Trans R Soc Trop Med Hyg* 1969;63(4):434–445.
144. Carrara AS, Gonzales G, Ferro C, et al. Venezuelan equine encephalitis virus infection of spiny rats. *Emerg Infect Dis* 2005;11(5):663–669.
145. Carrasco L, Sanz MA, Gonzalez-Almela E. The regulation of translation in alphavirus-infected cells. *Viruses* 2018;10(2).
146. Carrera JP, Bagamian KH, Travassos da Rosa AP, et al. Human and equine infection with alphaviruses and flaviviruses in Panama during 2010: a cross-sectional study of household contacts during an encephalitis outbreak. *Am J Trop Med Hyg* 2018;98(6):1798–1804.
147. Carrera JP, Forrester N, Wang E, et al. Eastern equine encephalitis in Latin America. *N Engl J Med* 2013;369(8):732–744.
148. Carter IW, Fraser JR, Cloonan MJ. Specific IgA antibody response in Ross River virus infection. *Immunol Cell Biol* 1987;65(Pt 6):511–513.
149. Carter IW, Smythe LD, Fraser JR, et al. Detection of Ross River virus immunoglobulin M antibodies by enzyme-linked immunosorbent assay using antibody class capture and comparison with other methods. *Pathology* 1985;17(3):503–508.
150. Carver S, Bestall A, Jardine A, et al. Influence of hosts on the ecology of arboviral transmission: potential mechanisms influencing dengue, Murray Valley encephalitis, and Ross River virus in Australia. *Vector Borne Zoonotic Dis* 2009;9(1):51–64.
151. Casals J. Antigenic variants of eastern equine encephalitis virus. *J Exp Med* 1964;119:547–565.
152. Casals J, Curnen EC, Thomas L. Venezuelan equine encephalomyelitis in man. *J Exp Med* 1943;77(6):521–530.
153. Casolari S, Briganti E, Zanotti M, et al. A fatal case of encephalitis associated with Chikungunya virus infection. *Scand J Infect Dis* 2008;40(11–12):995–996.
154. Castorena KM, Peltier DC, Peng W, et al. Maturation-dependent responses of human neuronal cells to western equine encephalitis virus infection and type I interferons. *Virology* 2008;372(1):208–220.
155. Causey OR, Casals J, Shope RE, et al. Aura and Una, two new group a arthropod-borne viruses. *Am J Trop Med Hyg* 1963;12:777–781.
156. Causey OR, Causey CE, Maroja OM, et al. The isolation of arthropod-borne viruses, including members of two hitherto undescribed serological groups, in the Amazon region of Brazil. *Am J Trop Med Hyg* 1961;10:227–249.
157. Causey OR, Maroja OM. Mayaro virus: a new human disease agent. III. Investigation of an epidemic of acute febrile illness on the river Guama in Para, Brazil, and isolation of Mayaro virus as causative agent. *Am J Trop Med Hyg* 1957;6(6):1017–1023.
158. Chamberlain RW, Rubin H, Kissling RE, et al. Recovery of virus of Eastern equine encephalomyelitis from a mosquito, Culiseta melanura (Coquillett). *Proc Soc Exp Biol Med* 1951;77(3):396–397.
159. Chanas AC, Ellis DS, Stamford S, et al. The interaction of monoclonal antibodies directed against envelope glycoprotein E1 of Sindbis virus with virus-infected cells. *Antiviral Res* 1982;2(4):191–201.
160. Chanock RM, Sabin AB. The hemagglutinin of western equine encephalitis virus: recovery, properties and use for diagnosis. *J Immunol* 1954;73(5):337–351.
161. Charles PC, Brown KW, Davis NL, et al. Mucosal immunity induced by parenteral immunization with a live attenuated Venezuelan equine encephalitis virus vaccine candidate. *Virology* 1997;228(2):153–160.
162. Charles PC, Trgovcich J, Davis NL, et al. Immunopathogenesis and immune modulation of Venezuelan equine encephalitis virus-induced disease in the mouse. *Virology* 2001;284(2):190–202.
163. Charles PC, Walters E, Margolis F, et al. Mechanism of neuroinvasion of Venezuelan equine encephalitis virus in the mouse. *Virology* 1995;208(2):662–671.
164. Chen CI, Clark DC, Pesavento P, et al. Comparative pathogenesis of epidemic and enzootic Chikungunya viruses in a pregnant Rhesus macaque model. *Am J Trop Med Hyg* 2010;83(6):1249–1258.
165. Chen W, Foo SS, Rulli NE, et al. Arthritogenic alphaviral infection perturbs osteoblast function and triggers pathologic bone loss. *Proc Natl Acad Sci U S A* 2014;111(16):6040–6045.
166. Chen G, Guo X, Lv F, et al. p72 DEAD box RNA helicase is required for optimal function of the zinc-finger antiviral protein. *Proc Natl Acad Sci U S A* 2008;105(11):4352–4357.
167. Chen R, Puri V, Fedorova N, et al. Comprehensive genome scale phylogenetic study provides new insights on the global expansion of chikungunya virus. *J Virol* 2016;90(23):10600–10611.
168. Chen R, Wang E, Tsetsarkin KA, et al. Chikungunya virus 3′ untranslated region: adaptation to mosquitoes and a population bottleneck as major evolutionary forces. *PLoS Pathog* 2013;9(8):e1003591.
169. Chen L, Wang M, Zhu D, et al. Implication for alphavirus host-cell entry and assembly indicated by a 3.5A resolution cryo-EM structure. *Nat Commun* 2018;9(1):5326.
170. Cheng RH, Kuhn RJ, Olson NH, et al. Nucleocapsid and glycoprotein organization in an enveloped virus. *Cell* 1995;80(4):621–630.
171. Chenier S, Cote G, Vanderstock J, et al. An eastern equine encephalomyelitis (EEE) outbreak in Quebec in the fall of 2008. *Can Vet J* 2010;51(9):1011–1015.
172. Chevillon C, Briant L, Renaud F, et al. The Chikungunya threat: an ecological and evolutionary perspective. *Trends Microbiol* 2008;16(2):80–88.
173. Chew-Lim M, Suckling AJ, Webb HE. Demyelination in mice after two or three infections with avirulent Semliki Forest virus. *Vet Pathol* 1977;14(1):62–72.
174. Chirathaworn C, Rianthavorn P, Wuttirattanakowit N, et al. Serum IL-18 and IL-18BP levels in patients with Chikungunya virus infection. *Viral Immunol* 2010;23(1):113–117.
175. Chompoosri J, Thavara U, Tawatsin A, et al. Vertical transmission of Indian Ocean Lineage of chikungunya virus in *Aedes aegypti* and *Aedes albopictus* mosquitoes. *Parasit Vectors* 2016;9:227.
176. Chow A, Her Z, Ong EK, et al. Persistent arthralgia induced by Chikungunya virus infection is associated with interleukin-6 and granulocyte macrophage colony-stimulating factor. *J Infect Dis* 2011;203(2):149–157.
177. Chua HH, Abdul Rashid K, Law WC, et al. A fatal case of chikungunya virus infection with liver involvement. *Med J Malaysia* 2010;65(1):83–84.
178. Chung BY, Firth AE, Atkins JF. Frameshifting in alphaviruses: a diversity of 3′ stimulatory structures. *J Mol Biol* 2010;397(2):448–456.
179. Chusri S, Siripaitoon P, Hirunpat S, et al. Case reports of neuro-Chikungunya in southern Thailand. *Am J Trop Med Hyg* 2011;85(2):386–389.
180. Cilnis MJ, Kang W, Weaver SC. Genetic conservation of Highlands J viruses. *Virology* 1996;218(2):343–351.
181. Cirimotich CM, Scott JC, Phillips AT, et al. Suppression of RNA interference increases alphavirus replication and virus-associated mortality in *Aedes aegypti* mosquitoes. *BMC Microbiol* 2009;9:49.
182. Claflin SB, Webb CE. Ross River virus: many vectors and unusual hosts make for an unpredictable pathogen. *PLoS Pathog* 2015;11(9):e1005070.
183. Clarris BJ, Doherty RL, Fraser JR, et al. Epidemic polyarthritis: a cytological, virological and immunochemical study. *Aust N Z J Med* 1975;5(5):450–457.
184. Coffey LL, Beeharry Y, Borderia AV, et al. Arbovirus high fidelity variant loses fitness in mosquitoes and mice. *Proc Natl Acad Sci U S A* 2011;108(38):16038–16043.
185. Coffey LL, Carrara AS, Paessler S, et al. Experimental Everglades virus infection of cotton rats (*Sigmodon hispidus*). *Emerg Infect Dis* 2004;10(12):2182–2188.
186. Coffey LL, Vasilakis N, Brault AC, et al. Arbovirus evolution in vivo is constrained by host alternation. *Proc Natl Acad Sci U S A* 2008;105(19):6970–6975.
187. Coffey LL, Vignuzzi M. Host alternation of chikungunya virus increases fitness while restricting population diversity and adaptability to novel selective pressures. *J Virol* 2011;85(2):1025–1035.
188. Contigiani MS, de Basualdo M, Camara A, et al. [Presence of antibodies against Venezuelan equine encephalitis virus subtype VI in patients with acute febrile illness]. *Rev Argent Microbiol* 1993;25(4):212–220.
189. Cook SH, Griffin DE. Luciferase imaging of a neurotropic viral infection in intact animals. *J Virol* 2003;77(9):5333–5338.
190. Cooper LA, Scott TW. Differential evolution of eastern equine encephalitis virus populations in response to host cell type. *Genetics* 2001;157(4):1403–1412.
191. Coppenhaver DH, Singh IP, Sarzotti M, et al. Treatment of intracranial alphavirus infections in mice by a combination of specific antibodies and an interferon inducer. *Am J Trop Med Hyg* 1995;52(1):34–40.
192. Couderc T, Chretien F, Schilte C, et al. A mouse model for Chikungunya: young age and inefficient type-I interferon signaling are risk factors for severe disease. *PLoS Pathog* 2008;4(2):e29.
193. Couderc T, Khandoudi N, Grandadam M, et al. Prophylaxis and therapy for Chikungunya virus infection. *J Infect Dis* 2009;200(4):516–523.
194. Couderc T, Lecuit M. Focus on Chikungunya pathophysiology in human and animal models. *Microbes Infect* 2009;11(14–15):1197–1205.
195. Cruz CC, Suthar MS, Montgomery SA, et al. Modulation of type I IFN induction by a virulence determinant within the alphavirus nsP1 protein. *Virology* 2010;399(1):1–10.
196. Cupp EW, Klingler K, Hassan HK, et al. Transmission of eastern equine encephalomyelitis virus in central Alabama. *Am J Trop Med Hyg* 2003;68(4):495–500.
197. Dal Canto MC, Rabinowitz SG. Central nervous system demyelination in Venezuelan equine encephalomyelitis infection. *J Neurol Sci* 1981;49(3):397–418.
198. Dalrymple JM, Young OP, Eldridge BF, et al. Ecology of arboviruses in a Maryland freshwater swamp. 3. Vertebrate hosts. *Am J Epidemiol* 1972;96(2):129–140.
199. Darman J, Backovic S, Dike S, et al. Viral-induced spinal motor neuron death is non-cell-autonomous and involves glutamate excitotoxicity. *J Neurosci* 2004;24(34):7566–7575.
200. Das T, Hoarau JJ, Jaffar Bandjee MC, et al. Multifaceted innate immune responses engaged by astrocytes, microglia and resident dendritic cells against Chikungunya neuroinfection. *J Gen Virol* 2015;96(Pt 2):294–310.
201. Davey MW, Dalgarno L. Semliki Forest virus replication in cultured *Aedes albopictus* cells: studies on the establishment of persistence. *J Gen Virol* 1974;24(3):453–463.
202. Davis NL, Fuller FJ, Dougherty WG, et al. A single nucleotide change in the E2 glycoprotein gene of Sindbis virus affects penetration rate in cell culture and virulence in neonatal mice. *Proc Natl Acad Sci U S A* 1986;83(18):6771–6775.
203. Davis NL, Powell N, Greenwald GF, et al. Attenuating mutations in the E2 glycoprotein gene of Venezuelan equine encephalitis virus: construction of single and multiple mutants in a full-length cDNA clone. *Virology* 1991;183(1):20–31.
204. Day JF, Stark LM. Eastern equine encephalitis transmission to emus (Dromaius novaehollandiae) in Volusia County, Florida: 1992 through 1994. *J Am Mosq Control Assoc* 1996;12(3 Pt 1):429–436.
205. de Andrade DC, Jean S, Clavelou P, et al. Chronic pain associated with the Chikungunya fever: long lasting burden of an acute illness. *BMC Infect Dis* 2010;10:31.
206. Delfraro A, Burgueno A, Morel N, et al. Fatal human case of Western equine encephalitis, Uruguay. *Emerg Infect Dis* 2011;17(5):952–954.
207. Deresiewicz RL, Thaler SJ, Hsu L, et al. Clinical and neuroradiographic manifestations of eastern equine encephalitis. *N Engl J Med* 1997;336(26):1867–1874.
208. Deretic V, Levine B. Autophagy, immunity, and microbial adaptations. *Cell Host Microbe* 2009;5(6):527–549.
209. Despres P, Griffin JW, Griffin DE. Antiviral activity of alpha interferon in Sindbis virus-infected cells is restored by anti-E2 monoclonal antibody treatment. *J Virol* 1995;69(11):7345–7348.
210. Despres P, Griffin JW, Griffin DE. Effects of anti-E2 monoclonal antibody on sindbis virus replication in AT3 cells expressing bcl-2. *J Virol* 1995;69(11):7006–7014.

211. Deuber SA, Pavlovic J. Virulence of a mouse-adapted Semliki Forest virus strain is associated with reduced susceptibility to interferon. *J Gen Virol* 2007;88(Pt 7):1952–1959.

212. Dhanushkodi NR, Mohankumar V, Raju R. Sindbis virus induced phosphorylation of IRF3 in human embryonic kidney cells is not dependent on mTOR. *Innate Immun* 2012;18(2):325–332.

213. Dhanwani R, Khan M, Lomash V, et al. Characterization of chikungunya virus induced host response in a mouse model of viral myositis. *PLoS One* 2014;9(3):e92813.

214. Dhileepan K, Azuolas JK, Gibson CA. Evidence of vertical transmission of Ross River and Sindbis viruses (Togaviridae: Alphavirus) by mosquitoes (Diptera: Culicidae) in southeastern Australia. *J Med Entomol* 1996;33(1):180–182.

215. Diallo M, Thonnon J, Traore-Lamizana M, et al. Vectors of Chikungunya virus in Senegal: current data and transmission cycles. *Am J Trop Med Hyg* 1999;60(2):281–286.

216. Diaz LA, Diaz Mdel P, Almiron WR, et al. Infection by UNA virus (Alphavirus; Togaviridae) and risk factor analysis in black howler monkeys (Alouatta caraya) from Paraguay and Argentina. *Trans R Soc Trop Med Hyg* 2007;101(10):1039–1041.

217. Diaz LA, Spinsanti LI, Almiron WR, et al. UNA virus: first report of human infection in Argentina. *Rev Inst Med Trop Sao Paulo* 2003;45(2):109–110.

218. Dietz WH Jr, Galindo P, Johnson KM. Eastern equine encephalomyelitis in Panama: the epidemiology of the 1973 epizootic. *Am J Trop Med Hyg* 1980;29(1):133–140.

219. Digoutte JP, Girault G. [The protective properties in mice of tonate virus and two strains of cabassou virus against neurovirulent everglades Venezuelan encephalitis virus (author's transl)]. *Ann Microbiol (Paris)* 1976;127B(3):429–437.

220. Doby PB, Schnurrenberger PR, Martin RJ, et al. Western encephalitis in Illinois horses and ponies. *J Am Vet Med Assoc* 1966;148(4):422–427.

221. Doherty RL, Barrett EJ, Gorman BM, et al. Epidemic polyarthritis in Eastern Australia, 1959-1970. *Med J Aust* 1971;1(1):5–8.

222. Doherty RL, Carley JG, Best JC. Isolation of Ross River virus from man. *Med J Aust* 1972;1(21):1083–1084.

223. Domingo-Gil E, Toribio R, Najera JL, et al. Diversity in viral anti-PKR mechanisms: a remarkable case of evolutionary convergence. *PLoS One* 2011;6(2):e16711.

224. Dong S, Balaraman V, Kantor AM, et al. Chikungunya virus dissemination from the midgut of *Aedes aegypti* is associated with temporal basal lamina degradation during bloodmeal digestion. *PLoS Negl Trop Dis* 2017;11(9):e0005976.

225. Dong S, Kantor AM, Lin J, et al. Infection pattern and transmission potential of chikungunya virus in two New World laboratory-adapted *Aedes aegypti* strains. *Sci Rep* 2016;6:24729.

226. Donnelly SM, Sheahan BJ, Atkins GJ. Long-term effects of Semliki Forest virus infection in the mouse central nervous system. *Neuropathol Appl Neurobiol* 1997;23(3):235–241.

227. Dryga SA, Dryga OA, Schlesinger S. Identification of mutations in a Sindbis virus variant able to establish persistent infection in BHK cells: the importance of a mutation in the nsP2 gene. *Virology* 1997;228(1):74–83.

228. Dubey SK, Shrinet J, Jain J, et al. *Aedes aegypti* microRNA miR-2b regulates ubiquitin-related modifier to control chikungunya virus replication. *Sci Rep* 2017;7(1):17666.

229. Dubrulle M, Mousson L, Moutailler S, et al. Chikungunya virus and Aedes mosquitoes: saliva is infectious as soon as two days after oral infection. *PLoS One* 2009;4(6):e5895.

230. Dubuisson J, Lustig S, Ruggli N, et al. Genetic determinants of Sindbis virus neuroinvasiveness. *J Virol* 1997;71(4):2636–2646.

231. Dubuisson J, Rice CM. Sindbis virus attachment: isolation and characterization of mutants with impaired binding to vertebrate cells. *J Virol* 1993;67(6):3363–3374.

232. Dulbecco R. Production of plaques in monolayer tissue cultures by single particles of an animal virus. *Proc Natl Acad Sci U S A* 1952;38(8):747–752.

233. Dupuy LC, Richards MJ, Ellefsen B, et al. A DNA vaccine for venezuelan equine encephalitis virus delivered by intramuscular electroporation elicits high levels of neutralizing antibodies in multiple animal models and provides protective immunity to mice and nonhuman primates. *Clin Vaccine Immunol* 2011;18(5):707–716.

234. Dupuy LC, Richards MJ, Reed DS, et al. Immunogenicity and protective efficacy of a DNA vaccine against Venezuelan equine encephalitis virus aerosol challenge in nonhuman primates. *Vaccine* 2010;28(46):7345–7350.

235. Durden LA, Linthicum KJ, Monath TP. Laboratory transmission of eastern equine encephalomyelitis virus to chickens by chicken mites (Acari: Dermanyssidae). *J Med Entomol* 1993;30(1):281–285.

236. Earnest MP, Goolishian HA, Calverley JR, et al. Neurologic, intellectual, and psychologic sequelae following western encephalitis. A follow-up study of 35 cases. *Neurology* 1971;21(9):969–974.

237. Economopoulou A, Dominguez M, Helynck B, et al. Atypical Chikungunya virus infections: clinical manifestations, mortality and risk factors for severe disease during the 2005-2006 outbreak on Reunion. *Epidemiol Infect* 2009;137(4):534–541.

238. Edelman R, Ascher MS, Oster CN, et al. Evaluation in humans of a new, inactivated vaccine for Venezuelan equine encephalitis virus (C-84). *J Infect Dis* 1979;140(5):708–715.

239. Edelman R, Tacket CO, Wasserman SS, et al. Phase II safety and immunogenicity study of live chikungunya virus vaccine TSI-GSD-218. *Am J Trop Med Hyg* 2000;62(6):681–685.

240. Ehrenkranz NJ, Ventura AK. Venezuelan equine encephalitis virus infection in man. *Annu Rev Med* 1974;25:9–14.

241. El-Bacha T, Menezes MM, Azevedo e Silva MC, et al. Mayaro virus infection alters glucose metabolism in cultured cells through activation of the enzyme 6-phosphofructo 1-kinase. *Mol Cell Biochem* 2004;266(1–2):191–198.

242. Elsinga J, Gerstenbluth I, van der Ploeg S, et al. Long-term chikungunya sequelae in Curacao: burden, determinants, and a novel classification tool. *J Infect Dis* 2017;216(5):573–581.

243. Elvin SJ, Bennett AM, Phillpotts RJ. Role for mucosal immune responses and cell-mediated immune functions in protection from airborne challenge with Venezuelan equine encephalitis virus. *J Med Virol* 2002;67(3):384–393.

244. Elvinger F, Liggett AD, Tang KN, et al. Eastern equine encephalomyelitis virus infection in swine. *J Am Vet Med Assoc* 1994;205(7):1014–1016.

245. Erasmus JH, Needham J, Raychaudhuri S, et al. Utilization of an Eilat virus-based chimera for serological detection of chikungunya infection. *PLoS Negl Trop Dis* 2015;9(10):e0004119.

246. Erasmus JH, Rossi SL, Weaver SC. Development of vaccines for chikungunya fever. *J Infect Dis* 2016;214(Suppl 5):S488–S496.

247. Erasmus JH, Seymour RL, Kaelber JT, et al. Novel insect-specific eilat virus-based chimeric vaccine candidates provide durable, mono- and multivalent, single-dose protection against lethal alphavirus challenge. *J Virol* 2018;92(4).

248. Eshoo MW, Whitehouse CA, Zoll ST, et al. Direct broad-range detection of alphaviruses in mosquito extracts. *Virology* 2007;368(2):286–295.

249. Espinosa BJ, Weaver SC, Paessler S, et al. Susceptibility of the Aotus nancymaae owl monkey to eastern equine encephalitis. *Vaccine* 2009;27(11):1729–1734.

250. Espmark A, Niklasson B. Ockelbo disease in Sweden: epidemiological, clinical, and virological data from the 1982 outbreak. *Am J Trop Med Hyg* 1984;33(6):1203–1211.

251. Estep LK, McClure CJ, Burkett-Cadena ND, et al. A multi-year study of mosquito feeding patterns on avian hosts in a southeastern focus of eastern equine encephalitis virus. *Am J Trop Med Hyg* 2011;84(5):718–726.

252. Estep LK, McClure CJ, Vander Kelen P, et al. Risk of exposure to eastern equine encephalomyelitis virus increases with the density of northern cardinals. *PLoS One* 2013;8(2):e57879.

253. Estrada-Franco JG, Navarro-Lopez R, Freier JE, et al. Venezuelan equine encephalitis virus, southern Mexico. *Emerg Infect Dis* 2004;10(12):2113–2121.

254. Faragher SG, Meek AD, Rice CM, et al. Genome sequences of a mouse-avirulent and a mouse-virulent strain of Ross River virus. *Virology* 1988;163(2):509–526.

255. Farber S, Hill A, Connerly ML, et al. Encephalitis in infants and children—Caused by the virus of the eastern variety of equine encephalitis. *J Am Med Assoc* 1940;114:1725–1731.

256. Favre D, Studer E, Michel MR. Semliki Forest virus capsid protein inhibits the initiation of translation by upregulating the double-stranded RNA-activated protein kinase (PKR). *Biosci Rep* 1996;16(6):485–511.

257. Fazakerley JK. Pathogenesis of Semliki Forest virus encephalitis. *J Neurovirol* 2002;8(Suppl 2):66–74.

258. Fazakerley JK, Amor S, Webb HE. Reconstitution of Semliki forest virus infected mice, induces immune mediated pathological changes in the CNS. *Clin Exp Immunol* 1983;52(1):115–120.

259. Fazakerley JK, Boyd A, Mikkola ML, et al. A single amino acid change in the nuclear localization sequence of the nsP2 protein affects the neurovirulence of Semliki Forest virus. *J Virol* 2002;76(1):392–396.

260. Feemster RF. Equine encephalitis in Massachusetts. *N Engl J Med* 1957;257(15):701–704.

261. Fensterl V, Sen GC. Interferon-induced Ifit proteins: their role in viral pathogenesis. *J Virol* 2015;89(5):2462–2468.

262. Ferguson MC, Saul S, Fragkoudis R, et al. Ability of the encephalitic arbovirus semliki forest virus to cross the blood-brain barrier is determined by the charge of the E2 glycoprotein. *J Virol* 2015;89(15):7536–7549.

263. Ferro C, Boshell J, Moncayo AC, et al. Natural enzootic vectors of Venezuelan equine encephalitis virus, Magdalena Valley, Colombia. *Emerg Infect Dis* 2003;9(1):49–54.

264. Ficken MD, Wages DP, Guy JS, et al. High mortality of domestic turkeys associated with Highlands J virus and eastern equine encephalitis virus infections. *Avian Dis* 1993;37(2):585–590.

265. Finley KH, Longshore WA Jr, Palmer RJ, et al. Western equine and St. Louis encephalitis; preliminary report of a clinical follow-up study in California. *Neurology* 1955;5(4):223–235.

266. Firth AE, Chung BY, Fleeton MN, et al. Discovery of frameshifting in alphavirus 6K resolves a 20-year enigma. *Virol J* 2008;5:108.

267. Flexman JP, Smith DW, Mackenzie JS, et al. A comparison of the diseases caused by Ross River virus and Barmah Forest virus. *Med J Aust* 1998;169(3):159–163.

268. Foo SS, Chen W, Taylor A, et al. Role of pentraxin 3 in shaping arthritogenic alphaviral disease: from enhanced viral replication to immunomodulation. *PLoS Pathog* 2015;11(2):e1004649.

269. Forrester NL, Guerbois M, Adams AP, et al. Analysis of intrahost variation in Venezuelan equine encephalitis virus reveals repeated deletions in the 6-kilodalton protein gene. *J Virol* 2011;85(17):8709–8717.

270. Forrester NL, Kenney JL, Deardorff E, et al. Western Equine Encephalitis submergence: lack of evidence for a decline in virus virulence. *Virology* 2008;380(2):170–172.

271. Forrester NL, Palacios G, Tesh RB, et al. Genome-scale phylogeny of the alphavirus genus suggests a marine origin. *J Virol* 2012;86(5):2729–2738.

272. Forrester NL, Wertheim JO, Dugan VG, et al. Evolution and spread of Venezuelan equine encephalitis complex alphavirus in the Americas. *PLoS Negl Trop Dis* 2017;11(8):e0005693.

273. Forshey BM, Guevara C, Laguna-Torres VA, et al. Arboviral etiologies of acute febrile illnesses in Western South America, 2000-2007. *PLoS Negl Trop Dis* 2010;4(8):e787.

274. Fothergill LD, Dingle JH, Fellow JJ. A fatal disease of pigeons caused by the virus of the eastern variety of equine encephalomyelitis. *Science* 1938;88(2293):549–550.

275. Fothergill LD, Holden M, Wyckoff RWG. Western equine encephalomyelitis in a laboratory worker. *J Am Med Assoc* 1939;113:206–207.

276. Fox JM, Diamond MS. Immune-mediated protection and pathogenesis of chikungunya virus. *J Immunol* 2016;197(11):4210–4218.

277. Fox JM, Long F, Edeling MA, et al. Broadly neutralizing alphavirus antibodies bind an epitope on E2 and inhibit entry and egress. *Cell* 2015;163(5):1095–1107.

278. Fragkoudis R, Breakwell L, McKimmie C, et al. The type I interferon system protects mice from Semliki Forest virus by preventing widespread virus dissemination in extraneural tissues, but does not mediate the restricted replication of avirulent virus in central nervous system neurons. *J Gen Virol* 2007;88(Pt 12):3373–3384.

279. Fragkoudis R, Chi Y, Siu RW, et al. Semliki Forest virus strongly reduces mosquito host defence signaling. *Insect Mol Biol* 2008;17(6):647–656.

280. Fragkoudis R, Tamberg N, Siu R, et al. Neurons and oligodendrocytes in the mouse brain differ in their ability to replicate Semliki Forest virus. *J Neurovirol* 2009;15(1):57–70.

281. Fraisier C, Koraka P, Belghazi M, et al. Kinetic analysis of mouse brain proteome alterations following Chikungunya virus infection before and after appearance of clinical symptoms. *PLoS One* 2014;9(3):e91397.

282. Francy DB, Jaenson TG, Lundstrom JO, et al. Ecologic studies of mosquitoes and birds as hosts of Ockelbo virus in Sweden and isolation of Inkoo and Batai viruses from mosquitoes. *Am J Trop Med Hyg* 1989;41(3):355–363.

283. Fraser JR. Epidemic polyarthritis and Ross River virus disease. *Clin Rheum Dis* 1986;12(2):369–388.

284. Fraser JR, Cunningham AL, Clarris BJ, et al. Cytology of synovial effusions in epidemic polyarthritis. *Aust N Z J Med* 1981;11(2):168–173.

285. Fraser JR, Ratnamohan VM, Dowling JP, et al. The exanthem of Ross River virus infection: histology, location of virus antigen and nature of inflammatory infiltrate. *J Clin Pathol* 1983;36(11):1256–1263.

286. Fritel X, Rollot O, Gerardin P, et al. Chikungunya virus infection during pregnancy, Reunion, France, 2006. *Emerg Infect Dis* 2010;16(3):418–425.

287. Froeschle JE, Reeves WC. Serologic epidemiology of western equine and St-Louis encephalitis-virus infection in California. 2. Analysis of inapparent infections in residents of an endemic area. *Am J Epidemiol* 1965;81(1):44–51.

288. Frolov I, Agapov E, Hoffman TA Jr, et al. Selection of RNA replicons capable of persistent noncytopathic replication in mammalian cells. *J Virol* 1999;73(5):3854–3865.

289. Frolova EI, Fayzulin RZ, Cook SH, et al. Roles of nonstructural protein nsP2 and Alpha/Beta interferons in determining the outcome of Sindbis virus infection. *J Virol* 2002;76(22):11254–11264.

290. Fros JJ, Liu WJ, Prow NA, et al. Chikungunya virus nonstructural protein 2 inhibits type I/II interferon-stimulated JAK-STAT signaling. *J Virol* 2010;84(20):10877–10887.

291. Fros JJ, Pijlman GP. Alphavirus infection: host cell shut-off and inhibition of antiviral responses. *Viruses* 2016;8(6).

292. Fulhorst CF, Hardy JL, Eldridge BF, et al. Natural vertical transmission of western equine encephalomyelitis virus in mosquitoes. *Science* 1994;263(5147):676–678.

293. Galindo P, Grayson MA. Culex (Melanoconion) aikenii: natural vector in Panama of endemic Venezuelan encephalitis. *Science* 1971;172(3983):594–595.

294. Gard G, Marshall ID, Woodroofe GM. Annually recurrent epidemic polyarthritis and Ross River virus activity in a coastal area of New South Wales. II. Mosquitoes, viruses, and wildlife. *Am J Trop Med Hyg* 1973;22(4):551–560.

295. Gardner J, Anraku I, Le TT, et al. Chikungunya virus arthritis in adult wild-type mice. *J Virol* 2010;84(16):8021–8032.

296. Gardner CL, Burke CW, Higgs ST, et al. Interferon-alpha/beta deficiency greatly exacerbates arthritogenic disease in mice infected with wild-type chikungunya virus but not with the cell culture-adapted live-attenuated 181/25 vaccine candidate. *Virology* 2012;425(2):103–112.

297. Gardner CL, Burke CW, Tesfay MZ, et al. Eastern and Venezuelan equine encephalitis viruses differ in their ability to infect dendritic cells and macrophages: impact of altered cell tropism on pathogenesis. *J Virol* 2008;82(21):10634–10646.

298. Gardner CL, Choi-Nurvitadhi J, Sun C, et al. Natural variation in the heparan sulfate binding domain of the eastern equine encephalitis virus E2 glycoprotein alters interactions with cell surfaces and virulence in mice. *J Virol* 2013;87(15):8582–8590.

299. Gardner CL, Ebel GD, Ryman KD, et al. Heparan sulfate binding by natural eastern equine encephalitis viruses promotes neurovirulence. *Proc Natl Acad Sci U S A* 2011;108(38):16026–16031.

300. Gardner J, Rudd PA, Prow NA, et al. Infectious Chikungunya Virus in the Saliva of Mice, Monkeys and Humans. *PLoS One* 2015;10(10):e0139481.

301. Gardner CL, Yin J, Burke CW, et al. Type I interferon induction is correlated with attenuation of a South American eastern equine encephalitis virus strain in mice. *Virology* 2009;390(2):338–347.

302. Garen PD, Tsai TF, Powers JM. Human eastern equine encephalitis: immunohistochemistry and ultrastructure. *Mod Pathol* 1999;12(6):646–652.

303. Garmashova N, Atasheva S, Kang W, et al. Analysis of Venezuelan equine encephalitis virus capsid protein function in the inhibition of cellular transcription. *J Virol* 2007;81(24):13552–13565.

304. Garmashova N, Gorchakov R, Frolova E, et al. Sindbis virus nonstructural protein nsP2 is cytotoxic and inhibits cellular transcription. *J Virol* 2006;80(12):5686–5696.

305. Garmashova N, Gorchakov R, Volkova E, et al. The Old World and New World alphaviruses use different virus-specific proteins for induction of transcriptional shutoff. *J Virol* 2007;81(5):2472–2484.

306. Gauci PJ, Wu JQ, Rayner GA, et al. Identification of Western equine encephalitis virus structural proteins that confer protection after DNA vaccination. *Clin Vaccine Immunol* 2010;17(1):176–179.

307. Gay N, Rousset D, Huc P, et al. Seroprevalence of Asian lineage chikungunya virus infection on Saint Martin Island, 7 months after the 2013 emergence. *Am J Trop Med Hyg* 2016;94(2):393–396.

308. Gerardin P, Barau G, Michault A, et al. Multidisciplinary prospective study of mother-to-child chikungunya virus infections on the island of La Reunion. *PLoS Med* 2008;5(3):e60.

309. Gerardin P, Couderc T, Bintner M, et al. Chikungunya virus-associated encephalitis: a cohort study on La Reunion Island, 2005–2009. *Neurology* 2016;86(1):94–102.

310. Gerardin P, Guernier V, Perrau J, et al. Estimating Chikungunya prevalence in La Reunion Island outbreak by serosurveys: two methods for two critical times of the epidemic. *BMC Infect Dis* 2008;8:99.

311. Giannakopoulos NV, Arutyunova E, Lai C, et al. ISG15 Arg151 and the ISG15-conjugating enzyme UbE1L are important for innate immune control of Sindbis virus. *J Virol* 2009;83(4):1602–1610.

312. Gibbons DL, Vaney MC, Roussel A, et al. Conformational change and protein-protein interactions of the fusion protein of Semliki Forest virus. *Nature* 2004;427(6972):320–325.

313. Gibney KB, Robinson S, Mutebi JP, et al. Eastern equine encephalitis: an emerging arboviral disease threat, Maine, 2009. *Vector Borne Zoonotic Dis* 2011;11(6):637–639.

314. Gifford GE, Mussett MV, Heller E. Comparative studies on the production and assay of interferon. *J Gen Microbiol* 1964;34:475–481.

315. Giry C, Roquebert B, Li-Pat-Yuen G, et al. Improved detection of genus-specific Alphavirus using a generic TaqMan(R) assay. *BMC Microbiol* 2017;17(1):164.

316. Glasgow GM, Killen HM, Liljestrom P, et al. A single amino acid change in the E2 spike protein of a virulent strain of Semliki Forest virus attenuates pathogenicity. *J Gen Virol* 1994;75(Pt 3):663–668.

317. Glasgow GM, McGee MM, Sheahan BJ, et al. Death mechanisms in cultured cells infected by Semliki Forest virus. *J Gen Virol* 1997;78(Pt 7):1559–1563.

318. Glasgow GM, McGee MM, Tarbatt CJ, et al. The Semliki Forest virus vector induces p53-independent apoptosis. *J Gen Virol* 1998;79(Pt 10):2405–2410.

319. Glasgow GM, Sheahan BJ, Atkins GJ, et al. Two mutations in the envelope glycoprotein E2 of Semliki Forest virus affecting the maturation and entry patterns of the virus alter pathogenicity for mice. *Virology* 1991;185(2):741–748.

320. Gleiser CA, Gochenour WS Jr, Berge TO, et al. The comparative pathology of experimental Venezuelan equine encephalomyelitis infection in different animal hosts. *J Infect Dis* 1962;110:80–97.

321. Goertz GP, McNally KL, Robertson SJ, et al. The methyltransferase-like domain of chikungunya virus nsP2 inhibits the interferon response by promoting the nuclear export of STAT1. *J Virol* 2018;92(17).

322. Goic B, Stapleford KA, Frangeul L, et al. Virus-derived DNA drives mosquito vector tolerance to arboviral infection. *Nat Commun* 2016;7:12410.

323. Goldfield M, Welsh JN, Taylor BF. The 1959 outbreak of Eastern encephalitis in New Jersey. 5. The inapparent infection:disease ratio. *Am J Epidemiol* 1968;87(1):32–33.

324. Gomez de Cedron M, Ehsani N, Mikkola ML, et al. RNA helicase activity of Semliki Forest virus replicase protein NSP2. *FEBS Lett* 1999;448(1):19–22.

325. Gonzalez-Salazar D, Estrada-Franco JG, Carrara AS, et al. Equine amplification and virulence of subtype IE Venezuelan equine encephalitis viruses isolated during the 1993 and 1996 Mexican epizootics. *Emerg Infect Dis* 2003;9(2):161–168.

326. Goodchild SA, O'Brien LM, Steven J, et al. A humanised murine monoclonal antibody with broad serogroup specificity protects mice from challenge with Venezuelan equine encephalitis virus. *Antiviral Res* 2011;90(1):1–8.

327. Gorbalenya AE, Koonin EV, Lai MM. Putative papain-related thiol proteases of positive-strand RNA viruses. Identification of rubi- and aphthovirus proteases and delineation of a novel conserved domain associated with proteases of rubi-, alpha- and coronaviruses. *FEBS Lett* 1991;288(1–2):201–205.

328. Gorchakov R, Frolova E, Frolov I. Inhibition of transcription and translation in Sindbis virus-infected cells. *J Virol* 2005;79(15):9397–9409.

329. Gorchakov R, Garmashova N, Frolova E, et al. Different types of nsP3-containing protein complexes in Sindbis virus-infected cells. *J Virol* 2008;82(20):10088–10101.

330. Gorchakov R, Wang E, Leal G, et al. Attenuation of Chikungunya virus vaccine strain 181/clone 25 is determined by two amino acid substitutions in the E2 envelope glycoprotein. *J Virol* 2012;86(11):6084–6096.

331. Gordon A, Gresh L, Ojeda S, et al. Differences in transmission and disease severity between 2 successive waves of chikungunya. *Clin Infect Dis* 2018;67(11):1760–1767.

332. Gorelkin L, Jahrling PB. Virus-initiated septic shock. Acute death of Venezuelan encephalitis virus-infected hamsters. *Lab Invest* 1975;32(1):78–85.

333. Gotte B, Liu L, McInerney GM. The enigmatic alphavirus non-structural protein 3 (nsP3) revealing its secrets at last. *Viruses* 2018;10(3).

334. Gould EA, Coutard B, Malet H, et al. Understanding the alphaviruses: recent research on important emerging pathogens and progress towards their control. *Antiviral Res* 2010;87(2):111–124.

335. Graham DA, Frost P, McLaughlin K, et al. A comparative study of marine salmonid alphavirus subtypes 1-6 using an experimental cohabitation challenge model. *J Fish Dis* 2011;34(4):273–286.

336. Graham SP, Hassan HK, Chapman T, et al. Serosurveillance of eastern equine encephalitis virus in amphibians and reptiles from Alabama, USA. *Am J Trop Med Hyg* 2012;86(3):540–544.

337. Grandadam M, Caro V, Plumet S, et al. Chikungunya virus, southeastern France. *Emerg Infect Dis* 2011;17(5):910–913.

338. Grandgirard D, Studer E, Monney L, et al. Alphaviruses induce apoptosis in Bcl-2-overexpressing cells: evidence for a caspase-mediated, proteolytic inactivation of Bcl-2. *EMBO J* 1998;17(5):1268–1278.

339. Granot T, Venticinque L, Tseng JC, et al. Activation of cytotoxic and regulatory functions of NK cells by Sindbis viral vectors. *PLoS One* 2011;6(6):e20598.

340. Grayson MA, Galindo P. Epidemiologic studies of Venezuelan equine encephalitis virus in Almirante, Panama. *Am J Epidemiol* 1968;88(1):80–96.

341. Greene IP, Lee EY, Prow N, et al. Protection from fatal viral encephalomyelitis: AMPA receptor antagonists have a direct effect on the inflammatory response to infection. *Proc Natl Acad Sci U S A* 2008;105(9):3575–3580.

342. Greene IP, Paessler S, Anishchenko M, et al. Venezuelan equine encephalitis virus in the guinea pig model: evidence for epizootic virulence determinants outside the E2 envelope glycoprotein gene. *Am J Trop Med Hyg* 2005;72(3):330–338.

343. Greene IP, Paessler S, Austgen L, et al. Envelope glycoprotein mutations mediate equine amplification and virulence of epizootic venezuelan equine encephalitis virus. *J Virol* 2005;79(14):9128–9133.

344. Greene IP, Wang E, Deardorff ER, et al. Effect of alternating passage on adaptation of Sindbis virus to vertebrate and invertebrate cells. *J Virol* 2005;79(22):14253–14260.

345. Greiser-Wilke I, Moenning V, Kaaden OR, et al. Most alphaviruses share a conserved epitopic region on their nucleocapsid protein. *J Gen Virol* 1989;70(Pt 3):743–748.

346. Grieder FB, Davis BK, Zhou XD, et al. Kinetics of cytokine expression and regulation of host protection following infection with molecularly cloned Venezuelan equine encephalitis virus. *Virology* 1997;233(2):302–312.

347. Grieder FB, Vogel SN. Role of interferon and interferon regulatory factors in early protection against Venezuelan equine encephalitis virus infection. *Virology* 1999;257(1):106–118.

348. Griffin DE. Role of the immune response in age-dependent resistance of mice to encephalitis due to Sindbis virus. *J Infect Dis* 1976;133(4):456–464.

349. Griffin DE. Immunoglobulins in the cerebrospinal fluid: changes during acute viral encephalitis in mice. *J Immunol* 1981;126(1):27–31.

350. Griffin DE. Alphavirus encephalomyelitis: mechanisms and approaches to prevention of neuronal damage. *Neurotherapeutics* 2016;13(3):455–460.

351. Griffin DE, Johnson RT. Cellular immune response to viral infection: in vitro studies of lymphocytes from mice infected with Sindbis virus. *Cell Immunol* 1973;9(3):426–434.

352. Griffin DE, Johnson RT. Role of the immune response in recovery from Sindbis virus encephalitis in mice. *J Immunol* 1977;118(3):1070–1075.

353. Griffin D, Levine B, Tyor W, et al. The role of antibody in recovery from alphavirus encephalitis. *Immunol Rev* 1997;159:155–161.

354. Griffin DE, Metcalf T. Clearance of virus infection from the CNS. *Curr Opin Virol* 2011;1(3):216–221.

355. Grimley PM, Friedman RM. Arboviral infection of voluntary striated muscles. *J Infect Dis* 1970;122(1):45–52.

356. Grivard P, Le Roux K, Laurent P, et al. Molecular and serological diagnosis of Chikungunya virus infection. *Pathol Biol (Paris)* 2007;55(10):490–494.

357. Grosfeld H, Velan B, Leitner M, et al. Semliki Forest virus E2 envelope epitopes induce a nonneutralizing humoral response which protects mice against lethal challenge. *J Virol* 1989;63(8):3416–3422.

358. Grywna K, Kupfer B, Panning M, et al. Detection of all species of the genus Alphavirus by reverse transcription-PCR with diagnostic sensitivity. *J Clin Microbiol* 2010;48(9):3386–3387.

359. Guo X, Carroll JW, Macdonald MR, et al. The zinc finger antiviral protein directly binds to specific viral mRNAs through the CCCH zinc finger motifs. *J Virol* 2004;78(23):12781–12787.

360. Guo X, Ma J, Sun J, et al. The zinc-finger antiviral protein recruits the RNA processing exosome to degrade the target mRNA. *Proc Natl Acad Sci U S A* 2007;104(1):151–156.

361. Guy JS, Ficken MD, Barnes HJ, et al. Experimental infection of young turkeys with eastern equine encephalitis virus and highlands J virus. *Avian Dis* 1993;37(2):389–395.

362. Guzman C, Calderon A, Martinez C, et al. Eco-epidemiology of the Venezuelan equine encephalitis virus in bats of Cordoba and Sucre, Colombia. *Acta Trop* 2019;191:178–184.

363. Gylfe A, Ribers A, Forsman O, et al. Mosquitoborne Sindbis Virus infection and long-term illness. *Emerg Infect Dis* 2018;24(6):1141–1142.

364. Hackbarth SA, Reinarz AB, Sagik BP. Age-dependent resistance of mice to sindbis virus infection: reticuloendothelial role. *J Reticuloendothel Soc* 1973;14(5):405–425.

365. Haddow AJ, Davies CW, Walker AJ. O'nyong-nyong fever: an epidemic virus disease in East Africa. I. Introduction. *Trans R Soc Trop Med Hyg* 1960;54:517–522.

366. Haese NN, Broeckel RM, Hawman DW, et al. Animal models of chikungunya virus infection and disease. *J Infect Dis* 2016;214(Suppl 5):S482–S487.

367. Hafer A, Whittlesey R, Brown DT, et al. Differential incorporation of cholesterol by Sindbis virus grown in mammalian or insect cells. *J Virol* 2009;83(18):9113–9121.

368. Hahn YS, Grakoui A, Rice CM, et al. Mapping of RNA- temperature-sensitive mutants of Sindbis virus: complementation group F mutants have lesions in nsP4. *J Virol* 1989;63(3):1194–1202.

369. Hahn CS, Lustig S, Strauss EG, et al. Western equine encephalitis virus is a recombinant virus. *Proc Natl Acad Sci U S A* 1988;85(16):5997–6001.

370. Haist KC, Burrack KS, Davenport BJ, et al. Inflammatory monocytes mediate control of acute alphavirus infection in mice. *PLoS Pathog* 2017;13(12):e1006748.

371. Halstead SB. Reappearance of chikungunya, formerly called dengue, in the Americas. *Emerg Infect Dis* 2015;21(4):557–561.

372. Hammon WM, Reeves WC, Brookman B, et al. Mosquitoes and encephalitis in the Yakima Valley, Washington I Arthropods tested and recovery of western equine and St Louis viruses from Culex tarsalis Coquillett. *J Infect Dis* 1942;70:263–266.

373. Hanson RP. An epizootic of equine encephalomyelitis that occurred in Massachusetts in 1831. *Am J Trop Med Hyg* 1957;6(5):858–862.

374. Hapuarachchi HC, Bandara KB, Sumanadasa SD, et al. Re-emergence of Chikungunya virus in South-east Asia: virological evidence from Sri Lanka and Singapore. *J Gen Virol* 2010;91(Pt 4):1067–1076.

375. Hardy JL. The ecology of western equine encephalomyelitis virus in the Central Valley of California, 1945-1985. *Am J Trop Med Hyg* 1987;37(3 Suppl):18S–32S.

376. Hardy JL, Presser SB, Chiles RE, et al. Mouse and baby chicken virulence of enzootic strains of western equine encephalomyelitis virus from California. *Am J Trop Med Hyg* 1997;57(2):240–244.

377. Harley D, Bossingham D, Purdie DM, et al. Ross River virus disease in tropical Queensland: evolution of rheumatic manifestations in an inception cohort followed for six months. *Med J Aust* 2002;177(7):352–355.

378. Harley D, Ritchie S, Bain C, et al. Risks for Ross River virus disease in tropical Australia. *Int J Epidemiol* 2005;34(3):548–555.

379. Harley D, Sleigh A, Ritchie S. Ross River virus transmission, infection, and disease: a cross-disciplinary review. *Clin Microbiol Rev* 2001;14(4):909–932, table of contents.

380. Havert MB, Schofield B, Griffin DE, et al. Activation of divergent neuronal cell death pathways in different target cell populations during neuroadapted sindbis virus infection of mice. *J Virol* 2000;74(11):5352–5356.

381. Hawkes RA, Boughton CR, Naim HM, et al. A major outbreak of epidemic polyarthritis in New South Wales during the summer of 1983/1984. *Med J Aust* 1985;143(8):330–333.

382. Hawman DW, Carpentier KS, Fox JM, et al. Mutations in the E2 glycoprotein and the 3' untranslated region enhance chikungunya virus virulence in mice. *J Virol* 2017;91(20).

383. Hawman DW, Fox JM, Ashbrook AW, et al. Pathogenic Chikungunya virus evades B cell responses to establish persistence. *Cell Rep* 2016;16(5):1326–1338.

384. Hawman DW, Stoermer KA, Montgomery SA, et al. Chronic joint disease caused by persistent Chikungunya virus infection is controlled by the adaptive immune response. *J Virol* 2013;87(24):13878–13888.

385. Hayes RO, Francy DB, Lazuick JS, et al. Role of cliff swallow bug (Oeciacus-Vicarius) in natural cycle of a western equine encephalitis-related alphavirus. *J Med Entomol* 1977;14(3):257–262.

386. Hayes CG, Wallis RC. Ecology of Western equine encephalomyelitis in the eastern United States. *Adv Virus Res* 1977;21:37–83.

387. He L, Piper A, Meilleur F, et al. The structure of Sindbis virus produced from vertebrate and invertebrate hosts as determined by small-angle neutron scattering. *J Virol* 2010;84(10):5270–5276.

388. Hefti HP, Frese M, Landis H, et al. Human MxA protein protects mice lacking a functional alpha/beta interferon system against La crosse virus and other lethal viral infections. *J Virol* 1999;73(8):6984–6991.

389. Helbig KJ, Beard MR. The role of viperin in the innate antiviral response. *J Mol Biol* 2014;426(6):1210–1219.

390. Helenius A, Kartenbeck J, Simons K, et al. On the entry of Semliki forest virus into BHK-21 cells. *J Cell Biol* 1980;84(2):404–420.

391. Helenius A, Kielian M, Wellsteed J, et al. Effects of monovalent cations on Semliki Forest virus entry into BHK-21 cells. *J Biol Chem* 1985;260(9):5691–5697.

392. Helenius A, Morein B, Fries E, et al. Human (HLA-A and HLA-B) and murine (H-2K and H-2D) histocompatibility antigens are cell surface receptors for Semliki Forest virus. *Proc Natl Acad Sci U S A* 1978;75(8):3846–3850.

393. Henderson BE, Chappell WA, Johnston JG Jr, et al. Experimental infection of horses with three strains of Venezuelan equine encephalomyelitis virus. I. Clinical and virological studies. *Am J Epidemiol* 1971;93(3):194–205.

394. Henderson JR, Karabatsos N, Bourke AT, et al. A survey for arthropod-borne viruses in south-central Florida. *Am J Trop Med Hyg* 1962;11:800–810.

395. Henss L, Yue C, Kandler J, et al. Establishment of an alphavirus-specific neutralization assay to distinguish infections with different members of the Semliki Forest complex. *Viruses* 2019;11(1).

396. Her Z, Kam YW, Lin RT, et al. Chikungunya: a bending reality. *Microbes Infect* 2009;11(14-15):1165–1176.

397. Her Z, Malleret B, Chan M, et al. Active infection of human blood monocytes by Chikungunya virus triggers an innate immune response. *J Immunol* 2010;184(10):5903–5913.

398. Her Z, Teng TS, Tan JJ, et al. Loss of TLR3 aggravates CHIKV replication and pathology due to an altered virus-specific neutralizing antibody response. *EMBO Mol Med* 2015;7(1):24–41.

399. Hermanns K, Zirkel F, Kopp A, et al. Discovery of a novel alphavirus related to Eilat virus. *J Gen Virol* 2017;98(1):43–49.

400. Hernandez R, Paredes A, Brown DT. Sindbis virus conformational changes induced by a neutralizing anti-E1 monoclonal antibody. *J Virol* 2008;82(12):5750–5760.

401. Herrero LJ, Lidbury BA, Bettadapura J, et al. Characterization of Barmah Forest virus pathogenesis in a mouse model. *J Gen Virol* 2014;95(Pt 10):2146–2154.

402. Herrero LJ, Nelson M, Srikiatkhachorn A, et al. Critical role for macrophage migration inhibitory factor (MIF) in Ross River virus-induced arthritis and myositis. *Proc Natl Acad Sci U S A* 2011;108(29):12048–12053.

403. Hesson JC, Verner-Carlsson J, Larsson A, et al. *Culex torrentium* mosquito role as major enzootic vector defined by rate of Sindbis Virus Infection, Sweden, 2009. *Emerg Infect Dis* 2015;21(5):875–878.

404. Hidmark AS, McInerney GM, Nordstrom EK, et al. Early alpha/beta interferon production by myeloid dendritic cells in response to UV-inactivated virus requires viral entry and interferon regulatory factor 3 but not MyD88. *J Virol* 2005;79(16):10376–10385.

405. Hiruma M, Ide S, Hohdatsu T, et al. Polymyositis in mice experimentally inoculated with Getah virus. *Nihon Juigaku Zasshi* 1990;52(4):767–772.

406. Ho K, Ang LW, Tan BH, et al. Epidemiology and control of chikungunya fever in Singapore. *J Infect* 2011;62(4):263–270.

407. Ho M, Breinig MK. Conditions for the production of an interferon appearing in chick cell cultures infected with Sindbis virus. *J Immunol* 1962;89:177–186.

408. Hoarau JJ, Jaffar Bandjee MC, Krejbich Trotot P, et al. Persistent chronic inflammation and infection by Chikungunya arthritogenic alphavirus in spite of a robust host immune response. *J Immunol* 2010;184(10):5914–5927.

409. Hodneland K, Bratland A, Christie KE, et al. New subtype of salmonid alphavirus (SAV), Togaviridae, from Atlantic salmon *Salmo salar* and rainbow trout *Oncorhynchus mykiss* in Norway. *Dis Aquat Organ* 2005;66(2):113–120.

410. Holzer GW, Coulibaly S, Aichinger G, et al. Evaluation of an inactivated Ross River virus vaccine in active and passive mouse immunization models and establishment of a correlate of protection. *Vaccine* 2011;29(24):4132–4141.

411. Hommel D, Heraud JM, Hulin A, et al. Association of Tonate virus (subtype IIIB of the Venezuelan equine encephalitis complex) with encephalitis in a human. *Clin Infect Dis* 2000;30(1):188–190.

412. Hopla CE, Francy DB, Calisher CH, et al. Relationship of cliff swallows, ectoparasites, and an alphavirus in west-central Oklahoma. *J Med Entomol* 1993;30(1):267–272.

413. Horling J, Vene S, Franzen C, et al. Detection of Ockelbo virus RNA in skin biopsies by polymerase chain reaction. *J Clin Microbiol* 1993;31(8):2004–2009.

414. Houk EJ, Arcus YM, Hardy JL, et al. Binding of western equine encephalomyelitis virus to brush border fragments isolated from mesenteronal epithelial cells of mosquitoes. *Virus Res* 1990;17(2):105–117.

415. Howitt BF. Equine encephalomyelitis. *J Infect Dis* 1932;51:493–510.

416. Howitt BF, Dodge HR, Bishop LK, et al. Recovery of the virus of eastern equine encephalomyelitis from mosquitoes (Mansonia perturbans) collected in Georgia. *Science* 1949;110(2849):141–142.

417. Hoz JM, Bayona B, Viloria S, et al. Fatal cases of Chikungunya virus infection in Colombia: diagnostic and treatment challenges. *J Clin Virol* 2015;69:27–29.

418. Hsieh P, Robbins PW. Regulation of asparagine-linked oligosaccharide processing. Oligosaccharide processing in *Aedes albopictus* mosquito cells. *J Biol Chem* 1984;259(4):2375–2382.

419. Hu J, Cai XF, Yan G. Alphavirus M1 induces apoptosis of malignant glioma cells via downregulation and nucleolar translocation of p21WAF1/CIP1 protein. *Cell Cycle* 2009;8(20):3328–3339.

420. Hu W, Clements A, Williams G, et al. Bayesian spatiotemporal analysis of socio-ecologic drivers of Ross River virus transmission in Queensland, Australia. *Am J Trop Med Hyg* 2010;83(3):722–728.

421. Hu WG, Phelps AL, Jager S, et al. A recombinant humanized monoclonal antibody completely protects mice against lethal challenge with Venezuelan equine encephalitis virus. *Vaccine* 2010;28(34):5558–5564.

422. Huang PY, Guo JH, Hwang LH. Oncolytic Sindbis virus targets tumors defective in the interferon response and induces significant bystander antitumor immunity in vivo. *Mol Ther* 2012;20(2):298–305.

423. Hunt AR, Bowen RA, Frederickson S, et al. Treatment of mice with human monoclonal antibody 24h after lethal aerosol challenge with virulent Venezuelan equine encephalitis virus prevents disease but not infection. *Virology* 2011;414(2):146–152.

424. Hunt AR, Johnson AJ, Roehrig JT. Synthetic peptides of Venezuelan equine encephalomyelitis virus E2 glycoprotein. I. Immunogenic analysis and identification of a protective peptide. *Virology* 1990;179(2):701–711.

425. Hunt AR, Roehrig JT. Biochemical and biological characteristics of epitopes on the E1 glycoprotein of western equine encephalitis virus. *Virology* 1985;142(2):334–346.

426. Hyde JL, Gardner CL, Kimura T, et al. A viral RNA structural element alters host recognition of nonself RNA. *Science* 2014;343(6172):783–787.

427. Inglis FM, Lee KM, Chiu KB, et al. Neuropathogenesis of Chikungunya infection: astrogliosis and innate immune activation. *J Neurovirol* 2016;22(2):140–148.

428. Inglot AD, Albin M, Chudzio T. Persistent infection of mouse cells with Sindbis virus: role of virulence of strains, auto-interfering particles and interferon. *J Gen Virol* 1973;20(1):105–110.

429. Irani DN, Griffin DE. Isolation of brain parenchymal lymphocytes for flow cytometric analysis. Application to acute viral encephalitis. *J Immunol Methods* 1991;139(2):223–231.

430. Irani DN, Griffin DE. Regulation of lymphocyte homing into the brain during viral encephalitis at various stages of infection. *J Immunol* 1996;156(10):3850–3857.

431. Irani DN, Prow NA. Neuroprotective interventions targeting detrimental host immune responses protect mice from fatal alphavirus encephalitis. *J Neuropathol Exp Neurol* 2007;66(6):533–544.

432. Jackson AC, Moench TR, Griffin DE, et al. The pathogenesis of spinal cord involvement in the encephalomyelitis of mice caused by neuroadapted Sindbis virus infection. *Lab Invest* 1987;56(4):418–423.

433. Jackson AC, Moench TR, Trapp BD, et al. Basis of neurovirulence in Sindbis virus encephalomyelitis of mice. *Lab Invest* 1988;58(5):503–509.

434. Jackson AC, Rossiter JP. Apoptotic cell death is an important cause of neuronal injury in experimental Venezuelan equine encephalitis virus infection of mice. *Acta Neuropathol* 1997;93(4):349–353.

435. Jacups SP, Whelan PI, Currie BJ. Ross River virus and Barmah Forest virus infections: a review of history, ecology, and predictive models, with implications for tropical northern Australia. *Vector Borne Zoonotic Dis* 2008;8(2):283–297.

436. Jacups SP, Whelan PI, Markey PG, et al. Predictive indicators for Ross River virus infection in the Darwin area of tropical northern Australia, using long-term mosquito trapping data. *Trop Med Int Health* 2008;13(7):943–952.

437. Jahrling PB. Virulence heterogeneity of a predominantly avirulent Western equine encephalitis virus population. *J Gen Virol* 1976;32(1):121–128.

438. Jahrling PB, Gorelkin L. Selective clearance of a benign clone of Venezuelan equine encephalitis virus from hamster plasma by hepatic reticuloendothelial cells. *J Infect Dis* 1975;132(6):667–676.

439. Jahrling PB, Hilmas DE, Heard CD. Vascular clearance of venezuelan equine encephalomyelitis viruses as a correlate to virulence for rhesus monkeys. *Arch Virol* 1977;55(1–2):161–164.

440. Jahrling PB, Navarro E, Scherer WF. Interferon induction and sensitivity as correlates to virulence of Venezuelan encephalitis viruses for hamsters. *Arch Virol* 1976;51(1–2):23–35.

441. Jahrling PB, Scherer WF. Growth curves and clearance rates of virulent and benign Venezuelan encephalitis viruses in hamsters. *Infect Immun* 1973;8(3):456–462.

442. Jahrling PB, Scherer F. Histopathology and distribution of viral antigens in hamsters infected with virulent and benign Venezuelan encephalitis viruses. *Am J Pathol* 1973;72(1):25–38.

443. Jahrling PB, Stephenson EH. Protective efficacies of live attenuated and formaldehyde-inactivated Venezuelan equine encephalitis virus vaccines against aerosol challenge in hamsters. *J Clin Microbiol* 1984;19(3):429–431.

444. Jain SK, DeCandido S, Kielian M. Processing of the p62 envelope precursor protein of Semliki Forest virus. *J Biol Chem* 1991;266(9):5756–5761.

445. Jan JT, Chatterjee S, Griffin DE. Sindbis virus entry into cells triggers apoptosis by activating sphingomyelinase, leading to the release of ceramide. *J Virol* 2000;74(14):6425–6432.

446. Jan JT, Griffin DE. Induction of apoptosis by Sindbis virus occurs at cell entry and does not require virus replication. *J Virol* 1999;73(12):10296–10302.

447. Jin J, Galaz-Montoya JG, Sherman MB, et al. Neutralizing antibodies inhibit chikungunya virus budding at the plasma membrane. *Cell Host Microbe* 2018;24(3):417–428 e415.

448. Jin J, Liss NM, Chen DH, et al. Neutralizing monoclonal antibodies block chikungunya virus entry and release by targeting an epitope critical to viral pathogenesis. *Cell Rep* 2015;13(11):2553–2564.

449. Joe AK, Ferrari G, Jiang HH, et al. Dominant inhibitory Ras delays Sindbis virus-induced apoptosis in neuronal cells. *J Virol* 1996;70(11):7744–7751.

450. Joe AK, Foo HH, Kleeman L, et al. The transmembrane domains of Sindbis virus envelope glycoproteins induce cell death. *J Virol* 1998;72(5):3935–3943.

451. Johnson RT, McFarland HF, Levy SE. Age-dependent resistance to viral encephalitis: studies of infections due to Sindbis virus in mice. *J Infect Dis* 1972;125(3):257–262.

452. Johnson BW, Russell BJ, Goodman CH. Laboratory diagnosis of chikungunya virus infections and commercial sources for diagnostic assays. *J Infect Dis* 2016;214(Suppl 5):S471–S474.

453. Johnson KM, Shelokov A, Peralta PH, et al. Recovery of Venezuelan equine encephalomyelitis virus in Panama. A fatal case in man. *Am J Trop Med Hyg* 1968;17(3):432–440.

454. Johnston LJ, Halliday GM, King NJ. Phenotypic changes in Langerhans' cells after infection with arboviruses: a role in the immune response to epidermally acquired viral infection? *J Virol* 1996;70(7):4761–4766.

455. Jones A, Lowry K, Aaskov J, et al. Molecular evolutionary dynamics of Ross River virus and implications for vaccine efficacy. *J Gen Virol* 2010;91(Pt 1):182–188.

456. Jones PH, Maric M, Madison MN, et al. BST-2/tetherin-mediated restriction of chikungunya (CHIKV) VLP budding is counteracted by CHIKV non-structural protein 1 (nsP1). *Virology* 2013;438(1):37–49.

457. Jonsson CB, Cao X, Lee J, et al. Efficacy of a ML336 derivative against Venezuelan and eastern equine encephalitis viruses. *Antiviral Res* 2019;167:25–34.

458. Jost H, Bialonski A, Storch V, et al. Isolation and phylogenetic analysis of Sindbis viruses from mosquitoes in Germany. *J Clin Microbiol* 2010;48(5):1900–1903.

459. Joubert PE, Werneke SW, de la Calle C, et al. Chikungunya virus-induced autophagy delays caspase-dependent cell death. *J Exp Med* 2012;209(5):1029–1047.

460. Journeaux SF, Brown WG, Aaskov JG. Prolonged infection of human synovial cells with Ross River virus. *J Gen Virol* 1987;68(Pt 12):3165–3169.

461. Julander JG, Bowen RA, Rao JR, et al. Treatment of Venezuelan equine encephalitis virus infection with (−)-carbodine. *Antiviral Res* 2008;80(3):309–315.

462. Julander JG, Siddharthan V, Blatt LM, et al. Effect of exogenous interferon and an interferon inducer on western equine encephalitis virus disease in a hamster model. *Virology* 2007;360(2):454–460.

463. Julander JG, Skirpstunas R, Siddharthan V, et al. C3H/HeN mouse model for the evaluation of antiviral agents for the treatment of Venezuelan equine encephalitis virus infection. *Antiviral Res* 2008;78(3):230–241.

464. Julander JG, Smee DF, Morrey JD, et al. Effect of T-705 treatment on western equine encephalitis in a mouse model. *Antiviral Res* 2009;82(3):169–171.

465. Junt T, Heraud JM, Lelarge J, et al. Determination of natural versus laboratory human infection with Mayaro virus by molecular analysis. *Epidemiol Infect* 1999;123(3):511–513.

466. Jupille HJ, Medina-Rivera M, Hawman DW, et al. A tyrosine-to-histidine switch at position 18 of the Ross River virus E2 glycoprotein is a determinant of virus fitness in disparate hosts. *J Virol* 2013;87(10):5970–5984.

467. Jupille HJ, Oko L, Stoermer KA, et al. Mutations in nsP1 and PE2 are critical determinants of Ross River virus-induced musculoskeletal inflammatory disease in a mouse model. *Virology* 2011;410(1):216–227.

468. Jupp PG, Blackburn NK, Thompson DL, et al. Sindbis and West Nile virus infections in the Witwatersrand-Pretoria region. *S Afr Med J* 1986;70(4):218–220.

469. Kam YW, Simarmata D, Chow A, et al. Early appearance of neutralizing immunoglobulin G3 antibodies is associated with chikungunya virus clearance and long-term clinical protection. *J Infect Dis* 2012;205(7):1147–1154.

470. Karabatsos N, Lewis AL, Calisher CH, et al. Identification of Highlands J virus from a Florida horse. *Am J Trop Med Hyg* 1988;39(6):603–606.

471. Kariuki Njenga M, Nderitu L, Ledermann JP, et al. Tracking epidemic Chikungunya virus into the Indian Ocean from East Africa. *J Gen Virol* 2008;89(Pt 11):2754–2760.

472. Karlsen M, Gjerset B, Hansen T, et al. Multiple introductions of salmonid alphavirus from a wild reservoir have caused independent and self-sustainable epizootics in aquaculture. *J Gen Virol* 2014;95(Pt 1):52–59.

473. Karpe YA, Aher PP, Lole KS. NTPase and 5'-RNA triphosphatase activities of Chikungunya virus nsP2 protein. *PLoS One* 2011;6(7):e22336.

474. Karpf AR, Brown DT. Comparison of Sindbis virus-induced pathology in mosquito and vertebrate cell cultures. *Virology* 1998;240(2):193–201.

475. Karpf AR, Lenches E, Strauss EG, et al. Superinfection exclusion of alphaviruses in three mosquito cell lines persistently infected with Sindbis virus. *J Virol* 1997;71(9):7119–7123.

476. Kay BH, Boyd AM, Ryan PA, et al. Mosquito feeding patterns and natural infection of vertebrates with Ross River and Barmah Forest viruses in Brisbane, Australia. *Am J Trop Med Hyg* 2007;76(3):417–423.

477. Keene KM, Foy BD, Sanchez-Vargas I, et al. RNA interference acts as a natural antiviral response to O'nyong-nyong virus (Alphavirus; Togaviridae) infection of *Anopheles gambiae*. *Proc Natl Acad Sci U S A* 2004;101(49):17240–17245.

478. Kelen PT, Downs JA, Burkett-Cadena ND, et al. Habitat associations of eastern equine encephalitis transmission in Walton County Florida. *J Med Entomol* 2012;49(3):746–756.

479. Kelser RA. Mosquitoes as vectors of the virus of equine encephalomyelitis. *J Am Vet Med Assoc* 1933;82:767–771.

480. Kempf C, Kohler U, Michel MR, et al. Semliki Forest virus-induced polykaryocyte formation is an ATP-dependent event. *Arch Virol* 1987;95(1–2):111–122.

481. Kennedy AC, Fleming J, Solomon L. Chikungunya viral arthropathy: a clinical description. *J Rheumatol* 1980;7(2):231–236.

482. Kerns JA, Emerman M, Malik HS. Positive selection and increased antiviral activity associated with the PARP-containing isoform of human zinc-finger antiviral protein. *PLoS Genet* 2008;4(1):e21.

483. Kerr PJ, Fitzgerald S, Tregear GW, et al. Characterization of a major neutralization domain of Ross River virus using anti-viral and anti-peptide antibodies. *Virology* 1992;187(1):338–342.

484. Kerr DA, Larsen T, Cook SH, et al. BCL-2 and BAX protect adult mice from lethal Sindbis virus infection but do not protect spinal cord motor neurons or prevent paralysis. *J Virol* 2002;76(20):10393–10400.

485. Kerr PJ, Weir RC, Dalgarno L. Ross River virus variants selected during passage in chick embryo fibroblasts: serological, genetic, and biological changes. *Virology* 1993;193(1):446–449.

486. Khalili-Shirazi A, Gregson N, Webb HE. Immunocytochemical evidence for Semliki Forest virus antigen persistence in mouse brain. *J Neurol Sci* 1988;85(1):17–26.

487. Khongwichit S, Wikan N, Abere B, et al. Cell-type specific variation in the induction of ER stress and downstream events in chikungunya virus infection. *Microb Pathog* 2016;101:104–118.

488. Khoo CC, Piper J, Sanchez-Vargas I, et al. The RNA interference pathway affects midgut infection- and escape barriers for Sindbis virus in *Aedes aegypti*. *BMC Microbiol* 2010;10:130.

489. Kim AS, Austin SK, Gardner CL, et al. Protective antibodies against Eastern equine encephalitis virus bind to epitopes in domains A and B of the E2 glycoprotein. *Nat Microbiol* 2019;4(1):187–197.

490. Kimura T, Griffin DE. The role of CD8(+) T cells and major histocompatibility complex class I expression in the central nervous system of mice infected with neurovirulent Sindbis virus. *J Virol* 2000;74(13):6117–6125.

491. Kimura T, Griffin DE. Extensive immune-mediated hippocampal damage in mice surviving infection with neuroadapted Sindbis virus. *Virology* 2003;311(1):28–39.

492. Kinney RM, Chang GJ, Tsuchiya KR, et al. Attenuation of Venezuelan equine encephalitis virus strain TC-83 is encoded by the 5'-noncoding region and the E2 envelope glycoprotein. *J Virol* 1993;67(3):1269–1277.

493. Kinney RM, Pfeffer M, Tsuchiya KR, et al. Nucleotide sequences of the 26S mRNAs of the viruses defining the Venezuelan equine encephalitis antigenic complex. *Am J Trop Med Hyg* 1998;59(6):952–964.

494. Kinney RM, Trent DW, France JK. Comparative immunological and biochemical analyses of viruses in the Venezuelan equine encephalitis complex. *J Gen Virol* 1983;64(Pt 1):135–147.

495. Kinney RM, Tsuchiya KR, Sneider JM, et al. Molecular evidence for the origin of the widespread Venezuelan equine encephalitis epizootic of 1969 to 1972. *J Gen Virol* 1992;73(Pt 12):3301–3305.

496. Kissling RE, Chamberlain RW, Eidson ME, et al. Studies on the North American arthropod-borne encephalitides. II. Eastern equine encephalitis in horses. *Am J Hyg* 1954;60(3):237–250.

497. Kissling RE, Chamberlain RW, Nelson DB, et al. Venezuelan equine encephalomyelitis in horses. *Am J Hyg* 1956;63(3):274–287.

498. Kiwanuka N, Sanders EJ, Rwaguma EB, et al. O'nyong-nyong fever in south-central Uganda, 1996–1997: clinical features and validation of a clinical case definition for surveillance purposes. *Clin Infect Dis* 1999;29(5):1243–1250.

499. Klapsing P, MacLean JD, Glaze S, et al. Ross River virus disease reemergence, Fiji, 2003–2004. *Emerg Infect Dis* 2005;11(4):613–615.

500. Klimstra WB, Nangle EM, Smith MS, et al. DC-SIGN and L-SIGN can act as attachment receptors for alphaviruses and distinguish between mosquito cell- and mammalian cell-derived viruses. *J Virol* 2003;77(22):12022–12032.

501. Klimstra WB, Ryman KD, Johnston RE. Adaptation of Sindbis virus to BHK cells selects for use of heparan sulfate as an attachment receptor. *J Virol* 1998;72(9):7357–7366.

502. Kokernot RH, Shinefield HR, Longshore WA Jr. The 1952 outbreak of encephalitis in California; differential diagnosis. *Calif Med* 1953;79(2):73–77.

503. Kolokoltsova OA, Domina AM, Kolokoltsov AA, et al. Alphavirus production is inhibited in neurofibromin 1-deficient cells through activated RAS signalling. *Virology* 2008;377(1):133–142.

504. Komar N, Dohm DJ, Turell MJ, et al. Eastern equine encephalitis virus in birds: relative competence of European starlings (*Sturnus vulgaris*). *Am J Trop Med Hyg* 1999;60(3):387–391.

505. Kono Y, Ho M. The role of the reticuloendothelial system in interferon formation in the rabbit. *Virology* 1965;25:163–166.

506. Kononchik JP Jr, Hernandez R, Brown DT. An alternative pathway for alphavirus entry. *Virol J* 2011;8:304.

507. Konopka JL, Thompson JM, Whitmore AC, et al. Acute infection with venezuelan equine encephalitis virus replicon particles catalyzes a systemic antiviral state and protects from lethal virus challenge. *J Virol* 2009;83(23):12432–12442.

508. Koonin EV, Dolja VV. Evolution and taxonomy of positive-strand RNA viruses: implications of comparative analysis of amino acid sequences. *Crit Rev Biochem Mol Biol* 1993;28(5):375–430.

509. Kostyuchenko VA, Jakana J, Liu X, et al. The structure of Barmah forest virus as revealed by cryo-electron microscopy at a 6-angstrom resolution has detailed transmembrane protein architecture and interactions. *J Virol* 2011;85(18):9327–9333.

510. Kramer LD, Fallah HM. Genetic variation among isolates of western equine encephalomyelitis virus from California. *Am J Trop Med Hyg* 1999;60(4):708–713.

511. Krejbich-Trotot P, Denizot M, Hoarau JJ, et al. Chikungunya virus mobilizes the apoptotic machinery to invade host cell defenses. *FASEB J* 2011;25(1):314–325.

512. Krejbich-Trotot P, Gay B, Li-Pat-Yuen G, et al. Chikungunya triggers an autophagic process which promotes viral replication. *Virol J* 2011;8:432.

513. Kubes V, Rios FA. The causative agent of infectious equine encephalomyelitis in Venezuela. *Science* 1939;90(2323):20–21.

514. Kuhn RJ, Griffin DE, Owen KE, et al. Chimeric Sindbis-Ross River viruses to study interactions between alphavirus nonstructural and structural regions. *J Virol* 1996;70(11):7900–7909.

515. Kulcsar KA, Baxter VK, Abraham R, et al. Distinct immune responses in resistant and susceptible strains of mice during neurovirulent alphavirus encephalomyelitis. *J Virol* 2015;89(16):8280–8291.

516. Kulcsar KA, Baxter VK, Greene IP, et al. Interleukin 10 modulation of pathogenic Th17 cells during fatal alphavirus encephalomyelitis. *Proc Natl Acad Sci U S A* 2014;111(45):16053–16058.

517. Kulcsar KA, Griffin DE. T cell-derived interleukin-10 is an important regulator of the Th17 response during lethal alphavirus encephalomyelitis. *J Neuroimmunol* 2016;295–296:60–67.

518. Kumar P, Sweeney TR, Skabkin MA, et al. Inhibition of translation by IFIT family members is determined by their ability to interact selectively with the 5'-terminal regions of cap0-, cap1- and 5'ppp- mRNAs. *Nucleic Acids Res* 2014;42(5):3228–3245.

519. Kuniholm MH, Wolfe ND, Huang CY, et al. Seroprevalence and distribution of *Flaviviridae*, *Togaviridae*, and *Bunyaviridae* arboviral infections in rural Cameroonian adults. *Am J Trop Med Hyg* 2006;74(6):1078–1083.

520. Kurkela S, Manni T, Myllynen J, et al. Clinical and laboratory manifestations of Sindbis virus infection: prospective study, Finland, 2002–2003. *J Infect Dis* 2005;191(11):1820–1829.

521. Kurkela S, Manni T, Vaheri A, et al. Causative agent of Pogosta disease isolated from blood and skin lesions. *Emerg Infect Dis* 2004;10(5):889–894.

522. Kurkela S, Ratti O, Huhtamo E, et al. Sindbis virus infection in resident birds, migratory birds, and humans, Finland. *Emerg Infect Dis* 2008;14(1):41–47.

523. Kurucz N, Markey P, Draper A, et al. Investigation into High Barmah Forest Virus Disease Case Numbers Reported in the Northern Territory, Australia in 2012-2013. *Vector Borne Zoonotic Dis* 2016;16(2):110–116.

524. La Linn M, Eble JA, Lubken C, et al. An arthritogenic alphavirus uses the alpha1beta1 integrin collagen receptor. *Virology* 2005;336(2):229–239.

525. La Linn M, Gardner J, Warrilow D, et al. Arbovirus of marine mammals: a new alphavirus isolated from the elephant seal louse, *Lepidophthirus macrorhini*. *J Virol* 2001;75(9):4103–4109.

526. Laakkonen P, Hyvonen M, Peranen J, et al. Expression of Semliki Forest virus nsP1-specific methyltransferase in insect cells and in *Escherichia coli*. *J Virol* 1994;68(11):7418–7425.

527. Labadie K, Larcher T, Joubert C, et al. Chikungunya disease in nonhuman primates involves long-term viral persistence in macrophages. *J Clin Invest* 2010;120(3):894–906.

528. LaBeaud AD, Banda T, Brichard J, et al. High rates of O'nyong nyong and Chikungunya virus transmission in coastal Kenya. *PLoS Negl Trop Dis* 2015;9(2):e0003436.

529. Labrada L, Liang XH, Zheng W, et al. Age-dependent resistance to lethal alphavirus encephalitis in mice: analysis of gene expression in the central nervous system and identification of a novel interferon-inducible protective gene, mouse ISG12. *J Virol* 2002;76(22):11688–11703.

530. Lambert AJ, Martin DA, Lanciotti RS. Detection of North American eastern and western equine encephalitis viruses by nucleic acid amplification assays. *J Clin Microbiol* 2003;41(1):379–385.

531. Lanciotti RS, Ludwig ML, Rwaguma EB, et al. Emergence of epidemic O'nyong-nyong fever in Uganda after a 35-year absence: genetic characterization of the virus. *Virology* 1998;252(1):258–268.

532. Landis H, Simon-Jodicke A, Kloti A, et al. Human MxA protein confers resistance to Semliki Forest virus and inhibits the amplification of a Semliki Forest virus-based replicon in the absence of viral structural proteins. *J Virol* 1998;72(2):1516–1522.

533. Laras K, Sukri NC, Larasati RP, et al. Tracking the re-emergence of epidemic chikungunya virus in Indonesia. *Trans R Soc Trop Med Hyg* 2005;99(2):128–141.

534. LaStarza MW, Lemm JA, Rice CM. Genetic analysis of the nsP3 region of Sindbis virus: evidence for roles in minus-strand and subgenomic RNA synthesis. *J Virol* 1994;68(9):5781–5791.

535. Lau C, Aubry M, Musso D, et al. New evidence for endemic circulation of Ross River virus in the Pacific Islands and the potential for emergence. *Int J Infect Dis* 2017;57:73–76.

536. Lavergne A, de Thoisy B, Lacoste V, et al. Mayaro virus: complete nucleotide sequence and phylogenetic relationships with other alphaviruses. *Virus Res* 2006;117(2):283–290.

537. Law LM, Albin OR, Carroll JW, et al. Identification of a dominant negative inhibitor of human zinc finger antiviral protein reveals a functional endogenous pool and critical homotypic interactions. *J Virol* 2010;84(9):4504–4512.

538. Lednicky J, De Rochars VM, Elbadry M, et al. Mayaro Virus in Child with Acute Febrile Illness, Haiti, 2015. *Emerg Infect Dis* 2016;22(11):2000–2002.

539. LeDuc JW, Suyemoto W, Eldridge BF, et al. Ecology of arboviruses in a Maryland freshwater swamp. II. Blood feeding patterns of potential mosquito vectors. *Am J Epidemiol* 1972;96(2):123–128.

540. Lee P, Knight R, Smit JM, et al. A single mutation in the E2 glycoprotein important for neurovirulence influences binding of Sindbis virus to neuroblastoma cells. *J Virol* 2002;76(12):6302–6310.

541. Lee E, Stocks C, Lobigs P, et al. Nucleotide sequence of the Barmah Forest virus genome. *Virology* 1997;227(2):509–514.

542. Lee MY, Sumpter R Jr, Zou Z, et al. Peroxisomal protein PEX13 functions in selective autophagy. *EMBO Rep* 2017;18(1):48–60.

543. Lee WW, Teo TH, Her Z, et al. Expanding regulatory T cells alleviates chikungunya virus-induced pathology in mice. *J Virol* 2015;89(15):7893–7904.

544. Lennette EH, Koprowski H. Human infection with Venezuelan equine encephalomyelitis virus—report on eight cases of infection acquired in the laboratory. *J Am Med Assoc* 1943;123:1088–1095.

545. Lenschow DJ, Giannakopoulos NV, Gunn LJ, et al. Identification of interferon-stimulated gene 15 as an antiviral molecule during Sindbis virus infection in vivo. *J Virol* 2005;79(22):13974–13983.

546. Lenschow DJ, Lai C, Frias-Staheli N, et al. IFN-stimulated gene 15 functions as a critical antiviral molecule against influenza, herpes, and Sindbis viruses. *Proc Natl Acad Sci U S A* 2007;104(4):1371–1376.

547. Leon CA. Sequelae of Venezuelan equine encephalitis in humans: a four year follow-up. *Int J Epidemiol* 1975;4(2):131–140.

548. Letson GW, Bailey RE, Pearson J, et al. Eastern equine encephalitis (EEE): a description of the 1989 outbreak, recent epidemiologic trends, and the association of rainfall with EEE occurrence. *Am J Trop Med Hyg* 1993;49(6):677–685.

549. Levine B, Goldman JE, Jiang HH, et al. Bcl-2 protects mice against fatal alphavirus encephalitis. *Proc Natl Acad Sci U S A* 1996;93(10):4810–4815.

550. Levine B, Griffin DE. Persistence of viral RNA in mouse brains after recovery from acute alphavirus encephalitis. *J Virol* 1992;66(11):6429–6435.

551. Levine B, Hardwick JM, Griffin DE. Persistence of alphaviruses in vertebrate hosts. *Trends Microbiol* 1994;2(1):25–28.

552. Levine B, Hardwick JM, Trapp BD, et al. Antibody-mediated clearance of alphavirus infection from neurons. *Science* 1991;254(5033):856–860.

553. Levine B, Huang Q, Isaacs JT, et al. Conversion of lytic to persistent alphavirus infection by the bcl-2 cellular oncogene. *Nature* 1993;361(6414):739–742.

554. Levine B, Kroemer G. Autophagy in the pathogenesis of disease. *Cell* 2008;132(1):27-42.

555. Levitt NH, Ramsburg HH, Hasty SE, et al. Development of an attenuated strain of chikungunya virus for use in vaccine production. *Vaccine* 1986;4(3):157–162.

556. Lewis J, Oyler GA, Ueno K, et al. Inhibition of virus-induced neuronal apoptosis by Bax. *Nat Med* 1999;5(7):832–835.

557. Lewis J, Wesselingh SL, Griffin DE, et al. Alphavirus-induced apoptosis in mouse brains correlates with neurovirulence. *J Virol* 1996;70(3):1828–1835.

558. Lhuillier M, Cunin P, Mazzariol MJ, et al. [A rural epidemic of Igbo Ora virus (with interhuman transmission) in the Ivory Coast 1984-1985]. *Bull Soc Pathol Exot Filiales* 1988;81(3):386–395.

559. Li L, Jose J, Xiang Y, et al. Structural changes of envelope proteins during alphavirus fusion. *Nature* 2010;468(7324):705–708.

560. Li XD, Qiu FX, Yang H, et al. Isolation of Getah virus from mosquitos collected on Hainan Island, China, and results of a serosurvey. *Southeast Asian J Trop Med Public Health* 1992;23(4):730–734.

561. Liang XH, Goldman JE, Jiang HH, et al. Resistance of interleukin-1beta-deficient mice to fatal Sindbis virus encephalitis. *J Virol* 1999;73(3):2563–2567.
562. Liang XH, Kleeman LK, Jiang HH, et al. Protection against fatal Sindbis virus encephalitis by beclin, a novel Bcl-2-interacting protein. *J Virol* 1998;72(11):8586–8596.
563. Lidbury BA, Rulli NE, Musso CM, et al. Identification and characterization of a Ross River virus variant that grows persistently in macrophages, shows altered disease kinetics in a mouse model, and exhibits resistance to type I interferon. *J Virol* 2011;85(11):5651–5663.
564. Lidbury BA, Rulli NE, Suhrbier A, et al. Macrophage-derived proinflammatory factors contribute to the development of arthritis and myositis after infection with an arthrogenic alphavirus. *J Infect Dis* 2008;197(11):1585–1593.
565. Lin KI, DiDonato JA, Hoffmann A, et al. Suppression of steady-state, but not stimulus-induced NF-kappaB activity inhibits alphavirus-induced apoptosis. *J Cell Biol* 1998;141(7):1479–1487.
566. Lindsay MD, Broom AK, Wright AE, et al. Ross River virus isolations from mosquitoes in arid regions of Western Australia: implication of vertical transmission as a means of persistence of the virus. *Am J Trop Med Hyg* 1993;49(6):686–696.
567. Lindsay M, Johansen C, Broom AK, et al. Emergence of Barmah Forest virus in Western Australia. *Emerg Infect Dis* 1995;1(1):22–26.
568. Lindsey NP, Staples JE, Fischer M. Eastern equine encephalitis virus in the United States, 2003–2016. *Am J Trop Med Hyg* 2018;98(5):1472–1477.
569. Linn ML, Mateo L, Gardner J, et al. Alphavirus-specific cytotoxic T lymphocytes recognize a cross-reactive epitope from the capsid protein and can eliminate virus from persistently infected macrophages. *J Virol* 1998;72(6):5146–5153.
570. Liu WJ, Rourke MF, Holmes EC, et al. Persistence of multiple genetic lineages within intrahost populations of Ross River virus. *J Virol* 2011;85(11):5674–5678.
571. Liu X, Tharmarajah K, Taylor A. Ross River virus disease clinical presentation, pathogenesis and current therapeutic strategies. *Microbes Infect* 2017;19(11):496–504.
572. Liu C, Voth DW, Rodina P, et al. A comparative study of the pathogenesis of western equine and eastern equine encephalomyelitis viral infections in mice by intracerebral and subcutaneous inoculations. *J Infect Dis* 1970;122(1):53–63.
573. Lobigs M, Zhao HX, Garoff H. Function of Semliki Forest virus E3 peptide in virus assembly: replacement of E3 with an artificial signal peptide abolishes spike heterodimerization and surface expression of E1. *J Virol* 1990;64(9):4346–4355.
574. Logue CH, Bosio CF, Welte T, et al. Virulence variation among isolates of western equine encephalitis virus in an outbred mouse model. *J Gen Virol* 2009;90(Pt 8):1848–1858.
575. Logue CH, Phillips AT, Mossel EC, et al. Treatment with cationic liposome-DNA complexes (CLDCs) protects mice from lethal Western equine encephalitis virus (WEEV) challenge. *Antiviral Res* 2010;87(2):195–203.
576. London WT, Levitt NH, Kent SG, et al. Congenital cerebral and ocular malformations induced in rhesus monkeys by Venezuelan equine encephalitis virus. *Teratology* 1977;16(3):285–285.
577. Long F, Fong RH, Austin SK, et al. Cryo-EM structures elucidate neutralizing mechanisms of anti-chikungunya human monoclonal antibodies with therapeutic activity. *Proc Natl Acad Sci U S A* 2015;112(45):13898–13903.
578. Long KC, Ziegler SA, Thangamani S, et al. Experimental transmission of Mayaro virus by *Aedes aegypti*. *Am J Trop Med Hyg* 2011;85(4):750–757.
579. Longshore WA Jr, Stevens IM, Hollister AC Jr, et al. Epidemiologic observations on acute infectious encephalitis in California, with special reference to the 1952 outbreak. *Am J Hyg* 1956;63(1):69–86.
580. Lu YE, Cassese T, Kielian M. The cholesterol requirement for sindbis virus entry and exit and characterization of a spike protein region involved in cholesterol dependence. *J Virol* 1999;73(5):4272–4278.
581. Lubelczyk C, Mutebi JP, Robinson S, et al. An epizootic of eastern equine encephalitis virus, Maine, USA in 2009: outbreak description and entomological studies. *Am J Trop Med Hyg* 2013;88(1):95–102.
582. Ludwig GV, Kondig JP, Smith JF. A putative receptor for Venezuelan equine encephalitis virus from mosquito cells. *J Virol* 1996;70(8):5592–5599.
583. Ludwig GV, Turell MJ, Vogel P, et al. Comparative neurovirulence of attenuated and non-attenuated strains of Venezuelan equine encephalitis virus in mice. *Am J Trop Med Hyg* 2001;64(1–2):49–55.
584. Luginbuhl RE, Satriano SF, Helmboldt CF, et al. Investigation of eastern equine encephalomyelitis. II. Outbreaks in Connecticut pheasants. *Am J Hyg* 1958;67(1):4–9.
585. Lukaszewski RA, Brooks TJ. Pegylated alpha interferon is an effective treatment for virulent venezuelan equine encephalitis virus and has profound effects on the host immune response to infection. *J Virol* 2000;74(11):5006–5015.
586. Lum FM, Teo TH, Lee WW, et al. An essential role of antibodies in the control of Chikungunya virus infection. *J Immunol* 2013;190(12):6295–6302.
587. Lumsden WH. An epidemic of virus disease in Southern Province, Tanganyika Territory, in 1952-53. II. General description and epidemiology. *Trans R Soc Trop Med Hyg* 1955;49(1):33–57.
588. Lundberg L, Carey B, Kehn-Hall K. Venezuelan equine encephalitis virus capsid—the clever caper. *Viruses* 2017;9(10).
589. Lundstrom JO. Mosquito-borne viruses in western Europe: a review. *J Vector Ecol* 1999;24(1):1–39.
590. Lundstrom JO, Lindstrom KM, Olsen B, et al. Prevalence of sindbis virus neutralizing antibodies among Swedish passerines indicates that thrushes are the main amplifying hosts. *J Med Entomol* 2001;38(2):289–297.
591. Lundstrom JO, Pfeffer M. Phylogeographic structure and evolutionary history of Sindbis virus. *Vector Borne Zoonotic Dis* 2010;10(9):889–907.
592. Lundstrom JO, Vene S, Saluzzo JF, et al. Antigenic comparison of Ockelbo virus isolates from Sweden and Russia with Sindbis virus isolates from Europe, Africa, and Australia: further evidence for variation among alphaviruses. *Am J Trop Med Hyg* 1993;49(5):531–537.
593. Lustig S, Halevy M, Ben-Nathan D, et al. A novel variant of Sindbis virus is both neurovirulent and neuroinvasive in adult mice. *Arch Virol* 1992;122(3–4):237–248.
594. Lustig S, Halevy M, Ben-Nathan D, et al. The role of host immunocompetence in neuroinvasion of Sindbis virus. *Arch Virol* 1999;144(6):1159–1171.
595. Lustig S, Jackson AC, Hahn CS, et al. Molecular basis of Sindbis virus neurovirulence in mice. *J Virol* 1988;62(7):2329–2336.
596. Lutwama JJ, Kayondo J, Savage HM, et al. Epidemic O'Nyong-nyong fever in southcentral Uganda, 1996-1997: entomologic studies in Bbaale village, Rakai District. *Am J Trop Med Hyg* 1999;61(1):158–162.
597. MacDonald GH, Johnston RE. Role of dendritic cell targeting in Venezuelan equine encephalitis virus pathogenesis. *J Virol* 2000;74(2):914–922.
598. MacDonald MR, Machlin ES, Albin OR, et al. The zinc finger antiviral protein acts synergistically with an interferon-induced factor for maximal activity against alphaviruses. *J Virol* 2007;81(24):13509–13518.
599. Mackenzie JS, Lindsay MD, Coelen RJ, et al. Arboviruses causing human disease in the Australasian zoogeographic region. *Arch Virol* 1994;136(3–4):447–467.
600. Mackenzie JS, Poidinger M, Lindsay MD, et al. Molecular epidemiology and evolution of mosquito-borne flaviviruses and alphaviruses enzootic in Australia. *Virus Genes* 1995;11(2–3):225–237.
601. Mackenzie-Liu D, Sokoloski KJ, Purdy S, et al. Encapsidated host factors in alphavirus particles influence midgut infection of *Aedes aegypti*. *Viruses* 2018;10(5).
602. Macnamara FN. The susceptibility of chicks to Semliki Forest virus (Kumba strain). *Ann Trop Med Parasitol* 1953;47(1):9–12.
603. Madan V, Sanz MA, Carrasco L. Requirement of the vesicular system for membrane permeabilization by Sindbis virus. *Virology* 2005;332(1):307–315.
604. Mahauad-Fernandez WD, Jones PH, Okeoma CM. Critical role for bone marrow stromal antigen 2 in acute Chikungunya virus infection. *J Gen Virol* 2014;95(Pt 11):2450–2461.
605. Malherbe H, Strickland-Cholmley M, Jackson AL. Sindbis virus infection in man. Report of a case with recovery of virus from skin lesions. *S Afr Med J* 1963;37:547–552.
606. Malvy D, Ezzedine K, Mamani-Matsuda M, et al. Destructive arthritis in a patient with chikungunya virus infection with persistent specific IgM antibodies. *BMC Infect Dis* 2009;9:200.
607. Mancini EJ, Clarke M, Gowen BE, et al. Cryo-electron microscopy reveals the functional organization of an enveloped virus, Semliki Forest virus. *Mol Cell* 2000;5(2):255–266.
608. Manimunda SP, Vijayachari P, Uppoor R, et al. Clinical progression of chikungunya fever during acute and chronic arthritic stages and the changes in joint morphology as revealed by imaging. *Trans R Soc Trop Med Hyg* 2010;104(6):392–399.
609. Manivannan S, Baxter VK, Schultz KL, et al. Protective effects of glutamine antagonist DON in mice with alphaviral encephalomyelitis. *J Virol* 2016;90(20):9251–9262.
610. Marcus PI, Fuller FJ. Interferon induction by viruses. II. Sindbis virus: interferon induction requires one-quarter of the genome—genes G and A. *J Gen Virol* 1979;44(1):169–177.
611. Marker SC, Connelly D, Jahrling PB. Receptor interaction between eastern equine encephalitis virus and chicken embryo fibroblasts. *J Virol* 1977;21(3):981–985.
612. Martin SS, Bakken RR, Lind CM, et al. Evaluation of formalin inactivated V3526 virus with adjuvant as a next generation vaccine candidate for Venezuelan equine encephalitis virus. *Vaccine* 2010;28(18):3143–3151.
613. Martinez MG, Snapp EL, Perumal GS, et al. Imaging the alphavirus exit pathway. *J Virol* 2014;88(12):6922–6933.
614. Mathews JH, Roehrig JT. Determination of the protective epitopes on the glycoproteins of Venezuelan equine encephalomyelitis virus by passive transfer of monoclonal antibodies. *J Immunol* 1982;129(6):2763–2767.
615. Mathiot CC, Grimaud G, Garry P, et al. An outbreak of human Semliki Forest virus infections in Central African Republic. *Am J Trop Med Hyg* 1990;42(4):386–393.
616. Mathur K, Anand A, Dubey SK, et al. Analysis of chikungunya virus proteins reveals that non-structural proteins nsP2 and nsP3 exhibit RNA interference (RNAi) suppressor activity. *Sci Rep* 2016;6:38065.
617. Mavale M, Parashar D, Sudeep A, et al. Venereal transmission of chikungunya virus by *Aedes aegypti* mosquitoes (Diptera: Culicidae). *Am J Trop Med Hyg* 2010;83(6):1242–1244.
618. Mayuri, Geders TW, Smith JL, Kuhn RJ. Role for conserved residues of sindbis virus nonstructural protein 2 methyltransferase-like domain in regulation of minus-strand synthesis and development of cytopathic infection. *J Virol* 2008;82(15):7284–7297.
619. McBride MP, Sims MA, Cooper RW, et al. Eastern equine encephalitis in a captive harbor seal (Phoca vitulina). *J Zoo Wildl Med* 2008;39(4):631–637.
620. McClain DJ, Pittman PR, Ramsburg HH, et al. Immunologic interference from sequential administration of live attenuated alphavirus vaccines. *J Infect Dis* 1998;177(3):634–641.
621. McFarland HF, Griffin DE, Johnson RT. Specificity of the inflammatory response in viral encephalitis. I. Adoptive immunization of immunosuppressed mice infected with Sindbis virus. *J Exp Med* 1972;136(2):216–226.
622. McInerney GM, Kedersha NL, Kaufman RJ, et al. Importance of eIF2alpha phosphorylation and stress granule assembly in alphavirus translation regulation. *Mol Biol Cell* 2005;16(8):3753–3763.
623. McIntosh BM, Worth CB, Kokernot RH. Isolation of Semliki Forest virus from Aedes (Aedimorphus) argenteopunctatus (Theobald) collected in Portuguese East Africa. *Trans R Soc Trop Med Hyg* 1961;55:192–198.
624. McKimmie CS, Johnson N, Fooks AR, et al. Viruses selectively upregulate Toll-like receptors in the central nervous system. *Biochem Biophys Res Commun* 2005;336(3):925–933.
625. McKnight KL, Simpson DA, Lin SC, et al. Deduced consensus sequence of Sindbis virus strain AR339: mutations contained in laboratory strains which affect cell culture and in vivo phenotypes. *J Virol* 1996;70(3):1981–1989.
626. McLean RG, Crans WJ, Caccamise DF, et al. Experimental infection of wading birds with eastern equine encephalitis virus. *J Wildl Dis* 1995;31(4):502–508.
627. McLoughlin MF, Graham DA. Alphavirus infections in salmonids—a review. *J Fish Dis* 2007;30(9):511–531.
628. McPherson RL, Abraham R, Sreekumar E, et al. ADP-ribosylhydrolase activity of Chikungunya virus macrodomain is critical for virus replication and virulence. *Proc Natl Acad Sci U S A* 2017;114(7):1666–1671.
629. Medovy H. Western equine encephalomyelitis in infants. *J Pediatr* 1943;22:308–318.
630. Meek AD, Faragher SG, Weir RC, et al. Genetic and phenotypic studies on Ross River virus variants of enhanced virulence selected during mouse passage. *Virology* 1989;172(2):399–407.

631. Mehta R, Soares CN, Medialdea-Carrera R, et al. The spectrum of neurological disease associated with Zika and chikungunya viruses in adults in Rio de Janeiro, Brazil: a case series. *PLoS Negl Trop Dis* 2018;12(2):e0006212.

632. Meissner JD, Huang CY, Pfeffer M, et al. Sequencing of prototype viruses in the Venezuelan equine encephalitis antigenic complex. *Virus Res* 1999;64(1):43–59.

633. Mendoza QP, Stanley J, Griffin DE. Monoclonal antibodies to the E1 and E2 glycoproteins of Sindbis virus: definition of epitopes and efficiency of protection from fatal encephalitis. *J Gen Virol* 1988;69(Pt 12):3015–3022.

634. Merits A, Vasiljeva L, Ahola T, et al. Proteolytic processing of Semliki Forest virus-specific non-structural polyprotein by nsP2 protease. *J Gen Virol* 2001;82(Pt 4):765–773.

635. Merour E, Lamoureux A, Bernard J, et al. A fully attenuated recombinant Salmonid alphavirus becomes pathogenic through a single amino acid change in the E2 glycoprotein. *J Virol* 2013;87(10):6027–6030.

636. Merrill MH, Lacaillade CW Jr, Broeck CT. Mosquito transmission of equine encephalomyelitis. *Science* 1934;80(2072):251–252.

637. Meshram CD, Agback P, Shiliaev N, et al. Multiple host factors interact with hypervariable domain of Chikungunya virus nsP3 and determine viral replication in cell-specific mode. *J Virol* 2018;92(16).

638. Metcalf TU, Baxter VK, Nilaratanakul V, et al. Recruitment and retention of B cells in the central nervous system in response to alphavirus encephalomyelitis. *J Virol* 2013;87(5):2420–2429.

639. Metcalf TU, Griffin DE. Alphavirus-induced encephalomyelitis: antibody-secreting cells and viral clearance from the nervous system. *J Virol* 2011;85(21):11490–11501.

640. Meyer KF, Haring CM, Howitt B. The etiology of epizootic encephalomyelitis of horses in the San Joaquin valley, 1930. *Science* 1931;74(1913):227–228.

641. Miller ML, Brown DT. Morphogenesis of Sindbis virus in three subclones of *Aedes albopictus* (mosquito) cells. *J Virol* 1992;66(7):4180–4190.

642. Milner AR, Marshall ID. Pathogenesis of in utero infections with abortogenic and non-abortogenic alphaviruses in mice. *J Virol* 1984;50(1):66–72.

643. Mims CA, Day MF, Marshall ID. Cytopathic effect of Semliki Forest virus in the mosquito *Aedes aegypti*. *Am J Trop Med Hyg* 1966;15(5):775–784.

644. Mims CA, Murphy FA, Taylor WP, et al. Pathogenesis of Ross River virus infection in mice. I. Ependymal infection, cortical thinning, and hydrocephalus. *J Infect Dis* 1973;127(2):121–128.

645. Mitchell CJ, Monath TP, Sabattini MS, et al. Arbovirus investigations in Argentina, 1977-1980. II. Arthropod collections and virus isolations from Argentine mosquitoes. *Am J Trop Med Hyg* 1985;34(5):945–955.

646. Mitchell CJ, Niebylski ML, Smith GC, et al. Isolation of eastern equine encephalitis virus from *Aedes albopictus* in Florida. *Science* 1992;257(5069):526–527.

647. Moench TR, Griffin DE. Immunocytochemical identification and quantitation of the mononuclear cells in the cerebrospinal fluid, meninges, and brain during acute viral meningoencephalitis. *J Exp Med* 1984;159(1):77–88.

648. Mohankumar V, Dhanushkodi NR, Raju R. Sindbis virus replication, is insensitive to rapamycin and torin1, and suppresses Akt/mTOR pathway late during infection in HEK cells. *Biochem Biophys Res Commun* 2011;406(2):262–267.

649. Mokhtarian F, Huan CM, Roman C, et al. Semliki Forest virus-induced demyelination and remyelination—involvement of B cells and anti-myelin antibodies. *J Neuroimmunol* 2003;137(1–2):19–31.

650. Mokhtarian F, Swoveland P. Predisposition to EAE induction in resistant mice by prior infection with Semliki Forest virus. *J Immunol* 1987;138(10):3264–3268.

651. Molaei G, Andreadis TG, Armstrong PM, et al. Vector-host interactions and epizootiology of eastern equine encephalitis virus in Massachusetts. *Vector Borne Zoonotic Dis* 2013;13(5):312–323.

652. Monath TP, Calisher CH, Davis M, et al. Experimental studies of rhesus monkeys infected with epizootic and enzootic subtypes of Venezuelan equine encephalitis virus. *J Infect Dis* 1974;129(2):194–200.

653. Monath TP, Kemp GE, Cropp CB, et al. Necrotizing myocarditis in mice infected with Western equine encephalitis virus: clinical, electrocardiographic, and histopathologic correlations. *J Infect Dis* 1978;138(1):59–66.

654. Monath TP, Lazuick JS, Cropp CB, et al. Recovery of Tonate virus ("Bijou Bridge" strain), a member of the Venezuelan equine encephalomyelitis virus complex, from Cliff Swallow nest bugs (Oeciacus vicarius) and nestling birds in North America. *Am J Trop Med Hyg* 1980;29(5):969–983.

655. Moore DL, Causey OR, Carey DE, et al. Arthropod-borne viral infections of man in Nigeria, 1964-1970. *Ann Trop Med Parasitol* 1975;69(1):49–64.

656. Moreira LA, Iturbe-Ormaetxe I, Jeffery JA, et al. A Wolbachia symbiont in *Aedes aegypti* limits infection with dengue, Chikungunya, and Plasmodium. *Cell* 2009;139(7):1268–1278.

657. Morgan IM, Schlesinger RW, Olitsky PK. Induced resistance of the central nervous system to experimental infection with equine encephalomyelitis virus: I. neutralizing antibody in the central nervous system in relation to cerebral resistance. *J Exp Med* 1942;76(4):357–369.

658. Moriishi K, Koura M, Matsuura Y. Induction of Bad-mediated apoptosis by Sindbis virus infection: involvement of pro-survival members of the Bcl-2 family. *Virology* 2002;292(2):258–271.

659. Morris MM, Dyson H, Baker D, et al. Characterization of the cellular and cytokine response in the central nervous system following Semliki Forest virus infection. *J Neuroimmunol* 1997;74(1–2):185–197.

660. Morris A, Tomkins PT, Maudsley DJ, et al. Infection of cultured murine brain cells by Semliki Forest virus: effects of interferon-alpha beta on viral replication, viral antigen display, major histocompatibility complex antigen display and lysis by cytotoxic T lymphocytes. *J Gen Virol* 1987;68(Pt 1):99–106.

661. Morrison TE, Fraser RJ, Smith PN, et al. Complement contributes to inflammatory tissue destruction in a mouse model of Ross River virus-induced disease. *J Virol* 2007;81(10):5132–5143.

662. Morrison TE, Oko L, Montgomery SA, et al. A mouse model of chikungunya virus-induced musculoskeletal inflammatory disease: evidence of arthritis, tenosynovitis, myositis, and persistence. *Am J Pathol* 2011;178(1):32–40.

663. Morrison TE, Simmons JD, Heise MT. Complement receptor 3 promotes severe Ross River virus-induced disease. *J Virol* 2008;82(22):11263–11272.

664. Morrison TE, Whitmore AC, Shabman RS, et al. Characterization of Ross River virus tropism and virus-induced inflammation in a mouse model of viral arthritis and myositis. *J Virol* 2006;80(2):737–749.

665. Mossel EC, Ledermann JP, Phillips AT, et al. Molecular determinants of mouse neurovirulence and mosquito infection for Western equine encephalitis virus. *PLoS One* 2013;8(3):e60427.

666. Mourao MP, Bastos Mde S, de Figueiredo RP, et al. Mayaro fever in the city of Manaus, Brazil, 2007-2008. *Vector Borne Zoonotic Dis* 2012;12(1):42–46.

667. Mourya DT, Ranadive SN, Gokhale MD, et al. Putative chikungunya virus-specific receptor proteins on the midgut brush border membrane of *Aedes aegypti* mosquito. *Indian J Med Res* 1998;107:10–14.

668. Mousson L, Martin E, Zouache K, et al. Wolbachia modulates Chikungunya replication in *Aedes albopictus*. *Mol Ecol* 2010;19(9):1953–1964.

669. Mudiganti U, Hernandez R, Brown DT. Insect response to alphavirus infection—establishment of alphavirus persistence in insect cells involves inhibition of viral polyprotein cleavage. *Virus Res* 2010;150(1–2):73–84.

670. Mudiganti U, Hernandez R, Ferreira D, et al. Sindbis virus infection of two model insect cell systems—a comparative study. *Virus Res* 2006;122(1–2):28–34.

671. Mullbacher A, Marshall ID, Blanden RV. Cross-reactive cytotoxic T cells to alphavirus infection. *Scand J Immunol* 1979;10(4):291–296.

672. Murphy FA, Harrison AK, Collin WK. The role of extraneural arbovirus infection in the pathogenesis of encephalitis. An electron microscopic study of Semliki Forest virus infection in mice. *Lab Invest* 1970;22(4):318–328.

673. Murphy AM, Sheahan BJ, Atkins GJ. Induction of apoptosis in BCL-2-expressing rat prostate cancer cells using the Semliki Forest virus vector. *Int J Cancer* 2001;94(4):572–578.

674. Murphy FA, Taylor WP, Mims CA, et al. Pathogenesis of Ross River virus infection in mice. II. Muscle, heart, and brown fat lesions. *J Infect Dis* 1973;127(2):129–138.

675. Murphy FA, Whitfield SG. Eastern equine encephalitis virus infection: electron microscopic studies of mouse central nervous system. *Exp Mol Pathol* 1970;13(2):131–146.

676. Mussgay M, Enzmann PJ, Horst J. Influence of an arbovirus infection (Sindbis virus) on the protein and ribonucleic acid synthesis of cultivated chick embryo cells. *Arch Gesamte Virusforsch* 1970;31(1):81–92.

677. Myles KM, Kelly CL, Ledermann JP, et al. Effects of an opal termination codon preceding the nsP4 gene sequence in the O'Nyong-Nyong virus genome on Anopheles gambiae infectivity. *J Virol* 2006;80(10):4992–4997.

678. Myles KM, Pierro DJ, Olson KE. Comparison of the transmission potential of two genetically distinct Sindbis viruses after oral infection of *Aedes aegypti* (Diptera: Culicidae). *J Med Entomol* 2004;41(1):95–106.

679. Myles KM, Wiley MR, Morazzani EM, et al. Alphavirus-derived small RNAs modulate pathogenesis in disease vector mosquitoes. *Proc Natl Acad Sci U S A* 2008;105(50):19938–19943.

680. Nagata LP, Hu WG, Masri SA, et al. Efficacy of DNA vaccination against western equine encephalitis virus infection. *Vaccine* 2005;23(17–18):2280–2283.

681. Nagata LP, Hu WG, Parker M, et al. Infectivity variation and genetic diversity among strains of Western equine encephalitis virus. *J Gen Virol* 2006;87(Pt 8):2353–2361.

682. Nair SR, Abraham R, Sundaram S, et al. Interferon regulated gene (IRG) expression-signature in a mouse model of chikungunya virus neurovirulence. *J Neurovirol* 2017;23(6):886–902.

683. Naish S, Hu W, Nicholls N, et al. Socio-environmental predictors of Barmah forest virus transmission in coastal areas, Queensland, Australia. *Trop Med Int Health* 2009;14(2):247–256.

684. Nargi-Aizenman JL, Havert MB, Zhang M, et al. Glutamate receptor antagonists protect from virus-induced neural degeneration. *Ann Neurol* 2004;55(4):541–549.

685. Nargi-Aizenman JL, Simbulan-Rosenthal CM, Kelly TA, et al. Rapid activation of poly (ADP-ribose) polymerase contributes to Sindbis virus and staurosporine-induced apoptotic cell death. *Virology* 2002;293(1):164–171.

686. Nasar F, Palacios G, Gorchakov RV, et al. Eilat virus, a unique alphavirus with host range restricted to insects by RNA replication. *Proc Natl Acad Sci U S A* 2012;109(36):14622–14627.

687. Nava VE, Rosen A, Veliuona MA, et al. Sindbis virus induces apoptosis through a caspase-dependent, CrmA-sensitive pathway. *J Virol* 1998;72(1):452–459.

688. Navarro JC, Medina G, Vasquez C, et al. Postepizootic persistence of Venezuelan equine encephalitis virus, Venezuela. *Emerg Infect Dis* 2005;11(12):1907–1915.

689. Neighbours LM, Long K, Whitmore AC, et al. Myd88-dependent toll-like receptor 7 signaling mediates protection from severe Ross River virus-induced disease in mice. *J Virol* 2012;86(19):10675–10685.

690. Nelson MA, Herrero LJ, Jeffery JA, et al. Role of envelope N-linked glycosylation in Ross River virus virulence and transmission. *J Gen Virol* 2016;97(5):1094–1106.

691. Nemoto M, Bannai H, Tsujimura K, et al. Getah virus infection among Racehorses, Japan, 2014. *Emerg Infect Dis* 2015;21(5):883–885.

692. Ng LF, Chow A, Sun YJ, et al. IL-1beta, IL-6, and RANTES as biomarkers of Chikungunya severity. *PLoS One* 2009;4(1):e4261.

693. Ng CG, Griffin DE. Acid sphingomyelinase deficiency increases susceptibility to fatal alphavirus encephalomyelitis. *J Virol* 2006;80(22):10989–10999.

694. Ng LC, Tan LK, Tan CH, et al. Entomologic and virologic investigation of Chikungunya, Singapore. *Emerg Infect Dis* 2009;15(8):1243–1249.

695. Nieva JL, Bron R, Corver J, et al. Membrane fusion of Semliki Forest virus requires sphingolipids in the target membrane. *EMBO J* 1994;13(12):2797–2804.

696. Niklasson B, Espmark A, Lundstrom J. Occurrence of arthralgia and specific IgM antibodies three to four years after Ockelbo disease. *J Infect Dis* 1988;157(4):832–835.

697. Nikonov A, Molder T, Sikut R, et al. RIG-I and MDA-5 detection of viral RNA-dependent RNA polymerase activity restricts positive-strand RNA virus replication. *PLoS Pathog* 2013;9(9):e1003610.

698. Nilaratanakul V, Chen J, Tran O, et al. Germ line IgM is sufficient, but not required, for antibody-mediated alphavirus clearance from the central nervous system. *J Virol* 2018;92(7):pii: e02081-17.

699. Nimmo JR. An unusual epidemic. *Med J Aust* 1928;1:549–550.
700. Nishimoto KP, Laust AK, Nelson EL. A human dendritic cell subset receptive to the Venezuelan equine encephalitis virus-derived replicon particle constitutively expresses IL-32. *J Immunol* 2008;181(6):4010–4018.
701. Nivitchanyong T, Tsai YC, Betenbaugh MJ, et al. An improved in vitro and in vivo Sindbis virus expression system through host and virus engineering. *Virus Res* 2009;141(1):1–12.
702. Noran HH. Chronic Equine Encephalitis. *Am J Pathol* 1944;20(2):259–267.
703. Noran HH, Baker AB. Sequels of equine encephalomyelitis. *Arch Neurol Psychiatr* 1943;49:398–413.
704. Noran HH, Baker AB. Western equine encephalitis—the pathogenesis of the pathological lesions. *J Neuropath Exper Neurol* 1945;4(3):269–276.
705. Noret M, Herrero L, Rulli N, et al. Interleukin 6, RANKL, and osteoprotegerin expression by chikungunya virus-infected human osteoblasts. *J Infect Dis* 2012;206(3):455–457; 457–459.
706. Oberste MS, Fraire M, Navarro R, et al. Association of Venezuelan equine encephalitis virus subtype IE with two equine epizootics in Mexico. *Am J Trop Med Hyg* 1998;59(1):100–107.
707. Oberste MS, Schmura SM, Weaver SC, et al. Geographic distribution of Venezuelan equine encephalitis virus subtype IE genotypes in Central America and Mexico. *Am J Trop Med Hyg* 1999;60(4):630–634.
708. O'Brien VA, Meteyer CU, Ip HS, et al. Pathology and virus detection in tissues of nestling house sparrows naturally infected with Buggy Creek virus (Togaviridae). *J Wildl Dis* 2010;46(1):23–32.
709. O'Brien VA, Moore AT, Young GR, et al. An enzootic vector-borne virus is amplified at epizootic levels by an invasive avian host. *Proc Biol Sci* 2011;278(1703):239–246.
710. Olaleye OD, Omilabu SA, Fagbami AH. Igbo-Ora virus (an alphavirus isolated in Nigeria): a serological survey for haemagglutination inhibiting antibody in humans and domestic animals. *Trans R Soc Trop Med Hyg* 1988;82(6):905–906.
711. Oldstone MB, Tishon A, Dutko FJ, et al. Does the major histocompatibility complex serve as a specific receptor for Semliki Forest virus? *J Virol* 1980;34(1):256–265.
712. Oliver KR, Fazakerley JK. Transneuronal spread of Semliki Forest virus in the developing mouse olfactory system is determined by neuronal maturity. *Neuroscience* 1998;82(3):867–877.
713. Oliver J, Lukacik G, Kokas J, et al. Twenty years of surveillance for Eastern equine encephalitis virus in mosquitoes in New York State from 1993 to 2012. *Parasit Vectors* 2018;11(1):362.
714. Oliver KR, Scallan MF, Dyson H, et al. Susceptibility to a neurotropic virus and its changing distribution in the developing brain is a function of CNS maturity. *J Neurovirol* 1997;3(1):38–48.
715. Olmsted RA, Meyer WJ, Johnston RE. Characterization of Sindbis virus epitopes important for penetration in cell culture and pathogenesis in animals. *Virology* 1986;148(2): 245–254.
716. Olson JG, Reeves WC, Emmons RW, et al. Correlation of Culex tarsalis population indices with the incidence of St. Louis encephalitis and western equine encephalomyelitis in California. *Am J Trop Med Hyg* 1979;28(2):335–343.
717. O'Neill K, Olson BJ, Huang N, et al. Rapid selection against arbovirus-induced apoptosis during infection of a mosquito vector. *Proc Natl Acad Sci U S A* 2015;112(10): E1152–E1161.
718. Ooi YS, Dube M, Kielian M. BST2/tetherin inhibition of alphavirus exit. *Viruses* 2015;7(4):2147–2167.
719. Ooi YS, Stiles KM, Liu CY, et al. Genome-wide RNAi screen identifies novel host proteins required for alphavirus entry. *PLoS Pathog* 2013;9(12):e1003835.
720. Orvedahl A, MacPherson S, Sumpter R, Jr., et al. Autophagy protects against Sindbis virus infection of the central nervous system. *Cell Host Microbe* 2010;7(2):115–127.
721. Orvedahl A, Sumpter R Jr, Xiao G, et al. Image-based genome-wide siRNA screen identifies selective autophagy factors. *Nature* 2011;480(7375):113–117.
722. Ovenden JR, Mahon RJ. Venereal transmission of Sindbis virus between individuals of Aedes australis (Diptera: Culicidae). *J Med Entomol* 1984;21(3):292–295.
723. Owen KE, Kuhn RJ. Identification of a region in the Sindbis virus nucleocapsid protein that is involved in specificity of RNA encapsidation. *J Virol* 1996;70(5):2757–2763.
724. Ozden S, Huerre M, Riviere JP, et al. Human muscle satellite cells as targets of Chikungunya virus infection. *PLoS One* 2007;2(6):e527.
725. Padhi A, Moore AT, Brown MB, et al. Phylogeographical structure and evolutionary history of two Buggy Creek virus lineages in the western Great Plains of North America. *J Gen Virol* 2008;89(Pt 9):2122–2131.
726. Paessler S, Aguilar P, Anishchenko M, et al. The hamster as an animal model for eastern equine encephalitis--and its use in studies of virus entrance into the brain. *J Infect Dis* 2004;189(11):2072–2076.
727. Paessler S, Rijnbrand R, Stein DA, et al. Inhibition of alphavirus infection in cell culture and in mice with antisense morpholino oligomers. *Virology* 2008;376(2):357–370.
728. Paessler S, Weaver SC. Vaccines for Venezuelan equine encephalitis. *Vaccine* 2009;27(Suppl 4):D80–D85.
729. Panday RS, Digoutte JP. Tonate and Guama-group viruses isolated from mosquitoes in both a savannah and coastal area in Surinam. *Trop Geogr Med* 1979;31(2):275–282.
730. Pandya J, Gorchakov R, Wang E, et al. A vaccine candidate for eastern equine encephalitis virus based on IRES-mediated attenuation. *Vaccine* 2012;30(7):1276–1282.
731. Park E, Griffin DE. Interaction of Sindbis virus non-structural protein 3 with poly (ADP-ribose) polymerase 1 in neuronal cells. *J Gen Virol* 2009;90(Pt 9):2073–2080.
732. Park E, Griffin DE. The nsP3 macro domain is important for Sindbis virus replication in neurons and neurovirulence in mice. *Virology* 2009;388(2):305–314.
733. Parker MD, Buckley MJ, Melanson VR, et al. Antibody to the E3 glycoprotein protects mice against lethal venezuelan equine encephalitis virus infection. *J Virol* 2010;84(24):12683–12690.
734. Parola P, de Lamballerie X, Jourdan J, et al. Novel chikungunya virus variant in travelers returning from Indian Ocean islands. *Emerg Infect Dis* 2006;12(10):1493–1499.
735. Parrott MM, Sitarski SA, Arnold RJ, et al. Role of conserved cysteines in the alphavirus E3 protein. *J Virol* 2009;83(6):2584–2591.
736. Pastorino B, Bessaud M, Grandadam M, et al. Development of a TaqMan RT-PCR assay without RNA extraction step for the detection and quantification of African Chikungunya viruses. *J Virol Methods* 2005;124(1–2):65–71.
737. Pastorino B, Muyembe-Tamfum JJ, Bessaud M, et al. Epidemic resurgence of Chikungunya virus in democratic Republic of the Congo: identification of a new central African strain. *J Med Virol* 2004;74(2):277–282.
738. Pathak S, Webb HE. Possible mechanisms for the transport of Semliki forest virus into and within mouse brain. An electron-microscopic study. *J Neurol Sci* 1974;23(2):175–184.
739. Pauvolid-Correa A, Tavares FN, Costa EV, et al. Serologic evidence of the recent circulation of Saint Louis encephalitis virus and high prevalence of equine encephalitis viruses in horses in the Nhecolandia sub-region in South Pantanal, Central-West Brazil. *Mem Inst Oswaldo Cruz* 2010;105(6):829–833.
740. Peng W, Peltier DC, Larsen MJ, et al. Identification of thieno[3,2-b] pyrrole derivatives as novel small molecule inhibitors of neurotropic alphaviruses. *J Infect Dis* 2009;199(7):950–957.
741. Peranen J, Rikkonen M, Liljestrom P, et al. Nuclear localization of Semliki forest virus-specific nonstructural protein nsP2. *J Virol* 1990;64(5):1888–1896.
742. Peranen J, Takkinen K, Kalkkinen N, et al. Semliki Forest virus-specific non-structural protein nsP3 is a phosphoprotein. *J Gen Virol* 1988;69(Pt 9):2165–2178.
743. Perri S, Driver DA, Gardner JP, et al. Replicon vectors derived from Sindbis virus and Semliki forest virus that establish persistent replication in host cells. *J Virol* 2000;74(20):9802–9807.
744. Petterson E, Sandberg M, Santi N. Salmonid alphavirus associated with Lepeophtheirus salmonis (Copepoda: Caligidae) from Atlantic salmon, *Salmo salar* L. *J Fish Dis* 2009;32(5):477–479.
745. Petterson E, Stormoen M, Evensen O, et al. Natural infection of Atlantic salmon (*Salmo salar* L.) with salmonid alphavirus 3 generates numerous viral deletion mutants. *J Gen Virol* 2013;94(Pt 9):1945–1954.
746. Pfeffer M, Foster JE, Edwards EA, et al. Phylogenetic analysis of Buggy Creek virus: evidence for multiple clades in the Western Great Plains, United States of America. *Appl Environ Microbiol* 2006;72(11):6886–6893.
747. Pfeffer M, Proebster B, Kinney RM, et al. Genus-specific detection of alphaviruses by a semi-nested reverse transcription-polymerase chain reaction. *Am J Trop Med Hyg* 1997;57(6):709–718.
748. Phillips DA, Murray JR, Aaskov JG, et al. Clinical and subclinical Barmah Forest virus infection in Queensland. *Med J Aust* 1990;152(9):463–466.
749. Phillips AT, Rico AB, Stauft CB, et al. Entry sites of Venezuelan and western equine encephalitis viruses in the mouse central nervous system following peripheral infection. *J Virol* 2016;90(12):5785–5796.
750. Phillips AT, Stauft CB, Aboellail TA, et al. Bioluminescent imaging and histopathologic characterization of WEEV neuroinvasion in outbred CD-1 mice. *PLoS One* 2013;8(1):e53462.
751. Pichlmair A, Lassnig C, Eberle CA, et al. IFIT1 is an antiviral protein that recognizes 5'-triphosphate RNA. *Nat Immunol* 2011;12(7):624–630.
752. Pichlmair A, Schulz O, Tan CP, et al. Activation of MDA5 requires higher-order RNA structures generated during virus infection. *J Virol* 2009;83(20):10761–10769.
753. Pierce JS, Strauss EG, Strauss JH. Effect of ionic strength on the binding of Sindbis virus to chick cells. *J Virol* 1974;13(5):1030–1036.
754. Pierro DJ, Powers EL, Olson KE. Genetic determinants of Sindbis virus mosquito infection are associated with a highly conserved alphavirus and flavivirus envelope sequence. *J Virol* 2008;82(6):2966–2974.
755. Pisano MB, Dantur MJ, Re VE, et al. Cocirculation of Rio Negro Virus (RNV) and Pixuna Virus (PIXV) in Tucuman province, Argentina. *Trop Med Int Health* 2010;15(7):865–868.
756. Pisano MB, Oria G, Beskow G, et al. Venezuelan equine encephalitis viruses (VEEV) in Argentina: serological evidence of human infection. *PLoS Negl Trop Dis* 2013;7(12):e2551.
757. Pisano MB, Re VE, Diaz LA, et al. Enzootic activity of pixuna and Rio Negro viruses (Venezuelan equine encephalitis complex) in a neotropical region of Argentina. *Vector Borne Zoonotic Dis* 2010;10(2):199–201.
758. Pittman PR, Liu CT, Cannon TL, et al. Immune interference after sequential alphavirus vaccine vaccinations. *Vaccine* 2009;27(36):4879–4882.
759. Pittman PR, Makuch RS, Mangiafico JA, et al. Long-term duration of detectable neutralizing antibodies after administration of live-attenuated VEE vaccine and following booster vaccination with inactivated VEE vaccine. *Vaccine* 1996;14(4):337–343.
760. Poddar S, Hyde JL, Gorman MJ, et al. The interferon-stimulated gene IFITM3 restricts infection and pathogenesis of arthritogenic and encephalitic alphaviruses. *J Virol* 2016;90(19):8780–8794.
761. Poidinger M, Roy S, Hall RA, et al. Genetic stability among temporally and geographically diverse isolates of Barmah Forest virus. *Am J Trop Med Hyg* 1997;57(2):230–234.
762. Poo YS, Rudd PA, Gardner J, et al. Multiple immune factors are involved in controlling acute and chronic chikungunya virus infection. *PLoS Negl Trop Dis* 2014;8(12):e3354.
763. Posey DL, O'Rourke T, Roehrig JT, et al. O'Nyong-nyong fever in West Africa. *Am J Trop Med Hyg* 2005;73(1):32.
764. Postic B, Schleupner CJ, Armstrong JA, et al. Two variants of Sindbis virus which differ in interferon induction and serum clearance. I. The phenomenon. *J Infect Dis* 1969;120(3):339–347.
765. Potter A, Johansen CA, Fenwick S, et al. The seroprevalence and factors associated with Ross River virus infection in western grey kangaroos (*Macropus fuliginosus*) in Western Australia. *Vector Borne Zoonotic Dis* 2014;14(10):740–745.
766. Powers AM, Aguilar PV, Chandler LJ, et al. Genetic relationships among Mayaro and Una viruses suggest distinct patterns of transmission. *Am J Trop Med Hyg* 2006;75(3): 461–469.
767. Powers AM, Brault AC, Kinney RM, et al. The use of chimeric Venezuelan equine encephalitis viruses as an approach for the molecular identification of natural virulence determinants. *J Virol* 2000;74(9):4258–4263.
768. Powers AM, Brault AC, Shirako Y, et al. Evolutionary relationships and systematics of the alphaviruses. *J Virol* 2001;75(21):10118–10131.

769. Powers AM, Brault AC, Tesh RB, et al. Re-emergence of Chikungunya and O'nyong-nyong viruses: evidence for distinct geographical lineages and distant evolutionary relationships. *J Gen Virol* 2000;81(Pt 2):471–479.

770. Powers AM, Logue CH. Changing patterns of chikungunya virus: re-emergence of a zoonotic arbovirus. *J Gen Virol* 2007;88(Pt 9):2363–2377.

771. Powers AM, Oberste MS, Brault AC, et al. Repeated emergence of epidemic/epizootic Venezuelan equine encephalitis from a single genotype of enzootic subtype ID virus. *J Virol* 1997;71(9):6697–6705.

772. Powers AM, Roehrig JT. Alphaviruses. *Methods Mol Biol* 2011;665:17–38.

773. Priya R, Patro IK, Parida MM. TLR3 mediated innate immune response in mice brain following infection with Chikungunya virus. *Virus Res* 2014;189:194–205.

774. Prow NA, Irani DN. The opioid receptor antagonist, naloxone, protects spinal motor neurons in a murine model of alphavirus encephalomyelitis. *Exp Neurol* 2007;205(2):461–470.

775. Prow NA, Tang B, Gardner J, et al. Lower temperatures reduce type I interferon activity and promote alphaviral arthritis. *PLoS Pathog* 2017;13(12):e1006788.

776. Przelomski MM, O'Rourke E, Grady GF, et al. Eastern equine encephalitis in Massachusetts: a report of 16 cases, 1970-1984. *Neurology* 1988;38(5):736–739.

777. Quetglas JI, Fioravanti J, Ardaiz N, et al. A Semliki forest virus vector engineered to express IFNalpha induces efficient elimination of established tumors. *Gene Ther* 2012;19(3):271–278.

778. Raghow RS, Grace TD, Filshie BK, et al. Ross River virus replication in cultured mosquito and mammalian cells: virus growth and correlated ultrastructural changes. *J Gen Virol* 1973;21:109–122.

779. Rainey SM, Martinez J, McFarlane M, et al. Wolbachia blocks viral genome replication early in infection without a transcriptional response by the endosymbiont or host small RNA pathways. *PLoS Pathog* 2016;12(4):e1005536.

780. Ramsey J, Mukhopadhyay S. Disentangling the frames, the state of research on the alphavirus 6K and TF proteins. *Viruses* 2017;9(8).

781. Rana J, Rajasekharan S, Gulati S, et al. Network mapping among the functional domains of Chikungunya virus nonstructural proteins. *Proteins* 2014;82(10):2403–2411.

782. Randall R, Maurer FD, Smadel JE. Immunization of laboratory workers with purified Venezuelan equine encephalomyelitis vaccine. *J Immunol* 1949;63(3):313–318.

783. Randall R, Mills JW. Fatal encephalitis in man due to the Venezuelan virus of equine encephalomyelitis in Trinidad. *Science* 1944;99(2568):225–226.

784. Randall R, Mills JW, Engel LL. The preparation and properties of a purified equine encephalomyelitis vaccine. *J Immunol* 1947;55(1):41–52.

785. Ratsitorahina M, Harisoa J, Ratovonjato J, et al. Outbreak of dengue and Chikungunya fevers, Toamasina, Madagascar, 2006. *Emerg Infect Dis* 2008;14(7):1135–1137.

786. Razumov IA, Khusainova AD, Agapov EV, et al. Analysis of the hemagglutination activity domains of the Venezuelan equine encephalomyelitis and eastern equine encephalomyelitis viruses. *Intervirology* 1994;37(6):356–360.

787. Reed DS, Glass PJ, Bakken RR, et al. Combined alphavirus replicon particle vaccine induces durable and cross-protective immune responses against equine encephalitis viruses. *J Virol* 2014;88(20):12077–12086.

788. Reed DS, Larsen T, Sullivan LJ, et al. Aerosol exposure to western equine encephalitis virus causes fever and encephalitis in cynomolgus macaques. *J Infect Dis* 2005;192(7):1173–1182.

789. Reed DS, Lind CM, Lackemeyer MG, et al. Genetically engineered, live, attenuated vaccines protect nonhuman primates against aerosol challenge with a virulent IE strain of Venezuelan equine encephalitis virus. *Vaccine* 2005;23(24):3139–3147.

790. Reed DS, Lind CM, Sullivan LJ, et al. Aerosol infection of cynomolgus macaques with enzootic strains of venezuelan equine encephalitis viruses. *J Infect Dis* 2004;189(6):1013–1017.

791. Reichert E, Clase A, Bacetty A, et al. Alphavirus antiviral drug development: scientific gap analysis and prospective research areas. *Biosecur Bioterror* 2009;7(4):413–427.

792. Reisen WK, Chiles RE. Prevalence of antibodies to western equine encephalomyelitis and St. Louis encephalitis viruses in residents of California exposed to sporadic and consistent enzootic transmission. *Am J Trop Med Hyg* 1997;57(5):526–529.

793. Reisen WK, Fang Y, Brault AC. Limited interdecadal variation in mosquito (Diptera: Culicidae) and avian host competence for Western equine encephalomyelitis virus (Togaviridae: Alphavirus). *Am J Trop Med Hyg* 2008;78(4):681–686.

794. Reisen WK, Hardy JL, Reeves WC, et al. Persistence of mosquito-borne viruses in Kern County, California, 1983-1988. *Am J Trop Med Hyg* 1990;43(4):419–437.

795. Reisen WK, Kramer LD, Chiles RE, et al. Simulated overwintering of encephalitis viruses in diapausing female Culex tarsalis (Diptera: Culicidae). *J Med Entomol* 2002;39(1):226–233.

796. Reisen WK, Lothrop HD, Hardy JL. Bionomics of Culex tarsalis (Diptera: Culicidae) in relation to arbovirus transmission in southeastern California. *J Med Entomol* 1995;32(3):316–327.

797. Reisen WK, Meyer RP, Presser SB, et al. Effect of temperature on the transmission of western equine encephalomyelitis and St. Louis encephalitis viruses by Culex tarsalis (Diptera: Culicidae). *J Med Entomol* 1993;30(1):151–160.

798. Reisen WK, Presser SB, Lin J, et al. Viremia and serological responses in adult chickens infected with western equine encephalomyelitis and St. Louis encephalitis viruses. *J Am Mosq Control Assoc* 1994;10(4):549–555.

799. Reisinger EC, Tschismarov R, Beubler E, et al. Immunogenicity, safety, and tolerability of the measles-vectored chikungunya virus vaccine MV-CHIK: a double-blind, randomised, placebo-controlled and active-controlled phase 2 trial. *Lancet* 2019;392(10165):2718–2727.

800. Reiter P, Fontenille D, Paupy C. Aedes albopictus as an epidemic vector of chikungunya virus: another emerging problem? *Lancet Infect Dis* 2006;6(8):463–464.

801. Renault P, Josseran L, Pierre V. Chikungunya-related fatality rates, Mauritius, India, and Reunion Island. *Emerg Infect Dis* 2008;14(8):1327.

802. Renault P, Solet JL, Sissoko D, et al. A major epidemic of chikungunya virus infection on Reunion Island, France, 2005-2006. *Am J Trop Med Hyg* 2007;77(4):727–731.

803. Reynaud JM, Kim DY, Atasheva S, et al. IFIT1 differentially interferes with translation and replication of alphavirus genomes and promotes induction of type I interferon. *PLoS Pathog* 2015;11(4):e1004863.

804. Rezza G. Chikungunya and West Nile virus outbreaks: what is happening in north-eastern Italy? *Eur J Public Health* 2009;19(3):236–237.

805. Rezza G, Chen R, Weaver SC. O'nyong-nyong fever: a neglected mosquito-borne viral disease. *Pathog Glob Health* 2017;111(6):271–275.

806. Rezza G, Weaver SC. Chikungunya as a paradigm for emerging viral diseases: Evaluating disease impact and hurdles to vaccine development. *PLoS Negl Trop Dis* 2019;13(1):e0006919.

807. Rico-Hesse R, Weaver SC, de Siger J, et al. Emergence of a new epidemic/epizootic Venezuelan equine encephalitis virus in South America. *Proc Natl Acad Sci U S A* 1995;92(12):5278–5281.

808. Rikkonen M. Functional significance of the nuclear-targeting and NTP-binding motifs of Semliki Forest virus nonstructural protein nsP2. *Virology* 1996;218(2):352–361.

809. Rikkonen M, Peranen J, Kaariainen L. ATPase and GTPase activities associated with Semliki Forest virus nonstructural protein nsP2. *J Virol* 1994;68(9):5804–5810.

810. Ritz N, Hufnagel M, Gerardin P. Chikungunya in children. *Pediatr Infect Dis J* 2015;34(7):789–791.

811. Rivas F, Diaz LA, Cardenas VM, et al. Epidemic Venezuelan equine encephalitis in La Guajira, Colombia, 1995. *J Infect Dis* 1997;175(4):828–832.

812. Robin S, Ramful D, Le Seach F, et al. Neurologic manifestations of pediatric chikungunya infection. *J Child Neurol* 2008;23(9):1028–1035.

813. Robinson MC. An epidemic of virus disease in Southern Province, Tanganyika Territory, in 1952-53. I. Clinical features. *Trans R Soc Trop Med Hyg* 1955;49(1):28–32.

814. Rodrigues Faria N, Lourenco J, Marques de Cerqueira E, et al. Epidemiology of chikungunya virus in Bahia, Brazil, 2014-2015. *PLoS Curr* 2016;8.

815. Roehrig JT, Day JW, Kinney RM. Antigenic analysis of the surface glycoproteins of a Venezuelan equine encephalomyelitis virus (TC-83) using monoclonal antibodies. *Virology* 1982;118(2):269–278.

816. Roehrig JT, Hunt AR, Chang GJ, et al. Identification of monoclonal antibodies capable of differentiating antigenic varieties of eastern equine encephalitis viruses. *Am J Trop Med Hyg* 1990;42(4):394–398.

817. Rose PP, Hanna SL, Spiridigliozzi A, et al. Natural resistance-associated macrophage protein is a cellular receptor for sindbis virus in both insect and mammalian hosts. *Cell Host Microbe* 2011;10(2):97–104.

818. Rosen A, Casciola-Rosen L, Ahearn J. Novel packages of viral and self-antigens are generated during apoptosis. *J Exp Med* 1995;181(4):1557–1561.

819. Rosen L, Gubler DJ, Bennett PH. Epidemic polyarthritis (Ross River) virus infection in the Cook Islands. *Am J Trop Med Hyg* 1981;30(6):1294–1302.

820. Rosenblum CI, Stollar V. SVMPA, a mutant of sindbis virus resistant to mycophenolic acid and ribavirin, shows an increased sensitivity to chick interferon. *Virology* 1999;259(1):228–233.

821. Ross RW. The Newala epidemic. III. The virus: isolation, pathogenic properties and relationship to the epidemic. *J Hyg* 1956;54(2):177–191.

822. Rossi SL, Russell-Lodrigue KE, Killeen SZ, et al. IRES-containing VEEV vaccine protects cynomolgus macaques from IE Venezuelan equine encephalitis virus aerosol challenge. *PLoS Negl Trop Dis* 2015;9(5):e0003797.

823. Rowell JF, Griffin DE. Contribution of T cells to mortality in neurovirulent Sindbis virus encephalomyelitis. *J Neuroimmunol* 2002;127(1–2):106–114.

824. Roy CJ, Reed DS, Wilhelmsen CL, et al. Pathogenesis of aerosolized Eastern Equine Encephalitis virus infection in guinea pigs. *Virol J* 2009;6:170.

825. Ruckert C, Weger-Lucarelli J, Garcia-Luna SM, et al. Impact of simultaneous exposure to arboviruses on infection and transmission by Aedes aegypti mosquitoes. *Nat Commun* 2017;8:15412.

826. Rudd PA, Wilson J, Gardner J, et al. Interferon response factors 3 and 7 protect against Chikungunya virus hemorrhagic fever and shock. *J Virol* 2012;86(18):9888–9898.

827. Rulli NE, Guglielmotti A, Mangano G, et al. Amelioration of alphavirus-induced arthritis and myositis in a mouse model by treatment with bindarit, an inhibitor of monocyte chemotactic proteins. *Arthritis Rheum* 2009;60(8):2513–2523.

828. Rulli NE, Rolph MS, Srikiatkhachorn A, et al. Protection from arthritis and myositis in a mouse model of acute chikungunya virus disease by bindarit, an inhibitor of monocyte chemotactic protein-1 synthesis. *J Infect Dis* 2011;204(7):1026–1030.

829. Rulli NE, Suhrbier A, Hueston L, et al. Ross River virus: molecular and cellular aspects of disease pathogenesis. *Pharmacol Ther* 2005;107(3):329–342.

830. Rumenapf T, Strauss EG, Strauss JH. Aura virus is a New World representative of Sindbis-like viruses. *Virology* 1995;208(2):621–633.

831. Ruotsalainen JJ, Kaikkonen MU, Niittykoski M, et al. Clonal variation in interferon response determines the outcome of oncolytic virotherapy in mouse CT26 colon carcinoma model. *Gene Ther* 2015;22(1):65–75.

832. Russell RC. Ross River virus: ecology and distribution. *Annu Rev Entomol* 2002;47:1–31.

833. Ryman KD, Klimstra WB. Host responses to alphavirus infection. *Immunol Rev* 2008;225:27–45.

834. Ryman KD, Klimstra WB, Nguyen KB, et al. Alpha/beta interferon protects adult mice from fatal Sindbis virus infection and is an important determinant of cell and tissue tropism. *J Virol* 2000;74(7):3366–3378.

835. Ryman KD, Meier KC, Gardner CL, et al. Non-pathogenic Sindbis virus causes hemorrhagic fever in the absence of alpha/beta and gamma interferons. *Virology* 2007;368(2):273–285.

836. Ryman KD, Meier KC, Nangle EM, et al. Sindbis virus translation is inhibited by a PKR/RNase L-independent effector induced by alpha/beta interferon priming of dendritic cells. *J Virol* 2005;79(3):1487–1499.

837. Ryman KD, White LJ, Johnston RE, et al. Effects of PKR/RNase L-dependent and alternative antiviral pathways on alphavirus replication and pathogenesis. *Viral Immunol* 2002;15(1):53–76.

838. Sabattini MS, Daffner JF, Monath TP, et al. Localized eastern equine encephalitis in Santiago del Estero Province, Argentina, without human infection. *Medicina (B Aires)* 1991;51(1):3–8.

839. Sabattini MS, Monath TP, Mitchell CJ, et al. Arbovirus investigations in Argentina, 1977-1980. I. Historical aspects and description of study sites. *Am J Trop Med Hyg* 1985;34(5):937–944.

840. Sabin AB. Hemagglutination by viruses affecting the human nervous system. *Fed Proc* 1951;10(2):573–578.
841. Sahu SP, Pedersen DD, Jenny AL, et al. Pathogenicity of a Venezuelan equine encephalomyelitis serotype IE virus isolate for ponies. *Am J Trop Med Hyg* 2003;68(4):485–494.
842. Saleh SM, Poidinger M, Mackenzie JS, et al. Complete genomic sequence of the Australian south-west genotype of Sindbis virus: comparisons with other Sindbis strains and identification of a unique deletion in the 3'-untranslated region. *Virus Genes* 2003;26(3):317–327.
843. Sammels LM, Coelen RJ, Lindsay MD, et al. Geographic distribution and evolution of Ross River virus in Australia and the Pacific Islands. *Virology* 1995;212(1):20–29.
844. Sammels LM, Lindsay MD, Poidinger M, et al. Geographic distribution and evolution of Sindbis virus in Australia. *J Gen Virol* 1999;80(Pt 3):739–748.
845. Samra JA, Hagood NL, Summer A, et al. clinical features and neurologic complications of children hospitalized with chikungunya virus in Honduras. *J Child Neurol* 2017;32(8):712–716.
846. Sanders EJ, Rwaguma EB, Kawamata J, et al. O'nyong-nyong fever in south-central Uganda, 1996-1997: description of the epidemic and results of a household-based seroprevalence survey. *J Infect Dis* 1999;180(5):1436–1443.
847. Sane J, Guedes S, Ollgren J, et al. Epidemic sindbis virus infection in Finland: a population-based case-control study of risk factors. *J Infect Dis* 2011;204(3):459–466.
848. Sane J, Kurkela S, Desdouits M, et al. Prolonged myalgia in Sindbis virus infection: case description and in vitro infection of myotubes and myoblasts. *J Infect Dis* 2012;206(3):407–414.
849. Sanmartin-Barberi C, Groot H, Osorno-Mesa E. Human epidemic in Colombia caused by the Venezuelan equine encephalomyelitis virus. *Am J Trop Med Hyg* 1954;3(2):283–293.
850. Santagati MG, Maatta JA, Roytta M, et al. The significance of the 3'-nontranslated region and E2 amino acid mutations in the virulence of Semliki Forest virus in mice. *Virology* 1998;243(1):66–77.
851. Sanz MA, Castello A, Ventoso I, et al. Dual mechanism for the translation of subgenomic mRNA from Sindbis virus in infected and uninfected cells. *PLoS One* 2009;4(3):e4772.
852. Sardelis MR, Dohm DJ, Pagac B, et al. Experimental transmission of eastern equine encephalitis virus by Ochlerotatus j. japonicus (Diptera: Culicidae). *J Med Entomol* 2002;39(3):480–484.
853. Sarid R, Ben-Moshe T, Kazimirsky G, et al. vFLIP protects PC-12 cells from apoptosis induced by Sindbis virus: implications for the role of TNF-alpha. *Cell Death Differ* 2001;8(12):1224–1231.
854. Sarver N, Stollar V. Sindbis virus-induced cytopathic effect in clones of *Aedes albopictus* (Singh) cells. *Virology* 1977;80(2):390–400.
855. Satriano SF, Luginbuhl RE, Wallis RC, et al. Investigation of eastern equine encephalomyelitis. IV. Susceptibility and transmission studies with virus of pheasant origin. *Am J Hyg* 1958;67(1):21–34.
856. Saul S, Ferguson M, Cordonin C, et al. Differences in Processing Determinants of Nonstructural Polyprotein and in the Sequence of Nonstructural Protein 3 Affect Neurovirulence of Semliki Forest Virus. *J Virol* 2015;89(21):11030–11045.
857. Sawicki D, Barkhimer DB, Sawicki SG, et al. Temperature sensitive shut-off of alphavirus minus strand RNA synthesis maps to a nonstructural protein, nsP4. *Virology* 1990;174(1):43–52.
858. Sawicki DL, Silverman RH, Williams BR, et al. Alphavirus minus-strand synthesis and persistence in mouse embryo fibroblasts derived from mice lacking RNase L and protein kinase R. *J Virol* 2003;77(3):1801–1811.
859. Saxton-Shaw KD, Ledermann JP, Borland EM, et al. O'nyong nyong virus molecular determinants of unique vector specificity reside in non-structural protein 3. *PLoS Negl Trop Dis* 2013;7(1):e1931.
860. Saxton-Shaw KD, Ledermann JP, Kenney JL, et al. The first outbreak of eastern equine encephalitis in Vermont: outbreak description and phylogenetic relationships of the virus isolate. *PLoS One* 2015;10(6):e0128712.
861. Scallan MF, Allsopp TE, Fazakerley JK. bcl-2 acts early to restrict Semliki Forest virus replication and delays virus-induced programmed cell death. *J Virol* 1997;71(2):1583–1590.
862. Scallan MF, Fazakerley JK. Aurothiolates enhance the replication of Semliki Forest virus in the CNS and the exocrine pancreas. *J Neurovirol* 1999;5(4):392–400.
863. Scherer WF, Anderson K. Antigenic and biologic characteristics of Venezuelan encephalitis virus strains including a possible new subtype, isolated from the Amazon region of Peru in 1971. *Am J Epidemiol* 1975;101(4):356–361.
864. Scherer WF, Campillo-Sainz C, de Mucha-Macias J, et al. Ecologic studies of Venezuelan encephalitis virus in southeastern Mexico. VII. Infection of man. *Am J Trop Med Hyg* 1972;21(2):79–85.
865. Schilte C, Buckwalter MR, Laird ME, et al. Cutting edge: independent roles for IRF-3 and IRF-7 in hematopoietic and nonhematopoietic cells during host response to Chikungunya infection. *J Immunol* 2012;188(7):2967–2971.
866. Schilte C, Couderc T, Chretien F, et al. Type I IFN controls chikungunya virus via its action on nonhematopoietic cells. *J Exp Med* 2010;207(2):429–442.
867. Schilte C, Staikowsky F, Couderc T, et al. Chikungunya virus-associated long-term arthralgia: a 36-month prospective longitudinal study. *PLoS Negl Trop Dis* 2013;7(3):e2137.
868. Schmaljohn AL, Kokubun KM, Cole GA. Protective monoclonal antibodies define maturational and pH-dependent antigenic changes in Sindbis virus E1 glycoprotein. *Virology* 1983;130(1):144–154.
869. Schoepp RJ, Johnston RE. Directed mutagenesis of a Sindbis virus pathogenesis site. *Virology* 1993;193(1):149–159.
870. Schuffenecker I, Iteman I, Michault A, et al. Genome microevolution of chikungunya viruses causing the Indian Ocean outbreak. *PLoS Med* 2006;3(7):e263.
871. Schultz KLW, Troisi EM, Baxter VK, et al. Interferon regulatory factors 3 and 7 have distinct roles in the pathogenesis of alphavirus encephalomyelitis. *J Gen Virol* 2019;100(1):46–62.
872. Schultz KL, Vernon PS, Griffin DE. Differentiation of neurons restricts Arbovirus replication and increases expression of the alpha isoform of IRF-7. *J Virol* 2015;89(1):48–60.
873. Schulz O, Pichlmair A, Rehwinkel J, et al. Protein kinase R contributes to immunity against specific viruses by regulating interferon mRNA integrity. *Cell Host Microbe* 2010;7(5):354–361.
874. Scott TW, Hildreth SW, Beaty BJ. The distribution and development of eastern equine encephalitis virus in its enzootic mosquito vector, *Culiseta melanura*. *Am J Trop Med Hyg* 1984;33(2):300–310.
875. Scott TW, Lorenz LH. Reduction of Culiseta melanura fitness by eastern equine encephalomyelitis virus. *Am J Trop Med Hyg* 1998;59(2):341–346.
876. Scott TW, Weaver SC. Eastern equine encephalomyelitis virus: epidemiology and evolution of mosquito transmission. *Adv Virus Res* 1989;37:277–328.
877. Seabaugh RC, Olson KE, Higgs S, et al. Development of a chimeric sindbis virus with enhanced per Os infection of *Aedes aegypti*. *Virology* 1998;243(1):99–112.
878. Seamer JH, Boulter EA, Zlotnik I. Delayed onset of encephalitis in mice passively immunised against Semliki Forest virus. *Br J Exp Pathol* 1971;52(4):408–414.
879. Seay AR, Griffin DE, Johnson RT. Experimental viral polymyositis: age dependency and immune responses to Ross River virus infection in mice. *Neurology* 1981;31(6):656–660.
880. Seay AR, Kern ER, Murray RS. Interferon treatment of experimental Ross River virus polymyositis. *Neurology* 1987;37(7):1189–1193.
881. Seay AR, Wolinsky JS. Ross River virus-induced demyelination: I. Pathogenesis and histopathology. *Ann Neurol* 1982;12(4):380–389.
882. Sellers RF, Maarouf AR. Trajectory analysis of winds and eastern equine encephalitis in USA, 1980-5. *Epidemiol Infect* 1990;104(2):329–343.
883. Sentsui H, Kono Y. An epidemic of Getah virus infection among racehorses: isolation of the virus. *Res Vet Sci* 1980;29(2):157–161.
884. Seo JY, Yaneva R, Cresswell P. Viperin: a multifunctional, interferon-inducible protein that regulates virus replication. *Cell Host Microbe* 2011;10(6):534–539.
885. Seymour RL, Rossi SL, Bergren NA, et al. The role of innate versus adaptive immune responses in a mouse model of O'nyong-nyong virus infection. *Am J Trop Med Hyg* 2013;88(6):1170–1179.
886. Shabman RS, Morrison TE, Moore C, et al. Differential induction of type I interferon responses in myeloid dendritic cells by mosquito and mammalian-cell-derived alphaviruses. *J Virol* 2007;81(1):237–247.
887. Shabman RS, Rogers KM, Heise MT. Ross River virus envelope glycans contribute to type I interferon production in myeloid dendritic cells. *J Virol* 2008;82(24):12374–12383.
888. Shang G, Seed CR, Gahan ME, et al. Duration of Ross River viraemia in a mouse model--implications for transfusion transmission. *Vox Sang* 2012;102(3):185–192.
889. Sharma A, Knollmann-Ritschel B. Current understanding of the molecular basis of venezuelan equine encephalitis virus pathogenesis and vaccine development. *Viruses* 2019;11(2).
890. Sherman LA, Griffin DE. Pathogenesis of encephalitis induced in newborn mice by virulent and avirulent strains of Sindbis virus. *J Virol* 1990;64(5):2041–2046.
891. Sherman MB, Weaver SC. Structure of the recombinant alphavirus Western equine encephalitis virus revealed by cryoelectron microscopy. *J Virol* 2010;84(19):9775–9782.
892. Shinefield HR, Townsend TE. Transplacental transmission of western equine encephalomyelitis. *J Pediatr* 1953;43(1):21–25.
893. Shirako Y, Niklasson B, Dalrymple JM, et al. Structure of the Ockelbo virus genome and its relationship to other Sindbis viruses. *Virology* 1991;182(2):753–764.
894. Shope RE, Causey OR, De Andrade AH. The Venezuelan equine encephalomyelitis complex of group a arthropod-borne viruses, including Mucambo and Pixuna from the Amazon region of Brazil. *Am J Trop Med Hyg* 1964;13:723–727.
895. Shope RE, de Andrade AH, Bensabath G, et al. The epidemiology of EEE WEE, SLE and Turlock viruses, with special reference to birds, in a tropical rain forest near Belem, Brazil. *Am J Epidemiol* 1966;84(3):467–477.
896. Shore H. O'nyong-nyong fever: an epidemic virus disease in East Africa. I. Some clinical and epidemiological observations in the Northern province of Uganda. *Trans R Soc Trop Med Hyg* 1961;55:361–373.
897. Sidwell RW, Smee DF. Viruses of the Bunya- and Togaviridae families: potential as bioterrorism agents and means of control. *Antiviral Res* 2003;57(1–2):101–111.
898. Sieczkarski SB, Whittaker GR. Differential requirements of Rab5 and Rab7 for endocytosis of influenza and other enveloped viruses. *Traffic* 2003;4(5):333–343.
899. Siegal FP, Kadowaki N, Shodell M, et al. The nature of the principal type 1 interferon-producing cells in human blood. *Science* 1999;284(5421):1835–1837.
900. Sigei F, Nindo F, Mukunzi S, et al. Evolutionary analyses of Sindbis virus strains isolated from mosquitoes in Kenya. *Arch Virol* 2018;163(9):2465–2469.
901. Silverman RH. Viral encounters with 2',5'-oligoadenylate synthetase and RNase L during the interferon antiviral response. *J Virol* 2007;81(23):12720–12729.
902. Silverman MA, Misasi J, Smole S, et al. Eastern equine encephalitis in children, Massachusetts and New Hampshire, USA, 1970–2010. *Emerg Infect Dis* 2013;19(2):194–201; quiz 352.
903. Sim C, Hong YS, Tsetsarkin KA, et al. *Anopheles gambiae* heat shock protein cognate 70B impedes o'nyong-nyong virus replication. *BMC Genomics* 2007;8:231.
904. Sim C, Hong YS, Vanlandingham DL, et al. Modulation of *Anopheles gambiae* gene expression in response to o'nyong-nyong virus infection. *Insect Mol Biol* 2005;14(5):475–481.
905. Simmons JD, White LJ, Morrison TE, et al. Venezuelan equine encephalitis virus disrupts STAT1 signaling by distinct mechanisms independent of host shutoff. *J Virol* 2009;83(20):10571–10581.
906. Simmons JD, Wollish AC, Heise MT. A determinant of Sindbis virus neurovirulence enables efficient disruption of Jak/STAT signaling. *J Virol* 2010;84(21):11429–11439.
907. Simpson DI, Smith CE, Marshall TF, et al. Arbovirus infections in Sarawak: the role of the domestic pig. *Trans R Soc Trop Med Hyg* 1976;70(1):66–72.
908. Sissoko D, Ezzedine K, Moendandze A, et al. Field evaluation of clinical features during chikungunya outbreak in Mayotte, 2005-2006. *Trop Med Int Health* 2010;15(5):600–607.
909. Sissoko D, Moendandze A, Malvy D, et al. Seroprevalence and risk factors of chikungunya virus infection in Mayotte, Indian Ocean, 2005-2006: a population-based survey. *PLoS One* 2008;3(8):e3066.
910. Siu RW, Fragkoudis R, Simmonds P, et al. Antiviral RNA interference responses induced by Semliki Forest virus infection of mosquito cells: characterization, origin, and frequency-dependent functions of virus derived small interfering RNAs. *J Virol* 2011;85(6):2907–2917.

911. Sjoberg M, Lindqvist B, Garoff H. Activation of the alphavirus spike protein is suppressed by bound E3. *J Virol* 2011;85(11):5644–5650.

912. Skabkin MA, Skabkina OV, Dhote V, et al. Activities of Ligatin and MCT-1/DENR in eukaryotic translation initiation and ribosomal recycling. *Genes Dev* 2010;24(16):1787–1801.

913. Smit JM, Bittman R, Wilschut J. Low-pH-dependent fusion of Sindbis virus with receptor-free cholesterol- and sphingolipid-containing liposomes. *J Virol* 1999;73(10):8476–8484.

914. Smith TJ, Cheng RH, Olson NH, et al. Putative receptor binding sites on alphaviruses as visualized by cryoelectron microscopy. *Proc Natl Acad Sci U S A* 1995;92(23):10648–10652.

915. Smith GC, Francy DB. Laboratory studies of a Brazilian strain of *Aedes albopictus* as a potential vector of Mayaro and Oropouche viruses. *J Am Mosq Control Assoc* 1991;7(1):89–93.

916. Smith JP, Morris-Downes M, Brennan FR, et al. A role for alpha4-integrin in the pathology following Semliki Forest virus infection. *J Neuroimmunol* 2000;106(1–2):60–68.

917. Smith SA, Silva LA, Fox JM, et al. Isolation and characterization of broad and ultrapotent human monoclonal antibodies with therapeutic activity against chikungunya virus. *Cell Host Microbe* 2015;18(1):86–95.

918. Smithburn KC, Haddow AJ. Semliki Forest virus I. Isolation and pathogenic properties. *J Immunol* 1944;49(3):141–157.

919. Smyth JM, Sheahan BJ, Atkins GJ. Multiplication of virulent and demyelinating Semliki Forest virus in the mouse central nervous system: consequences in BALB/c and SJL mice. *J Gen Virol* 1990;71(Pt 11):2575–2583.

920. Snow M. The contribution of molecular epidemiology to the understanding and control of viral diseases of salmonid aquaculture. *Vet Res* 2011;42:56.

921. Snow M, Black J, Matejusova I, et al. Detection of salmonid alphavirus RNA in wild marine fish: implications for the origins of salmon pancreas disease in aquaculture. *Dis Aquat Organ* 2010;91(3):177–188.

922. Snyder JE, Berrios CJ, Edwards TJ, et al. Probing the early temporal and spatial interaction of the Sindbis virus capsid and E2 proteins with reverse genetics. *J Virol* 2012;86(22):12372–12383.

923. Snyder JE, Kulcsar KA, Schultz KL, et al. Functional characterization of the alphavirus TF protein. *J Virol* 2013;87(15):8511–8523.

924. Soden M, Vasudevan H, Roberts B, et al. Detection of viral ribonucleic acid and histologic analysis of inflamed synovium in Ross River virus infection. *Arthritis Rheum* 2000;43(2):365–369.

925. Soilu-Hanninen M, Eralinna JP, Hukkanen V, et al. Semliki Forest virus infects mouse brain endothelial cells and causes blood-brain barrier damage. *J Virol* 1994;68(10):6291–6298.

926. Soilu-Hanninen M, Roytta M, Salmi AA, et al. Semliki Forest virus infection leads to increased expression of adhesion molecules on splenic T-cells and on brain vascular endothelium. *J Neurovirol* 1997;3(5):350–360.

927. Sokoloski KJ, Nease LM, May NA, et al. Identification of interactions between Sindbis virus capsid protein and cytoplasmic vRNA as novel virulence determinants. *PLoS Pathog* 2017;13(6):e1006473.

928. Somekh E, Glode MP, Reiley TT, et al. Multiple intracranial calcifications after western equine encephalitis. *Pediatr Infect Dis J* 1991;10(5):408–409.

929. Soumahoro MK, Gerardin P, Boelle PY, et al. Impact of Chikungunya virus infection on health status and quality of life: a retrospective cohort study. *PLoS One* 2009;4(11):e7800.

930. Sourisseau M, Schilte C, Casartelli N, et al. Characterization of reemerging chikungunya virus. *PLoS Pathog* 2007;3(6):e89.

931. Sousa IP Jr, Carvalho CAM, Mendes YS, et al. Fusion of a new world alphavirus with membrane microdomains involving partially reversible conformational changes in the viral spike proteins. *Biochemistry* 2017;56(43):5823–5830.

932. Sousa IP, Jr., Carvalho CA, Ferreira DF, et al. Envelope lipid-packing as a critical factor for the biological activity and stability of alphavirus particles isolated from mammalian and mosquito cells. *J Biol Chem* 2011;286(3):1730–1736.

933. Spertzel RO, Crabbs CL, Vaughn RE. Transplacental transmission of Venezuelan equine encephalomyelitis virus in mice. *Infect Immun* 1972;6(3):339–343.

934. Spotts DR, Reich RM, Kalkhan MA, et al. Resistance to alpha/beta interferons correlates with the epizootic and virulence potential of Venezuelan equine encephalitis viruses and is determined by the 5' noncoding region and glycoproteins. *J Virol* 1998;72(12):10286–10291.

935. Stanley J, Cooper SJ, Griffin DE. Monoclonal antibody cure and prophylaxis of lethal Sindbis virus encephalitis in mice. *J Virol* 1986;58(1):107–115.

936. Stec DS, Waddell A, Schmaljohn CS, et al. Antibody-selected variation and reversion in Sindbis virus neutralization epitopes. *J Virol* 1986;57(3):715–720.

937. Steele KE, Davis KJ, Stephan K, et al. Comparative neurovirulence and tissue tropism of wild-type and attenuated strains of Venezuelan equine encephalitis virus administered by aerosol in C3H/HeN and BALB/c mice. *Vet Pathol* 1998;35(5):386–397.

938. Steele KE, Twenhafel NA. REVIEW PAPER: pathology of animal models of alphavirus encephalitis. *Vet Pathol* 2010;47(5):790–805.

939. Stephenson EB, Peel AJ, Reid SA, et al. The non-human reservoirs of Ross River virus: a systematic review of the evidence. *Parasit Vectors* 2018;11(1):188.

940. Stevens TM. Arbovirus replication in mosquito cell lines (Singh) grown in monolayer or suspension culture. *Proc Soc Exp Biol Med* 1970;134(1):356–361.

941. Stollar V, Shenk TE. Homologous viral interference in *Aedes albopictus* cultures chronically infected with Sindbis virus. *J Virol* 1973;11(4):592–595.

942. Stollar V, Shenk TE, Koo R, et al. Observations of *Aedes albopictus* cell cultures persistently infected with Sindbis virus. *Ann N Y Acad Sci* 1975;266:214–231.

943. Storm N, Weyer J, Markotter W, et al. Human cases of Sindbis fever in South Africa, 2006-2010. *Epidemiol Infect* 2014;142(2):234–238.

944. Strauss JH, Strauss EG. The alphaviruses: gene expression, replication, and evolution. *Microbiol Rev* 1994;58(3):491–562.

945. Strizki JM, Repik PM. Differential reactivity of immune sera from human vaccinees with field strains of eastern equine encephalitis virus. *Am J Trop Med Hyg* 1995;53(5):564–570.

946. Subak-Sharpe I, Dyson H, Fazakerley J. In vivo depletion of CD8+ T cells prevents lesions of demyelination in Semliki Forest virus infection. *J Virol* 1993;67(12):7629–7633.

947. Suckling AJ, Jagelman S, Illavia SJ, et al. The effect of mouse strain on the pathogenesis of the encephalitis and demyelination induced by avirulent Semliki Forest virus infections. *Br J Exp Pathol* 1980;61(3):281–284.

948. Suckling AJ, Pathak S, Jagelman S, et al. Virus-associated demyelination. A model using avirulent Semliki Forest virus infection of mice. *J Neurol Sci* 1978;39(1):147–154.

949. Sudia WD, Newhouse VF. Epidemic Venezuelan equine encephalitis in North America: a summary of virus-vector-host relationships. *Am J Epidemiol* 1975;101(1):1–13.

950. Suhrbier A, La Linn M. Clinical and pathologic aspects of arthritis due to Ross River virus and other alphaviruses. *Curr Opin Rheumatol* 2004;16(4):374–379.

951. Sumpter R, Jr., Levine B. Autophagy and innate immunity: triggering, targeting and tuning. *Semin Cell Dev Biol* 2010;21(7):699–711.

952. Sumpter R, Jr., Sirasanagandla S, Fernandez AF, et al. Fanconi anemia proteins function in mitophagy and immunity. *Cell* 2016;165(4):867–881.

953. Suthar MS, Shabman R, Madric K, et al. Identification of adult mouse neurovirulence determinants of the Sindbis virus strain AR86. *J Virol* 2005;79(7):4219–4228.

954. Swayze RD, Bhogal HS, Barabe ND, et al. Envelope protein E1 as vaccine target for western equine encephalitis virus. *Vaccine* 2011;29(4):813–820.

955. Takemoto KK. Plaque mutants of animal viruses. *Prog Med Virol* 1966;8:314–348.

956. Talarmin A, Trochu J, Gardon J, et al. Tonate virus infection in French Guiana: clinical aspects and seroepidemiologic study. *Am J Trop Med Hyg* 2001;64(5–6):274–279.

957. Tamm K, Merits A, Sarand I. Mutations in the nuclear localization signal of nsP2 influencing RNA synthesis, protein expression and cytotoxicity of Semliki Forest virus. *J Gen Virol* 2008;89(Pt 3):676–686.

958. Tan Y, Tsan-Yuk Lam T, Heberlein-Larson LA, et al. Large scale complete genome sequencing and phylodynamic analysis of eastern equine encephalitis virus reveal source-sink transmission dynamics in the United States. *J Virol* 2018;92(12).

959. Tandale BV, Sathe PS, Arankalle VA, et al. Systemic involvements and fatalities during Chikungunya epidemic in India, 2006. *J Clin Virol* 2009;46(2):145–149.

960. Tang J, Jose J, Chipman P, et al. Molecular links between the E2 envelope glycoprotein and nucleocapsid core in Sindbis virus. *J Mol Biol* 2011;414(3):442–459.

961. Tappe D, Kapaun A, Emmerich P, et al. O'nyong-nyong virus infection imported to Europe from Kenya by a traveler. *Emerg Infect Dis* 2014;20(10):1766–1767.

962. Tarbatt CJ, Glasgow GM, Mooney DA, et al. Sequence analysis of the avirulent, demyelinating A7 strain of Semliki Forest virus. *J Gen Virol* 1997;78(Pt 7):1551–1557.

963. Tate CM, Howerth EW, Stallknecht DE, et al. Eastern equine encephalitis in a free-ranging white-tailed deer (Odocoileus virginianus). *J Wildl Dis* 2005;41(1):241–245.

964. Taylor RM, Hurlbut HS, Work TH, et al. Sindbis virus: a newly recognized arthropod-transmitted virus. *Am J Trop Med Hyg* 1955;4(5):844–862.

965. Taylor WP, Marshall ID. Adaptation studies with Ross River virus: laboratory mice and cell cultures. *J Gen Virol* 1975;28(1):59–72.

966. Telles JN, Le Roux K, Grivard P, et al. Evaluation of real-time nucleic acid sequence-based amplification for detection of Chikungunya virus in clinical samples. *J Med Microbiol* 2009;58(Pt 9):1168–1172.

967. Tenbroeck C, Hurst EW, Traub E. Epidemiology of equine encephalomyelitis in the eastern United States. *J Exp Med* 1935;62(5):677–685.

968. Teng TS, Foo SS, Simamarta D, et al. Viperin restricts chikungunya virus replication and pathology. *J Clin Invest* 2012;122(12):4447–4460.

969. Teng TS, Kam YW, Lee B, et al. A systematic meta-analysis of immune signatures in patients with acute chikungunya virus infection. *J Infect Dis* 2015;211(12):1925–1935.

970. Teo TH, Lum FM, Claser C, et al. A pathogenic role for CD4+ T cells during Chikungunya virus infection in mice. *J Immunol* 2013;190(1):259–269.

971. Tesfay MZ, Yin J, Gardner CL, et al. Alpha/beta interferon inhibits cap-dependent translation of viral but not cellular mRNA by a PKR-independent mechanism. *J Virol* 2008;82(6):2620–2630.

972. Tesh RB. Arthritides caused by mosquito-borne viruses. *Annu Rev Med* 1982;33:31–40.

973. Tesh RB, Gubler DJ, Rosen L. Variation among geographic strains of *Aedes albopictus* in susceptibility to infection with chikungunya virus. *Am J Trop Med Hyg* 1976;25(2):326–335.

974. Tesh RB, McLean RG, Shroyer DA, et al. Ross River virus (Togaviridae: Alphavirus) infection (epidemic polyarthritis) in American Samoa. *Trans R Soc Trop Med Hyg* 1981;75(3):426–431.

975. Tesh RB, Watts DM, Russell KL, et al. Mayaro virus disease: an emerging mosquito-borne zoonosis in tropical South America. *Clin Infect Dis* 1999;28(1):67–73.

976. Thach DC, Kimura T, Griffin DE. Differences between C57BL/6 and BALB/cBy mice in mortality and virus replication after intranasal infection with neuroadapted Sindbis virus. *J Virol* 2000;74(13):6156–6161.

977. Thach DC, Kleeberger SR, Tucker PC, et al. Genetic control of neuroadapted sindbis virus replication in female mice maps to chromosome 2 and associates with paralysis and mortality. *J Virol* 2001;75(18):8674–8680.

978. Thangamani S, Higgs S, Ziegler S, et al. Host immune response to mosquito-transmitted chikungunya virus differs from that elicited by needle inoculated virus. *PLoS One* 2010;5(8):e12137.

979. Thavara U, Tawatsin A, Pengsakul T, et al. Outbreak of chikungunya fever in Thailand and virus detection in field population of vector mosquitoes, *Aedes aegypti* (L.) and *Aedes albopictus* Skuse (Diptera: Culicidae). *Southeast Asian J Trop Med Public Health* 2009;40(5):951–962.

980. Tiwari M, Parida M, Santhosh SR, et al. Assessment of immunogenic potential of Vero adapted formalin inactivated vaccine derived from novel ECSA genotype of Chikungunya virus. *Vaccine* 2009;27(18):2513–2522.

981. Tomerini DM, Dale PE, Sipe N. Does mosquito control have an effect on mosquito-borne disease? The case of Ross River virus disease and mosquito management in Queensland, Australia. *J Am Mosq Control Assoc* 2011;27(1):39–44.

982. Tomori O, Monath TP, O'Connor EH, et al. Arbovirus infections among laboratory personnel in Ibadan, Nigeria. *Am J Trop Med Hyg* 1981;30(4):855–861.

983. Tong S, Dale P, Nicholls N, et al. Climate variability, social and environmental factors, and Ross River virus transmission: research development and future research needs. *Environ Health Perspect* 2008;116(12):1591–1597.

984. Tong S, Hayes JF, Dale P. Spatiotemporal variation of notified Barmah Forest virus infections in Queensland, Australia, 1993–2001. *Int J Environ Health Res* 2005;15(2):89–98.

985. Tooker P, Kennedy SI. Semliki Forest virus multiplication in clones of *Aedes albopictus* cells. *J Virol* 1981;37(2):589–600.

986. Toribio R, Ventoso I. Inhibition of host translation by virus infection in vivo. *Proc Natl Acad Sci U S A* 2010;107(21):9837–9842.

987. Torii S, Orba Y, Hang'ombe BM, et al. Discovery of Mwinilunga alphavirus: a novel alphavirus in Culex mosquitoes in Zambia. *Virus Res* 2018;250:31–36.

988. Torres JR, Cordova LG, Saravia V, et al. Nasal skin necrosis: an unexpected new finding in severe chikungunya fever. *Clin Infect Dis* 2016;62(1):78–81.

989. Torres JR, Falleiros-Arlant LH, Duenas L, et al. Congenital and perinatal complications of chikungunya fever: a Latin American experience. *Int J Infect Dis* 2016;51:85–88.

990. Torres JR, Russell KL, Vasquez C, et al. Family cluster of Mayaro fever, Venezuela. *Emerg Infect Dis* 2004;10(7):1304–1306.

991. Travassos da Rosa AP, Turell MJ, Watts DM, et al. Trocara virus: a newly recognized Alphavirus (Togaviridae) isolated from mosquitoes in the Amazon Basin. *Am J Trop Med Hyg* 2001;64(1–2):93–97.

992. Trgovcich J, Aronson JF, Eldridge JC, et al. TNFalpha, interferon, and stress response induction as a function of age-related susceptibility to fatal Sindbis virus infection of mice. *Virology* 1999;263(2):339–348.

993. Trobaugh DW, Gardner CL, Sun C, et al. RNA viruses can hijack vertebrate microRNAs to suppress innate immunity. *Nature* 2014;506(7487):245–248.

994. Trobaugh DW, Sun C, Dunn MD, et al. Rational design of a live-attenuated eastern equine encephalitis virus vaccine through informed mutation of virulence determinants. *PLoS Pathog* 2019;15(2):e1007584.

995. Tseng JC, Levin B, Hurtado A, et al. Systemic tumor targeting and killing by Sindbis viral vectors. *Nat Biotechnol* 2004;22(1):70–77.

996. Tseng JC, Zheng Y, Yee H, et al. Restricted tissue tropism and acquired resistance to Sindbis viral vector expression in the absence of innate and adaptive immunity. *Gene Ther* 2007;14(15):1166–1174.

997. Tsetsarkin KA, Chen R, Sherman MB, et al. Chikungunya virus: evolution and genetic determinants of emergence. *Curr Opin Virol* 2011;1(4):310–317.

998. Tsetsarkin KA, Chen R, Weaver SC. Interspecies transmission and chikungunya virus emergence. *Curr Opin Virol* 2016;16:143–150.

999. Tsetsarkin KA, Chen R, Yun R, et al. Multi-peaked adaptive landscape for chikungunya virus evolution predicts continued fitness optimization in *Aedes albopictus* mosquitoes. *Nat Commun* 2014;5:4084.

1000. Tsetsarkin KA, McGee CE, Higgs S. Chikungunya virus adaptation to *Aedes albopictus* mosquitoes does not correlate with acquisition of cholesterol dependence or decreased pH threshold for fusion reaction. *Virol J* 2011;8:376.

1001. Tsetsarkin KA, McGee CE, Volk SM, et al. Epistatic roles of E2 glycoprotein mutations in adaption of chikungunya virus to *Aedes albopictus* and *Ae. aegypti* mosquitoes. *PLoS One* 2009;4(8):e6835.

1002. Tucker PC, Griffin DE, Choi S, et al. Inhibition of nitric oxide synthesis increases mortality in Sindbis virus encephalitis. *J Virol* 1996;70(6):3972–3977.

1003. Tucker PC, Strauss EG, Kuhn RJ, et al. Viral determinants of age-dependent virulence of Sindbis virus for mice. *J Virol* 1993;67(8):4605–4610.

1004. Turell MJ. Effect of environmental temperature on the vector competence of Aedes taeniorhynchus for Rift Valley fever and Venezuelan equine encephalitis viruses. *Am J Trop Med Hyg* 1993;49(6):672–676.

1005. Turell MJ, Lundstrom JO, Niklasson B. Transmission of Ockelbo virus by *Aedes cinereus*, Ae. communis, and Ae. excrucians (Diptera: Culicidae) collected in an enzootic area in central Sweden. *J Med Entomol* 1990;27(3):266–268.

1006. Turell MJ, O'Guinn ML, Jones JW, et al. Isolation of viruses from mosquitoes (Diptera: Culicidae) collected in the Amazon Basin region of Peru. *J Med Entomol* 2005;42(5):891–898.

1007. Turell MJ, Tammariello RF, Spielman A. Nonvascular delivery of St. Louis encephalitis and Venezuelan equine encephalitis viruses by infected mosquitoes (Diptera: Culicidae) feeding on a vertebrate host. *J Med Entomol* 1995;32(4):563–568.

1008. Turunen M, Kuusisto P, Uggeldahl PE, et al. Pogosta disease: clinical observations during an outbreak in the province of North Karelia, Finland. *Br J Rheumatol* 1998;37(11):1177–1180.

1009. Tyor WR, Wesselingh S, Levine B, et al. Long term intraparenchymal Ig secretion after acute viral encephalitis in mice. *J Immunol* 1992;149(12):4016–4020.

1010. Tyzzer EE, Sellards AW. The pathology of equine encephalomyelitis in young chickens. *Am J Hyg* 1941;33(1/3):69–81.

1011. Ubol S, Levine B, Lee SH, et al. Roles of immunoglobulin valency and the heavy-chain constant domain in antibody-mediated downregulation of Sindbis virus replication in persistently infected neurons. *J Virol* 1995;69(3):1990–1993.

1012. Ubol S, Park S, Budihardjo I, et al. Temporal changes in chromatin, intracellular calcium, and poly (ADP-ribose) polymerase during Sindbis virus-induced apoptosis of neuroblastoma cells. *J Virol* 1996;70(4):2215–2220.

1013. Ubol S, Tucker PC, Griffin DE, et al. Neurovirulent strains of Alphavirus induce apoptosis in bcl-2-expressing cells: role of a single amino acid change in the E2 glycoprotein. *Proc Natl Acad Sci U S A* 1994;91(11):5202–5206.

1014. Uchime O, Fields W, Kielian M. The role of E3 in pH protection during alphavirus assembly and exit. *J Virol* 2013;87(18):10255–10262.

1015. Ulug ET, Garry RF, Bose HR Jr. The role of monovalent cation transport in Sindbis virus maturation and release. *Virology* 1989;172(1):42–50.

1016. Urban C, Rheme C, Maerz S, et al. Apoptosis induced by Semliki Forest virus is RNA replication dependent and mediated via Bak. *Cell Death Differ* 2008;15(9):1396–1407.

1017. Vaananen P, Kaariainen L. Fusion and haemolysis of erythrocytes caused by three togaviruses: Semliki Forest, Sindbis and rubella. *J Gen Virol* 1980;46(2):467–475.

1018. Vancini R, Wang G, Ferreira D, et al. Alphavirus genome delivery occurs directly at the plasma membrane in a time- and temperature-dependent process. *J Virol* 2013;87(8):4352–4359.

1019. Vaney MC, Duquerroy S, Rey FA. Alphavirus structure: activation for entry at the target cell surface. *Curr Opin Virol* 2013;3(2):151–158.

1020. Vanlandingham DL, Hong C, Klingler K, et al. Differential infectivities of o'nyong-nyong and chikungunya virus isolates in *Anopheles gambiae* and *Aedes aegypti* mosquitoes. *Am J Trop Med Hyg* 2005;72(5):616–621.

1021. Vanlandingham DL, Tsetsarkin K, Klingler KA, et al. Determinants of vector specificity of o'nyong nyong and chikungunya viruses in Anopheles and Aedes mosquitoes. *Am J Trop Med Hyg* 2006;74(4):663–669.

1022. Varjak M, Dietrich I, Sreenu VB, et al. Spindle-E acts antivirally against alphaviruses in mosquito cells. *Viruses* 2018;10(2):pii: E88.

1023. Vasiljeva L, Merits A, Auvinen P, et al. Identification of a novel function of the alphavirus capping apparatus. RNA 5'-triphosphatase activity of Nsp2. *J Biol Chem* 2000;275(23):17281–17287.

1024. Vazeille M, Moutailler S, Coudrier D, et al. Two Chikungunya isolates from the outbreak of La Reunion (Indian Ocean) exhibit different patterns of infection in the mosquito, *Aedes albopictus*. *PLoS One* 2007;2(11):e1168.

1025. Vazeille M, Zouache K, Vega-Rua A, et al. Importance of mosquito "quasispecies" in selecting an epidemic arthropod-borne virus. *Sci Rep* 2016;6:29564.

1026. Ventoso I. Adaptive changes in alphavirus mRNA translation allowed colonization of vertebrate hosts. *J Virol* 2012;86(17):9484–9494.

1027. Ventoso I, Sanz MA, Molina S, et al. Translational resistance of late alphavirus mRNA to eIF2alpha phosphorylation: a strategy to overcome the antiviral effect of protein kinase PKR. *Genes Dev* 2006;20(1):87–100.

1028. Vernon PS, Griffin DE. Characterization of an in vitro model of alphavirus infection of immature and mature neurons. *J Virol* 2005;79(6):3438–3447.

1029. Villoing S, Bearzotti M, Chilmonczyk S, et al. Rainbow trout sleeping disease virus is an atypical alphavirus. *J Virol* 2000;74(1):173–183.

1030. Vogel P, Abplanalp D, Kell W, et al. Venezuelan equine encephalitis in BALB/c mice: kinetic analysis of central nervous system infection following aerosol or subcutaneous inoculation. *Arch Pathol Lab Med* 1996;120(2):164–172.

1031. Vogel P, Kell WM, Fritz DL, et al. Early events in the pathogenesis of eastern equine encephalitis virus in mice. *Am J Pathol* 2005;166(1):159–171.

1032. Volk SM, Chen R, Tsetsarkin KA, et al. Genome-scale phylogenetic analyses of chikungunya virus reveal independent emergences of recent epidemics and various evolutionary rates. *J Virol* 2010;84(13):6497–6504.

1033. Voss JE, Vaney MC, Duquerroy S, et al. Glycoprotein organization of Chikungunya virus particles revealed by X-ray crystallography. *Nature* 2010;468(7324):709–712.

1034. Vrati S, Faragher SG, Weir RC, et al. Ross River virus mutant with a deletion in the E2 gene: properties of the virion, virus-specific macromolecule synthesis, and attenuation of virulence for mice. *Virology* 1986;151(2):222–232.

1035. Vrati S, Kerr PJ, Weir RC, et al. Entry kinetics and mouse virulence of Ross River virus mutants altered in neutralization epitopes. *J Virol* 1996;70(3):1745–1750.

1036. Wahlberg JM, Boere WA, Garoff H. The heterodimeric association between the membrane proteins of Semliki Forest virus changes its sensitivity to low pH during virus maturation. *J Virol* 1989;63(12):4991–4997.

1037. Walker DH, Harrison A, Murphy K, et al. Lymphoreticular and myeloid pathogenesis of Venezuelan equine encephalitis in hamsters. *Am J Pathol* 1976;84(2):351–370.

1038. Wang E, Barrera R, Boshell J, et al. Genetic and phenotypic changes accompanying the emergence of epizootic subtype IC Venezuelan equine encephalitis viruses from an enzootic subtype ID progenitor. *J Virol* 1999;73(5):4266–4271.

1039. Wang H, Blair CD, Olson KE, et al. Effects of inducing or inhibiting apoptosis on Sindbis virus replication in mosquito cells. *J Gen Virol* 2008;89(Pt 11):2651–2661.

1040. Wang E, Brault AC, Powers AM, et al. Glycosaminoglycan binding properties of natural venezuelan equine encephalitis virus isolates. *J Virol* 2003;77(2):1204–1210.

1041. Wang KS, Kuhn RJ, Strauss EG, et al. High-affinity laminin receptor is a receptor for Sindbis virus in mammalian cells. *J Virol* 1992;66(8):4992–5001.

1042. Wang E, Paessler S, Aguilar PV, et al. A novel, rapid assay for detection and differentiation of serotype-specific antibodies to Venezuelan equine encephalitis complex alphaviruses. *Am J Trop Med Hyg* 2005;72(6):805–810.

1043. Wang YF, Sawicki SG, Sawicki DL. Sindbis virus nsP1 functions in negative-strand RNA synthesis. *J Virol* 1991;65(2):985–988.

1044. Wang KS, Schmaljohn AL, Kuhn RJ, et al. Antiidiotypic antibodies as probes for the Sindbis virus receptor. *Virology* 1991;181(2):694–702.

1045. Wang KS, Strauss JH. Use of a lambda gt11 expression library to localize a neutralizing antibody-binding site in glycoprotein E2 of Sindbis virus. *J Virol* 1991;65(12):7037–7040.

1046. Wauquier N, Becquart P, Nkoghe D, et al. The acute phase of Chikungunya virus infection in humans is associated with strong innate immunity and T CD8 cell activation. *J Infect Dis* 2011;204(1):115–123.

1047. Way SJ, Lidbury BA, Banyer JL. Persistent Ross River virus infection of murine macrophages: an in vitro model for the study of viral relapse and immune modulation during long-term infection. *Virology* 2002;301(2):281–292.

1048. Weaver SC. Electron microscopic analysis of infection patterns for Venezuelan equine encephalomyelitis virus in the vector mosquito, Culex (Melanoconion) taeniopus. *Am J Trop Med Hyg* 1986;35(3):624–631.

1049. Weaver SC. Prediction and prevention of urban arbovirus epidemics: a challenge for the global virology community. *Antiviral Res* 2018;156:80–84.

1050. Weaver SC, Brault AC, Kang W, et al. Genetic and fitness changes accompanying adaptation of an arbovirus to vertebrate and invertebrate cells. *J Virol* 1999;73(5):4316–4326.

1051. Weaver SC, Charlier C, Vasilakis N, et al. Zika, chikungunya, and other emerging vector-borne viral diseases. *Annu Rev Med* 2018;69:395–408.

1052. Weaver SC, Ferro C, Barrera R, et al. Venezuelan equine encephalitis. *Annu Rev Entomol* 2004;49:141–174.

1053. Weaver SC, Forrester NL. Chikungunya: Evolutionary history and recent epidemic spread. *Antiviral Res* 2015;120:32–39.

1054. Weaver SC, Hagenbaugh A, Bellew LA, et al. Evolution of alphaviruses in the eastern equine encephalomyelitis complex. *J Virol* 1994;68(1):158–169.

1055. Weaver SC, Kang W, Shirako Y, et al. Recombinational history and molecular evolution of western equine encephalomyelitis complex alphaviruses. *J Virol* 1997;71(1):613–623.

1056. Weaver SC, Pfeffer M, Marriott K, et al. Genetic evidence for the origins of Venezuelan equine encephalitis virus subtype IAB outbreaks. *Am J Trop Med Hyg* 1999;60(3):441–448.

1057. Weaver SC, Powers AM, Brault AC, et al. Molecular epidemiological studies of veterinary arboviral encephalitides. *Vet J* 1999;157(2):123–138.

1058. Weaver SC, Salas R, Rico-Hesse R, et al. Re-emergence of epidemic Venezuelan equine encephalomyelitis in South America. VEE Study Group. *Lancet* 1996;348(9025):436–440.

1059. Weaver SC, Scherer WF, Taylor CA, et al. Laboratory vector competence of Culex (Melanoconion) cedecei for sympatric and allopatric Venezuelan equine encephalomyelitis viruses. *Am J Trop Med Hyg* 1986;35(3):619–623.

1060. Weaver SC, Scott TW, Lorenz LH. Patterns of eastern equine encephalomyelitis virus infection in Culiseta melanura (Diptera: Culicidae). *J Med Entomol* 1990;27(5):878–891.

1061. Weaver SC, Scott TW, Lorenz LH, et al. Togavirus-associated pathologic changes in the midgut of a natural mosquito vector. *J Virol* 1988;62(6):2083–2090.

1062. Weaver SC, Scott TW, Lorenz LH, et al. Detection of eastern equine encephalomyelitis virus deposition in Culiseta melanura following ingestion of radiolabeled virus in blood meals. *Am J Trop Med Hyg* 1991;44(3):250–259.

1063. Webster LT, Wright FH. Recovery of eastern equine encephalomyelitis virus from brain tissue of human cases of encephalitis in Massachusetts. *Science* 1938;88(2283):305–306.

1064. Weger-Lucarelli J, Ruckert C, Grubaugh ND, et al. Adventitious viruses persistently infect three commonly used mosquito cell lines. *Virology* 2018;521:175–180.

1065. Weiss B, Rosenthal R, Schlesinger S. Establishment and maintenance of persistent infection by Sindbis virus in BHK cells. *J Virol* 1980;33(1):463–474.

1066. Weiss CM, Trobaugh DW, Sun C, et al. The interferon-induced exonuclease ISG20 exerts antiviral activity through upregulation of type I interferon response proteins. *mSphere* 2018;3(5).

1067. Wenger F. Venezuelan equine encephalitis. *Teratology* 1977;16(3):359–362.

1068. Wengler G, Koschinski A, Wengler G, et al. Entry of alphaviruses at the plasma membrane converts the viral surface proteins into an ion-permeable pore that can be detected by electrophysiological analyses of whole-cell membrane currents. *J Gen Virol* 2003;84(Pt 1):173–181.

1069. Wengler G, Koschinski A, Wengler G, et al. During entry of alphaviruses, the E1 glycoprotein molecules probably form two separate populations that generate either a fusion pore or ion-permeable pores. *J Gen Virol* 2004;85(Pt 6):1695–1701.

1070. Wengler G, Wengler G, Rey FA. The isolation of the ectodomain of the alphavirus E1 protein as a soluble hemagglutinin and its crystallization. *Virology* 1999;257(2):472–482.

1071. Werneke SW, Schilte C, Rohatgi A, et al. ISG15 is critical in the control of Chikungunya virus infection independent of UbE1L mediated conjugation. *PLoS Pathog* 2011;7(10):e1002322.

1072. Wesselingh SL, Levine B, Fox RJ, et al. Intracerebral cytokine mRNA expression during fatal and nonfatal alphavirus encephalitis suggests a predominant type 2 T cell response. *J Immunol* 1994;152(3):1289–1297.

1073. Weston S, Czieso S, White IJ, et al. Alphavirus restriction by IFITM proteins. *Traffic* 2016;17(9):997–1013.

1074. Weston J, Villoing S, Bremont M, et al. Comparison of two aquatic alphaviruses, salmon pancreas disease virus and sleeping disease virus, by using genome sequence analysis, monoclonal reactivity, and cross-infection. *J Virol* 2002;76(12):6155–6163.

1075. Weston JH, Welsh MD, McLoughlin MF, et al. Salmon pancreas disease virus, an alphavirus infecting farmed Atlantic salmon, *Salmo salar* L. *Virology* 1999;256(2):188–195.

1076. White J, Helenius A. pH-dependent fusion between the Semliki Forest virus membrane and liposomes. *Proc Natl Acad Sci U S A* 1980;77(6):3273–3277.

1077. White G, Ottendorfer C, Graham S, et al. Competency of reptiles and amphibians for eastern equine encephalitis virus. *Am J Trop Med Hyg* 2011;85(3):421–425.

1078. White GS, Pickett BE, Lefkowitz EJ, et al. Phylogenetic analysis of eastern equine encephalitis virus isolates from Florida. *Am J Trop Med Hyg* 2011;84(5):709–717.

1079. White LK, Sali T, Alvarado D, et al. Chikungunya virus induces IPS-1-dependent innate immune activation and protein kinase R-independent translational shutoff. *J Virol* 2011;85(1):606–620.

1080. White LJ, Wang JG, Davis NL, et al. Role of alpha/beta interferon in Venezuelan equine encephalitis virus pathogenesis: effect of an attenuating mutation in the 5' untranslated region. *J Virol* 2001;75(8):3706–3718.

1081. Wiggins K, Eastmond B, Alto BW. Transmission potential of Mayaro virus in Florida *Aedes aegypti* and *Aedes albopictus* mosquitoes. *Med Vet Entomol* 2018;32(4):436–442.

1082. Willems WR, Kaluza G, Boschek CB, et al. Semliki forest virus: cause of a fatal case of human encephalitis. *Science* 1979;203(4385):1127–1129.

1083. Williams CR, Fricker SR, Kokkinn MJ. Environmental and entomological factors determining Ross River virus activity in the River Murray Valley of South Australia. *Aust N Z J Public Health* 2009;33(3):284–288.

1084. Williams MC, Woodall JP. O'nyong-nyong fever: an epidemic virus disease in East Africa. II. Isolation and some properties of the virus. *Trans R Soc Trop Med Hyg* 1961;55:135–141.

1085. Williams MC, Woodall JP, Corbet PS, et al. O'nyong-nyong fever: an epidemic virus disease in East Africa. 8. Virus isolations from anopheles mosquitoes. *Trans R Soc Trop Med Hyg* 1965;59:300–306.

1086. Williams MC, Woodall JP, Gillett JD. O'nyong-nyong fever; an epidemic virus disease in East Africa. VII. Virus isolations from man and serological studies up to July 1961. *Trans R Soc Trop Med Hyg* 1965;59:186–197.

1087. Win MK, Chow A, Dimatatac F, et al. Chikungunya fever in Singapore: acute clinical and laboratory features, and factors associated with persistent arthralgia. *J Clin Virol* 2010;49(2):111–114.

1088. Wolf S, Taylor A, Zaid A, et al. Inhibition of IL-1beta signaling by anakinra shows a critical role for bone loss in experimental arthritogenic alphavirus infections. *Arthritis Rheumatol* 2019;71(7):1185–1190.

1089. Wong HV, Vythilingam I, Sulaiman WY, et al. Detection of persistent Chikungunya virus RNA but not infectious virus in experimental vertical transmission in *Aedes aegypti* from Malaysia. *Am J Trop Med Hyg* 2016;94(1):182–186.

1090. Woodroofe G, Marshall ID, Taylor WP. Antigenically distinct strains of Ross River virus from north Queensland and coastal New South Wales. *Aust J Exp Biol Med Sci* 1977;55(1):79–97.

1091. Woodward TM, Miller BR, Beaty BJ, et al. A single amino acid change in the E2 glycoprotein of Venezuelan equine encephalitis virus affects replication and dissemination in *Aedes aegypti* mosquitoes. *J Gen Virol* 1991;72(Pt 10):2431–2435.

1092. Wressnigg N, van der Velden MV, Portsmouth D, et al. An inactivated Ross River virus vaccine is well tolerated and immunogenic in an adult population in a randomized phase 3 trial. *Clin Vaccine Immunol* 2015;22(3):267–273.

1093. Wu JQ, Barabe ND, Chau D, et al. Complete protection of mice against a lethal dose challenge of western equine encephalitis virus after immunization with an adenovirus-vectored vaccine. *Vaccine* 2007;25(22):4368–4375.

1094. Wu JQ, Barabe ND, Huang YM, et al. Pre- and post-exposure protection against Western equine encephalitis virus after single inoculation with adenovirus vector expressing interferon alpha. *Virology* 2007;369(1):206–213.

1095. Wust CJ, Nicholas JA, Fredin D, et al. Monoclonal antibodies that cross-react with the E1 glycoprotein of different alphavirus serogroups: characterization including passive protection in vivo. *Virus Res* 1989;13(2):101–112.

1096. Wyckoff RWG, Tesar WC. Equine encephalomyelitis in monkeys. *J Immunol* 1939;37(4):329–343.

1097. Yin J, Gardner CL, Burke CW, et al. Similarities and differences in antagonism of neuron alpha/beta interferon responses by Venezuelan equine encephalitis and Sindbis alphaviruses. *J Virol* 2009;83(19):10036–10047.

1098. Yoon IK, Alera MT, Lago CB, et al. High rate of subclinical chikungunya virus infection and association of neutralizing antibody with protection in a prospective cohort in the Philippines. *PLoS Negl Trop Dis* 2015;9(5):e0003764.

1099. Young NA, Johnson KM. Antigenic variants of Venezuelan equine encephalitis virus: their geographic distribution and epidemiologic significance. *Am J Epidemiol* 1969;89(3):286–307.

1100. Young DS, Kramer LD, Maffei JG, et al. Molecular epidemiology of eastern equine encephalitis virus, New York. *Emerg Infect Dis* 2008;14(3):454–460.

1101. Yun NE, Peng BH, Bertke AS, et al. CD4+ T cells provide protection against acute lethal encephalitis caused by Venezuelan equine encephalitis virus. *Vaccine* 2009;27(30):4064–4073.

1102. Zaid A, Rulli NE, Rolph MS, et al. Disease exacerbation by etanercept in a mouse model of alphaviral arthritis and myositis. *Arthritis Rheum* 2011;63(2):488–491.

1103. Zeng X, Mukhopadhyay S, Brooks CL III. Residue-level resolution of alphavirus envelope protein interactions in pH-dependent fusion. *Proc Natl Acad Sci U S A* 2015;112(7):2034–2039.

1104. Zhang Y, Burke CW, Ryman KD, et al. Identification and characterization of interferon-induced proteins that inhibit alphavirus replication. *J Virol* 2007;81(20):11246–11255.

1105. Zhang M, Fang Y, Brault AC, et al. Variation in western equine encephalomyelitis viral strain growth in mammalian, avian, and mosquito cells fails to explain temporal changes in enzootic and epidemic activity in California. *Vector Borne Zoonotic Dis* 2011;11(3):269–275.

1106. Zhang X, Fugere M, Day R, et al. Furin processing and proteolytic activation of Semliki Forest virus. *J Virol* 2003;77(5):2981–2989.

1107. Zhang W, Heil M, Kuhn RJ, et al. Heparin binding sites on Ross River virus revealed by electron cryo-microscopy. *Virology* 2005;332(2):511–518.

1108. Zhang R, Hryc CF, Cong Y, et al. 4.4 Å cryo-EM structure of an enveloped alphavirus Venezuelan equine encephalitis virus. *EMBO J* 2011;30(18):3854–3863.

1109. Zhang R, Kim AS, Fox JM, et al. Mxra8 is a receptor for multiple arthritogenic alphaviruses. *Nature* 2018;557(7706):570–574.

1110. Zhang W, Mukhopadhyay S, Pletnev SV, et al. Placement of the structural proteins in Sindbis virus. *J Virol* 2002;76(22):11645–11658.

1111. Zheng Y, Kielian M. Imaging of the alphavirus capsid protein during virus replication. *J Virol* 2013;87(17):9579–9589.

1112. Ziegler SA, Lu L, da Rosa AP, et al. An animal model for studying the pathogenesis of chikungunya virus infection. *Am J Trop Med Hyg* 2008;79(1):133–139.

1113. Zlotnik I, Batterha D, Grant DP, et al. Pathogenesis of western equine encephalitis-virus (WEE) in adult hamsters with special reference to long and short-term effects on CNS of tenuated clone 15 variant. *Br J Exp Pathol* 1972;53(1):59–77.

1114. Zlotnik I, Harris WJ. The changes in cell organelles of neurons in the brains of adult mice and hamsters during Semliki Forest virus and louping ill encephalitis. *Br J Exp Pathol* 1970;51(1):37–42.

1115. Zouache K, Michelland RJ, Failloux AB, et al. Chikungunya virus impacts the diversity of symbiotic bacteria in mosquito vector. *Mol Ecol* 2012;21(9):2297–2309.

1116. Zrachia A, Dobroslav M, Blass M, et al. Infection of glioma cells with Sindbis virus induces selective activation and tyrosine phosphorylation of protein kinase C delta. Implications for Sindbis virus-induced apoptosis. *J Biol Chem* 2002;277(26):23693–23701.

Flaviviridae: The Viruses and Their Replication

Brett D. Lindenbach • Glenn Randall • Ralf Bartenschlager • Charles M. Rice

INTRODUCTION

Yellow fever had been an endemic and emerging disease for centuries when, in 1901, Walter Reed demonstrated that this disease could be experimentally transferred via the filtered serum of an infected individual, the first identification of a human virus. It is now understood that yellow fever virus (YFV) is but one representative of a large family of related positive-strand RNA viruses, the *Flaviviridae* (from the Latin flavus, "yellow"). This family consists of four genera: *Flavivirus*, *Hepacivirus* (from the Greek *hepar*, "liver"), *Pegivirus* (for *pe*rsistent *G*B virus), and *Pestivirus* (from the Latin *pestis*, "plague").

Family Classification

The *Flaviviridae* exhibit diverse biological properties and limited serological cross-reactivity. Despite this diversity, viruses are classified within the *Flaviviridae* based on similarities in genome organization and shared phylogeny of essential viral replication enzymes. Currently, all members of the *Flaviviridae* share the following common features: (a) enveloped virus particles that are labile to detergents and organic solvents; (b) nonsegmented, positive-strand RNA genomes, 9.4 to 13.0 kb in length, which encode a large open reading frame (ORF); and (c) a common set of virus-encoded replication enzymes: nonstructural (NS) protein 3 (NS3) with serine protease and RNA helicase activities and NS5 (or NS5B) with RNA-dependent RNA polymerase (RdRP) activity. On larger evolutionary scales, the NS3 helicases share phylogenetic similarity to other superfamily 2 "DEx(D/H)" RNA helicases, including those of plant-infecting, positive-strand RNA potyviruses[447]; the NS5/NS5B RdRPs share phylogenetic similarity with a diverse set of "branch 3" positive-strand RNA viruses, including alphaviruses, nodaviruses, tombusviruses, and luteoviruses.[978]

Recent advances in virus discovery and metagenomics have led to profound reorganization and expansion of the *Flaviviridae*, including establishment of a new genus, *Pegivirus*, as well as the identification of new viruses within established genera with expanded host tropism, such as *Hepaciviruses* that infect rodents, bats, and nonhuman primates. All currently recognized members of the *Flaviviridae* are listed in Table 7.1; a molecular phylogeny of the *Flaviviridae*, based on conserved

TABLE 7.1   Taxonomy of the *Flaviviridae*

Taxonomic Unit	Member Species
Genus *Flavivirus*	
Mosquito-borne	*Aroa virus* (AROAV); *Bagaza virus* (BAGV); *Banzi virus* (BANV); *Bouboui virus* (BOUV); *Cacipacore virus* (CPCV); *Dengue virus*, types 1–4 (DENV-1 to DENV-4); *Edge Hill virus* (EHV); *Ilheus virus* (ILHV); *Israel turkey meningoencephalomyelitis virus* (ITV); *Japanese encephalitis virus* (JEV); *Jugra virus* (JUGV); *Kedougou virus* (KEDV); *Kokobera virus* (KOKV); *Koutango virus* (KOUV); *Murray Valley encephalitis virus* (MVEV); *Ntaya virus* (NTAV); *Saboya virus* (SABV); *Saint Louis encephalitis virus* (SLEV); *Sepik virus* (SEPV); *Tembusu virus* (TMUV); *Uganda S virus* (UGSV); *Usutu virus* (USUV); *Wesselsbron virus* (WESSV); *West Nile virus* (WNV); *Yaounde virus* (YAOV); *Yellow fever virus* (YFV); *Zika virus* (ZIKV)
Tick-borne	*Gadgets Gully virus* (GGYV); *Kadam virus* (KADV); *Kyasanur Forest disease virus* (KFDV); *Langat virus* (LGTV); *Louping ill virus* (LIV); *Meaban virus* (MEAV); *Omsk hemorrhagic fever virus* (OHFV); *Powassan virus* (POWV); *Royal Farm virus* (RFV); *Saumarez Reef virus* (SREV); *Tick-borne encephalitis virus* (TBEV-Eur); *Tyuleniy virus* (TYUV)
No known vector	*Apoi virus* (APOIV); *Bukalasa bat virus* (BBV); *Carey Island virus* (CIV); *Cowbone Ridge virus* (CRV); *Dakar bat virus* (DBV); *Entebbe bat virus* (ENTV); *Jutiapa virus* (JUTV); *Modoc virus* (MODV); *Montana myotis leukoencephalitis virus* (MMLV); *Phnom Penh bat virus* (PPBV); *Rio Bravo virus* (RBV); *Sal Vieja virus* (SVV); *San Perlita virus* (SPV); *Yokose virus* (YOKV)
Unclassified	*Aedes flavivirus* (AEFV), *Cell fusing agent virus* (CFAV); *Culex flavivirus* (CXFV); *Spondweni virus* (SPOV); *Tamana bat virus* (TABV), etc.
Genus *Hepacivirus*	*Hepacivirus A* (nonprimate hepacivirus, NHPV); *Hepacivirus B* (GB virusB, GBV-B); *Hepacivirus C* (hepatitis C virus; HCV, genotypes 1–7); *Hepacivirus D* (guereza hepacivirus, GHV); *Hepacivirus E* (rodent hepacivirus E, RHV-E); *Hepacivirus F* (rodent hepacivirus F; RHV-F); *Hepacivirus G* (Norway rat hepacivirus 1, NRHV1); *Hepacivirus H* (Norway rat hepacivirus 2, NRHV2); *Hepacivirus I* (rodent hepacivirus I, RHV-I); *Hepacivirus J* (rodent hepacivirus J, RHV-J); *Hepacivirus K* (bat hepacivirus K, BHV-K); *Hepacivirus L* (bat hepacivirus L, BHV-L); *Hepacivirus M* (bat hepacivirus M, BHV-M); *Hepacivirus N* (bovine hepacivirus N, BoHV)
Genus *Pegivirus*	*Pegivirus A* (simian pegivirus [formerly GB virus A], SPgV); *Pegivirus B* (GB virus-D, GBV-D); *Pegivirus C* (human pegivirus, HPgV); *Pegivirus D* (Theiler disease–associated virus, TDAV); *Pegivirus E* (equine pegivirus, EPgV); *Pegivirus F* (bat pegivirus F, BPgV-F); *Pegivirus G* (bat pegivirus G, BPgV-G); *Pegivirus H* (human hepegivirus, HHPgV); *Pegivirus I* (bat pegivirus I, BPgV-I); *Pegivirus J* (rodent pegivirus, RPgV); *Pegivirus K* (porcine pegivirus, PPgV)
Genus *Pestivirus*	*Pestivirus A* (bovine viral diarrhea virus 1, BVDV1); *Pestivirus B* (bovine viral diarrhea virus 2, BVDV2); *Pestivirus C* (classical swine fever virus [formerly hog cholera virus], CSFV); *Pestivirus D* (border disease virus, BDV); *Pestivirus E* (pronghorn antelope pestivirus, PAPeV); *Pestivirus F* (porcine pestivirus, PPeV); *Pestivirus G* (giraffe pestivirus, GPeV); *Pestivirus H* (HoBi-like pestivirus, HoBiPeV); *Pestivirus I* (Aydin-like pestivirus, AydinPeV); *Pestivirus J* (rat pestivirus, RPeV); *Pestivirus K* (atypical porcine pestivirus, APPeV)

Virus species and genera currently recognized by the International Committee on Taxonomy of Viruses are shown in italics; common names and abbreviations are shown in parentheses.

regions of viral RdRPs, is shown in Figure 7.1A. It should be noted that a number of *Flaviviridae* remain to be officially classified at the genus level, such as Tamana bat virus and, at the species level, such as several arthropod-specific flaviviruses. In addition, metagenomic surveys have identified several "flavi-like" viruses with very large (16–23 kb) monopartite genomes as well as "Jingmenviruses" with 10.5- to 11.0-kb multipartite genomes divided among four or five RNA segments that are independently encapsidated.[467,836] Jingmenviruses have been found in arthropod hosts but may be transmitted to humans and other primates, where they can cause febrile illness.[467,952] Although these latter virus groups have not been classified within the *Flaviviridae*, they do encode canonical NS3-like serine proteases/RNA helicases and NS5/NS5B–like RdRPs. Clearly the field is entering an exciting period of comparative studies and critical evaluation of essential features shared among the *Flaviviridae*.

Family Characteristics and Replication Cycle

This chapter is organized around common features of the family *Flaviviridae* life cycle (Fig. 7.2). The enveloped virions are composed of a lipid bilayer with two or more species of envelope (E) glycoprotein surrounding a nucleocapsid, which consists of a single-stranded, positive-sense RNA genome complexed with multiple copies of a small, basic capsid (C) protein. Binding and uptake are believed to involve receptor-mediated endocytosis, although bona fide entry receptors have only been positively identified for a few viruses. For the purposes of this chapter, we define virus entry factors as a general category of cellular molecules that contribute toward productive virus entry; attachment receptors are a subset of entry factors that bind to virus particles, often with low specificity, and thereby increase virus–cell avidity but may not be essential for virus entry; entry receptors are a distinct subset of virus-binding cell surface molecules that target the virus for essential steps in productive virus entry. Following endocytosis, the low pH of the endosome induces fusion of the virion envelope with cellular membranes. Following uncoating of the nucleocapsid, the RNA genome is released into the cytoplasm. The genome serves three discrete roles within the life cycle: as the messenger RNA (mRNA) for translation of all viral proteins, a template during RNA replication, and the genetic material packaged within new virus particles. The organization of the genome is similar for all genera. Viral proteins are produced as part of a single polyprotein that

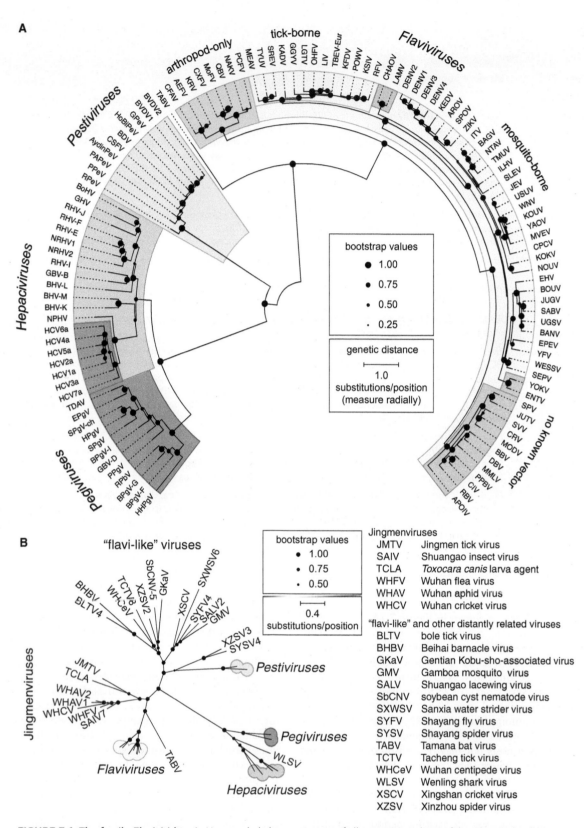

FIGURE 7.1 The family *Flaviviridae*. A: Unrooted phylogenetic tree of all current members of the *Flaviviridae*, based on maximum likelihood alignment of a conserved, 352-aa region of the RdRP domains, constructed by using previously described methodology.[836] Virus names are abbreviated as in Table 7.1 and the text, with clades of interest highlighted by colored arcs. TABV, which has not been officially classified as a *Flaviviridae*, was included as an outgroup. The linear scale bar represents genetic distance along the radial axis; circular scale bars represent bootstrap support values for each node (*n* = 1,000 iterations). We thank Anderson Brito and Nathan Grubaugh for assistance in sequence alignment and tree construction. **B:** Unrooted phylogenetic tree of unclassified viruses that resemble the *Flaviviridae*, based on maximum likelihood alignment of a conserved region of the RdRP domain, as above. We thank Mang Shi and Eddie Holmes for assistance in sequence alignment and tree construction.

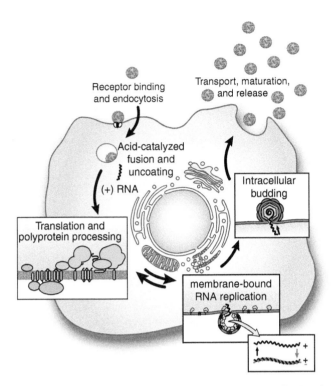

FIGURE 7.2 The life cycle of the *Flaviviridae*. See text for details.

is cleaved by a combination of host and viral proteases. The structural proteins are encoded in the N-terminal portion of the polyprotein with the NS proteins in the remainder. Sequence motifs characteristic of a serine protease, RNA helicase, and an RdRP are found in similar locations in the polyproteins of all four genera. RNA replication occurs entirely in the cytoplasm in close association with intracellular membranes; the synthesis of a genome-length minus-strand RNA provides the intermediate. Progeny virions assemble by budding into an intracellular membrane compartment, most likely the endoplasmic reticulum (ER), and then transit through the host secretory pathway and are released at the cell surface.

FLAVIVIRUSES

Background and Classification
The *Flavivirus* genus currently includes 56 virus species, many of which are arthropod-borne human pathogens. Flaviviruses cause a variety of human and animal diseases, including fever, encephalitis, and hemorrhagic fevers. Entities of major global concern include dengue virus (DENV)—with its associated dengue hemorrhagic fever (DHF) and dengue shock syndrome (DSS)—Japanese encephalitis virus (JEV), West Nile virus (WNV), YFV, and Zika virus (ZIKV).[959] Decreases in mosquito control efforts coupled with societal factors (e.g., increased transportation and dense urbanization) have contributed to several significant flavivirus outbreaks, including the reemergence of YFV in Africa and the Americas, reemergence of multiple DENV serotypes in the Americas, the introduction and spread of WNV in North America, and the emergence of ZIKV, notably linked to fetal birth defects, in South and Central America.

Mosquito-borne and tick-borne flaviviruses, although distinct, appear to have evolved via a common ancestral line

that diverged from viruses with no known arthropod vector. In addition, several arthropod-specific flaviviruses remain to be taxonomically classified within this genus. Flavivirus species are further categorized into antigenic complexes and subcomplexes based on serological criteria or into genetically related clusters and clades, according to molecular phylogenetics.[131,848] For instance, the JEV serocomplex includes eight virus species that are genetically and antigenically related. DENV, which is both a single virus species and a distinct serogroup, notably circulates as four distinct serotypes. Human antibody responses to one DENV serotype are poorly cross-protective and may even enhance pathogenesis during secondary infections with other DENV serotypes; one explanation for this immunopathology is through antibody-dependent enhancement (ADE) of virus entry into myeloid cells that express antibody Fc receptors.[333,413] Although DENV-specific antibodies can also enhance ZIKV infection in experimental models,[49,120,273,871] preexisting DENV immunity appears to afford partial cross-protection to ZIKV infection in humans.[775]

In 1937, Max Theiler developed a live attenuated yellow fever vaccine by extensive serial passage of a virulent YFV isolate in suckling mouse brain and chick embryo tissues. The resulting virus, YFV-17D, has been successfully used to prevent yellow fever in over 300 million people. Despite this early success, only a limited number of flavivirus vaccines are available, including both inactivated and live attenuated JEV for use in humans, inactivated TBEV for use in humans, and inactivated WNV for use in animals.[352] Development of effective DENV vaccines that exhibit cross-protection between serotypes remains particularly challenging. One recently approved tetravalent DENV vaccine, Dengvaxia, is based on four chimeric YFV-17D derivatives, each expressing the structural glycoproteins of one DENV serotype. However, Dengvaxia shows limited prophylaxis in DENV-naïve individuals and may enhance disease in natural infections.[773] Therefore, its use is currently limited to people aged 9 to 45 with prior DENV infection and who live in DENV endemic areas.

Structure and Physical Properties of the Virion
Infectious flavivirus particles are lipid enveloped, roughly spherical, and approximately 50 nm in diameter and lack prominent spikes (Fig. 7.3A–C). Viruses sediment between 170S and 210S and have buoyant densities of 1.19 to 1.23 g/cm^3 depending on the lipid composition, which varies by host.[793] The outer shell of the particle is made up of two viral proteins, envelope (E) and membrane (M). The E glycoprotein is the major antigenic determinant of the virion and mediates binding and fusion during virus entry. The M protein is a small proteolytic fragment of the precursor membrane (prM) protein and is produced during virus maturation within the secretory pathway. Removal of the lipid envelope with nonionic detergents reveals discrete nucleocapsids (120–140S; 1.30–1.31 g/cm^3), which consist of a single RNA genome and multiple copies of capsid (C) protein.[422]

Exquisite structural details of immature and mature flavivirus particles have been determined by cryo-electron microscopy and x-ray crystallography. Mature infectious particles display a relatively smooth, dimpled outer surface, with 90 antiparallel E glycoprotein dimers lying flat across the surface of the virion, tightly packed in a "herringbone" array that completely

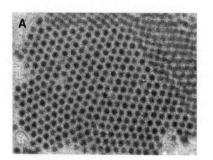
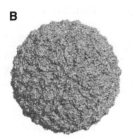
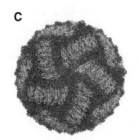
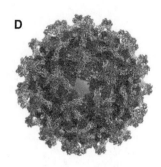

FIGURE 7.3 Flavivirus particles. A: Paracrystalline array of SLEV particles in the salivary gland of a *Culex pipiens* mosquito 25 days after blood meal feeding on an infected suckling mouse. (Courtesy of Sylvia G. Whitfield, Frederick A. Murphy, and W. Daniel Sudia.) **B:** Surface view of a symmetrical cryo-EM reconstruction of mature DENV-2 particles, at 3.5 Å resolution, as rendered from PDB 3J27.[1025] **C:** DENV-2 glycoproteins rendered on the same cryo-EM reconstruction in **panel B**, colored as in Figure 7.5: *red*, E glycoprotein domain I; *yellow*, E domain II; *blue*, E domain III; *green*, E membrane-proximal and transmembrane domains; *orange*, M protein; *slate*, envelope membrane. **D:** Symmetrical cryo-EM reconstruction of immature DENV-1 particles, at 6 Å resolution, as rendered from PDB 4B03.[449] Features are colored as in **panel C** except: *orange*, prM glycoprotein.

covers the lipid bilayer (Fig. 7.3C).[343] This packing involves two-, three-, and fivefold axes of symmetry, similar to a $T = 3$ icosahedral particle but lacking quasi-equivalence. Beneath this outer protein shell, the membrane-proximal and transmembrane domains of the M and E proteins interact with the membrane in orderly, regular intervals; beneath the lipid envelope, flavivirus nucleocapsids lack discernible symmetry and make intermittent contacts with the glycoprotein transmembrane domains.[908] Despite this seemingly well-ordered structure, flavivirus particles are not rigid, uniformly dimpled golf balls. Antibody neutralization studies have shown that the surface of DENV particles is conformationally dynamic and capable of strain- and temperature-dependent "breathing."[551] Moreover, a subset of flavivirus particles form with fewer than 180 copies of prM–E[908] and, as described below, mature virus particles display variable amounts of uncleaved prM.

Immature virions are larger than mature virions, 60 nm in diameter, and display 60 prominent spikes with icosahedral symmetry (Fig. 7.3D).[343] Each protrusion is composed of three prM–E heterodimers, with prM serving to protect the E fusion peptide against premature fusion during particle secretion. Within immature particles, the nucleocapsid appears as an asymmetric ovoid, displaced to one side of the virus particle.[908] As immature particles pass through the low pH environment of the *trans*-Golgi network, the 60 (prM–E)$_3$ complexes dissociate and reform as 90 (prM–E)$_2$ complexes, which lie flat against the envelope and give immature particles a smoother appearance.[1016] It is at this point that the trigger for fusion has been set, with E held in a pH-sensitive metastable conformation. Thereafter, prM is cleaved by the Golgi-resident host protease furin, leading to subsequent release of mature virions and free pr fragments. This process is imperfect: some flaviviruses, like DENV, release significant quantities of partially mature and immature particles.[761] Partially mature particles, which retain a mixture of M and uncleaved prM, can undergo attachment and fusion to initiate infection similar to fully mature particles. Released immature particles are incapable of triggering fusion and are noninfectious; however, immature particles opsonized by prM- or E-specific antibodies can infect Fc receptor–bearing cells.[268] The mechanisms of this antibody-dependent fusion are not well understood but may require cleavage of prM in the endosome. Importantly, immature and partially mature par-

ticles display envelope membrane and prM–E conformations that are not exposed in mature particles, pleiomorphisms that have significant implications for antibody neutralization, viral entry, and pathogenesis.[202,761]

Flavivirus-producing cells also secrete smaller, noninfectious subviral particles (SVPs), which contain E and M glycoproteins but lack nucleocapsids. SVPs complete the same maturation process as whole virions and can undergo fusion with target membranes; however due to lack of a genome-containing nucleocapsid, they are not infectious. Cells that express only prM and E release structurally similar "recombinant subviral particles" (RSPs), indicating that the viral glycoproteins are sufficient to drive the budding process.[19,810] RSPs are approximately 30 nm in diameter and less dense than infectious virus particles (1.14 g/cm³). RSPs have a markedly different arrangement of E glycoprotein, with only 30 E dimers lying flat against the surface in a $T = 1$ icosahedral shell rather than the herringbone pattern seen in mature virus particles.[258]

Binding and Entry

Flaviviruses enter target cells through receptor-mediated endocytosis, followed by intracellular membrane fusion. Bona fide flavivirus entry receptors have not been fully identified, although a number of important cellular entry factors have been characterized.[487,761] Binding of E glycoprotein to glycosaminoglycans (GAGs), such as heparan sulfate, can enhance cell surface attachment; however, cell culture–adapted flaviviruses with high affinities for GAGs are attenuated *in vivo*.[585] As mentioned above, ADE can lead to infection of Fc receptor–expressing cells with flavivirus particles opsonized with subneutralizing antibodies, which likely contributes to the pathogenesis of DSS and DHF in people previously exposed to other DENV serotypes.[334]

A number of C-type lectins, which bind mannose-rich glycans and are highly expressed on several myeloid-derived cell types, have been implicated in flavivirus attachment and entry. In particular, the C-type lectin DC-SIGN can function as an attachment receptor for DENV infection of dendritic cells[668,890]; this interaction may be particularly relevant when mosquito-produced virus particles, which display more high-mannose glycans and fewer complex glycans, encounter intradermal dendritic cells. In contrast, WNV preferentially binds DC-SIGNR, a related C-type lectin that is highly expressed on microvascular endothelial cells.[195] The mannose receptor, another C-type lectin, has been implicated in the endocytosis of DENV, JEV, and TBEV.[633] Interestingly, interaction of DENV particles with yet another C-type lectin, CLEC5A, does not mediate viral entry but can trigger the release of proinflammatory cytokines, which may contribute to dengue pathogenesis.[155]

Phosphatidylserine (PtdSer) receptors, which normally mediate recognition and phagocytosis of apoptotic cells, are another important class of flavivirus entry factors.[487,610,761] PtdSer, a phospholipid, is normally sequestered in the inner leaflet of the plasma membrane and membranes of the secretory pathway and only exposed to the extracellular milieu during apoptosis, when it serves as an "eat me" signal. Flaviviruses, which bud into the ER, may acquire envelope membranes enriched for PtdSer. Thus, when the viral envelope is exposed on the surface of immature, partially mature, and breathing flavivirus particles, it can be directly bound by T-cell immunoglobulin–mucin (TIM) proteins, a family of PtdSer receptors expressed on a variety of immune cells. Similarly, Tyro3, Axl, and Mer (TAM), a distinct family of PtdSer receptor–protein tyrosine kinases, can bind flavivirus particles indirectly via their soluble PtdSer-binding protein ligands Gas6 and ProS.[610] While TIMs and TAMs can contribute to flavivirus entry, they are not essential for virus infection[487]; thus, their specific roles in viral entry and pathogenesis require further study. Finally, the endoplasmic reticulum membrane complex (EMC) reportedly plays an important but undefined role in flavivirus entry, perhaps by modulating the trafficking of host factors needed for viral internalization.[805]

After binding to the appropriate receptor(s), flaviviruses are internalized by clathrin-mediated endocytosis and delivered to early or intermediate endosomes, which mature into late endosomes.[932] Fusion of the viral envelope with the bounding endosomal membranes occurs during endosomal trafficking, although the exact compartment where fusion occurs differs between flaviviruses, perhaps reflecting differences in pH optima.[932] In the acidic environment, E protein dimers dissociate and undergo an irreversible conformational change to become fusogenic trimers.[18,872] In this conformation, the fusion peptide, previously buried within the E homodimer interface, extends away from the viral envelope and inserts into the endosomal membrane (Video 7.1). The lipid composition of target membranes influences the pH threshold and efficiency of flavivirus fusion.[448,873,874,1020] Nevertheless, the flavivirus fusion mechanism is generally very rapid, complete within seconds after exposure to low pH.[149,718,932]

Flavivirus fusion is an active target of antiviral development, with a number of small molecules demonstrating potent virus-specific or broad activity against several flaviviruses.[718] Some of these compounds apparently target a hinge within the E glycoprotein that is needed to induce its conformational change into the fusogenic form. Other compounds may target the rate-limiting steps of trimer formation or fusion peptide extension.[148]

Following *in vitro* dissolution of the viral envelope, viral genomes are immediately accessible for translation, suggesting that capsids can spontaneously uncoat.[448] Indeed, nucleocapsids isolated from virions are unstable in high salt, disassembling into C protein dimers.[422] However, *in vivo*, it appears that postfusion capsid uncoating and genome translation require ubiquitylation of capsid protein.[129]

Genome Structure

As for other positive-strand RNA viruses, flavivirus genomes are infectious once delivered into the cytosol of target cells.[703] Several flavivirus infectious complementary DNA (cDNA) clones and replicons have been constructed, allowing the structure and function of the genome to be dissected via reverse genetics.[35,458,790] Flavivirus genomes consist of a single segment of positive-stranded RNA, approximately 11 kilobases (kb) in length (sedimentation, 42S), with a type 1 5′ cap, $^{m7}GpppA_mN$, and lacking a 3′ poly-A tail (Fig. 7.4).[171,970] The cap serves to initiate translation, stabilize viral RNA, and subvert innate antiviral defenses.[190,283] Genomes encode a single long open reading frame (ORF, ~3,400 codons) flanked by 5′ and 3′ noncoding regions (NCR) of approximately 100 nucleotides (nts) and 400 to 700 nts, respectively (Fig. 7.4A).[675] The NCRs contain *cis*-acting RNA structures and sequences important for viral gene expression, replication, and immune modulation.

Flavivirus 5′ and 3′ NCRs are poorly conserved across the genus, with particular divergence between mosquito-borne, tick-borne, and arthropod-specific flaviviruses and flaviviruses with no known vector, likely reflecting adaptation of these RNA structures to specific hosts.[941] Nevertheless, functionally important RNA structures and sequence motifs have been identified, including structurally conserved bifurcated 5′ stem–loop (SL) and large 3′ SL structures. A key unifying feature among flaviviruses is cyclization of their genomes via long-distance base pairing between the 5′ and 3′ ends.[331,538,941]

Because the study of flavivirus 5′ and 3′ NCRs is complicated by their inherent variability, a paucity of rigorously determined RNA structures, and differences in nomenclature, this discussion focuses on DENV, which is the best characterized model of flavivirus 5′ and 3′ NCR structures and genome cyclization. While the details differ between flaviviruses, the fundamental mechanisms elaborated with DENV appear to operate in other mosquito-borne flaviviruses and even extend to flaviviruses with other vector host ranges, despite low sequence similarity.[538,923,941] The DENV 5′SL, frequently termed SL-A, is followed by a small SL-B, just upstream of the translational start site, that includes a sequence termed the 5′ upstream AUG region (5′UAR) (Fig. 7.4A). Shortly within the capsid-coding region is another small SL, termed the capsid-coding region hairpin (cHP), followed by an unstructured 5′ cyclization sequence (5′CS) and additional small SLs.[941]

The DENV 3′ NCR consists of three functionally distinct regions. Region I is the most variable, with deletions and point mutations frequently arising in mosquito-adapted DENV isolates, suggesting that its function is particularly important in vertebrate hosts.[941] Region I typically folds into two SLs, xrRNA1 and xrRNA2 (sometimes called SLI and SLII), the loops of which can base-pair just downstream of each SL to form two adjacent pseudoknots (Fig. 7.4A). These pseudoknots are tightly packed, essentially threading the RNA backbone through the pseudoknot and rendering this region of flavivirus genomes resistant to the cellular 5′ to 3′ exonuclease XRN1 (inset, Fig. 7.4A).[11,150] Upon XRN1 degradation of the genome, the resulting subgenomic flavivirus RNAs (sfRNAs) have immunomodulatory properties.[856] Region II folds into two conserved dumbbell structures, DB1 and DB2, that also form pseudoknots with downstream adjacent regions. In particular, DB2 base-pairs to the 3′CS, which has complementarity to the

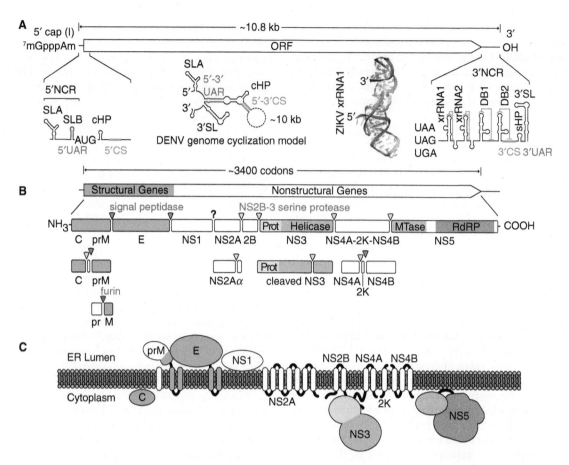

FIGURE 7.4 Flavivirus genome structure and polyprotein expression. A: Genome structure and RNA elements. The viral genome is depicted with the structural and nonstructural (NS) coding regions, the 5' cap, and the 5' and 3' noncoding regions (NCR) indicated. Functionally significant RNA structures within the DENV genome are illustrated, with pseudoknot base pairing indicated by *gray lines*. Insets include a model of DENV genome cyclization and the structure of the ZIKV xrRNA1 fragment, colored across the visible spectrum (5' blue–3' red), as rendered from PDB 5TPY.[11] **B:** Polyprotein processing and cleavage products. Boxes below the genome indicate precursors and mature proteins generated by the proteolytic processing cascade. Structural proteins are colored *blue*, while NS proteins are white or shaded according to their enzymatic subunits, as indicated. Cleavage sites for host signal peptidase, the viral NS2B-3 serine protease, furin, and an unknown protease (?) are indicated. **C:** Polyprotein membrane topology. The proposed membrane orientation of the flavivirus proteins is shown. The proteins are approximately to scale (areas are proportional to the number of amino acids) and arranged in order (*left* to *right*) of their appearance in the polyprotein.

5'CS, while DB1 can base-pair directly to the capsid-coding region. Region II can also tolerate variability, with mutations that stabilize DB1 or destabilize DB2 arising in mosquito-adapted DENV isolates.[196] Region III, the most conserved part of the DENV 3'NCR, consists of a small hairpin (sHP) followed by a large, structurally conserved terminal 3'SL; the base of sHP and 3'SL are formed from the 3'UAR sequence, which has complementarity to the 5'UAR.

The DENV genome exists in a dynamic equilibrium between competing linear and cyclized structures, formed by long-distance base pairing between the 5' to 3'UAR and 5' to 3'CS elements (inset, Fig. 7.4A). Mutations that disrupt or favor one conformation frequently select for reversions that restore this equilibrium.[940] The cyclized conformation is critical for RNA replication: SL-A binds the NS5 RdRP domain and positions it to initiate minus-strand synthesis from the 3' end, held proximal by genome cyclization.[265,266,546,1007] Genome cyclization also alters 5' and 3' secondary structures, leading to

occlusion of the translation start site. Thus, large-scale genome conformation may regulate the switch from translation to RNA replication. Consistent with this, *in vivo* SHAPE analysis of DENV and ZIKV RNA confirmed that viral genomes are highly structured, containing several conserved structural motifs and transient long-distance base-pairing interactions.[369]

Translation and Proteolytic Processing

The efficiency of genome translation is a primary determinant of flavivirus infectivity.[228] The viruses therefore use several mechanisms to ensure translational competence, including specialized structures within the 5' and 3' NCRs. Translation of flavivirus genomes is largely cap-dependent; 2'-O-methylation of the 5' nucleotide also helps to overcome innate antiviral defenses that down-regulate translation in infected cells.[190] While translation initiates via ribosomal scanning, many mosquito-borne flaviviruses lack a canonical Kozak initiation motif and contain several AUG codons near the correct start site.

To help ensure proper AUG selection, DENV uses a small RNA stem–loop embedded within the C gene to induce ribosomal pausing over the authentic initiation codon.[175]

In addition to canonical cap-dependent mechanisms of translation initiation, DENV and ZIKV 5′ NCRs are reported to have internal ribosome entry site (IRES) activity, capable of driving expression of a downstream reporter gene in bicistronic mRNAs within human cells, but not in mosquito cells.[861] Nevertheless, given that flavivirus genomes lacking a 5′ cap have approximately 1,000-fold reduced specific infectivity[764] and that flavivirus cap methylation activity is essential for RNA replication,[214,1034] it appears that flaviviruses are more dependent on cap-mediated translation than on IRES activity. Interestingly, mutations in the 5′ SL-A partially restored replication of a WNV genome containing lethal mutations in the NS5 methyltransferase active site[1024]; it will be interesting to see whether these mutations increase IRES activity. Thus, perhaps flaviviruses encode a proto-IRES, reflecting an evolutionary midpoint between capped and uncapped genomes within the family and allowing flaviviruses to maintain genome translation under conditions of translation-arresting stress in vertebrate cells. Indeed, flavivirus genomes remain efficiently translated even as the translation of host mRNAs is down-regulated during infection.[757,786] This preferential reprogramming of the translational apparatus involves activation of the MAPK-interacting Ser/Thr protein kinase 1, which phosphorylates eIF4E to enhance translation of capped mRNAs.[786] In addition, flaviviruses antagonize the formation of cytosolic RNA stress granules,[94,238,364] which inhibit virus genome translation and replication.[13]

Translation of the single, long ORF produces a large polyprotein that is co- and posttranslationally cleaved into at least 10 proteins (Fig. 7.4B). The N-terminal region of the polyprotein encodes the structural proteins C–prM–E, which are followed by the NS proteins NS1–NS2A–NS2B–NS3–NS4A–2K–NS4B–NS5.[138,765] Host signal peptidase is responsible for cleavages of C/prM, prM/E, E/NS1, and 2K/NS4B. Please note that dashes are used to refer to uncleaved polyproteins (e.g., NS4A-2K-NS4B) or to protein complexes (e.g., NS2B-3); slashes specifically refer to cleave sites within the polyprotein (e.g. C/prM). A virus-encoded serine protease, NS2B-3, processes at the NS2A/NS2B, NS2B/NS3, NS3/NS4A, NS4A/2K, and NS4B/NS5 junctions. The enzyme responsible for NS1-2A cleavage is presently unknown. The predicted topology of the flavivirus polyprotein is depicted in Figure 7.4C.

Features of the Structural Proteins

Capsid (C) Protein

The capsid (C) protein is a small (~12 kDa), positively charged protein that binds RNA with high affinity and low specificity; its major function is to encapsidate the viral genome within flavivirus particles. C is initially synthesized as an uncleaved C–prM precursor; processing of this intermediate occurs in two steps: cleavage by the viral serine protease on the cytosolic side of the transmembrane domain to release mature C, followed by signal peptidase cleavage on the lumenal side to generate the N-terminus of prM.[544] This coordinated cleavage results from the combination of a fairly short (14–22 aa) signal sequence, a suboptimal signalase cleavage site, and downstream regions of prM and E.[544,875] Mutations that uncouple signal peptidase cleavage from viral serine protease cleavage lead to increased production of empty virus particles.[495,545] Coordinated cleavage

therefore serves to delay structural protein processing until the viral serine protease has accumulated and replication is under way, which may limit the release of immunogenic but noninfectious SVPs early in infection. In addition, this delayed cleavage mechanism renders flaviviruses highly dependent on signal peptide complex protein SPCS1.[1026]

Mature C protein folds into a compact dimer with each monomer contributing four alpha helices that enwrap to form a wedge-like core (Fig. 7.5A). The N-terminal approximately 25 aa of C remains unstructured and encodes several basic residues; along with basic residues on the surface of α4, this region is involved in RNA binding.[128] On the opposite surface, α2 displays a hydrophobic surface that mediates membrane association of C.[128,572]

Despite its compact, well-ordered structure and essential function in virus particle formation, the flavivirus C protein is actually poorly conserved and demonstrates remarkable structural plasticity. YFV C retains its ability to package RNA even after deletion of nearly 40 residues from the N-terminus or 27 residues of the C-terminus; internal deletions of the hydrophobic sequence are less tolerated.[697] The TBEV C protein remains functional even after deletion of 16aa from the central hydrophobic helix, albeit with increased production of empty particles.[436] Mutants containing larger deletions are not viable but can be rescued by second-site changes that increase the hydrophobicity of downstream sequences.[437] WNV tolerates small deletions in hydrophobic helix α2 to various degrees; remarkably, infectivity of the deleted genomes was improved by even larger deletions—up to one-third of the C protein sequence—encompassing all of helix α3.[815] It is not yet clear how C protein dimers are organized within the apparently disordered nucleocapsids, but RNA or DNA can induce isolated C protein dimers to assemble into nucleocapsid-like particles *in vitro*.[422]

Small amounts of flavivirus C protein localize to the ER and to the outer surface of lipid droplets (LDs),[128,799] which are ER-derived cytosolic reservoirs of neutral fatty acids and cholesterol esters. However, a large fraction of C localizes to the nucleus and to the nucleolus in particular.[128,882] Since virus assembly occurs on the cytosolic surface of the ER, the function of nuclear localization is unclear. Nuclear localization (and LD localization) may serve to sequester C away from replication complexes until it is needed for virus assembly or may simply reflect the fact that clusters of basic residues, which are found in the RNA-binding regions of C, also serve as nuclear localization signals. On the other hand, DENV C can interact with histones and disrupt nucleosomes[182]; it also interacts with nucleolin, which may contribute to virus particle assembly.[44] In addition to these intranuclear interactions, YFV C reportedly inhibits RNA interference (RNAi) via its RNA-binding activity,[800] while the ZIKV C protein can enhance the replication of other RNA viruses without inhibiting RNAi.[934]

Precursor Membrane (prM) Glycoprotein

The glycoprotein precursor of M, prM (~26 kDa), functions as a chaperone for the E glycoprotein. The N-terminal pr region has a unique fold consisting of seven β strands, with six conserved, disulfide-linked cysteines, and one to three N-linked glycosylation sites[507]; prM folds rapidly after synthesis and assists in proper folding of the E glycoprotein.[445] In addition to interactions through their ectodomains, the C-terminal transmembrane domains of prM and E heterodimerize and act as an ER-retention signal for the prM–E complex.[687,689]

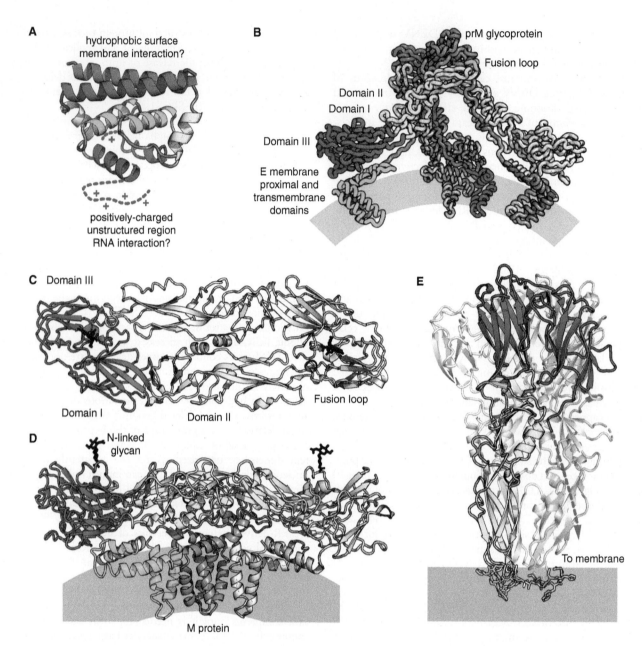

FIGURE 7.5 Flavivirus structural proteins. A: Flavivirus C protein structure. The WNV C protein dimer is shown, with helices colored sequentially N-blue, green, yellow, and red. Rendered from PDB 1SFK.[213] **B:** Structure of the trimeric prM–E glycoprotein complex on the surface of immature DENV-1 particles. One E monomer is colored *red* (domain I), *yellow* (domain II), *blue* (domain III), *cyan* (fusion loop), and *green* (membrane-proximal and transmembrane domains); one prM monomer is colored *orange*. Rendered from biological assembly 2 of PDB 4B03.[449] **C:** The structure of a mature ZIKV E glycoprotein dimer as viewed perpendicular to the lipid bilayer, with one monomer colored as in **(B)**, rendered from PDB 6CO8.[828] For simplicity, the E and M membrane-proximal and transmembrane domains are hidden from view. **D:** The structure of a mature ZIKV E glycoprotein dimer as viewed lateral to the lipid bilayer, colored as in **(B)**, as rendered from PDB 6CO8.[828] **E:** TBEV E protein trimers in their postfusion form, colored as in **(C)**. Rendered from PDB 1URZ.[114]

A key function of prM is to prevent E from undergoing premature acid-catalyzed fusion as virus particles transit through the secretory pathway.[326,353] In immature particles, the pr region sits at the tip of the E protein, forming the pr–E spike and shielding the fusion peptide from the cellular environment (Fig. 7.5C).[507] The acidity of the *trans*-Golgi compartment induces a global rearrangement of prM–E, exposing the furin cleavage site within prM.[864,1016,1029] After cleavage, the pr peptide remains associated with virus particles until exposure to neutral pH of the extracellular space.[864,1012,1016]

As a structural protein that sets the trigger for flavivirus fusion, prM is a key determinant of flavivirus pathogenesis. Incomplete furin cleavage of prM gives rise to partially mature virus particles that display different epitopes and the PtdSer-rich envelope membrane, which can influence cell entry and tropism.[761] This is particularly apparent for DENV prM, which features suboptimal furin cleavage[761]; indeed, prM-specific antibodies can contribute to ADE in secondary DENV infections.[202] Furthermore, a single point mutation on the surface of the pr region was reported to contribute to ZIKV pathogenesis in a murine model of microcephaly, although the epidemiological impact of this mutation on human infections is still under debate.[319,1017]

Envelope (E) Glycoprotein

Flavivirus E (~53 kDa) is the prototype class II fusion protein that, unlike class I and III fusion proteins, do not make preformed trimers. E mediates receptor binding and membrane fusion and is the major neutralizing antigen on the surface of flavivirus particles. E contains 12 conserved cysteines that form intramolecular disulfide bonds; it is anchored to the viral envelope by adjacent C-terminal transmembrane anchors; and in some viral species, E is N-glycosylated. Proper folding, ER retention, secretion, and acid stabilization of E is dependent on coexpression with prM.[445]

As originally isolated and crystallized in its prefusion conformation from mature TBEV particles,[760] E folds into an elongated β-sheet–rich structure, forming head-to-tail homodimers that lie parallel to the virus envelope (Fig. 7.5C, D). Each E monomer consists of three domains: DI, which forms an eight-stranded β-barrel; DII, a long, finger-like domain that projects along the virus surface; and DIII, which has an immunoglobulin-like fold. The interfaces between DI and DII and between DI and DIII, which contain conserved histidine residues, act as pH-sensitive hinges.[801] The DI–DII interface also contains a hydrophobic pocket that can accommodate a β-octylglucoside detergent molecule.[641] The fusion peptide is located at the tip of the DII finger, buried in a distinct hydrophobic pocket formed by DI and DIII of the partner monomer; this intermolecular interface is also where pr binds and is a major neutralizing epitope.[788] DIII, which slightly protrudes from the virion surface, is a determinant of host tropism and a target of neutralizing antibodies[241,762]; DIII is therefore postulated to bind receptors, although DIII-specific receptors have not yet been identified. Between the ectodomain of E and the membrane is a short but functionally important stem region composed of two α-helices that lie parallel to the plane of the membrane.[20,1023]

Upon exposure to low pH, the dimer-stabilizing histidine residues in E become protonated, causing E dimers to dissociate into monomeric subunits, which spontaneously reform as fusogenic trimers.[801] In its postfusion conformation (Fig. 7.5E), E is folded back onto itself, bringing the N-terminal fusion peptide (and target membrane) into proximity with the C-terminal transmembrane domain (and viral envelope).[642] To accomplish this, DII must rotate relative to DI, similar to the displacement of DII seen in crystals of native E protein grown in the presence of β-octylglucoside.[641,642] Furthermore, DIII must rotate and fold back more than 30 Å in relation to DI. Thus, flavivirus fusion is blocked by DIII-specific neutralizing antibodies or soluble, recombinant form of DIII, which inhibit these rearrangements.[520,680] Based on these mechanistic insights into the structure and function of E, a number of small molecules are under development as flavivirus fusion inhibitors and potential antiviral therapies.[148,718]

Features of the Nonstructural Proteins

NS1 Glycoprotein

NS1 (~46 kDa) is a high conserved, homodimeric glycoprotein that is retained within the early secretory pathway and also secreted from flavivirus-infected cells. NS1 has important roles in RNA replication and virus particle assembly; it is also a major humoral antigen, an immunomodulator, and a key determinant of flavivirus pathogenesis.

NS1 is cleaved from E by host signal peptidase; its C-terminus arises via cleavage at the NS1/NS2A junction by an unknown ER-resident host enzyme that requires the eight C-terminal residues of NS1 and an undefined portion of NS2A.[249,250] A report that NS1 has a C-terminal GPI-anchor has not held up to further scrutiny.[958,971] Flaviviruses in the JEV serogroup also express an elongated form of NS1, termed NS1′, which arises through a -1 ribosomal frameshifting event near the NS1-2A junction and terminates approximately 52 codons downstream.[267,596] NS1 contains 2 or 3 N-linked glycosylation sites and 12 conserved cysteines that are disulfide bonded.

Shortly after synthesis, NS1 forms stable homodimers that have an affinity for membranes. X-ray crystallography has revealed that NS1 consists of three domains: a small, N-terminal β-hairpin that interdigitates with the corresponding region of another NS1 monomer, forming a "β-roll" that drives stable dimer formation; a "wing" domain that includes a flexible loop and 2 N-linked glycans; and a long, C-terminal 9-stranded antiparallel β-sheet that forms an 18-rung "β-ladder" across the dimer interface (Fig. 7.6).[10] The near-planar arrangement of the wings and β-ladder render the NS1 dimer relatively flat, presenting one polar "outer" surface that displays epitopes and localized regions of variability, and one extended, hydrophobic

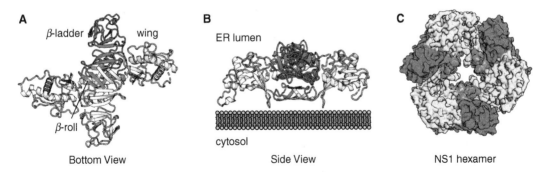

FIGURE 7.6 Flavivirus NS1 glycoprotein. A: Top view of ZIKV NS1 dimer, with one monomer colored to highlight the β-ladder (*red*), wing (*yellow*), and β-roll (*blue*). Rendered from PDB 5K6K.[119] **B:** Side view of ZIKV NS1 dimer, showing the inferred membrane-interaction surface, rendered as in (**A**). **C:** Model of the ZIKV NS1 hexamer, showing a central hydrophobic channel, rendered as in (**A**).

"inner" surface that mediates peripheral membrane interaction. Based on this membrane association, purified NS1 can coat liposomes and remodel them into smaller lipoprotein particles.[10] Although it is not yet clear if this membrane rearrangement activity is relevant for the formation flavivirus replication complexes, a recent study has shown that NS1 is essential for the formation of vesicle packets (VPs), which are the sites of viral RNA replication.[726]

Intracellular NS1 dimers are retained in the early secretory pathway and localize to the lumenal side of viral replication vesicles, where they play an essential but enigmatic role at an early stage of RNA replication.[528,576] As RNA synthesis occurs on the cytosolic side of these membranes, NS1 fulfills this essential function, at least in part, via interaction with two polytopic membrane proteins, NS4A and NS4B or the NS4A-2K-NS4B precursor.[532,726,1010] The intracellular form of NS1 also contributes to virus particle assembly via interactions with prM and E.[809,975]

Secreted NS1 (sNS1) forms soluble, hexameric lipoprotein particles of approximately 10 nm composed of three dimers held together in a barrel configuration surrounding a lipid core (Fig. 7.6C).[10,327] DENV sNS1 was originally identified as a soluble, complement-fixing antigen present at high levels during the acute phase of DENV infections[858,958]; indeed sNS1 is a diagnostic marker of flavivirus infections more broadly. Because of its abundance and multivalent structure, sNS1 is highly antigenic and induces strong humoral immune responses, including complement-fixing antibodies; NS1 can also directly inhibit thrombin and inhibit and/or stimulate components of the complement pathway.[958] While NS1-specific immune complex formation, reduced clotting activity, and complement activation all likely contribute to flavivirus pathogenesis, sNS1 also directly binds to and modulates relevant target cell types. For instance, DENV sNS1 is bound and internalized by hepatocytes, enhancing subsequent infection of these cells.[14] The mechanism whereby a secreted replication protein prepares cells for subsequent infection remains unclear but theoretically could enhance cross-species transmission. In fact, a genetic polymorphism in ZIKV correlates with higher sNS1 levels and increased ZIKV transmission to mosquitoes.[539] DENV sNS1 also binds to the innate immunity pattern recognition receptor TLR4 on the surface of monocytes, triggering release of proinflammatory cytokines, and on the surface of endothelial cells, triggering vascular leakage.[736,958] Surprisingly, sNS1 proteins from different flaviviruses disrupt endothelial barriers in a tissue-specific manner that resembles the tropism of the parental viruses.[736]

A fraction of NS1, presumably in dimeric form, is also expressed on the surface of infected cells via interaction with surface GAGs.[37] Cell surface–expressed NS1 can be recognized by NS1-specific antibodies, and NS1-specific antibodies can protect animals from lethal disease through direct complement-mediated lysis of infected cells, FcγR-mediated phagocytosis, or via complement- and FcγR-independent mechanisms.[958]

NS2A and NS2B Proteins

NS2A is a small (~22 kDa) polytopic membrane protein with important functions in RNA replication and virus assembly. While the NS1/2A junction is cleaved by an unidentified ER-resident protease, the NS2A C-terminus is generated by NS2B-3 serine protease cleavage in the cytosol, suggesting that NS2A

contains an odd number of transmembrane domains. NS2A contains eight membrane-interacting regions; its membrane topology has been inferred through genetic approaches although NS2A structure still awaits rigorous biochemical determination.[944,987] For some flaviviruses, the viral serine protease also cleaves at an internal site within NS2A to generate a C-terminally truncated form, NS2Aα.[671] Mutations at the YFV NS2Aα cleavage site have minimal effect on RNA replication but block virus particle production; these defects can be suppressed by a second mutation on the surface of the NS3 helicase domain.[459] Additional mutational analyses have identified NS2A residues critical for RNA replication, virus particle assembly, and interaction with NS2B and NS3, although the structure and function of NS2A remains elusive.[500,944,982,983,988]

Several flavivirus NS2A proteins have been reported to inhibit innate immunity. Mutations within the WNV NS2A gene enhance interferon-β promoter–driven transcription and attenuate WNV pathogenesis in mice, implying that the wild-type NS2A may function to inhibit this pathway.[536,542] Consistent with this, expression of DENV-2 NS2A inhibits interferon-β–stimulated gene induction and enhance the replication of an interferon-sensitive reporter virus.[660] Moreover, DENV NS2A inhibits TBK-1, a kinase that integrates input from several innate sensing pathways to phosphorylate IRF3.[191]

NS2B, a small (~14 kDa) membrane-associated protein, is an essential cofactor for the NS2B-3 serine protease activity and anchors this enzyme complex to cellular membranes.[174,251] NS2B's protease cofactor activity resides within a central peptide that intercalates within the fold of the serine protease domain.[242] DENV NS2B can target the human innate immune DNA sensor cGAS for lysosomal degradation, independent of its protease cofactor activity, thereby inhibiting innate immunity.[6] Mutational analysis has also identified determinants of RNA replication and virus particle assembly within the transmembrane domains of NS2B,[504] regions that were also found to interact with the SPCS1, a host-dependency factor for multiple flaviviruses.[573,1026]

NS3 Protein

NS3 is a large (~70 kDa) multifunctional protein, encoding enzymatic activities required for viral gene expression and RNA replication. The N-terminal third of the protein is the catalytic domain of the NS2B-3 serine protease, which has a chymotrypsin-like fold (Fig. 7.7A). X-ray crystallography revealed that the NS2B cofactor contributes one β-strand to an essential β-barrel of this protease fold.[242,563] The NS2B-3 serine protease cleaves substrates containing adjacent basic residues at the NS2A/NS2B, NS2B/NS3, NS3/NS4A, and NS4B/NS5 junctions.[141,142] Secondarily, the NS2B-3 serine protease generates the C-termini of capsid and NS4A proteins via delayed cleavage and cleaves internal sites within NS2A and NS3. DENV NS2B-3 can also cleave the human innate immune adaptor protein STING, inhibiting type I interferon induction.[7] Because NS2B-3 protease activity is essential for flavivirus gene expression, and because protease inhibitors have proven to be useful therapeutics against other viruses including hepatitis C virus (HCV) and human immunodeficiency virus, NS2B-3 is considered to be a high-priority target for antiviral development.[563]

As for other members of the *Flaviviridae*, NS3 encodes a C-terminal superfamily 2 nucleoside triphosphatase (NTPase)-RNA helicase.[302] *In vitro*, NS3 has demonstrated RNA-stimulated NTPase and RNA unwinding activities, and

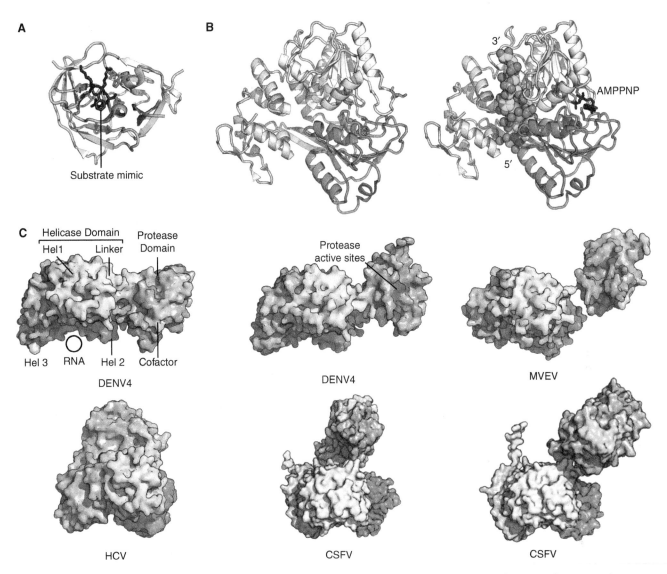

FIGURE 7.7 *Flaviviridae* **NS3 proteins. A:** The structure of the WNV NS2B-3 serine protease domain, with NS2B cofactor peptide (*green*), NS3 protease domain (*pink*), and a substrate-competitive inhibitor (*black*). Active site residues are shown in *red*. Rendered from PDB 2FP7.[242] **B:** Structure of the DENV-4 NS3 helicase domain with (*left*) or without (*right*) bound RNA substrate (*colored spheres*) and ATP analog (*black*). Note the ATPase active site (*red*) becomes structured at the interface of domain I (*cyan*) and domain II (*purple*) upon RNA binding. The RNA is bound within a cleft formed by the first two domains and domain III (*gold*). Rendered from PDBs 2JLQ and 2JLV.[566] **C:** Structural interdomain flexibility within full-length NS3. Shown are two conformations of full-length DENV-4 NS3 as rendered from PDBs 2VBC[565] and 2WHX[564], respectively; MVEV from PDB 2WV9[34]; HCV from PDB 1CU1[998]; and CSFV from PDB 5MZ4[223]. Helicases were structurally aligned, with molecular surfaces colored as in **panels (A)** and **(B)** and the protease–helicase linker peptide in *yellow*.

mutational analyses confirm that these activities are essential for RNA replication.[597,955,968] However, it is not yet clear what specific role the NTPase–RNA helicase performs in the viral life cycle, nor whether this enzyme unwinds double-stranded replicative intermediates (RI) *in vivo*. The helicase domain also exhibits RNA triphosphatase (RTPase) activity, which is presumed to remove the 5′ γ-phosphate, yielding 5′ dephosphorylated genomes for subsequent capping.[969] The NTPase, RNA helicase, and RTPase activities of NS3 all depend on the Walker B motif, indicating that all three nucleic acid–modifying activities utilize a common active site.[51,67] In addition to its essential but undefined role in RNA replication, the helicase domain of NS3 is also implicated in the assembly of virus particles.[289,459,698] This role in

virus assembly appears to be genetically separable from NS3's NTPase–RNA helicase activities[289,698] and may involve recruitment of the ESCRT pathway components to facilitate budding.[135] However, because flavivirus particle assembly is tightly coupled to RNA replication,[421] an additional role for helicase activity in virus assembly has not been formally excluded. In the context of full-length NS2B-3, the helicase also inhibits innate immunity, perhaps by unwinding double-stranded RNAs (dsRNAs).[827]

The NS3 helicase domain consists of three subdomains: two RecA-like subdomains that are conserved among all superfamily 2 helicases and an α-helix–rich C-terminal subdomain that is common to all *Flaviviridae* but structurally distinct between genera.[563,981,990] This latter region, subdomain 3, mediates critical interactions with NS5.[896] The NTP active site resides at the interface of the RecA-like subdomains 1 and 2, while RNA is bound in a cleft between subdomains 1 and 2 and subdomain 3 (Fig. 7.7).[563,566] Full-length NS3 structures have revealed both structural flexibility and coordination between the serine protease and helicase domains.[563–565] Thus, the flexible linker region likely plays an important role in coordinating these enzyme activities.

In addition to its enzymatic activities, DENV NS3 can also antagonize innate immunity by binding to the cellular 14-3-3ε protein.[143] Truncated forms of NS3, which result from NS2B-3 serine protease cleavage within the helicase domain, have been observed *in vitro* and *in vivo*.[31,737,904] The role of these cleavages is unclear, although it is possible that the products could have a distinct function. In this regard, replication defects caused by helicase domain mutations can be complemented in *trans*, while serine protease domain activities are required in *cis*.[394,420,541]

NS4A and NS4B Proteins

NS4A (~16 kDa) and NS4B (~27 kDa) are small, polytopic membrane proteins that contribute to RNA replication and subversion of innate immunity. These proteins are initially synthesized as a NS4A-2K-4B precursor that is cleaved by the NS2B-3 serine protease and host signal peptidase; similar to the coordinated processing of C protein, upstream cleavage by NS2B-3 at the NS4A/2K junction is a prerequisite for downstream cleavage by signal peptidase at the 2K/NS4B junction.[522,733] Expression of NS4A, NS4B, or NS4A-2K-4B has differing effects on cellular membranes[782]; thus, the coordinated cleavage of NS4A-2K-4B likely impacts the temporal assembly of membrane-bound replication complexes. In fact, mature NS4A, but not NS4A-2K, induces membrane alterations suggesting that removal of the 2K peptide is important for membrane activity.[634] The regulation of this cleavage is not fully understood, but it is interesting to note that in DENV-infected cells, NS1 selectively interacts with NS4A-2K-4B, but neither with mature NS4A nor NS4B.[726] Furthermore, NS2B-3 cleavage at the YFV NS3/4A and NS4A/2K junctions is highly dependent on DNAJC14, an Hsp40 cochaperone of Hsp70-mediated protein folding and a host factor required for the replication of multiple flaviviruses.[103,1003]

NS4A consists of an approximately 50-aa N-terminal cytosolic region, a transmembrane domain, a lumenal amphipathic helix, and a second transmembrane domain; a third transmembrane domain, 2K, is removed via NS2B-3 proteolysis.[634] NS4A forms higher-order structures via its first transmembrane domain, which mediates both homo-oligomerization and heterodimerization with NS4B.[496,1040] NS4A localizes to replication complexes and contributes to RNA replication via genetic interaction with NS1.[532,578,966] NS4A can also serve as a cofactor of the NS3 helicase, increasing the efficiency of NTPase activity.[844] Moreover, mutations in NS4A and 2K have been found to confer resistance to a potent inhibitor of flavivirus replication and to overcome superinfection exclusion, further implicating these proteins in RNA replication.[1038,1041]

NS4B consists of an N-terminal lumenal region, two transmembrane domains separated by a long cytoplasmic loop, and a third transmembrane domain that can posttranslationally insert across the membrane.[635,1039] For some flaviviruses, the N-terminal lumenal region is glycosylated on one or two asparagine residues; mutation of these glycosylation sites cause

defects in DENV RNA replication.[666] NS4B forms homodimers,[1039] localizes to sites of RNA synthesis,[635] and maintains critical interactions with several other replicase components, including NS1, NS3, and NS4A.[153,1010,1037,1040] The interaction of NS4B with NS3 may serve to enhance helicase activity.[929] The DENV NS1-NS4B complex was shown to interact with MAGT1, a subunit of the N-oligosaccharide transferase (OST) complex, and DENV replication is dependent on MAGT1 oxidoreductase activity.[524] This interaction may explain why OST is essential for the replication of several flaviviruses, independent of OST activity.[524,589,738]

Both NS4A and NS4B can inhibit innate immune activation. The DENV-2 NS4A protein binds mitochondrial antiviral-signaling (MAVS), a mitochondrial innate immune adaptor protein, inhibiting its activation by RIG-I.[348] DENV-1 NS4A also inhibits TBK-1,[191] and several flavivirus NS4B proteins potently antagonize TBK-1 as well as JAK/STAT1 signaling.[191,659,660] In addition, DENV NS4B counteracts innate immunity by dampening integrity of the mitochondria-associated membranes (MAMs) that serve as platforms for innate immune signaling.[152] Finally, WNV NS4A and NS4B expression cause ER stress, inducing an unfolded protein response that down-regulates JAK/STAT signaling through ATF-6.[23,24]

NS5 Protein

NS5 is a large (~103 kDa), highly conserved, and multifunctional protein essential for flavivirus RNA synthesis and capping. The N-terminal domain encodes RNA capping activities, while the C-terminal domain is the viral RdRP. In addition, NS5B modulates host gene expression and antagonizes innate immune activation.

The structure of the capping domain is shown within the context of full-length NS5 (Fig. 7.8A). Flaviviruses modify their genomes with a type 1 5′ RNA cap in a stepwise process: (a) removal of 5′ γ-phosphate from a triphosphorylated RNA substrate, presumably by the RTPase activity of the NS3 helicase domain[969]; (b) addition of a 5′ to 5′ guanosine cap (from GTP) by a guanylyltransferase activity within the NS5 capping domain[231,380]; (c) addition of a methyl group (from S-adenosylmethionine) to the N7 position of the guanylyl cap by NS5's methyltransferase (MTase) activity[231,754]; and (d) methylation at the 2′O position of the +1 nucleotide by a distinct NS5 MTase active site.[231,754] Thus, the capping of nascent viral RNAs requires coordination of the NS5 RdRP domain, the NS3 helicase domain, and the NS5 capping domain.[107] Mutational analyses showed that the cap methylation steps are separable and that N7 methylation is required for viral translation and replication, while 2′-O-methylation allows the virus to avoid innate antiviral defenses.[190,214,454,754,1034]

The C-terminal domain of NS5 contains conserved RdRP motifs and structurally resembles other RNA polymerases, forming a "right-hand" structure with palm, fingers, and thumb subdomains (Fig. 7.8A).[107,584,999] NS5 RNA polymerase activity has been confirmed with purified, recombinant protein.[2,885] The major product of *in vitro* RdRP reactions is often a self-primed copy-back RNA; however, NS5 can initiate *de novo* RNA synthesis, which likely reflects the authentic mechanism in infected cells.[2,679,1015] This unprimed RNA synthesis requires high concentrations of GTP, which binds within a GTP pocket much like a nascent RNA strand and helps to stabilize the initiating NTP.[107,679]

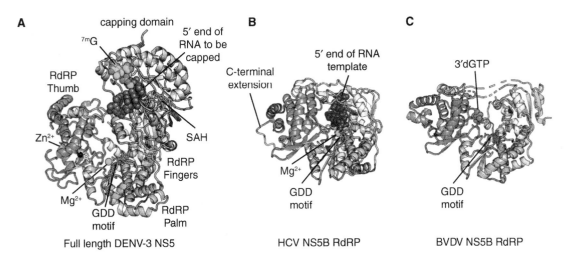

FIGURE 7.8 *Flaviviridae* NS5 and NS5B proteins. A: Full-length DENV-3 NS5 was labeled to highlight the capping domain (*wheat*) and the canonical RdRP fingers (*cyan*), palm (*pink*), and thumb (*blue*) domains. Catalytic Mg^{2+} and structural Zn^{2+} ions are indicated, as is ^{7m}G, the substrate for cap addition, and SAH (S-adenosyl-L-homocysteine), the by-product of the methylation reaction. Rendered from PDB 5DTO.[1028] **B:** The HCV NS5B RdRP is shown with bound template RNA; the HCV-specific C-terminal extension is shown in *yellow*. Rendered from PDB 1NB7.[681] **C:** The BVDV1 NS5B RdRP is shown modeled in the GTP-bound state by rendering PDB 2JCQ[160] and the GTP analog from 2J7W.[999] The pestivirus-specific N-terminal extension is shown in *green*.

Structures of full-length NS5 reveal flexibility in the linker between the capping and RdRP domains, with conserved interdomain interfaces and the potential to form functionally relevant homodimers.[107,127,430] NS3 presumably binds to the NS5 linker region in order to coordinate RNA synthesis with capping activities, and plausible models for NS3-NS5 interaction have been proposed, whereby nascent RNAs are modified and capped as they exit the RdRP,[107] very much like the capping assembly line originally described for bluetongue virus, a member of the *Reoviridae*.[878] NS5 does indeed form a complex with NS3 and stimulates its NTPase and RTPase activities.[188,1006] Cross-linking studies have shown that both proteins bind to the 3′ SL of the viral genome, which, together with genome cyclization, may serve to initiate minus-strand synthesis by 5′ SL-bound NS5.[154]

NS5 has been shown to localize to sites of viral RNA synthesis for only a few flaviviruses.[577,966] This is likely because only a small fraction of NS5 cofractionates biochemically with replicase activity[321,928]; rather, NS5 frequently localizes to the nucleus of flavivirus-infected cells, where it has been proposed to dysregulate gene expression and splicing.[121,198,608] Because the NS5 nuclear localization signals frequently overlap critical structures within the RdRP, it has been challenging to dissect the role of NS5's nuclear localization from its role in viral replication. Nevertheless, at least two groups have identified DENV mutants that replicate well with little or no nuclear NS5 localization.[456,897] In addition, NS5 has been shown to block the Jak/STAT pathway of IFN signaling by a variety of mechanisms.[79,80]

Ultrastructure and Biogenesis of the Flavivirus Replication Organelle

In flavivirus-infected cells, replicase activity is associated with membrane fractions that are enriched for most viral proteins.[167] Upon treatment of these membrane fractions with nonionic detergents, viral RNA and proteins are rendered sensitive to

degradation, arguing that membranes are protecting viral components against nucleolytic and proteolytic attack. Consistent with this observation, the flavivirus replication organelle consists of ER membrane invaginations toward the ER lumen,[184,294,399,636,683,966] giving rise to vesicles, which in the case of DENV have an average diameter of about 90 nm (Fig. 7.9). These vesicles are linked to the cytosol via a pore-like opening that has a diameter of around 11 nm (Fig. 7.9H). Thus, the lumen is topologically identical to the cytosol but provides a shielding environment, for example, to limit the access of pattern recognition receptors (PRRs) to viral RNA.[692,927] In 2D sections, these membrane invaginations appear as arrays of vesicles in ER tubes designated VPs.[576,966,972] VPs have been found in all flaviviruses studied thus far, including ZIKV, WNV, and TBEV.[184,294,399,636,683,966] Although several lines of evidence, including metabolic labeling of RNA, *in situ* hybridization, and immunodetection of dsRNA, suggest that VPs are the site of viral replication,[966,973] firm proof demonstrating *de novo* synthesis of viral RNA in the vesicle lumen is still lacking.

In addition to VPs, bundled smooth ER membranes, designated as convoluted membranes (CMs), are often found in close proximity to VPs and mitochondria (Fig. 7.9A). At least for WNV (subtype Kunjin), it has been proposed that CMs might be sites of polyprotein synthesis and cleavage by the NS2B-3 protease.[972,973] This assumption is based on the accumulation of viral proteins, but not dsRNA, in these membrane structures, but since CMs are largely devoid of ribosomes, this model is not easy to reconcile. Alternatively, CMs might serve as lipid stores or interfere with innate immunity. The latter might be mediated by disruption of MAMs, which play a critical role as signaling platforms to mount, for example, an interferon response or by sequestration of innate immune PRRs in CMs.[152] In any case, CMs appear to be dispensable for viral RNA replication as found for ZIKV, which induces CMs in human hepatoma cells, but not in human neuronal progenitor

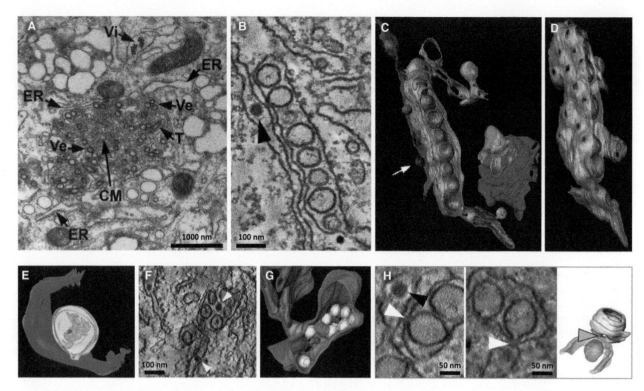

FIGURE 7.9 Flavivirus replication organelles. A: Membrane alterations induced in DENV-infected cells. Shown is a thin-section TEM image of DENV-infected, resin-embedded Huh-7 cells fixed at 24-hour postinfection. Ve, virus-induced vesicles; T, membrane tube; CM, convoluted membranes; Vi, clusters of virus particles. **B:** Single tomographic slice (~2 nm thick) showing DENV-induced vesicular invaginations toward the ER lumen. A virus particle (*black arrowhead*) is seen in the ER-proximal nuclear envelope. **C:** 3D reconstruction of vesicle packets and cellular membranes in close proximity. Virus particles (*white arrow*) are shown as *red spheres*. **D:** The vesicle-containing ER segment shown in **(C)**, rotated by 90 degrees around the y-axis to visualize the vesicle openings. **E:** 3D reconstruction of an ER-luminal vesicle in WNV-infected cells. An electron-dense structure assumed to correspond to viral RNA in the vesicle interior is shown in *red*. **F:** Membrane alterations induced by TBEV infection. The tomographic slice shows several vesicles in the ER lumen in close proximity to newly assembled virus particles residing in the same ER luminal compartment (*yellow arrowheads*). **G:** 3D surface rendering of the area in **(F)**, displaying TBEV-associated vesicles (*light yellow*) sharing the ER lumen with TBE virions (*dark red*) and surrounded by ER membranes (*light brown*). **H:** Single slices of tomograms showing DENV-induced vesicles as invaginations of the ER membrane (*white arrowheads*). Note the diffuse electron density at the cytosolic face of the vesicle openings and the tight apposition of vesicle openings to the opposing ER membrane containing a virus particle (*black arrowhead*). A 3D surface rendering of the ER/vesicle continuity (*yellow*) and the tightly apposed ER (*semitransparent*) containing a virus particle (*red*) are shown in the *right panel*. **(Panels (A–D)** and **(H)** were adapted from Welsch S, Miller S, Romero-Brey I, et al. Composition and three-dimensional architecture of the dengue virus replication and assembly sites. *Cell Host Microbe* 2009;5(4):365–375. Copyright © 2009 Elsevier. With permission. **Panel (E)** adapted from Gillespie LK, Hoenen A, Morgan G, et al. The endoplasmic reticulum provides the membrane platform for biogenesis of the flavivirus replication complex. *J Virol* 2010;84(20):10438–10447. doi: 10.1128/JVI.00986-10. With permission from American Society for Microbiology. **Panels (F)** and **(G)** adapted from Miorin L, Romero-Brey I, Maiuri P, et al. Three-dimensional architecture of tick-borne encephalitis virus replication sites and trafficking of the replicated RNA. *J Virol* 2013;87(11):6469–6481. doi: 10.1128/JVI.03456-12. With permission from American Society for Microbiology.)

cells, yet replicates comparably well in both cell types.[184] A third membrane structure found in infected cells is the "paracrystalline array," which appears to be a highly ordered form of CMs.[490]

While the overall 3D architecture of the flavivirus replication organelle is well established, surprisingly little is known about the mechanism underlying its biogenesis and the components involved. At least two viral proteins, NS4A and NS4B, appear to play critical roles in the formation of VPs.[415,634,782] Owing to their distinct membrane topology, both proteins should be capable of inducing negative membrane curvature. This property might be augmented by homo-oligomerization of the two viral proteins.[870,1039,1040] Interestingly, expression of NS4A lacking the carboxy-terminal 2K fragment induces the formation of cytoplasmic membrane alterations resembling CMs, whereas full-length NS4A containing the 2K fragment remains bound to the ER membrane but does not induce

membrane curvature.[634] Therefore, a regulated cleavage of the NS4A-2K-NS4B precursor appears to play a critical role in the formation of the replication organelle. However, the sole expression of NS4A or NS4B does not suffice to induce VP formation, arguing that additional viral components are required.

One likely component is NS1, which interacts with NS4A, NS4B, and the NS4A-2K-NS4B cleavage intermediate.[10,532,726,1010] In addition, NS1 binds to and remodels liposomes *in vitro* corroborating that this protein possesses membrane-altering properties.[10] Thus, NS1 is likely needed to induce VP formation. Moreover, by using a replication-independent expression system, NS1 was found to be essential for the formation of VPs.[726]

An additional viral component possibly contributing to replication organelle formation is NS2A, a small polytopic membrane protein. This protein can affect membrane permeability and might interact with the viral replicase complex as deduced from its enrichment at dsRNA-containing sites.[147,987] Based on these observations, a model for the biogenesis of VPs can be proposed in which NS4A and NS4B oligomers, perhaps supported by NS2A, induce negative curvature. This might be enhanced by NS1 binding to NS4A and NS4B from the luminal side of the ER membrane and inducing a positive curvature. Although an appealing model, firm proof requires a more detailed analysis of *cis*- and *trans*-acting factors involved in VP formation, including viral RNA that has been reported for other positive-strand RNA viruses to play a crucial role in VP/spherule formation.[243]

Induction of membrane curvature is an energetically unfavorable process that is facilitated by the insertion of lipids inducing membrane asymmetry and altering fluidity. In addition, assembly and functionality of membrane-resident macromolecular complexes are often enhanced by specific lipids such as cholesterol and sphingolipids, forming raft-like membrane microdomains. It is therefore not surprising that lipids play a central role for the flavivirus replication organelle. In infected cells, the lipid composition is very much altered.[164,611,708] For instance, ceramides, a family of lipids that are composed of sphingosine and a fatty acid, are increased in WNV-infected human cells and in DENV-infected mosquito cells.[592,708] Moreover, in the case of WNV, ceramides are redistributed to sites of replication. Of note, depletion of ceramide by extensive treatment with myriocin had opposing effects on these two flaviviruses, being suppressive in the case of WNV, but enhancing replication and virus production with DENV.[12] The sphingolipid biosynthetic pathway is also a critical factor for efficient DENV replication in the transmitting *Aedes aegypti* mosquito vector, but whether these lipids directly contribute to replication organelle formation or replicase activity, for example, by forming lipid rafts, is not known.[164] In any case, flavivirus replication is highly sensitive to inhibition or depletion of acetyl-CoA carboxylase and fatty acid synthase (FAS), key enzymes in the fatty acid biosynthetic pathway.[616] DENV NS3 interacts with FAS, thus recruiting this cellular enzyme to sites of virus replication and possibly promoting lipid biosynthesis for the sake of membrane expansion.[349,887] Along the same line, WNV increases the activity of 3-hydroxy-3-methylglutaryl-coenzyme A reductase (HMGCR), the rate-limiting enzyme in cholesterol biosynthesis, and alters subcellular distribution of cholesterol from the plasma membrane to replication organelles.[579] Also in the case of DENV, infection increases HMGCR activity and cholesterol accumulation at the ER, correlating with increased viral replication.[862] In addition, lipophagy, a type of selective autophagy that targets LDs, plays an important role in the DENV replication cycle. At early stages of infection, DENV induces autophagy and enhances autophagic flux, whereas later on, autophagosome–lysosome fusion and endolysosomal trafficking are suppressed.[606,621] This early elevated autophagosome formation appears to increase β-oxidation of lipids and ATP levels as well as turnover of triglycerides to promote viral replication.[350]

Apart from viral and host factors described above, several comprehensive screens and proteome analyses of viral proteins and complexes have identified candidate host cell factors promoting or restricting flavivirus replication or interacting with viral proteins.[672] It is likely that some of these factors contribute to replication organelle formation and the definition of their precise function will be an important future task.

RNA Replication

After the flavivirus genome is translated, the NS proteins must recruit the genome out of translation and into a replication complex. The mechanisms of this switch are not fully understood but likely involve genome cyclization, which favors RNA replication over translation.[538,941] Replication begins with the synthesis of a genome-length minus-strand RNA, which has been detected as early as 3 hours after infection[528]; minus strands then serve as templates for synthesizing new plus-strand genomes. Viral RNA synthesis is asymmetric, with approximately 10-fold more positive strands accumulating compared to minus strands.[172,528] Based on metabolic labeling, three major species of flavivirus RNAs have been described: the plus-strand genome, a double-stranded replicative form (RF), and a heterogeneous population of RI that most likely represent duplex regions and recently synthesized RNAs displaced by nascent strands undergoing elongation.[166,172] Pulse-chase analyses indicate that RF and RI are precursors to genome RNA, indicating semiconservative and asymmetric replication.[172]

In addition to genome-length products of RNA replication, 0.2 to 0.6 kb noncoding sfRNAs accumulate in infected cells.[523,930] sfRNAs are colinear with the 3′ end of the genome and are produced through stalled 5′ to 3′ degradation of the genome by the cellular 5′ exoribonuclease XRN1.[722] The XRN1 resistance of this region is due to conserved, pseudoknot structures located within the 3′ NCR, such that the RNA forms a tight, triple-helical "slip knot," making it difficult for enzymes like XRN1 to proceed in a 5′ to 3′ direction, but allowing enzymes like NS5 to proceed in a 3′ to 5′ direction (inset, Fig. 7.4A).[11,150,151,282] Mutant flaviviruses that do not produce sfRNAs are less cytopathic in cell culture and less pathogenic in mice; however, cytopathic effects were restored by supplying sfRNA in *trans*.[282,540,722] The accumulation of sfRNA has several proviral effects on host cells, including reduced XRN1 activity and dysregulated host mRNA turnover,[649] inhibited RIG-I activation,[588] reduced ISG expression,[81] and insensitivity to type I interferons.[821] While it may seem counterintuitive for a virus to employ a genome-destroying strategy for its own gain, flavivirus genomes are produced in vast excess; it is not yet clear whether a subset of nascent viral genomes are left uncapped to facilitate sfRNA formation.

Assembly and Release of Particles from Flavivirus-Infected Cells

Flavivirus particle assembly occurs in close association with intracellular membranes.[663] The assembly process is thought to commence by association of C protein dimers with genomic RNA, followed by budding into ER membranes containing the prM–E glycoprotein complex. As empty, preformed flavivirus capsids have never been observed, it is thought that nucleocapsid formation is tightly linked to envelopment. Immature virus particles pinch off into the ER lumen through noncanonical use of the ESCRT vesicle sorting and membrane scission machinery, with different component dependencies observed among flaviviruses.[881] Notably, the YFV NS3 protein interacts with Alix, which can recruit ESCRT III components.[135]

Electron tomography studies revealed that replication organelle pores are sometimes apposed to virus assembly sites, at least in the case of DENV and ZIKV, with clusters of virus particles being frequently observed in enlarged ER cisternae.[184,966] This close apposition of VPs and assembly sites provides a

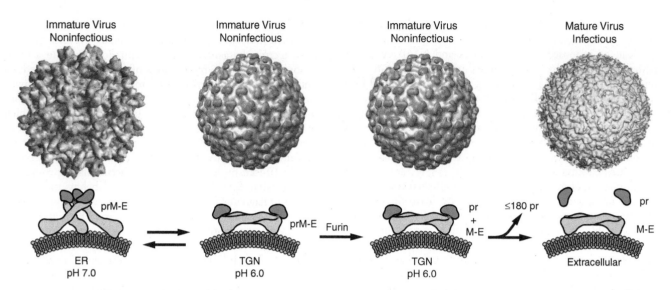

FIGURE 7.10 Flavivirus particle maturation. Nascent, noninfectious, immature particles undergo a pH-dependent conformational rearrangement of the viral glycoproteins E (*gray*) and prM (*blue*). Mature, infectious particles form upon furin cleavage of prM and release of the pr fragment. (Adapted from Perera and Kuhn[707] with permission from Elsevier Press.)

simple, yet so far largely hypothetical, explanation for the coupling of flavivirus replication and assembly.[421] Early in the replication cycle, when the amount of viral proteins, including C protein, are low, viral RNA released out of the vesicle interior might associate preferentially with ribosomes, thus promoting RNA translation. Newly produced viral proteins will enhance RNA replication, which in turn leads to an increase of viral proteins. Later in infection, when viral proteins accumulate to high abundance in the infected cell, *de novo* synthesized RNA might associate preferentially with the structural proteins, notably C protein, thus "competing" with ribosomes. In this way, viral RNA gets rapidly recruited into assembling virions that form by budding into the ER lumen in close vicinity to the vesicle pore, the presumed RNA exit site (Fig. 7.9H).

Following assembly, nascent virions are transported through the secretory pathway and released at the cell surface.[580] During transit through the reduced pH of the Golgi, immature particles undergo acid-induced prM–E rearrangement and prM cleavage (Fig. 7.10). Additional virion maturation steps occur during egress, including glycan modification of prM and E (for some flaviviruses) by trimming and terminal addition.[141,596] This implies that virions move through an exocytosis pathway similar to that used for host cell-surface glycoproteins and may traffic through recycling endosomes prior to release.[537] In at least one case, ZIKV was observed to be released in monolayer aggregate "sheets."[537]

HEPACIVIRUSES

Background and Classification

The existence of a novel blood-borne hepatitis virus, then called non-A, non-B hepatitis (NANBH), was first realized in the mid-1970s.[256,734] Early attempts to culture this agent proved to be frustrating and difficult to reproduce. It took another 14 years before HCV was formally identified through expression cloning of an immunoreactive cDNA from a NANBH-infected chimpanzee.[163] This discovery rapidly led to the development of

HCV diagnostics, which greatly reduced transmission through the blood supply.[462] Today, HCV is mainly transmitted via injection drug use, mother-to-infant care, and health care exposures and, infrequently, through sexual contact or unknown risk factors. Despite the recent development of highly effective HCV-specific direct-acting antivirals (DAAs), HCV currently infects 71 million people worldwide and remains a significant public health concern.[89] HCV causes chronic liver infections approximately 70% of the time, which can progress over decades to fibrosis, cirrhosis, and hepatocellular carcinoma (HCC). Despite slow disease progression, which can be accelerated by cofactors such as metabolic syndrome or alcohol consumption, mathematical models of HCV dynamics demonstrate robust replication in chronically infected individuals, with viral loads approximately 10^6 genomes per mL of serum, rapid viral clearance, and production of approximately 10^{12} virions per day.[706]

HCV is classified into seven genotypes, which differ from each other by greater than 30% at the nucleotide level.[664,859] These genotypes have distinct geographic distributions, disease progression, and susceptibility to some treatments. Intergenotypic recombinant HCV genomes, which presumably arise through coinfection, have been described.[203,400] The high level of sequence diversity between the HCV genotypes presents a formidable challenge for vaccine development.

Despite the lack of a vaccine, major advances in treatment have been made. The prior standard of care, pegylated interferon alpha and ribavirin, has been replaced by DAAs that have much higher cure rates with fewer side effects and shorter treatment durations. Effective DAA formulations typically combine at least two drugs targeting distinct HCV proteins. HCV drug development has culminated in the first pangenotypic DAAs, which cure more than 90% of HCV infections with each genotype.[257,271]

All genotypes of HCV are taxonomically classified as a single virus species, *Hepacivirus C*. For many years, HCV was the sole member of the *Hepacivirus* genus. The first non–HCV member of this genus, GB virus B (GBV-B; species name *Hepacivirus B*), was discovered in a human-derived, primate-passaged sample during a search for additional hepatitis viruses that ultimately led to the discovery of a related genus, the *Pegiviruses*. Recent advances in metagenomics have led to the discovery of a whole passel of additional *Hepaciviruses* (Table 7.1, Fig. 7.1A). The first of these was isolated from a canine with respiratory disease and was originally called canine hepacivirus. However, follow-up studies indicated that it is actually an equine virus causing acute and chronic hepatitis in horses; this virus has been renamed nonprimate hepacivirus (NPHV; species *Hepacivirus A*).[126,409] Several additional hepacivirus species have also been found, including several rodent hepaciviruses (RHV-E, species *Hepacivirus E*; RHV-F, species *Hepacivirus F*; NRHV1, species *Hepacivirus G*; NRHV2, species *Hepacivirus H*; RHV-I, species *Hepacivirus I*; RHV-J, species *Hepacivirus J*), bats (BHV-K, species *Hepacivirus K*; BHV-L, species *Hepacivirus L*), cows (BoHV, species *Hepacivirus M*), and colobus monkeys (guereza hepacivirus [GHV], species *Hepacivirus N*). Surprisingly, the closest relative to GBV-B is RHV-I, so the source of GBV-B in human- or primate-derived samples remains mysterious. Although it awaits official taxonomic classification, a hepaci-like virus has even been identified in the graceful shark, known as the Wenling shark virus (WLSV).[341]

Experimental Systems

Although HCV research was limited by the lack of replication systems for the first decade after its discovery, these challenges are now largely overcome. Once the correct 3′ end of the HCV genome was determined,[441,886] full-length HCV cDNAs were assembled, and synthetic transcripts were shown to be infectious by direct hepatic inoculation of chimpanzees in 1997.[440,995] These infectious cDNA clones were used to show that the viral enzymes, the p7 gene, and 3′ NCR are essential for HCV replication[442,797,996] and to study HCV immune response and viral evolution *in vivo*.[477] Unfortunately, RNAs from these clones failed to replicate in cultured cells.

The first useful cell culture system to study HCV replication was the genotype 1b (Con1) subgenomic replicon, developed in 1999.[549] The original replicons were bicistronic, wherein the HCV 5′ IRES promoted translation of the neomycin resistance gene and the encephalomyocarditis virus (EMCV) IRES promoted translation of the HCV NS2-5B or NS3-5B genes (see Fig. 7.12C). Upon transfection into the Huh-7 human hepatoma cell line, the first replicon RNAs replicated to low levels and transduced G418-resistance to rare HCV-supporting cells.[549] However, within these replicon-containing cell clones, HCV replicated to high levels. Based on the HCV sequences within surviving cell clones, cell culture–adaptive mutations were identified that increase transduction efficiency by up to 10,000-fold.[92,547] These efficient replicons enabled genetic, biochemical, and cell biological studies of intracellular stages in HCV replication and turbo-charged drug discovery efforts, but because the structural genes were not included, infectious virus particles were not produced. Surprisingly, full-length genomes containing these cell culture–adaptive mutations failed to produce infectious virions in cell culture and were attenuated *in vivo*, likely because these mutations enhance RNA replication but inhibited infectious virus production.[721]

The HCV pseudoparticle (HCVpp) system was developed to study viral entry. HCVpps are retrovirus particles displaying the HCV envelope glycoproteins, typically expressing a reporter gene to monitor viral entry and gene expression.[58,221,366] HCVpps reproduce many of the events in *bona fide* entry, such as receptor-dependent and clathrin-mediated endocytosis; however, significant differences between HCV and HCVpp entry exist.[139]

In 2003, a genotype 2a subgenomic replicon was identified that had the unusual feature of efficient cell culture replication without adaptive mutations.[411] This strain was isolated from a Japanese patient with fulminant hepatitis and was therefore named JFH-1. Full-length JFH-1 genomes produced the first infectious HCV in cell culture (HCVcc), albeit at relatively low levels.[945] High infectivity titers could be attained by passage and adaptation of JFH-1 or by engineering chimeric genomes with a related genotype 2a strain, HC-J6, that serendipitously encodes more efficient structural genes than the original JFH-1 strain.[529,719,1030] We now know that the efficiency of JFH-1 replication is due to optimal NS3 helicase and NS5B RNA polymerase activities, optimal 3′ NCR sequences, as well as a relative insensitivity of this strain to lipid peroxidation.[85,661,795,992] In the past several years, the variety of HCV replication systems has increased dramatically, including replicons for each genotype, infectious chimeric JFH-1 genomes that express structural genes from other genotypes, as well as infectious cell culture–adapted full-length clones for other genotypes.[747,1004] Infectious clones and replicon systems have also been developed for a number of nonhuman hepaciviruses.[199,200] Additionally, hepatoma cells that overexpress the cellular protein Sec14L2 were shown to support pangenotype HCV replication, including patient-derived virus.[795] Sec14L2, a carrier protein for vitamin E, enhances HCV replication most likely by reducing lipid peroxidation and protecting viral proteins from oxidative damage, to which they are sensitive.[992]

The chimpanzee is the only animal model that supports HCV replication, reproduces many clinical aspects of HCV infection, and is useful for studying HCV-specific immune responses and assessing drug efficacy.[477] However, due to ethical concerns, there is a moratorium on the experimental use of chimpanzees, which has increased the urgency for developing small animal models for HCV infection. Mice do not naturally support HCV entry or replication. One approach has been to partially deplete immunodeficient mice of hepatocytes and then engraft human hepatocytes to generate mice with chimeric livers.[87,615,622] The human hepatocytes within these chimeric livers support HCV infection; however, the utility of this model is limited by the immunocompromised nature of these mice. Immunocompromised mice engrafted with human hepatocytes and hematopoietic stem cells reconstitute both the hepatic and immune compartments and produce HCV-specific T-cell responses but do not support detectable viremia.[957]

Efforts to genetically humanize mice to make them permissive for HCV infection have provided incremental successes. Immunocompetent mice expressing the human HCV entry factors CD81 and occludin (OCLN) do support the early steps of HCV infection but greatly restrict viral replication.[216] HCV replication is improved by using mice genetically deficient in type I interferon signaling, suggesting that this pathway is critical in restricting viral replication.[215] An alternative approach has been to adapt HCV to use mouse host factors. HCV containing three mutations in the envelope glycoproteins can enter mouse hepatocytes *in vivo*; however, replication is not supported, suggesting additional incompatibilities.[943]

Given the challenges of studying HCV in immunocompetent mice, recent attention has turned to the related hepaciviruses that infect experimentally tractable animals. As the first non–HCV hepacivirus identified, GBV-B has been studied as a surrogate model system. It infects primary tamarin or marmoset hepatocytes[61,117,476] but replicates poorly in most immortalized cell lines.[122] Full-length GBV-B infectious clones have been assembled and produce hepatitis in tamarins, but not chimpanzees, suggesting that it does not infect apes, including humans.[124,591,807] More recently, *Hepacivirus G*, which naturally causes chronic infection in Norway rats, was found to cause acute infections in common laboratory mice and chronic infection in immunodeficient mice.[84,920] This model provides a powerful platform to evaluate strategies for hepacivirus vaccine development, recently confirming the role of vaccine-elicited CD4+ and CD8+ T cells in protecting rats from viral challenge.[342]

Structure and Physical Properties of the Virion

HCV particles derived from patients are heterogeneous in size, are 30 to 80 nm in diameter,[104,347,1018] and exhibit broad, unusually low buoyant densities of 1.03 to 1.10 g/mL.[105,359] Low-density virus particles have higher specific infectivity than high-density particles, suggesting that particle infectivity correlates with the degree of lipid association. HCVcc particles have relatively low specific infectivity (~1 infectious unit per 1,000 particles); most particles have a buoyant density of approximately 1.15 g/mL, while the peak infectivity is near 1.10 g/mL.[130,529,1030] The low specific infectivity of HCVcc particles likely reflects their physical properties when grown in Huh-7 cells, as specific infectivity improves upon passage in animals or primary hepatocyte cultures, but goes back down upon reculture.[530,728]

HCV particles are lipid enveloped, display an unknown number of viral envelope glycoproteins E1 and E2 on their surface, and contain a nucleocapsid composed of the core (C) protein and the viral RNA genome. A key feature of HCV particles is their propensity to associate with host-derived serum lipoproteins, which likely contribute to their low buoyant density.[25,676,735,912] HCV particles have similar lipid content as low-density lipoprotein (LDL) and very-low-density lipoprotein (VLDL) particles and associate with apolipoproteins, which are expressed on the surface of lipoproteins and function in their secretion and trafficking.[618] Serum-derived HCV associates with apolipoprotein AI (ApoAI), ApoB, ApoC1, and ApoE,[446,623,676,912] while HCVcc particles associate with ApoE and ApoC1.[146,618,623] ApoB is less consistently associated with HCVcc particles, leading to controversy about its role in HCV particle infectivity.[56] In any case, serum lipoproteins are thought to impact virion stability, enhance virus particle entry, and block antibody neutralization.[980] Because of their association with lipoproteins, HCV particles are sometimes referred to as "lipoviroparticles."[26,533] Although the structural basis for these interactions remain elusive, they may be mediated, at least in part, by interaction of ApoE (and possibly other apolipoproteins) with the E1–E2 envelope glycoprotein complex.[494] Proteomic analysis of purified HCVcc particles also identified other components, including the viral NS3 protein and several cellular proteins.[569]

Ultrastructural analyses of HCVcc or serum-derived HCV particles reveal pleiomorphic particles, 40 to 100 nm in diameter, lacking regularly discernible surface features (Fig. 7.11).[140,287,618,725,945] Due to this pleiomorphism, a key challenge has been to confirm that particle types observed through the microscope correspond to virus particles. In this regard, immunogold labeling has been used to identify the viral glycoproteins, ApoE, ApoAI, and occasionally ApoB, on the surface of putative HCVcc particles approximately 60 nm in diameter.[140,287,618,725] In one study, partial purification of HCVcc particles yielded two major particle classes.[287] One class, presumably infectious virus particles, were approximately 55 nm in diameter, contained a lipid bilayer and an electron-dense core and had a relatively smooth, featureless surface that reacted with E2- and ApoE-specific antibodies; the second class of particles, electron-dense structures approximately 45 nm in diameter, lack a lipid bilayer and are presumed to be naked nucleocapsids.[287] An independent study imaged tagged HCVcc particles directly capturing them on affinity matrices, revealing putative HCVcc particles of up to 85 nM in diameter.[140] A similar approach was taken to affinity capture serum-derived HCV particles, revealing pleiomorphic particles that range up to 150 nm in diameter, sparsely decorated on the surface with E2, ApoB, and ApoE.[725] Despite this progress, we still do not understand how HCV particles are organized, how the viral glycoproteins are arranged on the surface of virus particles, or the molecular basis of how HCV particles interact with serum lipoproteins.

Binding and Entry

The mechanisms of hepacivirus entry are best characterized for HCV; very little is known about the entry of non–HCV hepaciviruses. HCV enters its target hepatocyte via an unusually complex, dynamic process with distinct spatiotemporal steps. Blood-borne virus particles initially bind to the basolateral surface of hepatocytes via low-affinity interaction with GAGs[57,291] and possibly the LDL receptor (LDLR).[4,646] Virion-associated ApoE binds syndecans 1 and 4, core components of heparan sulfate proteoglycans, to enhance entry.[387,834] Following initial attachment, HCV entry requires coordination between several "early" host factors, including scavenger receptor class B type I (SCARB1),[808] CD81,[723] and EGFR on the basolateral surface,[567] and the "late" factors CLDN1; OCLN, which localizes to tight junctions; and the Niemann-Pick C1–like 1 (NPC1L1) cholesterol absorption receptor, which localizes to the apical surface.[245,727,796]

SCARB1, which is greatly enriched on hepatocytes, is normally involved in the uptake of cholesterol and phospholipids from serum lipoproteins. Because other HCV entry factors are expressed by multiple cell types, the liver-specific expression of SCARB1 might help to define the hepatotropism of HCV entry. The HCV E2 glycoprotein directly binds SCARB1 via its N-terminal hypervariable region 1 (HVR1).[808] As HVR1 occludes the CD81 binding site on E2, the interaction with SCARB1 may facilitate subsequent CD81 binding.[46] Consistent with this coordination, SCARB1- and CD81-specific antibodies inhibit HCV entry with similar postbinding kinetics.[405,1021] In addition to E2 binding, SCARB1's lipid transfer activity is involved in

HCV entry, perhaps by serving to reduce virus-associated lipoproteins.[192,1019] Interestingly, there appears to be some functional redundancy between SCARB1 and LDLR, such that SCARB1 is not essential for HCV infection when LDLR is expressed.[991]

As a tetraspanin, CD81 coordinates the interaction of multiple other proteins into larger complexes. During HCV entry, CD81 is thought to be an initial, postattachment, high-affinity receptor that directly interacts with E2 via its large extracellular loop.[357,713] CD81-bound virus particles are trafficked to tight junctions, where internalization occurs.[43,112] This trafficking requires EGFR and RAS signaling, as well as Rho GTPase activation and remodeling of cortical actin.[533] In addition to binding, CD81 has two other key functions in HCV entry. First, CD81 binding can induce conformational changes in the HCV glycoproteins, priming the virion for low pH-induced fusion.[830] Second, CD81 recruits the cytosolic serum response factor binding protein 1, which aids HCV entry by an unknown mechanism.[292]

Once HCV-CD81 complexes migrate to tight junctions, they colocalize with CLDN1 and OCLN, which are essential for HCV internalization.[533] Proper CLDN1 and OCLN localization and HCV entry depend on expression of E-cadherin and tumor-associated calcium signal transducer

2 (TACSTD2).[510,825] In the absence of CLDN1, some HCV isolates can use CLDN6 or CLDN9 for entry[332]; however, other strains require adaptive mutations in E1 in order to use alternate CLDNs, suggesting that E1 may mediate interaction with CLDNs.[363] In support of this finding, soluble E1–E2 specifically binds to CLDN1-expressing cells.[217] There is no evidence for direct binding of OCLN to HCV virion components.

The HCV-CD81-CLDN complex is internalized via clathrin-mediated endocytosis.[90,177,255,609] Interestingly, HCV endocytosis requires active EGFR signaling.[43] Once internalized, virus particles are delivered to early endosomes, where the low pH likely induces fusion.[366,922] HCV entry requires endosomal acidification, yet virus particles are resistant to low pH, indicating that during the initial steps of virus entry, perhaps via binding to one or more entry factors, a conformational change occurs that renders the virions pH sensitive. Available data suggest that this does not require proteolytic cleavage of the envelope glycoproteins but may involve isomerization of disulfides within the viral glycoproteins.[274] The mechanisms of HCV E1–E2 glycoprotein–mediated fusion are largely unknown.

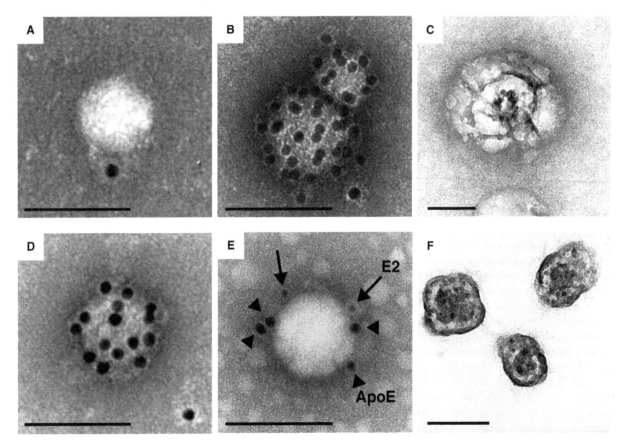

FIGURE 7.11 HCV particles. A: His-tagged HCVcc particles were affinity-captured on a Ni^{2+}-NTA–coated EM grid and immunogold labeled with antibodies specific for the HCV E2 glycoprotein. **B:** As in **panel (A)** but labeled with antibodies specific for ApoE. **C:** Human serum-derived HCV particles were affinity captured on the EM grid with the E2-antibody ARA3. **D:** As in **panel (B)** but labeled with antibodies specific for ApoA1. **E:** As in **panel (B)** but dual-labeled with antibodies specific for E2 and ApoE. **F:** Patient serum–derived HCV particles were affinity captured as in **(C)**. **(Panels (A, B, D)**, and **(E)** were adapted with permission from Catanese et al.[140]; **Panels (C)** and **(F)** were adapted with permission from Piver et al.[725] All scale bars, 100 nm.)

Genome Structure

Hepacivirus genomes are approximately 8.9 to 10.4 kb in length, with the HCV genome weighing in at approximately 9.6 kb, and lack 5′ caps or 3′ poly(A) tails. As for other members of the family, hepaciviruses encode single long ORFs (2,748–3,335 codons, with HCV at ~3,011 codons), flanked by highly conserved 5′ and 3′ NCRs (Fig. 7.11A). The HCV 5′ NCR is relatively compact, is 341 nt long, and folds into four major structural domains that have overlapping functions in both RNA translation and replication. The 5′ 125 nt serves as a minimal replication element,[278] although nearly the entire 5′ NCR (or the complementary 3′ end of the negative strand) contributes to the efficiency of RNA replication.[307,313] Domain I forms a 5′ SL that is dispensable for translation but essential for RNA replication; domains II and III function as an IRES to mediate cap-independent translation of the viral genome and also contain cryptic replication signals.[313,354] The 5′ NCRs of other hepaciviruses have similar overall organization but can range up to 445 nt in length, in the case of GBV-B. Despite this size difference, regions of the HCV and GBV-B 5′ NCRs can be functionally exchanged.[397,769,771]

The HCV 5′ NCR can bind two copies of the abundant, liver-specific microRNA (miR)-122, which regulates numerous hepatic mRNAs and is required for efficient viral replication.[395,502] One or two miR-122 binding sites are also found in similar genome locations of other hepaciviruses.[341] Numerous functions have been proposed for the HCV-miR-122 interaction, including translation of the viral genome, modulating the switch from RNA translation to RNA replication, or regulating RNA–protein or RNA–RNA interactions during replication.[803] One major effect of miR-122 binding is that it stabilizes HCV RNA from degradation.[575] In the absence of miR-122, the viral genome is processed by cellular triphosphatases DUSP11 and DOM3Z,[22,426] rendering a 5′ monophosphorylated genome that is sensitive to XRN 5′ to 3′ exonucleases.[508,824,841,909] Cells that lack DUSP11 support HCV infection in the absence of detectable miR-122, suggesting that miR-122 primarily acts to protect HCV RNA from degradation.[426] The HCV genome also acts as a miR-122 "sponge," causing derepression of cellular transcripts regulated by miR-122.[560] Small, miR-122–binding, locked nucleic acid "antagomirs" have shown antiviral efficacy in phase II clinical trials, leading to sustained virological responses in a subset of patients.[385]

The coding region of the HCV genome is extensively structured, containing several conserved RNA secondary structures, some of which have been shown to be critical for viral replication. For instance, nearly 90% of the core gene is base-paired into several discretely folding and interacting structures.[724] Mutations that disrupt these core-embedded structures, for example, SL588, can inhibit translation of viral RNA, RNA replication, or virus assembly.[607,724,936] However, since the HCV structural genes are dispensable for the replication of subgenomic replicons, these structural elements must function in concert with other structures. One structure in the NS4B-coding region, SL6038, can alternatively form a cloverleaf, which facilitates RNA replication, or a long SL, which inhibits RNA replication, suggesting that this region may act as a replication-mediating toggle.[724] Other RNA structures throughout the genome may serve to sequester UU/UA–rich sequences that are the preferred substrate of endoribonuclease RNaseL.[335,598]

The NS5B gene is particularly rich in functional RNA structures, including an essential *cis*-acting replication element (CRE), also termed 5BSL3.2.[1009] 5BSL3.2 can bind 40S ribosomal sub-

units[780] and also forms a critical long-distance base pairing with complementary sequences in the 3′ NCR (Fig. 7.12A).[277] This kissing-loop interaction, which influences translation, is competed by binding of the CRE to EWSR1, a cellular RNA-binding protein required for efficient HCV RNA replication.[682] Another loop within the CRE forms essential base pairing with a region approximately 200 nt upstream of the CRE.[211,925] The regions flanking the CRE also form competing long-distance base pairs with the CRE, as well as with the IRES region within the 5′ NCR.[780]

The HCV 3′ NCR consists of a ~40-nt, structured variable domain, a poly(U/UC) tract of at least 26 nt, and a highly conserved 98-nt 3′X domain.[441,677,886] The HCV 3′ NCR enhances translation of the viral genome, in part through binding of the poly(U/UC) region to the 40S ribosomal subunit, suggesting crosstalk between the 5′ and 3′ NCRs.[40] The 3′X domain, which may adopt configurations containing either two or three SLs,[275] is essential for both RNA replication and virus assembly.[276,833,996,1001,1008] In the two SL configuration, a dimer linkage sequence (DLS) within the upstream SL (Fig. 7.12A) can mediate genome dimerization, at least *in vitro*; it is unclear whether genome dimerization is functionally relevant, but it is enhanced by the HCV core protein.[186,382] In the three SL configuration, the middle SL interacts with 5BSL3.2 in the essential kissing-loop interaction.[277,677,832] This kissing interaction has been alternately reported to both enhance and inhibit translation, differences that may reflect specific reporter designs.[677] Nevertheless, these results further indicate cross talk between the 5′ and 3′ ends of the viral genome.

A number of studies have suggested that, similar to flaviviruses, the HCV genome can cyclize via long-distance base pairing between its 5′ and 3′ ends.[275,441,779] However, these predicted interactions have been difficult to validate given the complexity and density of functionally important RNA structures within these regions. Several cellular factors and complexes can bind to both the 5′ and 3′ ends, likely impacting such cross talk. These include RNA-binding proteins PCBP2, IGF2BP1, PTB/hnRNPL, and NF90/45.[677] Other factors bind specifically to the HCV 3′ NCR, including hnRNPC, GAPDH, and HuR.[514]

Among other hepaciviruses, the GBV-B 3′ NCR contains a short poly(U) tract followed by a unique 309-nt sequence.[124,806] Although this region lacks sequence homology to HCV, the terminal 82 nt is structurally similar to the HCV 3′X region. The NHPV 3′ NCR is also larger (~318 nt) than that of HCV and contains a short poly(A) tract, a variable region, a poly(U/UC) tract, a conserved structured region, a long poly(U) tract, and a conserved 3′X–like region.[811]

Translation and Proteolytic Processing

Hepaciviruses encode the prototype class IV IRES element,[593] which utilizes RNA structures to functionally replace a subset of translation initiation factors and drive cap-independent translation from a prepositioned AUG, that is, without scanning. Specifically, HCV IRES domains II, IIId to IIIf, and IV directly bind the 40S ribosome (Fig. 7.12A inset). The affinity of this interaction is largely driven by specific contacts between domains IIId to IIIf and the ES7 region of 18S rRNA.[744] Meanwhile, domain II forms an L-shaped structure that binds across the 40S subunit, reaching into the ribosomal intersubunit space to interact with the ribosomal E site, positioning the AUG within the P site, and inducing a conformational shift in the 40S subunit that helps to recruit the 60S subunit,[263,264,863] In addition, domain IIIb independently binds eIF3, thereby

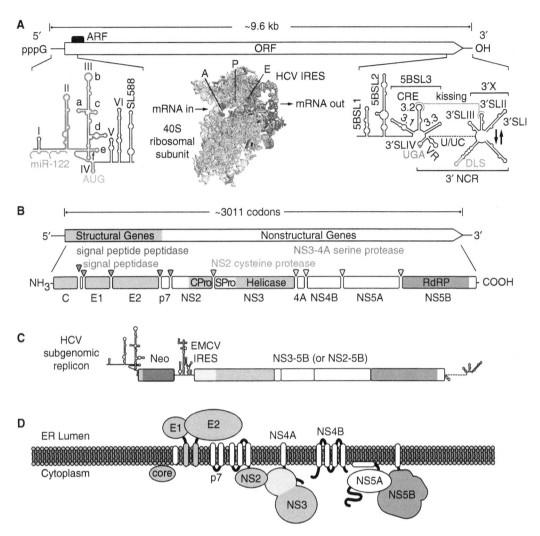

FIGURE 7.12 Hepacivirus genome structure and protein expression. A: HCV genome structure and RNA elements. Important RNA elements are indicated as in Figure 7.4. Two binding sites of miR-122 are indicated in *orange*; the ARF is indicated by a *black box*; the initiation (AUG) and termination (UGA) codons are indicated; and parts of the HCV IRES are color coded for interpretation of the inset, which shows the HCV IRES-40S human ribosomal subunit viewed from the perspective of an incoming 60S subunit and captured by cryo-EM at 3.9 Å resolution, as rendered from PDB 5A2Q.[744] For simplicity, the 18S rRNA is colored *white*, ribosomal proteins are colored *wheat*. The 18S rRNA residues nearest the tRNA anticodon are labeled within the ribosomal acceptor (A), peptidyl (P), and exit (E) sites. **B:** Polyprotein processing and cleavage products. Cleavage sites are indicated as in Figure 7.4 except the NS2/NS3 cleavage, which is mediated by the NS2 cysteine autoprotease. **C:** The design of the original G418-selectable HCV subgenomic replicon is illustrated. **D:** Polyprotein membrane topology. See the legend of Figure 7.4 for symbol definitions and the text for further details.

bypassing a requirement for the eIF4F 5′ cap-binding complex.[181,690,711,854,863] Recruitment of eIF2·GTP·Met-tRNA_i then forms a 48S preinitiation complex.[384,386,690] Upon 60S ribosomal joining, eIF2 hydrolyzes GTP, resulting in the dissociation of the initiation complex and producing an active 80S ribosome in which the initiating AUG codon is positioned within the ribosomal P site.[386,690,711] SLV and SLIV in the core-coding region also play important but unknown roles in translation initiation.[936] In addition to this canonical pathway, the HCV IRES can utilize alternative mechanisms to initiate translation under stress conditions.[475,905] For instance, when eIF2 is phosphorylated by the innate immune sensor kinase PKR, eIF5B can

recruit Met-tRNA_i, enabling translation initiation despite inactive eIF2. A number of cellular factors are reported to modulate HCV IRES activity, including miR-122 and RNA-binding proteins La, PSMA7, nucleolin, PCBP1, PCBP2, and PTB.[514]

Translation of the HCV genome produces a large (~3,011 aa) polyprotein that is cleaved by viral and host proteases to produce 10 viral proteins (Fig. 7.12B); these include the structural proteins core (C) and envelope glycoproteins E1 and E2, as well as the NS proteins p7, NS2, NS3, NS4A, NS4B, NS5A, and NS5B. The C/E1, E1/E2, E2/p7, and p7/NS2 junctions are cleaved by host signal peptidase, while the C-terminus of C is further processed by signal peptide peptidase (SPP) to remove the E1 signal peptide and generate mature C protein. NS2 contains a cysteine protease domain that cleaves the NS2/3 junction, while NS3-4A encodes a serine protease that cleaves all downstream NS junctions (Fig. 7.12B).

In addition to the large ORF, small alternative reading frame proteins (ARFPs) may be produced from a +1 reading frame located within the C gene. Different ARFP forms have been described, including ARFP/F (frameshift), ARFP/DF (double frameshift), or ARFP/S (short form). However, detection of these products varies greatly between HCV isolates and laboratories.[106] Evidence in support of ARFP expression include detection of protein products with ARFP-specific antibodies as well as the detection of ARFP-specific immune responses in HCV-infected patients. While it has been assumed that these products are produced via ribosomal frameshifting, alternate translational initiation sites may also be involved.[106] It is unclear what role ARFP expression plays in the virus life cycle. In addition, small amounts of an approximately 8-kDa "minicore" protein are reportedly expressed via initiation of translation at codon approximately 90 within the main ORF.[239] Given the mechanism of HCV IRES activity, it is unclear how the minicore start codon is recognized.

Features of the Structural Proteins

Core (C) Protein

C is a conserved, α-helix–rich RNA-binding protein that encapsidates the HCV genome within virus particles. While C lacks a well-defined structure, it does contain three functionally distinct domains. Domain I is approximately 120 aa in length, enriched in basic residues, binds structured RNAs, and is capable of forming nucleocapsid-like complexes in vitro.[461] Domain II is smaller, is approximately 55 aa, and forms two amphipathic helices that, together with palmitoylation at residue Cys 172, mediate peripheral membrane interaction.[100,583] Domain III is a transmembrane region that acts as a signal peptide for translocation of E1 into the ER; this region is only found on the 191-aa immature form of capsid because, following signal peptidase cleavage of the C/E1 junction, it is removed from mature core via SPP cleavage between residues 177 and 178.[569,686]

C forms native homodimers[102,558] that can be stabilized by disulfide bonding[463] and/or trans-glutamination.[558] C dimers also form higher-order, capsid-like structures in vitro.[428,461] These homotypic interactions may also mediate interaction with the E1 glycoprotein in cells,[543,667] although C does not appear to form preformed capsids prior to virus assembly. Domain II also contains a highly conserved YXXø motif that interacts with AP2M1 and is required for virion assembly.[674]

The peripheral membrane association of C allows it to traffic to ER-associated LDs,[47,100,605,652] where virus particles' assembly is thought to occur.[638,831] Trafficking of C to LDs requires the cytosolic phospholipase A2 and is enhanced by DGAT-1, an ER-resident enzyme that catalyzes triglyceride synthesis.[355,614] C also alters the size, distribution, and protein composition of LDs, in part by inhibiting adipose triglyceride lipase and causing lipid accumulation.[99,134,206] In humans, this accumulation likely contributes to hepatic steatosis that occurs during chronic HCV infection, particularly with genotype 3 viruses.[776] Mutations in C that disrupt LD trafficking greatly inhibit virus assembly,[101] although it is unclear why HCV prefers that C traffic to LDs. One possibility is that it serves to sequester C away from sites of viral translation and genome

replication, yet easily accessible for virus assembly. Indeed, C protein has been reported to both enhance and inhibit HCV IRES–mediated translation.[95,842]

In addition to the posttranslational modifications mentioned above, C can be phosphorylated by protein kinases A and C, which can alter C localization and down-regulates the ability of C to inhibit the replication of hepatitis B virus.[557,838] Furthermore, C has been reported to manipulate numerous cellular pathways, including signal transduction pathways, transcriptional control, apoptosis, and cellular transformation.[604,903]

Envelope Glycoproteins

Hepacivirus glycoproteins show limited but significant interspecies conservation,[745] with the HCV glycoproteins being the best characterized. HCV E1 (~30 kDa) and E2 (~70 kDa) are highly glycosylated type I transmembrane proteins that mediate virus attachment and membrane fusion. Each has a large lumenal domain and a single C-terminal transmembrane domain.[224,227,787] To generate this topology, both transmembrane regions contain charged residues, driving the formation of intramembrane hairpin structures during glycoprotein translocation.[688] Following signal peptidase cleavage, the lumenal C-termini reorient to face the cytoplasm, yielding tandem proteins each with a single-membrane anchor.[176] The transmembrane domains of E1 and E2 interact, contributing to heterodimerization, and also act as an ER retention signal of the E1–E2 complex.[168,169,252,688]

During folding in the ER, HCV E1–E2 heterodimer formation is slow and interdependent,[113,632,696] requiring the ER chaperone calnexin.[225] In addition to the transmembrane domains, heterodimerization involves interactions between the E1 and E2 ectodomains,[1002] as well as the membrane-proximal region of E2.[222] Although ER-localized E1 and E2 interact noncovalently, they form large covalent complexes stabilized by disulfide bonds in purified virions.[939] These linkages may contribute to the acid resistance of virus particles[922] and suggest that virus maturation may require disulfide bond isomerization. Analysis of virion-associated glycoproteins also indicates that E1 drives trimerization of E1–E2 heterodimers.[252]

The structures of E1 and E2 are not fully known, but it is clear that they have unique folds and do not resemble other known fusion proteins, including the corresponding flavivirus and pestivirus envelope glycoproteins. HCV E1 consists of four functional regions, including an ~80-aa N-terminal domain, a putative fusion peptide, an ~30-aa conserved region, and a C-terminal transmembrane domain (Fig. 7.13A). Crystallization of the N-terminal domain revealed a network of covalently linked homodimers with an intermolecular disulfide bridge (Fig. 7.13B).[234] Consistent with this, E1 can form stable trimers on HCVcc particles.[252] Mutations in the N-terminal domain influence the fidelity of virion assembly and CLDN specificity during entry,[330] consistent with the observation that mutations in E1 can influence CLDN utilization.[363] Intriguingly, the N-terminal domain has distant structural similarity to phosphatidylcholine transfer protein, which transfers phosphatidylcholine between membranes.[234] Given the complicated relationship(s) between HCV particles and lipids, it will be interesting to determine whether this observation is functionally relevant to the mechanisms of viral assembly and/or entry. Mutations in the putative fusion peptide inhibit E1–E2 heterodimerization and HCVcc assembly[657] and lead to

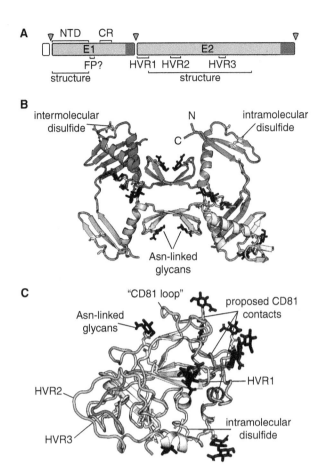

FIGURE 7.13 HCV glycoprotein structures. A: A map of the HCV E1–E2 glycoproteins is illustrated, showing the locations of the E1 N-terminal domain (NTD), putative fusion peptide (FP?), and conserved region (CR); the E2 hypervariable regions (HVRs) 1, 2, and 3 are shown. The cleavage sites for signal peptidase are shown, as in Figure 7.12. The regions for which structures are available are indicated; the C-terminal transmembrane domains are indicated with *dark purple*. **B:** Structure of the E1 N-terminal domain is shown, forming a disulfide-linked multimer. Four full N-terminal chains are shown in *purple*, *blue*, *green*, and *orange*; two partial chains within the asymmetric unit are shown in *pale yellow* and *red*; intramolecular and intermolecular disulfide bonds are shown in *yellow* and *green*, respectively. The view is looking down on the surface of the molecule, with N-linked glycans (*black*) pointing up from the page, as rendered from PDB 4UOI.[234] **C:** Structure of the partial E2 ectodomain is shown, highlighting spatial arrangement of the HVRs and CD81 loop around a compact globular core. Intramolecular disulfide bonds are indicated in *yellow*. The location of residues that, when mutated, disrupt CD81 interaction are shown in *orange*. The view is looking down on the surface of the molecule, with N-linked glycans (*black*) pointing up from the page, as rendered from PDB 6MEI.[269]

production of noninfectious HCVpp.[220] The function of the membrane-proximal conserved region is poorly understood. Mutations in this region primarily affect entry and the sensitivity of entry to CLDN1- and SCARB1-specific antibodies, suggesting possible interaction with these receptors.[657]

E2 is the HCV attachment protein, directly binding to CD81 and SCARB1 on target cells, and the major neutralizing antigen displayed on the surface of virus particles.[723,808] Structures of a minimal E2 "core" domain[419,444] or near–full-length E2

ectodomains[269] reveal a central β-sheet–rich, C2-set (e.g., CD2) immunoglobulin–like fold containing a hydrophobic core stabilized by intramolecular disulfide bridges and surrounded by extensive flexible loops, including three HVRs (Fig. 7.13C). This multifaceted structure presents distinct interaction surfaces, including the Ig-like β-sandwich, a conserved CD81-binding loop that projects from the β-sandwich, a glycan-rich "front" that is conformationally flexible, and a back surface. While the CD81-binding loop is the primary determinant of interaction with this receptor, CD81 actually interacts with a much larger conformationally defined surface on E2, including parts of the front layer and a major epitope, termed antigenic site 412.[269,419,444] Thus, the CD81-binding surface of E2 is a major target for broadly neutralizing antibodies.[339,489,926,935] As mentioned, HVR1 partially protects the CD81-binding region from neutralizing antibodies.[46,808] Thus, HVR1-specific antibodies can also neutralize virus infectivity[412,963] and protect chimpanzees from homologous challenge[254]; early induction of HVR1-specific antibodies also correlates with viral clearance in humans.[17,1035] Based on this immunologic selection pressure, HVR1 exhibits a high level of sequence variability even within individual patients.[253,601,647,964]

While the structure of the E1–E2 complex has not yet been experimentally determined, a computational model of this complex has been proposed, partially based on the existing E1 and E2 structures, mutational analysis, and immunoreactivity profiling.[137] This model predicts that E1–E2 forms a compact structure held together by an intermolecular disulfide bond. Clearly, solving the structure of the E1–E2 complex is a high priority for understanding the mechanisms of HCV entry and antibody-mediated neutralization.

Features of the Nonstructural Proteins

p7/p13 Proteins

The HCV p7 protein is a small (~7 kDa), 63-aa polytopic membrane protein with ion channel activity, often called a "viroporin."[316,559,648,702,732] While p7 is dispensable for RNA replication,[549] it plays important roles in virus particle assembly, virus particle release, and antagonism of type I interferons. Signal peptidase cleavage of E2–p7 and p7–NS2 are somewhat inefficient, leading to the accumulation of proteolytic processing intermediates, especially E2–p7, which may impose an inverted topology on p7.[375,525,640,720,826] The N-terminal α-helix of p7 is a major determinant of E2–p7 cleavage efficiency,[823] which in turn influences virus particle assembly.[205]

Structurally, p7 is predicted to contain two transmembrane domains, forming a membrane-bound hairpin with N- and C-termini that face the ER lumen, separated by a short, basic, cytoplasmic loop (Fig. 7.14A).[136] However, it is unlikely that p7 remains as a monomer and more likely that it functions through homo- and heterotypic interactions. Most notably, p7 ion channel activity requires homo-oligomerization.[581] EM and single particle reconstruction of p7 hexamers in detergent micelles revealed a flower-shaped oligomer with six petals protruding from a conical base (Fig. 7.14B).[559] However, the 16 Å resolution achieved was too low to definitively fit p7 monomers within this structure. Currently, two competing structural models of hexameric p7 have been proposed based on additional EM and NMR measurements of different HCV p7 proteins in various membrane-mimetic environments.[559,581,691] In one model, p7 hairpins interact with neighboring p7 hairpins

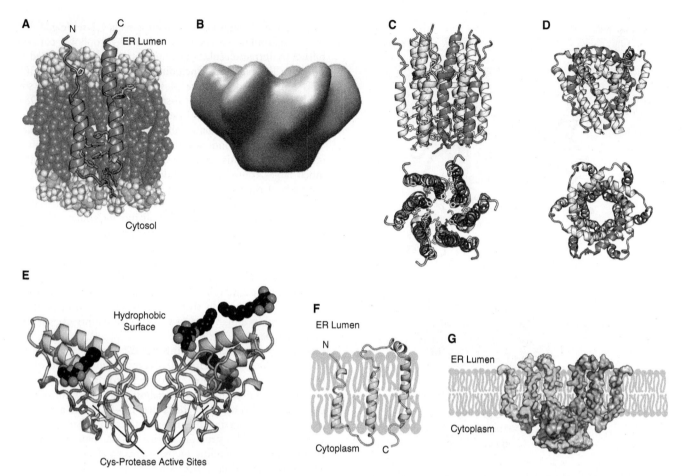

FIGURE 7.14 Structure of the HCV p7 and NS2 proteins. A: Model of the p7 monomer in a lipid bilayer.[648] Functionally important, conserved residues His 17 (*green*); Lys 33 and Arg 35 (*magenta*); Pro 58 (*yellow*); and Phe 26, Trp 30, Tyr 42, and Tyr 45 (*slate*) are shown. NMR coordinates and membrane modeling kindly provided by R. Montserret and F. Penin. **B:** EM reconstruction of a hexameric p7 conical flower, as rendered from EMD-1661.[559] **C:** The pinwheel model of a p7 hexamer as viewed from the side or from the ER lumen. Modeling coordinates kindly provided by R. Montserret and F. Penin. **D:** The conical flower model of a p7 hexamer as viewed from the side or from the ER lumen. Rendered from PDB 2M6X.[691] **E:** The dimeric NS2 cysteine protease domain. Monomeric subunits are colored *green* and *blue*; active site residues, *red*; C-terminal residues, *yellow*; cocrystallized detergent molecules are shown as *spheres*. Rendered from PDB 2HD0.[553] **F:** Model of NS2 TM domains, based on NMR data.[389] **G:** A model of the full-length NS2, based on the models presented in **(E)** and **(F)**.

around a common axis, much like a pinwheel (Fig. 7.14C).[559] In the other model, each p7 extends through the plane of the membrane to intercalate with all five other subunits to form a conical pore (Fig. 7.14D).[691] While this latter model can nicely account for the flower-like electron density observed via EM, it requires a more rigid structure that seems inconsistent with other considerations. For instance, molecular dynamics simulations predict that p7 can form structurally plastic, minimalist ion channels through multiple oligomeric configurations, and indeed p7 oligomers containing 4, 5, and 7 subunits have also been described.[144,170]

HCV p7 is essential for virus assembly in cell culture and for infectivity *in vivo*.[392,797,869] During virus particle assembly, p7 mediates critical interactions with NS2 and the viral glycoproteins.[97,389,571,938] There is also evidence that delayed E2-p7 cleavage allows for the N-terminus of p7 to be (at least transiently) cytosolic, where it may mediate interactions between NS2 and NS5A.[205] Indeed, genetic interactions link p7 and NS5A during virus assembly,[813] and additional genetic interac-

tions link p7 and NS5B in influencing the lipid composition and infectivity of virus particles.[16]

During HCV particle secretion, p7 has a critical role as a cation-selective, class IIa viroporin, modulating proton conductance to neutralize pH gradients in the secretory pathway, which may prevent premature acid-induced fusion of the viral glycoproteins.[979] In keeping with this model, the influenza A virus M2 viroporin can partially complement HCV mutants lacking p7 ion channel activity.[69,979] Two highly conserved basic residues located in the central cytosolic loop are required for p7 ion channel activity in vitro and for HCV infectivity *in vivo*.[317,797] Furthermore, inhibitors of p7 ion channel activity reduce virus particle release.[581]

In addition to its essential roles in virus assembly and release, p7 also has anti-inflammatory activities. Specifically, HCV p7 binds to the interferon γ-inducible DNA-binding protein IFI-16 and can prevent IFI-16 activation by modulating mitochondria membrane potentials, thereby subverting activation of the type I interferon system.[741] HCV p7 can also enhance cellular SOCS3 expression in a JAK/STAT- and MAPK-dependent manner, thereby reducing cellular response to TNF-α.[183]

Similar p7-like proteins are found in other hepaciviruses, although they can vary considerably in size. The largest and best characterized of these is the GBV-B p13 protein (~13 kDa), which has partial homology to HCV p7.[293] GBV-B p13 gene can be functionally replaced by HCV p7.[318] p13 is predicted to span the membrane four times and can be processed by signal peptidase into two tandem p7-like proteins.[293,884] The functional significance of the first half of p13 is unclear, since only the second half of p13, which has greater similarity to the HCV p7 gene, is required for infectivity in tamarins.[884]

NS2 Protein

NS2 (~23 kDa) is a polytopic membrane protein with cysteine protease activity and a key regulator of virus particle assembly.[312,358,553,820] NS2 contains three N-terminal transmembrane segments followed by a C-terminal cysteine protease domain.[388,389] The only known substrate of the NS2 protease is the NS2/3 junction, and NS2 is often referred to as an autoprotease.[312,358,553] NS2 has intrinsic protease activity[98] that can be stimulated by the N-terminal zinc–binding domain of NS3 and a conserved hydrophobic surface patch in the protease domain of NS3.[312,358,377,820] Mutation of this surface prevents RNA replication and NS5A hyperphosphorylation, suggesting that NS2-3 cleavage precedes functional replicase assembly.[377]

A crystal structure of the HCV NS2 catalytic domain revealed a homodimeric cysteine protease with two composite active sites (Fig. 7.14E–G).[553] One monomer contributes catalytic histidine and glutamate residues to each active site, with the nucleophilic cysteine supplied by the other monomer. This structure is supported by mutagenesis studies wherein HCV NS2 protease mutants can be complemented in *trans*, a feature that is conserved among other hepaciviruses.[98,312,756] The C-terminus of NS2 occludes the substrate-binding groove, suggesting that this protease is inactive following cleavage.

NS2 has several noncatalytic functions in HCV assembly and egress. It is a central organizer of virion assembly, coordinating interactions with E1–E2, p7, NS3–NS4A, NS5A, and host factors involved in virus assembly.[97,389,423,571,715,731,865] For instance, the interaction of NS2 with NS3–4A is critical for trafficking of C from the surface of LDs into nucleocapsids.[178,185] NS2 also interacts with E2 and signal peptidase complex subunit 1,[879] perhaps to facilitate E2-p7 cleavage required for virus assembly. In addition to its role as a matchmaker, bringing together virion components, NS2 also mediates envelopment. Specifically, the MARCH8 E3 ligase K63-polyubiquitylates NS2, which then recruits HGS, a component of the ESCRT0 pathway, to facilitate fission.[50,455] Finally, NS2 helps to mediate virus trafficking and release through interaction with the secretory vesicle coat adaptor complex proteins AP-1 and AP-4.[986] Consistent with this, some NS2 mutants display late, post-Golgi defects in virus particle egress.[197,587]

NS3 Protein

HCV NS3 is a large (~70 kDa) multifunctional protein, containing an N-terminal serine protease domain and a C-terminal RNA helicase/NTPase domain.[655] These enzyme activities play essential roles in virus gene expression, RNA replication, virus

particle assembly, and subversion of host innate defenses. The serine protease, in particular, was the first HCV protein successfully targeted via DAA development.[471] While the first generation of HCV serine protease inhibitors were generally genotype specific and resistance arose with low fitness barriers, newer third-generation protease inhibitors are effective tools in combating HCV replication without these caveats.[670]

NS3 belongs to the chymotrypsin-like superfamily of serine proteases. Structurally, it is composed of two β-barrels flanked by α-helices, with the central peptide of NS4A contributing one strand to one of the β-barrels (reviewed in Ref.[655]). Thus, NS4A is an essential cofactor of the serine protease.[52,248,526] The protease domain also has a Zn^{2+} coordination motif,[555] which has a structural role in protein folding, as well as an N-terminal amphipathic helix,[108] which contributes to the membrane association of the NS3-4A complex. The serine protease active site is composed of residues His 57, Asp 81, and Ser 139, surrounding a shallow substrate-binding surface located between the two β-barrels.[655] Cleavage sites within the HCV polyprotein have the consensus sequence (Asp/Glu)XXXX(Cys/Thr)/(Ser/Ala),[55] which is conserved among other hepaciviruses. In order to form the serine protease, NS3 must first cleave the NS3/4A junction in *cis*, before it can cleave the NS4A/4B, NS4B/5A, and NS5A/5B junctions in *cis* or in *trans*. The preferred order of cleavage is NS5A/5B > NS4A/4B > NS4B/5A.[655,868] Interestingly, the structure of a single-chain, full-length NS3 shows the C-terminus coordinated by the serine protease, as would be expected from the NS3-4A *cis*-cleavage reaction (Fig. 7.7).[998]

In addition to the canonical cleavage sites within the polyprotein, HCV NS3-4A also mediates internal cleavages within NS3, NS4B, and NS5A although the functional relevance of these cleavages are not yet known.[655] Many additional peptide sequences can also be cleaved by NS3-4A.[53,712,845] Given this low substrate specificity, it is unsurprising that NS3-4A has evolved to cleave cellular proteins of functional relevance, including MAVS, TRIF, PTPN2, TC-PTP, GPx8, DBB1, and Neuregulin 1.[402,654,655,822] MAVS is a mitochondrial membrane protein that transduces signals from cytoplasmic RNA sensors RIG-I and MDA5 to activate IRF3 and subsequent ISG expression. Several studies have demonstrated that NS3-4A cleavage removes MAVS from the mitochondria and attenuates ISG induction. In addition, HCV might also target TRIF, an adaptor molecule involved in the toll-like receptor 3 signaling, which senses endosomal dsRNA to initiate antiviral signaling. Thus, cleavage of MAVS and eventually TRIF serves to subvert innate antiviral defenses.[505,511,630]

Similar to other *Flaviviridae*, the C-terminal domain of hepacivirus NS3 proteins encode a superfamily 2 RNA helicase/NTPase. These enzymes are motor proteins, utilizing the energy derived from NTP hydrolysis to translocate along one strand of a nucleic acid substrate; if the substrate is double-stranded, this translocation leads to strand displacement and unwinding.[739]

Structurally, the HCV helicase domain contains two RecA-like subdomains, which bind and hydrolyze NTPs at their interface, as well as a third α-helix–rich subdomain. Nucleic acid substrates are bound in a cleft formed between the two RecA-like subdomains and subdomain 3.[425] NS3 can unwind RNA and DNA homo- and heteroduplexes by binding to an unpaired region of a template strand and translocating in a 3′ to 5′ direction, unwinding one base pair for each ATP hydrolyzed.[29,324,328]

Helicase activity and substrate recognition are stimulated by the NS3 serine protease domain and NS4A, and the helicase in turn stimulates NS3-4A serine protease activity.[70–72] Thus, the essential enzymatic activities of NS3-4A are tightly coordinated. Helicase activity can also be up-regulated by NS5B, presumably through interactions with the serine protease domain.[1022] Likewise, the NS3 helicase activity enhances NS5B RdRP activity.[717] NS3-4A helicase activity is also down-regulated by the cellular arginine methyltransferase PRMT1, which methylates residues within the NTPase active site.[226,763]

Although the precise roles of the NS3 helicase are not fully understood, the NTPase and helicase activities are essential for HCV replication and viral infectivity,[442,470] and the helicase domain has been implicated in virus particle assembly.[391,574,715] Furthermore, the NS3 helicase activity is required in *cis* for RNA replication, suggesting that it functions on the RNA from which it was translated; that is, it may play a role in recruiting RNA from translation into RNA replication.[416]

The nonenzymatic regions of NS3 have also been implicated in HCV particle assembly. A mutation in the N-terminal amphipathic helix enhances transfer of C protein from LDs to the ER, thereby increasing the efficiency of virus assembly.[994] Furthermore, mutations in the peptide linker that connects the protease and helicase domains selectively inhibit assembly without impacting enzymatic function, suggesting potential protein–protein interactions.[439] A likely candidate is NS2 that, via interaction with the NS3 protease domain, could bring together the replicase and the NS2-associated envelope glycoprotein complex.

NS4A and NS4B Proteins

NS4A (~7 kDa) is a small 54-aa protein with multiple functions. Its N-terminal transmembrane domain anchors NS3-4A to the ER and promotes NS4A dimerization, which is important for RNA replication and virus particle assembly.[438] As mentioned above, the central region of NS4A facilitates proper folding of the NS3 serine protease domain, thereby acting as a cofactor for serine protease activity. The acidic C-terminal domain of NS4A stimulates NS3 NTPase/helicase activity,[70] NS5A phosphorylation,[401,434,531] RNA replication,[531,662] and virus particle assembly.[662,716,774] NS4A also physically interacts with NS2, NS4B, NS5A, and uncleaved NS4B-5A.[32,527]

NS4B (~27 kDa) is an integral membrane protein with cytosolic N- and C-terminal regions flanking four transmembrane domains.[310] The N-terminal cytosolic region encodes two amphipathic helices, the second of which can insert in the membrane, thereby inverting the topology of the first helix.[310,561] NS4B helix insertion into the ER leaflet is likely to generate positive membrane curvature, which may contribute to forming the HCV replication organelle.[309] The C-terminus of NS4B also encodes two α-helices, the second of which is membrane-associated.[308] A key feature of NS4B is that it oligomerizes and plays a central role in organizing the membrane-bound replication complex.[311,700,1014] For instance, expression of NS4B is sufficient to induce membrane rearrangements resembling RNA replication compartments,[230,303] although other NS proteins (especially NS5A) are required for the formation of *bona fide* "membranous web" structures.[778] NS4B also binds to the cellular SAR1B GTP exchange factor, PREB, which is involved in COPII vesicle biogenesis and influences membranous web formation.[443] Cell culture–adaptive mutations have

been mapped to NS4B (reviewed in Ref.[55]) and NS4B has been genetically linked to virion assembly.[309,393]

In addition to its role in rearranging cellular membranes, NS4B also inhibits innate immune signaling. Specifically, it binds to the innate immune adaptor STING, preventing its interaction with TBK1 and subsequent ISG induction.[209,678] NS4B also induces TRIF degradation in a caspase 8–dependent manner.[516]

NS5A Protein

NS5A (~56–58 kDa) is a homodimeric phosphoprotein that plays multiple roles in the viral life cycle. NS5A is a multidomain protein that contains an N-terminal Zn^{2+}–binding domain I (DI), a central conserved domain II (DII), and a C-terminal variable domain III (DIII); these domains are separated by two short linkers of low-complexity sequence (LCS), as illustrated in Figure 7.15A.[900] The N-terminus of DI contains an amphipathic α-helix that mediates peripheral membrane association and LD localization.[109,235,705] The remainder of DI has been crystallized into two major homodimeric conformations. In one conformation, DI dimers form a claw-like structure containing a positively charged groove, which is postulated to bind RNA (Fig. 7.15B, C).[901] In the other conformation, two DI monomers bind along their length, forming a barrel-shaped dimeric structure (Fig. 7.15D).[554] Both dimer conformations bury extensive surface area (~1,000 Å[2]) and contain well-conserved residues at their interface, and mutations at these interfaces support the functional relevance of both dimer models in HCV replication.[829] NS5A DI has also been crystallized in two additional dimer conformations.[472] However, these latter models contain far less buried surface area and feature opposing membrane anchors, so their relevance remains unclear. It should be noted that several highly effective and potent NS5A-specific DAAs emerged from extensive compound library screening, for example, daclatasvir. The main line of evidence that these compounds target NS5A is that mutations conferring resistance map to NS5A DI, more precisely in the membrane-proximal region of the molecule and often in the linker connecting the N-terminal amphipathic α-helix and DI; however, the mechanisms of action of these compounds are not yet understood. A key feature of these compounds is their symmetry, consistent with models predicting that they bind at the NS5A dimer interface.[286,498] One intriguing hypothesis is that these compounds inhibit virus replication by locking NS5A in one dimer conformation.

Downstream of DI lies DII and DIII, which have natively unfolded structures that contain some α-helical content.[39,519,937] In line with this flexibility, DIII is tolerant of large deletions and insertions.[27,368,535,603,653,899] This conformational flexibility is also observed in other hepaciviruses, such as in GHV, which has an exceptionally long NS5A with a 521-aa C-terminal region.[485]

NS5A is phosphorylated by multiple cellular Ser/Thr kinases and can be found in basally phosphorylated (56 kDa) and hyperphosphorylated (58 kDa) forms. These designations, however, greatly oversimplify NS5A phosphorylation status, which is quite complex and can differ between genotypes. Interestingly, many of the cell culture–adaptive mutations in genotype 1b replicons lead to increased basal NS5A phosphorylation and promote RNA replication.[92,547] Basal phosphorylation involves a central region of NS5A and a large C-terminal

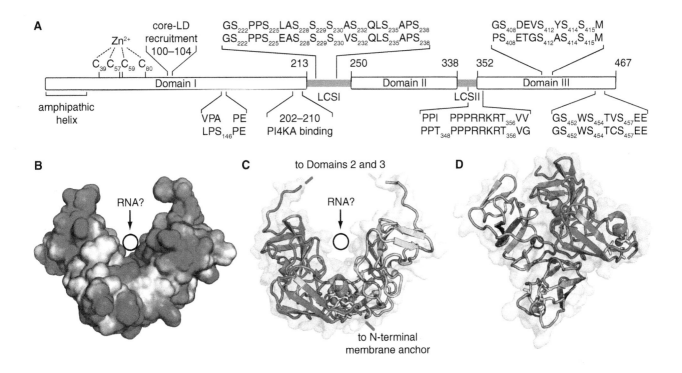

FIGURE 7.15 Structures of HCV NS5A protein. A: A map of NS5A is illustrated, highlighting structural features, including two low-complexity sequences (LCS), known interaction sites, and residue numbers of phosphorylated Ser and Thr residues. This figure is loosely based on prior analyses.[784,900] Sequences presented are genotype 1b (J4 isolate, upper sequence) and genotype 2a (JFH-1 isolate, lower sequence). **B:** Surface electrostatic potential of the dimeric NS5A zinc–binding domain, as rendered from PDB 1ZH1.[901] Negative charges are in *red* and positive charges in *blue*. **C:** The NS5A zinc–binding domain (PDB 1ZH1), with individual monomeric subunits colored *purple* and *green*. Zn[2+] ions are shown in *red*, and coordinating residues are shown in *yellow*. **D:** An alternative structure of the NS5A zinc–binding domain, as rendered from PDB 3FQM.[554] The *purple* subunit is structurally aligned the same as the *purple* subunit in **(C)**.

region of DIII.[889] Initial mutational analysis of genotype 1a HCV NS5A found that Ser residues within LCSI are required for hyperphosphorylation.[889] Subsequent analyses of genotype 2a HCV NS5A with phosphospecific antibodies or mass spectrometry definitively identified several phosphorylated residues, particularly in the LCS I region (Fig. 7.15A). Mutational analysis suggested that phosphorylation of Ser 225, Ser 229, Ser 232, and Ser 235 positively regulates RNA replication, whereas phosphorylation of Ser 222, Ser 242, and Ser 245 negatively regulates replication.[162,246,300,301,497,594,783,784]

Several NS5A kinases have been tentatively identified.[594,784] Basal phosphorylation likely involves phosphorylation at multiple sites by casein kinase II subunit α, protein kinase A subunit Cβ, and/or serine/threonine–protein kinase PLK1. Hyperphosphorylation is likely due to sequential, clustered phosphorylation of Ser 232→Ser 235→Ser 238 and (Ser 247 and Thr 244)→Thr 242 by casein kinase Iα.[365,784,814] NS5A hyperphosphorylation requires prior phosphorylation at positions Ser 225 and Ser 229,[365] coexpression of NS3-5A in *cis*,[434,669] and interaction between NS4A and NS5A[32,401]; in contrast, hyperphosphorylation is inhibited by interaction with PI4K.[758] In addition to phosphorylation on multiple Ser/Thr residues, NS5A is also phosphorylated on Tyr 93 by c-Src.[432] Thus, NS5A phosphorylation is complicated and hierarchical and integrates multiple interactions as inputs. Depending on the viral genotype and strain, outputs of this mechanism may be expressed as altered protein–protein or protein–RNA interactions, differences in NS5A localization, and efficiencies of RNA replication or virus assembly.[300,301,594,784,785]

NS5A plays two key roles in HCV RNA replication: first, it alters ER membranes to build replication organelles; second, it is a nonenzymatic component of the replicase. To build the RNA replication organelle, NS5A binds and activates PI4KA[75,76,759,883] which generates phosphatidylinositol 4-phosphate, PI4P. PI4P then recruits membrane effectors like oxysterol-binding protein (OSBP), which shuttles cholesterol between membranes in coordination with VAMP-associated protein A (VAPA), as described below. Interestingly, VAPA is also an important NS5A interaction partner, preferentially binding to hypophosphorylated NS5A and stimulating RNA replication.[244,300] Thus, NS5A phosphorylation status regulates replication complex assembly, and it should be noted that one particularly potent cell culture–adaptive mutation (S232I) coordinately abrogates hyperphosphorylation and enhances RNA replication of most HCV strains in Huh-7 cells but dampens the activation of PI4KA, which is overproduced in Huh-7 cells.[92,337]

Once replication organelles are formed, NS5A localizes to sites of viral RNA synthesis.[303] NS5A binds to NS5B and can modulate its RdRP activity *in vitro*,[843] including increased RdRP processivity,[586] and mutations in NS5A that block NS5B interaction are detrimental for HCV replication in cell culture.[840] The interaction between NS5A and NS5B requires c-Src, which binds to these proteins via its SH2 and SH3 domains, respectively.[714] NS5A also has RNA-binding activity, with the minimal RNA-binding domain in DI and LCSI,[371] although DII and DIII may also contribute to RNA binding.[272] The

RNA-binding ability of NS5A can be regulated by cyclophilin A, a cellular proline cis–trans isomerase that is essential for HCV replication.[784] Furthermore, NS5A phosphorylation is postulated to competitively inhibit RNA binding.[472]

NS5A plays an important role in virion assembly, primarily through trafficking to LDs and interaction with the viral C protein.[28,595,638] Recruitment of NS5A to LDs is mediated by determinants located in DI[638,1005] and enhanced by the cellular enzymes DGAT1[133] and Rab18.[798] DGAT1, a diacylglycerol acyltransferase, is important for LD formation; Rab18, a small GTPase, regulates protein trafficking to LDs. Further downstream, DIII contains determinants of virus particle assembly; deletion of these determinants selectively inhibits virus assembly with minimal effects on RNA replication.[28,898,1005] More specifically, virion assembly requires NS5A phosphorylation on Ser 457 by casein kinase IIα.[898] These findings have led to a model wherein the major assembly function of NS5A is to traffic genomic RNA from replication compartments to LDs for nucleocapsid assembly. In support of this model, the NS5A inhibitor daclatasvir prevents transfer of HCV RNA to sites of assembly.[96] In addition, NS5A DIII recruits annexin A2, a cellular phospholipid-binding protein that enhances virus assembly.[38] NS5A also reportedly interacts with ApoE,[68,189] which is essential for HCV particle assembly; however, it remains unclear how cytosolic NS5A interacts with this secreted glycoprotein.

NS5B Protein

NS5B (~68 kDa) is the hepacivirus RdRP, the enzyme responsible for viral RNA synthesis, and a major target of DAAs. NS5B is a tail-anchored membrane protein, posttranslationally inserting its C-terminal 21 aa into the ER membrane.[383,817] The tail anchor of GBV-B NS5B can functionally substitute for the tail anchor of HCV NS5B.[110] Deletion of this domain in HCV alters NS5B localization and inhibits replication in cell culture,[651] although it does not affect RdRP activity in vitro.[993] This truncated, active form of NS5B can be efficiently purified in soluble form, enabling biophysical and biochemical characterization.

Like other RdRPs, the structure of NS5B resembles a right hand with distinct finger, palm, and thumb domains, with nucleotidyltransferase active site residues located in the palm domain and a template-binding groove located within the fingers (Fig. 7.8B).[5,115,116,499] HCV NS5B has been crystallized in both inactive "open" and active "closed" conformations, featuring an enclosed active site with extensive interactions between the finger and thumb domains. An unusual β-hairpin protrudes from the thumb into the active site, where it serves to stabilize the intermediates of de novo initiation.[30,362,681,750] In some structures, a C-terminal regulatory motif occludes the binding of RNA templates and inhibits RdRP activity.[30,501,750] A recent breakthrough in the field was structural determination of stalled NS5B initiation and elongation complexes, highlighting the molecular basis of RNA synthesis via an in-line geometry of nucleotide attack, as well as conformational changes needed to clear the active site.[30]

Recombinant HCV NS5B is capable of in vitro synthesis of full-length HCV RNA with nucleotide incorporation rates of approximately 150 to 200 nt/minutes.[548,684,751] The rate-limiting step of NS5B RNA synthesis is de novo initiation: essentially, the synthesis of a 2-nt primer with a 5′ purine, which can be mono-, di-, or triphosphorylated.[64,562,749–752,839,1033]

The efficiency of de novo initiation is enhanced by an allosteric GTP binding site[340,550] and correlates with the efficiency of replication in cell culture, with thumb residue 405, near the thumb–finger interface, greatly impacting the efficiency of initiation.[818,847] In vitro synthesis generally prefers to initiate with a GTP; however, most HCV isolates terminate with a 3′ uridylate, suggesting that negative-strand RNA synthesis initiates with ATP in vivo. Optimal RNA templates for de novo initiation contain limited secondary structure and an unpaired 3′ end.[404] However, the HCV 3′ NCR terminates with a stable 3′SL, suggesting that it is a suboptimal template for initiation. Indeed, when the HCV 3′ NCR is used as a template for de novo RNA synthesis, only internally initiated negative strands are produced.[404,424,685,877] However, addition of a 2-nt 3′ extension leads to the production of template-length minus-strand products.[685] Thus, authentic initiation of HCV minus-strand synthesis may depend on the local unwinding of the terminal stem-loop, perhaps by the NS3-4A helicase.

NS5B RdRP activity depends on intramolecular interactions and is influenced by intermolecular interactions with other NS proteins. Important contacts between NS5B domains were revealed through structural studies with non-nucleoside RdRP inhibitors, which allosterically block polymerase activity.[88,158,173,208,323,556,917,918,949] Additionally, NS5B oligomerization can cooperatively stimulate polymerase activity.[742,946] NS3-4A, NS4B, and NS5A can all bind NS5B and influence its enzymatic activity in vitro.[717,843] Genetic studies indicate that NS5A primarily binds to NS5B via determinants located on the back of the thumb and inner surface of the fingers[742] and as mentioned above, c-Src mediates interaction between NS5A and NS5B.

In addition to RdRP activity, NS5B has terminal nucleotide transferase (TnTase) activity, adding a few untemplated nts to the 3′ end of an RNA substrate.[64,748,839] The TnTase activity of a highly purified NS5B preparation was shown to depend on RdRP active site residues; thus this activity is an inherent property of NS5B and not a contaminating enzyme.[748,753] Moreover, NS5B TnTase activity can convert an RNA lacking a correct 3′ end into a useful template for de novo initiation,[748] suggesting that this activity may act as a "telomerase" to maintain genome integrity.

As for many RNA viruses, only vanishingly small amounts of RdRP activity are needed to support hepacivirus replication. Indeed, protease protection experiments demonstrated that approximately 2.5% of NS5B protein resides inside membrane-bound replication compartments isolated from replicon-bearing cells yet fully accounts for all of the RdRP activity.[746] Thus, only a small fraction of NS5B may be actively involved in RNA synthesis at a given time; the other, larger fraction presumably may have other functions. Recently, mutations in p7 and NS5B were shown to cooperatively enhance the specific infectivity and lipid composition of a highly cell culture–adapted HCVcc,[16] suggesting that NS5B may also contribute to virus assembly.

Ultrastructure and Biogenesis of the HCV Replication Organelle

HCV RNA replication takes place in a membranous compartment. Consistently, viral RNA synthesis is resistant to protease and nuclease treatment unless membranes are permeabilized with detergents.[9,15,237,338,468,639,746,997] Membrane fractions containing HCV RNA and viral proteins are not solubilized by treatment with cold Triton X-100, arguing for replicase assembly in lipid rafts. In agreement, extraction of cholesterol from these membrane fractions inhibits replicase activity.[699] Isolated membranous replicase complexes can use endogenous viral RNA but do not accept exogenous templates. Thus, the predominant reaction product from these complexes is elongation of RNA strands initiated *in vivo*. However, the observed inhibition of RNA synthesis by treatment with heparin[338] and the shift of single-stranded into dsRNA observed in pulse-chase

experiments[468] suggest that a limited number of *de novo* initiation events do occur in these complexes.

Studies with liver biopsies and human hepatoma cells expressing viral proteins or containing a stably replicating subgenomic HCV replicon revealed small clusters of single-membrane vesicles embedded into an electron-dense matrix, designated as the membranous web (Fig. 7.16A, B).[230,303] In addition, enlarged ER and aberrant mitochondria were observed *in vivo*,

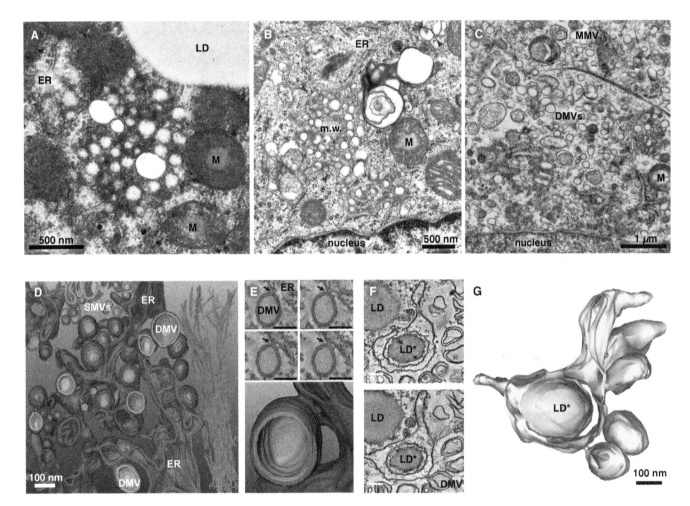

FIGURE 7.16 Hepacivirus replication organelles. A: Membrane rearrangements detected in the livers of a chronic HCV carrier. TEM image of a liver biopsy specimen showing a membranous web composed of small clusters of single-membrane vesicles. A representative cluster of 10 to 30 single-membrane vesicles residing close to the endoplasmic reticulum (ER), mitochondria, and a lipid droplet (LDs) are shown. **B:** Membranous web (m.w.) detected in a human hepatoma cell line containing a stably replicating subgenomic HCV replicon RNA. M, mitochondria. **C:** Membrane alterations induced in a human hepatoma cell line infected with a highly replication-competent HCV strain (JFH1) 36 hours after infection. DMVs, double-membrane vesicles; MMV, multimembrane vesicle; M, mitochondrium. **D:** 3D surface reconstruction of a dual axis tomogram obtained with human hepatoma cells infected with a JFH1 variant and fixed 16 hours after infection. ER, endoplasmic reticulum (*dark brown*); DMV, double-membraned vesicle (inner membrane in *yellowish brown*, outer membrane in semitransparent *light brown*); SMVs, single-membrane vesicles (*pink*). The Golgi apparatus is shown in green, intermediate filaments in *dark blue*. **E:** Single tomographic slices displaying a DMV and its link to the ER membrane are shown on the top. A 3D surface rendering of the DMV and its stalk-like connection to the ER is shown on the bottom. Color codes as in **(D)**. **F:** Single tomographic slice of an HCV-infected cell showing a lipid droplet staining positive or not for E2 as determined by light microscopy (LD* and LD, respectively). Note the tight wrapping of the E2-positive droplet (LD*) by an ER membrane, which is not the case with the E2-negative lipid droplet (LD). **G:** 3D surface rendering of the E2-positive lipid droplet in **(F)**. Note the DMVs emanating from the wrapping ER membrane. (Panel (A) was reproduced under a Creative Commons license from Blanchard and Roingeard.[91] **Panel (B)** is from Gosert R, Egger D, Lohmann V, et al. Identification of the hepatitis C virus RNA replication complex in Huh-7 cells harboring subgenomic replicons. *J Virol* 2003;77(9):5487–5492. doi: 10.1128/JVI.77.9.5487-5492.2003. Reproduced with permission from American Society for Microbiology.[303] **Panel (C)** is from Romero-Brey, I. and Bartenschlager, R., unpublished. **Panels (D)** and **(E)** are reproduced under a Creative Commons license from Romero-Brey et al.[778] **Panels (F)** and **(G)** are from Lee, J.-Y. and Bartenschlager, R., unpublished.)

which might be the result of a virus-induced stress response.[33,48] However, in hepatoma cell lines containing highly replication-competent HCV isolates, the predominant structures are double-membrane vesicles (DMVs) (Fig. 7.16C, D).[259,260,699,778] DMVs are heterogeneous in size (~150 nm diameter), enriched in the perinuclear region, and thought to be the site of HCV RNA replication because they contain active viral replicase and their abundance correlates with RNA replication.[699,778] In addition to DMVs, single-membrane vesicles are found in high-level HCV-replicating cells (Fig. 7.16D), and although they contain the majority of viral proteins as determined by immuno EM,[778] their role in RNA replication is unknown. It has been proposed that single-membrane vesicles might be precursors of DMVs,[259] similar to events occurring in poliovirus-infected cells where single-membrane structures originating from the *cis*-Golgi are later transformed into DMVs by membrane wrapping processes.[65] However, single- to double-membrane intermediates have not been observed in the case of HCV. Multimembrane vesicles (MMVs) are also found in HCV-infected cells (Fig. 7.16C), but since they become visible only after the formation of DMVs, MMVs are thought to be a by-product, for example, resulting from a cellular stress response, rather than contributing to RNA replication.[778]

While the origins of SMVs are unclear, DMVs are derived from the ER with the outer membrane often observed in connection to the ER membrane via a small "stalk" (Fig. 7.16E).[778] Thus, topologically DMVs correspond to exvaginations, ballooning out of the ER toward the cytosol, which is the opposite orientation found with flavivirus replication organelles (Fig. 7.16B–E). The exact site of HCV RNA replication within its membranous replication organelle is not firmly established and awaits a method to detect nascent viral RNA with high spatial resolution. However, the nuclease and protease resistance of HCV RNA and the reported exclusion of pattern recognition receptors from the membranous web suggest that HCV might shield its RNA in the lumen of DMVs.[673] In this case, only a small fraction of DMVs would be engaged in RNA replication because only approximately 8% of DMVs were found to have an opening toward the cytosol at a given time point.[778] Alternatively, HCV might generate a proteinaceous "pore" to allow passage of NTPs and RNA release from the vesicle lumen as originally proposed for *Coronaviridae*[433] or the viral replicase might reside on the DMV surface as proposed for the poliovirus.[83,229] Assuming that replication occurs within DMVs and a transport mechanism for viral RNA and membrane-impermeable metabolites would not exist, replication in these DMVs would cease upon vesicle closure, raising the question as to the turnover of these inactive DMVs. One possibility is the release of dsRNA-containing vesicles via the exocytic pathway.[125,218,322] Interestingly, in HCV-replicating cells, blocking the exocytic release of vesicles that occurs in an ESCRT-dependent manner induces TLR3-dependent interferon response suggesting that dsRNA release in the form of extracellular vesicles is a mechanism that dampens the activation of the interferon response in the HCV-infected cell.[322]

The striking structural similarity of DMVs to autophagosomes and their common origin from the ER suggest that HCV utilizes autophagy or components of this cellular machinery for membranous web formation. Indeed, activation of autophagy in HCV-infected cells has been reported by several groups, but the contribution of this cellular process to viral replication is controversial.[8,219,247,417,852,853,888] Several viral proteins, notably NS4B and NS5B, have been reported to activate autophagy.[325,876] In addition, formation of DMVs can be induced by the sole expression of NS5A.[777] However, efficiency of DMV formation by NS5A is low but strongly increased by coexpression of other NS proteins and profoundly blocked by clinically used NS5A inhibitors such as daclatasvir.[77] Thus, a concerted action of all HCV replicase factors, that is, NS3 to NS5B, is most likely required for efficient formation of the viral replication organelle.

Although DMVs are derived from the ER membrane, they have a different lipid composition. While ER membranes are low in cholesterol and sphingolipid, concentrations of these lipids are high in the case of DMVs.[699] A key mediator of this change in lipid composition is PI4KA, which is recruited, via binding to NS5A, to ER/DMV membranes.[75,503,759,883,921] There, the kinase synthesizes large amounts of PI4P, which are usually low in abundance at ER membranes but high in the Golgi and plasma membranes. In addition, NS5A, via association with VAPA/B, binds to and recruits nonvesicular transport proteins such as the cholesterol transfer protein OSBP.[950] By analogy to other cellular systems, we can assume that once recruited to the PI4P-enriched ER or DMV membrane, OSBP releases cholesterol into the ER/DMV membrane in exchange for PI4P.[619,620] Presumably by an analogous countercurrent mechanism, glycosphingolipids might be incorporated into membranes of the HCV replication organelle via the PI4P-dependent glucosylceramide transporter protein FAPP-2 that under normal conditions mediates the nonvesicular transport of glucosylceramide from the TGN to the plasma membrane.[418] Thus, by recruitment and activation of PI4KA, HCV sustains a PI4P gradient to enable the accumulation of distinct lipids in ER/DMV membranes. These lipids might provide building blocks for lipid rafts, promoting replicase assembly and/or activity. This conclusion is based on several observations. First, treatment with methyl-β-cyclodextrin, which extracts cholesterol from membranes, impairs replicase activity and causes DMVs to shrink in size.[699] Second, altering cholesterol metabolism pharmacologically leads to reduced geranylgeranylation, replicase disassembly, and inhibition of RNA replication.[406,1000] Third, the membranous web is poorly soluble in nonionic detergents, consistent with an enrichment of cholesterol and sphingolipids.[9,835] Fourth, genetic knockdown or pharmacological inhibition of PI4KA blocks HCV replication, concomitant with a clustering of DMVs that are reduced in size and rather homogenous.[759] Fifth, sphingolipids can stimulate HCV replicase activity.[361,967] Taken together, HCV might use components of the autophagy machinery to generate DMVs that are altered in lipid composition via a PI4KA-dependent lipid transfer pathway.

Although PI4KA is essential for HCV replication, the abundance of PI4P has to be kept within a certain range because high levels appear to be deleterious for replication. Some cell culture–adaptive mutations, which promote HCV replication in Huh-7 cells, are loss-of-function mutations that reduce PI4KA activation, thus lowering PI4P production.[337] Since Huh-7 cells express much higher levels of PI4KA than primary human hepatocytes, reducing the interaction with the kinase via cell culture-adaptive mutations compensates for high-level expression of the kinase in hepatoma cells. Furthermore, PI4KA inhibitors can also enhance replication of unadapted HCV strains and allow efficient replication of primary isolates in cell culture.[337]

Apart from local enrichment of distinct lipids within the replication organelle, HCV-infected cells contain high overall lipid content as a result of reduced VLDL secretion and activation of lipid synthesis pathways.[637,709] These include the sterol regulatory element–binding protein (SREBP) pathway, which can be induced by NS4B- or HCV-triggered ER stress,[695,953] and activation of DDX3X, a cytosolic RNA helicase that senses HCV RNA and induces, via the cellular transcriptional coactivator CBP-p300, expression of SREBP.[509] In either case, the expression of lipogenic genes is activated, including FAS and HMGCR, the rate-limiting enzyme of the isoprenoid pathway, which feeds into both cholesterol biosynthesis and protein lipidation. In addition, replication organelle formation might exploit LDs, which are highly enriched in triacylglycerol and cholesterol esters. Consistent with this, DMVs are often found in close proximity to LDs, with ER membranes wrapping around nearby LDs (Fig. 7.16F, G). These membranes are often decorated by DMVs, arguing for a close spatial coupling of HCV RNA replication and assembly (Fig. 7.16F, G).

HCV RNA replication is stimulated by increased availability of saturated and monounsaturated fatty acids and inhibited by polyunsaturated fatty acids (PUFAs) or inhibitors of fatty acid synthesis,[406] suggesting that specific lipids and/or membrane fluidity are important for the function of the membranous web. Moreover, lipid peroxidation arising from ROS-induced conversion of PUFAs, which leads to covalent adducts of modified lipids with proteins, suppresses HCV RNA replication.[367,992] This block can be overcome by mutations in the transmembrane and membrane-proximal regions of NS4A and NS5B and by lipophilic antioxidants, such as vitamin E. Interestingly, Sec14L2, a lipid transporter protein expressed in the liver but not in Huh-7 cells, was identified as a host cell factor that renders human hepatoma cells permissive for non–cell culture–adapted HCV strains.[795] Ectopic expression of Sec14L2 made Huh-7 cells permissive for primary HCV isolates in human serum and nonadapted viral strains. Although the precise mechanism is not known, SEC14L2 might enhance vitamin E–mediated protection of HCV against lipid peroxidation. Of note, the genotype 2a isolate JFH-1, which is the only isolate that replicates to high level in hepatoma cells without cell culture-adaptive mutations, is intrinsically resistant to lipid peroxidation.[992] To which extent this property contributes to its unique replication capacity remains to be determined.

RNA Replication

HCV genomes must be translated more frequently than they are replicated, since 1,000 viral proteins are produced per viral RNA at steady state.[746] Thus, only after an initial burst of translation is the hepacivirus genome recruited out of translation and into a replication complex. The mechanisms by which these processes are coordinated have not been elucidated but may involve crosstalk between the 5′ and 3′ ends.[677] For instance, the cellular PTB protein binds to the HCV 5′ NCR and C coding region, where it may modulate IRES activity[381,915] and to the 3′ NCR, where it may repress replication.[381,924] Another RNA-binding protein, HuR, competes with PTB for binding to the 3′ NCR and recruits La protein, which may promote genome cyclization.[457,846] Thus, it is plausible that hepacivirus genome cyclization may facilitate RNA replication. It has also been proposed that C protein contributes to the switch between translation and replication, enhancing IRES-mediated translation when C protein levels are low and inhibiting translation while C protein levels are high.[95,1027] However, this model does not explain the regulatory mechanisms of subgenomic replicons that do not express C protein. Finally, it has been noted that the RNA-binding and ATPase activities of the NS3 helicase domain are required in *cis* for HCV RNA replication.[416] One interpretation of these data is that the helicase binds to the RNA from which it was translated, perhaps to recruit the viral genome out of translation and into the replication compartment. This may parallel the role of the 1a RNA helicase protein of brome mosaic virus, another positive-strand RNA virus, in recruiting the viral genome into RNA replication.[947]

HCV RNA replication initiates with the synthesis of genome-length, negative-strand RNAs, which may be found as partially double-stranded RI or fully double-stranded RFs.[15] Negative-strand RNA then serves as a template for multiple rounds of positive-strand synthesis, leading to the asymmetric accumulation of nearly 10 positive strands for every negative strand.[9,639,746]

Virus Assembly

HCV particles bud directly into the ER, transit the secretory pathway, and are released through exocytosis. A notable difference from flaviviruses is that HCV does not undergo proteolytic maturation and is infectious upon envelopment. Following SPP cleavage, mature C localizes to cytoplasmic LDs, the presumed site of nucleocapsid assembly,[605,638] NS5A also localizes to LDs and is thought to relocalize genomic RNAs from replication compartments to assembly sites.[28] Localization of C and NS5A to LDs requires the cellular DGAT1 and Rab18 proteins.[355,798] NS5A localization to LDs also requires CK1-dependent hyperphosphorylation. Core is thought to recruit the membrane-associated replication complex through its interaction with NS5A.[28,595,638] NS2 is a major scaffolding protein of virion assembly, interacting with NS3-4A possibly for nucleocapsid assembly and p7 to recruit nucleocapsids to sites of envelopment where they interact with E1/E2.[97,389,571,715,731,865] NS4B and 5B also are required for efficient virion assembly.

HCV particle formation is associated with VLDL assembly, which also takes place in the secretory pathway of hepatocytes. Virions have a lipid composition similar to LDL and VLDL.[618] HCV particles also incorporate ApoA1, ApoB, ApoC, and ApoE and require Apos for infectivity (reviewed in Ref.[488]). It is unclear whether VLDL components are incorporated as a hybrid viral/host envelope or if they are tethered. The amphipathic α-helices of the apolipoproteins are important for supporting assembly and infectivity.[281] Interestingly, the apolipoproteins seem to be playing a role similar to NS1 for flaviviruses or E^{rns} for pestiviruses, as they can partially substitute for each other in virion assembly.[280]

HCV egresses through the secretory pathway, where the ion channel activity of p7 may protect nascent virions from premature fusion induced by the low pH of the secretory compartment although released virions are pH-resistant.[979] While intracellular HCV particles are infectious, their buoyant density becomes lower as they egress in a maturation process that parallels VLDL.[288] Virions are thought to undergo ER-to-Golgi transit in COPII vesicles, traffic through the *trans*-Golgi network and endosomal and recycling compartments in association with VAMP1-expressing vesicles, ultimately leading to secretion from the cell.[178,587,880] It is also clear that there is a distinct cell–cell spread pathway allowing the virus to spread between hepatocytes while avoiding antibody surveillance.[914] These pathways appear to be regulated in part by a NS2 inter-action with AP-1 and four clathrin adaptors that sort cargo for post-Golgi trafficking.[986]

In addition to these major egress pathways, HCV RNA can spread from cell to cell via exosomes, albeit at low levels.[125,552] ESCRT components have also been implicated, although they probably have noncanonical functions, as opposed to a classical role in membrane scission.[50] In addition to the VLDL secretory pathway, a number of other host factors have been implicated in HCV assembly, including the NS5A-interacting annexin A2, autophagy proteins ATG7 and Beclin-1, HSC70,TIP47, PLA2G4A, FIG 4, ABHD5, and CIDEB.[488]

PEGIVIRUSES

Background and Classification

In 1967, serum from a surgeon "GB" who had contracted acute hepatitis was inoculated into four marmosets, caus-ing hepatitis in all of them.[201] After 11 serial passages of the GB agent in tamarins, two viruses were eventually cloned in 1995 and named GBV-A and GBV-B.[851] Both viruses are similar to HCV yet genetically quite distinct.[658] Although GBV-A was initially thought to have originated from human serum, subsequent work showed that it is a cryptic monkey virus that was likely acquired during passage in tamarins.[123,492] GBV-B has not been reisolated, and its origin remains a mys-tery; nevertheless, GBV-B is now recognized as a member of the genus *Hepacivirus*, its closest relative being RHV-I.[910] A third related virus was identified in humans by two different groups and called GBV-C or hepatitis G virus.[534,850] A virus distantly related to GBV-A and GBV-C was then discovered in Old World frugivorous bats in Bangladesh and designated GBV-D.[240] Based on sequence relatedness and overall genome structure, GBVs have been classified as members of the family *Flaviviridae*, with GBV-A, GBV-C, and GBV-D classified as a separate genus, *Pegivirus*, indicating that they are *pe*rsistent *G*B viruses.[857,866] GBV-A and GBV-C have been renamed simian pegivirus (SPgV) and human pegivirus (HPgV), respectively. Currently, six genotypes of HPgV are recognized.

Virus discovery efforts have identified several additional pegiviruses in other animal species. Recently identified mam-malian pegiviruses include rodent pegivirus (RPgV); porcine pegivirus (PPgV); two pegiviruses of horses, equine pegivirus (EPgV) and Theiler disease–associated virus (TDAV); as well as three distinct rat pegiviruses (BPgV-F, BPgV-G, and BPgV-I). An additional human-infecting pegivirus is known as hepegi-virus (HHPgV) because it has some hepacivirus-like features yet classified as a pegivirus based on molecular phylogeny.[341,857] Pegiviruses generally produce subclinical, persistent infections. While TDAV was originally associated with acute hepatitis in equines, subsequent work identified a parvovirus as the etio-logic agent of hepatitis.[210]

Clinical Perspective

Human infection with HPgV is surprisingly common: approxi-mately 1% to 5% of blood donors in developed countries and approximately 20% in developing countries have detectable viremia. Nearly three-quarters of infections are cleared within 2 years,[74] with the remainder persisting for years without obvi-ous symptoms.[21] Clearance usually correlates with the appear-ance of antibodies against E2.[729] HPgV appears to be primarily lymphotropic *in vivo*,[482,483] although evidence also exists for hepatotropism.[270] This virus can be transmitted parenterally or sexually, with vertical transmission also likely.[78,729] HPgV infection is associated with increased risk of non-Hodgkin lym-phoma, although the underlying mechanisms of this linkage are unclear.[159] Surprisingly, HPgV may have beneficial effects to HPgV-HIV coinfected patients, with lower HIV titers, higher CD4+ T-cell counts, and slower HIV disease progression.[159] Based on these observations, as well as *in vitro* experiments, it has been proposed that HPgV interferes with HIV replication by altering expression of cytokines, chemokines, and chemokine receptors,[729,985] decreasing T-cell activation,[582] directly inhibit-ing HIV-1 entry,[356,398,435,644] and/or eliciting cross-reactive anti-bodies that neutralize HIV particles.[645] A causal relationship is not clear, however, since HPgV is lymphotropic and higher HPgV titers could correlate with higher lymphocyte count.[931] It is also notable that this relationship does not extend to other pegiviruses and lentiviruses: SPgV does not protect against SIV coinfection.[41]

HHPgV is much less prevalent than HPgV, infecting approximately 0.4% of healthy blood donors. HHPgV may also be parenterally spread, as the infection rates increase to approximately 2% in HCV-, HIV- or HCV/HIV–coinfected individuals.[73,407,631] HHPgV infection has not been linked to any specific clinical symptoms or changes in HIV disease progression.

SPgV has been detected in several species of New World monkeys in the absence of experimental infection or overt dis-ease.[123,491] Surprisingly, SPgV replicates to high titers without inducing an adaptive immune response[41] and exhibits remark-able genetic stability.[42]

Virion Structure and Entry

Similar to HCV, HPgV particles exhibit unusually low and heterogeneous buoyant density, with peaks near 1.08 and 1.17 g/mL.[612,804,984] A peculiarity of many pegiviruses is that they do not encode an obvious C gene, so it is unclear how nucleocapsids are formed. Treatment of virions with detergents to solubilize the viral envelope shifts the peak of viral RNA to a higher density form, suggesting that they may contain nucleo-capsids.[612,804,984] Little is known about the pegivirus entry mech-anisms, although it has been proposed that GBV-C utilizes the LDLR for entry.[4]

Genome Structure and Expression

Pegivirus genomes range from 9.4 to greater than 10.8 kb in length, containing long ORFs (2,973–3,469 codons) flanked by 5′ and 3′ NCRs (Fig. 7.17). Pegivirus 5′ NCRs can be consider-ably longer than their hepacivirus counterparts, up to 617 nt in length in the case of TDAV. Most pegiviruses, such as SPgV,[849] HHPgV,[849] and EPgV,[408] encode hepacivirus-like class IV IRES elements, while others, such as TDAV, lack structural similarity to known IRES elements.[145] Pegivirus 3′ NCRs also differ consid-erably from other genera within the family, lacking a poly(U/UC) tract, but do sometimes contain short poly(G) tracts, as well as repeated structural elements reminiscent of the flaviviruses.[187,410]

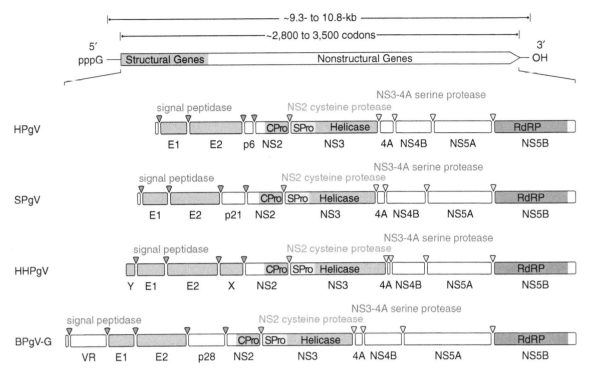

FIGURE 7.17 Pegivirus genome structure. The structural organization of several pegivirus genomes is illustrated. See text for details.

Structural Proteins

Several pegiviruses, like HPgV, SPgV, BPgV-I, EPgV, and TDAV, lack any obvious capsid- or core-like gene, initiating translation shortly upstream of a predicted signal peptide for E1.[534,658,857] Others, such as GBV-D and HHPgV, encode short (~57 and 60 aa, respectively), basic N-terminal peptides, which may function as capsid or core proteins (Fig. 7.17). In the case of HHPgV, this core-like protein has been called "Y protein" (Fig. 7.17).[407] Furthermore, some HPgV-infected individuals generate antibodies against a small basic peptide that can be translated from an in-frame, upstream AUG, suggesting that such a protein is expressed *in vivo*.[984] Finally, bat-infecting pegiviruses encode "variable region" (VR) proteins in place of the C gene; VR proteins are predicted to contain N-terminal signal peptides, ectodomains of 20 to 150 aa, and two to four transmembrane domains (Fig. 7.17).[745] While these proteins are basic (pI ~8.16–9.12), it is not clear whether they are structural proteins, nor whether their membrane anchoring and topology are compatible with nucleocapsid formation. Alternative explanations for the lack of a capsid-like protein include the possibilities that pegiviruses may usurp a capsid-like protein or other polycationic molecule from the host cell or a coinfecting virus or that additional pegivirus proteins may be involved. In this regard, a region of the HPgV NS5A gene that exhibits a bias against synonymous mutation has been noted to potentially encode a small basic protein (~10 kDa, pI 11.5) in an alternate reading frame.[701]

Pegiviruses encode two viral glycoproteins of unknown structure, E1 and E2, which presumably mediate binding and entry. Consistent with this, the presence of E2-specific antibodies correlates with protection from HPgV reinfection in the context of liver transplantation.[345,913] HPgV E2 does not bind CD81,[414] indicating that it likely uses different entry factors than HCV. One curious feature of HPgV E1 and E2 is that these glycoproteins reportedly inhibit HIV-1 replication via a variety of mechanisms.[232,297,644,951] In addition to E1 and E2, HHPgV and EPgV encode a third glycoprotein, known as X, located between E2 and NS2 (Fig. 7.17). The function of X is unknown and its classification as a virion structural protein remains tentative.

Nonstructural Proteins

Many pegiviruses encode a small polytopic membrane protein, similar to the hepacivirus p7 protein, immediately following the structural proteins. These range in size from the approximately 6-kDa p6 protein of HPgV to the approximately 28-kDa p28 protein of BPgV-G.[408,745] It is unclear whether these proteins are true orthologs of the HCV p7 protein or are capable of forming ion channels. Surprisingly, EPgV and HHPV lack p7-like proteins but do encode X glycoproteins between E2 and NS2. Given that p7 is essential for hepacivirus virus assembly and secretion, perhaps the X glycoprotein can functionally replace p7.

Of the remaining pegivirus NS genes, their overall architecture is remarkably similar to the hepaciviruses, although highly divergent at the amino acid level. Nevertheless, conserved active site and structural motifs are found in the corresponding locations for NS2 cysteine autoproteases, NS3 serine protease/NTPase–RNA helicases, NS4A membrane–bound serine protease cofactors, NS4B nucleotide–binding membrane proteins, NS5A Zn^{2+}–binding phosphoproteins, and NS5B RdRPs.[408,745] For HPgV, the membrane topology and autoprotease activity of NS2 have been confirmed,[66] the NS3-4A serine protease was shown to cleave MAVS and thereby inhibit type I interferon induction,[165] and the NS3 helicase domain possesses NTP-dependent RNA unwinding activity.[329,1032] One notable difference between pegiviruses and hepaciviruses is that their NS3-4A serine proteases have very different substrate recognition motifs. The HPgV NS3 serine protease is also reported to interfere with HIV-1 replication[290] and may bias infected T lymphocytes toward a Th1 phenotype.[794]

With no significant human or animal disease associations, the pegiviruses are woefully understudied, and virtually nothing is known about virus structure, virus entry, mechanisms of RNA replication, and virus assembly. From an evolutionary standpoint, it seems particularly interesting that some pegiviruses lack defined nucleocapsid-forming proteins, while others express VR and Y proteins; similarly, some pegiviruses lack p7-like proteins, while others encode p7-like proteins that are much larger than their hepacivirus counterparts. Clearly, these viruses are likely to exhibit interesting variations on virus assembly and release within the family.

PESTIVIRUSES

Background and Classification

Pestiviruses are animal pathogens of major economic importance, particularly for the livestock industry. They include the type member, bovine viral diarrhea virus 1 (BVDV1), classical swine fever virus (CSFV), border disease virus (BDV) of sheep, as well as several recently identified species that infect cows (BVDV2; HoBi-like pestivirus [HoBiPeV]), pigs and boars (porcine pestivirus [PPeV], also known as Bungowannah virus; atypical porcine pestivirus [APPeV]), sheep (Aydin-like pestivirus [AydinPeV]), giraffes (giraffe pestivirus [GPeV]), pronghorns (pronghorn antelope pestivirus [PAPeV]), and rodents (rat pestivirus [RPeV]).[860] A partially sequenced pesti-like virus from bats awaits classification, but it is notable that rats and bats are the only known natural hosts of pestiviruses outside the order Artiodactyla, that is, cloven-hooved animals. It is also notable that CSFV has been adapted to grow in rabbits; this strain is attenuated in pigs and has been used as a live vaccine in China for over 60 years.[157]

Pestiviruses can be cultured in the laboratory and several highly permissive cell lines have been identified. It is notable that BVDV is found in most commercially available lots of pooled fetal calf serum, so permissive cells stocks must be validated as BVDV-free and maintained under serum-free conditions or with serum from other species. In cell culture, pestiviruses are generally noncytopathic (ncp), although stable cytopathic (cp) biotypes have been identified based on their ability to induce cell death in cell culture. Infectious cDNA clones and replicons have been assembled for several pestiviruses, allowing all aspects of their life cycle to be dissected at the molecular level.

Pestiviruses produce a range of diseases in their respective hosts; the two most economically impactful are CSFV and BVDV. CSFV is one of the most severe infectious diseases of pigs, with mortality rates up to 90%. CSFV infections may have an acute course, with malaise and gastrointestinal distress progressing to fatal hemorrhagic and neurological syndromes within 4 weeks, or follow a chronic course, typically in immunologically immature newborn piglets, producing a more extended (1–3 months) but no less lethal course of disease.[93] BVDV1 usually causes only subclinical or mild symptoms in adult animals, while some strains of BVDV2 have been associated with a severe, acute hemorrhagic disease.[704] However, vertical transmission of BVDV1, BVDV2, or BDV can lead to chronic infections of newborn calves or lambs that invariably lead to fatal mucosal disease (MD); interestingly, both ncp and cp viral biotypes can be recovered from animals with MD.[894] Effective vaccine strategies have been developed for CSFV; however, the development of BVDV vaccines has proven to be more challenging due to the inherent antigenic diversity of these viruses.[643] One promising approach has been the development of live, recombinant cpBVDV strains containing in-frame deletions in the viral N^{pro} gene and inactivating mutations in the viral E^{rns} gene, which induce strain-specific immune responses but do not establish persistent infections or cause fetal death in immunized pregnant cows.[625]

Structure and Physical Properties of the Virion

Pestivirus particles are 40 to 60 nm in diameter, are lipid enveloped, and display viral envelope glycoproteins E^{rns}, E1, and E2 surrounding a nucleocapsid composed of the core (C) protein and viral RNA. Similar to HCV, pestiviruses are remarkably stable to low pH.[207,453] Virus particles are relatively featureless, although GPeV particles show an intriguing electron-lucent internal space to one side of the capsid (Fig. 7.18). Given the similarity of GPeV particle morphology to proposed HCV lipoviroparticle structures and that pestivirus particles have

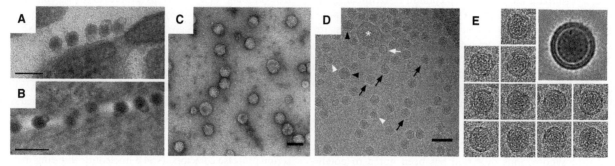

FIGURE 7.18 Pestivirus particles. A: Extracellular forms of GPeV by standard TEM, showing loosely attached envelope membranes. **B:** Extracellular GPV, as in **(A)**, imaged with electron tomography. (**Panels (A)** and **(B)** were adapted from Schmeiser S, Mast J, Thiel HJ, et al. Morphogenesis of pestiviruses: new insights from ultrastructural studies of strain Giraffe-1. J Virol 2014;88(5):2717–2724. doi: 10.1128/JVI.03237-13. With permission from American Society for Microbiology.[816]) **C:** Purified BVDV1 particles imaged by negative staining and standard TEM. **D:** Purified BVDV1 particles imaged by cryo-EM. As per Callens et al.,[132] "*Black arrows*: enveloped, capsid-containing particles of approximately 50 nm, *black arrowheads*: larger enveloped, capsid-containing particles, *white arrowheads*: nonenveloped, capsid-like particles, *white arrows*: small empty vesicles, *white asterisks*: large vesicles." **E:** BVDV1 particle (*large inset*) reconstructed by averaging from representative cryo-EM micrographs (*small insets*). (**Panels (C)** to **(E)** were reproduced under Creative Commons license from Callens et al.[132] All scale bars, 100 nm.)

relatively light buoyant densities, approximately 1.090 to 1.134 g/mL,[486,599] it is tempting to speculate that this extracapsular space may be filled with lipids. Consistent with this, BVDV1 particles were found to have a high cholesterol, sphingomyelin, and hexosylceramide content for a virus that buds into the ER, although extracapsular spaces were not prominent.[132]

Binding and Entry

Pestiviruses exhibit broad cell tropism *in vivo*. Both CSFV and ncpBVDV1 infect epithelia, B and T lymphocytes, monocytes, and bone marrow cells, causing marked lymphopenia and thrombocytopenia as well as hemorrhage in lymph nodes and Peyer patches.[590,933] Pestiviruses can initially attach to cells via interaction of the E[rns] glycoprotein with cell-surface GAGs.[372,373] However, only E1 and E2 are required for the entry of BVDV1 pseudoparticles, suggesting that E[rns] serves to enhance avidity in native virions.[781] Recombinant CSFV E2 can bind to cells and block infection of both CSFV and BVDV, suggesting that both viruses share a common entry receptor.[370] In contrast, the BDV E2 exhibits virus-specific tropism.[518] An early report that LDLR serves as a receptor for BVDV1 has not held up to further scrutiny.[452] One validated entry receptor for BVDV1 and BVDV2 entry into bovine cells is CD46, which binds to these viruses via its first complement control protein repeat.[451,599] BVDV1 and CSFV are internalized via clathrin-mediated endocytosis and delivered to endosomes, where low pH-dependent fusion occurs.[320,453,493,837] Similar to HCV, pestiviruses are acid stable and must be primed to respond to low pH. Combined treatment of BVDV1 with a reducing agent and low pH allowed "fusion-from-without," suggesting that one or more protein disulfide isomerases on the cell surface or endosomal compartments may contribute to priming.[453] The fusion process releases the nucleocapsid, which is presuma-

bly disassembled to release the viral genome. Interestingly, the growth of a unique CSFV mutant lacking core protein was highly restricted by ISG expression in target cells, suggesting that the nucleocapsid serves to protect the incoming genome from innate antiviral responses.[766]

Genome Structure

Pestivirus genomes are approximately 12.3 kb in length, lack a 5′ cap or 3′ poly(A) tail, and contain 5′ and 3′ NCRs of 372 to 385 and 185 to 273 nts, respectively, flanking one long ORF of approximately 3,900 codons (Fig. 7.19A).[118,180,650] Similar to hepaci- and pegiviruses, the 5′ NCRs of pestiviruses contain an IRES that directs cap-independent translation of the viral genome.[730] Upstream of the IRES are two 5′ SL structures (domains Ia and Ib in Fig. 7.19A) shown to be important for BVDV1 RNA replication.[279,1013] Surprisingly, all of domain Ia and part of Ib may be substituted or deleted; however, replication is strictly dependent on the 5′-terminal GUAU sequence.[62,279] Thus, pestiviruses and hepaciviruses differ in the organization of their 5′ signals needed for genome replication.[313]

Pestivirus 3′ NCRs contain a SL-containing variable region followed by a conserved region that contains two conserved SLs.[204,1011] Mutational analyses indicate that the 3′ variable region is important for translational termination and may coordinate translation and replication, while the 3′ conserved region is critical for RNA replication, likely to direct minus-strand initiation.[376,694,1011] A critical feature of the 3′ conserved region is to bind and sequester microRNAs miR-17 and let-7; these binding events are important for BVDV1 and CSFV RNA replication but also dysregulate expression of host genes dependent on miR-17 and let-7.[812] While miR-17 binds to one unstructured loop within the 3′ conserved region, let-7 can

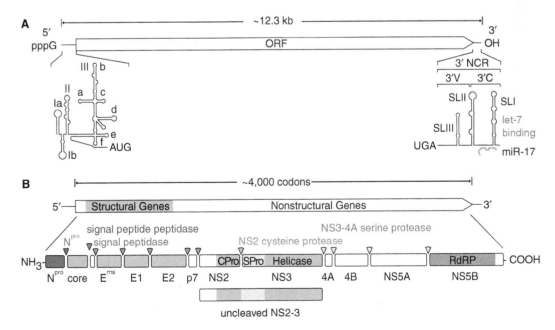

FIGURE 7.19 Pestivirus genome structure and protein expression. A: Genome structure and RNA elements. Important RNA elements are indicated as in Figure 7.4. **B:** Polyprotein processing and cleavage products. Symbols identifying proteolytic cleavages for the cpBVDV1 NADL strain are the same as those described in Figure 7.4 except for the autocatalytic cleavage releasing the N-terminal nonstructural protein N[pro] from the pestivirus polyprotein, which is indicated by a closed bullet. See text for details.

bind to several sequences located within secondary structures, presumably destabilizing them (Fig. 7.19A). Thus, these miRNAs may act as switches that stabilize or destabilize structures within the 3′ NCR, respectively.

Translation and Polyprotein Processing

The pestivirus IRES bears structural and functional similarity to that of hepaciviruses.[710,730,770] The minimal functional IRES includes 5′ NCR domains II and III, although its activity is influenced by RNA structures downstream of the initiation codon. Similar to hepaciviruses, the pestivirus IRES binds ribosomal 40S subunits without the need for translation initiation factors eIF4A, eIF4B, and eIF4F.[710,711,855] In fact, the CSFV IRES displaces eIF3 from its ribosomal position, so much so that eIF3 is held in the 43S subcomplex solely via its interaction with IRES domain III.[344]

The pestivirus polyprotein is proteolytically processed into individual viral proteins: Npro–C–Erns–E1–E2–p7–NS2–NS3–NS4A–NS4B–NS5A–NS5B (Fig. 7.19B). Unlike for other members of the family, the first pestivirus protein, Npro, is not a structural protein but a NS autoprotease responsible for cleavage at the Npro/C site.[867,976] The pestivirus structural proteins are cleaved by signal peptidase at the C/Erns, E1/E2, E2/p7, and p7/NS2 sites, with incomplete cleavage leading to accumulation of uncleaved E2–p7.[236,336,792] Similar to HCV, the pestivirus C protein is further processed by SPP, releasing mature C protein from the signal peptide.[351] The pestivirus Erns–E1 polyprotein is processed slowly by an unknown protease, most

likely signal peptidase.[86,792] In the NS region, the NS2 cysteine autoprotease cleaves the NS2/3 junction in a regulated manner,[465] while the NS3-4A serine protease cleaves the NS3/4A, NS4A/4B, NS4B/5A, and NS5A/5B junctions.[891,977,989] As will be discussed, the viral serine protease activity is reduced during late times of infection with ncp pestiviruses, leading to accumulation of uncleaved NS4A-B, NS4B-5A, and NS5A-B.[179,473] Genetic analysis suggest that NS4A-B is not essential for BVDV replication in cell culture.[284]

Npro Autoprotease

Npro is a bifunctional protein. The N-terminal region forms a cysteine protease with a unique fold and catalytic mechanism (dyad active site residues H49 and C69), classified as its own cysteine protease clade.[304,306,867,976,1036] This protease cleaves only once, at the Npro/C junction, as the C-terminal peptide of Npro remains tightly integrated in the protease structure once cleavage occurs (Fig. 7.20A).[306,1036] Upstream of the substrate peptide is a Zn^{2+}-binding TRASH domain, which binds to IRF3 and targets this immunoregulator for polyubiquitylation and proteasomal degradation, thereby inhibiting innate antiviral responses.[59,60,156,305,360,789,791] The mechanism by which Npro targets IRF3 for polyubiquitylation, including the identity of the relevant E3 ligase, remains obscure. Other cellular Npro-binding partners include IRF7 and IκBα, two immune transcription regulators; S100A9, a Ca^{2+}- and Zn^{2+}-binding immunomodulator; HAX1, a regulator of cortical actin and apoptosis; PCBP1, a single-stranded poly(rC)–binding protein;

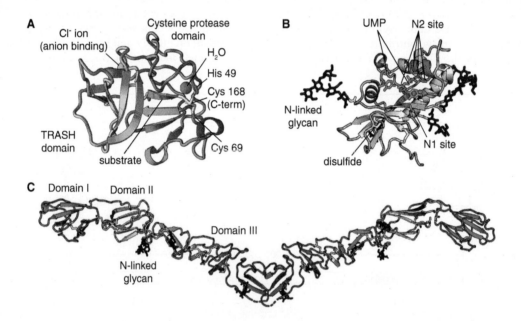

FIGURE 7.20 Pestivirus Npro and structural proteins. A: Structure of HoBiPeV Npro is shown, including the cysteine protease and TRASH domains. The molecule is in the postcleavage form, with the C-terminal residue, Cys 168 at the tip of the substrate peptide, and disulfide bonded to the catalytic Cys 69 residue. Catalytic moieties His 49 and H_2O are shown, as is an anion-binding pocket, postulated to bind an unknown ligand *in vivo*. Rendered from PDB 3ZFO.[1036] **B:** Structure of the BVDV1 Erns ectodomain is shown, including two uridine monophosphates (UMPs) as RNA-like substrates within the N1- and N2-binding pockets. Disulfides and N-linked glycans are labeled in *yellow* and *black*, respectively. Rendered from PDB 4DW4.[450] **C:** Structure of the BVDV1 E2 glycoprotein, which forms tail–tail disulfide-linked dimers. Domains I, II, and III are labeled; disulfides and N-linked glycans are labeled in *yellow* and *black*, respectively. Rendered from PDB 4ILD.[512]

and uS10, a 40S ribosomal protein involved in translational quality control.[194,212,262,390,506,570] N[pro] is dispensable for replication in cell culture but is required for pestivirus pathogenesis *in vivo*; as such, N[pro] deletion mutants have been tested as live vaccines.[600,919]

Pestivirus Structural Proteins

The capsid (C) protein (~14 kDa) is a positively charged, natively unfolded protein that binds RNA with low affinity and specificity.[382,665] Remarkably, C protein can tolerate deletions, duplications, and insertions; for one of these mutants, profound defects in virus assembly were suppressed by a second-site mutation in the NS3 helicase domain.[767,768]

E[rns] (44–48 kDa) is an unusual viral glycoprotein that forms disulfide-linked homodimers and is highly glycosylated on seven to nine Asn residues.[911] E[rns] peripherally associates with membranes via a C-terminal amphipathic helix[1,261,906] and is also secreted in soluble form from infected cells.[792,960] The most surprising feature of E[rns] is that it encodes ribonuclease activity with a RNase T2–like fold and specificity for uridine residues (Fig. 7.20B).[346,450,819] This RNase activity serves to inhibit host innate antiviral responses.[374,894] Viruses containing mutations in the E[rns] catalytic active site are attenuated *in vivo*,[624,942] and antibodies that inhibit RNA cleavage tend to neutralize virus infectivity.[974] RNase activity does not require disulfide linkage of E[rns] homodimers at C171, yet mutation of this residue gives rise to mutant viruses that are less virulent *in vivo*, suggesting that dimer formation contributes additional determinant(s) of pathogenesis.[907,974] E[rns] binds to cell-surface–expressed GAGs and may translocate across cellular membrane via its C-terminal amphipathic helix[478] or be taken up by clathrin-mediated endocytosis.[1042] A key *in vivo* target of E[rns] may be plasmacytoid dendritic cells, which abundantly produce type I interferons in response to CSFV-infected cells; this response is largely inhibited by E[rns].[740]

E1 (25–33 kDa) and E2 (53–55 kDa) are integral membrane glycoproteins that form disulfide-linked heterodimers and E2 homodimers.[911,961] Heterodimer formation is essential for viral entry and involves charge interactions within the E1 and E2 transmembrane domains.[781,948] E1 folds slowly and is poorly immunogenic, while E2 is immunodominant and has a well-defined structure. Surprisingly, E2 has a linear domain topology and forms tail-to-tail disulfide-linked homodimers that project out from the virus surface like opposing crane booms (Fig. 7.20C).[233,512] E2 lacks structural similarity to known fusion proteins and does not encode recognizable fusion peptides. Thus, E2 may only be involved in receptor binding, while E1 is the likely fusion protein. Indeed, E1 does contain two putative fusion peptides, although it is hard to reconcile the small size of this protein with known fusion protein mechanisms.[948]

Pestivirus Nonstructural Proteins

Pestiviruses encode a small p7 protein that is essentially a hairpin of two transmembrane domains flanking a central charged peptide. Similar to the HCV p7 protein, pestivirus p7 is dispensable for RNA replication[63] but required for the production of infectious virus particles[336,517] and appears to function as a viroporin with ion channel activity.[296,479–481,568]

The NS2 protein (~54 kDa) is a polytopic membrane protein with a C-terminal, cytosolic cysteine protease domain that is responsible for cleaving the NS2-3 precursor (~125 kDa).[464,466] This cleavage is temporally regulated in ncp pestiviruses,

leading to accumulation of uncleaved NS2-3 late in infection. Uncleaved NS2-3 has reduced NS3-4A serine protease activity and is incapable of supporting RNA replication but is important for virus assembly.[3,63,465,656] Remarkably, NS2 cysteine protease activity requires stable interaction with a cellular HSP40-family chaperone, DNAJC14 (originally identified as Jiv for J-domain protein interacting with viral protein), which is required for the replication of all pestiviruses examined to date.[379,464]

As for other members of this virus family, the NS3 protein (~80 kDa) encodes an N-terminal chymotrypsin-like serine protease domain and a C-terminal NTPase/RNA helicase domain (Fig. 7.7).[954,977] The NS3 serine protease requires NS4A as a cofactor[989]; cleaves between leucine and small uncharged amino acids, L↓(S/A/N)[891,989]; and is essential for virus viability.[989] Surprisingly, the protease retains activity when threonine is substituted for the serine nucleophile.[891] As for other members of the family, the pestivirus serine protease is also capable of internal autoproteolysis at one or two sites within NS3.[474] Interestingly, one of these cleavages releases a functional NS3-4A protease domain and a soluble helicase domain with unknown functions.

The pestivirus NS4A protein (~10 kDa) is functionally similar to the HCV NS4A protein, despite lack of sequence conservation. It has an N-terminal membrane anchor and an internal peptide that intercalates with the serine protease fold and is an essential cofactor for the NS3 serine protease activity.[223,892,989] NS4A also has an important but previously uncharacterized role in virus assembly.[223,517,656] Interestingly, structures of full-length CSFV NS3-4A reveal additional configurations between the serine protease and helicase domains previously not seen with other members of the family, as well as a molecular mechanism whereby interaction of the NS4A C-terminal peptide with the NS3 serine protease domain acts as a switch between RNA replication and virus assembly.[223]

NS4B (~38 kDa) is a polytopic membrane protein that associates with RNA replication complexes.[965] Like HCV, pestivirus NS4B proteins also encode an NTPase activity of unknown function.[295]

Similar to HCV NS5A, the pestivirus NS5A (~58 kDa) is a phosphoprotein that contains an N-terminal amphipathic helix mediating peripheral membrane association, a structured Zn²⁺-binding domain, and two downstream domains separated by LCSs.[111,378,802,902] Also similar to HCV NS5A, pestivirus NS5A is tolerant of insertions and deletions in its second domain; insertion of a mCherry fluorescent protein demonstrated that pestivirus NS5A, like HCV NS5A, is trafficked to LDs.[378] Furthermore, NS5A is phosphorylated by serine–threonine kinase(s) similar to the enzymes that phosphorylate flavivirus NS5 and hepacivirus NS5A.[755] Genetic analysis revealed that defects in the NS5A gene can be efficiently complemented in *trans*, whereas mutations in other pestivirus NS genes were not.[755] NS5A may also serve to antagonize GBP1, an interferon-induced GTPase that inhibits CSFV and other viruses.[515]

NS5B (~75 kDa) is the key driver of pestivirus RNA replication, the RdRP. *In vitro*, recombinant NS5B has been shown to extend template-primed RNA into double-stranded copy-back products[894,1031] or to catalyze *de novo* initiation from short, synthetic RNA or DNA templates, depending on the presence of sufficiently high GTP levels.[403,469] BVDV1 and CSFV NS5B are structurally similar to HCV NS5B, containing a canonical palm subdomain surrounded by finger and thumb subdomains but with some key differences (Fig. 7.8).[160,161,513] Notably, pestiviruses have a conserved, N-terminal approximately 90-aa extension not found in hepacivirus NS5B; structurally, this region has been captured in three different conformations interacting with the outer surface of the polymerase core. The function of the N-terminal domain is not clear; however, mutations or deletion of the N-terminal domain strongly impacts RNA synthesis, suggesting that it may regulate RdRp activity through allosteric mechanisms.[513]

RNA Replication

Pestivirus RNA replication requires NS3 through NS5B and is associated with cytosolic membranes, albeit without the profound membrane rearrangements described for flaviviruses or hepaciviruses.[63,816] Synthesis of new viral positive- and negative-strand RNAs is first detected between 4 and 6 hours of infection; at later times, viral RNAs are found in double-stranded RFs and partially duplex RIs, consistent with the asymmetric synthesis of excess positive-strand over negative-strand RNAs.[298,299,916,956]

The study of ncp and cpBVDV1 has provided key insights into the mechanisms of pestivirus RNA replication and virus assembly. A critical discovery was that ncp and cpBVDV1 isolates temporally differ in their expression of NS2-3, NS2, and NS3.[465] As mentioned above, uncleaved NS2-3 functions in virus assembly but not in RNA replication, and NS2-3 cleavage requires the cellular chaperone DNAJC14 to activate the latent cysteine protease within NS2. Thus, early in infection, when DNAJC14 is abundant, the NS2 protease is activated, leading to autocleavage of NS2-3, release of NS3, and enabling RNA replication. However, as DNAJC14 levels become rate limiting at later times, NS2-3 cleavage is greatly reduced, switching the life cycle of ncpBVDV1 from RNA replication to virus assembly.[379] cpBVDV viruses are able to promote continuous NS2-3 cleavage, despite limited DNAJC14 levels, through a variety of genetic rearrangements, as described below.

A second way that the study of cp versus ncp viruses has contributed to our understanding of pestivirus RNA replication is in RNA recombination. As will be discussed shortly, many cpBVDV have genetic insertions or rearrangements that must have arisen through RNA recombination, which led some groups to examine the molecular basis for these presumably rare but profoundly impactful events. One likely driver of RNA recombination is a copy-choice mechanism,[427] whereby an RdRP switches templates during minus-strand synthesis to produce chimeric transcripts that are consistent with the coding orientation of cellular inserts found in cpBVDV1 genomes. There is also evidence for the existence of one or more alternative mechanisms of RNA recombination that are independent of RNA synthesis. Namely, cotransfection of two BVDV1 transcripts, each lacking a different essential part of the genome, gave rise to viable viruses with signs of homologous and nonhomologous recombination.[284,285,429] Subsequent analysis of recombinants, and the factors influencing their biogenesis, suggested that this nonreplicative mechanism likely occurs via endoribonuclease activity and end-to-end ligation, presumably by cellular enzymes.[36]

Assembly and Release of Virus Particles

Pestivirus particles bud into the ER and transit through the secretory pathway.[82,314,816] Consistent with this, pestivirus envelope glycoproteins are retained within the secretory pathway,[315,962] and the secretion of virus particles, but not their assembly, is inhibited by brefeldin A, an inhibitor of ER–Golgi transport.[315,962] As the lipid content of purified virus particles greatly differ from the composition of the ER membrane, it appears that BVDV1 particles acquire additional lipids during their maturation.[132] Virus particles are sometimes observed in multivesicular bodies, suggesting that they may traffic through an endosomal compartment during their secretion.[816] Once released, it appears that BVDV1 is preferentially transmitted via cell-to-cell transmission, at least in cell culture.[617]

The assembly of pestivirus particles depends on several NS proteins, including uncleaved NS2-3, which accumulates during late times of infection. Indeed, chimeric BVDV1 genomes incapable of producing NS2-3 were found to be blocked in virus assembly[484]; further, genetic dissection of the chimeras identified additional determinants in the NS2 cysteine protease domain and NS3 serine protease domain that allowed BVDV1 growth in the absence of uncleaved NS2-3.[431] Intriguingly, this region of the serine protease interacts with the C-terminus of NS4A in crystal structures of full-length NS3-4A, and mutations that disrupt or stabilize this interaction switch between RNA replication and virus assembly.[223]

Pathogenesis of Mucosal Disease and the Generation of cp Pestiviruses

BVDV- and BDV-associated MD, which is universally lethal, has a fascinating etiology. MD arises only after *in utero* infection with ncp viruses between 40 and 125 days of gestation, leading to birth of immunotolerant calves or lambs that remain persistently infected for life. By the time MD symptoms appear, usually between 6 and 24 months of age, both cp and ncp viral biotypes can be isolated; this can reflect superinfection of ncp-infected dams with a cp virus.[193,602,894] However, most cp strains arise *de novo*, generated via RNA recombination from the coinfecting parental ncp strain; only rarely do cp strains lack obvious genome rearrangements.[704,894] These rearrangements lead to increased NS3 expression independent of cellular DNAJ14 expression, enhanced RNA replication, and cytopathic effects in cell culture.

Some of the remarkable genetic rearrangements discovered in cpBVDV are illustrated in Figure 7.21. Most cpBVDV genome rearrangements lead to increased NS3 production and enhanced RNA replication. For instance, the cpBVDV1 strain NADL contains an in-frame fragment of the cellular DNAJC14 gene (aka Jiv) inserted within NS2 (Fig. 7.21B).[613,772] As described above, DNAJC14 is essential for proper folding and activation of the NS2 cysteine protease, and overexpression of a critical 90-aa DNAJC14 subdomain enhances NS2-3 cleavage, regardless whether the fragment is provided in *cis* or in *trans*.[465] Surprisingly, the cpBVDV1 strain CP7 contains an even smaller insertion in NS2, a 27-nt out-of-frame duplication from an upstream region of NS2, which also leads to increased NS2-3 processing and the ncp phenotype (Fig. 7.21C).[626,893] Several other virus- or cell-derived insertions at or close to the same site in NS2 have been described for other cpBVDV1 isolates.[45] Given these observations, it is tempting to speculate that mutations in the NS2 gene of an ancient, NS2/3-cleaving cp pestivirus may have given rise to a ncp virus that became dependent on DNAJC14 but gained ecological fitness through reduced cytopathic effects and persistence. According to this model, insertions in NS2 may cause reversion of ncp viruses

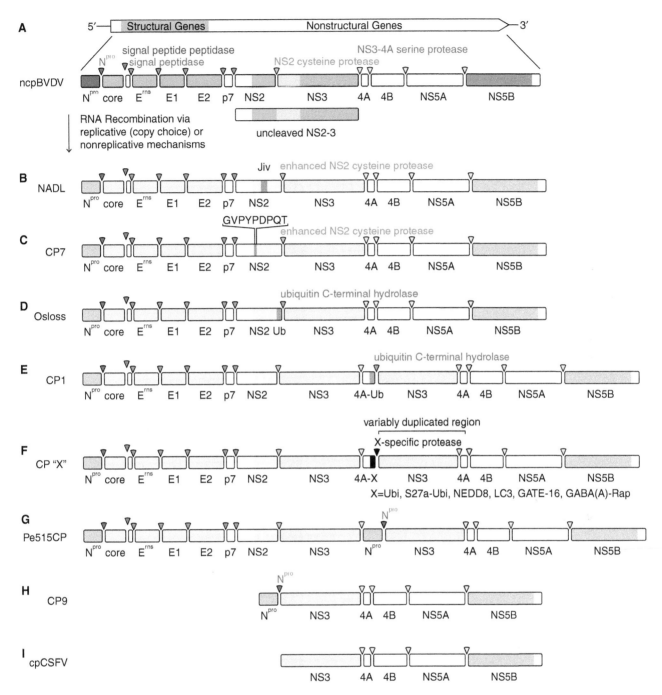

FIGURE 7.21 Pestivirus genome rearrangements associated with cp viruses. A: The polyprotein of a typical ncp pestivirus, for reference. **B:** The genome of cpBVDV1 strain NADL, showing the Jiv insertion within NS2. **C:** The genome of cpBVDV1 strain CP7, showing the nine-codon insertion within NS2. **D:** The genome of cpBVDV1 strain Osloss, showing insertion of the cellular ubiquitin (Ubi) gene at the 3' end of NS2. **E:** The genome of cpBVDV1 strain CP1, showing the insertion of the cellular ubiquitin gene at the 3' end of NS4A and duplication of the NS3-4A region. **F:** The genome organization of numerous cpBVDV isolates, similar to CP1, that have duplications in the NS3-4B region and insertion of ubiquitin or ubiquitin-like genes. **G:** The genome of cpBVDV1 strain Pe515CP, showing duplication of the NS3 gene, preceded by duplication of the N^pro gene. **H:** The genome of cpBVDV1 strain CP9, a naturally occurring DI genome that lacks the core–NS2 genes. **I:** The genome organization of numerous cpCSFV isolates, naturally occurring DI genomes that lack the N^pro–NS2 genes. As discussed in the text, these rearrangements increase NS3 expression relative to NS2-3 expression.

back to the cp biotype. Indeed, some cpBVDV isolates, such as BVDV1 strain Oregon, lack insertions or other genome arrangements yet retain NS2-3 autoprotease activity.[460] Thus, perhaps this strain cleaves NS2/3 like the putative ancestral cpBVDV isolate, without the need for insertions.

Another common rearrangement is the insertion of cellular ubiquitin (Ubi) or Ubi-like genes immediately upstream of NS3 (Fig. 7.21D), leading to NS2/3 cleavage by ubiquitin C-terminal hydrolase or related enzymes (e.g., BVDV1 strain Osloss).[627,894] For some viruses, like BVDV1 strain CP1, Ubi insertion is also accompanied by duplication in the NS3–4A region (Fig. 7.21E) or other genome rearrangements (Fig. 7.21F).[628] These duplications give rise to viruses encoding an intact NS2-3 region for virion morphogenesis and an NS3–NS5B cassette for efficient RNA replication.

In yet another recurring configuration, cp pestivirus genomes contain the N^pro autoprotease immediately upstream of NS3. For instance, N^pro is duplicated together with the NS3 and NS4A genes in BVDV1 strain Pe515CP (Fig. 7.21G).[628] Other isolates, such as cpBVDV1 strain CP9, contain a precise deletion of the C–NS2 coding region, resulting in the in-frame fusion of N^pro and NS3 (Fig. 7.21H).[895] These subgenomic DI RNAs are naturally occurring replicons, capable of autonomous RNA replication but requiring ncpBVDV helper viruses to provide packaging functions in *trans*.[63] Similarly, some cpCSFV subgenomic RNAs lack the entire coding sequence upstream of NS3 (Fig. 7.21I).[629]

The genome rearrangements in cp pestivirus genomes lead to increased NS3 expression, independence from cellular DNAJ14 expression, enhanced RNA replication, and cytopathic effects in cell culture. Efforts have been made to dissect these phenotypes and reveal the basis of viral cytopathic effects. For instance, a point mutation in NS2 confers a temperature-sensitive cp phenotype to the cpBVDV1 strain CP7; at higher temperatures, this mutant retains high NS3 expression but reduced RNA replication and cytopathic effects.[693] On the other hand, a point mutation in NS4B attenuates the cytopathic effect of cpBVDV1 strain NADL, which still produces NS3 and viral RNA at comparable levels to the cp parent.[743] Similarly, other ncpBVDV strains show changes in NS4B.[284] Given that NS4B is associated with membrane rearrangements,[965] and that cpBVDV causes ER stress,[396] one hypothesis is that the overcommitment of cellular membranes to viral replication may lead to cell death. In infected animals, viral cytopathic effects may enhance viral spread but induce widespread tissue injury and inflammation. Indeed, animals with MD have increased viral loads, greater distribution of viral antigens, and higher infected cell counts than animals persistently infected with ncp virus.[521] Another intriguing possibility is that viral tropism might be expanded by viral independence from DNAJ14 expression. Thus, enhanced cytopathology, increased tropism, and lack of immune control may all contribute to the severe pathogenesis observed in MD.

PERSPECTIVES

This is an incredible, exciting time to be studying the *Flaviviridae*. With widespread emerging and reemerging human DENV, YFV, JEV, WNV, and ZIKV infections, flaviviruses retain their high medical relevance, driving basic research and the development of novel vaccine and antiviral strategies. HCV research has come full circle, from humble beginnings as a veritable backwater lacking a culturable virus into one of the most well-studied, positive-strand RNA viruses and an advanced armamentarium of highly effective DAAs. While these successes have largely ended HCV drug discovery efforts, significant challenges remain in understanding the structure and function of the virus particle, improving animal models of HCV pathogenesis, and developing vaccines that can prevent or cure HCV infection.[54] Moreover, the discovery of related

hepaciviruses, pegiviruses, as well as segmented Jingmenviruses and large flavi-like viruses have raised far more questions than they have answered about the ecology, evolution, and molecular biology of this virus family. Some overarching questions include: How did the *Flaviviridae* evolve, particularly in relation to other positive-strand RNA virus families? How much diversity is still left to discover within this family? And, what threads link all members of this family together? Our field welcomes new talent and diverse, innovative approaches as we tackle these and other important questions.

REFERENCES

1. Aberle D, Oetter KM, Meyers G. Lipid binding of the amphipathic helix serving as membrane anchor of pestivirus glycoprotein Erns. *PLoS One* 2015;10(8):e0135680.
2. Ackermann M, Padmanabhan R. De novo synthesis of RNA by the dengue virus RNA-dependent RNA polymerase exhibits temperature dependence at the initiation but not elongation phase. *J Biol Chem* 2001;276(43):39926–39937.
3. Agapov EV, Murray CL, Frolov I, et al. Uncleaved NS2-3 is required for production of infectious bovine viral diarrhea virus. *J Virol* 2004;78(5):2414–2425.
4. Agnello V, Abel G, Elfahal M, et al. Hepatitis C virus and other Flaviviridae viruses enter cells via low density lipoprotein receptor. *Proc Natl Acad Sci U S A* 1999;96(22):12766–12771.
5. Ago H, Adachi T, Yoshida A, et al. Crystal structure of the RNA-dependent RNA polymerase of hepatitis C virus. *Structure* 1999;7(11):1417–1426.
6. Aguirre S, Luthra P, Sanchez-Aparicio MT, et al. Dengue virus NS2B protein targets cGAS for degradation and prevents mitochondrial DNA sensing during infection. *Nat Microbiol* 2017;2:17037.
7. Aguirre S, Maestre AM, Pagni S, et al. DENV inhibits type I IFN production in infected cells by cleaving human STING. *PLoS Pathog* 2012;8(10):e1002934.
8. Ait-Goughoulte M, Kanda T, Meyer K, et al. Hepatitis C virus genotype 1a growth and induction of autophagy. *J Virol* 2008;82(5):2241–2249.
9. Aizaki H, Lee KJ, Sung VM, et al. Characterization of the hepatitis C virus RNA replication complex associated with lipid rafts. *Virology* 2004;324(2):450–461.
10. Akey DL, Brown WC, Dutta S, et al. Flavivirus NS1 structures reveal surfaces for associations with membranes and the immune system. *Science* 2014;343(6173):881–885.
11. Akiyama BM, Laurence HM, Massey AR, et al. Zika virus produces noncoding RNAs using a multi-pseudoknot structure that confounds a cellular exonuclease. *Science* 2016;354(6316):1148–1152.
12. Aktepe TE, Pham H, Mackenzie JM. Differential utilisation of ceramide during replication of the flaviviruses West Nile and dengue virus. *Virology* 2015;484:241–250.
13. Albornoz A, Carletti T, Corazza G, et al. The stress granule component TIA-1 binds tick-borne encephalitis virus RNA and is recruited to perinuclear sites of viral replication to inhibit viral translation. *J Virol* 2014;88(12):6611–6622.
14. Alcon-LePoder S, Drouet MT, Roux P, et al. The secreted form of dengue virus non-structural protein NS1 is endocytosed by hepatocytes and accumulates in late endosomes: implications for viral infectivity. *J Virol* 2005;79(17):11403–11411.
15. Ali N, Tardif KD, Siddiqui A. Cell-free replication of the hepatitis C virus subgenomic replicon. *J Virol* 2002;76(23):12001–12007.
16. Aligeti M, Roder A, Horner SM. Cooperation between the Hepatitis C virus p7 and NS5B proteins enhances virion infectivity. *J Virol* 2015;89(22):11523–11533.
17. Allander T, Beyene A, Jacobson SH, et al. Patients infected with the same hepatitis C virus strain display different kinetics of the isolate-specific antibody response. *J Infect Dis* 1997;175(1):26–31.
18. Allison SL, Schalich J, Stiasny K, et al. Oligomeric rearrangement of tick-borne encephalitis virus envelope proteins induced by an acidic pH. *J Virol* 1995;69(2):695–700.
19. Allison SL, Stadler K, Mandl CW, et al. Synthesis and secretion of recombinant tick-borne encephalitis virus protein E in soluble and particulate form. *J Virol* 1995;69(9):5816–5820.
20. Allison SL, Stiasny K, Stadler K, et al. Mapping of functional elements in the stem-anchor region of tick-borne encephalitis virus envelope protein E. *J Virol* 1999;73(7):5605–5612.
21. Alter MJ, Gallagher M, Morris TT, et al. Acute non-A-E hepatitis in the United States and the role of hepatitis G virus infection. Sentinel Counties Viral Hepatitis Study Team. *N Engl J Med* 1997;336(11):741–746.
22. Amador-Canizares Y, Bernier A, Wilson JA, et al. miR-122 does not impact recognition of the HCV genome by innate sensors of RNA but rather protects the 5′ end from the cellular pyrophosphatases, DOM3Z and DUSP11. *Nucleic Acids Res* 2018;46(10):5139–5158.
23. Ambrose RL, Mackenzie JM. West Nile virus differentially modulates the unfolded protein response to facilitate replication and immune evasion. *J Virol* 2011;85(6):2723–2732.
24. Ambrose RL, Mackenzie JM. ATF6 signaling is required for efficient West Nile virus replication by promoting cell survival and inhibition of innate immune responses. *J Virol* 2013;87(4):2206–2214.
25. André P, Komurian-Pradel F, Deforges S, et al. Characterization of low- and very-low-density hepatitis C virus RNA-containing particles. *J Virol* 2002;76(14):6919–6928.
26. André P, Perlemuter G, Budkowska A, et al. Hepatitis C virus particles and lipoprotein metabolism. *Semin Liver Dis* 2005;25(1):93–104.
27. Appel N, Pietschmann T, Bartenschlager R. Mutational analysis of hepatitis C virus non-structural protein 5A: potential role of differential phosphorylation in RNA replication and identification of a genetically flexible domain. *J Virol* 2005;79(5):3187–3194.
28. Appel N, Zayas M, Miller S, et al. Essential role of domain III of nonstructural protein 5A for hepatitis C virus infectious particle assembly. *PLoS Pathog* 2008;4(3):e1000035.
29. Appleby TC, Anderson R, Fedorova O, et al. Visualizing ATP-dependent RNA translocation by the NS3 helicase from HCV. *J Mol Biol* 2011;405(5):1139–1153.

30. Appleby TC, Perry JK, Murakami E, et al. Viral replication. Structural basis for RNA replication by the hepatitis C virus polymerase. *Science* 2015;347(6223):771–775.
31. Arias CF, Preugschat F, Strauss JH. Dengue 2 virus NS2B and NS3 form a stable complex that can cleave NS3 within the helicase domain. *Virology* 1993;193:888–899.
32. Asabe SI, Tanji Y, Satoh S, et al. The N-terminal region of hepatitis C virus-encoded NS5A is important for NS4A-dependent phosphorylation. *J Virol* 1997;71(1):790–796.
33. Asselah T, Bieche I, Mansouri A, et al. In vivo hepatic endoplasmic reticulum stress in patients with chronic hepatitis C. *J Pathol* 2010;221(3):264–274.
34. Assenberg R, Mastrangelo E, Walter TS, et al. Crystal structure of a novel conformational state of the flavivirus NS3 protein: implications for polyprotein processing and viral replication. *J Virol* 2009;83(24):12895–12906.
35. Aubry F, Nougairede A, Gould EA, et al. Flavivirus reverse genetic systems, construction techniques and applications: a historical perspective. *Antiviral Res* 2015;114:67–85.
36. Austermann-Busch S, Becher P. RNA structural elements determine frequency and sites of nonhomologous recombination in an animal plus-strand RNA virus. *J Virol* 2012;86(13):7393–7402.
37. Avirutnan P, Zhang L, Punyadee N, et al. Secreted NS1 of dengue virus attaches to the surface of cells via interactions with heparan sulfate and chondroitin sulfate E. *PLoS Pathog* 2007;3(11):e183.
38. Backes P, Quinkert D, Reiss S, et al. Role of annexin A2 in the production of infectious hepatitis C virus particles. *J Virol* 2010;84(11):5775–5789.
39. Badillo A, Receveur-Brechot V, Sarrazin S, et al. Overall structural model of NS5A protein from hepatitis C virus and modulation by mutations conferring resistance of virus replication to cyclosporin A. *Biochemistry* 2017;56(24):3029–3048.
40. Bai Y, Zhou K, Doudna JA. Hepatitis C virus 3′UTR regulates viral translation through direct interactions with the host translation machinery. *Nucleic Acids Res* 2013;41(16):7861–7874.
41. Bailey AL, Buechler CR, Matson DR, et al. Pegivirus avoids immune recognition but does not attenuate acute-phase disease in a macaque model of HIV infection. *PLoS Pathog* 2017;13(10):e1006692.
42. Bailey AL, Lauck M, Mohns M, et al. Durable sequence stability and bone marrow tropism in a macaque model of human pegivirus infection. *Sci Transl Med* 2015;7(305):305ra144.
43. Baktash Y, Madhav A, Coller KE, et al. Single particle imaging of polarized hepatoma organoids upon hepatitis C virus infection reveals an ordered and sequential entry process. *Cell Host Microbe* 2018;23(3):382.e385–394.e385.
44. Balinsky CA, Schmeisser H, Ganesan S, et al. Nucleolin interacts with the dengue virus capsid protein and plays a role in formation of infectious virus particles. *J Virol* 2013;87(24):13094–13106.
45. Bálint A, Pálfi V, Belák S, et al. Viral sequence insertions and a novel cellular insertion in the NS2 gene of cytopathic isolates of bovine viral diarrhea virus as potential cytopathogenicity markers. *Virus Genes* 2005;30(1):49–58.
46. Bankwitz D, Steinmann E, Bitzegeio J, et al. Hepatitis C virus hypervariable region 1 modulates receptor interactions, conceals the CD81 binding site, and protects conserved neutralizing epitopes. *J Virol* 2010;84(11):5751–5763.
47. Barba G, Harper F, Harada T, et al. Hepatitis C virus core protein shows a cytoplasmic localization and associates to cellular lipid storage droplets. *Proc Natl Acad Sci U S A* 1997;94(4):1200–1205.
48. Barbaro G, Di Lorenzo G, Asti A, et al. Hepatocellular mitochondrial alterations in patients with chronic hepatitis C: ultrastructural and biochemical findings. *Am J Gastroenterol* 1999;94(8):2198–2205.
49. Bardina SV, Bunduc P, Tripathi S, et al. Enhancement of Zika virus pathogenesis by preexisting antiflavivirus immunity. *Science* 2017;356(6334):175–180.
50. Barouch-Bentov R, Neveu G, Xiao F, et al. Hepatitis C virus proteins interact with the endosomal sorting complex required for transport (ESCRT) machinery via ubiquitination to facilitate viral envelopment. *MBio* 2016;7(6).
51. Bartelma G, Padmanabhan R. Expression, purification, and characterization of the RNA 5′-triphosphatase activity of dengue virus type 2 nonstructural protein 3. *Virology* 2002;299(1):122–132.
52. Bartenschlager R, Ahlborn-Laake L, Mous J, et al. Kinetic and structural analyses of hepatitis C virus polyprotein processing. *J Virol* 1994;68(8):5045–5055.
53. Bartenschlager R, Ahlborn-Laake L, Yasargil K, et al. Substrate determinants for cleavage in cis and in trans by the hepatitis C virus NS3 proteinase. *J Virol* 1995;69(1):198–205.
54. Bartenschlager R, Baumert TF, Bukh J, et al. Critical challenges and emerging opportunities in hepatitis C virus research in an era of potent antiviral therapy: considerations for scientists and funding agencies. *Virus Res* 2018;248:53–62.
55. Bartenschlager R, Frese M, Pietschmann T. Novel insights into hepatitis C virus replication and persistence. *Adv Virus Res* 2004;63:71–180.
56. Bartenschlager R, Penin F, Lohmann V, et al. Assembly of infectious hepatitis C virus particles. *Trends Microbiol* 2011;19(2):95–103.
57. Barth H, Schafer C, Adah MI, et al. Cellular binding of hepatitis C virus envelope glycoprotein E2 requires cell surface heparan sulfate. *J Biol Chem* 2003;278(42):41003–41012.
58. Bartosch B, Dubuisson J, Cosset FL. Infectious hepatitis C virus pseudo-particles containing functional E1-E2 envelope protein complexes. *J Exp Med* 2003;197(5):633–642.
59. Bauhofer O, Summerfield A, McCullough KC, et al. Role of double-stranded RNA and N(pro) of classical swine fever virus in the activation of monocyte-derived dendritic cells. *Virology* 2005;343(1):93–105.
60. Bauhofer O, Summerfield A, Sakoda Y, et al. Classical swine fever virus N^{pro} interacts with interferon regulatory factor 3 and induces its proteasomal degradation. *J Virol* 2007;81(7):3087–3096.
61. Beames B, Chavez D, Guerra B, et al. Development of a primary tamarin hepatocyte culture system for GB virus-B: a surrogate model for hepatitis C virus. *J Virol* 2000;74(24):11764–11772.
62. Becher P, Orlich M, Thiel HJ. Mutations in the 5′ nontranslated region of bovine viral diarrhea virus result in altered growth characteristics. *J Virol* 2000;74(17):7884–7894.
63. Behrens SE, Grassmann CW, Thiel HJ, et al. Characterization of an autonomous subgenomic pestivirus RNA replicon. *J Virol* 1998;72(3):2364–2372.
64. Behrens SE, Tomei L, De Francesco R. Identification and properties of the RNA-dependent RNA polymerase of hepatitis C virus. *EMBO J* 1996;15(1):12–22.
65. Belov GA, Nair V, Hansen BT, et al. Complex dynamic development of poliovirus membranous replication complexes. *J Virol* 2012;86(1):302–312.
66. Belyaev AS, Chong S, Novikov A, et al. Hepatitis G virus encodes protease activities which can effect processing of the virus putative nonstructural proteins. *J Virol* 1998;72(1):868–872.
67. Benarroch D, Selisko B, Locatelli GA, et al. The RNA helicase, nucleotide 5′-triphosphatase, and RNA 5′-triphosphatase activities of Dengue virus protein NS3 are Mg2+-dependent and require a functional Walker B motif in the helicase catalytic core. *Virology* 2004;328(2):208–218.
68. Benga WJ, Krieger SE, Dimitrova M, et al. Apolipoprotein E interacts with hepatitis C virus nonstructural protein 5A and determines assembly of infectious particles. *Hepatology* 2010;51(1):43–53.
69. Bentham MJ, Foster TL, McCormick C, et al. Mutations in hepatitis C virus p7 reduce both the egress and infectivity of assembled particles via impaired proton channel function. *J Gen Virol* 2013;94(Pt 10):2236–2248.
70. Beran RK, Lindenbach BD, Pyle AM. The NS4A protein of hepatitis C virus promotes RNA-coupled ATP hydrolysis by the NS3 helicase. *J Virol* 2009;83(7):3268–3275.
71. Beran RK, Pyle AM. Hepatitis C viral NS3-4A protease activity is enhanced by the NS3 helicase. *J Biol Chem* 2008;283(44):29929–29937.
72. Beran RK, Serebrov V, Pyle AM. The serine protease domain of hepatitis C viral NS3 activates RNA helicase activity by promoting the binding of RNA substrate. *J Biol Chem* 2007;282(48):34913–34920.
73. Berg MG, Lee D, Coller K, et al. Discovery of a novel human pegivirus in blood associated with hepatitis C virus co-infection. *PLoS Pathog* 2015;11(12):e1005325.
74. Berg T, Müller AR, Platz KP, et al. Dynamics of GB virus C viremia early after orthotopic liver transplantation indicates extrahepatic tissues as the predominant site of GB virus C replication. *Hepatology* 1999;29(1):245–249.
75. Berger KL, Cooper JD, Heaton NS, et al. Roles for endocytic trafficking and phosphatidylinositol 4-kinase III alpha in hepatitis C virus replication. *Proc Natl Acad Sci U S A* 2009;106(18):7577–7582.
76. Berger KL, Kelly SM, Jordan TX, et al. Hepatitis C virus stimulates the phosphatidylinositol 4-kinase III alpha-dependent phosphatidylinositol 4-phosphate production that is essential for its replication. *J Virol* 2011;85(17):8870–8883.
77. Berger C, Romero-Brey I, Radujkovic D, et al. Daclatasvir-like inhibitors of NS5A block early biogenesis of hepatitis C virus-induced membranous replication factories, independent of RNA replication. *Gastroenterology* 2014;147(5):1094.e25–1105.e25.
78. Bernardin F, Operskalski E, Busch M, et al. Transfusion transmission of highly prevalent commensal human viruses. *Transfusion* 2010;50(11):2474–2483.
79. Best SM. The many faces of the flavivirus NS5 protein in antagonism of type I interferon signaling. *J Virol* 2017;91(3).
80. Best SM, Morris KL, Shannon JG, et al. Inhibition of interferon-stimulated JAK-STAT signaling by a tick-borne flavivirus and identification of NS5 as an interferon antagonist. *J Virol* 2005;79(20):12828–12839.
81. Bidet K, Dadlani D, Garcia-Blanco MA. G3BP1, G3BP2 and CAPRIN1 are required for translation of interferon stimulated mRNAs and are targeted by a dengue virus non-coding RNA. *PLoS Pathog* 2014;10(7):e1004242.
82. Bielefeldt-Ohmann H, Bloch B. Electron microscopic studies of bovine viral diarrhea virus in tissues of diseased calves and in cell cultures. *Arch Virol* 1982;71(1):57–74.
83. Bienz K, Egger D, Pfister T, et al. Structural and functional characterization of the poliovirus replication complex. *J Virol* 1992;66(5):2740–2747.
84. Billerbeck E, Wolfisberg R, Fahnoe U, et al. Mouse models of acute and chronic hepacivirus infection. *Science* 2017;357(6347):204–208.
85. Binder M, Quinkert D, Bochkarova O, et al. Identification of determinants involved in initiation of hepatitis C virus RNA synthesis by using intergenotypic replicase chimeras. *J Virol* 2007;81(10):5270–5283.
86. Bintintan I, Meyers G. A new type of signal peptidase cleavage site identified in an RNA virus polyprotein. *J Biol Chem* 2010;285(12):8572–8584.
87. Bissig KD, Wieland SF, Tran P, et al. Human liver chimeric mice provide a model for hepatitis B and C virus infection and treatment. *J Clin Invest* 2010;120(3):924–930.
88. Biswal BK, Cherney MM, Wang M, et al. Crystal structures of the RNA-dependent RNA polymerase genotype 2a of hepatitis C virus reveal two conformations and suggest mechanisms of inhibition by non-nucleoside inhibitors. *J Biol Chem* 2005;280(18):18202–18210.
89. Blach S, Zeuzem S, Manns M, et al. Global prevalence and genotype distribution of hepatitis C virus infection in 2015: a modelling study. *Lancet Gastroenterol Hepatol* 2017;2(3):161–176.
90. Blanchard E, Belouzard S, Goueslain L, et al. Hepatitis C virus entry depends on clathrin-mediated endocytosis. *J Virol* 2006;80(14):6964–6972.
91. Blanchard E, Roingeard P. The hepatitis C virus-induced membranous web in liver tissue. *Cells* 2018;7(11).
92. Blight KJ, Kolykhalov AA, Rice CM. Efficient initiation of HCV RNA replication in cell culture. *Science* 2000;290(5498):1972–1974.
93. Blome S, Staubach C, Henke J, et al. Classical swine fever-an updated review. *Viruses* 2017;9(4).
94. Bonenfant G, Williams N, Netzband R, et al. Zika virus subverts stress granules to promote and restrict viral gene expression. *J Virol* 2019;93.
95. Boni S, Lavergne JP, Boulant S, et al. Hepatitis C virus core protein acts as a trans-modulating factor on internal translation initiation of the viral RNA. *J Biol Chem* 2005;280(18):17737–17748.
96. Boson B, Denolly S, Turlure F, et al. Daclatasvir prevents hepatitis C virus infectivity by blocking transfer of the viral genome to assembly sites. *Gastroenterology* 2017;152(4):895.e814–907.e814.
97. Boson B, Granio O, Bartenschlager R, et al. A concerted action of hepatitis C virus p7 and nonstructural protein 2 regulates core localization at the endoplasmic reticulum and virus assembly. *PLoS Pathog* 2011;7(7):e1002144.

98. Boukadida C, Fritz M, Blumen B, et al. NS2 proteases from hepatitis C virus and related hepaciviruses share composite active sites and previously unrecognized intrinsic proteolytic activities. *PLoS Pathog* 2018;14(2):e1006863.
99. Boulant S, Douglas MW, Moody L, et al. Hepatitis C virus core protein induces lipid droplet redistribution in a microtubule- and Dynein-dependent manner. *Traffic* 2008;9(8):1268–1282.
100. Boulant S, Montserret R, Hope RG, et al. Structural determinants that target the hepatitis C virus core protein to lipid droplets. *J Biol Chem* 2006;281(31):22236–22247.
101. Boulant S, Targett-Adams P, McLauchlan J. Disrupting the association of hepatitis C virus core protein with lipid droplets correlates with a loss in production of infectious virus. *J Gen Virol* 2007;88(Pt 8):2204–2213.
102. Boulant S, Vanbelle C, Ebel C, et al. Hepatitis C virus core protein is a dimeric alpha-helical protein exhibiting membrane protein features. *J Virol* 2005;79(17):11353–11365.
103. Bozzacco L, Yi Z, Andreo U, et al. Chaperone-assisted protein folding is critical for yellow fever virus NS3/4A cleavage and replication. *J Virol* 2016;90(6):3212–3228.
104. Bradley DW, McCaustland KA, Cook EH, et al. Posttransfusion non-A, non-B hepatitis in Chimpanzees: physicochemical evidence that the tubule-forming agent is a small, enveloped virus. *Gastroenterology* 1985;88:773–779.
105. Bradley D, McCaustland K, Krawczynski K, et al. Hepatitis C virus: buoyant density of the factor VIII-derived isolate in sucrose. *J Med Virol* 1991;34:206–208.
106. Branch AD, Stump DD, Gutierrez JA, et al. The hepatitis C virus alternate reading frame (ARF) and its family of novel products: the alternate reading frame protein/F-protein, the double-frameshift protein, and others. *Semin Liver Dis* 2005;25(1):105–117.
107. Brand C, Bisaillon M, Geiss BJ. Organization of the flavivirus RNA replicase complex. *Wiley Interdiscip Rev RNA* 2017;8(6).
108. Brass V, Berke JM, Montserret R, et al. Structural determinants for membrane association and dynamic organization of the hepatitis C virus NS3-4A complex. *Proc Natl Acad Sci U S A* 2008;105(38):14545–14550.
109. Brass V, Bieck E, Montserret R, et al. An amino-terminal amphipathic alpha-helix mediates membrane association of the hepatitis C virus nonstructural protein 5A. *J Biol Chem* 2002;277(10):8130–8139.
110. Brass V, Gouttenoire J, Wahl A, et al. Hepatitis C virus RNA replication requires a conserved structural motif within the transmembrane domain of the NS5B RNA-dependent RNA polymerase. *J Virol* 2010;84(21):11580–11584.
111. Brass V, Pal Z, Sapay N, et al. Conserved determinants for membrane association of nonstructural protein 5A from hepatitis C virus and related viruses. *J Virol* 2007;81(6):2745–2757.
112. Brazzoli M, Bianchi A, Filippini S, et al. CD81 is a central regulator of cellular events required for hepatitis C virus infection of human hepatocytes. *J Virol* 2008;82(17):8316–8329.
113. Brazzoli M, Helenius A, Foung SK, et al. Folding and dimerization of hepatitis C virus E1 and E2 glycoproteins in stably transfected CHO cells. *Virology* 2005;332(1):438–453.
114. Bressanelli S, Stiasny K, Allison SL, et al. Structure of a flavivirus envelope glycoprotein in its low-pH-induced membrane fusion conformation. *EMBO J* 2004;23(4):728–738.
115. Bressanelli S, Tomei L, Rey FA, et al. Structural analysis of the hepatitis C virus RNA polymerase in complex with ribonucleotides. *J Virol* 2002;76(7):3482–3492.
116. Bressanelli S, Tomei L, Roussel A, et al. Crystal structure of the RNA-dependent RNA polymerase of hepatitis C virus. *Proc Natl Acad Sci U S A* 1999;96(23):13034–13039.
117. Bright H, Carroll AR, Watts PA, et al. Development of a GB virus B marmoset model and its validation with a novel series of hepatitis C virus NS3 protease inhibitors. *J Virol* 2004;78(4):2062–2071.
118. Brock KV, Deng R, Riblet SM. Nucleotide sequencing of 5′ and 3′ termini of bovine viral diarrhea virus by RNA ligation and PCR. *J Virol Methods* 1992;38(1):39–46.
119. Brown WC, Akey DL, Konwerski JR, et al. Extended surface for membrane association in Zika virus NS1 structure. *Nat Struct Mol Biol* 2016;23(9):865–867.
120. Brown JA, Singh G, Acklin JA, et al. Dengue virus immunity increases Zika virus-induced damage during pregnancy. *Immunity* 2019;50:751.e5–762.e5.
121. Buckley A, Gaidamovich S, Turchinskaya A, et al. Monoclonal antibodies identify the NS5 yellow fever virus non- structural protein in the nuclei of infected cells. *J Gen Virol* 1992;73(Pt 5):1125–1130.
122. Buckwold VE, Collins B, Hogan P, et al. Investigation into the ability of GB virus B to replicate in various immortalized cell lines. *Antiviral Res* 2005;66(2–3):165–168.
123. Bukh J, Apgar CL. Five new or recently discovered (GBV-A) virus species are indigenous to New World monkeys and may constitute a separate genus of the Flaviviridae. *Virology* 1997;229:429–436.
124. Bukh J, Apgar CL, Yanagi M. Toward a surrogate model for hepatitis C virus: an infectious molecular clone of the GB virus-B hepatitis agent. *Virology* 1999;262(2):470–478.
125. Bukong TN, Momen-Heravi F, Kodys K, et al. Exosomes from hepatitis C infected patients transmit HCV infection and contain replication competent viral RNA in complex with Ago2-miR122-HSP90. *PLoS Pathog* 2014;10(10):e1004424.
126. Burbelo PD, Dubovi EJ, Simmonds P, et al. Serology-enabled discovery of genetically diverse hepaciviruses in a new host. *J Virol* 2012;86(11):6171–6178.
127. Bussetta C, Choi KH. Dengue virus nonstructural protein 5 adopts multiple conformations in solution. *Biochemistry* 2012;51(30):5921–5931.
128. Byk LA, Gamarnik AV. Properties and functions of the dengue virus capsid protein. *Annu Rev Virol* 2016;3(1):263–281.
129. Byk LA, Iglesias NG, De Maio FA, et al. Dengue virus genome uncoating requires ubiquitination. *MBio* 2016;7(3):e00804.
130. Cai Z, Zhang C, Chang KS, et al. Robust production of infectious hepatitis C virus (HCV) from stably HCV cDNA-transfected human hepatoma cells. *J Virol* 2005;79(22):13963–13973.
131. Calisher CH, Karabatsos N, Dalrymple JM, et al. Antigenic relationships between flaviviruses as determined by cross-neutralization tests with polyclonal antisera. *J Gen Virol* 1989;70:37–43.
132. Callens N, Brugger B, Bonnafous P, et al. Morphology and molecular composition of purified bovine viral diarrhea virus envelope. *PLoS Pathog* 2016;12(3):e1005476.
133. Camus G, Herker E, Modi AA, et al. Diacylglycerol acyltransferase-1 localizes hepatitis C virus NS5A protein to lipid droplets and enhances NS5A interaction with the viral capsid core. *J Biol Chem* 2013;288(14):9915–9923.
134. Camus G, Schweiger M, Herker E, et al. The hepatitis C virus core protein inhibits adipose triglyceride lipase (ATGL)-mediated lipid mobilization and enhances the ATGL interaction with comparative gene identification 58 (CGI-58) and lipid droplets. *J Biol Chem* 2014;289(52):35770–35780.
135. Carpp LN, Galler R, Bonaldo MC. Interaction between the yellow fever virus nonstructural protein NS3 and the host protein Alix contributes to the release of infectious particles. *Microbes Infect* 2011;13(1):85–95.
136. Carrere-Kremer S, Montpellier-Pala C, Cocquerel L, et al. Subcellular localization and topology of the p7 polypeptide of hepatitis C virus. *J Virol* 2002;76(8):3720–3730.
137. Castelli M, Clementi N, Pfaff J, et al. A biologically-validated HCV E1E2 heterodimer structural model. *Sci Rep* 2017;7(1):214.
138. Castle E, Leidner U, Nowak T, et al. Primary structure of the West Nile flavivirus genome region coding for all nonstructural proteins. *Virology* 1986;149:10–26.
139. Catanese MT, Dorner M. Advances in experimental systems to study hepatitis C virus in vitro and in vivo. *Virology* 2015;479:221–233.
140. Catanese MT, Uryu K, Kopp M, et al. Ultrastructural analysis of hepatitis C virus particles. *Proc Natl Acad Sci U S A* 2013;110(23):9505–9510.
141. Chambers TJ, McCourt DW, Rice CM. Production of yellow fever virus proteins in infected cells: identification of discrete polyprotein species and analysis of cleavage kinetics using region-specific polyclonal antisera. *Virology* 1990;177:159–174.
142. Chambers TJ, Weir RC, Grakoui A, et al. Evidence that the N-terminal domain of nonstructural protein NS3 from yellow fever virus is a serine protease responsible for site-specific cleavages in the viral polyprotein. *Proc Natl Acad Sci U S A* 1990;87:8898–8902.
143. Chan YK, Gack MU. A phosphomimetic-based mechanism of dengue virus to antagonize innate immunity. *Nat Immunol* 2016;17(5):523–530.
144. Chandler DE, Penin F, Schulten K, et al. The p7 protein of hepatitis C virus forms structurally plastic, minimalist ion channels. *PLoS Comput Biol* 2012;8(9):e1002702.
145. Chandriani S, Skewes-Cox P, Zhong W, et al. Identification of a previously undescribed divergent virus from the Flaviviridae family in an outbreak of equine serum hepatitis. *Proc Natl Acad Sci U S A* 2013;110(15):E1407–E1415.
146. Chang KS, Jiang J, Cai Z, et al. Human apolipoprotein E is required for infectivity and production of hepatitis C virus in cell culture. *J Virol* 2007;81(24):13783–13793.
147. Chang YS, Liao CL, Tsao CH, et al. Membrane permeabilization by small hydrophobic nonstructural proteins of Japanese encephalitis virus. *J Virol* 1999;73(8):6257–6264.
148. Chao LH, Jang J, Johnson A, et al. How small-molecule inhibitors of dengue-virus infection interfere with viral membrane fusion. *Elife* 2018;7.
149. Chao LH, Klein DE, Schmidt AG, et al. Sequential conformational rearrangements in flavivirus membrane fusion. *Elife* 2014;3:e04389.
150. Chapman EG, Costantino DA, Rabe JL, et al. The structural basis of pathogenic subgenomic flavivirus RNA (sfRNA) production. *Science* 2014;344(6181):307–310.
151. Chapman EG, Moon SL, Wilusz J, et al. RNA structures that resist degradation by Xrn1 produce a pathogenic Dengue virus RNA. *Elife* 2014;3:e01892.
152. Chatel-Chaix L, Cortese M, Romero-Brey I, et al. Dengue virus perturbs mitochondrial morphodynamics to dampen innate immune responses. *Cell Host Microbe* 2016;20(3):342–356.
153. Chatel-Chaix L, Fischl W, Scaturro P, et al. A Combined Genetic-Proteomic Approach Identifies Residues within Dengue Virus NS4B Critical for Interaction with NS3 and Viral Replication. *J Virol* 2015;89(14):7170–7186.
154. Chen CJ, Kuo MD, Chien LJ, et al. RNA-protein interactions: involvement of NS3, NS5, and 3′ noncoding regions of Japanese encephalitis virus genomic RNA. *J Virol* 1997;71(5):3466–3473.
155. Chen ST, Lin YL, Huang MT, et al. CLEC5A is critical for dengue-virus-induced lethal disease. *Nature* 2008;453(7195):672–676.
156. Chen ZH, Rijnbrand R, Jangra RK, et al. Ubiquitination and proteasomal degradation of interferon regulatory factor-3 induced by N^{pro} from a cytopathic bovine viral diarrhea virus. *Virology* 2007;366(2):277–292.
157. Chenut G, Saintilan AF, Burger C, et al. Oral immunisation of swine with a classical swine fever vaccine (Chinese strain) and transmission studies in rabbits and sheep. *Vet Microbiol* 1999;64(4):265–276.
158. Chinnaswamy S, Murali A, Li P, et al. Regulation of de novo-initiated RNA synthesis in hepatitis C virus RNA-dependent RNA polymerase by intermolecular interactions. *J Virol* 2010;84(12):5923–5935.
159. Chivero ET, Stapleton JT. Tropism of human pegivirus (formerly known as GB virus C/hepatitis G virus) and host immunomodulation: insights into a highly successful viral infection. *J Gen Virol* 2015;96(Pt 7):1521–1532.
160. Choi KH, Gallei A, Becher P, et al. The structure of bovine viral diarrhea virus RNA-dependent RNA polymerase and its amino-terminal domain. *Structure* 2006;14(7): 1107–1113.
161. Choi KH, Groarke JM, Young DC, et al. The structure of the RNA-dependent RNA polymerase from bovine viral diarrhea virus establishes the role of GTP in de novo initiation. *Proc Natl Acad Sci U S A* 2004;101(13):4425–4430.
162. Chong WM, Hsu SC, Kao WT, et al. Phosphoproteomics identified an NS5A phosphorylation site involved in hepatitis C virus replication. *J Biol Chem* 2016;291(8):3918–3931.
163. Choo QL, Kuo G, Weiner AJ, et al. Isolation of a cDNA clone derived from a blood-borne non-A, non-B viral hepatitis genome. *Science* 1989;244:359–362.
164. Chotiwan N, Andre BG, Sanchez-Vargas I, et al. Dynamic remodeling of lipids coincides with dengue virus replication in the midgut of *Aedes aegypti* mosquitoes. *PLoS Pathog* 2018;14(2):e1006853.
165. Chowdhury AY, Tavis JE, George SL. Human pegivirus (GB virus C) NS3 protease activity inhibits induction of the type I interferon response and is not inhibited by HCV NS3 protease inhibitors. *Virology* 2014;456-457:300–309.
166. Chu PW, Westaway EG. Replication strategy of Kunjin virus: evidence for recycling role of replicative form RNA as template in semiconservative and asymmetric replication. *Virology* 1985;140:68–79.
167. Chu PW, Westaway EG. Molecular and ultrastructural analysis of heavy membrane fractions associated with the replication of Kunjin virus RNA. *Arch Virol* 1992;125(1–4):177–191.

168. Ciczora Y, Callens N, Montpellier C, et al. Contribution of the charged residues of hepatitis C virus glycoprotein E2 transmembrane domain to the functions of the E1E2 heterodimer. *J Gen Virol* 2005;86(Pt 10):2793–2798.

169. Ciczora Y, Callens N, Penin F, et al. Transmembrane domains of hepatitis C virus envelope glycoproteins: residues involved in E1E2 heterodimerization and involvement of these domains in virus entry. *J Virol* 2007;81(5):2372–2381.

170. Clarke D, Griffin S, Beales L, et al. Evidence for the formation of a heptameric ion channel complex by the hepatitis C virus p7 protein in vitro. *J Biol Chem* 2006;281(48):37057–37068.

171. Cleaves GR, Dubin DT. Methylation status of intracellular dengue type 2 40 S RNA. *Virology* 1979;96:159–165.

172. Cleaves GR, Ryan TE, Schlesinger RW. Identification and characterization of type 2 dengue virus replicative intermediate and replicative form RNAs. *Virology* 1981;111:73–83.

173. Clemente-Casares P, López-Jiménez AJ, Bellón-Echeverría I, et al. De novo polymerase activity and oligomerization of hepatitis C virus RNA-dependent RNA-polymerases from genotypes 1 to 5. *PLoS One* 2011;6(4):e18515.

174. Clum S, Ebner KE, Padmanabhan R. Cotranslational membrane insertion of the serine proteinase precursor NS2B-NS3(Pro) of dengue virus type 2 is required for efficient in vitro processing and is mediated through the hydrophobic regions of NS2B. *J Biol Chem* 1997;272(49):30715–30723.

175. Clyde K, Harris E. RNA secondary structure in the coding region of dengue virus type 2 directs translation start codon selection and is required for viral replication. *J Virol* 2006;80(5):2170–2182.

176. Cocquerel L, Op de Beeck A, Lambot M, et al. Topological changes in the transmembrane domains of hepatitis C virus envelope glycoproteins. *EMBO J* 2002;21(12):2893–2902.

177. Coller KE, Berger KL, Heaton NS, et al. RNA interference and single particle tracking analysis of hepatitis C virus endocytosis. *PLoS Pathog* 2009;5(12):e1000702.

178. Coller KE, Heaton NS, Berger KL, et al. Molecular determinants and dynamics of hepatitis C virus secretion. *PLoS Pathog* 2012;8(1):e1002466.

179. Collett MS, Larson R, Belzer SK, et al. Proteins encoded by bovine viral diarrhea virus: the genomic organization of a pestivirus. *Virology* 1988;165:200–208.

180. Collett MS, Larson R, Gold C, et al. Molecular cloning and nucleotide sequence of the pestivirus bovine viral diarrhea virus. *Virology* 1988;165:191–199.

181. Collier AJ, Gallego J, Klinck R, et al. A conserved RNA structure within the HCV IRES eIF3-binding site. *Nat Struct Biol* 2002;9(5):375–380.

182. Colpitts TM, Barthel S, Wang P, et al. Dengue virus capsid protein binds core histones and inhibits nucleosome formation in human liver cells. *PLoS One* 2011;6(9):e24365.

183. Convery O, Gargan S, Kickham M, et al. The hepatitis C virus (HCV) protein, p7, suppresses inflammatory responses to tumor necrosis factor (TNF)-alpha via signal transducer and activator of transcription (STAT)3 and extracellular signal-regulated kinase (ERK)-mediated induction of suppressor of cytokine signaling (SOCS)3. *FASEB J* 2019;33:8732–8744.

184. Cortese M, Goellner S, Acosta EG, et al. Ultrastructural characterization of Zika virus replication factories. *Cell Rep* 2017;18(9):2113–2123.

185. Counihan NA, Lindenbach BD. Gumming up the works: DNA polymers as HCV entry inhibitors. *Gastroenterology* 2009;137(2):427–430.

186. Cristofari G, Ivanyi-Nagy R, Gabus C, et al. The hepatitis C virus core protein is a potent nucleic acid chaperone that directs dimerization of the viral (+) strand RNA in vitro. *Nucleic Acids Res* 2004;32(8):2623–2631.

187. Cuceanu NM, Tuplin A, Simmonds P. Evolutionarily conserved RNA secondary structures in coding and non- coding sequences at the 3′ end of the hepatitis G virus/GB-virus C genome. *J Gen Virol* 2001;82(Pt 4):713–722.

188. Cui T, Sugrue RJ, Xu Q, et al. Recombinant dengue virus type 1 NS3 protein exhibits specific viral RNA binding and NTPase activity regulated by the NS5 protein. *Virology* 1998;246(2):409–417.

189. Cun W, Jiang J, Luo G. The C-terminal alpha-helix domain of apolipoprotein E is required for interaction with nonstructural protein 5A and assembly of hepatitis C virus. *J Virol* 2010;84(21):11532–11541.

190. Daffis S, Szretter KJ, Schriewer J, et al. 2′-O methylation of the viral mRNA cap evades host restriction by IFIT family members. *Nature* 2010;468(7322):452–456.

191. Dalrymple NA, Cimica V, Mackow ER. Dengue virus NS proteins inhibit RIG-I/MAVS signaling by blocking TBK1/IRF3 phosphorylation: dengue virus serotype 1 NS4A is a unique interferon-regulating virulence determinant. *MBio* 2015;6(3):e00553.

192. Dao Thi VL, Granier C, Zeisel MB, et al. Characterization of hepatitis C virus particle subpopulations reveals multiple usage of the scavenger receptor BI for entry steps. *J Biol Chem* 2012;287(37):31242–31257.

193. Darweesh MF, Rajput MK, Braun LJ, et al. Characterization of the cytopathic BVDV strains isolated from 13 mucosal disease cases arising in a cattle herd. *Virus Res* 2015;195:141–147.

194. Darweesh MF, Rajput MKS, Braun LJ, et al. BVDV Nᵖʳᵒ protein mediates the BVDV induced immunosuppression through interaction with cellular S100A9 protein. *Microb Pathog* 2018;121:341–349.

195. Davis CW, Nguyen HY, Hanna SL, et al. West Nile virus discriminates between DC-SIGN and DC-SIGNR for cellular attachment and infection. *J Virol* 2006;80(3):1290–1301.

196. de Borba L, Villordo SM, Marsico FL, et al. RNA structure duplication in the dengue virus 3′ UTR: redundancy or host specificity? *MBio* 2019;10(1).

197. de la Fuente C, Goodman Z, Rice CM. Genetic and functional characterization of the N-terminal region of the hepatitis C virus NS2 protein. *J Virol* 2013;87(8):4130–4145.

198. De Maio FA, Risso G, Iglesias NG, et al. The dengue virus NS5 protein intrudes in the cellular spliceosome and modulates splicing. *PLoS Pathog* 2016;12(8):e1005841.

199. De Tomassi A, Pizzuti M, Graziani R, et al. Cell clones selected from the Huh7 human hepatoma cell line support efficient replication of a subgenomic GB virus B replicon. *J Virol* 2002;76(15):7736–7746.

200. De Tomassi A, Pizzuti M, Traboni C. Hep3B human hepatoma cells support replication of the wild-type and a 5′-end deletion mutant GB virus B replicon. *J Virol* 2003;77(22):11875–11881.

201. Deinhardt F, Holmes AW, Capps RB, et al. Studies on the transmission of human viral hepatitis to marmoset monkeys. *J Exp Med* 1967;125:673–688.

202. Dejnirattisai W, Jumnainsong A, Onsirisakul N, et al. Cross-reacting antibodies enhance dengue virus infection in humans. *Science* 2010;328(5979):745–748.

203. Demetriou VL, Kyriakou E, Kostrikis LG. Near-full genome characterisation of two natural intergenotypic 2k/1b recombinant hepatitis C virus isolates. *Adv Virol* 2011;2011:710438.

204. Deng R, Brock KV. 5′ and 3′ untranslated regions of pestivirus genome: primary and secondary structure analyses. *Nucleic Acids Res* 1993;21(8):1949–1957.

205. Denolly S, Mialon C, Bourlet T, et al. The amino-terminus of the hepatitis C virus (HCV) p7 viroporin and its cleavage from glycoprotein E2-p7 precursor determine specific infectivity and secretion levels of HCV particle types. *PLoS Pathog* 2017;13(12):e1006774.

206. Depla M, Uzbekov R, Hourioux C, et al. Ultrastructural and quantitative analysis of the lipid droplet clustering induced by hepatitis C virus core protein. *Cell Mol Life Sci* 2010;67(18):3151–3161.

207. Depner K, Bauer T, Liess B. Thermal and pH stability of pestiviruses. *Rev Sci Tech* 1992;11(3):885–893.

208. Di Marco S, Volpari C, Tomei L, et al. Interdomain communication in hepatitis C virus polymerase abolished by small molecule inhibitors bound to a novel allosteric site. *J Biol Chem* 2005;280(33):29765–29770.

209. Ding Q, Cao X, Lu J, et al. Hepatitis C virus NS4B blocks the interaction of STING and TBK1 to evade host innate immunity. *J Hepatol* 2013;59(1):52–58.

210. Divers TJ, Tennant BC, Kumar A, et al. New parvovirus associated with serum hepatitis in horses after inoculation of common biological product. *Emerg Infect Dis* 2018;24(2):303–310.

211. Diviney S, Tuplin A, Struthers M, et al. A hepatitis C virus cis-acting replication element forms a long-range RNA-RNA interaction with upstream RNA sequences in NS5B. *J Virol* 2008;82(18):9008–9022.

212. Doceul V, Charleston B, Crooke H, et al. The Nᵖʳᵒ product of classical swine fever virus interacts with IkappaBalpha, the NF-kappaB inhibitor. *J Gen Virol* 2008;89(Pt 8):1881–1889.

213. Dokland T, Walsh M, Mackenzie JM, et al. West Nile virus core protein; tetramer structure and ribbon formation. *Structure* 2004;12(7):1157–1163.

214. Dong H, Chang DC, Xie X, et al. Biochemical and genetic characterization of dengue virus methyltransferase. *Virology* 2010;405(2):568–578.

215. Dorner M, Horwitz JA, Donovan BM, et al. Completion of the entire hepatitis C virus life cycle in genetically humanized mice. *Nature* 2013;501:237–241.

216. Dorner M, Horwitz JA, Robbins JB, et al. A genetically humanized mouse model for hepatitis C virus infection. *Nature* 2011;474(7350):208–211.

217. Douam F, Thi VL, Maurin G, et al. Critical interaction between E1 and E2 glycoproteins determines binding and fusion properties of hepatitis C virus during cell entry. *Hepatology* 2014;59(3):776–788.

218. Dreux M, Garaigorta U, Boyd B, et al. Short-range exosomal transfer of viral RNA from infected cells to plasmacytoid dendritic cells triggers innate immunity. *Cell Host Microbe* 2012;12(4):558–570.

219. Dreux M, Gastaminza P, Wieland SF, et al. The autophagy machinery is required to initiate hepatitis C virus replication. *Proc Natl Acad Sci U S A* 2009;106(33):14046–14051.

220. Drummer HE, Boo I, Poumbourios P. Mutagenesis of a conserved fusion peptide-like motif and membrane-proximal heptad-repeat region of hepatitis C virus glycoprotein E1. *J Gen Virol* 2007;88(Pt 4):1144–1148.

221. Drummer HE, Maerz A, Poumbourios P. Cell surface expression of functional hepatitis C virus E1 and E2 glycoproteins. *FEBS Lett* 2003;546(2–3):385–390.

222. Drummer HE, Poumbourios P. Hepatitis C virus glycoprotein E2 contains a membrane-proximal heptad repeat sequence that is essential for E1E2 glycoprotein heterodimerization and viral entry. *J Biol Chem* 2004;279(29):30066–30072.

223. Dubrau D, Tortorici MA, Rey FA, et al. A positive-strand RNA virus uses alternative protein-protein interactions within a viral protease/cofactor complex to switch between RNA replication and virion morphogenesis. *PLoS Pathog* 2017;13(2):e1006134.

224. Dubuisson J, Hsu HH, Cheung RC, et al. Formation and intracellular localization of hepatitis C virus envelope glycoprotein complexes expressed by recombinant vaccinia and Sindbis viruses. *J Virol* 1994;68(10):6147–6160.

225. Dubuisson J, Rice CM. Hepatitis C virus glycoprotein folding: disulfide bond formation and association with calnexin. *J Virol* 1996;70(2):778–786.

226. Duong FH, Christen V, Berke JM, et al. Upregulation of protein phosphatase 2Ac by hepatitis C virus modulates NS3 helicase activity through inhibition of protein arginine methyltransferase 1. *J Virol* 2005;79(24):15342–15350.

227. Duvet S, Cocquerel L, Pillez A, et al. Hepatitis C virus glycoprotein complex localization in the endoplasmic reticulum involves a determinant for retention and not retrieval. *J Biol Chem* 1998;273(48):32088–32095.

228. Edgil D, Diamond MS, Holden KL, et al. Translation efficiency determines differences in cellular infection among dengue virus type 2 strains. *Virology* 2003;317(2):275–290.

229. Egger D, Pasamontes L, Bolten R, et al. Reversible dissociation of the poliovirus replication complex: functions and interactions of its components in viral RNA synthesis. *J Virol* 1996;70(12):8675–8683.

230. Egger D, Wölk B, Gosert R, et al. Expression of hepatitis C virus proteins induces distinct membrane alterations including a candidate viral replication complex. *J Virol* 2002;76(12):5974–5984.

231. Egloff MP, Benarroch D, Selisko B, et al. An RNA cap (nucleoside-2′-O-)-methyltransferase in the flavivirus RNA polymerase NS5: crystal structure and functional characterization. *EMBO J* 2002;21(11):2757–2768.

232. Eissmann K, Mueller S, Sticht H, et al. HIV-1 fusion is blocked through binding of GB Virus C E2-derived peptides to the HIV-1 gp41 disulfide loop [corrected]. *PLoS One* 2013;8(1):e54452.

233. El Omari K, Iourin O, Harlos K, et al. Structure of a pestivirus envelope glycoprotein E2 clarifies its role in cell entry. *Cell Rep* 2013;3(1):30–35.

234. El Omari K, Iourin O, Kadlec J, et al. Unexpected structure for the N-terminal domain of hepatitis C virus envelope glycoprotein E1. *Nat Commun* 2014;5:4874.

235. Elazar M, Cheong KH, Liu P, et al. Amphipathic helix-dependent localization of NS5A mediates hepatitis C virus RNA replication. *J Virol* 2003;77(10):6055–6061.

236. Elbers K, Tautz N, Becher P, et al. Processing in the pestivirus E2-NS2 region: identification of proteins p7 and E2p7. *J Virol* 1996;70(6):4131–4135.

237. El-Hage N, Luo G. Replication of hepatitis C virus RNA occurs in a membrane-bound replication complex containing nonstructural viral proteins and RNA. *J Gen Virol* 2003;84(Pt 10):2761–2769.

238. Emara MM, Brinton MA. Interaction of TIA-1/TIAR with West Nile and dengue virus products in infected cells interferes with stress granule formation and processing body assembly. *Proc Natl Acad Sci U S A* 2007;104(21):9041–9046.

239. Eng FJ, Walewski JL, Klepper AL, et al. Internal initiation stimulates production of p8 minicore, a member of a newly discovered family of hepatitis C virus core protein isoforms. *J Virol* 2009;83(7):3104–3114.

240. Epstein JH, Quan PL, Briese T, et al. Identification of GBV-D, a novel GB-like flavivirus from old world frugivorous bats (Pteropus giganteus) in Bangladesh. *PLoS Pathog* 2010;6:e1000972.

241. Erb SM, Butrapet S, Moss KJ, et al. Domain-III FG loop of the dengue virus type 2 envelope protein is important for infection of mammalian cells and *Aedes aegypti* mosquitoes. *Virology* 2010;406(2):328–335.

242. Erbel P, Schiering N, D'Arcy A, et al. Structural basis for the activation of flaviviral NS3 proteases from dengue and West Nile virus. *Nat Struct Mol Biol* 2006;13(4):372–373.

243. Ertel KJ, Benefield D, Castano-Diez D, et al. Cryo-electron tomography reveals novel features of a viral RNA replication compartment. *Elife* 2017;6:e25940.

244. Evans MJ, Rice CM, Goff SP. Phosphorylation of hepatitis C virus nonstructural protein 5A modulates its protein interactions and viral RNA replication. *Proc Natl Acad Sci U S A* 2004;101(35):13038–13043.

245. Evans MJ, von Hahn T, Tscherne DM, et al. Claudin-1 is a hepatitis C virus co-receptor required for a late step in entry. *Nature* 2007;446(7137):801–805.

246. Eyre NS, Hampton-Smith RJ, Aloia AL, et al. Phosphorylation of NS5A Serine-235 is essential to hepatitis C virus RNA replication and normal replication compartment formation. *Virology* 2016;491:27–44.

247. Fahmy AM, Labonte P. The autophagy elongation complex (ATG5-12/16L1) positively regulates HCV replication and is required for wild-type membranous web formation. *Sci Rep* 2017;7:40351.

248. Failla C, Tomei L, De Francesco R. Both NS3 and NS4A are required for proteolytic processing of hepatitis C virus nonstructural proteins. *J Virol* 1994;68(6):3753–3760.

249. Falgout B, Chanock R, Lai C-J. Proper processing of dengue virus nonstructural glycoprotein NS1 requires the N-terminal hydrophobic signal sequence and the downstream nonstructural protein NS2a. *J Virol* 1989;63(5):1852–1860.

250. Falgout B, Markoff L. Evidence that flavivirus NS1-NS2A cleavage is mediated by a membrane-bound host protease in the endoplasmic reticulum. *J Virol* 1995;69(11):7232–7243.

251. Falgout B, Pethel M, Zhang Y-M, et al. Both nonstructural proteins NS2B and NS3 are required for the proteolytic processing of Dengue virus nonstructural proteins. *J Virol* 1991;65:2467–2475.

252. Falson P, Bartosch B, Alsaleh K, et al. Hepatitis C virus envelope glycoprotein E1 forms trimers at the surface of the virion. *J Virol* 2015;89:10333–10346.

253. Farci P, Shimoda A, Coiana A, et al. The outcome of acute hepatitis C predicted by the evolution of the viral quasispecies. *Science* 2000;288(5464):339–344.

254. Farci P, Shimoda A, Wong D, et al. Prevention of hepatitis C virus infection in chimpanzees by hyperimmune serum against the hypervariable region 1 of the envelope 2 protein. *Proc Natl Acad Sci U S A* 1996;93(26):15394–15399.

255. Farquhar MJ, Hu K, Harris HJ, et al. Hepatitis C virus induces CD81 and claudin-1 endocytosis. *J Virol* 2012;86(8):4305–4316.

256. Feinstone SM, Kapikian AZ, Purcell RH, et al. Transfusion-associated hepatitis not due to viral hepatitis type A or B. *N Engl J Med* 1975;292(15):767–770.

257. Feld JJ, Jacobson IM, Hezode C, et al. Sofosbuvir and Velpatasvir for HCV Genotype 1, 2, 4, 5, and 6 Infection. *N Engl J Med* 2015;373(27):2599–2607.

258. Ferlenghi I, Clarke M, Ruttan T, et al. Molecular organization of a recombinant subviral particle from tick- borne encephalitis virus. *Mol Cell* 2001;7(3):593–602.

259. Ferraris P, Beaumont E, Uzbekov R, et al. Sequential biogenesis of host cell membrane rearrangements induced by hepatitis C virus infection. *Cell Mol Life Sci* 2013;70(7):1297–1306.

260. Ferraris P, Blanchard E, Roingeard P. Ultrastructural and biochemical analyses of hepatitis C virus-associated host cell membranes. *J Gen Virol* 2010;91(Pt 9):2230–2237.

261. Fetzer C, Tews BA, Meyers G. The carboxy-terminal sequence of the pestivirus glycoprotein E(rns) represents an unusual type of membrane anchor. *J Virol* 2005;79(18):11901–11913.

262. Fiebach AR, Guzylack-Piriou L, Python S, et al. Classical swine fever virus N(pro) limits type I interferon induction in pDC by interacting with interferon regulatory factor 7. *J Virol* 2011;85:8002–8011.

263. Filbin ME, Kieft JS. HCV IRES domain IIb affects the configuration of coding RNA in the 40S subunit's decoding groove. *RNA* 2011;17(7):1258–1273.

264. Filbin ME, Vollmar BS, Shi D, et al. HCV IRES manipulates the ribosome to promote the switch from translation initiation to elongation. *Nat Struct Mol Biol* 2013;20(2):150–158.

265. Filomatori CV, Iglesias NG, Villordo SM, et al. RNA sequences and structures required for the recruitment and activity of the dengue virus polymerase. *J Biol Chem* 2011;286(9):6929–6939.

266. Filomatori CV, Lodeiro MF, Alvarez DE, et al. A 5' RNA element promotes dengue virus RNA synthesis on a circular genome. *Genes Dev* 2006;20(16):2238–2249.

267. Firth AE, Atkins JF. A conserved predicted pseudoknot in the NS2A-encoding sequence of West Nile and Japanese encephalitis flaviviruses suggests NS1' may derive from ribosomal frameshifting. *Virol J* 2009;6:14.

268. Flipse J, Wilschut J, Smit JM. Molecular mechanisms involved in antibody-dependent enhancement of dengue virus infection in humans. *Traffic* 2013;14(1):25–35.

269. Flyak AI, Ruiz S, Colbert MD, et al. HCV broadly neutralizing antibodies use a CDRH3 disulfide motif to recognize an E2 glycoprotein site that can be targeted for vaccine design. *Cell Host Microbe* 2018;24(5):703.e703–716.e703.

270. Fogeda M, López-Alcorocho JM, Bartolomé J, et al. Existence of distinct GB virus C/hepatitis G virus variants with different tropism. *J Virol* 2000;74(17):7936–7942.

271. Foster GR, Afdhal N, Roberts SK, et al. Sofosbuvir and velpatasvir for HCV genotype 2 and 3 infection. *N Engl J Med* 2015;373(27):2608–2617.

272. Foster TL, Belyaeva T, Stonehouse NJ, et al. All three domains of the hepatitis C virus nonstructural NS5A protein contribute to RNA binding. *J Virol* 2010;84(18):9267–9277.

273. Fowler AM, Tang WW, Young MP, et al. Maternally acquired Zika antibodies enhance dengue disease severity in mice. *Cell Host Microbe* 2018;24(5):743.e745–750.e745.

274. Fraser J, Boo I, Poumbourios P, et al. Hepatitis C virus (HCV) envelope glycoproteins E1 and E2 contain reduced cysteine residues essential for virus entry. *J Biol Chem* 2011;286(37):31984–31992.

275. Fricke M, Dunnes N, Zayas M, et al. Conserved RNA secondary structures and long-range interactions in hepatitis C viruses. *RNA* 2015;21(7):1219–1232.

276. Friebe P, Bartenschlager R. Genetic analysis of sequences in the 3' nontranslated region of hepatitis C virus that are important for RNA replication. *J Virol* 2002;76(11):5326–5338.

277. Friebe P, Boudet J, Simorre JP, et al. Kissing-loop interaction in the 3' end of the hepatitis C virus genome essential for RNA replication. *J Virol* 2005;79(1):380–392.

278. Friebe P, Lohmann V, Krieger N, et al. Sequences in the 5' nontranslated region of hepatitis C virus required for RNA replication. *J Virol* 2001;75(24):12047–12057.

279. Frolov I, McBride MS, Rice CM. cis-acting RNA elements required for replication of bovine viral diarrhea virus-hepatitis C virus 5' nontranslated region chimeras. *RNA* 1998;4(11):1418–1435.

280. Fukuhara T, Tamura T, Ono C, et al. Host-derived apolipoproteins play comparable roles with viral secretory proteins Erns and NS1 in the infectious particle formation of Flaviviridae. *PLoS Pathog* 2017;13(6):e1006475.

281. Fukuhara T, Wada M, Nakamura S, et al. Amphipathic alpha-helices in apolipoproteins are crucial to the formation of infectious hepatitis C virus particles. *PLoS Pathog* 2014;10(12):e1004534.

282. Funk A, Truong K, Nagasaki T, et al. RNA structures required for production of subgenomic flavivirus RNA. *J Virol* 2010;84(21):11407–11417.

283. Furuichi Y, Shatkin AJ. Viral and cellular mRNA capping: past and prospects. *Adv Virus Res* 2000;55:135–184.

284. Gallei A, Orlich M, Thiel HJ, et al. Noncytopathogenic pestivirus strains generated by nonhomologous RNA recombination: alterations in the NS4A/NS4B coding region. *J Virol* 2005;79(22):14261–14270.

285. Gallei A, Pankraz A, Thiel HJ, et al. RNA recombination in vivo in the absence of viral replication. *J Virol* 2004;78(12):6271–6281.

286. Gao M, Nettles RE, Belema M, et al. Chemical genetics strategy identifies an HCV NS5A inhibitor with a potent clinical effect. *Nature* 2010;465(7294):96–100.

287. Gastaminza P, Dryden KA, Boyd B, et al. Ultrastructural and biophysical characterization of hepatitis C virus particles produced in cell culture. *J Virol* 2010;84(21):10999–11009.

288. Gastaminza P, Kapadia SB, Chisari FV. Differential biophysical properties of infectious intracellular and secreted hepatitis C virus particles. *J Virol* 2006;80(22):11074–11081.

289. Gebhard LG, Iglesias NG, Byk LA, et al. A proline-rich N-terminal region of the dengue virus NS3 is crucial for infectious particle production. *J Virol* 2016;90(11):5451–5461.

290. George SL, Varmaz D, Tavis JE, et al. The GB virus C (GBV-C) NS3 serine protease inhibits HIV-1 replication in a CD4+ T lymphocyte cell line without decreasing HIV receptor expression. *PLoS One* 2012;7(1):e30653.

291. Germi R, Crance JM, Garin D, et al. Cellular glycosaminoglycans and low density lipoprotein receptor are involved in hepatitis C virus adsorption. *J Med Virol* 2002;68(2):206–215.

292. Gerold G, Meissner F, Bruening J, et al. Quantitative proteomics identifies serum response factor binding protein 1 as a host factor for hepatitis C virus entry. *Cell Rep* 2015;12(5):864–878.

293. Ghibaudo D, Cohen L, Penin F, et al. Characterization of GB virus B polyprotein processing reveals the existence of a novel 13-kDa protein with partial homology to hepatitis C virus p7 protein. *J Biol Chem* 2004;279(24):24965–24975.

294. Gillespie LK, Hoenen A, Morgan G, et al. The endoplasmic reticulum provides the membrane platform for biogenesis of the flavivirus replication complex. *J Virol* 2010;84(20):10438–10447.

295. Gladue DP, Gavrilov BK, Holinka LG, et al. Identification of an NTPase motif in classical swine fever virus NS4B protein. *Virology* 2011;411(1):41–49.

296. Gladue DP, Holinka LG, Largo E, et al. Classical swine fever virus p7 protein is a viroporin involved in virulence in swine. *J Virol* 2012;86(12):6778–6791.

297. Gomara MJ, Sanchez-Merino V, Paus A, et al. Definition of an 18-mer synthetic peptide derived from the GB virus C E1 protein as a new HIV-1 entry inhibitor. *Biochim Biophys Acta* 2016;1860(6):1139–1148.

298. Gong Y, Shannon A, Westaway EG, et al. The replicative intermediate molecule of bovine viral diarrhoea virus contains multiple nascent strands. *Arch Virol* 1998;143(2):399–404.

299. Gong Y, Trowbridge R, Macnaughton TB, et al. Characterization of RNA synthesis during a one-step growth curve and of the replication mechanism of bovine viral diarrhoea virus. *J Gen Virol* 1996;77 (Pt 11):2729–2736.

300. Goonawardane N, Gebhardt A, Bartlett C, et al. Phosphorylation of serine 225 in hepatitis C virus NS5A regulates protein-protein interactions. *J Virol* 2017;91(17).

301. Goonawardane N, Ross-Thriepland D, Harris M. Regulation of hepatitis C virus replication via threonine phosphorylation of the NS5A protein. *J Gen Virol* 2018;99(1):62–72.

302. Gorbalenya AE, Koonin EV, Donchenko AP, et al. Two related superfamilies of putative helicases involved in replication, recombination, repair and expression of DNA and RNA genomes. *Nucleic Acids Res* 1989;17(12):4713–4730.

303. Gosert R, Egger D, Lohmann V, et al. Identification of the hepatitis C virus RNA replication complex in Huh-7 cells harboring subgenomic replicons. *J Virol* 2003;77(9):5487–5492.

304. Gottipati K, Acholi S, Ruggli N, et al. Autocatalytic activity and substrate specificity of the pestivirus N-terminal protease N^pro. *Virology* 2014;452-453:303–309.

305. Gottipati K, Holthauzen LM, Ruggli N, et al. Pestivirus N^pro directly interacts with interferon regulatory factor 3 monomer and dimer. *J Virol* 2016;90(17):7740–7747.

306. Gottipati K, Ruggli N, Gerber M, et al. The structure of classical swine fever virus N(pro): a novel cysteine Autoprotease and zinc-binding protein involved in subversion of type I interferon induction. *PLoS Pathog* 2013;9(10):e1003704.

307. Gottwein JM, Bukh J. Cutting the gordian knot development and biological relevance of hepatitis C virus cell culture systems. *Adv Virus Res* 2008;71:51–133.

308. Gouttenoire J, Montserret R, Kennel A, et al. An amphipathic alpha-helix at the C terminus of hepatitis C virus nonstructural protein 4B mediates membrane association. *J Virol* 2009;83(21):11378–11384.
309. Gouttenoire J, Montserret R, Paul D, et al. Aminoterminal amphipathic alpha-helix AH1 of hepatitis C virus nonstructural protein 4B possesses a dual role in RNA replication and virus production. *PLoS Pathog* 2014;10(10):e1004501.
310. Gouttenoire J, Penin F, Moradpour D. Hepatitis C virus nonstructural protein 4B: a journey into unexplored territory. *Rev Med Virol* 2010;20(2):117–129.
311. Gouttenoire J, Roingeard P, Penin F, et al. Amphipathic alpha-helix AH2 is a major determinant for the oligomerization of hepatitis C virus nonstructural protein 4B. *J Virol* 2010;84(24):12529–12537.
312. Grakoui A, McCourt DW, Wychowski C, et al. A second hepatitis C virus-encoded proteinase. *Proc Natl Acad Sci U S A* 1993;90(22):10583–10587.
313. Grassmann CW, Yu H, Isken O, et al. Hepatitis C virus and the related bovine viral diarrhea virus considerably differ in the functional organization of the 5′ non-translated region: implications for the viral life cycle. *Virology* 2005;333(2):349–366.
314. Gray EW, Nettleton PF. The ultrastructure of cell cultures infected with border disease and bovine virus diarrhoea viruses. *J Gen Virol* 1987;68 (Pt 9):2339–2346.
315. Greiser-Wilke I, Dittmar KE, Liess B, et al. Immunofluorescence studies of biotype-specific expression of bovine viral diarrhoea virus epitopes in infected cells. *J Gen Virol* 1991;72 (Pt 8):2015–2019.
316. Griffin SD, Beales LP, Clarke DS, et al. The p7 protein of hepatitis C virus forms an ion channel that is blocked by the antiviral drug, Amantadine. *FEBS Lett* 2003;535(1–3):34–38.
317. Griffin SD, Harvey R, Clarke DS, et al. A conserved basic loop in hepatitis C virus p7 protein is required for amantadine-sensitive ion channel activity in mammalian cells but is dispensable for localization to mitochondria. *J Gen Virol* 2004;85(Pt 2):451–461.
318. Griffin S, Trowbridge R, Thommes P, et al. Chimeric GB virus B genomes containing hepatitis C virus p7 are infectious in vivo. *J Hepatol* 2008;49(6):908–915.
319. Grubaugh ND, Ishtiaq F, Setoh YX, et al. Misperceived Risks of Zika-related Microcephaly in India. *Trends Microbiol* 2019;27:381–383.
320. Grummer B, Grotha S, Greiser-Wilke I. Bovine viral diarrhoea virus is internalized by clathrin-dependent receptor-mediated endocytosis. *J Vet Med B Infect Dis Vet Public Health* 2004;51(10):427–432.
321. Grun JB, Brinton MA. Dissociation of NS5 from cell fractions containing West Nile virus-specific polymerase activity. *J Virol* 1987;61:3641–3644.
322. Grunvogel O, Colasanti O, Lee JY, et al. Secretion of hepatitis C virus replication intermediates reduces activation of toll-like receptor 3 in hepatocytes. *Gastroenterology* 2018;154(8):2237.e2216–2251.e2216.
323. Gu B, Johnston VK, Gutshall LL, et al. Arresting initiation of hepatitis C virus RNA synthesis using heterocyclic derivatives. *J Biol Chem* 2003;278(19):16602–16607.
324. Gu M, Rice CM. Three conformational snapshots of the hepatitis C virus NS3 helicase reveal a ratchet translocation mechanism. *Proc Natl Acad Sci U S A* 2010;107(2):521–528.
325. Guevin C, Manna D, Belanger C, et al. Autophagy protein ATG5 interacts transiently with the hepatitis C virus RNA polymerase (NS5B) early during infection. *Virology* 2010;405(1):1–7.
326. Guirakhoo F, Bolin RA, Roehrig JT. The Murray Valley encephalitis virus prM protein confers acid resistance to virus particles and alters the expression of epitopes within the R2 domain of E glycoprotein. *Virology* 1992;191(2):921–931.
327. Gutsche I, Coulibaly F, Voss JE, et al. Secreted dengue virus nonstructural protein NS1 is an atypical barrel-shaped high-density lipoprotein. *Proc Natl Acad Sci U S A* 2011;108(19):8003–8008.
328. Gwack Y, Kim DW, Han JH, et al. Characterization of RNA binding activity and RNA helicase activity of the hepatitis C virus NS3 protein. *Biochem Biophys Res Commun* 1996;225(2):654–659.
329. Gwack Y, Yoo H, Song I, et al. RNA-Stimulated ATPase and RNA helicase activities and RNA binding domain of hepatitis G virus nonstructural protein 3. *J Virol* 1999;73(4):2909–2915.
330. Haddad JG, Rouille Y, Hanoulle X, et al. Identification of novel functions for hepatitis C virus envelope glycoprotein E1 in virus entry and assembly. *J Virol* 2017;91(8).
331. Hahn CS, Hahn YS, Rice CM, et al. Conserved elements in the 3′ untranslated region of flavivirus RNAs and potential cyclization sequences. *J Mol Biol* 1987;198(1):33–41.
332. Haid S, Grethe C, Dill MT, et al. Isolate-dependent use of claudins for cell entry by hepatitis C virus. *Hepatology* 2014;59(1):24–34.
333. Halstead SB. Neutralization and antibody-dependent enhancement of dengue viruses. *Adv Virus Res* 2003;60:421–467.
334. Halstead SB, O'Rourke EJ. Dengue viruses and mononuclear phagocytes. I. Infection enhancement by non-neutralizing antibody. *J Exp Med* 1977;146(1):201–217.
335. Han JQ, Barton DJ. Activation and evasion of the antiviral 2′-5′ oligoadenylate synthetase/ribonuclease L pathway by hepatitis C virus mRNA. *RNA* 2002;8(4):512–525.
336. Harada T, Tautz N, Thiel HJ. E2-p7 region of the bovine viral diarrhea virus polyprotein: processing and functional studies. *J Virol* 2000;74(20):9498–9506.
337. Harak C, Meyrath M, Romero-Brey I, et al. Tuning a cellular lipid kinase activity adapts hepatitis C virus to replication in cell culture. *Nat Microbiol* 2016;2:16247.
338. Hardy RW, Marcotrigiano J, Blight KJ, et al. Hepatitis C virus RNA synthesis in a cell-free system isolated from replicon-containing hepatoma cells. *J Virol* 2003;77(3):2029–2037.
339. Harman C, Zhong L, Ma L, et al. A view of the E2-CD81 interface at the binding site of a neutralizing antibody against hepatitis C virus. *J Virol* 2015;89(1):492–501.
340. Harrus D, Ahmed-El-Sayed N, Simister PC, et al. Further insights into the roles of GTP and the C terminus of the hepatitis C virus polymerase in the initiation of RNA synthesis. *J Biol Chem* 2010;285(43):32906–32918.
341. Hartlage AS, Cullen JM, Kapoor A. The strange, expanding world of animal hepaciviruses. *Annu Rev Virol* 2016;3:53–75.
342. Hartlage AS, Murthy S, Kumar A, et al. Vaccination to prevent T cell subversion can protect against persistent hepacivirus infection. *Nat Commun* 2019;10(1):1113.
343. Hasan SS, Sevvana M, Kuhn RJ, et al. Structural biology of Zika virus and other flaviviruses. *Nat Struct Mol Biol* 2018;25(1):13–20.
344. Hashem Y, des Georges A, Dhote V, et al. Hepatitis-C-virus-like internal ribosome entry sites displace eIF3 to gain access to the 40S subunit. *Nature* 2013;503(7477):539–543.
345. Hassoba HM, Pessoa MG, Terrault NA, et al. Antienvelope antibodies are protective against GBV-C reinfection: evidence from the liver transplant model. *J Med Virol* 1998;56(3):253–258.
346. Hausmann Y, Roman-Sosa G, Thiel HJ, et al. Classical swine fever virus glycoprotein E rns is an endoribonuclease with an unusual base specificity. *J Virol* 2004;78(10):5507–5512.
347. He LF, Alling D, Popkin T, et al. Determining the size of non-A, non-B hepatitis virus by filtration. *J Infect Dis* 1987;156(4):636–640.
348. He Z, Zhu X, Wen W, et al. Dengue virus subverts host innate immunity by targeting adaptor protein MAVS. *J Virol* 2016;90(16):7219–7230.
349. Heaton NS, Perera R, Berger KL, et al. Dengue virus nonstructural protein 3 redistributes fatty acid synthase to sites of viral replication and increases cellular fatty acid synthesis. *Proc Natl Acad Sci U S A* 2010;107(40):17345–17350.
350. Heaton NS, Randall G. Dengue virus-induced autophagy regulates lipid metabolism. *Cell Host Microbe* 2010;8(5):422–432.
351. Heimann M, Roman-Sosa GR, Martoglio B, et al. Core protein of pestiviruses is processed at the C terminus by signal peptide peptidase. *J Virol* 2006;80(4):1915–1921.
352. Heinz FX, Stiasny K. Flaviviruses and flavivirus vaccines. *Vaccine* 2012;30(29):4301–4306.
353. Heinz FX, Stiasny K, Püschner-Auer G, et al. Structural changes and functional control of the tick-borne encephalitis virus glycoprotein E by the heterodimeric association with protein prM. *Virology* 1994;198(1):109–117.
354. Hellen CU. IRES-induced conformational changes in the ribosome and the mechanism of translation initiation by internal ribosomal entry. *Biochim Biophys Acta* 2009;1789(9-10):558–570.
355. Herker E, Harris C, Hernandez C, et al. Efficient hepatitis C virus particle formation requires diacylglycerol acyltransferase-1. *Nat Med* 2010;16(11):1295–1298.
356. Herrera E, Tenckhoff S, Gómara MJ, et al. Effect of synthetic peptides belonging to E2 envelope protein of GB virus C on human immunodeficiency virus type 1 infection. *J Med Chem* 2010;53(16):6054–6063.
357. Higginbottom A, Quinn ER, Kuo CC, et al. Identification of amino acid residues in CD81 critical for interaction with hepatitis C virus envelope glycoprotein E2. *J Virol* 2000;74(8):3642–3649.
358. Hijikata M, Mizushima H, Akagi T, et al. Two distinct proteinase activities required for the processing of a putative nonstructural precursor protein of hepatitis C virus. *J Virol* 1993;67(8):4665–4675.
359. Hijikata M, Shimizu YK, Kato H, et al. Equilibrium centrifugation studies of hepatitis C virus: evidence for circulating immune complexes. *J Virol* 1993;67(4):1953–1958.
360. Hilton L, Moganeradj K, Zhang G, et al. The NPro product of bovine viral diarrhea virus inhibits DNA binding by interferon regulatory factor 3 and targets it for proteasomal degradation. *J Virol* 2006;80(23):11723–11732.
361. Hirata Y, Ikeda K, Sudoh M, et al. Self-enhancement of hepatitis C virus replication by promotion of specific sphingolipid biosynthesis. *PLoS Pathog* 2012;8(8):e1002860.
362. Hong Z, Cameron CE, Walker MP, et al. A novel mechanism to ensure terminal initiation by hepatitis C virus NS5B polymerase. *Virology* 2001;285(1):6–11.
363. Hopcraft SE, Evans MJ. Selection of a hepatitis C virus with altered entry factor requirements reveals a genetic interaction between the E1 glycoprotein and claudins. *Hepatology* 2015;62(4):1059–1069.
364. Hou S, Kumar A, Xu Z, et al. Zika virus hijacks stress granule proteins and modulates the host stress response. *J Virol* 2017;91(16).
365. Hsu SC, Tsai CN, Lee KY, et al. Sequential S232/S235/S238 phosphorylation of the hepatitis C virus nonstructural protein 5A. *J Virol* 2018;92(20).
366. Hsu M, Zhang J, Flint M, et al. Hepatitis C virus glycoproteins mediate pH-dependent cell entry of pseudotyped retroviral particles. *Proc Natl Acad Sci U S A* 2003;100(12):7271–7276.
367. Huang H, Chen Y, Ye J. Inhibition of hepatitis C virus replication by peroxidation of arachidonate and restoration by vitamin E. *Proc Natl Acad Sci U S A* 2007;104(47):18666–18670.
368. Huang L, Hwang J, Sharma SD, et al. Hepatitis C virus nonstructural protein 5A (NS5A) is an RNA-binding protein. *J Biol Chem* 2005;280(43):36417–36428.
369. Huber RG, Lim XN, Ng WC, et al. Structure mapping of dengue and Zika viruses reveals functional long-range interactions. *Nat Commun* 2019;10(1):1408.
370. Hulst MM, Moormann RJ. Inhibition of pestivirus infection in cell culture by envelope proteins E(rns) and E2 of classical swine fever virus: E(rns) and E2 interact with different receptors. *J Gen Virol* 1997;78 (Pt 11):2779–2787.
371. Hwang J, Huang L, Cordek DG, et al. Hepatitis C virus nonstructural protein 5A: biochemical characterization of a novel structural class of RNA-binding proteins. *J Virol* 2010;84(24):12480–12491.
372. Iqbal M, Flick-Smith H, McCauley JW. Interactions of bovine viral diarrhoea virus glycoprotein E(rns) with cell surface glycosaminoglycans. *J Gen Virol* 2000;81(Pt 2):451–459.
373. Iqbal M, McCauley JW. Identification of the glycosaminoglycan-binding site on the glycoprotein E(rns) of bovine viral diarrhoea virus by site-directed mutagenesis. *J Gen Virol* 2002;83(Pt 9):2153–2159.
374. Iqbal M, Poole E, Goodbourn S, et al. Role for bovine viral diarrhea virus E^{rns} glycoprotein in the control of activation of beta interferon by double-stranded RNA. *J Virol* 2004;78(1):136–145.
375. Isherwood BJ, Patel AH. Analysis of the processing and transmembrane topology of the E2p7 protein of hepatitis C virus. *J Gen Virol* 2005;86(Pt 3):667–676.
376. Isken O, Grassmann CW, Yu H, et al. Complex signals in the genomic 3′ nontranslated region of bovine viral diarrhea virus coordinate translation and replication of the viral RNA. *RNA* 2004;10(10):1637–1652.
377. Isken O, Langerwisch U, Jirasko V, et al. A conserved NS3 surface patch orchestrates NS2 protease stimulation, NS5A hyperphosphorylation and HCV genome replication. *PLoS Pathog* 2015;11(3):e1004736.
378. Isken O, Langerwisch U, Schonherr R, et al. Functional characterization of bovine viral diarrhea virus nonstructural protein 5A by reverse genetic analysis and live cell imaging. *J Virol* 2014;88(1):82–98.

379. Isken O, Postel A, Bruhn B, et al. CRISPR/Cas9-mediated knockout of DNAJC14 verifies this chaperone as a pivotal host factor for RNA replication of pestiviruses. *J Virol* 2019;93(5).

380. Issur M, Geiss BJ, Bougie I, et al. The flavivirus NS5 protein is a true RNA guanylyltransferase that catalyzes a two-step reaction to form the RNA cap structure. *RNA* 2009;15(12):2340–2350.

381. Ito T, Lai MM. An internal polypyrimidine-tract-binding protein-binding site in the hepatitis C virus RNA attenuates translation, which is relieved by the 3'-untranslated sequence. *Virology* 1999;254(2):288–296.

382. Ivanyi-Nagy R, Lavergne JP, Gabus C, et al. RNA chaperoning and intrinsic disorder in the core proteins of *Flaviviridae*. *Nucleic Acids Res* 2008;36(3):712–725.

383. Ivashkina N, Wölk B, Lohmann V, et al. The hepatitis C virus RNA-dependent RNA polymerase membrane insertion sequence is a transmembrane segment. *J Virol* 2002;76(24):13088–13093.

384. Jaafar ZA, Oguro A, Nakamura Y, et al. Translation initiation by the hepatitis C virus IRES requires eIF1A and ribosomal complex remodeling. *Elife* 2016;5:e21198.

385. Janssen HLA, Reesink HW, Lawitz EJ, et al. Treatment of HCV infection by targeting microRNA. *N Engl J Med* 2013;368(18):1685–1694.

386. Ji H, Fraser CS, Yu Y, et al. Coordinated assembly of human translation initiation complexes by the hepatitis C virus internal ribosome entry site RNA. *Proc Natl Acad Sci U S A* 2004;101(49):16990–16995.

387. Jiang J, Cun W, Wu X, et al. Hepatitis C virus attachment mediated by apolipoprotein E binding to cell surface heparan sulfate. *J Virol* 2012;86(13):7256–7267.

388. Jirasko V, Montserret R, Appel N, et al. Structural and functional characterization of non-structural protein 2 for its role in hepatitis C virus assembly. *J Biol Chem* 2008;283(42):28546–28562.

389. Jirasko V, Montserret R, Lee JY, et al. Structural and functional studies of nonstructural protein 2 of the hepatitis C virus reveal its key role as organizer of virion assembly. *PLoS Pathog* 2010;6(12):e1001233.

390. Johns HL, Doceul V, Everett H, et al. The classical swine fever virus N-terminal protease N(pro) binds to cellular HAX-1. *J Gen Virol* 2010;91(Pt 11):2677–2686.

391. Jones DM, Atoom AM, Zhang X, et al. A genetic interaction between the core and NS3 proteins of hepatitis C virus is essential for production of infectious virus. *J Virol* 2011;85(23):12351–12361.

392. Jones CT, Murray CL, Eastman DK, et al. Hepatitis C virus p7 and NS2 proteins are essential for production of infectious virus. *J Virol* 2007;81(16):8374–8383.

393. Jones DM, Patel AH, Targett-Adams P, et al. The hepatitis C virus NS4B protein can *trans*-complement viral RNA replication and modulates production of infectious virus. *J Virol* 2009;83(5):2163–2177.

394. Jones CT, Patkar CG, Kuhn RJ. Construction and applications of yellow fever virus replicons. *Virology* 2005;331(2):247–259.

395. Jopling CL, Yi M, Lancaster AM, et al. Modulation of hepatitis C virus RNA abundance by a liver-specific MicroRNA. *Science* 2005;309(5740):1577–1581.

396. Jordan R, Wang L, Graczyk TM, et al. Replication of a cytopathic strain of bovine viral diarrhea virus activates PERK and induces endoplasmic reticulum stress-mediated apoptosis of MDBK cells. *J Virol* 2002;76(19):9588–9599.

397. Jubin R, Vantuno NE, Kieft JS, et al. Hepatitis C virus internal ribosome entry site (IRES) stem loop IIId contains a phylogenetically conserved GGG triplet essential for translation and IRES folding. *J Virol* 2000;74(22):10430–10437.

398. Jung S, Eichenmüller M, Donhauser N, et al. HIV entry inhibition by the envelope 2 glycoprotein of GB virus C. *AIDS* 2007;21(5):645–647.

399. Junjhon J, Pennington JG, Edwards TJ, et al. Ultrastructural characterization and three-dimensional architecture of replication sites in dengue virus-infected mosquito cells. *J Virol* 2014;88(9):4687–4697.

400. Kalinina O, Norder H, Mukomolov S, et al. A natural intergenotypic recombinant of hepatitis C virus identified in St. Petersburg. *J Virol* 2002;76(8):4034–4043.

401. Kaneko T, Tanji Y, Satoh S, et al. Production of two phosphoproteins from the NS5A region of the hepatitis C viral genome. *Biochem Biophys Res Commun* 1994;205(1):320–326.

402. Kang X, Chen X, He Y, et al. DDB1 is a cellular substrate of NS3/4A protease and required for hepatitis C virus replication. *Virology* 2013;435(2):385–394.

403. Kao CC, Del Vecchio AM, Zhong W. De novo initiation of RNA synthesis by a recombinant flaviviridae RNA-dependent RNA polymerase. *Virology* 1999;253(1):1–7.

404. Kao CC, Yang X, Kline A, et al. Template requirements for RNA synthesis by a recombinant hepatitis C virus RNA-dependent RNA polymerase. *J Virol* 2000;74(23):11121–11128.

405. Kapadia SB, Barth H, Baumert T, et al. Initiation of hepatitis C virus infection is dependent on cholesterol and cooperativity between CD81 and scavenger receptor B type I. *J Virol* 2007;81(1):374–383.

406. Kapadia SB, Chisari FV. Hepatitis C virus RNA replication is regulated by host geranylgeranylation and fatty acids. *Proc Natl Acad Sci U S A* 2005;102(7):2561–2566.

407. Kapoor A, Kumar A, Simmonds P, et al. Virome analysis of transfusion recipients reveals a novel human virus that shares genomic features with hepaciviruses and pegiviruses. *MBio* 2015;6(5):e01466.

408. Kapoor A, Simmonds P, Cullen JM, et al. Identification of a pegivirus (GB virus-like virus) that infects horses. *J Virol* 2013;87(12):7185–7190.

409. Kapoor A, Simmonds P, Gerold G, et al. Characterization of a canine homolog of hepatitis C virus. *Proc Natl Acad Sci U S A* 2011;108(28):11608–11613.

410. Kapoor A, Simmonds P, Scheel TK, et al. Identification of rodent homologs of hepatitis C virus and pegiviruses. *MBio* 2013;4(2):e00216.

411. Kato T, Date T, Miyamoto M, et al. Efficient replication of the genotype 2a hepatitis C virus subgenomic replicon. *Gastroenterology* 2003;125(6):1808–1817.

412. Kato N, Ootsuyama Y, Ohkoshi S, et al. Characterization of hypervariable regions in the putative envelope protein of hepatitis C virus. *Biochem Biophys Res Commun* 1992;189(1):119–127.

413. Katzelnick LC, Gresh L, Halloran ME, et al. Antibody-dependent enhancement of severe dengue disease in humans. *Science* 2017;358(6365):929–932.

414. Kaufman TM, McLinden JH, Xiang J, et al. The GBV-C envelope glycoprotein E2 does not interact specifically with CD81. *AIDS* 2007;21(8):1045–1048.

415. Kaufusi PH, Kelley JF, Yanagihara R, et al. Induction of endoplasmic reticulum-derived replication-competent membrane structures by West Nile virus non-structural protein 4B. *PLoS One* 2014;9(1):e84040.

416. Kazakov T, Yang F, Ramanathan HN, et al. Hepatitis C virus RNA replication depends on specific *cis*- and *trans*-acting activities of viral nonstructural proteins. *PLoS Pathog* 2015;11(4):e1004817.

417. Ke PY, Chen SS. Activation of the unfolded protein response and autophagy after hepatitis C virus infection suppresses innate antiviral immunity in vitro. *J Clin Invest* 2011;121(1):37–56.

418. Khan I, Katikaneni DS, Han Q, et al. Modulation of hepatitis C virus genome replication by glycosphingolipids and four-phosphate adaptor protein 2. *J Virol* 2014;88(21):12276–12295.

419. Khan AG, Whidby J, Miller MT, et al. Structure of the core ectodomain of the hepatitis C virus envelope glycoprotein 2. *Nature* 2014;509(7500):381–384.

420. Khromykh AA, Sedlak PL, Westaway EG. *cis*- and *trans*-acting elements in flavivirus RNA replication. *J Virol* 2000;74(7):3253–3263.

421. Khromykh AA, Varnavski AN, Sedlak PL, et al. Coupling between replication and packaging of flavivirus RNA: evidence derived from the use of DNA-based full-length cDNA clones of Kunjin virus. *J Virol* 2001;75(10):4633–4640.

422. Kiermayr S, Kofler RM, Mandl CW, et al. Isolation of capsid protein dimers from the tick-borne encephalitis flavivirus and in vitro assembly of capsid-like particles. *J Virol* 2004;78(15):8078–8084.

423. Kiiver K, Merits A, Ustav M, et al. Complex formation between hepatitis C virus NS2 and NS3 proteins. *Virus Res* 2006;117(2):264–272.

424. Kim M, Kim H, Cho SP, et al. Template requirements for de novo RNA synthesis by hepatitis C virus nonstructural protein 5B polymerase on the viral X RNA. *J Virol* 2002;76(14):6944–6956.

425. Kim JL, Morgenstern KA, Griffith JP, et al. Hepatitis C virus NS3 RNA helicase domain with a bound oligonucleotide: the crystal structure provides insights into the mode of unwinding. *Structure* 1998;6(1):89–100.

426. Kincaid RP, Lam VL, Chirayil RP, et al. RNA triphosphatase DUSP11 enables exonuclease XRN-mediated restriction of hepatitis C virus. *Proc Natl Acad Sci U S A* 2018;115(32):8197–8202.

427. Kirkegaard K, Baltimore D. The mechanism of RNA recombination in poliovirus. *Cell* 1986;47(3):433–443.

428. Klein KC, Polyak SJ, Lingappa JR. Unique features of hepatitis C virus capsid formation revealed by de novo cell-free assembly. *J Virol* 2004;78(17):9257–9269.

429. Kleine Büning M, Meyer D, Austermann-Busch S, et al. Nonreplicative RNA recombination of an animal plus-strand RNA virus in the absence of efficient translation of viral proteins. *Genome Biol Evol* 2017;9(4):817–829.

430. Klema VJ, Ye M, Hindupur A, et al. Dengue virus nonstructural protein 5 (NS5) assembles into a dimer with a unique methyltransferase and polymerase interface. *PLoS Pathog* 2016;12(2):e1005451.

431. Klemens O, Dubrau D, Tautz N. Characterization of the determinants of NS2-3-independent virion morphogenesis of pestiviruses. *J Virol* 2015;89(22):11668–11680.

432. Klinker S, Stindt S, Gremer L, et al. Phosphorylated tyrosine 93 of hepatitis C virus nonstructural protein 5A is essential for interaction with host c-Src and efficient viral replication. *J Biol Chem* 2019;294:7388–7402.

433. Knoops K, Kikkert M, Worm SH, et al. SARS-coronavirus replication is supported by a reticulovesicular network of modified endoplasmic reticulum. *PLoS Biol* 2008;6(9):e226.

434. Koch JO, Bartenschlager R. Modulation of hepatitis C virus NS5A hyperphosphorylation by nonstructural proteins NS3, NS4A, and NS4B. *J Virol* 1999;73(9):7138–7146.

435. Koedel Y, Eissmann K, Wend H, et al. Peptides derived from a distinct region of GB Virus C glycoprotein E2 mediate strain specific HIV-1 entry inhibition. *J Virol* 2011;85(14):7037–7047.

436. Kofler RM, Heinz FX, Mandl CW. Capsid protein C of tick-borne encephalitis virus tolerates large internal deletions and is a favorable target for attenuation of virulence. *J Virol* 2002;76(7):3534–3543.

437. Kofler RM, Leitner A, O'Riordain G, et al. Spontaneous mutations restore the viability of tick-borne encephalitis virus mutants with large deletions in protein C. *J Virol* 2003;77(1):443–451.

438. Kohlway A, Pirakitikulr N, Barrera FN, et al. Hepatitis C virus RNA replication and virus particle assembly require specific dimerization of the NS4A protein transmembrane domain. *J Virol* 2014;88(1):628–642.

439. Kohlway A, Pirakitikulr N, Ding SC, et al. The linker region of NS3 plays a critical role in the replication and infectivity of hepatitis C virus. *J Virol* 2014;88(18):10970–10974.

440. Kolykhalov AA, Agapov EV, Blight KJ, et al. Transmission of hepatitis C by intrahepatic inoculation with transcribed RNA. *Science* 1997;277(5325):570–574.

441. Kolykhalov AA, Feinstone SM, Rice CM. Identification of a highly conserved sequence element at the 3' terminus of hepatitis C virus genome RNA. *J Virol* 1996;70(6):3363–3371.

442. Kolykhalov AA, Mihalik K, Feinstone SM, et al. Hepatitis C virus-encoded enzymatic activities and conserved RNA elements in the 3' nontranslated region are essential for virus replication in vivo. *J Virol* 2000;74(4):2046–2051.

443. Kong L, Fujimoto A, Nakamura M, et al. Prolactin regulatory element binding protein is involved in hepatitis C virus replication by interaction with NS4B. *J Virol* 2016;90(6):3093–3111.

444. Kong L, Giang E, Nieusma T, et al. Hepatitis C virus E2 envelope glycoprotein core structure. *Science* 2013;342(6162):1090–1094.

445. Konishi E, Mason PW. Proper maturation of the Japanese encephalitis virus envelope glycoprotein requires cosynthesis with the premembrane protein. *J Virol* 1993;67(3):1672–1675.

446. Kono Y, Hayashida K, Tanaka H, et al. High-density lipoprotein binding rate differs greatly between genotypes 1b and 2a/2b of hepatitis C virus. *J Med Virol* 2003;70(1):42–48.

447. Koonin EV, Dolja VV. Evolution and taxonomy of positive-strand RNA viruses: implications of comparative analysis of amino acid sequences. *Crit Rev Biochem Mol Biol* 1993;28(5):375–430.

448. Koschinski A, Wengler G, Repp H. The membrane proteins of flaviviruses form ion-permeable pores in the target membrane after fusion: identification of the pores and analysis of their possible role in virus infection. *J Gen Virol* 2003;84(Pt 7):1711–1721.
449. Kostyuchenko VA, Zhang Q, Tan JL, et al. Immature and mature dengue serotype 1 virus structures provide insight into the maturation process. *J Virol* 2013;87(13):7700–7707.
450. Krey T, Bontems F, Vonrhein C, et al. Crystal structure of the pestivirus envelope glycoprotein E(rns) and mechanistic analysis of its ribonuclease activity. *Structure* 2012;20(5):862–873.
451. Krey T, Himmelreich A, Heimann M, et al. Function of bovine CD46 as a cellular receptor for bovine viral diarrhea virus is determined by complement control protein 1. *J Virol* 2006;80(8):3912–3922.
452. Krey T, Moussay E, Thiel HJ, et al. Role of the low-density lipoprotein receptor in entry of bovine viral diarrhea virus. *J Virol* 2006;80(21):10862–10867.
453. Krey T, Thiel HJ, Rümenapf T. Acid-resistant bovine pestivirus requires activation for pH-triggered fusion during entry. *J Virol* 2005;79(7):4191–4200.
454. Kroschewski H, Lim SP, Butcher RE, et al. Mutagenesis of the dengue virus type 2 NS5 methyltransferase domain. *J Biol Chem* 2008;283(28):19410–19421.
455. Kumar S, Barouch-Bentov R, Xiao F, et al. MARCH8 ubiquitinates the hepatitis C virus nonstructural 2 protein and mediates viral envelopment. *Cell Rep* 2019;26(7):1800.e1805–1814.e1805.
456. Kumar A, Buhler S, Selisko B, et al. Nuclear localization of dengue virus nonstructural protein 5 does not strictly correlate with efficient viral RNA replication and inhibition of type I interferon signaling. *J Virol* 2013;87(8):4545–4557.
457. Kumar A, Ray U, Das S. Human La protein interaction with GCAC near the initiator AUG enhances hepatitis C Virus RNA replication by promoting linkage between 5′ and 3′ untranslated regions. *J Virol* 2013;87(12):6713–6726.
458. Kümmerer BM. Establishment and application of flavivirus replicons. *Adv Exp Med Biol* 2018;1062:165–173.
459. Kümmerer BM, Rice CM. Mutations in the yellow fever virus nonstructural protein NS2A selectively block production of infectious particles. *J Virol* 2002;76(10):4773–4784.
460. Kümmerer BM, Stoll D, Meyers G. Bovine viral diarrhea virus strain Oregon: a novel mechanism for processing of NS2-3 based on point mutations. *J Virol* 1998;72(5):4127–4138.
461. Kunkel M, Lorinczi M, Rijnbrand R, et al. Self-assembly of nucleocapsid-like particles from recombinant hepatitis C virus core protein. *J Virol* 2001;75(5):2119–2129.
462. Kuo G, Choo QL, Alter HJ, et al. An assay for circulating antibodies to a major etiologic virus of human non-A, non-B hepatitis. *Science* 1989;244(4902):362–364.
463. Kushima Y, Wakita T, Hijikata M. A disulfide-bonded dimer of the core protein of hepatitis C virus is important for virus-like particle production. *J Virol* 2010;84(18):9118–9127.
464. Lackner T, Müller A, König M, et al. Persistence of bovine viral diarrhea virus is determined by a cellular cofactor of a viral autoprotease. *J Virol* 2005;79(15):9746–9755.
465. Lackner T, Müller A, Pankraz A, et al. Temporal modulation of an autoprotease is crucial for replication and pathogenicity of an RNA virus. *J Virol* 2004;78(19):10765–10775.
466. Lackner T, Thiel HJ, Tautz N. Dissection of a viral autoprotease elucidates a function of a cellular chaperone in proteolysis. *Proc Natl Acad Sci U S A* 2006;103(5):1510–1515.
467. Ladner JT, Wiley MR, Beitzel B, et al. A multicomponent animal virus isolated from mosquitoes. *Cell Host Microbe* 2016;20(3):357–367.
468. Lai VC, Dempsey S, Lau JY, et al. In vitro RNA replication directed by replicase complexes isolated from the subgenomic replicon cells of hepatitis C virus. *J Virol* 2003;77(3):2295–2300.
469. Lai VC, Kao CC, Ferrari E, et al. Mutational analysis of bovine viral diarrhea virus RNA-dependent RNA polymerase. *J Virol* 1999;73(12):10129–10136.
470. Lam AM, Frick DN. Hepatitis C virus subgenomic replicon requires an active NS3 RNA helicase. *J Virol* 2006;80(1):404–411.
471. Lamarre D, Anderson PC, Bailey M, et al. An NS3 protease inhibitor with antiviral effects in humans infected with hepatitis C virus. *Nature* 2003;426(6963):186–189.
472. Lambert SM, Langley DR, Garnett JA, et al. The crystal structure of NS5A domain 1 from genotype 1a reveals new clues to the mechanism of action for dimeric HCV inhibitors. *Protein Sci* 2014;23(6):723–734.
473. Lamp B, Riedel C, Roman-Sosa G, et al. Biosynthesis of classical swine fever virus nonstructural proteins. *J Virol* 2011;85(7):3607–3620.
474. Lamp B, Riedel C, Wentz E, et al. Autocatalytic cleavage within classical swine fever virus NS3 leads to a functional separation of protease and helicase. *J Virol* 2013;87(21):11872–11883.
475. Lancaster AM, Jan E, Sarnow P. Initiation factor-independent translation mediated by the hepatitis C virus internal ribosome entry site. *RNA* 2006;12(5):894–902.
476. Lanford RE, Chavez D, Notvall L, et al. Comparison of tamarins and marmosets as hosts for GBV-B infections and the effect of immunosuppression on duration of viremia. *Virology* 2003;311(1):72–80.
477. Lanford RE, Walker CM, Lemon SM. The chimpanzee model of viral hepatitis: advances in understanding the immune response and treatment of viral hepatitis. *Ilar J* 2017;58(2):172–189.
478. Langedijk JP. Translocation activity of C-terminal domain of pestivirus E^{rns} and ribotoxin L3 loop. *J Biol Chem* 2002;277(7):5308–5314.
479. Largo E, Gladue DP, Huarte N, et al. Pore-forming activity of pestivirus p7 in a minimal model system supports genus-specific viroporin function. *Antiviral Res* 2014;101:30–36.
480. Largo E, Gladue DP, Torralba J, et al. Mutation-induced changes of transmembrane pore size revealed by combined ion-channel conductance and single vesicle permeabilization analyses. *Biochim Biophys Acta Biomembr* 2018;1860(5):1015–1021.
481. Largo E, Verdia-Baguena C, Aguilella VM, et al. Ion channel activity of the CSFV p7 viroporin in surrogates of the ER lipid bilayer. *Biochim Biophys Acta* 2016;1858(1):30–37.
482. Laskus T, Radkowski M, Wang LF, et al. Lack of evidence for hepatitis G virus replication in the livers of patients coinfected with hepatitis C and G viruses. *J Virol* 1997;71(10):7804–7806.
483. Laskus T, Radkowski M, Wang LF, et al. Detection of hepatitis G virus replication sites by using highly strand-specific Tth-based reverse transcriptase PCR. *J Virol* 1998;72(4):3072–3075.
484. Lattwein E, Klemens O, Schwindt S, et al. Pestivirus virion morphogenesis in the absence of uncleaved nonstructural protein 2-3. *J Virol* 2012;86(1):427–437.
485. Lauck M, Sibley SD, Lara J, et al. A novel hepacivirus with an unusually long and intrinsically disordered NS5A protein in a wild old world primate. *J Virol* 2013;87(16):8971–8981.
486. Laude H, Gelfi J. Properties of Border disease virus as studied in a sheep cell line. *Arch Virol* 1979;62(4):341–346.
487. Laureti M, Narayanan D, Rodriguez-Andres J, et al. Flavivirus receptors: diversity, identity, and cell entry. *Front Immunol* 2018;9:2180.
488. Lavie M, Dubuisson J. Interplay between hepatitis C virus and lipid metabolism during virus entry and assembly. *Biochimie* 2017;141:62–69.
489. Lavie M, Sarrazin S, Montserret R, et al. Identification of conserved residues in hepatitis C virus envelope glycoprotein E2 that modulate virus dependence on CD81 and SRB1 entry factors. *J Virol* 2014;88(18):10584–10597.
490. Leary K, Blair CD. Sequential events in the morphogenesis of Japanese encephalitis virus. *J Ultrastruct Res* 1980;72:123–129.
491. Leary TP, Desai SM, Yamaguchi J, et al. Species-specific variants of GB virus A in captive monkeys [published erratum appears in J Virol 1997 Nov;71(11):8953]. *J Virol* 1996;70(12):9028–9030.
492. Leary TP, Muerhoff AS, Simons JN, et al. Sequence and genomic organization of GBV-C: a novel member of the Flaviviridae associated with human non-A-E hepatitis. *J Med Virol* 1996;48(1):60–67.
493. Lecot S, Belouzard S, Dubuisson J, et al. Bovine viral diarrhea virus entry is dependent on clathrin-mediated endocytosis. *J Virol* 2005;79(16):10826–10829.
494. Lee JY, Acosta EG, Stoeck IK, et al. Apolipoprotein E likely contributes to a maturation step of infectious hepatitis C virus particles and interacts with viral envelope glycoproteins. *J Virol* 2014;88(21):12422–12437.
495. Lee E, Stocks CE, Amberg SM, et al. Mutagenesis of the signal sequence of yellow fever virus prM protein: enhancement of signalase cleavage in vitro is lethal for virus production. *J Virol* 2000;74(1):24–32.
496. Lee CM, Xie X, Zou J, et al. Determinants of dengue virus NS4A protein oligomerization. *J Virol* 2015;89(12):6171–6183.
497. Lemay KL, Treadaway J, Angulo I, et al. A hepatitis C virus NS5A phosphorylation site that regulates RNA replication. *J Virol* 2013;87(2):1255–1260.
498. Lemm JA, Leet JE, O'Boyle DR, et al. Discovery of potent hepatitis C virus NS5A inhibitors with dimeric structures. *Antimicrob Agents Chemother* 2011;55(8):3795–3802.
499. Lesburg CA, Cable MB, Ferrari E, et al. Crystal structure of the RNA-dependent RNA polymerase from hepatitis C virus reveals a fully encircled active site. *Nat Struct Biol* 1999;6(10):937–943.
500. Leung JY, Pijlman GP, Kondratieva N, et al. Role of nonstructural protein NS2A in flavivirus assembly. *J Virol* 2008;82(10):4731–4741.
501. Lévêque VJ, Johnson RB, Parsons S, et al. Identification of a C-terminal regulatory motif in hepatitis C virus RNA-dependent RNA polymerase: structural and biochemical analysis. *J Virol* 2003;77(16):9020–9028.
502. Lewis AP, Jopling CL. Regulation and biological function of the liver-specific miR-122. *Biochem Soc Trans* 2010;38(6):1553–1557.
503. Li Q, Brass AL, Ng A, et al. A genome-wide genetic screen for host factors required for hepatitis C virus propagation. *Proc Natl Acad Sci U S A* 2009;106(38):16410–16415.
504. Li XD, Deng CL, Ye HQ, et al. Transmembrane domains of NS2B contribute to both viral RNA replication and particle formation in Japanese encephalitis virus. *J Virol* 2016;90(12):5735–5749.
505. Li K, Foy E, Ferreon JC, et al. Immune evasion by hepatitis C virus NS3/4A protease-mediated cleavage of the Toll-like receptor 3 adaptor protein TRIF. *Proc Natl Acad Sci U S A* 2005;102(8):2992–2997.
506. Li D, Li S, Sun Y, et al. Poly(C)-binding protein 1, a novel N(pro)-interacting protein involved in classical swine fever virus growth. *J Virol* 2013;87(4):2072–2080.
507. Li L, Lok SM, Yu IM, et al. The flavivirus precursor membrane-envelope protein complex: structure and maturation. *Science* 2008;319(5871):1830–1834.
508. Li Y, Masaki T, Yamane D, et al. Competing and noncompeting activities of miR-122 and the 5′ exonuclease Xrn1 in regulation of hepatitis C virus replication. *Proc Natl Acad Sci U S A* 2013;110(5):1881–1886.
509. Li Q, Pene V, Krishnamurthy S, et al. Hepatitis C virus infection activates an innate pathway involving IKK-alpha in lipogenesis and viral assembly. *Nat Med* 2013;19(6):722–729.
510. Li Q, Sodroski C, Lowey B, et al. Hepatitis C virus depends on E-cadherin as an entry factor and regulates its expression in epithelial-to-mesenchymal transition. *Proc Natl Acad Sci U S A* 2016;113(27):7620–7625.
511. Li XD, Sun L, Seth RB, et al. Hepatitis C virus protease NS3/4A cleaves mitochondrial antiviral signaling protein off the mitochondria to evade innate immunity. *Proc Natl Acad Sci U S A* 2005;102(49):17717–17722.
512. Li Y, Wang J, Kanai R, et al. Crystal structure of glycoprotein E2 from bovine viral diarrhea virus. *Proc Natl Acad Sci U S A* 2013;110(17):6805–6810.
513. Li W, Wu B, Soca WA, et al. Crystal structure of classical swine fever virus NS5B reveals a novel N-terminal domain. *J Virol* 2018;92(14).
514. Li Y, Yamane D, Masaki T, et al. The yin and yang of hepatitis C: synthesis and decay of hepatitis C virus RNA. *Nat Rev Microbiol* 2015;13(9):544–558.
515. Li LF, Yu J, Li Y, et al. Guanylate-binding protein 1, an interferon-induced gtpase, exerts an antiviral activity against classical swine fever virus depending on its GTPase activity. *J Virol* 2016;90(9):4412–4426.
516. Liang Y, Cao X, Ding Q, et al. Hepatitis C virus NS4B induces the degradation of TRIF to inhibit TLR3-mediated interferon signaling pathway. *PLoS Pathog* 2018;14(5):e1007075.
517. Liang D, Chen L, Ansari IH, et al. A replicon *trans*-packaging system reveals the requirement of nonstructural proteins for the assembly of bovine viral diarrhea virus (BVDV) virion. *Virology* 2009;387(2):331–340.
518. Liang D, Sainz IF, Ansari IH, et al. The envelope glycoprotein E2 is a determinant of cell culture tropism in ruminant pestiviruses. *J Gen Virol* 2003;84(Pt 5):1269–1274.
519. Liang Y, Ye H, Kang CB, et al. Domain 2 of nonstructural protein 5A (NS5A) of hepatitis C virus is natively unfolded. *Biochemistry* 2007;46(41):11550–11558.

520. Liao M, Kielian M. Domain III from class II fusion proteins functions as a dominant-negative inhibitor of virus membrane fusion. *J Cell Biol* 2005;171(1):111–120.

521. Liebler EM, Waschbüsch J, Pohlenz JF, et al. Distribution of antigen of noncytopathogenic and cytopathogenic bovine virus diarrhea virus biotypes in the intestinal tract of calves following experimental production of mucosal disease. *Arch Virol Suppl* 1991;3:109–124.

522. Lin C, Amberg SM, Chambers TJ, et al. Cleavage at a novel site in the NS4A region by the yellow fever virus NS2B-3 proteinase is a prerequisite for processing at the downstream 4A/4B signalase site. *J Virol* 1993;67(4):2327–2335.

523. Lin KC, Chang HL, Chang RY. Accumulation of a 3′-terminal genome fragment in Japanese encephalitis virus-infected mammalian and mosquito cells. *J Virol* 2004;78(10):5133–5138.

524. Lin DL, Cherepanova NA, Bozzacco L, et al. Dengue virus hijacks a noncanonical oxidoreductase function of a cellular oligosaccharyltransferase complex. *MBio* 2017;8(4).

525. Lin C, Lindenbach BD, Prágai BM, et al. Processing in the hepatitis C virus E2-NS2 region: identification of p7 and two distinct E2-specific products with different C termini. *J Virol* 1994;68(8):5063–5073.

526. Lin C, Thomson JA, Rice CM. A central region in the hepatitis C virus NS4A protein allows formation of an active NS3-NS4A serine proteinase complex in vivo and in vitro. *J Virol* 1995;69:4373–4380.

527. Lin C, Wu JW, Hsiao K, et al. The hepatitis C virus NS4A protein: interactions with the NS4B and NS5A proteins. *J Virol* 1997;71(9):6465–6471.

528. Lindenbach BD, Rice CM. trans-Complementation of yellow fever virus NS1 reveals a role in early RNA replication. *J Virol* 1997;71(12):9608–9617.

529. Lindenbach BD, Evans MJ, Syder AJ, et al. Complete replication of hepatitis C virus in cell culture. *Science* 2005;309(5734):623–626.

530. Lindenbach BD, Meuleman P, Ploss A, et al. Cell culture-grown hepatitis C virus is infectious in vivo and can be recultured in vitro. *Proc Natl Acad Sci U S A* 2006;103(10):3805–3809.

531. Lindenbach BD, Prágai BM, Montserret R, et al. The C terminus of hepatitis C virus NS4A encodes an electrostatic switch that regulates NS5A hyperphosphorylation and viral replication. *J Virol* 2007;81(17):8905–8918.

532. Lindenbach BD, Rice CM. Genetic interaction of flavivirus nonstructural proteins NS1 and NS4A as a determinant of replicase function. *J Virol* 1999;73(6):4611–4621.

533. Lindenbach BD, Rice CM. The ins and outs of hepatitis C virus entry and assembly. *Nat Rev Microbiol* 2013;11(10):688–700.

534. Linnen J, Wages J, Jr., Zhang-Keck ZY, et al. Molecular cloning and disease association of hepatitis G virus: a transfusion-transmissible agent. *Science* 1996;271(5248):505–508.

535. Liu S, Ansari IH, Das SC, et al. Insertion and deletion analyses identify regions of nonstructural protein 5A of Hepatitis C virus that are dispensable for viral genome replication. *J Gen Virol* 2006;87(Pt 2):323–327.

536. Liu WJ, Chen HB, Wang XJ, et al. Analysis of adaptive mutations in Kunjin virus replicon RNA reveals a novel role for the flavivirus nonstructural protein NS2A in inhibition of beta interferon promoter-driven transcription. *J Virol* 2004;78(22):12225–12235.

537. Liu J, Kline BA, Kenny TA, et al. A novel sheet-like virus particle array is a hallmark of Zika virus infection. *Emerg Microbes Infect* 2018;7(1):69.

538. Liu ZY, Li XF, Jiang T, et al. Viral RNA switch mediates the dynamic control of flavivirus replicase recruitment by genome cyclization. *Elife* 2016;5.

539. Liu Y, Liu J, Du S, et al. Evolutionary enhancement of Zika virus infectivity in *Aedes aegypti* mosquitoes. *Nature* 2017;545(7655):482–486.

540. Liu Y, Liu H, Zou J, et al. Dengue virus subgenomic RNA induces apoptosis through the Bcl-2-mediated PI3k/Akt signaling pathway. *Virology* 2014;448:15–25.

541. Liu WJ, Sedlak PL, Kondratieva N, et al. Complementation analysis of the flavivirus kunjin NS3 and NS5 proteins defines the minimal regions essential for formation of a replication complex and shows a requirement of NS3 in *cis* for virus assembly. *J Virol* 2002;76(21):10766–10775.

542. Liu WJ, Wang XJ, Clark DC, et al. A single amino acid substitution in the West Nile virus nonstructural protein NS2A disables its ability to inhibit alpha/beta interferon induction and attenuates virus virulence in mice. *J Virol* 2006;80(5):2396–2404.

543. Lo SY, Selby MJ, Ou JH. Interaction between hepatitis C virus core protein and E1 envelope protein. *J Virol* 1996;70(8):5177–51782.

544. Lobigs M. Flavivirus premembrane protein cleavage and spike heterodimer secretion requires the function of the viral proteinase NS3. *Proc Natl Acad Sci U S A* 1993;90:6218–6222.

545. Lobigs M, Lee E, Ng ML, et al. A flavivirus signal peptide balances the catalytic activity of two proteases and thereby facilitates virus morphogenesis. *Virology* 2010;401(1):80–89.

546. Lodeiro MF, Filomatori CV, Gamarnik AV. Structural and functional studies of the promoter element for dengue virus RNA replication. *J Virol* 2009;83(2):993–1008.

547. Lohmann V, Körner F, Dobierzewska A, et al. Mutations in hepatitis C virus RNAs conferring cell culture adaptation. *J Virol* 2001;75:1437–1449.

548. Lohmann V, Körner F, Herian U, et al. Biochemical properties of hepatitis C virus NS5B RNA-dependent RNA polymerase and identification of amino acid sequence motifs essential for enzymatic activity. *J Virol* 1997;71(11):8416–8428.

549. Lohmann V, Korner F, Koch JO, et al. Replication of subgenomic hepatitis C virus RNAs in a hepatoma cell line. *Science* 1999;285:110–113.

550. Lohmann V, Overton H, Bartenschlager R. Selective stimulation of hepatitis C virus and pestivirus NS5B RNA polymerase activity by GTP. *J Biol Chem* 1999;274(16):10807–10815.

551. Lok SM, Kostyuchenko V, Nybakken GE, et al. Binding of a neutralizing antibody to dengue virus alters the arrangement of surface glycoproteins. *Nat Struct Mol Biol* 2008;15(3):312–317.

552. Longatti A, Boyd B, Chisari FV. Virion-independent transfer of replication-competent hepatitis C virus RNA between permissive cells. *J Virol* 2015;89(5):2956–2961.

553. Lorenz IC, Marcotrigiano J, Dentzer TG, et al. Structure of the catalytic domain of the hepatitis C virus NS2-3 protease. *Nature* 2006;442(7104):831–835.

554. Love RA, Brodsky O, Hickey MJ, et al. Crystal structure of a novel dimeric form of NS5A domain I protein from hepatitis C virus. *J Virol* 2009;83(9):4395–4403.

555. Love RA, Parge H, Wickersham JA, et al. The crystal structure of hepatitis C virus NS3 proteinase reveals a trypsin-like fold and a structural zinc binding site. *Cell* 1996;87:331–342.

556. Love RA, Parge HE, Yu X, et al. Crystallographic identification of a noncompetitive inhibitor binding site on the hepatitis C virus NS5B RNA polymerase enzyme. *J Virol* 2003;77(13):7575–7581.

557. Lu W, Ou JH. Phosphorylation of hepatitis C virus core protein by protein kinase A and protein kinase C. *Virology* 2002;300(1):20–30.

558. Lu W, Strohecker A, Ou Jh JH. Post-translational modification of the hepatitis C virus core protein by tissue transglutaminase. *J Biol Chem* 2001;276(51):47993–47999.

559. Luik P, Chew C, Aittoniemi J, et al. The 3-dimensional structure of a hepatitis C virus p7 ion channel by electron microscopy. *Proc Natl Acad Sci U S A* 2009;106(31):12712–12716.

560. Luna JM, Scheel TK, Danino T, et al. Hepatitis C virus RNA functionally sequesters miR-122. *Cell* 2015;160(6):1099–1110.

561. Lundin M, Monné M, Widell A, et al. Topology of the membrane-associated hepatitis C virus protein NS4B. *J Virol* 2003;77(9):5428–5438.

562. Luo G, Hamatake RK, Mathis DM, et al. De novo initiation of RNA synthesis by the RNA-dependent RNA polymerase (NS5B) of hepatitis C virus. *J Virol* 2000;74(2):851–863.

563. Luo D, Vasudevan SG, Lescar J. The flavivirus NS2B-NS3 protease-helicase as a target for antiviral drug development. *Antiviral Res* 2015;118:148–158.

564. Luo D, Wei N, Doan DN, et al. Flexibility between the protease and helicase domains of the dengue virus NS3 protein conferred by the linker region and its functional implications. *J Biol Chem* 2010;285(24):18817–18827.

565. Luo D, Xu T, Hunke C, et al. Crystal structure of the NS3 protease-helicase from dengue virus. *J Virol* 2008;82(1):173–183.

566. Luo D, Xu T, Watson RP, et al. Insights into RNA unwinding and ATP hydrolysis by the flavivirus NS3 protein. *EMBO J* 2008;27(23):3209–3219.

567. Lupberger J, Zeisel MB, Xiao F, et al. EGFR and EphA2 are host factors for hepatitis C virus entry and possible targets for antiviral therapy. *Nat Med* 2011;17(5):589–595.

568. Luscombe CA, Huang Z, Murray MG, et al. A novel Hepatitis C virus p7 ion channel inhibitor, BIT225, inhibits bovine viral diarrhea virus in vitro and shows synergism with recombinant interferon-alpha-2b and nucleoside analogues. *Antiviral Res* 2010;86(2):144–153.

569. Lussignol M, Kopp M, Molloy K, et al. Proteomics of HCV virions reveals an essential role for the nucleoporin Nup98 in virus morphogenesis. *Proc Natl Acad Sci U S A* 2016;113(9):2484–2489.

570. Lv H, Dong W, Qian G, et al. uS10, a novel N^{pro}-interacting protein, inhibits classical swine fever virus replication. *J Gen Virol* 2017;98(7):1679–1692.

571. Ma Y, Anantpadma M, Timpe JM, et al. Hepatitis C virus NS2 protein serves as a scaffold for virus assembly by interacting with both structural and nonstructural proteins. *J Virol* 2011;85(1):86–97.

572. Ma L, Jones CT, Groesch TD, et al. Solution structure of dengue virus capsid protein reveals another fold. *Proc Natl Acad Sci U S A* 2004;101(10):3414–3419.

573. Ma L, Li F, Zhang JW, et al. Host factor SPCS1 regulates the replication of Japanese encephalitis virus through interactions with transmembrane domains of NS2B. *J Virol* 2018;92(12).

574. Ma Y, Yates J, Liang Y, et al. NS3 helicase domains involved in infectious intracellular hepatitis C virus particle assembly. *J Virol* 2008;82(15):7624–7639.

575. Machlin ES, Sarnow P, Sagan SM. Masking the 5′ terminal nucleotides of the hepatitis C virus genome by an unconventional microRNA-target RNA complex. *Proc Natl Acad Sci U S A* 2011;108(8):3193–3198.

576. Mackenzie JM, Jones MK, Young PR. Immunolocalization of the dengue virus nonstructural glycoprotein NS1 suggests a role in viral RNA replication. *Virology* 1996;220:232–240.

577. Mackenzie JM, Kenney MT, Westaway EG. West Nile virus strain Kunjin NS5 polymerase is a phosphoprotein localized at the cytoplasmic site of viral RNA synthesis. *J Gen Virol* 2007;88(Pt 4):1163–1168.

578. Mackenzie JM, Khromykh AA, Jones MK, et al. Subcellular localization and some biochemical properties of the flavivirus Kunjin nonstructural proteins NS2A and NS4A. *Virology* 1998;245(2):203–215.

579. Mackenzie JM, Khromykh AA, Parton RG. Cholesterol manipulation by West Nile virus perturbs the cellular immune response. *Cell Host Microbe* 2007;2(4):229–239.

580. Mackenzie JM, Westaway EG. Assembly and maturation of the flavivirus Kunjin virus appear to occur in the rough endoplasmic reticulum and along the secretory pathway, respectively. *J Virol* 2001;75(22):10787–10799.

581. Madan V, Bartenschlager R. Structural and functional properties of the hepatitis C virus p7 viroporin. *Viruses* 2015;7(8):4461–4481.

582. Maidana-Giret MT, Silva TM, Sauer MM, et al. GB virus type C infection modulates T-cell activation independently of HIV-1 viral load. *AIDS* 2009;23(17):2277–2287.

583. Majeau N, Fromentin R, Savard C, et al. Palmitoylation of hepatitis C virus core protein is important for virion production. *J Biol Chem* 2009;284(49):33915–33925.

584. Malet H, Egloff MP, Selisko B, et al. Crystal structure of the RNA polymerase domain of the West Nile virus non-structural protein 5. *J Biol Chem* 2007;282(14):10678–10689.

585. Mandl CW, Kroschewski H, Allison SL, et al. Adaptation of tick-borne encephalitis virus to BHK-21 cells results in the formation of multiple heparan sulfate binding sites in the envelope protein and attenuation in vivo. *J Virol* 2001;75(12):5627–5637.

586. Mani N, Yuzhakov A, Yuzhakov O, et al. Nonstructural protein 5A (NS5A) and human replication protein A increase the processivity of hepatitis C virus NS5B polymerase activity in vitro. *J Virol* 2015;89(1):165–180.

587. Mankouri J, Walter C, Stewart H, et al. Release of infectious hepatitis C virus from Huh7 cells occurs via a *trans*-Golgi network-to-endosome pathway independent of very-low-density lipoprotein secretion. *J Virol* 2016;90(16):7159–7170.

588. Manokaran G, Finol E, Wang C, et al. Dengue subgenomic RNA binds TRIM25 to inhibit interferon expression for epidemiological fitness. *Science* 2015;350(6257):217–221.

589. Marceau CD, Puschnik AS, Majzoub K, et al. Genetic dissection of Flaviviridae host factors through genome-scale CRISPR screens. *Nature* 2016;535(7610):159–163.

590. Marshall DJ, Moxley RA, Kelling CL. Distribution of virus and viral antigen in specific pathogen-free calves following inoculation with noncytopathic bovine viral diarrhea virus. *Vet Pathol* 1996;33(3):311–318.

591. Martin A, Bodola F, Sangar DV, et al. Chronic hepatitis associated with GB virus B persistence in a tamarin after intrahepatic inoculation of synthetic viral RNA. *Proc Natl Acad Sci U S A* 2003;100(17):9962–9967.

592. Martin-Acebes MA, Merino-Ramos T, Blazquez AB, et al. The composition of West Nile virus lipid envelope unveils a role of sphingolipid metabolism in flavivirus biogenesis. *J Virol* 2014;88(20):12041–12054.

593. Martinez-Salas E, Francisco-Velilla R, Fernandez-Chamorro J, et al. Insights into structural and mechanistic features of viral IRES elements. *Front Microbiol* 2017;8:2629.

594. Masaki T, Matsunaga S, Takahashi H, et al. Involvement of hepatitis C virus NS5A hyperphosphorylation mediated by casein kinase I-alpha in infectious virus production. *J Virol* 2014;88(13):7541–7555.

595. Masaki T, Suzuki R, Murakami K, et al. Interaction of hepatitis C virus nonstructural protein 5A with core protein is critical for the production of infectious virus particles. *J Virol* 2008;82(16):7964–7976.

596. Mason PW. Maturation of Japanese encephalitis virus glycoproteins produced by infected mammalian and mosquito cells. *Virology* 1989;169(2):354–364.

597. Matusan AE, Pryor MJ, Davidson AD, et al. Mutagenesis of the Dengue virus type 2 NS3 protein within and outside helicase motifs: effects on enzyme activity and virus replication. *J Virol* 2001;75(20):9633–9643.

598. Mauger DM, Golden M, Yamane D, et al. Functionally conserved architecture of hepatitis C virus RNA genomes. *Proc Natl Acad Sci U S A* 2015;112(12):3692–3697.

599. Maurer K, Krey T, Moennig V, et al. CD46 is a cellular receptor for bovine viral diarrhea virus. *J Virol* 2004;78(4):1792–1799.

600. Mayer D, Hofmann MA, Tratschin JD. Attenuation of classical swine fever virus by deletion of the viral N(pro) gene. *Vaccine* 2004;22(3-4):317–328.

601. McAllister J, Casino C, Davidson F, et al. Long-term evolution of the hypervariable region of hepatitis C virus in a common-source-infected cohort. *J Virol* 1998;72(6):4893–4905.

602. McClurkin AW, Bolin SR, Coria MF. Isolation of cytopathic and noncytopathic bovine viral diarrhea virus from the spleen of cattle acutely and chronically affected with bovine viral diarrhea. *J Am Vet Med Assoc* 1985;186(6):568–569.

603. McCormick CJ, Maucourant S, Griffin S, et al. Tagging of NS5A expressed from a functional hepatitis C virus replicon. *J Gen Virol* 2006;87(Pt 3):635–640.

604. McLauchlan J. Properties of the hepatitis C virus core protein: a structural protein that modulates cellular processes. *J Viral Hepat* 2000;7(1):2–14.

605. McLauchlan J, Lemberg MK, Hope G, et al. Intramembrane proteolysis promotes trafficking of hepatitis C virus core protein to lipid droplets. *EMBO J* 2002;21(15):3980–3988.

606. McLean JE, Wudzinska A, Datan E, et al. Flavivirus NS4A-induced autophagy protects cells against death and enhances virus replication. *J Biol Chem* 2011;286(25):22147–22159.

607. McMullan LK, Grakoui A, Evans MJ, et al. Evidence for a functional RNA element in the hepatitis C virus core gene. *Proc Natl Acad Sci U S A* 2007;104(8):2879–2884.

608. Medin CL, Fitzgerald KA, Rothman AL. Dengue virus nonstructural protein NS5 induces interleukin-8 transcription and secretion. *J Virol* 2005;79(17):11053–11061.

609. Meertens L, Bertaux C, Dragic T. Hepatitis C virus entry requires a critical postinternalization step and delivery to early endosomes via clathrin-coated vesicles. *J Virol* 2006;80(23):11571–11578.

610. Meertens L, Carnec X, Lecoin MP, et al. The TIM and TAM families of phosphatidylserine receptors mediate dengue virus entry. *Cell Host Microbe* 2012;12(4):544–557.

611. Melo CF, de Oliveira DN, Lima EO, et al. A lipidomics approach in the characterization of Zika-infected mosquito cells: potential targets for breaking the transmission cycle. *PLoS One* 2016;11(10):e0164377.

612. Melvin SL, Dawson GJ, Carrick RJ, et al. Biophysical characterization of GB virus C from human plasma. *J Virol Methods* 1998;71(2):147–157.

613. Mendez E, Ruggli N, Collett MS, et al. Infectious bovine viral diarrhea virus (strain NADL) RNA from stable cDNA clones: a cellular insert determines NS3 production and viral cytopathogenicity. *J Virol* 1998;72(6):4737–4745.

614. Menzel N, Fischl W, Hueging K, et al. MAP-kinase regulated cytosolic phospholipase A2 activity is essential for production of infectious hepatitis C virus particles. *PLoS Pathog* 2012;8(7):e1002829.

615. Mercer DF, Schiller DE, Elliott JF, et al. Hepatitis C virus replication in mice with chimeric human livers. *Nat Med* 2001;7(8):927–933.

616. Merino-Ramos T, Vazquez-Calvo A, Casas J, et al. Modification of the host cell lipid metabolism induced by hypolipidemic drugs targeting the acetyl coenzyme a carboxylase impairs West Nile virus replication. *Antimicrob Agents Chemother* 2016;60(1):307–315.

617. Merwaiss F, Czibener C, Alvarez DE. Cell-to-cell transmission is the main mechanism supporting bovine viral diarrhea virus spread in cell culture. *J Virol* 2019;93(3).

618. Merz A, Long G, Hiet MS, et al. Biochemical and morphological properties of hepatitis C virus particles and determination of their lipidome. *J Biol Chem* 2011;286(4):3018–3032.

619. Mesmin B, Bigay J, Moser von Filseck J, et al. A four-step cycle driven by PI(4)P hydrolysis directs sterol/PI(4)P exchange by the ER-Golgi tether OSBP. *Cell* 2013;155(4):830–843.

620. Mesmin B, Bigay J, Polidori J, et al. Sterol transfer, PI4P consumption, and control of membrane lipid order by endogenous OSBP. *EMBO J* 2017;36(21):3156–3174.

621. Metz P, Chiramel A, Chatel-Chaix L, et al. Dengue virus inhibition of autophagic flux and dependency of viral replication on proteasomal degradation of the autophagy receptor p62. *J Virol* 2015;89(15):8026–8041.

622. Meuleman P, Libbrecht L, De Vos R, et al. Morphological and biochemical characterization of a human liver in a uPA-SCID mouse chimera. *Hepatology* 2005;41(4):847–856.

623. Meunier JC, Russell RS, Engle RH, et al. Apolipoprotein C1 association with hepatitis C virus. *J Virol* 2008;82(19):9647–9656.

624. Meyer C, Von Freyburg M, Elbers K, et al. Recovery of virulent and RNase-negative attenuated type 2 bovine viral diarrhea viruses from infectious cDNA clones. *J Virol* 2002;76(16):8494–8503.

625. Meyers G, Ege A, Fetzer C, et al. Bovine viral diarrhea virus: prevention of persistent fetal infection by a combination of two mutations affecting E^{rns} RNase and N^{pro} protease. *J Virol* 2007;81(7):3327–3338.

626. Meyers G, Tautz N, Becher P, et al. Recovery of cytopathogenic and noncytopathogenic bovine viral diarrhea viruses from cDNA constructs. *J Virol* 1996;70(12):8606–8613.

627. Meyers G, Tautz N, Dubovi EJ, et al. Viral cytopathogenicity correlated with integration of ubiquitin-coding sequences. *Virology* 1991;180(2):602–616.

628. Meyers G, Tautz N, Stark R, et al. Rearrangement of viral sequences in cytopathogenic pestiviruses. *Virology* 1992;191(1):368–386.

629. Meyers G, Thiel HJ. Cytopathogenicity of classical swine fever virus caused by defective interfering particles. *J Virol* 1995;69(6):3683–3689.

630. Meylan E, Curran J, Hofmann K, et al. Cardif is an adaptor protein in the RIG-I antiviral pathway and is targeted by hepatitis C virus. *Nature* 2005;437(7062):1167–1172.

631. Miao Z, Gao L, Song Y, et al. Prevalence and clinical impact of human pegivirus-1 infection in HIV-1-infected individuals in Yunnan, China. *Viruses* 2017;9(2).

632. Michalak JP, Wychowski C, Choukhi A, et al. Characterization of truncated forms of hepatitis C virus glycoproteins. *J Gen Virol* 1997;78 (Pt 9):2299–2306.

633. Miller JL, de Wet BJ, Martinez-Pomares L, et al. The mannose receptor mediates dengue virus infection of macrophages. *PLoS Pathog* 2008;4(2):e17.

634. Miller S, Kastner S, Krijnse-Locker J, et al. The non-structural protein 4A of dengue virus is an integral membrane protein inducing membrane alterations in a 2K-regulated manner. *J Biol Chem* 2007;282(12):8873–8882.

635. Miller S, Sparacio S, Bartenschlager R. Subcellular localization and membrane topology of the dengue virus type 2 non-structural protein 4B. *J Biol Chem* 2006;281(13):8854–8863.

636. Miorin L, Romero-Brey I, Maiuri P, et al. Three-dimensional architecture of tick-borne encephalitis virus replication sites and trafficking of the replicated RNA. *J Virol* 2013;87(11):6469–6481.

637. Mirandola S, Bowman D, Hussain MM, et al. Hepatic steatosis in hepatitis C is a storage disease due to HCV interaction with microsomal triglyceride transfer protein (MTP). *Nutr Metab (Lond)* 2010;7:13.

638. Miyanari Y, Atsuzawa K, Usuda N, et al. The lipid droplet is an important organelle for hepatitis C virus production. *Nat Cell Biol* 2007;9(9):1089–1097.

639. Miyanari Y, Hijikata M, Yamaji M, et al. Hepatitis C virus non-structural proteins in the probable membranous compartment function in viral genome replication. *J Biol Chem* 2003;278(50):50301–50308.

640. Mizushima H, Hijikata M, Asabe S, et al. Two hepatitis C virus glycoprotein E2 products with different C termini. *J Virol* 1994;68(10):6215–6222.

641. Modis Y, Ogata S, Clements D, et al. A ligand-binding pocket in the dengue virus envelope glycoprotein. *Proc Natl Acad Sci U S A* 2003;100(12):6986–6991.

642. Modis Y, Ogata S, Clements D, et al. Structure of the dengue virus envelope protein after membrane fusion. *Nature* 2004;427(6972):313–319.

643. Moennig V, Becher P. Pestivirus control programs: how far have we come and where are we going? *Anim Health Res Rev* 2015;16(1):83–87.

644. Mohr EL, Stapleton JT. GB virus type C interactions with HIV: the role of envelope glycoproteins. *J Viral Hepat* 2009;16(11):757–768.

645. Mohr EL, Xiang J, McLinden JH, et al. GB virus type C envelope protein E2 elicits antibodies that react with a cellular antigen on HIV-1 particles and neutralize diverse HIV-1 isolates. *J Immunol* 2010;185(7):4496–4505.

646. Monazahian M, Böhme I, Bonk S, et al. Low density lipoprotein receptor as a candidate receptor for hepatitis C virus. *J Med Virol* 1999;57(3):223–229.

647. Mondelli MU, Cerino A, Lisa A, et al. Antibody responses to hepatitis C virus hypervariable region 1: evidence for cross-reactivity and immune-mediated sequence variation. *Hepatology* 1999;30(2):537–545.

648. Montserret R, Saint N, Vanbelle C, et al. NMR structure and ion channel activity of the p7 protein from hepatitis C virus. *J Biol Chem* 2010;285(41):31446–31461.

649. Moon SL, Anderson JR, Kumagai Y, et al. A noncoding RNA produced by arthropod-borne flaviviruses inhibits the cellular exoribonuclease XRN1 and alters host mRNA stability. *RNA* 2012;18(11):2029–2040.

650. Moormann RJ, Hulst MM. Hog cholera virus: identification and characterization of the viral RNA and the virus-specific RNA synthesized in infected swine kidney cells. *Virus Res* 1988;11(4):281–291.

651. Moradpour D, Brass V, Bieck E, et al. Membrane association of the RNA-dependent RNA polymerase is essential for hepatitis C virus RNA replication. *J Virol* 2004;78(23):13278–13284.

652. Moradpour D, Englert C, Wakita T, et al. Characterization of cell lines allowing tightly regulated expression of hepatitis C virus core protein. *Virology* 1996;222(1):51–63.

653. Moradpour D, Evans MJ, Gosert R, et al. Insertion of green fluorescent protein into nonstructural protein 5A allows direct visualization of functional hepatitis C virus replication complexes. *J Virol* 2004;78(14):7400–7409.

654. Morikawa K, Gouttenoire J, Hernandez C, et al. Quantitative proteomics identifies the membrane-associated peroxidase GPx8 as a cellular substrate of the hepatitis C virus NS3-4A protease. *Hepatology* 2014;59(2):423–433.

655. Morikawa K, Lange CM, Gouttenoire J, et al. Nonstructural protein 3-4A: the Swiss army knife of hepatitis C virus. *J Viral Hepat* 2011;18(5):305–315.

656. Moulin HR, Seuberlich T, Bauhofer O, et al. Nonstructural proteins NS2-3 and NS4A of classical swine fever virus: essential features for infectious particle formation. *Virology* 2007;365(2):376–389.

657. Moustafa RI, Haddad JG, Linna L, et al. Functional study of the C-terminal part of the hepatitis C virus E1 ectodomain. *J Virol* 2018;92(20).

658. Muerhoff AS, Leary TP, Simons JN, et al. Genomic organization of GB viruses A and B: two new members of the Flaviviridae associated with GB agent hepatitis. *J Virol* 1995;69(9):5621–5630.

659. Muñoz-Jordán JL, Laurent-Rolle M, Ashour J, et al. Inhibition of alpha/beta interferon signaling by the NS4B protein of flaviviruses. *J Virol* 2005;79(13):8004–8013.

660. Muñoz-Jordán JL, Sánchez-Burgos GG, Laurent-Rolle M, et al. Inhibition of interferon signaling by dengue virus. *Proc Natl Acad Sci U S A* 2003;100(24):14333–14338.

661. Murayama A, Date T, Morikawa K, et al. The NS3 helicase and NS5B-to-3'X regions are important for efficient hepatitis C virus strain JFH-1 replication in Huh7 cells. *J Virol* 2007;81(15):8030–8040.

662. Murayama A, Sugiyama N, Suzuki R, et al. Amino acid mutations in the NS4A region of hepatitis C virus contribute to viral replication and infectious virus production. *J Virol* 2017;91(4).

663. Murphy FA. Togavirus morphology and morphogenesis. In: Schlesinger RW, ed. *The Togaviruses: Biology, Structure, Replication.* New York: Academic Press; 1980:241–316.

664. Murphy DG, Willems B, Deschênes M, et al. Use of sequence analysis of the NS5B region for routine genotyping of hepatitis C virus with reference to C/E1 and 5' untranslated region sequences. *J Clin Microbiol* 2007;45(4):1102–1112.

665. Murray CL, Marcotrigiano J, Rice CM. Bovine viral diarrhea virus core is an intrinsically disordered protein that binds RNA. *J Virol* 2008;82(3):1294–1304.
666. Naik NG, Wu HN. Mutation of putative N-glycosylation sites on dengue virus NS4B decreases RNA replication. *J Virol* 2015;89(13):6746–6760.
667. Nakai K, Okamoto T, Kimura-Someya T, et al. Oligomerization of hepatitis C virus core protein is crucial for interaction with the cytoplasmic domain of E1 envelope protein. *J Virol* 2006;80(22):11265–11273.
668. Navarro-Sanchez E, Altmeyer R, Amara A, et al. Dendritic-cell-specific ICAM3-grabbing non-integrin is essential for the productive infection of human dendritic cells by mosquito-cell-derived dengue viruses. *EMBO Rep* 2003;4(7):723–728.
669. Neddermann P, Clementi A, De Francesco R. Hyperphosphorylation of the hepatitis C virus NS5A protein requires an active NS3 protease, NS4A, NS4B, and NS5A encoded on the same polyprotein. *J Virol* 1999;73(12):9984–9991.
670. Neelamkavil SF, Agrawal S, Bara T, et al. Discovery of MK-8831, A novel spiro-proline macrocycle as a pan-genotypic HCV-NS3/4a protease inhibitor. *ACS Med Chem Lett* 2016;7(1):111–116.
671. Nestorowicz A, Chambers TJ, Rice CM. Mutagenesis of the yellow fever virus NS2A/2B cleavage site: effects on proteolytic processing, viral replication and evidence for alternative processing of the NS2A protein. *Virology* 1994;199:114–123.
672. Neufeldt CJ, Cortese M, Acosta EG, et al. Rewiring cellular networks by members of the Flaviviridae family. *Nat Rev Microbiol* 2018;16(3):125–142.
673. Neufeldt CJ, Joyce MA, Van Buuren N, et al. The hepatitis C virus-induced membranous web and associated nuclear transport machinery limit access of pattern recognition receptors to viral replication sites. *PLoS Pathog* 2016;12(2):e1005428.
674. Neveu G, Barouch-Bentov R, Ziv-Av A, et al. Identification and targeting of an interaction between a tyrosine motif within hepatitis C virus core protein and AP2M1 essential for viral assembly. *PLoS Pathog* 2012;8(8):e1002845.
675. Ng WC, Soto-Acosta R, Bradrick SS, et al. The 5′ and 3′ untranslated regions of the flaviviral genome. *Viruses* 2017;9(6).
676. Nielsen SU, Bassendine MF, Burt AD, et al. Association between hepatitis C virus and very-low-density lipoprotein (VLDL)/LDL analyzed in iodixanol density gradients. *J Virol* 2006;80(5):2418–2428.
677. Niepmann M, Shalamova LA, Gerresheim GK, et al. Signals involved in regulation of hepatitis C virus RNA genome translation and replication. *Front Microbiol* 2018;9:395.
678. Nitta S, Sakamoto N, Nakagawa M, et al. Hepatitis C virus NS4B protein targets STING and abrogates RIG-I–mediated type I interferon-dependent innate immunity. *Hepatology* 2013;57(1):46–58.
679. Nomaguchi M, Teramoto T, Yu L, et al. Requirements for West Nile virus (−)- and (+)-strand subgenomic RNA synthesis in vitro by the viral RNA-dependent RNA polymerase expressed in Escherichia coli. *J Biol Chem* 2004;279(13):12141–12151.
680. Nybakken GE, Oliphant T, Johnson S, et al. Structural basis of West Nile virus neutralization by a therapeutic antibody. *Nature* 2005;437(7059):764–769.
681. O'Farrell D, Trowbridge R, Rowlands D, et al. Substrate complexes of hepatitis C virus RNA polymerase (HC-J4): structural evidence for nucleotide import and de-novo initiation. *J Mol Biol* 2003;326(4):1025–1035.
682. Oakland TE, Haselton KJ, Randall G. EWSR1 binds the hepatitis C virus *cis*-acting replication element and is required for efficient viral replication. *J Virol* 2013;87(12):6625–6634.
683. Offerdahl DK, Dorward DW, Hansen BT, et al. A three-dimensional comparison of tick-borne flavivirus infection in mammalian and tick cell lines. *PLoS One* 2012;7(10):e47912.
684. Oh JW, Ito T, Lai MM. A recombinant hepatitis C virus RNA-dependent RNA polymerase capable of copying the full-length viral RNA. *J Virol* 1999;73(9):7694–7702.
685. Oh JW, Sheu GT, Lai MM. Template requirement and initiation site selection by hepatitis C virus polymerase on a minimal viral RNA template. *J Biol Chem* 2000;275(23):17710–17717.
686. Okamoto K, Mori Y, Komoda Y, et al. Intramembrane processing by signal peptide peptidase regulates the membrane localization of hepatitis C virus core protein and viral propagation. *J Virol* 2008;82(17):8349–8361.
687. Op De Beeck A, Molenkamp R, Caron M, et al. Role of the transmembrane domains of prM and E proteins in the formation of yellow fever virus envelope. *J Virol* 2003;77(2):813–820.
688. Op De Beeck A, Montserret R, Duvet S, et al. The transmembrane domains of hepatitis C virus envelope glycoproteins E1 and E2 play a major role in heterodimerization. *J Biol Chem* 2000;275(40):31428–31437.
689. Op De Beeck A, Rouillé Y, Caron M, et al. The transmembrane domains of the prM and E proteins of yellow fever virus are endoplasmic reticulum localization signals. *J Virol* 2004;78(22):12591–12602.
690. Otto GA, Puglisi JD. The pathway of HCV IRES-mediated translation initiation. *Cell* 2004;119(3):369–380.
691. Ouyang B, Xie S, Berardi MJ, et al. Unusual architecture of the p7 channel from hepatitis C virus. *Nature* 2013;498:521–525.
692. Overby AK, Popov VL, Niedrig M, et al. Tick-borne encephalitis virus delays interferon induction and hides its double-stranded RNA in intracellular membrane vesicles. *J Virol* 2010;84(17):8470–8483.
693. Pankraz A, Preis S, Thiel HJ, et al. A single point mutation in nonstructural protein NS2 of bovine viral diarrhea virus results in temperature-sensitive attenuation of viral cytopathogenicity. *J Virol* 2009;83(23):12415–12423.
694. Pankraz A, Thiel HJ, Becher P. Essential and nonessential elements in the 3′ nontranslated region of Bovine viral diarrhea virus. *J Virol* 2005;79(14):9119–9127.
695. Park CY, Jun HJ, Wakita T, et al. Hepatitis C virus nonstructural 4B protein modulates sterol regulatory element-binding protein signaling via the AKT pathway. *J Biol Chem* 2009;284(14):9237–9246.
696. Patel J, Patel AH, McLauchlan J. The transmembrane domain of the hepatitis C virus E2 glycoprotein is required for correct folding of the E1 glycoprotein and native complex formation. *Virology* 2001;279(1):58–68.
697. Patkar CG, Jones CT, Chang YH, et al. Functional requirements of the yellow fever virus capsid protein. *J Virol* 2007;81(12):6471–6481.
698. Patkar CG, Kuhn RJ. Yellow Fever virus NS3 plays an essential role in virus assembly independent of its known enzymatic functions. *J Virol* 2008;82(7):3342–3352.
699. Paul D, Hoppe S, Saher G, et al. Morphological and biochemical characterization of the membranous hepatitis C virus replication compartment. *J Virol* 2013;87(19):10612–10627.
700. Paul D, Romero-Brey I, Gouttenoire J, et al. NS4B self-interaction through conserved C-terminal elements is required for the establishment of functional hepatitis C virus replication complexes. *J Virol* 2011;85(14):6963–6976.
701. Pavesi A. Detection of signature sequences in overlapping genes and prediction of a novel overlapping gene in hepatitis G virus. *J Mol Evol* 2000;50(3):284–295.
702. Pavlovíc D, Neville DC, Argaud O, et al. The hepatitis C virus p7 protein forms an ion channel that is inhibited by long-alkyl-chain iminosugar derivatives. *Proc Natl Acad Sci U S A* 2003;100(10):6104–6108.
703. Peleg J. Behaviour of infectious RNA from four different viruses in continuously subcultured *Aedes aegypti* mosquito embryo cells. *Nature* 1969;221(5176):193–194.
704. Pellerin C, van den Hurk J, Lecomte J, et al. Identification of a new group of bovine viral diarrhea virus strains associated with severe outbreaks and high mortalities. *Virology* 1994;203(2):260–268.
705. Penin F, Brass V, Appel N, et al. Structure and function of the membrane anchor domain of hepatitis C virus nonstructural protein 5A. *J Biol Chem* 2004;279(39):40835–40843.
706. Perelson AS, Herrmann E, Micol F, et al. New kinetic models for the hepatitis C virus. *Hepatology* 2005;42(4):749–754.
707. Perera R, Kuhn RJ. Structural proteomics of dengue virus. *Curr Opin Microbiol* 2008;11(4):369–377.
708. Perera R, Riley C, Isaac G, et al. Dengue virus infection perturbs lipid homeostasis in infected mosquito cells. *PLoS Pathog* 2012;8(3):e1002584.
709. Perlemuter G, Sabile A, Letteron P, et al. Hepatitis C virus core protein inhibits microsomal triglyceride transfer protein activity and very low density lipoprotein secretion: a model of viral-related steatosis. *FASEB J* 2002;16(2):185–194.
710. Pestova TV, Hellen CU. Internal initiation of translation of bovine viral diarrhea virus RNA. *Virology* 1999;258(2):249–256.
711. Pestova TV, Shatsky IN, Fletcher SP, et al. A prokaryotic-like mode of cytoplasmic eukaryotic ribosome binding to the initiation codon during internal translation initiation of hepatitis C and classical swine fever virus RNAs. *Genes Dev* 1998;12(1):67–83.
712. Pethe MA, Rubenstein AB, Khare SD. Data-driven supervised learning of a viral protease specificity landscape from deep sequencing and molecular simulations. *Proc Natl Acad Sci U S A* 2019;116(1):168–176.
713. Petracca R, Falugi F, Galli G, et al. Structure-function analysis of hepatitis C virus envelope-CD81 binding. *J Virol* 2000;74(10):4824–4830.
714. Pfannkuche A, Buther K, Karthe J, et al. c-Src is required for complex formation between the hepatitis C virus-encoded proteins NS5A and NS5B: a prerequisite for replication. *Hepatology* 2011;53(4):1127–1136.
715. Phan T, Beran RK, Peters C, et al. Hepatitis C virus NS2 protein contributes to virus particle assembly via opposing epistatic interactions with the E1-E2 glycoprotein and NS3-NS4A enzyme complexes. *J Virol* 2009;83(17):8379–8395.
716. Phan T, Kohlway A, Dimberu P, et al. The acidic domain of hepatitis C virus NS4A contributes to RNA replication and virus particle assembly. *J Virol* 2011;85(3):1193–1204.
717. Piccininni S, Varaklioti A, Nardelli M, et al. Modulation of the hepatitis C virus RNA-dependent RNA polymerase activity by the non-structural (NS) 3 helicase and the NS4B membrane protein. *J Biol Chem* 2002;277(47):45670–45679.
718. Pierson TC, Kielian M. Flaviviruses: braking the entering. *Curr Opin Virol* 2013;3(1):3–12.
719. Pietschmann T, Kaul A, Koutsoudakis G, et al. Construction and characterization of infectious intragenotypic and intergenotypic hepatitis C virus chimeras. *Proc Natl Acad Sci U S A* 2006;103(19):7408–7413.
720. Pietschmann T, Lohmann V, Kaul A, et al. Persistent and transient replication of full-length hepatitis C virus genomes in cell culture. *J Virol* 2002;76(8):4008–4021.
721. Pietschmann T, Zayas M, Meuleman P, et al. Production of infectious genotype 1b virus particles in cell culture and impairment by replication enhancing mutations. *PLoS Pathog* 2009;5(6):e1000475.
722. Pijlman GP, Funk A, Kondratieva N, et al. A highly structured, nuclease-resistant, noncoding RNA produced by flaviviruses is required for pathogenicity. *Cell Host Microbe* 2008;4(6):579–591.
723. Pileri P, Uematsu Y, Campagnoli S, et al. Binding of hepatitis C virus to CD81. *Science* 1998;282(5390):938–941.
724. Pirakitikulr N, Kohlway A, Lindenbach BD, et al. The coding region of the HCV genome contains a network of regulatory RNA structures. *Mol Cell* 2016;62(1):111–120.
725. Piver E, Boyer A, Gaillard J, et al. Ultrastructural organisation of HCV from the bloodstream of infected patients revealed by electron microscopy after specific immunocapture. *Gut* 2017;66(8):1487–1495.
726. Płaszczyca A, Scaturro P, Neufeldt CJ, et al. A novel interaction between dengue virus nonstructural protein 1 and the NS4A-2K-4B precursor is required for viral RNA replication but not for formation of the membranous replication organelle. *PLoS Pathog* 2019;15:e1007736.
727. Ploss A, Evans MJ, Gaysinskaya VA, et al. Human occludin is a hepatitis C virus entry factor required for infection of mouse cells. *Nature* 2009;457(7231):882–886.
728. Podevin P, Carpentier A, Pene V, et al. Production of infectious hepatitis C virus in primary cultures of human adult hepatocytes. *Gastroenterology* 2010;139(4):1355–1364.
729. Polgreen PM, Xiang J, Chang Q, et al. GB virus type C/hepatitis G virus: a non-pathogenic flavivirus associated with prolonged survival in HIV-infected individuals. *Microbes Infect* 2003;5(13):1255–1261.
730. Poole TL, Wang C, Popp RA, et al. Pestivirus translation initiation occurs by internal ribosome entry. *Virology* 1995;206(1):750–754.
731. Popescu CI, Callens N, Trinel D, et al. NS2 protein of hepatitis C virus interacts with structural and non-structural proteins towards virus assembly. *PLoS Pathog* 2011;7(2):e1001278.
732. Premkumar A, Wilson L, Ewart GD, et al. Cation-selective ion channels formed by p7 of hepatitis C virus are blocked by hexamethylene amiloride. *FEBS Lett* 2004;557(1–3):99–103.

733. Preugschat F, Strauss JH. Processing of nonstructural proteins NS4A and NS4B of dengue 2 virus in vitro and in vivo. *Virology* 1991;185:689–697.

734. Prince AM, Brotman B, Grady GF, et al. Long-incubation post-transfusion hepatitis without serological evidence of exposure to hepatitis B virus. *Lancet* 1974;2:241–246.

735. Prince AM, Huima-Byron T, Parker TS, et al. Visualization of hepatitis C virions and putative defective interfering particles isolated from low-density lipoproteins. *J Viral Hepat* 1996;3(1):11–17.

736. Puerta-Guardo H, Glasner DR, Espinosa DA, et al. Flavivirus NS1 triggers tissue-specific vascular endothelial dysfunction reflecting disease tropism. *Cell Rep* 2019;26(6):1598.e1598–1613.e1598.

737. Pugachev KV, Nomokonova NY, Morozova OV, et al. A short form of the tick-borne encephalitis virus NS3 protein. *FEBS Lett* 1992;297(1–2):67–69.

738. Puschnik AS, Marceau CD, Ooi YS, et al. A small-molecule oligosaccharyltransferase inhibitor with pan-flaviviral activity. *Cell Rep* 2017;21(11):3032–3039.

739. Pyle AM. Translocation and unwinding mechanisms of RNA and DNA helicases. *Annu Rev Biophys* 2008;37:317–336.

740. Python S, Gerber M, Suter R, et al. Efficient sensing of infected cells in absence of virus particles by plasmacytoid dendritic cells is blocked by the viral ribonuclease E(rns.). *PLoS Pathog* 2013;9(6):e1003412.

741. Qi H, Chu V, Wu NC, et al. Systematic identification of anti-interferon function on hepatitis C virus genome reveals p7 as an immune evasion protein. *Proc Natl Acad Sci U S A* 2017;114(8):2018–2023.

742. Qin W, Luo H, Nomura T, et al. Oligomeric interaction of hepatitis C virus NS5B is critical for catalytic activity of RNA-dependent RNA polymerase. *J Biol Chem* 2002;277(3):2132–2137.

743. Qu L, McMullan LK, Rice CM. Isolation and characterization of noncytopathic pestivirus mutants reveals a role for nonstructural protein NS4B in viral cytopathogenicity. *J Virol* 2001;75:10651–10662.

744. Quade N, Boehringer D, Leibundgut M, et al. Cryo-EM structure of Hepatitis C virus IRES bound to the human ribosome at 3.9-A resolution. *Nat Commun* 2015;6:7646.

745. Quan PL, Firth C, Conte JM, et al. Bats are a major natural reservoir for hepaciviruses and pegiviruses. *Proc Natl Acad Sci U S A* 2013;110(20):8194–8199.

746. Quinkert D, Bartenschlager R, Lohmann V. Quantitative analysis of the hepatitis C virus replication complex. *J Virol* 2005;79(21):13594–13605.

747. Ramirez S, Bukh J. Current status and future development of infectious cell-culture models for the major genotypes of hepatitis C virus: essential tools in testing of antivirals and emerging vaccine strategies. *Antiviral Res* 2018;158:264–287.

748. Ranjith-Kumar CT, Gajewski J, Gutshall L, et al. Terminal nucleotidyl transferase activity of recombinant Flaviviridae RNA-dependent RNA polymerases: implication for viral RNA synthesis. *J Virol* 2001;75(18):8615–8623.

749. Ranjith-Kumar CT, Gutshall L, Kim MJ, et al. Requirements for de novo initiation of RNA synthesis by recombinant flaviviral RNA-dependent RNA polymerases. *J Virol* 2002;76(24):12526–12536.

750. Ranjith-Kumar CT, Gutshall L, Sarisky RT, et al. Multiple interactions within the hepatitis C virus RNA polymerase repress primer-dependent RNA synthesis. *J Mol Biol* 2003;330(4):675–685.

751. Ranjith-Kumar CT, Kao CC. Biochemical activities of the HCV NS5B RNA-dependent RNA polymerase. In: Tan SL, ed. *Hepatitis C Viruses: Genomes and Molecular Biology*. Norfolk, UK: Horizon Bioscience; 2006.

752. Ranjith-Kumar CT, Kim YC, Gutshall L, et al. Mechanism of de novo initiation by the hepatitis C virus RNA-dependent RNA polymerase: role of divalent metals. *J Virol* 2002;76(24):12513–12525.

753. Ranjith-Kumar CT, Sarisky RT, Gutshall L, et al. De novo initiation pocket mutations have multiple effects on hepatitis C virus RNA-dependent RNA polymerase activities. *J Virol* 2004;78(22):12207–12217.

754. Ray D, Shah A, Tilgner M, et al. West Nile virus 5′-cap structure is formed by sequential guanine N-7 and ribose 2′-O methylations by nonstructural protein 5. *J Virol* 2006;80(17):8362–8370.

755. Reed KE, Gorbalenya AE, Rice CM. The NS5A/NS5 proteins of viruses from three genera of the family *Flaviviridae* are phosphorylated by associated serine/threonine kinases. *J Virol* 1998;72:6199–6206.

756. Reed KE, Grakoui A, Rice CM. Hepatitis C virus-encoded NS2-3 protease: cleavage-site mutagenesis and requirements for bimolecular cleavage. *J Virol* 1995;69(7):4127–4136.

757. Reid DW, Campos RK, Child JR, et al. Dengue virus selectively annexes endoplasmic reticulum-associated translation machinery as a strategy for co-opting host cell protein synthesis. *J Virol* 2018;92(7).

758. Reiss S, Harak C, Romero-Brey I, et al. The lipid kinase phosphatidylinositol–4 kinase III alpha regulates the phosphorylation status of hepatitis C virus NS5A. *PLoS Pathog* 2013;9(5):e1003359.

759. Reiss S, Rebhan I, Backes P, et al. Recruitment and activation of a lipid kinase by hepatitis C virus NS5A is essential for integrity of the membranous replication compartment. *Cell Host Microbe* 2011;9(1):32–45.

760. Rey FA, Heinz FX, Mandl C, et al. The envelope glycoprotein from tick-borne encephalitis virus at 2 A resolution. *Nature* 1995;375(6529):291–298.

761. Rey FA, Stiasny K, Heinz FX. Flavivirus structural heterogeneity: implications for cell entry. *Curr Opin Virol* 2017;24:132–139.

762. Rey FA, Stiasny K, Vaney MC, et al. The bright and the dark side of human antibody responses to flaviviruses: lessons for vaccine design. *EMBO Rep* 2018;19(2):206–224.

763. Rho J, Choi S, Seong YR, et al. The arginine-1493 residue in QRRGRTGR1493G motif IV of the hepatitis C virus NS3 helicase domain is essential for NS3 protein methylation by the protein arginine methyltransferase 1. *J Virol* 2001;75(17):8031–8044.

764. Rice CM, Grakoui A, Galler R, et al. Transcription of infectious yellow fever virus RNA from full-length cDNA templates produced by in vitro ligation. *New Biol* 1989;1:285–296.

765. Rice CM, Lenches EM, Eddy SR, et al. Nucleotide sequence of yellow fever virus: implications for flavivirus gene expression and evolution. *Science* 1985;229:726–733.

766. Riedel C, Lamp B, Hagen B, et al. The core protein of a pestivirus protects the incoming virus against IFN-induced effectors. *Sci Rep* 2017;7:44459.

767. Riedel C, Lamp B, Heimann M, et al. Characterization of essential domains and plasticity of the classical swine fever virus core protein. *J Virol* 2010;84(21):11523–11531.

768. Riedel C, Lamp B, Heimann M, et al. The core protein of classical Swine Fever virus is dispensable for virus propagation in vitro. *PLoS Pathog* 2012;8(3):e1002598.

769. Rijnbrand R, Thiviyanathan V, Kaluarachchi K, et al. Mutational and structural analysis of stem-loop IIIC of the hepatitis C virus and GB virus B internal ribosome entry sites. *J Mol Biol* 2004;343(4):805–817.

770. Rijnbrand R, van der Straaten T, van Rijn PA, et al. Internal entry of ribosomes is directed by the 5′ noncoding region of classical swine fever virus and is dependent on the presence of an RNA pseudoknot upstream of the initiation codon. *J Virol* 1997;71(1):451–457.

771. Rijnbrand R, Yang Y, Beales L, et al. A chimeric GB virus B with 5′ nontranslated RNA sequence from hepatitis C virus causes hepatitis in tamarins. *Hepatology* 2005;41(5):986–994.

772. Rinck G, Birghan C, Harada T, et al. A cellular J-domain protein modulates polyprotein processing and cytopathogenicity of a pestivirus. *J Virol* 2001;75(19):9470–9482.

773. Robinson ML, Durbin AP. Dengue vaccines: implications for dengue control. *Curr Opin Infect Dis* 2017;30(5):449–454.

774. Roder AE, Vazquez C, Horner SM. The acidic domain of the hepatitis C virus NS4A protein is required for viral assembly and envelopment through interactions with the viral E1 glycoprotein. *PLoS Pathog* 2019;15(2):e1007163.

775. Rodriguez-Barraquer I, Costa F, Nascimento EJM, et al. Impact of preexisting dengue immunity on Zika virus emergence in a dengue endemic region. *Science* 2019;363(6427):607–610.

776. Roingeard P, Hourioux C. Hepatitis C virus core protein, lipid droplets and steatosis. *J Viral Hepat* 2008;15(3):157–164.

777. Romero-Brey I, Berger C, Kallis S, et al. NS5A domain 1 and polyprotein cleavage kinetics are critical for induction of double-membrane vesicles associated with hepatitis C virus replication. *MBio* 2015;6(4):e00759.

778. Romero-Brey I, Merz A, Chiramel A, et al. Three-dimensional architecture and biogenesis of membrane structures associated with hepatitis C virus replication. *PLoS Pathog* 2012;8(12):e1003056.

779. Romero-Lopez C, Berzal-Herranz A. A long-range RNA-RNA interaction between the 5′ and 3′ ends of the HCV genome. *RNA* 2009;15(9):1740–1752.

780. Romero-Lopez C, Rios-Marco P, Berzal-Herranz B, et al. The HCV genome domains 5BSL3.1 and 5BSL3.3 act as managers of translation. *Sci Rep* 2018;8(1):16101.

781. Ronecker S, Zimmer G, Herrler G, et al. Formation of bovine viral diarrhea virus E1-E2 heterodimers is essential for virus entry and depends on charged residues in the transmembrane domains. *J Gen Virol* 2008;89(Pt 9):2114–2121.

782. Roosendaal J, Westaway EG, Khromykh A, et al. Regulated cleavages at the West Nile virus NS4A-2K-NS4B junctions play a major role in rearranging cytoplasmic membranes and Golgi trafficking of the NS4A protein. *J Virol* 2006;80(9):4623–4632.

783. Ross-Thriepland D, Harris M. Insights into the complexity and functionality of hepatitis C virus NS5A phosphorylation. *J Virol* 2014;88(3):1421–1432.

784. Ross-Thriepland D, Harris M. Hepatitis C virus NS5A: enigmatic but still promiscuous 10 years on! *J Gen Virol* 2015;96(Pt 4):727–738.

785. Ross-Thriepland D, Mankouri J, Harris M. Serine phosphorylation of the hepatitis C virus NS5A protein controls the establishment of replication complexes. *J Virol* 2015;89(6):3123–3135.

786. Roth H, Magg V, Uch F, et al. Flavivirus infection uncouples translation suppression from cellular stress responses. *MBio* 2017;8(1).

787. Rouillé Y, Helle F, Delgrange D, et al. Subcellular localization of hepatitis C virus structural proteins in a cell culture system that efficiently replicates the virus. *J Virol* 2006;80(6):2832–2841.

788. Rouvinski A, Guardado-Calvo P, Barba-Spaeth G, et al. Recognition determinants of broadly neutralizing human antibodies against dengue viruses. *Nature* 2015;520(7545):109–113.

789. Ruggli N, Bird BH, Liu L, et al. N(pro) of classical swine fever virus is an antagonist of double-stranded RNA-mediated apoptosis and IFN-alpha/beta induction. *Virology* 2005;340(2):265–276.

790. Ruggli N, Rice CM. Functional cDNA clones of the Flaviviridae: strategies and applications. *Adv Virus Res* 1999;53:183–207.

791. Ruggli N, Tratschin JD, Schweizer M, et al. Classical swine fever virus interferes with cellular antiviral defense: evidence for a novel function of N(pro). *J Virol* 2003;77(13):7645–7654.

792. Rümenapf T, Unger G, Strauss JH, et al. Processing of the envelope glycoproteins of pestiviruses. *J Virol* 1993;67(6):3288–3294.

793. Russell PK, Brandt WE, Dalrymple JM. Chemical and antigenic structure of flaviviruses. In: Schlesinger RW, ed. *The Togaviruses: Biology, Structure, Replication*. New York: Academic Press; 1980:503–529.

794. Rydze RT, Xiang J, McLinden JH, et al. GB virus type C infection polarizes T-cell cytokine gene expression toward a Th1 cytokine profile via NS5A protein expression. *J Infect Dis* 2012;206(1):69–72.

795. Saeed M, Andreo U, Chung HY, et al. SEC14L2 enables pan-genotype HCV replication in cell culture. *Nature* 2015;524:471–475.

796. Sainz B, Jr., Barretto N, Martin DN, et al. Identification of the Niemann-Pick C1-like 1 cholesterol absorption receptor as a new hepatitis C virus entry factor. *Nat Med* 2012;18(2):281–285.

797. Sakai A, Claire MS, Faulk K, et al. The p7 polypeptide of hepatitis C virus is critical for infectivity and contains functionally important genotype-specific sequences. *Proc Natl Acad Sci U S A* 2003;100(20):11646–11651.

798. Salloum S, Wang H, Ferguson C, et al. Rab18 binds to hepatitis C virus NS5A and promotes interaction between sites of viral replication and lipid droplets. *PLoS Pathog* 2013;9(8):e1003513.

799. Samsa MM, Mondotte JA, Iglesias NG, et al. Dengue virus capsid protein usurps lipid droplets for viral particle formation. *PLoS Pathog* 2009;5(10):e1000632.

800. Samuel GH, Wiley MR, Badawi A, et al. Yellow fever virus capsid protein is a potent suppressor of RNA silencing that binds double-stranded RNA. *Proc Natl Acad Sci U S A* 2016;113(48):13863–13868.

801. Sanchez-San Martin C, Liu CY, Kielian M. Dealing with low pH: entry and exit of alpha-viruses and flaviviruses. *Trends Microbiol* 2009;17(11):514–521.

802. Sapay N, Montserret R, Chipot C, et al. NMR structure and molecular dynamics of the in-plane membrane anchor of nonstructural protein 5A from bovine viral diarrhea virus. *Biochemistry* 2006;45(7):2221–2233.

803. Sarnow P, Sagan SM. Unraveling the mysterious interactions between hepatitis C virus RNA and liver-specific MicroRNA-122. *Annu Rev Virol* 2016;3:309–332.

804. Sato K, Tanaka T, Okamoto H, et al. Association of circulating hepatitis G virus with lipoproteins for a lack of binding with antibodies. *Biochem Biophys Res Commun* 1996;229(3):719–725.

805. Savidis G, McDougall WM, Meraner P, et al. Identification of Zika virus and dengue virus dependency factors using functional genomics. *Cell Rep* 2016;16(1):232–246.

806. Sbardellati A, Scarselli E, Tomei L, et al. Identification of a novel sequence at the 3′ end of the GB virus B genome. *J Virol* 1999;73(12):10546–10550.

807. Sbardellati A, Scarselli E, Verschoor E, et al. Generation of infectious and transmissible virions from a GB virus B full-length consensus clone in tamarins. *J Gen Virol* 2001; 82(Pt 10):2437–2448.

808. Scarselli E, Ansuini H, Cerino R, et al. The human scavenger receptor class B type I is a novel candidate receptor for the hepatitis C virus. *EMBO J* 2002;21(19):5017–5025.

809. Scaturro P, Cortese M, Chatel-Chaix L, et al. Dengue virus non-structural protein 1 modulates infectious particle production via interaction with the structural proteins. *PLoS Pathog* 2015;11(11):e1005277.

810. Schalich J, Allison SL, Stiasny K, et al. Recombinant subviral particles from tick-borne encephalitis virus are fusogenic and provide a model system for studying flavivirus envelope glycoprotein functions. *J Virol* 1996;70(7):4549–4557.

811. Scheel TKH, Kapoor A, Nishiuchi E, et al. Characterization of nonprimate hepacivirus and construction of a functional molecular clone. *Proc Natl Acad Sci U S A* 2015; 112(7):2192–2197.

812. Scheel TK, Luna JM, Liniger M, et al. A Broad RNA Virus Survey Reveals Both miRNA Dependence and Functional Sequestration. *Cell Host Microbe* 2016;19(3):409–423.

813. Scheel TK, Prentoe J, Carlsen TH, et al. Analysis of functional differences between hepatitis C virus NS5A of genotypes 1-7 in infectious cell culture systems. *PLoS Pathog* 2012;8(5):e1002696.

814. Schenk C, Meyrath M, Warnken U, et al. Characterization of a threonine-rich cluster in hepatitis C virus nonstructural protein 5A and its contribution to hyperphosphorylation. *J Virol* 2018;92(24).

815. Schlick P, Taucher C, Schittl B, et al. Helices alpha2 and alpha3 of West Nile virus capsid protein are dispensable for assembly of infectious virions. *J Virol* 2009;83(11):5581–5591.

816. Schmeiser S, Mast J, Thiel HJ, et al. Morphogenesis of pestiviruses: new insights from ultrastructural studies of strain Giraffe-1. *J Virol* 2014;88(5):2717–2724.

817. Schmidt-Mende J, Bieck E, Hugle T, et al. Determinants for membrane association of the hepatitis C virus RNA-dependent RNA polymerase. *J Biol Chem* 2001;276(47):44052–44063.

818. Schmitt M, Scrima N, Radujkovic D, et al. A comprehensive structure-function comparison of hepatitis C virus strain JFH1 and J6 polymerases reveals a key residue stimulating replication in cell culture across genotypes. *J Virol* 2011;85(6):2565–2581.

819. Schneider R, Unger G, Stark R, et al. Identification of a structural glycoprotein of an RNA virus as a ribonuclease. *Science* 1993;261(5125):1169–1171.

820. Schregel V, Jacobi S, Penin F, et al. Hepatitis C virus NS2 is a protease stimulated by cofactor domains in NS3. *Proc Natl Acad Sci U S A* 2009;106(13):5342–5347.

821. Schuessler A, Funk A, Lazear HM, et al. West Nile virus noncoding subgenomic RNA contributes to viral evasion of the type I interferon-mediated antiviral response. *J Virol* 2012;86(10):5708–5718.

822. Schwartz N, Pellach M, Glick Y, et al. Neuregulin 1 discovered as a cleavage target for the HCV NS3/4A protease by a microfluidic membrane protein array. *N Biotechnol* 2018;45:113–122.

823. Scull MA, Schneider WM, Flatley BR, et al. The N-terminal helical region of the hepatitis C virus p7 ion channel protein is critical for infectious virus production. *PLoS Pathog* 2015;11(11).

824. Sedano CD, Sarnow P. Hepatitis C virus subverts liver-specific miR-122 to protect the viral genome from exoribonuclease Xrn2. *Cell Host Microbe* 2014;16(2):257–264.

825. Sekhar V, Pollicino T, Diaz G, et al. Infection with hepatitis C virus depends on TACSTD2, a regulator of claudin-1 and occludin highly downregulated in hepatocellular carcinoma. *PLoS Pathog* 2018;14(3):e1006916.

826. Selby MJ, Glazer E, Masiarz F, et al. Complex processing and protein:protein interactions in the E2:NS2 region of HCV. *Virology* 1994;204(1):114–122.

827. Setoh YX, Periasamy P, Peng NYG, et al. Helicase domain of West Nile virus NS3 protein plays a role in inhibition of type I interferon signalling. *Viruses* 2017;9(11).

828. Sevvana M, Long F, Miller AS, et al. Refinement and analysis of the mature Zika virus cryo-EM structure at 3.1 A resolution. *Structure* 2018;26(9):1169.e1163–1177.e1163.

829. Shanmugam S, Nichols AK, Saravanabalaji D, et al. HCV NS5A dimer interface residues regulate HCV replication by controlling its self-interaction, hyperphosphorylation, subcellular localization and interaction with cyclophilin A. *PLoS Pathog* 2018;14(7):e1007177.

830. Sharma NR, Mateu G, Dreux M, et al. Hepatitis C virus is primed by CD81 protein for low pH-dependent fusion. *J Biol Chem* 2011;286(35):30361–30376.

831. Shavinskaya A, Boulant S, Penin F, et al. The lipid droplet binding domain of hepatitis C virus core protein is a major determinant for efficient virus assembly. *J Biol Chem* 2007;282(51):37158–37169.

832. Shetty S, Kim S, Shimakami T, et al. Hepatitis C virus genomic RNA dimerization is mediated via a kissing complex intermediate. *RNA* 2010;16(5):913–925.

833. Shi G, Ando T, Suzuki R, et al. Involvement of the 3′ untranslated region in encapsidation of the hepatitis C virus. *PLoS Pathog* 2016;12(2):e1005441.

834. Shi Q, Jiang J, Luo G. Syndecan-1 serves as the major receptor for attachment of hepatitis C virus to the surfaces of hepatocytes. *J Virol* 2013;87(12):6866–6875.

835. Shi ST, Lee KJ, Aizaki H, et al. Hepatitis C virus RNA replication occurs on a detergent-resistant membrane that cofractionates with caveolin-2. *J Virol* 2003;77(7):4160–4168.

836. Shi M, Lin XD, Vasilakis N, et al. Divergent viruses discovered in arthropods and vertebrates revise the evolutionary history of the *flaviviridae* and related viruses. *J Virol* 2016;90(2):659–669.

837. Shi BJ, Liu CC, Zhou J, et al. Entry of classical swine fever virus into PK-15 cells via a pH-, dynamin-, and cholesterol-dependent, clathrin-mediated endocytic pathway that requires Rab5 and Rab7. *J Virol* 2016;90(20):9194–9208.

838. Shih C-M, Chen C-M, Chen S-Y, et al. Modulation of the *trans*-suppression activity of hepatitis C virus core protein by phosphorylation. *J Virol* 1995;69:1160–1171.

839. Shim JH, Larson G, Wu JZ, et al. Selection of 3′-template bases and initiating nucleotides by hepatitis C virus NS5B RNA-dependent RNA polymerase. *J Virol* 2002;76(14):7030–7039.

840. Shimakami T, Hijikata M, Luo H, et al. Effect of interaction between hepatitis C virus NS5A and NS5B on hepatitis C virus RNA replication with the hepatitis C virus replicon. *J Virol* 2004;78(6):2738–2748.

841. Shimakami T, Yamane D, Jangra RK, et al. Stabilization of hepatitis C virus RNA by an Ago2-miR-122 complex. *Proc Natl Acad Sci U S A* 2012;109(3):941–946.

842. Shimoike T, Mimori S, Tani H, et al. Interaction of hepatitis C virus core protein with viral sense RNA and suppression of its translation. *J Virol* 1999;73(12):9718–9725.

843. Shirota Y, Luo H, Qin W, et al. Hepatitis C virus (HCV) NS5A binds RNA-dependent RNA polymerase (RdRP) NS5B and modulates RNA-dependent RNA polymerase activity. *J Biol Chem* 2002;277(13):11149–11155.

844. Shiryaev SA, Chernov AV, Aleshin AE, et al. NS4A regulates the ATPase activity of the NS3 helicase: a novel cofactor role of the non-structural protein NS4A from West Nile virus. *J Gen Virol* 2009;90(Pt 9):2081–2085.

845. Shiryaev SA, Thomsen ER, Cieplak P, et al. New details of HCV NS3/4A proteinase functionality revealed by a high-throughput cleavage assay. *PLoS One* 2012;7(4):e35759.

846. Shwetha S, Kumar A, Mullick R, et al. HuR displaces polypyrimidine tract binding protein to facilitate La binding to the 3′ untranslated region and enhances hepatitis C virus replication. *J Virol* 2015;89(22):11356–11371.

847. Simister P, Schmitt M, Geitmann M, et al. Structural and functional analysis of hepatitis C virus strain JFH1 polymerase. *J Virol* 2009;83(22):11926–11939.

848. Simmonds P, Becher P, Bukh J, et al. ICTV virus taxonomy profile: flaviviridae. *J Gen Virol* 2017;98(1):2–3.

849. Simons JN, Desai SM, Schultz DE, et al. Translation initiation in GB viruses A and C: evidence for internal ribosome entry and implications for genome organization. *J Virol* 1996;70(9):6126–6135.

850. Simons JN, Leary TP, Dawson GJ, et al. Isolation of novel virus-like sequences associated with human hepatitis. *Nat Med* 1995;1(6):564–569.

851. Simons JN, Pilot-Matias TJ, Leary TP, et al. Identification of two flavivirus-like genomes in the GB hepatitis agent. *Proc Natl Acad Sci U S A* 1995;92(8):3401–3405.

852. Sir D, Chen WL, Choi J, et al. Induction of incomplete autophagic response by hepatitis C virus via the unfolded protein response. *Hepatology* 2008;48(4):1054–1061.

853. Sir D, Kuo CF, Tian Y, et al. Replication of hepatitis C virus RNA on autophagosomal membranes. *J Biol Chem* 2012;287(22):18036–18043.

854. Siridechadilok B, Fraser CS, Hall RJ, et al. Structural roles for human translation factor eIF3 in initiation of protein synthesis. *Science* 2005;310(5753):1513–1515.

855. Sizova DV, Kolupaeva VG, Pestova TV, et al. Specific interaction of eukaryotic translation initiation factor 3 with the 5′ nontranslated regions of hepatitis C virus and classical swine fever virus RNAs. *J Virol* 1998;72(6):4775–4782.

856. Slonchak A, Khromykh AA. Subgenomic flaviviral RNAs: What do we know after the first decade of research. *Antiviral Res* 2018;159:13–25.

857. Smith DB, Becher P, Bukh J, et al. Proposed update to the taxonomy of the genera Hepacivirus and Pegivirus within the Flaviviridae family. *J Gen Virol* 2016;97:2894–2907.

858. Smith TJ, Brandt WE, Swanson JL, et al. Physical and biological properties of dengue-2 virus and associated antigens. *J Virol* 1970;5(4):524–532.

859. Smith DB, Bukh J, Kuiken C, et al. Expanded classification of hepatitis C virus into 7 genotypes and 67 subtypes: updated criteria and genotype assignment web resource. *Hepatology* 2014;59(1):318–327.

860. Smith DB, Meyers G, Bukh J, et al. Proposed revision to the taxonomy of the genus Pestivirus, family Flaviviridae. *J Gen Virol* 2017;98(8):2106–2112.

861. Song Y, Mugavero J, Stauft CB, et al. Dengue and Zika virus 5′-UTRs harbor IRES functions. *MBio* 2019;10(2).

862. Soto-Acosta R, Bautista-Carbajal P, Cervantes-Salazar M, et al. DENV up-regulates the HMG-CoA reductase activity through the impairment of AMPK phosphorylation: a potential antiviral target. *PLoS Pathog* 2017;13(4):e1006257.

863. Spahn CM, Kieft JS, Grassucci RA, et al. Hepatitis C virus IRES RNA-induced changes in the conformation of the 40s ribosomal subunit. *Science* 2001;291(5510):1959–1962.

864. Stadler K, Allison SL, Schalich J, et al. Proteolytic activation of tick-borne encephalitis virus by furin. *J Virol* 1997;71:8475–8481.

865. Stapleford KA, Lindenbach BD. Hepatitis C virus NS2 coordinates virus particle assembly through physical interactions with the E1-E2 glycoprotein and NS3-NS4A enzyme complexes. *J Virol* 2011;85(4):1706–1717.

866. Stapleton JT, Foung S, Muerhoff AS, et al. The GB viruses: a review and proposed classification of GBV-A, GBV-C (HGV), and GBV-D in genus Pegivirus within the family Flaviviridae. *J Gen Virol* 2011;92(Pt 2):233–246.

867. Stark R, Meyers G, Rümenapf T, et al. Processing of pestivirus polyprotein: cleavage site between autoprotease and nucleocapsid protein of classical swine fever virus. *J Virol* 1993;67(12):7088–7095.

868. Steinkühler C, Biasiol G, Brunetti M, et al. Product inhibition of the hepatitis C virus NS3 protease. *Biochemistry* 1998;37(25):8899–8905.

869. Steinmann E, Penin F, Kallis S, et al. Hepatitis C Virus p7 protein is crucial for assembly and release of infectious virions. *PLoS Pathog* 2007;3(7):e103.

870. Stern O, Hung YF, Valdau O, et al. An N-terminal amphipathic helix in dengue virus nonstructural protein 4A mediates oligomerization and is essential for replication. *J Virol* 2013;87(7):4080–4085.

871. Stettler K, Beltramello M, Espinosa DA, et al. Specificity, cross-reactivity, and function of antibodies elicited by Zika virus infection. *Science* 2016;353(6301):823–826.

872. Stiasny K, Allison SL, Marchler-Bauer A, et al. Structural requirements for low-pH-induced rearrangements in the envelope glycoprotein of tick-borne encephalitis virus. *J Virol* 1996;70(11):8142–8147.

873. Stiasny K, Heinz FX. Effect of membrane curvature-modifying lipids on membrane fusion by tick-borne encephalitis virus. *J Virol* 2004;78(16):8536–8542.

874. Stiasny K, Koessl C, Heinz FX. Involvement of lipids in different steps of the flavivirus fusion mechanism. *J Virol* 2003;77(14):7856–7862.

875. Stocks CE, Lobigs M. Signal peptidase cleavage at the flavivirus C-prM junction: dependence on the viral NS2B-3 protease for efficient processing requires determinants in C, the signal peptide, and prM. *J Virol* 1998;72(3):2141–2149.

876. Su WC, Chao TC, Huang YL, et al. Rab5 and class III phosphoinositide 3-kinase Vps34 are involved in hepatitis C virus NS4B-induced autophagy. *J Virol* 2011;85(20):10561–10571.

877. Sun XL, Johnson RB, Hockman MA, et al. De novo RNA synthesis catalyzed by HCV RNA-dependent RNA polymerase. *Biochem Biophys Res Commun* 2000;268(3):798–803.

878. Sutton G, Grimes JM, Stuart DI, et al. Bluetongue virus VP4 is an RNA-capping assembly line. *Nat Struct Mol Biol* 2007;14(5):449–451.

879. Suzuki R, Matsuda M, Watashi K, et al. Signal peptidase complex subunit 1 participates in the assembly of hepatitis C virus through an interaction with E2 and NS2. *PLoS Pathog* 2013;9(8):e1003589.

880. Syed GH, Khan M, Yang S, et al. Hepatitis C virus lipoviroparticles assemble in the endoplasmic reticulum (ER) and bud off from the ER to the golgi compartment in COPII vesicles. *J Virol* 2017;91(15).

881. Tabata K, Arimoto M, Arakawa M, et al. Unique requirement for ESCRT factors in flavivirus particle formation on the endoplasmic reticulum. *Cell Rep* 2016;16(9):2339–2347.

882. Tadano M, Makino Y, Fukunaga T, et al. Detection of dengue 4 virus core protein in the nucleus. I. A monoclonal antibody to dengue 4 virus reacts with the antigen in the nucleus and cytoplasm. *J Gen Virol* 1989;70 (Pt 6):1409–1415.

883. Tai AW, Benita Y, Peng LF, et al. A functional genomic screen identifies cellular cofactors of hepatitis C virus replication. *Cell Host Microbe* 2009;5(3):298–307.

884. Takikawa S, Engle RE, Emerson SU, et al. Functional analyses of GB virus B p13 protein: development of a recombinant GB virus B hepatitis virus with a p7 protein. *Proc Natl Acad Sci U S A* 2006;103(9):3345–3350.

885. Tan BH, Fu J, Sugrue RJ, et al. Recombinant dengue type 1 virus NS5 protein expressed in Escherichia coli exhibits RNA-dependent RNA polymerase activity. *Virology* 1996;216(2):317–325.

886. Tanaka T, Kato N, Cho MJ, et al. Structure of the 3′ terminus of the hepatitis C virus genome. *J Virol* 1996;70(5):3307–3312.

887. Tang WC, Lin RJ, Liao CL, et al. Rab18 facilitates dengue virus infection by targeting fatty acid synthase to sites of viral replication. *J Virol* 2014;88(12):6793–6804.

888. Tanida I, Fukasawa M, Ueno T, et al. Knockdown of autophagy-related gene decreases the production of infectious hepatitis C virus particles. *Autophagy* 2009;5(7):937–945.

889. Tanji Y, Kaneko T, Satoh S, et al. Phosphorylation of hepatitis C virus-encoded nonstructural protein NS5A. *J Virol* 1995;69(7):3980–3986.

890. Tassaneetrithep B, Burgess TH, Granelli-Piperno A, et al. DC-SIGN (CD209) mediates dengue virus infection of human dendritic cells. *J Exp Med* 2003;197(7):823–829.

891. Tautz N, Elbers K, Stoll D, et al. Serine protease of pestiviruses: determination of cleavage sites. *J Virol* 1997;71(7):5415–5422.

892. Tautz N, Kaiser A, Thiel HJ. NS3 serine protease of bovine viral diarrhea virus: characterization of active site residues, NS4A cofactor domain, and protease-cofactor interactions. *Virology* 2000;273(2):351–363.

893. Tautz N, Meyers G, Stark R, et al. Cytopathogenicity of a pestivirus correlates with a 27-nucleotide insertion. *J Virol* 1996;70(11):7851–7858.

894. Tautz N, Tews BA, Meyers G. The Molecular Biology of Pestiviruses. *Adv Virus Res* 2015;93:47–160.

895. Tautz N, Thiel HJ, Dubovi EJ, et al. Pathogenesis of mucosal disease: a cytopathogenic pestivirus generated by an internal deletion. *J Virol* 1994;68(5):3289–3297.

896. Tay MY, Saw WG, Zhao Y, et al. The C-terminal 50 amino acid residues of dengue NS3 protein are important for NS3-NS5 interaction and viral replication. *J Biol Chem* 2015;290(4):2379–2394.

897. Tay MY, Smith K, Ng IH, et al. The C-terminal 18 amino acid region of dengue virus NS5 regulates its subcellular localization and contains a conserved arginine residue essential for infectious virus production. *PLoS Pathog* 2016;12(9):e1005886.

898. Tellinghuisen TL, Foss KL, Treadaway J. Regulation of hepatitis C virion production via phosphorylation of the NS5A protein. *PLoS Pathog* 2008;4(3):e1000032.

899. Tellinghuisen TL, Foss KL, Treadaway JC, et al. Identification of residues required for RNA replication in domains II and III of the hepatitis C virus NS5A protein. *J Virol* 2008;82(3):1073–1083.

900. Tellinghuisen TL, Marcotrigiano J, Gorbalenya AE, et al. The NS5A protein of hepatitis C virus is a zinc metalloprotein. *J Biol Chem* 2004;279(47):48576–48587.

901. Tellinghuisen TL, Marcotrigiano J, Rice CM. Structure of the zinc-binding domain of an essential component of the hepatitis C virus replicase. *Nature* 2005;435(7040):374–379.

902. Tellinghuisen TL, Paulson MS, Rice CM. The NS5A protein of bovine viral diarrhea virus contains an essential zinc-binding site similar to that of the hepatitis C virus NS5A protein. *J Virol* 2006;80(15):7450–7458.

903. Tellinghuisen TL, Rice CM. Interaction between hepatitis C virus proteins and host cell factors. *Curr Opin Microbiol* 2002;5(4):419–427.

904. Teo KF, Wright PJ. Internal proteolysis of the NS3 protein specified by dengue virus 2. *J Gen Virol* 1997;78(Pt 2):337–341.

905. Terenin IM, Dmitriev SE, Andreev DE, et al. Eukaryotic translation initiation machinery can operate in a bacterial-like mode without eIF2. *Nat Struct Mol Biol* 2008;15(8):836–841.

906. Tews BA, Meyers G. The pestivirus glycoprotein E^rns is anchored in plane in the membrane via an amphipathic helix. *J Biol Chem* 2007;282(45):32730–32741.

907. Tews BA, Schürmann EM, Meyers G. Mutation of cysteine 171 of pestivirus E rns RNase prevents homodimer formation and leads to attenuation of classical swine fever virus. *J Virol* 2009;83(10):4823–4834.

908. Therkelsen MD, Klose T, Vago F, et al. Flaviviruses have imperfect icosahedral symmetry. *Proc Natl Acad Sci U S A* 2018;115(45):11608–11612.

909. Thibault PA, Huys A, Amador-Canizares Y, et al. Regulation of hepatitis C virus genome replication by Xrn1 and microRNA-122 binding to individual sites in the 5′ untranslated region. *J Virol* 2015;89(12):6294–6311.

910. Thiel H-J, Collett MS, Gould EA, et al. Family flaviviridae. In: Fauquet CM, Mayo MA, Maniloff J, et al., eds. *Virus Taxonomy. VIIIth Report of the International Committee on Taxonomy of Viruses.* San Diego: Academic Press; 2005:979 996.

911. Thiel HJ, Stark R, Weiland E, et al. Hog cholera virus: molecular composition of virions from a pestivirus. *J Virol* 1991;65(9):4705–4712.

912. Thomssen R, Bonk S, Propfe C, et al. Association of hepatitis C virus in human sera with beta-lipoprotein. *Med Microbiol Immunol* 1992;181(5):293–300.

913. Tillmann HL, Heringlake S, Trautwein C, et al. Antibodies against the GB virus C envelope 2 protein before liver transplantation protect against GB virus C de novo infection. *Hepatology* 1998;28(2):379–384.

914. Timpe JM, Stamataki Z, Jennings A, et al. Hepatitis C virus cell-cell transmission in hepatoma cells in the presence of neutralizing antibodies. *Hepatology* 2008;47(1):17–24.

915. Tischendorf JJ, Beger C, Korf M, et al. Polypyrimidine tract-binding protein (PTB) inhibits Hepatitis C virus internal ribosome entry site (HCV IRES)-mediated translation, but does not affect HCV replication. *Arch Virol* 2004;149(10):1955–1970.

916. Tomassini JE, Boots E, Gan L, et al. An in vitro Flaviviridae replicase system capable of authentic RNA replication. *Virology* 2003;313(1):274–285.

917. Tomei L, Altamura S, Bartholomew L, et al. Mechanism of action and antiviral activity of benzimidazole-based allosteric inhibitors of the hepatitis C virus RNA-dependent RNA polymerase. *J Virol* 2003;77(24):13225–13231.

918. Tomei L, Altamura S, Bartholomew L, et al. Characterization of the inhibition of hepatitis C virus RNA replication by nonnucleosides. *J Virol* 2004;78(2):938–946.

919. Tratschin JD, Moser C, Ruggli N, et al. Classical swine fever virus leader proteinase N^pro is not required for viral replication in cell culture. *J Virol* 1998;72(9):7681–7684.

920. Trivedi S, Murthy S, Sharma H, et al. Viral persistence, liver disease, and host response in a hepatitis C-like virus rat model. *Hepatology* 2018;68(2):435–448.

921. Trotard M, Lepere-Douard C, Regeard M, et al. Kinases required in hepatitis C virus entry and replication highlighted by small interference RNA screening. *FASEB J* 2009; 23(11):3780–3789.

922. Tscherne DM, Jones CT, Evans MJ, et al. Time- and temperature-dependent activation of hepatitis C virus for low-pH-triggered entry. *J Virol* 2006;80(4):1734–1741.

923. Tsetsarkin KA, Liu G, Shen K, et al. Kissing-loop interaction between 5′ and 3′ ends of tick-borne Langat virus genome "bridges the gap" between mosquito- and tick-borne flaviviruses in mechanisms of viral RNA cyclization: applications for virus attenuation and vaccine development. *Nucleic Acids Res* 2016;44(7):3330–3350.

924. Tsuchihara K, Tanaka T, Hijikata M, et al. Specific interaction of polypyrimidine tract-binding protein with the extreme 3′-terminal structure of the hepatitis C virus genome, the 3′X. *J Virol* 1997;71(9):6720–6726.

925. Tuplin A, Struthers M, Simmonds P, et al. A twist in the tail: SHAPE mapping of long-range interactions and structural rearrangements of RNA elements involved in HCV replication. *Nucleic Acids Res* 2012;40(14):6908–6921.

926. Tzarum N, Wilson IA, Law M. The neutralizing face of hepatitis C virus E2 envelope glycoprotein. *Front Immunol* 2018;9:1315.

927. Uchida L, Espada-Murao LA, Takamatsu Y, et al. The dengue virus conceals double-stranded RNA in the intracellular membrane to escape from an interferon response. *Sci Rep* 2014;4:7395.

928. Uchil PD, Satchidanandam V. Characterization of RNA synthesis, replication mechanism, and in vitro RNA-dependent RNA polymerase activity of Japanese encephalitis virus. *Virology* 2003;307(2):358–371.

929. Umareddy I, Chao A, Sampath A, et al. Dengue virus NS4B interacts with NS3 and dissociates it from single-stranded RNA. *J Gen Virol* 2006;87(Pt 9):2605–2614.

930. Urosevic N, van Maanen M, Mansfield JP, et al. Molecular characterization of virus-specific RNA produced in the brains of flavivirus-susceptible and -resistant mice after challenge with Murray Valley encephalitis virus. *J Gen Virol* 1997;78(Pt 1):23–29.

931. Van der Bij AK, Kloosterboer N, Prins M, et al. GB virus C coinfection and HIV-1 disease progression: the Amsterdam cohort study. *J Infect Dis* 2005;191(5):678–685.

932. van der Schaar HM, Rust MJ, Chen C, et al. Dissecting the cell entry pathway of dengue virus by single-particle tracking in living cells. *PLoS Pathog* 2008;4(12):e1000244.

933. Van Oirschot JT, De Jong D, Huffels ND. Effect of infections with swine fever virus on immune functions. II. Lymphocyte response to mitogens and enumeration of lymphocyte subpopulations. *Vet Microbiol* 1983;8(1):81–95.

934. Varjak M, Donald CL, Mottram TJ, et al. Characterization of the Zika virus induced small RNA response in *Aedes aegypti* cells. *PLoS Negl Trop Dis* 2017;11(10):e0006010.

935. Vasiliauskaite I, Owsianka A, England P, et al. Conformational flexibility in the immunoglobulin-like domain of the hepatitis C virus glycoprotein E2. *MBio* 2017;8(3).

936. Vassilaki N, Friebe P, Meuleman P, et al. Role of the hepatitis C virus core+1 open reading frame and core cis-acting RNA elements in viral RNA translation and replication. *J Virol* 2008;82(23):11503–11515.

937. Verdegem D, Badillo A, Wieruszeski JM, et al. Domain 3 of NS5A protein from the hepatitis C virus has intrinsic alpha-helical propensity and is a substrate of cyclophilin A. *J Biol Chem* 2011;286(23):20441–20454.

938. Vieyres G, Brohm C, Friesland M, et al. Subcellular localization and function of an epitope-tagged p7 viroporin in hepatitis C virus-producing cells. *J Virol* 2013;87(3):1664–1678.

939. Vieyres G, Thomas X, Descamps V, et al. Characterization of the envelope glycoproteins associated with infectious hepatitis C virus. *J Virol* 2010;84(19):10159–10168.

940. Villordo SM, Alvarez DE, Gamarnik AV. A balance between circular and linear forms of the dengue virus genome is crucial for viral replication. *RNA* 2010;16(12):2325–2335.

941. Villordo SM, Carballeda JM, Filomatori CV, et al. RNA structure duplications and flavivirus host adaptation. *Trends Microbiol* 2016;24(4):270–283.

942. von Freyburg M, Ege A, Saalmüller A, et al. Comparison of the effects of RNase-negative and wild-type classical swine fever virus on peripheral blood cells of infected pigs. *J Gen Virol* 2004;85(Pt 7):1899–1908.

943. von Schaewen M, Dorner M, Hueging K, et al. Expanding the host range of hepatitis C virus through viral adaptation. *Mbio* 2016;7(6).

944. Vossmann S, Wieseler J, Kerber R, et al. A basic cluster in the N terminus of yellow fever virus NS2A contributes to infectious particle production. *J Virol* 2015;89(9):4951–4965.
945. Wakita T, Pietschmann T, Kato T, et al. Production of infectious hepatitis C virus in tissue culture from a cloned viral genome. *Nat Med* 2005;11(7):791–796.
946. Wang QM, Hockman MA, Staschke K, et al. Oligomerization and cooperative RNA synthesis activity of hepatitis C virus RNA-dependent RNA polymerase. *J Virol* 2002;76(8):3865–3872.
947. Wang X, Lee WM, Watanabe T, et al. Brome mosaic virus 1a nucleoside triphosphatase/helicase domain plays crucial roles in recruiting RNA replication templates. *J Virol* 2005;79(21):13747–13758.
948. Wang J, Li Y, Modis Y. Structural models of the membrane anchors of envelope glycoproteins E1 and E2 from pestiviruses. *Virology* 2014;454-455:93–101.
949. Wang M, Ng KK, Cherney MM, et al. Non-nucleoside analogue inhibitors bind to an allosteric site on HCV NS5B polymerase. Crystal structures and mechanism of inhibition. *J Biol Chem* 2003;278(11):9489–9495.
950. Wang H, Perry JW, Lauring AS, et al. Oxysterol-binding protein is a phosphatidylinositol 4-kinase effector required for HCV replication membrane integrity and cholesterol trafficking. *Gastroenterology* 2014;146(5):1373–1385.e1–e11.
951. Wang C, Timmons CL, Shao Q, et al. GB virus type C E2 protein inhibits human immunodeficiency virus type 1 Gag assembly by downregulating human ADP-ribosylation factor 1. *Oncotarget* 2015;6(41):43293–43309.
952. Wang ZD, Wang B, Wei F, et al. A new segmented virus associated with human febrile illness in China. *N Engl J Med* 2019;380(22):2116–2125.
953. Waris G, Felmlee DJ, Negro F, et al. Hepatitis C virus induces proteolytic cleavage of sterol regulatory element binding proteins and stimulates their phosphorylation via oxidative stress. *J Virol* 2007;81(15):8122–8130.
954. Warrener P, Collett MS. Pestivirus NS3 (p80) protein possesses RNA helicase activity. *J Virol* 1995;69(3):1720–1726.
955. Warrener P, Tamura JK, Collett MS. RNA-stimulated NTPase activity associated with yellow fever virus NS3 protein expressed in bacteria. *J Virol* 1993;67:989–996.
956. Warrilow D, Lott WB, Greive S, et al. Properties of the bovine viral diarrhoea virus replicase in extracts of infected MDBK cells. *Arch Virol* 2000;145(10):2163–2171.
957. Washburn ML, Bility MT, Zhang LG, et al. A humanized mouse model to study hepatitis C virus infection, immune response, and liver disease. *Gastroenterology* 2011;140(4): 1334–1344.
958. Watterson D, Modhiran N, Young PR. The many faces of the flavivirus NS1 protein offer a multitude of options for inhibitor design. *Antiviral Res* 2016;130:7–18.
959. Weaver SC, Charlier C, Vasilakis N, et al. Zika, chikungunya, and other emerging vector-borne viral diseases. *Annu Rev Med* 2018;69:395–408.
960. Weiland E, Ahl R, Stark R, et al. A second envelope glycoprotein mediates neutralization of a pestivirus, hog cholera virus. *J Virol* 1992;66(6):3677–3682.
961. Weiland E, Stark R, Haas B, et al. Pestivirus glycoprotein which induces neutralizing antibodies forms part of a disulfide-linked heterodimer. *J Virol* 1990;64(8):3563–3569.
962. Weiland F, Weiland E, Unger G, et al. Localization of pestiviral envelope proteins E(rns) and E2 at the cell surface and on isolated particles. *J Gen Virol* 1999;80 (Pt 5):1157–1165.
963. Weiner AJ, Brauer MJ, Rosenblatt J, et al. Variable and hypervariable domains are found in the regions of HCV corresponding to the flavivirus envelope and NS1 proteins and the pestivirus envelope glycoproteins. *Virology* 1991;180(2):842–848.
964. Weiner AJ, Geysen HM, Christopherson C, et al. Evidence for immune selection of hepatitis C virus (HCV) putative envelope glycoprotein variants: potential role in chronic HCV infections. *Proc Natl Acad Sci U S A* 1992;89(8):3468–3472.
965. Weiskircher E, Aligo J, Ning G, et al. Bovine viral diarrhea virus NS4B protein is an integral membrane protein associated with Golgi markers and rearranged host membranes. *Virol J* 2009;6:185.
966. Welsch S, Miller S, Romero-Brey I, et al. Composition and three-dimensional architecture of the dengue virus replication and assembly sites. *Cell Host Microbe* 2009;5(4):365–375.
967. Weng L, Hirata Y, Arai M, et al. Sphingomyelin activates hepatitis C virus RNA polymerase in a genotype-specific manner. *J Virol* 2010;84(22):11761–11770.
968. Wengler G. The carboxy-terminal part of the NS3 protein of the West Nile flavivirus can be isolated as a soluble protein after proteolytic cleavage and represents an RNA-stimulated NTPase. *Virology* 1991;184:707–715.
969. Wengler G. The NS 3 nonstructural protein of flaviviruses contains an RNA triphosphatase activity. *Virology* 1993;197(1):265–273.
970. Wengler G, Gross HJ. Studies on virus-specific nucleic acids synthesized in vertebrate and mosquito cells infected with flaviviruses. *Virology* 1978;89:423–437.
971. Wengler G, Nowak T, Castle E. Description of a procedure which allows isolation of viral nonstructural proteins from BHK vertebrate cells infected with the West Nile flavivirus in a state which allows their direct chemical characterization. *Virology* 1990;177:795–801.
972. Westaway EG, Khromykh AA, Mackenzie JM. Nascent flavivirus RNA colocalized in situ with double-stranded RNA in stable replication complexes. *Virology* 1999;258(1):108–117.
973. Westaway EG, Mackenzie JM, Kenney MT, et al. Ultrastructure of Kunjin virus-infected cells: colocalization of NS1 and NS3 with double-stranded RNA, and of NS2B with NS3, in virus- induced membrane structures. *J Virol* 1997;71(9):6650–6661.
974. Windisch JM, Schneider R, Stark R, et al. RNase of classical swine fever virus: biochemical characterization and inhibition by virus-neutralizing monoclonal antibodies. *J Virol* 1996;70(1):352–358.
975. Winkelmann ER, Widman DG, Suzuki R, et al. Analyses of mutations selected by passaging a chimeric flavivirus identify mutations that alter infectivity and reveal an interaction between the structural proteins and the nonstructural glycoprotein NS1. *Virology* 2011;421(2):96–104.
976. Wiskerchen M, Belzer SK, Collett MS. Pestivirus gene expression: the first protein product of the bovine viral diarrhea virus large open reading frame, p20, possesses proteolytic activity. *J Virol* 1991;65(8):4508–4514.
977. Wiskerchen M, Collett MS. Pestivirus gene expression: protein p80 of bovine viral diarrhea virus is a proteinase involved in polyprotein processing. *Virology* 1991;184(1):341–350.
978. Wolf YI, Kazlauskas D, Iranzo J, et al. Origins and evolution of the global RNA virome. *MBio* 2018;9(6).
979. Wozniak AL, Griffin S, Rowlands D, et al. Intracellular proton conductance of the hepatitis C virus p7 protein and its contribution to infectious virus production. *PLoS Pathog* 2010;6(9):e1001087.
980. Wrensch F, Crouchet E, Ligat G, et al. Hepatitis C virus (HCV)-apolipoprotein interactions and immune evasion and their impact on HCV vaccine design. *Front Immunol* 2018;9:1436.
981. Wu J, Bera AK, Kuhn RJ, et al. Structure of the flavivirus helicase: implications for catalytic activity, protein interactions, and proteolytic processing. *J Virol* 2005;79(16):10268–10277.
982. Wu RH, Tsai MH, Chao DY, et al. Scanning mutagenesis studies reveal a potential intramolecular interaction within the C-terminal half of dengue virus NS2A involved in viral RNA replication and virus assembly and secretion. *J Virol* 2015;89(8):4281–4295.
983. Wu RH, Tsai MH, Tsai KN, et al. Mutagenesis of dengue virus protein NS2A revealed a novel domain responsible for virus-induced cytopathic effect and interactions between NS2A and NS2B transmembrane segments. *J Virol* 2017;91(12).
984. Xiang J, Klinzman D, McLinden J, et al. Characterization of hepatitis G virus (GB-C virus) particles: evidence for a nucleocapsid and expression of sequences upstream of the E1 protein. *J Virol* 1998;72(4):2738–2744.
985. Xiang J, McLinden JH, Chang Q, et al. Characterization of a peptide domain within the GB virus C NS5A phosphoprotein that inhibits HIV replication. *PLoS One* 2008;3(7):e2580.
986. Xiao F, Wang S, Barouch-Bentov R, et al. Interactions between the Hepatitis C virus nonstructural 2 protein and host adaptor proteins 1 and 4 orchestrate virus release. *MBio* 2018;9(2).
987. Xie X, Gayen S, Kang C, et al. Membrane topology and function of dengue virus NS2A protein. *J Virol* 2013;87(8):4609–4622.
988. Xie X, Zou J, Puttikhunt C, et al. Two distinct sets of NS2A molecules are responsible for dengue virus RNA synthesis and virion assembly. *J Virol* 2015;89(2):1298–1313.
989. Xu J, Mendez E, Caron PR, et al. Bovine viral diarrhea virus NS3 serine proteinase: polyprotein cleavage sites, cofactor requirements, and molecular model of an enzyme essential for pestivirus replication. *J Virol* 1997;71(7):5312–5322.
990. Xu T, Sampath A, Chao A, et al. Structure of the dengue virus helicase/nucleoside triphosphatase catalytic domain at a resolution of 2.4 A. *J Virol* 2005;79(16):10278–10288.
991. Yamamoto S, Fukuhara T, Ono C, et al. Lipoprotein receptors redundantly participate in entry of hepatitis C virus. *PLoS Pathog* 2016;12(5):e1005610.
992. Yamane D, McGivern DR, Wauthier E, et al. Regulation of the hepatitis C virus RNA replicase by endogenous lipid peroxidation. *Nat Med* 2014;20(8):927–935.
993. Yamashita T, Kaneko S, Shirota Y, et al. RNA-dependent RNA polymerase activity of the soluble recombinant hepatitis C virus NS5B protein truncated at the C-terminal region. *J Biol Chem* 1998;273(25):15479–15486.
994. Yan Y, He Y, Boson B, et al. A point mutation in the N-terminal amphipathic helix α_0 in NS3 promotes hepatitis C virus assembly by altering core localization to the endoplasmic reticulum and facilitating virus budding. *J Virol* 2017;91(6).
995. Yanagi M, Purcell RH, Emerson SU, et al. Transcripts from a single full-length cDNA clone of hepatitis C virus are infectious when directly transfected into the liver of a chimpanzee. *Proc Natl Acad Sci U S A* 1997;94(16):8738–8743.
996. Yanagi M, St Claire M, Emerson SU, et al. In vivo analysis of the 3′ untranslated region of the hepatitis C virus after in vitro mutagenesis of an infectious cDNA clone. *Proc Natl Acad Sci U S A* 1999;96(5):2291–2295.
997. Yang G, Pevear DC, Collett MS, et al. Newly synthesized hepatitis C virus replicon RNA is protected from nuclease activity by a protease-sensitive factor(s). *J Virol* 2004;78(18):10202–10205.
998. Yao N, Reichert P, Taremi SS, et al. Molecular views of viral polyprotein processing revealed by the crystal structure of the hepatitis C virus bifunctional protease-helicase. *Structure* 1999;7(11):1353–1363.
999. Yap TL, Xu T, Chen YL, et al. Crystal structure of the dengue virus RNA-dependent RNA polymerase catalytic domain at 1.85-angstrom resolution. *J Virol* 2007;81(9):4753–4765.
1000. Ye J, Wang C, Sumpter R Jr, et al. Disruption of hepatitis C virus RNA replication through inhibition of host protein geranylgeranylation. *Proc Natl Acad Sci U S A* 2003;100(26):15865–15870.
1001. Yi M, Lemon SM. 3′ nontranslated RNA signals required for replication of hepatitis C virus RNA. *J Virol* 2003;77(6):3557–3568.
1002. Yi M, Nakamoto Y, Kaneko S, et al. Delineation of regions important for heteromeric association of hepatitis C virus E1 and E2. *Virology* 1997;231(1):119–129.
1003. Yi Z, Sperzel L, Nürnberger C, et al. Identification and characterization of the host protein DNAJC14 as a broadly active flavivirus replication modulator. *PLoS Pathog* 2011;7(1):e1001255.
1004. Yi M, Villanueva RA, Thomas DL, et al. Production of infectious genotype 1a hepatitis C virus (Hutchinson strain) in cultured human hepatoma cells. *Proc Natl Acad Sci U S A* 2006;103(7):2310–2315.
1005. Yin C, Goonawardane N, Stewart H, et al. A role for domain I of the hepatitis C virus NS5A protein in virus assembly. *PLoS Pathog* 2018;14(1):e1006834.
1006. Yon C, Teramoto T, Mueller N, et al. Modulation of the nucleoside triphosphatase/RNA helicase and 5′-RNA triphosphatase activities of Dengue virus type 2 nonstructural protein 3 (NS3) by interaction with NS5, the RNA-dependent RNA polymerase. *J Biol Chem* 2005;280(29):27412–27419.
1007. You S, Padmanabhan R. A novel in vitro replication system for Dengue virus. Initiation of RNA synthesis at the 3′-end of exogenous viral RNA templates requires 5′- and 3′-terminal complementary sequence motifs of the viral RNA. *J Biol Chem* 1999;274(47): 33714–33722.
1008. You S, Rice CM. 3′ RNA elements in hepatitis C virus replication: kissing partners and long poly (U). *J Virol* 2008;82:184–195.
1009. You S, Stump DD, Branch AD, et al. A *cis*-acting replication element in the sequence encoding the NS5B RNA-dependent RNA polymerase is required for hepatitis C virus RNA replication. *J Virol* 2004;78(3):1352–1366.
1010. Youn S, Li T, McCune BT, et al. Evidence for a genetic and physical interaction between nonstructural proteins NS1 and NS4B that modulates replication of West Nile virus. *J Virol* 2012;86(13):7360–7371.

1011. Yu H, Grassmann CW, Behrens SE. Sequence and structural elements at the 3′ terminus of bovine viral diarrhea virus genomic RNA: functional role during RNA replication. *J Virol* 1999;73(5):3638–3648.

1012. Yu IM, Holdaway HA, Chipman PR, et al. Association of the pr peptides with dengue virus at acidic pH blocks membrane fusion. *J Virol* 2009;83(23):12101–12107.

1013. Yu H, Isken O, Grassmann CW, et al. A stem-loop motif formed by the immediate 5′ terminus of the bovine viral diarrhea virus genome modulates translation as well as replication of the viral RNA. *J Virol* 2000;74(13):5825–5835.

1014. Yu GY, Lee KJ, Gao L, et al. Palmitoylation and polymerization of hepatitis C virus NS4B protein. *J Virol* 2006;80(12):6013–6023.

1015. Yu L, Nomaguchi M, Padmanabhan R, et al. Specific requirements for elements of the 5′ and 3′ terminal regions in flavivirus RNA synthesis and viral replication. *Virology* 2008;374(1):170–185.

1016. Yu IM, Zhang W, Holdaway HA, et al. Structure of the immature dengue virus at low pH primes proteolytic maturation. *Science* 2008;319(5871):1834–1837.

1017. Yuan L, Huang XY, Liu ZY, et al. A single mutation in the prM protein of Zika virus contributes to fetal microcephaly. *Science* 2017;358(6365):933–936.

1018. Yuasa T, Ishikawa G, Manabe S, et al. The particle size of hepatitis C virus estimated by filtration through microporous regenerated cellulose fibre. *J Gen Virol* 1991;72 (Pt 8):2021–2024.

1019. Zahid MN, Turek M, Xiao F, et al. The postbinding activity of scavenger receptor class B type I mediates initiation of hepatitis C virus infection and viral dissemination. *Hepatology* 2013;57(2):492–504.

1020. Zaitseva E, Yang ST, Melikov K, et al. Dengue virus ensures its fusion in late endosomes using compartment-specific lipids. *PLoS Pathog* 2010;6(10).

1021. Zeisel MB, Koutsoudakis G, Schnober EK, et al. Scavenger receptor class B type I is a key host factor for hepatitis C virus infection required for an entry step closely linked to CD81. *Hepatology* 2007;46(6):1722–1731.

1022. Zhang C, Cai Z, Kim YC, et al. Stimulation of hepatitis C virus (HCV) nonstructural protein 3 (NS3) helicase activity by the NS3 protease domain and by HCV RNA-dependent RNA polymerase. *J Virol* 2005;79(14):8687–8697.

1023. Zhang PR, Corver J, et al. Visualization of membrane protein domains by cryo-electron microscopy of dengue virus. *Nat Struct Biol* 2003;10(11):907–912.

1024. Zhang B, Dong H, Zhou Y, et al. Genetic interactions among the West Nile virus methyltransferase, the RNA-dependent RNA polymerase, and the 5′ stem-loop of genomic RNA. *J Virol* 2008;82(14):7047–7058.

1025. Zhang X, Ge P, Yu X, et al. Cryo-EM structure of the mature dengue virus at 3.5-A resolution. *Nat Struct Mol Biol* 2013;20(1):105–110.

1026. Zhang R, Miner JJ, Gorman MJ, et al. A CRISPR screen defines a signal peptide processing pathway required by flaviviruses. *Nature* 2016;535(7610):164–168.

1027. Zhang J, Yamada O, Yoshida H, et al. Autogenous translational inhibition of core protein: implication for switch from translation to RNA replication in hepatitis C virus. *Virology* 2002;293(1):141–150.

1028. Zhao Y, Soh TS, Lim SP, et al. Molecular basis for specific viral RNA recognition and 2′-O-ribose methylation by the dengue virus nonstructural protein 5 (NS5). *Proc Natl Acad Sci U S A* 2015;112(48):14834–14839.

1029. Zheng A, Yuan F, Kleinfelter LM, et al. A toggle switch controls the low pH-triggered rearrangement and maturation of the dengue virus envelope proteins. *Nat Commun* 2014;5:3877.

1030. Zhong J, Gastaminza P, Cheng G, et al. Robust hepatitis C virus infection in vitro. *Proc Natl Acad Sci U S A* 2005;102(26):9294–9299.

1031. Zhong W, Gutshall LL, Del Vecchio AM. Identification and characterization of an RNA-dependent RNA polymerase activity within the nonstructural protein 5B region of bovine viral diarrhea virus. *J Virol* 1998;72(11):9365–9369.

1032. Zhong W, Ingravallo P, Wright-Minogue J, et al. Nucleoside triphosphatase and RNA helicase activities associated with GB virus B nonstructural protein 3. *Virology* 1999;261(2):216–226.

1033. Zhong W, Uss AS, Ferrari E, et al. De novo initiation of RNA synthesis by hepatitis C virus nonstructural protein 5B polymerase. *J Virol* 2000;74(4):2017–2022.

1034. Zhou Y, Ray D, Zhao Y, et al. Structure and function of flavivirus NS5 methyltransferase. *J Virol* 2007;81(8):3891–3903.

1035. Zibert A, Meisel H, Kraas W, et al. Early antibody response against hypervariable region 1 is associated with acute self-limiting infections of hepatitis C virus. *Hepatology* 1997;25(5):1245–1249.

1036. Zögg T, Sponring M, Schindler S, et al. Crystal structures of the viral protease N^pro imply distinct roles for the catalytic water in catalysis. *Structure* 2013;21(6):929–938.

1037. Zou J, Lee le T, Wang QY, et al. Mapping the interactions between the NS4B and NS3 proteins of dengue virus. *J Virol* 2015;89(7):3471–3483.

1038. Zou G, Puig-Basagoiti F, Zhang B, et al. A single-amino acid substitution in West Nile virus 2K peptide between NS4A and NS4B confers resistance to lycorine, a flavivirus inhibitor. *Virology* 2009;384(1):242–252.

1039. Zou J, Xie X, Lee le T, et al. Dimerization of flavivirus NS4B protein. *J Virol* 2014;88(6):3379–3391.

1040. Zou J, Xie X, Wang QY, et al. Characterization of dengue virus NS4A and NS4B protein interaction. *J Virol* 2015;89(7):3455–3470.

1041. Zou G, Zhang B, Lim PY, et al. Exclusion of West Nile virus superinfection through RNA replication. *J Virol* 2009;83(22):11765–11776.

1042. Zürcher C, Sauter KS, Mathys V, et al. Prolonged activity of the pestiviral RNase E^rns as an interferon antagonist after uptake by clathrin-mediated endocytosis. *J Virol* 2014;88(13):7235–7243.

Christopher Walker

HISTORY

Posttransfusion hepatitis that could not be attributed to hepatitis A virus (HAV) or hepatitis B virus (HBV) infection was first reported in the mid-1970s.[202,365,610] This disease entity, designated non-A, non-B hepatitis (NANBH), was marked by elevated hepatic transaminases in recipients of blood products. Transaminase elevations often persisted and were associated in many cases with chronic inflammatory liver disease and cirrhosis.[202,365,610] Passage of blood components to a variety of Old and New World monkey species failed to replicate the transaminase elevation observed in humans. Only a great ape, the common chimpanzee (*Pan troglodytes*), developed NANBH after transfusion with blood that caused hepatitis in human recipients.[22,292,732] Serial passage of NANBH between chimpanzees provided critical insight into the nature of the infectious agent. Physicochemical studies revealed that NANBH was caused by a small (80 nm) filterable virus with an envelope that was sensitive to treatment with organic solvents.[73,203]

Well-established approaches used to identify other hepatitis viruses were not effective in the search for the NANBH agent.[298] Virus particles were not visualized by electron microscopy in the liver or serum from patients with NANBH or in cultured primary and established hepatocyte cell lines after inoculation with these materials. Moreover, the cultured hepatocytes did not develop cytopathic effects or tubular ultrastructural alterations in hepatocyte endoplasmic reticulum that were diagnostic of NANBH.[298] Approximately 15 years after the first description of posttransfusion NANBH, a highly novel approach of blind immune screening was used to identify the infectious agent. This strategy, devised by Michael Houghton and his colleagues at Chiron Corporation, involved reverse transcription of nucleic acids from the liver and serum of infected humans and chimpanzees.[121] Recombinant λGT11 phage expression libraries constructed from the cDNA were then screened for recognition by radiolabeled IgG antibodies from NANBH patients. Tens of millions of λGT11 clones were screened over 2 years before a single positive clone designated 5-1-1 was identified.[121,298] This clone, derived from the serum of a chimpanzee with a high infectious titer of the NANBH agent, was extrachromosomal (i.e., not of host origin) and encoded a polypeptide recognized by antibodies from humans and chimpanzees with NANBH but not HAV or HBV infections.[121] Molecular cloning revealed that the newly identified hepatitis C virus (HCV) had a positive-strand RNA genome of approximately 10,000 nucleotides that is transcribed as a single open reading frame.[121] Based on these features and organization of structural and nonstructural proteins, HCV was classified as member of the *Flaviviridae* family.[122] Serologic assays that incorporated antigen 5-1-1 derived from HCV nonstructural protein 4 (NS4), and other structural and nonstructural antigens identified in the λGT11 library, were rapidly developed.[20,388] Seroepidemiology revealed that almost all transfusion-related and community-acquired hepatitis was caused by HCV.[20]

Discovery of HCV laid the groundwork for development of new direct-acting antivirals (DAA) that recently replaced type I interferon-based therapies for chronic hepatitis C. Almost all chronic infections, including those that were previously difficult to treat because of HCV genotype resistance or comorbidities, can now be cured by 8 to 12 weeks of therapy with an all oral, once-a-day DAA regimen (see Treatment). Elimination of HCV by 2030, 40 years after the discovery of

HCV, is now an objective of the World Health Organization (see www.who.int/hepatitis/strategies2016-2021/ghss-hep/en) that has gained support from many advisory and governmental agencies including the United States National Academy of Sciences[537] (see Public Health Measures).

INFECTIOUS AGENT

Classification

HCV is a genetically diverse virus that is classified into seven genotypes with a remarkable 35% nucleotide divergence between strains belonging to different genotypes. A total of 86 subtypes that differ in sequence by 25% are also distributed among the 7 genotypes (see http://talk.ictvonline.org/links/hcv/hcv-classification.html) (Fig. 8.1).[701]

HCV belongs to the *Hepacivirus* genus of the *Flaviviridae* family. The genus has expanded in recent years to include hepaciviruses isolated from a diverse array of animals including rats, bats, horses, and colobus monkeys.[165,700] Hepaciviruses are now classified into 14 discrete species (A–M) that vary largely by host range, with HCV genotypes grouped in *Hepacivirus* species C. The wide host range of the hepaciviruses is highlighted by the recent discovery of an unclassified, more divergent hepacivirus-like sequence assembled from liver tissue of a gracile shark.[681] Rodent and equine hepaciviruses that segregate into distinct species share only about 50% sequence homology with HCV and can also establish persistent infections in their hosts (Fig. 8.2). They have emerged as valuable animal models for the study of HCV infection and immunity (see Immune Responses).

HCV Particle Morphology

HCV exists in serum as lipoviral particles (LVPs) with a light buoyant density (≤1.055 g/mL) and diameter of 60 to 70 nm.[102,594] LVPs are formed around HCV core proteins that are in close association with the RNA genome of the virus. Ultrastructural studies of cell culture–derived LVP revealed that they are the most irregular members of the *Flaviviridae* family from a structural perspective, with spike-like projections and a heterogeneous size distribution.[102] They resemble very-low-density lipoproteins (VLDL) in structure and are associated with cholesterol esters, triglycerides, and host apolipoproteins, including apoE that is required for HCV infectivity.[107,149,303,326,492] They can associate with VLDL upon release from infected cells to form particle complexes.[39,819] Low-density particles recovered from patients were immunoreactive with antibodies against the HCV E1 and E2 envelope glycoproteins that are anchored in the particle membrane.[611] Moreover, LVPs recovered from the serum of persistently infected chimpanzees are highly infectious.[74]

The HCV Replication Cycle

Primary HCV isolates from humans replicate poorly, if at all, in cell culture models. Progress in unraveling the HCV replication cycle accelerated with development of viral pseudoparticles that display the HCV envelope glycoproteins,[47,300] subgenomic replicons,[63,441] and more recently viruses from all seven genotypes adapted for efficient replication in cell culture.[434,622,796,840] Chapter 7 provides a detailed description of HCV entry, replication, assembly, and egress from infected cells. Key features of this process relevant to understanding HCV pathogenesis, immunity, and antiviral therapy are discussed below.

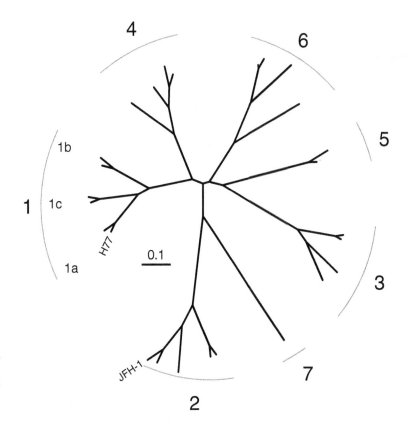

FIGURE 8.1 Phylogenetic tree of representative sequences from the seven proposed genotypes of hepatitis C virus (HCV). Full-genome nucleotide sequences were aligned and analyzed using a maximum likelihood model with estimation of invariant sites and modeling of variable rates using the gamma distribution, with bootstrap resampling to confirm support for each genotype cluster. Reference isolates H77 (AF009606) and JFH-1 (AB047639) are indicated. Subtypes of genotype 1 (1a, 1b, 1c) are indicated for illustration.

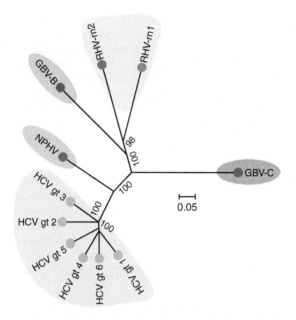

FIGURE 8.2 Evolutionary relationships and genetic distances between HCV, NPHV, GBV-B, rat hepacivirus (RHV), and GBV-C. A total of 629 amino acid positions of NS3 protein were aligned and used for comparative phylogenetic analysis using MEGA7 (1). The evolutionary history was inferred using the neighbor-joining method. The optimal tree with the sum of branch length = 2.07891938 is shown. The tree is drawn to scale, with branch lengths in the same units as those of the evolutionary distances used to infer the phylogenetic tree. The evolutionary distances were computed using the p-distance method and are in the units of the number of amino acid differences per site. The rate variation among sites was modeled with a gamma distribution (shape parameter = 1). The analysis involved 12 amino acid sequences. All ambiguous positions were removed for each sequence pair. Kindly provided by Dr. Amit Kapoor.

Entry of HCV into hepatocytes is mediated by the type I transmembrane E1 and E2 envelope glycoproteins proteins that are displayed on the surface of infectious virions as a cross-linked heterodimer (Fig. 8.3).[792] The initial step in entry is mediated by an interaction between apoE in the LVP and the heparan sulfate proteoglycans[149,325,400] and scavenger receptor class B type I (SR-BI) on hepatocytes.[141] Subsequent steps involve E2 binding to the CD81[591] and SR-BI[591,596] cellular receptors and clathrin-dependent internalization of particles into the endosome in a process mediated by two additional entry receptors, the tight junction proteins claudin-1[186] and occludin[596] (Fig. 8.3). Internalized HCV particles undergo membrane fusion in the acidified environment of the endosome in a process facilitated by the E1 envelope glycoprotein, resulting in release of HCV genomes into the hepatocyte cytoplasm (Fig. 8.3).[166,402,421,580,679,760]

Cap-independent translation of the HCV genome occurs on the rough endoplasmic reticulum and is directed by a type III internal ribosome entry site (IRES) located in the 5' nontranslated region (NTR) of the viral genome (Fig. 8.4).[550,766] Activity of the IRES is critically dependent on liver-specific microRNA 122 (miR-122) that recruits Argonaute 2 to stabilize and protect the HCV genome against the Xrn1 host cell exonuclease activity and to shift the balance between translation and transcription of genomes.[331,427,467,683,816] The product of translation is a single polyprotein of approximately 3,000 amino acids that is co- and posttranslationally processed by host and viral proteases. Junctional cleavage between the structural core, E1, and E2 proteins is mediated by host cell signal peptidase, while the seven nonstructural proteins are released from the polyprotein by viral proteases. HCV-encoded proteases include NS2 that mediates cleavage of the NS2–NS3 junction through C-terminal cysteine protease activity and NS3 with its membrane-anchoring NS4A cofactor that cut at the remaining junctional sites between NS proteins via serine protease activity (Fig. 8.4).[45,122]

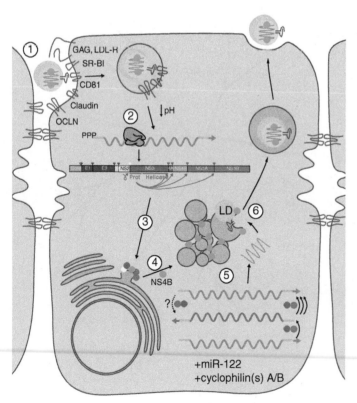

FIGURE 8.3 Life cycle of hepatitis C virus (HCV). Initial binding and internalization (*1*) probably involve glycosaminoglycans (GAGs) and low-density lipoprotein receptor (LDL-R), which may interact with viral envelope proteins or with virion-associated lipoproteins. Entry depends directly on binding of E2 with the tetraspanin CD81, as well as interactions with scavenger receptor BI (SR-BI) and tight junction proteins claudin-1 and occludin (OCLN). The viral genome is released from late endosomes (*2*) in a pH-dependent manner, followed by internal ribosome entry site (IRES)-dependent polyprotein synthesis (*3*) with initial cleavages among the structural proteins mediated by signalase and signal peptide peptidase followed by cleavage of the NS2–NS3 junction by NS2–NS3 cysteine protease; the remaining junctions are cleaved by the NS3–NS4A serine protease. NS4B recruits and rearranges endoplasmic reticulum (ER) membranes (*4*) to form a *membranous web*, the principal site of viral replication. Minus-strand and subsequent plus-strand RNA syntheses are affected by the NS5B RNA-dependent RNA polymerase (RdRp) (*5*) and depend on miR-122 and cyclophilin B, as well as conserved structural elements at the 5' and 3' ends of the genome. Core protein associates with lipid droplets (LDs) in the lipoprotein assembly pathway (*6*), linked to NS5A and other members of the replication complex by interaction with NS2. Viroporin p7 is necessary for production of stable viral particles coated with E1 and E2, which fold in a cooperative manner and are glycosylated in a manner consistent with ER but not Golgi processing.

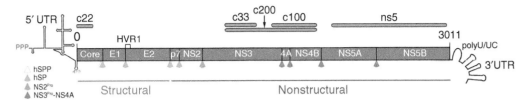

FIGURE 8.4 Map of the hepatitis C virus (HCV) genome. Structure of the HCV genome including the 5′ untranslated region (5′UTR), capsid core, envelope genes *E1* and *E2*, viroporin p7, membrane-anchored cysteine protease NS2, serine protease–helicase NS3, NS3 protease cofactor NS4A, membrane remodeling protein NS4B, phosphoprotein NS5A, RNA-dependent RNA polymerase NS5B, and the 3′UTR. Depicted as green bars are recombinant protein segments used as antigens in HCV enzyme immune assay (EIA) and recombinant immunoblot assay (RIBA). Cleavage of the polyprotein is due to the action of host signal peptidase (*solid orange*), signal peptide peptidase (*open orange*), NS2 cysteine autoprotease (*green*) and NS3-NS4A serine protease (*blue*).

Released NS proteins are organized into replicase complexes on a membranous web formed from 150-nm double-membrane vesicles (DMV) that are derived from the hepatocyte endoplasmic reticulum.[642] This structure concentrates cellular and viral factors required for replication and may also sequester HCV proteins and genomes from host innate sensors (see Innate Immunity). Web formation is directed by the membrane-associated NS4B and NS5A proteins.[641,642] NS4B is essential for HCV replication, but its functions are not well understood. It induces host cell membrane alterations[172] and may be involved in recruitment of autophagic factors into the membranous web.[190,269,690,737] NS5A, a phosphoprotein, serves several functions including binding of HCV RNA genomes,[218,301] regulation of the NS5B polymerase,[644,688] and recruitment of multiple host proteins including cyclophilin A[112,450] and phosphatidylinositol 4-kinase IIIα (PI4P)[53] that are required for HCV replication. The NS5B RNA-dependent RNA polymerase (RdRp) directs synthesis of negative-stranded RNA templates and new positive-stranded RNA genomes within the replicase complex where required NS3-mediated RNA helicase and NTPase functions are localized.

Virion assembly occurs near replication complexes at sites that are in close proximity to lipid droplets (Fig. 8.3).[191,511] This complex process involving multiple NS proteins (p7, NS2, NS4B, NS5A) is still poorly understood, in part because it is tightly linked to liver lipid metabolism that may not be fully recapitulated in cell culture models. The p7 and NS2 proteins are thought to be enriched at cytosolic sites where they coordinate assembly of the core, E1 and E2 structural proteins.[72,150,328,449,600,711,830] NS5A has a key role in the transition from replication to assembly, in part by chaperoning newly synthesized RNA genomes to the assembly sites.[72,830] Components of the cellular VLDL lipoprotein assembly pathway, including microsomal transfer protein,[303] apoB,[303] and DGAT1,[287] are thought to be usurped for formation and possibly release of HCV particles. As noted above, apoE is an essential component of HCV particles and contributes to particle maturation, release, and infectivity.[411] LVP maturation occurs during transit through the secretory pathway that is regulated by the ESCRT system[30,191,207] and continues at a post-egress step.[207] HCV particles may also be released from cells in exosomes as part of the autophagy response to infection.[690,737] The function of HCV proteins and membranous structures in regulation or evasion of the innate immune response and development of antiviral inhibitors targeting the NS3/4A protease, NS5A replicase factor, and NS5B RdRp are described later in this chapter.

Genetic Diversity and Evolution

HCV replication within an infected host results in a mixture of highly diverse variants that are genetically distinct.[395,459] This swarm, called a quasispecies, is generated by low-fidelity transcription of the HCV genome by the NS5B RdRp that lacks a proofreading mechanism. The estimated error rate is approximately 2 × 10⁻⁵ substitutions per nucleotide and round of replication of the 10-kB genome.[44,637] With daily production of about 10¹² virions,[547] each progeny genome is likely unique, and every possible combination of two mutations is generated within an infected individual every day. The HCV replication strategy is therefore highly adapted for rapid evasion of selection pressure exerted by immune responses and antiviral drugs (see Immune Responses and Treatment). Analysis of quasispecies evolution during the acute phase of infection revealed two sequential population bottlenecks. The first occurred upon transmission of HCV from a donor to recipient.[85,798] Infection is initiated by a very small number of HCV genomes, with an estimated median of four founder genomes in a study of 17 acutely infected humans.[424] Single-genome sequencing revealed that HCV diversifies rapidly by a model of simple random evolution during the early phase of acute infection.[3,425] A second bottleneck several weeks later coincides with the onset of adaptive immune responses (see Immunity).[85] Envelope glycoproteins diversify more rapidly than do other regions of the genome,[258] reflecting selection pressure from neutralizing antibodies. Within nonstructural proteins, the rate of nonsynonymous mutation is higher within class I restricted epitopes targeted by CD8+ T cells when compared with flanking nontargeted sequences.[94] Diversification of the nonstructural proteins slows with the transition to chronic infection,[94,208,387] which is thought to reflect functional exhaustion of the T-cell response. Other forces shaping the HCV genome during infection include emergence of compensatory mutations to restore fitness[548,646] and reversion of nontargeted sequences to a subtype consensus sequence considered more fit for replication.[387,654] A transmission bottleneck has also been identified after vertical transmission of HCV from mother to child.[200] The second immune-related bottleneck does occur, but is delayed until about 1 year postinfection when maternal antibodies decline. This timing of diversification is consistent with delayed onset of adaptive immunity to HCV in very young children.[200] Additional detail on HCV mutational escape from immune responses and antiviral drugs is provided in Immune Responses and Treatment sections.

PATHOGENESIS AND PATHOLOGY

Spread

The mode of spread of HCV throughout the liver is poorly understood. Only 10% to 20% of hepatocytes harbor HCV genomes in the chronic phase of infection despite high replication and viremia.[430,714,808] The infection status of single hepatocytes within liver specimens from chronically infected patients has been assessed using laser capture microdissection.[335] Creation of a viral infection landscape by assessing the intracellular HCV RNA content of adjacent individual cells revealed that infected hepatocytes occur in small clusters of 4 to 50 cells.[335] Moreover, the HCV RNA content in a cluster formed a gradient, from the presumptive founder hepatocyte to cells at the periphery.[257] Mathematical modeling suggested that hepatocytes within the cluster were infected for about 5 days.[257] Clustering is consistent with a model of random hepatocyte seeding from blood followed by local spread that could occur by cell-free or direct cell-to-cell mechanisms. Cell-to-cell spread of HCV infection has been documented in cell culture models[759,811] and may involve cellular receptors that partially overlap with those required for cell-free spread.[192] Why infection is restricted to small hepatocyte clusters is not known. Localized cell-to-cell spread of HCV may be favored as it provides protection from neutralizing antibodies in cell culture models.[77,759] Infection also triggers a strong interferon-stimulated gene response that could render neighboring cells resistant to infection (see Innate Immunity), although there is as yet no direct evidence to support this possibility.

Entry into the Host

As discussed in the Transmission section later (under Epidemiology), the primary route of HCV entry is percutaneous, although permucosal infection has also been described. Experimentally, HCV infection can be achieved by intravenous injection of HCV virions or intrahepatic injection of HCV genomic RNA.[371,818]

Cell and Tissue Tropism

HCV replication occurs primarily or exclusively in hepatocytes, the major parenchymal cell of the liver. The basis for this tropism is likely to be multifactorial. Entry receptors may be a key restriction factor. SR-BI, as an example, is preferentially expressed at high levels on hepatocytes.[591,596] Expression of other entry receptors such as CD81,[591] claudin-I,[186] occludin,[596] and cyclophilins[112,450] is not restricted to hepatocytes. Nonetheless, multiple receptors may be uniquely situated or patterned within subcellular spaces of the liver to support the dynamic, multistep entry process utilized by HCV. Dependence on liver-specific miR-122 for efficient replication of the HCV genome,[330,331] and utilization of the lipoprotein assembly pathway for virion production, may also contribute to hepatotropism of HCV.[303] Productive infection of cell types other than hepatocytes is controversial. HCV negative-strand replicative intermediates have been detected in cells of hematopoietic origin,[109,417,831] and compartmentalization of sequence variants has been described.[540,664] Apparent replication of HCV in cultured B and T cells has been described.[699,726] Viral dynamic modeling of data from the anhepatic phase of liver transplantation suggested that in a subset of patients with end-stage liver disease, an extrahepatic compartment exists that contributes no more than 3% to 4% of plasma viremia.[139,601]

Immune Response

Innate Immune Responses

Acute HCV infection induces potent innate immune defenses, including inflammasome activation,[110] expression of interferon-stimulated genes (ISG),[123,661] and expansion of natural killer (NK) cells. These responses are often persistent into the chronic phase of infection, indicating that HCV can deploy a multilayered defense that ensures ongoing viral replication in hepatocytes.

Inflammasome activation

Acute hepatitis C is characterized by elevated serum titers of IL-1β and IL-18, proinflammatory cytokines that are a product of inflammasome activation.[111,542,691] Cell culture models have demonstrated that the inflammasome response in macrophages and monocytes is triggered by direct binding of HCV to the toll-like receptor 7 (TLR7) innate sensor located in the endosome of these mononuclear cells. Inflammasome activation in this model was independent of virus replication[110,542] and the IFN-driven ISG response.[110] Activation of proinflammatory mediators like CXCL10 via an interferon-independent mechanisms involving NF-κB has also been described.[79] This process may also contribute to progressive liver injury, as macrophages exposed to HCV also activate inflammasome and fibrosis markers in cocultured stellate cells through a mechanism involving the chemokine CCL5.[660]

Interferon-stimulated gene responses

ISG responses are initiated when cellular sensors bind HCV RNA in the form of double-stranded structures and replicative intermediates.[123,661] Activation of toll-like receptor 3 (TLR3) sensors located in the endosome, or the retinoic acid–inducible gene-1 (RIG-I) and melanoma differentiation antigen 5 (MDA-5) sensors located in the cytosol,[123,284,422] results in a signaling cascade to the nucleus and expression of type I (IFN-α and IFN-β) and type III (IFN-λ1, IFN-λ2, IFN-λ3, and IFN-λ4) interferons that drive ISG gene expression[284,422,661] (Fig. 8.5).

Type III IFN gene expression is dominant in the liver during acute[570,753] and chronic[24,155,551] HCV infection, and in HCV-infected cultured hepatocytes,[312,466,570,753] indicating that IFN-λ proteins are the major driver of hepatic ISG activity. Plasmacytoid and myeloid dendritic cells cocultured with HCV-infected hepatocytes produce type I[164,733] and III[715,827,837] IFN, but their contribution to ISG induction in the infected liver remains to be determined. Several hundred hepatic ISG are up-regulated, some more than 100-fold, within hours or days of HCV infection (Fig. 8.6).[284,422] ISG expression increases sharply in liver and peripheral blood mononuclear cells in parallel with viremia during acute infection.[58,719] The response normalizes after several weeks in spontaneously resolving infections,[643] with a transition to an IFN-γ gene signature that marks the onset of adaptive immune responses.[58,59,156,719,748] Hepatic ISG activity is sustained through the chronic phase of infection in humans[32,113,656] and chimpanzees[59,719] and provides no apparent control of persistent HCV replication (Fig. 8.6). Intensity of hepatic ISG activity is variable between chronically infected individuals.[32,58,113,656,719] High-level ISG expression predicts a poor response to treatment with pegIFN/riba as detailed below.[113,206,294,656]

Type III IFN polymorphisms

Polymorphisms in the *IFNL* gene locus determine the strength of the ISG response in the HCV-infected liver. *IFNL* haplotype and ISG activity are in turn associated with the outcome of acute HCV infection and treatment of chronic hepatitis C with pegIFN/riba.[554] More recent studies demonstrated that viral

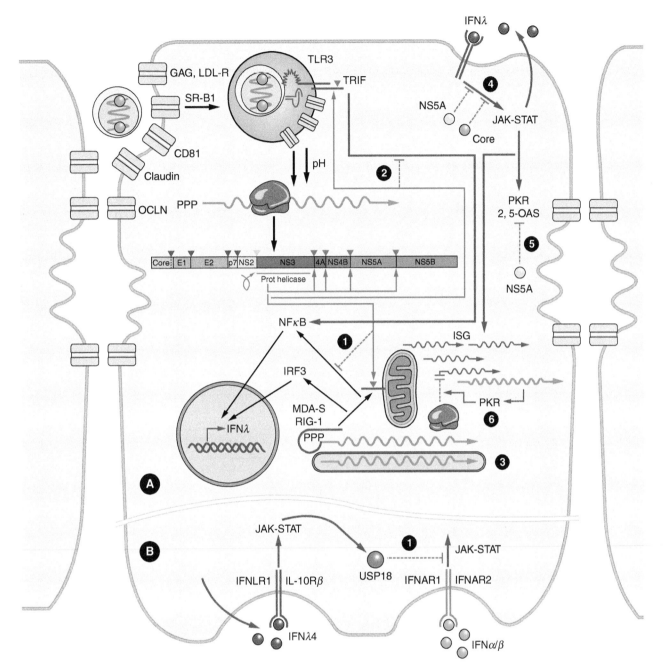

FIGURE 8.5 Interferon responses to hepatitis C virus (HCV) and their evasion by the virus. (A) Cytoplasmic HCV RNA genomes can be sensed by RIG-I and MDA-5 (*1*), resulting in signaling through mitochondrial antiviral signaling protein (MAVS) and subsequent nuclear translocation of nuclear factor (NF)-κB and phosphorylated IRF3 that activate an antiviral program. Signaling through this pathway can induce expression of type I (IFN-α and IFN-β) and type III (IFN-λ1, IFN-λ2, IFN-λ3, and IFN-λ4) interferons (IFN), but only the latter are detected in HCV-infected hepatocytes. HCV NS3-NS4A protease cleaves MAVS to block downstream signaling. (*2*) HCV RNA genomes are sequestered from RIG-I and MDA-5 detection in exosomes, vesicles generated by autophagy or the membranous web where HCV replicates. (*3*) HCV RNA may be sensed in endosomes by toll-like receptor 3 (TLR3), which signals via the adapter molecule TIR domain–containing adapter-inducing interferon-β (TRIF), resulting in nuclear translocation of NF-κB and IFN gene expression; the NS3-NS4A protease cleaves TRIF, interfering with this response. Ectopic expression of HCV proteins in cultured cells can inhibit the (*4*) JAK-STAT pathway that transduces signals from IFN type I and III receptors to the nucleus for interferon-stimulated gene (ISG) expression and (*5*) antiviral activity of induced ISG including protein kinase R (PKR) and 2′,5′-oligoadenylate synthetase (2,5-OAS). HCV RNA in infected hepatocytes activates PKR, impairing cap-dependent translation of antiviral ISG but not IRES-mediated translation of the HCV genome (*6*). (B) IFN-λ4 induced in individuals with the *IFNL4* rs386234815-ΔG polymorphism stimulates a robust and sustained antiviral ISG response including ubiquitin-specific protease 18 (USP18) that impairs JAK-STAT signaling through the type I IFN heterodimeric (IFNAR1/IFNAR2) receptor but not the type III (IFNLR1/IL10R2) receptor. Further details and additional innate responses and evasive mechanisms are described in the text.

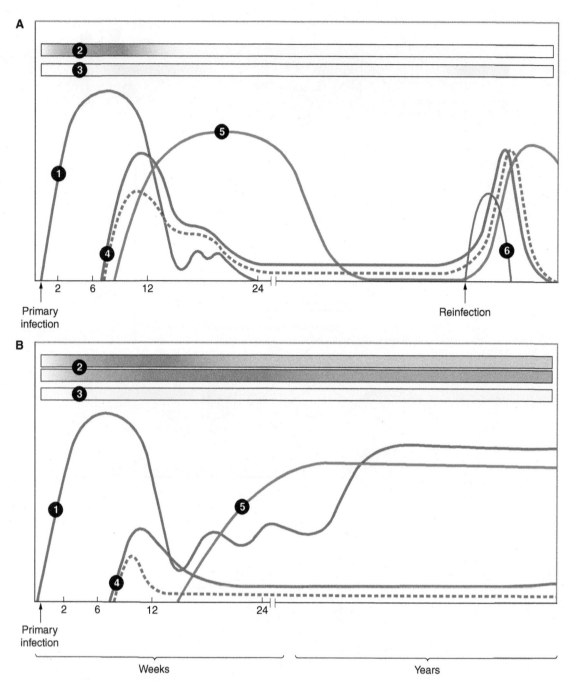

FIGURE 8.6 Profile of HCV replication, liver disease, and immune responses. A: Spontaneous resolution of infection. HCV viremia (*1*) and elevated hepatic interferon-stimulated gene (ISG) activity (*2*) are observed within days of infection. The ISG response closely tracks viremia and normalizes with termination of virus replication. A sharp decline in viremia is typically observed after approximately 8 to 12 weeks of infection and is coincident with elevation of serum aminotransferases and signs and symptoms of hepatitis (*3*). CD4+ (*dashed*) and CD8+ (solid) T-cell (*4*) and neutralizing antibody responses (*5*) are also observed in this time frame. Time to resolution of infection is variable; low, oscillating level viremia can be detected for about 1 year in some cases. ISG expression normalizes after resolution of infection, and adaptive immune responses decline but are rapidly recalled upon reexposure to the virus (*6*). **B:** Persistent infection. Viremia (*1*) typically declines after 8 to 12 weeks of infection, but can remain high with no apparent control in some acute persisting infections (not depicted). Partial control of HCV replication for several months is not uncommon, but high (10^5 to 10^7 RNA genomes/mL serum) stable viremia is characteristic of chronic infection. Hepatic ISG activity remains persistently high in individuals carrying the unfavorable (ΔG) (*2*, bottom bar) versus favorable (TT) (*2*, top bar) *IFNL4* polymorphism rs368234815 (*2*). Signs and symptoms of chronic liver disease are typically evident after years to decades of infection (*3*). T-cell responses fail before resolution of infection (*4*); CD4+ T cells (*dashed line*) lose function and disappear from circulation, and CD8+ T cells gradually exhaust, losing effector functions. Neutralizing antibody responses are delayed when compared with resolving infections but persist at high titer through chronic infection (*5*).

decay kinetics and risk of relapse in DAA-treated patients are also associated with *IFNL* genotype[485,553] (see Treatment section). Two polymorphisms located in *IFNL4* are important from a functional perspective (Fig. 8.7). A compound dinucleotide polymorphism, rs368234815-ΔG or rs368234815-ΔG-TT, located in exon 1 of *IFNL4*, is determinative of gene expression.[612] Frameshifting of the *IFNL4* gene caused by the TT variant results in premature termination and non–sense-mediated RNA decay, while rs368234815-ΔG encodes a full-length 179–amino acid IFN-λ4 protein (Fig. 8.7).[612] Spontaneous clearance of acute HCV infection is much more likely in individuals who carry the loss of function rs368234815-TT allele when compared with those who carry a functional ΔG allele encoding IFN-λ4.[16,612] Hepatic ISG activity is higher in chronically infected patients who carry a rs368234815-ΔG allele, and

the response to pegIFN/riba therapy is poor.[294,377,772] The favorable TT allele is much less common in individuals of African versus European or Asian ancestry, providing an explanation for racial disparities in the response to pegIFN/riba therapy.[612] The second polymorphism, rs117648444 located in exon 2 of the functional *IFNL4* (rs368234815-ΔG) gene, encodes serine (S) or proline (G) at amino acid 70 of IFN-λ4.[612] The IFN-λ4-S70 (rs117648444-A) variant elicits an inferior ISG response in cultured cells when compared with IFN-λ4-P70, perhaps because of reduced protein stability.[744]

Homozygosity for rs117648444-A is associated with lower hepatic ISG levels and an intermediate response to pegIFN/riba therapy (Fig. 8.7).[744] Additional polymorphisms in the *IFNL* locus associated with a positive treatment response[239,727,736] and spontaneous clearance of HCV infection[623,754] were identified

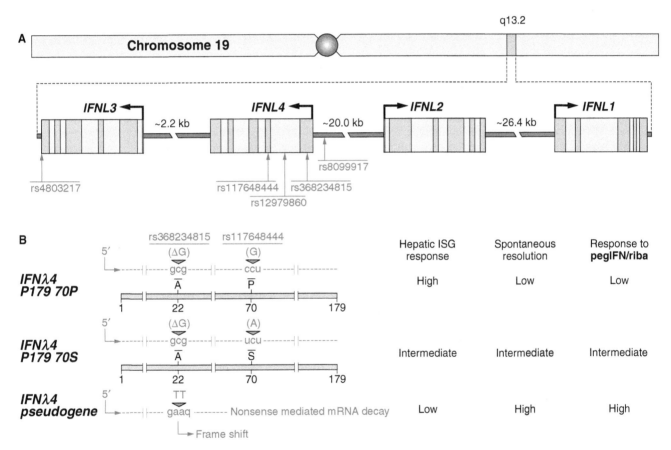

FIGURE 8.7 Influence of type III interferon on HCV infection outcome and treatment. A: Genomic organization and polymorphisms in the type III interferon locus located on human chromosome 19q13. Four genes (*IFNL1*, *IFNL2*, *IFNL3*, and *IFNL4*) express IFN-λ proteins in the indicated orientation. Polymorphisms associated with HCV infection outcome and treatment response are indicated. Polymorphisms rs8099917 (noncoding, upstream of *IFNL4*) and rs12979860 (noncoding, *IFNL4* intron 1) were associated with responsiveness to pegIFN/riba treatment[239,727,736] and infection outcome[623,754] by GWAS analysis. Polymorphisms rs368234815 (coding, *IFNL4* exon 1) and rs117648444 (coding, *IFNL4* exon 2) were identified with discovery of the *IFNL4* gene.[612] These polymorphisms are in strong linkage disequilibrium.[554] Polymorphism rs4803217 is located in a regulatory domain of the *IFNL3* gene. It is in linkage disequilibrium with rs12979860, and gene expression may be modulated by HCV infection.[476] **B:** *IFNL4* polymorphisms and consequences for gene expression and HCV infection and treatment. The *IFNL4* exon 1 polymorphism (rs368234815; ΔG/TT) results in expression of a 179–amino acid IFN-λ4 protein (ΔG) or a frameshifting loss of function variant (TT dinucleotide) that results in a premature stop codon and nonsense-mediated mRNA decay. The polymorphism in *IFNL4* exon 2 (rs117648444; G/A) determines expression of proline (G) or serine (S) at IFN-λ4 position 70. The *IFNL4* rs368234815:rs117648444 haplotype ΔG:G is associated with the highest levels of liver ISG expression and the lowest probability of a positive response to pegIFN/riba therapy and spontaneous clearance of infection. The ΔG:A haplotype is associated with intermediate ISG expression and treatment response or infection outcome. ISG activity is lowest in individuals carrying the rs368234815-TT loss of function variant and associated with higher rates of treatment response and spontaneous clearance of infection.

by genome-wide association studies (GWAS). These polymorphisms have less predictive power, and their association with HCV clearance is explained by strong linkage disequilibrium (LD) with rs368234815-ΔG/ rs368234815-TT.[554] As an example, one SNP (rs12979860-C or rs12979860-T) identified by GWAS is located in intron 1 of *IFNL4*, and the unfavorable variant (rs12979860-C) is almost always inherited with rs368234815-ΔG.[612] One additional polymorphism (rs4803217) is located in a 3′ untranslated region of *IFNL3* (Fig. 8.7).[476] The unfavorable allele is repressed by HCV-induced cellular microRNA species that destabilize or decay *IFNL3* mRNA.[476] The contribution of this mechanism to HCV infection outcome is not yet clear as the polymorphism is in strong linkage disequilibrium with rs12979860.

How expression of IFN-λ4 in individuals carrying the unfavorable rs368234815-ΔG allele impairs spontaneous clearance of acute infection and type I IFN-based antiviral therapy is not understood. IFN-λ4 mRNA is detected in the HCV-infected liver,[24,155] although at low levels perhaps because of posttranscriptional or posttranslational control of gene expression.[296] IFN-λ4 binds to the same heterodimeric (IL-10Rβ/IFNLR1) cellular receptor as other IFN-λ proteins[278] and elicits a robust ISG response in primary human hepatocytes.[193,396,477,552] One notable feature of the ISG response is strong induction of negative regulatory factors including ubiquitin-specific protease 18 (USP18). USP18 blocks type I IFN signaling through the IFNAR1/IFNAR2 receptor,[193,552,724,725] but has no impact on type III IFN signaling through the IL-10Rβ/IFNLR1 receptor.[65] Silencing of USP18 expression in IFN-λ4–treated hepatocytes restores type I IFN signaling,[193,725] suggesting a role for negative regulatory mechanisms in the poor responsiveness to pegIFN/riba therapy. Consistent with this possibility, USP18 is selectively up-regulated in the liver of chronically infected patients with a preactivated ISG response associated with the rs386234815-ΔG haplotype.[113,156,552]

Constitutive ISG activity in the liver of persistently infected patients normalizes with initiation of DAA treatment.[17,86,99,620] These observations provide additional evidence that strong ISG activity in the chronically infected liver is driven directly by HCV replication. As noted above, unfavorable *IFNL* haplotypes are associated with a slower early decay in viremia during DAA treatment[485] and an increased risk of relapse.[553] Whether *IFNL* haplotype influences the timing or magnitude of ISG recovery, with effects on HCV decay and clearance during DAA treatment, remains to be determined. Intriguingly, two studies have demonstrated that an unfavorable *IFNL4* haplotype may exert pressure against HCV, selecting for amino acid substitutions in the HCV NS5A protein that could potentially facilitate virus replication in an environment of strong ISG activity or affect susceptibility to DAA inhibitors.[27,826]

Evasion of the type I/III IFN responses

ISG induced by HCV infection have the potential to interfere with every stage of the viral replication cycle, including entry, replication, and release.[494,495,662,663,839] Viral evasion mechanisms that subvert the innate antiviral response were investigated by ectopic expression of individual HCV proteins in transformed cells lines and with replicons and HCV isolates adapted for replication in hepatocyte cell lines (Fig. 8.5).[169,422] More recently, mice repopulated with human hepatocytes have been infected with genetically modified HCV isolates to demonstrate the

importance of viral proteins like NS5A in evasion of the interferon response.[289] Although these approaches have limitations, they suggest the possibility of a multilayered defense against antiviral effector mechanisms. Failure of cellular sensors to detect HCV RNA is a potential first line of defense. Consistent with this possibility, cytosolic receptors are excluded from the membranous web of rearranged cytoplasmic vesicles where HCV replicative intermediates are generated.[546] HCV RNA is also sequestered in DMV produced by autophagy[209] and in extracellular vesicles that are exported from cells via a pathway that bypasses the endosome and TLR3 detection (Fig. 8.5).[263] Blockade of signaling pathways downstream of the TLR and RLR receptors HCV proteins provides an additional defensive layer.[169,422] The NS3/4A protease targets the adaptor proteins MAVS[426,500] and TRIF[419] for cleavage in infected cells, effectively blocking ISG responses. TRIF may also be degraded by HCV NS4B through a caspase 8–dependent mechanism.[428] Reduced stability of transcripts encoding IFN-λ2 and IFN-λ3[476] or the type I IFN receptor[320] by microRNAs induced in hepatocytes by HCV has been described. Signaling from the type I and III IFN receptors through the JAK-STAT pathway may also be blocked by HCV proteins E2 and NS5A when expressed in cell lines.[169,422] HCV infection may also alter activation of the ISG PKR. On one hand, NS5A protein expressed in cultured cells and in transgenic mice bound to PKR and prevented activation of its antiviral ISG activity (Fig. 8.5).[229,381] However, it was also reported that HCV activates PKR to block cap-dependent translation of host effector ISG proteins,[31,234] an evasion mechanism that would not impair IRES-mediated translation of the HCV genome (Fig. 8.5). It is possible that blockade of PKR activation in the early stage of infection during initial translation of the RNA genome is advantageous for replication. A transition to PKR activation at a later stage in the replication cycle would impair translation of antiviral ISG effector proteins and perhaps provide an explanation for the paradoxical coexpression of HCV RNA genomes and ISG mRNA in infected hepatocytes.[808] Finally, NS4A-mediated MAVS cleavage has been visualized *in situ* in infected hepatocytes, suggesting that this evasion mechanism is active in the liver.[419,500] Whether other evasion mechanisms defined in cell culture models contribute to evasion of innate immune responses or persistence of HCV remains to be established. Sustained HCV replication through the acute and chronic phases of infection, especially in subjects with high constitutive ISG activity associated with rs368234815-ΔG and related polymorphisms, cannot be fully explained by these models. Molecular mechanisms that contribute to evasion of the response may require a more detailed understanding of ISG activity in the membranous web where HCV genome replication and assembly occur (see Chapter 7). Differences in ISG kinetics, susceptibility to negative regulation, and the hepatic antiviral environment induced by one or more of the IFN-λ proteins are also likely to be important factors in understanding why innate IFN responses are ineffective at HCV control.[65,68,327,552,680]

NK cell responses and HCV evasion

NK cells with enhanced cytotoxic activity and production of antiviral cytokines are detected in blood during the acute hepatitis C.[23,370,575] NK cell activation is driven by direct binding of cytokines like type I IFN and IL-12 that are produced as part of the strong acute phase ISG response elicited by HCV.

Monocytes also contribute to NK cell activation during acute hepatitis C through inflammasome-dependent secretion of IL-18.[677] NK cell mediated suppression of HCV replication through killing of infected hepatocytes and production of IFN-γ and TNF-α that provide noncytolytic control of HCV replication was documented in cell culture models.[370,380,385,712] Their role in providing complete or partial control of HCV replication in patients with acute HCV infection is uncertain. This analysis has been hampered by limited access to the liver, where NK cells constitute one-third to one-half of all intrahepatic lymphocytes.[385] The timing and strength of the circulating NK- and HCV-specific T-cell responses appear to be linked in individuals with a robust pattern of acute phase HCV replication.[23,370,575] It is therefore difficult to separate the relative contribution of these innate and adaptive populations to virus control.[23,370,575] NK cell activation also occurs in individuals exposed to very low HCV inocula through intravenous drug use or occupational needlestick injuries. Indeed, NK activation may be a very sensitive marker of exposure to HCV as it has been observed in cases where virus inoculum was low and there was no virologic evidence of infection. NK cells might contribute to an abortive or highly attenuated course of HCV infection in this setting. In support of this possibility, immunogenetic studies revealed that homozygosity for genes encoding the inhibitory KIR2DL3 receptor on NK cells and the HLA-C1 ligand on target cells increased the probability of spontaneous resolution of HCV infection.[356,751] The effect of this compound genotype on infection outcome was most apparent in injection drug users[246,356,720,751] and in cases of needlestick injury,[805] where a lower NK cell activation threshold may be advantageous in rapidly containing infections established with a low HCV inoculum. Other host factors may also regulate NK cell function in acute hepatitis C. For example, acute phase NK cell effector functions were enhanced in individuals with *IFNL* genotypes that favor virus control.[151] Because NK cells lack type III IFN receptors,[151,522] any effect of this cytokine family on activation or effector function must be indirect.

Chronic HCV infection has a pervasive effect on the NK cell compartment. Circulating NK cells are clearly activated in the chronic phase of infection as assessed by enhanced expression of HLA-DR, CD69, and multiple NK cytotoxicity receptors.[633] They are also skewed toward cytotoxic activity with decreased production of IFN-γ and TNF-α.[13,284,518,557,633,675] The repertoire of inhibitory and activating NK receptors is also altered in chronic infection.[718] NK cell activation and polarization toward cytotoxicity in the chronic phase of infection most likely reflect continuous stimulation by innate cytokines. Type I IFN is likely a key driver of this NK cell phenotype in chronic hepatitis C.[171,510] This mechanism is supported by the observation that the STAT1, an ISG that is essential for signaling and induced by type I IFN stimulation, is increased in NK cells from patients with chronic hepatitis C.[171,510] As with ISG responses,[17,86,99,620] NK cell function and responsiveness to type I IFN therapy are normalized by successful DAA therapy,[675,676] although alterations to the NK receptor repertoire imposed by chronic HCV infection are more durable and perhaps not reversible.[718]

Mechanisms to subvert NK cell effector function and recognition of HCV-infected target cells have been identified using cell culture models. Expression of class I HLA-C and HLA-E molecules, which are ligands for inhibitory NK cell receptors,

may be stabilized on the surface of infected hepatocytes by peptides derived from structural and nonstructural HCV proteins.[445,532,538] A direct inhibitory effect of HCV-infected cell lines, virions, and recombinant proteins on cultured NK cells has also been described.[136,633,765,820,824] HCV virions and component proteins could act by altering NK signaling or function, for instance, through cross-linking of cellular receptors,[136,765] but relevance of the mechanisms to evasion of the response in the liver remains to be established.

Cellular Immune Responses

Circulating HCV-specific CD4+ helper and CD8+ cytotoxic T cells are detected approximately 8 to 12 weeks after infection in humans and experimentally infected chimpanzees (Fig. 8.6).[129,410,506,689,748,749] The initial delay in generating a T-cell response, which is not yet explained, is a feature of most acute infections regardless of whether they resolve or persist. In overview, onset of the response is kinetically associated with a sharp decline in viremia and in some individuals with acute hepatitis (Fig. 8.6).[7,129,293,410,506,689,748,749] Resolution of acute infection requires a multifunctional CD4+[154,240,444,666,673] and CD8+[132,261,409] T-cell response that is sustained until after termination of HCV replication; premature loss of functional CD4+ T cell help is highly predictive of a persistent outcome.[7,293] Durable CD4+ and CD8+ T-cell memory is generated in humans and chimpanzees with infections that spontaneously resolve.[6,7,293,559,689,735] Reinfection elicits an accelerated memory T-cell response that is temporally associated with a sharply reduced duration and magnitude of viremia and a decreased risk of a persistent outcome when compared with primary HCV infection in humans[15,259,484,559] and chimpanzees (Fig. 8.6).[48,256,455,536,689] Antibody-mediated depletion of CD4+ helper[256] or CD8+ cytotoxic cells[689] from chimpanzees with naturally acquired immunity to HCV resulted in prolonged or persistent infection after rechallenge with the virus. Collectively, these observations provide a strong argument that sustained HCV-specific T-cell immunity is critical for spontaneous resolution of acute primary infections and secondary infections in immune individuals who are reexposed to the virus.

T-cell immunity in acute resolving and persisting infections

At least three functionally distinct HCV-specific CD4+ T-cell populations that provide help for CD8+ T-cell or B-cell responses are detected in blood during acute resolving infection. Help for the CD8+ T-cell response is provided by HCV-specific CD4+ T helper 1 (Th1)[221,673,770] and T helper 17 (Th17)[339] populations. A sustained response by CD4+ T cells that produce the signature Th1 cytokine IL-2 is associated with functional antiviral CD8+ T-cell immunity and resolution of HCV infection.[221,673,770] HCV-specific Th17 CD4+ T cells that produce IL-21, a cytokine that also supports development of effector CD8+ T-cell responses, are primed during acute infection.[339] Elevated serum IL-21 titers are associated with stronger circulating CD8+ T-cell responses and resolution of acute HCV infection.[339] Antiviral CD4+ T cells with a T follicular helper (Tfh) phenotype are also visualized in blood during acute HCV infection.[629] This response, which directs germinal center formation that is essential for humoral immunity, was associated with development of HCV-specific antibodies.[629] Premature loss of the CD4+ T-cell response is a defining feature of acute infections that persist.[215,221,506,705,774,813] Breadth of the response, defined by the number of HLA class II epitopes targeted by circulating CD4+ T cells, is not necessarily a determinant of infection outcome.[666] Approximately 10 class II epitopes (range 2–26) located predominately in NS proteins (particularly NS3 and NS4) were detected in the early phase of acute resolving infection, and this pattern was not significantly different in time-matched samples from infections that persisted.[666] HCV antigen–driven proliferation and cytokine production by early acute phase CD4+ T cells are, however, comparatively poor in infections that persist.[7,293,666] Failure of the response is marked by a progressive decline in CD4+ T-cell frequencies and a narrowing repertoire of targeted HCV epitopes.[132,143,409,666]

CD8+ T cells are multifunctional in infections that resolve. They degranulate, indicating the potential for cytotoxic killing of infected hepatocytes, and produce antiviral cytokines like IFN-γ and TNF-α.[132,262,338,506,749,774] The response is also considered broad, targeting on average 9 to 10 epitopes localized mostly to NS proteins but with no obvious pattern of dominance.[397,399,706] CD8+ T cells in acute resolving infections follow a typical pattern of differentiation with transient expression of programmed cell death 1 (PD-1), a marker of T-cell activation during acute infection,[342,685] transcription factor T-bet (T-box expressed in T cells) that regulates effector functions,[389] and the antiapoptotic transcription factor BCL-2.[685] With resolution of infection, CD8+ T cells gain expression of CD127, a component of the IL-7 receptor that facilitates homeostatic proliferation required for maintenance of the memory response.[672,685,749,774] Progressive loss of CD8+ T-cell function, including HCV antigen–driven proliferation, cytotoxic activity, and production of antiviral cytokines, leads to transient and incomplete control of HCV replication.[132,262,338,506,749,774] Circulating CD8+ T cells can target multiple class I epitopes in the early phase of acute infection, but the repertoire typically narrows as persistence is established.[132,253,398,409] Intrahepatic CD8+ T cells do persist in the chronically infected liver, and the response is multispecific in some humans and chimpanzees.[254,379,499,544]

Evasion of T-cell immunity

CD4+ T-cell failure compromises CD8+ T-cell and B-cell responses, but the cause is unknown. CD4+ T-cell proliferation and cytokine production are impaired by HCV core protein binding to the cellular C1qR complement receptor[362] and HCV RNA genome binding to toll-like receptor 7 (TLR7).[486] All CD4+ T cells express C1qR and TLR7, however, and so these mechanisms are difficult to reconcile with a defect that is HCV specific. Host genetics may be a factor. Certain HLA class II alleles have been associated with spontaneous clearance (for instance, *HLA-DQB1*03:01, DRB1*01:01, DRB1*03:01,* and *HLA-DRB1*11:01*) or persistence (*DQB1*02:01*) of HCV infection.[167,238,280,503,750,790] There is as yet no clear evidence that the encoded class II molecules present dominant HCV epitopes that are more or less protective against persistence. Mutational escape in HCV class II epitopes driven by CD4+ T-cell selection pressure appears to be uncommon. Nonsynonymous polymorphisms in the HCV genome have been associated with shared class II HLA haplotypes in populations of chronically infected humans.[443] While these HLA-related polymorphisms in the viral genome are consistent with CD4+ T-cell selection pressure, emergence of escape mutations in known dominant class II epitopes is difficult to discern in individual

humans[213,577,666] and chimpanzees,[228] especially when compared with the very visible evidence of HCV evolution in epitopes targeted by CD8+ T cells and antibodies as described below. A mechanism by which CD4+ T cells exert direct selection pressure against HCV, for example, by cytolysis of virus-infected hepatocytes, has not yet been described. Many HCV-specific CD4+ T-cell populations detected in blood during the early acute phase of persisting infections drop below the threshold for detection. It is possible that they are deleted from the CD4+ T-cell repertoire, but localization of some populations to the chronically infected liver cannot be excluded.[577] HCV-specific CD4+ T cells that circulate in the chronic phase of infection express multiple inhibitory receptors, including PD-1, CTLA-4, CD305, and CD200R.[630] Th1 and Th17 helper function has been restored by antibody-mediated blockade of inhibitory receptor signaling in cell culture models.[339,630,776] Nonetheless, it is not yet clear if this mechanism fully explains functional silencing of CD4+ T cells. Other suppressive pathways may be operational, including T regulatory (Treg) activity that acts through production-suppressive cytokines like IL-10 and TGF-β.[630]

HCV-specific CD8+ T cells are maintained in the chronically infected liver for decades but provide no apparent control of persistent virus replication. Direct viral interference with antigen-processing machinery or class I MHC expression could protect infected hepatocytes from CD8+ T-cell recognition as demonstrated in cell culture models.[336,358] Enhanced regulatory T-cell activity during the acute and chronic phases of infection could also suppress CD8+ T-cell proliferation and effector functions,[67,89,339,721] but an association with infection outcome has not been observed. As detailed below, evasion of the CD8+ T-cell response in chronically infected humans and chimpanzees occurs by (a) mutational escape of HCV class I epitopes and (b) functional exhaustion.

Mutational escape of class I HCV epitopes occurs in humans[84,133,747,756,758] and chimpanzees[180] who develop chronic infections. Multiple cross-sectional studies have also demonstrated enrichment of amino acid changes in predicted or confirmed class I epitopes among chronically infected individuals with who share HLA alleles.[212,237,394,625,647,757] Approximately 25% to 50% of class I epitopes in the dominant NS proteins acquire escape mutations, although this frequency is variable between individuals and studies.[132,387,489,647,758] Escape mutations are a consequence of CD8+ T-cell selection pressure as the rate of nonsynonymous mutation is significantly higher in class I restricted epitopes when compared with the remainder of the HCV genome.[84,94,180,387,589] The rate of mutation within class I epitopes slows as persistence is established.[67,94,133,208,387] This is consistent with stability of class I escape mutations over years of persistent HCV replication.[647,654,769] Mutation of intact epitopes during chronic infection has been described but is uncommon.[133,794] Failure to generate an effective CD8+ T-cell response against a class I escape variant may be due in some instances to a gap in the human T-cell repertoire.[812] In most cases, however, it almost certainly reflects impaired generation of new mutant-specific CD8+ T cells in an environment of inadequate HCV-specific CD4+ T-cell help and high antigen load. From a functional perspective, escape mutations within epitopes can impair class I MHC binding[133,756] or CD8+ T-cell receptor recognition.[758,812] Mutations in sequences adjacent to or within an epitope can also alter proteasome processing of the HCV polyprotein, resulting in epitope destruction.[360,671,797] Replicative fitness of HCV can be impaired by escape mutations.[144,654,769] An iterative process of amino acid replacement to efficiently balance replication and escape from CD8+ T-cell recognition can occur in the acute phase of infection while the epitope is still under selection pressure.[769] Impaired replication during the chronic phase of infection can also be offset by compensatory mutations that are sometimes distant from the epitope that contains an escape mutation.[212,548,558] Mutational escape of epitopes may spare cognate CD8+ T cells from a complete loss of function. They maintain the ability to proliferate in response to antigen stimulation, and expression of CD127 indicates a status that more closely resembles memory than exhaustion.[341,648] Effector function is sufficient to maintain selection pressure against some escaped epitopes in the chronic phase of infection.[295,756,832] As an example, reversion of HCV escape mutations was observed in chronically infected women during pregnancy, a setting where immune function is transiently attenuated.[295] Escape mutations were reacquired in the postpartum period with transient resurgence of a functional HCV-specific T-cell response.[295]

Class I epitopes that remain intact induce a more profound state of CD8+ T-cell exhaustion when compared with escaped epitopes.[51,341,648,773] A transcriptional signature characteristic of exhaustion is evident in the early acute phase of infection (Fig. 8.8). Using integrative systems analysis, coordinated expression and rapid down-regulation of gene modules associated with metabolic function were observed in HCV-specific CD8+ T cells from patients with acute persisting but not resolving infections.[813] An early but transient transcriptional burst related to oxidative phosphorylation occurred within the first 12 to 18 weeks of infection and was linked to a pervasive effect on gene modules associated with nucleosomal regulation of transcription and T-cell differentiation and inflammatory pathways (Fig. 8.8). The unfavorable pattern of metabolic gene transcription in CD8+ T cells was also associated with loss of HCV-specific CD4+ T helper cells from circulation.[813] The exhausted phenotype in chronic infection is defined by low or no CD127 and sustained expression of PD-1 and other inhibitory receptors including cytotoxic T lymphocyte–associated antigen 4 (CTLA-4), T-cell immunoglobulin- and mucin-domain-containing molecule 3 (TIM-3), the NK receptor 2B4.[51,247,341,342,482,534,563,617,618,648,773,774]

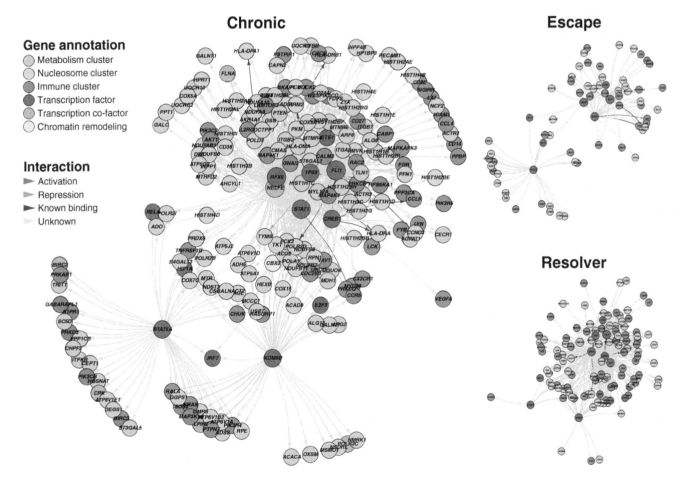

FIGURE 8.8 Transcriptional analysis of HCV-specific CD8+ T cells in acute resolving and persisting HCV infection. Transcriptional activity was compared in HCV-specific CD8 T cells isolated at different time points from patients with resolving (resolver) and persisting HCV infections.[813] CD8+ T cells from chronically infected patients were further subclassified as (chronic) if they recognized intact class I HCV epitopes or escaped if they did not receive TCR signal due to viral escape mutations. A transcriptional network constructed from a weighted gene coexpression network analysis (WGCNA) is shown.[813] Dysregulated gene modules identified in the chronic but not resolver or escaped CD8+ T-cell populations were related to cell metabolism (most notably oxidative phosphorylation), nucleosomal regulation, and known immune response functions. Dysregulated gene modules were connected by coregulated transcription factors, demonstrating that the path to T-cell exhaustion is most likely an integrated process affecting different molecular pathways simultaneously and in a coordinated manner. (From Wolski, Foote, Chen, et. al. Early transcriptional divergence marks virus-specific primary human CD8(+) T cells in chronic versus acute infection. *Immunity* 2017; 47(4):648, with permission.)

These CD8+ T cells also express eomesodermin (Eomes),[568] a transcription factor associated with exhaustion, and chromatin structure is more open at exhaustion regions than memory regions of the CD8+ T-cell genome.[674] Terminally differentiated CD8+ T cells are enriched in the chronically infected liver and programmed for death.[384,617–619] Of note, exhausted CD8+ T cells are continuously replenished from a pool of self-renewing HCV-specific CD8+ T cells that are defined by expression of the CD127 memory marker and the transcription factor T-cell factor 1 (TCF1) that is important in formation and maintenance of immunological memory.[807]

Function can be restored to exhausted HCV-specific CD8+ T cells in culture models by antibody-mediated blockade of PD-1 signaling.[247,578,617,775] Anti–PD-1 antibodies have also been administered to persistently infected humans and chimpanzees. A greater than 4 log reduction in viremia was observed in 15% of subjects (3/20) who received the highest dose of a fully humanized IgG4 anti–PD-1 monoclonal antibody with no serious side effects.[236] By comparison, HCV viremia rarely varies by more than 0.5 log in the chronic phase of infection. An apparent cure of chronic HCV infection was achieved in one subject with an unfavorable *IFNL4* genotype who had previously failed type I IFN therapy.[236] Recovery of HCV-specific T-cell function was not assessed in these patients. Transient reduction of viremia and restoration of functional HCV-specific CD4+ and CD8+ T-cell immunity were also observed in one of three persistently infected chimpanzees treated with a humanized anti–PD-1 monoclonal antibody.[227] These studies provide direct evidence that signaling through coinhibitory receptor(s) contributes to CD8+ T-cell exhaustion in chronic hepatitis C. Failure of most treated individuals to respond to PD-1 blockade cannot yet be explained. Cell culture models have demonstrated that restoration of T-cell function may require blockade of additional inhibitory receptors like CTLA-4 or TIM-3.[482,533,563] Restoration of function to exhausted HCV-specific CD8+ T cells in cell culture may also be highly individualized as no clear hierarchy or dominance of inhibitory receptor usage has been observed.[563] Finally, anti–PD-1 antibodies probably act on the small pool of self-renewing CD8+ T cells[807] that are the source of exhausted, terminally differentiated CD8+ T cells. Success of inhibitory receptor blockade may depend on the size of the self-renewing pool, the repertoire of HCV epitopes they target, and the capacity of blocking antibodies to promote effector activity instead of exhaustion.

Recovery of T-cell immunity after antiviral therapy

T-cell immunity does not recover after successful treatment of chronic hepatitis C with pegIFN/riba.[5,7,293,507] DAA cure of infection leads to partial recovery of CD8+ T-cell effector function.[460,807] Termination of persistent HCV replication leads to loss of exhausted CD8+ T cells. CD8+ T cells that survive after DAA cure are derived from the TCF1+ memory-like population. They proliferate after stimulation with escaped and intact epitopes, indicating that even the most profoundly exhausted populations can recover from this self-renewing progenitor population.[460] Production of IFN-γ and TNF-α was weak, however, especially when compared with memory CD8+ T cells generated by resolution of acute infection.[807] To date, there have been few studies to assess the capacity of CD8+ T

cells to control virus replication in a post-DAA setting. The question is of practical importance as reinfection after DAA cure has been documented.[461–463,501,592,665] In one study, 15/77 participants were reinfected at 18 months posttreatment, yielding a reinfection rate of 21.5/100 person-years, close to a recent estimated rate of HCV incidence among recent injectors (past 6 months) in the same community.[665]

Relapse of HCV replication in one subject 12 weeks after termination of DAA therapy resulted in expansion of memory-like TCF1+ CD8+ T cells that reacquired an exhausted phenotype as persistent infection was reestablished. In a second case study, CD8+ T cells targeting intact and escaped class I epitopes persisted in a chimpanzee for 2 years after DAA cure but failed to prevent a second chronic infection after experimental HCV rechallenge.[95] In summary, these early studies indicate that T-cell exhaustion is a pervasive and persistent mechanism of immune evasion that may be partially but not completely reversed after DAA cure.

Humoral Immune Response

The HCV E1 and E2 envelope glycoproteins elicit an acute phase antibody response in all infected humans with normal immune function, regardless of whether the infection resolves or persists. Seroconversion measured by E1 and E2 antibody-binding assays occurs several weeks to months after infection,[115,545] a delay that may reflect the slow onset of CD4+ T-cell help during acute hepatitis C (Fig. 8.6) (discussed in Cellular Immune Response). Anti-E1 and anti-E2 antibodies persist for life in infections that become chronic.[545] Antibody titers decline after spontaneous resolution of infection in individuals without ongoing exposure to HCV (Fig. 8.6).[373,513,670,735] Seroreversion occurs over a period of years in a subset of these cases,[373,670,735] as illustrated by a single-source HCV transmission accident in the former East Germany, where HCV-specific T cells but not antibodies were detected in about 40% of subjects 18 to 20 years after spontaneous recovery from acute hepatitis C.[735] Reinfection can occur in humans[259,484] and chimpanzees[48,195,609] after spontaneous resolution of acute hepatitis C (Fig. 8.6), indicating that antibody-mediated sterilizing protection is uncommon, if it occurs at all.

Neutralizing function of serum antibodies is assessed using hepatitis C virus pseudoparticles (HCVpp) bearing HCV E1 and E2 envelope glycoproteins[47,300] and hepatitis C virus cell culture (HCVcc) adapted viruses[796] that facilitate analysis of the kinetic, titer, and breadth of the response. HCV E1 and E2 sequence diversity, which ranges from approximately 30% between genotypes to 10% between subtypes,[701] is an important consideration in measuring neutralizing responses. Further complexity is observed within individuals, where HCV circulates as an evolving swarm of distinct strains that may differ in susceptibility to antibody neutralization.[194,459] Because E1 and E2 sequences vary and can evolve rapidly during acute infection, neutralizing antibody activity within HCV-infected individuals is measured against HCVpp bearing E1 and E2 glycoproteins from cocirculating (i.e., autologous) viruses. Neutralizing antibodies are not necessarily required for control of acute phase virus replication; spontaneous resolution can occur in cases of primary immune deficiency affecting B-cell development[10] and in chimpanzees where seroconversion is often not observed at the time of virus control.[49] These are exceptional circumstances, however, and accumulating evidence is consistent with a role for neutralizing antibodies in limiting HCV replication and spread in the liver. Antibodies that neutralize HCVpp infectivity appear at about the time of seroconversion,[163,401,585] and an early and broad response has been associated with spontaneous clearance of acute infection.[36,184,560,585] Single-source outbreaks of HCV infection have provided important insight into the acute phase neutralizing antibody response.[401,585] As an example, control of acute hepatitis was associated with rapid induction of neutralizing antibodies against the infecting virus in pregnant women treated with anti-D immunoglobulins contaminated with a single HCV strain.[585] Neutralizing antibody responses were absent or of low titer in subjects following a chronic course.[585] Antibody responses that broadly neutralize infectivity of HCVpp bearing multiple, diverse genotype 1 envelope glycoproteins are also associated with resolution of acute primary infection.[560] Rapid recall of broadly neutralizing antibodies may also contribute to the much shorter duration and magnitude of viremia, and decreased likelihood of HCV persistence, in individuals who are reexposed to the virus after spontaneous clearance of infection (Fig. 8.6).[559]

Patterns of antibody neutralization against genetically diverse E1 and E2 species were defined using HCVpp and HCVcc panels representative of different genotypes and subtypes. These studies revealed that HCV genotypes and subtypes do not correspond to neutralization serotypes.[560,740] Sensitivity to neutralization instead varies widely for isolates within HCV genotypes and subtypes, as determined with HCVpp panels that encompass most of the known global diversity of HCV genotype 1 envelope sequences.[37,98,777] Mechanistic insight into antibody-mediated neutralization has advanced with resolution of the HCV E2 ectodomain structure by x-ray crystallography[357,375] and development of murine and recombinant human monoclonal antibodies against E1 and E2.[36,78,244,329,353,498,561,562,581] Neutralizing epitopes map to the E1 and E2 glycoproteins and the E1/E2 complex that is cross-linked on the virion surface.[352,767,792] Neutralizing responses against E1 and the E1/E2 complex are the least well characterized. Two epitopes have been defined in E1,[332,349,498] including one that is recognized by monoclonal antibodies that neutralize several HCV genotypes.[498] Conservation of this epitope sequence across several genotypes indicates that E1 has an important but still undefined role in the HCV entry process. E2 is the dominant target of antibodies that neutralize HCV entry at a post-attachment step.[652,791] This heavily glycosylated and compact globular structure is composed of β-strands and random coils flanked by two small α-helices.[357,375] It binds at least two entry receptors on hepatocytes, the CD81 tetraspanin and the high-density lipoprotein receptor scavenger receptor class B type I (SR-BI) (see Fig. 8.3).[101] The neutralizing antibody response is directed predominately against epitope clusters on the exposed surface of E2 (Fig. 8.9). The clusters localize to the conserved neutralizing face of E2 and hypervariable region 1 (HVR1; aa 384–410). HVR1 is functionally important for HCV entry as it guides or modulates E2 interaction with the SR-B1 cellular receptor,[606] but is under few structural constraints and readily tolerant of amino acid substitutions. Neutralizing antibodies directed against HVR1 are often isolate or strain specific and exert selection pressure leading to emergence of escape variants.[163,198,395] Broadly neutralizing antibodies recognize epitopes

in the conserved, mostly hydrophobic neutralizing face of E2 that is essential for CD81 binding (Fig. 8.9).[36,329,561,562,581] The neutralizing face is composed predominately of the E2 front layer (amino acids 421–459) and CD81 binding loop (amino acids 519–535), structures that are highly flexible[376] and not obstructed by glycans. Epitopes within the neutralizing face localize to three overlapping or adjacent clusters that are essential for CD81 binding, as determined by mapping with murine and recombinant human monoclonal antibodies that cross-neutralize viruses from different HCV genotypes (Fig. 8.9). One cluster, designated antigenic site 412 (AS412) or domain E, spans amino acids 412 to 423 immediately downstream of HVR1.[352,767] Immunogenicity of the AS412 E2 region is poor in natural infection, as broadly neutralizing antibodies are detected in only 2% to 15% of infected humans.[351,739,741] The other two epitope clusters within the neutralization face are composed of amino acids in the E2 front layer (aa 434–446, designated AS434 or domain D) and discontinuous amino acids from the front layer (aa 426–443) and CD81 binding loop (aa 529–531) (designated antigen region 3, AR3) brought together by the overall fold of the E2 protein (Fig. 8.9).[352,767] Passive transfer of broadly neutralizing monoclonal antibodies targeting epitopes in AS412,[152] AS434,[350] and AR3[244,404] protected humanized mice from challenge with HCV, including a complex quasispecies in one study.[404] Termination of an established infection in a humanized mouse was also observed after infusion of monoclonal antibodies against AR3 epitopes.[146] Broadly neutralizing monoclonal antibodies targeting conserved AS412 epitopes in the neutralizing face also prevented or modified the course of HCV infection in chimpanzees and humans.[124,517,702]

Common features of broadly neutralizing human monoclonal antibodies that recognize epitopes in the E2 neutralizing face have emerged. Those targeting the AS434 and AR3 epitopes utilize immunoglobulin heavy chains with a V_H1-69 encoded variable segment.[36,490] A detailed analysis of monoclonal antibodies from two subjects who spontaneously cleared HCV infection suggests that antibody genes contain few somatic mutations, but those that do appear are important for efficient neutralization of the cocirculating HCV quasispecies swarm late in acute infection.[36,361] Of note, broadly neutralizing antibodies with these features also appear in individuals with chronic hepatitis C.[352,767] It is likely that they appear too late in the course of acute infection to limit virus replication, but differences in their physical interaction with conserved epitopes in highly flexible E2 structures can't be excluded.

HVR1 is susceptible to selection pressure by neutralizing antibodies because of its highly flexible structure and tolerance of amino acid substitutions (Fig. 8.10).[344,738,802] Timing of the first appearance of antibody-driven mutations first appears in HVR1, and the consequence for infection outcome may depend on the kinetics and breadth of the acute phase neutralizing response.[163,198,395] An early, rapid pace of nonsynonymous mutation in HVR1 is associated with spontaneous resolution of infection[437] and marks the coincident onset of a broadly neutralizing antibody response targeting HVR1 and epitopes in the conserved neutralizing face of E2 that are constrained from mutation.[163,361,560,585]

Onset of the neutralizing antibody response and HVR1 diversification is typically delayed in acute infections that persist.[300,440,496,585,713] The pace of HVR1 diversification accelerates

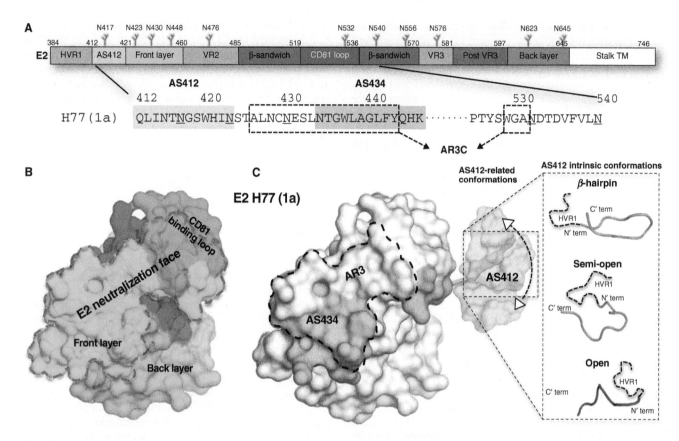

FIGURE 8.9 The HCV E2 neutralizing face and localization of epitopes. The x-ray crystallographic structure of an HCV genotype 1a (H77) E2 envelope glycoprotein complexed with an antibody against the AR3 region. **A:** E2 ectodomain schematic (aa 384–746, based on the prototypic isolate H77 numbering). Structural components including variable regions (*gray*), AS412 (domain E) (*pink*), front layer (*cyan*), β-sandwich (*red*), CD81 binding loop (*blue*), back layer (*green*), and the stalk and transmembrane regions (*white*) are shown. The AS412, antigenic region 3 (AR3), and AS434 neutralization epitopes are marked in *pink*, *dashed rectangle*, and wheat. The N-linked glycosylation sites surrounding the neutralizing face (N417, N423, N430, N532, and N540) are underlined. **B:** Surface representation of the E2 structure[375] with the structural components colored as in (**A**). The neutralizing face is marked by a *red dashed line*. **C:** Neutralizing epitopes on the E2 structure. The conformational flexibility of AS412[376] related to E2 is schematically shown. The three known AS412 conformations (β-hairpin, semiopen, and open) for neutralization are shown on the right. (From Tzarum N, Wilson IA, Law M. The neutralizing face of hepatitis C virus E2 envelope glycoprotein. *Front Immunol* 2018;9:1315, with permission.)

with the transition to chronic infection.[436] Nonsynonymous mutation continues through the chronic phase of infection and provides escape from neutralization[46,440,496,794] as illustrated by longitudinal study of a patient through 25 years of acute and chronic infection.[794] Narrowly focused acute phase neutralizing activity broadened significantly in chronic infection to neutralize distant genotypes and autologous viruses present at earlier acute and chronic time points. Serum antibodies did not, however, neutralize contemporaneous viruses, and resistance was associated with ongoing nonsynonymous mutation within HVR1.[794] Escape mutations do occur in conserved epitopes of the neutralization face, but appear to be uncommon[559,639] and can impair HCV fitness because of their proximity to CD81 binding residues.[348,361] As an example, accumulation of polymorphisms in the E2 front region and VR2 caused a partial resistance to early, broadly neutralizing antibodies targeting the conserved AR3 region.[361] Resolution of acute HCV infection was associated with reduced E2 binding affinity for CD81 and SR-B1 and progressive loss of HCV replicative fitness.[361]

Extraepitopic mutations can also impair recognition of E2 by broadly neutralizing antibodies,[37,175,347] in some instances by modulating the use of SR-BI and CD81 in virus entry (Fig. 8.10).[175] Nonneutralizing antibodies that bind HRV1 and other E2 domains may also sterically interfere with recognition of the neutralizing face by broadly neutralizing antibodies.[346,838] The E2 neutralization face is also physically shielded by HVR1,[608] extensive glycosylation,[285] and lipoproteins that associate with the virion (Fig. 8.10).[40,102,201,607] Direct cell-to-cell transmission of HCV may also sequester the virus from broadly neutralizing antibody responses, as demonstrated in cell culture models.[77,759,811]

Immunity and Animal Models of Infection

The common chimpanzee was the only model of HCV that recapitulated most features of human infection. The model was essential for the initial discovery of HCV and provided key insights into pathogenesis and immunity but is no longer used in research.[392] A number of rodent models were engineered for

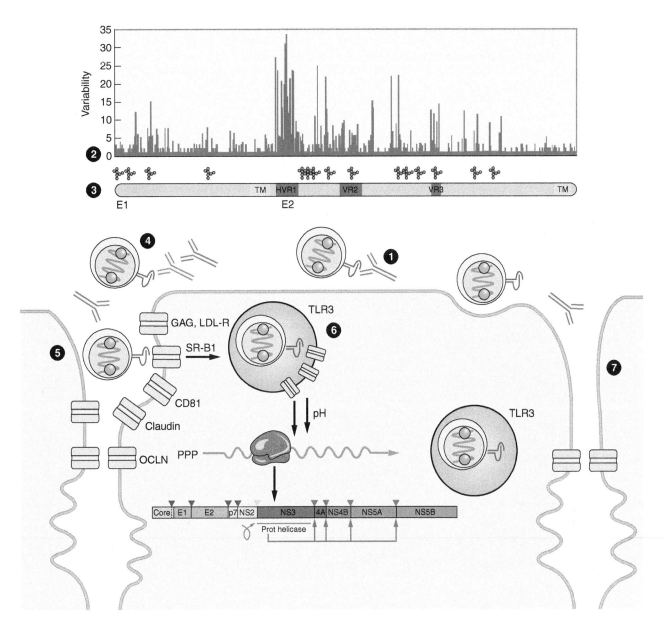

FIGURE 8.10 Evasion of anti–hepatitis C virus (HCV) antibody-mediated responses. Neutralization of HCV by antibodies can block infection of the cell (*1*). Binding of neutralizing antibodies (*red*) can be evaded by variability in the envelope proteins (*2*) illustrated here in a plot of Wu-Kabat amino acid variability[815] and by dense glycosylation at approximately 15 positions (*3*). Nonneutralizing antibodies (*4, green*) and lipoproteins (*5*) may hinder neutralizing antibody binding to HCV envelope glycoproteins, and delayed exposure of conserved domains until late in the entry process may prevent their recognition on free virions (*6*). Cell-to-cell transfer of virions is resistant to neutralizing antibodies *in vitro*, suggesting an additional mode of escape for local spread of infection (*7*). Along the envelope gene map are indicated transmembrane regions (TMs), hypervariable region 1 (HVR1), and variable regions 2 (VR2) and 3 (VR3, the intergenotypic variable regions IgVR).

susceptibility to HCV infection.[306,491,596,801] Examples include mice with a severe combined immunodeficiency phenotype reconstituted with human liver by ectopic implantation under the kidney capsule,[306] immunodeficient mice transgenic for the urokinase plasminogen activator (uPA) gene that facilitates reconstitution with human hepatocytes,[491] and genetically humanized mice that express murine CD81 and SR-BI and human claudin-I and occludin required for HCV entry.[596] These animals permit the study of HCV entry and antibody-mediated neutralization of HCV infectivity (see Humoral

Immunity) but are limited by other species restrictions on HCV replication or a functioning adaptive immune response.

Newly discovered equine and rodent hepaciviruses have great potential to provide new insight into mechanisms of immune control and failure leading to persistence. A nonprimate equine *Hepacivirus* is hepatotropic in horses[586] and like HCV has an NS3/4A protease that cleaves MAVS.[25,569] Experimental challenge of horses results in spontaneously resolving and persisting infections. Importantly, horses that resolved acute infection had very transient viremia upon reinfection, indicating immune protection similar to that observed in reinfected humans and chimpanzees.[588] Hepaciviruses isolated from rats are hepatotropic, have the potential to persist in their host species, and have a dependence on miR-122 for replication.[764] Transmission of the rat *Hepacivirus* to mice resulted in transient infection that persisted with antibody-mediated depletion of CD4+ T cells.[60] Natural persistence of the virus in rats was associated with a defect in acute phase T-cell immunity. Importantly, vaccination with a recombinant adenovirus expressing the nonstructural proteins protected most rats from persistence, and antibody-mediated depletion of CD4+ and CD8+ T cell abrogated protection or delayed resolution.[282] These models are emerging as an important new approach for understanding defects in immunity that lead to persistence and how they can be circumvented by vaccination.

EPIDEMIOLOGY

Morbidity and Mortality

Morbidity and mortality caused by HCV infection are related primarily to liver failure and/or liver cancer as a result of chronic infection. In the Unites States, the Centers for Disease Control and Prevention estimates that chronic HCV infection contributes to 15,000 deaths per year, is the leading cause of liver failure leading to transplantation, and in 2007 superseded HIV as a cause of death.[187,448,810] By 2012 to 2013, the annual number of HCV-related deaths exceeded 60 other nationally notifiable infectious diseases combined (Fig. 8.11).[446] HCV-related liver morbidity and mortality increase with older age and greater duration of HCV infection and are expected to rise in the coming decades. HCV-related liver failure and cancer are predicted to increase until 2020–2023 without widespread treatment.[142] This trend may be exacerbated by failure to identify and treat patients with advanced liver diseases including fibrosis and cirrhosis.[250,364,515] Liver-related mortality is predicted to rise from 146,667 cases in 2000–2009 to 283,378 in 2020–2029 in the United States. Global estimates of HCV-related disease burden at the level of individual countries are emerging.[105] They suggest a trend similar to the one predicted for the United States, where mortality associated with HCV infection continues to increase through 2030 with the exception of a small number of countries with higher DAA treatment rates.[105]

HCV-infected persons are at increased risk of mortality from causes other than liver failure. In one study, 10,259 HCV antibody–positive blood donors were compared to donors matched by year of donation, age, gender, and zip code and followed for a mean of 7.7 years.[271] Compared to the HCV-uninfected donors, the risk of death was 3.13-fold higher in HCV-infected donors, who were more likely to die of not just liver-related but also drug/alcohol-related events, trauma/suicide, and cardiovascular causes. Persons with HCV infection are also at much higher risk of some medical conditions such as mixed cryoglobulinemic vasculitis and porphyria cutanea tarda (PCT) (see Clinical Features).[147] The degree to which HCV infection contributes to less specific medical syndromes such as chronic fatigue/arthritis or mental illness is more difficult to establish.

Prevalence and Seroepidemiology

Transmission

Percutaneous exposure to contaminated blood is by far the most common mode of HCV transmission globally. Surveys of epidemiological literature have established that inadequate infection control measures including reuse of needles for medical and nonmedical practices are a significant risk for HCV transmission in many developing regions of the world.[131,355,692] Injection drug use is a dominant mode of HCV transmission globally, especially in countries with well-established screening programs for blood products and a low incidence of infection.[131,355,692] The size of the transmitted inoculum is a significant factor that determines whether infection is established. HCV RNA titers range from 5 to 7 $\log_{10}$ copies/mL of serum or plasma, and so almost all transfusion events with large volumes of contaminated blood products result in infection.[183,795] The risk of infection with a very small inoculum is apparent from chimpanzee studies, where low amounts of HCV RNA (~10–100 copies) similar to what might be found in a contaminated needle is sufficient to initiate productive infection.[87,343,455,787] The risk of HCV seroconversion after percutaneous accident involving health care workers in the United States has been estimated at 1.8%,[768] although a more recent analysis of 1,361 mucocutaneous and percutaneous exposures among health care workers at a large academic medical center over 13 years provided a lower seroconversion rate of 0.1% related to blood transmission. In addition to the quantity and titer of infectious material transferred, seroconversion is also determined by

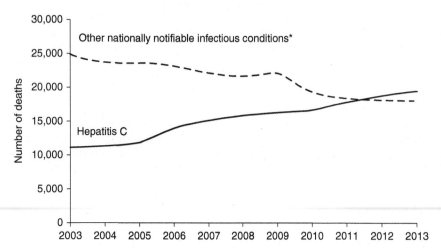

FIGURE 8.11 Annual number of deaths associated with hepatitis C virus and all other nationally notifiable infectious conditions* listed as multiple causes of death in the United States between 2003 and 2013. *Identified in the absence of hepatitis C. The list of 60 other nationally notifiable infectious conditions was obtained from the Centers for Disease Control and Prevention National Notifiable Diseases Surveillance System Web site. (From Ly KN, Hughes EM, Jiles RB, et al. Rising mortality associated with hepatitis C virus in the United States, 2003–2013. *Clin Infect Dis* 2016;62(10):1287–1288, with permission.)

the type of injury (superficial or deep) and use of hollow-bore needles and syringes with low or high dead space volume.[363,821] In one study of percutaneous accidents involving health care workers, the risk of HCV infection was 11-fold higher in those exposed to an inoculum of greater than 10^6 RNA versus less than 10^4 genomes/mL of serum.[821] More recently, mathematical modeling has demonstrated how the minimum estimated HCV inoculum size required for infection via IDU needle sharing varies with frequency of exposure and changing virus load through the acute and chronic phases of infection.[454] Other simulations have demonstrated that HCV titers decline in syringes over time, but virus infectivity can be maintained for weeks.[61,158,566,567] HCV RNA is stable for weeks in body fluids other than blood[587] and is detected in tears, seminal fluid, and CSF by sensitive molecular techniques.[210,488,799] There is no evidence that HCV RNA is present in these fluids at a titer sufficient for transmission of infection.[587] Nonmedical percutaneous exposures such as body piercing, tattooing, and other cultural practices emerge as plausible risks for HCV transmission in some regions of the world.[692]

The frequency by which HCV is transmitted sexually is controversial. Transmission is relatively rare among long-term monogamous partners of individuals with HCV infection. HCV prevalence among partners was 4% in one cross-sectional study of 500 anti–HCV-positive, human immunodeficiency virus-negative index subjects and their long-term heterosexual partners.[745] Of the 20 infections detected, nine couples had concordant genotypes. Viral isolates in three couples (0.6%) were highly related, consistent with transmission of virus within the couple. The maximum incidence rate of HCV transmission by sex was 0.07% per year, or approximately 1 per 190,000 sexual contacts.[745] HCV infection does occur in persons

acknowledging high-risk sexual practices with no other risk factor such as injection drug use.[782] Transmission between HIV-infected and HIV-uninfected men who have high-risk sexual exposures with other men is well established and is thought to result from traumatic sexual practices.[439,621,779–781,804]

The rate of vertical HCV transmission is estimated at 2% to 10%.[470,636,829] How and when infection occurs in this setting is not known, but risk is increased by maternal HIV infection and/or high HCV RNA levels, prolonged rupture of membranes, and internal fetal monitoring.[235,473,763]

Global Burden, Incidence, and Prevalence

An estimated 71 million people, or 1% of the human population, are infected with HCV globally as defined by viremia.[597] HCV prevalence varies widely between regions and countries (Fig. 8.12).[80,597] In an analysis of 16 countries by literature search and expert consensus, viremic prevalence estimates ranged from 0.3% in Austria, England, and Germany to 8.5% in Egypt.[80] The largest viremic populations were in Egypt, with 6,358,000 cases in 2008, and Brazil with 2,106,000 cases in 2007.[80]

The high prevalence in Egypt has historical roots in a campaign to eradicate schistosomiasis infection by intravenously administering tartar emetic to millions of citizens.[717] The effort, commended at the time as a public health model, occurred before there was widespread appreciation for blood-borne transmission of infectious agents. HCV was transmitted extensively because of the widespread reuse of insufficiently cleaned injection equipment.[222] Consequently, the prevalence of HCV infection can exceed 50% in persons alive during that campaign while being 1% to 2% in those born after. In addition, more than 90% of HCV infections in Egypt are genotype 4, which make up less than 10% of genotypes in most other

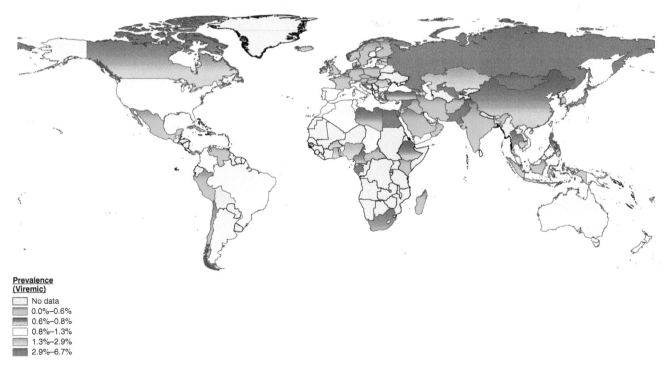

Prevalence (Viremic)
- No data
- 0.0%–0.6%
- 0.6%–0.8%
- 0.8%–1.3%
- 1.3%–2.9%
- 2.9%–6.7%

FIGURE 8.12 Map depicting geographic variation in the relative prevalence of hepatitis C virus (HCV) infection. Shading of country indicates prevalence. (Reprinted from Global prevalence and genotype distribution of hepatitis C virus infection in 2015: a modelling study. *Lancet Gastroenterol Hepatol* 2017;2(3):161–176. Copyright © 2017 Elsevier. With permission.)

regions of the world.[624] Of note, Egypt is now at the forefront of national programs to eliminate HCV through a combination of public health measures as well as identification and treatment of infections (see Prevention and Control).[682] Diagnostic testing programs for HCV infection are highly refined and on track to identify and treat millions of people who are unaware of chronic HCV infection.[174]

United States Prevalence and Incidence

An estimated 1% of the US population, or 2.1 million people, were HCV RNA–positive in a survey that spanned 2013–2016.[291] Approximately 4.1 million were seropositive for antibodies against HCV.[291] Of note, this estimate was generated by combining data from the National Health and Nutrition Examination Survey (NHANES) that estimates infection rates among noninstitutionalized civilian populations and a literature review to define prevalence in incarcerated and unsheltered homeless populations, active duty military, and nursing home residents. Inclusion of the populations who were not surveyed by NHANES increased the number of viremic (actively infected) individuals by 0.25 million.[291] Disparities associated with sex and race have been noted. Estimated HCV RNA prevalence is 1.5 to 2.5 times higher in males when compared with females.[276] When stratified by race, HCV RNA prevalence is highest among the non-Hispanic Black population (2.43), followed by non-Hispanic White (1.05) and Hispanic/other (0.74) populations.[276] Genotype distribution also differs by race and geography,[251] a consideration in DAA treatment with some non–pan-genotypic regimens.

Prevalence among the civilian noninstitutionalized population estimated from the most recent NHANES spanning 2013 to 2016 (0.9%)[291] is lower than the estimate from the 2003 to 2010 survey (1%).[148] This difference may reflect continued mortality (HCV-related and all-cause) and an impact of DAA therapy. Reductions associated with mortality and treatment may be offset by a changing epidemic of HCV transmission in the United States.[374,728,843] The annual incidence of acute HCV infection rose from 0.3 to 0.7 cases per 100,000 from 2004 to 2014, an increase in the overall rate of 133% (Fig. 8.13).[843] The greatest increase, and cause for concern, occurred among non-Hispanic Whites and Hispanics in the 18 to 29 (400%) and 30 to 39 (325%) age groups.[843] This increase was directly related to an epidemic of opioid and heroin drug use (Fig. 8.13).[843] A survey of data from the National Notifiable Diseases Surveillance System also documented a doubling of the number of reproductive-aged women with acute or past or present HCV infection between 2006 and 2014.[447] Estimated HCV prevalence was 3.2 times higher for children aged 2 to 3 years when compared with the 12- to 13-year age group.[447] Reasons for this disparity are not known, but may reflect in part a decrease in testing frequency among older children once HCV status is established, or spontaneous clearance of infection that occurs at an older age in children.[447]

Global Molecular Epidemiology and Origin

The seven HCV genotypes are not uniformly distributed globally or regionally (Fig. 8.14).[493,597] Genotype 1 is prevalent worldwide. HCV prevalence is highest, and genetically most diverse, in Africa.[493] Genotype 3 is dominant in the Asia South region. Genotype 4 is found almost exclusively in the North Africa/Middle East and sub-Saharan Africa Central and

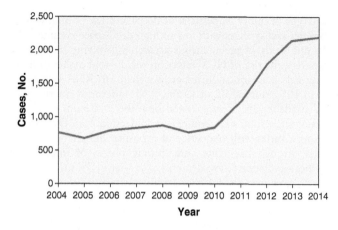

FIGURE 8.13 Cases of HCV infection by year reported to the National Notifiable Disease Surveillance System, United States. The annual incidence rate of acute HCV infection increased by 133% from 2004 to 2014 due to an epidemic of opioid use. (From Zibbell JE, Asher AK, Patel RC, et al. Increases in acute hepatitis C virus infection related to a growing opioid epidemic and associated injection drug use, United States, 2004 to 2014. *Am J Public Health* 2018;108(2):175–181, with permission.)

Eastern regions.[493] The global distribution of HCV genotypes and subtypes has been shaped by human migration, catastrophic events including war, and early widespread adoption of medical practices like transfusion before infectious diseases risks were appreciated. Of the 86 recognized HCV subtypes, only a few that represent a small fraction of HCV diversity account for the overwhelming majority of infections worldwide.[493,695] Epidemic subtypes 1a, 1b, 2a, and 3a spread rapidly in most regions of the world over the past 50 to 100 years with the development of practices that promoted parenteral exposure.[314,614,695] Bayesian evolutionary analysis has provided insight into the spatiotemporal spread and probable causes of epidemic transmission of these subtypes. Most studies are consistent with spread of genotype 1 viruses, the most widely dispersed globally, from approximately 1940 until a plateau was reached about 4 to 5 decades later. Phylodynamic analyses are consistent with global expansion of subtype 1b in the early decades by iatrogenic transmission through transfusion, reuse of needles, and other procedures that caused exposure to contaminated blood. Spread of genotype 1a in later decades was likely facilitated by injection drug use until harm reduction practices for PWID became commonplace.[125,451,614] The impact of widespread use of nonsterile needles on HCV spread in the middle of the 20th century is exemplified by campaigns to treat schistosomiasis in Japan and later Egypt.[512] For example, the extremely high prevalence of HCV genotype 4a in Egypt that persists until today can be traced to mass distribution of antischistosomal medication with unsterilized injection equipment between 1930 and 1950.[512,615]

Endemic spread of HCV genotypes is also apparent from phylogenetic studies that demonstrated highly divergent subtypes of the same genotype in geographically contiguous areas. By this measure, HCV genotype 2 is considered endemic in West Africa, genotypes 1 and 4 in Central Africa and the Middle East, and genotype 6 in Asia.[97,321,487,541,613] This pattern is consistent with circulation of a given genotype in a defined geographic location for hundreds or thousands of years long-standing

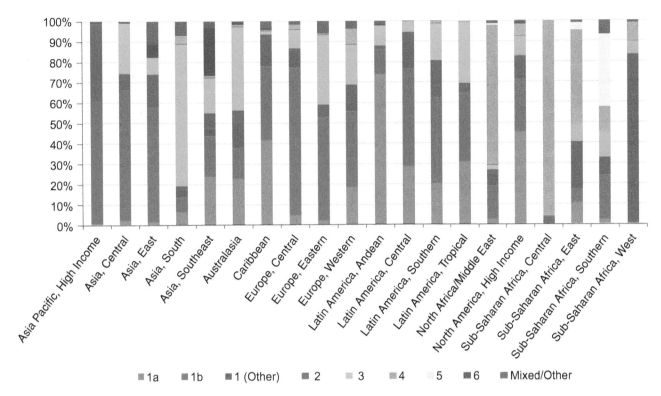

FIGURE 8.14 Global distribution of medically relevant HCV genotypes. HCV prevalence is highest, and genetically most diverse, in Africa. Genotype 1 is prevalent worldwide. Genotype 3 is dominant in the Asia, South region. Genotype 4 is found almost exclusively found in the North Africa/Middle East and sub-Saharan Africa Central and Eastern regions. (Reprinted from Global prevalence and genotype distribution of hepatitis C virus infection in 2015: a modelling study. *Lancet Gastroenterol Hepatol* 2017;2(3):161–176. Copyright © 2017 Elsevier. With permission.)

association of the virus with human populations.[694] This concept is supported by recent estimates of the time to most recent common ancestor (tMRCA) for these endemic genotypes. The tMRCA for genotype 3 in South Asia and the ancestor of genotypes 1 and 4 in Central Africa were estimated to be in the 800 BCE to 700 CE range, while genotype 6 endemic in Southeast Asia had an estimated origin of at least 2,000 years ago.[216]

Estimates of tMRCA for the seven HCV genotypes range from approximately 1,000 to 3,000 years ago.[216,423,442,614,695,704] These estimates for HCV genotypes are in the same time frame (or perhaps slightly earlier) than the tMRCA of CE 1100–1800 estimate for equine hepaciviruses.[216,616] These estimates do support the concept that HCV entered human populations relatively recently, although it must be acknowledged that extrapolation of short-term substitution rates to longer evolutionary periods has limitations. It is conceivable that human HCV originated from a cross-species transmission event, a possibility that seems plausible with the recent isolation of hepaciviruses from a variety of disparate species. From an evolutionary perspective, however, the animal hepaciviruses discovered to date are probably too distant from the diverse constellation of HCV genotypes and subtypes found in humans to have an ancestral relationship.

CLINICAL FEATURES

Acute HCV

Acute HCV infection is usually asymptomatic,[134,524] though a minority of persons will present with more typical symptoms of acute viral hepatitis (malaise, fatigue, anorexia, nausea, abdominal pain, jaundice, dark urine, and sometimes pale stool). While HCV can cause fulminant hepatitis, this presentation is rare.[196,249,334,814,817,825] In general, the latent period (from exposure to symptoms or laboratory abnormalities) is approximately 7 weeks (range 1–16 weeks) (Fig. 8.6).[524] In many cases, the only sign of acute infection may be elevation of hepatic transaminases.[1,134,793]

Most exposures that result in HCV infection are percutaneous (see Transmission), after which hematogenous infection of the liver is presumed to occur. Viremia is detectable within days[524] and reaches levels of 10^5 to 10^7 IU/mL within weeks (Fig. 8.6). A decrease in viremia 1 to 2 weeks later is associated with expansion of HCV-specific T cells and in some individuals a sharp rise in hepatic transaminase levels in blood (see Immune Responses) (Fig. 8.6). This sharp ALT increase is thought to result from immune-mediated cytolysis by adaptive responses as the virus is not considered to be directly cytopathic.[9,134,197,524,684] HCV-specific cytotoxic CD8+ T cells are detected individuals who clear infection regardless of whether a sharp transaminase increase is observed.[748] This suggests that control of infection may be mediated in some individuals by noncytotoxic mechanisms involving production of antiviral cytokines.[748] The mechanism of acute phase liver injury, when it is observed, is likely to be complex. One recent study established an association between host *IFNL4* genotype and symptoms of acute hepatitis C that could explain the higher spontaneous clearance observed in some patients with symptomatic disease.[565]

A low oscillating pattern of viremia can persist for up to a year until resolution (Fig. 8.6).[275,479] Protective sterilizing immunity is uncommon after spontaneous resolution of infection, if it occurs at all. Reinfection is associated with a reduced duration and magnitude of viremia, and the risk of persistent infection is decreased (Fig. 8.6).[138,260,484,559,653] A similar drop in viremia is observed in many acute persisting infections (Fig. 8.6). After several months, it reaches a higher set point that is stable or increases gradually over a lifetime of persistent HCV replication (Fig. 8.6).[274] Transient partial control of HCV replication is not observed in some individuals following a chronic course, suggesting an absence of apparent immune control during the acute phase of infection (see Immune Responses). Late spontaneous resolution has been observed[619] but is rare when treatment is not initiated and spontaneous clearance does not occur within 12 months.

Predictors of Spontaneous Clearance

Spontaneous clearance of HCV RNA usually occurs within 6 months of infection and is associated with having overt symptoms of hepatitis, non-African descent, and lack of HIV infection.[241,793] GWAS have identified significant associations between spontaneous clearance of HCV infection and the *IFNL* locus.[554,623,754] The compound dinucleotide polymorphism rs368234815-ΔG or rs368234815-TT located in exon 1 of *IFNL4* is most notable from a functional perspective, as a ΔG/ΔG haplotype results in production of IFN-*λ*4 and a higher risk of persistent infection (see Innate Immunity).[612] The protective IFNL genotypes are also more frequently found in Asians and least frequently among persons with African ancestry, in keeping with the clinically observed effect of race.[554,623,754] HLA class I and II associations with the outcome of acute infection have also been observed.[167,211,238,280,481,503,750,790,844] Specific class II alleles that associate with spontaneous clearance (*HLA-DQB1*03:01*, *DRB1*01:01*, *DRB1*03:01*, and *HLA-DRB1*11:01*) or persistence (*DQB1*02:01*) have been identified in multiple studies.[167,238,280,503,750,790] The *IFNL* and MHC association has been confirmed by meta-analysis, including one study that provided a dense multiracial GWAS analysis that included individuals of African ancestry.[790] This study provided an additional association with G-protein–coupled receptor 158 gene (GPR158). These three loci (IFNL, MHC, and GPR18) had independent, additive effects on HCV clearance. Persons of African or European ancestry carrying all six clearance-associated variants were 24-fold and 11-fold, respectively, more likely to clear HCV infection when compared with individuals carrying one or none of them.[464]

Chronic HCV

The level of HCV RNA in the blood tends to be stable over long periods of time in chronic hepatitis C, within 1 $\log_{10}$ of 10^6 IU/mL in 90% of individuals. Conditions associated with modest increases include HIV infection, male gender, and increasing age and body mass index, whereas lower levels may be found in those with ongoing HBV infection and more advanced stage of liver disease.[21,127,308,752,755,761] Chronic HCV infection is a heterogeneous condition, with highly individual manifestations and rates of progression (Fig. 8.15).[248] Associated morbidity and mortality occur almost exclusively when the disease progresses to cirrhosis and end-stage liver disease that may manifest as hepatocellular carcinoma (HCC). Chronic HCV infection is characterized by high-level viremia and fluctuating hepatic inflammation and transaminase levels,[363,582,809] yet chronically infected people typically have few symptoms that are directly attributable to HCV infection. It is difficult to establish a causal

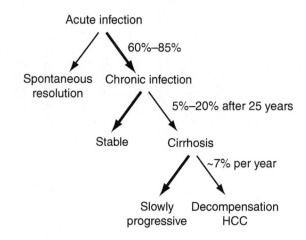

FIGURE 8.15 Progression of hepatitis C virus (HCV) infection. Most HCV infections are persistent and stable, but a minority will progress to cirrhosis within 20 to 30 years. Of those with cirrhosis, most are slowly progressive, but 7% per year will develop either hepatocellular carcinoma (HCC) or decompensated liver disease.

relation between HCV and nonspecific symptoms, though they do tend to improve after successful therapy.[56,220]

Chronic HCV infection is associated with varying degrees of chronic inflammation and steatosis. Lymphocytic infiltrates are typically found in periportal regions of the liver (Fig. 8.16),

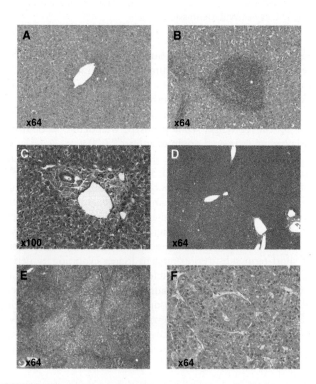

FIGURE 8.16 Histology illustrating progression of hepatitis C virus (HCV)-related liver disease. A: Normal portal tract (hematoxylin and eosin [H&E] stain). **B:** Portal inflammation (H&E stain). **C:** No fibrosis (trichrome stain). **D:** Bridging fibrosis (trichrome stain). **E:** Cirrhosis (trichrome stain). **F:** Hepatocellular carcinoma (HCC) (H&E stain). (Courtesy of Michael Torbenson, MD.)

though these do not correlate strongly with liver disease progression.[678] For reasons that are not clear, many individuals will not develop significant fibrosis despite decades of high-level viral infection, while others have more production than resorption of collagen, also initially in the periportal region. This process may be stable or progress to formation of septa that expand to form bridges between lobules, and further expansion may result in the severe scarring and regeneration that characterize cirrhosis. Increasing portal venous pressure may lead to portal hypertension, and neoplastic transformation may lead to HCC, hallmarks of end-stage liver disease.

The risk of fibrosis is associated with *IFNL4* genotype through viral and/or nonviral mechanisms that have not yet been identified,[14,66,181,182] but extend the pervasive effect of polymorphisms linked to IFN-*λ*4 production on HCV pathogenesis. Studies demonstrating that the *IFNL4* CC genotype (associated with clearance of infection) is linked to more severe fibrosis in those who are chronically infected[66,182] are consistent with higher rates of chronic infection with milder inflammation and slower progression of fibrosis among people of African descent.[135,746]

Of note, liver disease progresses slowly in children with vertically transmitted HCV. Liver inflammation with no or very mild fibrosis is often evident in children who were infected as infants. Only 1% to 2% develop cirrhosis,[270,324] but it is likely that they will develop serious liver disease over a lifetime of persistent HCV replication if untreated.[286,514,529]

Alcohol consumption is frequent in persons with chronic HCV and is strongly associated with liver disease progression.[18,584] Along with its well-known hepatotoxicity, alcohol use is associated with reduced access to and early discontinuation of HCV treatment.[584] Elimination of alcohol consumption should be attempted to reduce complications in all persons with chronic HCV.[242,243,508,710,822]

Chronic HCV infection is also associated with metabolic dysfunction including insulin resistance, type 2 diabetes, lipid derangement, and steatosis that may be more common in (but not exclusive to) persons infected with HCV genotype 3.[130,304,469,483,543] This association is stronger for HCV than for HBV, suggesting that the mechanism may be specific to HCV.[687,806] Potential contributing mechanisms to metabolic dysfunction in HCV include down-regulation of hepatocyte insulin receptor substrate 1[71] and glucose transporter 2[340] and up-regulation of PP2A.[55,168] Flares of hepatitis (with elevated serum transaminases and/or bilirubin), common in HBV infection,[583] are rare in chronic HCV and should prompt a search for other causes. For example, acute HAV infection during chronic HCV infection may be associated with severe acute hepatitis, including liver failure[789]; for this reason, persons with chronic HCV infection should be vaccinated for HAV and HBV if susceptible.

Hepatocellular Carcinoma

HCC is a growing problem in countries like the United States with relatively recent HCV epidemics and is a major established problem in countries like Japan and Egypt where the epidemic of HCV infection occurred 10 to 20 years earlier. This is consistent with studies demonstrating a lag of approximately 40 years between onset of transfusion-associated chronic hepatitis C and HCC diagnosis.[333] Chronic HCV infection is strongly associated with development of HCC.[176,429,696] The

risk of HCC is increased approximately 17-fold in individuals with chronic hepatitis C when compared with uninfected controls.[160] Moreover, serologic or virologic evidence of HCV infection is found in serum and liver tissue in approximately 40% of patients with HCC.[8]

Successful eradication of HCV with IFN-based therapy dramatically reduced but did not eliminate risk of HCC.[38,177,516,531,555] There is now sufficient experience to conclude that IFN- and ribavirin-free DAA treatment also does not increase,[593,697] but instead substantially decreases, the probability of developing liver cancer by more than 70%.[100,310,337] Importantly, after SVR, the absolute risk of developing HCC remains high at approximately 1% per year in patients with established cirrhosis, so continued monitoring is recommended. This may reflect persistence of epigenetic alterations associated with liver cancer after a sustained virologic response (SVR).[277] Two small uncontrolled trials suggested a higher rate of HCC recurrence in DAA-treated patients,[128,634] but larger studies have so far not confirmed this effect.[26,117,302,530] From these studies, it can be concluded that DAA treatment should be undertaken before development of cirrhosis.

Mechanisms of hepatocarcinogenesis in chronic hepatitis C are not known. Repeated cycles of hepatocyte destruction and regenerative cell proliferation caused by the chronic inflammatory process could promote tumorigenesis. This mechanism is consistent with significantly higher rates of HCC (~1%–4% per year) in patients after several years of inflammatory liver disease leading to cirrhosis.[81,82,199,277,429,655,696] The possibility that HCV contributes directly to development of HCC can't be excluded, but it should be emphasized that HCV has no potential for integration of viral RNA sequences into the host genome. Induction of protooncogenes and suppression of apoptosis have been observed by overexpression of the core protein under control of a strong promoter in rodent models.[108,114,116,471,626–628,726,842] HCC developed in the absence of inflammation, suggesting a direct oncogenic effect of the transgenic HCV core.[416,519] As noted above, HCC in the absence of cirrhosis is a rare occurrence, and it is perhaps more likely that the virus acts by altering the intracellular environment through activation of protooncogenes like *β*-catenin or disruption of tumor suppressor pathways involving retinoblastoma protein Rb and the RNA helicase DDX3.[106,504,527] Function of the tumor suppressor proteins like p53 may also be modulated through direct interaction with HCV proteins[527] or as a function of PKR activation in the infected cell.[509] Model systems suggest that HCV may also act by induction of reactive oxygen species and oxidative stress.[520]

Insights from human studies are limited. Activation of the telomerase reverse transcriptase promoter may be a frequent early neoplastic event in HCC, including cases associated with chronic HCV infection.[539] Hepatic epigenetic changes associated with liver cancer risk have been reported to persist after DAA treatment of chronic hepatitis C.[277] Genetic variants associated with HCC risk in patients with chronic hepatitis C have been assessed by GWAS. For instance, polymorphism rs17047200 in the tolloid like gene 1 (*TLL1*) was associated with development of HCC after SVR.[472] Other polymorphisms in or near HCP5, PNPLA3, DEPDC5, and MHC loci have been associated with progression to or protection from cirrhosis or HCC.[386,393,412,502,771,778] The mechanistic significance of these polymorphisms is not yet understood.

Extrahepatic Manifestations

Chronic HCV infection is associated with a wide variety of extrahepatic manifestations that are mostly inflammatory in nature.[90] A common feature of these conditions is chronic inflammation. Essential mixed cryoglobulinemia, a condition in which cold-precipitating immune complexes are deposited in multiple organ systems, is strongly associated with HCV infection, though other inflammatory conditions may be implicated. Manifestations often include purpuric rash, weakness, and joint pain but may also include Raynaud syndrome and vasculitis complicated by membranoproliferative glomerulonephritis and neuropathy.[91,458,505] The chronic stimulation of B cells implicated in HCV-related cryoglobulinemia[651] may also explain the elevated risk of non-Hodgkin lymphoma.[140] PCT, characterized primarily by disorders of the skin (blistering, hyperpigmentation) and nails (onycholysis) worsened by sun exposure and complicated by scarring, is associated with liver disease and is caused by reduced activity of uroporphyrinogen decarboxylase. It is a multifactorial disease, potentiated by mutations in the *HFE* gene (associated with hereditary hemochromatosis and found in 15% of persons with PCT), as well as HCV infection, alcohol, and estrogen use—all of which should be evaluated in persons presenting with PCT.[69] Thyroiditis and antithyroid antibodies have been associated with chronic hepatitis C by meta-analysis, though the mechanism remains unclear.[28]

SVR following DAA therapy can provide relief from mixed cyroglobulinemia.[92,126,179,255,650] Clinical and immunological improvements may not be immediate, however.[179] Approximately 60% of patients had complete or partial resolution of mixed cryoglobulinemia 12 weeks after completion of therapy in one study.[179] Consistent with gradual improvement after SVR, clinical outcomes improve with longer follow-up.[126,179] Recovery of affected organ systems may not be uniform, with less success in resolving renal and neurologic complications.[126,179] Regression and prevention of relapse of non-Hodgkin lymphoma associated with DAA therapy has been reported (reviewed in Ref.[309])

DIAGNOSIS

HCV infection is suspected in persons with otherwise unexplained liver disease. In asymptomatic persons, this infection should be suspected in any person reporting risk factors for infection (see Epidemiology) or having elevated hepatic transaminases even in the absence of known risk factors, because the infection is highly prevalent. Because of shared risk factors and increased severity of disease, the U.S. Public Health Service recommends HCV testing for all HIV-infected persons upon entry into health care.[703] Because more than two-thirds of persons with HCV infection in the United States were born between 1945 and 1965, the U.S. Public Health Service has recommended that everyone in that "birth cohort" be tested once for HCV infection.[703] The cost-effectiveness of birth cohort testing has already been demonstrated.[635] Retrospective analysis demonstrated that 68% of persons with HCV infection would have been identified with a birth cohort testing strategy whereas only 27% would have been screened with the risk-based approach.[452] A recent survey of screening practices in 51 high-income countries in the top quartile of the United

Nations Human Development Index (HDI) countries revealed consistent risk and age-based recommendations similar to those in place in the United States.[311] Screening recommendations may be reconsidered in the near future for additional populations. Simulations indicate that expanded screening for those greater than 18 years of age is cost-effective.[43] Screening pregnant women is also under debate given the sharp increase in new HCV infections associated with opioid use and risk of vertical transmission.[104,323]

Differential Diagnosis

Other viral causes of acute hepatitis (described in Clinical Features) include the named hepatitis viruses (HAV, HBV with or without the delta hepatitis agent, or hepatitis E virus), yellow fever virus, and a wide range of viruses with broader tropism including Epstein-Barr virus and cytomegalovirus. In immunocompromised hosts, adenovirus and other agents with broad tropism can also cause hepatitis. Nonviral causes of acute hepatitis include leptospirosis, tuberculosis, rickettsia and rickettsia-like organisms, numerous toxins (alcohol, acetaminophen, isoniazid, and *Amanita phalloides* toxin being prominent), anoxia/hypoperfusion, and autoimmune disease. Chronic hepatitis may be caused by HBV and occasionally HEV (in immunocompromised hosts), as well as nonviral etiologies (e.g., toxoplasmosis, autoimmune hepatitis, and nonalcoholic steatohepatitis).

Laboratory

Algorithms for laboratory diagnosis of HCV infection are available for guidance on use and interpretation of assays to detect serologic responses and viral genomes.[103] Most persons recommended for HCV screening are tested initially for serum antibodies against HCV.[103,185] A laboratory-based enzyme immunoassay (EIA) incorporating HCV proteins is most commonly used.[2,185] Rapid diagnostic assays that detect antibodies in whole blood by finger-stick capillary or oral (cervicular) fluid are also available, avoiding venipuncture and costly blood processing procedures. One point-of-care assay that delivers a result in 20 minutes with sensitivity and specificity similar to the EIA is available in the United States.[413]

A positive test result for HCV antibody indicates either current infection that is acute or chronic, past infection that has resolved, or a false-positive result.[572] An HCV nucleic acid test (NAT) to detect viremia is necessary to confirm active HCV infection and guide clinical management, including initiation of HCV treatment. HCV RNA testing is recommended for persons with a negative HCV antibody test who either are immunocompromised (e.g., persons receiving chronic hemodialysis) or might have been exposed to HCV within the last 6 months because these persons may be HCV antibody negative. An HCV RNA test is also required to detect reinfection in HCV antibody–positive persons after previous spontaneous or treatment-related viral clearance or in vertically exposed infants prior to loss of transplacentally acquired maternal antibodies. Quantitative or qualitative NAT with a detection limit of 15 to 25 IU/mL or lower is used to detect HCV RNA.

HCV genotype is an important variable in DAA treatment decisions, particularly in patients with prior treatment experience or cirrhosis who will not be treated with a pan-genotypic regimen.[2,185] Genotyping is performed with an assay (typically line probe) that targets the 5′ NTR to accurately discriminate subtype 1a from 1b.[118] A second target, from either core or NS5B coding region, is also incorporated into the test.[118]

Prevention and Control

Treatment

Antiviral therapy for chronic HCV infection has undergone revolutionary change since 2013. Type I interferon alpha (IFN-α), the cornerstone of HCV therapy for almost 30 years, has been replaced by combinations of two or more DAA that inhibit function of the HCV NS3/4A protease, NS5A replicase factor, and/or NS5B RNA-dependent polymerase required for virus replication. A brief recounting of major milestones in the type I IFN treatment era provides a baseline for understanding the transition to a rapid cycle of DAA development, licensure, and replacement over the past 6 to 7 years (Fig. 8.17). The first study of IFN-α monotherapy for NANBH was initiated in 1984, well before discovery of HCV in 1989.[297] Sustained normalization of liver function and resolution of hepatitis were observed only in a subset of patients after discontinuation of therapy.[297] With development of assays for detection and quantification of HCV genomes, it was apparent that infection was cured in less than 20% of treated patients with chronic genotype 1 HCV infections.[686] Cure rates increased gradually over the next 2 decades with addition of the broad-spectrum antiviral agent ribavirin to the treatment regimen,[480,602] pegylation of IFN-α to extend its half-life,[435,833] and monitoring of the early virologic response to guide decisions on the duration or early discontinuation of therapy (Fig. 8.17).[170] Approximately 80% of previously untreated genotype 2 and 3 infections could be cured with these modifications to therapy, but the success rate for most genotype 1 infections was a very unsatisfactory 40% even with 48 weeks of treatment.[272]

Tolerability of IFN-α–based therapy was limited by fatigue, headache, nausea, pyrexia, and a number of other adverse effects. Other variables that reduced the cure rate and complicated pegIFN-α–based therapies included the stage of liver disease (cirrhosis less responsive than early stage) and obesity and host factors such as sex (males less responsive than females), age (>40 years less

responsive), and race (most notably African ancestry). As detailed in Innate Immunity, the influence of race on pegIFN-α treatment outcome was associated with polymorphisms in *IFNL* genes just as the transition to the DAA era began (Fig. 8.13).[239,727,736]

The end of this treatment era was presaged by new therapies that combined pegIFN-α, ribavirin, and a DAA. Combination therapy with pegIFN-α, ribavirin, and a first-generation NS3/4A protease inhibitor (telaprevir or boceprevir) received FDA approval in 2011 for treatment of chronic HCV genotype 1 infections (Fig. 8.18).[170,242] Triple therapy that included one of these protease inhibitors increased the cure rate to approximately 70% compared with 40% for pegIFN-α and ribavirin alone. Other DAA subsequently approved for use with pegIFN-α and ribavirin in the United States or Europe in 2013 included a third protease inhibitor (simeprevir)[315,456] and the first inhibitors of the HCV NS5A (daclatasvir)[162,288] and NS5B (sofosbuvir)[406,407] proteins. As an example, triple combination therapy with pegIFN-α, ribavirin and sofosbuvir yielded an overall cure rate of 92% in patients without cirrhosis after only 12 weeks of therapy.[406,407] Treatment failures were not due to selection of NS5B resistance variants.

Based on this very promising profile, the first trials of IFN-α–free therapy were undertaken with sofosbuvir in combination with ribavirin, simeprevir, or daclatasvir. These early studies provided proof that pegIFN-α could be eliminated from treatment regimens, but also revealed that outcome was influenced by HCV genotype, patient treatment history, and/or severity of liver disease. Development and licensing of new DAA combinations that overcome these limitations has continued at a stunning pace since 2013 (Fig. 8.17). As detailed below, therapy is now converging on newly licensed DAA combinations that cure almost all treatment-naïve patients with chronic HCV infection, regardless of genotype, with a single pill taken daily for 8 or 12 weeks. Options for difficult-to-treat patients with decompensated cirrhosis, prior treatment failure, or renal impairment have also expanded. This almost certainly represents one of the most impressive triumphs of antiviral drug development in recent history.

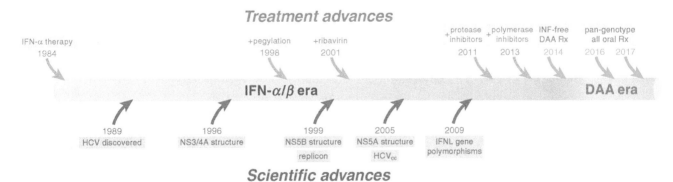

FIGURE 8.17 Timeline of scientific and treatment advances leading to highly effective pan-genotypic direct-acting antiviral therapy. The first exploratory trial of type IFN for cure of non-A, non-B hepatitis was initiated in 1984, 5 years before the discovery of HCV as the causative agent. Treatment response rates improved gradually over 30 years, with pegylation to improve IFN half-life (1998), addition of ribavirin as a second antiviral (2001) and direct-acting antivirals targeting the NS3/4A protease (2011) and NS5B polymerase (2013). The first IFN-free DAA formulation was approved for use in 2014. All oral, pan-genotypic DAA combinations taken as single tablet once a day were approved for use in 2016 and 2017. Scientific advances after discovery of HCV in 1989 that drove DAA development include crystallization of nonstructural proteins NS3, NS5A, and NS5B, the targets of current therapeutic agents. Development of the HCV replicon system (2000) and HCVcc replication system (2005) were also essential for DAA characterization. Association of IFN lambda (*IFNL*) gene polymorphisms with type IFN treatment outcome in 2009 provided predictive power and remains relevant given an unexpected influence on DAA therapy.

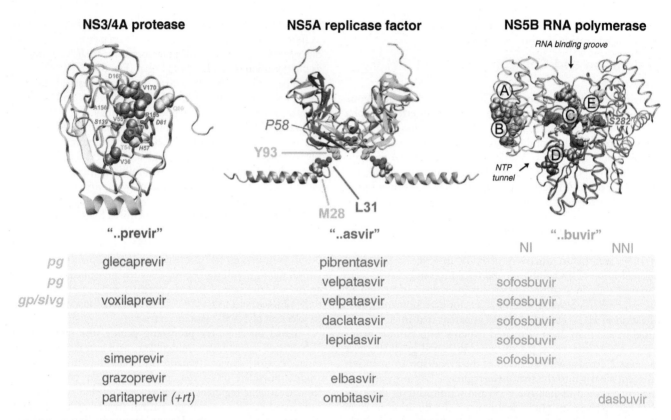

FIGURE 8.18 Direct-acting antiviral (DAA) combinations approved for use in Europe and the United States. Three DAA classes are used in therapy of chronic HCV infection targeting the NS3/4A serine protease (suffix *previr*), NS5A replicase factor (suffix *asvir*), and NS5A RNA-dependent RNA polymerase (suffix *buvir*). Ribbon diagrams illustrating the structure of the targeted HCV proteins and location of resistance-associated substitutions (RAS) are shown (see Chapter 7 for structural detail). The NS3 protease domain (left) is shown with the central NS4A activation domain (yellow) and the catalytic triad (His57, Asp81, Ser139) diagrammed as red sticks. Mutations that confer resistance to protease inhibitors are shown with side chains as colored van der Waals spheres. Side view of the NS5A D1 dimer structure with RAS sites (center). Pro58 mutations are associated with secondary resistance to daclatasvir but do not confer resistance on their own.[226] Structure of the NS5B RNA polymerase is shown with the RNA binding groove, NTP tunnel (right). Five distinct sites (A–E) targeted by nonnucleotide inhibitors are shown with side chains of some amino acid residues that confer resistance to NNI. The position of the major resistance mutation for nucleotide/nucleoside inhibitors (Ser252) is indicated. Three DAA combinations that are effective against all HCV genotypes and subtypes are highlighted (pan-genotypic, *pg*). One pan-genotypic combination (SOF:VEL:VOX) is approved for salvage (*slvg*) therapy in cases of prior treatment failure with DAA. Effectiveness of the protease inhibitor paritaprevir is boosted with ritonavir (*+rt*) as indicated. Updates to approved combinations and guidelines for use are provided by the European Association for the Study of the Liver (EASL)[185] and the American Association for the Study of Liver Diseases (AASLD).[2] A Web-based resource is also provided by AASLD (HCVguidelines.org). (Adapted from Bartenschlager R, Lohmann V, Penin F. The molecular and structural basis of advanced antiviral therapy for hepatitis C virus infection. *Nat Rev Microbiol* 2013;11(7):482–496, with permission. Ribbon diagrams of targeted HCV proteins with RAS were kindly provided by Dr. Ralf Bartenschlager, the University of Heidelberg.)

Treatment endpoints and goals

The endpoint of antiviral therapy is to permanently clear HCV RNA from circulation. Undetectable HCV RNA genomes in serum or plasma at 12 weeks (SVR12) or 24 weeks (SVR24) after completion of DAA therapy are considered a cure as the risk of relapse is less than 1%.[457] Quantitative or qualitative NAT assays with a lower detection limit of 15 international units (IU) (or less) of HCV RNA per ml of serum or plasma are the standard for determining SVR.[465] SVR24 can also be established using an EIA for circulating HCV core antigen if it is measurable in patients before initiation of treatment.[11,119,120,224]

The goal of antiviral therapy is to reverse or arrest chronic progressive liver disease related to HCV infection. Benefits to health and quality of life afforded by cure of chronic HCV

infection were established in the era of type I IFN-based therapy. Termination of chronic infection by antiviral therapy decreases liver necroinflammation and fibrosis in patients without cirrhosis.[603] Patients with advanced fibrosis remain at increased risk for serious liver diseases,[784] but progression of fibrosis and clinical manifestations including portal hypertension and splenomegaly improve.[603] Resolution of cirrhosis is observed in approximately half of cured infections, and a sharp reduction (>70%) in the risk of liver cancer is a consistent finding across studies.[35,366,516,603] Extrahepatic diseases associated with chronic HCV infection such as cyroglobulinemia[189,390,453,698] and lymphoproliferative disorders[245,474,734] also improve with antiviral cure (see Extrahepatic Manifestations). The benefit of curative antiviral therapy is underscored by dramatic reductions in the risk of liver-related and all-cause mortality[81,531,785] and markedly improved quality of life.[70,828] It is now apparent that DAA therapy expands the health benefits of antiviral cure to chronically infected patients with severe liver disease who were often poor responders to pegIFN/riba therapy.[100,366,378,571,783] In one large study of patients with advanced liver disease and comorbidities followed for almost 3 years after DAA cure, a significant reduction in liver-related and all-cause mortality and HCC was observed.[100] As noted above, approved DAA regimens are remarkably safe, and so far no direct long-term impact on health has been observed except for an increased risk of HBV reactivation in some coinfected patients that is as yet not fully unexplained.[62,525]

Current treatment landscape

DAA therapies are approved for all adults and children 12 years of age or older with chronic hepatitis C. Several studies have demonstrated safety and effectiveness of IFN- and ribavirin-free DAA regimens in children as young as 3 years old.[4,19,178,528,564,667] Approval of these therapies for children under 12 years of age is expected in the near future.[556] Treatment is highly cost-effective when compared with deferral until chronic infection is established.[57]

Treatment of chronic HCV infection is based upon a complex matrix of factors that must be considered when selecting effective DAA combinations.[2,185] Patient-related factors of importance include HCV genotype or subtype, treatment history with early-generation DAA that may have selected for resistant variants, pregnancy, and comorbidities such as compensated or decompensated cirrhosis, impaired kidney function, and HCV/HBV coinfection.[2,185] These factors must be considered when selecting the optimal DAA combination and duration of therapy to maximize the probability of achieving SVR while minimizing health risks in those with comorbidities. This complexity, along with the rapid cycle of DAA approval and withdrawal and refinements to therapy duration, precludes a detailed description of treatment options for chronic hepatitis C. Treatment of acute hepatitis C, defined as the first 6 months of infection, is recommended to prevent progression to chronic hepatitis C, onward transmission of the virus, or loss to follow-up. The reader is directed to evidence-based guidelines provided by the European Association for the Study of the Liver (EASL),[185] the American Association for the Study of Liver Diseases (AASLD), and the Infectious Diseases Society of America (IDSA) who jointly publish updates[2] and provide detailed web-based guidance for pre- and on-treatment assessment, DAA regimen selection, and posttreament follow-up where required (www.HCVGuidelines.org). The World Health Organization also publishes guidance for treatment of chronic hepatitis C (www.who.int/hepatitis/publications/hepatitis-c-guidelines-2018).

Eleven single or coformulated DAA were available for use in the United States at the close of 2018 (Fig. 8.18). DAA carry a suffix that identify inhibitors targeting the NS3/4A protease (*previr*), the NS5A replicase factor (*asvir*), or the NS5B RNA polymerase (*buvir*) (Fig. 8.18). Some DAA combinations have restricted use because they are not active against certain HCV genotypes, are toxic in the setting of advanced liver or kidney disease, interact with other drugs, or are ineffective in the setting of retreatment. As an example, genotype 3 infections are more difficult to cure for reasons that are not understood and fewer DAA regimens are available for treatment.

Two DAA combinations approved for use in 2016 (sofosbuvir and velpatasvir, SOF:VEL) and 2017 (glecaprevir and pibrentasvir, GLE:PIB) provided a significant advance in treatment of HCV infection. Both have pan-genotypic antiviral activity and cure almost all chronic HCV infections when taken orally as a single pill once per day. In open-label trials (POLARIS-2 and POLARIS-3) of SOF:VEL for 12 weeks, 96% to 98% of patients representing all HCV genotypes with and without compensated cirrhosis achieved an SVR.[317] Shortening therapy to 8 weeks failed to show noninferior efficacy,[188] and so this pan-genotypic combination is currently approved for 12-week regimens. Efficacy of the GLE:PIB combination was established in a series of 8- to 16-week treatment trials involving patients with and without comorbidities (cirrhosis and kidney disease) and inclusive of six HCV genotypes. SVR rates approaching 100% were observed against most genotypes (ENDURANCE 1, 2 and 4; SURVEYOR-1),[33,834] including those with compensated cirrhosis (EXPEDITION-1)[217] and severe kidney disease (EXPEDITION-4)[230] reflecting the limited metabolic activity of GLE and PIB in the liver and kidney. Very high SVR rates were also documented in liver and kidney transplant recipients with chronic hepatitis C (Magellan-2).[631] GLE:PIB is currently approved for 8 weeks of therapy in noncirrhotic patients infected with any HCV genotype. A longer (12-week) course of therapy is recommended under several circumstances including compensated cirrhosis, kidney disease, and liver and kidney transplant. Prior treatment experience with NS5A and NS3/4A DAA also adds complexity for GLE:PIB and SOF:VEL (see www.HCVGuidelines.org for details). A third pan-genotypic regimen approved in 2017 (SOF:VEL plus voxilaprevir, VOX) provides salvage therapy for those who failed prior DAA treatment due to emergence of stable resistant variants (Fig. 8.18). Importantly, large-scale postlicensure studies have demonstrated that the very high DAA cure rates observed in clinical trials are mostly replicated in a real-world setting, with low rates of discontinuation or adverse events.[34,83,93] Improved real-world SVR rates also extend to patients with advanced liver disease[632] and genotype 2 or 3 infections[205,803] who were difficult to cure with early-generation DAA combinations.

Mechanism of DAA action and resistance

The structure of HCV NS3 protease and NS5B polymerase proteins, how they function within the virus replication cycle, and DAA inhibition of enzymatic function are now well defined.[45,264] NS5A lacks enzymatic activity, and the functions that are impaired by DAA to achieve viral suppression remain somewhat less certain. The requirement for combination therapy with at least two classes of current-generation DAA underscores the tremendous potential of HCV for adaptive mutation and susceptibility of all three targeted NS proteins to resistance mutations. The rapid response of the HCV quasispecies to DAA selection pressure is explained by a high inherent replication rate, the error-prone replicase function of NS5B, and capacity for compensating mutations elsewhere in the viral genome (see Infectious Agent for details). Substitutions in the HCV genome that confer resistance to antiviral agents are termed resistance-associated substitutions (RAS).[573] HCV quasispecies populations that carry RAS are defined as resistant variants (RAV).[573] Emergence of RAV while on treatment is termed a virological breakthrough, while resurgence of virus replication after cessation of therapy is called a relapse. There is a consensus that baseline (i.e., pretreatment) RAS do not have an impact on DAA treatment outcome if present at a frequency of less than 15%, which is approximately equivalent to the lower limit of sensitivity (10%–25%) for the widely used Sanger sequencing method.[573] As noted above, the importance of RAS testing before treatment has diminished for current frontline pan-genotypic therapies.[2,185] The structure and function of the NS3/4A protease, NS5A replicase factor, and NS5B polymerase in the HCV replication cycle are detailed in Chapter 7 but are reviewed briefly below to provide a foundation for understanding the current concepts of inhibitor function and antiviral resistance. RAS active against each inhibitor class have been catalogued.[709] Use of DAA to suppress HCV replication in cell culture models has provided important insight into the emergence and fitness of RAS,[279,590] as well as antiviral potency[369] and the virus replication cycle.[52,478]

Virologic response to DAA treatment. A detailed profile of HCV RNA decline in serum after treatment with pegIFN/riba was obtained by frequent sampling of patients after initiation of therapy.[547] A delay of about 8 hours observed before the initial decline in viremia was attributed to the time required for IFN to initiate an ISG response. A rapid decline in HCV RNA from serum over the 1st day occurs with a calculated half-life of approximately 2.7 hours.[547] From the decay kinetic, virus production was calculated as 10^{11} to 10^{12} virions per day to maintain the typical viral titers of 10^6 RNA genomes/mL of serum observed during untreated chronic infection.[547] A much slower decline after day 2 is attributed to gradual loss of infected cells that are not replaced.[547]

A decline in viremia is observed within 2 hours of initiating DAA therapy, and the first and second phases of viral decline are substantially shorter than for pegIFN/riba therapy.[233] The analysis of viral decay kinetics on DAA therapy has provided insight into the mechanism of action of different DAA classes and to predict duration of treatment. As an example, the first phase of viral decline is much faster during treatment with NS5A inhibitors when compared with NS5B inhibitors or pegIFN/riba.[233,266,267] A 1,000-fold decline in serum HCV RNA titer 12 hours observed after a single dose of the NS5A inhibitor daclatasvir[233] would predict a half-life of 45 minutes[265] versus the estimated 2 to 3 hours based on the response to IFN-based therapy.[547] As noted below, studies of NS5A antiviral mechanisms[52,54,72,478] and mathematical modeling[265] demonstrated that accelerated decay is due to a dual mode of action that includes rapid inhibition of viral export from infected cells in addition to suppression of HCV RNA replication.

The shortened second phase of viral decline under DAA treatment may not be explained by cell death alone. Cure of infected hepatocytes by highly effective drugs is an alternate explanation that is consistent with elimination of replicating HCV genomes from cultured cells by prolonged treatment with protease or polymerase inhibitors.[64,638] Decay kinetics can also be employed to estimate the duration of DAA therapy required to cure infection. From a theoretical perspective, cure is defined as less than 1 virus particle in extracellular body fluid or less than one infected cell, a concept known as the cure boundary.[268,707] The decay kinetic of viremia in patients treated with combined protease and polymerase inhibitors yielded an estimate of approximately 8 to 12 weeks to cure in the absence of viral breakthrough.[231] This estimate is consistent with the

recommended minimum duration of treatment for the two pan-genotypic DAA combinations that have a high barrier to resistance (8 weeks for GLE:PIB and 12 weeks for SOF:VEL in treatment-naïve patients). Low SVR rates in patients treated with 4- or 6-week ultrashort DAA regimens further support this estimate.[345,367,368]

Inhibitors of the NS3/NS4a protease. The HCV NS3 protein has protease and helicase activities, but only the former has been targeted for antiviral development because of structural similarities between NS3 and cellular helicases.[45] NS3 protease function requires a physical association with the NS4A cofactor for tethering to the membranous web where HCV replicates and for stabilization of the NS3 protease domain and substrate recognition site.[45,75,359] The active site of the NS3 serine protease is a cleft formed by two β-barrel subdomains with a chymotrypsin-like structural fold (Fig. 8.18).[45,75,359] Specificity of the protease is defined by a substrate motif consisting of an acidic residue at position P6 (6 amino acids N-terminal of the cleavage site), a cysteine residue at position P1, and small amino acid side chain at the P1' site (immediately after the cleavage site).[372] Low substrate specificity imparted by this motif and weak interactions along an extended surface of the protease active site may facilitate cleavage of adapter proteins MAVS and TRIF to impair interferon signaling pathways (see Innate Immunity section). It also posed challenges for antiviral design. Early inhibitor design capitalized on the observation that an N-terminal hexapeptide product (DDIVPC-OH) derived from cleavage of the NS3-4A junction inhibited protease function.[307,438] Mutagenesis and single amino acid substitutions led to development of the first peptide inhibitors of HCV protease function.[307,438] Protease inhibitors act by blocking the NS3 catalytic site and fall into two major classes based on physicochemical and structural properties. Boceprevir and telaprevir, the two first-generation FDA-licensed protease inhibitors that are now discontinued, were linear ketoamide peptides that acted by reversible covalent binding to the NS3 protease site.[433,788] All subsequent protease inhibitors are macrocyclic (P1-P3 or P2-P4) or linear acyclic peptides that bind noncovalently to NS3.[475] The potential for emergence of NS3 RAV is illustrated by studies of monotherapy with protease inhibitors.[432,658] In one early study, telaprevir caused a rapid initial decline in viremia, but virologicial breakthrough was evident before cessation of drug dosing at day 14.[658] RAV were replaced by wild-type virus within 3 to 7 months after withdrawal of therapy,[658] a finding common to all generations of protease inhibitors under conditions of functional monotherapy.[88,415,723] Resistance in patients is caused by a complex pattern of distinct but overlapping NS3 RAS that can vary by HCV genotype, replication rate, and fitness as well as drug potency,[659] an observation that has been recapitulated in cell culture models with a large panel of protease inhibitors assessed against multiple HCV genotypes.[322] Three mutations at NS3 positions 155Arg(Lys/Thr/Gln), 156Ala(ValThr), and 168Asp(Ala/Val/Thr/His) are in general the most fit across genotypes[322] and were identified as major drivers of resistance to early-generation NS3 inhibitors (Fig. 8.18). Improvement in protease inhibitor function has been directed toward reducing toxicity and RAS susceptibility while enhancing potency and pan-genotypic activity. For example, the protease inhibitor grazoprevir is not inhibited by RAS Arg155 because of structural modifications that alter its interaction with the NS3 active site.[640] Importantly, baseline

NS3 RAS have no impact on effectiveness of protease inhibitors glecaprevir and voxilaprevir incorporated into the recently approved pan-genotypic regimens,[382,657] and they are effective against common RAS engineered into HCV replicons representing six genotypes.[279,590]

Inhibitors of the NS5A replicase factor. HCV NS5A is a multifunctional phosphoprotein important for replication of viral genome, assembly and egress of virions, as well as interaction with many cellular proteins essential for virus replication including cyclophilin A and the phosphatidylinositol 4-kinase IIIα (see Infectious Agent).[29,50,219,431,644] It is composed of three domains (D1–D3) separated by low-complexity sequences anchored to intracellular membrane layers by an N-terminal amphipathic α-helix (Fig. 8.18).[576,644,743] The three domains are involved in RNA binding and replication as well as assembly and transport of infectious particles through interaction with lipid droplets.[468,644,742,823] NS5A proteins exist as multiple phosphovariants and form dimers or perhaps oligomers to tether HCV RNA genomes to the membranous web.[45,644,823] NS5A was not an obvious target for antiviral drug development given its lack of enzymatic activity and complex interaction with HCV proteins and genomes as well as cellular proteins. HCV replicon models facilitated a chemical genetics strategy to identify NS5A inhibitors.[233] A screen of large compound libraries revealed a small molecule, daclatasvir, that suppressed HCV replication and selected for mutations in NS5A.[233] Several NS5A inhibitors are now used in combination with a NS3/4A protease and/or NS5B polymerase inhibitors for treatment of chronic infection (Fig. 8.18). How these inhibitors suppress HCV replication is poorly understood, but they may have a pervasive effect on patterns of NS5A phosphorylation[226] and subcellular localization.[414] Although they were initially identified as inhibitors of HCV replication, it is now apparent that they also act through additional mechanisms including a rapid independent block of viral assembly[54,478] and transfer of genomic RNA to assembly sites.[72] A mode of action targeting virion assembly or export in addition to inhibition of RNA replication is also consistent with accelerated decay of viremia in patients treated with NS5A inhibitors[233] and provided the best fit for mathematical models seeking to explain the viral dynamics.[265] Further analysis of NS5A antiviral activity in cell culture models demonstrated that replicase complex stability is variable between viruses and is determined by sequence differences in NS5A proteins.[52] As a class, these inhibitors have pan-genotypic antiviral activity that may be facilitated by binding to a conserved site on NS5A monomers or dimers that stabilizes their structure, preventing further conformational changes important for virus replication.[54,233] NS5A RAS are detected in the HCV quasispecies before treatment and amplify under selection pressure from inhibitors. The most potent RAS that provide resistance across four or more genotypes are located within NS5A D1 domain (93Tyr) or the linker sequence between D1 and the N-terminal α-helix (31Leu) (Fig. 8.18).[45] Genotype and even subtype differences in RAS diversity and barrier to resistance have been described[836] and may be related to differences in evolutionary pathways to inhibitor resistance observed in genotype 1a versus 1b infections during a short course of monotherapy with an NS5a inhibitor (elbasvir).[841] NS5A RAV that emerged under selection pressure due to treatment failure with earlier-generation DAA combinations are very stable for years.[383,826] As noted above, persistence of NS5A RAV is

an important consideration in selection of DAA for retreatment. The high SVR rate with current pan-genotypic DAA combinations may reflect in part a higher barrier to resistance for pibrentasvir and velpatasvir. When compared with earlier-generation NS5A inhibitors, pibrentasvir and velpatasvir had high uniform antiviral activity against all seven HCV genotypes in a cell culture model of virus replication.[252] Three days of monotherapy with these inhibitors selected for RAS in some patients but the barrier to resistance was generally higher. Unlike other NS5A inhibitors, resistance usually required replacement of amino acids at more than one position, and fitness for replication was impaired.[405,549]

Inhibitors of the NS5B RNA-dependent RNA polymerase. Synthesis of HCV RNA genomes by the membrane-anchored NS5B RdRp is mediated by a catalytic core with right-handed "finger, palm, thumb" subdomains (Fig. 8.18).[12,45,76,418] Structural studies and comparison with other viral RdRps indicate that the catalytic core is closely tethered to the membrane in a closed conformation for initiation of synthesis with a single-stranded RNA template.[281,693] Conversion to an open conformation with a large cavity accommodates double-stranded RNA for the elongation process (Fig. 8.18).[45,523] Polymerase inhibitors fall into two major classes based on mode of action. The nucleotide and nucleoside inhibitors (NI) are mimics of ribonucleosides or ribonucleotides that competitively inhibit binding of the natural substrate to the HCV RdRp active site. Once incorporated into the catalytic site during transcription, NI 2′-C-methyl or 5′-fluoro groups sterically hinder further incorporation of nucleotides resulting in chain termination.[145] As a class, NI are nonphosphorylated prodrugs that must be converted into the active nucleoside 5′ triphosphate by cellular enzymes, an inefficient and rate-limiting process. Sofosbuvir (SOF), the only NI approved for treatment of chronic hepatitis C, is a ProTide that overcomes this limitation by adding one phosphate during synthesis.[708] All NI including SOF have pan-genotypic antiviral activity and a high barrier to resistance because they bind the functionally conserved catalytic pocket of the polymerase.[316,407] One RAS, Ser282Thr, provides escape from SOF in a cell culture model, but it substantially impairs virus replication (Fig. 8.18).[408] Selection of RAS including Ser282Thr by SOF is rarely observed in clinical studies.[159,406,729] Nonnucleoside inhibitors (NNI) bind allosteric sites in the NS5B thumb and palm domains outside of the catalytic pocket. They act noncompetitively by preventing RdRp conformational changes after binding to one of five allosteric sites outside of the catalytic grove (Fig. 8.18).[45] The only NNI licensed for treatment of chronic hepatitis C is dasbuvir that binds a site at the junction of the palm and thumb subdomains to block a step before RNA chain elongation.[599] Unlike NI, NNI readily select for RAS that do not impose a high fitness for HCV replication. Failure to achieve SVR with early DAA combinations containing dasbuvir was associated with emergence of NS5B RAS Met414Thr and Ser556Gly in genotype 1a viruses (Fig. 8.18).[204,598,835] Several NS5B NNI RAS occur naturally at high frequency.[153] For instance, the RAS Ser556Gly was found in approximately 8% of HCV-1b sequences and a remarkable 97% (genotype 4) to 100% (genotypes 2, 3, 5) of other clinically significant genotypes.[153]

Host-targeting agents

HCV has a pervasive impact on the infected hepatocyte, subverting and repurposing multiple cellular pathways to support entry, translation and replication, assembly, and export of virions. Development of host-targeting agents (HTA) to inhibit HCV replication has occurred in parallel with DAA development, with the objective of finding alternative or complementary pan-genotypic antivirals with a high barrier to resistance. HTA designed to block almost every stage of the virus replication cycle have been developed, and a small number were assessed in clinical studies. They include small molecules designed to block HCV binding to the SR-BI entry receptor,[645,722] the cyclophilin A:NS5A interaction required for replication and membranous web formation,[535,574] and core protein trafficking to lipid droplets.[232] None were sufficiently potent against HCV when compared with DAA combinations. One potential exception is an inhibitor of miRNA-122 designated miravirsen (SPC3549). Miravirsen is an antisense locked nucleic acid–modified phosphorothiate oligonucleotide that demonstrated strong pan-genotypic suppression of HCV replication in cell culture models.[330,331,420] Weekly dosing of patients with chronic hepatitis C demonstrated that the compound is safe, an important consideration given the role of miR-122 in host lipid metabolism. It was highly effective in dose-dependent suppression of HCV replication. Virological relapse within 14 weeks of completing treatment and wide variation in patient responsiveness indicated that miravirsen will only be effective in combination with other agents.[318,786]

Public Health Measures and Treatment to Reduce Transmission

A global strategy to eliminate HCV and HBV by 2030 was adopted by the World Health Organization (WHO) in 2016 (see www.who.int/hepatitis/strategies2016-2021/ghss-hep/en). This goal is aligned with a 2017 recommendation from the National Academy of Sciences to undertake elimination of these viruses in the United States.[537] Elimination of infection is distinct from eradication and is defined as the reduction of infection and/or disease in a given geographic area through deliberate control efforts that must be continued indefinitely to prevent reemergence. The 2030 elimination target for viral hepatitis is a 90% reduction in new chronic infections caused by HCV and HBV and a 65% reduction in deaths when compared with a 2015 baseline. HCV elimination programs have been initiated in a number of countries but are most advanced in Egypt, Georgia, Iceland, and Australia.[161,173,669]

Safety of the blood supply has improved dramatically with implementation of effective screening measures for HCV antibodies and nucleic acid testing to identify contaminated units. In countries with effective screening measures, the estimated risk of HCV infection from blood transfusion is now 1:1,900,000 donated units, a dramatic reduction from the era before the discovery of HCV when the risk was approximately 1:10.[157,319,605] Further progress in reducing transfusion-associated infections in low-income countries will require more uniform adoption of effective blood screening measures.[137] Unsafe injection practices caused by reuse of needles and an absence of sterile equipment in medical settings also continue to be a source of HCV infections in many parts of the world despite improvement.[305,579,604] As noted above (Epidemiology), new HCV infections are increasing globally and in the United States because of needle sharing associated with injection of opioids and heroin. Needle exchange and opioid substitution therapy sharply reduce the risk of HCV transmission,[521,595] but these programs have not been instituted in much of the

world. Regional disparities in availability exist in many developed countries including those in Europe and the United States.[223,649,800] Availability of DAA to treat HCV safely and with fewer side effects can reduce prevalence.[291,313] It also has the potential to interrupt transmission,[283,526] but will require a commitment to diagnosis and treatment in many regions of the world where new HCV infections still outpace cure of chronic hepatitis C.[290] Expanded treatments, along with other harm reduction strategies discussed above, are cornerstones of national elimination programs in Egypt, Australia, Iceland, and Georgia that may provide models for the future.[161,173,283,669]

Vaccines

Vaccines to prevent and treat chronic HCV infection have been a major research focus since discovery of the virus. Therapeutic vaccines directed at restoring HCV-specific T-cell immunity were assessed in chronically infected humans, but they provided no significant control of persistent virus replication.[41,762] Two studies demonstrated the challenge in restoring T-cell immunity under conditions of persistent HCV infection. Chronically infected chimpanzees that received a genetic vaccine expressing HCV nonstructural proteins NS3-NS5B while viremia was transiently suppressed with DAA failed to clear the virus.[96] The HCV genes, delivered by priming and boosting with recombinant adenoviruses, elicited a CD8+ T-cell response against epitopes that were unique to the vaccine or had acquired escape mutations earlier in infection.[96] The same highly immunogenic vaccine also failed to elicit CD8+ T cells targeting the circulating virus in humans treated with pegIFN/riba.[354,731] Therapeutic vaccines are no longer a priority with the advent of DAA therapy.

A preventive vaccine is considered a high priority for prevention of primary infection and reinfection after DAA cure, especially in those who remain at risk for reexposure to the virus.[461,462,501,592] Modeling studies indicate that even a partially effective vaccine would reduce HCV transmission[273,454,668,716] and contribute directly to the goal of global HCV elimination that for now relies entirely on public health measures and expanded access to DAA therapies.

The objective of vaccination is to prevent persistent infection. As detailed above (see Clinical Features), acute hepatitis C is often subclinical, and so there is no apparent requirement to induce sterilizing immunity by vaccination. Two observations support the concept that a vaccine to prevent persistence, but not necessarily infection, is feasible. Most importantly, spontaneous resolution of infection elicits long-lasting adaptive immunity that responds rapidly upon reexposure to the virus. Duration and magnitude of viremia are reduced, and the risk of persistent infection is sharply lower in individuals with naturally acquired immunity. Protection against an array of HCV genotypes has been observed in chimpanzees after clearance of primary infeciton.[391] In addition, there is clear evidence that control of acute primary and secondary infection is associated with onset of sustained HCV-specific neutralizing antibody and T-cell responses (discussed in detail in Immune Responses).

Two parallel approaches to vaccine development have been pursued. The first is immunization with envelope glycoproteins to induce protective humoral immunity. This approach is exemplified by immunization with recombinant HCV genotype 1a envelope glycoproteins E1 and E2 produced in CHO cells and formulated in an oil/water emulsion adjuvant (designated MF59) for induction of neutralizing antibodies.[299] This strategy, developed at Chiron Corporation, elicited antibodies that provided apparent sterilizing immunity to HCV challenge in some chimpanzees.[299] Breakthrough infections were observed, but virus replication was attenuated and spontaneous resolution was more likely when compared with mock vaccination controls.[299] The vaccine induced strong CD4+ T-cell immunity and antibodies that had broad neutralizing activity against most HCV genotypes in cell culture studies.[497] Safety and immunogenicity of this vaccine was assessed in human volunteers with no risk factors for HCV infection. Pan-genotypic neutralizing antibodies and robust CD4+ T-cell memory were also elicited in the human volunteers.[225,403] Expanded immunogenicity and efficacy trials have not yet been undertaken.

The second approach to preventive vaccination involves induction of T-cell immunity with a nonstructural NS-NS5B gene cassette delivered using a prime boost strategy with virus vectors. This vaccine is unlike others developed for protection against virus infections, as it was designed to prime CD4+ and CD8+ T cells that are resistant to exhaustion during acute infection. Preclinical studies demonstrated that this vaccine elicited strong memory T-cell immunity in chimpanzees that was rapidly recalled upon HCV challenge.[214] A typical pattern of robust acute phase HCV replication observed in mock-vaccinated animals was suppressed by several orders of magnitude in the group that received the vaccine.[214] Safety and immunogenicity of this vaccine was assessed in human volunteers. Vaccinees who received two immunizations with serologically distinct adenovirus vectors developed robust T-cell immunity targeting class I and II epitopes encoded by the NS3-NS5B gene cassette.[42] The second adenovirus vector was replaced with a modified vaccinia Ankara (MVA) vector in a immunogenicity second trial. The MVA vector provided substantially stronger boosting of HCV-specific T-cell immunity.[730] The combination of adenovirus and MVA vectors containing the HCV NS3-NS5B gene cassette has been assessed in a staged phase I/II clinical trial in Baltimore, San Francisco, and Santa Fe, New Mexico (see Clinical Trials.gov NCT01436357). The objective of the trial was to assess protection from HCV persistence in participants who are HCV-naïve but at risk for infection. An initial report of results was provided on the ClinicalTrials.gov Web site (NCT01436357) in 2019. The frequency of incident persistent infections (5.1%) was identical in the vaccine and placebo arms. Analysis of a subset of subjects in both arms revealed that HCV-specific immune responses were present in 97% of vaccinees versus 4% of subjects who received the placebo. Why this vaccine failed to protect against HCV persistence is not known. A detailed analysis of immunogenicity in vaccinated subjects at risk of HCV exposure, as well as the nature of the recall response in those who were infected, sequencing matching between the vaccine and circulating virus, and evolution of HCV genomes in acute and chronic phases of infection should provide critical insight into this question.

PERSPECTIVE

The landscape of HCV research and treatment has changed dramatically over the past 6 to 7 years. From a research perspective, the discovery of new rodent and equine hepaciviruses provides new opportunities to study key elements of the host–virus relationship that are difficult to approach in humans. Important unanswered questions about *Hepacivirus* subversion of hepatic innate and adaptive immune responses can be addressed in these tractable animal models. Whether immune responses recover or afford protection after DAA cure is also unknown and will be assessed in humans and possibly the new animal models. Understanding failure and recovery of virus-specific T cells is likely to provide general knowledge relevant to other persistent human infections and diseases where immune exhaustion is a barrier to cure.

The rapid evolution of DAA to pan-genotypic regimens of 8- to 12-week duration with a single daily pill has revolutionized treatment for chronic HCV infection. It has also made the concept of HCV elimination a possibility, although it is clear that the task will be difficult with enhanced public health measures and antiviral treatment alone. Mathematical modeling indicates that a vaccine with 30% efficacy would have a measurable impact on transmission.[273,454,668,716] A detailed understanding of why the first efficacy trial of a preventive HCV vaccine failed is an imperative. New animal models may also provide guidance on the critical unanswered question of what constitutes protective immunity. Success will ultimately also require a sustained commitment to assess vaccines in humans, and to learn from setbacks, in an era of highly effective DAA therapy.

REFERENCES

1. Aach RD, Stevens CE, Hollinger FB, et al. Hepatitis C virus infection in post-transfusion hepatitis. An analysis with first- and second-generation assays. *N Engl J Med* 1991;325(19):1325–1329.
2. AASLD-IDSA HCV Guidance Panel. Hepatitis C Guidance 2018 Update: AASLD-IDSA recommendations for testing, managing, and treating hepatitis C virus infection. *Clin Infect Dis* 2018;67(10):1477–1492.
3. Abayasingam A, Leung P, Eltahla A, et al. Genomic characterization of hepatitis C virus transmitted founder variants with deep sequencing. *Infect Genet Evol* 2019;71:36–41.
4. Abdel Ghaffar TY, El Naghi S, Abdel Gawad M, et al. Safety and efficacy of combined sofosbuvir/daclatasvir treatment of children and adolescents with chronic hepatitis C Genotype 4. *J Viral Hepat* 2019;26(2):263–270.
5. Abdel-Hakeem MS, Bedard N, Badr G, et al. Comparison of immune restoration in early versus late alpha interferon therapy against hepatitis C virus. *J Virol* 2010;84(19):10429–10435.
6. Abdel-Hakeem MS, Bedard N, Murphy D, et al. Signatures of protective memory immune responses during hepatitis C virus reinfection. *Gastroenterology* 2014;147(4):870–881.e878.
7. Abdel-Hakeem MS, Shoukry NH. Protective immunity against hepatitis C: many shades of gray. *Front Immunol* 2014;5:274.
8. Abe K, Edamoto Y, Park YN, et al. In situ detection of hepatitis B, C, and G virus nucleic acids in human hepatocellular carcinoma tissues from different geographic regions. *Hepatology* 1998;28(2):568–572.
9. Abe K, Inchauspe G, Shikata T, et al. Three different patterns of hepatitis C virus infection in chimpanzees. *Hepatology* 1992;15(4):690–695.
10. Adams G, Kuntz S, Rabalais G, et al. Natural recovery from acute hepatitis C virus infection by agammaglobulinemic twin children. *Pediatr Infect Dis J* 1997;16(5):533–534.
11. Aghemo A, Degasperi E, De Nicola S, et al. Quantification of core antigen monitors efficacy of direct-acting antiviral agents in patients with chronic hepatitis C virus infection. *Clin Gastroenterol Hepatol* 2016;14(9):1331–1336.
12. Ago H, Adachi T, Yoshida A, et al. Crystal structure of the RNA-dependent RNA polymerase of hepatitis C virus. *Structure* 1999;7(11):1417–1426.
13. Ahlenstiel G, Titerence RH, Koh C, et al. Natural killer cells are polarized toward cytotoxicity in chronic hepatitis C in an interferon-alfa-dependent manner. *Gastroenterology* 2010;138(1):325–335.e321–322.
14. Aiken T, Garber A, Thomas D, et al. Donor IFNL4 genotype is associated with early post-transplant fibrosis in recipients with hepatitis C. *PLoS One* 2016;11(11):e0166998.
15. Aitken CK, Tracy SL, Revill P, et al. Consecutive infections and clearances of different hepatitis C virus genotypes in an injecting drug user. *J Clin Virol* 2008;41(4):293–296.
16. Aka PV, Kuniholm MH, Pfeiffer RM, et al. Association of the IFNL4-DeltaG allele with impaired spontaneous clearance of hepatitis C virus. *J Infect Dis* 2014;209(3):350–354.
17. Alao H, Cam M, Keembiyehetty C, et al. Baseline intrahepatic and peripheral innate immunity are associated with hepatitis C virus clearance during direct-acting antiviral therapy. *Hepatology* 2018;68(6):2078–2088.
18. Alemy-Carreau M, Durbec JP, Giordanella J, et al. Lack of interaction between hepatitis C virus and alcohol in the pathogenesis of cirrhosis. A statistical study. *J Hepatol* 1996;25(5):627–632.
19. Alkaaby BA, Al-Ethawi AE. The effectiveness of oral antiviral (Sofosbuvir/Ledipasvir) in treating children with HCV infection. *Pak J Med Sci* 2018;34(6):1353–1356.
20. Alter MJ. Epidemiology of hepatitis C. *Hepatology* 1997;26(3 Suppl 1):62S–65S.

This chapter represents a revised and updated version of the chapter from the Sixth Edition of Fields Virology written by Stuart C. Ray, Justin R. Bailey, and David L. Thomas. Some of the figures and tables, as well as portions of the text have been carried forward from previous editions.

21. Alter MJ, Margolis HS, Krawczynski K, et al. The natural history of community-acquired hepatitis C in the United States. The Sentinel Counties Chronic non-A, non-B Hepatitis Study Team. *N Engl J Med* 1992;327(27):1899–1905.

22. Alter HJ, Purcell RH, Holland PV, et al. Transmissible agent in non-A, non-B hepatitis. *Lancet* 1978;1(8062):459–463.

23. Amadei B, Urbani S, Cazaly A, et al. Activation of natural killer cells during acute infection with hepatitis C virus. *Gastroenterology* 2010;138(4):1536–1545.

24. Amanzada A, Kopp W, Spengler U, et al. Interferon-lambda4 (IFNL4) transcript expression in human liver tissue samples. *PLoS One* 2013;8(12):e84026.

25. Anggakusuma, Brown RJP, Banda DH, et al. Hepacivirus NS3/4A proteases interfere with MAVS signaling in both their cognate animal hosts and humans: implications for zoonotic transmission. *J Virol* 2016;90(23):10670–10681.

26. ANRS collaborative study group on hepatocellular carcinoma (ANRS CO22 HEPATHER, CO12 CirVir and CO23 CUPILT cohorts). Lack of evidence of an effect of direct-acting antivirals on the recurrence of hepatocellular carcinoma: data from three ANRS cohorts. *J Hepatol* 2016;65(4):734–740.

27. Ansari MA, Pedergnana V, L CI p C, et al. Genome-to-genome analysis highlights the effect of the human innate and adaptive immune systems on the hepatitis C virus. *Nat Genet* 2017;49(5):666–673.

28. Antonelli A, Ferri C, Fallahi P, et al. Thyroid disorders in chronic hepatitis C virus infection. *Thyroid* 2006;16(6):563–572.

29. Appel N, Zayas M, Miller S, et al. Essential role of domain III of nonstructural protein 5A for hepatitis C virus infectious particle assembly. *PLoS Pathog* 2008;4(3):e1000035.

30. Ariumi Y, Kuroki M, Maki M, et al. The ESCRT system is required for hepatitis C virus production. *PLoS One* 2011;6(1):e14517.

31. Arnaud N, Dabo S, Maillard P, et al. Hepatitis C virus controls interferon production through PKR activation. *PLoS One* 2010;5(5):e10575.

32. Asselah T, Bieche I, Narguet S, et al. Liver gene expression signature to predict response to pegylated interferon plus ribavirin combination therapy in patients with chronic hepatitis C. *Gut* 2008;57(4):516–524.

33. Asselah T, Kowdley KV, Zadeikis N, et al. Efficacy of glecaprevir/pibrentasvir for 8 or 12 weeks in patients with hepatitis C virus genotype 2, 4, 5, or 6 infection without cirrhosis. *Clin Gastroenterol Hepatol* 2018;16(3):417–426.

34. Backus LI, Belperio PS, Shahoumian TA, et al. Real-world effectiveness and predictors of sustained virological response with all-oral therapy in 21,242 hepatitis C genotype-1 patients. *Antivir Ther* 2017;22(6):481–493.

35. Backus LI, Boothroyd DB, Phillips BR, et al. A sustained virologic response reduces risk of all-cause mortality in patients with hepatitis C. *Clin Gastroenterol Hepatol* 2011;9(6):509–516. e501.

36. Bailey JR, Flyak AI, Cohen VJ, et al. Broadly neutralizing antibodies with few somatic mutations and hepatitis C virus clearance. *JCI Insight* 2017;2(9).

37. Bailey JR, Wasilewski LN, Snider AE, et al. Naturally selected hepatitis C virus polymorphisms confer broad neutralizing antibody resistance. *J Clin Invest* 2015;125(1):437–447.

38. Bang CS, Song IH. Impact of antiviral therapy on hepatocellular carcinoma and mortality in patients with chronic hepatitis C: systematic review and meta-analysis. *BMC Gastroenterol* 2017;17(1):46.

39. Bankwitz D, Doepke M, Hueging K, et al. Maturation of secreted HCV particles by incorporation of secreted ApoE protects from antibodies by enhancing infectivity. *J Hepatol* 2017;67(3):480–489.

40. Bankwitz D, Steinmann E, Bitzegeio J, et al. Hepatitis C virus hypervariable region 1 modulates receptor interactions, conceals the CD81 binding site, and protects conserved neutralizing epitopes. *J Virol* 2010;84(11):5751–5763.

41. Barnes E. Therapeutic vaccines in HBV: lessons from HCV. *Med Microbiol Immunol* 2015;204(1):79–86.

42. Barnes E, Folgori A, Capone S, et al. Novel adenovirus-based vaccines induce broad and sustained T cell responses to HCV in man. *Sci Transl Med* 2012;4(115):115ra111.

43. Barocas JA, Tasillo A, Eftekhari Yazdi G, et al. Population-level outcomes and cost-effectiveness of expanding the recommendation for age-based hepatitis C testing in the United States. *Clin Infect Dis* 2018;67(4):549–556.

44. Bartenschlager R, Lohmann V. Replication of hepatitis C virus. *J Gen Virol* 2000;81 (Pt 7):1631–1648.

45. Bartenschlager R, Lohmann V, Penin F. The molecular and structural basis of advanced antiviral therapy for hepatitis C virus infection. *Nat Rev Microbiol* 2013;11(7):482–496.

46. Bartosch B, Bukh J, Meunier JC, et al. In vitro assay for neutralizing antibody to hepatitis C virus: evidence for broadly conserved neutralization epitopes. *Proc Natl Acad Sci U S A* 2003;100(24):14199–14204.

47. Bartosch B, Dubuisson J, Cosset FL. Infectious hepatitis C virus pseudo-particles containing functional E1-E2 envelope protein complexes. *J Exp Med* 2003;197(5):633–642.

48. Bassett SE, Guerra B, Brasky K, et al. Protective immune response to hepatitis C virus in chimpanzees rechallenged following clearance of primary infection. *Hepatology* 2001;33(6):1479–1487.

49. Bassett SE, Thomas DL, Brasky KM, et al. Viral persistence, antibody to E1 and E2, and hypervariable region 1 sequence stability in hepatitis C virus-inoculated chimpanzees. *J Virol* 1999;73(2):1118–1126.

50. Benga WJ, Krieger SE, Dimitrova M, et al. Apolipoprotein E interacts with hepatitis C virus nonstructural protein 5A and determines assembly of infectious particles. *Hepatology* 2010;51(1):43–53.

51. Bengsch B, Seigel B, Ruhl M, et al. Coexpression of PD-1, 2B4, CD160 and KLRG1 on exhausted HCV-specific CD8+ T cells is linked to antigen recognition and T cell differentiation. *PLoS Pathog* 2010;6(6):e1000947.

52. Benzine T, Brandt R, Lovell WC, et al. NS5A inhibitors unmask differences in functional replicase complex half-life between different hepatitis C virus strains. *PLoS Pathog* 2017;13(6):e1006343.

53. Berger KL, Cooper JD, Heaton NS, et al. Roles for endocytic trafficking and phosphatidylinositol 4-kinase III alpha in hepatitis C virus replication. *Proc Natl Acad Sci U S A* 2009;106(18):7577–7582.

54. Berger C, Romero-Brey I, Radujkovic D, et al. Daclatasvir-like inhibitors of NS5A block early biogenesis of hepatitis C virus-induced membranous replication factories, independent of RNA replication. *Gastroenterology* 2014;147(5):1094–1105.e1025.

55. Bernsmeier C, Duong FH, Christen V, et al. Virus-induced over-expression of protein phosphatase 2A inhibits insulin signalling in chronic hepatitis C. *J Hepatol* 2008;49(3):429–440.

56. Bernstein D, Kleinman L, Barker CM, et al. Relationship of health-related quality of life to treatment adherence and sustained response in chronic hepatitis C patients. *Hepatology* 2002;35(3):704–708.

57. Bethea ED, Chen Q, Hur C, et al. Should we treat acute hepatitis C? A decision and cost-effectiveness analysis. *Hepatology* 2018;67(3):837–846.

58. Bigger CB, Brasky KM, Lanford RE. DNA microarray analysis of chimpanzee liver during acute resolving hepatitis C virus infection. *J Virol* 2001;75(15):7059–7066.

59. Bigger CB, Guerra B, Brasky KM, et al. Intrahepatic gene expression during chronic hepatitis C virus infection in chimpanzees. *J Virol* 2004;78(24):13779–13792.

60. Billerbeck E, Wolfisberg R, Fahnoe U, et al. Mouse models of acute and chronic hepacivirus infection. *Science* 2017;357(6347):204–208.

61. Binka M, Paintsil E, Patel A, et al. Survival of hepatitis c virus in syringes is dependent on the design of the syringe-needle and dead space volume. *PLoS One* 2015;10(11):e0139737.

62. Blackard JT, Sherman KE. Hepatitis B virus (HBV) reactivation-The potential role of direct-acting agents for hepatitis C virus (HCV). *Rev Med Virol* 2018;28(4):e1984.

63. Blight KJ, Kolykhalov AA, Rice CM. Efficient initiation of HCV RNA replication in cell culture. *Science* 2000;290(5498):1972–1974.

64. Blight KJ, McKeating JA, Rice CM. Highly permissive cell lines for subgenomic and genomic hepatitis C virus RNA replication. *J Virol* 2002;76(24):13001–13014.

65. Blumer T, Coto-Llerena M, Duong FHT, et al. SOCS1 is an inducible negative regulator of interferon lambda (IFN-lambda)-induced gene expression in vivo. *J Biol Chem* 2017;292(43):17928–17938.

66. Bochud PY, Bibert S, Kutalik Z, et al. IL28B alleles associated with poor hepatitis C virus (HCV) clearance protect against inflammation and fibrosis in patients infected with non-1 HCV genotypes. *Hepatology* 2012;55(2):384–394.

67. Boettler T, Spangenberg HC, Neumann-Haefelin C, et al. T cells with a CD4+CD25+ regulatory phenotype suppress in vitro proliferation of virus-specific CD8+ T cells during chronic hepatitis C virus infection. *J Virol* 2005;79(12):7860–7867.

68. Bolen CR, Ding S, Robek MD, et al. Dynamic expression profiling of type I and type III interferon-stimulated hepatocytes reveals a stable hierarchy of gene expression. *Hepatology* 2014;59(4):1262–1272.

69. Bonkovsky HL, Poh-Fitzpatrick M, Pimstone N, et al. Porphyria cutanea tarda, hepatitis C, and HFE gene mutations in North America. *Hepatology* 1998;27(6):1661–1669.

70. Boscarino JA, Lu M, Moorman AC, et al. Predictors of poor mental and physical health status among patients with chronic hepatitis C infection: the Chronic Hepatitis Cohort Study (CHeCS). *Hepatology* 2015;61(3):802–811.

71. Bose SK, Shrivastava S, Meyer K, et al. Hepatitis C virus activates the mTOR/S6K1 signaling pathway in inhibiting IRS-1 function for insulin resistance. *J Virol* 2012;86(11):6315–6322.

72. Boson B, Denolly S, Turlure F, et al. Daclatasvir prevents hepatitis C virus infectivity by blocking transfer of the viral genome to assembly sites. *Gastroenterology* 2017;152(4):895–907.e814.

73. Bradley DW, McCaustland KA, Cook EH, et al. Posttransfusion non-A, non-B hepatitis in chimpanzees. Physicochemical evidence that the tubule-forming agent is a small, enveloped virus. *Gastroenterology* 1985;88(3):773–779.

74. Bradley D, McCaustland K, Krawczynski K, et al. Hepatitis C virus: buoyant density of the factor VIII-derived isolate in sucrose. *J Med Virol* 1991;34(3):206–208.

75. Brass V, Berke JM, Montserret R, et al. Structural determinants for membrane association and dynamic organization of the hepatitis C virus NS3-4A complex. *Proc Natl Acad Sci U S A* 2008;105(38):14545–14550.

76. Bressanelli S, Tomei L, Roussel A, et al. Crystal structure of the RNA-dependent RNA polymerase of hepatitis C virus. *Proc Natl Acad Sci U S A* 1999;96(23):13034–13039.

77. Brimacombe CL, Grove J, Meredith LW, et al. Neutralizing antibody-resistant hepatitis C virus cell-to-cell transmission. *J Virol* 2011;85(1):596–605.

78. Broering TJ, Garrity KA, Boatright NK, et al. Identification and characterization of broadly neutralizing human monoclonal antibodies directed against the E2 envelope glycoprotein of hepatitis C virus. *J Virol* 2009;83(23):12473–12482.

79. Brownell J, Bruckner J, Wagoner J, et al. Direct, interferon-independent activation of the CXCL10 promoter by NF-kappaB and interferon regulatory factor 3 during hepatitis C virus infection. *J Virol* 2014;88(3):1582–1590.

80. Bruggmann P, Berg T, Ovrehus AL, et al. Historical epidemiology of hepatitis C virus (HCV) in selected countries. *J Viral Hepat* 2014;21 (Suppl 1):5–33.

81. Bruno S, Di Marco V, Iavarone M, et al. Survival of patients with HCV cirrhosis and sustained virologic response is similar to the general population. *J Hepatol* 2016;64(6):1217–1223.

82. Bruno S, Silini E, Crosignani A, et al. Hepatitis C virus genotypes and risk of hepatocellular carcinoma in cirrhosis: a prospective study. *Hepatology* 1997;25(3):754–758.

83. Buggisch P, Vermehren J, Mauss S, et al. Real-world effectiveness of 8-week treatment with ledipasvir/sofosbuvir in chronic hepatitis C. *J Hepatol* 2018;68(4):663–671.

84. Bull RA, Leung P, Gaudieri S, et al. Transmitted/founder viruses rapidly escape from CD8+ T Cell responses in acute hepatitis C virus infection. *J Virol* 2015;89(10):5478–5490.

85. Bull RA, Luciani F, McElroy K, et al. Sequential bottlenecks drive viral evolution in early acute hepatitis C virus infection. *PLoS Pathog* 2011;7(9):e1002243.

86. Burchill MA, Roby JA, Crochet N, et al. Rapid reversal of innate immune dysregulation in blood of patients and livers of humanized mice with HCV following DAA therapy. *PLoS One* 2017;12(10):e0186213.

87. Busch MP, Murthy KK, Kleinman SH, et al. Infectivity in chimpanzees (Pan troglodytes) of plasma collected before HCV RNA detectability by FDA-licensed assays: implications for transfusion safety and HCV infection outcomes. *Blood* 2012;119(26):6326–6334.

88. Buti M, Gordon SC, Zuckerman E, et al. Grazoprevir, elbasvir, and ribavirin for chronic hepatitis C virus genotype 1 infection after failure of pegylated interferon and ribavirin with an earlier-generation protease inhibitor: final 24-week results from C-SALVAGE. *Clin Infect Dis* 2016;62(1):32–36.

89. Cabrera R, Tu Z, Xu Y, et al. An immunomodulatory role for CD4(+)CD25(+) regulatory T lymphocytes in hepatitis C virus infection. *Hepatology* 2004;40(5):1062–1071.

90. Cacoub P, Comarmond C, Domont F, et al. Extrahepatic manifestations of chronic hepatitis C virus infection. *Ther Adv Infect Dis* 2016;3(1):3–14.

91. Cacoub P, Saadoun D, Limal N, et al. Hepatitis C virus infection and mixed cryoglobulinaemia vasculitis: a review of neurological complications. *AIDS* 2005;19(Suppl 3):S128–S134.

92. Cacoub P, Si Ahmed SN, Ferfar Y, et al. Long-term efficacy of interferon-free antiviral treatment regimens in patients with hepatitis C virus-associated cryoglobulinemia vasculitis. *Clin Gastroenterol Hepatol* 2019;17(3):518–526.

93. Calleja JL, Crespo J, Rincon D, et al. Effectiveness, safety and clinical outcomes of direct-acting antiviral therapy in HCV genotype 1 infection: results from a Spanish real-world cohort. *J Hepatol* 2017;66(6):1138–1148.

94. Callendret B, Bukh J, Eccleston HB, et al. Transmission of clonal hepatitis C virus genomes reveals the dominant but transitory role of CD8(+) T cells in early viral evolution. *J Virol* 2011;85(22):11833–11845.

95. Callendret B, Eccleston HB, Hall S, et al. T-cell immunity and hepatitis C virus reinfection after cure of chronic hepatitis C with an interferon-free antiviral regimen in a chimpanzee. *Hepatology* 2014;60(5):1531–1540.

96. Callendret B, Eccleston HB, Satterfield W, et al. Persistent hepatitis C viral replication despite priming of functional CD8+ T cells by combined therapy with a vaccine and a direct-acting antiviral. *Hepatology* 2016;63(5):1442–1454.

97. Candotti D, Temple J, Sarkodie F, et al. Frequent recovery and broad genotype 2 diversity characterize hepatitis C virus infection in Ghana, West Africa. *J Virol* 2003;77(14):7914–7923.

98. Carlsen TH, Pedersen J, Prentoe JC, et al. Breadth of neutralization and synergy of clinically relevant human monoclonal antibodies against HCV genotypes 1a, 1b, 2a, 2b, 2c, and 3a. *Hepatology* 2014;60(5):1551–1562.

99. Carlton-Smith C, Holmes JA, Naggie S, et al. IFN-free therapy is associated with restoration of type I IFN response in HIV-1 patients with acute HCV infection who achieve SVR. *J Viral Hepat* 2018;25(5):465–472.

100. Carrat F, Fontaine H, Dorival C, et al. Clinical outcomes in patients with chronic hepatitis C after direct-acting antiviral treatment: a prospective cohort study. *Lancet* 2019;393(10179):1453–1464.

101. Cashman SB, Marsden BD, Dustin LB. The humoral immune response to HCV: understanding is key to vaccine development. *Front Immunol* 2014;5:550.

102. Catanese MT, Uryu K, Kopp M, et al. Ultrastructural analysis of hepatitis C virus particles. *Proc Natl Acad Sci U S A* 2013;110(23):9505–9510.

103. Centers for Disease Control and Prevention (CDC). Testing for HCV infection: an update of guidance for clinicians and laboratorians. *MMWR Morb Mortal Wkly Rep* 2013;62(18):362–365.

104. Chaillon A, Rand EB, Reau N, et al. Cost-effectiveness of universal hepatitis C virus screening of pregnant women in the United States. *Clin Infect Dis* 2019;69(11):1888–1895.

105. Chan HLY, Chen CJ, Omede O, et al. The present and future disease burden of hepatitis C virus infections with today's treatment paradigm: Volume 4. *J Viral Hepat* 2017;24 (Suppl 2):25–43.

106. Chang PC, Chi CW, Chau GY, et al. DDX3, a DEAD box RNA helicase, is deregulated in hepatitis virus-associated hepatocellular carcinoma and is involved in cell growth control. *Oncogene* 2006;25(14):1991–2003.

107. Chang KS, Jiang J, Cai Z, et al. Human apolipoprotein e is required for infectivity and production of hepatitis C virus in cell culture. *J Virol* 2007;81(24):13783–13793.

108. Chang SC, Yen JH, Kang HY, et al. Nuclear localization signals in the core protein of hepatitis C virus. *Biochem Biophys Res Commun* 1994;205(2):1284–1290.

109. Chang TT, Young KC, Yang YJ, et al. Hepatitis C virus RNA in peripheral blood mononuclear cells: comparing acute and chronic hepatitis C virus infection. *Hepatology* 1996;23(5):977–981.

110. Chattergoon MA, Latanich R, Quinn J, et al. HIV and HCV activate the inflammasome in monocytes and macrophages via endosomal Toll-like receptors without induction of type 1 interferon. *PLoS Pathog* 2014;10(5):e1004082.

111. Chattergoon MA, Levine JS, Latanich R, et al. High plasma interleukin-18 levels mark the acute phase of hepatitis C virus infection. *J Infect Dis* 2011;204(11):1730–1740.

112. Chatterji U, Bobardt M, Tai A, et al. Cyclophilin and NS5A inhibitors, but not other antihepatitis C virus (HCV) agents, preclude HCV-mediated formation of double-membrane-vesicle viral factories. *Antimicrob Agents Chemother* 2015;59(5):2496–2507.

113. Chen L, Borozan I, Feld J, et al. Hepatic gene expression discriminates responders and nonresponders in treatment of chronic hepatitis C viral infection. *Gastroenterology* 2005;128(5):1437–1444.

114. Chen SY, Kao CF, Chen CM, et al. Mechanisms for inhibition of hepatitis B virus gene expression and replication by hepatitis C virus core protein. *J Biol Chem* 2003;278(1):591–607.

115. Chen M, Sallberg M, Sonnerborg A, et al. Limited humoral immunity in hepatitis C virus infection. *Gastroenterology* 1999;116(1):135–143.

116. Chen CM, You LR, Hwang LH, et al. Direct interaction of hepatitis C virus core protein with the cellular lymphotoxin-beta receptor modulates the signal pathway of the lymphotoxin-beta receptor. *J Virol* 1997;71(12):9417–9426.

117. Cheung MCM, Walker AJ, Hudson BE, et al. Outcomes after successful direct-acting antiviral therapy for patients with chronic hepatitis C and decompensated cirrhosis. *J Hepatol* 2016;65(4):741–747.

118. Chevaliez S, Bouvier-Alias M, Brillet R, et al. Hepatitis C virus (HCV) genotype 1 subtype identification in new HCV drug development and future clinical practice. *PLoS One* 2009;4(12):e8209.

119. Chevaliez S, Feld J, Cheng K, et al. Clinical utility of HCV core antigen detection and quantification in the diagnosis and management of patients with chronic hepatitis C receiving an all-oral, interferon-free regimen. *Antivir Ther* 2018;23(3):211–217.

120. Chevaliez S, Soulier A, Poiteau L, et al. Clinical utility of hepatitis C virus core antigen quantification in patients with chronic hepatitis C. *J Clin Virol* 2014;61(1):145–148.

121. Choo QL, Kuo G, Weiner AJ, et al. Isolation of a cDNA clone derived from a blood-borne non-A, non-B viral hepatitis genome. *Science* 1989;244(4902):359–362.

122. Choo QL, Richman KH, Han JH, et al. Genetic organization and diversity of the hepatitis C virus. *Proc Natl Acad Sci U S A* 1991;88(6):2451–2455.

123. Chow KT, Gale M Jr, Loo YM. RIG-I and other RNA sensors in antiviral immunity. *Annu Rev Immunol* 2018;36:667–694.

124. Chung RT, Gordon FD, Curry MP, et al. Human monoclonal antibody MBL-HCV1 delays HCV viral rebound following liver transplantation: a randomized controlled study. *Am J Transplant* 2013;13(4):1047–1054.

125. Cochrane A, Searle B, Hardie A, et al. A genetic analysis of hepatitis C virus transmission between injection drug users. *J Infect Dis* 2002;186(9):1212–1221.

126. Comarmond C, Garrido M, Pol S, et al. Direct-acting antiviral therapy restores immune tolerance to patients with hepatitis C virus-induced cryoglobulinemia vasculitis. *Gastroenterology* 2017;152(8):2052–2062.e2052.

127. Conry-Cantilena C, VanRaden M, Gibble J, et al. Routes of infection, viremia, and liver disease in blood donors found to have hepatitis C virus infection. *N Engl J Med* 1996;334(26):1691–1696.

128. Conti F, Buonfiglioli F, Scuteri A, et al. Early occurrence and recurrence of hepatocellular carcinoma in HCV-related cirrhosis treated with direct-acting antivirals. *J Hepatol* 2016;65(4):727–733.

129. Cooper S, Erickson AL, Adams EJ, et al. Analysis of a successful immune response against hepatitis C virus. *Immunity* 1999;10(4):439–449.

130. Corey KE, Kane E, Munroe C, et al. Hepatitis C virus infection and its clearance alter circulating lipids: implications for long-term follow-up. *Hepatology* 2009;50(4):1030–1037.

131. Cornberg M, Razavi HA, Alberti A, et al. A systematic review of hepatitis C virus epidemiology in Europe, Canada and Israel. *Liver Int* 2011;31(Suppl 2):30–60.

132. Cox AL, Mosbruger T, Lauer GM, et al. Comprehensive analyses of CD8+ T cell responses during longitudinal study of acute human hepatitis C. *Hepatology* 2005;42(1):104–112.

133. Cox AL, Mosbruger T, Mao Q, et al. Cellular immune selection with hepatitis C virus persistence in humans. *J Exp Med* 2005;201(11):1741–1752.

134. Cox AL, Netski DM, Mosbruger T, et al. Prospective evaluation of community-acquired acute-phase hepatitis C virus infection. *Clin Infect Dis* 2005;40(7):951–958.

135. Crosse K, Umeadi OG, Anania FA, et al. Racial differences in liver inflammation and fibrosis related to chronic hepatitis C. *Clin Gastroenterol Hepatol* 2004;2(6):463–468.

136. Crotta S, Stilla A, Wack A, et al. Inhibition of natural killer cells through engagement of CD81 by the major hepatitis C virus envelope protein. *J Exp Med* 2002;195(1):35–41.

137. Custer B, Zou S, Glynn SA, et al. Addressing gaps in international blood availability and transfusion safety in low- and middle-income countries: a NHLBI workshop. *Transfusion* 2018;58(5):1307–1317.

138. Dahari H, Feinstone SM, Major ME. Meta-analysis of hepatitis C virus vaccine efficacy in chimpanzees indicates an importance for structural proteins. *Gastroenterology* 2010;139(3):965–974.

139. Dahari H, Feliu A, Garcia-Retortillo M, et al. Second hepatitis C replication compartment indicated by viral dynamics during liver transplantation. *J Hepatol* 2005;42(4):491–498.

140. Dal Maso L, Franceschi S. Hepatitis C virus and risk of lymphoma and other lymphoid neoplasms: a meta-analysis of epidemiologic studies. *Cancer Epidemiol Biomarkers Prev* 2006;15(11):2078–2085.

141. Dao Thi VL, Granier C, Zeisel MB, et al. Characterization of hepatitis C virus particle subpopulations reveals multiple usage of the scavenger receptor BI for entry steps. *J Biol Chem* 2012;287(37):31242–31257.

142. Davis GL, Alter MJ, El-Serag H, et al. Aging of hepatitis C virus (HCV)-infected persons in the United States: a multiple cohort model of HCV prevalence and disease progression. *Gastroenterology* 2010;138(2):513–521, 521.e511–516.

143. Day CL, Lauer GM, Robbins GK, et al. Broad specificity of virus-specific CD4+ T-helper-cell responses in resolved hepatitis C virus infection. *J Virol* 2002;76(24):12584–12595.

144. Dazert E, Neumann-Haefelin C, Bressanelli S, et al. Loss of viral fitness and cross-recognition by CD8+ T cells limit HCV escape from a protective HLA-B27-restricted human immune response. *J Clin Invest* 2009;119(2):376–386.

145. De Clercq E. Curious (old and new) antiviral nucleoside analogues with intriguing therapeutic potential. *Curr Med Chem* 2015;22(34):3866–3880.

146. de Jong YP, Dorner M, Mommersteeg MC, et al. Broadly neutralizing antibodies abrogate established hepatitis C virus infection. *Sci Transl Med* 2014;6(254):254ra129.

147. DeCastro M, Sanchez J, Herrera JF, et al. Hepatitis C virus antibodies and liver disease in patients with porphyria cutanea tarda. *Hepatology* 1993;17(4):551–557.

148. Denniston MM, Jiles RB, Drobeniuc J, et al. Chronic hepatitis C virus infection in the United States, National Health and Nutrition Examination Survey 2003 to 2010. *Ann Intern Med* 2014;160(5):293–300.

149. Denolly S, Granier C, Fontaine N, et al. A serum protein factor mediates maturation and apoB-association of HCV particles in the extracellular milieu. *J Hepatol* 2019;70(4):626–638.

150. Denolly S, Mialon C. The amino-terminus of the hepatitis C virus (HCV) p7 viroporin and its cleavage from glycoprotein E2-p7 precursor determine specific infectivity and secretion levels of HCV particle types. *PLoS Pathog* 2017;13(12):e1006774.

151. Depla M, Pelletier S, Bedard N, et al. IFN-lambda3 polymorphism indirectly influences NK cell phenotype and function during acute HCV infection. *Immun Inflamm Dis* 2016;4(3):376–388.

152. Desombere I, Fafi-Kremer S, Van Houtte F, et al. Monoclonal anti-envelope antibody AP33 protects humanized mice against a patient-derived hepatitis C virus challenge. *Hepatology* 2016;63(4):1120–1134.

153. Di Maio VC, Cento V, Mirabelli C, et al. Hepatitis C virus genetic variability and the presence of NS5B resistance-associated mutations as natural polymorphisms in selected genotypes could affect the response to NS5B inhibitors. *Antimicrob Agents Chemother* 2014;58(5):2781–2797.

154. Diepolder HM, Zachoval R, Hoffmann RM, et al. Possible mechanism involving T-lymphocyte response to non-structural protein 3 in viral clearance in acute hepatitis C virus infection. *Lancet* 1995;346(8981):1006–1007.

155. Dill MT, Duong FH, Vogt JE, et al. Interferon-induced gene expression is a stronger predictor of treatment response than IL28B genotype in patients with hepatitis C. *Gastroenterology* 2011;140(3):1021–1031.

156. Dill MT, Makowska Z, Duong FHT, et al. Interferon-gamma-stimulated genes, but not USP18, are expressed in livers of patients with acute hepatitis C. *Gastroenterology* 2012;143(3):777–786.e776.

157. Dodd RY, Notari EPt, Stramer SL. Current prevalence and incidence of infectious disease markers and estimated window-period risk in the American Red Cross blood donor population. *Transfusion* 2002;42(8):975–979.

158. Doerrbecker J, Behrendt P, Mateu-Gelabert P, et al. Transmission of hepatitis C virus among people who inject drugs: viral stability and association with drug preparation equipment. *J Infect Dis* 2013;207(2):281–287.

159. Donaldson EF, Harrington PR, O'Rear JJ, et al. Clinical evidence and bioinformatics characterization of potential hepatitis C virus resistance pathways for sofosbuvir. *Hepatology* 2015;61(1):56–65.

160. Donato F, Boffetta P, Puoti M. A meta-analysis of epidemiological studies on the combined effect of hepatitis B and C virus infections in causing hepatocellular carcinoma. *Int J Cancer* 1998;75(3):347–354.

161. Dore GJ, Hajarizadeh B. Elimination of hepatitis C virus in Australia: laying the foundation. *Infect Dis Clin North Am* 2018;32(2):269–279.

162. Dore GJ, Lawitz E, Hezode C, et al. Daclatasvir plus peginterferon and ribavirin is noninferior to peginterferon and ribavirin alone, and reduces the duration of treatment for HCV genotype 2 or 3 infection. *Gastroenterology* 2015;148(2):355–366.e351.

163. Dowd KA, Netski DM, Wang XH, et al. Selection pressure from neutralizing antibodies drives sequence evolution during acute infection with hepatitis C virus. *Gastroenterology* 2009;136(7):2377–2386.

164. Dreux M, Garaigorta U, Boyd B, et al. Short-range exosomal transfer of viral RNA from infected cells to plasmacytoid dendritic cells triggers innate immunity. *Cell Host Microbe* 2012;12(4):558–570.

165. Drexler JF, Corman VM, Muller MA, et al. Evidence for novel hepaciviruses in rodents. *PLoS Pathog* 2013;9(6):e1003438.

166. Drummer HE, Boo I, Poumbourios P. Mutagenesis of a conserved fusion peptide-like motif and membrane-proximal heptad-repeat region of hepatitis C virus glycoprotein E1. *J Gen Virol* 2007;88(Pt 4):1144–1148.

167. Duggal P, Thio CL, Wojcik GL, et al. Genome-wide association study of spontaneous resolution of hepatitis C virus infection: data from multiple cohorts. *Ann Intern Med* 2013;158(4):235–245.

168. Duong FH, Filipowicz M, Tripodi M, et al. Hepatitis C virus inhibits interferon signaling through up-regulation of protein phosphatase 2A. *Gastroenterology* 2004;126(1):263–277.

169. Dustin LB. Innate and adaptive immune responses in chronic HCV infection. *Curr Drug Targets* 2017;18(7):826–843.

170. EASL Clinical Practice Guidelines: management of hepatitis C virus infection. *J Hepatol* 2011;55(2):245–264.

171. Edlich B, Ahlenstiel G, Zabaleta Azpiroz A, et al. Early changes in interferon signaling define natural killer cell response and refractoriness to interferon-based therapy of hepatitis C patients. *Hepatology* 2012;55(1):39–48.

172. Egger D, Wolk B, Gosert R, et al. Expression of hepatitis C virus proteins induces distinct membrane alterations including a candidate viral replication complex. *J Virol* 2002;76(12):5974–5984.

173. El Kassas M, Elbaz T, Elsharkawy A, et al. HCV in Egypt, prevention, treatment and key barriers to elimination. *Expert Rev Anti Infect Ther* 2018;16(4):345–350.

174. El-Akel W, El-Sayed MH, El Kassas M, et al. National treatment programme of hepatitis C in Egypt: hepatitis C virus model of care. *J Viral Hepat* 2017;24(4):262–267.

175. El-Diwany R, Cohen VJ, Mankowski MC, et al. Extra-epitopic hepatitis C virus polymorphisms confer resistance to broadly neutralizing antibodies by modulating binding to scavenger receptor B1. *PLoS Pathog* 2017;13(2):e1006235.

176. El-Serag HB. Hepatocellular carcinoma and hepatitis C in the United States. *Hepatology* 2002;36(5 Suppl 1):S74–S83.

177. El-Serag HB, Kanwal F, Richardson P, et al. Risk of hepatocellular carcinoma after sustained virological response in Veterans with hepatitis C virus infection. *Hepatology* 2016;64(1):130–137.

178. El-Shabrawi MHF, Kamal NM, El-Khayat HR, et al. A pilot single arm observational study of sofosbuvir/ledipasvir (200 + 45 mg) in 6- to 12- year old children. *Aliment Pharmacol Ther* 2018;47(12):1699–1704.

179. Emery JS, Kuczynski M, La D, et al. Efficacy and safety of direct acting antivirals for the treatment of mixed cryoglobulinemia. *Am J Gastroenterol* 2017;112(8):1298–1308.

180. Erickson AL, Kimura Y, Igarashi S, et al. The outcome of hepatitis C virus infection is predicted by escape mutations in epitopes targeted by cytotoxic T lymphocytes. *Immunity* 2001;15(6):883–895.

181. Eslam M, Hashem AM, Leung R, et al. Interferon-lambda rs12979860 genotype and liver fibrosis in viral and non-viral chronic liver disease. *Nat Commun* 2015;6:6422.

182. Eslam M, McLeod D, Kelaeng KS, et al. IFN-lambda3, not IFN-lambda4, likely mediates IFNL3-IFNL4 haplotype-dependent hepatic inflammation and fibrosis. *Nat Genet* 2017;49(5):795–800.

183. Esteban JI, Lopez-Talavera JC, Genesca J, et al. High rate of infectivity and liver disease in blood donors with antibodies to hepatitis C virus. *Ann Intern Med* 1991;115(6):443–449.

184. Esteban-Riesco L, Depaulis F, Moreau A, et al. Rapid and sustained autologous neutralizing response leading to early spontaneous recovery after HCV infection. *Virology* 2013;444(1–2):90–99.

185. European Association for the Study of the Liver. EASL recommendations on treatment of hepatitis C 2018. *J Hepatol* 2018;69(2):461–511.

186. Evans MJ, von Hahn T, Tscherne DM, et al. Claudin-1 is a hepatitis C virus co-receptor required for a late step in entry. *Nature* 2007;446(7137):801–805.

187. Everhart JE, Ruhl CE. Burden of digestive diseases in the United States Part III: liver, biliary tract, and pancreas. *Gastroenterology* 2009;136(4):1134–1144.

188. Everson GT, Towner WJ, Davis MN, et al. Sofosbuvir with velpatasvir in treatment-naive noncirrhotic patients with genotype 1 to 6 hepatitis C virus infection: a randomized trial. *Ann Intern Med* 2015;163(11):818–826.

189. Fabrizi F, Dixit V, Messa P. Antiviral therapy of symptomatic HCV-associated mixed cryoglobulinemia: meta-analysis of clinical studies. *J Med Virol* 2013;85(6):1019–1027.

190. Fahmy AM, Labonte P. The autophagy elongation complex (ATG5–12/16L1) positively regulates HCV replication and is required for wild-type membranous web formation. *Sci Rep* 2017;7:40351.

191. Falcon V, Acosta-Rivero N, Gonzalez S, et al. Ultrastructural and biochemical basis for hepatitis C virus morphogenesis. *Virus Genes* 2017;53(2):151–164.

192. Fan H, Qiao L, Kang KD, et al. Attachment and postattachment receptors important for hepatitis C virus infection and cell-to-cell transmission. *J Virol* 2017;91(13).

193. Fan W, Xie S, Zhao X, et al. IFN-lambda4 desensitizes the response to IFN-alpha treatment in chronic hepatitis C through long-term induction of USP18. *J Gen Virol* 2016;97(9):2210–2220.

194. Farci P. New insights into the HCV quasispecies and compartmentalization. *Semin Liver Dis* 2011;31(4):356–374.

195. Farci P, Alter HJ, Govindarajan S, et al. Lack of protective immunity against reinfection with hepatitis C virus. *Science* 1992;258(5079):135–140.

196. Farci P, Alter HJ, Shimoda A, et al. Hepatitis C virus-associated fulminant hepatic failure. *N Engl J Med* 1996;335(9):631–634.

197. Farci P, Alter HJ, Wong D, et al. A long-term study of hepatitis C virus replication in non-A, non-B hepatitis. *N Engl J Med* 1991;325(2):98–104.

198. Farci P, Shimoda A, Coiana A, et al. The outcome of acute hepatitis C predicted by the evolution of the viral quasispecies. *Science* 2000;288(5464):339–344.

199. Fattovich G, Giustina G, Degos F, et al. Morbidity and mortality in compensated cirrhosis type C: a retrospective follow-up study of 384 patients. *Gastroenterology* 1997;112(2):463–472.

200. Fauteux-Daniel S, Larouche A, Calderon V, et al. Vertical transmission of hepatitis C virus: variable transmission bottleneck and evidence of midgestation in utero infection. *J Virol* 2017;91(23).

201. Fauvelle C, Felmlee DJ, Crouchet E, et al. Apolipoprotein E mediates evasion from hepatitis C virus neutralizing antibodies. *Gastroenterology* 2016;150(1):206–217.e204.

202. Feinstone SM, Kapikian AZ, Purcell RH, et al. Transfusion-associated hepatitis not due to viral hepatitis type A or B. *N Engl J Med* 1975;292(15):767–770.

203. Feinstone SM, Mihalik KB, Kamimura T, et al. Inactivation of hepatitis B virus and non-A, non-B hepatitis by chloroform. *Infect Immun* 1983;41(2):816–821.

204. Feld JJ, Kowdley KV, Coakley E, et al. Treatment of HCV with ABT-450/r-ombitasvir and dasabuvir with ribavirin. *N Engl J Med* 2014;370(17):1594–1603.

205. Feld JJ, Maan R, Zeuzem S, et al. Effectiveness and safety of sofosbuvir-based regimens for chronic HCV genotype 3 infection: results of the HCV-TARGET study. *Clin Infect Dis* 2016;63(6):776–783.

206. Feld JJ, Nanda S, Huang Y, et al. Hepatic gene expression during treatment with peginterferon and ribavirin: identifying molecular pathways for treatment response. *Hepatology* 2007;46(5):1548–1563.

207. Felmlee DJ, Coilly A, Chung RT, et al. New perspectives for preventing hepatitis C virus liver graft infection. *Lancet Infect Dis* 2016;16(6):735–745.

208. Fernandez J, Taylor D, Morhardt DR, et al. Long-term persistence of infection in chimpanzees inoculated with an infectious hepatitis C virus clone is associated with a decrease in the viral amino acid substitution rate and low levels of heterogeneity. *J Virol* 2004;78(18):9782–9789.

209. Ferraris P, Blanchard E, Roingeard P. Ultrastructural and biochemical analyses of hepatitis C virus-associated host cell membranes. *J Gen Virol* 2010;91(Pt 9):2230–2237.

210. Fiore RJ, Potenza D, Monno L, et al. Detection of HCV RNA in serum and seminal fluid from HIV-1 co-infected intravenous drug addicts. *J Med Virol* 1995;46(4):364–367.

211. Fitzmaurice K, Hurst J, Dring M, et al. Additive effects of HLA alleles and innate immune genes determine viral outcome in HCV infection. *Gut* 2015;64(5):813–819.

212. Fitzmaurice K, Petrovic D, Ramamurthy N, et al. Molecular footprints reveal the impact of the protective HLA-A*03 allele in hepatitis C virus infection. *Gut* 2011;60(11):1563–1571.

213. Fleming VM, Harcourt G, Barnes E, et al. Virological footprint of CD4+ T-cell responses during chronic hepatitis C virus infection. *J Gen Virol* 2010;91(Pt 6):1396–1406.

214. Folgori A, Capone S, Ruggeri L, et al. A T-cell HCV vaccine eliciting effective immunity against heterologous virus challenge in chimpanzees. *Nat Med* 2006;12(2):190–197.

215. Folgori A, Spada E, Pezzanera M, et al. Early impairment of hepatitis C virus specific T cell proliferation during acute infection leads to failure of viral clearance. *Gut* 2006;55(7):1012–1019.

216. Forni D, Cagliani R, Pontremoli C, et al. Evolutionary analysis provides insight into the origin and adaptation of HCV. *Front Microbiol* 2018;9:854.

217. Forns X, Lee SS, Valdes J, et al. Glecaprevir plus pibrentasvir for chronic hepatitis C virus genotype 1, 2, 4, 5, or 6 infection in adults with compensated cirrhosis (EXPEDITION-1): a single-arm, open-label, multicentre phase 3 trial. *Lancet Infect Dis* 2017;17(10):1062–1068.

218. Foster TL, Belyaeva T, Stonehouse NJ, et al. All three domains of the hepatitis C virus nonstructural NS5A protein contribute to RNA binding. *J Virol* 2010;84(18):9267–9277.

219. Foster TL, Gallay P, Stonehouse NJ, et al. Cyclophilin A interacts with domain II of hepatitis C virus NS5A and stimulates RNA binding in an isomerase-dependent manner. *J Virol* 2011;85(14):7460–7464.

220. Foster GR, Goldin RD, Thomas HC. Chronic hepatitis C virus infection causes a significant reduction in quality of life in the absence of cirrhosis. *Hepatology* 1998;27(1):209–212.

221. Francavilla V, Accapezzato D, De Salvo M, et al. Subversion of effector CD8+ T cell differentiation in acute hepatitis C virus infection: exploring the immunological mechanisms. *Eur J Immunol* 2004;34(2):427–437.

222. Frank C, Mohamed MK, Strickland GT, et al. The role of parenteral antischistosomal therapy in the spread of hepatitis C virus in Egypt. *Lancet* 2000;355(9207):887–891.

223. Fraser H, Martin NK, Brummer-Korvenkontio H, et al. Model projections on the impact of HCV treatment in the prevention of HCV transmission among people who inject drugs in Europe. *J Hepatol* 2018;68(3):402–411.

224. Freiman JM, Tran TM, Schumacher SG, et al. Hepatitis C core antigen testing for diagnosis of hepatitis C virus infection: a systematic review and meta-analysis. *Ann Intern Med* 2016;165(5):345–355.

225. Frey SE, Houghton M, Coates S, et al. Safety and immunogenicity of HCV E1E2 vaccine adjuvanted with MF59 administered to healthy adults. *Vaccine* 2010;28(38):6367–6373.

226. Fridell RA, Qiu D, Wang C, et al. Resistance analysis of the hepatitis C virus NS5A inhibitor BMS-790052 in an in vitro replicon system. *Antimicrob Agents Chemother* 2010;54(9):3641–3650.

227. Fuller MJ, Callendret B, Zhu B, et al. Immunotherapy of chronic hepatitis C virus infection with antibodies against programmed cell death-1 (PD-1). *Proc Natl Acad Sci U S A* 2013;110(37):15001–15006.

228. Fuller MJ, Shoukry NH, Gushima T, et al. Selection-driven immune escape is not a significant factor in the failure of CD4 T cell responses in persistent hepatitis C virus infection. *Hepatology* 2010;51(2):378–387.

229. Gale MJ Jr, Korth MJ, Katze MG. Repression of the PKR protein kinase by the hepatitis C virus NS5A protein: a potential mechanism of interferon resistance. *Clin Diagn Virol* 1998;10(2–3):157–162.

230. Gane E, Lawitz E, Pugatch D, et al. Glecaprevir and pibrentasvir in patients with HCV and severe renal impairment. *N Engl J Med* 2017;377(15):1448–1455.

231. Gane EJ, Roberts SK, Stedman CA, et al. Oral combination therapy with a nucleoside polymerase inhibitor (RG7128) and danoprevir for chronic hepatitis C genotype 1 infection (INFORM-1): a randomised, double-blind, placebo-controlled, dose-escalation trial. *Lancet* 2010;376(9751):1467–1475.

232. Gane E, Stedman C, Dole K, et al. A diacylglycerol transferase 1 inhibitor is a potent hepatitis C antiviral in vitro but not in patients in a randomized clinical trial. *ACS Infect Dis* 2017;3(2):144–151.

233. Gao M, Nettles RE, Belema M, et al. Chemical genetics strategy identifies an HCV NS5A inhibitor with a potent clinical effect. *Nature* 2010;465(7294):96–100.

234. Garaigorta U, Chisari FV. Hepatitis C virus blocks interferon effector function by inducing protein kinase R phosphorylation. *Cell Host Microbe* 2009;6(6):513–522.

235. Garcia-Tejedor A, Maiques-Montesinos V, Diago-Almela VJ, et al. Risk factors for vertical transmission of hepatitis C virus: a single center experience with 710 HCV-infected mothers. *Eur J Obstet Gynecol Reprod Biol* 2015;194:173–177.

236. Gardiner D, Lalezari J, Lawitz E, et al. A randomized, double-blind, placebo-controlled assessment of BMS-936558, a fully human monoclonal antibody to programmed death-1 (PD-1), in patients with chronic hepatitis C virus infection. *PLoS One* 2013;8(5):e63818.

237. Gaudieri S, Rauch A, Park LP, et al. Evidence of viral adaptation to HLA class I-restricted immune pressure in chronic hepatitis C virus infection. *J Virol* 2006;80(22):11094–11104.

238. Gauthiez E, Habfast-Robertson I, Rueger S, et al. A systematic review and meta-analysis of HCV clearance. *Liver Int* 2017;37(10):1431–1445.

239. Ge D, Fellay J, Thompson AJ, et al. Genetic variation in IL28B predicts hepatitis C treatment-induced viral clearance. *Nature* 2009;461(7262):399–401.

240. Gerlach JT, Diepolder HM, Jung MC, et al. Recurrence of hepatitis C virus after loss of virus-specific CD4(+) T-cell response in acute hepatitis C. *Gastroenterology* 1999;117(4):933–941.

241. Gerlach JT, Diepolder HM, Zachoval R, et al. Acute hepatitis C: high rate of both spontaneous and treatment-induced viral clearance. *Gastroenterology* 2003;125(1):80–88.

242. Ghany MG, Nelson DR, Strader DB, et al. An update on treatment of genotype 1 chronic hepatitis C virus infection: 2011 practice guideline by the American Association for the Study of Liver Diseases. *Hepatology* 2011;54(4):1433–1444.

243. Ghany MG, Strader DB, Thomas DL, et al. Diagnosis, management, and treatment of hepatitis C: an update. *Hepatology* 2009;49(4):1335–1374.

244. Giang E, Dorner M, Prentoe JC, et al. Human broadly neutralizing antibodies to the envelope glycoprotein complex of hepatitis C virus. *Proc Natl Acad Sci U S A* 2012;109(16):6205–6210.

245. Gisbert JP, Garcia-Buey L, Pajares JM, et al. Systematic review: regression of lymphoproliferative disorders after treatment for hepatitis C infection. *Aliment Pharmacol Ther* 2005;21(6):653–662.

246. Golden-Mason L, Cox AL, Randall JA, et al. Increased natural killer cell cytotoxicity and NKp30 expression protects against hepatitis C virus infection in high-risk individuals and inhibits replication in vitro. *Hepatology* 2010;52(5):1581–1589.

247. Golden-Mason L, Palmer B, Klarquist J, et al. Upregulation of PD-1 expression on circulating and intrahepatic hepatitis C virus-specific CD8+ T cells associated with reversible immune dysfunction. *J Virol* 2007;81(17):9249–9258.

248. Goodman ZD, Ishak KG. Histopathology of hepatitis C virus infection. *Semin Liver Dis* 1995;15(1):70–81.

249. Gordon FD, Anastopoulos H, Khettry U, et al. Hepatitis C infection: a rare cause of fulminant hepatic failure. *Am J Gastroenterol* 1995;90(1):117–120.

250. Gordon SC, Lamerato LE, Rupp LB, et al. Prevalence of cirrhosis in hepatitis C patients in the Chronic Hepatitis Cohort Study (CHeCS): a retrospective and prospective observational study. *Am J Gastroenterol* 2015;110(8):1169–1177; quiz 1178.

251. Gordon SC, Trudeau S, Li J, et al. Race, age, and geography impact hepatitis C genotype distribution in the United States. *J Clin Gastroenterol* 2019;53(1):40–50.

252. Gottwein JM, Pham LV, Mikkelsen LS, et al. Efficacy of NS5A inhibitors against hepatitis C virus genotypes 1–7 and escape variants. *Gastroenterology* 2018;154(5):1435–1448.

253. Gottwein JM, Scheel TK, Callendret B, et al. Novel infectious cDNA clones of hepatitis C virus genotype 3a (strain S52) and 4a (strain ED43): genetic analyses and in vivo pathogenesis studies. *J Virol* 2010;84(10):5277–5293.

254. Grabowska AM, Lechner F, Klenerman P, et al. Direct ex vivo comparison of the breadth and specificity of the T cells in the liver and peripheral blood of patients with chronic HCV infection. *Eur J Immunol* 2001;31(8):2388–2394.

255. Gragnani L, Visentini M, Fognani E, et al. Prospective study of guideline-tailored therapy with direct-acting antivirals for hepatitis C virus-associated mixed cryoglobulinemia. *Hepatology* 2016;64(5):1473–1482.

256. Grakoui A, Shoukry NH, Woollard DJ, et al. HCV persistence and immune evasion in the absence of memory T cell help. *Science* 2003;302(5645):659–662.

257. Graw F, Balagopal A, Kandathil AJ, et al. Inferring viral dynamics in chronically HCV infected patients from the spatial distribution of infected hepatocytes. *PLoS Comput Biol* 2014;10(11):e1003934.

258. Gray RR, Parker J, Lemey P, et al. The mode and tempo of hepatitis C virus evolution within and among hosts. *BMC Evol Biol* 2011;11:131.

259. Grebely J, Conway B, Raffa JD, et al. Hepatitis C virus reinfection in injection drug users. *Hepatology* 2006;44(5):1139–1145.

260. Grebely J, Prins M, Hellard M, et al. Hepatitis C virus clearance, reinfection, and persistence, with insights from studies of injecting drug users: towards a vaccine. *Lancet Infect Dis* 2012;12(5):408–414.

261. Gruener NH, Lechner F, Jung MC, et al. Sustained dysfunction of antiviral CD8+ T lymphocytes after infection with hepatitis C virus. *J Virol* 2001;75(12):5550–5558.

262. Gruner NH, Gerlach TJ, Jung MC, et al. Association of hepatitis C virus-specific CD8+ T cells with viral clearance in acute hepatitis C. *J Infect Dis* 2000;181(5):1528–1536.

263. Grunvogel O, Colasanti O, Lee JY, et al. Secretion of hepatitis C virus replication intermediates reduces activation of toll-like receptor 3 in hepatocytes. *Gastroenterology* 2018;154(8):2237–2251.e2216.

264. Gu M, Rice CM. Structures of hepatitis C virus nonstructural proteins required for replicase assembly and function. *Curr Opin Virol* 2013;3(2):129–136.

265. Guedj J, Dahari H, Rong L, et al. Modeling shows that the NS5A inhibitor daclatasvir has two modes of action and yields a shorter estimate of the hepatitis C virus half-life. *Proc Natl Acad Sci U S A* 2013;110(10):3991–3996.

266. Guedj J, Dahari H, Shudo E, et al. Hepatitis C viral kinetics with the nucleoside polymerase inhibitor mericitabine (RG7128). *Hepatology* 2012;55(4):1030–1037.

267. Guedj J, Pang PS, Denning J, et al. Analysis of hepatitis C viral kinetics during administration of two nucleotide analogues: sofosbuvir (GS-7977) and GS-0938. *Antivir Ther* 2014;19(2):211–220.

268. Guedj J, Perelson AS. Second-phase hepatitis C virus RNA decline during telaprevir-based therapy increases with drug effectiveness: implications for treatment duration. *Hepatology* 2011;53(6):1801–1808.

269. Guevin C, Manna D, Belanger C, et al. Autophagy protein ATG5 interacts transiently with the hepatitis C virus RNA polymerase (NS5B) early during infection. *Virology* 2010;405(1):1–7.

270. Guido M, Bortolotti F, Leandro G, et al. Fibrosis in chronic hepatitis C acquired in infancy: is it only a matter of time? *Am J Gastroenterol* 2003;98(3):660–663.

271. Guiltinan AM, Kaidarova Z, Custer B, et al. Increased all-cause, liver, and cardiac mortality among hepatitis C virus-seropositive blood donors. *Am J Epidemiol* 2008;167(6):743–750.

272. Hadziyannis SJ, Sette H Jr, Morgan TR, et al. Peginterferon-alpha2a and ribavirin combination therapy in chronic hepatitis C: a randomized study of treatment duration and ribavirin dose. *Ann Intern Med* 2004;140(5):346–355.

273. Hahn JA, Wylie D, Dill J, et al. Potential impact of vaccination on the hepatitis C virus epidemic in injection drug users. *Epidemics* 2009;1(1):47–57.

274. Hajarizadeh B, Grady B, Page K, et al. Patterns of hepatitis C virus RNA levels during acute infection: the InC3 study. *PLoS One* 2015;10(4):e0122232.

275. Hajarizadeh B, Grebely J, Applegate T, et al. Dynamics of HCV RNA levels during acute hepatitis C virus infection. *J Med Virol* 2014;86(10):1722–1729.

276. Hall EW, Rosenberg ES, Sullivan PS. Estimates of state-level chronic hepatitis C virus infection, stratified by race and sex, United States, 2010. *BMC Infect Dis* 2018;18(1):224.

277. Hamdane N, Juhling F, Crouchet E, et al. HCV-induced epigenetic changes associated with liver cancer risk persist after sustained virologic response. *Gastroenterology* 2019;156(8):2313–2329.e7.

278. Hamming OJ, Terczynska-Dyla E, Vieyres G, et al. Interferon lambda 4 signals via the IFNlambda receptor to regulate antiviral activity against HCV and coronaviruses. *EMBO J* 2013;32(23):3055–3065.

279. Han B, Parhy B, Zhou E, et al. In vitro susceptibility of HCV genotype 1 through 6 clinical isolates to the pan-genotypic NS3/4A inhibitor voxilaprevir. *J Clin Microbiol* 2019;57(4):e01844-18.

280. Harris RA, Sugimoto K, Kaplan DE, et al. Human leukocyte antigen class II associations with hepatitis C virus clearance and virus-specific CD4 T cell response among Caucasians and African Americans. *Hepatology* 2008;48(1):70–79.

281. Harrus D, Ahmed-El-Sayed N, Simister PC, et al. Further insights into the roles of GTP and the C terminus of the hepatitis C virus polymerase in the initiation of RNA synthesis. *J Biol Chem* 2010;285(43):32906–32918.

282. Hartlage AS, Murthy S, Kumar A, et al. Vaccination to prevent T cell subversion can protect against persistent hepacivirus infection. *Nat Commun* 2019;10(1):1113.

283. Heffernan A, Cooke GS, Nayagam S, et al. Scaling up prevention and treatment towards the elimination of hepatitis C: a global mathematical model. *Lancet* 2019;393(10178):1319–1329.

284. Heim MH, Thimme R. Innate and adaptive immune responses in HCV infections. *J Hepatol* 2014;61(1S):S14–S25.

285. Helle F, Duverlie G, Dubuisson J. The hepatitis C virus glycan shield and evasion of the humoral immune response. *Viruses* 2011;3(10):1909–1932.

286. Henderson WA, Shankar R, Feld JJ, et al. Symptomatic and pathophysiologic predictors of hepatitis C virus progression in pediatric patients. *Pediatr Infect Dis J* 2009;28(8):724–727.

287. Herker E, Harris C, Hernandez C, et al. Efficient hepatitis C virus particle formation requires diacylglycerol acyltransferase-1. *Nat Med* 2010;16(11):1295–1298.

288. Hezode C, Hirschfield GM, Ghesquiere W, et al. Daclatasvir plus peginterferon alfa and ribavirin for treatment-naive chronic hepatitis C genotype 1 or 4 infection: a randomised study. *Gut* 2015;64(6):948–956.

289. Hiet MS, Bauhofer O, Zayas M, et al. Control of temporal activation of hepatitis C virus-induced interferon response by domain 2 of nonstructural protein 5A. *J Hepatol* 2015;63(4):829–837.

290. Hill AM, Nath S, Simmons B. The road to elimination of hepatitis C: analysis of cures versus new infections in 91 countries. *J Virus Erad* 2017;3(3):117–123.

291. Hofmeister MG, Rosenthal EM, Barker LK, et al. Estimating prevalence of hepatitis C virus infection in the United States, 2013–2016. *Hepatology* 2019;69(3):1020–1031.

292. Hollinger FB, Gitnick GL, Aach RD, et al. Non-A, non-B hepatitis transmission in chimpanzees: a project of the transfusion-transmitted viruses study group. *Intervirology* 1978;10(1):60–68.

293. Holz L, Rehermann B. T cell responses in hepatitis C virus infection: historical overview and goals for future research. *Antiviral Res* 2014.
294. Honda M, Sakai A, Yamashita T, et al. Hepatic ISG expression is associated with genetic variation in interleukin 28B and the outcome of IFN therapy for chronic hepatitis C. *Gastroenterology* 2010;139(2):499–509.
295. Honegger JR, Kim S, Price AA, et al. Loss of immune escape mutations during persistent HCV infection in pregnancy enhances replication of vertically transmitted viruses. *Nat Med* 2013;19(11):1529–1533.
296. Hong M, Schwerk J, Lim C, et al. Interferon lambda 4 expression is suppressed by the host during viral infection. *J Exp Med* 2016;213(12):2539–2552.
297. Hoofnagle JH, Mullen KD, Jones DB, et al. Treatment of chronic non-A, non-B hepatitis with recombinant human alpha interferon. A preliminary report. *N Engl J Med* 1986;315(25):1575–1578.
298. Houghton M. Discovery of the hepatitis C virus. *Liver Int* 2009;29(Suppl 1):82–88.
299. Houghton M. Prospects for prophylactic and therapeutic vaccines against the hepatitis C viruses. *Immunol Rev* 2011;239(1):99–108.
300. Hsu M, Zhang J, Flint M, et al. Hepatitis C virus glycoproteins mediate pH-dependent cell entry of pseudotyped retroviral particles. *Proc Natl Acad Sci U S A* 2003;100(12):7271–7276.
301. Huang L, Hwang J, Sharma SD, et al. Hepatitis C virus nonstructural protein 5A (NS5A) is an RNA-binding protein. *J Biol Chem* 2005;280(43):36417–36428.
302. Huang AC, Mehta N, Dodge JL, et al. Direct-acting antivirals do not increase the risk of hepatocellular carcinoma recurrence after local-regional therapy or liver transplant waitlist dropout. *Hepatology* 2018;68(2):449–461.
303. Huang H, Sun F, Owen DM, et al. Hepatitis C virus production by human hepatocytes dependent on assembly and secretion of very low-density lipoproteins. *Proc Natl Acad Sci U S A* 2007;104(14):5848–5853.
304. Hui JM, Sud A, Farrell GC, et al. Insulin resistance is associated with chronic hepatitis C virus infection and fibrosis progression [corrected]. *Gastroenterology* 2003;125(6):1695–1704.
305. Hutin YJ, Bulterys M, Hirnschall GO. How far are we from viral hepatitis elimination service coverage targets? *J Int AIDS Soc* 2018;21(Suppl 2):e25050.
306. Ilan E, Arazi J, Nussbaum O, et al. The hepatitis C virus (HCV)-Trimera mouse: a model for evaluation of agents against HCV. *J Infect Dis* 2002;185(2):153–161.
307. Ingallinella P, Altamura S, Bianchi E, et al. Potent peptide inhibitors of human hepatitis C virus NS3 protease are obtained by optimizing the cleavage products. *Biochemistry* 1998;37(25):8906–8914.
308. Inglesby TV, Rai R, Astemborski J, et al. A prospective, community-based evaluation of liver enzymes in individuals with hepatitis C after drug use. *Hepatology* 1999;29(2):590–596.
309. Ioannou GN, Feld JJ. What are the benefits of a sustained virologic response to direct-acting antiviral therapy for hepatitis C virus infection? *Gastroenterology* 2019;156(2):446–460.e442.
310. Ioannou GN, Green PK, Berry K. HCV eradication induced by direct-acting antiviral agents reduces the risk of hepatocellular carcinoma. *J Hepatol* 2018;68:25–32.
311. Irvin R, Ward K, Agee T, et al. Comparison of hepatitis C virus testing recommendations in high-income countries. *World J Hepatol* 2018;10(10):743–751.
312. Israelow B, Narbus CM, Sourisseau M, et al. HepG2 cells mount an effective antiviral interferon-lambda based innate immune response to hepatitis C virus infection. *Hepatology* 2014;60(4):1170–1179.
313. Iversen J, Dore GJ, Catlett B, et al. Association between rapid utilisation of direct hepatitis C antivirals and decline in the prevalence of viremia among people who inject drugs in Australia. *J Hepatol* 2019;70(1):33–39.
314. Jackowiak P, Kuls K, Budzko L, et al. Phylogeny and molecular evolution of the hepatitis C virus. *Infect Genet Evol* 2014;21:67–82.
315. Jacobson IM, Dore GJ, Foster GR, et al. Simeprevir with pegylated interferon alfa 2a plus ribavirin in treatment-naive patients with chronic hepatitis C virus genotype 1 infection (QUEST-1): a phase 3, randomised, double-blind, placebo-controlled trial. *Lancet* 2014;384(9941):403–413.
316. Jacobson IM, Gordon SC, Kowdley KV, et al. Sofosbuvir for hepatitis C genotype 2 or 3 in patients without treatment options. *N Engl J Med* 2013;368(20):1867–1877.
317. Jacobson IM, Lawitz E, Gane EJ, et al. Efficacy of 8 weeks of sofosbuvir, velpatasvir, and voxilaprevir in patients with chronic HCV infection: 2 phase 3 randomized trials. *Gastroenterology* 2017;153(1):113–122.
318. Janssen HL, Reesink HW, Lawitz EJ, et al. Treatment of HCV infection by targeting microRNA. *N Engl J Med* 2013;368(18):1685–1694.
319. Janssen MP, van Hulst M, Custer B. An assessment of differences in costs and health benefits of serology and NAT screening of donations for blood transfusion in different Western countries. *Vox Sang* 2017;112(6):518–525.
320. Jarret A, McFarland AP, Horner SM, et al. Hepatitis-C-virus-induced microRNAs dampen interferon-mediated antiviral signaling. *Nat Med* 2016;22(12):1475–1481.
321. Jeannel D, Fretz C, Traore Y, et al. Evidence for high genetic diversity and long-term endemicity of hepatitis C virus genotypes 1 and 2 in West Africa. *J Med Virol* 1998;55(2):92–97.
322. Jensen SB, Serre SB, Humes DG, et al. Substitutions at NS3 residue 155, 156, or 168 of hepatitis C virus genotypes 2 to 6 induce complex patterns of protease inhibitor resistance. *Antimicrob Agents Chemother* 2015;59(12):7426–7436.
323. Jhaveri R, Broder T, Bhattacharya D, et al. Universal screening of pregnant women for hepatitis C: the time is now. *Clin Infect Dis* 2018;67(10):1493–1497.
324. Jhaveri R, Swamy GK. Hepatitis C virus in pregnancy and early childhood: current understanding and knowledge deficits. *J Pediatric Infect Dis Soc* 2014;3 (Suppl 1):S13–S18.
325. Jiang J, Cun W, Wu X, et al. Hepatitis C virus attachment mediated by apolipoprotein E binding to cell surface heparan sulfate. *J Virol* 2012;86(13):7256–7267.
326. Jiang J, Luo G. Apolipoprotein E but not B is required for the formation of infectious hepatitis C virus particles. *J Virol* 2009;83(24):12680–12691.
327. Jilg N, Lin W, Hong J, et al. Kinetic differences in the induction of interferon stimulated genes by interferon-alpha and interleukin 28B are altered by infection with hepatitis C virus. *Hepatology* 2014;59(4):1250–1261.
328. Jirasko V, Montserret R, Appel N, et al. Structural and functional characterization of nonstructural protein 2 for its role in hepatitis C virus assembly. *J Biol Chem* 2008;283(42):28546–28562.
329. Johansson DX, Voisset C, Tarr AW, et al. Human combinatorial libraries yield rare antibodies that broadly neutralize hepatitis C virus. *Proc Natl Acad Sci U S A* 2007;104(41):16269–16274.
330. Jopling CL, Schutz S, Sarnow P. Position-dependent function for a tandem microRNA miR-122-binding site located in the hepatitis C virus RNA genome. *Cell Host Microbe* 2008;4(1):77–85.
331. Jopling CL, Yi M, Lancaster AM, et al. Modulation of hepatitis C virus RNA abundance by a liver-specific MicroRNA. *Science* 2005;309(5740):1577–1581.
332. Kachko A, Kochneva G, Sivolobova G, et al. New neutralizing antibody epitopes in hepatitis C virus envelope glycoproteins are revealed by dissecting peptide recognition profiles. *Vaccine* 2011;30(1):69–77.
333. Kamitsukasa H, Harada H, Tanaka H, et al. Late liver-related mortality from complications of transfusion-acquired hepatitis C. *Hepatology* 2005;41(4):819–825.
334. Kanamori H, Fukawa H, Maruta A, et al. Case report: fulminant hepatitis C viral infection after allogeneic bone marrow transplantation. *Am J Med Sci* 1992;303(2):109–111.
335. Kandathil AJ, Graw F, Quinn J, et al. Use of laser capture microdissection to map hepatitis C virus-positive hepatocytes in human liver. *Gastroenterology* 2013;145(6):1404–1413. e1401–1410.
336. Kang W, Sung PS, Park SH, et al. Hepatitis C virus attenuates interferon-induced major histocompatibility complex class I expression and decreases CD8+ T cell effector functions. *Gastroenterology* 2014;146(5):1351–1360.e1351–1354.
337. Kanwal F, Kramer J, Asch SM, et al. Risk of hepatocellular cancer in HCV patients treated with direct-acting antiviral agents. *Gastroenterology* 2017;153(4):996–1005.e1001.
338. Kaplan DE, Sugimoto K, Newton K, et al. Discordant role of CD4 T-cell response relative to neutralizing antibody and CD8 T-cell responses in acute hepatitis C. *Gastroenterology* 2007;132(2):654–666.
339. Kared H, Fabre T, Bedard N, et al. Galectin-9 and IL-21 mediate cross-regulation between Th17 and Treg cells during acute hepatitis C. *PLoS Pathog* 2013;9(6):e1003422.
340. Kasai D, Adachi T, Deng L, et al. HCV replication suppresses cellular glucose uptake through down-regulation of cell surface expression of glucose transporters. *J Hepatol* 2009;50(5):883–894.
341. Kasprowicz V, Kang YH, Lucas M, et al. Hepatitis C virus (HCV) sequence variation induces an HCV-specific T-cell phenotype analogous to spontaneous resolution. *J Virol* 2010;84(3):1656–1663.
342. Kasprowicz V, Schulze Zur Wiesch J, Kuntzen T, et al. High level of PD-1 expression on hepatitis C virus (HCV)-specific CD8+ and CD4+ T cells during acute HCV infection, irrespective of clinical outcome. *J Virol* 2008;82(6):3154–3160.
343. Katayama K, Kumagai J, Komiya Y, et al. Titration of hepatitis C virus in chimpanzees for determining the copy number required for transmission. *Intervirology* 2004;47(1):57–64.
344. Kato N, Sekiya H, Ootsuyama Y, et al. Humoral immune response to hypervariable region 1 of the putative envelope glycoprotein (gp70) of hepatitis C virus. *J Virol* 1993;67(7):3923–3930.
345. Kattakuzhy S, Wilson E, Sidharthan S, et al. Moderate sustained virologic response rates with 6-week combination directly acting anti-hepatitis C virus therapy in patients with advanced liver disease. *Clin Infect Dis* 2016;62(4):440–447.
346. Keck ZY, Girard-Blanc C, Wang W, et al. Antibody response to hypervariable region 1 interferes with broadly neutralizing antibodies to hepatitis C virus. *J Virol* 2016;90(6):3112–3122.
347. Keck ZY, Li SH, Xia J, et al. Mutations in hepatitis C virus E2 located outside the CD81 binding sites lead to escape from broadly neutralizing antibodies but compromise virus infectivity. *J Virol* 2009;83(12):6149–6160.
348. Keck ZY, Saha A, Xia J, et al. Mapping a region of hepatitis C virus E2 that is responsible for escape from neutralizing antibodies and a core CD81-binding region that does not tolerate neutralization escape mutations. *J Virol* 2011;85(20):10451–10463.
349. Keck ZY, Sung VM, Perkins S, et al. Human monoclonal antibody to hepatitis C virus E1 glycoprotein that blocks virus attachment and viral infectivity. *J Virol* 2004;78(13): 7257–7263.
350. Keck ZY, Wang Y, Lau P, et al. Affinity maturation of a broadly neutralizing human monoclonal antibody that prevents acute hepatitis C virus infection in mice. *Hepatology* 2016;64(6):1922–1933.
351. Keck Z, Wang W, Wang Y, et al. Cooperativity in virus neutralization by human monoclonal antibodies to two adjacent regions located at the amino terminus of hepatitis C virus E2 glycoprotein. *J Virol* 2013;87(1):37–51.
352. Keck ML, Wrensch F, Pierce BG, et al. Mapping determinants of virus neutralization and viral escape for rational design of a hepatitis C virus vaccine. *Front Immunol* 2018;9:1194.
353. Keck ZY, Xia J, Wang Y, et al. Human monoclonal antibodies to a novel cluster of conformational epitopes on HCV E2 with resistance to neutralization escape in a genotype 2a isolate. *PLoS Pathog* 2012;8(4):e1002653.
354. Kelly C, Swadling L, Capone S, et al. Chronic hepatitis C viral infection subverts vaccine-induced T-cell immunity in humans. *Hepatology* 2016;63(5):1455–1470.
355. Kershenobich D, Razavi HA, Sanchez-Avila JF, et al. Trends and projections of hepatitis C virus epidemiology in Latin America. *Liver Int* 2011;31(Suppl 2):18–29.
356. Khakoo SI, Thio CL, Martin MP, et al. HLA and NK cell inhibitory receptor genes in resolving hepatitis C virus infection. *Science* 2004;305(5685):872–874.
357. Khan AG, Whidby J, Miller MT, et al. Structure of the core ectodomain of the hepatitis C virus envelope glycoprotein 2. *Nature* 2014;509(7500):381–384.
358. Kim AY, Kuntzen T, Timm J, et al. Spontaneous control of HCV is associated with expression of HLA-B 57 and preservation of targeted epitopes. *Gastroenterology* 2011;140(2): 686–696. e681.
359. Kim JL, Morgenstern KA, Lin C, et al. Crystal structure of the hepatitis C virus NS3 protease domain complexed with a synthetic NS4A cofactor peptide. *Cell* 1996;87(2):343–355.
360. Kimura Y, Gushima T, Rawale S, et al. Escape mutations alter proteasome processing of major histocompatibility complex class I-restricted epitopes in persistent hepatitis C virus infection. *J Virol* 2005;79(8):4870–4876.
361. Kinchen VJ, Zahid MN, Flyak AI, et al. Broadly neutralizing antibody mediated clearance of human hepatitis C virus infection. *Cell Host Microbe* 2018;24(5):717–730.e715.
362. Kittlesen DJ, Chianese-Bullock KA, Yao ZQ, et al. Interaction between complement receptor gC1qR and hepatitis C virus core protein inhibits T-lymphocyte proliferation. *J Clin Invest* 2000;106(10):1239–1249.

363. Kiyosawa K, Sodeyama T, Tanaka E, et al. Hepatitis C in hospital employees with needle-stick injuries. *Ann Intern Med* 1991;115(5):367–369.
364. Klevens RM, Canary L, Huang X, et al. The burden of hepatitis C infection-related liver fibrosis in the United States. *Clin Infect Dis* 2016;63(8):1049–1055.
365. Knodell RG, Conrad ME, Dienstag JL, et al. Etiological spectrum of post-transfusion hepatitis. *Gastroenterology* 1975;69(6):1278–1285.
366. Kobayashi M, Suzuki F, Fujiyama S, et al. Sustained virologic response by direct antiviral agents reduces the incidence of hepatocellular carcinoma in patients with HCV infection. *J Med Virol* 2017;89(3):476–483.
367. Kohli A, Kattakuzhy S, Sidharthan S, et al. Four-week direct-acting antiviral regimens in noncirrhotic patients with hepatitis C virus genotype 1 infection: an open-label, nonrandomized trial. *Ann Intern Med* 2015;163(12):899–907.
368. Kohli A, Osinusi A, Sims Z, et al. Virological response after 6 week triple-drug regimens for hepatitis C: a proof-of-concept phase 2A cohort study. *Lancet* 2015;385(9973):1107–1113.
369. Koizumi Y, Ohashi H, Nakajima S, et al. Quantifying antiviral activity optimizes drug combinations against hepatitis C virus infection. *Proc Natl Acad Sci U S A* 2017;114(8): 1922–1927.
370. Kokordelis P, Kramer B, Korner C, et al. An effective interferon-gamma-mediated inhibition of hepatitis C virus replication by natural killer cells is associated with spontaneous clearance of acute hepatitis C in human immunodeficiency virus-positive patients. *Hepatology* 2014;59(3):814–827.
371. Kolykhalov AA, Agapov EV, Blight KJ, et al. Transmission of hepatitis C by intrahepatic inoculation with transcribed RNA. *Science* 1997;277(5325):570–574.
372. Kolykhalov AA, Agapov EV, Rice CM. Specificity of the hepatitis C virus NS3 serine protease: effects of substitutions at the 3/4A, 4A/4B, 4B/5A, and 5A/5B cleavage sites on polyprotein processing. *J Virol* 1994;68(11):7525–7533.
373. Kondili LA, Chionne P, Costantino A, et al. Infection rate and spontaneous seroreversion of anti-hepatitis C virus during the natural course of hepatitis C virus infection in the general population. *Gut* 2002;50(5):693–696.
374. Koneru A, Nelson N, Hariri S, et al. Increased hepatitis C virus (HCV) detection in women of childbearing age and potential risk for vertical transmission—United States and Kentucky, 2011–2014. *MMWR Morb Mortal Wkly Rep* 2016;65(28):705–710.
375. Kong L, Giang E, Nieusma T, et al. Hepatitis C virus E2 envelope glycoprotein core structure. *Science* 2013;342(6162):1090–1094.
376. Kong L, Lee DE, Kadam RU, et al. Structural flexibility at a major conserved antibody target on hepatitis C virus E2 antigen. *Proc Natl Acad Sci U S A* 2016;113(45):12768–12773.
377. Konishi H, Motomura T, Matsumoto Y, et al. Interferon-lambda4 genetic polymorphism is associated with the therapy response for hepatitis C virus recurrence after a living donor liver transplant. *J Viral Hepat* 2014;21(6):397–404.
378. Kozbial K, Moser S, Al-Zoairy R, et al. Follow-up of sustained virological responders with hepatitis C and advanced liver disease after interferon/ribavirin-free treatment. *Liver Int* 2018;38(6):1028–1035.
379. Koziel MJ, Wong DK, Dudley D, et al. Hepatitis C virus-specific cytolytic T lymphocyte and T helper cell responses in seronegative persons. *J Infect Dis* 1997;176(4):859–866.
380. Kramer B, Korner C, Kebschull M, et al. Natural killer p46High expression defines a natural killer cell subset that is potentially involved in control of hepatitis C virus replication and modulation of liver fibrosis. *Hepatology* 2012;56(4):1201–1213.
381. Kriegs M, Burckstummer T, Himmelsbach K, et al. The hepatitis C virus non-structural NS5A protein impairs both the innate and adaptive hepatic immune response in vivo. *J Biol Chem* 2009;284(41):28343–28351.
382. Krishnan P, Pilot-Matias T, Schnell G, et al. Pooled resistance analysis in patients with hepatitis C virus genotype 1 to 6 infection treated with glecaprevir-pibrentasvir in phase 2 and 3 clinical trials. *Antimicrob Agents Chemother* 2018;62(10).
383. Krishnan P, Schnell G, Tripathi R, et al. Analysis of hepatitis C virus genotype 1b resistance variants in japanese patients treated with paritaprevir-ritonavir and ombitasvir. *Antimicrob Agents Chemother* 2016;60(2):1106–1113.
384. Kroy DC, Ciuffreda D, Cooperrider JH, et al. Liver environment and HCV replication affect human T-cell phenotype and expression of inhibitory receptors. *Gastroenterology* 2014;146(2):550–561.
385. Kubes P, Jenne C. Immune responses in the liver. *Annu Rev Immunol* 2018;36:247–277.
386. Kumar V, Kato N, Urabe Y, et al. Genome-wide association study identifies a susceptibility locus for HCV-induced hepatocellular carcinoma. *Nat Genet* 2011;43(5):455–458.
387. Kuntzen T, Timm J, Berical A, et al. Viral sequence evolution in acute hepatitis C virus infection. *J Virol* 2007;81(21):11658–11668.
388. Kuo G, Choo QL, Alter HJ, et al. An assay for circulating antibodies to a major etiologic virus of human non-A, non-B hepatitis. *Science* 1989;244(4902):362–364.
389. Kurktschiev PD, Raziorrouh B, Schraut W, et al. Dysfunctional CD8+ T cells in hepatitis B and C are characterized by a lack of antigen-specific T-bet induction. *J Exp Med* 2014;211(10):2047–2059.
390. Landau DA, Scerra S, Sene D, et al. Causes and predictive factors of mortality in a cohort of patients with hepatitis C virus-related cryoglobulinemic vasculitis treated with antiviral therapy. *J Rheumatol* 2010;37(3):615–621.
391. Lanford RE, Guerra B, Chavez D, et al. Cross-genotype immunity to hepatitis C virus. *J Virol* 2004;78(3):1575–1581.
392. Lanford RE, Walker CM, Lemon SM. The chimpanzee model of viral hepatitis: advances in understanding the immune response and treatment of viral hepatitis. *ILAR J* 2017;58(2):172–189.
393. Lange CM, Bibert S, Dufour JF, et al. Comparative genetic analyses point to HCP5 as susceptibility locus for HCV-associated hepatocellular carcinoma. *J Hepatol* 2013;59(3): 504–509.
394. Lange CM, Roomp K, Dragan A, et al. HLA class I allele associations with HCV genetic variants in patients with chronic HCV genotypes 1a or 1b infection. *J Hepatol* 2010;53(6):1022–1028.
395. Laskus T, Wilkinson J, Gallegos-Orozco JF, et al. Analysis of hepatitis C virus quasispecies transmission and evolution in patients infected through blood transfusion. *Gastroenterology* 2004;127(3):764–776.
396. Lauber C, Vieyres G, Terczynska-Dyla E, et al. Transcriptome analysis reveals a classical interferon signature induced by IFNlambda4 in human primary cells. *Genes Immun* 2015;16(6):414–421.
397. Lauer GM, Barnes E, Lucas M, et al. High resolution analysis of cellular immune responses in resolved and persistent hepatitis C virus infection. *Gastroenterology* 2004;127(3): 924–936.
398. Lauer GM, Lucas M, Timm J, et al. Full-breadth analysis of CD8+ T-cell responses in acute hepatitis C virus infection and early therapy. *J Virol* 2005;79(20):12979–12988.
399. Lauer GM, Ouchi K, Chung RT, et al. Comprehensive analysis of CD8(+)-T-cell responses against hepatitis C virus reveals multiple unpredicted specificities. *J Virol* 2002;76(12): 6104–6113.
400. Lavie M, Dubuisson J. Interplay between hepatitis C virus and lipid metabolism during virus entry and assembly. *Biochimie* 2017;141:62–69.
401. Lavillette D, Morice Y, Germanidis G, et al. Human serum facilitates hepatitis C virus infection, and neutralizing responses inversely correlate with viral replication kinetics at the acute phase of hepatitis C virus infection. *J Virol* 2005;79(10):6023–6034.
402. Lavillette D, Pecheur EI, Donot P, et al. Characterization of fusion determinants points to the involvement of three discrete regions of both E1 and E2 glycoproteins in the membrane fusion process of hepatitis C virus. *J Virol* 2007;81(16):8752–8765.
403. Law JL, Chen C, Wong J, et al. A hepatitis C virus (HCV) vaccine comprising envelope glycoproteins gpE1/gpE2 derived from a single isolate elicits broad cross-genotype neutralizing antibodies in humans. *PLoS One* 2013;8(3):e59776.
404. Law M, Maruyama T, Lewis J, et al. Broadly neutralizing antibodies protect against hepatitis C virus quasispecies challenge. *Nat Med* 2008;14(1):25–27.
405. Lawitz EJ, Dvory-Sobol H, Doehle BP, et al. Clinical resistance to velpatasvir (GS-5816), a novel pan-genotypic inhibitor of the hepatitis C virus NS5A protein. *Antimicrob Agents Chemother* 2016;60(9):5368–5378.
406. Lawitz E, Lalezari JP, Hassanein T, et al. Sofosbuvir in combination with peginterferon alfa-2a and ribavirin for non-cirrhotic, treatment-naive patients with genotypes 1, 2, and 3 hepatitis C infection: a randomised, double-blind, phase 2 trial. *Lancet Infect Dis* 2013;13(5):401–408.
407. Lawitz E, Mangia A, Wyles D, et al. Sofosbuvir for previously untreated chronic hepatitis C infection. *N Engl J Med* 2013;368(20):1878–1887.
408. Le Pogam S, Jiang WR, Leveque V, et al. In vitro selected Con1 subgenomic replicons resistant to 2′-C-methyl-cytidine or to R1479 show lack of cross resistance. *Virology* 2006;351(2):349–359.
409. Lechner F, Gruener NH, Urbani S, et al. CD8+ T lymphocyte responses are induced during acute hepatitis C virus infection but are not sustained. *Eur J Immunol* 2000;30(9): 2479–2487.
410. Lechner F, Wong DK, Dunbar PR, et al. Analysis of successful immune responses in persons infected with hepatitis C virus. *J Exp Med* 2000;191(9):1499–1512.
411. Lee JY, Acosta EG, Stoeck IK, et al. Apolipoprotein E likely contributes to a maturation step of infectious hepatitis C virus particles and interacts with viral envelope glycoproteins. *J Virol* 2014;88(21):12422–12437.
412. Lee MH, Huang YH, Chen HY, et al. Human leukocyte antigen variants and risk of hepatocellular carcinoma modified by hepatitis C virus genotypes: a genome-wide association study. *Hepatology* 2017;67(2):651–661.
413. Lee SR, Kardos KW, Schiff E, et al. Evaluation of a new, rapid test for detecting HCV infection, suitable for use with blood or oral fluid. *J Virol Methods* 2011;172(1–2):27–31.
414. Lee C, Ma H, Hang JQ, et al. The hepatitis C virus NS5A inhibitor (BMS-790052) alters the subcellular localization of the NS5A non-structural viral protein. *Virology* 2011;414(1):10–18.
415. Lenz O, Verbinnen T, Fevery B, et al. Virology analyses of HCV isolates from genotype 1-infected patients treated with simeprevir plus peginterferon/ribavirin in Phase IIb/III studies. *J Hepatol* 2015;62(5):1008–1014.
416. Lerat H, Honda M, Beard MR, et al. Steatosis and liver cancer in transgenic mice expressing the structural and nonstructural proteins of hepatitis C virus. *Gastroenterology* 2002;122(2):352–365.
417. Lerat H, Rumin S, Habersetzer F, et al. In vivo tropism of hepatitis C virus genomic sequences in hematopoietic cells: influence of viral load, viral genotype, and cell phenotype. *Blood* 1998;91(10):3841–3849.
418. Lesburg CA, Cable MB, Ferrari E, et al. Crystal structure of the RNA-dependent RNA polymerase from hepatitis C virus reveals a fully encircled active site. *Nat Struct Biol* 1999;6(10):937–943.
419. Li K, Foy E, Ferreon JC, et al. Immune evasion by hepatitis C virus NS3/4A protease-mediated cleavage of the Toll-like receptor 3 adaptor protein TRIF. *Proc Natl Acad Sci U S A* 2005;102(8):2992–2997.
420. Li YP, Gottwein JM, Scheel TK, et al. MicroRNA-122 antagonism against hepatitis C virus genotypes 1–6 and reduced efficacy by host RNA insertion or mutations in the HCV 5′ UTR. *Proc Natl Acad Sci U S A* 2011;108(12):4991–4996.
421. Li HF, Huang CH, Ai LS, et al. Mutagenesis of the fusion peptide-like domain of hepatitis C virus E1 glycoprotein: involvement in cell fusion and virus entry. *J Biomed Sci* 2009;16:89.
422. Li K, Lemon SM. Innate immune responses in hepatitis C virus infection. *Semin Immunopathol* 2013;35(1):53–72.
423. Li C, Lu L, Murphy DG, et al. Origin of hepatitis C virus genotype 3 in Africa as estimated through an evolutionary analysis of the full-length genomes of nine subtypes, including the newly sequenced 3d and 3e. *J Gen Virol* 2014;95(Pt 8):1677–1688.
424. Li H, Stoddard MB, Wang S, et al. Elucidation of hepatitis C virus transmission and early diversification by single genome sequencing. *PLoS Pathog* 2012;8(8):e1002880.
425. Li H, Stoddard MB, Wang S, et al. Single-genome sequencing of hepatitis C virus in donor-recipient pairs distinguishes modes and models of virus transmission and early diversification. *J Virol* 2016;90(1):152–166.
426. Li XD, Sun L, Seth RB, et al. Hepatitis C virus protease NS3/4A cleaves mitochondrial antiviral signaling protein off the mitochondria to evade innate immunity. *Proc Natl Acad Sci U S A* 2005;102(49):17717–17722.

427. Li Y, Yamane D, Lemon SM. Dissecting the roles of the 5′ exoribonucleases Xrn1 and Xrn2 in restricting hepatitis C virus replication. *J Virol* 2015;89(9):4857–4865.

428. Liang Y, Cao X, Ding Q, et al. Hepatitis C virus NS4B induces the degradation of TRIF to inhibit TLR3-mediated interferon signaling pathway. *PLoS Pathog* 2018;14(5):e1007075.

429. Liang TJ, Heller T. Pathogenesis of hepatitis C-associated hepatocellular carcinoma. *Gastroenterology* 2004;127(5 Suppl 1):S62–S71.

430. Liang Y, Shilagard T, Xiao SY, et al. Visualizing hepatitis C virus infections in human liver by two-photon microscopy. *Gastroenterology* 2009;137(4):1448–1458.

431. Lim YS, Hwang SB. Hepatitis C virus NS5A protein interacts with phosphatidylinositol 4-kinase type IIIalpha and regulates viral propagation. *J Biol Chem* 2011;286(13):11290–11298.

432. Lim SR, Qin X, Susser S, et al. Virologic escape during danoprevir (ITMN-191/RG7227) monotherapy is hepatitis C virus subtype dependent and associated with R155K substitution. *Antimicrob Agents Chemother* 2012;56(1):271–279.

433. Lin C, Kwong AD, Perni RB. Discovery and development of VX-950, a novel, covalent, and reversible inhibitor of hepatitis C virus NS3.4A serine protease. *Infect Disord Drug Targets* 2006;6(1):3–16.

434. Lindenbach BD, Evans MJ, Syder AJ, et al. Complete replication of hepatitis C virus in cell culture. *Science* 2005;309(5734):623–626.

435. Lindsay KL, Trepo C, Heintges T, et al. A randomized, double-blind trial comparing pegylated interferon alfa-2b to interferon alfa-2b as initial treatment for chronic hepatitis C. *Hepatology* 2001;34(2):395–403.

436. Liu L, Fisher BE, Dowd KA, et al. Acceleration of hepatitis C virus envelope evolution in humans is consistent with progressive humoral immune selection during the transition from acute to chronic infection. *J Virol* 2010;84(10):5067–5077.

437. Liu L, Fisher BE, Thomas DL, et al. Spontaneous clearance of primary acute hepatitis C virus infection correlated with high initial viral RNA level and rapid HVR1 evolution. *Hepatology* 2012;55(6):1684–1691.

438. Llinas-Brunet M, Bailey M, Fazal G, et al. Peptide-based inhibitors of the hepatitis C virus serine protease. *Bioorg Med Chem Lett* 1998;8(13):1713–1718.

439. Lockart I, Matthews GV, Danta M. Sexually transmitted hepatitis C infection: the evolving epidemic in HIV-positive and HIV-negative MSM. *Curr Opin Infect Dis* 2019;32(1):31–37.

440. Logvinoff C, Major ME, Oldach D, et al. Neutralizing antibody response during acute and chronic hepatitis C virus infection. *Proc Natl Acad Sci U S A* 2004;101(27):10149–10154.

441. Lohmann V, Korner F, Dobierzewska A, et al. Mutations in hepatitis C virus RNAs conferring cell culture adaptation. *J Virol* 2001;75(3):1437–1449.

442. Lu L, Li C, Xu Y, et al. Full-length genomes of 16 hepatitis C virus genotype 1 isolates representing subtypes 1c, 1d, 1e, 1g, 1h, 1i, 1j and 1k, and two new subtypes 1m and 1n, and four unclassified variants reveal ancestral relationships among subtypes. *J Gen Virol* 2014;95(Pt 7):1479–1487.

443. Lucas M, Deshpande P, James I, et al. Evidence of CD4(+) T cell-mediated immune pressure on the hepatitis C virus genome. *Sci Rep* 2018;8(1):7224.

444. Lucas M, Ulsenheimer A, Pfafferot K, et al. Tracking virus-specific CD4+ T cells during and after acute hepatitis C virus infection. *PLoS One* 2007;2(7):e649.

445. Lunemann S, Martrus G, Holzemer A, et al. Sequence variations in HCV core-derived epitopes alter binding of KIR2DL3 to HLA-C *03:04 and modulate NK cell function. *J Hepatol* 2016;65(2):252–258.

446. Ly KN, Hughes EM, Jiles RB, et al. Rising mortality associated with hepatitis C virus in the United States, 2003–2013. *Clin Infect Dis* 2016;62(10):1287–1288.

447. Ly KN, Jiles RB, Teshale EH, et al. Hepatitis C virus infection among reproductive-aged women and children in the United States, 2006 to 2014. *Ann Intern Med* 2017;166(11):775–782.

448. Ly KN, Xing J, Klevens RM, et al. The increasing burden of mortality from viral hepatitis in the United States between 1999 and 2007. *Ann Intern Med* 2012;156(4):271–278.

449. Ma Y, Anantpadma M, Timpe JM, et al. Hepatitis C virus NS2 protein serves as a scaffold for virus assembly by interacting with both structural and nonstructural proteins. *J Virol* 2011;85(1):86–97.

450. Madan V, Paul D, Lohmann V, et al. Inhibition of HCV replication by cyclophilin antagonists is linked to replication fitness and occurs by inhibition of membranous web formation. *Gastroenterology* 2014;146(5):1361–1372.e1361–1369.

451. Magiorkinis G, Magiorkinis E, Paraskevis D, et al. The global spread of hepatitis C virus 1a and 1b: a phylodynamic and phylogeographic analysis. *PLoS Med* 2009;6(12):e1000198.

452. Mahajan R, Liu SJ, Klevens RM, et al. Indications for testing among reported cases of HCV infection from enhanced hepatitis surveillance sites in the United States, 2004–2010. *Am J Public Health* 2013;103(8):1445–1449.

453. Mahale P, Engels EA, Li R, et al. The effect of sustained virological response on the risk of extrahepatic manifestations of hepatitis C virus infection. *Gut* 2018;67(3):553–561.

454. Major M, Gutfraind A, Shekhtman L, et al. Modeling of patient virus titers suggests that availability of a vaccine could reduce hepatitis C virus transmission among injecting drug users. *Sci Transl Med* 2018;10(449).

455. Major ME, Mihalik K, Puig M, et al. Previously infected and recovered chimpanzees exhibit rapid responses that control hepatitis C virus replication upon rechallenge. *J Virol* 2002;76(13):6586–6595.

456. Manns MP, Fried MW, Zeuzem S, et al. Simeprevir with peginterferon/ribavirin for treatment of chronic hepatitis C virus genotype 1 infection: pooled safety analysis from Phase IIb and III studies. *J Viral Hepat* 2015;22(4):366–375.

457. Manns MP, McHutchison JG, Gordon SC, et al. Peginterferon alfa-2b plus ribavirin compared with interferon alfa-2b plus ribavirin for initial treatment of chronic hepatitis C: a randomised trial. *Lancet* 2001;358(9286):958–965.

458. Marcellin P, Descamps V, Martinot-Peignoux M, et al. Cryoglobulinemia with vasculitis associated with hepatitis C virus infection. *Gastroenterology* 1993;104(1):272–277.

459. Martell M, Esteban JI, Quer J, et al. Hepatitis C virus (HCV) circulates as a population of different but closely related genomes: quasispecies nature of HCV genome distribution. *J Virol* 1992;66(5):3225–3229.

460. Martin B, Hennecke N, Lohmann V, et al. Restoration of HCV-specific CD8+ T cell function by interferon-free therapy. *J Hepatol* 2014;61(3):538–543.

461. Martin TC, Martin NK, Hickman M, et al. Hepatitis C virus reinfection incidence and treatment outcome among HIV-positive MSM. *AIDS* 2013;27(16):2551–2557.

462. Martinello M, Grebely J, Petoumenos K, et al. HCV reinfection incidence among individuals treated for recent infection. *J Viral Hepat* 2017;24(5):359–370.

463. Martinello M, Hajarizadeh B, Grebely J, et al. HCV cure and reinfection among people with HIV/HCV coinfection and people who inject drugs. *Curr HIV/AIDS Rep* 2017;14(3):110–121.

464. Martinez-Bauer E, Forns X, Armelles M, et al. Hospital admission is a relevant source of hepatitis C virus acquisition in Spain. *J Hepatol* 2008;48(1):20–27.

465. Martinot-Peignoux M, Stern C, Maylin S, et al. Twelve weeks posttreatment follow-up is as relevant as 24 weeks to determine the sustained virologic response in patients with hepatitis C virus receiving pegylated interferon and ribavirin. *Hepatology* 2010;51(4):1122–1126.

466. Marukian S, Andrus L, Sheahan TP, et al. Hepatitis C virus induces interferon-lambda and interferon-stimulated genes in primary liver cultures. *Hepatology* 2011;54(6):1913–1923.

467. Masaki T, Arend KC, Li Y, et al. miR-122 stimulates hepatitis C virus RNA synthesis by altering the balance of viral RNAs engaged in replication versus translation. *Cell Host Microbe* 2015;17(2):217–228.

468. Masaki T, Suzuki R, Murakami K, et al. Interaction of hepatitis C virus nonstructural protein 5A with core protein is critical for the production of infectious virus particles. *J Virol* 2008;82(16):7964–7976.

469. Mason AL, Lau JY, Hoang N, et al. Association of diabetes mellitus and chronic hepatitis C virus infection. *Hepatology* 1999;29(2):328–333.

470. Mast EE, Hwang LY, Seto DS, et al. Risk factors for perinatal transmission of hepatitis C virus (HCV) and the natural history of HCV infection acquired in infancy. *J Infect Dis* 2005;192(11):1880–1889.

471. Matsumoto M, Hsieh TY, Zhu N, et al. Hepatitis C virus core protein interacts with the cytoplasmic tail of lymphotoxin-beta receptor. *J Virol* 1997;71(2):1301–1309.

472. Matsuura K, Sawai H, Ikeo K, et al. Genome-wide association study identifies TLL1 variant associated with development of hepatocellular carcinoma after eradication of hepatitis C virus infection. *Gastroenterology* 2017;152(6):1383–1394.

473. Mavilia MG, Wu GY. Mechanisms and prevention of vertical transmission in chronic viral hepatitis. *J Clin Transl Hepatol* 2017;5(2):119–129.

474. Mazzaro C, Little D, Pozzato G. Regression of splenic lymphoma after treatment of hepatitis C virus infection. *N Engl J Med* 2002;347(26):2168–2170; author reply 2168–2170.

475. McCauley JA, Rudd MT. Hepatitis C virus NS3/4a protease inhibitors. *Curr Opin Pharmacol* 2016;30:84–92.

476. McFarland AP, Horner SM, Jarret A, et al. The favorable IFNL3 genotype escapes mRNA decay mediated by AU-rich elements and hepatitis C virus-induced microRNAs. *Nat Immunol* 2014;15(1):72–79.

477. McGilvray I, Feld JJ, Chen L, et al. Hepatic cell-type specific gene expression better predicts HCV treatment outcome than IL28B genotype. *Gastroenterology* 2012;142(5):1122–1131.e1121.

478. McGivern DR, Masaki T, Williford S, et al. Kinetic analyses reveal potent and early blockade of hepatitis C virus assembly by NS5A inhibitors. *Gastroenterology* 2014;147(2):453–462.e457.

479. McGovern BH, Birch CE, Bowen MJ, et al. Improving the diagnosis of acute hepatitis C virus infection with expanded viral load criteria. *Clin Infect Dis* 2009;49(7):1051–1060.

480. McHutchison JG, Gordon SC, Schiff ER, et al. Interferon alfa-2b alone or in combination with ribavirin as initial treatment for chronic hepatitis C. Hepatitis Interventional Therapy Group. *N Engl J Med* 1998;339(21):1485–1492.

481. McKiernan SM, Hagan R, Curry M, et al. Distinct MHC class I and II alleles are associated with hepatitis C viral clearance, originating from a single source. *Hepatology* 2004;40(1):108–114.

482. McMahan RH, Golden-Mason L, Nishimura MI, et al. Tim-3 expression on PD-1+ HCV-specific human CTLs is associated with viral persistence, and its blockade restores hepatocyte-directed in vitro cytotoxicity. *J Clin Invest* 2010;120(12):4546–4557.

483. Mehta SH, Brancati FL, Strathdee SA, et al. Hepatitis C virus infection and incident type 2 diabetes. *Hepatology* 2003;38(1):50–56.

484. Mehta SH, Cox A, Hoover DR, et al. Protection against persistence of hepatitis C. *Lancet* 2002;359(9316):1478–1483.

485. Meissner EG, Bon D, Prokunina-Olsson L, et al. IFNL4-DeltaG genotype is associated with slower viral clearance in hepatitis C, genotype-1 patients treated with sofosbuvir and ribavirin. *J Infect Dis* 2014;209(11):1700–1704.

486. Mele D, Mantovani S, Oliviero B, et al. Hepatitis C virus inhibits CD4 T cell function via binding to Toll-like receptor 7. *Antiviral Res* 2017;137:108–111.

487. Mellor J, Holmes EC, Jarvis LM, et al. Investigation of the pattern of hepatitis C virus sequence diversity in different geographical regions: implications for virus classification. The International HCV Collaborative Study Group. *J Gen Virol* 1995;76(Pt 10):2493–2507.

488. Mendel I, Muraine M, Riachi G, et al. Detection and genotyping of the hepatitis C RNA in tear fluid from patients with chronic hepatitis C. *J Med Virol* 1997;51(3):231–233.

489. Merani S, Petrovic D, James I, et al. Effect of immune pressure on hepatitis C virus evolution: insights from a single-source outbreak. *Hepatology* 2011;53(2):396–405.

490. Merat SJ, Molenkamp R, Wagner K, et al. Hepatitis C virus broadly neutralizing monoclonal antibodies isolated 25 years after spontaneous clearance. *PLoS One* 2016;11(10):e0165047.

491. Mercer DF, Schiller DE, Elliott JF, et al. Hepatitis C virus replication in mice with chimeric human livers. *Nat Med* 2001;7(8):927–933.

492. Merz A, Long G, Hiet MS, et al. Biochemical and morphological properties of hepatitis C virus particles and determination of their lipidome. *J Biol Chem* 2011;286(4):3018–3032.

493. Messina JP, Humphreys I, Flaxman A, et al. Global distribution and prevalence of hepatitis C virus genotypes. *Hepatology* 2015;61(1):77–87.

494. Metz P, Dazert E, Ruggieri A, et al. Identification of type I and type II interferon-induced effectors controlling hepatitis C virus replication. *Hepatology* 2012;56(6):2082–2093.

495. Metz P, Reuter A, Bender S, et al. Interferon-stimulated genes and their role in controlling hepatitis C virus. *J Hepatol* 2013;59(6):1331–1341.
496. Meunier JC, Engle RE, Faulk K, et al. Evidence for cross-genotype neutralization of hepatitis C virus pseudo-particles and enhancement of infectivity by apolipoprotein C1. *Proc Natl Acad Sci U S A* 2005;102(12):4560–4565.
497. Meunier JC, Gottwein JM, Houghton M, et al. Vaccine-induced cross-genotype reactive neutralizing antibodies against hepatitis C virus. *J Infect Dis* 2011;204(8):1186–1190.
498. Meunier JC, Russell RS, Goossens V, et al. Isolation and characterization of broadly neutralizing human monoclonal antibodies to the e1 glycoprotein of hepatitis C virus. *J Virol* 2008;82(2):966–973.
499. Meyer-Olson D, Shoukry NH, Brady KW, et al. Limited T cell receptor diversity of HCV-specific T cell responses is associated with CTL escape. *J Exp Med* 2004;200(3):307–319.
500. Meylan E, Curran J, Hofmann K, et al. Cardif is an adaptor protein in the RIG-I antiviral pathway and is targeted by hepatitis C virus. *Nature* 2005;437(7062):1167–1172.
501. Midgard H, Bjoro B, Maeland A, et al. Hepatitis C reinfection after sustained virological response. *J Hepatol* 2016;64(5):1020–1026.
502. Miki D, Ochi H, Hayes CN, et al. Variation in the DEPDC5 locus is associated with progression to hepatocellular carcinoma in chronic hepatitis C virus carriers. *Nat Genet* 2011;43(8):797–800.
503. Miki D, Ochi H, Takahashi A, et al. HLA-DQB1*03 confers susceptibility to chronic hepatitis C in Japanese: a genome-wide association study. *PLoS One* 2013;8(12):e84226.
504. Milward A, Mankouri J, Harris M. Hepatitis C virus NS5A protein interacts with beta-catenin and stimulates its transcriptional activity in a phosphoinositide-3 kinase-dependent fashion. *J Gen Virol* 2010;91(Pt 2):373–381.
505. Misiani R, Bellavita P, Fenili D, et al. Hepatitis C virus infection in patients with essential mixed cryoglobulinemia. *Ann Intern Med* 1992;117(7):573–577.
506. Missale G, Bertoni R, Lamonaca V, et al. Different clinical behaviors of acute hepatitis C virus infection are associated with different vigor of the anti-viral cell-mediated immune response. *J Clin Invest* 1996;98(3):706–714.
507. Missale G, Pilli M, Zerbini A, et al. Lack of full CD8 functional restoration after antiviral treatment for acute and chronic hepatitis C virus infection. *Gut* 2012;61(7):1076–1084.
508. Mitchell AE, Colvin HM, Palmer Beasley R. Institute of Medicine recommendations for the prevention and control of hepatitis B and C. *Hepatology* 2010;51(3):729–733.
509. Mitchell JK, Midkiff BR, Israelow B, et al. Hepatitis C virus indirectly disrupts DNA damage-induced p53 responses by activating protein kinase R. *MBio* 2017;8(2).
510. Miyagi T, Takehara T, Nishio K, et al. Altered interferon-alpha-signaling in natural killer cells from patients with chronic hepatitis C virus infection. *J Hepatol* 2010;53(3):424–430.
511. Miyanari Y, Atsuzawa K, Usuda N, et al. The lipid droplet is an important organelle for hepatitis C virus production. *Nat Cell Biol* 2007;9(9):1089–1097.
512. Mizokami M, Tanaka Y, Miyakawa Y. Spread times of hepatitis C virus estimated by the molecular clock differ among Japan, the United States and Egypt in reflection of their distinct socioeconomic backgrounds. *Intervirology* 2006;49(1–2):28–36.
513. Mizukoshi E, Eisenbach C, Edlin BR, et al. Hepatitis C virus (HCV)-specific immune responses of long-term injection drug users frequently exposed to HCV. *J Infect Dis* 2008;198(2):203–212.
514. Mohan P, Colvin C, Glymph C, et al. Clinical spectrum and histopathologic features of chronic hepatitis C infection in children. *J Pediatr* 2007;150(2):168–174, 174.e161.
515. Moorman AC, Rupp LB, Gordon SC, et al. Long-term liver disease, treatment, and mortality outcomes among 17,000 persons diagnosed with chronic hepatitis C virus infection: current Chronic Hepatitis Cohort Study status and review of findings. *Infect Dis Clin North Am* 2018;32(2):253–268.
516. Morgan RL, Baack B, Smith BD, et al. Eradication of hepatitis C virus infection and the development of hepatocellular carcinoma: a meta-analysis of observational studies. *Ann Intern Med* 2013;158(5 Pt 1):329–337.
517. Morin TJ, Broering TJ, Leav BA, et al. Human monoclonal antibody HCV1 effectively prevents and treats HCV infection in chimpanzees. *PLoS Pathog* 2012;8(8):e1002895.
518. Morishima C, Paschal DM, Wang CC, et al. Decreased NK cell frequency in chronic hepatitis C does not affect ex vivo cytolytic killing. *Hepatology* 2006;43(3):573–580.
519. Moriya K, Fujie H, Shintani Y, et al. The core protein of hepatitis C virus induces hepatocellular carcinoma in transgenic mice. *Nat Med* 1998;4(9):1065–1067.
520. Moriya K, Nakagawa K, Santa T, et al. Oxidative stress in the absence of inflammation in a mouse model for hepatitis C virus-associated hepatocarcinogenesis. *Cancer Res* 2001;61(11):4365–4370.
521. Morris MD, Shiboski S, Bruneau J, et al. Geographic differences in temporal incidence trends of hepatitis C virus infection among people who inject drugs: the InC3 collaboration. *Clin Infect Dis* 2017;64(7):860–869.
522. Morrison MH, Keane C, Quinn LM, et al. IFNL cytokines do not modulate human or murine NK cell functions. *Hum Immunol* 2014;75(9):996–1000.
523. Mosley RT, Edwards TE, Murakami E, et al. Structure of hepatitis C virus polymerase in complex with primer-template RNA. *J Virol* 2012;86(12):6503–6511.
524. Mosley JW, Operskalski EA, Tobler LH, et al. Viral and host factors in early hepatitis C virus infection. *Hepatology* 2005;42(1):86–92.
525. Mucke MM, Backus LI, Mucke VT, et al. Hepatitis B virus reactivation during direct-acting antiviral therapy for hepatitis C: a systematic review and meta-analysis. *Lancet Gastroenterol Hepatol* 2018;3(3):172–180.
526. Muljono DH. Effective drugs on the road to HCV elimination and a therapeutic gap to close. *Lancet Gastroenterol Hepatol* 2019;4(2):86–88.
527. Munakata T, Liang Y, Kim S, et al. Hepatitis C virus induces E6AP-dependent degradation of the retinoblastoma protein. *PLoS Pathog* 2007;3(9):1335–1347.
528. Murray KF, Balistreri WF, Bansal S, et al. Safety and efficacy of Ledipasvir-Sofosbuvir with or without ribavirin for chronic hepatitis C in children ages 6–11. *Hepatology* 2018;68(6):2158–2166.
529. Murray KF, Finn LS, Taylor SL, et al. Liver histology and alanine aminotransferase levels in children and adults with chronic hepatitis C infection. *J Pediatr Gastroenterol Nutr* 2005;41(5):634–638.
530. Nagata H, Nakagawa M, Asahina Y, et al. Effect of interferon-based and -free therapy on early occurrence and recurrence of hepatocellular carcinoma in chronic hepatitis C. *J Hepatol* 2017;67(5):933–939.
531. Nahon P, Bourcier V, Layese R, et al. Eradication of hepatitis C virus infection in patients with cirrhosis reduces risk of liver and non-liver complications. *Gastroenterology* 2017;152(1):142–156.e142.
532. Naiyer MM, Cassidy SA, Magri A, et al. KIR2DS2 recognizes conserved peptides derived from viral helicases in the context of HLA-C. *Sci Immunol* 2017;2(15).
533. Nakamoto N, Cho H, Shaked A, et al. Synergistic reversal of intrahepatic HCV-specific CD8 T cell exhaustion by combined PD-1/CTLA-4 blockade. *PLoS Pathog* 2009;5(2):e1000313.
534. Nakamoto N, Kaplan DE, Coleclough J, et al. Functional restoration of HCV-specific CD8 T cells by PD-1 blockade is defined by PD-1 expression and compartmentalization. *Gastroenterology* 2008;134(7):1927–1937, 1937.e1921–1922.
535. Naoumov NV. Cyclophilin inhibition as potential therapy for liver diseases. *J Hepatol* 2014;61(5):1166–1174.
536. Nascimbeni M, Mizukoshi E, Bosmann M, et al. Kinetics of CD4+ and CD8+ memory T-cell responses during hepatitis C virus rechallenge of previously recovered chimpanzees. *J Virol* 2003;77(8):4781–4793.
537. National Academies of Sciences, Engineering, and Medicine, Health and Medicine Division; Board on Population Health and Public Health Practice; Committee on a National Strategy for the Elimination of Hepatitis B and C. In: Strom BL, Buckley GJ, eds. *A National Strategy for the Elimination of Hepatitis B and C: Phase Two Report*. Washington (DC): National Academies Press (US). Copyright 2017 by the National Academy of Sciences. All rights reserved; 2017.
538. Nattermann J, Nischalke HD, Hofmeister V, et al. The HLA-A2 restricted T cell epitope HCV core 35–44 stabilizes HLA-E expression and inhibits cytolysis mediated by natural killer cells. *Am J Pathol* 2005;166(2):443–453.
539. Nault JC, Mallet M, Pilati C, et al. High frequency of telomerase reverse-transcriptase promoter somatic mutations in hepatocellular carcinoma and preneoplastic lesions. *Nat Commun* 2013;4:2218.
540. Navas S, Martin J, Quiroga JA, et al. Genetic diversity and tissue compartmentalization of the hepatitis C virus genome in blood mononuclear cells, liver, and serum from chronic hepatitis C patients. *J Virol* 1998;72(2):1640–1646.
541. Ndjomou J, Pybus OG, Matz B. Phylogenetic analysis of hepatitis C virus isolates indicates a unique pattern of endemic infection in Cameroon. *J Gen Virol* 2003;84 (Pt 9):2333–2341.
542. Negash AA, Ramos HJ, Crochet N, et al. IL-1beta production through the NLRP3 inflammasome by hepatic macrophages links hepatitis C virus infection with liver inflammation and disease. *PLoS Pathog* 2013;9(4):e1003330.
543. Negro F. Abnormalities of lipid metabolism in hepatitis C virus infection. *Gut* 2010; 59(9):1279–1287.
544. Nelson DR, Marousis CG, Davis GL, et al. The role of hepatitis C virus-specific cytotoxic T lymphocytes in chronic hepatitis C. *J Immunol* 1997;158(3):1473–1481.
545. Netski DM, Mosbruger T, Depla E, et al. Humoral immune response in acute hepatitis C virus infection. *Clin Infect Dis* 2005;41(5):667–675.
546. Neufeldt CJ, Joyce MA, Van Buuren N, et al. The hepatitis C virus-induced membranous web and associated nuclear transport machinery limit access of pattern recognition receptors to viral replication sites. *PLoS Pathog* 2016;12(2):e1005428.
547. Neumann AU, Lam NP, Dahari H, et al. Hepatitis C viral dynamics in vivo and the antiviral efficacy of interferon-alpha therapy. *Science* 1998;282(5386):103–107.
548. Neumann-Haefelin C, Oniangue-Ndza C, Kuntzen T, et al. Human leukocyte antigen B27 selects for rare escape mutations that significantly impair hepatitis C virus replication and require compensatory mutations. *Hepatology* 2011;54(4):1157–1166.
549. Ng TI, Pilot-Matias T, Tripathi R, et al. Resistance analysis of a 3-day monotherapy study with glecaprevir or pibrentasvir in patients with chronic hepatitis C virus genotype 1 infection. *Viruses* 2018;10(9).
550. Niepmann M, Shalamova LA, Gerresheim GK, et al. Signals involved in regulation of hepatitis C virus RNA genome translation and replication. *Front Microbiol* 2018;9:395.
551. Noureddin M, Rotman Y, Zhang F, et al. Hepatic expression levels of interferons and interferon-stimulated genes in patients with chronic hepatitis C: a phenotype-genotype correlation study. *Genes Immun* 2015;16(5):321–329.
552. Obajemu AA, Rao N, Dilley KA, et al. IFN-lambda4 attenuates antiviral responses by enhancing negative regulation of IFN signaling. *J Immunol* 2017;199(11):3808–3820.
553. O'Brien TR, Kottilil S, Pfeiffer RM. IFNL4 genotype is associated with virologic relapse after 8-week treatment with sofosbuvir, velpatasvir, and voxilaprevir. *Gastroenterology* 2017;153(6):1694–1695.
554. O'Brien TR, Yang HI, Groover S, et al. Genetic factors that affect spontaneous clearance of hepatitis C or B virus, response to treatment, and disease progression. *Gastroenterology* 2019;156(2):400–417.
555. Ogawa E, Furusyo N, Kajiwara E, et al. Efficacy of pegylated interferon alpha-2b and ribavirin treatment on the risk of hepatocellular carcinoma in patients with chronic hepatitis C: a prospective, multicenter study. *J Hepatol* 2013;58(3):495–501.
556. Ohmer S, Honegger J. New prospects for the treatment and prevention of hepatitis C in children. *Curr Opin Pediatr* 2016;28(1):93–100.
557. Oliviero B, Varchetta S, Paudice E, et al. Natural killer cell functional dichotomy in chronic hepatitis B and chronic hepatitis C virus infections. *Gastroenterology* 2009;137(3): 1151–1160, 1160.e1151–1157.
558. Oniangue-Ndza C, Kuntzen T, Kemper M, et al. Compensatory mutations restore the replication defects caused by cytotoxic T lymphocyte escape mutations in hepatitis C virus polymerase. *J Virol* 2011;85(22):11883–11890.
559. Osburn WO, Fisher BE, Dowd KA, et al. Spontaneous control of primary hepatitis C virus infection and immunity against persistent reinfection. *Gastroenterology* 2010;138(1):315–324.
560. Osburn WO, Snider AE, Wells BL, et al. Clearance of Hepatitis C infection is associated with early appearance of broad neutralizing antibody responses. *Hepatology* 2014;59(6): 2140–2151.
561. Owsianka A, Tarr AW, Juttla VS, et al. Monoclonal antibody AP33 defines a broadly neutralizing epitope on the hepatitis C virus E2 envelope glycoprotein. *J Virol* 2005;79(17): 11095–11104.

562. Owsianka AM, Tarr AW, Keck ZY, et al. Broadly neutralizing human monoclonal antibodies to the hepatitis C virus E2 glycoprotein. *J Gen Virol* 2008;89(Pt 3):653–659.
563. Owusu Sekyere S, Suneetha PV, Kraft AR, et al. A heterogeneous hierarchy of co-regulatory receptors regulates exhaustion of HCV-specific CD8 T cells in patients with chronic hepatitis C. *J Hepatol* 2015;62(1):31–40.
564. Padhi S, Maharshi S, Gupta GK, et al. Efficacy and safety of direct acting antiviral therapy for chronic hepatitis C in thalassemic children. *J Pediatr Hematol Oncol* 2018;40(7):511–514.
565. Page K, Mirzazadeh A, Rice TM, et al. Interferon Lambda 4 genotype is associated with jaundice and elevated aminotransferase levels during acute hepatitis C virus infection: findings from the InC3 collaborative. *Open Forum Infect Dis* 2016;3(1):ofw024.
566. Paintsil E, Binka M, Patel A, et al. Hepatitis C virus maintains infectivity for weeks after drying on inanimate surfaces at room temperature: implications for risks of transmission. *J Infect Dis* 2014;209(8):1205–1211.
567. Paintsil E, He H, Peters C, et al. Survival of hepatitis C virus in syringes: implication for transmission among injection drug users. *J Infect Dis* 2010;202(7):984–990.
568. Paley MA, Kroy DC, Odorizzi PM, et al. Progenitor and terminal subsets of CD8+ T cells cooperate to contain chronic viral infection. *Science* 2012;338(6111):1220–1225.
569. Parera M, Martrus G, Franco S, et al. Canine hepacivirus NS3 serine protease can cleave the human adaptor proteins MAVS and TRIF. *PLoS One* 2012;7(8):e42481.
570. Park H, Serti E, Eke O, et al. IL-29 is the dominant type III interferon produced by hepatocytes during acute hepatitis C virus infection. *Hepatology* 2012;56(6):2060–2070.
571. Pascasio JM, Vinaixa C, Ferrer MT, et al. Clinical outcomes of patients undergoing antiviral therapy while awaiting liver transplantation. *J Hepatol* 2017;67(6):1168–1176.
572. Pawlotsky JM. Use and interpretation of virological tests for hepatitis C. *Hepatology* 2002;36(5 Suppl 1):S65–S73.
573. Pawlotsky JM. Hepatitis C virus resistance to direct-acting antiviral drugs in interferon-free regimens. *Gastroenterology* 2016;151(1):70–86.
574. Pawlotsky JM, Flisiak R, Sarin SK, et al. Alisporivir plus ribavirin, interferon free or in combination with pegylated interferon, for hepatitis C virus genotype 2 or 3 infection. *Hepatology* 2015;62(4):1013–1023.
575. Pelletier S, Drouin C, Bedard N, et al. Increased degranulation of natural killer cells during acute HCV correlates with the magnitude of virus-specific T cell responses. *J Hepatol* 2010;53(5):805–816.
576. Penin F, Brass V, Appel N, et al. Structure and function of the membrane anchor domain of hepatitis C virus nonstructural protein 5A. *J Biol Chem* 2004;279(39):40835–40843.
577. Penna A, Missale G, Lamonaca V, et al. Intrahepatic and circulating HLA class II-restricted, hepatitis C virus-specific T cells: functional characterization in patients with chronic hepatitis C. *Hepatology* 2002;35(5):1225–1236.
578. Penna A, Pilli M, Zerbini A, et al. Dysfunction and functional restoration of HCV-specific CD8 responses in chronic hepatitis C virus infection. *Hepatology* 2007;45(3):588–601.
579. Pepin J, Abou Chakra CN, Pepin E, et al. Evolution of the global use of unsafe medical injections, 2000–2010. *PLoS One* 2013;8(12):e80948.
580. Perin PM, Haid S, Brown RJ, et al. Flunarizine prevents hepatitis C virus membrane fusion in a genotype-dependent manner by targeting the potential fusion peptide within E1. *Hepatology* 2016;63(1):49–62.
581. Perotti M, Mancini N, Diotti RA, et al. Identification of a broadly cross-reacting and neutralizing human monoclonal antibody directed against the hepatitis C virus E2 protein. *J Virol* 2008;82(2):1047–1052.
582. Perrillo RP. The role of liver biopsy in hepatitis C. *Hepatology* 1997;26(3 Suppl 1):57s–61s.
583. Perrillo RP. Acute flares in chronic hepatitis B: the natural and unnatural history of an immunologically mediated liver disease. *Gastroenterology* 2001;120(4):1009–1022.
584. Pessione F, Degos F, Marcellin P, et al. Effect of alcohol consumption on serum hepatitis C virus RNA and histological lesions in chronic hepatitis C. *Hepatology* 1998; 27(6):1717–1722.
585. Pestka JM, Zeisel MB, Blaser E, et al. Rapid induction of virus-neutralizing antibodies and viral clearance in a single-source outbreak of hepatitis C. *Proc Natl Acad Sci U S A* 2007;104(14):6025–6030.
586. Pfaender S, Cavalleri JM, Walter S, et al. Clinical course of infection and viral tissue tropism of hepatitis C virus-like nonprimate hepaciviruses in horses. *Hepatology* 2015;61(2):447–459.
587. Pfaender S, Helfritz FA, Siddharta A, et al. Environmental stability and infectivity of hepatitis C virus (HCV) in different human body fluids. *Front Microbiol* 2018;9:504.
588. Pfaender S, Walter S, Grabski E, et al. Immune protection against reinfection with nonprimate hepacivirus. *Proc Natl Acad Sci U S A* 2017;114(12):e2430–e2439.
589. Pfafferott K, Gaudieri S, Ulsenheimer A, et al. Constrained pattern of viral evolution in acute and early HCV infection limits viral plasticity. *PLoS One* 2011;6(2):e16797.
590. Pham LV, Jensen SB, Fahnoe U, et al. HCV genotype 1–6 NS3 residue 80 substitutions impact protease inhibitor activity and promote viral escape. *J Hepatol* 2019;70(3):388–397.
591. Pileri P, Uematsu Y, Campagnoli S, et al. Binding of hepatitis C virus to CD81. *Science* 1998;282(5390):938–941.
592. Pineda JA, Nunez-Torres R, Tellez F, et al. Hepatitis C virus reinfection after sustained virological response in HIV-infected patients with chronic hepatitis C. *J Infect* 2015;71(5):571–577.
593. Pinero F, Mendizabal M, Ridruejo E, et al. Treatment with direct-acting antivirals for HCV decreases but does not eliminate the risk of hepatocellular carcinoma. *Liver Int* 2019;39(6):1033–1043.
594. Piver E, Boyer A, Gaillard J, et al. Ultrastructural organisation of HCV from the bloodstream of infected patients revealed by electron microscopy after specific immunocapture. *Gut* 2017;66(8):1487–1495.
595. Platt L, Minozzi S, Reed J, et al. Needle and syringe programmes and opioid substitution therapy for preventing HCV transmission among people who inject drugs: findings from a Cochrane Review and meta-analysis. *Addiction* 2018;113(3):545–563.
596. Ploss A, Evans MJ, Gaysinskaya VA, et al. Human occludin is a hepatitis C virus entry factor required for infection of mouse cells. *Nature* 2009;457(7231):882–886.
597. Polaris Observatory HCV Collaborators. Global prevalence and genotype distribution of hepatitis C virus infection in 2015: a modelling study. *Lancet Gastroenterol Hepatol* 2017;2(3):161–176.
598. Poordad F, Hezode C, Trinh R, et al. ABT-450/r-ombitasvir and dasabuvir with ribavirin for hepatitis C with cirrhosis. *N Engl J Med* 2014;370(21):1973–1982.
599. Poordad F, Lawitz E, Kowdley KV, et al. Exploratory study of oral combination antiviral therapy for hepatitis C. *N Engl J Med* 2013;368(1):45–53.
600. Popescu CI, Callens N, Trinel D, et al. NS2 protein of hepatitis C virus interacts with structural and non-structural proteins towards virus assembly. *PLoS Pathog* 2011;7(2):e1001278.
601. Powers KA, Ribeiro RM, Patel K, et al. Kinetics of hepatitis C virus reinfection after liver transplantation. *Liver Transpl* 2006;12(2):207–216.
602. Poynard T, Marcellin P, Lee SS, et al. Randomised trial of interferon alpha2b plus ribavirin for 48 weeks or for 24 weeks versus interferon alpha2b plus placebo for 48 weeks for treatment of chronic infection with hepatitis C virus. International Hepatitis Interventional Therapy Group (IHIT). *Lancet* 1998;352(9138):1426–1432.
603. Poynard T, McHutchison J, Manns M, et al. Impact of pegylated interferon alfa-2b and ribavirin on liver fibrosis in patients with chronic hepatitis C. *Gastroenterology* 2002; 122(5):1303–1313.
604. Pozzetto B, Memmi M, Garraud O, et al. Health care-associated hepatitis C virus infection. *World J Gastroenterol* 2014;20(46):17265–17278.
605. Prati D. Transmission of viral hepatitis by blood and blood derivatives: current risks, past heritage. *Dig Liver Dis* 2002;34(11):812–817.
606. Prentoe J, Bukh J. Hypervariable region 1 in envelope protein 2 of hepatitis C virus: a linchpin in neutralizing antibody evasion and viral entry. *Front Immunol* 2018;9:2146.
607. Prentoe J, Jensen TB, Meuleman P, et al. Hypervariable region 1 differentially impacts viability of hepatitis C virus strains of genotypes 1 to 6 and impairs virus neutralization. *J Virol* 2011;85(5):2224–2234.
608. Prentoe J, Velazquez-Moctezuma R, Foung SK, et al. Hypervariable region 1 shielding of hepatitis C virus is a main contributor to genotypic differences in neutralization sensitivity. *Hepatology* 2016;64(6):1881–1892.
609. Prince AM. Immunity in hepatitis C virus infection. *Vox Sang* 1994;67(Suppl 3):227–228.
610. Prince AM, Brotman B, Grady GF, et al. Long-incubation post-transfusion hepatitis without serological evidence of exposure to hepatitis-B virus. *Lancet* 1974;2(7875):241–246.
611. Prince AM, Huima-Byron T, Parker TS, et al. Visualization of hepatitis C virions and putative defective interfering particles isolated from low-density lipoproteins. *J Viral Hepat* 1996;3(1):11–17.
612. Prokunina-Olsson L, Muchmore B, Tang W, et al. A variant upstream of IFNL3 (IL28B) creating a new interferon gene IFNL4 is associated with impaired clearance of hepatitis C virus. *Nat Genet* 2013;45(2):164–171.
613. Pybus OG, Barnes E, Taggart R, et al. Genetic history of hepatitis C virus in East Asia. *J Virol* 2009;83(2):1071–1082.
614. Pybus OG, Charleston MA, Gupta S, et al. The epidemic behavior of the hepatitis C virus. *Science* 2001;292(5525):2323–2325.
615. Pybus OG, Drummond AJ, Nakano T, et al. The epidemiology and iatrogenic transmission of hepatitis C virus in Egypt: a Bayesian coalescent approach. *Mol Biol Evol* 2003;20(3):381–387.
616. Pybus OG, Theze J. Hepacivirus cross-species transmission and the origins of the hepatitis C virus. *Curr Opin Virol* 2016;16:1–7.
617. Radziewicz H, Ibegbu CC, Fernandez ML, et al. Liver-infiltrating lymphocytes in chronic human hepatitis C virus infection display an exhausted phenotype with high levels of PD-1 and low levels of CD127 expression. *J Virol* 2007;81(6):2545–2553.
618. Radziewicz H, Ibegbu CC, Hon H, et al. Impaired hepatitis C virus (HCV)-specific effector CD8+ T cells undergo massive apoptosis in the peripheral blood during acute HCV infection and in the liver during the chronic phase of infection. *J Virol* 2008; 82(20):9808–9822.
619. Raghuraman S, Park H, Osburn WO, et al. Spontaneous clearance of chronic hepatitis C virus infection is associated with appearance of neutralizing antibodies and reversal of T-cell exhaustion. *J Infect Dis* 2012;205(5):763–771.
620. Ramamurthy N, Marchi E, Ansari MA, et al. Impact of IFNL4 genotype on interferon-stimulated gene expression during DAA therapy for hepatitis C. *Hepatology* 2018;68(3):859–871.
621. Ramiere C, Charre C, Miailhes P, et al. Patterns of HCV transmission in HIV-infected and HIV-negative men having sex with men. *Clin Infect Dis* 2019.
622. Ramirez S, Bukh J. Current status and future development of infectious cell-culture models for the major genotypes of hepatitis C virus: essential tools in testing of antivirals and emerging vaccine strategies. *Antiviral Res* 2018;158:264–287.
623. Rauch A, Kutalik Z, Descombes P, et al. Genetic variation in IL28B is associated with chronic hepatitis C and treatment failure: a genome-wide association study. *Gastroenterology* 2010;138(4):1338–1345, 1345.e1331–1337.
624. Ray SC, Arthur RR, Carella A, et al. Genetic epidemiology of hepatitis C virus throughout egypt. *J Infect Dis* 2000;182(3):698–707.
625. Ray SC, Fanning L, Wang XH, et al. Divergent and convergent evolution after a common-source outbreak of hepatitis C virus. *J Exp Med* 2005;201(11):1753–1759.
626. Ray RB, Lagging LM, Meyer K, et al. Hepatitis C virus core protein cooperates with ras and transforms primary rat embryo fibroblasts to tumorigenic phenotype. *J Virol* 1996;70(7):4438–4443.
627. Ray RB, Meyer K, Ray R. Suppression of apoptotic cell death by hepatitis C virus core protein. *Virology* 1996;226(2):176–182.
628. Ray RB, Steele R, Meyer K, et al. Transcriptional repression of p53 promoter by hepatitis C virus core protein. *J Biol Chem* 1997;272(17):10983–10986.
629. Raziorrouh B, Sacher K, Tawar RG, et al. Virus-specific CD4+ T cells have functional and phenotypic characteristics of follicular T-helper cells in patients with acute and chronic HCV infections. *Gastroenterology* 2016;150(3):696–706.e693.
630. Raziorrouh B, Ulsenheimer A, Schraut W, et al. Inhibitory molecules that regulate expansion and restoration of HCV-specific CD4+ T cells in patients with chronic infection. *Gastroenterology* 2011;141(4):1422–1431, 1431.e1421–1426.
631. Reau N, Kwo PY, Rhee S, et al. Glecaprevir/pibrentasvir treatment in liver or kidney transplant patients with hepatitis C virus infection. *Hepatology* 2018;68(4):1298–1307.
632. Reddy KR, Lim JK, Kuo A, et al. All-oral direct-acting antiviral therapy in HCV-advanced liver disease is effective in real-world practice: observations through HCV-TARGET database. *Aliment Pharmacol Ther* 2017;45(1):115–126.

633. Rehermann B. Natural killer cells in viral hepatitis. *Cell Mol Gastroenterol Hepatol* 2015;1(6):578–588.
634. Reig M, Marino Z, Perello C, et al. Unexpected high rate of early tumor recurrence in patients with HCV-related HCC undergoing interferon-free therapy. *J Hepatol* 2016; 65(4):719–726.
635. Rein DB, Smith BD, Wittenborn JS, et al. The cost-effectiveness of birth-cohort screening for hepatitis C antibody in U.S. primary care settings. *Ann Intern Med* 2012;156(4):263–270.
636. Resti M, Azzari C, Mannelli F, et al. Mother to child transmission of hepatitis C virus: prospective study of risk factors and timing of infection in children born to women seronegative for HIV-1. Tuscany Study Group on hepatitis C virus infection. *BMJ* 1998;317(7156):437–441.
637. Ribeiro RM, Li H, Wang S, et al. Quantifying the diversification of hepatitis C virus (HCV) during primary infection: estimates of the in vivo mutation rate. *PLoS Pathog* 2012;8(8):e1002881.
638. Robinson M, Yang H, Sun SC, et al. Novel hepatitis C virus reporter replicon cell lines enable efficient antiviral screening against genotype 1a. *Antimicrob Agents Chemother* 2010;54(8):3099–3106.
639. Rodrigo C, Walker MR, Leung P, et al. Limited naturally occurring escape in broadly neutralizing antibody epitopes in hepatitis C glycoprotein E2 and constrained sequence usage in acute infection. *Infect Genet Evol* 2017;49:88–96.
640. Romano KP, Ali A, Aydin C, et al. The molecular basis of drug resistance against hepatitis C virus NS3/4A protease inhibitors. *PLoS Pathog* 2012;8(7):e1002832.
641. Romero-Brey I, Berger C, Kallis S, et al. NS5A domain 1 and polyprotein cleavage kinetics are critical for induction of double-membrane vesicles associated with hepatitis C virus replication. *MBio* 2015;6(4):e00759.
642. Romero-Brey I, Merz A, Chiramel A, et al. Three-dimensional architecture and biogenesis of membrane structures associated with hepatitis C virus replication. *PLoS Pathog* 2012;8(12):e1003056.
643. Rosenberg BR, Depla M, Freije CA, et al. Longitudinal transcriptomic characterization of the immune response to acute hepatitis C virus infection in patients with spontaneous viral clearance. *PLoS Pathog* 2018;14(9):e1007290.
644. Ross-Thriepland D, Harris M. Hepatitis C virus NS5A: enigmatic but still promiscuous 10 years on! *J Gen Virol* 2015;96(Pt 4):727–738.
645. Rowe IA, Tully DC, Armstrong MJ, et al. Effect of scavenger receptor class B type I antagonist ITX5061 in patients with hepatitis C virus infection undergoing liver transplantation. *Liver Transpl* 2016;22(3):287–297.
646. Ruhl M, Chhatwal P, Strathmann H, et al. Escape from a dominant HLA-B*15-restricted CD8+ T cell response against hepatitis C virus requires compensatory mutations outside the epitope. *J Virol* 2012;86(2):991–1000.
647. Ruhl M, Knuschke T, Schewior K, et al. CD8+ T-cell response promotes evolution of hepatitis C virus nonstructural proteins. *Gastroenterology* 2011;140(7):2064–2073.
648. Rutebemberwa A, Ray SC, Astemborski J, et al. High-programmed death-1 levels on hepatitis C virus-specific T cells during acute infection are associated with viral persistence and require preservation of cognate antigen during chronic infection. *J Immunol* 2008;181(12):8215–8225.
649. Saab S, Le L, Saggi S, et al. Toward the elimination of hepatitis C in the United States. *Hepatology* 2018;67(6):2449–2459.
650. Saadoun D, Pol S, Ferfar Y, et al. Efficacy and safety of sofosbuvir plus daclatasvir for treatment of HCV-associated cryoglobulinemia vasculitis. *Gastroenterology* 2017;153(1):49–52.e45.
651. Saadoun D, Rosenzwajg M, Landau D, et al. Restoration of peripheral immune homeostasis after rituximab in mixed cryoglobulinemia vasculitis. *Blood* 2008;111(11):5334–5341.
652. Sabo MC, Luca VC, Prentoe J, et al. Neutralizing monoclonal antibodies against hepatitis C virus E2 protein bind discontinuous epitopes and inhibit infection at a postattachment step. *J Virol* 2011;85(14):7005–7019.
653. Sacks-Davis R, Grebely J, Dore GJ, et al. Hepatitis C virus reinfection and spontaneous clearance of reinfection—the InC3 study. *J Infect Dis* 2015;212(9):1407–1419.
654. Salloum S, Oniangue-Ndza C, Neumann-Haefelin C, et al. Escape from HLA-B*08-restricted CD8 T cells by hepatitis C virus is associated with fitness costs. *J Virol* 2008;82(23):11803–11812.
655. Sangiovanni A, Prati GM, Fasani P, et al. The natural history of compensated cirrhosis due to hepatitis C virus: A 17-year cohort study of 214 patients. *Hepatology* 2006;43(6):1303–1310.
656. Sarasin-Filipowicz M, Oakeley EJ, Duong FH, et al. Interferon signaling and treatment outcome in chronic hepatitis C. *Proc Natl Acad Sci U S A* 2008;105(19):7034–7039.
657. Sarrazin C, Cooper CL, Manns MP, et al. No impact of resistance-associated substitutions on the efficacy of sofosbuvir, velpatasvir, and voxilaprevir for 12 weeks in HCV DAA-experienced patients. *J Hepatol* 2018;69(6):1221–1230.
658. Sarrazin C, Kieffer TL, Bartels D, et al. Dynamic hepatitis C virus genotypic and phenotypic changes in patients treated with the protease inhibitor telaprevir. *Gastroenterology* 2007;132(5):1767–1777.
659. Sarrazin C, Zeuzem S. Resistance to direct antiviral agents in patients with hepatitis C virus infection. *Gastroenterology* 2010;138(2):447–462.
660. Sasaki R, Devhare PB, Steele R, et al. Hepatitis C virus-induced CCL5 secretion from macrophages activates hepatic stellate cells. *Hepatology* 2017;66(3):746–757.
661. Schneider WM, Chevillotte MD, Rice CM. Interferon-stimulated genes: a complex web of host defenses. *Annu Rev Immunol* 2014;32:513–545.
662. Schoggins JW, Rice CM. Innate immune responses to hepatitis C virus. *Curr Top Microbiol Immunol* 2013;369:219–242.
663. Schoggins JW, Wilson SJ, Panis M, et al. A diverse range of gene products are effectors of the type I interferon antiviral response. *Nature* 2011;472(7344):481–485.
664. Schramm F, Soulier E, Royer C, et al. Frequent compartmentalization of hepatitis C virus with leukocyte-related amino acids in the setting of liver transplantation. *J Infect Dis* 2008;198(11):1656–1666.
665. Schulkind J, Stephens B, Ahmad F, et al. High response and re-infection rates among people who inject drugs treated for hepatitis C in a community needle and syringe programme. *J Viral Hepat* 2019;26(5):519–528.
666. Schulze Zur Wiesch J, Ciuffreda D, Lewis-Ximenez L, et al. Broadly directed virus-specific CD4+ T cell responses are primed during acute hepatitis C infection, but rapidly disappear from human blood with viral persistence. *J Exp Med* 2012;209(1):61–75.
667. Schwarz KB, Rosenthal P, Murray KF, et al. Ledipasvir -Sofosbuvir for 12 weeks in children 3 to <6 years old with chronic hepatitis C. *Hepatology* 2019.
668. Scott N, McBryde E, Vickerman P, et al. The role of a hepatitis C virus vaccine: modelling the benefits alongside direct-acting antiviral treatments. *BMC Med* 2015;13:198.
669. Scott N, Olafsson S, Gottfreethsson M, et al. Modelling the elimination of hepatitis C as a public health threat in Iceland: a goal attainable by 2020. *J Hepatol* 2018;68(5):932–939.
670. Seeff LB, Hollinger FB, Alter HJ, et al. Long-term mortality and morbidity of transfusion-associated non-A, non-B, and type C hepatitis: a National Heart, Lung, and Blood Institute collaborative study. *Hepatology* 2001;33(2):455–463.
671. Seifert U, Liermann H, Racanelli V, et al. Hepatitis C virus mutation affects proteasomal epitope processing. *J Clin Invest* 2004;114(2):250–259.
672. Seigel B, Bengsch B, Lohmann V, et al. Factors that determine the antiviral efficacy of HCV-specific CD8(+) T cells ex vivo. *Gastroenterology* 2013;144(2):426–436.
673. Semmo N, Day CL, Ward SM, et al. Preferential loss of IL-2-secreting CD4+ T helper cells in chronic HCV infection. *Hepatology* 2005;41(5):1019–1028.
674. Sen DR, Kaminski J, Barnitz RA, et al. The epigenetic landscape of T cell exhaustion. *Science* 2016;354(6316):1165–1169.
675. Serti E, Chepa-Lotrea X, Kim YJ, et al. Successful interferon-free therapy of chronic hepatitis C virus infection normalizes natural killer cell function. *Gastroenterology* 2015;149(1):190–200.e192.
676. Serti E, Park H, Keane M, et al. Rapid decrease in hepatitis C viremia by direct acting antivirals improves the natural killer cell response to IFNalpha. *Gut* 2017;66(4):724–735.
677. Serti E, Werner JM, Chattergoon M, et al. Monocytes activate natural killer cells via inflammasome-induced interleukin 18 in response to hepatitis C virus replication. *Gastroenterology* 2014;147(1):209–220.e203.
678. Shakil AO, Conry-Cantilena C, Alter HJ, et al. Volunteer blood donors with antibody to hepatitis C virus: clinical, biochemical, virologic, and histologic features. The Hepatitis C Study Group. *Ann Intern Med* 1995;123(5):330–337.
679. Sharma NR, Mateu G, Dreux M, et al. Hepatitis C virus is primed by CD81 protein for low pH-dependent fusion. *J Biol Chem* 2011;286(35):30361–30376.
680. Sheahan T, Imanaka N, Marukian S, et al. Interferon lambda alleles predict innate antiviral immune responses and hepatitis C virus permissiveness. *Cell Host Microbe* 2014;15(2):190–202.
681. Shi M, Lin XD, Vasilakis N, et al. Divergent viruses discovered in arthropods and vertebrates revise the evolutionary history of the flaviviridae and related viruses. *J Virol* 2016;90(2):659–669.
682. Shiha G, Metwally AM, Soliman R, et al. An educate, test, and treat programme towards elimination of hepatitis C infection in Egypt: a community-based demonstration project. *Lancet Gastroenterol Hepatol* 2018;3(11):778–789.
683. Shimakami T, Yamane D, Jangra RK, et al. Stabilization of hepatitis C virus RNA by an Ago2-miR-122 complex. *Proc Natl Acad Sci U S A* 2012;109(3):941–946.
684. Shimizu YK, Weiner AJ, Rosenblatt J, et al. Early events in hepatitis C virus infection of chimpanzees. *Proc Natl Acad Sci U S A* 1990;87(16):6441–6444.
685. Shin EC, Park SH, Nascimbeni M, et al. The frequency of CD127(+) hepatitis C virus (HCV)-specific T cells but not the expression of exhaustion markers predicts the outcome of acute HCV infection. *J Virol* 2013;87(8):4772–4777.
686. Shindo M, Di Bisceglie AM, Cheung L, et al. Decrease in serum hepatitis C viral RNA during alpha-interferon therapy for chronic hepatitis C. *Ann Intern Med* 1991; 115(9):700–704.
687. Shintani Y, Fujie H, Miyoshi H, et al. Hepatitis C virus infection and diabetes: direct involvement of the virus in the development of insulin resistance. *Gastroenterology* 2004;126(3):840–848.
688. Shirota Y, Luo H, Qin W, et al. Hepatitis C virus (HCV) NS5A binds RNA-dependent RNA polymerase (RdRP) NS5B and modulates RNA-dependent RNA polymerase activity. *J Biol Chem* 2002;277(13):11149–11155.
689. Shoukry NH, Grakoui A, Houghton M, et al. Memory CD8+ T cells are required for protection from persistent hepatitis C virus infection. *J Exp Med* 2003;197(12):1645–1655.
690. Shrivastava S, Devhare P, Sujijantarat N, et al. Knockdown of autophagy inhibits infectious hepatitis C virus release by the exosomal pathway. *J Virol* 2016;90(3):1387–1396.
691. Shrivastava S, Mukherjee A, Ray R, et al. Hepatitis C virus induces interleukin-1beta (IL-1beta)/IL-18 in circulatory and resident liver macrophages. *J Virol* 2013;87(22):12284–12290.
692. Sievert W, Altraif I, Razavi HA, et al. A systematic review of hepatitis C virus epidemiology in Asia, Australia and Egypt. *Liver Int* 2011;31(Suppl 2):61–80.
693. Simister P, Schmitt M, Geitmann M, et al. Structural and functional analysis of hepatitis C virus strain JFH1 polymerase. *J Virol* 2009;83(22):11926–11939.
694. Simmonds P. Genetic diversity and evolution of hepatitis C virus—15 years on. *J Gen Virol* 2004;85(Pt 11):3173–3188.
695. Simmonds P. The origin of hepatitis C virus. *Curr Top Microbiol Immunol* 2013;369:1–15.
696. Simonetti RG, Camma C, Fiorello F, et al. Hepatitis C virus infection as a risk factor for hepatocellular carcinoma in patients with cirrhosis. A case-control study. *Ann Intern Med* 1992;116(2):97–102.
697. Singal AG, Rich NE, Mehta N, et al. Direct-acting antiviral therapy not associated with recurrence of hepatocellular carcinoma in a multicenter North American Cohort Study. *Gastroenterology* 2019;156(6):1683–1692.e1.
698. Sise ME, Bloom AK, Wisocky J, et al. Treatment of hepatitis C virus-associated mixed cryoglobulinemia with direct-acting antiviral agents. *Hepatology* 2016;63(2):408–417.
699. Skardasi G, Chen AY, Michalak TI. Authentic patient-derived hepatitis C virus infects and productively replicates in primary CD4(+) and CD8(+) T lymphocytes in vitro. *J Virol* 2018;92(3).
700. Smith DB, Becher P, Bukh J, et al. Proposed update to the taxonomy of the genera Hepacivirus and Pegivirus within the Flaviviridae family. *J Gen Virol* 2016;97(11):2894–2907.
701. Smith DB, Bukh J, Kuiken C, et al. Expanded classification of hepatitis C virus into 7 genotypes and 67 subtypes: updated criteria and genotype assignment web resource. *Hepatology* 2014;59(1):318–327.
702. Smith HL, Chung RT, Mantry P, et al. Prevention of allograft HCV recurrence with peri-transplant human monoclonal antibody MBL-HCV1 combined with a single oral direct-acting antiviral: a proof-of-concept study. *J Viral Hepat* 2017;24(3):197–206.

703. Smith BD, Morgan RL, Beckett GA, et al. Recommendations for the identification of chronic hepatitis C virus infection among persons born during 1945–1965. *MMWR Recomm Rep* 2012;61(Rr-4):1–32.

704. Smith DB, Pathirana S, Davidson F, et al. The origin of hepatitis C virus genotypes. *J Gen Virol* 1997;78(Pt 2):321–328.

705. Smyk-Pearson S, Tester IA, Klarquist J, et al. Spontaneous recovery in acute human hepatitis C virus infection: functional T-cell thresholds and relative importance of CD4 help. *J Virol* 2008;82(4):1827–1837.

706. Smyk-Pearson S, Tester IA, Lezotte D, et al. Differential antigenic hierarchy associated with spontaneous recovery from hepatitis C virus infection: implications for vaccine design. *J Infect Dis* 2006;194(4):454–463.

707. Snoeck E, Chanu P, Lavielle M, et al. A comprehensive hepatitis C viral kinetic model explaining cure. *Clin Pharmacol Ther* 2010;87(6):706–713.

708. Sofia MJ, Bao D, Chang W, et al. Discovery of a beta-d-2′-deoxy-2′-alpha-fluoro-2′-beta-C-methyluridine nucleotide prodrug (PSI-7977) for the treatment of hepatitis C virus. *J Med Chem* 2010;53(19):7202–7218.

709. Sorbo MC, Cento V, Di Maio VC, et al. Hepatitis C virus drug resistance associated substitutions and their clinical relevance: update 2018. *Drug Resist Updat* 2018;37:17–39.

710. Soriano V, Puoti M, Sulkowski M, et al. Care of patients coinfected with HIV and hepatitis C virus: 2007 updated recommendations from the HCV-HIV International Panel. *AIDS* 2007;21(9):1073–1089.

711. Stapleford KA, Lindenbach BD. Hepatitis C virus NS2 coordinates virus particle assembly through physical interactions with the E1-E2 glycoprotein and NS3-NS4A enzyme complexes. *J Virol* 2011;85(4):1706–1717.

712. Stegmann KA, Bjorkstrom NK, Veber H, et al. Interferon-alpha-induced TRAIL on natural killer cells is associated with control of hepatitis C virus infection. *Gastroenterology* 2010;138(5):1885–1897.

713. Steinmann D, Barth H, Gissler B, et al. Inhibition of hepatitis C virus-like particle binding to target cells by antiviral antibodies in acute and chronic hepatitis C. *J Virol* 2004;78(17):9030–9040.

714. Stiffler JD, Nguyen M, Sohn JA, et al. Focal distribution of hepatitis C virus RNA in infected livers. *PLoS One* 2009;4(8):e6661.

715. Stone AE, Giugliano S, Schnell G, et al. Hepatitis C virus pathogen associated molecular pattern (PAMP) triggers production of lambda-interferons by human plasmacytoid dendritic cells. *PLoS Pathog* 2013;9(4):e1003316.

716. Stone J, Martin NK, Hickman M, et al. The potential impact of a hepatitis C vaccine for people who inject drugs: is a vaccine needed in the age of direct-acting antivirals? *PLoS One* 2016;11(5):e0156213.

717. Strickland GT. Liver disease in Egypt: hepatitis C superseded schistosomiasis as a result of iatrogenic and biological factors. *Hepatology* 2006;43(5):915–922.

718. Strunz B, Hengst J, Deterding K, et al. Chronic hepatitis C virus infection irreversibly impacts human natural killer cell repertoire diversity. *Nat Commun* 2018;9(1):2275.

719. Su AI, Pezacki JP, Wodicka L, et al. Genomic analysis of the host response to hepatitis C virus infection. *Proc Natl Acad Sci U S A* 2002;99(24):15669–15674.

720. Sugden PB, Cameron B, Mina M, et al.; HITS investigators. Protection against hepatitis C infection via NK cells in highly-exposed uninfected injecting drug users. *J Hepatol* 2014;61(4):738–745.

721. Sugimoto K, Ikeda F, Stadanlick J, et al. Suppression of HCV-specific T cells without differential hierarchy demonstrated ex vivo in persistent HCV infection. *Hepatology* 2003;38(6):1437–1448.

722. Sulkowski MS, Kang M, Matining R, et al. Safety and antiviral activity of the HCV entry inhibitor ITX5061 in treatment-naive HCV-infected adults: a randomized, double-blind, phase 1b study. *J Infect Dis* 2014;209(5):658–667.

723. Sullivan JC, De Meyer S, Bartels DJ, et al. Evolution of treatment-emergent resistant variants in telaprevir phase 3 clinical trials. *Clin Infect Dis* 2013;57(2):221–229.

724. Sung PS, Cheon H, Cho CH, et al. Roles of unphosphorylated ISGF3 in HCV infection and interferon responsiveness. *Proc Natl Acad Sci U S A* 2015;112(33):10443–10448.

725. Sung PS, Hong SH, Chung JH, et al. IFN-lambda4 potently blocks IFN-alpha signalling by ISG15 and USP18 in hepatitis C virus infection. *Sci Rep* 2017;7(1):3821.

726. Sung VM, Shimodaira S, Doughty AL, et al. Establishment of B-cell lymphoma cell lines persistently infected with hepatitis C virus in vivo and in vitro: the apoptotic effects of virus infection. *J Virol* 2003;77(3):2134–2146.

727. Suppiah V, Moldovan M, Ahlenstiel G, et al. IL28B is associated with response to chronic hepatitis C interferon-alpha and ribavirin therapy. *Nat Genet* 2009;41(10):1100–1104.

728. Suryaprasad AG, White JZ, Xu F, et al. Emerging epidemic of hepatitis C virus infections among young nonurban persons who inject drugs in the United States, 2006–2012. *Clin Infect Dis* 2014;59(10):1411–1419.

729. Svarovskaia ES, Dvory-Sobol H, Parkin N, et al. Infrequent development of resistance in genotype 1–6 hepatitis C virus-infected subjects treated with sofosbuvir in phase 2 and 3 clinical trials. *Clin Infect Dis* 2014;59(12):1666–1674.

730. Swadling L, Capone S, Antrobus RD, et al. A human vaccine strategy based on chimpanzee adenoviral and MVA vectors that primes, boosts, and sustains functional HCV-specific T cell memory. *Sci Transl Med* 2014;6(261):261ra153.

731. Swadling L, Halliday J, Kelly C, et al. Highly-immunogenic virally-vectored T-cell vaccines cannot overcome subversion of the T-cell response by HCV during chronic infection. *Vaccines* 2016;4(3).

732. Tabor E, Gerety RJ, Drucker JA, et al. Transmission of non-A, non-B hepatitis from man to chimpanzee. *Lancet* 1978;1(8062):463–466.

733. Takahashi K, Asabe S, Wieland S, et al. Plasmacytoid dendritic cells sense hepatitis C virus-infected cells, produce interferon, and inhibit infection. *Proc Natl Acad Sci U S A* 2010;107(16):7431–7436.

734. Takahashi K, Nishida N, Kawabata H, et al. Regression of Hodgkin lymphoma in response to antiviral therapy for hepatitis C virus infection. *Intern Med* 2012;51(19):2745–2747.

735. Takaki A, Wiese M, Maertens G, et al. Cellular immune responses persist and humoral responses decrease two decades after recovery from a single-source outbreak of hepatitis C. *Nat Med* 2000;6(5):578–582.

736. Tanaka Y, Nishida N, Sugiyama M, et al. Genome-wide association of IL28B with response to pegylated interferon-alpha and ribavirin therapy for chronic hepatitis C. *Nat Genet* 2009;41(10):1105–1109.

737. Tanida I, Fukasawa M, Ueno T, et al. Knockdown of autophagy-related gene decreases the production of infectious hepatitis C virus particles. *Autophagy* 2009;5(7):937–945.

738. Taniguchi S, Okamoto H, Sakamoto M, et al. A structurally flexible and antigenically variable N-terminal domain of the hepatitis C virus E2/NS1 protein: implication for an escape from antibody. *Virology* 1993;195(1):297–301.

739. Tarr AW, Owsianka AM, Jayaraj D, et al. Determination of the human antibody response to the epitope defined by the hepatitis C virus-neutralizing monoclonal antibody AP33. *J Gen Virol* 2007;88(Pt 11):2991–3001.

740. Tarr AW, Urbanowicz RA, Hamed MR, et al. Hepatitis C patient-derived glycoproteins exhibit marked differences in susceptibility to serum neutralizing antibodies: genetic subtype defines antigenic but not neutralization serotype. *J Virol* 2011;85(9):4246–4257.

741. Tarr AW, Urbanowicz RA, Jayaraj D, et al. Naturally occurring antibodies that recognize linear epitopes in the amino terminus of the hepatitis C virus E2 protein confer noninterfering, additive neutralization. *J Virol* 2012;86(5):2739–2749.

742. Tellinghuisen TL, Foss KL, Treadaway JC, et al. Identification of residues required for RNA replication in domains II and III of the hepatitis C virus NS5A protein. *J Virol* 2008;82(3):1073–1083.

743. Tellinghuisen TL, Marcotrigiano J, Gorbalenya AE, et al. The NS5A protein of hepatitis C virus is a zinc metalloprotein. *J Biol Chem* 2004;279(47):48576–48587.

744. Terczynska-Dyla E, Bibert S, Duong FH, et al. Reduced IFNlambda4 activity is associated with improved HCV clearance and reduced expression of interferon-stimulated genes. *Nat Commun* 2014;5:5699.

745. Terrault NA, Dodge JL, Murphy EL, et al. Sexual transmission of hepatitis C virus among monogamous heterosexual couples: the HCV partners study. *Hepatology* 2013;57(3):881–889.

746. Terrault NA, Im K, Boylan R, et al. Fibrosis progression in African Americans and Caucasian Americans with chronic hepatitis C. *Clin Gastroenterol Hepatol* 2008;6(12):1403–1411.

747. Tester I, Smyk-Pearson S, Wang P, et al. Immune evasion versus recovery after acute hepatitis C virus infection from a shared source. *J Exp Med* 2005;201(11):1725–1731.

748. Thimme R, Bukh J, Spangenberg HC, et al. Viral and immunological determinants of hepatitis C virus clearance, persistence, and disease. *Proc Natl Acad Sci U S A* 2002;99(24):15661–15668.

749. Thimme R, Oldach D, Chang KM, et al. Determinants of viral clearance and persistence during acute hepatitis C virus infection. *J Exp Med* 2001;194(10):1395–1406.

750. Thio CL, Thomas DL, Goedert JJ, et al. Racial differences in HLA class II associations with hepatitis C virus outcomes. *J Infect Dis* 2001;184(1):16–21.

751. Thoens C, Berger C, Trippler M, et al. KIR2DL3(+)NKG2A(−) natural killer cells are associated with protection from productive hepatitis C virus infection in people who inject drugs. *J Hepatol* 2014;61(3):475–481.

752. Thomas DL, Astemborski J, Vlahov D, et al. Determinants of the quantity of hepatitis C virus RNA. *J Infect Dis* 2000;181(3):844–851.

753. Thomas E, Gonzalez VD, Li Q, et al. HCV infection induces a unique hepatic innate immune response associated with robust production of type III interferons. *Gastroenterology* 2012;142(4):978–988.

754. Thomas DL, Thio CL, Martin MP, et al. Genetic variation in IL28B and spontaneous clearance of hepatitis C virus. *Nature* 2009;461(7265):798–801.

755. Ticehurst JR, Hamzeh FM, Thomas DL. Factors affecting serum concentrations of hepatitis C virus (HCV) RNA in HCV genotype 1-infected patients with chronic hepatitis. *J Clin Microbiol* 2007;45(8):2426–2433.

756. Timm J, Lauer GM, Kavanagh DG, et al. CD8 epitope escape and reversion in acute HCV infection. *J Exp Med* 2004;200(12):1593–1604.

757. Timm J, Li B, Daniels MG, et al. Human leukocyte antigen-associated sequence polymorphisms in hepatitis C virus reveal reproducible immune responses and constraints on viral evolution. *Hepatology* 2007;46(2):339–349.

758. Timm J, Walker CM. Mutational escape of CD8+ T cell epitopes: implications for prevention and therapy of persistent hepatitis virus infections. *Med Microbiol Immunol* 2015;204(1):29–38.

759. Timpe JM, Stamataki Z, Jennings A, et al. Hepatitis C virus cell-cell transmission in hepatoma cells in the presence of neutralizing antibodies. *Hepatology* 2008;47(1):17–24.

760. Tong Y, Chi X, Yang W, et al. Functional analysis of hepatitis C virus (HCV) envelope protein E1 using a trans-complementation system reveals a dual role of a putative fusion peptide of E1 in both HCV entry and morphogenesis. *J Virol* 2017;91(7).

761. Tong MJ, el-Farra NS, Reikes AR, et al. Clinical outcomes after transfusion-associated hepatitis C. *N Engl J Med* 1995;332(22):1463–1466.

762. Torresi J, Johnson D, Wedemeyer H. Progress in the development of preventive and therapeutic vaccines for hepatitis C virus. *J Hepatol* 2011;54(6):1273–1285.

763. Tovo PA, Calitri C, Scolfaro C, et al. Vertically acquired hepatitis C virus infection: correlates of transmission and disease progression. *World J Gastroenterol* 2016;22(4):1382–1392.

764. Trivedi S, Murthy S, Sharma H, et al. Viral persistence, liver disease, and host response in a hepatitis C-like virus rat model. *Hepatology* 2018;68(2):435–448.

765. Tseng CT, Klimpel GR. Binding of the hepatitis C virus envelope protein E2 to CD81 inhibits natural killer cell functions. *J Exp Med* 2002;195(1):43–49.

766. Tsukiyama-Kohara K, Iizuka N, Kohara M, et al. Internal ribosome entry site within hepatitis C virus RNA. *J Virol* 1992;66(3):1476–1483.

767. Tzarum N, Wilson IA, Law M. The neutralizing face of hepatitis C virus E2 envelope glycoprotein. *Front Immunol* 2018;9:1315.

768. U.S. Public Health Service. Updated U.S. Public Health Service guidelines for the management of occupational exposures to HBV, HCV, and HIV and recommendations for postexposure prophylaxis. *MMWR Recomm Rep* 2001;50(RR-11):1–52.

769. Uebelhoer L, Han JH, Callendret B, et al. Stable cytotoxic T cell escape mutation in hepatitis C virus is linked to maintenance of viral fitness. *PLoS Pathog* 2008;4(9):e1000143.

770. Ulsenheimer A, Lucas M, Seth NP, et al. Transient immunological control during acute hepatitis C virus infection: ex vivo analysis of helper T-cell responses. *J Viral Hepat* 2006;13(10):708–714.

771. Urabe Y, Ochi H, Kato N, et al. A genome-wide association study of HCV-induced liver cirrhosis in the Japanese population identifies novel susceptibility loci at the MHC region. *J Hepatol* 2013;58(5):875–882.
772. Urban TJ, Thompson AJ, Bradrick SS, et al. IL28B genotype is associated with differential expression of intrahepatic interferon-stimulated genes in patients with chronic hepatitis C. *Hepatology* 2010;52(6):1888–1896.
773. Urbani S, Amadei B, Cariani E, et al. The impairment of CD8 responses limits the selection of escape mutations in acute hepatitis C virus infection. *J Immunol* 2005;175(11):7519–7529.
774. Urbani S, Amadei B, Fisicaro P, et al. Outcome of acute hepatitis C is related to virus-specific CD4 function and maturation of antiviral memory CD8 responses. *Hepatology* 2006;44(1):126–139.
775. Urbani S, Amadei B, Tola D, et al. PD-1 expression in acute hepatitis C virus (HCV) infection is associated with HCV-specific CD8 exhaustion. *J Virol* 2006;80(22):11398–11403.
776. Urbani S, Amadei B, Tola D, et al. Restoration of HCV-specific T cell functions by PD-1/PD-L1 blockade in HCV infection: effect of viremia levels and antiviral treatment. *J Hepatol* 2008;48(4):548–558.
777. Urbanowicz RA, McClure CP, Brown RJ, et al. A diverse panel of hepatitis C virus glycoproteins for use in vaccine research reveals extremes of monoclonal antibody neutralization resistance. *J Virol* 2015;90(7):3288–3301.
778. Valenti L, Rumi M, Galmozzi E, et al. Patatin-like phospholipase domain-containing 3 I148M polymorphism, steatosis, and liver damage in chronic hepatitis C. *Hepatology* 2011;53(3):791–799.
779. van de Laar TJ, Matthews GV, Prins M, et al. Acute hepatitis C in HIV-infected men who have sex with men: an emerging sexually transmitted infection. *AIDS* 2010;24(12):1799–1812.
780. van de Laar TJ, Paxton WA, Zorgdrager F, et al. Sexual transmission of hepatitis C virus in human immunodeficiency virus-negative men who have sex with men: a series of case reports. *Sex Transm Dis* 2011;38(2):102–104.
781. van de Laar T, Pybus O, Bruisten S, et al. Evidence of a large, international network of HCV transmission in HIV-positive men who have sex with men. *Gastroenterology* 2009;136(5):1609–1617.
782. van de Laar TJ, van der Bij AK, Prins M, et al. Increase in HCV incidence among men who have sex with men in Amsterdam most likely caused by sexual transmission. *J Infect Dis* 2007;196(2):230–238.
783. van der Meer AJ, Berenguer M. Reversion of disease manifestations after HCV eradication. *J Hepatol* 2016;65(1 Suppl):S95–S108.
784. van der Meer AJ, Feld JJ, Hofer H, et al. Risk of cirrhosis-related complications in patients with advanced fibrosis following hepatitis C virus eradication. *J Hepatol* 2017;66(3):485–493.
785. van der Meer AJ, Veldt BJ, Feld JJ, et al. Association between sustained virological response and all-cause mortality among patients with chronic hepatitis C and advanced hepatic fibrosis. *JAMA* 2012;308(24):2584–2593.
786. van der Ree MH, van der Meer AJ, de Bruijne J, et al. Long-term safety and efficacy of microRNA-targeted therapy in chronic hepatitis C patients. *Antiviral Res* 2014;111:53–59.
787. Veerapu NS, Park SH, Tully DC, et al. Trace amounts of sporadically reappearing HCV RNA can cause infection. *J Clin Invest* 2014;124(8):3469–3478.
788. Venkatraman S, Bogen SL, Arasappan A, et al. Discovery of (1R,5S)-N-[3-amino-1-(cyclobutylmethyl)-2,3-dioxopropyl]-3-[2(S)-[[[(1,1-dimethylethyl)amino]carbonyl]amino]-3,3-dimethyl-1-oxobutyl]- 6,6-dimethyl-3-azabicyclo[3.1.0]hexan-2(S)-carboxamide (SCH 503034), a selective, potent, orally bioavailable hepatitis C virus NS3 protease inhibitor: a potential therapeutic agent for the treatment of hepatitis C infection. *J Med Chem* 2006;49(20):6074–6086.
789. Vento S, Garofano T, Renzini C, et al. Fulminant hepatitis associated with hepatitis A virus superinfection in patients with chronic hepatitis C. *N Engl J Med* 1998;338(5):286–290.
790. Vergara C, Thio CL, Johnson E, et al. Multi-Ancestry Genome-Wide Association Study of spontaneous clearance of hepatitis C virus. *Gastroenterology* 2019;156(5):1496–1507.e7.
791. Vieyres G, Dubuisson J, Patel AH. Characterization of antibody-mediated neutralization directed against the hypervariable region 1 of hepatitis C virus E2 glycoprotein. *J Gen Virol* 2011;92(Pt 3):494–506.
792. Vieyres G, Thomas X, Descamps V, et al. Characterization of the envelope glycoproteins associated with infectious hepatitis C virus. *J Virol* 2010;84(19):10159–10168.
793. Villano SA, Vlahov D, Nelson KE, et al. Persistence of viremia and the importance of long-term follow-up after acute hepatitis C infection. *Hepatology* 1999;29(3):908–914.
794. von Hahn T, Yoon JC, Alter H, et al. Hepatitis C virus continuously escapes from neutralizing antibody and T-cell responses during chronic infection in vivo. *Gastroenterology* 2007;132(2):667–678.
795. Vrielink H, van der Poel CL, Reesink HW, et al. Look-back study of infectivity of anti-HCV ELISA-positive blood components. *Lancet* 1995;345(8942):95–96.
796. Wakita T, Pietschmann T, Kato T, et al. Production of infectious hepatitis C virus in tissue culture from a cloned viral genome. *Nat Med* 2005;11(7):791–796.
797. Walker A, Skibbe K, Steinmann E, et al. Distinct escape pathway by hepatitis C virus genotype 1a from a dominant CD8+ T cell response by selection of altered epitope processing. *J Virol* 2016;90(1):33–42.
798. Wang GP, Sherrill-Mix SA, Chang KM, et al. Hepatitis C virus transmission bottlenecks analyzed by deep sequencing. *J Virol* 2010;84(12):6218–6228.
799. Wang JT, Wang TH, Sheu JC, et al. Hepatitis C virus RNA in saliva of patients with posttransfusion hepatitis and low efficiency of transmission among spouses. *J Med Virol* 1992;36(1):28–31.
800. Ward JW, Hinman AR. What is needed to eliminate hepatitis B virus and hepatitis C virus as global health threats. *Gastroenterology* 2019;156(2):297–310.
801. Washburn ML, Bility MT, Zhang L, et al. A humanized mouse model to study hepatitis C virus infection, immune response, and liver disease. *Gastroenterology* 2011;140(4):1334–1344.
802. Weiner AJ, Geysen HM, Christopherson C, et al. Evidence for immune selection of hepatitis C virus (HCV) putative envelope glycoprotein variants: potential role in chronic HCV infections. *Proc Natl Acad Sci U S A* 1992;89(8):3468–3472.
803. Welzel TM, Nelson DR, Morelli G, et al. Effectiveness and safety of sofosbuvir plus ribavirin for the treatment of HCV genotype 2 infection: results of the real-world, clinical practice HCV-TARGET study. *Gut* 2017;66(10):1844–1852.
804. Werner RN, Gaskins M, Nast A, et al. Incidence of sexually transmitted infections in men who have sex with men and who are at substantial risk of HIV infection—a meta-analysis of data from trials and observational studies of HIV pre-exposure prophylaxis. *PLoS One* 2018;13(12):e0208107.
805. Werner JM, Heller T, Gordon AM, et al. Innate immune responses in hepatitis C virus-exposed healthcare workers who do not develop acute infection. *Hepatology* 2013;58(5):1621–1631.
806. White DL, Ratziu V, El-Serag HB. Hepatitis C infection and risk of diabetes: a systematic review and meta-analysis. *J Hepatol* 2008;49(5):831–844.
807. Wieland D, Kemming J, Schuch A, et al. TCF1(+) hepatitis C virus-specific CD8(+) T cells are maintained after cessation of chronic antigen stimulation. *Nat Commun* 2017;8:15050.
808. Wieland S, Makowska Z, Campana B, et al. Simultaneous detection of hepatitis C virus and interferon stimulated gene expression in infected human liver. *Hepatology* 2014;59(6):2121–2130.
809. Wilson LE, Torbenson M, Astemborski J, et al. Progression of liver fibrosis among injection drug users with chronic hepatitis C. *Hepatology* 2006;43(4):788–795.
810. Wise M, Bialek S, Finelli L, et al. Changing trends in hepatitis C-related mortality in the United States, 1995–2004. *Hepatology* 2008;47(4):1128–1135.
811. Witteveldt J, Evans MJ, Bitzegeio J, et al. CD81 is dispensable for hepatitis C virus cell-to-cell transmission in hepatoma cells. *J Gen Virol* 2009;90(Pt 1):48–58.
812. Wolfl M, Rutebemberwa A, Mosbruger T, et al. Hepatitis C virus immune escape via exploitation of a hole in the T cell repertoire. *J Immunol* 2008;181(9):6435–6446.
813. Wolski D, Foote PK, Chen DY, et al. Early transcriptional divergence marks virus-specific primary human CD8(+) T cells in chronic versus acute infection. *Immunity* 2017;47(4):648–663.e648.
814. Wright TL, Hsu H, Donegan E, et al. Hepatitis C virus not found in fulminant non-A, non-B hepatitis. *Ann Intern Med* 1991;115(2):111–112.
815. Wu TT, Kabat EA. An analysis of the sequences of the variable regions of Bence Jones proteins and myeloma light chains and their implications for antibody complementarity. *J Exp Med* 1970;132(2):211–250.
816. Yamane D, Selitsky SR, Shimakami T, et al. Differential hepatitis C virus RNA target site selection and host factor activities of naturally occurring miR-122 3 variants. *Nucleic Acids Res* 2017;45(8):4743–4755.
817. Yanagi M, Kaneko S, Unoura M, et al. Hepatitis C virus in fulminant hepatic failure. *N Engl J Med* 1991;324(26):1895–1896.
818. Yanagi M, Purcell RH, Emerson SU, et al. Transcripts from a single full-length cDNA clone of hepatitis C virus are infectious when directly transfected into the liver of a chimpanzee. *Proc Natl Acad Sci U S A* 1997;94(16):8738–8743.
819. Yang Z, Wang X, Chi X, et al. Neglected but important role of apolipoprotein E exchange in hepatitis C virus infection. *J Virol* 2016;90(21):9632–9643.
820. Yang CM, Yoon JC, Park JH, et al. Hepatitis C virus impairs natural killer cell activity via viral serine protease NS3. *PLoS One* 2017;12(4):e0175793.
821. Yazdanpanah Y, De Carli G, Migueres B, et al. Risk factors for hepatitis C virus transmission to health care workers after occupational exposure: a European case-control study. *Clin Infect Dis* 2005;41(10):1423–1430.
822. Yee HS, Currie SL, Darling JM, et al. Management and treatment of hepatitis C viral infection: recommendations from the Department of Veterans Affairs Hepatitis C Resource Center program and the National Hepatitis C Program office. *Am J Gastroenterol* 2006;101(10):2360–2378.
823. Yin C, Goonawardane N, Stewart H, et al. A role for domain 1 of the hepatitis C virus NS5A protein in virus assembly. *PLoS Pathog* 2018;14(1):e1006834.
824. Yoon JC, Yang CM, Song Y, et al. Natural killer cells in hepatitis C: current progress. *World J Gastroenterol* 2016;22(4):1449–1460.
825. Yoshiba M, Dehara K, Inoue K, et al. Contribution of hepatitis C virus to non-A, non-B fulminant hepatitis in Japan. *Hepatology* 1994;19(4):829–835.
826. Yoshimi S, Imamura M, Murakami E, et al. Long term persistence of NS5A inhibitor-resistant hepatitis C virus in patients who failed daclatasvir and asunaprevir therapy. *J Med Virol* 2015;87(11):1913–1920.
827. Yoshio S, Kanto T, Kuroda S, et al. Human blood dendritic cell antigen 3 (BDCA3)(+) dendritic cells are a potent producer of interferon-lambda in response to hepatitis C virus. *Hepatology* 2013;57(5):1705–1715.
828. Younossi ZM, Stepanova M, Afdhal N, et al. Improvement of health-related quality of life and work productivity in chronic hepatitis C patients with early and advanced fibrosis treated with ledipasvir and sofosbuvir. *J Hepatol* 2015;63(2):337–345.
829. Zanetti AR, Tanzi E, Paccagnini S, et al. Mother-to-infant transmission of hepatitis C virus. Lombardy Study Group on Vertical HCV Transmission. *Lancet* 1995;345(8945):289–291.
830. Zayas M, Long G, Madan V, et al. Coordination of hepatitis C virus assembly by distinct regulatory regions in nonstructural protein 5A. *PLoS Pathog* 2016;12(1):e1005376.
831. Zehender G, Meroni L, De Maddalena C, et al. Detection of hepatitis C virus RNA in CD19 peripheral blood mononuclear cells of chronically infected patients. *J Infect Dis* 1997;176(5):1209–1214.
832. Zehn D, Utzschneider DT, Thimme R. Immune-surveillance through exhausted effector T-cells. *Curr Opin Virol* 2016;16:49–54.
833. Zeuzem S, Feinman SV, Rasenack J, et al. Peginterferon alfa-2a in patients with chronic hepatitis C. *N Engl J Med* 2000;343(23):1666–1672.
834. Zeuzem S, Foster GR, Wang S, et al. Glecaprevir-pibrentasvir for 8 or 12 weeks in HCV genotype 1 or 3 infection. *N Engl J Med* 2018;378(4):354–369.
835. Zeuzem S, Jacobson IM, Baykal T, et al. Retreatment of HCV with ABT-450/r-ombitasvir and dasabuvir with ribavirin. *N Engl J Med* 2014;370(17):1604–1614.
836. Zeuzem S, Mizokami M, Pianko S, et al. NS5A resistance-associated substitutions in patients with genotype 1 hepatitis C virus: prevalence and effect on treatment outcome. *J Hepatol* 2017;66(5):910–918.

837. Zhang S, Kodys K, Li K, et al. Human type 2 myeloid dendritic cells produce interferon-lambda and amplify interferon-alpha in response to hepatitis C virus infection. *Gastroenterology* 2013;144(2):414–425. e417.

838. Zhang P, Zhong L, Struble EB, et al. Depletion of interfering antibodies in chronic hepatitis C patients and vaccinated chimpanzees reveals broad cross-genotype neutralizing activity. *Proc Natl Acad Sci U S A* 2009;106(18):7537–7541.

839. Zhao H, Lin W, Kumthip K, et al. A functional genomic screen reveals novel host genes that mediate interferon-alpha's effects against hepatitis C virus. *J Hepatol* 2012;56(2):326–333.

840. Zhong J, Gastaminza P, Cheng G, et al. Robust hepatitis C virus infection in vitro. *Proc Natl Acad Sci U S A* 2005;102(26):9294–9299.

841. Zhou S, Williford SE, McGivern DR, et al. Evolutionary pathways to NS5A inhibitor resistance in genotype 1 hepatitis C virus. *Antiviral Res* 2018;158:45–51.

842. Zhu N, Khoshnan A, Schneider R, et al. Hepatitis C virus core protein binds to the cytoplasmic domain of tumor necrosis factor (TNF) receptor 1 and enhances TNF-induced apoptosis. *J Virol* 1998;72(5):3691–3697.

843. Zibbell JE, Asher AK, Patel RC, et al. Increases in acute hepatitis C virus infection related to a growing opioid epidemic and associated injection drug use, United States, 2004 to 2014. *Am J Public Health* 2018;108(2):175–181.

844. Ziegler S, Ruhl M, Tenckhoff H, et al. Susceptibility to chronic hepatitis C virus infection is influenced by sequence differences in immunodominant CD8+ T cell epitopes. *J Hepatol* 2013;58(1):24–30.

Flaviviruses: Dengue, Zika, West Nile, Yellow Fever and Other Flaviviruses

Theodore C. Pierson • Helen M. Lazear • Michael S. Diamond

Flaviviruses acquired their name from the jaundice associated with the liver dysfunction caused by yellow fever virus (YFV) infections. YFV played an important historical role in defining the nature of viruses. Seminal studies by Walter Reed and colleagues demonstrated that the etiology of yellow fever was a filterable agent that could be transmitted through the bite of a mosquito, confirming the postulates of Carlos Finlay.[1064] YFV was the first flavivirus isolated (in 1927), the first flavivirus to be propagated *in vitro*,[1073,1113] and the first flavivirus for which a vaccine was developed and deployed.[770] Experiments with louping-ill virus (LIV) in 1931 established that ticks also could transmit viruses associated with human disease.[152] The discovery that flavivirus-immune sera could be cross-reactive with other flaviviruses that caused similar diseases (e.g., encephalitis) provided a method to investigate relatedness among these viruses.[167–169,1188] These evolutionary concepts were refined further with new serologic assays that allowed them to be distinguished from alphaviruses.[168] Advances in the molecular genetics of flaviviruses confirmed and advanced an understanding of the evolution, biology, pathogenesis, and immunity to these viruses. Fifty-four species within the *Flavivirus* genus have since been defined by the International Committee on Taxonomy of Viruses.

FLAVIVIRUS EVOLUTION, DIVERSITY, AND DISTRIBUTION

Molecular Phylogeny and Evolution

Phylogenetic relationships among viruses within the *Flavivirus* genus reflect key features of the biology and ecology of these viruses (Fig. 9.1). Four groups of flaviviruses cluster according to their natural host and mode of transmission, including tick-borne flaviviruses (TBFVs), mosquito-borne flaviviruses (MBFVs), those with no known vector (NKV), and insect-specific flaviviruses (ISFs).[577,701,948] Flaviviruses have an African origin. Efforts to determine the date of the appearance of the first flavivirus using molecular clock approaches vary considerably depending on analysis parameters, including the event used for calibration in time.[379,795] For example, a recent study hypothesized the introduction of the TBFV Powassan virus (POWV) into North America occurred 11 to 15 thousand years (kyr) ago and was linked to use of the Beringian land bridge that once connected Alaska and Asia. Analysis of the timing of the origin of flaviviruses with respect to this reference led to the conclusion that flaviviruses are older than previously appreciated and

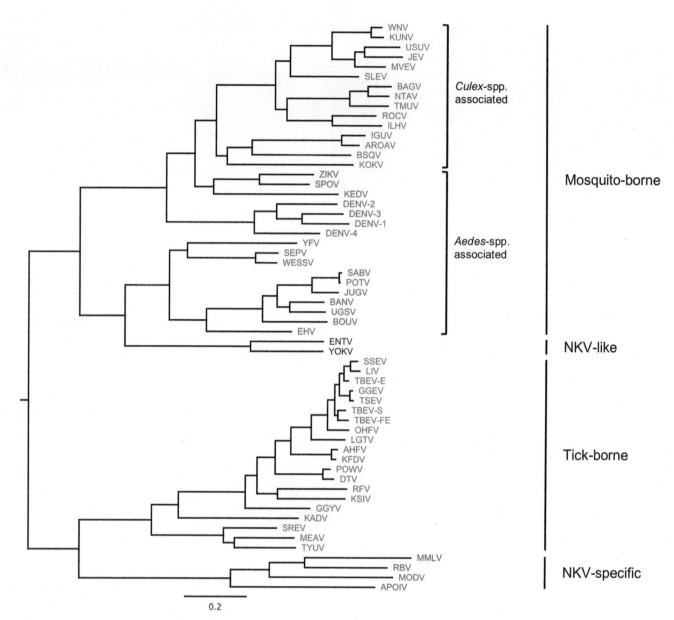

0.2

FIGURE 9.1 Phylogenetic tree of viruses in the *Flavivirus* genus. A maximum-likelihood (ML) tree was generated using the complete polyprotein amino acid sequence of the indicated flaviviruses. The polyprotein amino acid sequence alignment was generated using Clustal W2 provided in Geneious v11.1.2, and the ML tree was constructed using PhyML v3.2.2. The tree is midpoint rooted, and vertical length is arbitrary. The scale bar represents substitutions per site. The viral taxa are abbreviated and colored according to their mode of transmission. Apoi virus; MODV, Modoc virus; RBV, Rio Bravo virus; MMLV, Montana myotis leukoencephalitis virus; TYUV, Tyuleniy virus; MEAV, Meaban virus; SREV, Saumarez Reef virus; KADV, Kadam virus; GGYV, Gadgets Gully virus; KSIV, Karshi virus; RFV, Royal Farm virus; DTV, deer tick virus; POWV, Powassan virus; KFDV, Kyasanur Forest disease virus; AHFV, Alkhurma hemorrhagic fever virus; LGTV, Langat virus; OHFV, Omsk hemorrhagic fever virus; TBEV-FE, tick-borne encephalitis virus Far Eastern subtype; TBEV-S, tick-borne encephalitis virus-Siberian subtype; TSEV, Turkish sheep encephalitis virus; GGEV, Greek goat encephalomyelitis virus; TBEV-E, tick-borne encephalitis virus-European subtype; LIV, louping ill virus; SSEV, Spanish sheep encephalomyelitis virus; YOKV, Yokose virus; ENTV, Entebbe bat virus; EHV, Edge Hill virus; BOUV, Bouboui virus; UGSV, Uganda S virus; BANV, Banzi virus; JUGV, Jugra virus; POTV, Potiskum virus; SABV, Saboya virus; WESSV, Wesselsbron virus; SEPV, Sepik virus; YFV, yellow fever virus; DENV-4, dengue virus serotype 4; DENV-1, dengue virus serotype 1; DENV-3, dengue virus serotype 3; DENV-2, dengue virus serotype 2; KEDV, Kedougou virus; SPOV, Spondweni virus; ZIKV, Zika virus; KOKV, Kokobera virus; BSQV, Bussuquara virus; AROAV, Aroa virus; IGUV, Iguape virus; ILHV, Ilheus virus; ROCV, Rocio virus; TMUV, Tembusu virus; NTAV, Ntaya virus; BAGV, Bagaza virus; SLEV, St. Louis encephalitis virus; MVEV, Murray Valley encephalitis virus; JEV, Japanese encephalitis virus; USUV, Usutu virus; KUNV, Kunjin virus; WNV, West Nile virus; NKV, species with no known vector. The tree was created by Ms. Katherine Burgomaster (NIAID, NIH).

emerged approximately 80 kyr.[872] Flaviviruses diverged from an ancestor that was not vectored by arthropods into groups containing the TBFV and MBFV; two groups of NKV viruses cluster among both branches of the phylogenic tree, as detailed below.[380]

Mosquito-Borne Flaviviruses

MBFVs diverged early into two lineages that principally use *Aedes* or *Culex* genus mosquitoes as vectors[389,536] (Fig. 9.1). Viruses in these two MBFV clades generally cause hemorrhagic disease or encephalitis, respectively, in humans and livestock. While many of the viruses in the *Culex* clade infect avian hosts, *Aedes* viruses do not. Conversely, *Culex* viruses are not maintained in infection cycles involving primates. Viruses of the *Aedes* clade are a paraphyletic group thought to predate and give rise to the *Culex* viruses.[380,389] One branch of the MBFV phylogenic tree includes viruses of the YFV group, the recently proposed Edge Hill virus (EHV) group, and three NKV viruses discussed in detail below. The YFV group includes Wesselsbron virus (WESSV), Sepik virus (SEPV), and YFV. WESSV is a veterinary pathogen transmitted by *Aedes* mosquitoes that causes a nonfatal febrile illness in humans. Very little is known about the clinical significance and vector biology of SEPV infection. Both SEPV and WESSV are found in Africa and Asia.[389] YFV biology and pathogenesis are detailed below. The seven viruses of the EHV group are transmitted predominantly by *Aedes* mosquitoes, found primarily in Africa (except for EHV, which is present in Australia), and share the unique property of encoding five (instead of six) disulfide bridges in the envelope (E) glycoprotein. Among this group, human cases have been associated only with Banzi virus (BANV) infection.[389] The second branch of the MBFV phylogenic tree contains dengue viruses (DENV), which are transmitted by *Aedes* mosquitoes, a large group of viruses vectored by *Culex* mosquitoes (e.g., Japanese encephalitis virus [JEV], West Nile virus [WNV]), and a group of *Aedes*-vectored viruses closely related to the *Culex* flaviviruses including Spondweni virus (SPOV) and Zika virus (ZIKV).[536] The biology, pathogenesis, and diversity of viruses in the JEV serocomplex, ZIKV, and DENV are described in detail below.

Tick-Borne Flavivirus

The TBFVs include three groups that differ with respect to their vertebrate host and tick vectors.[390,536] The largest group of TBFVs infect mammalian hosts (typically rodents), are vectored by *Ixodes* ticks, and can cause encephalitis (e.g., tick-borne encephalitis viruses [TBEVs]) or hemorrhagic fever (e.g., Kyasanur Forest disease virus [KFDV]) in humans. Mammalian TBFVs that are not linked to human disease include Royal Farm virus (RFV), Karshi virus (KSIV), and Gadgets Gully virus (GGYV). Analysis of the evolution of viruses of the TBEV serocomplex has demonstrated that the rate of nonsynonymous nucleotide changes in the E protein correlates with geographic distance from the point of origin of these viruses.[1237] This is reflected by the asymmetrical, stepwise branching pattern of the phylogenetic tree of the mammalian viruses[1238] (Fig. 9.1). This pattern of evolution has been confirmed using larger datasets.[453] These studies conclude that TBFVs evolved from a common ancestor in Africa approximately 28 kyr ago. The subsequent distribution and spread of early TBEVs, such as GGYV and POWV, may have been constrained by climate conditions

of Asia until the glacial retreat at the outset of the Holocene epoch. POWV diverged further in North America into two lineages, which now includes deer tick virus (DTV).[458] These two viruses remain the only autochthonous TBFVs in the New World. Viruses of the TBEV serocomplex emerged into central Russia approximately 5 to 7 kyr ago, at which time they spread and diversified in eastward and westward directions.[453]

The second group of TBFVs replicates within seabirds and ornithophilic ticks but does not cause disease in humans. Viruses in this group include Meaban virus (MEAV), Saumarez Reef virus (SREV), and Tyuleniy virus (TYUV).[153] These viruses have a broad geographic range that presumably reflects the migratory patterns of their avian hosts.[380,390] A serological surveillance study for MEAV-reactive antibodies in residents of southern France, where the virus was first discovered, proved negative,[180] whereas SREV and TYUV may be capable of causing mild disease in humans.[701]

The TBFV Kadam virus (KADV) is the sole representative of a third lineage that arose early in the evolution of these viruses. An understanding of the relationship between KADV and other members of the TBFVs has emerged. While KADV was assigned to both the mammalian and seabird groups of flaviviruses, a more recent analysis of the complete coding sequence of TBFVs places KADV in its own group, which is supported by unique features of its E protein and the fact that it encodes a polyprotein that is smaller than the rest of the TBFV.[390,453] KADV is found in Africa, vectored by hard ticks that feed on mammals, and typically infects livestock.[380] KADV has not been associated with human infections.

No Known Vector Flavivirus

In comparison to the vector-borne flaviviruses, relatively little is known about viruses of the NKV group. These flaviviruses are reviewed comprehensively by Blitvich and Firth.[103] The 14 known NKV-like viruses are found in rodents or bats, in which they do not appear to cause disease or a high viremia. NKV viruses of rodents are found only in the New World, whereas those infecting bats are found globally.[379] Several NKV viruses can cause human disease following occupational exposure, and while natural infection resulting in clinical illness has been reported, it appears uncommon. Two groups of NKV flaviviruses have been defined. The first cluster forms a clade that is more closely associated with TBFV than those vectored by mosquitoes and may contain the common ancestor from which both groups arose. This group of NKV flaviviruses can be divided further into two lineages that define those infecting rodents and bats.

The Entebbe bat virus group (Yokose virus [YOKV], Sokoluk virus [SOKV], and Entebbe bat virus [ENTV]) forms a lineage within the *Aedes*-vectored MBFV from which the YFV and EHV groups may have evolved. That some of these viruses can replicate in mosquito cell cultures raises the possibility that they, or their ancestors, were once transmitted by mosquitoes and then lost this trait[379,576,1097] (Fig. 9.1). This concept is supported by sequence features in the untranslated regions (UTR) of the viral genome that are similar to those present in MBFVs. However, one study reported the isolation of SOKV from a field-caught tick, suggesting that a capacity to replicate in arthropods has not been lost completely. A recent analysis of dinucleotide frequency among viruses of this group suggests greater adaptation to arthropods than mammals.[103] The natural history and vector competence of this group require further study to reconcile these observations.

Insect-Specific Flavivirus

The last 15 years has brought progress in the identification of ISF and insights into their biology.[212] The first ISF cell-fusing agent virus (CFAV) was discovered in 1975 as the causative agent of cytopathology in insect cell cultures occurring when exposed to materials derived from other mosquito cells.[1075] The isolation of Kamiti River virus (KRV) from *Aedes* mosquitoes in Kenya in 2003[967] was the first discovery of ISFs from mosquito populations. A detailed discussion of the molecular phylogeny is provided by Moureau and colleagues.[795]

Global Distribution

Flaviviruses are found on six continents where they are responsible for endemic and epidemic disease each year (Fig. 9.2). The geographic distribution of flaviviruses has proven dynamic, enabling emergence in new areas and with increased disease incidence.[685] Many examples of flavivirus emergence with impacts on global health have occurred. The recent materialization of ZIKV from a virus of minimal clinical significance in Africa to a pathogen of global health concern following its introduction into the Americas in 2015 is a clear demonstration of the threat posed by the shifting distributions of flaviviruses. Likewise, it took only 4 years for WNV to spread across the United States, where it is now an endemic pathogen, following its introduction into New York City in 1999.[943] The contribution of human activity toward the spread of flaviviruses is significant.[380] Prior to the development of rapid intercontinental transportation, the movement of flaviviruses between the Old World and New World was uncommon. YFV (and potentially the *Aedes aegypti* mosquito) was introduced into the Americas during the slave trade 300 to 400 years ago.[137] The distribution of DENV was enhanced as a consequence of the large-scale troop movements during World War II.[399] The continued spread of flaviviruses globally due to enhanced travel, urbanization, and climate change presents a persistent threat and highlights a need for the countermeasures against this genus of viruses.

FLAVIVIRUS COMPOSITION

Flavivirus Structural Proteins

Flaviviruses encapsulate a positive-stranded RNA genome encoding a single open reading frame flanked by two structured UTRs. The single viral polyprotein is processed by host and viral proteases into three structural (capsid [C], premembrane [prM], and E) and seven nonstructural proteins (NS1, NS2A, NS2B, NS3, NS4A, NS4B, and NS5), the latter of which mediate genome replication, viral polyprotein processing, and modulation of the host response. Flavivirus virions are spherical particles composed of three viral structural proteins, an approximately 11-kb genomic RNA, and a lipid envelope. The E protein is an approximately 53-kDa structural protein that functions in multiple steps of the virus replication cycle including virion assembly and budding, attachment of the virus to target cells, and viral membrane fusion (reviewed by Ref.[444]) It is also the major target of neutralizing antibodies

(reviewed by Ref.[1044]) The E protein ectodomain structure has been solved for several flaviviruses, revealing an elongated finger-like protein composed of three domains connected by flexible hinges (Fig. 9.3). This structural organization is similar to other class II viral fusion proteins, such as alphavirus E1 proteins.[924] The E protein domain I (E-DI; shown in red) is an eight-stranded β-barrel located in the center of the E protein molecule. This central domain contains two of the six disulfide bonds present in the E protein, as well as a site for the addition of an asparagine-linked (N-linked) carbohydrate. E protein domain II (E-DII; shown in yellow) is an elongated structure that mediates dimerization of E proteins on the mature virion. A glycine-rich loop composed of 13 amino acids is located at the tip of E-DII, called the E-DII fusion loop (E-DII-FL; shown in green). In the context of the E protein dimers present on mature virions, the E-DII-FL sits in a hydrophobic pocket formed at the interface of E-DI and E protein domain III (E-DIII; shown in blue). The highly conserved fusion loop plays a key role in viral membrane fusion by inserting into the membranes of target cells.[19,123,758] The introduction of mutations into the fusion loop blocks fusion between virions and the membranes of synthetic liposomes.[215] For some flaviviruses, E-DII contains a second N-linked glycosylation site, which facilitates attachment to host lectins during virus entry. E-DIII adopts an immunoglobulin-like fold and is stabilized by a single disulfide bridge. The E protein ectodomain is tethered to the viral membrane by a helical stem (the stem anchor) and two antiparallel transmembrane domains.[20,1244]

The precursor to membrane protein (prM) is an approximately 20-kDa protein that facilitates E protein folding and trafficking.[668] Interactions with the E protein also prevent the adventitious fusion of the virus during egress.[452] Virion maturation is regulated by the proteolytic cleavage of prM, which results in the formation of a "pr" protein and is ultimately released from the virion, and an approximately 8-kDa membrane associated M peptide. The structure of the "pr" peptide has been solved at the atomic level and is composed of seven β-strands held together by three disulfide bonds.[623] prM interacts with the E protein near the tip of E-DII adjacent to the E-DII-FL.[1245,1248] prM is anchored into the viral membrane via two antiparallel transmembrane domains.[797,1244]

The flavivirus capsid (C) protein is an approximately 12-kDa protein that orchestrates the encapsidation of the viral genome into the virus particle during morphogenesis.[146] The C protein contains four helical domains that interact as homodimers.[273,498,683,1017] In this arrangement, one surface is highly basic and capable of interacting with membranes.[702] The opposite face of the protein is concave, is positively charged, and binds nucleic acids.[524] The amino terminus of the protein exists in an ensemble of different states.[108] Flavivirus capsid proteins also have other roles in the replication cycle including interactions with host lipid droplets,[962] modulations of host signaling,[11] and antagonism of innate immune responses.[1160]

Flavivirus Assembly and Structure

Flaviviruses assemble on a network of highly organized virus-induced membranes derived from the endoplasmic

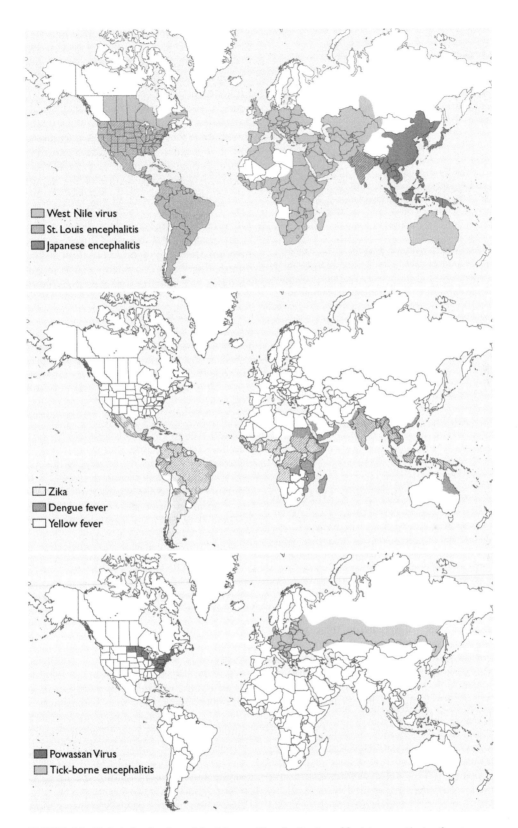

FIGURE 9.2 Global distribution of flaviviruses. The distribution of flaviviruses with significant impact on global health.

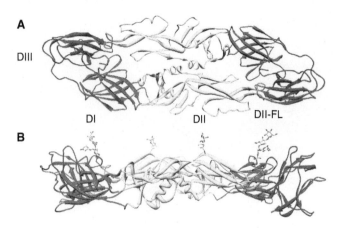

FIGURE 9.3 Structure of the flavivirus E protein. The envelope (E) proteins of flaviviruses are elongated class II viral fusion proteins composed of three structurally distinct domains. **A:** Ribbon diagram of the DENV E protein dimer as seen from the top; individual domains of each E protein monomer are indicated (domain I, E-DI, *red*; domain II, E-DII, *yellow*; and domain III, E-DIII, *blue*). The fusion loop at the tip of E-DII is shown in *green*. **B:** DENV E protein as viewed from the side. The stem anchor connecting the E protein to the viral membrane is not shown. The two N-linked carbohydrate modifications at positions Asn67 and Asn154 are shown. We thank Mr. Phong Lee (NIAID, NIH) for preparation of the figure.

reticulum (Fig. 9.4). Virions bud into the lumen of these membrane structures as immature virus particles on which E and prM proteins interact as trimers of prM-E dimers that project as spikes away from the viral membrane. The structure of the immature noninfectious form of the virion has been solved at high resolution for WNV, YFV, DENV, and ZIKV.[554,892,1234,1245,1248] These studies reveal that each virus particle contains 60 trimers arranged with icosahedral symmetry (Fig. 9.5). Analysis of the immature virion structure using methods that do not assume symmetry demonstrates that the capsid core of the virion is not located in the center of the virus particle, but positioned close to one side, with a disruption of the structural protein shell on the opposing pole. Although further studies are required to explore the functional significance of these "imperfections" in symmetry, these features may have implications for mechanisms of virus assembly and fusion.[1117] Transit of the immature virion through the acidic compartments of the trans-Golgi network (TGN) triggers an extensive rearrangement of E proteins on the immature virion. Under these conditions, E proteins lie flat against the viral membrane as antiparallel dimers, analogous to the arrangement of E proteins on the mature virions discussed below.[1234] In this configuration, prM remains associated with the fusion loop and protrudes as a bump from the surface of an otherwise smooth virus particle. This pH-dependent conformational change exposes a cleavage site on prM recognized by host serine furin-like proteases.[1061] Cleavage of prM by furin-like proteases is the hallmark of the virion maturation process and a required step in the virus replication cycle.[302] The release of the virion into the neutral conditions of the extracellular milieu results in the dissociation of the pr peptide.[623,1234]

Pioneering cryoelectron microscopic studies of DENV by the Kuhn and Rossmann laboratories revealed that mature virions are relatively smooth in appearance and incorporate 180 copies of the E protein arranged in a herringbone pattern (Fig. 9.5).[563]

Subsequent studies of WNV, JEV, and ZIKV confirmed this organization, and advances in cryoelectron microscopy now allow the interactions among structural proteins of the virion to be viewed with atomic resolution.[552,553,1013,1041,1172,1247] One striking structural feature of the virion is that virtually the entire surface of the membrane is covered by viral proteins. This dense arrangement likely is linked to the structural mechanisms that orchestrate viral fusion but presents unresolved steric challenges for host factors that bind directly to the viral lipid envelope during virion attachment, such as TIM-1 or Gas6 as detailed below. A second key feature of the mature virion structure is that E proteins are not arranged with true icosahedral symmetry. The significance of this is that E proteins of the virion exist in three chemically distinct dimer environments defined by their proximity to the two-, three-, or fivefold symmetry axes. An important biological implication of this arrangement is that antibodies[833] and host factors may be capable of engaging only a subset of E proteins that constitute the virion.

Subviral Particles

Expression of the flavivirus structural proteins prM and E is sufficient for the production of subviral particles (SVPs) that share many functional and antigenic features with infectious virions.[981] SVP expression systems have been used to examine the cell biology of structural protein folding and trafficking, virus particle morphogenesis, mechanisms of viral membrane fusion, and antibody epitope mapping.[221,668,669,981] The atomic structure of SVPs remains uncertain. Early cryoelectron microscopic reconstruction studies of TBEV SVPs revealed an icosahedral structure of roughly 30 nm in diameter composed of 30 antiparallel E protein dimers.[319] A similar structure was recently reported for a variant of DENV SVPs that encoded an optimized furin cleavage site.[1020] However, other studies demonstrate SVPs are heterogeneous in structure and size.[21] Because SVPs are used as vaccine candidates for multiple flaviviruses,[331,549,550,561,710,880] a more detailed understanding of the structures of these virus-like particles is needed.

Virion Heterogeneity and Dynamics
Implications of Inefficient prM Cleavage

While atomic resolution structures of the mature virion exist, it is now clear these images do not capture all biologically active forms of the infectious virus.[876] Cleavage of prM is a required step in the flavivirus replication cycle; mutation of the RRXR/S motif in prM recognized by furin-like proteases renders TBEV noninfectious.[302] However, biochemical studies of preparations of flaviviruses produced *in vitro* indicate that a substantial amount of prM remains uncleaved; greater than 90% of DENV virions could be precipitated with anti-prM antibodies.[500] Electron microscopy studies identified virus particles with structural features of both mature and immature virions (hereafter referred to as "partially mature virions").[887] Several lines of evidence indicate that partially mature virions are infectious: (a) virions that retain significant uncleaved prM are less sensitive to inactivation by acid pH conditions sufficient to trigger the E-protein rearrangements that drive viral membrane fusion, presumably because pH-mediated changes in the arrangement of E protein are reversible when in complex with prM[401]; (b) uncleaved prM can modify the efficiency and mechanism of virion attachment to cells[241,253,796]; (c) antibodies that target prM can enhance virus infection *in vitro* and *in vivo*[52,251,1240]; and

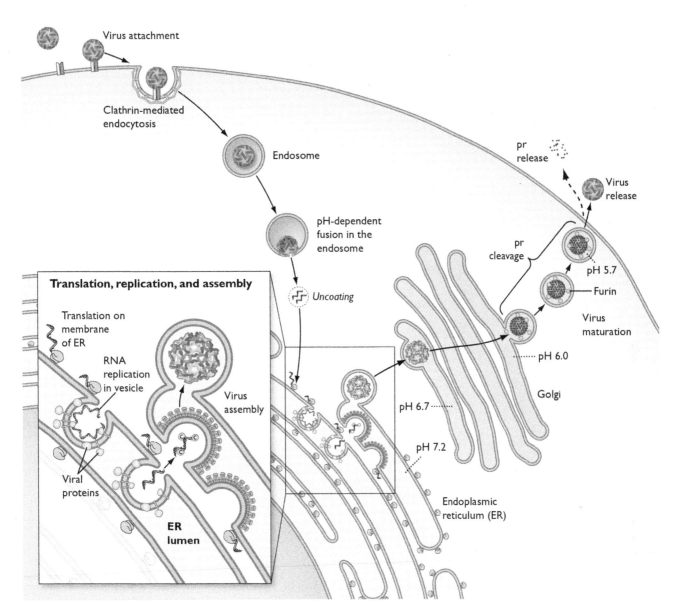

FIGURE 9.4 The replication cycle of flaviviruses. Flaviviruses bind cells via interactions with one or more cell-surface molecules. Viruses are internalized via clathrin-mediated endocytosis and fuse with membranes of the late endosome in a pH-dependent manner. Viral RNA replication begins shortly thereafter in association with cellular membranes. Infected cells reveal striking host membrane rearrangements thought to coordinate the processes of genomic RNA replication and virus assembly. Virus particles assemble at and bud into the endoplasmic reticulum and are secreted from the cell. During egress, virion maturation occurs in the acidic compartments of the Golgi and is characterized by cleavage of the prM protein by a furin-like protease. The cleaved "pr" peptide is released from the virus particle once released into the neutral pH of the extracellular space.

(d) the efficiency of prM cleavage may influence the sensitivity of virions to neutralization by antibodies targeting the E protein.[281,818] Although these studies demonstrate that virions containing prM may be infectious, the stoichiometric requirements of prM cleavage have not yet been determined. Thus, virion infectivity, antibody recognition, and host–factor interactions have the potential to be influenced by levels of uncleaved prM. The efficiency of prM cleavage *in vivo* remains an important question and should be considered for both vector and mammalian hosts. Of interest, recent analysis of DENV serotype one (DENV-1) isolates from human plasma demonstrated that viruses in this compartment are largely mature.[914]

Implications of Dynamic Virions

Flaviviruses present a dynamic antigenic surface that is not fully captured by static models of virion structure. It has long been appreciated that proteins are in constant motion and sample an ensemble of conformations at equilibrium.[106] Proteins incorporated into virus particles also are structurally dynamic.[493,1207] Conformational dynamics, or virus "breathing," has been demonstrated for several unrelated classes of viruses[112,614,801] and may affect antibody recognition.[441,627,1226] The first example of the impact of conformational dynamics on the structure of flaviviruses arose from studies of the recognition of a DENV serotype 2 (DENV-2) virus by a

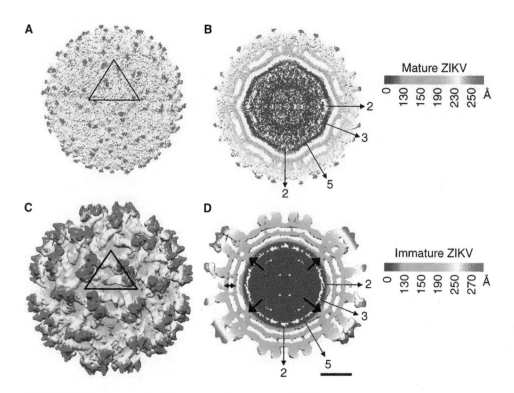

FIGURE 9.5 The structure of flaviviruses. Flaviviruses assemble as immature virus particles decorated by trimers of prM-E dimers. During virion egress, prM is cleaved by a host furin-like serine protease in a pH-dependent process. Release of the virus particle into the neutral environment of the extracellular space results in the disassociation of the cleaved "pr" fragment and formation of the mature virion. Surface and cross-sectional view of the structure of the mature ZIKV **(A and B)**. The thin black arrows depict the three symmetry axes of the herringbone arrangement of E proteins on the relatively smooth surface of the virion. The virion is colored radially. Surface and cross-sectional view of the structure of the immature ZIKV virion **(C and D)**. The thick black arrows highlight the interactions between the core of the virion and the inner leaflet of the virion, whereas double-ended arrows mark the inner and outer layers of the viral membrane. (This image was published by Prasad VM, Miller AS, Klose T, et al. Structure of the immature Zika virus at 9 A resolution. *Nat Struct Mol Biol* 2017;24:184–186, and included with permission.)

neutralizing E-DIII–reactive monoclonal antibody (mAb) 1A1D-2.[664] Analysis of the binding interface of 1A1D-2 suggested occupancy of this site would be prevented by steric clashes arising from the dense arrangement of E proteins on the virion. Binding of 1A1D-2 Fab fragments was possible only at physiological temperatures. Cryoelectron microscopic reconstruction of mature DENV-2 bound by the 1A1D-2 Fab fragment revealed changes in the arrangement and orientation of E proteins on the surface of the virus particle, suggesting antibodies can trap the virion in states distinct from the herringbone arrangement found on mature virions. Subsequent structural studies of this strain at physiological temperatures in the absence of mAb revealed a heterogeneous population of virions that included an expanded "bumpy" conformation more permissive for 1A1D-2 recognition,[324,1249] although not all DENV strains adopt this configuration. Neutralization studies with multiple flaviviruses suggest that the conformational dynamics of virions frequently contributes to the efficiency of antibody recognition, although the degree to which this is observed correlates with the accessibility of the antibody epitope on the mature virus particle.[279,281] Virions that retain prM also sample multiple states at equilibrium.[281,950] That temperature, viral strain, and even single amino acid substitutions influence the structural ensemble of flaviviruses highlights the importance of understanding how interactions among viral structural proteins determine the average state of the virion, its stability, antigenicity, and capacity for fusion.[278,373] The recent application of hydrogen/deuterium exchange mass spectrometry (HDX-MS) to explore these issues is a promising technical advance.[636,637]

CLINICAL AND PATHOLOGIC SYNDROMES OF THE FLAVIVIRUSES

Dengue Virus

History, Global Distribution, and Epidemic Cycle

The natural cycle of epidemic DENV infection is between the mosquito vector (*Aedes aegypti* or *Aedes albopictus*) and humans (Fig. 9.6). After mosquito inoculation, DENV infection causes a spectrum of clinical disease ranging from self-limited dengue fever (DF) to a life-threatening hemorrhagic and capillary leak

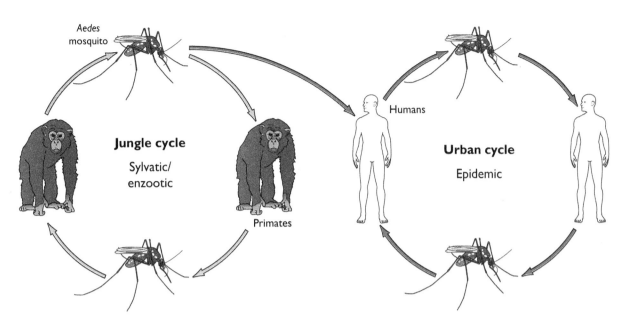

FIGURE 9.6 Life cycle of dengue virus. DENV circulates in nature in two relatively distinct transmission cycles vectored by *Aedes* spp. mosquitoes. DENV infection of humans results in a sufficiently high viremia to support infection of feeding mosquitoes; DENV transmission cycles do not require an enzootic amplifying host. DENV may also replicate in a sylvatic cycle. While incompletely understood, the contribution of sylvatic strains of DENV to human infections appears minimal.

syndrome (dengue hemorrhagic fever [DHF]/dengue shock syndrome [DSS], now termed "severe dengue"). Globally, there is significant diversity among DENV strains, including four serotypes (DENV-1, DENV-2, DENV-3, and DENV-4) that differ at the amino acid level in the viral envelope proteins by 25% to 40%. DENV causes an estimated 390 million infections and 500,000 cases of DHF/DSS per year worldwide, with 2.5 billion people at risk.[90,419,765]

Although a dengue-like syndrome may have occurred in China several times during the first millennium AD, the initial description of a DENV epidemic is attributed to Benjamin Rush, a physician in Philadelphia, in his article reporting a febrile outbreak in 1780.[951] Primary DENV infection and epidemics were common in North America, the Caribbean, Asia, and Australia during the 18th and 19th centuries, presumably due to the widespread distribution of the mosquito vectors. During World War II, DENV spread to and through Southeast Asia. Troop movement and the destruction of the environment and human settlements are believed to have promoted the spread of DENV and their mosquito vectors.[575] Since 1950, the number of people infected has risen steadily, such that today dengue is the most prevalent arthropod-borne viral disease in the world. With the spread and cocirculation of multiple DENV serotypes, secondary infection with heterologous serotypes and epidemic DHF/DSS emerged 50 years ago in Southeast Asia[435] and more recently in the Americas in 1981[556] and South Asia in 1989.[740] Since the 1950s, epidemics involving thousands of people with multiple DENV serotypes and strains occur annually in multiple parts of the world including the Americas, Asia, Africa, and Australia, in essence wherever the primary mosquito vector *Aedes aegypti* is present. Indeed, after an outbreak of DENV in Key West, Florida, in 2009, a serosurvey conducted by the CDC reported that 5.4%

of households had evidence of recent DENV infection.[28] As a reflection of this, the global incidence of DHF/DSS has increased over 500-fold, with more than 100 countries affected by outbreaks of dengue.[585]

DENV Diversity

Globally, there is significant diversity among DENV strains. The four serotypes of DENV (DENV-1, DENV-2, DENV-3, and DENV-4) are genetically distinct but cause similar diseases and share epidemiological features. All DENV strains are members of the dengue antigenic complex; inclusion of a strain as DENV is based on antigen cross-reactivity, sequence homology, and genomeorganization.[153] The four serotypes of DENV were historically distinguished by limited cross-neutralization or hemagglutination inhibition using serum from infected individuals. Subsequent sequencing analysis revealed that individual serotypes of DENV can differ from one another at the amino acid level significantly with 30% to 40% variation in the viral envelope proteins. Thus, individual DENV serotypes (e.g., DENV-1 vs. DENV-4) vary far more than distinct viruses in the Japanese encephalitis serocomplex (e.g., WNV and JEV vary by 10%–15% at the amino acid level), which has led some to consider DENV as a group of four different viruses that are linked by serology, epidemiology, and disease pathogenesis. Notwithstanding these sequence differences, recent analysis suggests that some DENV strains have greater antigenic resemblance to viruses of a different serotype than to some viruses of the same serotype, which has implications for clinical disease and DENV evolution.[511] Differences in severity associated with individual serotypes or particular sequences of serotypes in sequential infection have been observed, and it still is unclear whether some serotypes are inherently more pathogenic than others. DENV-2 viruses are most commonly associated with DHF/DSS,[49,142,1115] as are DENV-1 and DENV-3.[384,442,740] In comparison, DENV-4 appears more commonly to be clinically mild, although it can cause severe disease.[829]

Genetic variation of DENV, however, is not limited to serotype. Geographic variants within a serotype were initially identified by RNAse fingerprint assays.[923,1154] Subsequently, nucleic acid sequencing confirmed differences within each serotype, allowing for classification of genotypes that vary further by up to approximately 6% and 3% at the nucleotide and amino acid levels, respectively.[470,931] DENV genotype classification originally was defined by sequence variation within a given genomic region (e.g., E and NS1 sequences). More recent analysis has used full-genome sequencing to assign a phylogenetic classification. Although there remains some dissonance among investigators because of a lack of defined, formal definitions,[226] most classification schemes include five DENV-1 genotypes, four or five DENV-2 genotypes, four DENV-3 genotypes, and two or three DENV-4 genotypes.[932,1186] Beyond serotype and genotype, two further types of DENV complexity should be mentioned: strain variation and quasispecies. DENV strain variation refers to the limited amino acid change that occurs among isolates of a given genotype. Strain variation may be functionally important as it can affect antibody neutralization, presumably due to changes at key sites within or that affect the display of antigenic epitopes.[124,1078,1162,1258]

In addition to serotype, genotype, and strain variation, DENV has the capacity to accumulate variation rapidly within an individual host. Viral quasispecies is composed of a cloud of variants that are linked by a spectrum of mutations. It is observed during infection by many RNA viruses (e.g., HCV, HIV, and influenza) and creates the diversity that allows a viral population to adapt rapidly to dynamic environments and evolve resistance to immune responses, vaccines, and antiviral drugs.[598,1155] DENV (and other flaviviruses) exist as a collection of highly similar variants forming a quasispecies[1173] by virtue of its error-prone NS5 polymerase, which has an estimated mutation rate of 10^3 to 10^5 substitutions per nucleotide copied per round of replication.[179,1137] DENV intrahost diversity in humans appears to be driven by immune pressures as well as replicative success in cells.[859] Hot spots for intrahost variation were identified in the viral E and prM/M proteins and appeared to be immune escape variants. In other studies, DENV quasispecies generation was associated with the development of rapid drug resistance against nucleoside inhibitors of the RNA-dependent RNA polymerase.[712] Apart from these reports, the study of genetic and intrahost diversity for DENV is still in its relative infancy, and thus more analysis is warranted to define how mutation and variation impact fitness, tropism, and drug or immune system resistance.

Clinical Features of Acute Dengue Fever: Primary DENV Infection

DENV infection of humans after mosquito inoculation causes a spectrum of clinical disease ranging from inapparent disease (~50% of infections[50,142,304]) and self-limited DF to severe dengue. A classical presentation of DF is an abrupt onset of a debilitating febrile illness characterized by headache, retroorbital pain, myalgias, arthralgias, and a maculopapular rash that occurs 2 to 7 days after mosquito inoculation.[956] Some individuals experience severe bone and joint pain ("breakbone fever") and develop petechial hemorrhages that are associated with mild to severe thrombocytopenia. There is no specific

constellation of signs or symptoms to differentiate DF from other acute flu-like viral syndromes, so a health care provider must have a high index of suspicion for diagnosis in the setting of the appropriate epidemiology. DF also may present in a less classical form as an undifferentiated febrile illness with rash along with mild upper respiratory symptoms (cough, pharyngitis, rhinitis), particularly in children. DF is usually self-limited, lasting 1 to 2 weeks, although some (up to 25% of hospitalized patients) experience a prolonged postinfectious fatigue and depression syndrome that can persist for weeks, akin to that seen after Epstein-Barr virus infection and mononucleosis.[1006] Because of the debilitating fever and musculoskeletal symptoms, the morbidity toll is high in clinically apparent DF, although the mortality rate is exceedingly low.

Clinical Features of Severe Dengue: Secondary and Infant DENV Infection

The incidence of severe dengue (which includes DHF/DSS) varies considerably between primary and secondary infections. A secondary DENV infection results when a person previously infected with one serotype is exposed to a different serotype and is the single most important risk factor for severe dengue disease.[142,304,412,428] Epidemiologic data in Thailand have shown greater than 10-fold higher rates of DHF/DSS during secondary compared to the primary infection of children.[1148] It should be pointed out that even during secondary infection, severe dengue is quite rare, with only 0.5% of secondary infections progressing to this disease. Severe dengue is characterized by rapid onset of capillary leakage accompanied by thrombocytopenia and mild to moderate liver damage reflected by increases in serum levels of hepatic enzyme (e.g., aspartate aminotransferase and alanine aminotransferase).[422] Severe dengue usually occurs as a second phase of the illness, after a short period of defervescence from the initial fever. Hemorrhagic manifestations are observed in a subset of cases and include petechiae, epistaxis, gastrointestinal bleeding (hematemesis or melena), menorrhagia, and a positive tourniquet test. Use of the term hemorrhagic fever instead of dengue capillary leak syndrome has led many to anticipate that bleeding is the greatest threat. Rather, fluid loss into tissue spaces with hemoconcentration and hypotension can result in shock, which carries the highest risk of mortality.[822] From a diagnostic standpoint, an elevated hematocrit and upper abdominal ultrasonogram showing a thickened gallbladder wall, hepatomegaly, ascites, or pleural effusions are evidence of fluid shifts associated with a capillary leak syndrome.

Whereas severe dengue occurs largely after secondary infection by a different DENV serotype in children and adults,[384] in infants less than age 1 born to dengue-immune mothers, a primary infection can cause significant morbidity and mortality.[428,486,1038] In clinical studies, maternal anti–dengue neutralization antibody titers and age of the infant correlated with disease. The actual age at which severe dengue occurs in infants (peak at 7 months) corresponds to the age at which serum antibodies most efficiently enhance the infection of primary monocytes observed in vitro via a mechanism called antibody-dependent enhancement (ADE) of infection, described below.[538] Clinical manifestations of severe dengue are more prevalent in infants,[436] and there is an approximately fourfold higher mortality rate compared to other age groups.[506] Infants represent approximately 5% of children hospitalized with severe dengue in many parts of Southeast Asia.[183,384,425] The more prevalent or severe clinical manifestations associated with infant dengue include seizures, hepatic dysfunction, thrombocytopenia, high-grade fever, diffuse rash, peripheral edema, ascites, and frank shock.[486]

More recent clinical studies have suggested that severe DENV infection also can have neurological manifestations including transverse myelitis, Guillain-Barré syndrome (GBS), encephalitis, and encephalopathy,[1051,1145] occurring in as many as 1% to 6% of severe dengue cases.[157,455,624] In contrast to other encephalitic flaviviruses (e.g., JEV, WNV, or TBEV), DENV historically has not been considered as neuroinvasive. However, the discovery of DENV and anti-dengue IgM in the cerebrospinal fluid of patients with encephalopathy suggests that it may be capable of causing central nervous system infection as part of a severe syndrome, at least in a subset of individuals.[677,1051] In support of this, focal imaging abnormalities have been detected in brain MRI scans of DENV-infected patients.[157,1184] Although it is increasingly appreciated that neurological involvements of DENV in the CNS peripheral nervous system can occur,[624] a more complete understanding of the molecular determinants of neurotropism remains to be defined.

Pathological Features of Severe Dengue

Although DENV is the most prevalent mosquito-transmitted viral infection in the world, there are few detailed autopsy series of patients who succumbed to severe dengue, and fewer performed with newer molecular techniques and markers. Detailed histopathological studies that might inform a basic understanding of DENV pathogenesis are rare because much of the lethal disease occurs in regions lacking sophisticated laboratory infrastructure, highly trained personnel, and repositories for long-term tissue storage. Forensic studies also are complicated by the lack of standardization of histological procedures and variation in the quality of specimen preparation and storage.

A summary of the autopsy literature from a total of 160 fatal DHF/DSS cases occurring primarily in children and adolescents has been published.[705] Pathological findings in the liver include centrilobular necrosis, changes in fatty tissue, inflammatory leukocyte infiltration, and Kupffer cell hyperplasia.[89,141] Gross macroscopic examination revealed multiple hemorrhagic foci. Microscopic analysis has shown increased inflammatory infiltrates around the portal vessels, sinusoidal congestion, small hemorrhages, midzonal hepatocyte necrosis, and microvesicular steatosis.[309,411] In other tissues (spleen or lung), hemorrhage, tissue edema, and plasma leakage have been observed.[66]

A key to understanding the pathogenesis of severe DENV infection is defining the cellular tropism of infection, which could influence the host inflammatory response that results in the capillary leak syndrome. Autopsy series have shown the presence of DENV antigen or nucleic acid in cells of the skin, liver, spleen, lymph nodes, kidney, lung, thymus, or brain.[51,66,216,411,508,525,744,945] However, several of these studies used *in situ* hybridization or RT-PCR–based assays and thus have not definitively shown that infectious virus is produced in a given cell of a target tissue. Infectious virus can be isolated reliably from blood, lymphoid tissues, and the liver, although the cellular source of the virus remains controversial. Studies in humans, nonhuman primates, and small animal models support a role for infection of myeloid cells (blood monocytes, tissue macrophages, Kupffer cells) and possibly other cells including hepatocytes[417] and endothelial cells.[66,1240]

Zika Virus

History, Global Distribution, and Epidemic Cycle

ZIKV was first isolated in 1947 in the Zika Forest of Uganda.[266,267,1004] Over the next 60 years, ZIKV was isolated from mosquitoes in East Africa, West Africa, and Southeast Asia, and serological surveys suggested that ZIKV circulated sporadically in humans in these regions (reviewed in Ref.[1203]). Despite evidence of ZIKV circulation, reports of human cases were rare, with the first known significant ZIKV outbreak occurring in 2007, in Micronesia.[287,592] The introduction of ZIKV into a small island population without prior immunity may have provided an opportunity to observe ZIKV disease that went unnoticed in endemic transmission settings. This outbreak marked the emergence of ZIKV as a globally significant human pathogen, as over the next decade the virus spread throughout Oceania, causing a large outbreak in French Polynesia,[160] and then in Latin America. The first autochthonous ZIKV cases in the Americas were reported in Northeast Brazil in 2015, though the virus most likely was introduced at least 1 year prior.[158,317,741,1236] Within a year of the first reports, the virus had spread throughout Latin America and the Caribbean, in explosive fashion with infection rates of 50% to 90% in many areas. With more than 200,000 confirmed cases and more than 500,000 suspected cases from 2015 to 2017, and only approximately 25% to 50% of ZIKV infections being symptomatic,[36,287,671,754] it is likely that millions of people were infected. The rapid and intense spread of ZIKV in the Western Hemisphere likely was enabled by an abundance of *Aedes aegypti* mosquito vectors and immunologically naïve populations in urban areas. While ZIKV transmission has waned in the Americas (possibly due to herd immunity), infections continue to occur in Africa and Asia[334,459,1039,1220]; the attention resulting from the emergence of ZIKV in the Americas is likely to bring greater recognition of ZIKV-associated disease in areas where it previously went unnoticed.

ZIKV initially was isolated from a sentinel rhesus macaque, an Asian monkey not necessarily representative of primate hosts native to the Zika Forest. ZIKV subsequently was isolated from *Aedes africanus* mosquitoes, and multiple monkey species in the Zika Forest were found seropositive for ZIKV, implying that ZIKV circulates in a sylvatic cycle between mosquitoes and monkeys.[415,722] Small mammals in the Zika Forest did not show serological evidence of ZIKV infection.[415] Other historical studies have reported ZIKV seropositivity in a variety of vertebrate species, but analyses that detect antibody binding (e.g., hemagglutination inhibition, complement fixation, or ELISA) should be interpreted with caution, as antigenic cross-reactivity between flaviviruses can make it difficult to ascertain specificity, particularly in areas where multiple flaviviruses co-circulate. Recent work using more specific serological assays found ZIKV-seropositive grivets and ZIKV-seropositive baboons in Tanzania and the Gambia.[139] Altogether, these studies are consistent with a model in which primates (both humans and monkeys) are the primary vertebrate hosts for ZIKV.

Both Old World and New World primates can be infected with ZIKV experimentally (see "Animal Models"). However, it remains an open question whether ZIKV will establish a nonhuman primate reservoir in Latin America, as did YFV. Alternatively, ZIKV may behave more like DENV, which has a sylvatic cycle in Old World monkeys but in Latin America is maintained exclusively through transmission between humans and mosquitoes.

ZIKV Diversity

ZIKV is classified in the Spondweni serogroup, and to date, these two viruses are the only members of this clade. ZIKV strains form a single serotype[277] but are genetically divided into African and Asian lineages. The African lineage includes the prototype strain isolated in 1947, as well as strains isolated from mosquitoes in Senegal and the Central African Republic in the 1970s and 1980s. This lineage continues to circulate, as African lineage strains were detected in contemporary samples from West Africa.[459] Asian lineage strains include ZIKV strains isolated from Southeast Asia and all outbreak strains from Oceania and Latin America.[317,741] Following the emergence of ZIKV in the Americas, Asian lineage strains were detected in individuals in Africa, suggesting that both Asian and African lineage strains now may circulate in Africa.[973] Furthermore, while American ZIKV strains have been reintroduced to Asia by travelers, Asian lineage strains distinct from those in the Americas continue to circulate in Southeast Asia and were responsible for a 2016 outbreak in Singapore and a 2018 outbreak in India.[1039,1099,1220] ZIKV strains associated with disease in the Americas, particularly congenital Zika syndrome (CZS), have genetic differences compared to earlier African and Asian

strains not associated with significant disease. The causal role for these variants in ZIKV pathogenesis remains unclear, but they may have the potential to enhance neurovirulence or the efficiency of mosquito transmission.[184,659,1235]

ZIKV Transmission

ZIKV endemic and epidemic transmission can be sustained by direct transmission between humans and *Aedes aegypti* mosquitoes in an urban/peridomestic cycle without a requirement for other vertebrate animals as amplifying hosts (Fig. 9.7). ZIKV has been isolated from many species of *Aedes* mosquito, but only a subset are competent vectors for transmission (reviewed in Ref.[305]). *Aedes aegypti* is a key vector for ZIKV transmission because of its high competence, abundance throughout the tropics and subtropics, and anthropophilic nature. During the emergence of ZIKV in the Americas, autochthonous transmission in the United States occurred in southern Florida and Texas, where *Aedes aegypti* mosquitoes are found.[397,634] Subsequent spread to regions where *Aedes albopictus* mosquitoes dominate did not occur, but it is difficult to ascertain whether this was because *Aedes albopictus* is not an efficient ZIKV vector or because interventions that limit mosquito exposure prevented extensive spread.

ZIKV outbreaks are driven by mosquito transmission. However, ZIKV is unusual compared to other flaviviruses in also being transmitted directly between humans through sexual contact. While ZIKV sexual transmission became evident through travel-associated cases in the Americas,[274,780] the first

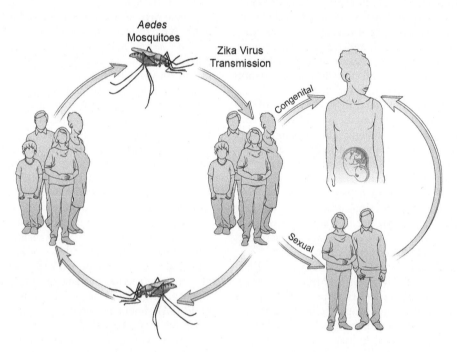

FIGURE 9.7 Transmission cycle of Zika virus. ZIKV infection in humans produces sufficiently high viremia to allow direct transmission between humans and *Aedes* spp. mosquitoes; this transmission mechanism is similar to other *Aedes*-borne flaviviruses and is responsible for most ZIKV infections. Unlike other flaviviruses, ZIKV also can be transmitted directly between humans through congenital and sexual routes. These vector-independent transmission mechanisms are notable because they involve distinct tissue tropism compared to mosquito-borne transmission and can produce distinct disease outcomes, most notably neurodevelopmental defects in infants infected *in utero* (congenital Zika syndrome).

reported case predates this epidemic and resulted from ZIKV infection in Africa.[334] Even with decades of comparable travel-associated DENV cases,[171,490,933,1204] there is no evidence of DENV sexual transmission. As it is difficult to evaluate ZIKV sexual transmission in regions that also support mosquito transmission, the epidemiologic significance of ZIKV sexual transmission remains uncertain. However, vector-independent transmission may broaden the geographic area over which ZIKV outbreaks can be sustained. The mechanisms that enable ZIKV sexual transmission are unknown, but likely include tropism for tissues in the male and female reproductive tracts. ZIKV infects human testicular cells in culture[716,1035] and targets the testes in mouse models.[382,684,1140] However, sexual transmission from vasectomized men and mice implies that tissues other than the testis contribute to the presence of ZIKV in semen.[33,288,338] ZIKV RNA can be detected in semen for months following the resolution of acute infection,[726,825,863,1135] suggesting that ZIKV infection may persist in the testes or other tissues of the male reproductive tract. ZIKV also has been detected in vaginal secretions of infected women[805,863,867] and replicates in the vaginal epithelium of experimentally inoculated mice and macaques.[149,165,1103,1229]

ZIKV can traverse the placental barrier and cause fetal infections, producing congenital ZIKV syndrome (CZS) in a subset of exposed pregnancies. While other arboviruses are known to be teratogenic in livestock,[272] and other flaviviruses have been associated with adverse pregnancy outcomes,[853] ZIKV is the first example of a flavivirus with clear evidence of teratogenicity in humans. Congenital infection is a transmission dead end for arboviruses, so fetal/placental infection likely is an incidental outcome rather than an adaptive trait. However, congenital infection is associated with prolonged maternal viremia,[283,727,842,1005] potentially extending the period during which infected individuals can transmit the virus to mosquitoes.

Clinical Features of ZIKV Infection

Most ZIKV infections are asymptomatic, with approximately 25% to 50% progressing to febrile illness. Maculopapular rash is the most common manifestation of ZIKV infection, along with fever, headache, myalgia, and conjunctivitis.[754,807] Symptoms typically manifest within 3 to 7 days of a mosquito bite and usually are self-limited. Prior to its emergence in the Western Hemisphere, ZIKV was considered a benign infection, but large-scale outbreaks after 2013 revealed more serious disease manifestations. ZIKV infection has been associated with GBS, a postinfectious autoimmune peripheral neuropathy.[118,159,835] There also are isolated reports of more severe manifestations of ZIKV including meningitis, encephalitis, and thrombocytopenia, usually in individuals who are immunocompromised or have other comorbidities.[166,509] ZIKV also can target tissues in the eye, leading to uveitis and other ophthalmological diseases.[341,545,739] ZIKV also targets tissues in the male reproductive tract, allowing for sexual transmission and causing urogenital disease including hematospermia.[334,808] Although ZIKV generally is considered to be an acute illness, infection of immune-privileged tissues such as the eye and male reproductive tract allows for viral persistence.[10,466,726,825,863,1135]

Although ZIKV infection in adults rarely causes significant or durable morbidity, infection during pregnancy can result in intrauterine growth restriction and a spectrum of neurodevelopmental defects.[218] The teratogenic effects of ZIKV were first noted in 2015 in Northeast Brazil as an increase in cases of microcephaly following the ZIKV outbreak in that region.[855] Subsequently, microcephaly and other neurodevelopmental defects were associated with the ZIKV outbreak throughout Latin America,[156,197,245,247,248,335,471,605,755,851,971] and retrospective studies found an increase in similar outcomes associated with the 2013 to 2014 ZIKV outbreak in French Polynesia.[85,170] Studies in nonhuman primates corroborate the teratogenic effects of ZIKV during pregnancy.[4,5,209,286,408,465,687,708,761,823,1007] Though the mechanisms that cause congenital anomalies are still being determined, ZIKV appears to target neural progenitor cells in the developing brain,[440,625,1101] eliciting a range of neurological effects including microcephaly, seizures, impaired motor function, vision and hearing loss, arthrogryposis, and cognitive impairment. Neural progenitor cells could be damaged directly by viral infection or indirectly by inflammatory responses, which can inhibit cell proliferation, trafficking, and differentiation.[678] ZIKV infection also can damage the placenta, resulting in intrauterine growth restriction and impaired fetal development.[465,830,908,916,1096] The long-term effects of ZIKV exposure *in utero* remain to be determined, but the 2-year follow-up of the earliest cohorts of CZS cases has found severe motor impairment, seizure disorders, hearing and vision abnormalities, and sleep difficulties; these children are developmentally delayed and likely will require long-term support.[794,974] Congenital ZIKV infection also may result in subtle cognitive or functional deficits that could become apparent as affected children develop. The rate at which ZIKV infection during pregnancy results in CZS is still under investigation, as are the factors modulating this risk, with one study identifying rates as high as 42% of ZIKV-infected pregnant women[117] and other studies finding rates of approximately 5%.[1018] ZIKV infection at any gestational stage can result in CZS, although exposure earlier in pregnancy seems to produce more severe manifestations. Fetal outcome does not depend on maternal disease severity, and even asymptomatic maternal infection can result in CZS. Although ZIKV can circumvent the placental barrier and access the fetal compartment, the mechanism by which it does so remains unclear.[218] ZIKV can infect placental macrophages,[908] but the syncytiotrophoblasts, which form the interface between the placenta and maternal circulation, do not support viral replication.[68,214] ZIKV may access susceptible cytotrophoblasts at sites of placental implantation into the decidua,[1096] or the maternal immune response may compromise the integrity of the placental barrier.

The extensive antigenic cross-reactivity between ZIKV and DENV creates the possibility that prior DENV exposure could modulate the outcome of ZIKV infection. The emergence of ZIKV in regions with high DENV seroprevalence implies that prior DENV infection does not provide durable protection against ZIKV. However, cross-reactive immunity may provide short-term protection or reduce disease severity.[374,393,779,940] Although cross-reactive nonneutralizing antibody responses between different DENV serotypes can exacerbate DENV disease via ADE,[512] currently there is no evidence that DENV antibodies enhance ZIKV infection in humans or nonhuman primates.[374,779,858] A greater risk may be that cross-reactive antibodies from a prior ZIKV infection could exacerbate subsequent DENV infection, which will become apparent now that the two viruses are coendemic in Latin America and Southeast Asia.

Pathological Features

Since ZIKV disease in adults typically is self-limited and benign, it is not generally associated with significant pathology beyond erythematous maculopapular lesions and petechiae.[271] Although the range of manifestations that constitute CZS is not fully known, pathological features have been described, particularly for severe presentations.[197,245,706] Overall, the pathological features of CZS are similar to other congenital infection syndromes, such as those caused by human cytomegalovirus or rubella virus. The brains of severely affected fetuses and infants exhibit lissencephaly, hypoplasia, calcifications, and ventriculomegaly, most often seen when ZIKV exposure occurred early in gestation. Other commonly reported lesions include microglial nodules, gliosis, neurodegeneration, and necrosis. Affected fetuses also may exhibit microphthalmia, and infants may present with ophthalmological disease including focal pigment mottling, chorioretinal atrophy, and optic nerve atrophy.[248,322,1151] The ophthalmological effects of ZIKV infection may not be limited to *in utero* exposure, as ZIKV-associated uveitis has been reported in adults, including chorioretinal lesions.[545,739] Congenital ZIKV infection is associated with placental damage, which likely is an additional source of fetal damage beyond direct viral-induced pathology.[197,245,706] Placental findings include chronic villitis, stromal fibrosis and calcifications, and chorionic vasculitis. In a subset of affected fetuses, ZIKV RNA and antigens have been detected by *in situ* hybridization and immunohistochemistry.

Yellow Fever Virus

History, Global Distribution, and Epidemic Cycle

Several reviews have described the historical details and epidemiology of YFV infection.[57,299,348] The causative agent of yellow fever (YF), YFV, was first isolated (strain Asibi) in 1927 after inoculation of a rhesus monkey with the blood of a patient from Ghana.[1074] YFV originated in Africa, was imported into the Americas during the slave trade, and had the first reported epidemic in the Yucatan in 1648.[61] Historically, large epidemics of YF disease occurred beyond these regions and were described in the 17th through 20th centuries as far north in the Americas as Canada, as well as in parts of Europe including Spain, Italy, France, and England.[764] Despite the presence of an effective vaccine (17D strain), with more than 500 million doses administered to humans,[348] YFV infection has remained a public health threat in some parts of the world. Currently, YFV is endemic in tropical regions of Africa and the Americas, infects humans and nonhuman primates, and is transmitted by mosquitoes including *Aedes aegypti*. The WHO estimates an incidence of 200,000 YF cases per year, leading to approximately 30,000 to 60,000 deaths with the majority occurring in sub-Saharan Africa.[846] Overall, 47 countries in Africa and the Americas are considered within the modern YFV-endemic zone, with 600 to 700 million people at risk of infection.[299,348]

The sylvatic or jungle cycle of YFV in which transmission occurs between mosquitoes and monkeys explains why extensive vaccination campaigns have reduced but not eradicated infection. In East Africa, YFV infection is maintained in monkey transmission cycles in the jungle with the *Aedes africanus* mosquito vector. Periodically, infection may cross into humans during an intermediate savannah cycle, with transmission by several different *Aedes* mosquito species (e.g., *Aedes bromeliae*). Indeed, in the Americas, most cases appear to be a result of humans exposed to the jungle cycle of YFV.[63] Epidemic YFV infection (human–mosquito–human cycle) ensues in urban or domestic areas with *Aedes aegypti* as the principal mosquito vector. Rapid urbanization in Africa and the Americas with population shifts from rural to urban settings combined with the collapse of mosquito eradication programs has allowed the *Aedes aegypti* vector to repopulate many parts of the world and caused YFV to be classified as a reemerging threat.[348]

Unfortunately, dramatic increases in YFV incidence have occurred recently in areas that had been considered essentially free of YF.[59,350] In 2013, YFV infection resulted in 130,000 cases and 78,000 deaths in Africa.[350] In Uganda and Brazil in 2016, YFV infections and deaths were associated with a lack of vaccination and likely were due to sylvatic transmission.[316,583] In 2016, urban YF occurred in Angola and the Democratic Republic of the Congo and was difficult to contain due to vaccine shortages.[1055]

YFV Diversity

YFV does not belong to an antigenic subgroup based on plaque reduction neutralization assays,[153] but shows greater genetic relationship to other African flaviviruses including Banzi, Wesselsbron, and Bouboui viruses. Indeed, cross-protection against YFV infection in monkeys has been shown after immunization with some of these related viruses.[456] Although there is only one serotype of YFV, there is significant diversity within the genus. Seven genotypes have been proposed including two West African genotypes, a single Central/South African genotype, two East African genotypes, and two South American genotypes.[299] These genotypes of YFV were originally defined based on nucleotide variation of greater than 9% in the prM, E, and 3′ UTR gene regions[810,1182] and have been confirmed with full-genome sequencing of YFV isolates.[1159] Phylogenic studies suggest that YFV originated in East or Central Africa and was introduced subsequently into West Africa and South America.[809,810] Beyond genotypes, sequence analysis of 135 YFV strains isolated from 1935 to 2016 in Brazil revealed further strain divergence into clades that differ at the nucleotide and amino acid level by up to 7% and 5%, respectively.[1146] The physiological basis for genotype-specific amino acid variation between YFV isolates remains uncertain although it is likely that selection confers a phenotypic advantage in a given host.

Clinical Features of YFV Infection

In humans, YFV infection causes a variable clinical syndrome ranging from no symptoms to mild febrile flu-like illness to fulminate and possibly fatal disease. Approximately 15% of people who become infected develop a severe visceral disease, and in this group, there is a 20% to 50% case fatality rate.[767] Symptoms occur within 3 to 6 days of mosquito inoculation and include an abrupt onset of fever, chills, myalgia, back pain, and headache during the initial period of infection, which usually lasts 3 days and corresponds to peak viremia. During this phase, individuals are infectious to mosquitoes. In some, this stage may be followed by a short "period of remission," with defervescence and improvement of clinical sign and symptoms. Shortly after, in a subset (20%) of patients, fever and symptoms worsen ("period of intoxication") with vomiting, epigastric pain, and jaundice; this is associated with YFV replication in the liver, an absence of viremia, and measurable anti-YFV antibodies in serum. As time progresses, severe YFV infection evolves into a hemorrhagic fever characterized by severe hepatitis, renal failure, hemorrhage, shock, and multiorgan failure. A bleeding diathesis manifests with melena, hematemesis, epistaxis, ecchymosis, menorrhagia, petechial hemorrhages, and blood oozing from mucus membranes. Renal failure is associated with an abrupt decrease in urine output and albuminuria. Laboratory tests show leukopenia, thrombocytopenia, and a coagulopathy. Death occurs on the 7th to 10th day of illness and is preceded by hemodynamic and cardiovascular instability, acute liver failure, hypothermia, hypoglycemia, and coma. For those individuals surviving severe YFV infection, convalescence is prolonged with hepatitis and associated constitutional symptoms persisting sometimes for months.

Pathological Features of YFV Infection

Macroscopic gross pathology of tissues from YFV infection autopsy studies shows an enlarged and icteric liver and edematous and enlarged kidneys and heart. Microscopic pathologic analyses of the liver reveal six major features,[348,541,768] which occur primarily during the "period of intoxication": (a) eosinophilic degeneration of hepatocytes and Kupffer cells; (b) midzonal hepatocellular swelling and necrosis, with sparing of the cells in the portal area; (c) the presence of Councilman bodies coincident with hepatocyte cell death; (d) absence of leukocyte inflammatory infiltrates; (e) microvesicular fatty changes and lipid accumulation, likely secondary to decreased apoprotein synthesis by hepatocytes; and (f) retention of the reticulin structure. YFV antigen and RNA are demonstrable in hepatocytes by immunohistochemistry or *in situ* hybridization,[244] and this, coupled with the absence of inflammation, suggests that cell death is mediated directly by virus infection, likely via an apoptotic mechanism.[768,905]

In the kidney, severe eosinophilic degeneration and a microvesicular fatty change of renal tubular epithelium are observed, analogous to that seen in the liver. Viral antigen can be detected by immunohistochemistry in renal tubular cells.[244] Glomerular damage and albuminuria with changes in the basement membrane and degeneration of cells lining the Bowman capsule may be due to direct viral injury[768] or secondary to decreased blood flow during the sepsis syndrome.[348] The spleen shows an overall loss of lymphocytes, hyperplasia of the follicle, appearance of large mononuclear tissue histiocytes, and degeneration of cells with accumulation of fragmented nuclei.[542] In monkeys, necrosis of B-cell follicular areas of the spleen is more apparent.[769] In the heart, myocardial cells also undergo apoptotic changes as in other organs, in the absence of a significant cellular inflammatory response. Patchy lesions have been described in the sinoatrial (SA) node and bundle of His,[662] which could explain the paradoxical bradycardia and late cardiac death observed in some severe YFV cases.

Hemorrhagic manifestations and plasma leakage from capillaries are characteristic findings of severe YFV infection.[768] The bleeding manifestations are attributed to decreased synthesis of vitamin K–dependent coagulation factors by the injured liver, disseminated intravascular coagulation, and reduced platelet numbers and function. Beyond direct bleeding, there is additional vascular dysfunction, with pleural and peritoneal effusions, and edema of several other organs, including the brain. At present, the precise pathogenesis of the vascular leakage syndrome associated with YFV remains unknown, although highly elevated levels of proinflammatory and vasoactive cytokines are observed.[1108]

West Nile Virus

History, Global Distribution, and Epidemic cycle

WNV was first isolated in 1937 in the West Nile district of Uganda from a woman with an undiagnosed febrile illness.[1048] Historically, WNV caused sporadic outbreaks of a mild febrile illness in regions of Africa, the Middle East, Asia, and Australia. Indeed, in the 1950s, detailed studies of WNV showed recurrent outbreaks in Israel[83,366] and high levels of seroconversion in adults from Egypt[482,736]; these outbreaks and others in Africa generally were not associated with severe human disease. However, in the 1990s, the epidemiology of infection changed. New outbreaks in Eastern Europe were associated with higher rates of neurological disease.[478] In 1999, WNV entered North America and caused seven human fatalities in the New York area as well a large number of avian and equine deaths. Since then, WNV has been present throughout the continental United States as well in parts of Canada, Mexico, the Caribbean, and South America. Because of the increased range, the number of human cases has continued to rise: in the United States between 1999 and 2019, 51,684 cases were confirmed (48% of which were neuroinvasive) and associated with 2,374 deaths (https://www.cdc.gov/westnile/statsmaps/index.html). The highest incidence (3.4 cases per 100,000 individuals) of WNV infection in the United States has occurred in South Dakota.

WNV cycles in nature between *Culex* mosquitoes and birds but also infects and causes disease in humans, horses, and other mammals (Fig. 9.8). Although its enzootic cycle is overwhelmingly between mosquitoes and birds, with mammals serving as "dead-end" hosts because of low-level and transient viremia, nonviremic transmission of WNV between cofeeding mosquitoes[462] suggests that mammals could act as reservoirs for mosquito infection. Most (~85%) human infections in the Northern Hemisphere occur in the late summer with a peak number of cases in August and September. This reflects the seasonal activity of *Culex* mosquito vectors and a requirement for virus amplification in the late spring and early summer in avian hosts. In warmer parts of the world, virtually year-round transmission is observed. Although more than 100 avian species are susceptible to WNV infection, in the United States, some are particularly vulnerable with a large number of deaths in crows, jays, and hawks. Ecology studies suggest that *Culex pipiens*, the dominant enzootic (bird-to-bird) and bridge (bird-to-human) vector of WNV in urbanized areas in the northeast and north central United States, shifts its feeding preferences from birds to humans during the late summer and early fall, coincident with the dispersal of its preferred host, the American robin (*Turdus migratorius*).[526]

WNV Diversity

Sequencing and phylogenic analysis of full-length genomes have resulted in a division of WNV strains into four or more distinct lineages.[84,492,591,681] However, most severe neuroinvasive WNV infections are attributed to strains from lineages 1 and 2. Lineage 1 strains are separated into three clades (1a, 1b, and 1c). Clade 1a is composed of isolates from Europe, the Middle East, Russia, and the Americas and includes all strains from

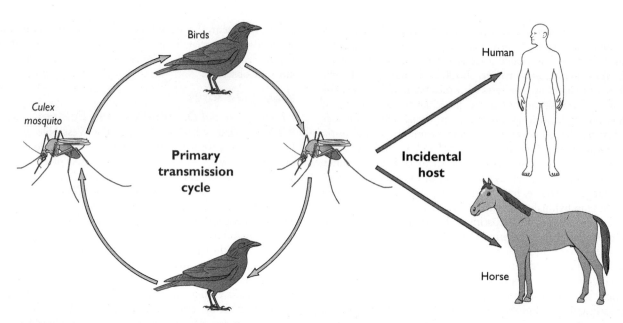

FIGURE 9.8 Transmission cycle of West Nile virus. WNV is maintained in nature in an enzootic transmission cycle between mosquitoes and birds. Many vertebrate species, including humans, may also be infected as "dead-end" hosts for WNV. The resulting transient low-level viremia in mammalian hosts does not support sufficient infection of the mosquito vector to continue the transmission cycle.

the United States and Canada. Clade 1b contains the naturally attenuated Australian variant, Kunjin virus, which forms a tight cluster with approximately 2% to 3% difference at the amino acid level from North American WNV strains.[985] Clade 1c is composed only of isolates from India, sometimes referred to as lineage 5 strains. Historically, lineage 2 isolates were isolated from sub-Saharan Africa and Madagascar and generally showed less ability to cause disease in humans and animals[71,478]; lineage 2 isolates now circulate in parts of Eastern Europe[306] where they have caused severe neurological disease and fatalities.[111] There are fewer sequenced strains from lineage 3 and 4 WNV, with only one lineage 3 isolate from Austria in 1997[45] and several lineage 4 isolates[681] from Russia between 2002 and 2006. A putative 6th WNV lineage has been described from Spain and is based on a small gene fragment.[1150] Koutango virus, which was initially classified as a different virus, is now considered a 7th lineage of WNV; it is unusual, as it has been isolated from ticks and rodents.[313] Within a given ecological niche, possibly because of its enzootic cycle, WNV has remarkable genetic stability despite its error-prone RNA-dependent RNA polymerase; full-length sequencing analysis of North American isolates over the past decade has revealed a rate of approximately 5 nucleotide and less than 1 amino acid mutation per genome per year, with little geographic subdivision.[240,1102]

Clinical Features of WNV Infection

Seroprevalence studies suggest that most (~80%) cases are subclinical, without significant symptoms. Among clinical cases, many develop a self-limiting illness termed "WNV fever." This syndrome begins after a 2- to 14-day incubation period and is characterized by fever accompanied with myalgia, arthralgia, headache, fatigue, gastrointestinal complaints (nausea, vomiting, and diarrhea), maculopapular rash, or lymphadenopathy. This nonneuroinvasive form of WNV infection can be severe as 38% of patients with WNV fever were hospitalized with a

mean length stay of 5.4 days.[480] A subset of the symptomatic cases progress to the neuroinvasive forms of WNV infection, including acute flaccid paralysis, meningitis, encephalitis, and ocular manifestations[46,1010]; in many instances, a combination of these syndromes is present. Overall, about 1 in 150 WNV infections result in the most severe and potentially lethal form of the disease. During an epidemic, the seroconversion rate is approximately 3%,[792,1132] and the attack rate for severe disease during an epidemic is approximately 7 per 100,000.[480] The risk of severe WNV infection is greatest in the elderly.[201,814,1132] At least two studies have estimated a 20-fold increased risk of neuroinvasive disease and death in those over 50 years of age.[480,814] Persistent movement disorders, cognitive complaints, and functional disability may occur after West Nile neuroinvasive disease. West Nile poliomyelitis-like disease may result in limb weakness or paralysis. Moreover, even patients with apparently mild cases of acute disease have sustained subjective and somatic sequelae following WNV infection. Thus, the neurological and functional disability associated with WNV infection represents a considerable source of morbidity in patients long after their recovery from acute illness.[1008–1011]

Although most human WNV infections occur after the bite of an infected *Culex* mosquito, other routes have been reported including via transfusion, organ transplantation, congenital, and breast milk transmission. In 2002, 23 cases of WNV infection were identified after transfusion of blood products.[864] These cases led to the development and implementation of nucleic acid amplification tests, which have been used to identify infected pools or individual blood product samples[143,871] and largely prevent transmission by transfusion. Nucleic acid screening of blood donors has not completely eliminated transfusion-transmitted WNV infections as "breakthrough" infections have occurred and were attributed to units that had levels of viremia below the sensitivity of the screening assay.[144] In addition to transfusion-associated WNV infection, organ transplantation–associated cases have been reported.[566,570] Because of the relatively low incidence of WNV infection in organ transplantation and risk of false positives that can occur with wide-scale testing, screening is not mandated.

Pathological Features of WNV Infection

WNV causes encephalitis in several vertebrate species including humans, horses, and birds, by virtue of its ability to infect and cause injury to neurons through direct (viral-induced) and indirect (immune response induced) mechanisms.[172] Pathologic observations in humans, however, are limited by the small number of autopsy studies on individuals succumbing to WNV infection. Gross macroscopic examination of organs (brain, lung, kidney, and spleen) tends to be unremarkable.[843] Microscopic examination of the brain in humans and other animals reveals histological changes that are consistent with the clinical disease.[298,843] This includes neuronal cell death, activation of resident microglia and infiltrating macrophages, perivascular and parenchymal accumulation of CD4[+] and CD8[+] lymphocytes and CD138[+] plasma cells, and the formation of microglial nodules. These lesions, which tend to be patchy in distribution, occur in the brainstem, cerebral cortex, hippocampus, thalamus, and cerebellum.[843] Additionally, overt meningitis with cellular infiltrates in the meninges can be apparent. In some cases, destruction of vascular structures with focal hemorrhage is present, suggestive of a vasculitis; this may be associated with local compromise of the blood–brain barrier.[262,1180] Immunohistochemical analysis and *in situ* hybridization confirm that WNV antigen and RNA are present in neurons from multiple regions of the brain, although other cells (e.g., astrocytes or CD11b[+] myeloid cells) may be infected to lesser degrees.[228,270]

WNV infection also causes a poliomyelitis-like syndrome of acute flaccid paralysis.[365,613] Patients show markedly decreased motor responses in the paretic limbs, preserved sensory responses, and widespread asymmetric muscle denervation without evidence of demyelination or myopathy.[613] Microscopically, in the spinal cord, an intense inflammatory infiltrate around large and small blood vessels is observed with large numbers of microglia in the ventral horn. Anterior horn motor neurons are targeted by WNV,[613,1028] and studies suggest that axonal transport from peripheral neurons can mediate WNV entry into the spinal cord and induce acute flaccid paralysis.[964]

A recent study in mice suggested that WNV infection in pregnancy, similar to ZIKV, might have the potential to cause congenital anomalies in fetuses. WNV replicated efficiently in human placental explants and caused similar levels of placental infection, transplacental transmission, and fetal demise in immunocompetent mice.[885] Several prior studies examined small cohorts of women infected with WNV during pregnancy and their offspring,[838,893,1042] including one study of 77 pregnant women. Among infants born to WNV-infected mothers, two had microcephaly, one had lissencephaly, and eight exhibited abnormal postnatal growth, suggesting a microcephaly rate of 2.6% in this group of WNV-infected neonates. Although a statistically significant link between congenital WNV infection and microcephaly was not established given the small numbers, more study of this possibility may be warranted.

Although most mammalian WNV infections are cleared by the adaptive immune response, persistence in the kidney has been described, albeit infrequently. Hamsters experimentally infected with WNV developed chronic renal infection and viruria for up to 8 months despite clearance from blood and the appearance of neutralizing antibodies. Although minimal histopathology was reported, WNV antigen staining was detected in the renal epithelium, interstitial cells, and tubules.[1110] Interestingly, these persistent viruses evolved genetically and no longer caused neuroinvasive disease on challenge of naïve animals.[1212] Analogous to the studies in hamsters, WNV RNA was demonstrated in 5 of 25 urine samples from convalescent humans 1.6 to 6.7 years after the initial infection, although infectious virus was not successfully isolated.[806] In separate studies, higher viral RNA copy numbers were measured in the urine samples compared with the serum sample from the same patient during the acute phase,[813] although only a small fraction tested positive approximately 5 months later.[67]

Persistent WNV infection in the CNS also has been suggested by experimental infection studies in monkeys, hamsters, and mice. In monkeys, WNV persisted at least 5.5 months after initial infection and was isolated in the cerebellum and cerebral subcortical ganglia but had lost its neurovirulence and cytopathic properties.[889] In hamsters, persistent WNV RNA and foci of WNV antigen–positive cells were identified in the CNS of hamsters between 28 and 86 days after infection,[1033] and this was associated with long-term neurological sequelae. In mice, infectious WNV persisted in the brains of wild-type animals up to 4 months, and viral RNA could be detected at 6 months in up 12% of mice, even in animals with subclinical infection.[30] Consistent with this observation, a model of persistent WNV disease was identified in a panel of genetically diverse mice, with virus in the brain observed for approximately 2 months.[386] The authors postulated that regulatory T-cell responses restrained the immune response, preventing clearance of the infection.

Japanese Encephalitis Virus

History, Global Distribution, and Epidemic Cycle

JEV is a mosquito-transmitted flavivirus and the prototype virus of the JEV antigenic serocomplex. JEV causes severe neurological disease, primarily in Asia, where it accounts for approximately 35,000 to 50,000 cases and 10,000 to 15,000 deaths annually.[1129] JEV epidemics originally were described in Japan in the 1870s, and the virus initially was recovered in 1935 from the brain of an infected human in Tokyo; this isolate was established as the prototype JEV strain (Nakayama).[615] While most human infections are asymptomatic, greater than 50% of the symptomatic cases are fatal or result in devastating long-term neurological sequelae.[1001] Moreover, as JEV-induced disease largely occurs in children living in rural areas, it is likely vastly underreported in most regions of Asia.[1001,1050]

The enzootic cycle of JEV is between waterbirds (e.g., egrets and herons) and mosquitoes, with pigs also serving as an amplifying host. JEV is transmitted primarily by *Culex* mosquitoes (principally *Culex tritaeniorhynchus*) that breed in rice fields and stagnant water. Humans are considered incidental targets and dead-end hosts, as they do not produce a viremia sufficient to infect mosquitoes. Two epidemiological patterns are observed: in northern temperate areas, JEV infections occur during the summer months, whereas as in tropical climates, year-round transmission of JEV has been described.[381]

Globally, despite the introduction of several inactivated and live attenuated vaccines (see below), JEV remains an important cause of arthropod-transmitted viral encephalitis. Disease caused by JEV is widely distributed in Asia with outbreaks occurring in Japan, China, Taiwan, Korea, the Philippines, India, parts of Southeast Asia, and the Far Eastern region of Russia. While cases in China appear to be declining, possibly due to vaccination campaigns, epidemic activity in India, Nepal, and other parts of Southeast Asia appears to be escalating. More recently, JEV has been described in Pakistan, Papua New Guinea, and Australia, suggesting that its geographic range may be expanding.[438,439]

JEV Diversity

Phylogenetic analysis suggests that JEV evolved from an ancestral flavivirus in Africa, within the last few centuries.[377] Based on sequence analysis primarily of the viral structural genes, JEV was initially classified into a single serotype with four genotypes (I–IV),[192,193,1134] with as much as 12% variation at the nucleotide level. These divisions have been confirmed by full-length genome sequencing on a subset of isolates. Genotype I includes isolates from Thailand, Cambodia, Korea, China, Japan, Vietnam, Taiwan, and Australia from 1967 to the present. Genotype II includes strains from Thailand, Malaysia, Indonesia, Papa New Guinea, and Australia from 1951 to 1999. Genotype III includes isolates recovered from mostly temperate areas of Asia including Japan, China, Taiwan, the Philippines, and the Asian subcontinent between 1935 and the present. Finally, genotype IV includes strains from Indonesia that were isolated only in 1980 and 1981. A fifth, more divergent genotype (V) was defined based on full-genome sequencing of a 1952 isolate from a patient in the Muar region of Malaysia[760] and a second isolate from *Culex tritaeniorhynchus* mosquitoes from 2011.[621] Genotype V strains have approximately 20% and 9% nucleotide and amino acid divergence, respectively, and showed significant variation with respect to neutralization by JEV-specific monoclonal antibodies.[445] Additional sequence fragments of genotype V strains have been detected more recently in Korea,[527] suggesting the possible emergence of this more diverse JEV clade.

Because genotypes I and III largely were isolated in epidemic regions, and genotypes II and IV were associated with endemic transmission, differences in strain virulence were hypothesized to explain the epidemiological patterns of JEV.[193] However, as the geographic range of JEV has expanded, there are now several examples in which strains of individual genotypes cause either epidemic or endemic disease depending on the region or country.[1054]

Clinical Features of JEV Infection

In humans, JEV infection can be asymptomatic or produce a range of syndromes including a mild nonspecific febrile illness, aseptic meningitis, seizures, encephalitis, and poliomyelitis-like flaccid paralysis. Disease onset usually begins with a 1- to 2-week period of flu-like symptoms including headache, fever, cough, and upper respiratory symptoms as well as gastrointestinal complaints such as nausea, vomiting, and diarrhea. In infants and young children, the disease can progress rapidly as the virus invades the CNS and infects and injures neurons. CNS invasion is heralded by nuchal rigidity, photophobia, and altered mental status. JEV infection in the CNS can share features with Parkinson disease including mask-like facies, hypertonia, tremor, and cogwheel rigidity. Other CNS symptoms include seizures (more common in children than adults), ataxia, involuntary movements (e.g., choreoathetosis, facial grimacing,

and lip smacking), and cranial nerve palsies. Associated with this are elevated white blood cell counts and pressure in the CSF and abnormal EEG examinations. Imaging studies in the brain have revealed thalamic and basal ganglia abnormalities during the acute phase of the disease.[1050] Upper rather than lower extremity paralysis is more common, and lower motor neuron disease of the spinal cord can develop. Death can occur, especially in children, within 3 to 5 days of CNS symptoms or much later due to complications associated with hospitalization or cardiopulmonary status. A prospective study evaluated the clinical features and long-term prognosis of 118 children with encephalitis due to JEV in Malaysia.[845] Only 44% of patients had a full recovery, with 8% dying during the acute phase of the illness and 31% having persistent and severe neurological sequelae. These included chronic seizures, motor dysfunction, and neuropsychiatric symptoms such as mental retardation and psychiatric disorders.

Pathological Features of JEV Infection

JEV infection in the brain results in neuronal degeneration, necrosis, microglial nodule formation, and perivascular and parenchymal leukocyte infiltrates as well as focal hemorrhage. Parenchymal damage in the CNS is attributed to both direct cytopathic effect of the virus in nonrenewing populations of neurons and the resultant inflammatory state induced by activated microglia and infiltrating leukocytes. While these histological findings can occur throughout the brain, they usually are more restricted to the gray matter in the cortex, midbrain, and brainstem, providing anatomical correlates for the tremor and dystonias associated with CNS infection. Focal lesions are seen predominantly in the thalamus and cerebral peduncles but also are observed in the substantia nigra, cerebral and cerebellar cortices, and the anterior horn of the spinal cord,[1050] the latter of which is associated with a poliomyelitis-like acute flaccid paralysis.[1053] In patients that die rapidly, there may be little histological evidence of inflammation, but instead, high levels of JEV antigen can be detected in morphologically intact neurons.[494]

St. Louis Encephalitis Virus

History, Global Distribution, and Epidemic Cycle

St. Louis encephalitis virus (SLEV) is a mosquito-borne member of the JEV serocomplex capable of causing severe neurological disease in humans. SLEV was first discovered in 1933 following a large epidemic of encephalitis in St. Louis, Missouri (1,095 cases and 225 deaths).[242,679,919] More than 10,000 cases of severe illness and 1,000 deaths have since been attributed to SLEV infection, reflecting annual endemic transmission (~50 cases/year) punctuated by epidemic periods that occur every 5 to 15 years.[763] At least 41 epidemics of SLEV have occurred in the United States since 1933,[242] the largest of these in 1975.[220] During this epidemic, SLEV cases were reported in 29 states and the District of Columbia; the greatest number of illnesses occurred in Ohio, Mississippi, Indiana, and Illinois. Roughly 1,500 confirmed cases were reported, resulting in 171 fatalities. The most recent large outbreak of SLEV occurred in central Florida during 1990, resulting in 222 laboratory-confirmed cases and 14 deaths.[728] A more contemporary study reviewed the SLEV surveillance data in the United States for 2003 through 2017, including human disease cases and nonhuman infections.[225] Over the 15-year period, 198 counties from 33 states reported SLEV activity; 94 of those counties reported SLEV activity only in nonhuman species and 193 human SLEV infections were documented, including 148 cases of neuroinvasive disease. Among these cases, clusters of infections were reported in Arizona and California in 2015.[1198]

SLEV distribution ranges from Canada to Argentina and across North America.[919] SLEV is maintained in nature in enzootic cycles between *Culex* mosquitoes and birds (primarily songbirds and pigeons). The transmission cycle of this virus varies by region due to differences in the biology of the primary vector mosquitoes.[919] In the eastern and central United States, the principal vectors of SLEV are *Culex pipiens* and *Culex quinquefasciatus* mosquitoes. *Culex tarsalis* is the primary vector for SLEV in Western states, whereas *Culex nigripalpus* transmits SLEV in Florida. The avian hosts of SLEV in these transmission cycles include house finches, house sparrows, and mourning doves. The mechanism of virus transmission and amplification in South and Central America is less clear. SLEV has been isolated from 11 different mosquito genera, many of which feed primarily on mammals.

Both WNV and SLEV are antigenically related members of the JEV serogroup that share a similar transmission cycle between *Culex* mosquitoes and birds. How the introduction of WNV in North America has impacted the epidemiology of SLEV is of significant interest. Analysis of the number of neuroinvasive cases attributed to SLEV reported to the CDC between 1999 and 2007 revealed a threefold reduction by comparison to data in the pre-WNV era.[918] Interpretation of this finding is complicated by changes in the intensity of surveillance and local testing for arboviral diseases in the years after the introduction of WNV. Because major epidemics of SLEV have occurred infrequently in the past, the modest number of clinical cases may simply reflect a nadir in the natural cycle of this virus. Alternatively, the existence of cross-reactive antibodies in WNV-immune avian reservoirs may disrupt the transmission cycle of SLEV via competition for avian hosts. While the infection of house finches with WNV has been shown to confer protection from subsequent infection by SLEV, the reciprocal is not true. Prior exposure of finches to SLEV prevents mortality following WNV infection but not the level of viremia that is sufficient for transmission of WNV.[314] Similar findings were reported in a golden hamster model of infection.[1111] The disappearance of SLEV from regions of California following the introduction of WNV is consistent with the notion that competition may allow for the local displacement of the virus from historically endemic areas.[920]

SLEV Diversity

Phylogenetic studies grouped SLEV isolates into seven genetic lineages (I–VII), many of which were divided further into clades of related genotypes.[558,717] These groups correspond roughly to the geographic distribution of each lineage of SLEV.[1126] For example, lineage I includes viruses isolated in the western United States, whereas lineage V contains South American strains and an isolate from Trinidad. However, the relationship between phylogenetic relatedness and geographic region is imperfect. SLEV strains vary considerably with respect to virulence in avian and mammalian hosts; these differences correlate roughly with geographic distribution.[114,772] In addition to

regional persistence, sequence analysis reveals that SLEV may be transported between regions.[558]

Clinical and Pathological Features of SLEV Infection

As is the case for both WNV and JEV, the majority of SLEV infections of humans are clinically asymptomatic. The ratio of apparent to inapparent infections has been reported to range from 1:16 to 1:425.[763] Increasing age is a significant factor influencing susceptibility to severe illness. Symptomatic illness is noted after an incubation period of 5 to 15 days and is characterized by mild malaise, fever, headache, nausea, myalgia, sore throat, and cough.[128] Severe neurological manifestations including encephalitis and aseptic meningitis may occur and can be fatal. Case fatality rates for SLEV range from 5% to 20%, with fatalities increasing in the elderly.[919] While most SLEV cases resolve spontaneously and without sequelae, many patients (30%–50%) experience an extended convalescence lasting up to 3 years. This phase is characterized by headache, depression, memory loss, and weakness.[128,919]

Tick-Borne Encephalitis Viruses
History, Global Distribution, and Epidemic Cycle

TBEV causes a fatal neurological syndrome that primarily occurs in northern China and Japan, through Russia, to parts of Northern Europe.[698] TBEV infection was first described in 1931 after a pattern of seasonal meningoencephalitis cases in Austria.[992] In 1939, experiments confirmed that this seasonal encephalitis in humans was caused by a virus transmitted by the tick, *Ixodes persulcatus*.[1256] Although a highly effective formalin-inactivated vaccine has been implemented in some European countries (e.g., Austria) with marked reductions in case numbers,[451] TBEV-induced morbidity and mortality continue to rise.[1086] Between 1990 and 2012, over 65,500 cases of TBE were reported in 18 European countries.[1242] TBEV is believed to cause several thousand human cases per year, the majority of which occur in parts of Russia.[395] This increase is thought to be due to changes in climate, population dynamics and range of permissive ticks, and shifts in land usage. Seroprevalence in domestic animals in Eastern Europe has shown good spatial correlation with TBEV incidence in humans.[483] Within Russia, Siberia has the highest number of TBEV cases, whereas outside of Russia, the Czech Republic has the greatest incidence.[698] The relative virulence of TBEV increases with its eastward spread, with the Far Eastern subtype having a case fatality rate of almost 40%.

In the enzootic cycle, TBEV is maintained between ticks and different vertebrate hosts, with humans as incidental hosts (Fig. 9.9). TBEV is primarily transmitted by the hard tick *Ixodes ricinus*, although in Eastern Europe and Russia, the principal vector is *Ixodes persulcatus*. Infection is seasonal, usually occurring between March and November,[504] and coincides with peaks of feeding activity of the particular tick vector. TBEV is endemic from Central Europe to Far East Asia with cases reported in 34 countries.[1085] Ticks can become chronically infected after ingesting viremic blood or by transstadial or transovarial transmission. In addition, infected ticks can transmit virus to uninfected ticks during cofeeding on rodents.[395,587] This is because the local skin environment supports TBEV replication, and migratory infected cells transport virus within the skin allowing for transmission in the absence of viremia.[586]

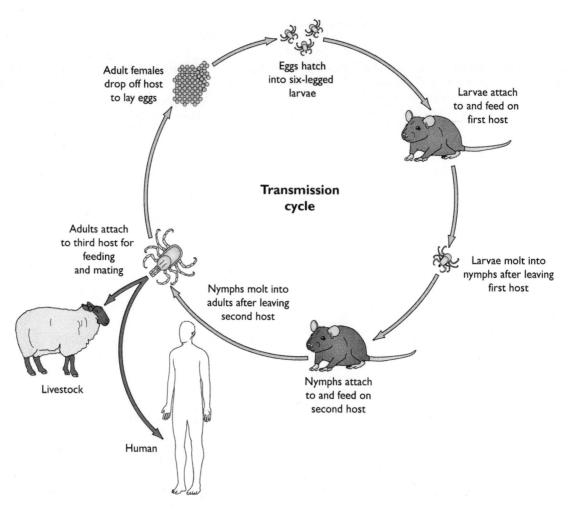

FIGURE 9.9 Transmission cycle of tick–borne encephalitis virus. TBEV transmission is connected to the life cycle of the vector due to a requirement for the tick to feed prior to transition through each of its developmental stage. Ticks are infected during this blood meal, molt, and then may infect a mammalian host. Nonviremic transmission between cofeeding ticks has also been shown to be an important mechanism of transmission and is not pictured.

One exception to TBEV transmission by tick inoculation is the syndrome of biphasic milk fever, which results from oral infection and was first identified in Russia between 1947 and 1951. During milk fever epidemics, whole families contracted TBEV infection, and this was associated with the consumption of goat milk. Goats develop subclinical TBEV infection after tick bite and become the source of infectious virus after secretion into milk. Analogously, TBEV transmission to humans has been reported after consumption of unpasteurized cow or sheep milk or dairy products.[395] These findings are supported by experiments in mice in which TBEV infection was established after oral feeding.[888]

TBEV Diversity

Based on sequence similarity, three main subtypes of TBEV exist: the Far Eastern genotype 1 (previously Russian spring and summer encephalitis), European genotype 2 (previously Central European encephalitis), and Siberian genotype 3 (previously West Siberian). Within these three genotypes, there is approximately 1.2% to 1.7% difference at the amino acid level. The Far Eastern, European, and Siberian genotypes 1, 2, and 3 differ from each other by approximately 5% to 7% at the amino

acid level. In addition to these three TBEV genotypes, two additional genotypes (4 and 5) have been described based on nucleotide and amino acid differences.[255] Other viruses that are antigenically related across Europe, Asia, and North America are classified as part of the TBEV serocomplex,[151] also termed the mammalian group of TBFVs. Besides TBEV, this group includes Omsk hemorrhagic fever virus (OHFV), louping-ill virus, Langat virus (LGTV), Powassan virus (POWV), Kyasanur Forest disease virus (KFDV), Kadam virus (KADV), Royal Farm virus (RFV), Gadgets Gully virus (GGYV), Alkhurma hemorrhagic fever virus (AHFV), and Karshi virus (KSIV). Of these viruses, TBEV, LIV, and POWV cause encephalitis in humans and animals, whereas OHFV, KFDV, and AHFV cause hemorrhagic fever.[396,952] LGTV is a naturally occurring avirulent virus (analogous to Kunjin virus among WNV strains), and no clinical disease has been reported for KSIV, RFV, or GGYV.

Clinical Features of TBEV Infection

About one-third of patients after inoculation by an infected tick will become symptomatic,[504] with men affected twice as frequently as women, although this could reflect exposure bias. The incubation period for TBEV infection in humans varies but for most individuals is approximately 1 to 2 weeks. A prodrome of fatigue, musculoskeletal pain, and headache lasts a few days and is followed by an abrupt onset of fever, nausea, vomiting, and myalgia; this phase is associated with thrombocytopenia, leukopenia, and mildly elevated levels of liver enzymes in the serum. Subsequent to this, several clinical syndromes of TBEV infection develop, as reviewed previously[395,504]: (a) *Febrile syndrome.* This illness is characterized by high fever (39°C) with no evidence of neuroinvasion. It lasts from 1 to 5 days, and upon defervescence, patients recover completely; (b) *Meningitis.* This is the most common form of clinically apparent TBEV infection occurring in approximately 50% of individuals. After the onset of fever, symptoms worsen with progressive headache, nausea, vomiting, and photophobia. Patients exhibit cerebrospinal fluid leukocyte pleocytosis after lumbar puncture. Fever lasts 1 to 2 weeks, with gradual recovery; (c) *Meningoencephalitis.* This form occurs in approximately 10% of cases, is more severe, and is associated with damage to the CNS. Individuals become weak and lethargic and develop focal signs of disease including hemiparesis, hemiplegia, seizures, and autonomic instability. Up to 30% of these cases are fatal, and survivors have long-term neurological sequelae with slow convalescence; (d) *Poliomyelitis-like disease.* This is characterized by a prodrome of limb weakness or numbness that progresses to paralysis. Paralysis occurs more frequently in the upper limbs, with the proximal segments affected more often. Recovery is slow, is partial, and occurs in only one-half of patients, with the remainder showing progressive deterioration; (e) *Polyradiculitis.* This syndrome has a biphasic course with fever, headache, and myalgia followed by defervescence. Approximately one week later the second phase starts and is characterized by pain and damage in peripheral nerves, sometimes coupled with meningitis. Recovery from this form of TBEV infection is usually complete; (f) *Chronic or persistent infection.* This form has been described in Siberia and Far East Russia although not in Europe and is believed to associate uniquely with the Siberian subtype of TBEV. Chronic or persistent infection is characterized by a late phase (months or even years later) deterioration of the neurological sequelae that developed during the acute illness. Alternatively, chronic TBEV infection can begin with the acute phase of disease, such that neurological symptoms occur years after a tick bite. Clinical symptoms can include epilepsy, parkinsonian movement and cognitive disorders, and progressive muscle atrophy, ultimately with dementia and death ensuing. Although infectious virus has not been routinely recovered in autopsy studies, a TBEV strain was isolated from a patient who died of a progressive (2-year) form of tick-borne encephalitis 10 years after experiencing a tick bite[394]; and (g) *Postencephalitic syndrome.* Both retrospective and prospective clinical trials have shown that TBEV infection is associated with a slow recovery period that has considerable long-term morbidity.[403,503,746] This postencephalitic syndrome occurs in approximately 40% to 60% of patients and includes memory disturbances, headache, and affective and gait disorders. The frequency of these symptoms was proportionately higher in more severe cases.

Pathological Features of TBEV Infection

Gross pathologic analysis of the brain of humans who succumb to lethal TBEV infection shows edema and hyperemia. Microscopic lesions occur in a patchy distribution throughout the CNS but are most prominent in the brainstem, basal ganglia, thalamus, cerebellum, and spinal cord. The cerebral and spinal meninges show a diffuse leukocyte infiltration, predominantly with lymphocytes. In the parenchyma of the brain and spinal cord, perivascular infiltrates, microglial nodules, and necrosis of neurons are observed. Notably, Purkinje cell neurons in the cerebellum and anterior horn motor neurons in the spinal cord are preferentially targeted and injured by TBEV.[504] Immunohistochemical analysis of brains from 28 autopsy cases[353] showed prominent TBEV antigen staining in Purkinje cells, neurons of the dentate gyrus, the brainstem, and basal ganglia, with T lymphocytes detected in direct apposition to TBEV-infected neurons.

Emergence of POWV in the United States

POWV is a tick-borne flavivirus that was first isolated from the brain of a child who died of encephalitis in Powassan, Ontario, in 1958.[719] Human cases of POWV have been reported in the United States, Canada, and Russia.[458] Although POWV infections are relatively rare, they can cause severe neuroinvasive disease including meningitis and encephalitis. Approximately 10% of neuroinvasive POWV cases are fatal, and 50% of survivors suffer long-term neurological sequelae.[458] POWV is emerging, as increasing numbers of cases have been diagnosed in the United States over the past decade[562] and up to 3% to 5% of *Ixodes scapularis* ticks isolated in parts of the United States now test positive for POWV.[18,543]

Two genetic lineages of POWV circulate in North America, lineage I and lineage II (also called deer-tick virus [DTV]), that share at least 96% amino acid identity in their E proteins.[296] POWV lineage I strains are predominantly maintained in *Ixodes cookei* ticks and include isolates from New York and Canada, whereas lineage II strains are found in *Ixodes scapularis* deer ticks and include strains from regions infested by these ticks.[296] Although POWV has been found predominantly in north central and northeastern parts of the United States in *Ixodes* species ticks, POWV also has been isolated from *Dermacentor andersoni* ticks, indicating the vector and geographical range may be larger than estimated.

PATHOGENESIS AND IMMUNITY

Virus Attachment

Flavivirus entry into cells is mediated by the E proteins and can be considered in three discrete steps (Fig. 9.10). The first step involves the attachment of the virion to the target cell. Collisions between virions and target cells are not always productive. "Attachment factors" promote infection by increasing the duration of contact between the virion and cell surface and thereby increase the likelihood that subsequent steps in the virus entry pathway will occur. Attachment factors are not strictly required for infection. In contrast, interactions with viral "receptors" promote required events during virus entry. While the distinction between these two types of cellular factors is clear for some viruses (e.g., HIV), the cell biology of flavivirus entry remains poorly understood, as no cellular factor is required for fusion between the virion and membranes once exposed to an acidic environment.[215,369] Several cellular factors have been shown to function as attachment factors or receptors during the flavivirus entry as discussed below.

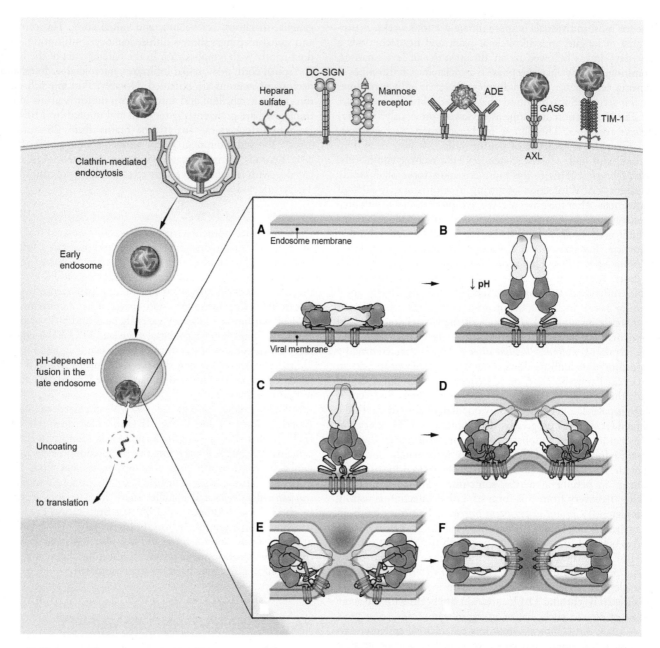

FIGURE 9.10 Flavivirus entry into cells. The entry of flaviviruses into mammalian cells is mediated by interactions with a variety of cell surface–expressed host factors. These include heparan sulfate, C-type lectins (DC-SIGN, DC-SIGNR, and mannose receptor), and members of the phosphatidylserine receptor family including TIM-1 and AXL. Viruses complexed with antibodies also efficiently attach to cells expressing Fc receptors. Flaviviruses enter cells via clathrin-mediated endocytosis and then traffic to endosomal compartments in which fusion occurs. The mechanism of fusion is depicted in the **inset**. Exposure of the E protein dimers present on mature virions **(A)** to a mildly acid environment results in their disassociation and a conformational change that projects E-DII away from the virion membrane **(B)**. This orients the E-DII-FL in a position where it may insert in the target cell membrane. E proteins in this extended conformation next form trimers **(C)**. The stem anchor packs into grooves of the core trimer **(D–F)** as the molecule folds back on itself and pulls viral and host membranes into proximity. Antibodies have the potential to block multiple steps in this virus entry pathway. (This figure was modified from Pierson TC, Kielian M. Flaviviruses: braking the entering. *Curr Opin Virol* 2013;3:3–12.)

Glycosaminoglycans

The interactions between flaviviruses and glycosaminoglycans (GAGs) have been documented.[191,464,609,694] The binding site on the virion for these sulfated polysaccharides has been mapped to positively charged surfaces of the E protein.[191,694] GAGs promote more efficient attachment to cells via electrostatic interactions with the virus particle. Passage of virus in cell culture selects for variants that bind more efficiently to GAGs,

although this adaptation appears to be associated with reduced fitness *in vivo*.[608,610,694] Treatment of cells with soluble heparin sulfate can inhibit infection.[191,612,647]

Lectins

The prM and E proteins of flaviviruses may be modified by the addition of one or two N-linked complex- or high-mannose–type sugars. Host lectins may contribute to more efficient virion attachment through interactions with these viral sugars. CD209 (DC-SIGN) is a calcium-dependent (C-type) lectin that serves as an attachment factor for several classes of viruses (reviewed in Ref.[1142]), including some flaviviruses.[241,817,1104] CD209 is expressed *in vivo* on a subset of dendritic cells (DCs) and macrophages.[1142] The infectivity of DCs by DENV correlates with CD209 expression; immature DCs express CD209 and are more permissive to infection than mature DCs expressing lower levels of CD209.[1104,1210] Antibodies against CD209 or soluble forms of this lectin can block DENV infection of DCs.[817,1104] Experiments with truncated forms of CD209 suggest that internalization of CD209 is not required to increase the efficiency of virus attachment to selected cell types.[670] CD209L (DC-SIGNR)[241,1104] and the mannose receptor (MR)[747] also have been identified as attachment factors for flaviviruses. The genetic linkage between DENV disease severity and polymorphisms in the CD209 promoter is consistent with a role for this attachment factor in humans.[850]

Phosphatidylserine Receptor Family

Genetic complementation experiments first identified members of two phosphatidylserine receptor families as capable of enhancing interactions of flaviviruses with target cells.[729] These molecules bind negatively charged phosphatidylserine lipids incorporated into the inner leaflet of the plasma membrane that become exposed on the outer leaflet during the process of apoptosis.[310] Incorporation of phosphatidylserine into the lipid envelopes of viruses allows virions to hijack this pathway via a process referred to as apoptotic mimicry.[22] Many viruses exploit this pathway.[491] Molecules in the T-cell immunoglobulin domain and mucin domain (TIM) family of receptors bind phosphatidylserine directly and have been shown to facilitate virus entry, including TIM-1 and TIM-4. These molecules are expressed on lymphocytes and antigen-presenting cells (macrophages and dendritic cells) of the immune system and function as signaling molecules that coordinate immune functions. TYRO3 and AXL of the TAM (*TYRO3, AXL, MERTK*) family of tyrosine kinases indirectly mediate virus attachment through interactions with phosphatidylserine-binding proteins Gas6 or protein S. AXL is expressed widely and plays multiple roles in immune regulation, and in human diseases, including cancer and autoimmunity, when dysregulated. The signaling functions of TAM receptors are required to promote more efficient virus infection, although virus binding remains unaffected.[729,870]

A role for host factors of the TIM/TAM family in flavivirus infection *in vivo* was studied extensively in the wake of the emergence of ZIKV. Multiple studies demonstrated that expression of AXL enhanced ZIKV infection *in vitro*,[433,730] and this molecule was expressed on target cells *in vivo* with the potential to contribute to the unique pathogenesis of ZIKV.[568,831] Studies in knockout mice demonstrated that AXL was not required for ZIKV infection in mice deficient in interferon (IFN) receptor signaling[448,626,1181] or for WNV infection in mice with intact IFN signaling.[751] A role for AXL in pathogenesis may relate to its capacity to dampen the innate immune response in target cells or affect the blood–brain barrier.[194,751] It remains possible that human AXL may have a more significant role in flavivirus infectivity than its mouse ortholog.[926,975]

The Cell Biology of Flavivirus Entry

Flaviviruses enter cells via clathrin-mediated endocytosis.[3,202,368,560,1141] Single-particle tracking studies of DENV suggest that virions move across the surface of cells until they encounter preformed clathrin-coated pits. Virus particles are then internalized and traffic into endosomal compartments where viral fusion occurs. Fusion between viral and cellular membranes is triggered by the acidic environment of endosomes. The conformational changes in the E proteins that orchestrate membrane fusion have been studied using biochemical and structural approaches (reviewed in Ref.[877]).

Flavivirus Tropism

The molecular basis for the tropism of flaviviruses is incompletely understood. A wide variety of cell lines representing different lineages and species can be infected *in vitro*. This suggests that cellular factors involved in virus entry are either highly conserved (from arthropods to vertebrate hosts) or redundant. Alternatively, the adaptation of cell lines to continuous culture may select for expression of host factors used by virions *in vitro* distinct from those used *in vivo*. Targets for flavivirus infection *in vivo* appear more restricted. Target cell types infected by flaviviruses include monocytes, macrophages, DCs, hepatocytes, neurons, and endothelial cells.[51,963] Insights that followed emergence and unique pathogenesis of ZIKV identified the importance of placental cells and those of the male and female reproductive tract as important targets of infection.[149,382] Tropism may be regulated at a postentry level through the activities of IFN and IFN-stimulated genes (ISGs).[149,963]

Mechanisms of Dissemination

Viscerotropic Viruses

For both viscerotropic (e.g., DENV, ZIKV, and YFV) and encephalitic (e.g., WNV, JEV, and TBEV) flaviviruses, the skin is the likely initial infection site after vector inoculation, with resident dendritic cells[147,703] or epidermal keratinocytes[635] believed to be the primary target cells. Subsequently, recruitment of monocytes and monocyte-derived dendritic cells to the underlying dermis may provide additional targets for infection.[881,991] The dose of virus inoculated by mosquitoes under conditions of natural infection is not known precisely, but likely ranges from 10^3 to 10^5 plaque-forming units (PFU),[995,1076] depending on the flavivirus and vector species. Active WNV replication can be detected at the subcutaneous site of infection within one day of inoculation,[133] and viral spread to the lymph node occurs in animals infected by mosquitoes or with mosquito salivary extracts.[995,1077] Factors in mosquito saliva alter cytokine levels and other components of innate immunity, leading to local immunosuppression or dysregulation,[993] and enhanced viral spread and replication. One exception to this paradigm is the sexual transmission of ZIKV, where epithelial cells in the vagina (male-to-female) or rectum (male-to-male) likely are the initial targets of infection.

Flaviviruses disseminate to local lymph nodes either associated with migratory infected dendritic cells[900] or as free virus that transudates directly into lymphatic fluid.[501] Macrophages on the floor of the subcapsular sinus and in the medulla of lymph nodes capture viral particles, serving as additional targets of virus amplification and initiators of innate and adaptive immune responses.[501] Virus produced in the draining lymph nodes likely spreads to intravascular venous compartments via efferent lymphatic drainage. Virus in the bloodstream can directly infect blood cells or visceral tissues, which can result in further dissemination and secondary viremia.

The infectivity of flaviviruses in plasma, the fluid component of blood, appears remarkably short, with a half-life in mice ranging from 2 to 10 minutes for DENV and WNV, respectively.[339] The loss of infectivity is due in part to complement (C3 and C4 components) opsonization via mannose-binding lectin (MBL) recognition of N-linked glycans on the surface of virions[339] and binding by antibodies. The short half-life of an infectious flavivirus in plasma may also reflect sequestration and removal by different visceral organs.[485] Alternatively, flaviviruses may transit rapidly into the cellular compartment of blood. One study of patients with DENV infections of different disease severity showed DENV antigen (prM and NS3) predominantly in cells of monocyte (CD14+, CD32+) lineage, with up to 80% to 90% of cells of expressing viral antigen.[292] Analogously, CD14+ monocytes are principal targets of ZIKV infection in peripheral blood mononuclear cells.[332,745] The finding of DENV in blood monocytes is consistent with prior literature[699] but contrasts with studies in rhesus macaques suggesting that platelets become positive for dengue antigen during the course of infection.[844] Finally, another explanation for the rapid drop of plasma infectivity is that flaviviruses adhere readily to erythrocytes in whole blood.[934]

Neurotropic Viruses

Flavivirus neuropathogenesis requires neuroinvasiveness, the capacity to enter the CNS, and neurotropism, the ability to propagate efficiently within cells of the CNS. In classical studies, phenotypic distinctions were made among different arthropod-borne viruses on the basis of replication efficiency and pathogenic potential in peripheral versus CNS tissues.[13] A main principle was the relationship between peripheral viral burden and propensity for neuroinvasion. Viruses with a low capacity to replicate in the periphery generally had less neuroinvasive potential, regardless of their intrinsic neurovirulence. Aerosol-acquired infections are possible exceptions, as these may use alternate routes of CNS entry (e.g., accessing the olfactory bulb via the cribriform plate). Also, in the context of ZIKV vertical transmission, the viral burden in the mother likely facilitates infection of the maternal decidua, seeding of the fetally derived placenta, and dissemination to the fetal brain.[218]

Data from several studies indicate that the time of onset, magnitude, and duration of viremia, as well as the integrity of the host immune system, influences the risk of entry into the CNS. Thus, the neuropathogenic potential of most flaviviruses is a balance between replication efficiency and the effectiveness of early host defenses in clearing viremia. Neuroinvasiveness is affected by both viral and host factors. Based on genetic analysis of virulent and attenuated strains of JEV, TBEV, YFV, ZIKV, and WNV, viral determinants of neuroinvasiveness generally map to the E protein.[71,73,173,724,826,827] However, NS1 also may contribute to neuroinvasiveness of certain flaviviruses by modulating endothelial barrier function in a tissue-specific manner and influencing virus dissemination across tissue barriers.[896] The precise mechanisms associated with these viral genetic determinants have not been determined but are believed to relate to increased viral infectivity of key target cells through enhanced binding and penetration or induction of proinflammatory cytokines and disruption of the endothelial glycocalyx-like layer.[361]

Animal models of infection of encephalitic flaviviruses have begun to define factors that govern virus entry into the CNS. Blood–brain barrier (BBB) crossing likely occurs through a hematogenous route, as increased viral burden in the serum correlates with earlier and enhanced neuroinvasion.[265] Accordingly, changes in endothelial barrier permeability may facilitate CNS entry; these may be triggered by vasoactive cytokines (e.g., TNF-α)[680,1180] or activation of matrix metalloproteinases that degrade the BBB extracellular matrix.[1152,1169] Nonetheless, other cytokines and signaling pathways, including type I and III IFNs and TAM receptors, can tighten the BBB and prevent virus and immune cell crossing.[236,599,751] Additional mechanisms may contribute to CNS infection of flaviviruses, including (a) direct infection of or passive transport through the endothelium[284,654,1153]; (b) infection of olfactory neurons and rostral spread from the olfactory bulb.[133] Access through the olfactory bulb is believed to occur after infection by aerosol or intranasal routes[812,828,909] as well as in the context of peripheral inoculation.[725] The olfactory bulb is vulnerable to direct infection because of the exposure of its nerve terminals within the olfactory mucosa; (c) virus is transported by infected immune cells trafficking into the CNS[1183]; (d) Access to the CNS after breakdown of BBB integrity[182,544]; and (e) Retrograde axonal transport from infected peripheral neurons.[481,786,964,1179] Although much has been learned from infection studies in mice and hamsters, the precise mechanisms of CNS entry of encephalitic flaviviruses in humans and other animals require additional study.

Mechanisms of Immune Control—Innate Immunity

Cellular Innate Immunity

Monocytes and macrophages

Monocytes and macrophages play key roles in orchestrating control of flaviviruses but also can become targets and reservoirs of infection. Recent studies of human patients infected with ZIKV showed that CD14+CD16+ monocytes are principal targets of infection in peripheral blood.[745] Because monocytes can infiltrate many tissues, they may act as "Trojan horses" for the spread of infection across tissue compartments. Analogously, after DENV infection, sorting of peripheral blood mononuclear cells revealed that CD14+ monocytes were infected with DENV and produced the inhibitory cytokine IL-10.[1040] In a mouse model of primary infection, Ly6C^{hi} monocytes were recruited to the DENV-infected dermis and differentiated to monocyte-derived DCs, which then became targets for DENV replication.[991] During secondary DENV infection, DENV can be opsonized with non- or subneutralizing antibody levels that augment entry and infection of monocytes through activating Fc-gamma receptors (FcγRs).[426,539] In this context of enhanced infection, DENV immune complexes activate Syk to mediate elevated secretion of proinflammatory cytokines including IL-1β.[154]

Macrophages can limit infection through direct viral clearance, enhanced antigen presentation to B and T cells, and production of proinflammatory or antiviral cytokines and chemokines.[564,700] The protective role of macrophages is highlighted by studies in mice, which demonstrated exacerbated WNV, TBEV, DENV, or YFV disease after selective macrophage depletion.[81,136,326,522,900,1257] Macrophages may control flaviviruses through the production of nitric oxide (NO) and other reactive oxygen intermediates after stimulation of inducible nitric oxide synthase (NOS2).[559,646,978,979] Activation of macrophages in response to flavivirus infection also promotes the release of type I IFN, TNF-α, IL-1β, IL-8, and other cytokines, some of which have antiviral activity.[1031] Despite their protective role in innate defense, macrophages and microglia also are targets of infection by some flaviviruses[548,584,936] and have the potential to contribute to pathogenesis through ADE mediated by Fcγ and complement receptors.[162,367,866] The macrophage cell-surface receptor CLEC5A has been reported to interact with DENV and JEV directly, resulting in DAP12 phosphorylation, activation of the NLRP3 inflammasome, and the release of proinflammatory cytokines.[189,190,1209] Anti-CLEC5A mAb inhibited JEV-induced proinflammatory cytokine release from microglia and prevented bystander damage to neuronal cells. Thus, in some circumstances, macrophages can contribute to flavivirus-induced disease, although the contribution to clearance versus pathogenesis may vary depending on the specific virus, the presence of preexisting nonneutralizing antibodies, and the specific proinflammatory molecules that are produced.

Neutrophils

Although neutrophils are among the first circulating leukocytes to respond to infection or inflammatory stimuli, their function in flavivirus infection remains uncertain. While some studies suggest a protective function, others indicate that neutrophils can contribute to flavivirus pathogenesis. A protective role was reported in the context of WNV infection, as macrophages produced neutrophil chemoattractive chemokines (CXCL1 and CXCL2), neutrophils rapidly migrated to the site of infection, and mice depleted of neutrophils 1 or 2 days after virus infection developed higher viremia and experienced earlier death.[43] Paradoxically, if neutrophils were depleted prior to infection, viremia was reduced and survival was enhanced.[43] Analogously, depletion of neutrophils resulted in prolonged survival and decreased mortality in Murray Valley encephalitis virus–infected mice, and neutrophil infiltration and disease correlated with iNOS expression within the CNS.[26] Moreover, WNV burden, proinflammatory cytokines, and apoptotic cells in the CNS of *Il22*$^{-/-}$ mice were reduced, and this was associated with decreased neutrophil migration into the brain.[1168] Finally, transcriptional gene signatures from whole blood showed a greater abundance of neutrophil transcripts in patients who progressed to severe dengue, a finding supported by higher plasma levels of proteins associated with neutrophil degranulation.[468] Although further studies are warranted, neutrophils may prevent or promote flavivirus disease, depending on the specific virus and immunological context.

Dendritic cells

Human peripheral blood contains two major classes of dendritic cells (DCs), plasmacytoid DCs (pDCs) and myeloid DCs (mDCs), which can be distinguished based on function and surface markers. pDCs lack phagocytic capacity, are less efficient in capturing and presenting antigens to T cells, but produce extraordinarily high levels of type I IFN in the presence of viruses or bacteria,[1034] and are thus considered to have a crucial sentinel role in antiviral immunity.[1090,1091] In pDCs, flaviviruses can stimulate either TLR7 or RIG-I signaling in the same cell, depending on how its nucleic acid content is delivered (i.e., via internalization or active replication).[135]

Low levels of DENV replication are observed in pDC, but proinflammatory cytokines are produced rapidly and can accumulate to high levels. This cytokine response was not dependent on viral replication, but was dependent on endosomal TLR7, and could be induced by purified DENV RNA.[1083,1174] Immature virus particles, which carry viral RNA to the endolysosome-localized TLR7 sensor, may contribute to progression of dengue disease by eliciting a strong innate immune response in pDCs.[250] In prospective clinical studies, the absolute number of circulating pDC remained stable early in moderately ill children with dengue fever or other nondengue, febrile illnesses. However, there was an early decrease in circulating pDC in children who subsequently developed DHF, as a blunted blood pDC response was associated with an altered innate immune response, higher viremia levels, and severe disease.[874] Interestingly, the host origin of the flavivirus influences the response generated by pDC as WNV grown in mammalian cells was a potent inducer of IFN-α secretion in pDCs, whereas pDCs failed to produce IFN-α when exposed to WNV grown in mosquito cells.[1037]

mDCs reside and circulate throughout the body, enabling them to transport antigens from the periphery to lymphoid tissues. They are professional antigen-presenting cells that transmit incoming infectious signals to B and T cells, to orchestrate rapid and efficient adaptive immune responses.[1067] mDCs are more readily infected by flaviviruses *ex vivo* and are thought to contribute to viral spread and early immune system priming depending on the particular virus. For example, WNV efficiently infects mouse mDCs and induces a type I IFN and proinflammatory cytokine response through RIG-I–like pattern recognition receptors (PRRs) and MAVS-dependent signaling cascade.[231,1088] In comparison, JEV induced impaired responses in mice through MyD88-dependent and MyD88-independent pathways, with blunted costimulatory molecule expression and production of the anti-inflammatory cytokine IL-10, which resulted in poor T-cell priming.[15] DENV productively infects human mDCs and induces the release of high levels of chemokines and proinflammatory cytokines, with the notable exception of type I IFN,[941,942] although this latter finding has not been observed with all strains of DENV.[47,630] As an example, DENV-4 replication peaks earlier and promotes stronger innate immune responses, with increased expression of DC activation and migration markers and increased cytokine production, compared with DENV-2.[434] Apart from this, mature mDCs were capable of supporting ADE of DENV, whereas immature DC, due to the expression of higher levels of DC-SIGN, did not support ADE.[110]

Despite an accumulating wealth of data on purified mDCs *ex vivo*, few studies have assessed their direct function *in vivo* in the context of flavivirus infection. Selective genetic deletion of *Batf3* or *Wdfy4*, which affect CD8α^+ mDC (DC1) homeostasis or function, resulted in defective cross presentation and virus-specific CD8$^+$ T-cell responses to WNV in mice.[463,1116] However, JEV infection appears to actively suppress *in vivo* cross presentation of soluble and cell-associated antigens, resulting in diminished CD8$^+$ T-cell responses.[17]

Natural killer cells

Natural killer (NK) cells are innate immune lymphocytes that serve as a first line of defense against a variety of infections.[95] NK cells mediate protection through the recognition and killing of target cells and the production of immunomodulatory cytokines, particularly IFN-γ, which enhances innate immunity and shapes the subsequent adaptive immune response.[213] Unlike adaptive T and B lymphocytes, NK cells do not rearrange their receptor genes somatically but rely on inhibitory and activating cell receptors that recognize MHC class I and class I–like molecules, as well as other ligands.[138] The function of NK cells in flavivirus infection remains uncertain. Some *in vitro* studies suggest that human NK cells can inhibit WNV infection through both cytolytic (ADCC) and noncytolytic (IFN-γ) activities.[1246] The activating human NK cell receptor, NKp44, has been reported to bind directly to domain III of DENV and WNV E proteins. This interaction induced IFN-γ secretion and lysis of WNV-infected targets by NK cells.[460] However, flavivirus infection may inhibit NK cell killing by increasing the cell-surface expression of class I MHC molecules,[276,360,461,532] which sends an inhibitory signal to NK cells.[497] *In vivo*, the function of NK cells in flavivirus infection also remains unclear. While NK cells expand and become activated in YFV- and DENV-infected humans and mice,[183,820,1022] antibody depletion of NK cells in mice did not alter morbidity or mortality after WNV infection.[1029] In humans infected with TBEV, highly differentiated CD57+ NK cells were activated, but this was associated with decreased expression of perforin and granzyme B, as well as diminished NK cell responses to target cells.[104] However, in *ex vivo* experiments, the combination of type I IFN, TNF-α, and cell-surface receptor engagement with DCs enabled NK cells to overcome immune evasion by DENV.[643]

γδ T cells

γδ T cells contribute to the innate defense against several viruses by virtue of their abundance in epithelial and mucosal tissues and ability to respond rapidly to nonpeptide antigens by secreting proinflammatory cytokines and chemokines. As they lack classical MHC restriction, γδ T cells can react with viral antigens in the absence of conventional antigen processing.[1065] γδ T cells are divided into functionally distinct subsets, which have disparate effects on host immunity to pathogen infection.[715] As an example, Vγ4+ γδ T cells enhance Th1 cell activation through IFN-γ– and CD1-dependent mechanisms.[479] To date, much of the initial analysis of γδ T-cell function during flavivirus infection has focused on studies with WNV in mice, although recent studies confirm that human and monkey γδ T cells also are activated rapidly after YFV infection.[258,821] Mice deficient in γδ T cells were more susceptible to WNV infection,[1177] and this was in part due to their ability to produce IFN-γ, which has direct antiviral effects.[1030] Moreover, mice depleted of Vγ1+ γδ T cells have enhanced viremia and higher WNV mortality, whereas the opposite is observed with depletion of Vγ4+ γδ T cells.[1194] Subsequent work showed that γδ T cells also contribute to the development of a protective CD8+ T-cell response against WNV as TCRδ−/− mice were more susceptible than wild-type mice to secondary WNV challenge.[1170] This priming effect may reflect DC maturation (increased expression of surface costimulatory and class II MHC molecules and secretion of IL-12) that is promoted by γδ T cells after activation by WNV.[315]

Mast cells

Mast cells contribute to a variety of inflammatory reactions and host defense against pathogens by secreting chemokines, cytokines, and inflammatory lipid mediators and granule-associated products.[692] Mast cells express Fc receptors, reside primarily in tissues, and associate closely with vascular beds.[1012] Infection or activation of mast cells by DENV can promote viral clearance[1060] or have immunopathological consequences that contribute to the vasculopathy associated with secondary infection. DENV infection of mast cells *ex vivo* resulted in increased secretion of chemokines including CCL5 without inducing degranulation,[531] and production of vasoactive cytokines was enhanced in the presence of subneutralizing concentrations of antibody that promote ADE.[533] Mast cells also are targets of DENV in human skin, and this induces degranulation and alters cytokine expression profiles.[1128] Antibody-enhanced DENV infection of mast cells in culture also resulted in significant production of TNF-α that can stimulate endothelial cells[131] as well as massive mast cell apoptosis that occurs via global caspase activation.[132] Preexisting anti-DENV IgG can enhance both mast cell degranulation and vascular leakage during DENV infection.[1092] Thus, mast cells may contribute to a second mechanism of antibody-enhanced immune pathology during DENV infection that is dependent not on enhanced virus replication but on FcγR-mediated augmented degranulation responses. Drugs (e.g., ketotifen or leukotriene receptor antagonists) that stabilize mast cells diminished metabolic dysregulation, complement activation, and inflammation associated with DENV infection and pathogenesis in mice.[790,1059]

Cell-Intrinsic Immunity

Recognition and control of flaviviruses by host sensors

IFN responses are an essential host defense program against many viruses, including flaviviruses. IFNs are produced during the earliest stages of viral infection after recognition of pathogen-associated molecular patterns (PAMPs) by specific PRRs. Mammalian cells primarily detect and respond to RNA virus infection by recognizing non-self viral RNA or viral RNA structural elements through several distinct PRRs including the cell-surface and endosomal RNA sensors toll-like receptors 3 and 7 (TLR3 and TLR7) and the cytoplasmic RNA sensors retinoic acid–inducible gene I (RIG-I) and melanoma differentiation–associated gene 5 (MDA5) (Fig. 9.11). Binding of single- and/or double-stranded viral RNA to PRRs results in downstream activation of transcription factors, such as IFN-regulatory factors 3 and 7 (IRF3 and IRF7) and NF-κB, and induction of IFN-α and β. Secretion of IFNs followed by engagement of the IFN-αβ receptor (IFNAR) in an autocrine and paracrine fashion activates JAK–STAT-dependent and JAK–STAT-independent signal transduction cascades[622] that induce the expression of hundreds of ISGs, a subset of which have antiviral activity against flaviviruses (Fig. 9.12).[998]

RIG-I and MDA5 contribute to the induction of host IFN and antiviral response to flaviviruses. The highly structured 5′ region of the DENV and ZIKV genomes are recognized by RIG-I.[185] Fibroblasts deficient in RIG-I and MDA5 showed decreased IRF3 activation, delayed induction of IFN and ISG responses, and augmented WNV and DENV replication.[336,337,667,815] RIG-I primes the early type I IFN response, whereas MDA5 has a role in a second phase of ISG expression that occurs later in the course of infection, possibly due to accumulation of dsRNA replication intermediates. A genetic deficiency of MAVS, an essential RIG-I and MDA5 adaptor molecule that is anchored to mitochondria, completely

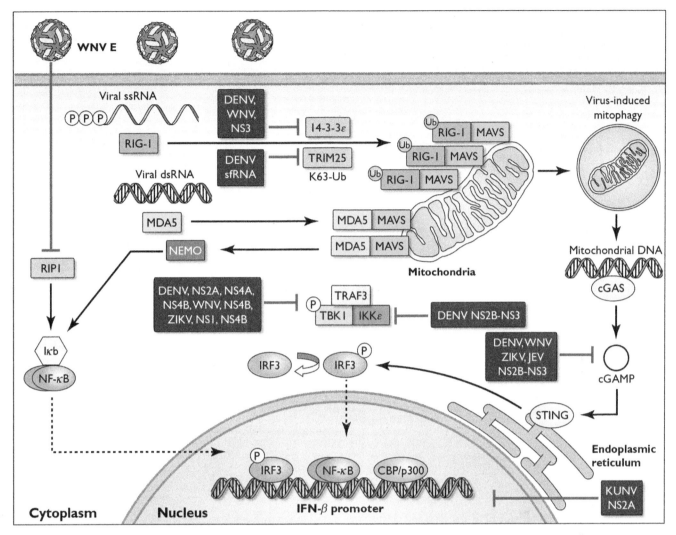

FIGURE 9.11 Detection of flavivirus RNA by cytosolic pathogen recognition receptors (PRRs) and mechanisms of viral evasion. Cytoplasmic PRR and signaling cascade. Infection by flaviviruses produces dsRNA replication intermediates that display motifs recognized by RIG-I and MDA5. Binding of viral RNA promotes an interaction with MAVS that results in recruitment of signaling proteins (NEMO and TRAF3) that activate IRF3 and NF-κB. These transcription factors translocate to the nucleus and bind to the promoter region of the IFN-β gene leading to transcription and translation. Mechanisms of evasion by flaviviruses include the following: (a) a delay in recognition of WNV RNA by RIG-I; (b) impairment of RIP-1 signaling by high-mannose carbohydrates on the structural E protein; (c) reduction in IFN-β gene transcription by the KUNV NS2A protein; (d) reduction of type I IFN production by catalytically active DENV NS2B-NS3 protein; and (e) viral dsRNA intermediates localize to specialized membrane vesicles, which prevent rapid detection by intracellular sensors such as RIG-I.

disabled the IFN response in fibroblasts[231,337] and was associated with enhanced WNV lethality and dysregulated immune responses in mice.[1088] RIG-I–dependent signaling appears dominant in mice as animals deficient in RIG-I were more vulnerable to JEV infection,[510] and a deficiency of proteins that regulate the TRIM25-mediated ubiquitination and activation of RIG-I resulted in enhanced WNV replication and mortality.[1167] Consistent with this, JEV and DENV induce the type I IFN response through a mechanism involving RIG-I/IRF3 and NF-κB.[176] Nonetheless, higher mortality rates, altered CD8+ T-cell responses, and increased viral infection in primary macrophages were observed after WNV infection in mice and cells lacking MDA5.[307,602] Despite data suggesting that RIG-I and MDA5 recognize flavivirus RNA and induce type I IFN

responses, IFN-α and IFN-β production in some cell types appears independent of MAVS[1088] or the downstream transcription factor IRF3.[113,227,230]

TLR3, which is expressed on the surface of fibroblasts and in the endosomes of myeloid cells, promotes IRF3 phosphorylation after binding double-stranded viral RNA through a signaling cascade that includes recruitment of TRIF and activation of the kinases TBK1 and IKKε.[714,999] Initial studies with TRIF-deficient fibroblasts suggested that TLR3 may be dispensable for recognition of flaviviruses in cells,[336] although subsequent cell culture studies showed a proinflammatory and protective effect of TLR3 after DENV infection.[815,1130] Experiments in *Tlr3*−/− mice have had conflicting results. *Tlr3*−/− mice injected by an intraperitoneal route paradoxically showed decreased

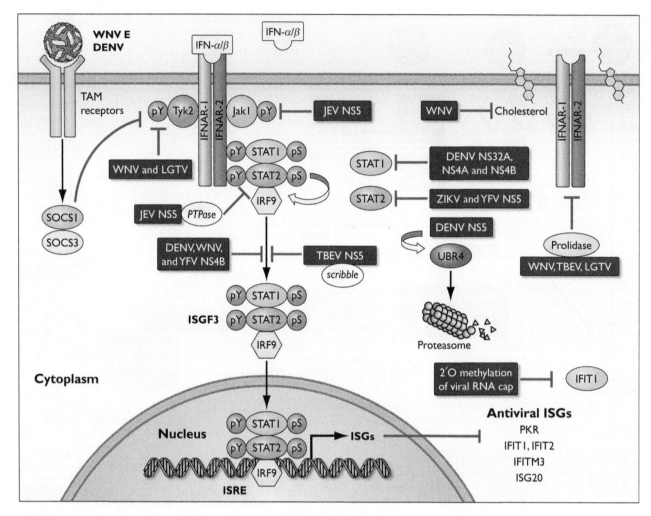

FIGURE 9.12 Type I interferon (IFN) signaling and mechanisms of disruption by flaviviruses. Secretion of IFN by a flavivirus-infected cell results in autocrine and paracrine signaling through the heterodimeric IFN-αβ receptor (IFNAR). IFN binding results in activation and tyrosine phosphorylation of JAK family members (JAK1 and Tyk2) and the cytoplasmic tail of IFNAR. This promotes recruitment of STAT1 and STAT2, which themselves become phosphorylated by the JAKs. Phosphorylated STAT1 and STAT2 proteins heterodimerize, associate with IRF9, and translocate to the nucleus, where they bind ISRE sequences to induce expression of hundreds of interferon-stimulated genes (ISGs). Mechanisms of evasion by flaviviruses include the following: blockade of phosphorylation of (a) Tyk2 and (b) JAK1 by flavivirus NS5; (c) activation of a phosphotyrosine phosphatase by JEV NS5; (d) reduction in STAT2 gene and protein expression by DENV and YFV NS5; (e) attenuation of STAT signaling by flavivirus NS4B; (f) down-regulation of IFNAR through virus-induced redistribution of cellular cholesterol; and (g) antagonism of IFIT family gene effector functions by 2'-O-methylation of flavivirus RNA.

WNV lethality despite higher peripheral viral titers, presumably because of blunted cytokine responses (e.g., TNF-α) that normally facilitate neuroinvasion.[1180] Consistent with a possible pathological role, preliminary studies suggest a functional TLR3 allele is a risk factor for severe human TBEV infection.[530] In comparison, other studies with *Tlr3*⁻/⁻ mice and a different WNV strain or with JEV showed increased viral burden in the brain and enhanced lethality,[228,437] as might be anticipated for a PRR that triggers a protective host immune response. *Ex vivo* and *in vivo* experiments suggest a cell-specific role of TLR3, as it protected against WNV largely by restricting replication in neurons. More recent studies have defined a link between ZIKV-mediated TLR3 activation, perturbed cell fate, and a reduction in the volume of cerebral organoid cultures, which suggests TLR3 activation may lead to disrupted neurogenesis.[235]

Although TLR4 is a PRR best known for its ability to recognize lipopolysaccharide present in many gram-negative bacteria, it may functionally impact flavivirus infection, immunity, and pathogenesis. A possible pathogenic role of TLR4 was suggested in studies with JEV, as *Tlr4*⁻/⁻ mice showed enhanced resistance to infection.[437] Genetic ablation of TLR4 resulted in enhanced type I IFN, humoral, and T-cell responses, which were mediated by increased numbers of pDCs and NK cells and reduced numbers of Tregs in lymphoid tissues. A second pathogenic role of TLR4 signaling was suggested when studies showed that DENV NS1 devoid of bacterial endotoxin activity directly activated human peripheral blood mononuclear and endothelial cells via TLR4, which induced the release of proinflammatory cytokines and chemokines. The importance of TLR4 activation *in vivo* was confirmed by the reduction in capillary leakage by a TLR4 antagonist in a mouse model of

DENV infection[756,757] and suggested by analysis of *TLR4* gene polymorphisms in human DENV patients.[1019] However, a second group did not corroborate these findings and observed that DENV NS1 induced vascular leakage in Tlr4-/- mice at similar levels to wild-type animals.[362]

TLR7 is an endosomal PRR that detects guanosine- and uridine-rich single-stranded RNA[268] and activates IRF7 via the adaptor molecule MyD88 IRF7 was identified as a primary regulator of antiviral gene induction after YFV infection,[351] with some of this activation occurring through TLR7 recognition of viral RNA.[906,907,1083,1174] Similarly, DENV stimulates IFN production in pDC in a TLR7-dependent manner after virus uncoating.[1174] The antiviral IFN-α response against WNV is primarily mediated by IRF7,[229] and at least some of this signal is attributed to recognition of viral RNA by TLR7. Indeed, both *Tlr7*[−/−] and *Myd88*[−/−] mice show increased susceptibility to WNV infection, and this was associated with increased local infection and yet decreased production of IL-1β, IL-6, IL-12 and IL-23 and several chemokines, which altered leukocyte trafficking and control in several tissues.[1094,1124,1195] Studies in aged mice showed that dysregulation of TLR7 signaling contributes to impaired innate and adaptive T-cell responses and an enhanced vulnerability in old mice during WNV infection.[1216]

In addition to using RNA sensors to detect flaviviruses, immune cells use the DNA-sensing machinery to detect intracellular damage generated early during infection by flaviviruses.[6] DENV infection induces mislocalization of mitochondrial DNA into the cytoplasm of infected cells.[7] The leaked mitochondrial DNA is detected by the DNA sensor cyclic GMP–AMP synthase (cGAS), which triggers the stimulator of IFN genes (STING) pathway and induction of type I IFN production. This mechanism likely explains why *cGAS*[−/−] and *STING*[−/−] mice and cells showed greater susceptibility to WNV infection.[997,1230]

Type I IFN signaling pathway

Type I IFNs induce an antiviral state by up-regulating genes with both direct and indirect inhibitory functions.[884] In humans and mice, there are multiple IFN-α genes (13 in humans, 14 in mice) and one IFN-β gene, in addition to multiple other subtypes.[1143] IFN-α and IFN-β are considered the dominant functional type I IFNs in humans and are secreted by many cell types following virus infection. Type I IFN primes adaptive immune responses through stimulation of DCs, through activation of B and T cells, and by prolonging survival of recently activated T cells.[603,604,1068] Pretreatment of cells with IFN-α or IFN-β inhibits flavivirus replication *in vitro*,[87,264,649,673,1157] but treatment after infection is less effective.[25,219,264,963,1062] Although flaviviruses can antagonize IFN-induced responses after infection, IFN still restricts replication and spread *in vivo*. Mice lacking the type I IFN receptor (*Ifnar1*[−/−]) or downstream signaling components (e.g., STAT1 or STAT2) show enhanced lethality and replication after WNV,[517,963] DENV,[1023] YFV,[735] ZIKV,[600,1127] or MVEV[663] infections. Increased replication occurred in normally resistant cell populations and tissues after flavivirus infection of *Ifnar1*[−/−] mice, suggesting that IFN acts in part to restrict viral tropism. The importance of type I IFN in controlling flavivirus infection has been confirmed in therapeutic disease models. Pretreatment of animals with IFN-α or inducers of IFN-α attenuates infection by SLEV, WNV, YFV, and Modoc viruses.[130,499,616,617,883,1105] The relevance of these pathways has been confirmed *in vivo*, as transcriptomic analyses show that animals or primary cells infected with flaviviruses produce a potent innate antiviral transcriptional signature characterized by ISGs.[47,468,906,970]

Type I IFN-induced genes that control flavivirus infection

Substantial progress has been made in defining the specific IFN-induced antiviral genes that limit flavivirus infection (reviewed in Ref.[996]) (Fig. 9.12). Initial studies showed that dsRNA-dependent protein kinase (PKR) and 2′-5′-oligoadenylate synthase (Oas) proteins mediate intrinsic cell resistance to WNV.[965] PKR is activated by binding dsRNA and phosphorylates the eukaryotic translation initiation factor 2 (eIF2-α) resulting in attenuation of protein synthesis.[743] PKR also may have independent antiviral effects by activating signaling pathways that augment type I IFN production[64,356] and directly regulating IFN-α mRNA stability.[1003] RNase L is activated by 2′-5′-linked oligoadenylates that are synthesized by Oas enzymes. RNase L inhibits viral infections by functioning as an endoribonuclease that cleaves viral RNA[1253,1254] and by generating small self-RNA PAMPs that amplify antiviral immunity through a RIG-I– and MDA5-dependent pathway.[690,691] *Rnasel*[−/−] fibroblasts and macrophages support increased WNV replication *in vitro*,[965,983] and knockdown of RNase L enhanced infection in human cells.[651] Moreover, mice deficient in RNase L showed increased lethality following WNV infection, with higher viral loads in peripheral tissues at early time points after infection.[965]

Flavivirus resistance is one of the earliest examples of a genetic determinant of pathogen susceptibility defined in mice. In 1937, flavivirus resistance was shown to be inherited in a single-gene autosomal dominant manner.[1187] In 2002, susceptibility to flaviviruses in mice was mapped to a mutation in the gene *Oas1b* (found in most common laboratory mouse strains), resulting in the expression of a nonfunctional truncated Oas1b isoform.[709,868] Oas1b restricts flavivirus replication by a cell-intrinsic post-entry mechanism independent of RNase L[983] and the type I IFN signaling pathway.[129] Knock-in of the wild-type Oas1b allele into a flavivirus-susceptible mouse generated a resistant phenotype,[982] and murine cells that ectopically expressed Oas1b resisted WNV infection by preventing viral RNA accumulation inside infected cells.[505] While biochemical studies have shown that Oas1b itself is an inactive 2′-5′-Oas, other experiments suggest that Oas1b inhibits Oas1a activity resulting in reduced 2′-5′-oligoA production in response to poly(I:C).[297] Negative regulation of 2′-5′-Oas by inactive Oas1b proteins may tune the RNase L response that could cause significant damage in cells, if it were not tightly controlled. OAS orthologs in other species also restrict flavivirus replication, and *OAS1* polymorphisms are associated with WNV disease in humans[94,639] and horses.[639,869,935]

Ectopic expression and siRNA or knockdown or CRISPR-Cas9 gene editing have been used to identify novel ISGs that restrict infection of multiple different flaviviruses.[927,997,998] The ISG viperin has inhibitory activity against TBEV, WNV, DENV, and ZIKV (reviewed in Ref.[652]). Viperin inhibits flavivirus infection and virulence by diminishing RNA synthesis and replication,[1139] inducing assembly of defective virions,[1160] and targeting the NS3 protein for proteasomal degradation.[857] JEV appears to counteract the antiviral actions of viperin by targeting it for proteasomal degradation.[174] The interferon-inducible transmembrane (IFITM) proteins inhibit multiple enveloped viruses, including flaviviruses.[119] IFITM3 suppressed WNV replication in nonneuronal cells, and *Ifitm3⁻/⁻* mice were vulnerable to lethal WNV infection.[376] Cell culture studies have shown that IFITM3 can restrict infection and cell death associated with ZIKV infection[776,976] and that IFITM3 contributed to both the baseline and IFN-induced inhibition of DENV infection and entry.[1255] Members of the IFI-6-16 family of ISGs (e.g., human *IFI-6*; mouse *Ifi27l2a*) also have antiviral activity against multiple flaviviruses. Ifi27l2a initially was identified in neuronal subsets as antiviral gene against SLEV and WNV.[199] Consistent with these data, *Ifi27l2a⁻/⁻* mice were more susceptible to lethal WNV infection and sustained higher viral burden in specific brain regions.[675] A CRISPR-Cas9 screen identified the human ortholog, IFI-6, as an inhibitor of WNV, ZIKV, YFV, and DENV infections by preventing the formation of virus-induced ER membrane invaginations required for replication.[927] Cholesterol 25-hydroxylase is an ISG that catalyzes the formation of 25-hydroxycholesterol (25-HC) from cholesterol and was shown to block entry of ZIKV, DENV, YFV, and WNV.[618] Studies in nonhuman primates and mice showed that 25-HC treatment suppressed ZIKV-induced viremia and infection and tissue damage in the embryonic brain of mice.[618] Although the field is rapidly advancing with respect to identifying antiviral ISGs against flaviviruses, definitive studies in genetically deficient animals may be required to establish the cell- and tissue-specific nonredundant effects of individual ISGs in controlling flavivirus infection in the context of a robust type I IFN response.

Type III IFN signaling pathway

Recent studies have identified important immunomodulatory and antiviral effects of the type III (IFN-λ) signaling pathway against flaviviruses. IFN-λ functions at barrier surfaces and is induced downstream of pathogen recognition receptor sensing and activation of MAVS.[601] IFN-λ binds to and signals through a selectively expressed heterodimeric receptor (IFNLR1/IL10Rβ), distinguishing it from type I IFNs, which bind to the more broadly expressed IFNAR1/IFNAR2 heterodimeric receptor. IFN-λ has antiviral functions against ZIKV in the context of infection of the maternally derived decidua and fetally derived placenta during pregnancy in mice and humans.[68,188,214,484] A K154E coding variant of human IFN-λ4, which is restricted to certain African populations, remarkably has greatly enhanced *in vitro* activity against ZIKV infection.[53] Apart from its direct antiviral effects,[682] IFN-λ also inhibited neuroinvasion and infection of WNV and YFV by tightening the blood–brain barrier.[275,599]

Inflammasome

The NOD-like receptors (NLRs) detect danger signals within cells, leading to formation of the inflammasome signaling complex and secretion of proinflammatory cytokines of the IL-1β family.[972] Pathogens can be detected by NLRs NLRP3 or AIM2, which leads to activation of caspase-1 via multiprotein complexes known as inflammasomes. Activation of procaspase 1 enables processing of pro–IL-1β and pro–IL-18 and subsequent release of the proinflammatory cytokines IL-1β and IL-18 from cells.[707] WNV, DENV, and ZIKV infections of humans are associated with elevated levels of systemic IL-1β, suggesting that flavivirus infection can activate inflammasome signaling.[911,1171] In mice, IL-1β signaling and the NLRP3 inflammasome are involved in control of viral replication and CNS disease

associated with WNV infection, and WNV infection triggers production of IL-1β from cortical neurons.[911] Consistent with these observations, mice deficient in the inflammasome adaptor protein ASC, which is essential for IL-1β production, showed reduced survival and enhanced WNV replication in peripheral tissues and the CNS.[571] Subsequent studies showed that IL-1R1 signaling promotes control of WNV infection within the CNS via modulation of local DC-mediated T-cell reactivation and T-cell localization.[294,295]

Inflammasome activation also has been implicated in enhancing protective immune responses or contributing to immunopathology of other flaviviruses including DENV and ZIKV. Type I IFNs and IL-18 regulate the antiviral response of primary human γδ T cells against DCs infected with DENV, and antagonizing inflammasome activation significantly inhibited the anti-DENV IFN-γ response of γδ T cells.[1131] In macrophages, the cell-surface signaling receptor, CLEC5a, appears to be important for DENV-induced inflammasome activation, which might contribute to the febrile syndrome in DENV patients.[1209] Platelets appear to enhance the vascular permeability associated with DENV infection through inflammasome-dependent release of IL-1β.[472] In the context of ZIKV infection, silencing of NLRP3 in cells and knockout of NLRP3 in mice inhibited IL-1β secretion, indicating an essential role for NLRP3 in ZIKV-induced IL-1β activation and inflammatory responses in the brain and peripheral organs.[1171] ZIKV NS5 protein reportedly facilitates the assembly of the NLRP3 inflammasome complex, leading to IL-1β activation through interaction with NLRP3 and induction of reactive oxygen species production.[449] ZIKV NS1 recruits the host deubiquitinase USP8 to cleave polyubiquitin chains from caspase-1 to inhibit its degradation by the proteasome.[1252] An analysis of the neural parenchyma from ZIKV-positive microcephaly cases found higher expression levels of NLRs NLRP1, NLRP3, and AIM2; cytokines IL-1β, IL-18, and IL-33; and enzymes caspase-1, iNOS, and arginase 1 compared to healthy controls. These results suggest that inflammasome activation might cause damaging neuroinflammatory responses that contribute to CZS.[249]

Chemokines

Depending on the specific flavivirus infection, individual chemokines and cytokines can either protect or contribute to pathogenesis. For encephalitic flaviviruses, production of inflammatory chemokines in the brain by neuronal and nonneuronal cells coordinates recruitment of lymphocytes for clearance of viral infection. Chemokines that have been detected in the brain or CSF after WNV, JEV, or TBEV infection of mice include CXCL9 (MIG), CXCL10 (IP-10), CXCL11 (I-TAC), CCL2 (MCP-1), CCL3 (MIP-1α), CCL4 (MIP-1β), and CCL5 (RANTES).[347,406,537,1021,1121] WNV infection in the brain is associated with the early expression of the T-cell chemoattractant CXCL10 by infected neurons[537]; this expression proceeds in a caudal to rostral direction with higher levels detected in the cerebellum. This regional heterogeneity in CXCL10 expression is due to differential regulation by WNV-infected cortical versus cerebellar granule cell neurons and leads to enhanced trafficking of WNV-specific T cells that express the CXCL10 receptor CXCR3 into the cerebellum.[1243] Loss of CXCL10 or CXCR3 via targeted deletion or neutralizing antibody administration leads to decreased recruitment of WNV-specific CD8⁺ T cells into the CNS, especially within the cerebellum, increased viral loads, and enhanced mortality.[537,1243] In contrast, antagonism of polarized CXCR4–CXCL12 interactions along the BBB improved survival from lethal WNV infection through enhanced intraparenchymal migration of WNV-specific CD8+ T cells within the brain, leading to reduced viral loads and decreased immunopathology.[721]

A genetic deficiency in CCR2, a chemokine receptor on inflammatory monocytes and other leukocyte subtypes, resulted in markedly increased WNV-induced mortality in mice[642] and was associated with a selective reduction of monocyte accumulation in the brain. Subsequent experiments showed that CCR2 mediates selective peripheral blood monocytosis in the context of WNV infection, and this is critical for accumulation of protective monocytes in the brain. While a protective role for CCL2–CCR2 interactions was observed with a virulent WNV strain, an opposing phenotype was seen after infection with an attenuated strain; neutralization of CCL2 reduced the number of microglia in the brain during WNV infection but prolonged the life of infected animals.[355] Thus, depending on the virulence of the strain, CCL2-CCR2-dependent monocyte accumulation and migration may differentially affect disease outcome after WNV infection. Although both CCR2 ligands CCL2 and CCL7 are required for monocytosis and monocyte accumulation in the CNS, only CCL7 deficiency resulted in increased WNV burden in the brain and enhanced mortality. The enhanced susceptibility in *Ccl7*−/− mice was associated with the delayed migration of neutrophils and CD8+ T cells into the CNS.[56]

Additional studies have established that the chemokines CCL3, CCL4, and CCL5, all of which bind to the chemokine receptor CCR5, are strongly induced within the brain after WNV infection.[363,537,1021] Moreover, targeted deletion of CCR5 is associated with depressed leukocyte trafficking, increased viral burden, and enhanced mortality.[363] In humans, homozygosity for a defective CCR5 allele (*CCR5Δ32*) correlates with an increased risk of symptomatic WNV and TBEV disease.[364,529,640,641] Because the mouse studies examined the entire brain with regard to expression and leukocyte trafficking and the human studies did not report on specific neurological symptoms, it remains unclear whether CCR5-expressing leukocytes also exhibit regional specificity during CNS recruitment.

For viscerotropic flaviviruses such as DENV, the function of chemokine interaction with their receptors remains less certain. Although DENV-infected wild-type mice produce high levels of chemokines CCL2, CCL3, and CCL5 in their spleen and liver, Ccr1−/− mice had a phenotype similar to wild-type mice, whereas infection of Ccr2−/− or Ccr4−/− mice showed attenuated lethality, liver damage, leukocyte activation, and levels of IL-6 and IFN-γ without significant differences in viral load.[398] Thus, chemokine–chemokine receptor interactions in the context of DENV infection appear to contribute to the development of disease. Nevertheless, in an encephalitic mouse model of DENV infection, CXCL10 interaction with CXCR3 was required for clearance and resistance to infection.[473] Finally, a case of YFV vaccine-associated viscerotropic disease was associated with polymorphisms in both CCR5 and CCL5 genes.[899]

Complement Activation and Flaviviruses
The complement system is a family of serum and cell-surface proteins that recognize PAMPs, altered-self ligands, and immune complexes. Although complement activation inhibits infection of many viruses (reviewed in Refs.[40,1072]), it has both protective and pathogenic roles in flavivirus infection depending on the specific virus, phase of the infection, and immune status of the host.[40,211] Activation of the complement cascade triggers several antiviral functions including pathogen opsonization and/or lysis and priming of adaptive immune responses. Complement is activated through the classical, lectin, and alternative pathways depending on specific recognition molecules.[1165,1166] Classical pathway activity is triggered by C1q binding to antigen–antibody complexes on the surface of pathogens. The lectin pathway is initiated by MBL or ficolin recognition of carbohydrate structures on the surface of microbes or apoptotic cells. The alternative pathway is constitutively active at low levels through the spontaneous hydrolysis of C3 and also amplifies activation of the classical and lectin pathways. Deposition of C3 and C4 fragments (C3b and C4b) on a pathogen facilitates binding and phagocytosis by complement receptors (CR1, CR3, CR4, and CRIg), a process called opsonization, which helps to clear microbial infections.[164]

Protective activity of complement on flavivirus infection
Complement can limit flavivirus infection by stimulating adaptive immune responses or by directly neutralizing infection. In support of an immune-priming role for complement, *C3*−/− mice are more susceptible to lethal WNV infection and show greater viral burden and reduced antiviral antibody titers.[734] Infection studies with mice lacking C1q, MBL, C4, or factor B establish that all complement activation pathways protect against WNV infection.[340,732] However, each activation pathway exerts distinct effects in response to WNV infection. Humoral IgM responses to WNV depend upon activation of C3 by the lectin recognition pathway. In contrast, both the lectin and alternative pathways appear necessary for efficient T-cell priming as *C4*−/−, factor B−/−, and factor D−/− mice exhibited reduced WNV-specific CD8+ T-cell responses.[732] The T-cell defects in C4−/− mice may be indirect as depressed IgM responses could affect viral opsonization and antigen presentation. The terminal lytic complement components (C5–C9) do not appear to serve a major function in protection, as C5 neither contributed to protection against WNV pathogenesis nor augmented the neutralizing efficacy of complement-fixing anti–WNV-neutralizing antibodies in mice.[733] Flaviviruses directly trigger complement activation, which can inhibit infectivity. Increasing concentrations of serum complement neutralize WNV or DENV in cell culture and *in vivo* in the absence of antibody, and this depends on recognition of N-linked glycans on the surface of the virion by MBL.[339] Complement activation by flaviviruses occurs *in vivo* as C3 and C4 consumption occurs prior to the induction of a specific antibody response.[732] Complement augments antibody-mediated neutralization of flaviviruses, including YFV, DENV, and WNV.[254,734,1057] The C1q component of complement is sufficient to enhance the potency of antibody neutralization as it reduces the number of antibodies that must bind the virion to neutralize infectivity.[733] The protective efficacy of flavivirus-neutralizing antibodies *in vivo* correlates with IgG subclasses that efficiently fix complement.[733,989]

Pathologic effects of complement on flavivirus infection
In myeloid cells that express complement receptors, antibody-dependent complement activation paradoxically may

enhance viral infection.[162,163] Blockade of complement receptor-3 (CD11b/CD18) abrogated the complement-dependent enhancement of WNV infection in this model system. Thus, under certain circumstances, antibody and complement-dependent opsonization of flaviviruses may increase infection in myeloid cells. During WNV infection, a complement-microglial axis promoted synapse loss in brain neurons and was associated with memory impairment in mice.[1147] C1q was up-regulated and localized to microglia, infected neurons, and presynaptic terminals during WNV neuroinvasive disease. Microglial engulfment of presynaptic terminals in hippocampal neurons in the context of acute and subacute WNV infection occurred through a complement-dependent process.[1147] A pathological role for complement activation has been proposed for the vascular leakage syndrome that accompanies severe dengue.[41,107] In early clinical studies, reduced levels of C3, C4, and factor B and increased catabolic rates of C3 and C1q were observed, particularly in patients with severe DENV disease.[107] Additionally, C3 breakdown products and anaphylatoxins accumulated in the circulation of severely ill patients and peaked at the day of maximum vascular leakage.[206,689] Circulating immune complexes formed by virions and DENV-specific antibodies have been hypothesized to cause pathological complement activation.[107] One alternative hypothesis is that infected cells express sufficient amounts of DENV antigens (E or NS1 proteins) on their surface facilitating immune complex formation and complement deposition.[88] Indeed, in DENV-infected endothelial cells, lower factor H compared to factor B production and greater C3b and C5b-9 deposition was observed, which might contribute to enhanced vascular permeability.[39,41,148] In some human populations, factor H gene polymorphisms and haplotypes with higher levels of expression are associated with protection against severe DENV disease.[557,862]

Humoral Immunity

Humoral immunity contributes significantly to the protective host response to flavivirus infection (reviewed by Ref.[1044]). Passive administration of flavivirus-reactive monoclonal antibodies (mAbs), purified polyclonal γ-globulin, or immune sera confers significant protection in animal models of flavivirus infection.[303,358,516] Moreover, the administration of γ-globulin has been used therapeutically.[80,915] Advances in antibody sequencing and isolation techniques enabled isolation of potently neutralizing human antibodies with therapeutic potential.[320,839] Although neutralizing antibody titers correlate with protection by several flavivirus vaccines,[78,451,711,774] this relationship is imperfect.[99,1106] Antibodies also exert protective effects via effector functions coordinated by the Fc portion of the immunoglobulin heavy-chain molecule, including complement fixation, antibody-mediated cellular cytotoxicity, and facilitating virus clearance.[733,989,990] Furthermore, anti-flavivirus antibodies may be protective even when targeting nonstructural proteins, such as NS1.[44,282,513]

Mechanisms of Neutralization

Antibody-mediated neutralization is defined as a reduction in the ability of viruses to productively infect cells as a direct result of antibody occupancy of the virion. Antibody-mediated neutralization of flaviviruses occurs when individual virions are engaged by antibody with a stoichiometry that exceeds a required threshold (reviewed in Ref.[282]). The number of antibodies decorating the virion at any antibody concentration is controlled by the functional avidity of antibody binding and epitope accessibility on the virion. As detailed above, the dense arrangement and dynamics of E proteins on the virus particle, combined with structural heterogeneity arising from incomplete prM cleavage, define the accessibility of viral surfaces for antibody recognition and neutralization.[279,818] While some antibodies target poorly accessible epitopes with limited or no capacity to neutralize infection, other classes recognize quaternary epitopes displayed on the surface of infectious virions, as detailed below. Advances in defining structure–function relationships of antibodies elicited by flavivirus infection or vaccination have improved understanding of neutralization mechanisms, potency, and vaccine antigen design.

Antibodies block infection via mechanisms that act at distinct steps in the flavivirus replication cycle (Fig. 9.10). Antibodies can block flavivirus attachment to host cells.[223,450,833] At present, it is unknown whether antibodies that block attachment to cells do so by interfering with specific receptor interactions on the target cells or via a general steric hindrance mechanism. Flavivirus-reactive antibodies also block infection after the virus attachment step. Seminal studies by Gollins and Porterfield demonstrated that antibodies could block the uncoating and infectivity of WNV even when added after virions attached to cells. Furthermore, they demonstrated that antibodies could directly block fusion of virions to synthetic liposomes.[370] These observations have been expanded greatly to include other flaviviruses and antibodies.[944,1119] Analysis of the ability of a large panel of TBEV-reactive antibodies to block liposomal fusion revealed mAbs capable of blocking fusion completely (25% of antibodies tested), partially (58% of antibodies tested), or not at all (17% of antibodies tested).[1070] These results suggest an ability to block fusion is a relatively common functional property of neutralizing antibodies. Structural studies illustrate different ways in which antibodies block fusion. Experiments with anti-WNV mAb E16 suggest this antibody blocks the radial expansion of the virus particle and traps it in an intermediate step of the fusion process following exposure of the virus to acidic pH conditions (Fig. 9.10).[514] Alternatively, some antibodies prevent the disassociation of E protein dimers at the onset of fusion through the recognition of epitopes composed of features on more than one E protein. Multiple antibodies that inhibit fusion via this type of quaternary recognition have been described including those targeting WNV, DENV, and ZIKV.[323,325,443,515,1107] Individual mAbs may be capable of blocking infection at more than one step of the virus entry pathway. Factors with the potential to impact neutralization mechanism include antibody concentration, virion maturation state, and host immune factors such as C1q and Fc receptors.[254,733,734,1057]

Antibody-Dependent Enhancement of Infection

ADE of infection describes the marked increase in the efficiency of infection of cells expressing Fc receptors by viruses–antibody complexes.[429,430] While ADE has been demonstrated for several families of viruses *in vitro*, a role for enhancing antibodies in the pathogenesis of human disease has been demonstrated in limited contexts, including secondary DENV infection.[538,539] Aspects of the complex pathogenesis of secondary DENV infection have been recapitulated in animal models. Passive transfer of DENV-reactive antibodies increases viral burden and exacerbates disease in an IFN-$\alpha\beta\gamma$ receptor-deficient mice[52,1240] and increases viremia in primates.[371,418] A recent study of serum collected from a longitudinal cohort identified a narrow range of pre-existing anti-DENV antibody titers as a predictor of risk for severe dengue.[512] ADE has also been suggested as a cause for adverse outcomes in the context of the Dengvaxia® tetravalent vaccine in children, as detailed below.

The mechanism of ADE has been studied extensively. The phenomenon of ADE is controlled by the number of antibody molecules, which serve to more efficiently attach viral immune complexes to cells expressing Fcγ or complement receptors.[421] Almost all antibodies have the capacity to support ADE, although exceptions have been reported.[922] Antibody concentrations that support ADE are bounded at the upper end by the neutralization threshold and at lower concentrations by the minimal number of antibodies required for durable attachment to Fcγ receptors. This window of enhancing concentrations is modulated by antibody isotype, Fc receptor subtype, and complement.[731,1221] Interactions between viral immune complexes and Fcγ receptors are determined by the constant region of the antibody heavy chain and influenced by the single conserved N-linked glycan at position N297 of the IgG heavy chain. ADE can be inhibited by antibodies that block Fcγ–receptor interactions,[865] enzymatic removal of the heavy chain of the antibody molecule,[1240] and removal of the N-linked glycan on IgG molecules.[52,371,878] A recent study suggested the composition of the N-linked sugar on anti-DENV antibodies correlated with disease outcome,[1178] providing a new mechanistic link between antibody effector activities and DENV pathogenesis. Two Fc receptor–independent mechanisms of ADE have also been described. Haslwanter and colleagues demonstrated that the binding of an antibody at the TBEV E protein dimer interface of mature virions caused displacement of the E-DII-FL resulting in more efficient binding to lipid membranes.[446] A DENV-reactive antibody that is cross-reactive with a cell-surface–expressed host protein has been shown to promote ADE in the absence of Fc receptors because it is capable of simultaneously binding both the virion and target cell.[477]

The mechanisms of ADE also may promote more efficient viral replication and spread at a postentry step. The ligation of monocyte or macrophage Fcγ receptors by IgG immune complexes, rather than aiding host defenses, has been hypothesized to suppress innate immunity, increase production of IL-10, and bias T-helper cell responses, leading to increased infectious output by infected cells.[427,791] Initial studies with the unrelated Ross River alphavirus in RAW 264.7 macrophage-like cells showed that infection by ADE suppressed expression of CXCL10, NOS2, IRF1, TNF-α, and IFN-γ.[633,688] Subsequent experiments with DENV in the THP-1 monocytic cell line confirmed that ADE attenuated innate immune responses by down-regulating the RIG-I/MDA5 signaling pathway and decreasing production of type I IFN and ISGs.[1138] However, more recent experiments with DENV infection and primary human monocytes[109,555] did not demonstrate suppressed production of inhibitory or immunomodulatory cytokines in the context of ADE. One caveat to this concept of intrinsic ADE is that enhanced viral entry and infectivity (via DENV immune complex interaction with Fcγ receptor) yield higher levels of viral nonstructural proteins in a cell, which themselves independently suppress innate immunity[259,260] irrespective of Fcγ receptor signaling. Although the idea that intrinsic ADE of

infection suppresses innate immunity and modulates disease severity of DENV infection is appealing,[427] it remains to be distinguished from the enhanced infectivity *per se* and confirmed in a physiologically relevant setting.

The Antigenic Structure of Flaviviruses

Flaviviruses were first classified according to serological reactivity by arbovirus-immune sera.[168,246] Flavivirus-reactive antibodies continue to be classified with respect to their capacity to discriminate between the antigens of viruses within and between related serological groups of viruses.[1125] For example, mAbs that react with DENV may be type-specific (one DENV serotype), sub–complex-specific (more than one DENV serotype), complex-reactive (all DENV viruses), or flavivirus group–reactive (multiple flaviviruses).[454] The extensive cross-reactivity among flaviviruses complicates the use of serological diagnostics to manage flavivirus outbreaks and disease. Large panels of murine and human mAbs against DENV, WNV, ZIKV, TBEV, and JEV have been developed and characterized.[1044] These efforts reveal that virtually every exposed surface of the flavivirus virion may be targeted by antibodies.

E protein epitopes recognized by neutralizing antibodies

The majority of neutralizing antibodies bind epitopes on the E protein.[1044] Early studies distinguished epitopes on the E protein based on the biochemical and functional properties of mAbs, including a capacity to bind and compete for viral antigens, neutralize virus, and inhibit hemagglutination of red blood cells. Epitopes are now cataloged using structural methods, saturation mutagenesis, and neutralization escape studies. A nonexhaustive catalogue of well-characterized flavivirus epitopes is detailed below:

1. *DIII-LR*. The DIII-LR epitope is an accessible surface of DIII composed of three discontinuous loops and the amino-terminal region. Multiple DIII-LR–reactive neutralizing antibodies have been described. As an example, mAb E16 is a type-specific WNV-reactive MAb that neutralizes at picomolar concentrations *in vitro* and protects mice from lethal challenge when administered 5 days after infection.[783,784,839] The molecular basis for E16 recognition on E-DIII and mature virions has been detailed using structural and functional approaches.[611,833] Type-specific mAbs that bind the DIII-LR of DENV, JEV, TBEV, and ZIKV have been described.[124,321,516,938,1079,1222,1251] While antibodies of this specificity are common in the repertoire of murine antibodies elicited by infection, their contribution to the human repertoire of antibodies elicited by WNV or DENV is limited.[79,818,1120,1163] In contrast, the contribution of DIII-reactive antibodies to the neutralizing activity of ZIKV-immune sera is significant.[938,1233]

2. *DII-FL*. Antibodies that bind the E-DII-FL are highly cross-reactive.[221,224,841,1071] The accessibility of this epitope is very sensitive to the maturation state of the virion; antibodies that bind this conserved structure have a limited capacity to bind mature virions.[841,1071] Passive transfer of E-DII-FL antibodies in mice reveals they may be protective, have limited potency, and may be dependent on Fc-dependent mechanisms.[1080,1158] While mutation of E-DII-FL residues reduces antibody binding, other adjacent structures also

may contribute to the fine specificity of binding and the functional properties of these antibodies.[233,372,841] The structure of the E-DII-FL antibody mAb E53 bound to soluble E proteins was solved.[196] Residues shown to be important antibody contacts for this antibody include those of the fusion loop (residues 104–107 and 109–110) as well as residues of the BC loop of E-DII.[841] The DENV 1C19 mAb binds a similar epitope, including the BC loop, and was remarkably potent *in vitro* and in murine models.[1046] Other modes of E-DII-FL recognition have been documented. DII-FL antibodies are common in humans.[79,252,840,1069,1120]

3. *Quaternary epitopes.* Many antibodies have been described that recognize quaternary epitopes unique to the surface of mature virions (reviewed by Ref.[1044]). Antibodies with these properties typically are identified by their inability to bind soluble E proteins despite efficient recognition of the virus particle. One well-studied example is the E-dimer epitope (EDE).[253,320,950] Antibodies that bind the EDE interact with residues on E-DI and E-DIII of one E protein subunit and a conserved patch of E-DII on the opposing E protein of the dimer, including the E-DII-FL. Some EDE antibodies also contact the N-linked sugar of E-DII.[950] The EDE footprint largely overlaps the surface contacted by prM on immature virions at low pH.[950] EDE antibodies potently neutralize infection and are cross-reactive; antibodies elicited by DENV infection have been shown to neutralize both ZIKV and SPOV and are cross-protective in animal models[960] Unexpectedly, EDE antibodies bind virions in a manner insensitive to the presence of uncleaved prM, despite the quaternary nature of the epitope, and overlap between the EDE and prM binding footprints.[950] These data suggest partially mature virions exist in a dynamic equilibrium that allows antibody to displace uncleaved prM and trap E proteins in antiparallel dimers.

Antibodies that bind the prM protein
Antibodies that bind prM protein have been described.[79,155,251,311,1047,1149] Generally, these antibodies are characterized by limited neutralizing activity *in vitro*. Studies of the memory B-cell antibody repertoire indicated that DENV prM-reactive antibodies are relatively common.[243,251] These antibodies are typically cross-reactive among DENV viral serotypes. prM-specific antibodies have been hypothesized to contribute to the pathogenesis of DENV infection due to their capacity to readily support ADE.[251,939] A recent demonstration that DENV-1 circulates as mature virions *in vivo* raises questions about the role of partially mature viruses in the pathogenesis of DENV.[914]

NS1-reactive antibodies
The nonstructural protein NS1 of some flaviviruses is secreted at high levels into the extracellular environment during flavivirus infection, predominantly as a hexamer,[330] with significant accumulation (up to 50 μg/mL) in the sera of DENV-infected patients.[14,41,631,1231] NS1 plays multiple roles in flavivirus pathogenesis including the inhibition of complement by binding the negative regulator factor H or by promoting C4 degradation.[37,203] NS1 has been hypothesized to play a mechanistic role in severe dengue (reviewed by Ref.[361]). NS1 interactions with the vascular endothelium increase permeability by disrupting tight junctions.[897] NS1 also promotes dysregulated cytokine production following TLR4-dependent interactions with mononuclear

cells, indirectly contributing to vascular leakage.[757] Autoreactive NS1-binding antibodies may contribute to pathogenic features of secondary DENV infections through multiple mechanisms including the activation and complement-mediated opsonization of platelets, decreasing anticoagulation factors, and promoting inflammation and apoptosis.[1082,1084] Many NS1-reactive mAbs have been characterized. Passive transfer of mAbs against NS1 can protect mice against lethal infection by DENV, WNV, YFV, and ZIKV,[44,204,588,987] and this requires an intact Fc moiety.[204,205,989,990] Protective anti-NS1 MAbs have been shown to recognize cell-surface–associated NS1 and trigger Fcγ receptor-dependent phagocytosis and clearance of WNV-infected cells.[205] NS1 has been developed as a vaccine target for multiple flaviviruses with promising results.[74,120,257,312,902,986,988] Because NS1-reactive antibodies do not bind virus particles, a conceptual advantage of this vaccine platform is that antibodies are incapable of contributing to ADE.

The Repertoire of Antibodies Elicited In Vivo
The composition of the polyclonal antibody response elicited by infection has been studied using multiple techniques, yielding many important insights (reviewed in Refs.[343,1044]). Analysis of the specificity of antibodies in the memory B-cell compartment provided insight into surfaces recognized by antibodies, antibody ontogeny, and identified the importance of quaternary modes of recognition. Biochemical studies with recombinant proteins and virus particles incorporating mutations in the fusion loop suggest antibodies that bind the E-DII-FL are a considerable portion of circulating antibodies.[221,222,590,650,840] Cross-reactive human E-DII-FL mAbs are frequently isolated from the memory B-cell compartment.[79,251,252,1120] Serum antibody depletion experiments using intact virions or soluble dimeric E proteins suggest the majority of circulating neutralizing antibodies bind epitopes contained within and/or among E protein dimers on mature virions.[488,1161] Numerous human mAbs that bind complex quaternary epitopes have been described (reviewed by Ref.[343]). The use of molecular clone technology to transplant selected quaternary epitopes recognized by type-specific DENV antibodies among DENV strains has provided insight into the specificity of the neutralizing antibody response to infection and vaccination.[343,344]

T-Cell–Mediated Control
CD8+ T Cells
CD8+ T cells, by virtue of their ability to lyse infected target cells and produce inflammatory cytokines (e.g., IFN-γ and TNF-α), can have either protective or pathologic effects depending on the context. Depending on the flavivirus strain and experimental system, beneficial or adverse functions of CD8+ T cells have been reported. Experiments in small animal models and *in vitro* demonstrate that CD8+ T lymphocytes can be an essential component of protection against infection by several flaviviruses, including WNV, DENV, YFV, ZIKV, and JEV.[97,125–127,655,802,803,901,917,1026,1043,1196,1223,1225] Consistent with this, individuals with hematologic malignancies and impaired T-cell function have an increased risk of neuroinvasive WNV infection.[804,895] Upon recognition of a flavivirus-infected cell that expresses class I MHC molecules, antigen-restricted cytotoxic T lymphocytes (CTL) proliferate, release proinflammatory cytokines,[126,276,520,564,901] and lyse cells directly through the delivery of

perforin and granzymes A and B, or via Fas–Fas-ligand interactions. In WNV infection, mice deficient in CD8+ T cells have higher and sustained WNV burdens in the spleen and CNS and increased mortality.[1026,1175] CD8+ T cells require perforin and Fas ligand interactions to control infection of virulent WNV strains as mice deficient in these molecules had increased CNS viral burdens and lethality.[1027,1029] Moreover, adoptive transfer of wild-type but not perforin- or Fas-ligand–deficient CD8+ T cells decreased CNS viral burden and enhanced survival. The net function of CD8+ T cells in infection by other encephalitic flaviviruses (e.g., JEV or MVEV) also varies. Initial reports showed that JEV-specific cytotoxic CD8+ T cells could reduce production of infectious virus from infected macrophage and neuronal-like cells *in vitro*.[802] Moreover, adoptive transfer of anti-JEV CD8+ T cells by an intracerebral route protected adult but not newborn or suckling BALB/c mice against lethal JEV challenge.[803] However, in vaccine immunization studies, challenge experiments in mice deficient in CD8+ T cells indicate that CD8+ T cells are dispensable, and immune antibody was the most critical component of protection.[856] CD8+ T cells may have a lesser role *in vivo* in JEV infection because of active subversion of the antigen-presentation pathway by the virus; JEV infection can lead to active depletion and impairment of CD8α+CD11c+ dendritic cells,[15,16] which are the cells that dominantly mediate cross presentation of antigen and priming of CD8+ T-cell responses *in vivo*.[463] With MVEV infection, effector CD8+ T cells in the brain appear pathological as mice deficient in granule exocytosis (perforin or granzyme B) or Fas-mediated cytotoxicity showed delayed and reduced mortality.[632]

For DENV, which generally does not cause encephalitis, the protective or pathologic function of CD8+ T cells still is not fully resolved. During primary infection of mice, depletion of CD8+ T cells before infection resulted in significantly higher viral loads. DENV-specific CD8+ T cells produced IFN-γ and TNF-α and exhibited cytotoxic activity *in vivo*.[1225] In comparison, a pathogenic role of CD8+ T cells has been reported during secondary DENV infection. Due to the significant amino acid sequence homology among the four serotypes, there is a high potential for T-cell cross-reactivity during secondary heterologous DENV infection. Serotype cross-reactive CD8+ T cells are preferentially activated during secondary infection in humans in a phenomenon termed "original antigenic sin".[777] These cross-reactive CD8+ T cells exhibit altered cytokine production and reduced cytolytic activity.[65,75,695,778] Aberrant cytokine production by T cells could contribute to severe DENV disease, as higher levels of proinflammatory mediators may contribute to endothelial cell dysfunction or damage, leading to plasma leakage.[713]

More recent studies that have profiled antigen-specific CD8+ T-cell responses against DENV have suggested that immune imprinting contributes to a protective response. An analysis of CD8+ T-cell responses from human subjects in Sri Lanka challenges the original antigenic sin theory.[1189] Although skewing toward primary infecting DENV was detected, this was not associated with qualitative or quantitative impairment of responses. Higher magnitude and more polyfunctional responses for HLA alleles were associated with decreased susceptibility to severe disease, suggesting that CD8+ T cells are protective against DENV disease.[1189,1191] Consistent with these results, in studies with HLA transgenic mice although cross-reactive DENV CD8+ T-cell responses were lower than

responses elicited by serotype-specific T cells, immunization with either serotype-specific or variant peptide epitopes enhanced viral clearance, demonstrating that both serotype-specific and cross-reactive CD8+ T cells can contribute to *in vivo* protection against DENV infection.[300] Finally, primary DENV infection induces antigen-specific CD8+ T cells that are highly activated and proliferating, exhibit antiviral effector functions, and home to the skin.[937]

In the context of the intensive study of ZIKV pathogenesis, much has been learned about CD8+ T-cell responses to ZIKV from animal and human studies, which suggest these immune cells are largely protective. In mice, polyfunctional, cytotoxic CD8+ T cells become activated and can reduce ZIKV burden, whereas their depletion or genetic absence resulted in greater ZIKV infection and mortality,[301] and adoptive transfer of ZIKV-immune CD8+ T cells protects against ZIKV infection.[476] Another study showed that both ZIKV-specific and ZIKV/DENV cross-reactive CD8+ T cells can protect against ZIKV infection,[1196] and prior DENV immunity can protect against ZIKV infection during pregnancy in mice, and CD8+ T cells mediate this cross protection.[917] Whereas in most cases, CD8+ T cells have conferred protective activity against ZIKV in mice, pathological consequences in the CNS have been described as well.[502,693]

Less is known about human CD8+ T-cell responses to ZIKV. Initial studies showed that CD8+ T cells were highly activated during the viremic phase, and tetramer-positive ZIKV-specific CD8+ T cells could be detected in blood.[589,925] More recent studies have shown that ZIKV-specific CD8+ T cells have a polyfunctional IFN-γ signature with up-regulation of TNF-α, cell activation markers (e.g., CD69), and cytotoxic proteins.[392]

CD4+ T Cells

CD4+ T cells can restrict or contribute to pathogenesis depending on the flavivirus and whether the response is primary or anamnestic. Studies in mice have shown that CD4+ T cells restrict pathogenesis of primary WNV infection. A genetic or acquired deficiency of CD4+ T-cell function resulted in protracted WNV infection in the CNS that culminated in uniform lethality by 50 days after infection. CD4+ T cells protect against primary WNV infection by providing help for antibody responses, sustaining WNV-specific CD8+ T-cell responses in the CNS that enable viral clearance, producing antiviral cytokines, and directly killing cells.[127,1043] A protective role for CD4+ T cells against lethal JEV infection in mice was observed as depletion reduced and adoptive transfer promoted survival.[97] Moreover, in humans, impaired JEV-specific CD4+ T-cell function (e.g., IFN-γ secretion) was seen preferentially in patients with encephalitis and neurological sequelae,[572] and a high-quality, polyfunctional CD4+ T-cell response was associated with recovery from JEV.[1136] Consistent with these data, CD4-/- mice also showed greater susceptibility to CNS infection by a neuroadapted strain of YFV.[655] In comparison, depletion of CD4+ T cells prior to DENV infection in mice had no effect on tissue viral burden, DENV-specific antibody titers or neutralizing activity, or CD8+ T-cell responses.[1223]

Memory CD4+ T cells can have protective or pathological consequences depending on the context. For DENV, immunization schemes that elicit antigen-specific CD4+ T cells prior to infection of mice resulted in significantly lower viral burden after challenge with homologous DENV.[1223] Moreover, in humans, highly polarized cytotoxic CD4+ T cells were associated with protective immunity.[1190] A megapool of 180 different peptides has been developed to effectively measure *ex vivo* CD4+ T-cell responses irrespective of DENV serotype or geographical location.[391] Under certain conditions, induction of CD4+ T cells can contribute to viral clearance and reduced pathogenesis. However, during heterologous secondary DENV infection, cross-reactive CD4+ memory T cells may be stimulated by antigen from the secondary infection. These CD4+ T cells then augment the response of memory CD8+ T cells, which can result in an overexuberant production of inflammatory cytokines and an increased risk for severe DENV disease.[75]

Experiments with ZIKV also have established protective functions of CD4+ T cells. In studies with *Ifnar1−/−* mice, a neutralizing antibody response was dependent on CD4+ T cells and associated with reduced viral load in the brain and mortality. Adoptive transfer of purified CD4+ T cells prevented infection-associated weight loss and protected all animals against a lethal ZIKV infection.[447,674] A polyfunctional and polyclonal CD4+ T-cell response can prevent ZIKV neuroinvasion and infection within the CNS. Moreover, DENV-specific memory CD4+ T cells display antiviral effector capacity toward ZIKV, suggesting a potential beneficial effect in humans of preexisting T-cell immunity to DENV upon ZIKV infection.[638]

CD4+CD25+FoxP3+ Regulatory T Cells

Regulatory CD4+ T cells (Tregs) are a subset of CD4+ T cells that can suppress effector T cells to control reactivity to self-antigens and pathogens.[959,1089] These cells blunt inflammation and maintain antigen-specific T-cell homeostasis.[565,836] Tregs control the development of symptomatic WNV infection in humans and mice.[594] Symptomatic WNV-infected mice and humans had lower Treg frequencies compared with asymptomatic cohorts, and Treg-deficient mice developed lethal WNV infection at a higher rate than controls. Using the genetic variation of mice from the Collaborative Cross, one group established a model of chronic, persistent WNV infection, and this was associated with a strong immunoregulatory signature upon infection that correlated with restraint of the WNV-directed cytolytic responses.[386] Moreover, Treg-dependent production of TGF-β shaped the resident memory CD8+ T-cell response in the brain after WNV infection.[383] Interestingly, in severe DENV infection in humans, although Tregs expand and function normally, their relative frequencies are insufficient to control the immunopathology of severe disease.[676] Indeed, a separate study showed that although FoxP3+ Tregs expand in acute dengue, they predominantly consist of naïve Tregs, with poor suppressive capacity.[489] A more detailed study is needed to clarify the role of Tregs in preventing or promoting flavivirus pathogenesis.

Flavivirus Immune Evasion

Evasion of the Type I IFN Pathway

Flaviviruses have evolved several strategies to avoid and/or attenuate induction of type I IFN and its effector responses. In cell culture, flaviviruses are largely resistant to the antiviral effects of IFN once infection is established.[264] This may explain, in part, the relatively modest therapeutic window for IFN-α administration that has been observed clinically in animal models

or humans infected with JEV, SLEV, and WNV.[178,507,910,1052] Experiments by several groups have demonstrated that individual flaviviruses attenuate IFN signaling at distinct and multiple steps in the cascade. Excellent recent reviews can be accessed for further mechanistic detail.[86,342,753]

Inhibition of IFN-β gene induction

Three mechanisms have been described by which flaviviruses minimize the induction of IFN-β (Fig. 9.11):

1. *PRR detection.* Highly pathogenic WNV strains evade IRF3-dependent recognition pathways without actively antagonizing the host defense signaling pathways.[336] Virulent WNV strains delay activation of PRR, such as RIG-I, through uncertain mechanisms to provide the virus with a kinetic advantage in the infected cell to elude host detection during replication at early times after infection.[518] In contrast, less pathogenic strains of WNV induce greater levels of IFN at early time points.[517] One strategy that DENV and WNV likely use to prevent RLRs from accessing viral RNA in the cytoplasm is the formation of separate replication compartments. Flaviviruses replicate in ER-convoluted membrane vesicles, also called viroplasm-like structures,[357,1193] which may function as a physical barrier to conceal dsRNA from cytoplasmic RLR sensors and delay IFN induction. As a second strategy, DENV and ZIKV NS4B induces elongation of mitochondria, which physically contact the ER-associated membranes that are sites of replication. This restructuring attenuates RIG-I–dependent activation of IFN responses.[181]

2. *PRR signaling.* Individual flaviviruses interfere with specific steps in PRR signaling pathways to inhibit IFN-β induction. DENV sfRNA, a noncoding RNA derived from the 3′ UTR of viral genomic RNA that contributes to pathogenicity and evasion of the type I IFN response,[1000] can inhibit TRIM25-dependent activation of RIG-I.[696] Multiple flavivirus NS3 proteins (e.g., DENV and WNV) can compete with RIG-I for 14-3-3ε binding to inhibit the translocation of RIG-I to mitochondria.[175] The strong binding affinity of NS3 for 14-3-3ε was attributed to a highly conserved 4–amino acid motif 64-R-X-E-P-67, in which the central E66 glutamic acid residue mimics the phosphorylated Ser/Thr residue of cellular 14-3-3–binding motifs. ZIKV, DENV, WNV, and JEV, but not YFV NS2B/3 proteases, cleave STING, thereby preventing type I IFN induction mediated by cGAS, possibly downstream of virus-induced DNA damage or mitophagy.[8,269,1232] As the cleavage sites for DENV and ZIKV NS2B/3 are present in human STING, but not in the murine ortholog, STING likely functions as a species-specific restriction factor for these viruses.

3. *Downstream of PRR signaling.* The NS2B/3 protease of DENV can bind to IKKε and block its kinase activity, thereby inhibiting IRF3 phosphorylation and its nuclear translocation.[27] Ectopic expression of NS2A and NS4B from DENV-1, DENV-2, and DENV-4, as well as NS4B of WNV, inhibited the autophosphorylation-dependent activation of TBK1.[234] The NS4A protein from DENV-1, but not other DENV serotypes, also inhibited TBK1, suggesting that DENV-1 contains additional IFN-regulating virulence determinants. ZIKV NS1 and NS4B also appear to inhibit IFN-β induction at the level of TBK1 activation.[1213] The high-mannose carbohydrates on the E protein

may independently block the production of IFN-β, IL-6, and TNF-α that is induced by dsRNA in macrophages. This effect was not directly dependent on TLR3 but instead occurred downstream at the level of the signaling intermediate and NF-κB activator, receptor-interacting protein (RIP)-1.[31] Based on studies with macrophages from different age cohorts, this E protein–dependent inhibitory pathway may be dysregulated in elderly humans, leading to a pathogenic cytokine response.[548] Although the mechanistic basis for how specific forms of the E protein alter antiviral signaling programs remains uncertain, glycosylated E proteins can potentially signal through multiple cell-surface lectins including the mannose receptor[747] and CLEC5a.[189]

4. *IFN-β gene transcription and translation.* Studies with KUNV have identified the nonstructural protein NS2A as an inhibitor of IFN-β gene transcription.[656,660] Incorporation of an A30P mutation of NS2A into a KUNV genome resulted in a virus that elicits more rapid and sustained synthesis of type I IFN; infection of this mutant virus *in vitro* and *in vivo* was highly attenuated. The exact cellular target of NS2A and its mechanism of inhibition remain unknown. More recent studies with ZIKV suggest that flaviviruses also may independently inhibit IFN-β translation in human dendritic cells and neuroprogenitor cells through an as yet uncharacterized mechanism that may depend on motifs in the viral NS4B protein.[116,375]

Impaired IFNAR pathway signaling

In addition to antagonizing induction of IFN-β, several flaviviruses target the JAK–STAT signaling pathway for evasion to prevent the induction of antiviral ISGs (Fig. 9.12). Thus, even when type I IFN is produced, it may not achieve its optimal inhibitory effect because of attenuated signaling capacity. As the nonstructural proteins NS2A, NS3, NS4A, NS4B, and NS5 mediate many of the viral evasion mechanisms described below, these countermeasures are largely intrinsic to infected cells.

1. *Phosphorylation of JAKs.* Studies with LGTV and WNV found interference with phosphorylation of both JAK1 and Tyk2.[87,405] A variation on this was observed with JEV, which showed complete inhibition of phosphorylation of Tyk2 with little effect on JAK1 phosphorylation.[649] Expression of a subgenomic replicon or infection of cells with DENV also inhibited Tyk2 phosphorylation and had no effect on IFNAR expression.[467] However, there may be cell- or virus-specific effects, as JEV also inhibits STAT1 and STAT2 activation in the setting of normal levels of Tyk2 phosphorylation.[645]

2. *STAT1 and STAT2 protein expression and function.* Another important evasion strategy employed by several different flaviviruses is the direct antagonism of STAT1 and/or STAT2. Ectopic expression studies in A549 cells with DENV showed that NS2A, NS4A, or NS4B enhanced replication of an IFN-sensitive virus by blocking nuclear localization of STAT1.[800] Subsequent experiments showed that NS4B of DENV, WNV, and YFV partially blocks STAT1 activation and ISG induction.[799] Mutagenesis studies have identified a sequence determinant on WNV NS4B (E22/K24) that controls IFN resistance in cells expressing subgenomic replicons.[308]

The nonstructural proteins of WNV, DENV, ZIKV, and YFV potently block STAT2 activation through different mechanisms.[34,388,567,596,661,718] The NS5 protein of DENV recruits the host factor UBR4, which induces the proteasomal degradation of STAT2.[789] Although ZIKV similarly promoted proteasomal degradation of STAT2, it did not require UBR4.[388] Both DENV and ZIKV NS5 interact with human STAT2, but not mouse Stat2,[35,388] indicating that STAT2 also contributes to the species-specific restriction of DENV and ZIKV infection. Introduction of either the structural (capsid and E proteins) or nonstructural (NS1–5) proteins from a pathogenic WNV strain (Texas 2002) into an attenuated strain (Madagascar 1978) led to more potent IFN-antagonistic activity and pathogenesis, suggesting that both structural and nonstructural proteins of WNV contribute to efficient STAT1/2 inhibition.[1087] Antagonism of STAT2 by YFV has some unique features. For example, the binding of YFV NS5 to STAT2 depends on stimulation of cells with type I or III IFNs.[597] Type I IFN signaling promotes TRIM23-dependent K63-linked ubiquitination of YFV NS5 that enables its association with STAT2.[597] Unlike DENV or ZIKV, STAT2 binding by YFV NS5 does not promote degradation but rather inhibits interaction of ISGF3 to promoter elements to prevent ISG transcription.

While NS5 attenuates JAK–STAT signaling after TBEV, LGTV, and JEV infection, the mechanism of NS5 inhibition appears to have virus-specific characteristics. For TBEV, a sequence in the methyltransferase domain of NS5 binds the PDZ protein scribble to inhibit JAK–STAT signaling.[1197] For LGTV, the JAK–STAT inhibitory domain was mapped to sites within the RNA-dependent RNA polymerase domain.[861] For JEV, the N-terminal 83 residues of NS5 inhibit JAK–STAT signaling through a protein tyrosine phosphatase–dependent mechanism.[644]

3. *Cholesterol redistribution.* Flavivirus infection can promote relocalization of cholesterol to intracellular membranous sites of replication. This redistribution diminishes the formation of cholesterol-rich lipid rafts in the plasma membrane and attenuates the IFN antiviral signaling response.[686]

4. *Up-regulating negative regulators.* WNV, JEV, and TBEV can block IFNAR-dependent signal transduction by up-regulating the expression of suppressors of cytokine signaling (SOCS) 1 and 3,[574,697] which dampen JAK1 activity. Subsequent mechanistic studies showed that WNV and also other enveloped viruses that incorporate phosphatidylserine lipids into their virions induce SOCS1/3 gene expression by binding to inhibitory TAM (Tyro3/Axl/Mer) receptors on dendritic cells, thereby blunting the antiviral IFN response.[91]

5. *IFNAR expression.* TBEV and WNV antagonize type I IFN signaling by inhibiting surface expression of IFNAR1. Loss of IFNAR1 was associated with binding of the viral NS5 protein to prolidase, a cellular dipeptidase. Prolidase was required for IFNAR1 maturation and accumulation, activation of IFN-β–stimulated gene induction, and type I IFN-dependent control of viral infection.[672]

Impaired IFN effector functions

Although flaviviruses devote a significant segment of their genome to inhibiting JAK–STAT signaling, they also target individual downstream antiviral effector molecules. Viperin is a an antiviral ISG that inhibits hepatitis C, influenza, HIV, and

Sindbis viruses, possibly because of its ability to alter lipid raft formation. JEV, however, counteracts viperin by promoting rapid proteasome-dependent degradation.[174] The mechanism of this inhibition remains unclear, as transfection of individual JEV proteins failed to explain the phenotype suggesting a combined effect of viral proteins or replication is required. Viperin also restricts WNV pathogenesis[1093] and inhibits replication of TBEV and ZIKV by targeting NS3 for proteasomal degradation.[857] Viperin also attenuates flavivirus replication by catalyzing the production of a chain-terminator ribonucleotide.[359]

All pathogenic flaviviruses (e.g., WNV, DENV, JEV, ZIKV, TBEV, and YFV) encode methyltransferases as part of their NS5 proteins to modify the 5′ cap structure of their viral mRNAs, thereby mimicking eukaryotic cap 1 (m7GpppNm) structures. Flavivirus 2′-O-methyltransferase activity evades viral RNA detection by IFIT proteins,[232,1259] which can block viral protein synthesis by binding preferentially to non–2′-O-methylated cap 0 (m7GpppN-RNA) structures and competing for eIF4e binding.[413,528] A recombinant WNV encoding an NS5 E218A mutant protein that is defective in 2′-O-methyltransferase activity was more sensitive to the antiviral action of IFIT family members.[232,1095] Similarly, ablation of the 2′-O-methyltransferase activity from JEV and DENV led to growth attenuation of the mutant viruses in the context of cellular innate immune responses.[620,1260] Recent studies have suggested that in addition to enhanced recognition by IFIT1, flavivirus RNA lacking 2′-O-methylation also may act as a PAMP for induction of multiple innate immune genes.[620,1259]

Evasion of the Complement Pathway by NS1

To minimize recognition and/or destruction by complement, viruses have evolved strategies to evade or exploit complement to establish infection.[40,1072] Flavivirus NS1 is expressed on cell surfaces, secreted from infected cells, and accumulates in the serum of infected individuals, with high circulating levels correlating with severe DENV disease.[41,629] WNV NS1 attenuates complement activation of the alternative pathway by enhancing the cofactor activity of factor H for factor I–mediated cleavage of C3b to iC3b, which decreases deposition of C3b and the C5b to C9 membrane attack complex on cell surfaces.[203] As an additional mechanism by which flaviviruses can evade complement, NS1 also binds to C4 and C1s, which enhanced the cleavage of C4 to C4b and reduced C4b and C3b deposition on cell surfaces.[37] NS1 also protects DENV from neutralization in solution by binding to MBL and inhibiting complement deposition.[1118] Soluble NS1 has also been reported to bind the complement regulatory factors C4bp,[38] vitronectin, and clusterin, the latter two of which inhibit the formation of the C5b to C9 membrane attack complex.[210,581]

Class I MHC and NK Cell Evasion

Because of their capacity to directly kill virally infected cells or produce inflammatory cytokines that control early stages of infection, NK cells are an important initial defense against many viruses. NK cells lyse infected cells by releasing cytotoxic granules that contain perforin and granzymes or by binding to cell death–inducing receptors on target cells. NK cell activation is finely regulated through a balance of activating (Ly49D, Ly49H, and NKG2D) and inhibitory cell-surface receptors (killer cell immunoglobulin-like receptors [KIR],

immunoglobulin-like inhibitory receptors [ILT], and CD94-NKG2A). To control the consequences of untoward activation of NK cells, inhibitory receptors are expressed constitutively, some of which bind to host MHC class I molecules on opposing cells and transmit inhibitory signals through intracellular tyrosine-based inhibitory motifs in their cytoplasmic domains. A decrease in expression of class I MHC molecules on a cell may prompt NK cell activation by attenuating the inhibitory signals. Thus, NK cell target recognition occurs after ligation of activating receptors and repression of inhibitory receptors on the cell surface.

Although many DNA viruses attempt to avoid NK responses by a variety of mechanisms including expressing MHC class I homologs, flaviviruses may evade NK cell cytotoxicity by increasing surface expression of class I MHC molecules.[532,657,658] Expression of class I MHC molecules is stimulated by increasing the transport activity of TAP[762,798] and by NF-kB–dependent transcriptional activation of MHC class I genes.[521] The rapid increase in expression of MHC class I suggests that early in the course of infection, flaviviruses may overcome susceptibility to NK cell–mediated lysis, even if it is at the expense of later recognition by an adaptive CD8+ T-cell response. Consistent with this, splenocytes from WNV-immunized mice had poor NK cell lytic activity,[762] and mice with acquired deficiencies in NK cells demonstrated no increased morbidity or mortality compared to wild-type controls.[1029]

ANIMAL MODELS OF FLAVIVIRUS PATHOGENESIS AND DISEASE

Animal models of viral infections are used to address fundamental questions that are difficult to answer in human studies. These investigations are often directed toward defining basic mechanisms of viral pathogenesis (tropism, dissemination, and virulence) and host immune responses (protective and pathologic), but also are important for determining relative efficacy of candidate vaccines and antiviral agents. In general, the most useful surrogate models mimic features of human disease, are reproducible, and have the capacity for high-throughput experimentation. The weakness of many animal models is they often do not fully recapitulate human disease with respect to kinetics, viral replication and spread, or disease phenotype, and thus restraint is required in applying these results to the human condition. Animal models of flavivirus infection are varied in their fidelity to human disease and, thus, utility in providing basic insight into pathogenesis, immune control, and likely efficacy of vaccines or antiviral agents. This section will review the strengths and weaknesses of key animal models and what investigators in the field have learned by using them.

Dengue Virus

One of the major limitations in identifying and working with animal models of DENV infection is that humans are the only known host to develop disease after infection. A second consideration is that severe dengue and its plasma leakage syndrome are associated with preexisting maternal antibody in infants and secondary infection in children and adults, suggesting an immunopathogenesis mechanism, which has been difficult to recapitulate in animals. While each of the animal models described below has been informative for understanding DENV infection, their inability to mimic human disease has limited the insight on human DENV infection.

Nonhuman Primate Model of DENV Infection

Although humans are the natural host for DENV, serological data support the existence of a sylvatic cycle between mosquitoes and nonhuman primates (NHPs).[1176] Several species of NHP (e.g., chimpanzees and rhesus macaques) have been infected experimentally with DENV and develop viremia and adaptive immune responses,[431,432,984] although in most cases, there is limited evidence of the severe disease seen in humans. One study in macaques showed thrombocytopenia, transiently reduced complement levels, and enhanced peak viremia after secondary infection with heterologous DENV serotype although only 1 of 44 animals developed a syndrome that shared features of severe human disease.[432] Features of severe dengue were observed in six rhesus macaques after high-dose (10^7 PFU per animal) intravenous infection with a DENV-2 strain including neutropenia, thrombocytopenia, clotting abnormalities, and petechial hemorrhage.[844]

NHPs also have been used as a model to study ADE and its consequences. Enhancement of viremia was observed in juvenile rhesus monkeys after passive transfer of antibody and heterologous DENV challenge.[418] Analogously, an approximately 100-fold increase of DENV-4 viremia was demonstrated in juvenile rhesus monkeys that received a cross-reactive mAb recognizing the fusion loop in DII.[371] In neither model, however, was evidence of severe vascular leakage observed despite the increase in DENV replication. NHPs also have been used to evaluate adaptive immune response and protection of live attenuated or subunit-based DENV vaccine candidates.[207,289,551]

Mouse Models

The utility and clinical features of individual mouse models of DENV infection have been described in great detail.[1224,1241] Below, we describe some features of the more commonly used models in the field. In general, there are several hurdles to establishing mouse models of DENV disease pathogenesis: (a) the majority of models are not ideal because most mice do not develop the same clinical disease as humans; (b) it has been difficult to infect mice reliably and reproducibly with low passage clinical and mosquito isolates. Hence, many studies are performed with laboratory- or mouse-adapted strains that have uncertain relevance to the strains that cause human disease; and (c) DENV is virulent in humans because it has evolved specific countermeasures to evade the human immune response.[260] In mice, these evasion mechanisms do not function, resulting in rapid control.

IFN signaling–deficient mice

Because of the importance of STAT2 and the IFN response in restricting DENV infection, mice lacking receptors for both type I (IFN-α/β) and type II (IFN-γ) (e.g., AG129) were tested and shown vulnerable to intraperitoneal (IP) infection with a mouse-adapted (New Guinea C) DENV-2 strain[495] or intravenous (IV) infection with a laboratory-adapted (PL046) DENV-2 strain.[1023] In these studies, however, mice succumbed to DENV infection because of rapid spread to the CNS, resulting in encephalitis and paralysis, which are not common

features of human disease. Similar results were observed in Stat1$^{-/-}$ and Stat2$^{-/-}$ mice,[35,1025] although in some cases hemorrhage was observed after inoculation at multiple sites.[189] Other studies identified mouse-adapted (DENV-2 D2S10) and non-adapted strains (DENV-2 Y98P) that cause rapid death of AG129 mice associated with some characteristics of human disease, including cytokine storm, vascular leakage, and high TNF-α levels[1024,1098] after IV or IP infection.

AG129 mice have been used as a model to test antiviral candidates[195,1002,1066] or to explore the role of ADE in disease severity. Preexisting cross-reactive monoclonal or polyclonal antibodies facilitate ADE *in vivo* and promote more severe DENV disease including vascular leakage.[52,1240] Importantly, when the Fc fragment was eliminated by proteolysis or modified genetically, enhanced replication and disease were no longer observed, thus confirming that ADE via Fcγ receptor engagement can cause severe disease in an animal.[420,1205] Cellular and tissue tropisms have been examined in the ADE model in AG129 mice[52,1240]; the virus targets are similar to that described in human autopsy studies with antigen present in the lymph node, spleen, and bone marrow, with infection in myeloid cells, and possibly with sinusoidal endothelial cells in the liver. Although the comparative data are intriguing, the absence of IFN in mice independently broadens cellular and tissue tropism of flaviviruses,[963] and thus, some caution in interpretation is warranted. Some of this concern was mitigated through the use of mice with cell-type–specific gene deletions of IFNAR1. For example, *LysM* Cre$^+$ *Ifnar1*$^{fl/fl}$ mice, which lack Ifnar1 expression only in myeloid cells, sustained high levels of DENV infection and disease, including plasma leakage, hypercytokinemia, liver injury, hemoconcentration, and thrombocytopenia.[882]

Immunocompetent mice

The successful infection of immunocompetent mice with DENV strains would allow more detailed analysis of the kinetics and function of protective immune responses. Although most DENV strains replicate poorly in wild-type laboratory strains of mice, recent reports suggest that infection may be possible, with the development of a spectrum of disease. Subcutaneous and systemic hemorrhage was induced in wild-type C57BL/6 mice after intradermal (ID) infection with a laboratory-passaged DENV-2 16681 strain.[186] With this strain, C57BL/6 and BALB/c mice also developed thrombocytopenia, elevated levels of systemic TNF-α, and liver damage.[187,852] These experiments did not show evidence of vascular leakage, the hallmark of severe DENV disease in humans. However, wild-type mice experimentally inoculated with a DENV clinical isolate (DENV-2, Eden strain) experienced a rise in hematocrit values that remained increased over naïve mice for 4 days postinfection, demonstrating some evidence of increased vascular permeability.[1059]

Mouse–human chimeras

Because most mouse strains do not sustain DENV replication after infection, mouse–human chimeras have been developed. Early studies using severe combined immunodeficient (SCID) mice engrafted with human peripheral blood lymphocytes showed marginal infection with a DENV-1 strain.[1211] Subsequent studies engrafted human tumor cells (K562, HepG2, Huh-7),[23,98,648] which supported DENV replication but caused CNS disease and not a vascular leakage syndrome.

Nonobese diabetic (NOD)/SCID or NOD/SCID IL2R$\gamma^{-/-}$ mice have been engrafted with CD34$^+$ human cord blood hematopoietic progenitor cells. After infection with DENV-2, these chimeric mice developed some of the signs of severe human disease including fever, rash, and thrombocytopenia.[82,487,793] In an analogous model, Rag2$^{-/-}$ x γ chain$^{-/-}$ mice engrafted with CD34$^+$ human fetal liver stem cells and inoculated with DENV-2 developed viremia and fever and produced human specific anti-DENV antibody responses.[582] While engraftment of human cells is advantageous as the response of human cells, pathogenesis, and possibly tropism can be analyzed, the chimeric models have limitations: (a) the disease phenotype recapitulates only some of the features of severe DENV; (b) the mouse-to-mouse level of chimerism is variable, making phenotypic analysis challenging; (c) the throughput of experiments is low, making these models less practical for vaccine or antiviral testing; and (d) the immune cross talk between human and mouse cells within an animal may be altered, limiting interpretation of effects on immunity.

Zika Virus

Prior to the emergence of ZIKV in Latin America, few studies had evaluated ZIKV pathogenesis in animals.[77,266,1185] However, the explosive growth of ZIKV research since 2015 has spurred the development of new animal models, revealing pathogenic mechanisms and providing systems for evaluating therapeutic interventions. The most significant models of ZIKV infection are nonhuman primates and mice (reviewed in Ref.[788]), but ZIKV disease also has been studied in guinea pigs, hamsters, tree shrews, and swine.[93,237,238,256,569,748,1032,1200,1250] Early ZIKV isolates were maintained by serial passage in suckling mouse brains, which likely selected variants with improved replication in this tissue. Thus, historical studies (as well as contemporary studies using historical strains) may overestimate the neurotropism of ZIKV relative to strains circulating in humans and mosquitoes.

Nonhuman Primate Models

Rhesus macaques serve as valuable models for ZIKV pathogenesis research, owing to their physiological similarity to humans and a significant preexisting research infrastructure resulting from their use in models of other infectious diseases. Rhesus macaques recapitulate key features of ZIKV infection in humans including transient viremia; fever and rash; viral RNA in saliva, urine, and semen; viral replication in tissues such as the eye and testis; susceptibility via subcutaneous, intravenous, or intravaginal inoculation; and commonly asymptomatic infection.[165,285,414,466,619,849] Experimental ZIKV infection in cynomolgus and pigtail macaques is similar to rhesus.[42,256,414,546,834,849] ZIKV also infects baboons, which may better represent the sylvatic reservoir of ZIKV as they are African monkeys and have been found to be ZIKV seropositive in nature.[139,407] Marmosets, squirrel monkeys, and owl monkeys also are susceptible to experimental ZIKV infection, which may be relevant to the establishment of a sylvatic reservoir in New World primates.[198,1144]

Mouse Models

Mice offer advantages in terms of cost, scale, speed, and genetic tractability, enabling mechanistic studies that are not feasible in nonhuman primate models. A disadvantage of mouse models is that ZIKV replicates poorly in immunocompetent mice and thus does not exhibit the tissue tropism and disease phenotypes characteristic of human infection. Mice lacking type I interferon (IFN-$\alpha\beta$) production or responses succumb to ZIKV infection and exhibit broad tissue tropism, implying that the innate antiviral response is a key barrier to ZIKV replication and pathogenesis in mice.[600,947] Mice lacking the IFN-$\alpha\beta$ receptor (alone or also lacking the IFN-γ receptor) have provided models for studying ZIKV disease phenotypes including congenital infection (below), sexual transmission, and ocular infection, as well as for evaluating vaccines and antivirals.[288,382,723,752,928,1103,1251] The restriction of ZIKV replication in mice results in part from an inability of ZIKV NS5 to degrade murine Stat2, and therefore ZIKV cannot inhibit IFN signaling in mice by the same mechanism used in human cells.[388,567] Indeed, *Stat2*$^{-/-}$ mice succumb to ZIKV infection, and transgenic wild-type mice expressing human STAT2 can develop disease in the context of ZIKV strains with additional mouse-adaptive mutations.[375,1127] In addition, the ZIKV NS2B-NS3 protease targets human but not murine STING, resulting in sustained IFN production and diminished viral replication in mouse cells.[269] However, mice lacking STING were not more susceptible to ZIKV than wild-type mice,[269,600] implying that STING is a contributing but not dominant factor restricting ZIKV infection in mice.

Human Tissue Models

ZIKV replicates in a variety of human cell types in culture, with monocytes being key targets in humans and macaques.[332,466,745,834,849] Recent advances in brain organoid culture systems, as well as studies of neural progenitor cells in culture and in mice, have revealed a tropism for neuronal subsets in the developing brain that likely contributes to the neurodevelopmental defects caused by ZIKV infection *in utero*.[235,346,440,625,903,904,1101] Cellular mechanisms that may contribute to ZIKV neuropathogenesis include neural progenitor death and dysregulated proliferation,[1101] the ability of Musashi-1 to bind the 3′ UTR of the ZIKV genome and promote viral replication in neural progenitors,[184] and the ability of ZIKV sfRNA to antagonize fragile X mental retardation protein, which has important functions in neurodevelopment.[1056] The mechanisms of ZIKV congenital disease also have been advanced by *ex vivo* culture systems that model infection at the maternal–fetal interface. These systems include cultures of syncytiotrophoblasts from term placentas as well as explants of midgestation chorionic villi, both of which have revealed that syncytiotrophoblasts are resistant to ZIKV infection whereas cytotrophoblasts are susceptible, and suggest that constitutive cytokine production contributes to antiviral immunity in the placenta.[68,214,484,1096]

Pregnancy and Vertical Transmission Models

Physiological similarity to humans, including in placental architecture, has made nonhuman primate systems the most faithful models of ZIKV vertical transmission and congenital disease. ZIKV infection in pregnant macaques recapitulates key features of CZS in humans including placental inflammation and calcifications, disrupted brain development, ophthalmological pathology, and fetal demise.[4,5,209,286,465,687,708,761,823] ZIKV infection in pregnant macaques also produces sustained maternal viremia similar to that observed in pregnant women.[687,708,823] As in humans, only a subset of ZIKV-exposed macaque pregnancies develops CZS and the manifestation of disease is variable, making it challenging to design studies with a feasible number of animals. Baboons offer advantages as pregnancy models because they breed year-round and their estrous phase is externally evident, facilitating timed infection experiments, though research facilities for baboons are more limited.[408] Marmosets provide an interesting system for studying congenital ZIKV infection because their pregnancies typically are dizygotic twins, allowing assessment of independent transplacental transmission events in each infected dam[1007]; such studies support observations in humans finding concordant CZS outcomes in monozygotic twins and discordant outcomes in dizygotic twins exposed to ZIKV *in utero*.[150,969]

While NHPs have provided valuable systems for understanding the manifestations of CZS, limitations in terms of experimental size and cost have meant that mice have emerged as a key model for studying the mechanisms that control transplacental transmission and fetal pathology. Mouse and human placentas are both hemochorial, although other anatomic differences as well as developmental differences between 3-week mouse and 40-week human pregnancies require caveats when translating effects in mouse pregnancy systems to humans.[24] Most ZIKV congenital infection models use dams with impaired IFN-$\alpha\beta$ signaling, commonly transgenic mice lacking the IFN-$\alpha\beta$ receptor or administration of an IFN-$\alpha\beta$ receptor-blocking monoclonal antibody. In these systems, fetuses become infected and exhibit growth restriction or demise, with infection at earlier gestational stages associated with more severe fetal pathology.[484,750,1229] IFN-$\alpha\beta$ signaling plays a key role in restricting ZIKV replication and thereby controlling transplacental transmission, but this antiviral response itself also elicits placental and fetal pathology, pointing to immune pathology as a potential contributing factor to CZS.[1228]

Yellow Fever Virus

Despite the fact that YFV was isolated in 1927 and that a vaccine was developed 10 years later, our understanding of the mechanisms underlying the pathogenesis of virulent YFV remains limited. Analogous to DENV, part of this stems from the lack of a small animal model that recapitulates the viscerotropism of human infection. Given the reemergence of YFV, an improved understanding of its pathogenesis and a vehicle for testing novel vaccines and antiviral agents through the use of existing and new animal models of disease is now a research priority.

Human Vaccine Model

Vaccination with the attenuated 17D strain of YFV has conferred protection on hundreds of millions of humans worldwide. Recent prospective analyses have examined the interaction of 17D YFV with the innate immune system and how this might be important for triggering long-term protective adaptive immunity.[898] A systems biology approach defined early gene signatures that predicted immune responses in humans vaccinated with yellow fever vaccine YFV-17D. Computational analyses identified induction of genes (e.g., complement protein C1qB, TNFRS17, and eukaryotic translation initiation factor 2 alpha kinase 4) that correlated with and predicted protective B- and T-cell responses with high accuracy in an independent, blinded trial.[906]

Nonhuman Primate Model of Severe YFV Infection

YFV cycles in nature as part of a sylvatic cycle between *Aedes* mosquitoes and wild monkeys. Rhesus and cynomologus monkeys develop viscerotropic disease, analogous to humans, ranging from mild to fulminant hepatitis, whereas African and New World NHPs generally have milder or silent infections,[768] with some exceptions.[781] The pathogenesis of YFV infection in rhesus monkeys resembles severe human disease with the development of jaundice, acute renal failure, coagulopathy, and shock,[769] although the course is more severe, not biphasic, produces markedly higher viral burden, and is also associated with severe necrosis of lymphoid tissue.[542,769] The coagulopathy in monkeys is associated with a global decrease in synthesis of clotting factors secondary to direct hepatic damage and impaired hemostasis associated with abnormalities of platelet function.[768]

In contrast to that described for DENV, preexisting immunity to heterologous flaviviruses results in protection rather than enhanced pathogenesis of YFV in NHP. Rhesus monkeys that were infected previously with DENV were protected against YFV challenge, and recipients of anti-DENV antibodies by passive transfer showed no evidence of enhanced disease.[768,1112] Monkeys immunized with other flaviviruses,[456] similar to humans with prior exposure to flaviviruses,[771] manifest a lower incidence of severe YFV disease.

Rodent Models of YFV Infection

Historical infection studies in mice and hamsters with nonadapted YFV did not cause viscerotropic disease. Syrian golden hamsters, however, did develop disease more closely resembling human YFV infection (hepatitis, hepatic necrosis, splenic necrosis), but this phenotype requires serial passage of YFV *in vivo*, and renal disease was not observed.[720,1215] In comparison, peripheral infection of wild-type mice does not cause viscerotropic disease. However, YFV-induced encephalitis can be induced in suckling mice after IP or IC inoculation, in adult mice if the blood–brain barrier is disturbed, or if mouse-adapted strains are used.[60,328,329,768,977] Because these models do not cause viscerotropism, they are of limited relevance to understanding the pathophysiology of human YFV infection and have been largely restricted to vaccine and antiviral testing. Subcutaneous infection studies of mice deficient in IFN signaling revealed viscerotropic YFV infection and disease (liver and spleen necrosis) without a requirement for virus adaptation.[735] This study suggests that nonadapted YFV has little ability to evade the antiviral activity of IFN-α/β in mice, whereas species-specific antagonism of IFN-α/β antiviral activity in primate hosts may contribute to infection outcome.

West Nile Virus

WNV and other encephalitic flaviviruses are generally more promiscuous in their ability to infect and cause disease in different species of animals. Beyond its endemic cycle in multiple species of birds, WNV causes severe disease in horses and occasionally can infect other mammals sometimes with severe consequences.[115] Although the molecular basis for its broad animal tropism remains uncharacterized, as a result of this, it has been easier to develop small animal models of infection that recapitulate features of human disease using low passage field isolates. However, the frequency of neuroinvasive disease may vary significantly among animal species, making some models preferred for studying pathogenesis and disease outcome.

Nonhuman Primate Model of WNV Infection

Nonhuman primate models of WNV infection are important because of their potential for use in evaluating vaccine and therapeutic candidates. In one study of five intradermally infected rhesus macaques, the clinical course, level and duration of viremia, and antibody response were similar to that occurring in uncomplicated human WNV infection, although it was unclear whether virus entered the brain in these animals.[913] This model of sustained viremia and measurable immune responses has been used to evaluate the efficacy of WNV vaccine candidates.[1201] Analogously, in baboons, after intradermal infection, WNV accumulated to high levels in blood and was associated with a transient macular rash, but failed to cause encephalitis or other severe clinical signs.[1208] Although these NHP models do not develop WNV encephalitis, it remains possible that the frequency of neuroinvasive disease parallels human infection (1:150) and thus would require much larger studies to identify severe cases. In contrast to infection via a peripheral route, intracerebral inoculation of rhesus monkeys with different African and Asian WNV strains results in persistent viral infection in the CNS and other organs.[889] These animals sustained a prolonged infection course and showed evidence of fatal encephalitis with diffuse neuronal degeneration and necrosis and inflammation. Similar severe clinical manifestations (fever, tremors, and spasticity) were observed in rhesus macaques challenged via a frontal lobe injection with the New York 1999 strain of WNV.[32]

Hamster Model

Syrian golden hamsters are an excellent small animal model for studying WNV pathogenesis, vaccine efficacy, and antiviral screening. Intraperitoneal or even oral infection of WNV results in viremia of 5 to 6 days in duration, followed by the development of virus-specific antibodies.[980,1214] Clinical signs of encephalitis (weakness, tremor, ataxia, and paralysis) were apparent within 6 to 7 days of infection with an approximately 50% mortality rate. WNV disease correlated with the detection of viral antigen and neuronal degeneration in several regions of the brain including the cerebral cortex, basal ganglia, hippocampus, cerebellum, and brain stem. Because of their larger size relative to mice, hamsters have been used to elucidate particular aspects of neuropathogenesis. WNV spread to the CNS can occur through a retrograde axonal transport mechanism, as the virus moves from peripheral motor neurons into the spinal cord.[964,1179] Electrophysiology studies have shown that respiratory distress associated with WNV infection is caused by diaphragmatic suppression through lesions in the brain stem and cervical spinal cord or altered vagal afferent function.[785]

In the hamster model, infectious WNV can be cultured from the brains of hamsters up to 53 days after initial infection,[1214] suggesting that persistent replication occurs. Persistent WNV infection in the spinal cord causes continued neuronal dysfunction, chronic neuropathological lesions, and poliomyelitis-like disease and can be measured using electrophysiological approaches.[1033] Hamsters also develop persistent viruria, as infectious WNV can be cultured from urine for several weeks.[1122]

The hamster model has been used to evaluate candidate therapeutics or vaccines against WNV disease. Studies with small molecule inhibitors,[787] antiviral cytokines,[782] synthetic oligonucleotides,[1123] and humanized monoclonal antibodies[783] have been performed with varying efficacy, especially when administered as postexposure therapy.[261] Analogously, immunization with single-cycle,[1202] recombinant subunit,[1036] or live attenuated[1109] vaccines has elicited durable protective immunity and, thus, has provided a robust preclinical small animal model for assessment and comparison of the surrogate markers of protection.

Mouse Models

Infection studies in several inbred laboratory strains of mice have provided insight into the fundamental mechanisms of WNV dissemination, pathogenesis, and immune system control. Most studies have been performed with North American WNV strains and wild-type and immunodeficient C57BL/6 mice. The strengths of this particular model include (a) depending on the dose of virus and age of mice, a subset of wild-type mice develop neuroinvasive disease, whereas the remainder are infected with minimal or limited spread to the CNS. Thus, the mechanisms by which the immune system restricts viral entry or facilitates viral clearance can be studied; (b) many features of pathogenesis and neuropathology appear remarkably similar to that observed in humans; (c) non-adapted low passage WNV isolates cause disease in wild-type mice. Thus, this model can be used to define the genetics of virus attenuation; (d) there are many transgenic, knockout, and conditional knockout mice available from academic laboratories and public consortia to study the role of specific genes or cells in pathogenesis; and (e) genes (e.g., CCR5 and OAS1b) that predict susceptibility in mice have been corroborated as risk factors for human WNV disease.[263] Nonetheless, there are limitations to the model including the compressed disease time course, the difficulty in obtaining CSF samples in live animals because of size, and a rather flat virus dose–response curve after peripheral infection.

Following peripheral inoculation of mice, initial WNV replication is thought to occur in skin Langerhans dendritic cells,[147] with mosquito saliva modulating the local proinflammatory cytokine response.[994] Dendritic cells migrate to and seed draining lymph nodes, resulting in a primary viremia and subsequent infection of peripheral tissues such as the spleen and, occasionally, the kidney. By the end of the first week, WNV is largely cleared from the serum and peripheral organs, and infection in the CNS is observed in a subset of immunocompetent animals. Mice that succumb to infection develop CNS pathology similar to that observed in human WNV cases, including infection and injury of brain stem, hippocampal, and spinal cord neurons.[1028] WNV infection is detected in at much lower levels in nonneuronal CNS cell populations, such as CD11b+ cells[228,1124] or astrocytes.[270] In most surviving wild-type mice, infectious WNV is cleared from all tissue compartments within 2 to 3 weeks after infection. However, persistent WNV infection in the brains of class II MHC,[1043] CD8+ T-cell,[1026] or perforin-deficient mice[1029] was routinely observed. Analogously, a small subset of wild-type mice sustained WNV persistence in the CNS even in the setting of a robust antibody response and inflammation.[30] More recent studies in mice of the Collaborative Cross with greater genetic heterogeneity have described a larger range of clinical phenotypes and their associations with particular genes and immune signatures.[385–387]

FLAVIVIRUS VACCINES

Successful vaccination programs have reduced the clinical impact of flavivirus infections dramatically. More than 500 million doses of vaccine to prevent YFV infection have been administered since its development in 1937.[348] This landmark achievement effectively blunted the impact of this virus on global health. However, decades later, limited vaccine availability to combat the emergence of YFV in Africa and South America highlights a need for continued innovation in vaccine design and manufacturing.[816] Furthermore, safe and effective vaccines are not yet available for many flaviviruses with a sustained or emergent potential to significantly impact public health. This section will provide a noncomprehensive overview of flavivirus vaccine platforms and vaccine development efforts, focused principally on efforts that have yielded licensed vaccines or those in advanced clinical trials.

Flavivirus Vaccine Platforms

Numerous vaccine strategies have been evaluated in preclinical and clinical studies to protect against flaviviruses (Fig. 9.13). While most vaccines seek to present the E protein to the immune system, several approaches employing the nonstructural protein NS1 as an antigen also have been utilized.[120,628]

Live Attenuated Vaccines

Live attenuated flavivirus vaccines have been created by extensive passage, including the earliest efforts to produce a vaccine against DENV by Sabin and colleagues.[957] Multiple licensed vaccine products have been created using this approach including countermeasures for YFV and JEV, as detailed below. The development of molecular clone technology for flaviviruses enabled the design and evaluation of multiple strategies to rationally attenuate infectious viruses, including deletions in the 3′-untranslated region,[737,1015] inhibiting the activity of the 2′-*O*-methyltransferase involved in modulating the host response to viral RNA in the cytoplasm,[1261] and removing N-linked sugars on the NS1 protein.[930] Furthermore, noninfectious self-replicating RNAs derived from the genome designed to express SVPs have also shown promise in preclinical studies.[177,819,1201,1202]

Inactivated Vaccines

Virus inactivation is a proven approach to create safe and protective vaccines. Vaccines produced from JEV-infected mouse brains have been effective at controlling JEV in many parts of Asia, including Japan, South Korea, Taiwan, and Thailand.[327] Inactivated TBEVs are also successful vaccines.[921] This conceptually straightforward pathway to vaccine design and production prompted several groups to create inactivated vaccine candidates for ZIKV.[1,759] Inactivation of live attenuated vaccine candidates has also been evaluated as new vaccine products, conferring an additional layer of safety.[327]

Subunit Vaccines

Subunit vaccines have been evaluated in preclinical and clinical studies. Soluble forms of the E protein have been proposed for several viruses.[607] Soluble DIII and E proteins can be relatively straightforward to express at high levels, manufacture, combine with increasingly powerful adjuvant technologies, and optimally dose. However, the discovery that many potently neutralizing and protective antibodies recognize complex epitopes that include features of multiple E proteins on the virion may limit the utility of this approach.[950] To address this limitation, several groups have designed stabilized E protein dimers as immunogens.[742,949] Numerous approaches to immunize with recombinant SVPs have been reported and show promise in animal models.[550,738,961]

Nucleic Acid Vaccines

Nucleic acid vaccines have several desirable features as vaccine platforms including a completely synthetic manufacturing process, rapid ability to design antigens, capacity to

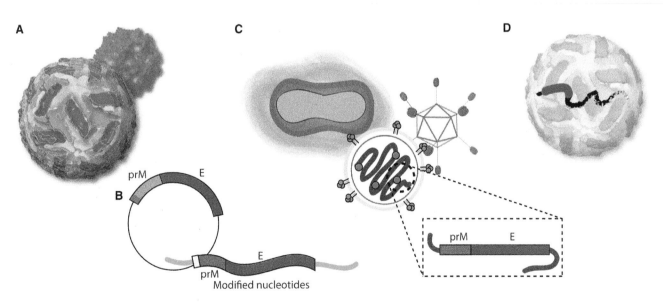

FIGURE 9.13 Flavivirus vaccine platforms. Multiple vaccine platforms have been evaluated in preclinical and clinical studies as vaccine candidates to protect against flaviviruses. These include subunit and subviral particle vaccines **(A)**, nucleic acid vaccines **(B)**, viral vectors **(C)**, and live attenuated viruses **(D)**.

simultaneously deliver multiple antigens, and, in the case of DNA vaccines, a well-established safety profile in humans. DNA vaccine constructs have been developed and evaluated in the clinic for several flaviviruses, including WNV, DENV, and ZIKV.[76,352,606,704,1106]

Nucleoside-modified mRNAs (mRNAs) are synthetic RNA molecules delivered as lipid nanoparticles or complexed with lipids of varied composition.[1192] This technology is capable of producing protein at high level *in vivo* and is being evaluated as a vaccine platform for several unrelated virus families, cancer, and as a therapeutic to address other human diseases. mRNA design includes multiple features thought to avoid recognition by host sensors including a 5′ cap, modified nucleosides, and optimized UTR.[1192] mRNAs expressing ZIKV antigens were evaluated as part of the rapid response to the 2015 epidemic and subsequently as a potential countermeasure to the increased prevalence of POWV in North America.[496]

Yellow Fever Virus

The live attenuated YF-17D vaccine is considered among the most safe and effective vaccines ever developed, an achievement for which Max Theiler was awarded the Nobel Prize in 1951 (the only one awarded for the development of a viral vaccine).[770] The current YFV vaccine was derived from a virus isolated in 1927 from a West African man suffering from a mild febrile illness (the Asibi strain).[1074] The Asibi strain was passaged 176 times in the embryonic tissue of mice and chickens to yield the YF-17D virus with considerably reduced neuro- and viscero-tropic properties.[766,1114] Vaccines currently in use are substrains of YF-17D; strain YF-17DD is used in vaccines produced for South America (passage 287–289), whereas the YF-17D-204 strain (passages 235–240) is distributed elsewhere, including the United States.[62,1063] The consensus sequence of the vaccine strains differs from the parent Asibi strain by approximately 20 amino acids as well as four nucleotide changes in the 3′ UTR.[766] Vaccine is produced in chicken embryos, lyophilized, and administered by subcutaneous injection following reconstitution in saline. A single dose of YFV vaccine contains roughly 10^4 to 10^6 PFU,[62] but administration of a 1/5 fractional dose confers similar protection and allows vaccine supplies to be extended during an outbreak.[58]

The Immune Response to YF-17D Infection

The host response to YF-17D infection involves both the innate and adaptive arms of the immune system.[770] Multiple studies highlight the significance of the innate immune response to YF-17D in shaping the adaptive immune response to vaccination.[351,898,907] YF-17D activates mDC and pDC through multiple TLR proteins, including TLR2, TLR7, TLR8, and TLR9, resulting in the induction of proinflammatory cytokines and IFN-α.[906,907] Of interest, a capacity to interact with multiple TLR pathways does not appear redundant; these interactions tune the adaptive response by influencing the balance of Th1 and Th2 cytokines and the quality of the anti-YFV T-cell response.[907] Indeed, YF-17D infection induces a mixture of Th1 and Th2 cytokines *in vivo*,[351,968] and YF-17D–infected DCs present viral antigen to T cells despite inefficient replication in these cells.[54,854]

YF-17D vaccination induces a low transient viremia that peaks 5 days postvaccination.[766] Defervescence is coincident with a reduction in viremia and the detection of cellular and humoral responses. YF-17D infection induces a polyfunctional CD8+ T-cell response of considerable magnitude (2%–13% of CD8+ T cells) that peaks roughly 2 weeks postimmunization.[9] Analysis of the breadth of this response demonstrates that all 10 viral proteins contain epitopes recognized by CD8+ T cells; reactivity with epitopes in E, NS3, and NS5 proteins was most common.[12,351] The virus-specific CD8+ T-cell response contracts at approximately day 30 postinfection to a size that corresponds to approximately 5% to 10% of the magnitude of the original response, with memory CD8+ T cells persisting for years.[12,749]

Vaccination with YF-17D also elicits a neutralizing antibody response in virtually all recipients.[78,873] Kinetic analysis of vaccinated adults revealed that approximately 87% had neutralizing antibodies at 2 weeks postvaccination, with virtually 100% of subjects developing neutralizing antibody by day 28.[593] YFV-reactive IgM can be detected by day 9, peaks between days 14 and 17, and persists for more than 1 year. YFV-specific IgG is detected between days 10 and 17 and peaks approximately 1 month postvaccination.[770] Neutralizing antibodies that correlate with protection persist for decades.[78,711,770,774] More than 90% of vaccinated subjects had neutralizing antibody when examined 16 to 19 years postimmunization.[946] Indeed, neutralizing antibody was detected in 80% of vaccinated US military personnel when assayed 30 to 35 years after receiving YF-17D.[890]

Adverse Events Arising from YF-17D Vaccination

More than 500 million doses of YF-17D have been administered to humans with a high track record of safety.[348] The most common side effects from YF-17D vaccination are transient headache, myalgia, and low-grade fever.[1063] Severe adverse events (SAE) following vaccination have been reported, albeit at a very low frequency. The risk of SAE following vaccination increases with age; the incidence of SAE in vaccine recipients greater than 70 years of age is roughly 10-fold higher than that for individuals aged 19 to 29.[523] Three main classes of SAE have been reported: (a) anaphylactic reactions are infrequent (1 in 135,000) and likely are a result of allergic responses to components of the vaccine including egg and chicken proteins, gelatin, and latex.[519,1063] (b) Yellow fever vaccine–associated neurological disease (YEL-AND) is associated with invasion of the CNS by the vaccine strain. This SAE was most commonly reported prior to the establishment of the vaccine seed system (in 1945) and in infants prior to changes in the recommendations for vaccination of children less than 6 months old (in 1960).[766] The mechanism underlying the increased risk of YEL-AND in infants remains uncertain, but may reflect differences in the level or duration of viremia, the integrity of the BBB, or a failure to mount an effective immune response.[770] Twenty-nine cases of YEL-AND have been reported since 1990 with a case fatality ratio of 6.9%[770] with an incidence of 0.4 to 0.8 per 100,000 doses.[653,1063] (c) Yellow fever vaccine–associated viscerotropic disease (YEL-AVD) is a SAE that mimics aspects of naturally acquired YFV infection. It is characterized by high fever (within 2–5 days of vaccination), malaise, and myalgia that is followed by jaundice, oliguria, cardiovascular instability, and hemorrhage. Analysis of the sequence of viruses recovered from vaccine recipients with YEL-AVD failed to identity mutations associated with this SAE.[62] Risk factors for YEL-AVD include advanced age and a history of thymus disease or thymectomy.

As of 2010, 57 cases of YEL-AVD have been reported with a case fatality rate of 64%. In the United States, the incidence is estimated as 0.3 to 0.5 per 100,000 doses.[1063]

Dengue Virus

Three live attenuated tetravalent DENV vaccines have been evaluated in advanced clinical trials. Two methods of attenuation were employed to create the four replicating viruses used in combination with each vaccine candidate. The 3′ UTR of flaviviruses folds into RNA structures that regulate genomic RNA replication, translation, and cytopathic properties.[208,879] The introduction of a 30-nucleotide deletion into the 3′ UTR yielded a markedly attenuated virus *in vivo*, which still elicited a robust humoral response in monkeys and humans.[289,737] Vaccination of humans with a DENV-4Δ30 virus resulted in low-level viremia (~1.6 logs) in 70% of recipients,[289] which is not sufficient for blood meal transmission of the vaccine to mosquito vectors. Similar results have been reported with a DENV-1Δ30 virus constructed from the Western Pacific 1974 strain.[291] While introduction of this deletion was not sufficient for attenuating all DENV strains,[100,101] further iterations of this concept, including additional deleted regions, were successful.[102] ZIKV was attenuated using similar strategies, as detailed below. The attenuating mechanism of deletions in the 3′ UTR was mapped to changes in the abundance of the sfRNA involved in modulating the host innate immune response.[145,1045]

The creation of chimeric flaviviruses encoding the structural genes of heterologous viruses is a second attenuation approach that has yielded promising vaccine candidates. The first chimeric viruses were constructed by introducing the C, prM, and E genes of DENV-1 or DENV-2 into the genetic background of DENV-4.[121] These viruses were immunogenic and attenuated as immunization of monkeys elicited neutralizing antibodies and reduced viremia following challenge with a homologous wild-type strain.[122] These early studies established that the structural proteins conferred the serological specificity of chimeric DENV. Chimeric vaccine candidates encoding the heterologous C-prM-E and prM-E cassettes have been characterized; viruses constructed using the latter replicated more efficiently than those encoding all three structural genes, perhaps due to a requirement for interaction between RNA elements in the capsid gene and the 3′ UTR.[122] Three tetravalent chimeric flavivirus vaccine candidates in advanced stages of clinical development are detailed below.

NIAID Tetravalent Vaccine Candidate

A tetravalent DENV vaccine consisting of live viruses bearing a combination of both full-length and chimeric genomes is being developed by the National Institute of Allergy and Infectious Diseases and National Institutes of Health.[1199] At the core of this vaccine platform are viruses attenuated by a Δ30 deletion in the UTR. Chimeric viruses were constructed using the DENV-4Δ30 background and prM-E cassettes from the other DENV serotypes. While a large number of different configurations were evaluated in preclinical studies, nine were tested as monovalent vaccine candidates in phase I clinical studies. Testing individual components in healthy subjects confirmed the infectivity of each candidate and simplified the optimization of a tetravalent formulation in humans.[290] The original combination of this vaccine is called TV003 and dosing includes 10^3 PFU each of a DENV-1Δ30 virus, a chimeric

DENV-2/DENV-4Δ30 virus encoding DENV-2 prM-E, a DENV-3Δ30/31 virus containing both a Δ30 and Δ31 deletions, and a DENV-4Δ30 virus.[534] An additional combination, TV005, also was prepared and included an increased dose (10^4 PFU) of the chimeric DENV-2/4Δ30 virus component. Administration of TV003 or TV005 is safe and immunogenic; at 90 days postvaccination, 90% of the TV005 recipients had circulating antibody capable of neutralizing all four DENV serotypes. Of interest, administration of a second dose of vaccine 6 months later does not result in the mild rash associated with primary TV005 vaccination nor an anamnestic neutralizing antibody response (defined by an increase in titer by more than fourfold). These data suggest TV005 is capable of eliciting sterilizing immunity and the possibility that a single vaccine dose may be sufficient.[534] A controlled human challenge study has demonstrated the protective capacity of TV003 against DENV-2,[535] and additional studies are underway with TV005 and DENV-3. Phase III clinical studies are ongoing.

Takeda Tetravalent Vaccine Candidate

A second chimeric tetravalent DENV vaccine candidate has been developed using an attenuated DENV-2 strain as the backbone.[474,475] This vaccine, called TDV, includes three chimeric viruses encoding the prM-E of DENV-1, DENV-3, and DENV-4 as well as the highly passaged DENV-2 strain PDK-50. Three mutations in this DENV-2 backbone contribute to the attenuation of each component of the vaccine. Preclinical studies revealed TDV elicited a balanced neutralizing antibody response that was protective in mouse and NHP challenge models.[848] Clinical studies of TDV administered via a subcutaneous or intradermal route in two doses 90 days apart revealed 90% to 93% of volunteers were capable of neutralizing at least three DENV serotypes.[354,847] A phase II study of a high-dose formulation confirmed the immunogenicity of this vaccine in a DENV-endemic setting, with the highest responses observed after the second vaccine dose.[958] Phase III clinical studies are underway.

Sanofi Pasteur Tetravalent Vaccine Candidate

Because of the well-established safety profile of the YF-17D vaccine, a tetravalent chimeric DENV vaccine, Dengvaxia®, was constructed by replacing prM-E of YF-17D with those of four low passage primary DENV strains.[400,409] Three doses of vaccine are administered in humans at 6-month intervals. The immunogenicity and efficacy of CYD-TVD have been evaluated in multiple advanced clinical studies (reviewed in Ref.[410]). Multiple phase III clinical trials demonstrated Dengvaxia® confers protection in DENV-experienced subjects 9 to 45 years of age. Dengvaxia® was the first anti-DENV vaccine licensed. However, the use of Dengvaxia® in DENV-seronegative individuals is not recommended, as discussed below.

Complications Associated with DENV Vaccine Deployment

The severe clinical outcomes that occurred following some secondary DENV infections highlighted a risk that vaccine-elicited antibodies might contribute to pathogenesis under some circumstances. While the goal of tetravalent vaccine development efforts was to create a balanced tetravalent response protective against all four DENV serotypes, uniform immunogenicity has been difficult to achieve. In the phase IIb study of Dengvaxia® in approximately 4,000 healthy Thai schoolchildren, three doses of vaccine failed to protect against DENV-2 challenge, whereas efficacy against other DENV serotypes ranged from 56% to 100%.[953] Changes to the formulation of tetravalent vaccine to adjust the dose of individual components to achieve a more balanced response were only straightforward in instances where each monovalent component was tested independently in clinical trials, as reflected by the evolution of the NIH vaccine candidate from the TV003 to TV005 formulation.[534]

The clinical development of Dengvaxia® identified possible disease enhancement in vaccine-elicited immunity, reinforcing a need for greater insight into the complexities of immunity to DENV. Two large phase III studies of this vaccine conducted in Asia[161] or Latin America[1156] revealed an overall efficacy of 56% to 60.8% against virologically confirmed symptomatic dengue. These studies noted that the vaccine was most effective in individuals with prior exposure to DENV and less so in younger age groups. Long-term follow-up revealed that the protection conferred by Dengvaxia® was restricted to individuals greater than 9 years of age.[416] Dengvaxia® was subsequently licensed for use in 20 countries for individuals 9 years of age and older. This recommendation was based in part on the finding that vaccinated children aged 2 to 5 in the Asia study detailed above were at greater risk of hospitalization as compared to controls.[29] Serological studies later demonstrated that DENV-immune status was an important predictor of vaccine efficacy.[1058] Individuals who were DENV seropositive at the time of vaccine administration experienced benefit from Dengvaxia® for at least 5 years, whereas DENV-naïve individuals were at increased risk over this interval, independent of age.[423] Recommendations for vaccine use were changed to exclude DENV-seronegative subjects. It has been suggested that Dengvaxia® sensitizes an immune response to secondary infections in a manner analogous to the primary exposure to authentic DENV.[318] Further follow-up is required to evaluate the public health impact of the use of this vaccine candidate on children since its licensure.

While antibody cross-reactivity among flaviviruses is common, more severe disease following a secondary infection in humans has been limited to DENV infections. The unusual pathogenesis of ZIKV in DENV-endemic settings led to the hypothesis that antibodies elicited by DENV might play a role in exacerbating ZIKV disease. The infection of ZIKV can be enhanced *in vitro* by cross-reactive antibodies in some circumstances.[252] However, ADE can be demonstrated in cell culture with virtually all flaviviruses and has not proven to correlate with clinical disease outcomes. Several studies have shown the passive transfer of antibodies into mouse models of ZIKV infection can exacerbate disease.[55,134,912] The relevance of these models to human disease remains to be established; passive transfer of mAbs into mice also exacerbates disease caused by YFV, MVEV, and JEV.[378,1164] Studies of DENV in similar murine models demonstrate that the presence of T cells limits ADE in similar circumstances.[1239] Enhanced ZIKV disease in DENV convalescent mice was not observed, although more severe DENV following ZIKV challenge was possible.[333] Ultimately, a role for prior DENV in ZIKV pathogenesis will be addressed by epidemiological studies in the field. So far, two large studies suggest prior DENV was protective against ZIKV in the 2015 outbreak.[374,940]

Japanese Encephalitis Virus

JEV is a principal cause of pediatric encephalitis in Asia and has been a focus of vaccine development efforts since before World War II.[424] Inactivated suspensions of JEV-infected mouse brains were administered to military personnel in response to an outbreak of Japanese B virus (now recognized as JEV) on Okinawa in 1945.[954] While circumstances did not permit a complete evaluation of efficacy, this vaccine elicited neutralizing antibodies in a subset of vaccinated subjects at titers that protected mice from lethal infection.[955] Since that time, considerable progress has been made toward developing a safe and effective JEV vaccine. Multiple vaccination approaches have reduced the incidence of JEV in countries with the means to utilize them.

Mouse Brain–Derived JEV Vaccines

Vaccines produced from JEV-infected mouse brains have been effective at controlling JEV in many parts of Asia, including Japan, South Korea, Taiwan, and Thailand.[327] The Research Foundation for Microbial Diseases of Osaka University (BIKEN) produced the majority of mouse brain–derived JEV vaccine licensed for international use between 1954 and 2005. This vaccine platform uses genotype III Nakayama or Beijing-1 strains for different markets.[70] Brain tissue from intracranially infected mice is homogenized, and virus is purified by ultracentrifugation and filtration steps and inactivated by formalin.[469] These vaccines were used primarily in Japan, Korea, Thailand, Malaysia, Sri Lanka, and Vietnam to protect against endemic JEV.[70] The BIKEN vaccine was licensed for travelers in the United States and elsewhere and marketed as JE-VAX™.[327] Efficacy studies of mouse brain–derived JEV vaccines suggest they are modestly immunogenic and require multiple boosts. A placebo-controlled, double-blinded evaluation of monovalent (Nakayama strain) or bivalent (Nakayama and Beijing strains) formulations of JE-VAX conducted in Thailand revealed an efficacy of 91% in children receiving two doses of vaccine 7 days apart.[469] However, interpretation of these studies is complicated by the prevalence of individuals with prior flavivirus experience in JEV-endemic regions. Studies of the immunogenicity of two doses of JE-VAX in flavivirus-naïve subjects revealed only 33% seroconversion at 26 weeks post vaccination; however, near-complete seroconversion was achieved using a third dose.[891,966] Attempts to measure the durability of antibody responses elicited by mouse brain–derived vaccine in endemic regions have been complicated by the potential boosting by naturally acquired flavivirus infection. Studies of military vaccine recipients suggest that neutralizing antibodies may persist for at least 3 years.[345] Vaccine is typically administered in two doses separated by 1 to 4 weeks, followed by a booster 1 to 2 years later. Travelers require a rapid three-dose vaccination regimen (days 0, 7, and 30).[327] Although mouse brain–derived JEV vaccines have efficacy in humans, roughly 20% of JE-VAX recipients experience local adverse events including swelling, redness, and pain at the injection site and mild systemic symptoms. Severe allergic and neurological complications of vaccination have been observed (10–260 and 0.1–2 per 100,000 vaccinees, respectively).[70,327] Vaccine-related fatalities resulted in cessation of production of JE-VAX in 2005 in favor of newer vaccines with more favorable safety profiles.

Live Attenuated JEV Vaccines

SA14-14-2 is a live attenuated JEV vaccine that has been administered to more than 300 million individuals.[424] The parental SA14 strain was isolated from the larvae of *Culex pipiens* mosquitoes collected in China in 1954 and causes lethality when inoculated into weanling mice via the intracranial route. The attenuated strain was developed after extensive passaging of the SA14 strain in cell culture and in hamsters and suckling mice.[824,1218] A single dose of SA14-14-2 induces a neutralizing antibody response in 85% to 100% of nonimmune recipients.[1049,1133,1218] Case-controlled studies demonstrated that a single dose of SA14-14-2 vaccine provided considerable protection (80%–99%),[96,457,573,837] which was durable even after 5 years.[1100] SA-14-14-2 was licensed for use in China in 1988 and subsequently distributed in Nepal, South Korea, Sri Lanka, Thailand, and India.

ChimeriVax-JE (also known as JE-CV or IMOJEV) is a promising live attenuated vaccine constructed using the YF-17D backbone described above (reviewed in Ref.[72]). ChimeriVax-JE was constructed by replacing the prM-E genes of YF-17D with SA-14-14-2 prM-E. Vaccination with ChimeriVax-JE elicits a protective response in mice and primates.[72,402,775] Clinical studies in humans reveal the vaccine is well tolerated and elicits a durable neutralizing antibody response (reviewed in Ref.[200]). This vaccine is licensed in 14 countries including Australia and Thailand.

Inactivated JEV Vaccines Produced in Cell Culture

The IC51 (or IXIARO) vaccine is a formalin-inactivated vaccine produced in Vero cells under serum-free conditions and adjuvanted with aluminum hydroxide.[327] IC51 uses the SA14-14-2 JEV strain[547] and is administered in two doses 28 days apart, each containing approximately 6 mg of purified virus. Licensure was granted based on a noninferiority immunogenicity study comparing the response of recipients receiving IC51 to those vaccinated with a three-dose regimen of JEVAX. While a single dose of IC51 was poorly immunogenic (41% seroconversion), 4 weeks after the second dose, 96% of recipients had detectable neutralizing antibodies, and these persisted in most subjects 6 months after vaccination.[547] No significant local or systemic adverse events were associated with vaccination; rare events await a more detailed analysis of larger populations of vaccine recipients. IC51 was licensed for use in the United States as a traveler's vaccine in 2009 for individuals over 17 years of age. An inactivated JEV vaccine derived from the genotype III P3 strain and produced in hamster cell cultures also has been used extensively in China, with as many as 70 million doses of this vaccine administered each year.[424]

Tick-Borne Encephalitis Virus

Two inactivated TBEV vaccines are used to prevent infection in Europe, but are not licensed in the United States.[921] Kunz and colleagues developed the first licensed vaccine in 1973 using the Austrian Neudörfl strain of TBEV grown in chick embryo fibroblasts, after inactivation with formalin and adjuvanting with aluminum hydroxide.[578,579] Today, this vaccine is distributed as FSME-IMMUN by Baxter Biosciences. A second vaccine, produced by Novartis and marketed as Encepur,[105,540] was licensed in 1991. It is produced using similar methods except the German K23 strain of TBEV is substituted. Both inactivated TBEV vaccines are administered in three doses and require boosting. The conventional schedule requires three vaccinations at 0, 1 to 3 months, and 9 to 12 months, a booster at 3 years, followed by additional booster vaccinations every 5 years. These vaccines are immunogenic; virtually, 100% of vaccinated subjects develop neutralizing antibody titers following their third dose,[578] and antibodies persist for at least 5 years.[886,1206] The effectiveness of current TBEV vaccines in the field has been estimated at approximately 99%.[1070] Despite the availability of effective vaccine, TBEV incidence in parts of Europe has increased, coincident with poor vaccine coverage.[580]

Zika Virus

The emergence of ZIKV in the Americas and its linkage to congenital disease in 2015 prompted vaccine development efforts using multiple vaccine platform technologies detailed below.

Inactivated Vaccines

The first ZIKV vaccine development efforts were initiated even before the epidemic in the Americas. A formalin-inactivated adjuvanted vaccinate candidate using an African strain of ZIKV was shown to be protective in mice and advanced to clinical trials in India; the results of these studies are not yet available.[1081] The Walter Reed Army Institute of Research (WRAIR) developed a ZIKV-purified inactivated vaccine (ZPIV) using a Puerto Rican ZIKV isolate that was highly successful in animal models[1] and subsequently evaluated in multiple clinical studies.[759] The ZPIV vaccine was licensed by Sanofi Pasteur but not developed further. The development of similar vaccine products by the Takeda Pharmaceuticals[48] and Emergent BioSolutions is ongoing.

Nucleic Acid Vaccines

Numerous DNA vaccine candidates encoding ZIKV prM-E have been developed and evaluated in preclinical studies.[280,349,811,1227] The sequence of these vaccine candidates differed with respect to the plasmid background, codon optimization method, strain selection, signal sequence of prM, and presence of an N-linked glycosylation site. A DNA vaccine candidate that lacks the "pr" peptide of prM (called M-E) also showed promise in animal models despite being incapable of SVP production.[1,595] Three prM-E encoding DNA vaccine candidates were evaluated in phase I clinical studies.[352,1106] These studies revealed a varying capacity to elicit neutralizing antibodies. For example, the administration of three doses of vaccine VRC5283 by needle-free injection elicited antibodies with a geometric mean titer of 1/304 12 weeks after administration of the first dose. In contrast, while most recipients of the vaccine candidate GLS-5700 generated ZIKV E protein–binding antibodies in response to vaccination, only a fraction of the vaccine-immune sera from these individuals showed neutralizing activity. Of interest, passive transfer of these antibodies into a lethal mouse model was protective, highlighting a need for a more detailed understanding of the protective mechanisms of vaccine-elicited antibodies. VRC5283 is currently being evaluated in a placebo-controlled phase II clinical trial at multiple sites in the Americas. ZIKV mRNA vaccines encoding prM-E were shown to be highly immunogenic and protective in mice and NHP models.[860,929,930] mRNA vaccine candidates are being evaluated in clinical studies, but data describing these vaccine development efforts have not yet been published. The short timeline (>4 months) between the identification of an appropriate vaccine candidate sequence and the initiation of clinical trials highlights the potential for synthetic vaccines as a rapid first response to emerging threats.

Live Attenuated Vaccines

Multiple live attenuated vaccines for ZIKV are being developed and have been evaluated in mice and NHP models.[1014,1016,1217] These platforms protect against viremia in animal models, prevent damage to the male reproductive tract, and inhibit congenital disease. These constructs employ multiple modes to attenuate the viruses using information obtained from both vaccine development programs for other flaviviruses[737,1015] and more fundamental studies of flavivirus biology.[930] A chimeric DENV-2 virus encoding ZIKV prM-E genes is being evaluated in phase I clinical studies by scientists at NIAID.

Viral Vectors

Numerous viral vectors have constructed to express ZIKV genes as vaccine candidates and shown to confer immunity.[120,894,986] Multiple adenovirus-based vectors, using different rhesus and human adenovirus strains, have been evaluated as ZIKV vaccine platforms.[140,404,1219] Adenovirus vectors expressing ZIKV M-E have been studied extensively and this antigen and vaccine platform is being evaluated in clinical trials.[1,217] Administration of a rhesus adenovirus 52 vaccine candidate elicited neutralizing antibodies and a protective immune response in mice and NHP models. Subsequent studies revealed remarkably durable protection from viremia in NHPs 1-year postadministration of a single vaccine dose.[1,2,595] A ZIKV vaccine utilizing a live attenuated measles strain to express prM and a soluble form of the E protein has been described.[832] Administration of this vaccine candidate reduced viral loads and protected against congenital disease in a mouse model.

West Nile Virus

While there is no WNV vaccine licensed for use in humans, several platforms have been developed (reviewed in Ref.[69]). Live attenuated flavivirus chimeras were developed for WNV using the strategies described above. ChimeriVax WNV vaccine candidates were constructed by replacing the prM-E genes of the YF-17D virus with those of WNV.[409] ChimeriVax-WN01 encodes unmodified prM-E sequence of the NY99 strain and was developed as a veterinary vaccine that has been used in horses since 2006.[665,666] ChimeriVax-WN02 differs from the veterinary vaccine by three amino acid substitutions in the E protein introduced to reduce neurovirulence and a fourth adventitious substitution that arose during adaptation of the vaccine lot to growth on Vero cells.[409] ChimeriVax-WN02 was safe and immunogenic in phase I and II clinical trials in humans.[92,773] In addition, a third chimeric WNV vaccine candidate was developed using the DENV-4Δ30 backbone included in the TV-005 DENV vaccine and shown to be safe and immunogenic in clinical studies.[293,875]

DNA vaccination has also shown promise for WNV vaccination. DNA vaccine constructs typically express genes encoding prM-E. Two phase I clinical studies of a WNV nucleic acid vaccine have been performed.[239,606,704] These trials demonstrated that three doses of vaccine were well tolerated and capable of eliciting both a T-cell and neutralizing antibody response.

A similar construct has proven to be efficacious at reducing WNV incidence in horses and a variety of birds.[69]

ACKNOWLEDGMENTS

We thank Mr. Ethan Tyler and Mrs. Erina He (OD, NIH) for preparation of Figures 9.2, 9.4, and 9.6 to 9.13. This work was supported by the NIAID Division of Intramural Research (TCP) and NIAID Grants R01 AI073755, R01 AI127828, P01 AI106695, R01 AI125202 and R01 HD091218 to MSD and R01 AI139512 to HML.

REFERENCES

1. Abbink P, Larocca RA, De La Barrera RA, et al. Protective efficacy of multiple vaccine platforms against Zika virus challenge in rhesus monkeys. *Science* 2016;353:1129–1132.
2. Abbink P, Larocca RA, Visitsunthorn K, et al. Durability and correlates of vaccine protection against Zika virus in rhesus monkeys. *Sci Transl Med* 2017;9.
3. Acosta EG, Castilla V, Damonte EB. Functional entry of dengue virus into Aedes albopictus mosquito cells is dependent on clathrin-mediated endocytosis. *J Gen Virol* 2008;89:474–484.
4. Adams Waldorf KM, Nelson BR, Stencel-Baerenwald JE, et al. Congenital Zika virus infection as a silent pathology with loss of neurogenic output in the fetal brain. *Nat Med* 2018;24:368–374.
5. Adams Waldorf KM, Stencel-Baerenwald JE, Kapur RP, et al. Fetal brain lesions after subcutaneous inoculation of Zika virus in a pregnant nonhuman primate. *Nat Med* 2016;22:1256–1259.
6. Aguirre S, Fernandez-Sesma A. Collateral damage during dengue virus infection: making sense of DNA by cGAS. *J Virol* 2017;91.
7. Aguirre S, Luthra P, Sanchez-Aparicio MT, et al. Dengue virus NS2B protein targets cGAS for degradation and prevents mitochondrial DNA sensing during infection. *Nat Microbiol* 2017;2:17037.
8. Aguirre S, Maestre AM, Pagni S, et al. DENV inhibits type I IFN production in infected cells by cleaving human STING. *PLoS Pathog* 2012;8:e1002934.
9. Ahmed R, Akondy RS. Insights into human CD8(+) T-cell memory using the yellow fever and smallpox vaccines. *Immunol Cell Biol* 2011;89:340–345.
10. Aid M, Abbink P, Larocca RA, et al. Zika virus persistence in the central nervous system and lymph nodes of Rhesus monkeys. *Cell* 2017;169:610–620, e614.
11. Airo AM, Urbanowski MD, Lopez-Orozco J, et al. Expression of flavivirus capsids enhance the cellular environment for viral replication by activating Akt-signalling pathways. *Virology* 2018;516:147–157.
12. Akondy RS, Monson ND, Miller JD, et al. The yellow fever virus vaccine induces a broad and polyfunctional human memory CD8+ T cell response. *J Immunol* 2009;183:7919–7930.
13. Albrecht P. Pathogenesis of neurotropic arbovirus infections. *Curr Top Microbiol Immunol* 1968;43:44–91.
14. Alcon S, Talarmin A, Debruyne M, et al. Enzyme-linked immunosorbent assay specific to Dengue virus type 1 nonstructural protein NS1 reveals circulation of the antigen in the blood during the acute phase of disease in patients experiencing primary or secondary infections. *J Clin Microbiol* 2002;40:376–381.
15. Aleyas AG, George JA, Han YW, et al. Functional modulation of dendritic cells and macrophages by Japanese encephalitis virus through MyD88 adaptor molecule-dependent and -independent pathways. *J Immunol* 2009;183:2462–2474.
16. Aleyas AG, Han YW, George JA, et al. Multifront assault on antigen presentation by Japanese encephalitis virus subverts CD8+ T cell responses. *J Immunol* 2010;185:1429–1441.
17. Aleyas AG, Han YW, Patil AM, et al. Impaired cross-presentation of CD8alpha+ CD11c+ dendritic cells by Japanese encephalitis virus in a TLR2/MyD88 signal pathway-dependent manner. *Eur J Immunol* 2012;42:2655–2666.
18. Aliota MT, Dupuis AP II, Wilczek MP, et al. The prevalence of zoonotic tick-borne pathogens in Ixodes scapularis collected in the Hudson Valley, New York State. *Vector Borne Zoonotic Dis* 2014;14:245–250.
19. Allison SL, Schalich J, Stiasny K, et al. Mutational evidence for an internal fusion peptide in flavivirus envelope protein E. *J Virol* 2001;75:4268–4275.
20. Allison SL, Stiasny K, Stadler K, et al. Mapping of functional elements in the stem-anchor region of tick-borne encephalitis virus envelope protein E. *J Virol* 1999;73:5605–5612.
21. Allison SL, Tao YJ, O'Riordain G, et al. Two distinct size classes of immature and mature subviral particles from tick-borne encephalitis virus. *J Virol* 2003;77:11357–11366.
22. Amara A, Mercer J. Viral apoptotic mimicry. *Nat Rev Microbiol* 2015;13:461–469.
23. An J, Kimura-Kuroda J, Hirabayashi Y, et al. Development of a novel mouse model for dengue virus infection. *Virology* 1999;263:70–77.
24. Ander SE, Diamond MS, Coyne CB. Immune responses at the maternal-fetal interface. *Sci Immunol* 2019;4.
25. Anderson JF, Rahal JJ. Efficacy of interferon alpha-2b and ribavirin against West Nile virus in vitro. *Emerg Infect Dis* 2002;8:107–108.
26. Andrews DM, Matthews VB, Sammels LM, et al. The severity of murray valley encephalitis in mice is linked to neutrophil infiltration and inducible nitric oxide synthase activity in the central nervous system. *J Virol* 1999;73:8781–8790.
27. Anglero-Rodriguez YI, Pantoja P, Sariol CA. Dengue virus subverts the interferon induction pathway via NS2B/3 protease-IkappaB kinase epsilon interaction. *Clin Vaccine Immunol* 2014;21:29–38.

28. Anonymous. Locally acquired Dengue--Key West, Florida, 2009–2010. *MMWR Morb Mortal Wkly Rep* 2010;59:577–581.

29. Anonymous. Addendum to report of the Global Advisory Committee on Vaccine Safety (GACVS), 10–11 June 2015(1). Safety of CYD-TDV dengue vaccine. *Wkly Epidemiol Rec* 2015;90:421–423.

30. Appler KK, Brown AN, Stewart BS, et al. Persistence of West Nile virus in the central nervous system and periphery of mice. *PLoS One* 2010;5:e10649.

31. Arjona A, Ledizet M, Anthony K, et al. West Nile virus envelope protein inhibits dsRNA-induced innate immune responses. *J Immunol* 2007;179:8403–8409.

32. Arroyo J, Miller C, Catalan J, et al. ChimeriVax-West Nile virus live-attenuated vaccine: pre-clinical evaluation of safety, immunogenicity, and efficacy. *J Virol* 2004;78:12497–12507.

33. Arsuaga M, Bujalance SG, Diaz-Menendez M, et al. Probable sexual transmission of Zika virus from a vasectomised man. *Lancet Infect Dis* 2016;16:1107.

34. Ashour J, Laurent-Rolle M, Shi PY, et al. NS5 of dengue virus mediates STAT2 binding and degradation. *J Virol* 2009;83:5408–5418.

35. Ashour J, Morrison J, Laurent-Rolle M, et al. Mouse STAT2 restricts early dengue virus replication. *Cell Host Microbe* 2010;8:410–421.

36. Aubry M, Teissier A, Huart M, et al. Zika virus seroprevalence, French polynesia, 2014–2015. *Emerg Infect Dis* 2017;23:669–672.

37. Avirutnan P, Fuchs A, Hauhart RE, et al. Antagonism of the complement component C4 by flavivirus nonstructural protein NS1. *J Exp Med* 2010;207:793–806.

38. Avirutnan P, Hauhart RE, Somnuke P, et al. Binding of flavivirus nonstructural protein NS1 to C4b binding protein modulates complement activation. *J Immunol* 2011;187:424–433.

39. Avirutnan P, Malasit P, Seliger B, et al. Dengue virus infection of human endothelial cells leads to chemokine production, complement activation, and apoptosis. *J Immunol* 1998;161:6338–6346.

40. Avirutnan P, Mehlhop E, Diamond MS. Complement and its role in protection and pathogenesis of flavivirus infections. *Vaccine* 2008;26(Suppl 8):I100–I107.

41. Avirutnan P, Punyadee N, Noisakran S, et al. Vascular leakage in severe dengue virus infections: a potential role for the nonstructural viral protein NS1 and complement. *J Infect Dis* 2006;193:1078–1088.

42. Azar SR, Rossi SL, Haller SH, et al. ZIKV demonstrates minimal pathologic effects and mosquito infectivity in viremic cynomolgus macaques. *Viruses* 2018;10.

43. Bai F, Kong KF, Dai J, et al. A paradoxical role for neutrophils in the pathogenesis of West Nile virus. *J Infect Dis* 2010;202:1804–1812.

44. Bailey MJ, Duehr J, Dulin H, et al. Human antibodies targeting Zika virus NS1 provide protection against disease in a mouse model. *Nat Commun* 2018;9:4560.

45. Bakonyi T, Hubalek Z, Rudolf I, et al. Novel flavivirus or new lineage of West Nile virus, central Europe. *Emerg Infect Dis* 2005;11:225–231.

46. Bakri SJ, Kaiser PK. Ocular manifestations of West Nile virus. *Curr Opin Ophthalmol* 2004;15:537–540.

47. Balas C, Kennel A, Deauvieau F, et al. Different innate signatures induced in human monocyte-derived dendritic cells by wild-type dengue 3 virus, attenuated but reactogenic dengue 3 vaccine virus, or attenuated nonreactogenic dengue 1–4 vaccine virus strains. *J Infect Dis* 2011;203:103–108.

48. Baldwin WR, Livengood JA, Giebler HA, et al. Purified inactivated Zika vaccine candidates afford protection against lethal challenge in mice. *Sci Rep* 2018;8:16509.

49. Balmaseda A, Hammond SN, Perez L, et al. Serotype-specific differences in clinical manifestations of dengue. *Am J Trop Med Hyg* 2006;74:449–456.

50. Balmaseda A, Hammond SN, Tellez Y, et al. High seroprevalence of antibodies against dengue virus in a prospective study of schoolchildren in Managua, Nicaragua. *Trop Med Int Health* 2006;11:935–942.

51. Balsitis SJ, Coloma J, Castro G, et al. Tropism of dengue virus in mice and humans defined by viral nonstructural protein 3-specific immunostaining. *Am J Trop Med Hyg* 2009;80:416–424.

52. Balsitis SJ, Williams KL, Lachica R, et al. Lethal antibody enhancement of dengue disease in mice is prevented by Fc modification. *PLoS Pathog* 2010;6:e1000790.

53. Bamford CGG, Aranday-Cortes E, Filipe IC, et al. A polymorphic residue that attenuates the antiviral potential of interferon lambda 4 in hominid lineages. *PLoS Pathog* 2018;14:e1007307.

54. Barba-Spaeth G, Longman RS, Albert ML, et al. Live attenuated yellow fever 17D infects human DCs and allows for presentation of endogenous and recombinant T cell epitopes. *J Exp Med* 2005;202:1179–1184.

55. Bardina SV, Bunduc P, Tripathi S, et al. Enhancement of Zika virus pathogenesis by preexisting antiflavivirus immunity. *Science* 2017;356:175–180.

56. Bardina SV, Michlmayr D, Hoffman KW, et al. Differential Roles of Chemokines CCL2 and CCL7 in Monocytosis and Leukocyte Migration during West Nile virus infection. *J Immunol* 2015;195:4306–4318.

57. Barnett ED. Yellow fever: epidemiology and prevention. *Clin Infect Dis* 2007;44:850–856.

58. Barrett ADT. Yellow fever live attenuated vaccine: a very successful live attenuated vaccine but still we have problems controlling the disease. *Vaccine* 2017;35:5951–5955.

59. Barrett ADT. The reemergence of yellow fever. *Science* 2018;361:847–848.

60. Barrett AD, Gould EA. Comparison of neurovirulence of different strains of yellow fever virus in mice. *J Gen Virol* 1986;67(Pt 4):631–637.

61. Barrett AD, Monath TP. Epidemiology and ecology of yellow fever virus. *Adv Virus Res* 2003;61:291–315.

62. Barrett AD, Teuwen DE. Yellow fever vaccine—how does it work and why do rare cases of serious adverse events take place? *Curr Opin Immunol* 2009;21:308–313.

63. Barros ML, Boecken G. Jungle yellow fever in the central Amazon. *Lancet* 1996;348:969–970.

64. Barry G, Breakwell L, Fragkoudis R, et al. PKR acts early in infection to suppress Semliki Forest virus production and strongly enhances the type I interferon response. *J Gen Virol* 2009;90:1382–1391.

65. Bashyam HS, Green S, Rothman AL. Dengue virus-reactive CD8+ T cells display quantitative and qualitative differences in their response to variant epitopes of heterologous viral serotypes. *J Immunol* 2006;176:2817–2824.

66. Basilio-de-Oliveira CA, Aguiar GR, Baldanza MS, et al. Pathologic study of a fatal case of dengue-3 virus infection in Rio de Janeiro, Brazil. *Braz J Infect Dis* 2005;9:341–347.

67. Baty SA, Gibney KB, Staples JE, et al. Evaluation for West Nile Virus (WNV) RNA in urine of patients within 5 months of WNV infection. *J Infect Dis* 2012;205:1476–1477.

68. Bayer A, Lennemann NJ, Ouyang Y, et al. Type III interferons produced by human placental trophoblasts confer protection against Zika virus infection. *Cell Host Microbe* 2016;19:705–712.

69. Beasley DW. Vaccines and immunotherapeutics for the prevention and treatment of infections with West Nile virus. *Immunotherapy* 2011;3:269–285.

70. Beasley DW, Lewthwaite P, Solomon T. Current use and development of vaccines for Japanese encephalitis. *Expert Opin Biol Ther* 2008;8:95–106.

71. Beasley DW, Li L, Suderman MT, et al. Mouse neuroinvasive phenotype of West Nile virus strains varies depending upon virus genotype. *Virology* 2002;296:17–23.

72. Beasley DW, Li L, Suderman MT, et al. Protection against Japanese encephalitis virus strains representing four genotypes by passive transfer of sera raised against ChimeriVax-JE experimental vaccine. *Vaccine* 2004;22:3722–3726.

73. Beasley DW, Whiteman MC, Zhang S, et al. Envelope protein glycosylation status influences mouse neuroinvasion phenotype of genetic lineage 1 West Nile virus strains. *J Virol* 2005;79:8339–8347.

74. Beatty PR, Puerta-Guardo H, Killingbeck SS, et al. Dengue virus NS1 triggers endothelial permeability and vascular leak that is prevented by NS1 vaccination. *Sci Transl Med* 2015;7:304ra141.

75. Beaumier CM, Rothman AL. Cross-reactive memory CD4+ T cells alter the CD8+ T-cell response to heterologous secondary dengue virus infections in mice in a sequence-specific manner. *Viral Immunol* 2009;22:215–219.

76. Beckett CG, Tjaden J, Burgess T, et al. Evaluation of a prototype dengue-1 DNA vaccine in a Phase 1 clinical trial. *Vaccine* 2011;29:960–968.

77. Bell TM, Field EJ, Narang HK. Zika virus infection of the central nervous system of mice. *Arch Gesamte Virusforsch* 1971;35:183–193.

78. Belmusto-Worn VE, Sanchez JL, McCarthy K, et al. Randomized, double-blind, phase III, pivotal field trial of the comparative immunogenicity, safety, and tolerability of two yellow fever 17D vaccines (Arilvax and YF-VAX) in healthy infants and children in Peru. *Am J Trop Med Hyg* 2005;72:189–197.

79. Beltramello M, Williams KL, Simmons CP, et al. The human immune response to Dengue virus is dominated by highly cross-reactive antibodies endowed with neutralizing and enhancing activity. *Cell Host Microbe* 2010;8:271–283.

80. Ben-Nathan D, Gershoni-Yahalom O, Samina I, et al. Using high titer West Nile intravenous immunoglobulin from selected Israeli donors for treatment of West Nile virus infection. *BMC Infect Dis* 2009;9:18.

81. Ben-Nathan D, Huitinga I, Lustig S, et al. West Nile virus neuroinvasion and encephalitis induced by macrophage depletion in mice. *Arch Virol* 1996;141:459–469.

82. Bente DA, Melkus MW, Garcia JV, et al. Dengue fever in humanized NOD/SCID mice. *J Virol* 2005;79:13797–13799.

83. Bernkopf H, Levine S, Nerson R. Isolation of West Nile virus in Israel. *J Infect Dis* 1953;93:207–218.

84. Berthet FX, Zeller HG, Drouet MT, et al. Extensive nucleotide changes and deletions within the envelope glycoprotein gene of Euro-African West Nile viruses. *J Gen Virol* 1997;78(Pt 9):2293–2297.

85. Besnard M, Eyrolle-Guignot D, Guillemette-Artur P, et al. Congenital cerebral malformations and dysfunction in fetuses and newborns following the 2013 to 2014 Zika virus epidemic in French Polynesia. *Euro Surveill* 2016;21.

86. Best SM. The many faces of the flavivirus NS5 protein in antagonism of type I interferon signaling. *J Virol* 2017;91.

87. Best SM, Morris KL, Shannon JG, et al. Inhibition of interferon-stimulated JAK-STAT signaling by a tick-borne flavivirus and identification of NS5 as an interferon antagonist. *J Virol* 2005;79:12828–12839.

88. Bhakdi S, Kazatchkine MD. Pathogenesis of dengue: an alternative hypothesis. *Southeast Asian J Trop Med Public Health* 1990;21:652–657.

89. Bhamarapravati N, Tuchinda P, Boonyapaknavik V. Pathology of Thailand haemorrhagic fever: a study of 100 autopsy cases. *Ann Trop Med Parasitol* 1967;61:500–510.

90. Bhatt S, Gething PW, Brady OJ, et al. The global distribution and burden of dengue. *Nature* 2013;496:504–507.

91. Bhattacharyya S, Zagorska A, Lew ED, et al. Enveloped viruses disable innate immune responses in dendritic cells by direct activation of TAM receptors. *Cell Host Microbe* 2013;14:136–147.

92. Biedenbender R, Bevilacqua J, Gregg AM, et al. Phase II, randomized, double-blind, placebo-controlled, multicenter study to investigate the immunogenicity and safety of a West Nile virus vaccine in healthy adults. *J Infect Dis* 2011;203:75–84.

93. Bierle CJ, Fernandez-Alarcon C, Hernandez-Alvarado N, et al. Assessing Zika virus replication and the development of Zika-specific antibodies after a mid-gestation viral challenge in guinea pigs. *PLoS One* 2017;12:e0187720.

94. Bigham AW, Buckingham KJ, Husain S, et al. Host genetic risk factors for West Nile virus infection and disease progression. *PLoS One* 2011;6:e24745.

95. Biron CA, Brossay L. NK cells and NKT cells in innate defense against viral infections. *Curr Opin Immunol* 2001;13:458–464.

96. Bista MB, Banerjee MK, Shin SH, et al. Efficacy of single-dose SA 14–14–2 vaccine against Japanese encephalitis: a case control study. *Lancet* 2001;358:791–795.

97. Biswas SM, Ayachit VM, Sapkal GN, et al. Japanese encephalitis virus produces a CD4+ Th2 response and associated immunoprotection in an adoptive-transfer murine model. *J Gen Virol* 2009;90:818–826.

98. Blaney JE Jr, Johnson DH, Manipon GG, et al. Genetic basis of attenuation of dengue virus type 4 small plaque mutants with restricted replication in suckling mice and in SCID mice transplanted with human liver cells. *Virology* 2002;300:125–139.

99. Blaney JE Jr, Matro JM, Murphy BR, et al. Recombinant, live-attenuated tetravalent dengue virus vaccine formulations induce a balanced, broad, and protective neutralizing antibody response against each of the four serotypes in rhesus monkeys. *J Virol* 2005;79:5516–5528.

100. Blaney JE Jr, Hanson CT, Firestone CY, et al. Genetically modified, live attenuated dengue virus type 3 vaccine candidates. *Am J Trop Med Hyg* 2004;71:811–821.

101. Blaney JE Jr, Hanson CT, Hanley KA, et al. Vaccine candidates derived from a novel infectious cDNA clone of an American genotype dengue virus type 2. *BMC Infect Dis* 2004;4:39.

102. Blaney JE Jr, Sathe NS, Goddard L, et al. Dengue virus type 3 vaccine candidates generated by introduction of deletions in the 3′ untranslated region (3′-UTR) or by exchange of the DENV-3 3′-UTR with that of DENV-4. *Vaccine* 2008;26:817–828.

103. Blitvich BJ, Firth AE. A review of Flaviviruses that have no known arthropod vector. *Viruses* 2017;9.

104. Blom K, Braun M, Pakalniene J, et al. NK cell responses to human Tick-Borne Encephalitis virus infection. *J Immunol* 2016;197:2762–2771.

105. Bock HL, Klockmann U, Jungst C, et al. A new vaccine against tick-borne encephalitis: initial trial in man including a dose-response study. *Vaccine* 1990;8:22–24.

106. Boehr DD, Wright PE. Biochemistry. How do proteins interact? *Science* 2008;320:1429–1430.

107. Bokisch VA, Top FH Jr, Russell PK, et al. The potential pathogenic role of complement in dengue hemorrhagic shock syndrome. *N Engl J Med* 1973;289:996–1000.

108. Boon PLS, Saw WG, Lim XX, et al. Partial intrinsic disorder governs the dengue capsid protein conformational ensemble. *ACS Chem Biol* 2018;13:1621–1630.

109. Boonnak K, Dambach KM, Donofrio GC, et al. Cell type specificity and host genetic polymorphisms influence antibody-dependent enhancement of dengue virus infection. *J Virol* 2011;85:1671–1683.

110. Boonnak K, Slike BM, Burgess TH, et al. Role of dendritic cells in antibody-dependent enhancement of dengue virus infection. *J Virol* 2008;82:3939–3951.

111. Botha EM, Markotter W, Wolfaardt M, et al. Genetic determinants of virulence in pathogenic lineage 2 West Nile virus strains. *Emerg Infect Dis* 2008;14:222–230.

112. Bothner B, Dong XF, Bibbs L, et al. Evidence of viral capsid dynamics using limited proteolysis and mass spectrometry. *J Biol Chem* 1998;273:673–676.

113. Bourne N, Scholle F, Silva MC, et al. Early production of type I interferon during West Nile virus infection: role for lymphoid tissues in IRF3-independent interferon production. *J Virol* 2007;81:9100–9108.

114. Bowen GS, Monath TP, Kemp GE, et al. Geographic variation among St. Louis encephalitis virus strains in the viremic responses of avian hosts. *Am J Trop Med Hyg* 1980;29:1411–1419.

115. Bowen RA, Nemeth NM. Experimental infections with West Nile virus. *Curr Opin Infect Dis* 2007;20:293–297.

116. Bowen JR, Quicke KM, Maddur MS, et al. Zika virus antagonizes type I interferon responses during infection of human dendritic cells. *PLoS Pathog* 2017;13:e1006164.

117. Brasil P, Pereira JP Jr, Moreira ME, et al. Zika virus infection in pregnant women in Rio de Janeiro. *N Engl J Med* 2016;375:2321–2334.

118. Brasil P, Sequeira PC, Freitas AD, et al. Guillain-Barre syndrome associated with Zika virus infection. *Lancet* 2016;387:1482.

119. Brass AL, Huang IC, Benita Y, et al. The IFITM proteins mediate cellular resistance to influenza A H1N1 virus, West Nile virus, and dengue virus. *Cell* 2009;139:1243–1254.

120. Brault AC, Domi A, McDonald EM, et al. A Zika vaccine targeting NS1 protein protects immunocompetent adult mice in a lethal challenge model. *Sci Rep* 2017;7:14769.

121. Bray M, Lai CJ. Construction of intertypic chimeric dengue viruses by substitution of structural protein genes. *Proc Natl Acad Sci U S A* 1991;88:10342–10346.

122. Bray M, Men R, Lai CJ. Monkeys immunized with intertypic chimeric dengue viruses are protected against wild-type virus challenge. *J Virol* 1996;70:4162–4166.

123. Bressanelli S, Stiasny K, Allison SL, et al. Structure of a flavivirus envelope glycoprotein in its low-pH-induced membrane fusion conformation. *EMBO J* 2004;23:728–738.

124. Brien JD, Austin SK, Sukupolvi-Petty S, et al. Genotype specific neutralization and protection by antibodies against dengue virus type 3. *J Virol* 2010;84:10630–10643.

125. Brien JD, Uhrlaub JL, Hirsch A, et al. Key role of T cell defects in age-related vulnerability to West Nile virus. *J Exp Med* 2009;206:2735–2745.

126. Brien JD, Uhrlaub JL, Nikolich-Zugich J. Protective capacity and epitope specificity of CD8(+) T cells responding to lethal West Nile virus infection. *Eur J Immunol* 2007;37:1855–1863.

127. Brien JD, Uhrlaub JL, Nikolich-Zugich J. West Nile virus-specific CD4 T cells exhibit direct antiviral cytokine secretion and cytotoxicity and are sufficient for antiviral protection. *J Immunol* 2008;181:8568–8575.

128. Brinker KR, Monath TP. The acute disease. In: Monath TP, ed. *St Louis Encephalitis*. Washington DC: American Public Health Association; 1980:503–534.

129. Brinton MA. Characterization of West Nile virus persistent infections in genetically resistant and susceptible mouse cells. I. Generation of defective nonplaquing virus particles. *Virology* 1982;116:84–98.

130. Brooks TJ, Phillpotts RJ. Interferon-alpha protects mice against lethal infection with St Louis encephalitis virus delivered by the aerosol and subcutaneous routes. *Antiviral Res* 1999;41:57–64.

131. Brown MG, Hermann LL, Issekutz AC, et al. Dengue virus infection of mast cells triggers endothelial cell activation. *J Virol* 2011;85:1145–1150.

132. Brown MG, Huang YY, Marshall JS, et al. Dramatic caspase-dependent apoptosis in antibody-enhanced dengue virus infection of human mast cells. *J Leukoc Biol* 2009;85:71–80.

133. Brown AN, Kent KA, Bennett CJ, et al. Tissue tropism and neuroinvasion of West Nile virus do not differ for two mouse strains with different survival rates. *Virology* 2007;368:422–430.

134. Brown JA, Singh G, Acklin JA, et al. Dengue virus immunity increases Zika virus-induced damage during pregnancy. *Immunity* 2019;50(3):751–762.e5. doi:10.1016/j.immuni.2019.01.005.

135. Bruni D, Chazal M, Sinigaglia L, et al. Viral entry route determines how human plasmacytoid dendritic cells produce type I interferons. *Sci Signal* 2015;8:ra25.

136. Bryan MA, Giordano D, Draves KE, et al. Splenic macrophages are required for protective innate immunity against West Nile virus. *PLoS One* 2018;13:e0191690.

137. Bryant JE, Holmes EC, Barrett AD. Out of Africa: a molecular perspective on the introduction of yellow fever virus into the Americas. *PLoS Pathog* 2007;3:e75.

138. Bryceson YT, Long EO. Line of attack: NK cell specificity and integration of signals. *Curr Opin Immunol* 2008;20:344–352.

139. Buechler CR, Bailey AL, Weiler AM, et al. Seroprevalence of Zika virus in wild African Green Monkeys and Baboons. *mSphere* 2017;2.

140. Bullard BL, Corder BN, Gorman MJ, et al. Efficacy of a T cell-biased adenovirus vector as a Zika virus vaccine. *Sci Rep* 2018;8:18017.

141. Burke T. Dengue haemorrhagic fever: a pathological study. *Trans R Soc Trop Med Hyg* 1968;62:682–692.

142. Burke DS, Nisalak A, Johnson DE, et al. A prospective study of dengue infections in Bangkok. *Am J Trop Med Hyg* 1988;38:172–180.

143. Busch MP, Caglioti S, Robertson EF, et al. Screening the blood supply for West Nile virus RNA by nucleic acid amplification testing. *N Engl J Med* 2005;353:460–467.

144. Busch MP, Tobler LH, Saldanha J, et al. Analytical and clinical sensitivity of West Nile virus RNA screening and supplemental assays available in 2003. *Transfusion* 2005;45:492–499.

145. Bustos-Arriaga J, Gromowski GD, Tsetsarkin KA, et al. Decreased accumulation of subgenomic RNA in human cells infected with vaccine candidate DEN4Delta30 increases viral susceptibility to type I interferon. *Vaccine* 2018;36:3460–3467.

146. Byk LA, Gamarnik AV. Properties and functions of the dengue virus capsid protein. *Annu Rev Virol* 2016;3:263–281.

147. Byrne SN, Halliday GM, Johnston LJ, et al. Interleukin-1beta but not tumor necrosis factor is involved in West Nile virus-induced Langerhans cell migration from the skin in C57BL/6 mice. *J Invest Dermatol* 2001;117:702–709.

148. Cabezas S, Bracho G, Aloia AL, et al. Dengue virus induces increased activity of the complement alternative pathway in infected cells. *J Virol* 2018;92.

149. Caine EA, Scheaffer SM, Arora N, et al. Interferon lambda protects the female reproductive tract against Zika virus infection. *Nat Commun* 2019;10:280.

150. Caires-Junior LC, Goulart E, Melo US, et al. Discordant congenital Zika syndrome twins show differential in vitro viral susceptibility of neural progenitor cells. *Nat Commun* 2018;9:475.

151. Calisher CH. Antigenic classification and taxonomy of flaviviruses (family Flaviviridae) emphasizing a universal system for the taxonomy of viruses causing tick-borne encephalitis. *Acta Virol* 1988;32:469–478.

152. Calisher CH, Gould EA. Taxonomy of the virus family Flaviviridae. *Adv Virus Res* 2003;59:1–19.

153. Calisher CH, Karabatsos N, Dalrymple JM, et al. Antigenic relationships between flaviviruses as determined by cross-neutralization tests with polyclonal antisera. *J Gen Virol* 1989;70(Pt 1):37–43.

154. Callaway JB, Smith SA, McKinnon KP, et al. Spleen Tyrosine Kinase (Syk) mediates IL-1beta induction by primary human monocytes during antibody-enhanced dengue virus infection. *J Biol Chem* 2015;290:17306–17320.

155. Calvert AE, Kalantarov GF, Chang GJ, et al. Human monoclonal antibodies to West Nile virus identify epitopes on the prM protein. *Virology* 2011;410:30–37.

156. Calvet G, Aguiar RS, Melo ASO, et al. Detection and sequencing of Zika virus from amniotic fluid of fetuses with microcephaly in Brazil: a case study. *Lancet Infect Dis* 2016;16:653–660.

157. Cam BV, Fonsmark L, Hue NB, et al. Prospective case-control study of encephalopathy in children with dengue hemorrhagic fever. *Am J Trop Med Hyg* 2001;65:848–851.

158. Campos GS, Bandeira AC, Sardi SI. Zika virus outbreak, Bahia, Brazil. *Emerg Infect Dis* 2015;21:1885–1886.

159. Cao-Lormeau VM, Blake A, Mons S, et al. Guillain-Barre Syndrome outbreak associated with Zika virus infection in French Polynesia: a case-control study. *Lancet* 2016;387:1531–1539.

160. Cao-Lormeau VM, Roche C, Teissier A, et al. Zika virus, French Polynesia, South pacific, 2013. *Emerg Infect Dis* 2014;20:1085–1086.

161. Capeding MR, Tran NH, Hadinegoro SR, et al. Clinical efficacy and safety of a novel tetravalent dengue vaccine in healthy children in Asia: a phase 3, randomised, observer-masked, placebo-controlled trial. *Lancet* 2014;384:1358–1365.

162. Cardosa MJ, Gordon S, Hirsch S, et al. Interaction of West Nile virus with primary murine macrophages: role of cell activation and receptors for antibody and complement. *J Virol* 1986;57:952–959.

163. Cardosa MJ, Porterfield JS, Gordon S. Complement receptor mediates enhanced flavivirus replication in macrophages. *J Exp Med* 1983;158:258–263.

164. Carroll MC. The complement system in regulation of adaptive immunity. *Nat Immunol* 2004;5:981–986.

165. Carroll T, Lo M, Lanteri M, et al. Zika virus preferentially replicates in the female reproductive tract after vaginal inoculation of rhesus macaques. *PLoS Pathog* 2017;13:e1006537.

166. Carteaux G, Maquart M, Bedet A, et al. Zika virus associated with meningoencephalitis. *N Engl J Med* 2016;374:1595–1596.

167. Casals J. Immunological relationships among central nervous system viruses. *J Exp Med* 1944;79:341–359.

168. Casals J, Brown LV. Hemagglutination with arthropod-borne viruses. *J Exp Med* 1954;99:429–449.

169. Casals J, Webster LT. Relationship of the virus of louping ill in sheep and the virus of russian spring-summer encephalitis in man. *J Exp Med* 1944;79:45–63.

170. Cauchemez S, Besnard M, Bompard P, et al. Association between Zika virus and microcephaly in French Polynesia, 2013–15: a retrospective study. *Lancet* 2016;387:2125–2132.

171. Centers for Disease Control and Prevention. Travel-associated Dengue surveillance—United States, 2006–2008. *MMWR Morb Mortal Wkly Rep* 2010;59:715–719.

172. Chambers TJ, Diamond MS. Pathogenesis of flavivirus encephalitis. In: Chambers TJ, Monath TP, eds. *The Flaviviruses: Current Molecular Aspects of Evolution, Biology, and Disease Prevention*, vol. 60. San Diego: Academic Press; 2003:273–342.

173. Chambers TJ, Droll DA, Walton AH, et al. West Nile 25A virus infection of B-cell-deficient ((micro)MT) mice: characterization of neuroinvasiveness and pseudoreversion of the viral envelope protein. *J Gen Virol* 2008;89:627–635.

174. Chan YL, Chang TH, Liao CL, et al. The cellular antiviral protein viperin is attenuated by proteasome-mediated protein degradation in Japanese encephalitis virus-infected cells. *J Virol* 2008;82:10455–10464.

175. Chan YK, Gack MU. A phosphomimetic-based mechanism of dengue virus to antagonize innate immunity. *Nat Immunol* 2016;17:523–530.
176. Chang TH, Liao CL, Lin YL. Flavivirus induces interferon-beta gene expression through a pathway involving RIG-I-dependent IRF-3 and PI3K-dependent NF-kappaB activation. *Microbes Infect* 2006;8:157–171.
177. Chang DC, Liu WJ, Anraku I, et al. Single-round infectious particles enhance immunogenicity of a DNA vaccine against West Nile virus. *Nat Biotechnol* 2008;26:571–577.
178. Chan-Tack KM, Forrest G. Failure of interferon alpha-2b in a patient with West Nile virus meningoencephalitis and acute flaccid paralysis. *Scand J Infect Dis* 2005;37:944–946.
179. Chao DY, King CC, Wang WK, et al. Strategically examining the full-genome of dengue virus type 3 in clinical isolates reveals its mutation spectra. *Virol J* 2005;2:72.
180. Chastel C, Main AJ, Guiguen C, et al. The isolation of Meaban virus, a new Flavivirus from the seabird tick Ornithodoros (Alectorobius) maritimus in France. *Arch Virol* 1985;83:129–140.
181. Chatel-Chaix L, Cortese M, Romero-Brey I, et al. Dengue Virus Perturbs Mitochondrial Morphodynamics to Dampen Innate Immune Responses. *Cell Host Microbe* 2016;20:342–356.
182. Chaturvedi UC, Dhawan R, Khanna M, et al. Breakdown of the blood-brain barrier during dengue virus infection of mice. *J Gen Virol* 1991;72(Pt 4):859–866.
183. Chau TN, Quyen NT, Thuy TT, et al. Dengue in Vietnamese infants--results of infection-enhancement assays correlate with age-related disease epidemiology, and cellular immune responses correlate with disease severity. *J Infect Dis* 2008;198:516–524.
184. Chavali PL, Stojic L, Meredith LW, et al. Neurodevelopmental protein Musashi-1 interacts with the Zika genome and promotes viral replication. *Science* 2017;357:83–88.
185. Chazal M, Beauclair G, Gracias S, et al. RIG-I recognizes the 5′ region of dengue and Zika virus genomes. *Cell Rep* 2018;24:320–328.
186. Chen HC, Hofman FM, Kung JT, et al. Both virus and tumor necrosis factor alpha are critical for endothelium damage in a mouse model of dengue virus-induced hemorrhage. *J Virol* 2007;81:5518–5526.
187. Chen HC, Lai SY, Sung JM, et al. Lymphocyte activation and hepatic cellular infiltration in immunocompetent mice infected by dengue virus. *J Med Virol* 2004;73:419–431.
188. Chen J, Liang Y, Yi P, et al. Outcomes of congenital Zika disease depend on timing of infection and maternal-fetal interferon action. *Cell Rep* 2017;21:1588–1599.
189. Chen ST, Lin YL, Huang MT, et al. CLEC5A is critical for dengue-virus-induced lethal disease. *Nature* 2008;453:672–676.
190. Chen ST, Liu RS, Wu MF, et al. CLEC5A regulates Japanese encephalitis virus-induced neuroinflammation and lethality. *PLoS Pathog* 2012;8:e1002655.
191. Chen Y, Maguire T, Hileman RE, et al. Dengue virus infectivity depends on envelope protein binding to target cell heparan sulfate. *Nat Med* 1997;3:866–871.
192. Chen WR, Rico-Hesse R, Tesh RB. A new genotype of Japanese encephalitis virus from Indonesia. *Am J Trop Med Hyg* 1992;47:61–69.
193. Chen WR, Tesh RB, Rico-Hesse R. Genetic variation of Japanese encephalitis virus in nature. *J Gen Virol* 1990;71(Pt 12):2915–2922.
194. Chen J, Yang YF, Yang Y, et al. AXL promotes Zika virus infection in astrocytes by antagonizing type I interferon signalling. *Nat Microbiol* 2018;3:302–309.
195. Chen YL, Yin Z, Lakshminarayana SB, et al. Inhibition of dengue virus by an ester prodrug of an adenosine analog. *Antimicrob Agents Chemother* 2010;54:3255–3261.
196. Cherrier MV, Kaufmann B, Nybakken GE, et al. Structural basis for the preferential recognition of immature flaviviruses by a fusion-loop antibody. *EMBO J* 2009;28:3269–3276.
197. Chimelli L, Melo ASO, Avvad-Portari E, et al. The spectrum of neuropathological changes associated with congenital Zika virus infection. *Acta Neuropathol* 2017;133:983–999.
198. Chiu CY, Sanchez-San Martin C, Bouquet J, et al. Experimental Zika virus inoculation in a New World monkey model reproduces key features of the human infection. *Sci Rep* 2017;7:17126.
199. Cho H, Proll SC, Szretter KJ, et al. Differential innate immune response programs in neuronal subtypes determine susceptibility to infection in the brain by positive-stranded RNA viruses. *Nat Med* 2013;19:458–464.
200. Chotpitayasunondh T, Pruekprasert P, Puthanakit T, et al. Post-licensure, phase IV, safety study of a live attenuated Japanese encephalitis recombinant vaccine in children in Thailand. *Vaccine* 2017;35:299–304.
201. Chowers MY, Lang R, Nassar F, et al. Clinical characteristics of the West Nile fever outbreak, Israel, 2000. *Emerg Infect Dis* 2001;7:675–678.
202. Chu JJ, Ng ML. Infectious entry of West Nile virus occurs through a clathrin-mediated endocytic pathway. *J Virol* 2004;78:10543–10555.
203. Chung KM, Liszewski MK, Nybakken G, et al. West Nile virus non-structural protein NS1 inhibits complement activation by binding the regulatory protein factor H. *Proc Natl Acad Sci U S A* 2006;103:19111–19116.
204. Chung KM, Nybakken GE, Thompson BS, et al. Antibodies against West Nile Virus nonstructural protein NS1 prevent lethal infection through Fc gamma receptor-dependent and -independent mechanisms. *J Virol* 2006;80:1340–1351.
205. Chung KM, Thompson BS, Fremont DH, et al. Antibody recognition of cell surface-associated NS1 triggers Fc-gamma receptor-mediated phagocytosis and clearance of West Nile Virus-infected cells. *J Virol* 2007;81:9551–9555.
206. Churdboonchart V, Bhamarapravati N, Futrakul P. Crossed immunoelectrophoresis for the detection of split products of the third complement in dengue hemorrhagic fever. I. Observations in patients' plasma. *Am J Trop Med Hyg* 1983;32:569–576.
207. Clements DE, Coller BA, Lieberman MM, et al. Development of a recombinant tetravalent dengue virus vaccine: immunogenicity and efficacy studies in mice and monkeys. *Vaccine* 2010;28:2705–2715.
208. Clyde K, Harris E. RNA secondary structure in the coding region of dengue virus type 2 directs translation start codon selection and is required for viral replication. *J Virol* 2006;80:2170–2182.
209. Coffey LL, Keesler RI, Pesavento PA, et al. Intraamniotic Zika virus inoculation of pregnant rhesus macaques produces fetal neurologic disease. *Nat Commun* 2018;9:2414.
210. Conde JN, da Silva EM, Allonso D, et al. Inhibition of the membrane attack complex by dengue virus NS1 through interaction with vitronectin and terminal complement proteins. *J Virol* 2016;90:9570–9581.
211. Conde JN, Silva EM, Barbosa AS, et al. The complement system in flavivirus infections. *Front Microbiol* 2017;8:213.
212. Cook S, Moureau G, Kitchen A, et al. Molecular evolution of the insect-specific flaviviruses. *J Gen Virol* 2012;93:223–234.
213. Cooper MA, Colonna M, Yokoyama WM. Hidden talents of natural killers: NK cells in innate and adaptive immunity. *EMBO Rep* 2009;10:1103–1110.
214. Corry J, Arora N, Good CA, et al. Organotypic models of type III interferon-mediated protection from Zika virus infections at the maternal-fetal interface. *Proc Natl Acad Sci U S A* 2017;114:9433–9438.
215. Corver J, Ortiz A, Allison SL, et al. Membrane fusion activity of tick-borne encephalitis virus and recombinant subviral particles in a liposomal model system. *Virology* 2000;269:37–46.
216. Couvelard A, Marianneau P, Bedel C, et al. Report of a fatal case of dengue infection with hepatitis: demonstration of dengue antigens in hepatocytes and liver apoptosis. *Hum Pathol* 1999;30:1106–1110.
217. Cox F, van der Fits L, Abbink P, et al. Adenoviral vector type 26 encoding Zika virus (ZIKV) M-Env antigen induces humoral and cellular immune responses and protects mice and nonhuman primates against ZIKV challenge. *PLoS One* 2018;13:e0202820.
218. Coyne CB, Lazear HM. Zika virus—reigniting the TORCH. *Nat Rev Microbiol* 2016;14:707–715.
219. Crance JM, Scaramozzino N, Jouan A, et al. Interferon, ribavirin, 6-azauridine and glycyrrhizin: antiviral compounds active against pathogenic flaviviruses. *Antiviral Res* 2003;58:73–79.
220. Creech WB. St Louis encephalitis in the United States, 1975. *J Infect Dis* 1977;135:1014–1016.
221. Crill WD, Chang GJ. Localization and characterization of flavivirus envelope glycoprotein cross-reactive epitopes. *J Virol* 2004;78:13975–13986.
222. Crill WD, Hughes HR, Delorey MJ, et al. Humoral immune responses of dengue fever patients using epitope-specific serotype-2 virus-like particle antigens. *PLoS One* 2009;4:e4991.
223. Crill WD, Roehrig JT. Monoclonal antibodies that bind to domain III of dengue virus E glycoprotein are the most efficient blockers of virus adsorption to Vero cells. *J Virol* 2001;75:7769–7773.
224. Crill WD, Trainor NB, Chang GJ. A detailed mutagenesis study of flavivirus cross-reactive epitopes using West Nile virus-like particles. *J Gen Virol* 2007;88:1169–1174.
225. Curren EJ, Lindsey NP, Fischer M, et al. St. Louis encephalitis virus disease in the United States, 2003–2017. *Am J Trop Med Hyg* 2018;99:1074–1079.
226. Cuypers L, Libin PJK, Simmonds P, et al. Time to Harmonize Dengue Nomenclature and Classification. *Viruses* 2018;10.
227. Daffis S, Samuel MA, Keller BC, et al. Cell-specific IRF-3 responses protect against West Nile virus infection by interferon-dependent and independent mechanisms. *PLoS Pathog* 2007;3:e106.
228. Daffis S, Samuel MA, Suthar MS, et al. Toll-like receptor 3 has a protective role against West Nile virus infection. *J Virol* 2008;82:10349–10358.
229. Daffis S, Samuel MA, Suthar MS, et al. Interferon regulatory factor IRF-7 induces the antiviral alpha interferon response and protects against lethal West Nile virus infection. *J Virol* 2008;82:8465–8475.
230. Daffis S, Suthar MS, Gale M Jr, et al. Measure and countermeasure: type I IFN (IFN-alpha/beta) antiviral response against West Nile virus. *J Innate Immun* 2009;1:435–445.
231. Daffis S, Suthar MS, Szretter KJ, et al. Induction of IFN-beta and the innate antiviral response in myeloid cells occurs through an IPS-1-dependent signal that does not require IRF-3 and IRF-7. *PLoS Pathog* 2009;5:e1000607.
232. Daffis S, Szretter KJ, Schriewer J, et al. 2′-O methylation of the viral mRNA cap evades host restriction by IFIT family members. *Nature* 2010;468:452–456.
233. Dai L, Song J, Lu X, et al. Structures of the Zika Virus envelope protein and its complex with a flavivirus broadly protective antibody. *Cell Host Microbe* 2016;19:696–704.
234. Dalrymple NA, Cimica V, Mackow ER. Dengue virus NS proteins inhibit RIG-I/MAVS signaling by blocking TBK1/IRF3 phosphorylation: dengue virus serotype 1 NS4A is a unique interferon-regulating virulence determinant. *MBio* 2015;6:e00553–00515.
235. Dang J, Tiwari SK, Lichinchi G, et al. Zika virus depletes neural progenitors in human cerebral organoids through activation of the innate immune receptor TLR3. *Cell Stem Cell* 2016;19:258–265.
236. Daniels BP, Holman DW, Cruz-Orengo L, et al. Viral pathogen-associated molecular patterns regulate blood-brain barrier integrity via competing innate cytokine signals. *MBio* 2014;5:e01476-14.
237. Darbellay J, Cox B, Lai K, et al. Zika virus causes persistent infection in porcine conceptuses and may impair health in offspring. *EBioMedicine* 2017;25:73–86.
238. Darbellay J, Lai K, Babiuk S, et al. Neonatal pigs are susceptible to experimental Zika virus infection. *Emerg Microbes Infect* 2017;6:e6.
239. Davis BS, Chang GJ, Cropp B, et al. West Nile virus recombinant DNA vaccine protects mouse and horse from virus challenge and expresses in vitro a noninfectious recombinant antigen that can be used in enzyme-linked immunosorbent assays. *J Virol* 2001;75:4040–4047.
240. Davis CT, Li L, May FJ, et al. Genetic stasis of dominant West Nile virus genotype, Houston, Texas. *Emerg Infect Dis* 2007;13:601–604.
241. Davis CW, Nguyen HY, Hanna SL, et al. West Nile virus discriminates between DC-SIGN and DC-SIGNR for cellular attachment and infection. *J Virol* 2006;80:1290–1301.
242. Day JF. Predicting St. Louis encephalitis virus epidemics: lessons from recent, and not so recent, outbreaks. *Annu Rev Entomol* 2001;46:111–138.
243. de Alwis R, Beltramello M, Messer WB, et al. In-depth analysis of the antibody response of individuals exposed to primary dengue virus infection. *PLoS Negl Trop Dis* 2011;5:e1188.
244. De Brito T, Siqueira SA, Santos RT, et al. Human fatal yellow fever. Immunohistochemical detection of viral antigens in the liver, kidney and heart. *Pathol Res Pract* 1992;188:177–181.
245. de Fatima Vasco Aragao M, van der Linden V, Brainer-Lima AM, et al. Clinical features and neuroimaging (CT and MRI) findings in presumed Zika virus related congenital infection and microcephaly: retrospective case series study. *BMJ* 2016;353:i1901.
246. De Madrid AT, Porterfield JS. The flaviviruses (group B arboviruses): a cross-neutralization study. *J Gen Virol* 1974;23:91–96.
247. de Oliveira WK, de Franca GVA, Carmo EH, et al. Infection-related microcephaly after the 2015 and 2016 Zika virus outbreaks in Brazil: a surveillance-based analysis. *Lancet* 2017;390:861–870.

248. de Paula Freitas B, de Oliveira Dias JR, Prazeres J, et al. Ocular findings in infants with microcephaly associated with presumed Zika virus congenital infection in Salvador, Brazil. *JAMA Ophthalmol* 2016;134(5):529–535. doi:10.1001/jamaophthalmol.2016.0267.
249. de Sousa JR, Azevedo R, Martins Filho AJ, et al. In situ inflammasome activation results in severe damage to the central nervous system in fatal Zika virus microcephaly cases. *Cytokine* 2018;111:255–264.
250. Decembre E, Assil S, Hillaire ML, et al. Sensing of immature particles produced by dengue virus infected cells induces an antiviral response by plasmacytoid dendritic cells. *PLoS Pathog* 2014;10:e1004434.
251. Dejnirattisai W, Jumnainsong A, Onsirisakul N, et al. Cross-reacting antibodies enhance dengue virus infection in humans. *Science* 2010;328:745–748.
252. Dejnirattisai W, Supasa P, Wongwiwat W, et al. Dengue virus sero-cross-reactivity drives antibody-dependent enhancement of infection with Zika virus. *Nat Immunol* 2016;17:1102–1108.
253. Dejnirattisai W, Wongwiwat W, Supasa S, et al. A new class of highly potent, broadly neutralizing antibodies isolated from viremic patients infected with dengue virus. *Nat Immunol* 2015;16:170–177.
254. Della-Porta AJ, Westaway EG. Immune response in rabbits to virion and nonvirion antigens of the Flavivirus kunjin. *Infect Immun* 1977;15:874–882.
255. Demina TV, Dzhioev YP, Verkhozina MM, et al. Genotyping and characterization of the geographical distribution of tick-borne encephalitis virus variants with a set of molecular probes. *J Med Virol* 2010;82:965–976.
256. Deng YQ, Zhang NN, Li XF, et al. Intranasal infection and contact transmission of Zika virus in guinea pigs. *Nat Commun* 2017;8:1648.
257. Despres P, Dietrich J, Girard M, et al. Recombinant baculoviruses expressing yellow fever virus E and NS1 proteins elicit protective immunity in mice. *J Gen Virol* 1991;72(Pt 11): 2811–2816.
258. Devilder MC, Allain S, Dousset C, et al. Early triggering of exclusive IFN-gamma responses of human Vgamma9Vdelta2 T cells by TLR-activated myeloid and plasmacytoid dendritic cells. *J Immunol* 2009;183:3625–3633.
259. Diamond MS. Evasion of innate and adaptive immunity by flaviviruses. *Immunol Cell Biol* 2003;81:196–206.
260. Diamond MS. Mechanisms of evasion of the type I interferon antiviral response by flaviviruses. *J Interferon Cytokine Res* 2009;29:521–530.
261. Diamond MS. Progress on the development of therapeutics against West Nile virus. *Antiviral Res* 2009;83:214–227.
262. Diamond MS, Klein RS. West Nile virus: crossing the blood-brain barrier. *Nat Med* 2004;10:1294–1295.
263. Diamond MS, Klein RS. A genetic basis for human susceptibility to West Nile virus. *Trends Microbiol* 2006;14:287–289.
264. Diamond MS, Roberts T, Edgil D, et al. Modulation of dengue virus infection in human cells by alpha, beta, and gamma interferons. *J Virol* 2000;74:4957–4966.
265. Diamond MS, Shrestha B, Marri A, et al. B cells and antibody play critical roles in the immediate defense of disseminated infection by West Nile encephalitis virus. *J Virol* 2003;77:2578–2586.
266. Dick GW. Zika virus. II. Pathogenicity and physical properties. *Trans R Soc Trop Med Hyg* 1952;46:521–534.
267. Dick GW, Kitchen SF, Haddow AJ. Zika virus. I. Isolations and serological specificity. *Trans R Soc Trop Med Hyg* 1952;46:509–520.
268. Diebold SS, Kaisho T, Hemmi H, et al. Innate antiviral responses by means of TLR7-mediated recognition of single-stranded RNA. *Science* 2004;303:1529–1531.
269. Ding Q, Gaska JM, Douam F, et al. Species-specific disruption of STING-dependent antiviral cellular defenses by the Zika virus NS2B3 protease. *Proc Natl Acad Sci U S A* 2018;115:E6310-E6318.
270. Diniz JA, Da Rosa AP, Guzman H, et al. West Nile virus infection of primary mouse neuronal and neuroglial cells: the role of astrocytes in chronic infection. *Am J Trop Med Hyg* 2006;75:691–696.
271. Dobson JS, Levell NJ. Spotting Zika spots: descriptive features of the rash used in 66 published cases. *Clin Exp Dermatol* 2019;44:4–12.
272. Doceul V, Lara E, Sailleau C, et al. Epidemiology, molecular virology and diagnostics of Schmallenberg virus, an emerging orthobunyavirus in Europe. *Vet Res* 2013;44:31.
273. Dokland T, Walsh M, Mackenzie JM, et al. West Nile virus core protein; tetramer structure and ribbon formation. *Structure* 2004;12:1157–1163.
274. D'Ortenzio E, Matheron S, Yazdanpanah Y, et al. Evidence of Sexual Transmission of Zika Virus. *N Engl J Med* 2016;374:2195–2198.
275. Douam F, Soto Albrecht YE, Hrebikova G, et al. Type III interferon-mediated signaling is critical for controlling live attenuated yellow fever virus infection in vivo. *MBio* 2017;8.
276. Douglas MW, Kesson AM, King NJ. CTL recognition of West Nile virus-infected fibroblasts is cell cycle dependent and is associated with virus-induced increases in class I MHC antigen expression. *Immunology* 1994;82:561–570.
277. Dowd KA, DeMaso CR, Pelc RS, et al. Broadly neutralizing activity of Zika virus-immune sera identifies a single viral serotype. *Cell Rep* 2016;16:1485–1491.
278. Dowd KA, DeMaso CR, Pierson TC. Genotypic differences in dengue virus neutralization are explained by a single amino acid mutation that modulates virus breathing. *MBio* 2015;6:e01559–01515.
279. Dowd KA, Jost CA, Durbin AP, et al. A dynamic landscape for antibody binding modulates antibody-mediated neutralization of west nile virus. *PLoS Pathog* 2011;7:e1002111.
280. Dowd KA, Ko SY, Morabito KM, et al. Rapid development of a DNA vaccine for Zika virus. *Science* 2016;354:237–240.
281. Dowd KA, Mukherjee S, Kuhn RJ, et al. Combined effects of the structural heterogeneity and dynamics of flaviviruses on antibody recognition. *J Virol* 2014;88:11726–11737.
282. Dowd KA, Pierson TC. Antibody-mediated neutralization of flaviviruses: a reductionist view. *Virology* 2011;411:306–315.
283. Driggers RW, Ho CY, Korhonen EM, et al. Zika virus infection with prolonged maternal viremia and fetal brain abnormalities. *N Engl J Med* 2016;374:2142–2151.
284. Dropulic B, Masters CL. Entry of neurotropic arboviruses into the central nervous system: an in vitro study using mouse brain endothelium. *J Infect Dis* 1990;161:685–691.
285. Dudley DM, Aliota MT, Mohr EL, et al. A rhesus macaque model of Asian-lineage Zika virus infection. *Nat Commun* 2016;7:12204.
286. Dudley DM, Van Rompay KK, Coffey LL, et al. Miscarriage and stillbirth following maternal Zika virus infection in nonhuman primates. *Nat Med* 2018;24:1104–1107.
287. Duffy MR, Chen TH, Hancock WT, et al. Zika virus outbreak on Yap Island, Federated States of Micronesia. *N Engl J Med* 2009;360:2536–2543.
288. Duggal NK, Ritter JM, Pestorius SE, et al. Frequent Zika virus sexual transmission and prolonged viral RNA shedding in an immunodeficient mouse model. *Cell Rep* 2017;18:1751–1760.
289. Durbin AP, Karron RA, Sun W, et al. Attenuation and immunogenicity in humans of a live dengue virus type-4 vaccine candidate with a 30 nucleotide deletion in its 3′-untranslated region. *Am J Trop Med Hyg* 2001;65:405–413.
290. Durbin AP, Kirkpatrick BD, Pierce KK, et al. A single dose of any of four different live attenuated tetravalent dengue vaccines is safe and immunogenic in flavivirus-naive adults: a randomized, double-blind clinical trial. *J Infect Dis* 2013;207:957–965.
291. Durbin AP, McArthur J, Marron JA, et al. The live attenuated dengue serotype 1 vaccine rDEN1Delta30 is safe and highly immunogenic in healthy adult volunteers. *Hum Vaccin* 2006;2:167–173.
292. Durbin AP, Vargas MJ, Wanionek K, et al. Phenotyping of peripheral blood mononuclear cells during acute dengue illness demonstrates infection and increased activation of monocytes in severe cases compared to classic dengue fever. *Virology* 2008;376:429–435.
293. Durbin AP, Wright PF, Cox A, et al. The live attenuated chimeric vaccine rWN/DEN4Delta30 is well-tolerated and immunogenic in healthy flavivirus-naive adult volunteers. *Vaccine* 2013;31:5772–5777.
294. Durrant DM, Daniels BP, Klein RS. IL-1R1 signaling regulates CXCL12-mediated T cell localization and fate within the central nervous system during West Nile virus encephalitis. *J Immunol* 2014;193:4095–4106.
295. Durrant DM, Robinette ML, Klein RS. IL-1R1 is required for dendritic cell-mediated T cell reactivation within the CNS during West Nile virus encephalitis. *J Exp Med* 2013;210:503–516.
296. Ebel GD, Spielman A, Telford SR III. Phylogeny of North American Powassan virus. *J Gen Virol* 2001;82:1657–1665.
297. Elbahesh H, Jha BK, Silverman RH, et al. The Flvr-encoded murine oligoadenylate synthetase 1b (Oas1b) suppresses 2–5A synthesis in intact cells. *Virology* 2011;409:262–270.
298. Eldadah AH, Nathanson N. Pathogenesis of West Nile Virus encepahlitis in mice and rats. II. Virus multiplication, evolution of immunofluorescence, and development of histological lesions in the brain. *Am J Epidemiol* 1967;86:776–790.
299. Ellis BR, Barrett AD. The enigma of yellow fever in East Africa. *Rev Med Virol* 2008;18:331–346.
300. Elong Ngono A, Chen HW, Tang WW, et al. Protective role of cross-reactive CD8 T cells against dengue virus infection. *EBioMedicine* 2016;13:284–293.
301. Elong Ngono A, Vizcarra EA, Tang WW, et al. Mapping and role of the CD8(+) T cell response during primary Zika virus infection in mice. *Cell Host Microbe* 2017;21:35–46.
302. Elshuber S, Allison SL, Heinz FX, et al. Cleavage of protein prM is necessary for infection of BHK-21 cells by tick-borne encephalitis virus. *J Gen Virol* 2003;84:183–191.
303. Elsterova J, Palus M, Sirmarova J, et al. Tick-borne encephalitis virus neutralization by high dose intravenous immunoglobulin. *Ticks Tick Borne Dis* 2017;8:253–258.
304. Endy TP, Chunsuttiwat S, Nisalak A, et al. Epidemiology of inapparent and symptomatic acute dengue virus infection: a prospective study of primary school children in Kamphaeng Phet, Thailand. *Am J Epidemiol* 2002;156:40–51.
305. Epelboin Y, Talaga S, Epelboin L, et al. Zika virus: an updated review of competent or naturally infected mosquitoes. *PLoS Negl Trop Dis* 2017;11:e0005933.
306. Erdelyi K, Ursu K, Ferenczi E, et al. Clinical and pathologic features of lineage 2 West Nile virus infections in birds of prey in Hungary. *Vector Borne Zoonotic Dis* 2007;7:181–188.
307. Errett JS, Suthar MS, McMillan A, et al. The essential, nonredundant roles of RIG-I and MDA5 in detecting and controlling West Nile virus infection. *J Virol* 2013;87:11416–11425.
308. Evans JD, Seeger C. Differential effects of mutations in NS4B on WNV replication and inhibition of interferon signaling. *J Virol* 2007;81:11809–11816.
309. Fabre A, Couvelard A, Degott C, et al. Dengue virus induced hepatitis with chronic calcific changes. *Gut* 2001;49:864–865.
310. Fadok VA, de Cathelineau A, Daleke DL, et al. Loss of phospholipid asymmetry and surface exposure of phosphatidylserine is required for phagocytosis of apoptotic cells by macrophages and fibroblasts. *J Biol Chem* 2001;276:1071–1077.
311. Falconar AK. Identification of an epitope on the dengue virus membrane (M) protein defined by cross-protective monoclonal antibodies: design of an improved epitope sequence based on common determinants present in both envelope (E and M) proteins. *Arch Virol* 1999;144:2313–2330.
312. Falgout B, Bray M, Schlesinger JJ, et al. Immunization of mice with recombinant vaccinia virus expressing authentic dengue virus nonstructural protein NS1 protects against lethal dengue virus encephalitis. *J Virol* 1990;64:4356–4363.
313. Fall G, Di Paola N, Faye M, et al. Biological and phylogenetic characteristics of West African lineages of West Nile virus. *PLoS Negl Trop Dis* 2017;11:e0006078.
314. Fang Y, Reisen WK. Previous infection with West Nile or St. Louis encephalitis viruses provides cross protection during reinfection in house finches. *Am J Trop Med Hyg* 2006;75:480–485.
315. Fang H, Welte T, Zheng X, et al. gammadelta T cells promote the maturation of dendritic cells during West Nile virus infection. *FEMS Immunol Med Microbiol* 2010;59:71–80.
316. Faria NR, Kraemer MUG, Hill SC, et al. Genomic and epidemiological monitoring of yellow fever virus transmission potential. *Science* 2018;361:894–899.
317. Faria NR, Quick J, Claro IM, et al. Establishment and cryptic transmission of Zika virus in Brazil and the Americas. *Nature* 2017;546:406–410.
318. Ferguson NM, Rodriguez-Barraquer I, Dorigatti I, et al. Benefits and risks of the Sanofi-Pasteur dengue vaccine: modeling optimal deployment. *Science* 2016;353:1033–1036.
319. Ferlenghi I, Clarke M, Ruttan T, et al. Molecular organization of a recombinant subviral particle from tick-borne encephalitis virus. *Mol Cell* 2001;7:593–602.
320. Fernandez E, Dejnirattisai W, Cao B, et al. Human antibodies to the dengue virus E-dimer epitope have therapeutic activity against Zika virus infection. *Nat Immunol* 2017;18: 1261–1269.
321. Fernandez E, Kose N, Edeling MA, et al. Mouse and human monoclonal antibodies protect against infection by multiple genotypes of Japanese encephalitis virus. *MBio* 2018;9.

322. Fernandez MP, Parra Saad E, Ospina Martinez M, et al. Ocular histopathologic features of congenital Zika syndrome. *JAMA Ophthalmol* 2017;135:1163–1169.
323. Fibriansah G, Ibarra KD, Ng TS, et al. DENGUE VIRUS. Cryo-EM structure of an antibody that neutralizes dengue virus type 2 by locking E protein dimers. *Science* 2015;349:88–91.
324. Fibriansah G, Ng TS, Kostyuchenko VA, et al. Structural changes in dengue virus when exposed to a temperature of 37 degrees C. *J Virol* 2013;87:7585–7592.
325. Fibriansah G, Tan JL, Smith SA, et al. A highly potent human antibody neutralizes dengue virus serotype 3 by binding across three surface proteins. *Nat Commun* 2015;6:6341.
326. Fink K, Ng C, Nkenfou C, et al. Depletion of macrophages in mice results in higher dengue virus titers and highlights the role of macrophages for virus control. *Eur J Immunol* 2009;39:2809–2821.
327. Fischer M, Lindsey N, Staples JE, et al. Japanese encephalitis vaccines: recommendations of the Advisory Committee on Immunization Practices (ACIP). *MMWR Recomm Rep* 2010;59:1–27.
328. Fitzgeorge R, Bradish CJ. Differentiation of strains of yellow fever virus in gamma-irradiated mice. *J Gen Virol* 1980;50:345–356.
329. Fitzgeorge R, Bradish CJ. The in vivo differentiation of strains of yellow fever virus in mice. *J Gen Virol* 1980;46:1–13.
330. Flamand M, Megret F, Mathieu M, et al. Dengue virus type 1 nonstructural glycoprotein NS1 is secreted from mammalian cells as a soluble hexamer in a glycosylation-dependent fashion. *J Virol* 1999;73:6104–6110.
331. Fonseca BA, Pincus S, Shope RE, et al. Recombinant vaccinia viruses co-expressing dengue-1 glycoproteins prM and E induce neutralizing antibodies in mice. *Vaccine* 1994;12:279–285.
332. Foo SS, Chen W, Chan Y, et al. Asian Zika virus strains target CD14(+) blood monocytes and induce M2-skewed immunosuppression during pregnancy. *Nat Microbiol* 2017;2:1558–1570.
333. Fowler AM, Tang WW, Young MP, et al. Maternally acquired Zika antibodies enhance dengue disease severity in mice. *Cell Host Microbe* 2018;24:743–750, e745.
334. Foy BD, Kobylinski KC, Chilson Foy JL, et al. Probable non-vector-borne transmission of Zika virus, Colorado, USA. *Emerg Infect Dis* 2011;17:880–882.
335. Franca GV, Schuler-Faccini L, Oliveira WK, et al. Congenital Zika virus syndrome in Brazil: a case series of the first 1501 livebirths with complete investigation. *Lancet* 2016;388: 891–897.
336. Fredericksen BL, Gale M Jr. West Nile virus evades activation of interferon regulatory factor 3 through RIG-I-dependent and -independent pathways without antagonizing host defense signaling. *J Virol* 2006;80:2913–2923.
337. Fredericksen BL, Keller BC, Fornek J, et al Establishment and maintenance of the innate antiviral response to West Nile virus involves both RIG-I and MDA5 signaling through IPS-1. *J Virol* 2008;82:609–616.
338. Froeschl G, Huber K, von Sonnenburg F, et al. Long-term kinetics of Zika virus RNA and antibodies in body fluids of a vasectomized traveller returning from Martinique: a case report. *BMC Infect Dis* 2017;17:55.
339. Fuchs A, Lin TY, Beasley DW, et al. Direct complement restriction of Flavivirus infection requires glycan recognition by Mannose Binding Lectin. *Cell Host Microbe* 2010;8:186–195.
340. Fuchs A, Pinto AK, Schwaeble WJ, et al. The lectin pathway of complement activation contributes to protection from West Nile virus infection. *Virology* 2011;412:101–109.
341. Furtado JM, Esposito DL, Klein TM, et al. Uveitis associated with Zika virus infection. *N Engl J Med* 2016;375:394–396.
342. Gack MU, Diamond MS. Innate immune escape by Dengue and West Nile viruses. *Curr Opin Virol* 2016;20:119–128.
343. Gallichotte EN, Baric RS, de Silva AM. The molecular specificity of the human antibody response to dengue virus infections. *Adv Exp Med Biol* 2018;1062:63–76.
344. Gallichotte EN, Widman DG, Yount BL, et al. A new quaternary structure epitope on dengue virus serotype 2 is the target of durable type-specific neutralizing antibodies. *MBio* 2015;6:e01461–01415.
345. Gambel JM, DeFraites R, Hoke C Jr, et al. Japanese encephalitis vaccine: persistence of antibody up to 3 years after a three-dose primary series. *J Infect Dis* 1995;171:1074.
346. Garcez PP, Loiola EC, Madeiro da Costa R, et al. Zika virus impairs growth in human neurospheres and brain organoids. *Science* 2016;352:816–818.
347. Garcia-Tapia D, Hassett DE, Mitchell WJ Jr, et al. West Nile virus encephalitis: sequential histopathological and immunological events in a murine model of infection. *J Neurovirol* 2007;13:130–138.
348. Gardner CL, Ryman KD. Yellow fever: a reemerging threat. *Clin Lab Med* 2010;30:237–260.
349. Garg H, Sedano M, Plata G, et al. Development of virus-like-particle vaccine and reporter assay for Zika virus. *J Virol* 2017;91.
350. Garske T, Van Kerkhove MD, Yactayo S, et al. Yellow Fever in Africa: estimating the burden of disease and impact of mass vaccination from outbreak and serological data. *PLoS Med* 2014;11:e1001638.
351. Gaucher D, Therrien R, Kettaf N, et al. Yellow fever vaccine induces integrated multilineage and polyfunctional immune responses. *J Exp Med* 2008;205(13):3119–3131.
352. Gaudinski MR, Houser KV, Morabito KM, et al. Safety, tolerability, and immunogenicity of two Zika virus DNA vaccine candidates in healthy adults: randomised, open-label, phase 1 clinical trials. *Lancet* 2017;391(10120):552–562. doi:10.1016/S0140-6736(17)33105-7.
353. Gelpi E, Preusser M, Garzuly F, et al. Visualization of Central European tick-borne encephalitis infection in fatal human cases. *J Neuropathol Exp Neurol* 2005;64:506–512.
354. George SL, Wong MA, Dube TJ, et al. Safety and immunogenicity of a live attenuated tetravalent dengue vaccine candidate in flavivirus-naive adults: a randomized, double-blinded phase 1 clinical trial. *J Infect Dis* 2015;212:1032–1041.
355. Getts DR, Matsumoto I, Muller M, et al. Role of IFN-gamma in an experimental murine model of West Nile virus-induced seizures. *J Neurochem* 2007;103(3):1019–1030.
356. Gilfoy FD, Mason PW. West Nile virus-induced IFN production is mediated by the double-stranded RNA-dependent protein kinase, PKR. *J Virol* 2007;81:11148–11158.
357. Gillespie LK, Hoenen A, Morgan G, et al. The endoplasmic reticulum provides the membrane platform for biogenesis of the flavivirus replication complex. *J Virol* 2010;84: 10438–10447.
358. Giordano D, Draves KE, Young LB, et al. Protection of mice deficient in mature B cells from West Nile virus infection by passive and active immunization. *PLoS Pathog* 2017;13: e1006743.
359. Gizzi AS, Grove TL, Arnold JJ, et al. A naturally occurring antiviral ribonucleotide encoded by the human genome. *Nature* 2018;558:610–614.
360. Glasner A, Oiknine-Djian E, Weisblum Y, et al. Zika Virus escapes NK cell detection by upregulating major histocompatibility complex class I molecules. *J Virol* 2017;91.
361. Glasner DR, Puerta-Guardo H, Beatty PR, et al. The Good, the bad, and the shocking: the multiple roles of dengue virus nonstructural protein 1 in protection and pathogenesis. *Annu Rev Virol* 2018;5:227–253.
362. Glasner DR, Ratnasiri K, Puerta-Guardo H, et al. Dengue virus NS1 cytokine-independent vascular leak is dependent on endothelial glycocalyx components. *PLoS Pathog* 2017;13:e1006673.
363. Glass WG, Lim JK, Cholera R, et al. Chemokine receptor CCR5 promotes leukocyte trafficking to the brain and survival in West Nile virus infection. *J Exp Med* 2005;202: 1087–1098.
364. Glass WG, McDermott DH, Lim JK, et al. CCR5 deficiency increases risk of symptomatic West Nile virus infection. *J Exp Med* 2006;203:35–40.
365. Glass JD, Samuels O, Rich MM. Poliomyelitis due to West Nile virus. *N Engl J Med* 2002;347:1280–1281.
366. Goldblum N, Sterk VV, Paderski B. West Nile fever; the clinical features of the disease and the isolation of West Nile virus from the blood of nine human cases. *Am J Hyg* 1954;59:89–103.
367. Gollins S, Porterfield J. Flavivirus infection enhancement in macrophages: radioactive and biological studies on the effect of antibody and viral fate. *J Gen Virol* 1984;65:1261–1272.
368. Gollins SW, Porterfield JS. Flavivirus infection enhancement in macrophages: an electron microscopic study of viral cellular entry. *J Gen Virol* 1985;66(Pt 9):1969–1982.
369. Gollins SW, Porterfield JS. pH-dependent fusion between the flavivirus West Nile and liposomal model membranes. *J Gen Virol* 1986;67:157–166.
370. Gollins SW, Porterfield JS. A new mechanism for the neutralization of enveloped viruses by antiviral antibody. *Nature* 1986;321:244–246.
371. Goncalvez AP, Engle RE, St Claire M, et al. Monoclonal antibody-mediated enhancement of dengue virus infection in vitro and in vivo and strategies for prevention. *Proc Natl Acad Sci U S A* 2007;104:9422–9427.
372. Goncalvez AP, Purcell RH, Lai CJ. Epitope determinants of a chimpanzee Fab antibody that efficiently cross-neutralizes dengue type 1 and type 2 viruses map to inside and in close proximity to fusion loop of the dengue type 2 virus envelope glycoprotein. *J Virol* 2004;78:12919–12928.
373. Goo L, VanBlargan LA, Dowd KA, et al. A single mutation in the envelope protein modulates flavivirus antigenicity, stability, and pathogenesis. *PLoS Pathog* 2017;13:e1006178.
374. Gordon A, Gresh L, Ojeda S, et al. Prior dengue virus infection and risk of Zika: a pediatric cohort in Nicaragua. *PLoS Med* 2019;16:e1002726.
375. Gorman MJ, Caine EA, Zaitsev K, et al. An immunocompetent mouse model of Zika virus infection. *Cell Host Microbe* 2018;23:672–685, e676.
376. Gorman MJ, Poddar S, Farzan M, et al. The interferon-stimulated gene Ifitm3 restricts West Nile virus infection and pathogenesis. *J Virol* 2016;90:8212–8225.
377. Gould EA. Evolution of the Japanese encephalitis serocomplex viruses. *Curr Top Microbiol Immunol* 2002;267:391–404.
378. Gould EA, Buckley A. Antibody-dependent enhancement of yellow fever and Japanese encephalitis virus neurovirulence. *J Gen Virol* 1989;70(Pt 6):1605–1608.
379. Gould EA, de Lamballerie X, Zanotto PM, et al. Evolution, epidemiology, and dispersal of flaviviruses revealed by molecular phylogenies. *Adv Virus Res* 2001;57:71–103.
380. Gould EA, de Lamballerie X, Zanotto PM, et al. Origins, evolution, and vector/host coadaptations within the genus Flavivirus. *Adv Virus Res* 2003;59:277–314.
381. Gould DJ, Edelman R, Grossman RA, et al. Study of Japanese encephalitis virus in Chiangmai Valley, Thailand. IV. Vector studies. *Am J Epidemiol* 1974;100:49–56.
382. Govero J, Esakky P, Scheaffer SM, et al. Zika virus infection damages the testes in mice. *Nature* 2016;540:438–442.
383. Graham JB, Da Costa A, Lund JM. Regulatory T cells shape the resident memory T cell response to virus infection in the tissues. *J Immunol* 2014;192:683–690.
384. Graham RR, Juffrie M, Tan R, et al. A prospective seroepidemiologic study on dengue in children four to nine years of age in Yogyakarta, Indonesia I. studies in 1995–1996. *Am J Trop Med Hyg* 1999;61:412–419.
385. Graham JB, Swarts JL, Thomas S, et al. Immune correlates of protection from West Nile virus neuroinvasion and disease. *J Infect Dis* 2019;219:1162–1171.
386. Graham JB, Swarts JL, Wilkins C, et al. A mouse model of chronic West Nile virus disease. *PLoS Pathog* 2016;12:e1005996.
387. Graham JB, Thomas S, Swarts J, et al. Genetic diversity in the collaborative cross model recapitulates human West Nile virus disease outcomes. *MBio* 2015;6:e00493–00415.
388. Grant A, Ponia SS, Tripathi S, et al. Zika virus targets human STAT2 to inhibit type I interferon signaling. *Cell Host Microbe* 2016;19:882–890.
389. Grard G, Moureau G, Charrel RN, et al. Genomics and evolution of Aedes-borne flaviviruses. *J Gen Virol* 2010;91:87–94.
390. Grard G, Moureau G, Charrel RN, et al. Genetic characterization of tick-borne flaviviruses: new insights into evolution, pathogenetic determinants and taxonomy. *Virology* 2007;361:80–92.
391. Grifoni A, Angelo MA, Lopez B, et al. Global assessment of dengue virus-specific CD4(+) T cell responses in dengue-endemic areas. *Front Immunol* 2017;8:1309.
392. Grifoni A, Costa-Ramos P, Pham J, et al. Cutting Edge: transcriptional profiling reveals multifunctional and cytotoxic antiviral responses of Zika virus-specific CD8(+) T cells. *J Immunol* 2018;201:3487–3491.
393. Grifoni A, Pham J, Sidney J, et al. Prior Dengue virus exposure shapes T cell immunity to Zika virus in humans. *J Virol* 2017;91(24). doi:10.1128/JVI.01469-17.
394. Gritsun TS, Frolova TV, Zhankov AI, et al. Characterization of a Siberian virus isolated from a patient with progressive chronic tick-borne encephalitis. *J Virol* 2003;77:25–36.
395. Gritsun TS, Lashkevich VA, Gould EA. Tick-borne encephalitis. *Antiviral Res* 2003;57:129–146.

396. Gritsun TS, Nuttall PA, Gould EA. Tick-borne flaviviruses. *Adv Virus Res* 2003;61:317–371.
397. Grubaugh ND, Ladner JT, Kraemer MUG, et al. Genomic epidemiology reveals multiple introductions of Zika virus into the United States. *Nature* 2017;546:401–405.
398. Guabiraba R, Marques RE, Besnard AG, et al. Role of the chemokine receptors CCR1, CCR2 and CCR4 in the pathogenesis of experimental dengue infection in mice. *PLoS One* 2010;5:e15680.
399. Gubler DJ. Dengue/dengue haemorrhagic fever: history and current status. *Novartis Found Symp* 2006;277:3–16; discussion 16–22, 71–13, 251–253.
400. Guirakhoo F, Arroyo J, Pugachev KV, et al. Construction, safety, and immunogenicity in nonhuman primates of a chimeric yellow fever-dengue virus tetravalent vaccine. *J Virol* 2001;75:7290–7304.
401. Guirakhoo F, Bolin RA, Roehrig JT. The Murray Valley encephalitis virus prM protein confers acid resistance to virus particles and alters the expression of epitopes within the R2 domain of E glycoprotein. *Virology* 1992;191:921–931.
402. Guirakhoo F, Zhang ZX, Chambers TJ, et al. Immunogenicity, genetic stability, and protective efficacy of a recombinant, chimeric yellow fever-Japanese encephalitis virus (ChimeriVax-JE) as a live, attenuated vaccine candidate against Japanese encephalitis. *Virology* 1999;257:363–372.
403. Gunther G, Haglund M, Lindquist L, et al. Tick-bone encephalitis in Sweden in relation to aseptic meningo-encephalitis of other etiology: a prospective study of clinical course and outcome. *J Neurol* 1997;244:230–238.
404. Guo Q, Chan JF, Poon VK, et al. Immunization with a novel human type 5 Adenovirus-vectored vaccine expressing the premembrane and envelope proteins of Zika virus provides consistent and sterilizing protection in multiple immunocompetent and immunocompromised animal models. *J Infect Dis* 2018;218(3):365–377. doi:10.1093/infdis/jiy187.
405. Guo JT, Hayashi J, Seeger C. West Nile virus inhibits the signal transduction pathway of alpha interferon. *J Virol* 2005;79:1343–1350.
406. Gupta N, Lomash V, Rao PV. Expression profile of Japanese encephalitis virus induced neuroinflammation and its implication in disease severity. *J Clin Virol* 2010;49:4–10.
407. Gurung S, Preno AN, Dubaut JP, et al. Translational model of Zika virus disease in baboons. *J Virol* 2018;92(16). doi:10.1128/JVI.00186–18.
408. Gurung S, Reuter N, Preno A, et al. Zika virus infection at mid-gestation results in fetal cerebral cortical injury and fetal death in the olive baboon. *PLoS Pathog* 2019;15:e1007507.
409. Guy B, Guirakhoo F, Barban V, et al. Preclinical and clinical development of YFV 17D-based chimeric vaccines against dengue, West Nile and Japanese encephalitis viruses. *Vaccine* 2010;28:632–649.
410. Guy B, Noriega F, Ochiai RL, et al. A recombinant live attenuated tetravalent vaccine for the prevention of dengue. *Expert Rev Vaccines* 2017;16:1–13.
411. Guzman MG, Alvarez M, Rodriguez R, et al. Fatal dengue hemorrhagic fever in Cuba, 1997. *Int J Infect Dis* 1999;3:130–135.
412. Guzman MG, Kouri G, Valdes L, et al. Enhanced severity of secondary dengue-2 infections: death rates in 1981 and 1997 Cuban outbreaks. *Rev Panam Salud Publica* 2002;11:223–227.
413. Habjan M, Hubel P, Lacerda L, et al. Sequestration by IFIT1 impairs translation of 2′O-unmethylated capped RNA. *PLoS Pathog* 2013;9:e1003663.
414. Haddow AD, Nalca A, Rossi FD, et al. High infection rates for adult Macaques after intravaginal or intrarectal inoculation with Zika virus. *Emerg Infect Dis* 2017;23:1274–1281.
415. Haddow AJ, Williams MC, Woodall JP, et al. Twelve isolations of Zika virus from Aedes (Stegomyia) Africanus (Theobald) taken in and above a Uganda forest. *Bull World Health Organ* 1964;31:57–69.
416. Hadinegoro SR, Arredondo-Garcia JL, Capeding MR, et al. Efficacy and long-term safety of a dengue vaccine in regions of endemic disease. *N Engl J Med* 2015;373:1195–1206.
417. Hall WC, Crowell TP, Watts DM, et al. Demonstration of yellow fever and dengue antigens in formalin-fixed paraffin-embedded human liver by immunohistochemical analysis. *Am J Trop Med Hyg* 1991;45:408–417.
418. Halstead SB. In vivo enhancement of dengue virus infection in rhesus monkeys by passively transferred antibody. *J Infect Dis* 1979;140:527–533.
419. Halstead SB. Pathogenesis of dengue: challenges to molecular biology. *Science* 1988;239:476–481.
420. Halstead SB. Antibody, macrophages, dengue virus infection, shock, and hemorrhage: a pathogenetic cascade. *Rev Infect Dis* 1989;11 Suppl 4:S830–S839.
421. Halstead SB. Neutralization and antibody-dependent enhancement of dengue viruses. *Adv Virus Res* 2003;60:421–467.
422. Halstead SB. Dengue. *Lancet* 2007;370:1644–1652.
423. Halstead SB. Dengvaxia sensitizes seronegatives to vaccine enhanced disease regardless of age. *Vaccine* 2017;35:6355–6358.
424. Halstead SB, Jacobson J. Japanese encephalitis vaccines. In: Plotkin SA, Orenstein WA, Offit PA, eds. *Vaccines*, 5th ed. Philadelphia: Saunders Elsevier. 2008:311–352.
425. Halstead SB, Lan NT, Myint TT, et al. Dengue hemorrhagic fever in infants: research opportunities ignored. *Emerg Infect Dis* 2002;8:1474–1479.
426. Halstead SB, Larsen K, Kliks S, et al. Comparison of P388D1 mouse macrophage cell line and human monocytes for assay of dengue-2 infection-enhancing antibodies. *Am J Trop Med Hyg* 1983;32:157–163.
427. Halstead SB, Mahalingam S, Marovich MA, et al. Intrinsic antibody-dependent enhancement of microbial infection in macrophages: disease regulation by immune complexes. *Lancet Infect Dis* 2010;10:712–722.
428. Halstead SB, Nimmannitya S, Cohen SN. Observations related to pathogenesis of dengue hemorrhagic fever. IV. Relation of disease severity to antibody response and virus recovered. *Yale J Biol Med* 1970;42:311–328.
429. Halstead SB, O'Rourke EJ. Antibody-enhanced dengue virus infection in primate leukocytes. *Nature* 1977;265:739–741.
430. Halstead SB, O'Rourke EJ. Dengue viruses and mononuclear phagocytes. I. Infection enhancement by non-neutralizing antibody. *J Exp Med* 1977;146:201–217.
431. Halstead SB, Shotwell H, Casals J. Studies on the pathogenesis of dengue infection in monkeys. I. Clinical laboratory responses to primary infection. *J Infect Dis* 1973;128:7–14.
432. Halstead SB, Shotwell H, Casals J. Studies on the pathogenesis of dengue infection in monkeys. II. Clinical laboratory responses to heterologous infection. *J Infect Dis* 1973;128:15–22.
433. Hamel R, Dejarnac O, Wichit S, et al. Biology of Zika virus infection in human skin cells. *J Virol* 2015;89:8880–8896.
434. Hamlin RE, Rahman A, Pak TR, et al. High-dimensional CyTOF analysis of dengue virus-infected human DCs reveals distinct viral signatures. *JCI Insight* 2017;2.
435. Hammon WM, Rudnick A, Sather GE. Viruses associated with epidemic hemorrhagic fevers of the Philippines and Thailand. *Science* 1960;131:1102–1103.
436. Hammond SN, Balmaseda A, Perez L, et al. Differences in dengue severity in infants, children, and adults in a 3-year hospital-based study in Nicaragua. *Am J Trop Med Hyg* 2005;73:1063–1070.
437. Han YW, Choi JY, Uyangaa E, et al. Distinct dictation of Japanese encephalitis virus-induced neuroinflammation and lethality via triggering TLR3 and TLR4 signal pathways. *PLoS Pathog* 2014;10:e1004319.
438. Hanna JN, Ritchie SA, Phillips DA, et al. Japanese encephalitis in north Queensland, Australia, 1998. *Med J Aust* 1999;170:533–536.
439. Hanna JN, Ritchie SA, Phillips DA, et al. An outbreak of Japanese encephalitis in the Torres Strait, Australia, 1995. *Med J Aust* 1996;165:256–260.
440. Hanners NW, Eitson JL, Usui N, et al. Western Zika virus in human fetal neural progenitors persists long term with partial cytopathic and limited immunogenic effects. *Cell Rep* 2016;15:2315–2322.
441. Hansman GS, Taylor DW, McLellan JS, et al. Structural basis for broad detection of genogroup II noroviruses by a monoclonal antibody that binds to a site occluded in the viral particle. *J Virol* 2012;86:3635–3646.
442. Harris E, Videa E, Perez L, et al. Clinical, epidemiologic, and virologic features of dengue in the 1998 epidemic in Nicaragua. *Am J Trop Med Hyg* 2000;63:5–11.
443. Hasan SS, Miller A, Sapparapu G, et al. A human antibody against Zika virus crosslinks the E protein to prevent infection. *Nat Commun* 2017;8:14722.
444. Hasan SS, Sevvana M, Kuhn RJ, et al. Structural biology of Zika virus and other flaviviruses. *Nat Struct Mol Biol* 2018;25:13–20.
445. Hasegawa H, Yoshida M, Fujita S, et al. Comparison of structural proteins among antigenically different Japanese encephalitis virus strains. *Vaccine* 1994;12:841–844.
446. Haslwanter D, Blaas D, Heinz FX, et al. A novel mechanism of antibody-mediated enhancement of flavivirus infection. *PLoS Pathog* 2017;13:e1006643.
447. Hassert M, Wolf KJ, Schwetye KE, et al. CD4+T cells mediate protection against Zika associated severe disease in a mouse model of infection. *PLoS Pathog* 2018;14:e1007237.
448. Hastings AK, Yockey LJ, Jagger BW, et al. TAM receptors are not required for Zika virus infection in mice. *Cell Rep* 2017;19:558–568.
449. He Z, Chen J, Zhu X, et al. NLRP3 Inflammasome activation mediates Zika virus-associated inflammation. *J Infect Dis* 2018;217:1942–1951.
450. He RT, Innis BL, Nisalak A, et al. Antibodies that block virus attachment to Vero cells are a major component of the human neutralizing antibody response against dengue virus type 2. *J Med Virol* 1995;45:451–461.
451. Heinz FX, Holzmann H, Essl A, et al. Field effectiveness of vaccination against tick-borne encephalitis. *Vaccine* 2007;25:7559–7567.
452. Heinz FX, Stiasny K, Puschner-Auer G, et al. Structural changes and functional control of the tick-borne encephalitis virus glycoprotein E by the heterodimeric association with protein prM. *Virology* 1994;198:109–117.
453. Heinze DM, Gould EA, Forrester NL. Revisiting the clinical concept of evolution and dispersal for the tick-borne flaviviruses by using phylogenetic and biogeographic analyses. *J Virol* 2012;86:8663–8671.
454. Henchal EA, Gentry MK, McCown JM, et al. Dengue virus-specific and flavivirus group determinants identified with monoclonal antibodies by indirect immunofluorescence. *Am J Trop Med Hyg* 1982;31:830–836.
455. Hendarto SK, Hadinegoro SR. Dengue encephalopathy. *Acta Paediatr Jpn* 1992;34:350–357.
456. Henderson BE, Cheshire PP, Kirya GB, et al. Immunologic studies with yellow fever and selected African group B arboviruses in rhesus and vervet monkeys. *Am J Trop Med Hyg* 1970;19:110–118.
457. Hennessy S, Liu Z, Tsai TF, et al. Effectiveness of live-attenuated Japanese encephalitis vaccine (SA14–14–2): a case-control study. *Lancet* 1996;347:1583–1586.
458. Hermance ME, Thangamani S. Powassan virus: an emerging arbovirus of public health concern in North America. *Vector Borne Zoonotic Dis* 2017;17:453–462.
459. Herrera BB, Chang CA, Hamel DJ, et al. Continued transmission of Zika virus in humans in West Africa, 1992–2016. *J Infect Dis* 2017;215:1546–1550.
460. Hershkovitz O, Rosental B, Rosenberg LA, et al. NKp44 receptor mediates interaction of the envelope glycoproteins from the West Nile and dengue viruses with NK cells. *J Immunol* 2009;183:2610–2621.
461. Hershkovitz O, Zilka A, Bar-Ilan A, et al. Dengue virus replicon expressing the nonstructural proteins suffices to enhance membrane expression of HLA class I and inhibit lysis by human NK cells. *J Virol* 2008;82:7666–7676.
462. Higgs S, Schneider BS, Vanlandingham DL, et al. Nonviremic transmission of West Nile virus. *Proc Natl Acad Sci U S A* 2005;102:8871–8874.
463. Hildner K, Edelson BT, Purtha WE, et al. Batf3 deficiency reveals a critical role for CD8alpha+ dendritic cells in cytotoxic T cell immunity. *Science* 2008;322:1097–1100.
464. Hilgard P, Stockert R. Heparan sulfate proteoglycans initiate dengue virus infection of hepatocytes. *Hepatology* 2000;32:1069–1077.
465. Hirsch AJ, Roberts VHJ, Grigsby PL, et al. Zika virus infection in pregnant rhesus macaques causes placental dysfunction and immunopathology. *Nat Commun* 2018;9:263.
466. Hirsch AJ, Smith JL, Haese NN, et al. Zika Virus infection of rhesus macaques leads to viral persistence in multiple tissues. *PLoS Pathog* 2017;13:e1006219.
467. Ho LJ, Hung LF, Weng CY, et al. Dengue virus type 2 antagonizes IFN-alpha but not IFN-gamma antiviral effect via down-regulating Tyk2-STAT signaling in the human dendritic cell. *J Immunol* 2005;174:8163–8172.
468. Hoang LT, Lynn DJ, Henn M, et al. The early whole-blood transcriptional signature of dengue virus and features associated with progression to dengue shock syndrome in Vietnamese children and young adults. *J Virol* 2010;84:12982–12994.
469. Hoke CH, Nisalak A, Sangawhipa N, et al. Protection against Japanese encephalitis by inactivated vaccines. *N Engl J Med* 1988;319:608–614.
470. Holmes EC, Twiddy SS. The origin, emergence and evolutionary genetics of dengue virus. *Infect Genet Evol* 2003;3:19–28.

471. Honein MA, Dawson AL, Petersen EE, et al. Birth defects among fetuses and infants of US women with evidence of possible Zika virus infection during pregnancy. *JAMA* 2017;317: 59–68.
472. Hottz ED, Lopes JF, Freitas C, et al. Platelets mediate increased endothelium permeability in dengue through NLRP3-inflammasome activation. *Blood* 2013;122:3405–3414.
473. Hsieh MF, Lai SL, Chen JP, et al. Both CXCR3 and CXCL10/IFN-inducible protein 10 are required for resistance to primary infection by dengue virus. *J Immunol* 2006;177:1855–1863.
474. Huang CY, Butrapet S, Pierro DJ, et al. Chimeric dengue type 2 (vaccine strain PDK-53)/dengue type 1 virus as a potential candidate dengue type 1 virus vaccine. *J Virol* 2000;74: 3020–3028.
475. Huang CY, Butrapet S, Tsuchiya KR, et al. Dengue 2 PDK-53 virus as a chimeric carrier for tetravalent dengue vaccine development. *J Virol* 2003;77:11436–11447.
476. Huang H, Li S, Zhang Y, et al. CD8(+) T cell immune response in immunocompetent mice during Zika virus infection. *J Virol* 2017;91.
477. Huang KJ, Yang YC, Lin YS, et al. The dual-specific binding of dengue virus and target cells for the antibody-dependent enhancement of dengue virus infection. *J Immunol* 2006;176:2825–2832.
478. Hubalek Z, Halouzka J. West Nile fever—a reemerging mosquito-borne viral disease in Europe. *Emerg Infect Dis* 1999;5:643–650.
479. Huber SA, Graveline D, Newell MK, et al. V gamma 1+ T cells suppress and V gamma 4+ T cells promote susceptibility to coxsackievirus B3-induced myocarditis in mice. *J Immunol* 2000;165:4174–4181.
480. Huhn GD, Austin C, Langkop C, et al. The emergence of West Nile Virus during a large outbreak in Illinois in 2002. *Am J Trop Med Hyg* 2005;72:768–776.
481. Hunsperger EA, Roehrig JT. Temporal analyses of the neuropathogenesis of a West Nile virus infection in mice. *J Neurovirol* 2006;12:129–139.
482. Hurlbut HS, Rizk F, Taylor RM, et al. A study of the ecology of West Nile virus in Egypt. *Am J Trop Med Hyg* 1956;5:579–620.
483. Imhoff M, Hagedorn P, Schulze Y, et al. Review: sentinels of tick-borne encephalitis risk. *Ticks Tick Borne Dis* 2015;6:592–600.
484. Jagger BW, Miner JJ, Cao B, et al. Gestational stage and IFN-lambda signaling regulate ZIKV infection in utero. *Cell Host Microbe* 2017;22:366–376, e363.
485. Jahrling PB, Hesse RA, Anderson AO, et al. Opsonization of alphaviruses in hamsters. *J Med Virol* 1983;12:1–16.
486. Jain A, Chaturvedi UC. Dengue in infants: an overview. *FEMS Immunol Med Microbiol* 2010;59:119–130.
487. Jaiswal S, Pearson T, Friberg H, et al. Dengue virus infection and virus-specific HLA-A2 restricted immune responses in humanized NOD-scid IL2rgammanull mice. *PLoS One* 2009;4:e7251.
488. Jarmer J, Zlatkovic J, Tsouchnikas G, et al. Variation of the specificity of the human antibody responses after tick-borne encephalitis virus infection and vaccination. *J Virol* 2014;88:13845–13857.
489. Jayaratne HE, Wijeratne D, Fernando S, et al. Regulatory T-cells in acute dengue viral infection. *Immunology* 2018;154:89–97.
490. Jelinek T, Muhlberger N, Harms G, et al Epidemiology and clinical features of imported dengue fever in Europe: sentinel surveillance data from TropNetEurop. *Clin Infect Dis* 2002;35:1047–1052.
491. Jemielity S, Wang JJ, Chan YK, et al. TIM-family proteins promote infection of multiple enveloped viruses through virion-associated phosphatidylserine. *PLoS Pathog* 2013;9: e1003232.
492. Jia XY, Briese T, Jordan I, et al. Genetic analysis of West Nile New York 1999 encephalitis virus. *Lancet* 1999;354:1971–1972.
493. Johnson JE. Virus particle dynamics. *Adv Protein Chem* 2003;64:197–218.
494. Johnson RT, Burke DS, Elwell M, et al. Japanese encephalitis: immunocytochemical studies of viral antigen and inflammatory cells in fatal cases. *Ann Neurol* 1985;18:567–573.
495. Johnson AJ, Roehrig JT. New mouse model for dengue virus vaccine testing. *J Virol* 1999;73:783–786.
496. Johnson B, VanBlargan LA, Xu W, et al. Human IFIT3 modulates IFIT1 RNA binding specificity and protein stability. *Immunity* 2018;48:487–499, e485.
497. Joncker NT, Raulet DH. Regulation of NK cell responsiveness to achieve self-tolerance and maximal responses to diseased target cells. *Immunol Rev* 2008;224:85–97.
498. Jones CT, Ma L, Burgner JW, et al. Flavivirus capsid is a dimeric alpha-helical protein. *J Virol* 2003;77:7143–7149.
499. Julander JG, Morrey JD, Blatt LM, et al. Comparison of the inhibitory effects of interferon alfacon-1 and ribavirin on yellow fever virus infection in a hamster model. *Antiviral Res* 2007;73:140–146.
500. Junjhon J, Edwards TJ, Utaipat U, et al. Influence of pr-M cleavage on the heterogeneity of extracellular dengue virus particles. *J Virol* 2010;84:8353–8358.
501. Junt T, Moseman EA, Iannacone M, et al. Subcapsular sinus macrophages in lymph nodes clear lymph-borne viruses and present them to antiviral B cells. *Nature* 2007;450:110–114.
502. Jurado KA, Yockey LJ, Wong PW, et al. Antiviral CD8 T cells induce Zika-virus-associated paralysis in mice. *Nat Microbiol* 2018;3:141–147.
503. Kaiser R. The clinical and epidemiological profile of tick-borne encephalitis in southern Germany 1994–98: a prospective study of 656 patients. *Brain* 1999;122 (Pt 11):2067–2078.
504. Kaiser R. Tick-borne encephalitis. *Infect Dis Clin North Am* 2008;22:561–575, x.
505. Kajaste-Rudnitski A, Mashimo T, Frenkiel MP, et al. The 2′,5′-oligoadenylate synthetase 1b is a potent inhibitor of West Nile virus replication inside infected cells. *J Biol Chem* 2006;281:4624–4637.
506. Kalayanarooj S, Nimmannitya S. Clinical presentations of dengue hemorrhagic fever in infants compared to children. *J Med Assoc Thai* 2003;86 Suppl 3:S673–S680.
507. Kalil AC, Devetten MP, Singh S, et al. Use of interferon-alpha in patients with West Nile encephalitis: report of 2 cases. *Clin Infect Dis* 2005;40:764–766.
508. Kangwanpong D, Bhamarapravati N, Lucia HL. Diagnosing dengue virus infection in archived autopsy tissues by means of the in situ PCR method: a case report. *Clin Diagn Virol* 1995;3:165–172.
509. Karimi O, Goorhuis A, Schinkel J, et al. Thrombocytopenia and subcutaneous bleedings in a patient with Zika virus infection. *Lancet* 2016;387:939–940.
510. Kato H, Takeuchi O, Sato S, et al. Differential roles of MDA5 and RIG-I helicases in the recognition of RNA viruses. *Nature* 2006;441:101–105.
511. Katzelnick LC, Fonville JM, Gromowski GD, et al. Dengue viruses cluster antigenically but not as discrete serotypes. *Science* 2015;349:1338–1343.
512. Katzelnick LC, Gresh L, Halloran ME, et al. Antibody-dependent enhancement of severe dengue disease in humans. *Science* 2017;358:929–932.
513. Kaufman BM, Summers PL, Dubois DR, et al. Monoclonal antibodies for dengue virus prM glycoprotein protect mice against lethal dengue infection. *Am J Trop Med Hyg* 1989;41:576–580.
514. Kaufmann B, Chipman PR, Holdaway HA, et al. Capturing a flavivirus pre-fusion intermediate. *PLoS Pathog* 2009;5:e1000672.
515. Kaufmann B, Vogt MR, Goudsmit J, et al. Neutralization of West Nile virus by cross-linking of its surface proteins with Fab fragments of the human monoclonal antibody CR4354. *Proc Natl Acad Sci U S A* 2010;107:18950–18955.
516. Keeffe JR, Van Rompay KKA, Olsen PC, et al. A combination of two human monoclonal antibodies prevents Zika virus escape mutations in non-human primates. *Cell Rep* 2018;25:1385–1394, e1387.
517. Keller BC, Fredericksen BL, Samuel MA, et al. Resistance to alpha/beta interferon is a determinant of West Nile virus replication fitness and virulence. *J Virol* 2006;80:9424–9434.
518. Keller BC, Johnson CL, Erickson AK, et al. Innate immune evasion by hepatitis C virus and West Nile virus. *Cytokine Growth Factor Rev* 2007;18:535–544.
519. Kelso JM, Mootrey GT, Tsai TF. Anaphylaxis from yellow fever vaccine. *J Allergy Clin Immunol* 1999;103:698–701.
520. Kesson AM, Blanden RV, Mullbacher A. The primary in vivo murine cytotoxic T cell response to the flavivirus, West Nile. *J Gen Virol* 1987;68:2001–2006.
521. Kesson AM, King NJ. Transcriptional regulation of major histocompatibility complex class I by flavivirus West Nile is dependent on NF-kappaB activation. *J Infect Dis* 2001;184:947–954.
522. Khozinsky VV, Semenov BF, Gresikova M, et al. Role of macrophages in the pathogenesis of experimental tick-borne encephalitis in mice. *Acta Virol* 1985;29:194–202.
523. Khromava AY, Eidex RB, Weld LH, et al. Yellow fever vaccine: an updated assessment of advanced age as a risk factor for serious adverse events. *Vaccine* 2005;23:3256–3263.
524. Khromykh AA, Westaway EG. RNA binding properties of core protein of the flavivirus Kunjin. *Arch Virol* 1996;141:685–699.
525. Killen H, O'Sullivan MA. Detection of dengue virus by in situ hybridization. *J Virol Methods* 1993;41:135–146.
526. Kilpatrick AM, Kramer LD, Jones MJ, et al. West Nile virus epidemics in North America are driven by shifts in mosquito feeding behavior. *PLoS Biol* 2006;4:e82.
527. Kim H, Cha GW, Jeong YE, et al. Detection of Japanese encephalitis virus genotype V in Culex orientalis and Culex pipiens (Diptera: Culicidae) in Korea. *PLoS One* 2015;10:e0116547.
528. Kimura T, Katoh H, Kayama H, et al. Ifit1 inhibits Japanese encephalitis virus replication through binding to 5′ capped 2′-O unmethylated RNA. *J Virol* 2013;87:9997–10003.
529. Kindberg E, Mickiene A, Ax C, et al. A deletion in the chemokine receptor 5 (CCR5) gene is associated with tickborne encephalitis. *J Infect Dis* 2008;197:266–269.
530. Kindberg E, Vene S, Mickiene A, et al. A functional Toll-like receptor 3 gene (TLR3) may be a risk factor for tick-borne encephalitis virus (TBEV) infection. *J Infect Dis* 2011;203:523–528.
531. King CA, Anderson R, Marshall JS. Dengue virus selectively induces human mast cell chemokine production. *J Virol* 2002;76:8408–8419.
532. King NJ, Kesson AM. Interferon-independent increases in class I major histocompatibility complex antigen expression follow flavivirus infection. *J Gen Virol* 1988;69:2535–2543.
533. King CA, Marshall JS, Alshurafa H, et al. Release of vasoactive cytokines by antibody-enhanced dengue virus infection of a human mast cell/basophil line. *J Virol* 2000;74:7146–7150.
534. Kirkpatrick BD, Durbin AP, Pierce KK, et al. Robust and balanced immune responses to all 4 dengue virus serotypes following administration of a single dose of a live attenuated tetravalent dengue vaccine to healthy, flavivirus-naive adults. *J Infect Dis* 2015;212:702–710.
535. Kirkpatrick BD, Whitehead SS, Pierce KK, et al. The live attenuated dengue vaccine TV003 elicits complete protection against dengue in a human challenge model. *Sci Transl Med* 2016;8:330ra336.
536. Kitchen A, Shackelton LA, Holmes EC. Family level phylogenies reveal modes of macroevolution in RNA viruses. *Proc Natl Acad Sci U S A* 2011;108:238–243.
537. Klein RS, Lin E, Zhang B, et al. Neuronal CXCL10 directs CD8+ T cell recruitment and control of West Nile virus encephalitis. *J Virol* 2005;79:11457–11466.
538. Kliks SC, Nimmanitya S, Nisalak A, et al. Evidence that maternal dengue antibodies are important in the development of dengue hemorrhagic fever in infants. *Am J Trop Med Hyg* 1988;38:411–419.
539. Kliks SC, Nisalak A, Brandt WE, et al. Antibody-dependent enhancement of dengue virus growth in human monocytes as a risk factor for dengue hemorrhagic fever. *Am J Trop Med Hyg* 1989;40:444–451.
540. Klockmann U, Bock HL, Franke V, et al. Preclinical investigations of the safety, immunogenicity and efficacy of a purified, inactivated tick-borne encephalitis vaccine. *J Biol Stand* 1989;17:331–342.
541. Klotz O, Belt TH. The pathology of the Liver in Yellow Fiver. *Am J Pathol* 1930;6: 663–688, 661.
542. Klotz O, Belt TH. The pathology of the spleen in yellow fever. *Am J Pathol* 1930;6: 655–662, 653.
543. Knox KK, Thomm AM, Harrington YA, et al. Powassan/Deer Tick Virus and Borrelia Burgdorferi infection in Wisconsin Tick populations. *Vector Borne Zoonotic Dis* 2017;17:463–466.
544. Kobiler D, Lustig S, Gozes Y, et al. Sodium dodecylsulphate induces a breach in the blood-brain barrier and enables a West Nile virus variant to penetrate into mouse brain. *Brain Res* 1989;496:314–316.
545. Kodati S, Palmore TN, Spellman FA, et al. Bilateral posterior uveitis associated with Zika virus infection. *Lancet* 2017;389:125–126.

546. Koide F, Goebel S, Snyder B, et al. Development of a Zika virus infection model in cynomolgus macaques. *Front Microbiol* 2016;7:2028.

547. Kollaritsch H, Paulke-Korinek M, Dubischar-Kastner K. IC51 Japanese encephalitis vaccine. *Expert Opin Biol Ther* 2009;9:921–931.

548. Kong KF, Delroux K, Wang X, et al. Dysregulation of TLR3 impairs the innate immune response to West Nile virus in the elderly. *J Virol* 2008;82:7613–7623.

549. Konishi E, Fujii A. Dengue type 2 virus subviral extracellular particles produced by a stably transfected mammalian cell line and their evaluation for a subunit vaccine. *Vaccine* 2002;20:1058–1067.

550. Konishi E, Pincus S, Paoletti E, et al. Mice immunized with a subviral particle containing the Japanese encephalitis virus prM/M and E proteins are protected from lethal JEV infection. *Virology* 1992;188:714–720.

551. Koraka P, Benton S, van Amerongen G, et al. Efficacy of a live attenuated tetravalent candidate dengue vaccine in naive and previously infected cynomolgus macaques. *Vaccine* 2007;25:5409–5416.

552. Kostyuchenko VA, Chew PL, Ng TS, et al. Near-atomic resolution cryo-electron microscopic structure of dengue serotype 4 virus. *J Virol* 2014;88:477–482.

553. Kostyuchenko VA, Lim EX, Zhang S, et al. Structure of the thermally stable Zika virus. *Nature* 2016;533:425–428.

554. Kostyuchenko VA, Zhang Q, Tan JL, et al. Immature and mature dengue serotype 1 virus structures provide insight into the maturation process. *J Virol* 2013;87:7700–7707.

555. Kou Z, Lim JY, Beltramello M, et al. Human antibodies against dengue enhance dengue viral infectivity without suppressing type I interferon secretion in primary human monocytes. *Virology* 2011;410:240–247.

556. Kouri GP, Guzman MG, Bravo JR, et al. Dengue haemorrhagic fever/dengue shock syndrome: lessons from the Cuban epidemic, 1981. *Bull World Health Organ* 1989;67:375–380.

557. Kraivong R, Vasanawathana S, Limpitikul W, et al. Complement alternative pathway genetic variation and Dengue infection in the Thai population. *Clin Exp Immunol* 2013;174:326–334.

558. Kramer LD, Chandler LJ. Phylogenetic analysis of the envelope gene of St. Louis encephalitis virus. *Arch Virol* 2001;146:2341–2355.

559. Kreil TR, Eibl MM. Nitric oxide and viral infection: NO antiviral activity against a flavivirus in vitro, and evidence for contribution to pathogenesis in experimental infection in vivo. *Virology* 1996;219:304–306.

560. Krishnan MN, Sukumaran B, Pal U, et al. Rab 5 is required for the cellular entry of dengue and West Nile viruses. *J Virol* 2007;81:4881–4885.

561. Kroeger MA, McMinn PC. Murray Valley encephalitis virus recombinant subviral particles protect mice from lethal challenge with virulent wild-type virus. *Arch Virol* 2002;147:1155–1172.

562. Krow-Lucal ER, Lindsey NP, Fischer M, et al. Powassan Virus Disease in the United States, 2006–2016. *Vector Borne Zoonotic Dis* 2018;18:286–290.

563. Kuhn RJ, Zhang W, Rossmann MG, et al. Structure of dengue virus: implications for flavivirus organization, maturation, and fusion. *Cell* 2002;108:717–725.

564. Kulkarni AB, Mullbacher A, Blanden RV. In vitro T-cell proliferative response to the flavivirus, west Nile. *Viral Immunol* 1991;4:73–82.

565. Kumar V. Homeostatic control of immunity by TCR peptide-specific Tregs. *J Clin Invest* 2004;114:1222–1226.

566. Kumar D, Drebot MA, Wong SJ, et al. A seroprevalence study of west nile virus infection in solid organ transplant recipients. *Am J Transplant* 2004;4:1883–1888.

567. Kumar A, Hou S, Airo AM, et al. Zika virus inhibits type-I interferon production and downstream signaling. *EMBO Rep* 2016;17:1766–1775.

568. Kumar A, Jovel J, Lopez-Orozco J, et al. Human Sertoli cells support high levels of Zika virus replication and persistence. *Sci Rep* 2018;8:5477.

569. Kumar M, Krause KK, Azouz F, et al. A guinea pig model of Zika virus infection. *Virol J* 2017;14:75.

570. Kumar D, Prasad GV, Zaltzman J, et al. Community-acquired West Nile virus infection in solid-organ transplant recipients. *Transplantation* 2004;77:399–402.

571. Kumar M, Roe K, Orillo B, et al. Inflammasome adaptor protein Apoptosis-associated speck-like protein containing CARD (ASC) is critical for the immune response and survival in west Nile virus encephalitis. *J Virol* 2013;87:3655–3667.

572. Kumar P, Sulochana P, Nirmala G, et al. Impaired T helper 1 function of nonstructural protein 3-specific T cells in Japanese patients with encephalitis with neurological sequelae. *J Infect Dis* 2004;189:880–891.

573. Kumar R, Tripathi P, Rizvi A. Effectiveness of one dose of SA 14–14–2 vaccine against Japanese encephalitis. *N Engl J Med* 2009;360:1465–1466.

574. Kundu K, Dutta K, Nazmi A, et al. Japanese encephalitis virus infection modulates the expression of suppressors of cytokine signaling (SOCS) in macrophages: implications for the hosts' innate immune response. *Cell Immunol* 2013;285:100–110.

575. Kuno G. Research on dengue and dengue-like illness in East Asia and the Western Pacific during the First Half of the 20th century. *Rev Med Virol* 2007;17:327–341.

576. Kuno G, Chang GJ. Characterization of Sepik and Entebbe bat viruses closely related to yellow fever virus. *Am J Trop Med Hyg* 2006;75:1165–1170.

577. Kuno G, Chang GJ, Tsuchiya KR, et al. Phylogeny of the genus Flavivirus. *J Virol* 1998;72:73–83.

578. Kunz C. TBE vaccination and the Austrian experience. *Vaccine* 2003;21 Suppl 1:S50–S55.

579. Kunz C, Heinz FX, Hofmann H. Immunogenicity and reactogenicity of a highly purified vaccine against tick-borne encephalitis. *J Med Virol* 1980;6:103–109.

580. Kunze U. Conference report of the 10th meeting of the international scientific working group on tick-borne encephalitis (ISW-TBE): combating tick-borne encephalitis: vaccination rates on the rise. *Vaccine* 2008;26:6738–6740.

581. Kurosu T, Chaichana P, Yamate M, et al. Secreted complement regulatory protein clusterin interacts with dengue virus nonstructural protein 1. *Biochem Biophys Res Commun* 2007;362:1051–1056.

582. Kuruvilla JG, Troyer RM, Devi S, et al. Dengue virus infection and immune response in humanized RAG2(-/-)gamma(c)(-/-) (RAG-hu) mice. *Virology* 2007;369:143–152.

583. Kwagonza L, Masiira B, Kyobe-Bosa H, et al. Outbreak of yellow fever in central and southwestern Uganda, February-may 2016. *BMC Infect Dis* 2018;18:548.

584. Kyle JL, Beatty PR, Harris E. Dengue virus infects macrophages and dendritic cells in a mouse model of infection. *J Infect Dis* 2007;195:1808–1817.

585. Kyle JL, Harris E. Global spread and persistence of dengue. *Annu Rev Microbiol* 2008;62:71–92.

586. Labuda M, Austyn JM, Zuffova E, et al. Importance of localized skin infection in tick-borne encephalitis virus transmission. *Virology* 1996;219:357–366.

587. Labuda M, Jones LD, Williams T, et al. Efficient transmission of tick-borne encephalitis virus between cofeeding ticks. *J Med Entomol* 1993;30:295–299.

588. Lai YC, Chuang YC, Liu CC, et al. Antibodies against modified NS1 wing domain peptide protect against dengue virus infection. *Sci Rep* 2017;7:6975.

589. Lai L, Rouphael N, Xu Y, et al. Innate, T-, and B-cell responses in acute human zika patients. *Clin Infect Dis* 2018;66:1–10.

590. Lai CY, Williams KL, Wu YC, et al. Analysis of cross-reactive antibodies recognizing the fusion loop of envelope protein and correlation with neutralizing antibody titers in Nicaraguan dengue cases. *PLoS Negl Trop Dis* 2013;7:e2451.

591. Lanciotti RS, Ebel GD, Deubel V, et al. Complete genome sequences and phylogenetic analysis of West Nile virus strains isolated from the United States, Europe, and the Middle East. *Virology* 2002;298:96–105.

592. Lanciotti RS, Kosoy OL, Laven JJ, et al. Genetic and serologic properties of Zika virus associated with an epidemic, Yap State, Micronesia, 2007. *Emerg Infect Dis* 2008;14:1232–1239.

593. Lang J, Zuckerman J, Clarke P, et al. Comparison of the immunogenicity and safety of two 17D yellow fever vaccines. *Am J Trop Med Hyg* 1999;60:1045–1050.

594. Lanteri MC, O'Brien KM, Purtha WE, et al. Tregs control the development of symptomatic West Nile virus infection in humans and mice. *J Clin Invest* 2009;119:3266–3277.

595. Larocca RA, Abbink P, Peron JP, et al. Vaccine protection against Zika virus from Brazil. *Nature* 2016;536:474–478.

596. Laurent-Rolle M, Boer EF, Lubick KJ, et al. The NS5 protein of the virulent West Nile virus NY99 strain is a potent antagonist of type I interferon-mediated JAK-STAT signaling. *J Virol* 2010;84:3503–3515.

597. Laurent-Rolle M, Morrison J, Rajsbaum R, et al. The interferon signaling antagonist function of yellow fever virus NS5 protein is activated by type I interferon. *Cell Host Microbe* 2014;16:314–327.

598. Lauring AS, Andino R. Quasispecies theory and the behavior of RNA viruses. *PLoS Pathog* 2010;6:e1001005.

599. Lazear HM, Daniels BP, Pinto AK, et al. Interferon-lambda restricts West Nile virus neuroinvasion by tightening the blood-brain barrier. *Sci Transl Med* 2015;7:284ra259.

600. Lazear HM, Govero J, Smith AM, et al. A mouse model of Zika virus pathogenesis. *Cell Host Microbe* 2016;19:720–730.

601. Lazear HM, Nice TJ, Diamond MS. Interferon-lambda: immune functions at barrier surfaces and beyond. *Immunity* 2015;43:15–28.

602. Lazear HM, Pinto AK, Ramos HJ, et al. Pattern recognition receptor MDA5 modulates CD8+ T cell-dependent clearance of West Nile virus from the central nervous system. *J Virol* 2013;87:11401–11415.

603. Le Bon A, Thompson C, Kamphuis E, et al. Cutting edge: enhancement of antibody responses through direct stimulation of B and T cells by type I IFN. *J Immunol* 2006;176:2074–2078.

604. Le Bon A, Tough DF. Links between innate and adaptive immunity via type I interferon. *Curr Opin Immunol* 2002;14:432–436.

605. Leal MC, Muniz LF, Ferreira TS, et al. Hearing loss in infants with microcephaly and evidence of congenital Zika virus infection - Brazil, November 2015-May 2016. *MMWR Morb Mortal Wkly Rep* 2016;65:917–919.

606. Ledgerwood JE, Pierson TC, Hubka SA, et al. A West Nile virus DNA vaccine utilizing a modified promoter induces neutralizing antibody in younger and older healthy adults in a phase I clinical trial. *J Infect Dis* 2011;203:1396–1404.

607. Ledizet M, Kar K, Foellmer HG, et al. A recombinant envelope protein vaccine against West Nile virus. *Vaccine* 2005;23:3915–3924.

608. Lee E, Hall RA, Lobigs M. Common E protein determinants for attenuation of glycosaminoglycan-binding variants of Japanese encephalitis and West Nile viruses. *J Virol* 2004;78:8271–8280.

609. Lee E, Lobigs M. Substitutions at the putative receptor-binding site of an encephalitic flavivirus alter virulence and host cell tropism and reveal a role for glycosaminoglycans in entry. *J Virol* 2000;74:8867–8875.

610. Lee E, Lobigs M. Mechanism of virulence attenuation of glycosaminoglycan-binding variants of Japanese encephalitis virus and Murray Valley encephalitis virus. *J Virol* 2002;76:4901–4911.

611. Lee PD, Mukherjee S, Edeling MA, et al. The Fc region of an antibody impacts the neutralization of West Nile viruses in different maturation states. *J Virol* 2013;87:13729–13740.

612. Lee E, Pavy M, Young N, et al. Antiviral effect of the heparan sulfate mimetic, PI-88, against dengue and encephalitic flaviviruses. *Antiviral Res* 2006;69:31–38.

613. Leis AA, Fratkin J, Stokic DS, et al. West Nile poliomyelitis. *Lancet Infect Dis* 2003;3:9–10.

614. Lewis JK, Bothner B, Smith TJ, et al. Antiviral agent blocks breathing of the common cold virus. *Proc Natl Acad Sci U S A* 1998;95:6774–6778.

615. Lewis L, Taylor HG, et al. Japanese B encephalitis; clinical observations in an outbreak on Okinawa Shima. *Arch Neurol Psychiatry* 1947;57:430–463.

616. Leyssen P, Drosten C, Paning M, et al. Interferons, interferon inducers, and interferon-ribavirin in treatment of flavivirus-induced encephalitis in mice. *Antimicrob Agents Chemother* 2003;47:777–782.

617. Leyssen P, Van Lommel A, Drosten C, et al. A novel model for the study of the therapy of flavivirus infections using the Modoc virus. *Virology* 2001;279:27–37.

618. Li C, Deng YQ, Wang S, et al. 25-Hydroxycholesterol protects host against Zika virus infection and its associated microcephaly in a mouse model. *Immunity* 2017;46:446–456.

619. Li XF, Dong HL, Huang XY, et al. Characterization of a 2016 clinical isolate of Zika virus in non-human primates. *EBioMedicine* 2016;12:170–177.

620. Li SH, Dong H, Li XF, et al. Rational design of a flavivirus vaccine by abolishing viral RNA 2′-O methylation. *J Virol* 2013;87:5812–5819.

621. Li MH, Fu SH, Chen WX, et al. Genotype v Japanese encephalitis virus is emerging. *PLoS Negl Trop Dis* 2011;5:e1231.

622. Li H, Gade P, Xiao W, et al. The interferon signaling network and transcription factor C/EBP-beta. *Cell Mol Immunol* 2007;4:407–418.
623. Li L, Lok SM, Yu IM, et al. The flavivirus precursor membrane-envelope protein complex: structure and maturation. *Science* 2008;319:1830–1834.
624. Li GH, Ning ZJ, Liu YM, et al. Neurological manifestations of dengue infection. *Front Cell Infect Microbiol* 2017;7:449.
625. Li H, Saucedo-Cuevas L, Regla-Nava JA, et al. Zika virus infects neural progenitors in the adult mouse brain and alters proliferation. *Cell Stem Cell* 2016;19:593–598.
626. Li F, Wang PR, Qu LB, et al. AXL is not essential for Zika virus infection in the mouse brain. *Emerg Microbes Infect* 2017;6:e16.
627. Li Q, Yafal AG, Lee YM, et al. Poliovirus neutralization by antibodies to internal epitopes of VP4 and VP1 results from reversible exposure of these sequences at physiological temperature. *J Virol* 1994;68:3965–3970.
628. Li A, Yu J, Lu M, et al. A Zika virus vaccine expressing premembrane-envelope-NS1 polyprotein. *Nat Commun* 2018;9:3067.
629. Libraty DH, Endy TP, Houng HS, et al. Differing influences of virus burden and immune activation on disease severity in secondary dengue-3 virus infections. *J Infect Dis* 2002;185:1213–1221.
630. Libraty DH, Pichyangkul S, Ajariyakhajorn C, et al. Human dendritic cells are activated by dengue virus infection: enhancement by gamma interferon and implications for disease pathogenesis. *J Virol* 2001;75:3501–3508.
631. Libraty DH, Young PR, Pickering D, et al. High circulating levels of the dengue virus nonstructural protein NS1 early in dengue illness correlate with the development of dengue hemorrhagic fever. *J Infect Dis* 2002;186:1165–1168.
632. Licon Luna RM, Lee E, Mullbacher A, et al. Lack of both Fas ligand and perforin protects from flavivirus-mediated encephalitis in mice. *J Virol* 2002;76:3202–3211.
633. Lidbury BA, Mahalingam S. Specific ablation of antiviral gene expression in macrophages by antibody-dependent enhancement of Ross River virus infection. *J Virol* 2000;74:8376–8381.
634. Likos A, Griffin I, Bingham AM, et al. Local mosquito-borne transmission of Zika virus - Miami-Dade and Broward Counties, Florida, June-August 2016. *MMWR Morb Mortal Wkly Rep* 2016;65:1032–1038.
635. Lim PY, Behr MJ, Chadwick CM, et al. Keratinocytes are cell targets of West Nile virus in vivo. *J Virol* 2011;85(10):5197–5201. doi: JVI.02692–10 [pii]10.1128/JVI.02692–10.
636. Lim XX, Chandramohan A, Lim XY, et al. Conformational changes in intact dengue virus reveal serotype-specific expansion. *Nat Commun* 2017;8:14339.
637. Lim XX, Chandramohan A, Lim XE, et al. Epitope and paratope mapping reveals temperature-dependent alterations in the dengue-antibody interface. *Structure* 2017;25:1391–1402, e1393.
638. Lim MQ, Kumaran EAP, Tan HC, et al. Cross-reactivity and anti-viral function of dengue capsid and NS3-specific memory T cells toward Zika virus. *Front Immunol* 2018;9:2225.
639. Lim JK, Lisco A, McDermott DH, et al. Genetic variation in OAS1 is a risk factor for initial infection with West Nile virus in man. *PLoS Pathog* 2009;5:e1000321.
640. Lim JK, Louie CY, Glaser C, et al. Genetic deficiency of chemokine receptor CCR5 is a strong risk factor for symptomatic West Nile virus infection: a meta-analysis of 4 cohorts in the US epidemic. *J Infect Dis* 2008;197:262–265.
641. Lim JK, McDermott DH, Lisco A, et al. CCR5 deficiency is a risk factor for early clinical manifestations of West Nile virus infection but not for viral transmission. *J Infect Dis* 2010;201:178–185.
642. Lim JK, Obara CJ, Rivollier A, et al. Chemokine receptor Ccr2 is critical for monocyte accumulation and survival in West Nile virus encephalitis. *J Immunol* 2011;186:471–478.
643. Lim DS, Yawata N, Selva KJ, et al. The combination of type I IFN, TNF-alpha, and cell surface receptor engagement with dendritic cells enables NK cells to overcome immune evasion by dengue virus. *J Immunol* 2014;193:5065–5075.
644. Lin RJ, Chang BL, Yu HP, et al. Blocking of interferon-induced Jak-Stat signaling by Japanese encephalitis virus NS5 through a protein tyrosine phosphatase-mediated mechanism. *J Virol* 2006;80:5908–5918.
645. Lin CW, Cheng CW, Yang TC, et al. Interferon antagonist function of Japanese encephalitis virus NS4A and its interaction with DEAD-box RNA helicase DDX42. *Virus Res* 2008;137:49–55.
646. Lin YL, Huang YL, Ma SH, et al. Inhibition of Japanese encephalitis virus infection by nitric oxide: antiviral effect of nitric oxide on RNA virus replication. *J Virol* 1997;71:5227–5235.
647. Lin YL, Lei HY, Lin YS, et al. Heparin inhibits dengue-2 virus infection of five human liver cell lines. *Antiviral Res* 2002;56:93–96.
648. Lin YL, Liao CL, Chen LK, et al. Study of Dengue virus infection in SCID mice engrafted with human K562 cells. *J Virol* 1998;72:9729–9737.
649. Lin RJ, Liao CL, Lin E, et al. Blocking of the alpha interferon-induced Jak-Stat signaling pathway by Japanese Encephalitis Virus. *J Virol* 2004;78:9285–9294.
650. Lin HE, Tsai WY, Liu IJ, et al. Analysis of epitopes on dengue virus envelope protein recognized by monoclonal antibodies and polyclonal human sera by a high throughput assay. *PLoS Negl Trop Dis* 2012;6:e1447.
651. Lin RJ, Yu HP, Chang BL, et al. Distinct antiviral roles for human 2′,5′-oligoadenylate synthetase family members against dengue virus infection. *J Immunol* 2009;183:8035–8043.
652. Lindqvist R, Overby AK. The Role of Viperin in Antiflavivirus Responses. *DNA Cell Biol* 2018;37:725–730.
653. Lindsey NP, Schroeder BA, Miller ER, et al. Adverse event reports following yellow fever vaccination. *Vaccine* 2008;26:6077–6082.
654. Liou ML, Hsu CY. Japanese encephalitis virus is transported across the cerebral blood vessels by endocytosis in mouse brain. *Cell Tissue Res* 1998;293:389–394.
655. Liu T, Chambers TJ. Yellow fever virus encephalitis: properties of the brain-associated T-cell response during virus clearance in normal and gamma interferon- deficient mice and requirement for CD4+ lymphocytes. *J Virol* 2001;75:2107–2118.
656. Liu WJ, Chen HB, Wang XJ, et al. Analysis of adaptive mutations in kunjin virus replicon RNA reveals a novel role for the flavivirus nonstructural protein NS2A in inhibition of beta interferon promoter-driven transcription. *J Virol* 2004;78:12225–12235.
657. Liu Y, King N, Kesson A, et al. West Nile virus infection modulates the expression of class I and class II MHC antigens on astrocytes in vitro. *Ann N Y Acad Sci* 1988;540:483–485.
658. Liu Y, King N, Kesson A, et al. Flavivirus infection up-regulates the expression of class I and class II major histocompatibility antigens on and enhances T cell recognition of astrocytes in vitro. *J Neuroimmunol* 1989;21:157–168.
659. Liu Y, Liu J, Du S, et al. Evolutionary enhancement of Zika virus infectivity in Aedes aegypti mosquitoes. *Nature* 2017;545:482–486.
660. Liu WJ, Wang XJ, Clark DC, et al. A single amino acid substitution in the West Nile virus nonstructural protein NS2A disables its ability to inhibit alpha/beta interferon induction and attenuates virus virulence in mice. *J Virol* 2006;80:2396–2404.
661. Liu WJ, Wang XJ, Mokhonov VV, et al. Inhibition of interferon signaling by the New York 99 strain and Kunjin subtype of West Nile virus involves blockage of STAT1 and STAT2 activation by nonstructural proteins. *J Virol* 2005;79:1934–1942.
662. Lloyd W. The myocardium in yellow fever. II. The myocardial lesions in experimental yellow fever. *Am Heart J* 1931;6:504.
663. Lobigs M, Mullbacher A, Wang Y, et al. Role of type I and type II interferon responses in recovery from infection with an encephalitic flavivirus. *J Gen Virol* 2003;84:567–572.
664. Lok SM, Kostyuchenko V, Nybakken GE, et al. Binding of a neutralizing antibody to dengue virus alters the arrangement of surface glycoproteins. *Nat Struct Mol Biol* 2008;15:312–317.
665. Long MT, Gibbs EP, Mellencamp MW, et al. Efficacy, duration, and onset of immunogenicity of a West Nile virus vaccine, live Flavivirus chimera, in horses with a clinical disease challenge model. *Equine Vet J* 2007;39:491–497.
666. Long MT, Gibbs EP, Mellencamp MW, et al. Safety of an attenuated West Nile virus vaccine, live Flavivirus chimera in horses. *Equine Vet J* 2007;39:486–490.
667. Loo YM, Fornek J, Crochet N, et al Distinct RIG-I and MDA5 signaling by RNA viruses in innate immunity. *J Virol* 2008;82:335–345.
668. Lorenz IC, Allison SL, Heinz FX, et al. Folding and dimerization of tick-borne encephalitis virus envelope proteins prM and E in the endoplasmic reticulum. *J Virol* 2002;76:5480–5491.
669. Lorenz IC, Kartenbeck J, Mezzacasa A, et al. Intracellular assembly and secretion of recombinant subviral particles from tick-borne encephalitis virus. *J Virol* 2003;77:4370–4382.
670. Lozach PY, Burleigh L, Staropoli I, et al. Dendritic cell-specific intercellular adhesion molecule 3-grabbing non-integrin (DC-SIGN)-mediated enhancement of dengue virus infection is independent of DC-SIGN internalization signals. *J Biol Chem* 2005;280:23698–23708.
671. Lozier MJ, Burke RM, Lopez J, et al. Differences in prevalence of symptomatic Zika virus infection, by age and sex—Puerto Rico, 2016. *J Infect Dis* 2018;217:1678–1689.
672. Lubick KJ, Robertson SJ, McNally KL, et al. Flavivirus antagonism of type I interferon signaling reveals prolidase as a regulator of IFNAR1 surface expression. *Cell Host Microbe* 2015;18:61–74.
673. Luby JP. Sensitivities of neurotropic arboviruses to human interferon. *J Infect Dis* 1975;132:361–367.
674. Lucas CGO, Kitoko JZ, Ferreira FM, et al. Critical role of CD4(+) T cells and IFNgamma signaling in antibody-mediated resistance to Zika virus infection. *Nat Commun* 2018;9:3136.
675. Lucas TM, Richner JM, Diamond MS. The interferon-stimulated gene Ifi27l2a restricts West Nile virus infection and pathogenesis in a cell-type- and region-specific manner. *J Virol* 2015;90:2600–2615.
676. Luhn K, Simmons CP, Moran E, et al. Increased frequencies of CD4+ CD25(high) regulatory T cells in acute dengue infection. *J Exp Med* 2007;204:979–985.
677. Lum LC, Lam SK, Choy YS, et al. Dengue encephalitis: a true entity? *Am J Trop Med Hyg* 1996;54:256–259.
678. Lum FM, Low DK, Fan Y, et al. Zika Virus infects human fetal brain microglia and induces inflammation. *Clin Infect Dis* 2017;64:914–920.
679. Lumsden LL. St. Louis encephalitis in 1933; observations on epidemiological features. *Public Health Rep* 1958;73:340–353.
680. Lustig S, Danenberg HD, Kafri Y, et al. Viral neuroinvasion and encephalitis induced by lipopolysaccharide and its mediators. *J Exp Med* 1992;176:707–712.
681. Lvov DK, Butenko AM, Gromashevsky VL, et al. West Nile virus and other zoonotic viruses in Russia: examples of emerging-reemerging situations. *Arch Virol Suppl* 2004;(18):85–96.
682. Ma D, Jiang D, Qing M, et al. Antiviral effect of interferon lambda against West Nile virus. *Antiviral Res* 2009;83:53–60.
683. Ma L, Jones CT, Groesch TD, et al. Solution structure of dengue virus capsid protein reveals another fold. *Proc Natl Acad Sci U S A* 2004;101:3414–3419.
684. Ma W, Li S, Ma S, et al. Zika virus causes testis damage and leads to male infertility in mice. *Cell* 2016;167:1511–1524, e1510.
685. Mackenzie JS, Gubler DJ, Petersen LR. Emerging flaviviruses: the spread and resurgence of Japanese encephalitis, West Nile and dengue viruses. *Nat Med* 2004;10:S98–S109.
686. Mackenzie JM, Khromykh AA, Parton RG. Cholesterol manipulation by West Nile virus perturbs the cellular immune response. *Cell Host Microbe* 2007;2:229–239.
687. Magnani DM, Rogers TF, Maness NJ, et al. Fetal demise and failed antibody therapy during Zika virus infection of pregnant macaques. *Nat Commun* 2018;9:1624.
688. Mahalingam S, Lidbury BA. Suppression of lipopolysaccharide-induced antiviral transcription factor (STAT-1 and NF-kappa B) complexes by antibody-dependent enhancement of macrophage infection by Ross River virus. *Proc Natl Acad Sci U S A* 2002;99:13819–13824.
689. Malasit P. Complement and dengue haemorrhagic fever/shock syndrome. *Southeast Asian J Trop Med Public Health* 1987;18:316–320.
690. Malathi K, Dong B, Gale M Jr, et al. Small self-RNA generated by RNase L amplifies antiviral innate immunity. *Nature* 2007;448:816–819.
691. Malathi K, Saito T, Crochet N, et al. RNase L releases a small RNA from HCV RNA that refolds into a potent PAMP. *RNA* 2010;16:2108–2119.
692. Malaviya R, Ikeda T, Ross E, et al. Mast cell modulation of neutrophil influx and bacterial clearance at sites of infection through TNF-alpha. *Nature* 1996;381:77–80.
693. Manangeeswaran M, Ireland DD, Verthelyi D. Zika (PRVABC59) infection is associated with T cell infiltration and neurodegeneration in CNS of immunocompetent neonatal C57Bl/6 mice. *PLoS Pathog* 2016;12:e1006004.
694. Mandl CW, Kroschewski H, Allison SL, et al. Adaptation of tick-borne encephalitis virus to BHK-21 cells results in the formation of multiple heparan sulfate binding sites in the envelope protein and attenuation in vivo. *J Virol* 2001;75:5627–5637.

695. Mangada MM, Endy TP, Nisalak A, et al. Dengue-specific T cell responses in peripheral blood mononuclear cells obtained prior to secondary dengue virus infections in Thai schoolchildren. *J Infect Dis* 2002;185:1697–1703.
696. Manokaran G, Finol E, Wang C, et al. Dengue subgenomic RNA binds TRIM25 to inhibit interferon expression for epidemiological fitness. *Science* 2015;350:217–221.
697. Mansfield KL, Johnson N, Cosby SL, et al. Transcriptional upregulation of SOCS 1 and suppressors of cytokine signaling 3 mRNA in the absence of suppressors of cytokine signaling 2 mRNA after infection with West Nile virus or tick-borne encephalitis virus. *Vector Borne Zoonotic Dis* 2010;10:649–653.
698. Mansfield KL, Johnson N, Phipps LP, et al. Tick-borne encephalitis virus—a review of an emerging zoonosis. *J Gen Virol* 2009;90:1781–1794.
699. Marchette NJ, Halstead SB, Falkler WA Jr, et al. Studies on the pathogenesis of dengue infection in monkeys. 3. Sequential distribution of virus in primary and heterologous infections. *J Infect Dis* 1973;128:23–30.
700. Marianneau P, Steffan AM, Royer C, et al. Infection of primary cultures of human Kupffer cells by dengue virus: no viral progeny synthesis, but cytokine production is evident. *J Virol* 1999;73:5201–5206.
701. Marin MS, Zanotto PM, Gritsun TS, et al. Phylogeny of TYU, SRE, and CFA virus: different evolutionary rates in the genus Flavivirus. *Virology* 1995;206:1133–1139.
702. Markoff L, Falgout B, Chang A. A conserved internal hydrophobic domain mediates the stable membrane integration of the dengue virus capsid protein. *Virology* 1997;233:105–117.
703. Marovich M, Grouard-Vogel G, Louder M, et al. Human dendritic cells as targets of dengue virus infection. *J Investig Dermatol Symp Proc* 2001;6:219–224.
704. Martin JE, Pierson TC, Hubka S, et al. A West Nile virus DNA vaccine induces neutralizing antibody in healthy adults during a phase 1 clinical trial. *J Infect Dis* 2007;196:1732–1740.
705. Martina BE, Koraka P, Osterhaus AD. Dengue virus pathogenesis: an integrated view. *Clin Microbiol Rev* 2009;22:564–581.
706. Martines RB, Bhatnagar J, de Oliveira Ramos AM, et al. Pathology of congenital Zika syndrome in Brazil: a case series. *Lancet* 2016;388:898–904.
707. Martinon F, Burns K, Tschopp J. The inflammasome: a molecular platform triggering activation of inflammatory caspases and processing of proIL-beta. *Mol Cell* 2002;10:417–426.
708. Martinot AJ, Abbink P, Afacan O, et al. Fetal Neuropathology in Zika virus-infected pregnant female Rhesus Monkeys. *Cell* 2018;173:1111–1122, e1110.
709. Mashimo T, Lucas M, Simon-Chazottes D, et al. A nonsense mutation in the gene encoding 2′-5′-oligoadenylate synthetase/L1 isoform is associated with West Nile virus susceptibility in laboratory mice. *Proc Natl Acad Sci U S A* 2002;99:11311–11316.
710. Mason PW, Pincus S, Fournier MJ, et al. Japanese encephalitis virus-vaccinia recombinants produce particulate forms of the structural membrane proteins and induce high levels of protection against lethal JEV infection. *Virology* 1991;180:294–305.
711. Mason RA, Tauraso NM, Spertzel RO, et al. Yellow fever vaccine: direct challenge of monkeys given graded doses of 17D vaccine. *Appl Microbiol* 1973;25:539–544.
712. Mateo R, Nagamine CM, Kirkegaard K. Suppression of drug resistance in dengue virus. *MBio* 2015;6:e01960–01915.
713. Mathew A, Rothman AL. Understanding the contribution of cellular immunity to dengue disease pathogenesis. *Immunol Rev* 2008;225:300–313.
714. Matsumoto M, Funami K, Oshiumi H, et al. Toll-like receptor 3: a link between toll-like receptor, interferon and viruses. *Microbiol Immunol* 2004;48:147–154.
715. Matsuzaki G, Yamada H, Kishihara K, et al. Mechanism of murine Vgamma1+ gamma delta T cell-mediated innate immune response against Listeria monocytogenes infection. *Eur J Immunol* 2002;32:928–935.
716. Matusali G, Houzet L, Satie AP, et al. Zika virus infects human testicular tissue and germ cells. *J Clin Invest* 2018;128:4697–4710.
717. May FJ, Li L, Zhang S, et al. Genetic variation of St. Louis encephalitis virus. *J Gen Virol* 2008;89:1901–1910.
718. Mazzon M, Jones M, Davidson A, et al. Dengue virus NS5 inhibits interferon-alpha signaling by blocking signal transducer and activator of transcription 2 phosphorylation. *J Infect Dis* 2009;200:1261–1270.
719. Mc LD, Donohue WL. Powassan virus: isolation of virus from a fatal case of encephalitis. *Can Med Assoc J* 1959;80:708–711.
720. McArthur MA, Suderman MT, Mutebi JP, et al. Molecular characterization of a hamster viscerotropic strain of yellow fever virus. *J Virol* 2003;77:1462–1468.
721. McCandless EE, Zhang B, Diamond MS, et al. CXCR4 antagonism increases T cell trafficking in the central nervous system and improves survival from West Nile virus encephalitis. *Proc Natl Acad Sci U S A* 2008;105:11270–11275.
722. McCrae AW, Kirya BG. Yellow fever and Zika virus epizootics and enzootics in Uganda. *Trans R Soc Trop Med Hyg* 1982;76:552–562.
723. McDonald EM, Duggal NK, Ritter JM, et al. Infection of epididymal epithelial cells and leukocytes drives seminal shedding of Zika virus in a mouse model. *PLoS Negl Trop Dis* 2018;12:e0006691.
724. McMinn PC. The molecular basis of virulence of the encephalitogenic flaviviruses. *J Gen Virol* 1997;78(Pt 11):2711–2722.
725. McMinn PC, Dalgarno L, Weir RC. A comparison of the spread of Murray Valley encephalitis viruses of high or low neuroinvasiveness in the tissues of Swiss mice after peripheral inoculation. *Virology* 1996;220:414–423.
726. Mead PS, Duggal NK, Hook SA, et al. Zika virus shedding in semen of symptomatic infected men. *N Engl J Med* 2018;378:1377–1385.
727. Meaney-Delman D, Oduyebo T, Polen KN, et al. Prolonged detection of Zika virus RNA in pregnant women. *Obstet Gynecol* 2016;128:724–730.
728. Meehan PJ, Wells DL, Paul W, et al. Epidemiological features of and public health response to a St. Louis encephalitis epidemic in Florida, 1990–1. *Epidemiol Infect* 2000;125:181–188.
729. Meertens L, Carnec X, Lecoin MP, et al. The TIM and TAM families of phosphatidylserine receptors mediate dengue virus entry. *Cell Host Microbe* 2012;12:544–557.
730. Meertens L, Labeau A, Dejarnac O, et al. Axl mediates ZIKA virus entry in human glial cells and modulates innate immune responses. *Cell Rep* 2017;18:324–333.
731. Mehlhop E, Ansarah-Sobrinho C, Johnson S, et al. Complement protein C1q inhibits antibody-dependent enhancement of flavivirus infection in an IgG subclass-specific manner. *Cell Host Microbe* 2007;2:417–426.
732. Mehlhop E, Diamond MS. Protective immune responses against West Nile virus are primed by distinct complement activation pathways. *J Exp Med* 2006;203:1371–1381.
733. Mehlhop E, Nelson S, Jost CA, et al. Complement protein C1q reduces the stoichiometric threshold for antibody-mediated neutralization of West Nile virus. *Cell Host Microbe* 2009;6:381–391.
734. Mehlhop E, Whitby K, Oliphant T, et al. Complement activation is required for the induction of a protective antibody response against West Nile virus infection. *J Virol* 2005;79:7466–7477.
735. Meier KC, Gardner CL, Khoretonenko MV, et al. A mouse model for studying viscerotropic disease caused by yellow fever virus infection. *PLoS Pathog* 2009;5:e1000614.
736. Melnick JL, Paul JR, Riordan JT, et al. Isolation from human sera in Egypt of a virus apparently identical to West Nile virus. *Proc Soc Exp Biol Med* 1951;77:661–665.
737. Men R, Bray M, Clark D, et al. Dengue type 4 virus mutants containing deletions in the 3′ noncoding region of the RNA genome: analysis of growth restriction in cell culture and altered viremia pattern and immunogenicity in rhesus monkeys. *J Virol* 1996;70:3930–3937.
738. Merino-Ramos T, Blazquez AB, Escribano-Romero E, et al. Protection of a single dose west nile virus recombinant subviral particle vaccine against lineage 1 or 2 strains and analysis of the cross-reactivity with Usutu virus. *PLoS One* 2014;9:e108056.
739. Merle H, Najioullah F, Chassery M, et al. Zika-related bilateral hypertensive anterior acute uveitis. *JAMA Ophthalmol* 2017;135:284–285.
740. Messer WB, Vitarana UT, Sivananthan K, et al. Epidemiology of dengue in Sri Lanka before and after the emergence of epidemic dengue hemorrhagic fever. *Am J Trop Med Hyg* 2002;66:765–773.
741. Metsky HC, Matranga CB, Wohl S, et al. Zika virus evolution and spread in the Americas. *Nature* 2017;546:411–415.
742. Metz SW, Gallichotte EN, Brackbill A, et al. In vitro assembly and stabilization of dengue and Zika virus envelope protein homo-dimers. *Sci Rep* 2017;7:4524.
743. Meurs EF, Watanabe Y, Kadereit S, et al. Constitutive expression of human double-stranded RNA-activated p68 kinase in murine cells mediates phosphorylation of eukaryotic initiation factor 2 and partial resistance to encephalomyocarditis virus growth. *J Virol* 1992;66:5804–5814.
744. Miagostovich MP, Ramos RG, Nicol AF, et al. Retrospective study on dengue fatal cases. *Clin Neuropathol* 1997;16:204–208.
745. Michlmayr D, Andrade P, Gonzalez K, et al. CD14(+)CD16(+) monocytes are the main target of Zika virus infection in peripheral blood mononuclear cells in a paediatric study in Nicaragua. *Nat Microbiol* 2017;2:1462–1470.
746. Mickiene A, Laiskonis A, Gunther G, et al. Tickborne encephalitis in an area of high endemicity in Lithuania: disease severity and long-term prognosis. *Clin Infect Dis* 2002;35:650–658.
747. Miller JL, de Wet BJ, Martinez-Pomares L, et al. The mannose receptor mediates dengue virus infection of macrophages. *PLoS Pathog* 2008;4:e17.
748. Miller LJ, Nasar F, Schellhase CW, et al. Zika virus infection in Syrian Golden Hamsters and Strain 13 Guinea Pigs. *Am J Trop Med Hyg* 2018;98:864–867.
749. Miller JD, van der Most RG, Akondy RS, et al. Human effector and memory CD8+ T cell responses to smallpox and yellow fever vaccines. *Immunity* 2008;28:710–722.
750. Miner JJ, Cao B, Govero J, et al. Zika virus infection during pregnancy in mice causes placental damage and fetal demise. *Cell* 2016;165:1081–1091.
751. Miner JJ, Daniels BP, Shrestha B, et al. The TAM receptor Mertk protects against neuroinvasive viral infection by maintaining blood-brain barrier integrity. *Nat Med* 2015;21:1464–1472.
752. Miner JJ, Sene A, Richner JM, et al. Zika virus infection in mice causes panuveitis with shedding of virus in tears. *Cell Rep* 2016;16:3208–3218.
753. Miorin L, Maestre AM, Fernandez-Sesma A, et al. Antagonism of type I interferon by flaviviruses. *Biochem Biophys Res Commun* 2017;492:587–596.
754. Mitchell PK, Mier YT-RL, Biggerstaff BJ, et al. Reassessing serosurvey-based estimates of the symptomatic proportion of Zika virus infections. *Am J Epidemiol* 2019;188:206–213.
755. Mlakar J, Korva M, Tul N, et al. Zika virus associated with microcephaly. *N Engl J Med* 2016;374:951–958.
756. Modhiran N, Watterson D, Blumenthal A, et al. Dengue virus NS1 protein activates immune cells via TLR4 but not TLR2 or TLR6. *Immunol Cell Biol* 2017;95:491–495.
757. Modhiran N, Watterson D, Muller DA, et al. Dengue virus NS1 protein activates cells via Toll-like receptor 4 and disrupts endothelial cell monolayer integrity. *Sci Transl Med* 2015;7:304ra142.
758. Modis Y, Ogata S, Clements D, et al. Structure of the dengue virus envelope protein after membrane fusion. *Nature* 2004;427:313–319.
759. Modjarrad K, Lin L, George SL, et al. Preliminary aggregate safety and immunogenicity results from three trials of a purified inactivated Zika virus vaccine candidate: phase 1, randomised, double-blind, placebo-controlled clinical trials. *Lancet* 2018;391:563–571.
760. Mohammed MA, Galbraith SE, Radford AD, et al. Molecular phylogenetic and evolutionary analyses of Muar strain of Japanese encephalitis virus reveal it is the missing fifth genotype. *Infect Genet Evol* 2011;11:855–862.
761. Mohr EL, Block LN, Newman CM, et al. Ocular and uteroplacental pathology in a macaque pregnancy with congenital Zika virus infection. *PLoS One* 2018;13:e0190617.
762. Momburg F, Mullbacher A, Lobigs M. Modulation of transporter associated with antigen processing (TAP)-mediated peptide import into the endoplasmic reticulum by flavivirus infection. *J Virol* 2001;75:5663–5671.
763. Monath TP. Epidemiology. In: Monath TP, ed. *St Louis Encephalitis*. Washington DC: American Public Health Association; 1980:239–312.
764. Monath TP. Yellow fever: Victor, Victoria? Conqueror, conquest? Epidemics and research in the last forty years and prospects for the future. *Am J Trop Med Hyg* 1991;45:1–43.
765. Monath TP. Dengue: the risk to developed and developing countries. *Proc Natl Acad Sci U S A* 1994;91:2395–2400.
766. Monath TP. Yellow fever vaccine. *Expert Rev Vaccines* 2005;4:553–574.
767. Monath TP. Treatment of yellow fever. *Antiviral Res* 2008;78:116–124.
768. Monath TP, Barrett AD. Pathogenesis and pathophysiology of yellow fever. *Adv Virus Res* 2003;60:343–395.
769. Monath TP, Brinker KR, Chandler FW, et al. Pathophysiologic correlations in a rhesus monkey model of yellow fever with special observations on the acute necrosis of B cell areas of lymphoid tissues. *Am J Trop Med Hyg* 1981;30:431–443.
770. Monath TP, Cetron MS, Teuwen DE. Yellow fever vaccine. In: Plotkin SA, Orenstein WA, Offit PA, eds. *Vaccines*, 5th ed. Philadelphia Saunders Elsevier; 2008:959–1055.

771. Monath TP, Craven RB, Adjukiewicz A, et al. Yellow fever in the Gambia, 1978–1979: epidemiologic aspects with observations on the occurrence of orungo virus infections. *Am J Trop Med Hyg* 1980;29:912–928.
772. Monath TP, Cropp CB, Bowen GS, et al. Variation in virulence for mice and rhesus monkeys among St. Louis encephalitis virus strains of different origin. *Am J Trop Med Hyg* 1980;29:948–962.
773. Monath TP, Liu J, Kanesa-Thasan N, et al. A live, attenuated recombinant West Nile virus vaccine. *Proc Natl Acad Sci U S A* 2006;103:6694–6699.
774. Monath TP, Nichols R, Archambault WT, et al. Comparative safety and immunogenicity of two yellow fever 17D vaccines (ARILVAX and YF-VAX) in a phase III multicenter, double-blind clinical trial. *Am J Trop Med Hyg* 2002;66:533–541.
775. Monath TP, Soike K, Levenbook I, et al. Recombinant, chimaeric live, attenuated vaccine (ChimeriVax) incorporating the envelope genes of Japanese encephalitis (SA14–14–2) virus and the capsid and nonstructural genes of yellow fever (17D) virus is safe, immunogenic and protective in non-human primates. *Vaccine* 1999;17:1869–1882.
776. Monel B, Compton AA, Bruel T, et al. Zika virus induces massive cytoplasmic vacuolization and paraptosis-like death in infected cells. *EMBO J* 2017;36:1653–1668.
777. Mongkolsapaya J, Dejnirattisai W, Xu XN, et al. Original antigenic sin and apoptosis in the pathogenesis of dengue hemorrhagic fever. *Nat Med* 2003;9:921–927.
778. Mongkolsapaya J, Duangchinda T, Dejnirattisai W, et al. T cell responses in dengue hemorrhagic fever: are cross-reactive T cells suboptimal? *J Immunol* 2006;176:3821–3829.
779. Montoya M, Collins M, Dejnirattisai W, et al. Longitudinal analysis of antibody cross-neutralization following Zika virus and dengue virus infection in Asia and the Americas. *J Infect Dis* 2018;218:536–545.
780. Moreira J, Peixoto TM, Siqueira AM, et al. Sexually acquired Zika virus: a systematic review. *Clin Microbiol Infect* 2017;23:296–305.
781. Moreno ES, Agostini I, Holzmann I, et al. Yellow fever impact on brown howler monkeys (Alouatta guariba clamitans) in Argentina: a metamodelling approach based on population viability analysis and epidemiological dynamics. *Mem Inst Oswaldo Cruz* 2015;110:865–876.
782. Morrey JD, Day CW, Julander JG, et al. Effect of interferon-alpha and interferon-inducers on West Nile virus in mouse and hamster animal models. *Antivir Chem Chemother* 2004;15:101–109.
783. Morrey JD, Siddharthan V, Olsen AL, et al. Humanized monoclonal antibody against West Nile virus E protein administered after neuronal infection protects against lethal encephalitis in hamsters. *J Infect Dis* 2006;194:1300–1308.
784. Morrey JD, Siddharthan V, Olsen AL, et al. Defining limits of treatment with humanized neutralizing monoclonal antibody for West Nile virus neurological infection in a hamster model. *Antimicrob Agents Chemother* 2007;51:2396–2402.
785. Morrey JD, Siddharthan V, Wang H, et al. Neurological suppression of diaphragm electromyographs in hamsters infected with West Nile virus. *J Neurovirol* 2010;16:318–329.
786. Morrey JD, Siddharthan V, Wang H, et al. West Nile virus-induced acute flaccid paralysis is prevented by monoclonal antibody treatment when administered after infection of spinal cord neurons. *J Neurovirol* 2008;14:152–163.
787. Morrey JD, Taro BS, Siddharthan V, et al. Efficacy of orally administered T-705 pyrazine analog on lethal West Nile virus infection in rodents. *Antiviral Res* 2008;80:377–379.
788. Morrison TE, Diamond MS. Animal models of Zika virus infection, pathogenesis, and immunity. *J Virol* 2017;91.
789. Morrison J, Laurent-Rolle M, Maestre AM, et al. Dengue virus co-opts UBR4 to degrade STAT2 and antagonize type I interferon signaling. *PLoS Pathog* 2013;9:e1003265.
790. Morrison J, Rathore APS, Mantri CK, et al. Transcriptional profiling confirms the therapeutic effects of mast cell stabilization in a dengue disease model. *J Virol* 2017;91.
791. Mosser DM, Edwards JP. Exploring the full spectrum of macrophage activation. *Nat Rev Immunol* 2008;8:958–969.
792. Mostashari F, Bunning ML, Kitsutani PT, et al. Epidemic West Nile encephalitis, New York, 1999: results of a household-based seroepidemiological survey. *Lancet* 2001;358:261–264.
793. Mota J, Rico-Hesse R. Humanized mice show clinical signs of dengue fever according to infecting virus genotype. *J Virol* 2009;83:8638–8645.
794. Moura da Silva AA, Ganz JS, Sousa PD, et al. Early growth and neurologic outcomes of infants with probable congenital zika virus syndrome. *Emerg Infect Dis* 2016;22:1953–1956.
795. Moureau G, Cook S, Lemey P, et al. New insights into flavivirus evolution, taxonomy and biogeographic history, extended by analysis of canonical and alternative coding sequences. *PLoS One* 2015;10:e0117849.
796. Mukherjee S, Dowd KA, Manhart CJ, et al. Mechanism and significance of cell type-dependent neutralization of flaviviruses. *J Virol* 2014;88:7210–7220.
797. Mukhopadhyay S, Kuhn RJ, Rossmann MG. A structural perspective of the flavivirus life cycle. *Nat Rev Microbiol* 2005;3:13–22.
798. Mullbacher A, Lobigs M. Up-regulation of MHC class I by flavivirus-induced peptide translocation into the endoplasmic reticulum. *Immunity* 1995;3:207–214.
799. Munoz-Jordan JL, Laurent-Rolle M, Ashour J, et al. Inhibition of alpha/beta interferon signaling by the NS4B protein of flaviviruses. *J Virol* 2005;79:8004–8013.
800. Munoz-Jordan JL, Sanchez-Burgos GG, Laurent-Rolle M, et al. Inhibition of interferon signaling by dengue virus. *Proc Natl Acad Sci U S A* 2003;100:14333–14338.
801. Munro JB, Gorman J, Ma X, et al. Conformational dynamics of single HIV-1 envelope trimers on the surface of native virions. *Science* 2014;346:759–763.
802. Murali-Krishna K, Ravi V, Manjunath R. Cytotoxic T lymphocytes raised against Japanese encephalitis virus: effector cell phenotype, target specificity and in vitro virus clearance. *J Gen Virol* 1994;75:799–807.
803. Murali-Krishna K, Ravi V, Manjunath R. Protection of adult but not newborn mice against lethal intracerebral challenge with Japanese encephalitis virus by adoptively transferred virus-specific cytotoxic T lymphocytes: requirement for L3T4+ T cells. *J Gen Virol* 1996;77:705–714.
804. Murray K, Baraniuk S, Resnick M, et al. Risk factors for encephalitis and death from West Nile virus infection. *Epidemiol Infect* 2006;134:1325–1332.
805. Murray KO, Gorchakov R, Carlson AR, et al. Prolonged detection of Zika virus in vaginal secretions and whole blood. *Emerg Infect Dis* 2017;23:99–101.
806. Murray K, Walker C, Herrington E, et al. Persistent infection with West Nile virus years after initial infection. *J Infect Dis* 2010;201:2–4.
807. Musso D, Bossin H, Mallet HP, et al. Zika virus in French Polynesia 2013–14: anatomy of a completed outbreak. *Lancet Infect Dis* 2018;18:e172–e182.
808. Musso D, Roche C, Robin E, et al. Potential sexual transmission of Zika virus. *Emerg Infect Dis* 2015;21:359–361.
809. Mutebi JP, Rijnbrand RC, Wang H, et al. Genetic relationships and evolution of genotypes of yellow fever virus and other members of the yellow fever virus group within the Flavivirus genus based on the 3′ noncoding region. *J Virol* 2004;78:9652–9665.
810. Mutebi JP, Wang H, Li L, et al. Phylogenetic and evolutionary relationships among yellow fever virus isolates in Africa. *J Virol* 2001;75:6999–7008.
811. Muthumani K, Griffin BD, Agarwal S, et al. In vivo protection against ZIKV infection and pathogenesis through passive antibody transfer and active immunisation with a prMEnv DNA vaccine. *npj Vaccines* 2016;1:16021.
812. Myint KS, Raengsakulrach B, Young GD, et al. Production of lethal infection that resembles fatal human disease by intranasal inoculation of macaques with Japanese encephalitis virus. *Am J Trop Med Hyg* 1999;60:338–342.
813. Nagy A, Ban E, Nagy O, et al. Detection and sequencing of West Nile virus RNA from human urine and serum samples during the 2014 seasonal period. *Arch Virol* 2016;161:1797–1806.
814. Nash D, Mostashari F, Fine A, et al. The outbreak of West Nile virus infection in the New York City area in 1999. *N Engl J Med* 2001;344:1807–1814.
815. Nasirudeen AM, Wong HH, Thien P, et al. RIG-I, MDA5 and TLR3 synergistically play an important role in restriction of dengue virus infection. *PLoS Negl Trop Dis* 2011;5:e926.
816. Nathan N, Barry M, Van Herp M, et al. Shortage of vaccines during a yellow fever outbreak in Guinea. *Lancet* 2001;358:2129–2130.
817. Navarro-Sanchez E, Altmeyer R, Amara A, et al. Dendritic-cell-specific ICAM3-grabbing non-integrin is essential for the productive infection of human dendritic cells by mosquito-cell-derived dengue viruses. *EMBO Rep* 2003;4:723–728.
818. Nelson S, Jost CA, Xu Q, et al. Maturation of West Nile virus modulates sensitivity to antibody-mediated neutralization. *PLoS Pathog* 2008;4:e1000060.
819. Nelson MH, Winkelmann E, Ma Y, et al. Immunogenicity of RepliVAX WN, a novel single-cycle West Nile virus vaccine. *Vaccine* 2010;29:174–182.
820. Neves PC, Matos DC, Marcovistz R, et al. TLR expression and NK cell activation after human yellow fever vaccination. *Vaccine* 2009;27:5543–5549.
821. Neves PC, Rudersdorf RA, Galler R, et al. CD8+ gamma-delta TCR+ and CD4+ T cells produce IFN-gamma at 5–7 days after yellow fever vaccination in Indian rhesus macaques, before the induction of classical antigen-specific T cell responses. *Vaccine* 2010;28:8183–8188.
822. Ngo NT, Cao XT, Kneen R, et al. Acute management of dengue shock syndrome: a randomized double-blind comparison of 4 intravenous fluid regimens in the first hour. *Clin Infect Dis* 2001;32:204–213.
823. Nguyen SM, Antony KM, Dudley DM, et al. Highly efficient maternal-fetal Zika virus transmission in pregnant rhesus macaques. *PLoS Pathog* 2017;13:e1006378.
824. Ni H, Barrett AD. Molecular differences between wild-type Japanese encephalitis virus strains of high and low mouse neuroinvasiveness. *J Gen Virol* 1996;77(Pt 7):1449–1455.
825. Nicastri E, Castilletti C, Liuzzi G, et al. Persistent detection of Zika virus RNA in semen for six months after symptom onset in a traveller returning from Haiti to Italy, February 2016. *Euro Surveill* 2016;21.
826. Nickells J, Cannella M, Droll DA, et al. Neuroadapted yellow fever virus strain 17D: a charged locus in domain III of the E protein governs heparin binding activity and neuroinvasiveness in the SCID mouse model. *J Virol* 2008;82:12510–12519.
827. Nickells M, Chambers TJ. Neuroadapted yellow fever virus 17D: determinants in the envelope protein govern neuroinvasiveness for SCID mice. *J Virol* 2003;77:12232–12242.
828. Nir Y, Beemer A, Goldwasser RA. West Nile Virus infection in mice following exposure to a viral aerosol. *Br J Exp Pathol* 1965;46:443–449.
829. Nisalak A, Endy TP, Nimmannitya S, et al. Serotype-specific dengue virus circulation and dengue disease in Bangkok, Thailand from 1973 to 1999. *Am J Trop Med Hyg* 2003;68:191–202.
830. Noronha L, Zanluca C, Azevedo ML, et al. Zika virus damages the human placental barrier and presents marked fetal neurotropism. *Mem Inst Oswaldo Cruz* 2016;111:287–293.
831. Nowakowski TJ, Pollen AA, Di Lullo E, et al. Expression analysis highlights AXL as a candidate Zika virus entry receptor in neural stem cells. *Cell Stem Cell* 2016;18:591–596.
832. Nurnberger C, Bodmer BS, Fiedler AH, et al. A measles virus-based vaccine candidate mediates protection against Zika Virus in an allogeneic mouse pregnancy model. *J Virol* 2019;93.
833. Nybakken GE, Oliphant T, Johnson S, et al. Structural basis of West Nile virus neutralization by a therapeutic antibody. *Nature* 2005;437:764–769.
834. O'Connor MA, Tisoncik-Go J, Lewis TB, et al. Early cellular innate immune responses drive Zika viral persistence and tissue tropism in pigtail macaques. *Nat Commun* 2018;9:3371.
835. Oehler E, Watrin L, Larre P, et al. Zika virus infection complicated by Guillain-Barre syndrome—case report, French Polynesia, December 2013. *Euro Surveill* 2014;19.
836. O'Garra A, Vieira P. Regulatory T cells and mechanisms of immune system control. *Nat Med* 2004;10:801–805.
837. Ohrr H, Tandan JB, Sohn YM, et al. Effect of single dose of SA 14–14–2 vaccine 1 year after immunisation in Nepalese children with Japanese encephalitis: a case-control study. *Lancet* 2005;366:1375–1378.
838. O'Leary DR, Kuhn S, Kniss KL, et al. Birth outcomes following West Nile Virus infection of pregnant women in the United States: 2003–2004. *Pediatrics* 2006;117:e537–e545.
839. Oliphant T, Engle M, Nybakken G, et al. Development of a humanized monoclonal antibody with therapeutic potential against West Nile virus. *Nat Med* 2005;11:522–530.
840. Oliphant T, Nybakken GE, Austin SK, et al. The induction of epitope-specific neutralizing antibodies against West Nile virus. *J Virol* 2007;81:11828–11839.
841. Oliphant T, Nybakken GE, Engle M, et al. Antibody recognition and neutralization determinants on domains I and II of West Nile Virus envelope protein. *J Virol* 2006;80:12149–12159.
842. Oliveira DB, Almeida FJ, Durigon EL, et al. Prolonged shedding of Zika virus associated with congenital infection. *N Engl J Med* 2016;375:1202–1204.
843. Omalu BI, Shakir AA, Wang G, et al. Fatal fulminant pan-meningo-polioencephalitis due to West Nile virus. *Brain Pathol* 2003;13:465–472.

844. Onlamoon N, Noisakran S, Hsiao HM, et al. Dengue virus-induced hemorrhage in a nonhuman primate model. *Blood* 2010;115:1823–1834.
845. Ooi MH, Lewthwaite P, Lai BF, et al. The epidemiology, clinical features, and long-term prognosis of Japanese encephalitis in central Sarawak, Malaysia, 1997–2005. *Clin Infect Dis* 2008;47:458–468.
846. World Health Organization. WHO report on global surveillance of epidemic-prone infectious diseases. *WHO/CDS/CSR/ISR/2001* 2000;2000:1–15.
847. Osorio JE, Velez ID, Thomson C, et al. Safety and immunogenicity of a recombinant live attenuated tetravalent dengue vaccine (DENVax) in flavivirus-naive healthy adults in Colombia: a randomised, placebo-controlled, phase 1 study. *Lancet Infect Dis* 2014;14:830–838.
848. Osorio JE, Wallace D, Stinchcomb DT. A recombinant, chimeric tetravalent dengue vaccine candidate based on a dengue virus serotype 2 backbone. *Expert Rev Vaccines* 2016;15:497–508.
849. Osuna CE, Lim SY, Deleage C, et al. Zika viral dynamics and shedding in rhesus and cynomolgus macaques. *Nat Med* 2016;22:1448–1455.
850. Pabalan N, Chaisri S, Tabunhan S, et al. Associations of DC-SIGN (CD209) promoter -336G/A polymorphism (rs4804803) with dengue infection: a systematic review and meta-analysis. *Acta Trop* 2018;177:186–193.
851. Pacheco O, Beltran M, Nelson CA, et al. Zika virus disease in Colombia—preliminary report. *N Engl J Med* 2016. doi:10.1056/NEJMoa1604037.
852. Paes MV, Pinhao AT, Barreto DF, et al. Liver injury and viremia in mice infected with dengue-2 virus. *Virology* 2005;338:236–246.
853. Paixao ES, Teixeira MG, Costa M, et al. Dengue during pregnancy and adverse fetal outcomes: a systematic review and meta-analysis. *Lancet Infect Dis* 2016;16:857–865.
854. Palmer DR, Fernandez S, Bisbing J, et al. Restricted replication and lysosomal trafficking of yellow fever 17D vaccine virus in human dendritic cells. *J Gen Virol* 2007;88:148–156.
855. Pan American Health Organization. *Epidemiological alert: increase of microcephaly in the northeast of Brazil.* 2015.
856. Pan CH, Chen HW, Huang HW, et al. Protective mechanisms induced by a Japanese encephalitis virus DNA vaccine: requirement for antibody but not CD8(+) cytotoxic T-cell responses. *J Virol* 2001;75:11457–11463.
857. Panayiotou C, Lindqvist R, Kurhade C, et al. Viperin restricts Zika virus and Tick-Borne encephalitis virus replication by targeting NS3 for proteasomal degradation. *J Virol* 2018;92.
858. Pantoja P, Perez-Guzman EX, Rodriguez IV, et al. Zika virus pathogenesis in rhesus macaques is unaffected by pre-existing immunity to dengue virus. *Nat Commun* 2017;8:15674.
859. Parameswaran P, Wang C, Trivedi SB, et al. Intrahost selection pressures drive rapid dengue virus microevolution in acute human infections. *Cell Host Microbe* 2017;22:400–410 e405.
860. Pardi N, Hogan MJ, Pelc RS, et al. Zika virus protection by a single low-dose nucleoside-modified mRNA vaccination. *Nature* 2017;543:248–251.
861. Park GS, Morris KL, Hallett RG, et al. Identification of residues critical for the interferon antagonist function of Langat virus NS5 reveals a role for the RNA-dependent RNA polymerase domain. *J Virol* 2007;81:6936–6946.
862. Pastor AF, Rodrigues Moura L, Neto JW, et al. Complement factor H gene (CFH) polymorphisms C-257T, G257A and haplotypes are associated with protection against severe dengue phenotype, possible related with high CFH expression. *Hum Immunol* 2013;74:1225–1230.
863. Paz-Bailey G, Rosenberg ES, Doyle K, et al. Persistence of Zika virus in body fluids—final report. *N Engl J Med* 2018;379:1234–1243.
864. Pealer LN, Marfin AA, Petersen LR, et al. Transmission of West Nile virus through blood transfusion in the United States in 2002. *N Engl J Med* 2003;349:1236–1245.
865. Peiris JS, Gordon S, Unkeless JC, et al. Monoclonal anti-Fc receptor IgG blocks antibody enhancement of viral replication in macrophages. *Nature* 1981;289:189–191.
866. Peiris JS, Porterfield JS. Antibody-mediated enhancement of Flavivirus replication in macrophage-like cell lines. *Nature* 1979;282:509–511.
867. Penot P, Brichler S, Guilleminot J, et al. Infectious Zika virus in vaginal secretions from an HIV-infected woman, France, August 2016. *Euro Surveill* 2017;22.
868. Perelygin AA, Scherbik SV, Zhulin IB, et al. Positional cloning of the murine flavivirus resistance gene. *Proc Natl Acad Sci U S A* 2002;99:9322–9327.
869. Perelygin AA, Zharkikh AA, Scherbik SV, et al. The mammalian 2′-5′ oligoadenylate synthetase gene family: evidence for concerted evolution of paralogous Oas1 genes in Rodentia and Artiodactyla. *J Mol Evol* 2006;63:562–576.
870. Persaud M, Martinez-Lopez A, Buffone C, et al. Infection by Zika viruses requires the transmembrane protein AXL, endocytosis and low pH. *Virology* 2018;518:301–312.
871. Petersen LR, Epstein JS. Problem solved? West Nile virus and transfusion safety. *N Engl J Med* 2005;353:516–517.
872. Pettersson JH, Fiz-Palacios O. Dating the origin of the genus Flavivirus in the light of Beringian biogeography. *J Gen Virol* 2014;95:1969–1982.
873. Pfister M, Kursteiner O, Hilfiker H, et al. Immunogenicity and safety of BERNA-YF compared with two other 17D yellow fever vaccines in a phase 3 clinical trial. *Am J Trop Med Hyg* 2005;72:339–346.
874. Pichyangkul S, Endy TP, Kalayanarooj S, et al. A blunted blood plasmacytoid dendritic cell response to an acute systemic viral infection is associated with increased disease severity. *J Immunol* 2003;171:5571–5578.
875. Pierce KK, Whitehead SS, Kirkpatrick BD, et al. A live attenuated Chimeric West Nile virus vaccine, rWN/DEN4Delta30, is well tolerated and immunogenic in flavivirus-naive older adult volunteers. *J Infect Dis* 2017;215:52–55.
876. Pierson TC, Diamond MS. Degrees of maturity: the complex structure and biology of flaviviruses. *Curr Opin Virol* 2012;2:168–175.
877. Pierson TC, Kielian M. Flaviviruses: braking the entering. *Curr Opin Virol* 2013;3:3–12.
878. Pierson TC, Xu Q, Nelson S, et al. The stoichiometry of antibody-mediated neutralization and enhancement of West Nile virus infection. *Cell Host Microbe* 2007;1:135–145.
879. Pijlman GP, Funk A, Kondratieva N, et al. A highly structured, nuclease-resistant, noncoding RNA produced by flaviviruses is required for pathogenicity. *Cell Host Microbe* 2008;4:579–591.
880. Pincus S, Mason PW, Konishi E, et al. Recombinant vaccinia virus producing the prM and E proteins of yellow fever virus protects mice from lethal yellow fever encephalitis. *Virology* 1992;187:290–297.
881. Pingen M, Bryden SR, Pondeville E, et al. Host inflammatory response to mosquito bites enhances the severity of arbovirus infection. *Immunity* 2016;44:1455–1469.
882. Pinto AK, Brien JD, Lam CY, et al. Defining new therapeutics using a more immunocompetent mouse model of antibody-enhanced dengue virus infection. *MBio* 2015;6:e01316–01315.
883. Pinto AJ, Morahan PS, Brinton M, et al. Comparative therapeutic efficacy of recombinant interferons-alpha, -beta, and -gamma against alphatogavirus, bunyavirus, flavivirus, and herpesvirus infections. *J Interferon Res* 1990;10:293–298.
884. Platanias LC. Mechanisms of type-I- and type-II-interferon-mediated signalling. *Nat Rev Immunol* 2005;5:375–386.
885. Platt DJ, Smith AM, Arora N, et al. Zika virus-related neurotropic flaviviruses infect human placental explants and cause fetal demise in mice. *Sci Transl Med* 2018;10.
886. Plentz A, Jilg W, Schwarz TF, et al. Long-term persistence of tick-borne encephalitis antibodies in adults 5 years after booster vaccination with Encepur Adults. *Vaccine* 2009;27:853–856.
887. Plevka P, Battisti AJ, Junjhon J, et al. Maturation of flaviviruses starts from one or more icosahedrally independent nucleation centres. *EMBO Rep* 2011;12:602–606.
888. Pogodina VV. [An experimental study on the pathogenesis of tick-borne encephalitis following alimentary infection. Part 1. The dynamics of distribution of the virus in white mice infected by the enteral route]. *Vopr Virusol* 1960;5:272–279.
889. Pogodina VV, Frolova MP, Malenko GV, et al. Study on West Nile virus persistence in monkeys. *Arch Virol* 1983;75:71–86.
890. Poland JD, Calisher CH, Monath TP, et al. Persistence of neutralizing antibody 30–35 years after immunization with 17D yellow fever vaccine. *Bull World Health Organ* 1981;59:895–900.
891. Poland JD, Cropp CB, Craven RB, et al. Evaluation of the potency and safety of inactivated Japanese encephalitis vaccine in US inhabitants. *J Infect Dis* 1990;161:878–882.
892. Prasad VM, Miller AS, Klose T, et al. Structure of the immature Zika virus at 9 A resolution. *Nat Struct Mol Biol* 2017;24:184–186.
893. Pridjian G, Sirois PA, McRae S, et al. Prospective study of pregnancy and newborn outcomes in mothers with West nile illness during pregnancy. *Birth Defects Res A Clin Mol Teratol* 2016;106:716–723.
894. Prow NA, Liu L, Nakayama E, et al. A vaccinia-based single vector construct multi-pathogen vaccine protects against both Zika and chikungunya viruses. *Nat Commun* 2018;9:1230.
895. Pruitt AA. Central nervous system infections in cancer patients. *Semin Neurol* 2004;24:435–452.
896. Puerta-Guardo H, Glasner DR, Espinosa DA, et al. Flavivirus NS1 triggers tissue-specific vascular endothelial dysfunction reflecting disease tropism. *Cell Rep* 2019;26:1598–1613.e8.
897. Puerta-Guardo H, Glasner DR, Harris E. Dengue virus NS1 disrupts the endothelial glycocalyx, leading to hyperpermeability. *PLoS Pathog* 2016;12:e1005738.
898. Pulendran B. Learning immunology from the yellow fever vaccine: innate immunity to systems vaccinology. *Nat Rev Immunol* 2009;9:741–747.
899. Pulendran B, Miller J, Querec TD, et al. Case of yellow fever vaccine--associated viscerotropic disease with prolonged viremia, robust adaptive immune responses, and polymorphisms in CCR5 and RANTES genes. *J Infect Dis* 2008;198:500–507.
900. Purtha WE, Chachu KA, Virgin HW, et al. Early B-cell activation after West Nile virus infection requires alpha/beta interferon but not antigen receptor signaling. *J Virol* 2008;82:10964–10974.
901. Purtha WE, Myers N, Mitaksov V, et al. Antigen-specific cytotoxic T lymphocytes protect against lethal West Nile virus encephalitis. *Eur J Immunol* 2007;37:1845–1854.
902. Putnak JR, Schlesinger JJ. Protection of mice against yellow fever virus encephalitis by immunization with a vaccinia virus recombinant encoding the yellow fever virus nonstructural proteins, NS1, NS2a and NS2b. *J Gen Virol* 1990;71(Pt 8):1697–1702.
903. Qian X, Nguyen HN, Jacob F, et al. Using brain organoids to understand Zika virus-induced microcephaly. *Development* 2017;144:952–957.
904. Qian X, Nguyen HN, Song MM, et al. Brain-region-specific organoids using mini-bioreactors for modeling ZIKV exposure. *Cell* 2016;165:1238–1254.
905. Quaresma JA, Barros VL, Pagliari C, et al. Revisiting the liver in human yellow fever: virus-induced apoptosis in hepatocytes associated with TGF-beta, TNF-alpha and NK cells activity. *Virology* 2006;345:22–30.
906. Querec TD, Akondy RS, Lee EK, et al. Systems biology approach predicts immunogenicity of the yellow fever vaccine in humans. *Nat Immunol* 2009;10:116–125.
907. Querec T, Bennouna S, Alkan S, et al. Yellow fever vaccine YF-17D activates multiple dendritic cell subsets via TLR2, 7, 8, and 9 to stimulate polyvalent immunity. *J Exp Med* 2006;203:413–424.
908. Quicke KM, Bowen JR, Johnson EL, et al. Zika virus infects human placental macrophages. *Cell Host Microbe* 2016;20:83–90.
909. Raengsakulrach B, Nisalak A, Gettayacamin M, et al. An intranasal challenge model for testing Japanese encephalitis vaccines in rhesus monkeys. *Am J Trop Med Hyg* 1999;60:329–337.
910. Rahal JJ, Anderson J, Rosenberg C, et al. Effect of interferon-alpha2b therapy on St. Louis viral meningoencephalitis: clinical and laboratory results of a pilot study. *J Infect Dis* 2004;190:1084–1087.
911. Ramos HJ, Lanteri MC, Blahnik G, et al. IL-1beta signaling promotes CNS-intrinsic immune control of West Nile virus infection. *PLoS Pathog* 2012;8:e1003039.
912. Rathore APS, Saron WAA, Lim T, et al. Maternal immunity and antibodies to dengue virus promote infection and Zika virus-induced microcephaly in fetuses. *Sci Adv* 2019;5:eaav3208.
913. Ratterree MS, Gutierrez RA, Travassos da Rosa AP, et al. Experimental infection of rhesus macaques with West Nile virus: level and duration of viremia and kinetics of the antibody response after infection. *J Infect Dis* 2004;189:669–676.
914. Raut R, Corbett KS, Tennekoon RN, et al. Dengue type 1 viruses circulating in humans are highly infectious and poorly neutralized by human antibodies. *Proc Natl Acad Sci U S A* 2019;116:227–232.
915. Rayamajhi A, Nightingale S, Bhatta NK, et al. A preliminary randomized double blind placebo-controlled trial of intravenous immunoglobulin for Japanese encephalitis in Nepal. *PLoS One* 2015;10:e0122608.

916. Reagan-Steiner S, Simeone R, Simon E, et al. Evaluation of placental and fetal tissue specimens for Zika virus infection - 50 States and District of Columbia, January-December, 2016. *MMWR Morb Mortal Wkly Rep* 2017;66:636–643.

917. Regla-Nava JA, Elong Ngono A, Viramontes KM, et al. Cross-reactive Dengue virus-specific CD8(+) T cells protect against Zika virus during pregnancy. *Nat Commun* 2018;9:3042.

918. Reimann CA, Hayes EB, DiGuiseppi C, et al. Epidemiology of neuroinvasive arboviral disease in the United States, 1999–2007. *Am J Trop Med Hyg* 2008;79:974–979.

919. Reisen WK. Epidemiology of St. Louis encephalitis virus. *Adv Virus Res* 2003;61:139–183.

920. Reisen WK, Lothrop HD, Wheeler SS, et al. Persistent West Nile virus transmission and the apparent displacement St. Louis encephalitis virus in southeastern California, 2003–2006. *J Med Entomol* 2008;45:494–508.

921. Rendi-Wagner P. Advances in vaccination against tick-borne encephalitis. *Expert Rev Vaccines* 2008;7:589–596.

922. Renner M, Flanagan A, Dejnirattisai W, et al. Characterization of a potent and highly unusual minimally enhancing antibody directed against dengue virus. *Nat Immunol* 2018;19:1248–1256.

923. Repik PM, Dalrymple JM, Brandt WE, et al. RNA fingerprinting as a method for distinguishing dengue 1 virus strains. *Am J Trop Med Hyg* 1983;32:577–589.

924. Rey FA, Stiasny K, Heinz FX. Flavivirus structural heterogeneity: implications for cell entry. *Curr Opin Virol* 2017;24:132–139.

925. Ricciardi MJ, Magnani DM, Grifoni A, et al. Ontogeny of the B- and T-cell response in a primary Zika virus infection of a dengue-naive individual during the 2016 outbreak in Miami, FL. *PLoS Negl Trop Dis* 2017;11:e0006000.

926. Richard AS, Shim BS, Kwon YC, et al. AXL-dependent infection of human fetal endothelial cells distinguishes Zika virus from other pathogenic flaviviruses. *Proc Natl Acad Sci U S A* 2017;114:2024–2029.

927. Richardson RB, Ohlson MB, Eitson JL, et al. A CRISPR screen identifies IFI6 as an ER-resident interferon effector that blocks flavivirus replication. *Nat Microbiol* 2018;3:1214–1223.

928. Richner JM, Himansu S, Dowd KA, et al. Modified mRNA vaccines protect against Zika virus infection. *Cell* 2017;169:176.

929. Richner JM, Himansu S, Dowd KA, et al. Modified mRNA vaccines protect against Zika virus infection. *Cell* 2017;168:1114–1125.e1110.

930. Richner JM, Jagger BW, Shan C, et al. Vaccine mediated protection against Zika virus-induced congenital disease. *Cell* 2017;170:273–283, e212.

931. Rico-Hesse R. Molecular evolution and distribution of dengue viruses type 1 and 2 in nature. *Virology* 1990;174:479–493.

932. Rico-Hesse R. Microevolution and virulence of dengue viruses. *Adv Virus Res* 2003;59:315–341.

933. Rigau-Perez JG, Gubler DJ, Vorndam AV, et al. Dengue: a literature review and case study of travelers from the United States, 1986–1994. *J Travel Med* 1997;4:65–71.

934. Rios M, Daniel S, Chancey C, et al. West Nile virus adheres to human red blood cells in whole blood. *Clin Infect Dis* 2007;45:181–186.

935. Rios JJ, Fleming JG, Bryant UK, et al. OAS1 polymorphisms are associated with susceptibility to West Nile encephalitis in horses. *PLoS One* 2010;5:e10537.

936. Rios M, Zhang MJ, Grinev A, et al. Monocytes-macrophages are a potential target in human infection with West Nile virus through blood transfusion. *Transfusion* 2006;46:659–667.

937. Rivino L, Kumaran EA, Thein TL, et al. Virus-specific T lymphocytes home to the skin during natural dengue infection. *Sci Transl Med* 2015;7:278ra235.

938. Robbiani DF, Bozzacco L, Keeffe JR, et al. Recurrent potent human neutralizing antibodies to Zika virus in Brazil and Mexico. *Cell* 2017;169:597–609, e511.

939. Rodenhuis-Zybert IA, van der Schaar HM, da Silva Voorham JM, et al. Immature dengue virus: a veiled pathogen? *PLoS Pathog* 2010;6:e1000718.

940. Rodriguez-Barraquer I, Costa F, Nascimento EJM, et al. Impact of preexisting dengue immunity on Zika virus emergence in a dengue endemic region. *Science* 2019;363:607–610.

941. Rodriguez-Madoz JR, Belicha-Villanueva A, Bernal-Rubio D, et al. Inhibition of the type I interferon response in human dendritic cells by dengue virus infection requires a catalytically active NS2B3 complex. *J Virol* 2010;84:9760–9774.

942. Rodriguez-Madoz JR, Bernal-Rubio D, Kaminski D, et al. Dengue virus inhibits the production of type I interferon in primary human dendritic cells. *J Virol* 2010;84:4845–4850.

943. Roehrig JT. West nile virus in the United States—a historical perspective. *Viruses* 2013;5:3088–3108.

944. Roehrig JT, Bolin RA, Kelly RG. Monoclonal antibody mapping of the envelope glycoprotein of the dengue 2 virus, Jamaica. *Virology* 1998;246:317–328.

945. Rosen L, Drouet MT, Deubel V. Detection of dengue virus RNA by reverse transcription-polymerase chain reaction in the liver and lymphoid organs but not in the brain in fatal human infection. *Am J Trop Med Hyg* 1999;61:720–724.

946. Rosenzweig EC, Babione RW, Wisseman CL Jr. Immunological studies with group B arthropod-borne viruses. IV. Persistence of yellow fever antibodies following vaccination with 17D strain yellow fever vaccine. *Am J Trop Med Hyg* 1963;12:230–235.

947. Rossi SL, Tesh RB, Azar SR, et al. Characterization of a Novel Murine Model to study Zika virus. *Am J Trop Med Hyg* 2016;94:1362–1369.

948. Roundy CM, Azar SR, Rossi SL, et al. Insect-specific viruses: a historical overview and recent developments. *Adv Virus Res* 2017;98:119–146.

949. Rouvinski A, Dejnirattisai W, Guardado-Calvo P, et al. Covalently linked dengue virus envelope glycoprotein dimers reduce exposure of the immunodominant fusion loop epitope. *Nat Commun* 2017;8:15411.

950. Rouvinski A, Guardado-Calvo P, Barba-Spaeth G, et al. Recognition determinants of broadly neutralizing human antibodies against dengue viruses. *Nature* 2015;520:109–113.

951. Rush AB. An account of the bilious remitting fever, as it appeared in Philadelphia in the summer and autumn of the year 1780. *Medical Enquiries and Observations* 1789:104–117.

952. Ruzek D, Yakimenko VV, Karan LS, et al. Omsk haemorrhagic fever. *Lancet* 2010;376:2104–2113.

953. Sabchareon A, Wallace D, Sirivichayakul C, et al. Protective efficacy of the recombinant, live-attenuated, CYD tetravalent dengue vaccine in Thai schoolchildren: a randomised, controlled phase 2b trial. *Lancet* 2012;380:1559–1567.

954. Sabin AB. Epidemic encephalitis in military personnel; isolation of Japanese B virus on Okinawa in 1945, serologic diagnosis, clinical manifestations, epidemiologic aspects and use of mouse brain vaccine. *J Am Med Assoc* 1947;133:281–293.

955. Sabin AB. Antibody response of people of different ages to two doses of uncentrifuged Japanese B encephalitis vaccine. *Proc Soc Exp Biol Med* 1947;65:127–130.

956. Sabin AB. Research on dengue during World War II. *Am J Trop Med Hyg* 1952;1:30–50.

957. Sabin AB, Schlesinger RW. Production of immunity to dengue with virus modified by propagation in mice. *Science* 1945;101:640–642.

958. Saez-Llorens X, Tricou V, Yu D, et al. Safety and immunogenicity of one versus two doses of Takeda's tetravalent dengue vaccine in children in Asia and Latin America: interim results from a phase 2, randomised, placebo-controlled study. *Lancet Infect Dis* 2017;17:615–625.

959. Sakaguchi S. Naturally arising Foxp3-expressing CD25+CD4+ regulatory T cells in immunological tolerance to self and non-self. *Nat Immunol* 2005;6:345–352.

960. Salazar V, Jagger BW, Mongkolsapaya J, et al. Dengue and Zika virus cross-reactive human monoclonal antibodies protect against spondweni virus infection and pathogenesis in mice. *Cell Rep* 2019;26:1585–1597, e1584.

961. Salvo MA, Kingstad-Bakke B, Salas-Quinchucua C, et al. Zika virus like particles elicit protective antibodies in mice. *PLoS Negl Trop Dis* 2018;12:e0006210.

962. Samsa MM, Mondotte JA, Iglesias NG, et al. Dengue virus capsid protein usurps lipid droplets for viral particle formation. *PLoS Pathog* 2009;5:e1000632.

963. Samuel MA, Diamond MS. Type I IFN protects against lethal West Nile Virus infection by restricting cellular tropism and enhancing neuronal survival. *J Virol* 2005;79:13350–13361.

964. Samuel MA, Wang H, Siddharthan V, et al. Axonal transport mediates West Nile virus entry into the central nervous system and induces acute flaccid paralysis. *Proc Natl Acad Sci U S A* 2007;104:17140–17145.

965. Samuel MA, Whitby K, Keller BC, et al. PKR and RNAse L contribute to protection against lethal West Nile virus infection by controlling early viral spread in the periphery and replication in neurons. *J Virol* 2006;80:7009–7019.

966. Sanchez JL, Hoke CH, McCown J, et al. Further experience with Japanese encephalitis vaccine. *Lancet* 1990;335:972–973.

967. Sang RC, Gichogo A, Gachoya J, et al. Isolation of a new flavivirus related to cell fusing agent virus (CFAV) from field-collected flood-water Aedes mosquitoes sampled from a dambo in central Kenya. *Arch Virol* 2003;148:1085–1093.

968. Santos AP, Matos DC, Bertho AL, et al. Detection of Th1/Th2 cytokine signatures in yellow fever 17DD first-time vaccinees through ELISpot assay. *Cytokine* 2008;42:152–155.

969. Santos VS, Oliveira SJG, Gurgel RQ, et al. Case report: microcephaly in twins due to the Zika virus. *Am J Trop Med Hyg* 2017;97:151–154.

970. Sariol CA, Munoz-Jordan JL, Abel K, et al. Transcriptional activation of interferon-stimulated genes but not of cytokine genes after primary infection of rhesus macaques with dengue virus type 1. *Clin Vaccine Immunol* 2007;14:756–766.

971. Sarno M, Sacramento GA, Khouri R, et al. Zika virus infection and stillbirths: a case of hydrops fetalis, hydranencephaly and fetal demise. *PLoS Negl Trop Dis* 2016;10:e0004517.

972. Sarvestani ST, McAuley JL. The role of the NLRP3 inflammasome in regulation of antiviral responses to influenza A virus infection. *Antiviral Res* 2017;148:32–42.

973. Sassetti M, Ze-Ze L, Franco J, et al. First case of confirmed congenital Zika syndrome in continental Africa. *Trans R Soc Trop Med Hyg* 2018;112:458–462.

974. Satterfield-Nash A, Kotzky K, Allen J, et al. Health and development at age 19–24 months of 19 children who were born with microcephaly and laboratory evidence of congenital zika virus infection during the 2015 Zika virus outbreak - Brazil, 2017. *MMWR Morb Mortal Wkly Rep* 2017;66:1347–1351.

975. Savidis G, McDougall WM, Meraner P, et al. Identification of Zika virus and dengue virus dependency factors using functional genomics. *Cell Rep* 2016;16:232–246.

976. Savidis G, Perreira JM, Portmann JM, et al. The IFITMs inhibit Zika virus replication. *Cell Rep* 2016;15:2323–2330.

977. Sawyer WA, Lloyd W. The use of mice in tests of immunity against yellow fever. *J Exp Med* 1931;54:533–555.

978. Saxena SK, Mathur A, Srivastava RC. Induction of nitric oxide synthase during Japanese encephalitis virus infection: evidence of protective role. *Arch Biochem Biophys* 2001;391:1–7.

979. Saxena SK, Singh A, Mathur A. Antiviral effect of nitric oxide during Japanese encephalitis virus infection. *Int J Exp Pathol* 2000;81:165–172.

980. Sbrana E, Tonry JH, Xiao SY, et al. Oral transmission of West Nile virus in a hamster model. *Am J Trop Med Hyg* 2005;72:325–329.

981. Schalich J, Allison SL, Stiasny K, et al. Recombinant subviral particles from tick-borne encephalitis virus are fusogenic and provide a model system for studying flavivirus envelope glycoprotein functions. *J Virol* 1996;70:4549–4557.

982. Scherbik SV, Kluetzman K, Perelygin AA, et al. Knock-in of the Oas1b(r) allele into a flavivirus-induced disease susceptible mouse generates the resistant phenotype. *Virology* 2007;368:232–237.

983. Scherbik SV, Paranjape JM, Stockman BM, et al. RNase L plays a role in the antiviral response to West Nile virus. *J Virol* 2006;80:2987–2999.

984. Scherer WF, Russell PK, Rosen L, et al. Experimental infection of chimpanzees with dengue viruses. *Am J Trop Med Hyg* 1978;27:590–599.

985. Scherret JH, Poidinger M, Mackenzie JS, et al. The relationships between West Nile and Kunjin viruses. *Emerg Infect Dis* 2001;7:697–705.

986. Schlesinger JJ, Brandriss MW, Cropp CB, et al. Protection against yellow fever in monkeys by immunization with yellow fever virus nonstructural protein NS1. *J Virol* 1986;60:1153–1155.

987. Schlesinger JJ, Brandriss MW, Walsh EE. Protection against 17D yellow fever encephalitis in mice by passive transfer of monoclonal antibodies to the nonstructural glycoprotein gp48 and by active immunization with gp48. *J Immunol* 1985;135:2805–2809.

988. Schlesinger JJ, Brandriss MW, Walsh EE. Protection of mice against dengue 2 virus encephalitis by immunization with the dengue 2 virus non-structural glycoprotein NS1. *J Gen Virol* 1987;68(Pt 3):853–857.

989. Schlesinger JJ, Chapman S. Neutralizing F (ab')2 fragments of protective monoclonal antibodies to yellow fever virus (YF) envelope protein fail to protect mice against lethal YF encephalitis. *J Gen Virol* 1995;76(Pt 1):217–220.

990. Schlesinger JJ, Foltzer M, Chapman S. The Fc portion of antibody to yellow fever virus NS1 is a determinant of protection against YF encephalitis in mice. *Virology* 1993;192:132–141.

991. Schmid MA, Harris E. Monocyte recruitment to the dermis and differentiation to dendritic cells increases the targets for dengue virus replication. *PLoS Pathog* 2014;10:e1004541.

992. Schneider H. An acute epidemic of serosal meningitis (in German). *Wien Klin Wochenschr* 1931;44.

993. Schneider BS, Higgs S. The enhancement of arbovirus transmission and disease by mosquito saliva is associated with modulation of the host immune response. *Trans R Soc Trop Med Hyg* 2008;102:400–408.

994. Schneider BS, Soong L, Coffey LL, et al. Aedes aegypti saliva alters leukocyte recruitment and cytokine signaling by antigen-presenting cells during West Nile virus infection. *PLoS One* 2010;5:e11704.

995. Schneider BS, Soong L, Girard YA, et al. Potentiation of West Nile encephalitis by mosquito feeding. *Viral Immunol* 2006;19:74–82.

996. Schoggins JW. Recent advances in antiviral interferon-stimulated gene biology. *F1000Res* 2018;7:309.

997. Schoggins JW, MacDuff DA, Imanaka N, et al. Pan-viral specificity of IFN-induced genes reveals new roles for cGAS in innate immunity. *Nature* 2014;505:691–695.

998. Schoggins JW, Wilson SJ, Panis M, et al. A diverse range of gene products are effectors of the type I interferon antiviral response. *Nature* 2011;472:481–485.

999. Schroder M, Bowie AG. TLR3 in antiviral immunity: key player or bystander? *Trends Immunol* 2005;26:462–468.

1000. Schuessler A, Funk A, Lazear HM, et al. West Nile virus noncoding subgenomic RNA contributes to viral evasion of the type I interferon-mediated antiviral response. *J Virol* 2012;86:5708–5718.

1001. Schuh AJ, Tesh RB, Barrett AD. Genetic characterization of Japanese encephalitis virus genotype II strains isolated from 1951 to 1978. *J Gen Virol* 2011;92:516–527.

1002. Schul W, Liu W, Xu HY, et al. A dengue fever viremia model in mice shows reduction in viral replication and suppression of the inflammatory response after treatment with antiviral drugs. *J Infect Dis* 2007;195:665–674.

1003. Schulz O, Pichlmair A, Rehwinkel J, et al. Protein kinase R contributes to immunity against specific viruses by regulating interferon mRNA integrity. *Cell Host Microbe* 2010;7:354–361.

1004. Schwartz DA. The origins and emergence of Zika Virus, the newest TORCH infection: what's old is new again. *Arch Pathol Lab Med* 2017;141:18–25.

1005. Schwartz KL, Chan T, Rai N, et al. Zika virus infection in a pregnant Canadian traveler with congenital fetal malformations noted by ultrasonography at 14-weeks gestation. *Trop Dis Travel Med Vaccines* 2018;4:2.

1006. Seet RC, Quek AM, Lim EC. Post-infectious fatigue syndrome in dengue infection. *J Clin Virol* 2007;38:1–6.

1007. Seferovic M, Sanchez-San Martin C, Tardif SD, et al. Experimental Zika virus infection in the pregnant common marmoset induces spontaneous fetal loss and neurodevelopmental abnormalities. *Sci Rep* 2018;8:6851.

1008. Sejvar JJ. The long-term outcomes of human West Nile virus infection. *Clin Infect Dis* 2007;44:1617–1624.

1009. Sejvar JJ, Bode AV, Marfin AA, et al. West Nile Virus-associated flaccid paralysis outcome. *Emerg Infect Dis* 2006;12:514–516.

1010. Sejvar JJ, Haddad MB, Tierney BC, et al. Neurologic manifestations and outcome of West Nile virus infection. *JAMA* 2003;290:511–515.

1011. Sejvar JJ, Lindsey NP, Campbell GL. Primary causes of death in reported cases of fatal West Nile fever, United States, 2002–2006. *Vector Borne Zoonotic Dis* 2011;11(2):161–164. doi:10.1089/vbz.2009.0086.

1012. Selye H. Mast cells and necrosis. *Science* 1966;152:1371–1372.

1013. Sevvana M, Long F, Miller AS, et al. Refinement and analysis of the mature Zika virus cryo-EM structure at 3.1 a resolution. *Structure* 2018;26:1169–1177, e1163.

1014. Shan C, Muruato AE, Jagger BW, et al. A single-dose live-attenuated vaccine prevents Zika virus infection, pregnancy transmission, and testis damage. *Nat Commun* 2017;8(1):676.

1015. Shan C, Muruato AE, Jagger BW, et al. A single-dose live-attenuated vaccine prevents Zika virus pregnancy transmission and testis damage. *Nat Commun* 2017;8:676.

1016. Shan C, Muruato AE, Nunes BTD, et al. A live-attenuated Zika virus vaccine candidate induces sterilizing immunity in mouse models. *Nat Med* 2017;23:763–767.

1017. Shang Z, Song H, Shi Y, et al. Crystal structure of the capsid protein from Zika virus. *J Mol Biol* 2018;430:948–962.

1018. Shapiro-Mendoza CK, Rice ME, Galang RR, et al. Pregnancy outcomes after maternal Zika virus infection during pregnancy—U.S. territories, January 1, 2016-April 25, 2017. *MMWR Morb Mortal Wkly Rep* 2017;66:615–621.

1019. Sharma S, Singh SK, Kakkar K, et al. Analysis of TLR4 (Asp299Gly and Thr399Ile) gene polymorphisms and mRNA level in patients with dengue infection: a case-control study. *Infect Genet Evol* 2016;43:412–417.

1020. Shen WF, Galula JU, Liu JH, et al. Epitope resurfacing on dengue virus-like particle vaccine preparation to induce broad neutralizing antibody. *Elife* 2018;7.

1021. Shirato K, Kimura T, Mizutani T, et al. Different chemokine expression in lethal and non-lethal murine West Nile virus infection. *J Med Virol* 2004;74:507–513.

1022. Shresta S, Kyle JL, Robert Beatty P, et al. Early activation of natural killer and B cells in response to primary dengue virus infection in A/J mice. *Virology* 2004;319:262–273.

1023. Shresta S, Kyle JL, Snider HM, et al. Interferon-dependent immunity is essential for resistance to primary dengue virus infection in mice, whereas T- and B-cell-dependent immunity are less critical. *J Virol* 2004;78:2701–2710.

1024. Shresta S, Sharar KL, Prigozhin DM, et al. Murine model for dengue virus-induced lethal disease with increased vascular permeability. *J Virol* 2006;80:10208–10217.

1025. Shresta S, Sharar KL, Prigozhin DM, et al. Critical roles for both STAT1-dependent and STAT1-independent pathways in the control of primary dengue virus infection in mice. *J Immunol* 2005;175:3946–3954.

1026. Shrestha B, Diamond MS. The role of CD8+ T cells in the control of West Nile virus infection. *J Virol* 2004;78:8312–8321.

1027. Shrestha B, Diamond MS. Fas Ligand interactions contribute to CD8+ T cell-mediated control of West Nile virus infection in the central nervous system. *J Virol* 2007;81:11749–11757.

1028. Shrestha B, Gottlieb DI, Diamond MS. Infection and injury of neurons by West Nile Encephalitis virus. *J Virol* 2003;77:13203–13213.

1029. Shrestha B, Samuel MA, Diamond MS. CD8+ T cells require perforin to clear West Nile virus from infected neurons. *J Virol* 2006;80:119–129.

1030. Shrestha B, Wang T, Samuel MA, et al. Gamma interferon plays a crucial early antiviral role in protection against West Nile virus infection. *J Virol* 2006;80:5338–5348.

1031. Shrestha B, Zhang B, Purtha WE, et al. Tumor necrosis factor alpha protects against lethal West Nile virus infection by promoting trafficking of mononuclear leukocytes into the central nervous system. *J Virol* 2008;82:8956–8964.

1032. Siddharthan V, Van Wettere AJ, Li R, et al. Zika virus infection of adult and fetal STAT2 knock-out hamsters. *Virology* 2017;507:89–95.

1033. Siddharthan V, Wang H, Motter NE, et al. Persistent west nile virus associated with a neurological sequela in hamsters identified by motor unit number estimation. *J Virol* 2009;83:4251–4261.

1034. Siegal FP, Kadowaki N, Shodell M, et al. The nature of the principal type 1 interferon-producing cells in human blood. *Science* 1999;284:1835–1837.

1035. Siemann DN, Strange DP, Maharaj PN, et al. Zika virus infects human Sertoli cells and modulates the integrity of the in vitro Blood-Testis Barrier Model. *J Virol* 2017;91.

1036. Siirin MT, Travassos da Rosa AP, Newman P, et al. Evaluation of the efficacy of a recombinant subunit West Nile vaccine in Syrian golden hamsters. *Am J Trop Med Hyg* 2008;79:955–962.

1037. Silva MC, Guerrero-Plata A, Gilfoy FD, et al. Differential activation of human monocyte-derived and plasmacytoid dendritic cells by West Nile virus generated in different host cells. *J Virol* 2007;81:13640–13648.

1038. Simmons CP, Chau TN, Thuy TT, et al. Maternal antibody and viral factors in the pathogenesis of dengue virus in infants. *J Infect Dis* 2007;196:416–424.

1039. Singapore Zika Study G. Outbreak of Zika virus infection in Singapore: an epidemiological, entomological, virological, and clinical analysis. *Lancet Infect Dis* 2017;17:813–821.

1040. Singla M, Kar M, Sethi T, et al. Immune response to dengue virus infection in pediatric patients in New Delhi, India—association of viremia, inflammatory mediators and monocytes with disease severity. *PLoS Negl Trop Dis* 2016;10:e0004497.

1041. Sirohi D, Chen Z, Sun L, et al. The 3.8 A resolution cryo-EM structure of Zika virus. *Science* 2016;352:467–470.

1042. Sirois PA, Pridjian G, McRae S, et al. Developmental outcomes in young children born to mothers with West Nile illness during pregnancy. *Birth Defects Res A Clin Mol Teratol* 2014;100:792–796.

1043. Sitati E, Diamond MS. CD4+ T Cell responses are required for clearance of West Nile Virus from the central nervous system. *J Virol* 2006;80:12060–12069.

1044. Slon Campos JL, Mongkolsapaya J, Screaton GR. The immune response against flaviviruses. *Nat Immunol* 2018;19:1189–1198.

1045. Slonchak A, Khromykh AA. Subgenomic flaviviral RNAs: what do we know after the first decade of research. *Antiviral Res* 2018;159:13–25.

1046. Smith SA, de Alwis AR, Kose N, et al. The potent and broadly neutralizing human dengue virus-specific monoclonal antibody 1C19 reveals a unique cross-reactive epitope on the bc loop of domain II of the envelope protein. *MBio* 2013;4:e00873–00813.

1047. Smith SA, Nivarthi UK, de Alwis R, et al. Dengue virus prM-specific human monoclonal antibodies with virus replication-enhancing properties recognize a single immunodominant antigenic site. *J Virol* 2016;90:780–789.

1048. Smithburn KC, Hughes TP, Burke AW, et al. A neurotropic virus isolated from the blood of a native of Uganda. *Am J Trop Med Hyg* 1940;20:471–492.

1049. Sohn YM, Park MS, Rho HO, et al. Primary and booster immune responses to SA14-14–2 Japanese encephalitis vaccine in Korean infants. *Vaccine* 1999;17:2259–2264.

1050. Solomon T, Dung NM, Kneen R, et al. Japanese encephalitis. *J Neurol Neurosurg Psychiatry* 2000;68:405–415.

1051. Solomon T, Dung NM, Vaughn DW, et al. Neurological manifestations of dengue infection. *Lancet* 2000;355:1053–1059.

1052. Solomon T, Dung NM, Wills B, et al. Interferon alfa-2a in Japanese encephalitis: a randomised double-blind placebo-controlled trial. *Lancet* 2003;361:821–826.

1053. Solomon T, Kneen R, Dung NM, et al. Poliomyelitis-like illness due to Japanese encephalitis virus. *Lancet* 1998;351:1094–1097.

1054. Solomon T, Ni H, Beasley DW, et al. Origin and evolution of Japanese encephalitis virus in southeast Asia. *J Virol* 2003;77:3091–3098.

1055. Song R, Guan S, Lee SS, et al. Late or Lack of Vaccination linked to importation of yellow fever from Angola to China. *Emerg Infect Dis* 2018;24.

1056. Soto-Acosta R, Xie X, Shan C, et al. Fragile X mental retardation protein is a Zika virus restriction factor that is antagonized by subgenomic flaviviral RNA. *Elife* 2018;7.

1057. Spector SL, Tauraso NM. Yellow fever virus. II. Factors affecting the plaque neutralization test. *Appl Microbiol* 1969;18:736–743.

1058. Sridhar S, Luedtke A, Langevin E, et al. Effect of dengue serostatus on dengue vaccine safety and efficacy. *N Engl J Med* 2018;379:327–340.

1059. St John AL, Rathore AP, Raghavan B, et al. Contributions of mast cells and vasoactive products, leukotrienes and chymase, to dengue virus-induced vascular leakage. *Elife* 2013;2:e00481.

1060. St John AL, Rathore AP, Yap H, et al. Immune surveillance by mast cells during dengue infection promotes natural killer (NK) and NKT-cell recruitment and viral clearance. *Proc Natl Acad Sci U S A* 2011;108(22):9190–9195. doi:1105079108 [pii] 10.1073/pnas.1105079108.

1061. Stadler K, Allison SL, Schalich J, et al. Proteolytic activation of tick-borne encephalitis virus by furin. *J Virol* 1997;71:8475–8481.

1062. Stancek D. The role of interferon in tick-borne encephalitis virus-infected L cells. IV. Origin of insusceptibility of persistently infected L cells to the action of exogenous interferon. *Acta Virol* 1965;9:409–415.

1063. Staples JE, Gershman M, Fischer M. Yellow fever vaccine: recommendations of the Advisory Committee on Immunization Practices (ACIP). *MMWR Recomm Rep* 2010;59:1–27.

1064. Staples JE, Monath TP. Yellow fever: 100 years of discovery. *JAMA* 2008;300:960–962.

1065. Steele CR, Oppenheim DE, Hayday AC. Gamma (delta) T cells: non-classical ligands for non-classical cells. *Curr Biol* 2000;10:R282–R285.

1066. Stein DA, Huang CY, Silengo S, et al. Treatment of AG129 mice with antisense morpholino oligomers increases survival time following challenge with dengue 2 virus. *J Antimicrob Chemother* 2008;62:555–565.

1067. Steinbrink K, Mahnke K, Grabbe S, et al. Myeloid dendritic cell: from sentinel of immunity to key player of peripheral tolerance? *Hum Immunol* 2009;70:289–293.

1068. Stetson DB, Medzhitov R. Type I interferons in host defense. *Immunity* 2006;25:373–381.

1069. Stettler K, Beltramello M, Espinosa DA, et al. Specificity, cross-reactivity, and function of antibodies elicited by Zika virus infection. *Science* 2016;353:823–826.

1070. Stiasny K, Brandler S, Kossl C, et al. Probing the flavivirus membrane fusion mechanism by using monoclonal antibodies. *J Virol* 2007;81:11526–11531.

1071. Stiasny K, Kiermayr S, Holzmann H, et al. Cryptic properties of a cluster of dominant flavivirus cross-reactive antigenic sites. *J Virol* 2006;80:9557–9568.

1072. Stoermer KA, Morrison TE. Complement and viral pathogenesis. *Virology* 2011;411:362–373.

1073. Stokes A, Bauer JH, Hudson NP. The transmission of yellow fever to macacus rhesus. *J Am Med Assoc* 1928;90:253–254.

1074. Stokes A, Bauer JH, Hudson JH. Transmission of yellow fever to Macacus rhesus, preliminary note. *JAMA* 1928;90:253–254.

1075. Stollar V, Thomas VL. An agent in the Aedes aegypti cell line (Peleg) which causes fusion of Aedes albopictus cells. *Virology* 1975;64:367–377.

1076. Styer LM, Bernard KA, Kramer LD. Enhanced early West Nile virus infection in young chickens infected by mosquito bite: effect of viral dose. *Am J Trop Med Hyg* 2006;75:337–345.

1077. Styer LM, Lim PY, Louie KL, et al. Mosquito saliva causes enhancement of West Nile virus infection in mice. *J Virol* 2011;85:1517–1527.

1078. Sukupolvi-Petty S, Austin SK, Engle M, et al. Structure and function analysis of therapeutic monoclonal antibodies against dengue virus type 2. *J Virol* 2010;84:9227–9239.

1079. Sukupolvi-Petty S, Austin SK, Purtha WE, et al. Type- and subcomplex-specific neutralizing antibodies against domain III of dengue virus type 2 envelope protein recognize adjacent epitopes. *J Virol* 2007;81:12816–12826.

1080. Sultana H, Foellmer HG, Neelakanta G, et al. Fusion loop peptide of the West Nile virus envelope protein is essential for pathogenesis and is recognized by a therapeutic cross-reactive human monoclonal antibody. *J Immunol* 2009;183:650–660.

1081. Sumathy K, Kulkarni B, Gondu RK, et al. Protective efficacy of Zika vaccine in AG129 mouse model. *Sci Rep* 2017;7:46375.

1082. Sun DS, Chang YC, Lien TS, et al. Endothelial cell sensitization by death receptor fractions of an anti-dengue nonstructural protein 1 antibody induced plasma leakage, coagulopathy, and mortality in mice. *J Immunol* 2015;195:2743–2753.

1083. Sun P, Fernandez S, Marovich MA, et al. Functional characterization of ex vivo blood myeloid and plasmacytoid dendritic cells after infection with dengue virus. *Virology* 2009;383:207–215.

1084. Sun DS, King CC, Huang HS, et al. Antiplatelet autoantibodies elicited by dengue virus non-structural protein 1 cause thrombocytopenia and mortality in mice. *J Thromb Haemost* 2007;5:2291–2299.

1085. Suss J. Epidemiology and ecology of TBE relevant to the production of effective vaccines. *Vaccine* 2003;21(Suppl 1):S19–S35.

1086. Suss J. Tick-borne encephalitis in Europe and beyond—the epidemiological situation as of 2007. *Euro Surveill* 2008;13.

1087. Suthar MS, Brassil MM, Blahnik G, et al Infectious clones of novel lineage 1 and lineage 2 West Nile virus strains WNV-TX02 and WNV-Madagascar. *J Virol* 2012;86:7704–7709.

1088. Suthar MS, Ma DY, Thomas S, et al. IPS-1 is essential for the control of West Nile virus infection and immunity. *PLoS Pathog* 2010;6:e1000757.

1089. Suvas S, Kumaraguru U, Pack CD, et al. CD4+CD25+ T cells regulate virus-specific primary and memory CD8+ T cell responses. *J Exp Med* 2003;198:889–901.

1090. Swiecki M, Colonna M. Accumulation of plasmacytoid DC: roles in disease pathogenesis and targets for immunotherapy. *Eur J Immunol* 2010;40:2094–2098.

1091. Swiecki M, Gilfillan S, Vermi W, et al. Plasmacytoid dendritic cell ablation impacts early interferon responses and antiviral NK and CD8(+) T cell accrual. *Immunity* 2010;33:955–966.

1092. Syenina A, Jagaraj CJ, Aman SA, et al. Dengue vascular leakage is augmented by mast cell degranulation mediated by immunoglobulin Fcgamma receptors. *Elife* 2015;4.

1093. Szretter KJ, Brien JD, Thackray LB, et al. The interferon-inducible gene viperin restricts West Nile virus pathogenesis. *J Virol* 2011;85:11557–11566.

1094. Szretter KJ, Daffis S, Patel J, et al. The innate immune adaptor molecule MyD88 restricts West Nile replication and spread in neurons of the central nervous system. *J Virol* 2010;84(23):12125–12138.

1095. Szretter KJ, Daniels BP, Cho H, et al. 2'-O methylation of the viral mRNA cap by West Nile virus evades ifit1-dependent and -independent mechanisms of host restriction in vivo. *PLoS Pathog* 2012;8:e1002698.

1096. Tabata T, Petitt M, Puerta-Guardo H, et al. Zika virus targets different primary human placental cells, suggesting two routes for vertical transmission. *Cell Host Microbe* 2016;20:155–166.

1097. Tajima S, Takasaki T, Matsuno S, et al. Genetic characterization of Yokose virus, a flavivirus isolated from the bat in Japan. *Virology* 2005;332:38–44.

1098. Tan GK, Ng JK, Trasti SL, et al. A non mouse-adapted dengue virus strain as a new model of severe dengue infection in AG129 mice. *PLoS Negl Trop Dis* 2010;4:e672.

1099. Tan CH, Tan LK, Hapuarachchi HC, et al. Viral and antibody kinetics, and mosquito infectivity of an imported case of Zika fever due to Asian Genotype (American Strain) in Singapore. *Viruses* 2018;10.

1100. Tandan JB, Ohrr H, Sohn YM, et al. Single dose of SA 14–14–2 vaccine provides long-term protection against Japanese encephalitis: a case-control study in Nepalese children 5 years after immunization. drjbtandan@yahoo.com. *Vaccine* 2007;25:5041–5045.

1101. Tang H, Hammack C, Ogden SC, et al. Zika virus infects human cortical neural progenitors and attenuates their growth. *Cell Stem Cell* 2016;18:587–590.

1102. Tang Y, Liu B, Hapip CA, et al. Genetic analysis of West Nile virus isolates from US blood donors during 2002–2005. *J Clin Virol* 2008;43:292–297.

1103. Tang WW, Young MP, Mamidi A, et al. A mouse model of Zika virus sexual transmission and vaginal viral replication. *Cell Rep* 2016;17:3091–3098.

1104. Tassaneetrithep B, Burgess TH, Granelli-Piperno A, et al. DC-SIGN (CD209) mediates dengue virus infection of human dendritic cells. *J Exp Med* 2003;197:823–829.

1105. Taylor JL, Schoenherr C, Grossberg SE. Protection against Japanese encephalitis virus in mice and hamsters by treatment with carboxymethylacridanone, a potent interferon inducer. *J Infect Dis* 1980;142:394–399.

1106. Tebas P, Roberts CC, Muthumani K, et al. Safety and immunogenicity of an anti-Zika virus DNA vaccine—preliminary report. *N Engl J Med* 2017. doi:10.1056/NEJMoa1708120.

1107. Teoh EP, Kukkaro P, Teo EW, et al. The structural basis for serotype-specific neutralization of dengue virus by a human antibody. *Sci Transl Med* 2012;4:139ra183.

1108. ter Meulen J, Sakho M, Koulemou K, et al. Activation of the cytokine network and unfavorable outcome in patients with yellow fever. *J Infect Dis* 2004;190:1821–1827.

1109. Tesh RB, Arroyo J, Travassos Da Rosa AP, et al. Efficacy of killed virus vaccine, live attenuated chimeric virus vaccine, and passive immunization for prevention of West Nile virus encephalitis in hamster model. *Emerg Infect Dis* 2002;8:1392–1397.

1110. Tesh RB, Siirin M, Guzman H, et al. Persistent West Nile virus infection in the golden hamster: studies on its mechanism and possible implications for other flavivirus infections. *J Infect Dis* 2005;192:287–295.

1111. Tesh RB, Travassos da Rosa AP, Guzman H, et al. Immunization with heterologous flaviviruses protective against fatal West Nile encephalitis. *Emerg Infect Dis* 2002;8:245–251.

1112. Theiler M, Anderson CR. The relative resistance of dengue-immune monkeys to yellow fever virus. *Am J Trop Med Hyg* 1975;24:115–117.

1113. Theiler M, Smith HH. The use of yellow fever virus modified by in vitro cultivation for human immunization. *J Exp Med* 1937;65:787–800.

1114. Theiler M, Smith HH. The effect of prolonged cultivation in vitro upon the pathogenicity of yellow fever virus. *J Exp Med* 1937;65:767–786.

1115. Thein S, Aung MM, Shwe TN, et al. Risk factors in dengue shock syndrome. *Am J Trop Med Hyg* 1997;56:566–572.

1116. Theisen DJ, Davidson JT 4th, Briseno CG, et al. WDFY4 is required for cross-presentation in response to viral and tumor antigens. *Science* 2018;362:694–699.

1117. Therkelsen MD, Klose T, Vago F, et al. Flaviviruses have imperfect icosahedral symmetry. *Proc Natl Acad Sci U S A* 2018;115:11608–11612.

1118. Thiemmeca S, Tamdet C, Punyadee N, et al. Secreted NS1 protects dengue virus from mannose-binding lectin-mediated neutralization. *J Immunol* 2016;197:4053–4065.

1119. Thompson BS, Moesker B, Smit JM, et al. A therapeutic antibody against west nile virus neutralizes infection by blocking fusion within endosomes. *PLoS Pathog* 2009;5:e1000453.

1120. Throsby M, Geuijen C, Goudsmit J, et al. Isolation and characterization of human monoclonal antibodies from individuals infected with West Nile Virus. *J Virol* 2006;80:6982–6992.

1121. Tigabu B, Juelich T, Holbrook MR. Comparative analysis of immune responses to Russian spring-summer encephalitis and Omsk hemorrhagic fever viruses in mouse models. *Virology* 2010;408:57–63.

1122. Tonry JH, Xiao SY, Siirin M, et al. Persistent shedding of West Nile virus in urine of experimentally infected hamsters. *Am J Trop Med Hyg* 2005;72:320–324.

1123. Torrence PF, Gupta N, Whitney C, et al. Evaluation of synthetic oligonucleotides as inhibitors of West Nile virus replication. *Antiviral Res* 2006;70:60–65.

1124. Town T, Bai F, Wang T, et al. Toll-like receptor 7 mitigates lethal West Nile encephalitis via interleukin 23-dependent immune cell infiltration and homing. *Immunity* 2009;30:242–253.

1125. Trent DW. Antigenic characterization of flavivirus structural proteins separated by isoelectric focusing. *J Virol* 1977;22:608–618.

1126. Trent DW, Monath TP, Bowen GS, et al. Variation among strains of St. Louis encephalitis virus: basis for a genetic, pathogenetic, and epidemiologic classification. *Ann N Y Acad Sci* 1980;354:219–237.

1127. Tripathi S, Balasubramaniam VR, Brown JA, et al. A novel Zika virus mouse model reveals strain specific differences in virus pathogenesis and host inflammatory immune responses. *PLoS Pathog* 2017;13:e1006258.

1128. Troupin A, Shirley D, Londono-Renteria B, et al. A role for human skin mast cells in dengue virus infection and systemic spread. *J Immunol* 2016;197:4382–4391.

1129. Tsai TF. New initiatives for the control of Japanese encephalitis by vaccination: minutes of a WHO/CVI meeting, Bangkok, Thailand, 13–15 October 1998. *Vaccine* 2000;18 Suppl 2:1–25.

1130. Tsai YT, Chang SY, Lee CN, et al. Human TLR3 recognizes dengue virus and modulates viral replication in vitro. *Cell Microbiol* 2009;11:604–615.

1131. Tsai CY, Liong KH, Gunalan MG, et al. Type I IFNs and IL-18 regulate the antiviral response of primary human gammadelta T cells against dendritic cells infected with Dengue virus. *J Immunol* 2015;194:3890–3900.

1132. Tsai TF, Popovici F, Cernescu C, et al. West Nile encephalitis epidemic in southeastern Romania. *Lancet* 1998;352:767–771.

1133. Tsai TF, Yu YX, Jia LL, et al. Immunogenicity of live attenuated SA14–14–2 Japanese encephalitis vaccine--a comparison of 1- and 3-month immunization schedules. *J Infect Dis* 1998;177:221–223.

1134. Tsarev SA, Sanders ML, Vaughn DW, et al. Phylogenetic analysis suggests only one serotype of Japanese encephalitis virus. *Vaccine* 2000;18 Suppl 2:36–43.

1135. Turmel JM, Abgueguen P, Hubert B, et al. Late sexual transmission of Zika virus related to persistence in the semen. *Lancet* 2016;387:2501.

1136. Turtle L, Bali T, Buxton G, et al. Human T cell responses to Japanese encephalitis virus in health and disease. *J Exp Med* 2016;213:1331–1352.

1137. Twiddy SS, Holmes EC, Rambaut A. Inferring the rate and time-scale of dengue virus evolution. *Mol Biol Evol* 2003;20:122–129.

1138. Ubol S, Phuklia W, Kalayanarooj S, et al. Mechanisms of immune evasion induced by a complex of dengue virus and preexisting enhancing antibodies. *J Infect Dis* 2010;201:923–935.

1139. Upadhyay AS, Vonderstein K, Pichlmair A, et al. Viperin is an iron-sulfur protein that inhibits genome synthesis of tick-borne encephalitis virus via radical SAM domain activity. *Cell Microbiol* 2014;16:834–848.

1140. Uraki R, Hwang J, Jurado KA, et al. Zika virus causes testicular atrophy. *Sci Adv* 2017;3:e1602899.

1141. van der Schaar HM, Rust MJ, Chen C, et al. Dissecting the cell entry pathway of dengue virus by single-particle tracking in living cells. *PLoS Pathog* 2008;4:e1000244.

1142. van Kooyk Y, Geijtenbeek TB. DC-SIGN: escape mechanism for pathogens. *Nat Rev Immunol* 2003;3:697–709.

1143. van Pesch V, Lanaya H, Renauld JC, et al. Characterization of the murine alpha interferon gene family. *J Virol* 2004;78:8219–8228.

1144. Vanchiere JA, Ruiz JC, Brady AG, et al. Experimental Zika virus infection of neotropical primates. *Am J Trop Med Hyg* 2018;98:173–177.

1145. Varatharaj A. Encephalitis in the clinical spectrum of dengue infection. *Neurol India* 2010;58:585–591.

1146. Vasconcelos PF, Bryant JE, da Rosa TP, et al. Genetic divergence and dispersal of yellow fever virus, Brazil. *Emerg Infect Dis* 2004;10:1578–1584.

1147. Vasek MJ, Garber C, Dorsey D, et al. A complement-microglial axis drives synapse loss during virus-induced memory impairment. *Nature* 2016;534:538–543.

1148. Vaughn DW, Green S, Kalayanarooj S, et al. Dengue viremia titer, antibody response pattern, and virus serotype correlate with disease severity. *J Infect Dis* 2000;181:2–9.

1149. Vazquez S, Guzman MG, Guillen G, et al. Immune response to synthetic peptides of dengue prM protein. *Vaccine* 2002;20:1823–1830.

1150. Vazquez A, Sanchez-Seco MP, Ruiz S, et al. Putative new lineage of west nile virus, Spain. *Emerg Infect Dis* 2010;16:549–552.

1151. Ventura CV, Maia M, Travassos SB, et al. Risk factors associated with the ophthalmoscopic findings identified in infants with presumed Zika virus congenital infection. *JAMA Ophthalmol* 2016;134:912–918.

1152. Verma S, Kumar M, Gurjav U, et al. Reversal of West Nile virus-induced blood-brain barrier disruption and tight junction proteins degradation by matrix metalloproteinases inhibitor. *Virology* 2010;397:130–138.

1153. Verma S, Lo Y, Chapagain M, et al. West Nile virus infection modulates human brain microvascular endothelial cells tight junction proteins and cell adhesion molecules: transmigration across the in vitro blood-brain barrier. *Virology* 2009;385:425–433.

1154. Vezza AC, Rosen L, Repik P, et al. Characterization of the viral RNA species of prototype dengue viruses. *Am J Trop Med Hyg* 1980;29:643–652.

1155. Vignuzzi M, Stone JK, Arnold JJ, et al. Quasispecies diversity determines pathogenesis through cooperative interactions in a viral population. *Nature* 2006;439:344–348.

1156. Villar L, Dayan GH, Arredondo-Garcia JL, et al. Efficacy of a tetravalent dengue vaccine in children in Latin America. *N Engl J Med* 2015;372:113–123.

1157. Vithanomsat S, Wasi C, Harinasuta C, et al. The effect of interferon on flaviviruses in vitro: a preliminary study. *Southeast Asian J Trop Med Public Health* 1984;15:27–31.

1158. Vogt MR, Dowd KA, Engle M, et al. Poorly neutralizing cross-reactive antibodies against the fusion loop of West Nile virus envelope protein protect in vivo via Fcgamma receptor and complement-dependent effector mechanisms. *J Virol* 2011;85:11567–11580.

1159. von Lindern JJ, Aroner S, Barrett ND, et al. Genome analysis and phylogenetic relationships between east, central and west African isolates of Yellow fever virus. *J Gen Virol* 2006;87:895–907.

1160. Vonderstein K, Nilsson E, Hubel P, et al. Viperin targets flavivirus virulence by inducing assembly of non-infectious capsid particles. *J Virol* 2017;92(1). doi:10.1128/JVI.01751–17.

1161. Vratskikh O, Stiasny K, Zlatkovic J, et al. Dissection of antibody specificities induced by yellow fever vaccination. *PLoS Pathog* 2013;9:e1003458.

1162. Wahala WM, Donaldson EF, de Alwis R, et al. Natural strain variation and antibody neutralization of Dengue serotype 3 viruses. *PLoS Pathog* 2010;6:e1000821.

1163. Wahala WM, Huang C, Butrapet S, et al. Recombinant dengue type 2 viruses with altered e protein domain III epitopes are efficiently neutralized by human immune sera. *J Virol* 2012;86:4019–4023.

1164. Wallace MJ, Smith DW, Broom AK, et al. Antibody-dependent enhancement of Murray Valley encephalitis virus virulence in mice. *J Gen Virol* 2003;84:1723–1728.

1165. Walport MJ. Complement. Second of two parts. *N Engl J Med* 2001;344:1140–1144.

1166. Walport MJ. Complement. First of two parts. *N Engl J Med* 2001;344:1058–1066.

1167. Wang P, Arjona A, Zhang Y, et al. Caspase-12 controls West Nile virus infection via the viral RNA receptor RIG-I. *Nat Immunol* 2010;11:912–919.

1168. Wang P, Bai F, Zenewicz LA, et al. IL-22 signaling contributes to West Nile encephalitis pathogenesis. *PLoS One* 2012;7:e44153.

1169. Wang P, Dai J, Bai F, et al. Matrix metalloproteinase 9 facilitates West Nile virus entry into the brain. *J Virol* 2008;82:8978–8985.

1170. Wang T, Gao Y, Scully E, et al. Gamma delta T cells facilitate adaptive immunity against West Nile virus infection in mice. *J Immunol* 2006;177:1825–1832.

1171. Wang W, Li G, De W, et al. Zika virus infection induces host inflammatory responses by facilitating NLRP3 inflammasome assembly and interleukin-1beta secretion. *Nat Commun* 2018;9:106.

1172. Wang X, Li SH, Zhu L, et al. Near-atomic structure of Japanese encephalitis virus reveals critical determinants of virulence and stability. *Nat Commun* 2017;8:14.

1173. Wang WK, Lin SR, Lee CM, et al. Dengue type 3 virus in plasma is a population of closely related genomes: quasispecies. *J Virol* 2002;76:4662–4665.

1174. Wang JP, Liu P, Latz E, et al. Flavivirus activation of plasmacytoid dendritic cells delineates key elements of TLR7 signaling beyond endosomal recognition. *J Immunol* 2006;177:7114–7121.

1175. Wang Y, Lobigs M, Lee E, et al. CD8+ T cells mediate recovery and immunopathology in West Nile virus encephalitis. *J Virol* 2003;77:13323–13334.

1176. Wang E, Ni H, Xu R, et al. Evolutionary relationships of endemic/epidemic and sylvatic dengue viruses. *J Virol* 2000;74:3227–3234.

1177. Wang T, Scully E, Yin Z, et al. IFN-g-producing gd T cells help control murine West Nile virus infection. *J Immunol* 2003;171:2524–2531.

1178. Wang TT, Sewatanon J, Memoli MJ, et al. IgG antibodies to dengue enhanced for FcgammaRIIIA binding determine disease severity. *Science* 2017;355:395–398.

1179. Wang H, Siddharthan V, Hall JO, et al. West Nile virus preferentially transports along motor neuron axons after sciatic nerve injection of hamsters. *J Neurovirol* 2009;15:293–299.

1180. Wang T, Town T, Alexopoulou L, et al. Toll-like receptor 3 mediates West Nile virus entry into the brain causing lethal encephalitis. *Nat Med* 2004;10:1366–1373.

1181. Wang ZY, Wang Z, Zhen ZD, et al. Axl is not an indispensable factor for Zika virus infection in mice. *J Gen Virol* 2017;98:2061–2068.

1182. Wang E, Weaver SC, Shope RE, et al. Genetic variation in yellow fever virus: duplication in the 3' noncoding region of strains from Africa. *Virology* 1996;225:274–281.

1183. Wang S, Welte T, McGargill M, et al. Drak2 contributes to West Nile virus entry into the brain and lethal encephalitis. *J Immunol* 2008;181:2084–2091.

1184. Wasay M, Channa R, Jumani M, et al. Encephalitis and myelitis associated with dengue viral infection clinical and neuroimaging features. *Clin Neurol Neurosurg* 2008;110:635–640.

1185. Way JH, Bowen ET, Platt GS. Comparative studies of some African arboviruses in cell culture and in mice. *J Gen Virol* 1976;30:123–130.

1186. Weaver SC, Vasilakis N. Molecular evolution of dengue viruses: contributions of phylogenetics to understanding the history and epidemiology of the preeminent arboviral disease. *Infect Genet Evol* 2009;9:523–540.

1187. Webster LT. Inheritance of resistance of mice to enteric bacterial and neurotropic virus infections. *J Exp Med* 1937;65:261–286.

1188. Webster LT. Japanese B encephalitis virus: its differentiation from St. Louis encephalitis virus and relationship to louping Ill virus. *J Exp Med* 1938;67:609–618.

1189. Weiskopf D, Angelo MA, de Azeredo EL, et al. Comprehensive analysis of dengue virus-specific responses supports an HLA-linked protective role for CD8+ T cells. *Proc Natl Acad Sci U S A* 2013;110:E2046–E2053.

1190. Weiskopf D, Bangs DJ, Sidney J, et al. Dengue virus infection elicits highly polarized CX3CR1+ cytotoxic CD4+ T cells associated with protective immunity. *Proc Natl Acad Sci U S A* 2015;112:E4256–E4263.

1191. Weiskopf D, Sette A. T-cell immunity to infection with dengue virus in humans. *Front Immunol* 2014;5:93.

1192. Weissman D. mRNA transcript therapy. *Expert Rev Vaccines* 2015;14:265–281.

1193. Welsch S, Miller S, Romero-Brey I, et al. Composition and three-dimensional architecture of the dengue virus replication and assembly sites. *Cell Host Microbe* 2009;5:365–375.

1194. Welte T, Lamb J, Anderson JF, et al. Role of two distinct gammadelta T cell subsets during West Nile virus infection. *FEMS Immunol Med Microbiol* 2008;53:275–283.

1195. Welte T, Reagan K, Fang H, et al. Toll-like receptor 7-induced immune response to cutaneous West Nile virus infection. *J Gen Virol* 2009;90:2660–2668.

1196. Wen J, Elong Ngono A, Regla-Nava JA, et al. Dengue virus-reactive CD8(+) T cells mediate cross-protection against subsequent Zika virus challenge. *Nat Commun* 2017;8:1459.

1197. Werme K, Wigerius M, Johansson M. Tick-borne encephalitis virus NS5 associates with membrane protein scribble and impairs interferon-stimulated JAK-STAT signalling. *Cell Microbiol* 2008;10:696–712.

1198. White GS, Symmes K, Sun P, et al. Reemergence of St. Louis encephalitis virus, California, 2015. *Emerg Infect Dis* 2016;22:2185–2188.

1199. Whitehead SS. Development of TV003/TV005, a single dose, highly immunogenic live attenuated dengue vaccine; what makes this vaccine different from the Sanofi-Pasteur CYD vaccine? *Expert Rev Vaccines* 2016;15:509–517.

1200. Wichgers Schreur PJ, van Keulen L, Anjema D, et al. Microencephaly in fetal piglets following in utero inoculation of Zika virus. *Emerg Microbes Infect* 2018;7:42.

1201. Widman DG, Ishikawa T, Giavedoni LD, et al. Evaluation of RepliVAX WN, a single-cycle flavivirus vaccine, in a non-human primate model of West Nile virus infection. *Am J Trop Med Hyg* 2010;82:1160–1167.

1202. Widman DG, Ishikawa T, Winkelmann ER, et al. RepliVAX WN, a single-cycle flavivirus vaccine to prevent West Nile disease, elicits durable protective immunity in hamsters. *Vaccine* 2009;27:5550–5553.

1203. Wikan N, Smith DR. Zika virus: history of a newly emerging arbovirus. *Lancet Infect Dis* 2016;16:e119–e126.

1204. Wilder-Smith A, Schwartz E. Dengue in travelers. *N Engl J Med* 2005;353:924–932.

1205. Williams KL, Sukupolvi-Petty S, Beltramello M, et al. Therapeutic efficacy of antibodies lacking Fcgamma receptor binding against lethal dengue virus infection is due to neutralizing potency and blocking of enhancing antibodies [corrected]. *PLoS Pathog* 2013;9:e1003157.

1206. Wittermann C, Petri E, Zent O. Long-term persistence of tick-borne encephalitis antibodies in children 5 years after first booster vaccination with Encepur Children. *Vaccine* 2009;27:1585–1588.

1207. Witz J, Brown F. Structural dynamics, an intrinsic property of viral capsids. *Arch Virol* 2001;146:2263–2274.

1208. Wolf RF, Papin JF, Hines-Boykin R, et al. Baboon model for West Nile virus infection and vaccine evaluation. *Virology* 2006;355:44–51.

1209. Wu MF, Chen ST, Yang AH, et al. CLEC5A is critical for dengue virus-induced inflammasome activation in human macrophages. *Blood* 2013;121:95–106.

1210. Wu SJ, Grouard-Vogel G, Sun W, et al. Human skin Langerhans cells are targets of dengue virus infection. *Nat Med* 2000;6:816–820.

1211. Wu SJ, Hayes CG, Dubois DR, et al. Evaluation of the severe combined immunodeficient (SCID) mouse as an animal model for dengue viral infection. *Am J Trop Med Hyg* 1995;52:468–476.

1212. Wu X, Lu L, Guzman H, et al. Persistent infection and associated nucleotide changes of West Nile virus serially passaged in hamsters. *J Gen Virol* 2008;89:3073–3079.

1213. Xia H, Luo H, Shan C, et al. An evolutionary NS1 mutation enhances Zika virus evasion of host interferon induction. *Nat Commun* 2018;9:414.

1214. Xiao SY, Guzman H, Zhang H, et al. West Nile virus infection in the golden hamster (Mesocricetus auratus): a model for West Nile encephalitis. *Emerg Infect Dis* 2001;7:714–721.

1215. Xiao SY, Zhang H, Guzman H, et al. Experimental Yellow fever virus infection in the Golden Hamster (Mesocricetus auratus). II. Pathology. *J Infect Dis* 2001;183:1437–1444.

1216. Xie G, Luo H, Pang L, et al. Dysregulation of Toll-Like receptor 7 compromises innate and adaptive T cell responses and host resistance to an attenuated West Nile virus infection in old mice. *J Virol* 2016;90:1333–1344.

1217. Xie X, Yang Y, Muruato AE, et al. Understanding Zika virus stability and developing a Chimeric vaccine through functional analysis. *MBio* 2017;8.

1218. Xin YY, Ming ZG, Peng GY, et al. Safety of a live-attenuated Japanese encephalitis virus vaccine (SA14–14–2) for children. *Am J Trop Med Hyg* 1988;39:214–217.

1219. Xu K, Song Y, Dai L, et al. Recombinant chimpanzee adenovirus vaccine AdC7-M/E protects against Zika virus infection and testis damage. *J Virol* 2018;92.

1220. Yadav PD, Malhotra B, Sapkal G, et al. Zika virus outbreak in Rajasthan, India in 2018 was caused by a virus endemic to Asia. *Infect Genet Evol* 2019;69:199–202.

1221. Yamanaka A, Kosugi S, Konishi E. Infection-enhancing and -neutralizing activities of mouse monoclonal antibodies against dengue type 2 and 4 viruses are controlled by complement levels. *J Virol* 2008;82:927–937.

1222. Yang X, Qi J, Peng R, et al. Molecular basis of a protective/neutralizing monoclonal antibody targeting envelope proteins of both tick-borne encephalitis virus and louping ill virus. *J Virol* 2019;93(8). doi:10.1128/JVI.02132–18.

1223. Yauch LE, Prestwood TR, May MM, et al. CD4+ T cells are not required for the induction of dengue virus-specific CD8+ T cell or antibody responses but contribute to protection after vaccination. *J Immunol* 2010;185:5405–5416.

1224. Yauch LE, Shresta S. Mouse models of dengue virus infection and disease. *Antiviral Res* 2008;80:87–93.

1225. Yauch LE, Zellweger RM, Kotturi MF, et al. A protective role for dengue virus-specific CD8+ T cells. *J Immunol* 2009;182:4865–4873.

1226. Yewdell JW, Taylor A, Yellen A, et al. Mutations in or near the fusion peptide of the influenza virus hemagglutinin affect an antigenic site in the globular region. *J Virol* 1993;67:933–942.

1227. Yi G, Xu X, Abraham S, et al. A DNA vaccine protects human immune cells against Zika virus infection in humanized mice. *EBioMedicine* 2017;25:87–94.

1228. Yockey LJ, Jurado KA, Arora N, et al. Type I interferons instigate fetal demise after Zika virus infection. *Sci Immunol* 2018;3.

1229. Yockey LJ, Varela L, Rakib T, et al. vaginal exposure to Zika Virus during pregnancy leads to fetal brain infection. *Cell* 2016;166:1247–1256, e1244.

1230. You F, Wang P, Yang L, et al. ELF4 is critical for induction of type I interferon and the host antiviral response. *Nat Immunol* 2013;14:1237–1246.

1231. Young PR, Hilditch PA, Bletchly C, et al. An antigen capture enzyme-linked immunosorbent assay reveals high levels of the dengue virus protein NS1 in the sera of infected patients. *J Clin Microbiol* 2000;38:1053–1057.

1232. Yu CY, Chang TH, Liang JJ, et al. Dengue virus targets the adaptor protein MITA to subvert host innate immunity. *PLoS Pathog* 2012;8:e1002780.

1233. Yu L, Wang R, Gao F, et al. Delineating antibody recognition against Zika virus during natural infection. *JCI Insight* 2017;2.

1234. Yu IM, Zhang W, Holdaway HA, et al. Structure of the immature dengue virus at low pH primes proteolytic maturation. *Science* 2008;319:1834–1837.

1235. Yuan L, Huang XY, Liu ZY, et al. A single mutation in the prM protein of Zika virus contributes to fetal microcephaly. *Science* 2017;358:933–936.

1236. Zanluca C, Melo VC, Mosimann AL, et al. First report of autochthonous transmission of Zika virus in Brazil. *Mem Inst Oswaldo Cruz* 2015;110:569–572.

1237. Zanotto PM, Gao GF, Gritsun T, et al. An arbovirus cline across the northern hemisphere. *Virology* 1995;210:152–159.

1238. Zanotto PM, Gould EA, Gao GF, et al. Population dynamics of flaviviruses revealed by molecular phylogenies. *Proc Natl Acad Sci U S A* 1996;93:548–553.

1239. Zellweger RM, Eddy WE, Tang WW, et al. CD8+ T cells prevent antigen-induced antibody-dependent enhancement of dengue disease in mice. *J Immunol* 2014;193:4117–4124.

1240. Zellweger RM, Prestwood TR, Shresta S. Enhanced infection of liver sinusoidal endothelial cells in a mouse model of antibody-induced severe dengue disease. *Cell Host Microbe* 2010;7:128–139.

1241. Zellweger RM, Shresta S. Mouse models to study dengue virus immunology and pathogenesis. *Front Immunol* 2014;5:151.

1242. Zeman P. Cyclic patterns in the central European tick-borne encephalitis incidence series. *Epidemiol Infect* 2017;145:358–367.

1243. Zhang B, Chan YK, Lu B, et al. CXCR3 mediates region-specific antiviral T cell trafficking within the central nervous system during West Nile virus encephalitis. *J Immunol* 2008;180:2641–2649.

1244. Zhang W, Chipman PR, Corver J, et al. Visualization of membrane protein domains by cryo-electron microscopy of dengue virus. *Nat Struct Biol* 2003;10:907–912.

1245. Zhang Y, Corver J, Chipman PR, et al. Structures of immature flavivirus particles. *EMBO J* 2003;22:2604–2613.

1246. Zhang M, Daniel S, Huang Y, et al. Anti-West Nile virus activity of in vitro expanded human primary natural killer cells. *BMC Immunol* 2010;11:3.

1247. Zhang X, Ge P, Yu X, et al. Cryo-EM structure of the mature dengue virus at 3.5-A resolution. *Nat Struct Mol Biol* 2013;20:105–110.

1248. Zhang Y, Kaufmann B, Chipman PR, et al. Structure of immature West Nile virus. *J Virol* 2007;81:6141–6145.

1249. Zhang X, Sheng J, Plevka P, et al. Dengue structure differs at the temperatures of its human and mosquito hosts. *Proc Natl Acad Sci U S A* 2013;110:6795–6799.

1250. Zhang NN, Zhang L, Deng YQ, et al. Zika virus infection in Tupaia belangeri causes dermatological manifestations and confers protection against secondary infection. *J Virol* 2019;93(8). doi:10.1128/JVI.01982–18.

1251. Zhao H, Fernandez E, Dowd KA, et al. Structural basis of Zika virus-specific antibody protection. *Cell* 2016;166:1016–1027.

1252. Zheng B, Liu Q, Wu Y, et al. Zika virus elicits inflammation to evade antiviral response by cleaving cGAS via NS1-caspase-1 axis. *EMBO J* 2018;37.

1253. Zhou A, Hassel BA, Silverman RH. Expression cloning of 2–5A-dependent RNAase: a uniquely regulated mediator of interferon action. *Cell* 1993;72:753–765.

1254. Zhou A, Paranjape J, Brown TL, et al. Interferon action and apoptosis are defective in mice devoid of 2′,5′- oligoadenylate-dependent RNase L. *EMBO J* 1997;16:6355–6363.

1255. Zhu X, He Z, Yuan J, et al. IFITM3-containing exosome as a novel mediator for anti-viral response in dengue virus infection. *Cell Microbiol* 2015;17:105–118.

1256. Zilber L. Spring-summer tick-borne encephalitis (in Russian). *Arkhiv Niol Nauk* 1939;56:255–261.

1257. Zisman B, Wheelock EF, Allison AC. Role of macrophages and antibody in resistance of mice against yellow fever virus. *J Immunol* 1971;107:236–243.

1258. Zulueta A, Martin J, Hermida L, et al. Amino acid changes in the recombinant Dengue 3 Envelope domain III determine its antigenicity and immunogenicity in mice. *Virus Res* 2006;121:65–73.

1259. Zust R, Cervantes-Barragan L, Habjan M, et al. Ribose 2′-O-methylation provides a molecular signature for the distinction of self and non-self mRNA dependent on the RNA sensor Mda5. *Nat Immunol* 2011;12:137–143.

1260. Zust R, Dong H, Li XF, et al. Rational design of a live attenuated dengue vaccine: 2′-o-methyltransferase mutants are highly attenuated and immunogenic in mice and macaques. *PLoS Pathog* 2013;9:e1003521.

1261. Zust R, Li SH, Xie X, et al. Characterization of a candidate tetravalent vaccine based on 2′-O-methyltransferase mutants. *PLoS One* 2018;13:e0189262.

Coronaviridae: The Viruses and Their Replication

Stanley Perlman • Paul S. Masters

HISTORY

Coronaviruses are enveloped RNA viruses that are broadly distributed among humans, other mammals, and birds, causing acute and persistent infections. Members of this family were isolated as early as the 1930s as the causative agents of infectious bronchitis in chickens, transmissible gastroenteritis in pigs, and severe hepatitis and neurologic disease in mice. It was not until the 1960s, however, that these viruses and certain human respiratory viruses[10,285] were recognized to share characteristics that merited grouping them together. Their most notable common feature, revealed by electron microscopy, was a fringe of widely spaced, club-shaped spikes that were morphologically distinct from similar surface projections of ortho- and paramyxoviruses. The halo of spikes, giving the viral particle the appearance of the solar corona, prompted the name that was adopted for this virus group.[404]

Over the next 40 years, coronaviruses were studied mainly because they cause economically significant respiratory and gastrointestinal diseases in domestic animals and because they provide unique models for viral pathogenesis. The only two recognized human coronaviruses (HCoVs) were found to be responsible for a substantial fraction of common colds, particularly those that circulate in winter months. This situation changed dramatically in 2002 with the emergence and worldwide spread of a devastating new human disease, severe acute respiratory syndrome (SARS), which was caused by a previously unknown coronavirus.[127,222,334] Although the SARS epidemic was extinguished within a year, research stimulated by the outbreak led to great strides in our understanding of coronaviruses. By 2005, two additional, widespread human respiratory coronaviruses were discovered.[425,455] Moreover, searches for animal virus reservoirs have nearly tripled the number of identified coronaviruses and defined an entire new genus,[289,457,459] although most of the recently discovered species are known only as genomic sequences and have yet to be isolated or propagated experimentally. This increased comprehension of coronaviruses bore fruit in 2012, when another zoonotic coronavirus crossed species from camels to cause the often-fatal human disease, Middle East respiratory syndrome (MERS),[474] which currently persists on the Arabian peninsula. The etiological coronavirus, its genome sequence, and its host cell receptor were all identified within 6 months, based on knowledge gained from the SARS epidemic.

CLASSIFICATION

The coronaviruses are the largest group within the *Nidovirales* (Fig. 10.1), a taxonomic order that comprises the families *Coronaviridae*, *Arteriviridae*, *Roniviridae*, and *Mesoniviridae*. The arteriviruses[225] consist of five genera of mammalian pathogens. The roniviruses,[99] which infect shrimp, and the mosquito-borne

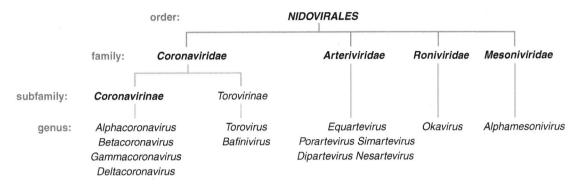

FIGURE 10.1 Taxonomy of the order *Nidovirales*.

mesoniviruses[313] are the only members of the order that have invertebrate hosts. Nidoviruses are membrane-enveloped, nonsegmented positive-strand RNA viruses that are set apart from other RNA viruses by certain distinctive characteristics.[152] Their most significant common features are (a) an invariant general genomic organization, with a very large replicase gene upstream of the structural protein genes; (b) the expression of the replicase–transcriptase polyprotein by means of ribosomal frameshifting; (c) a collection of unique enzymatic activities contained within the replicase–transcriptase protein products; and (d) the expression of downstream genes via transcription of multiple 3′-nested subgenomic mRNAs. It should be noted that the replicative similarities among the four nidovirus families are offset by marked differences in the numbers, types, and sizes of their structural proteins and great variation among the morphologies of their virions and nucleocapsids.

Coronaviruses are classified as one of two subfamilies (*Coronavirinae*) in the family *Coronaviridae* (Fig. 10.1). The other subfamily, *Torovirinae*, contains the toroviruses, which are pathogens of cattle, horses, and swine,[398] and the bafiniviruses, the only nidoviruses currently known to infect fish.[375] This chapter will concentrate almost exclusively on the *Coronavirinae*.

Coronaviruses were originally divided into three serological groups. More recently they have been arranged into four genera: the alpha-, beta-, gamma- and deltacoronaviruses (Fig. 10.1). This sorting is based on rooted phylogenetic clustering and pairwise evolutionary distances in seven key domains of the replicase–transcriptase polyprotein.[106,152,188] Within a genus, viruses are classified as the same species if they share more than 90% amino acid sequence identity in the conserved replicase domains. As a consequence, some viruses historically considered to be separate species are currently recognized as a single species, for example, alphacoronavirus 1 or betacoronavirus 1 (Table 10.1).

Although they have tremendous potential for interspecies transmission, coronaviruses are generally confined to a single

TABLE 10.1	Classification of coronaviruses	
Species[a]	**GenBank Accession[b]**	**Viruses Included Within Species**
Genus *Alphacoronavirus*		
Alphacoronavirus 1	AJ271965	Transmissible gastroenteritis virus (TGEV)
	EU186072	Feline coronavirus type I (FCoV-I)
	AY994055	Feline infectious peritonitis virus (FIPV)
	GQ477367	Canine coronavirus (CCoV)
Human coronavirus 229E (HCoV-229E)	AF304460	
Human coronavirus NL63 (HCoV-NL63)	AY567487	
Porcine epidemic diarrhea virus (PEDV)	AF353511	
Mink coronavirus 1 (MCoV 1)	HM245925	
Wénchéng shrew virus (WESV)	KY967735	
Lucheng Rn rat coronavirus (LRNV)	KF294380	
Rhinolophus bat coronavirus HKU2 (*Rh*-BatCoV HKU2)	EF203067	
Scotophilus bat coronavirus 512 (*Sc*-BatCoV 512)	DQ648858	
Miniopterus bat coronavirus 1 (*Mi*-BatCoV 1)	EU420138	
Miniopterus bat coronavirus HKU8 (*Mi*-BatCoV HKU8)	EU420139	
Bat coronavirus HKU10 (BatCoV HKU10)	JQ989266	
Bat coronavirus CDPHE15 (BatCoV CDPHE15)	KF430219	

(continued)

TABLE 10.1   Classification of coronaviruses *(Continued)*

Species[a]	GenBank Accession[b]	Viruses Included Within Species
Genus *Betacoronavirus*		
Betacoronavirus 1	U00735	Bovine coronavirus (BCoV)
	EF446615	Equine coronavirus (EqCoV)
	AY903460	Human coronavirus OC43 (HCoV-OC43)
	DQ011855	Porcine hemagglutinating encephalomyelitis virus (PHEV)
	KF906249	Dromedary camel coronavirus HKU23 (DcCoV HKU23)
Murine coronavirus	AY700211	Mouse hepatitis virus (MHV)
	FJ938068	Rat coronavirus (RCoV)
Human coronavirus HKU1 (HCoV-HKU1)	AY597011	
Severe acute respiratory syndrome–related coronavirus (SARSr-CoV)	AY278741	Human SARS coronavirus (SARS-CoV)
	DQ071615	SARS-related *Rhinolophus* bat coronavirus Rp3 (SARSr-*Rh*-BatCoV Rp3)
Middle East respiratory syndrome–related coronavirus (MERS-CoV)	JX869059	
Hedgehog coronavirus (EriCoV)	KC545383	
Tylonycteris bat coronavirus HKU4 (*Ty*-BatCoV HKU4)	EF065505	
Pipistrellus bat coronavirus HKU5 (*Pi*-BatCoV HKU5)	EF065509	
Rousettus bat coronavirus HKU9 (*Ro*-BatCoV HKU9)	EF065513	
Genus *Gammacoronavirus*		
Avian coronavirus	AJ311317	Infectious bronchitis virus (IBV)
	EU022526	Turkey coronavirus (TuCoV)
Cetacean coronavirus	EU111742	Beluga whale coronavirus SW1 (BWCoV SW1)
	KF793824	Bottlenose dolphin coronavirus HKU22 (BdCoV HKU22)
Genus *Deltacoronavirus*		
Porcine deltacoronavirus (PDCoV)	JQ065042	
Munia coronavirus HKU13 (MuCoV HKU13)	FJ376622	
Bulbul coronavirus HKU11 (BuCoV HKU11)	FJ376620	
Thrush coronavirus HKU12 (ThCoV HKU12)	FJ376621	
White-eye coronavirus HKU16 (WECoV HKU16)	JQ065044	
Common-moorhen coronavirus HKU21 (CMCoV HKU21)	JQ065049	
Widgeon coronavirus HKU20 (WiCoV HKU20)	JQ065048	
Night heron coronavirus HKU19 (NHCoV HKU19)	JQ065047	

[a]Only viruses for which there are complete genome sequences are listed.
[b]Representative GenBank accession numbers are given; in most cases, multiple genomic sequences for a given virus are available.

host or a small set of related hosts. The alpha- and betacoronaviruses almost exclusively infect mammals. In contrast, the gamma- and deltacoronaviruses, with few exceptions, have avian hosts. Many of the viruses listed in Table 10.1 have been studied for decades, specifically those included in the species alphacoronavirus 1, betacoronavirus 1, murine coronavirus, and avian coronavirus. The focus of research on these viruses came about largely because they were amenable to isolation and growth in tissue culture.

However, since 2004, molecular surveillance and metagenomics efforts initiated in the wake of the SARS epidemic have led to the discovery of a multitude of previously unknown coronaviruses in a variety of hosts. Notably, most of the newly recognized species were identified in bats, which form one of the largest orders of mammals. Diverse alpha- and betacoronaviruses have been described in bats from every continent except Antarctica; these viruses include the likely immediate predecessors of SARS-CoV,[179,287] as well as more distant relatives of ancestors of other HCoVs.[92,94,272] Birds have also proven to be a rich source of novel coronaviruses that are so highly divergent as to constitute a separate genus—the deltacoronaviruses.[238,457] It has been proposed that bats and birds are ideally suited as reservoirs for the incubation, spread, and evolution of coronaviruses, owing to their common ability to fly and their propensity to roost and flock.[456]

Six of the viruses in Table 10.1 are associated with human disease. The most categorically harmful of these, SARS-CoV, is not currently present in the human population but has the unabated potential to reemerge from animal sources. By contrast, MERS-CoV, which is discussed at length later in this chapter, continues to cause human infections with an alarmingly high case fatality rate. To date, however, this virus has remained geographically confined and has not evolved the high ability that SARS-CoV had for human-to-human transmission. The remaining four HCoVs, the alphacoronaviruses HCoV-229E and HCoV-NL63 and the betacoronaviruses HCoV-OC43 and HCoV-HKU1, typically cause common colds. Remarkably, HCoV-NL63 and HCoV-HKU1 were discovered in the post-SARS era,[425,455] despite the fact that each was subsequently found to be prevalent worldwide and to have been in circulation for a long time. Although generally associated with upper respiratory tract (URT) infections, the four endemic HCoVs can cause lower respiratory tract infections and have more serious consequences in the young, the elderly, and immunocompromised individuals.

VIRION STRUCTURE

Virus and Nucleocapsid

Virions of coronaviruses are roughly spherical and moderately pleomorphic. In early investigations, viral particles were reported to have average diameters of 80 to 120 nm but ranged from extremes of 50 to 200 nm.[284] Some of the variation in particle size and shape was likely attributable to distortions introduced by virion purification or negative staining of samples for electron microscopy. The characteristic spikes of coronaviruses, typically described as club-like or petal-shaped, were seen to emerge from the virion surface as stalks with bulb-like distal termini. More recent studies, employing cryoelectron microscopy and cryoelectron tomography,[28,36,307,310] have produced images, such as those shown in Figure 10.2A, in which virion size and shape were observed to be far more regular, although still pleomorphic. These studies, which examined a number of alpha- and betacoronaviruses, converge on mean particle diameters of 118 to 136 nm, including the contributions of the spikes, which protrude some 16 to 21 nm from the virion envelope.

Enclosed within the virion envelope is the nucleocapsid, a ribonucleoprotein containing the viral genome. The structure of this component is relatively obscure in whole virions, but its makeup can be discerned in some electron micrographs of virions spontaneously disrupted or solubilized with nonionic detergents.[57,104,144,205,277] Such studies revealed another distinguishing characteristic of coronaviruses: they have helically symmetric nucleocapsids. While helical symmetry is the rule for nucleocapsids of negative-strand RNA viruses, it is highly unusual for positive-strand RNA animal viruses, almost all of which have icosahedral capsids. The best-resolved images of a coronavirus nucleocapsid, that of HCoV-229E, showed filamentous structures with a diameter of 9 to 13 nm and a 3- to 4-nm-wide central canal[57]; these filaments were noted to be narrower and less sharply segmented than paramyxovirus nucleocapsids. However, varying and sometimes discrepant parameters have been reported for the nucleocapsids of other coronaviruses,[281] emphasizing the need for much further work to clearly define the dimensions, symmetry, and protein–RNA stoichiometry of this virion component in isolation. More recent coronavirus ultrastructural studies suggest that, when packaged within the virion envelope, the helical nucleocapsid is quite flexible, forming coils and other structures that fold back on themselves.[28,307]

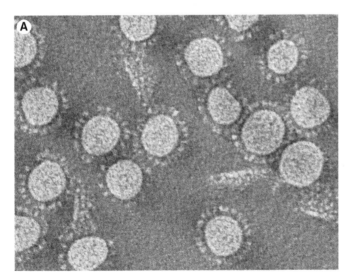
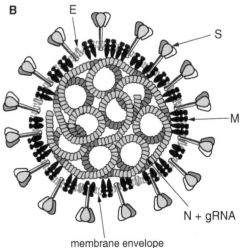

FIGURE 10.2 Coronavirus structure. A: Cryoelectron tomographic image of purified virions of mouse hepatitis virus (MHV), reconstructed as described in Neuman BW, Kiss G, Kunding AH, et al. A structural analysis of M protein in coronavirus assembly and morphology. *J Struct Biol* 2011;174:11–22. (Image provided by Benjamin Neuman, David Bhella, and Stanley Sawicki.) **B:** Schematic showing the major structural proteins of the coronavirus virion: S, spike protein; M, membrane protein; E, envelope protein; and N, nucleocapsid protein.

Virion Structural Proteins

Coronaviruses contain a canonical set of four major structural proteins: the spike (S), membrane (M), and envelope (E) proteins, all of which are located in the membrane envelope, and the nucleocapsid (N) protein, which is found in the ribonucleoprotein core (Fig. 10.2B).

The distinctive surface spikes of coronaviruses are composed of trimers of S molecules[36,119] that bind to host cell receptors and mediate the earliest steps of infection.[86] In some cases, S protein can also induce cell–cell fusion late in infection. S is a class I viral fusion protein,[46] in common with several RNA virus spike proteins, of which the influenza HA protein is the best-studied example.[168] The S monomer is a transmembrane protein containing a very large ectodomain and a tiny endodomain. Its mass ranges from 126 to 168 kDa, with glycosylation increasing this by some 40 kDa. The roughly equal-sized amino-terminal and carboxy-terminal subunits of the molecule are denoted S1 and S2, respectively (Fig. 10.3). S1 subunits display extremely low sequence homology across the four genera and often diverge considerably among different isolates of a single species.[326,441] By contrast, S2 subunits are more highly conserved.[107] High-resolution cryoelectron microscopic (EM) structures have recently been determined for the S protein ectodomains of at least one representative virus from each genus: SARS-CoV (Fig. 10.3),[473] MHV,[436] HCoV-HKU1,[214] HCoV-NL63,[437] MERS-CoV,[473] PDCoV,[379,465] and IBV.[380] These exhibit a remarkable unity in their architecture. S ectodomains extend 130 to 160 Å in length, from the base at the membrane envelope to the top of the spike. Viewed from above, the S trimer has a triangular cross section, tapering from a diameter of 115 to 140 Å at the membrane-distal head to 50 to 70 Å at the membrane-proximal base. In the S protein trimer, the S1 subunits make up the

bulbous, receptor-binding portion of the spike. Despite the high amino acid sequence variability of S1, all of the bulb structures are quite similar. S1 subunits each consist of an amino-terminal and a carboxy-terminal domain (NTD and CTD), as well as one to three smaller subdomains at differing locations. S1 NTDs have a fold like that of galectins, a family of cellular β-galactoside–binding proteins. Particular variations in the packing arrangements of S1 NTDs and CTDs within the trimer suggest that alpha- and deltacoronavirus S proteins are more closely related to each other than to other S proteins[379,465]; likewise, the beta- and gammacoronavirus S proteins bear more of a resemblance to each other than to S proteins of the other two genera.[380] The S2 subunit trimers constitute the narrower stalk of the spike, distancing the bulb from the membrane. S2 structures are highly similar across all four genera and are principally composed of multiple long α-helices, including those within two heptad repeat regions (HR1 and HR2).

During synthesis, the S protein is inserted, via a cleaved signal peptide,[59] into the endoplasmic reticulum (ER), where it becomes modified by N-linked glycosylation.[175,363] Comprehensive mapping of glycosylation sites has been carried out for the S proteins of HCoV-NL63[437] and PDCoV,[465] revealing that N-linked glycans occupy nearly all of the consensus NXS/T sites in the S1 and S2 subunits. The early steps of glycosylation occur cotranslationally, and this alteration assists monomer folding and proper oligomerization; terminal glycosylation is then completed subsequent to trimerization.[119] The shield formed by glycans covers a significant fraction of the surface of the S trimer and may mask epitopes, thereby contributing to evasion of immune surveillance.[437] S protein monomer folding is also accompanied by the formation of intrasubunit disulfide bonds among a subset of the cysteine residues of the

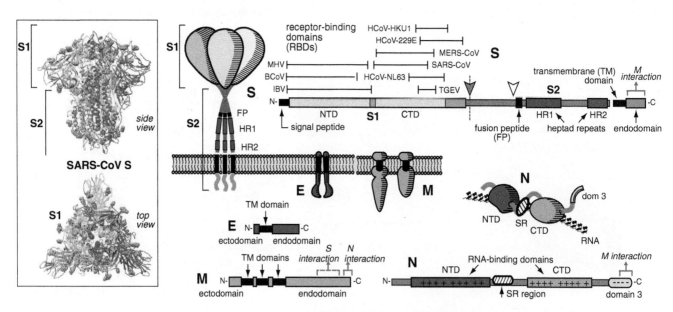

FIGURE 10.3 Virion structural proteins. Folded and linear representations of the spike (S), membrane (M), envelope (E), and nucleocapsid (N) proteins. Also shown (*boxed*) are side and top views of a cryo-EM model of the SARS-CoV S protein ectodomain. (From Yuan Y, Cao D, Zhang Y, et al. Cryo-EM structures of MERS-CoV and SARS-CoV spike glycoproteins reveal the dynamic receptor binding domains. *Nat Commun* 2017;8:15092.) In the model, each S monomer is colored differently; *blue spheres* represent N-linked glycans. The size scale for the linear diagram of S is half of that for the other proteins. In the linear diagram of S, *solid* and *open arrowheads* indicate the S1/S2 and S2′ cleavage sites, respectively. In the linear diagrams S, M, and N, *red brackets* indicate mapped regions involved in assembly interactions (see *Assembly and Release of Virions*)

ectodomain.[321] Most of the disulfide linkages have been mapped for the S trimer structures of MHV[436] and PDCoV.[465]

In many coronaviruses, the S protein is partially or completely cleaved by a furin-like host cell protease,[59,275] separating the S1 and S2 subunits (Fig. 10.3). This cleavage is a late event in virion assembly and release from infected cells. Another type of S protein cleavage (S2′), thought to be essential for all coronaviruses, takes place during the initiation of infection and activates the molecule for membrane fusion.[34] Generally, each type of S proteolytic processing occurs immediately downstream of a highly basic peptide motif.[290] The differing functions of S1 and S2, and the role of proteolysis, are discussed later (see *Viral Entry and Uncoating*).

The most abundant structural protein in coronaviruses, the M protein,[405] gives the virion envelope its shape. The M monomer, which ranges from 25 to 30 kDa, is a polytopic membrane protein that is embedded in the envelope by three transmembrane domains.[174,362] At its amino terminus is a very small ectodomain; the carboxy-terminal endodomain of M accounts for the major part of the molecule and is situated in the interior of the virion or on the cytoplasmic face of intracellular membranes (Fig. 10.3). Although it is inserted cotranslationally into the ER membrane, the M protein generally does not bear an amino-terminal signal peptide.[59,362] For IBV and MHV, it was found that either the first or the third transmembrane domain of M alone sufficed as a signal for insertion and anchoring of the protein in its native membrane orientation.[174,267,276] Anomalously, M proteins of the alphacoronavirus 1 species do contain cleavable amino-terminal signal peptides, but it is not clear whether these are necessary for membrane insertion.[201] The ectodomain of M is modified by glycosylation, which is usually N-linked.[174,195,300] However, a subset of betacoronavirus M proteins, and possibly some deltacoronavirus M proteins, exhibit O-linked glycosylation.[111] Glycosylation of M has been shown to influence both organ tropism and the interferon (IFN)-inducing capacity of certain coronaviruses.[109,240]

M proteins are moderately well conserved within each coronavirus genus, but they diverge considerably across genera. The most variable part of the molecule is the ectodomain. By contrast, a 22–amino acid endodomain segment immediately downstream of the third transmembrane domain exhibits a high degree of sequence conservation. As yet, the M protein has been refractory to crystallization, but cryo-EM and tomographic reconstructions have provided a glimpse of the structure of this protein within the virion envelope.[28,307,310] These studies reveal that the large carboxy terminus of M extends some 6 to 8 nm into the viral particle and is compressed into a globular domain, consistent with early work showing that the endodomain is very resistant to proteases.[58,362] The observed M structures are likely to be dimers, the monomers of which are associated through multiple interacting regions. M dimers appear to adopt two different conformations: a compact form that promotes greater membrane curvature and a more elongated form that contacts the nucleocapsid.[310]

The E protein is a small polypeptide, of 8 to 12 kDa, that is found in limited amounts in the virion envelope.[174,281] Despite its minor presence, no wild-type coronavirus has been discovered to lack this protein. Engineered knockout or deletion of the E gene has effects ranging from moderate,[115] to severe,[228,232] to lethal.[7,322] Thus, although E is not always essential, it is critical for coronavirus infectivity (see *Assembly and*

Release of Virions). E proteins have widely divergent sequences, but all share a common architecture: a short hydrophilic amino terminus, followed by a large hydrophobic region and, lastly, a large hydrophilic carboxy-terminal tail (Fig. 10.3). E is an integral membrane protein, but it does not have a cleavable signal peptide and is not glycosylated.[96,174,432] Beta- and gammacoronavirus E proteins have been shown to be palmitoylated on cysteine residues downstream and adjacent to the hydrophobic region.[44,97,268] The membrane topology of E is not completely resolved.[97,174,364,432] Most evidence indicates that this polypeptide transits the membrane once, with an amino-terminal exodomain and a carboxy-terminal endodomain. Contrary to this are reports that E has a hairpin conformation, with both termini on the cytoplasmic face of membranes, or that E can have multiple membrane topologies. E protein has been observed to assemble into homo-oligomers, ranging from dimers through hexamers,[174,452] and a pentameric α-helical bundle structure has been solved for the hydrophobic region of SARS-CoV E.[339] Oligomerization is consistent with the ion channel activity of this protein, but the monomeric form of E may also play a separate role[446] (see *Assembly and Release of Virions*).

Residing in the interior of the virion, the N protein is the sole protein constituent of the helical nucleocapsid.[174] Monomers of this 38- to 52-kDa protein bind along the RNA genome in a beads-on-a-string configuration common to other helical viral nucleocapsids (Fig. 10.2B). However, unlike the nucleoproteins of rhabdo- and paramyxoviruses, the coronavirus N protein provides little or no protection for its genome against the action of ribonucleases.[277,304] The bulk of the N protein monomer is made up of two independently folding domains, which are called the N-terminal domain (NTD) and the C-terminal domain (CTD), although neither includes its respective terminus of the N molecule (Fig. 10.3). With the exception of a highly conserved stretch of 30 amino acids within the NTD,[282] there is only a moderate degree of primary sequence homology among N proteins across all genera. However, high structural homology is evident among the crystal or solution structures that have been determined for the NTDs and CTDs of multiple coronaviruses.[68,73,137,157] Flanking the NTD and CTD are three spacer segments, the central one of which contains a serine- and arginine-rich tract (the SR region). The remaining functionally distinct region of N, the carboxy-terminal domain 3, has been defined genetically.[186,219] The spacer segments and domain 3 are each likely to be intrinsically disordered polypeptides.[68,69] Most of the N molecule, including the NTD and CTD, is highly basic; by contrast, domain 3 is acidic.

The N protein is a phosphoprotein,[174] modified at a limited number of serine and threonine residues. Phosphorylation sites have been mapped for TGEV, IBV, and MHV (representing three of the four genera), and collectively, targeted sites can fall in any domain or spacer region of the N molecule.[51,74,447] Thus, a general pattern for N protein phosphorylation cannot yet be discerned, nor have all responsible kinases been identified, although there is evidence linking glycogen synthase kinase-3 to phosphorylation of the SR region of MHV N.[460] The role of phosphorylation is not clearly established, but it has long been thought to have regulatory impact. Phosphorylation has been suggested to trigger a conformational change in N protein,[402] and it may modulate RNA-binding affinity, transcription elongation, or N oligomerization.[68,460]

The most salient function of the N protein is to bind to viral RNA. Nucleocapsid formation must involve both sequence-specific and nonspecific modes of RNA binding. Specific RNA substrates that have been identified for N protein include the transcription-regulating sequence (TRS)[157,281] (see *Viral RNA Synthesis*), polyadenylate,[421] and the genomic RNA packaging signal (PS)[87,293] (see *Assembly and Release of Virions*). The NTD and the CTD are each separately capable of binding to RNA ligands *in vitro*, and the (unbound) structures of these domains offer some clues as to how this is accomplished. The NTD consists of a U-shaped β-platform with an extruding β-hairpin, which presents a putative RNA-binding groove rich in basic and aromatic amino acid residues.[68,137,157] The tightly interconnected CTD dimer forms a rectangular slab, one face of which exhibits a potential RNA-binding groove lined by basic α-helices.[68,73] Some work suggests that, in the intact N protein, optimal RNA binding requires concerted contributions from both the NTD and the CTD, as well as other regions of the molecule.[69,184] In addition to RNA binding, a significant component of nucleocapsid stability results from interactions among N monomers.[304] A major part of this is generally attributed to dimerization and higher-order oligomerization of the CTD,[67,68,137] but additional regions of N–N association have been mapped to the NTD and to domain 3.[89,137,184] Another crucial interaction of the N protein is to bind to M protein.[136,405] This capability is provided by the carboxy-terminal domain 3 of N.[186,231,433]

A fifth prominent structural protein, the hemagglutinin–esterase (HE) protein, is found only in lineage A betacoronaviruses, which include MHV, BCoV, HCoV-OC43, and HCoV-HKU1. In virions of these species, HE forms a secondary set of short projections, of some 5 to 10 nm, arrayed beneath the canopy of S protein spikes.[105,162] The 48-kDa HE monomer is made up almost entirely of an amino-terminal ectodomain, which acquires an additional 17 kDa of N-linked glycosylation during synthesis. The mature protein is a disulfide-linked homodimer.[173] As its name indicates, the HE protein is a hemagglutinin; that is, it is able to bind to sialic acid moieties found on cell-surface glycoproteins and glycolipids.[105] Further, HE possesses acetylesterase activity, specific for either 9-O- or 4-O-acetylated sialic acids. These characteristics are thought to allow HE to act as a cofactor for S protein, assisting attachment of virus to host cells, as well as expediting the travel of virus through the extracellular mucosa. Consistent with this notion, the presence of HE in MHV dramatically enhances neurovirulence in the mouse host.[203] Conversely, in HCoV-OC43, which had a relatively recent zoonotic origin, the hemagglutinin activity of HE was lost by counterselection as the virus evolved to accommodate the sialoglycan composition of the human respiratory tract.[26] The two activities of the HE protein are strikingly similar to the receptor-binding and receptor-destroying activities found in influenza C virus. Remarkably, the coronavirus HE gene is clearly related to the influenza C virus HEF gene.[273] Moreover, toroviruses also possess a homolog of the HE gene,[95] raising the possibility that all three of these virus groups evolved from a common ancestor.[273,394] This kinship is further corroborated by the crystal structure of the BCoV HE protein, which reveals separate receptor-binding and acetylesterase domains perched atop a truncated membrane-proximal region.[476] The coronavirus HE protein thus resembles a squat version of its influenza virus counterpart.

GENOME STRUCTURE AND ORGANIZATION

Basic and Accessory Genes

The coronavirus genome, which ranges from 25 to 32 kb, is among the largest of those of all RNA viruses, including RNA viruses that have segmented genomes. This exceptional RNA molecule acts in at least three capacities[152]: as the initial mRNA of the infectious cycle (see *Expression of the Replicase–Transcriptase Complex*), as the template for RNA replication and transcription (see *Viral RNA Synthesis*), and as the substrate for packaging into progeny viruses (see *Assembly and Release of Virions*). Consistent with its role as an mRNA, the coronavirus genome has a canonical eukaryotic 5′-terminal cap 1 structure and a 3′ polyadenylate tail.[153] The genome comprises a basic set of genes in the invariant order 5′-replicase-S-E-M-N-3′, with the huge replicase gene occupying two-thirds of the available coding capacity (Fig. 10.4). The replicase–transcriptase is the only protein translated from the genome; the products of all downstream open reading frames (ORFs) are derived from subgenomic mRNAs. The 5′-most position of the replicase gene is dictated by the requirement for expression of the replicase to set in motion all subsequent events of infection. The organization of the other basic genes, however, does not seem to reflect any underlying principle, since engineered rearrangement of the downstream gene order is completely tolerated.[113]

Dispersed among the basic genes, there are from one to as many as eight additional ORFs, designated accessory genes, which tend to be specific to various lineages within each genus[281,303] (Fig. 10.4). These can fall in any of the intergenic intervals downstream of the replicase gene,[456] except, curiously, never between the E and M genes. In some cases, an accessory gene can be partially or entirely embedded as an alternate reading frame within another gene, for example, the internal (I) gene of MHV or the 3b gene of SARS-CoV. By convention, accessory genes are numbered according to the smallest transcript in which they fall. Consequently, there is usually no relatedness among identically named accessory genes in coronaviruses of different genera, for example, the 3a genes of SARS-CoV, FCoV, and IBV (Fig. 10.4). Some of these extra ORFs are thought to have been acquired through ancestral recombination with RNA from host or heterologous viral sources. The HE gene is the best supported example of this type of horizontal gene transfer.[273] Two other such candidates are the 2a gene found in MHV and HCoV-OC43, which encodes a 2′,5′-phosphodiesterase,[151] and gene 10 of beluga whale coronavirus, which encodes a putative uridine–cytidine kinase.[289] Notably, the 2a protein is structurally and functionally homologous to the MERS-CoV 4b protein,[416] to a module of the torovirus replicase,[394] and to the mouse AKAP7 protein.[151] This strongly suggests that the ancestral 2a gene was captured from a host mRNA. The origins of most accessory genes, however, remain an open question, as most have no identifiable orthologs in protein databases. Some others have ORFs with multiple disruptions and are likely to be relics of genes lost during evolution.

Almost all intact accessory genes that have been examined are expressed during infection, although the functions of only a handful are well resolved. The protein products of most accessory genes are nonstructural, but the HE protein is a clear

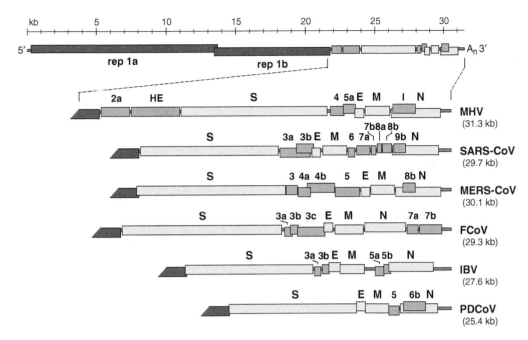

FIGURE 10.4 Coronavirus genome organization. A schematic of the entire genome of MHV is shown at the top. The replicase gene constitutes two ORFs, rep 1a and rep 1b, which are expressed by a ribosomal frame-shifting mechanism (see *Expression of the Replicase–Transcriptase Complex*). The expanded region shows the downstream genes of three betacoronaviruses (MHV, SARS-CoV, and MERS-CoV), an alphacoronavirus (FCoV), a gammacoronavirus (IBV), and a deltacoronavirus (PDCoV). The total genome size is given for each virus. The sizes and positions of accessory genes are indicated, relative to the basic genes S, E, M, and N.

exception to this rule,[173] and a few other accessory proteins have been shown to be components of virions.[303] Mutational knockout or deletion of accessory genes has not yet revealed any that are essential for viral replication in tissue culture. Conversely, accessory gene ablation,[101,110,203] or transfer to another virus,[411] can have profound effects on viral pathogenesis. In some cases, the basis for this is understood to result from interactions with host defenses, particularly innate immune mechanisms (see *Immune Response and Viral Evasion of the Immune Response*). For other accessory genes, though, potential *in vivo* functions have not been elucidated.

Coronavirus Genetics

Classical coronavirus genetics focused principally on two types of mutants: first, naturally arising viral isolates, particularly deletion mutants, which offered clues to the genetic basis of different pathogenic traits, and second, temperature-sensitive mutants isolated from MHV by chemical mutagenesis.[235] Some of the latter proved valuable in analyses of the functions of structural proteins.[219,274,282] However, owing to the large target size of the replicase gene, the majority of such randomly generated mutants had conditional–lethal, RNA-negative phenotypes. These are currently sorted into five complementation groups, yielding one approach to examining the multiplicity of functions encompassed by the viral replicase–transcriptase.[29,371,403]

The development of coronavirus reverse genetics proceeded in two phases.[120] Initially, a method called targeted RNA recombination was devised at a time when it was uncertain whether the construction of full-length infectious cDNA clones of coronavirus genomes would become technically feasible. With this scheme, a synthetic donor RNA bearing mutations of interest

is transfected into cells that have been infected with a recipient parent virus possessing some characteristic that can be selected against.[219] In its current form, for manipulation of MHV, the technique uses a chimeric recipient parent virus designated fMHV. The fMHV chimera is a mutant of MHV that contains the S protein ectodomain from feline infectious peritonitis virus (FIPV), a feline coronavirus, and can therefore only grow in feline cells (see *Virion Attachment to Host Cells*). The restoration of its ability to grow in murine cells, via recombination with donor RNA containing the MHV S gene, enables a powerful selection for viruses bearing site-specific mutations.[227,283] Analogous chimeras have been generated for construction of recombinants of FIPV, IBV, and PEDV. However, the utility of targeted RNA recombination is restricted to the 3′ third of the genome.

To obtain access to the coronavirus replicase gene, it was necessary to create full-length cDNAs. Three innovative strategies were developed to overcome the inherent barriers presented by the huge size of the replicase gene and the high instability of its various regions when propagated in bacterial clones.[9,120] In the first strategy, a full-length cDNA copy of a coronavirus genome is assembled downstream of the CMV promoter in a bacterial artificial chromosome (BAC) vector, which is stable by virtue of its low copy number.[8] The BAC can be manipulated by standard cloning techniques or, more recently, by λ phage–based homologous recombination in bacteria[140] or homologous recombination in yeast.[316] Viral infection is then launched from transfected BAC DNA, through transcription of infectious coronavirus RNA by host RNA polymerase II. This method of initiating infection obviates potential limitations of *in vitro* capping and synthesis of genomic RNA. In the second strategy, a full-length genomic cDNA is assembled by *in vitro* ligation of smaller cloned cDNA fragments, some of the boundaries of which have been chosen so as to interrupt regions of instability.[120,471] The ligation occurs in a directed order that is dictated by the use of asymmetric restriction sites. Infectious genomic RNA is then transcribed *in vitro* and used to transfect susceptible host cells. An extension of this method has demonstrated the construction entirely from synthetic cDNAs of the genome for a hypothetical progenitor of an extant coronavirus.[33] In the third strategy, the genome of vaccinia virus is used as the cloning vector for a full-length coronavirus cDNA that is generated by long-range RT-PCR.[415] The cDNA is then amenable to manipulation by the repertoire of techniques available for poxvirus reverse genetics.[9] Infections are launched from *in vitro*–synthesized RNA or, alternatively, from transfected cDNA transcribed *in vivo* by T7 RNA polymerase encoded by fowlpox helper virus.[54] Collectively, these systems developed for complete reverse genetics have provided an essential pathway toward unraveling the complexities of the coronavirus replicase.

CORONAVIRUS REPLICATION

Virion Attachment to Host Cells

Coronavirus infection is initiated by virion binding to a cellular receptor (Fig. 10.5). There then follows a series of events culminating in the delivery of the nucleocapsid to the cytoplasm, where the viral genome becomes available for translation. Individual coronaviruses usually infect only one or a few closely related hosts. The interaction between the viral S protein and its cognate receptor constitutes the principal determinant governing coronavirus host species range and tissue tropism.

This has been most convincingly shown in two ways. First, the expression of a particular receptor in nonpermissive cells of a heterologous species renders those cells permissive for the corresponding coronavirus.[117,130,253,258,355,420,442,470] Second, the engineered replacement of the S protein ectodomain changes the host cell species specificity or tissue tropism of a coronavirus in a predictable fashion.[165,227,341,368,424] The more variable subunit, S1, is the part of the spike protein that binds to receptor. Binding leads to large conformational changes, mediated by the more conserved S2 subunit, that result in the fusion of virion and cell membranes. The region of S1 that contacts the receptor, the receptor-binding domain (RBD), has been mapped to the CTD of S1 for SARS-CoV,[453] MERS-CoV,[270,443] HCoV-HKU1,[352] HCoV-NL63,[262] TGEV,[147] and HCoV-229E.[40] By contrast, the RBD for MHV maps to the NTD of its S1 subunit[224]; this galectin-like domain of S1 is often reserved by other coronaviruses for binding to carbohydrate attachment factors.[249,335,348] The RBD is usually found in a "lying" state, buried in the S trimer structure, and it must undergo a transition to a "standing" state to become accessible to the receptor.[380,473] It is not yet clear what governs this conformational change.

The known cellular receptors for coronaviruses are listed in Table 10.2. The MHV receptor, mCEACAM1, was the first discovered coronavirus receptor (as well as one of the first receptors defined for *any* virus).[450,451] That this molecule is the only biologically relevant receptor for MHV was made clear by the demonstration that homozygous *Ceacam1*[−/−] knockout mice are totally resistant to infection by high doses of MHV.[170] CEACAM1 is a member of the carcinoembryonic antigen (CEA) family within the immunoglobulin (Ig) superfamily, and, in its full-length form, CEACAM1 contains four Ig-like domains.[130] A diversity of two– and four–Ig domain

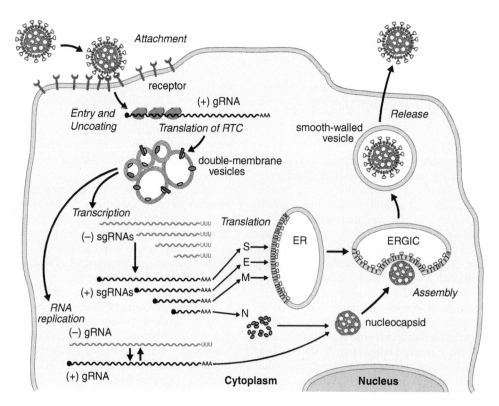

FIGURE 10.5 Overview of coronavirus replication (see text for details).

TABLE 10.2 Coronavirus receptors

Virus[a]	Receptor	References
Alphacoronaviruses		
TGEV	Porcine aminopeptidase N[b] (pAPN)	117
PRCoV	Porcine aminopeptidase N (pAPN)	118
PEDV	(Unknown, but *not* pAPN)	386,257
FCoV-II, FIPV	Feline aminopeptidase N (fAPN)	420
FCoV-I	(Unknown, but *not* fAPN)	131
CCoV	Canine aminopeptidase N (cAPN)	35
HCoV-229E	Human aminopeptidase N (hAPN)	470
HCoV-NL63	Angiotensin-converting enzyme 2 (ACE2)	172
Betacoronaviruses		
MHV	Murine carcinoembryonic antigen–related adhesion molecule 1 (mCEACAM1)	450
BCoV	*N*-Acetyl-9-*O*-acetylneuraminic acid[e]	374
HCoV-OC43	*N*-Acetyl-9-*O*-acetylneuraminic acid[e]	226
SARS-CoV	Angiotensin-converting enzyme 2 (ACE2)[c]	258
MERS-CoV	Dipeptidyl peptidase 4 (DPP4)[d]	355
Gammacoronaviruses		
IBV	Alpha-2,3-linked sialic acid[e]	348
Deltacoronaviruses		
PDCoV	Porcine aminopeptidase N (pAPN)	253,442

[a]All virus abbreviations are as given in Table 10.1.
[b]Mammalian aminopeptidase N is also known as CD13.
[c]Human CD209L (L-SIGN), a lectin family member, can also act as a receptor for SARS-CoV but with much lower efficiency than ACE2.[197]
[d]DPP4 is also known as CD26.
[e]It is not yet known whether BCoV, HCoV-OC43, and IBV also have protein receptors.

isoforms are generated by multiple alleles and alternative splicing variants of *Ceacam1*.[129] The wide range of pathogenicity of MHV in mice is thus thought to be strongly affected by the interactions of S proteins of different virus strains with the array of receptor isoforms that are expressed in mice of different genetic backgrounds.[408] The solved structure of the MHV RBD-mCEACAM1 complex has allowed the identification of key residues at the S protein–receptor interface and has also revealed why the closely related S protein of BCoV cannot bind the MHV receptor.[248]

Many alphacoronaviruses and one deltacoronavirus use aminopeptidase N (APN) of their respective hosts as a receptor (Table 10.2).[117,118,253,420,442,470] APN (also called CD13) is a cell-surface, zinc-binding protease that is resident in respiratory and enteric epithelia and in neural tissue. The APN molecule is a heavily glycosylated homodimer. In general, the alphacoronavirus receptor activities of APN homologs are not interchangeable among species.[35,116] In line with this specificity, structures

of RBD–APN complexes show that PRCoV and HCoV-229E have evolved to bind to different sites on pAPN and hAPN, respectively.[35,357,454] By contrast, the deltacoronavirus PDCoV is able to exploit as a receptor APN homologs from multiple mammalian and avian species.[253] This suggests that the S protein of this virus recognizes highly conserved determinants on APN, in accord with its postulated recent switch from an avian to a mammalian host.

The receptor for SARS-CoV, angiotensin-converting enzyme 2 (ACE2), was rapidly discovered following the isolation of the virus.[258] ACE2 is a cell-surface, zinc-binding carboxypeptidase involved in regulation of cardiac function and blood pressure. It is expressed in epithelial cells of the lung and the small intestine, the primary targets of SARS-CoV, as well as in heart, kidney, and other tissues. The crystal structure of the SARS-CoV S protein RBD in complex with ACE2 shows the RBD cradling one lobe of the claw-like catalytic domain of its receptor.[248,255] The cryo-EM structure of the complete S trimer bound to ACE2 indicates that receptor binding induces a conformational change in the RBD and may trigger the release of S1 subunits from S2 subunits.[396] Remarkably, ACE2 also serves as the receptor for the alphacoronavirus HCoV-NL63,[172] and the corresponding structural complex for that virus reveals that the HCoV-NL63 RBD binds to the very same motifs of ACE2 as are contacted by the SARS-CoV RBD.[248] Since the SARS-CoV and HCoV-NL63 RBDs have neither sequence nor structural homology, this finding strongly supports the notion that they have independently evolved to bind to the same hot spot on the ACE2 surface. Analysis of the SARS-CoV RBD–ACE2 interface and structure-guided mutational investigations demonstrated the basis for the final jump of SARS-CoV from palm civets to human hosts (see *Epidemiology*). These studies found that mutation of merely two key RBD residues facilitated civet-to-human transmission and subsequent human-to-human transmission.[248]

Shortly following the isolation of MERS-CoV, its receptor was found to be dipeptidyl peptidase 4 (DPP4, also called CD26).[355] DPP4 is a membrane-bound exoprotease with a wide tissue distribution; it cleaves dipeptides from hormones, chemokines, and cytokines and carries out multiple other physiological functions. The DPP4 molecule comprises a carboxy-terminal catalytic domain and an amino-terminal eight-blade β-propeller domain. The structure of the MERS-CoV RBD–DPP4 complex shows that the interacting surface of the RBD is a four-stranded β-sheet that contacts blades 4 and 5 of the DPP4 propeller domain.[248,270] Notably, critical residues in this region of the receptor are well conserved between DPP4 of humans and camels, the source of zoonotic transmission of MERS-CoV.[248] While it is intriguing that DPP4, like APN and ACE2, is a protease, catalytic site mutational analyses and inhibitor studies of all three of these molecules have shown that their enzymatic activities are not required for receptor function.[116,248,258,355]

Viral Entry and Uncoating

The entry of virions into cells results from large-scale rearrangements of the S protein that lead to the fusion of viral and cellular membranes.[46] Coronaviruses can enter cells either by an "early" pathway of fusion at the plasma membrane or by a "late" pathway of receptor-mediated endocytosis followed by fusion with membranes of acidified endosomes. The rearrangements of S are triggered by some combination of proteolytic cleavage, receptor binding, and possibly also exposure to acidic pH.[169,290] Upon synthesis, S protein initially folds into a stable configuration, to prevent its premature activation prior to contacting target cells. Thus, during the entry steps of infection, S requires at least one encounter with a protease in order to separate the receptor-binding and fusion components of the spike and to expose its fusion peptide. There are two main types of proteolytic cleavage of S. The first is a preliminary activation at the S1/S2 junction, which occurs in many coronaviruses but is not obligatory. This cleavage often takes place as virions exit from cells (in the previous round of infection), but it can also occur at the cell surface during receptor binding. The second type of cleavage happens at a locus (S2′) within the S2 subunit, upstream of the fusion peptide (Fig. 10.3).[34] This event can take place either at the cell surface or in endosomes. It is enhanced by prior S1/S2 cleavage and likely follows conformational changes in S that result from receptor binding. The gathering consensus is that S2′ cleavage occurs in all coronaviruses and is essential for fusion.[290] The exact assignment of the S2 fusion peptide is not agreed upon[46,290,323]; however, the best candidate is a region containing a highly conserved motif, IEDLLF, immediately downstream of the S2′ cleavage site.[291] High-resolution structures show that this putative fusion peptide is accessible on the periphery of the S trimer[214,436]; accordingly, S2′ cleavage would free its amino terminus for host cell membrane insertion.

The details of proteolytic activation are still incompletely understood but have been best studied for SARS-CoV. In most tissue culture cell types, entry of this virus is dependent upon cathepsins, which are acid-activated endosomal proteases. The infectivity of SARS-CoV, as well as many other coronaviruses, is thus suppressed by cathepsin inhibitors or by lysosomotropic agents.[388] It remains unresolved, however, whether neutralization of lysosomal pH prevents some required S protein conformational change or if its sole effect is to forestall the activation of endosomal proteases. Alternatively, cell-bound SARS-CoV can be activated by treatment with extracellular proteases, such as trypsin or elastase, greatly enhancing its infectivity and allowing the virus to enter from the cell surface.[290] This diversity of mechanisms of activation raises the question of which best reflects conditions during host infection. Recent studies suggest that for the SARS-CoV S protein, the most biologically relevant protease is TMPRSS2.[291,387] This transmembrane serine protease, which is expressed in pneumocytes, colocalizes with and binds to ACE2. In cells expressing TMPRSS2, SARS-CoV enters at the cell surface and is insensitive to cathepsin inhibitors and lysosomotropic agents. Similarly, there is evidence that "early" entry at the cell surface is also the most pertinent mechanism for initiation of MERS-CoV infection *in vivo*. In this case, it was found that TMPRSS2 is linked to the receptor DPP4 by a scaffold protein, tetraspanin CD9.[132] Likewise, TMPRSS2-dependent "early" entry appears to be the main pathway followed by clinical (rather than cell culture-adapted) isolates of HCoV-229E, HCoV-OC43, and HCoV-HKU1.[384,385]

The coronavirus S protein is a class I viral fusion protein with domains structurally and functionally homologous to those of the fusion proteins of phylogenetically distant RNA viruses, such as influenza virus, HIV, and Ebola virus, but on a much larger scale.[46,47,168,249] As in those other viral fusion proteins, the coronavirus S2 moiety contains two separated heptad repeats, HR1 and HR2, with the fusion peptide upstream of HR1 and the transmembrane domain immediately downstream of HR2 (Fig. 10.3). Conformational changes brought about by receptor binding and S2′ cleavage release the fusion peptide, allowing its insertion into the host cell membrane. Concomitant dissociation of the S1 subunit effectively unlocks the S2 trimer, triggering major rearrangements.[250] The result is an irreversible folding that brings together the heptad repeats to form a six-helix bundle, juxtaposing viral and cellular membranes in sufficient proximity to allow lipid bilayer mixing and deposition of the virion nucleocapsid into the cytoplasm. The six-helix bundle is an extremely stable, rod-like complex. Highly similar crystallographic structures for this complex from the S proteins of MHV, SARS-CoV, MERS-CoV, and HCoV-NL63 all show the three longer HR1 helices forming a central, coiled-coil core. Arrayed around this, in an antiparallel orientation, the three shorter HR2 helices pack into the grooves between the HR1 monomers via hydrophobic interactions.[249] The high-resolution cryo-EM model of the MHV postfusion S2 trimer[438] depicts a 180-Å-long cone-shaped structure (taller than the entire prefusion S1/S2 ectodomain) with the six-helix bundle at its apex. Notably, the multiple α-helices that make up HR1 and adjacent regions in each monomer of the prefusion structure[436] have refolded into unusually long single helices in the central coiled coil of the postfusion structure.

Expression of the Replicase–Transcriptase Complex

Following delivery of the viral nucleocapsid to the cytoplasm, the next event of infection is the translation of the replicase gene from genomic RNA. This gene consists of two large ORFs, rep 1a and rep 1b, which share a small region of overlap (Fig. 10.4). Translation of the entire replicase depends upon a mechanism called ribosomal frameshifting, whereby, with some probability, a translating ribosome shifts one nucleotide in the −1 direction, from the rep 1a reading frame into the rep 1b reading frame.[281] This repositioning is programmed by two RNA elements (Fig. 10.6A), embedded near the region of overlap, which were discovered in studies of IBV.[49] The first element is a heptanucleotide slippery sequence, 5′-UUUAAAC -3′, which is identical for all known coronaviruses and has apparently been selected as optimal for its role.[344] The second element, located a short distance downstream of the slippery sequence, is an extensively characterized RNA pseudoknot structure.[50] This latter component was initially thought to be a classic H-type pseudoknot, but analyses of SARS-CoV frameshifting support a more elaborate structure that includes a third stem-loop (SL) within pseudoknot loop 2.[343]

The two elements act together to produce the coterminal polyproteins pp1a and pp1ab. During most rounds of translation, the elongating ribosome unwinds the pseudoknot, and translation terminates at the rep 1a stop codon, yielding the smaller product, pp1a. In some fraction of the time, however, the pseudoknot blocks the mRNA entrance channel of the ribosome.[301] This allows the simultaneous slippage of the P- and A-site tRNAs into the rep 1b reading frame, resulting in the synthesis of pp1ab. It is not clear whether slippage is brought about by pausing required for the ribosome to melt out the mRNA structure[49] or without pausing, by mechanical deformation of the P-site tRNA.[190,301] Studies of reporter gene expression suggest that the incidence of coronaviral ribosomal frameshifting is as high as 25% to 30%[281] and an estimate of the *in vivo* frequency in infected cells accords with this high rate.[190] The role of programmed frameshifting is thought to be to provide a fixed ratio of translation products for assembly into a macromolecular complex.[344] It is also possible that frameshifting frequency is regulated to forestall expression of the enzymatic products of rep 1b until a suitable environment for RNA synthesis has been prepared by the products of rep 1a.

Polyproteins pp1a (402–502 kDa) and pp1ab (700–811 kDa) are autoproteolytically processed into mature products that are designated nsp1 to nsp16 (except in the gamma- and deltacoronaviruses, which do not have a counterpart of nsp1)[486] (Fig. 10.6B). Processing also generates many long-lived partial

proteolytic products, which may have functional importance. There are two types of polyprotein cleavage activity. One or two papain-like proteases (PLpro), which are situated within nsp3, carry out the relatively specialized separations of nsp1, nsp2, and nsp3.[288] Many PLpro also have deubiquitinase activity, which can block some host antiviral defenses. The main protease (Mpro), nsp5, performs the remaining 11 cleavage events.[15,399] Mpro is often designated the 3C-like protease (3CLpro) to point out its distant relationship to the 3C proteins of picornaviruses. Because of their pivotal roles early in infection, PLpro and Mpro present attractive targets for antiviral drug design.[288,467]

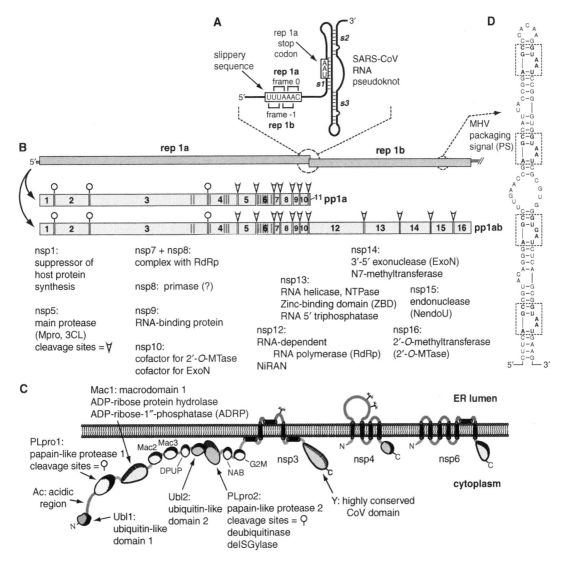

FIGURE 10.6 Coronavirus replicase gene and protein products. A: Ribosomal frameshifting elements of the SARS-CoV replicase gene.[343] Pseudoknot stems are indicated as s1, s2, and s3. **B:** Polyprotein pp1a and pp1ab processing scheme for alpha- and betacoronaviruses. The gammacoronavirus processing scheme is identical, except for the absence of nsp1. Known functions and properties of nsp1 to nsp16 are listed; nsp11 is an oligopeptide generated when ribosomal frameshifting does not occur. Transmembrane domains in nsp3, nsp4, and nsp6 are indicated by *red vertical lines*.[200,320] **C:** Schematic of the three membrane-bound replicase components. Known functions of modules of nsp3 are listed.[309] Modules not found in all coronaviruses are shown in *gray*; in coronaviruses with a single PLpro, its position is that of PLpro2. **D:** The RNA packaging signal (PS) located in the nsp15-encoding region of the MHV genome.[77] This element is found only in a subset of the betacoronaviruses (MHV, betacoronavirus 1, and HCoV-HKU1); repeat units are *boxed*.

The processed nsps assemble to form the coronavirus replicase, which is also called the replicase–transcriptase complex (RTC).[308] The challenge of defining the roles of the many nsp components of the RTC was initially addressed by foundational studies in bioinformatics,[154,487] a discipline that continues to inform the analysis of this intricate molecular machinery.[244,309,392] Besides PLpro and Mpro, the products of rep 1a contain several activities that establish cellular conditions favorable for infection. Some of these are directly linked to RNA synthesis. Others are nonessential for viral replication in tissue culture, but they can have major effects on virus–host interactions (see *Immune Response and Viral Evasion of the Immune Response*). The very first polyprotein product, nsp1, exhibits a broad set of antagonistic activities that selectively inhibit host gene expression.[305] For different viruses, this is accomplished by diverse mechanisms, some of which operate by nsp1 associating with the small ribosomal subunit and recruiting a cellular endonuclease that cleaves host mRNAs. As yet, no function has been demonstrated for the next polyprotein product, nsp2.[308]

Nsp3 is by far the largest of the RTC proteins. It consists of a concatenation of individual structural modules that are arranged as globular domains separated by flexibly disordered linkers[246,309] (Fig. 10.6C). At the amino terminus of nsp3 are a ubiquitin-like domain (Ubl1) and a hypervariable acidic region (Ac). Ubl1 interacts with the SR region of the N protein,[185,187,204] and it is proposed that this interaction tethers the genome to the assembling RTC, in order to allow formation of the initiation complex for RNA synthesis. Also located within nsp3, as noted above, are one or two PLpro modules. Downstream of the Ac region or PLpro1, all coronaviruses contain a conserved macrodomain (Mac1). Mac1 exhibits ADP-ribose-1″-phosphatase (ADRP) activity, but recent work suggests that its physiologically relevant role is as an ADP-ribose-protein hydrolase.[251] Although Mac1 is nonessential for viral replication, it is critical for *in vivo* pathogenesis.[140] At the carboxy terminus of nsp3 is a highly conserved region, designated the Y domain, containing three metal-binding clusters of cysteine and histidine residues.[309,487] The functions of other domains of nsp3 (Mac2, Mac3, DPUP, NAB, and G2M),[246,309,392] which appear only in various subsets of coronaviruses, remain to be elucidated.

Notably, the rep 1a products nsp3, nsp4, and nsp6 each contain multiple transmembrane helices that anchor the RTC to intracellular membranes (Fig. 10.6C).[200,320] These proteins are responsible for remodeling membranes to form organelles that are dedicated to viral RNA synthesis.[306] Cryoelectron tomographic imaging has revealed an extensive network of convoluted membranes, double-membraned vesicles (DMVs), and vesicle packets, all continuous with the ER, that are induced by coronavirus infection[216] (Fig. 10.7). Formation of these structures requires expression of nsp3, nsp4, and possibly also nsp6.[16,324] Apposition of paired membranes in DMVs may be promoted by interactions between the lumenal loops of nsp3 and nsp4.[164] Anchorage and compartmentalization of the RTC is thought to provide a scaffold for recruitment of soluble nsps, to offer protection from ribonucleases, and to sequester double-stranded viral RNA intermediates and other molecular signatures that can activate host innate immunity (see *Immune Response and Viral Evasion of the Immune Response*).

The most carboxy-terminal products of pp1a are a cluster of essential small proteins, nsp7 to nsp10,[121,393] that act as regulatory subunits for components generated further downstream.

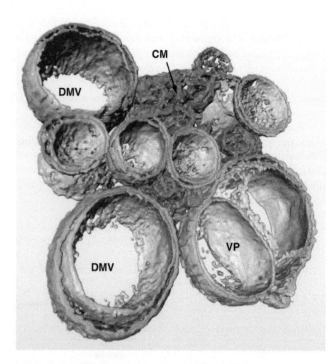

FIGURE 10.7 Membranous compartments for RNA replication and transcription induced by coronavirus infection. Shown is a cryoelectron tomographic reconstruction of the network of intracellular membrane rearrangements found in SARS-CoV–infected Vero cells. The three types of structures are convoluted membranes (CM), which are the major sites of nsp accumulation; double-membraned vesicles (DMVs), which appear to be the sites of active RNA synthesis; and vesicle packets (VP), which are formed by the merger of DMV. (From Knoops K, Kikkert M, Worm SH, et al. SARS-coronavirus replication is supported by a reticulovesicular network of modified endoplasmic reticulum. *PLoS Biol* 2008;6:e226.)

The processed products encoded by rep 1b contain a collection of well-studied enzymatic activities, including many that are common to all positive-strand RNA viruses. Most prominent in the latter class is the coronavirus RNA–dependent RNA polymerase (RdRp), which is contained in nsp12. *In vitro* expression and characterization of nsp12 RdRp activity has been difficult, and there is not complete agreement among the results of different biochemical studies of this enzyme.[347] Addition of nsp7 and nsp8 has been shown to greatly enhance RNA binding by nsp12 and to potentiate its polymerase activity and processivity.[407] Consistent with this, a structure of nsp12 in complex with nsp7 and nsp8 has very recently been determined.[215] The coronavirus RdRp contains the finger, palm, and thumb domains characteristic of many viral polymerases and most closely resembles the RdRps of picornaviruses. In this model, a heterodimer of nsp7 and nsp8 is seen to bind to the RdRp thumb domain, forming interfaces with nsp12 that are supported by previous mutagenesis studies.[407] Additionally, nsp12 has an unusually large amino-terminal domain, unique to the order *Nidovirales*, named nidovirus RdRp–associated nucleotidyltransferase (NiRAN), which appears able to form monophosphate adducts with either GTP or UTP.[244] Evidence has been presented both for primer-dependent and de novo initiation of RNA synthesis by nsp12 alone or by the nsp12-nsp7-nsp8 complex.[393] A strong candidate for a prospective primase is nsp8, which, in some reports, possesses independent RdRp activity capable of synthesizing short RNA oligomers.[347] Alternatively, protein priming is one speculative role for the nsp12 NiRAN activity.

Another enzyme crucial to RNA synthesis is nsp13, a helicase falling in superfamily 1.[154] *In vitro*, nsp13 has RNA-stimulated NTPase activity and unwinds RNA duplexes in the 5'-to-3' direction,[193] but its exact *in vivo* role remains to be established.[393] A multinuclear zinc-binding domain (ZBD) at the amino terminus of nsp13 governs helicase activity[245] and may also mediate interactions with other molecular partners.[167] Like the NiRAN domain of nsp12, the ZBD of nsp13 is a unique marker of nidoviruses.

In common with many RNA viruses, coronaviruses produce machinery to catalyze multiple steps of the pathway for synthesis of the 5'-terminal cap structure of mRNA.[378,393] RNA 5'-triphosphatase, required for the first step of capping, is likely provided by nsp13, which possesses this in addition to its helicase and NTPase activities.[193] Intriguingly, the guanylyltransferase needed for the next step has thus far not been identified among the nsps, and it cannot be ruled out that this enzyme is appropriated from the host. For the final cap modifications, the nsp14 carboxy terminus and nsp16, respectively, harbor N7-methyltransferase and 2'-*O*-methyltransferase activities.[72,114] These enzymes operate in an obligatory sequential manner, with guanosine N7 methylation preceding ribose 2'-*O*-methylation. Activation of the nsp16 methyltransferase requires nsp10 as a cofactor, and the crystal structure of a heterodimer of these two proteins suggests that nsp10 serves as a platform to stabilize nsp16.[378]

Finally, there are two rep 1b–encoded activities that are not found outside the order *Nidovirales*[152,392,393]; surprisingly, both are ribonucleases. The first is an endonuclease, designated NendoU, which resides in nsp15. NendoU hydrolyzes both single- and double-stranded RNA and specifically cleaves downstream of uridylate residues, producing 2'-3' cyclic phosphates.[122,192] Although it bears homology to XendoU, an enzyme involved in snoRNA processing and remodeling of the ER, the role of NendoU in coronavirus RNA synthesis, if any, is far from clear. However, NendoU catalytic mutants are profoundly attenuated due to activation of host innate immunity.[122] The second atypical activity is ExoN, a 3'-5' exonuclease that is contained in the amino-terminal portion of nsp14.[292] Interestingly, the ExoN activity of nsp14 (but not the N7-methyltransferase) is stimulated by nsp10, and the nsp10-nsp14 complex is most active on a double-stranded RNA substrate with a 3'-end mismatch.[48] Moreover, nsp14 associates *in vitro* with the nsp7-nsp8-nsp12 RNA polymerase complex.[407] ExoN is not essential for viral replication, but nsp14 mutants have a greatly enhanced mutation rate.[133] All of these properties support the model that ExoN provides a proofreading function for the coronavirus RdRp. Such a corrective activity may be essential for maintenance of the stability of the exceptionally large coronavirus genome.

Viral RNA Synthesis

Expression and assembly of the RTC sets the stage for viral RNA synthesis (Fig. 10.5), a process resulting in the replication of genomic RNA and the transcription of multiple subgenomic RNAs (sgRNAs).[281] The latter species serve as mRNAs for the genes downstream of the replicase gene. Each sgRNA consists of a leader RNA of 70 to 100 nucleotides, which is identical to the 5' end of the genome, joined to a body RNA, which is identical to a segment of the 3' end of the genome. The fusion of the leader RNA to body RNAs occurs at short motifs called TRSs, examples of which are listed in Figure 10.8. Like the genome, the sgRNAs have 5' caps and 3' polyadenylate tails. Together, these transcripts form a 3'-nested set, the single most distinctive feature of the order *Nidovirales*.[152] Synthesis of both genomic RNA and sgRNAs proceeds through negative-strand intermediates.[31,377] The negative-sense RNAs, which possess 5' oligouridylate tracts[462] and 3' antileaders,[376] are roughly a 10th to a 100th as abundant as their positive-sense counterparts.

At their 5' and 3' termini, coronavirus genomes contain *cis*-acting RNA elements that allow their selective recognition as templates for the RTC and play essential roles in RNA synthesis (Fig. 10.8). The initial localization of these elements was carried out in studies of defective interfering (DI) RNAs, which are extensively deleted genomic variants that propagate by competing for the viral RNA synthesis machinery. Manipulations of natural and artificially constructed DI RNAs, evaluated by transfection into helper virus–infected cells, made possible the mapping of sequences that are critical for the replication and transcription of DI RNA and, presumably, also for genomic RNA.[281] More recently, *cis*-acting RNA elements have been dissected through reverse genetics of the intact viral genome, complemented by *in vitro* biochemical and structural analyses.[278,466]

The most completely characterized 5'-terminal structures are those of the betacoronaviruses MHV and BCoV (Fig. 10.8), although structural and functional counterparts of some of these are found in SARS-CoV and in the alphacoronaviruses HCoV-229E and HCoV-NL63.[278,279] For MHV and BCoV, the elements that participate in viral RNA synthesis extend beyond the 5' untranslated region (5' UTR) into the replicase coding region, making up a series of at least eight SL.[160,466] One of these sequesters the start codon of the rep 1a gene within its stem and joins with two other SLs in a four-way junction formed by a long-range interaction between the 5' UTR and the nsp1-coding region.[159] Mutations or deletions in many of these elements have been found to debilitate or kill the virus or to abrogate DI RNA replication. Many, but not all, of these structures can be exchanged among the genomes of different betacoronaviruses.[160,199] Significantly, functional analyses have shown that either the stability[159,160] or the instability[254] of a given RNA stem can be critical for viral fitness, suggesting that these structures operate in a dynamic manner during RNA synthesis.

At the 3' end of the genome, *cis*-acting RNA structures are confined entirely to the 3' UTR[148] and, again, have been most thoroughly studied in MHV and BCoV. These elements consist of a bulged stem-loop (BSL)[281] and an adjacent pseudoknot[449] (Fig. 10.8) that have each been demonstrated to be essential for viral replication. The identical structures appear in other betacoronaviruses and are functionally interchangeable between MHV and either BCoV[281] or SARS-CoV.[150] The same structures are also found in the 3' UTRs of the deltacoronaviruses; however, alpha- or gammacoronaviruses possess only counterparts of the pseudoknot or the BSL, respectively.[150,278] Further downstream in the betacoronavirus 3' UTR is a hypervariable region, which is completely dispensable for viral replication but yet harbors an octanucleotide motif, 5'-GGAAGAGC-3', that is almost universally conserved in coronaviruses.[149] Notably, the BSL and the pseudoknot partially overlap, and they therefore cannot fold up simultaneously. The two structures are thus thought to constitute a molecular switch between

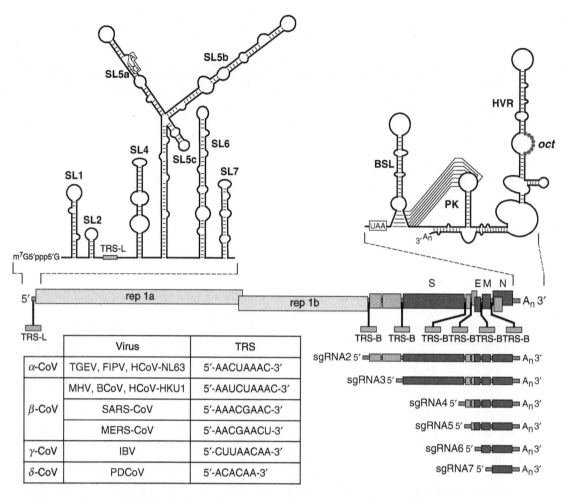

FIGURE 10.8 Coronavirus RNA synthesis. Shown are a schematic of MHV genomic RNA and the nested set of transcribed subgenomic RNA (sgRNA) species that are a defining feature of the order *Nidovirales*. The leader and body copies of the transcription-regulating sequence (TRS-L and TRS-B, respectively) are denoted by *green boxes*. At the left are listed examples of consensus TRSs for representative viruses of each genus. Expanded regions above the genome depict *cis*-acting RNA structures at the genome termini. The structures shown are those characterized for MHV. Homologous structures exist in the BCoV and SARS-CoV genomes, and counterparts of some of these elements appear in other coronaviruses.[278,466] The 5' expanded region represents the 210-nt 5' UTR and the first 281 nt of the rep 1a gene.[466] The elements shown are eight stem–loops (SL); TRS-L is denoted in *green*; the start codon of rep 1a is *boxed* in SL5a. The 3' expanded region represents the 301-nt 3' UTR.[493] The elements shown are the bulged stem–loop (BSL), the pseudoknot (PK), the hypervariable region (HVR), and the conserved coronavirus octanucleotide motif (*oct*); the stop codon for the upstream N gene is *boxed*.

different steps of RNA synthesis.[148] In addition, the first loop of the pseudoknot forms a duplex with the extreme 3' end of the genome and genetically interacts with the RTC subunits nsp8 and nsp9.[493] On this basis, a model has been proposed in which alternate RNA conformations of the 3' UTR facilitate the transition between initiation of negative-strand RNA synthesis by the nsp8 primase and elongation by the nsp12 RdRp. However, this scheme does not yet incorporate potential cross talk between the 5' and 3' ends of the genome,[254] and much remains to be learned about how *cis*-acting RNA elements are recognized by, and cooperate with, the RTC.

A central issue in coronavirus RNA synthesis is how the leader RNA becomes attached to the body segments of the sgRNAs. It became clear from early work that transcription involves a discontinuous process.[281] UV transcriptional mapping demonstrated that sgRNAs are not processed from a genome-length precursor, and mixed infections with two

different strains of MHV showed that leader RNAs could reassort between separate sgRNA body segments. It was also clearly established by DI RNA studies, and later confirmed by genomic reverse genetics,[490] that the TRSs play key roles in sgRNA formation. The efficiency of fusion at an individual body TRS (TRS-B) is, in part, governed by how closely it conforms to the leader TRS (TRS-L).[395] Nonetheless, factors such as the local sequence context of the TRS, the position of the TRS relative to the 3' end of the genome, and long-distance RNA–RNA interactions can also profoundly influence transcription levels.

It is now recognized that the leader-to-body fusion event takes place through a mechanism of discontinuous extension of negative-strand RNA synthesis.[370,490] In this model, both genomic and subgenomic negative-strand RNAs are initiated by the RTC at the 3' end of the (positive-strand) genome template (Fig. 10.9). A pause in RNA synthesis occurs when the RdRp crosses a TRS-B. At this point, the RdRp may continue

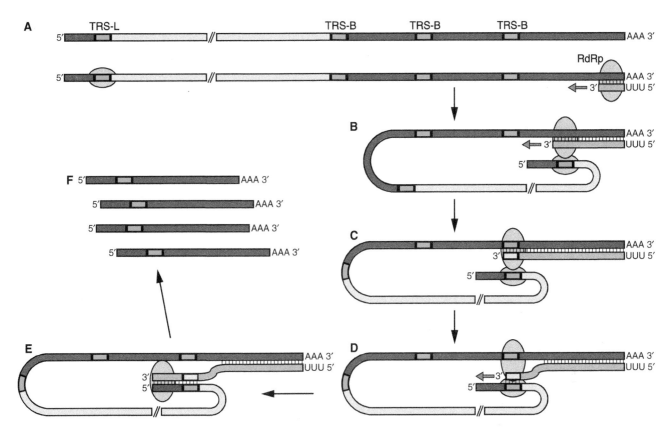

FIGURE 10.9 Coronavirus transcription through discontinuous extension of negative-strand RNA synthesis. A, B: Negative-strand sgRNA synthesis initiates at the 3' end of the positive-strand genomic RNA template. In the version of the model shown here, the genomic template loops out in such a way as to allow a component of the RTC to constantly monitor the potential complementarity of the 3' end of the nascent negative-strand RNA with the TRS-L. **C:** Transcription pauses at a TRS-B. At this point, elongation may resume, thereby bypassing the TRS-B. **D:** Alternatively, the nascent negative strand may switch templates, binding to the TRS-L. **E:** Resumption of elongation results in completion of synthesis of an antileader-containing negative-strand sgRNA. **F:** The resulting complex of genome and negative-strand sgRNA acts as template for the synthesis of multiple copies of the corresponding positive-strand sgRNA. (Adapted from Zúñiga S, Sola I, Alonso S, et al. Sequence motifs involved in the regulation of discontinuous coronavirus subgenomic RNA synthesis. *J Virol* 2004;78:980–994.)

to elongate the growing negative strand. Alternatively, it may switch to the leader at the 5' end of the genome template, guided by the complementarity between the 3' end of the nascent negative strand and the TRS-L of the genome. The resulting negative-strand sgRNA, in partial duplex with positive-strand gRNA, then serves as the template for synthesis of multiple copies of the corresponding positive-strand sgRNA.

Leader-to-body fusion during negative-strand synthesis is amply supported by accumulated experimental results both with coronaviruses and the closely related arteriviruses. First, as necessitated by the model, negative-strand sgRNAs contain antileaders at their 3' ends.[376] Second, in infected cells, there exist transcription intermediates containing negative-strand sgRNAs in association with the genome. These complexes actively participate in transcription[31,369] and can be biochemically separated from replication intermediates containing genome-length negative-strand RNAs.[372] Finally, as would be predicted for discontinuous negative-strand synthesis, engineered (or naturally occurring) variant nucleotides incorporated into the TRS-B, rather than the TRS-L, end up in the leader–body junction of the resulting sgRNA.[329,428,490] There remains, however, considerable further work to be done to elucidate the details of the model. It is not clear how the transcribing RdRp might continuously monitor the ability of its nascent product to base-pair to the TRS-L. Additionally, the synthesis of genome-length negative strands would require the RdRp to bypass all of the TRS-B sites in the genome template. This may come about through a stochastic process, or it may be actively promoted by some RTC component or by N protein[460] under certain conditions. These and other questions will need to be addressed, possibly with the aid of a robust *in vitro* viral RNA synthesizing system.[427] Such a system would also be decisive in assessing the potential roles of host factors in transcription and replication. A number of cellular proteins that bind *in vitro* to genomic RNA segments, including hnRNP A1, polypyrimidine tract–binding protein, and polyadenylate-binding protein, have been proposed to take part in coronavirus RNA synthesis.[281,347,395] However, it has been difficult to convincingly demonstrate their specific involvement in viral processes. As yet, only a single candidate host factor has been shown to be required for *in vitro* viral RNA synthesis.[427]

In addition to its central role in sgRNA formation, template switching is also at the heart of RNA recombination, another prominent feature of coronavirus RNA synthesis. Significant rates of both homologous and nonhomologous RNA recombination have been found among selected and unselected markers during the course of infection.[281] It is presumed, but remains to be formally demonstrated, that coronavirus RNA recombination results from a copy-choice mechanism. In MHV, recombination has been shown to take place at an estimated frequency of 1% per 1.3 kb (almost 25% over the entire genome), the highest rate observed for any RNA virus.[29] On a fine scale, the sites of crossover are random,[27] although selective pressures can generate the appearance of local clustering of recombinational hot spots. This facility for RdRp strand-switching may make a major contribution to the ability of the huge coronavirus genome to circumvent the accumulation of deleterious mutations. It may also serve as a driver of evolution by horizontal gene transfer[182,273] (see *Basic and Accessory Genes*).

Assembly and Release of Virions

The immediate outcome of transcription is to enable translation of the proteins that build progeny viruses. The membrane-bound proteins M, S, and E are initially inserted into the ER, and from there, they transit to the site of virion assembly, the endoplasmic reticulum–Golgi intermediate compartment (ERGIC). Here, nucleocapsids composed of progeny genomes encapsidated by N protein coalesce with the envelope components to form virions, which bud into the ERGIC[112,174] (Fig. 10.5).

Coronavirus assembly occurs through a network of cooperative interactions, most of which involve M protein. However, despite its central role, M is not assembly-competent by itself. Expression of M protein alone does not result in virion-like structures, and M traverses the secretory pathway beyond the budding site, as far as the *trans*-Golgi.[174,276,423] The first virus-like particle (VLP) systems developed for coronaviruses led to the key finding that coexpression of E protein with M protein is sufficient to yield the formation of particles that are released from cells and appear morphologically identical to coronavirus envelopes.[43,432] More recently, it has been shown that the additional coexpression of N protein substantially increases the efficiency of VLP formation[44,390] and can even compensate for mutational defects in M.[23] Other viral structural proteins, in particular S protein, are gathered into virions but are not specifically required for the assembly process. Since virions and VLPs contain very little E protein, this indicates that lateral interactions between M molecules provide the driving force for envelope morphogenesis. Investigations of the ability of M protein mutants to support VLP assembly concluded that M–M interactions occur via multiple contacts throughout the molecule, especially between the transmembrane domains.[112] Cryoelectron tomographic reconstructions of whole virions suggest that the M protein forms dimers that are maintained through multiple monomer–monomer contacts, while dimer–dimer interactions occur among the globular endodomains.[310]

It is incompletely understood how E protein critically assists M in envelope formation. E protein localizes to the ERGIC and *cis*-Golgi[96,315,430] and somehow secures localization of M protein at the budding site. Some evidence suggests that E protein promotes assembly by inducing membrane curvature.[174,432] Other work indicates a role for E in maintaining M protein in an assembly-competent state by preventing its nonproductive aggregation, a function that is crucially dependent on palmitoylation of E.[44] Such a chaperone-like role would be

consistent with demonstrations that diverse heterologous E proteins, and even truncated versions of M protein, can functionally replace E protein in MHV.[228,233] Additionally, there are reports that point to a need for E protein to facilitate the release of virions from infected cells.[365] These multiple roles are not mutually exclusive, and mutational studies have begun to assign individual functions to various regions of the E molecule. The carboxy-terminal endodomain of the IBV E protein has been shown to govern Golgi localization[96,97] and, when linked to a heterologous transmembrane domain, can support VLP and virion assembly.[365] Conversely, the transmembrane domain of IBV E disassembles the Golgi complex in a manner that promotes release of infectious virus, but it is unclear whether this is a general property of other coronavirus E proteins.[364] It is also presently unresolved which roles of E protein correlate with its state of oligomerization or require its function as an ion channel.[417,446]

The dispensability of S protein for VLP formation is consistent with earlier observations that spikeless (noninfectious) virions were formed by infected cells treated with the glycosylation inhibitor tunicamycin[175,363] or by cells infected with particular S mutants.[274] S protein thus appears to play a passive role in assembly, but during its passage through the secretory pathway, it is captured by M protein for virion incorporation.[112] For some S proteins, localization at or near the budding compartment is abetted by targeting signals contained in the endodomain.[423] The cysteine- and charge-rich S endodomain is also the region of the protein that interacts with M during assembly[45,469] (Fig. 10.3). The locus of M protein that reciprocally interacts with S has yet to be precisely mapped.[174]

Virion assembly is completed by condensation of the nucleocapsid with the envelope components. This is brought about principally by N and M protein interactions, which have been mapped, respectively, to the carboxy-terminal domain 3 of N[186,433] and to the carboxy terminus of the M endodomain[136,231] (Fig. 10.3). These interacting regions likely account for the thread-like connections that have been visualized between the M protein endodomain and the nucleocapsid in virion reconstructions.[28,310] Nucleocapsid formation is presumed to be concomitant with genome replication, but the details of how the nucleocapsid traffics to the budding compartment are not known. It is also only partially understood how coronaviruses selectively package genomic RNA from among the many positive- and negative-strand viral RNA species that are synthesized during infection. For MHV, DI RNA analyses mapped the genomic PS to a small span of RNA sequence embedded in the region of the replicase gene that encodes a surface loop of nsp15[281] (Fig. 10.6D). Highly homologous structures exist in the genomes of the related betacoronaviruses BCoV and HCoV-HKU1.[77,87] However, the PSs for most coronaviruses, including the betacoronaviruses SARS-CoV and MERS-CoV, are clearly not situated at the same locus.[234] The only other mapped PS, that of the alphacoronavirus TGEV, falls near the 5′ end of the genome.[135,295] The mechanism by which MHV packaging operates is undetermined. Some work demonstrates that M protein, in the absence of N, acts as the discriminatory factor for PS recognition.[281,302] Other studies have shown that the MHV PS is specifically bound by N protein *in vitro*[87,293] and that PS recognition during infection requires a coordinated interaction of both the CTD and domain 3 of the N protein.[229,230] Unexpectedly, it has also been found that selective genomic RNA packaging is required for MHV evasion of the innate immune response.[24]

Following assembly and budding, progeny virions are exported from infected cells by transport to the plasma membrane in smooth-walled vesicles and are released by exocytosis. This is currently a poorly characterized stage of the replication cycle. It remains to be more clearly defined whether coronaviruses follow the constitutive pathway for post-Golgi transport of large cargo or, alternatively, if specialized cellular machinery must be diverted for their exit.[174] The ion channel property of E protein has been implicated in this process, but many further details await elucidation.[365]

For some coronaviruses, contingent upon the nature of S endodomain intracellular retention signals,[423] a fraction of S protein that has not been assembled into virions transits to the plasma membrane. Here, S can mediate fusion between infected cells and adjacent, uninfected cells. This cell–cell fusion depends upon S1/S2 cleavage late in infection (see *Viral Entry and Uncoating*) and occurs by a mechanism distinct from that of virus–cell fusion.[169] The resultant formation of large, multinucleate syncytia enables the rapid spread of infection by a route that does not rely on an extracellular phase of completely assembled virions.

PATHOGENESIS AND PATHOLOGY OF CORONAVIRUS INFECTIONS

General Principles

Most coronaviruses spread to susceptible hosts by respiratory or fecal–oral routes of infection, with replication first occurring in epithelial cells (Table 10.3). Some, including

TABLE 10.3 Representative coronaviruses and associated diseases

Virus[a]	Host Species	Sites of Infection	Clinical Disease
Alphacoronaviruses			
CCoV	Canine	GI tract	Gastroenteritis
FeCoV	Felidae	GI tract, respiratory	Gastroenteritis
FIPV	Felidae	Systemic disease	Peritonitis, wasting disease
HCoV-229E	Human	Respiratory	Upper respiratory tract infection
HCoV-NL63	Human	Respiratory	Upper respiratory tract infection, croup
PEDV	Swine	GI tract	Gastroenteritis
TGEV	Swine	GI tract, respiratory	Gastroenteritis
BatCoV	Bat	GI tract, respiratory	Unknown
Rabbit CoV	Rabbit	Heart, GI tract, respiratory	Enteritis, myocarditis
SADS-CoV	Swine	GI tract	Gastroenteritis
Betacoronaviruses			
BCoV	Bovine, ruminants	GI tract, respiratory	Enteritis, upper and lower respiratory tract infection
HCoV-OC43	Human	Respiratory	Upper respiratory tract infection
HCoV-HKU1	Human	Respiratory	Upper and lower respiratory tract infection
MHV	Mouse, rat	GI tract, liver, brains, lung	Gastroenteritis, hepatitis, encephalitis, chronic demyelination
PHEV	Swine	Respiratory, brain	Vomiting, wasting, encephalomyelitis
RCoV	Rat	Respiratory, salivary and lachrymal glands, urogenital tract	Respiratory tract infection, metritis, sialodacryoadenitis
SARS-CoV	Human	Respiratory, GI tract	Pneumonia (SARS)
MERS-CoV	Camel, human	Respiratory tract	Pneumonia (MERS)
BatCoV	Bat	GI tract, respiratory tract	Unknown
Gammacoronaviruses			
IBV	Chicken	Respiratory, kidney	Bronchitis, nephritis
TuCoV	Turkey	GI tract	Gastroenteritis
BWCoV	Beluga whale	Respiratory tract	Pneumonia, hepatitis
Deltacoronaviruses			
ThCoV	Thrush	Respiratory, GI tract	Unknown
PDCoV	Swine	GI tract	Gastroenteritis

[a]All virus abbreviations as in Table 10.1.

HCoV-OC43, HCoV-229E, HCoV-NL63, HCoV-HKU1, and PRCoV, replicate principally in respiratory epithelial cells, where they produce virus and symptoms confined to the URT. Other coronaviruses, including TGEV, BCoV, PHEV, CCoV, FCoV, and enteric strains of MHV, infect epithelial cells of the enteric tract. Some of these viruses, such as TGEV, PEDV, and porcine deltacoronavirus (PDCoV), cause diarrhea that is particularly severe, and sometimes fatal, in young animals.[198,243] Inapparent enteric infection of adult animals maintains the virus in the population.[88] In addition to local infection of the upper respiratory or enteric tracts, several coronaviruses cause severe disease. For example, SARS-CoV and MERS-CoV spread from the upper airway to cause a severe lower respiratory tract infection, while FIPV spreads systemically to cause a generalized wasting disease in felines.[20,183,414] Rat coronavirus strains cause respiratory infection or sialodacryoadenitis due to infection of the salivary and lacrimal glands[337] but can also interfere with reproduction by infecting the female urogenital tract. PHEV of swine predominantly causes enteric infection but is also neurotropic.[252] Infection spreads to nerves that innervate the stomach of infected piglets and prevents gastric emptying, resulting in vomiting and wasting disease. The ability to cause localized versus systemic disease is mirrored in polarized tissue culture cells. Thus, coronaviruses such as mouse hepatitis virus, which can cause systemic disease, enter the apical side of cells and exit the basolateral side, whereas others, like HCoV-229E or SARS-CoV, which cause infection largely localized to the respiratory tract, enter and exit the cell apically.[90] In contrast, MERS-CoV enters and exits via both the apical and basolateral sides even though it causes mostly respiratory tract disease.[412]

Animal Coronavirus Infections

Several coronavirus infections have been extensively studied in their natural hosts. Here, we will focus on murine and feline coronavirus infections.

Mouse Hepatitis Virus

MHV, which until the advent of SARS and MERS was the most widely studied coronavirus, causes enteric, hepatic, and neurological infections of susceptible strains of rodents. Remarkably, closely related strains of MHV, all of which use the same host cell receptor for entry,[450] infect different organs. Enteric strains, such as MHV-Y and MHV-RI, are a major problem in animal research facilities.[88] These viruses spread within infected colonies to young, uninfected animals. They do not generally cause symptomatic disease but may subtly impair the host immune response to other pathogens and immunological stimuli.[88] Studies of MHV pathogenesis predominantly use the neurotropic JHM and A59 strains of virus (JHMV and MHV-A59), in part because they cause a demyelinating encephalomyelitis with similarities to the human disease multiple sclerosis (MS). Originally isolated from a mouse with hind limb paralysis,[25] JHMV became progressively more virulent on passage in mice, resulting in widespread neuronal infection.[445] Subsequently, most studies have used either attenuated JHMV variants or the mildly neurovirulent MHV-A59 strain for studies of demyelination. Infection with these viruses results in minimal infection of neurons, with oligodendrocytes, microglia, and astrocytes commonly infected.[401] Myelin destruction is largely immune-mediated, occurring during virus clearance from infected glia.[444,461] Thus, irradiated mice or congenitally immunodeficient mice

(mice with severe combined immunodeficiency [SCID] or with a disrupted recombination activation gene 1 [RAG1$^{-/-}$]) do not develop demyelination after JHMV infection. When these mice are reconstituted with virus-specific T cells, demyelination rapidly develops[444,461] (Fig. 10.10). Demyelination is accompanied by infiltration of macrophages and activated microglia into the white matter of the spinal cord. Both CD4 and CD8 T cells are required for virus clearance from the central nervous system (CNS), with CD8 T cells considered most important in this process. CD8 T cells eliminate virus from infected astrocytes and microglia by perforin-dependent pathways, while clearance from oligodendrocytes is IFNγ-dependent.[264,327] However, T-cell–mediated virus clearance is not complete, and antivirus antibody is required to prevent virus recrudescence.[263] Coronaviruses may become persistent. In one example, viruses mutated in an immunodominant CD8 T-cell epitope are selected, resulting in evasion of the cytotoxic T-cell immune response and persistence.[340] Further, antivirus CD4 T cells, while critical for virus clearance, may also be immunopathogenic. Thus, infection with MHV mutated in an immunodominant CD4 T-cell epitope causes attenuated clinical disease, while enhancement of the antivirus CD4 T-cell response increases disease severity.[17]

Other strains of MHV, including MHV-A59, MHV-2, and MHV-3, infect both the liver and the CNS. Most notably, MHV-3 causes a fulminant hepatitis in susceptible strains of mice and chronic neurological infections in semi-susceptible strains.[401] In susceptible strains, MHV-3 infects macrophages, resulting in upregulation of several proinflammatory cytokines, including IL-1β and fibrinogen-like protein 2 (FGL2), a transmembrane procoagulant molecule. Expression of FGL2 results in prothrombin cleavage, with consequent disseminated intravascular coagulation (DIC) and hepatic hypoperfusion and necrosis.[280] Levels of FGL2 are better predictors of a fatal outcome than are virus titers. Like JHMV, MHV-3 also infects the CNS, but infection of this organ occurs only in strains that do not develop a fulminant hepatitis. MHV-3 does not cause a demyelinating disease, but rather, ependymitis, hydrocephalus, encephalitis, and thrombotic vasculitis.[401] The pathogenesis of these entities is not well studied but appears to be immune-mediated. Unlike most other strains of MHV, MHV-3 directly infects T and B cells, resulting in lymphocyte apoptosis and lymphopenia. Lymphopenia, with consequent immunosuppression, facilitates virus persistence and its immunopathological consequences.

Feline Enteric Coronaviruses (FCoV) and FIPV

FCoV commonly cause mild or asymptomatic infections in domestic cats and other felines. Two serotypes of FCoV are recognized, with serotype II strains arising by recombination of serotype I FCoV with canine coronavirus in dually infected animals.[414] In some cats infected persistently with FCoV, mutations in the virus occur, resulting in the development of a lethal disease called feline infectious peritonitis (FIP); the virulent strain of FCoV is termed FIPV. Virulence correlates with the ability of the virus to replicate in macrophages. The nature of the mutations required for transition from FCoV to FIPV is not well understood, although for serotype II viruses, virulence maps in part to the surface glycoprotein.[414] This was shown using reverse genetics, in which S proteins from virulent and avirulent strains were swapped and tested for their ability to cause severe disease in cats. FIPV causes a multiphasic disease with relapses that result, ultimately, in immunosuppression, weight

Myelin	Macrophages	Virus	Axons

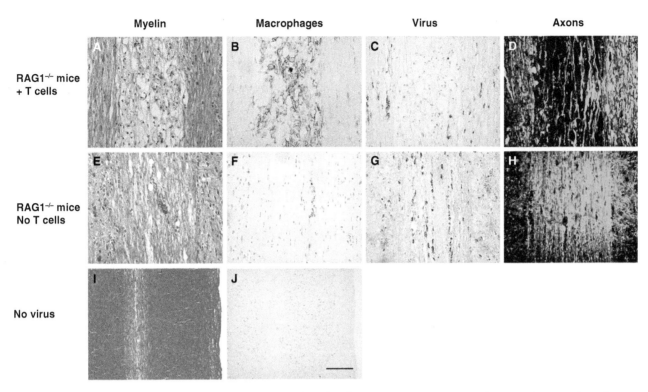

FIGURE 10.10 Immune-mediated demyelination in mice infected with a neurotropic MHV. RAG1[−/−] mice, lacking T and B cells, were either infected with a neurotropic coronavirus[461] (**A–H**) or uninfected (**I,J**). Four days later, some mice received adoptively transferred spleen cells from a wild-type C57Bl/6 mouse that was previously immunized intraperitoneally with MHV (**A–D**). All mice were sacrificed 8 days later and analyzed for demyelination (**A,E,I**), macrophage infiltration (**B,F,J**), viral antigen (**C,G**), and intact axons (**D,H**). Demyelination, macrophage infiltration, and axon destruction (**A,B,D**) were observed only in mice that received transferred MHV-immune cells showing that myelin destruction is largely mediated by T cells during the process of virus clearance (**C**).

loss, and death (Fig. 10.11). Each episode is characterized by increased virus replication, fever, and lymphopenia.[108] FIPV does not directly infect lymphocytes. Rather, lymphopenia is believed to be a consequence of infection and activation of macrophages and dendritic cells. Subsequent lymphocyte depletion occurs when cells are exposed to high levels of proinflammatory cytokines, such as tumor necrosis factor, released by these infected cells. Virus dissemination occurs when infected macrophages traffic throughout the body and are deposited in the vasculature. Infected macrophages provoke a pyogranulomatous reaction, which is responsible for many disease manifestations of FIP, such as peritonitis and serositis. Another consequence of immune dysregulation is hypergammaglobulinemia. Antibody–antigen complex formation commonly occurs in FIPV-infected cats and may contribute to vascular injury.[196] However, its precise role in pathogenesis remains uncertain because it is a late manifestation of disease and may make only a minor contribution to disease progression. Infection of macrophages by FIPV is enhanced by neutralizing antibody directed against the S glycoprotein. Enhanced macrophage infection is mediated by virus entry through Fcγ receptors. This phenomenon has been demonstrated *in vitro* using isolated macrophages and in cats that were previously immunized with vectors that express the S glycoprotein.[431] Although the potential occurrence of antibody-enhanced disease has hindered vaccine development, it has never been demonstrated in the natural feline infection. In fact, cats infected with FCoV often develop only low antivirus neutralizing antibody titers.[176]

Human Coronavirus Infections

Human Coronaviruses, Other Than SARS-CoV and MERS-CoV, Associated with Respiratory and Enteric Disease

Prior to 2003, HCoVs were primarily considered to be agents of URT disease and to cause little mortality. In general, while coronaviruses were readily isolated from infected birds and other animal species, and serially propagated in continuous cell lines, isolation of HCoVs from infected individuals was only rarely achieved. HCoV-229E and HCoV-OC43 were isolated from patients with URT infections in the 1960s.[284] There are striking differences in extent of genetic variability when isolates of HCoV-OC43 and HCoV-229E are compared. HCoV-229E isolated at geographically distinct locations show little evidence of variability.[79] In contrast, isolates of HCoV-OC43 from the same geographic area but isolated in different years show considerable sequence variations with emergence of novel recombinants.[237] The ability of HCoV-OC43 to tolerate mutations probably accounts for its ability to grow in mouse cells and infect the mouse brain as well as its ability to cross species (see *Epidemiology*). In contrast, HCoV-229E does not readily cross species and does not infect mice. Even in mice that are transgenic for expression of the HCoV-229E host cell receptor (hAPN), the virus does not readily grow or cause clinical disease.[236]

Two new HCoVs were isolated from the respiratory tracts of patients in the post-SARS era. HCoV-NL63, which causes mild respiratory disease, displays homology with HCoV-229E.

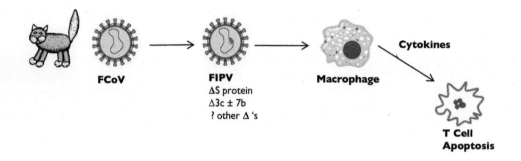

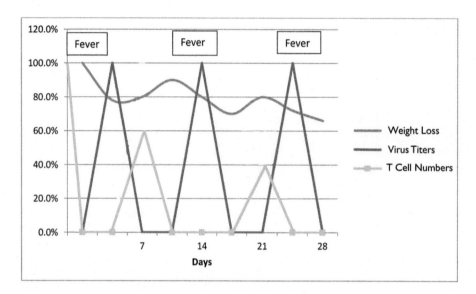

FIGURE 10.11 **Recurrent feline infectious peritonitis (FIP).** FIPV, the etiologic agent of FIP, occurs in felines persistently infected with feline coronaviruses. *Upper panels*: Mutations in the S glycoprotein and the ORF3b and 7b proteins occur as virus gains the ability to replicate in macrophages. Infected macrophages serve to transport the virus to sites in the host distant from the initial infection. These infected cells also express several cytokines that are believed to contribute to T-cell apoptosis. *Lower panel*: Clinical disease is characterized by recurrent bouts of virus replication accompanied by fever and clinical disease. Lymphopenia subsequently occurs as disease progresses. The pattern of disease shown in the figure is representative of progressive disease, but the rate and extent of recurrence of virus replication and the rate of weight loss and of development of lymphopenia are variable from animal to animal. (Adapted from de Groot-Mijnes JD, van Dun JM, van der Most RG, et al. Natural history of a recurrent feline coronavirus infection and the role of cellular immunity in survival and disease. *J Virol* 2005;79:1036–1044.)[108]

Phylogenetic analyses suggest that HCoV-NL63 and HCoV-229E diverged approximately 1,000 years ago.[350] A novel feature of HCoV-NL63 is that, unlike HCoV-229E, HCoV-NL63 does not use hAPN as a receptor. Rather, infection of cells is mediated by angiotensin-converting enzyme 2 (ACE2), the same molecule that is used by SARS-CoV, an unrelated betacoronavirus.[172,258] However, unlike SARS-CoV, HCoV-NL63 does not use cathepsin L or require endosomal acidification to infect ACE2-expressing cells[180] and does not cause severe respiratory disease. HCoV-HKU1, isolated from an adult patient in Hong Kong with pneumonia, also generally causes mild respiratory disease.[458]

A role for HCoVs in the etiology of the human disease MS was postulated, based on the ability of murine coronaviruses to cause chronic demyelinating diseases. Coronavirus-like particles have occasionally been detected in the CNS of patients with MS. HCoV-229E RNA was detected in about 44% (40 of 90) of human brains tested, with similar frequencies in brains from

MS patients and patients who died from other neurological diseases or normal control subjects.[22] HCoV-OC43 sequences were detected in 23% (21 of 90) of the brains tested, with 36% incidence in brains from MS patients and 14% in that of controls. HCoV-OC43 has been associated with fatal encephalitis in a severely immunodeficient 11-month-old patient.[296] Together, these results are intriguing, but the role of non–SARS-CoV HCoVs in diseases outside the respiratory tract, especially in CNS diseases such as MS, requires further investigation.

SARS-CoV Infections

SARS-CoV, which causes severe respiratory disease, infects both upper airway and alveolar epithelial cells, resulting in mild to severe lung injury.[332] Virus or viral products are also detected in other organs, such as the kidney, liver, and small intestine, and in stool. Although the lung is recognized as the organ most severely affected by SARS-CoV, the exact mechanism of lung injury is controversial. Levels of infectious virus appear to diminish as clinical disease worsens, consistent with an immunopathological mechanism.[331] However, this conclusion must be tempered because specimens were obtained from nasopharyngeal aspirates, not from the lungs or other organs. The SARS-CoV spike protein may also directly contribute to disease severity. Administration of the SARS-CoV S protein to mice with preexisting lung injury enhanced disease severity.[223] ACE2 appears to have a protective role in animals with lung injury, and S protein may exacerbate disease by causing its downregulation.

Pathological findings in patients who died from SARS were nonspecific. Cells in the upper airway were initially infected, resulting in cell sloughing but relatively little epithelial cell damage. However, virus rapidly spread to the alveoli, causing diffuse alveolar damage. This was characterized by pneumocyte desquamation, alveolar edema, inflammatory cell infiltration, and hyaline membrane formation (Fig. 10.12). Over time, alveolar damage progressed, eventually resulting in pathological signs of ALI (acute lung injury) and, in the most severe cases, ARDS (acute respiratory distress syndrome). Most notably, multinucleated giant cells, originating either from macrophages or respiratory epithelial cells, were detected in autopsy specimens. Although virus could be cultured from infected patients for several weeks, viral antigen was rarely detected in lung autopsy samples after 10 days postinfection.[314]

Like other coronaviruses, such as MHV and FIPV, SARS-CoV infects macrophages and dendritic cells, but unlike these two animal coronaviruses, it causes an abortive infection in these cells.[76,242,397] Several proinflammatory cytokines and chemokines, such as IP-10 (CXCL10), MCP-1 (CCL2), MIP-1a (CCL3), RANTES (CCL5), MCP-2 (CCL8), TNF, and IL-6, are expressed by infected dendritic cells; many of these molecules were also expressed at elevated levels in the serum of SARS-CoV–infected patients.[76] Lymphopenia and neutrophilia

were detected in infected patients and were likely to be primarily cytokine driven.[76] A potentially confounding factor is that many SARS patients were treated with corticosteroids,[400] and steroids are a well-known cause of lymphopenia.

Understanding the mechanism of SARS-CoV–mediated human lung disease is impossible to address in patients since SARS has not recurred since 2004, necessitating the use of animal models. SARS-CoV infects several species of animals, including mice, ferrets, hamsters, cats, and monkeys,[406] but most of these animals develop either mild or no clinical disease, making them not useful for studies of lethal SARS. More useful for these studies was the isolation of rodent-adapted strains that cause severe disease in some strains of mice and rats.[359] Importantly, rodent-adapted strains cause an age-dependent increase in clinical severity,[360,480] paralleling the age-dependent severity observed in infected patients.[126] Animals with severe disease show pathological signs of ALI, increased levels of proinflammatory chemokines and cytokines, and diminished T-cell responses. These observations suggest that immune dysregulation contributes to severe disease, paralleling pathological changes observed in infected humans. Elevated levels of type I interferon (IFN-I) were found in SARS patients with poor outcomes in the 2003 epidemic,[52] but its role in outcomes was not clear. However, mice infected with a lethal dose of SARS-CoV were protected if IFN-I expression was genetically deleted or if IFN signaling was blocked with antibody, suggesting that IFN-I contributed to severe disease.[70]

MERS-CoV Infections
MERS-CoV was first isolated in 2012 from a patient in the Kingdom of Saudi Arabia (KSA) with severe human respiratory disease.[474] MERS cases are confined to the Arabian peninsula and to travelers from the Middle East. In a notable example

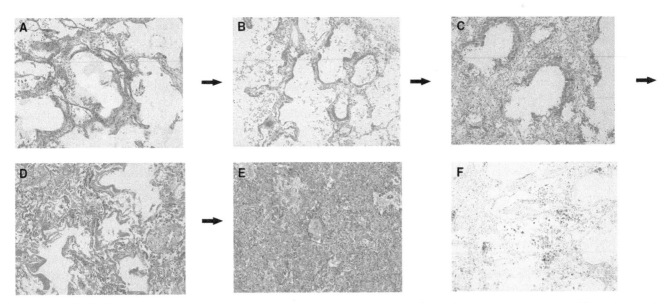

FIGURE 10.12 Pathological changes in lungs of patients with SARS. Lung samples obtained on autopsy were examined for pathological changes following SARS-CoV infection. **A–E:** Hematoxylin and eosin stain showing the progression of SARS pneumonia. Early stages of the SARS infection show edema and early hyaline membrane formation (**A**), hyaline membrane formation (**B**), and increased inflammatory cell infiltration and pneumocyte hyperplasia (**C**). As the disease progresses, fibrotic changes become apparent (**D**). Late manifestations include obliteration of the alveolar volume by fibrous tissue, reactive pneumocytes, and inflammatory cells (**E**). **F:** Viral antigen is detected most prominently during early stages of the infection in macrophages and alveolar pneumocytes. (Figure kindly provided by Dr. John Nicholls, University of Hong Kong. Magnification: ×100.)

of the latter, a single patient who contracted MERS on the Arabian peninsula returned to South Korea, infecting 186 patients.[81] In endemic areas, MERS-CoV appears to be periodically introduced into human populations from infected camels, which are considered the major if not the only zoonotic source of infection.[366] Similar to SARS, the infection begins in the URT with spread to the lower airway. Patients are most contagious after developing pneumonia. Less is known about pathological changes in MERS patients when compared to those with SARS, in large part because only a few autopsies have been performed.[12,311] Like SARS, the mortality rate in MERS is very high, but unlike SARS, a fraction of infected patients develop subclinical disease.[20,183] As in the SARS epidemic, health care workers taking care of MERS patients are at high risk of developing infection. The number of cases decreased substantially as improved infection control measures were introduced in hospitals and emergency rooms.[183]

MERS-CoV primarily infects airway and epithelial cells and poorly infects human macrophages and conventional and plasmacytoid dendritic cells (pDCs). Infection of macrophages and dendritic cells results in a strong inflammatory molecule response.[373,422,482] Furthermore, MERS-CoV actively replicates in activated human T cells,[84] which may contribute to poor immune responses and severe outcomes. Because of the small number of autopsy specimens, animal models of MERS are required for pathogenesis studies. MERS-CoV causes mild disease in experimentally infected camels, macaques, and rabbits but does not infect mice or rats.[65] Notably, experimentally infected camels develop rhinitis with high virus titers,[2] consistent with their role in camel–camel and camel–human transmission. Mice become susceptible to MERS-CoV infection if the human receptor is provided exogenously, either by transfection with adenovirus expressing hDPP4,[479] by transgenic expression of hDPP4,[4] or by replacement of mouse DPP4 with human DPP4 or a chimeric molecule.[85,259,328] Serial virus passage resulted in a lethal disease, making these mice useful for pathogenesis studies.[85,259] Similar to SARS-CoV–infected mice, mice with MERS developed pathological evidence of ALI, proinflammatory molecule expression, and diminished T-cell responses.

Immune Response and Viral Evasion of the Immune Response

As in most viral infections, both the innate and adaptive arms of the immune response are required for successful virus clearance and must be appropriate to minimize bystander immunopathological damage. One of the first steps in the host immune response to a coronavirus infection is the production of type 1 IFN (IFN-α/β). pDCs are the source for most IFN-α/β produced in coronavirus-infected hosts, although other cells, such as macrophages, also express IFN.[62,361] pDC expression of IFN is mediated by signaling through a TLR7- and IRF7-dependent pathway. The importance of IFN signaling in the initial immune response to coronaviruses was shown using mice defective in expression of the IFN-α/β receptor (IFNAR$^{-/-}$).[61,189] Infection of IFNAR$^{-/-}$ mice with mildly virulent strains of MHV results in rapid and uniformly fatal diseases. Additionally, the importance of the IFN response is also evidenced by the multiple IFN evasive mechanisms that coronaviruses employ, as described below. While the importance of the IFN response is well established, less is known about which specific IFN-stimulated genes (ISGs) are most critical for

protection. RNase L, a well-described ISG, has a protective role in mice infected with MHV[478] or MERS-CoV.[416]

Once the initial IFN response is induced, virus clearance requires expression of proinflammatory cytokines and chemokines and their receptors, such as CCL2, CXCL9, CXCL10, and CCL3, to mediate T-cell and macrophage trafficking to sites of infection.[37] Infection of the CNS also requires breakdown of the blood–brain barrier, which is partially neutrophil-dependent. In the absence of neutrophils or of neutrophil chemoattractants, such as CXCL1 and CXCL2, breakdown does not occur, resulting in more severe disease. A robust T-cell response is required for destruction of infected cells and clearance of infectious virus. T-cell responses are poor in felines with progressive FIP (Fig. 10.11) and in mice with severe SARS or MERS.[108,259,481] Virus is not cleared in MHV- or SARS-CoV–infected mice that lack T cells, again demonstrating the importance of the response in clearance.[381,461] Both CD4 and CD8 T-cell epitopes have been identified in mice infected with MHV, SARS-CoV, and MERS-CoV and in SARS patients. The vast majority of epitopes are located on the N, M, and S proteins.[75,266,336,338,479] Once virus has been cleared, the proinflammatory response must be controlled to prevent immunopathology. In MHV-infected mice, regulatory CD4 T cells, characterized by Foxp3 expression, are important for dampening a potentially pathogenic immune response.[418] IL-10, another anti-inflammatory factor important for minimizing immunopathological changes in MHV-infected mice, is expressed predominantly by virus-specific CD4 and CD8 T cells in the infected brain.[419] T cells are responsible for initial virus clearance, but an effective antivirus antibody response is required to prevent virus recrudescence.[263] Similarly, a robust neutralizing antibody response was detected in survivors during the 2002–2003 SARS outbreak[52] and in MERS survivors who had severe disease.[13]

Coronaviruses use several approaches, both active and passive, to evade the host IFN response and thereby establish a productive infection (Table 10.4). Coronaviruses replicate in double-membraned vesicles (DMVs) (Fig. 10.7), which may shield viral RNA from recognition by intracellular sensor molecules, such as RIG-I, MDA5, and TLR3. Thus, in fibroblasts or conventional DCs infected with MHV or SARS-CoV, no IFN is induced.[434,484] However, the IFN response does not appear to be actively blocked in these cells, because infection with *Sendai virus* or exposure to poly I–C induces IFN. In some cells, such as macrophages, microglia, and oligodendrocytes, coronaviruses induce an IFN response by signaling through MDA5 and, in oligodendrocytes, RIG-I.[256] To counter IFN induction through activation of MDA5, all coronaviruses express a 2'-O-methyltransferase (nsp16, see *Expression of the Replicase–Transcriptase Complex*). In the absence of 2'-O-methylation, viral RNA induces a potent MDA5-dependent IFN response, which limits replication in wild-type animals but not in those deficient in IFNAR expression[491] (Table 10.4). Additionally, SARS-CoV, but not MHV PLpro inhibits, inhibits IFN induction by antagonizing IRF3 and NF-κB function.[124,142] Another component of nsp3, ADP-ribose-1''-monophosphatase (also termed macrodomain 1), prevents IFN induction by countering host-derived ADP ribosylation.[141] Nsp15, an endoribonuclease encoded by all coronaviruses, probably has a role in virus replication but also inhibits MDA5 induction and IFN expression.[123,212]

TABLE 10.4 Coronavirus proteins with immunoevasive properties

Protein	Virus Source[a]	Function	References
nsp1	MHV, SARS-CoV, SARSr-BatCoV Rp3, BatCoV HKU4, BatCoV HKU9, TGEV, MERS-CoV	1. Suppresses host protein expression through direct inhibition of translation or by promoting degradation of host mRNA, including IFN mRNA	213,298
		2. Inhibits IFN induction and signaling	492
nsp3 (PLpro)	SARS-CoV, HCoV-NL63, MHV	Blocks IRF3 activation and NF-κB signaling	246
nsp3 (Mac2, Mac3, PLpro)	SARS-CoV, HCoV-NL63, MERS-CoV	Blocks p53 action	246
nsp3 (ADRP)	SARS-CoV, HCoV-229E, MHV	1. Interferes with IFN-induced antiviral activity 2. Enhances host proinflammatory cytokine expression	246,141
nsp5	PDCoV	Inhibits IFN induction	485
nsp14	MHV, TGEV	Interferes with IFN-induced antiviral activity	32,55
nsp15	MHV, HCoV-229E	Evades RNA sensing	123,212
nsp16	MHV	Evades MDA5 activation, evades IFIT recognition	491,103
ORF 3b protein	SARS-CoV	Inhibits IFN synthesis and signaling	220
ORF 6 protein	SARS-CoV	Inhibits STAT1 nuclear translocation	143
ORF 5a protein	MHV	Interferes with IFN-induced antiviral activity	218
ORF 7 protein	TGEV	Interferes with PKR and 2′-5′ OAS/RNase L activities	100
ORF 4a protein	MERS-CoV	Binds dsRNA and inhibits IFN induction, inhibits stress granule formation	391,299,353
ORF 4b protein	MERS-CoV	Inhibits NF-κB signaling, IFN induction, and RNase L activation	416,53,468
ORF 5 protein	MERS-CoV	Modulates NF-κB signaling	286
NS6 protein	PDCoV	Inhibits IFN induction	138
N protein	MHV, SARS-CoV, MERS-CoV	Inhibits IFN induction; interferes with 2′-5′ OAS/RNase L activity	213,125,178
M protein	SARS-CoV, MERS-CoV	Inhibits IRF3 activation	271,389
ORFX protein	SARSr-CoV WIV1	Inhibits IFN induction	475

[a]All virus abbreviations as in Table 29.1.

Once IFNs are expressed, they bind to IFNAR, resulting in the upregulation of a large number of ISGs. Several coronaviral proteins inhibit either IFN signaling or specific ISGs (Table 10.4). In addition to inhibiting IFN induction, the nsp16 2′-O-methyltransferase counters the ability of IFN-induced proteins IFIT1 and IFIT2 (also called ISG56 and ISG54) to inhibit translation of viral mRNA.[103] N protein inhibits IFN signaling, as do SARS-CoV, MHV, TGEV and MERS-CoV nsp1, and SARS-CoV ORF3b and ORF6 proteins. MERS-CoV ORF4a and ORF4b inhibit IFN expression.[213] The mechanism of action of some of these proteins has been elucidated. Nsp1 enhances host cell mRNA degradation and inhibits host cell protein synthesis, with specific effects on IFN signaling.[213] The karyopherin complex is required for nuclear import of STAT1, a critical component of the IFN signaling pathway, as well as the import of many other host proteins. SARS-CoV ORF6, by binding karyopherin-α2, sequesters karyopherin-β1 in the cytoplasm, indirectly inhibiting nuclear translocation of STAT1.[213] MERS-CoV 4b, by binding karyopherin-α4, inhibits NF-κB transport into the nucleus,[53] whereas ORF 4a binds to PACT, inhibiting MDA5 and RIG-I activation.[391] It should be noted that the

role of some of these proteins in the natural infection requires additional study because many of them were analyzed as isolated proteins in transient expression assays. Further, in MERS-CoV–infected camels and humans, some of these immunoevasive genes are deleted without apparent changes in virulence.[83,330,463]

EPIDEMIOLOGY

Human Coronaviruses Other Than SARS-CoV and MERS-CoV

Four known coronaviruses, HCoV-OC43, HCoV-229E, HCoV-NL63, and HCoV-HKU1, are endemic in human populations. HCoV-OC43 and HCoV-229E cause up to 30% of all URT infections, based on several prospective studies.[208,284,429] The variable range of detection reflects year-to-year variability, detection methods, season, and age of subjects. These studies also suggest that peak activity occurs every 2 to 4 years.[145,294] In temperate climates, infections occur predominantly in the winter and early spring. HCoV-OC43 and HCoV-229E have also been associated with severe pneumonia in neonates and aged populations, especially those with underlying illnesses, such as chronic obstructive pulmonary disease or those requiring intensive care.[155,429,439] The high rate of human coronavirus infections early in life and the pattern of infections during outbreaks demonstrate that HCoVs are efficiently transmitted in human populations, most likely via large and, to a lesser extent, small droplets. Infection may also occur via contact with contaminated surfaces.[41] Serologic studies suggest that infection with HCoV-229E and HCoV-OC43 frequently occurs in young children and then repeatedly throughout life.[191,202] Neutralizing antibodies against HCoV-OC43 or HCoV-229E have been detected in about 50% of school-age children and up to 80% of adults.[202,284,345]

HCoV-NL63 and HCoV-HKU1 also have worldwide distributions, causing up to 10% of respiratory tract infections.[1,349] Initial reports suggested that HCoV-NL63 was associated with

severe respiratory disease but subsequent population-based studies showed that most patients developed mild disease, similar to those infected with HCoV-229E or HCoV-OC43.[429] HCoV-NL63 is also an important etiological agent of acute laryngotracheitis (croup).[349] HCoV-HKU1 was initially identified in an elderly patient with severe pneumonia, but subsequent studies indicated that it is associated with both mild and severe respiratory infections.[349,458] HCoV-NL63 and HCoV-229E may have evolved from bat coronaviruses.[413]

Severe Acute Respiratory Syndrome

During the 2002–2003 epidemic, SARS-CoV was isolated from several exotic animals, including Himalayan palm civets (*Paguma larvata*) and raccoon dogs (*Nyctereutes procyonoides*), in wet markets in Guangdong Province in China[161] (Fig. 10.13). Subsequent investigations showed that SARS-CoV

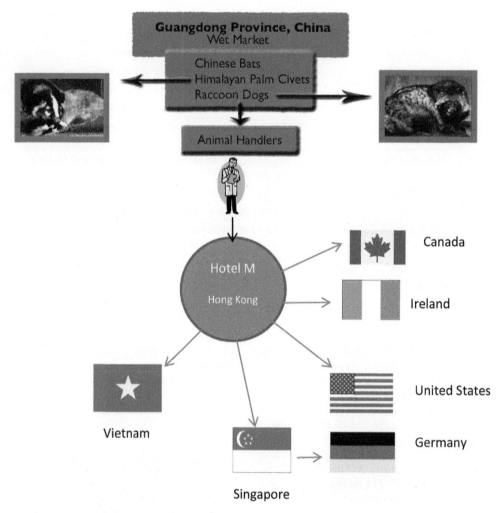

FIGURE 10.13 SARS-CoV spread from infected bats to infect humans in wet markets in Guangdong Province, China. SARS-related coronaviruses were detected in horseshoe bats and other bat species in China. The virus spread to human populations, likely animal handlers, in wet markets in Guangdong Province. Spread occurred either indirectly, via infection of exotic animals such as Himalayan palm civets, or directly, with subsequent human transmission to Himalayan palm civets and other exotic animals. This transmission occurred more than once, because a fraction of the animal handlers was positive for anti–SARS-CoV antibody.[161] In one episode, a physician taking care of an animal handler became infected. He then flew to Hong Kong and stayed at Hotel M, where he inadvertently infected several other people staying at the hotel, probably via superspreading events. These infected individuals then flew to other countries, resulting in the international outbreak.

could not be detected in these animals in the wild but SARS-related coronaviruses (SARSr-CoV) could be isolated from wild bats in China[146,179] (Table 10.1). Bats are now considered to be the ultimate source for SARS-CoV, with probable infection of human populations occurring after initial adaptation to animals in Chinese wet markets. The isolation of bat SARS-like coronaviruses that use ACE2, the same receptor as used by SARS-CoV, provides strong support for this conclusion.[146]

Serologic studies demonstrated that SARS-CoV did not circulate to a significant extent in humans prior to the outbreak in 2002–2003.[66,247] However, some persons working in wild animal wet markets in China had serologic evidence of a SARS-CoV–like infection acquired before the 2003 outbreak but reported no SARS-like respiratory illness.[161] Thus, virus may have circulated in these wild animal markets for a few years, with the SARS outbreak occurring only when a confluence of factors facilitated spread into larger populations. Although non-primate animals were the original source of SARS, its global spread occurred by human-to-human transmission. Transmission occurred through close contact, that is, direct person-to-person contact, fomites, or infectious droplets, and probably aerosols in some instances.[332] Because transmission usually only occurred after onset of illness and most efficiently after the patient was sufficiently ill to be hospitalized, most spread occurred in household and health care settings but infrequently in other settings.[334] A large number of susceptible persons were infected in superspreading events, but only a minority of infected individuals were involved in this type of spread[265,358] (Fig. 10.14). Superspreading events, which occur when a single individual infects multiple susceptible contacts, may have resulted from high virus burdens or a tendency for these individuals to aerosolize virus more efficiently than most infected persons. Most infected individuals spread the virus to only one or a few susceptible persons, suggesting that virus spread was relatively inefficient. Since the SARS outbreak was controlled in June 2003, only 17 cases of SARS were subsequently confirmed, and none of these occurred after June 2004.[260,261] Thirteen of

these 17 cases resulted from laboratory exposures, including 7 secondary cases associated with one of the cases.

Middle East Respiratory Syndrome

MERS-CoV has been isolated from the majority of camels in the Arabian peninsula, Africa, and parts of Asia[139] (Fig. 10.15). In addition, banked camel sera from the early 1980s show evidence of prior MERS-CoV infection. However, human infections have been identified primarily, if not solely, on the Arabian peninsula and even at this location, only since 2012. This difference in prevalence of camel and human infection remains unexplained and may relate to differences in human–camel interactions in countries on the Arabian peninsula compared to elsewhere. MERS-CoV likely originated in bats since MERS-like CoV have been detected in bats in Africa and elsewhere.[94,319] MERS-CoV itself has not been isolated yet from any bat species, reflecting, perhaps, its transmission to camels several years ago and evolution within camel populations. MERS-CoV may be continuing to evolve in camels, since there are distinct clades of MERS-CoV isolated in Africa and the Arabian peninsula.[83,366] Most strikingly, MERS-CoV isolated from camels in West Africa are variably deleted in ORFs3, 4a and 4b,[83] indicating that these genes, which are believed to encode proteins involved in immune evasion, are not required for virulence in camels. Camels in the KSA are largely seropositive for MERS-CoV, with virus maintained by infection of juvenile camels, which become susceptible after maternal antibody has waned. High antibody titers in adult camels suggest that they are periodically exposed to MERS-CoV, boosting antibody titers. Humans in contact with camels have higher MERS-CoV–specific antibody titers than the general population but do not have clinical signs of MERS.[297] In the early years of the KSA outbreak and in the 2016 Korean outbreak, a majority of patients acquired MERS in nosocomial settings.[20,183] This was particularly striking in the Korean outbreak, in which a single traveler from the Middle East sought medical attention in several hospital emergency rooms before a diagnosis of

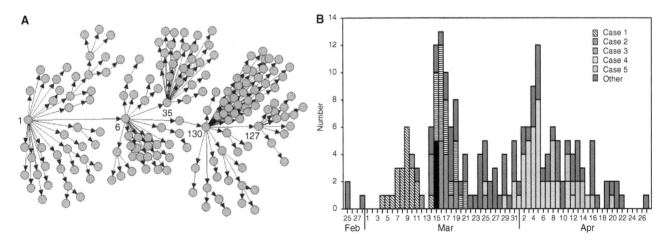

FIGURE 10.14 Role of superspreading events in SARS-CoV epidemics. SARS-CoV spread in Singapore in 2003, illustrated here, via superspreading and non-superspreading events. Most infected persons transmitted virus to less than five susceptible contacts. However, in a few instances, infected individuals were highly contagious, resulting in infection of larger numbers of contacts. The basis for superspreading events is not known but likely is a manifestation of larger virus burdens in a few infected patients. **A:** Probable cases of SARS by reported source of infection. **B:** Number of probable cases of SARS, by date of onset of fever and probable source of infection. (Originally published in Morbidity and Mortality Report, CDC, Atlanta, GA.)

* Human only
*Camel only
*Camel + Human

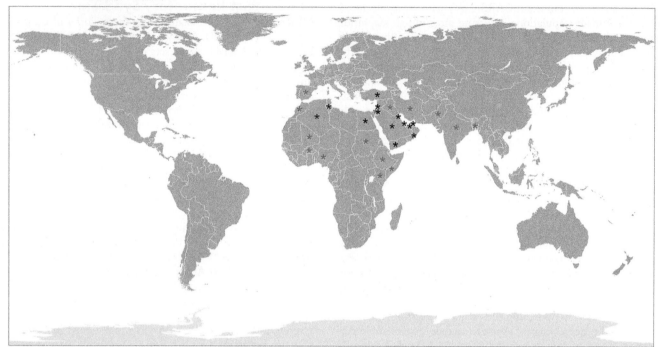

FIGURE 10.15 Global distribution of human and dromedary camel MERS cases.[139] *Black asterisks*—countries with human and camel MERS cases. *Red asterisks*—countries with camel cases only. *Green asterisks*—countries with only human MERS cases. Note that MERS-CoV was detected in camels in the Canary Islands, not in mainland Spain.

MERS was made.[81] The delay in diagnosis resulted in infection of 186 individuals, with a 20% mortality. Increased recognition of the infection and better infection control measures have decreased the number of hospital-acquired infections so that at least 30% of patients are now considered primary.[91] However, only 50% of these patients have a history of camel contact. MERS-CoV is not very contagious in community settings (R_0 < 1) but spreads readily in hospitals to patients with underlying conditions such as chronic pulmonary or cardiac disease, renal failure, or an immunocompromised state.[56,82] One possible explanation for these disparate results is that MERS-CoV is circulating at low levels in some populations and that clinical cases occur occasionally, most often if patients with comorbidities become infected. Although not proven, this would be consistent with the lack of camel contact described by many primary cases. Within hospitals, virus is transmitted via contact and during aerosol-generating procedures.[11] Fomite or aerosol spread may also occur since MERS-CoV RNA (and virus in some studies) can be detected in the air and on environmental surfaces in hospitals for several days.[38,209]

Remarkably, given the recent transmission to humans, there is little evidence for evolution of MERS-CoV in human populations, unlike SARS-CoV, which underwent extensive mutation as it adapted to humans.[80,98] Additionally, deletions in ORFs 3, 4a, 4b, and 5 have been detected in patients,[330,463] suggesting that these immune evasion genes are not critical for human disease. Further, viruses isolated from some patients in Korea were mutated in the S glycoprotein, resulting in lower binding affinity for the DPP4 receptor.[210] Surprisingly,

decreased affinity did not appear to affect clinical disease severity.

Genetic Diversity of Coronaviruses

The SARS and MERS outbreaks demonstrated the ability of coronaviruses to cross species. Initially predicted from studies of coronavirus-infected cultured cells,[30] the ability of coronaviruses to cross species was also demonstrated when the betacoronaviruses HCoV-OC43, porcine hemagglutinating encephalomyelitis virus (PHEV), and BCoV were analyzed[435] (Fig. 10.16). It is estimated that PHEV diverged from HCoV-OC43 and BCoV 100 to 200 years ago, while HCoV-OC43 and BCoV diverged about 100 years ago. More recently, BCoV has crossed species to infect many ruminants, including elks, giraffes, and antelopes.[5] Other phylogenetic studies suggest that the porcine alphacoronavirus TGEV resulted from cross species transmission of a canine coronavirus.[269] In other examples, a bat coronavirus, HKU2, was shown to cross species to cause gastroenteritis in pigs (swine acute diarrheal syndrome [SADS]),[483] and a virus similar to HCoV-229E was isolated from camels.[93] PDCoV, a cause of swine diarrhea, is classified as a deltacoronavirus, a genus comprised of avian viruses. PDCoV appeared to cross from avian to mammalian species, using APN as a receptor and raising the possibility that it could similarly cross species to infect a variety of species, including humans.[253]

In addition to their ability to cross species, coronaviruses readily undergo recombination (see *Viral RNA Synthesis*). Recombination events between canine (CCoV-I) and feline (FCoV-I) coronaviruses and an unknown coronavirus

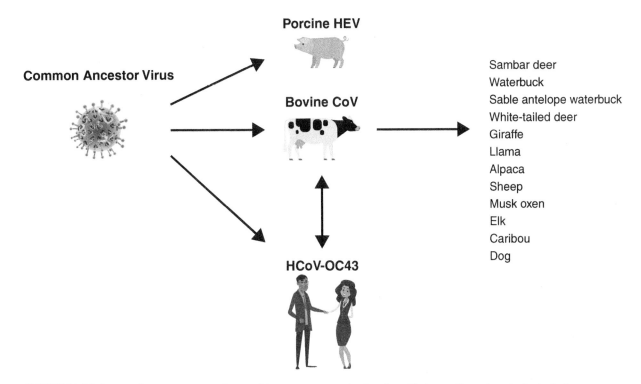

FIGURE 10.16 Coronaviruses mutate and recombine to cross species barriers. Phylogenetic analyses indicate that HCoV-OC43, BCoV, and porcine hemagglutinating encephalomyelitis virus (PHEV) shared a common ancestor and diverged about 200 years ago. More recently (100–130 years ago), HCoV-OC43 and BCoV diverged, but it is not known whether BCoV infected human populations or HCoV-OC43 crossed species barriers to infect bovids. BCoV then spread to many ruminants and to dogs, probably via contact with infected domesticated cows.

resulted in the appearance of two novel viruses (CCoV-II and FCoV-II).[269] In another illustration, new strains of IBV have been detected in chicken populations and appear to have resulted from recombination between circulating vaccine and wild-type IBV strains.[221] This propensity for recombination has raised concerns about the use of live attenuated coronavirus vaccines (see *Prevention*).

CLINICAL FEATURES

Human Coronaviruses Other Than SARS-CoV and MERS-CoV

HCoVs cause respiratory disease, including its most severe manifestations, SARS and MERS. Coronaviruses have occasionally been implicated in human enteric disease, particularly in newborns, with virus identified using electron microscopy because culture of infectious virus has been unsuccessful.[206] EM detection of coronavirus particles is not considered conclusive because other particles in stool specimens can have similar morphology to coronaviruses. However, RT-PCR assays designed to detect coronavirus RNA sequences in pathological specimens should clarify the role of coronaviruses in enteric diseases.

Clinical features of respiratory infections in humans follow two distinct patterns, one for non–SARS-CoV/MERS-CoV (i.e., HCoV-229E, HCoV-NL63, HCoV-OC43, HCoV-HKU1) and one for the zoonotic coronaviruses, SARS-CoV and MERS-CoV. HCoV-229E and HCoV-OC43 were extensively

characterized in volunteer studies in the 1960s.[284] Human volunteers inoculated intranasally with respiratory coronaviruses developed symptoms that included fever, headache, malaise, chills, rhinorrhea, sore throat, and cough with peak infection observed 3 to 4 days following infection. About half of the volunteers challenged with virus developed illness, and approximately 30% were asymptomatically infected, as indicated by detection of virus in the URT. Symptoms lasted for a mean of 7 days, with a range of 3 to 18 days. Natural infection in both adults and children is also usually associated with a common cold–like illness.[284] Natural infection is probably acquired in a fashion similar to that for many other respiratory viruses (i.e., inoculation of infectious secretions from infected persons or fomites onto mucous membranes of the URT or inhalation of infectious droplets), with primary infection of ciliated epithelial cells in the nasopharynx.[3] Destruction of these cells, combined with exuberant production of chemokines and cytokines by resident and infiltrating cells, results in signs and symptoms of clinical illness.

Non–SARS-CoV/MERS-CoV infections are occasionally associated with lower respiratory tract disease in children and adults.[155,409,429,439] One caveat is that coronaviruses are also sometimes detected in well, control patients, and, thus, the presence of virus may not be etiologically related to the illness. Studies using polymerase chain reaction (PCR) to detect viral RNA in middle ear fluids suggest that coronaviruses, like other respiratory viruses, can cause otitis media.[342] HCoV-NL63 and HCoV-HKU1 have also been detected in persons with acute upper and lower respiratory tract illness,[1,166,349] and

HCoV-NL63 is associated with croup in children under the age of 3.[426] Studies of natural infection and volunteer studies showed that reinfection with coronaviruses is common, indicating that infection does not induce stable protective immunity.[191,284] For example, previously infected volunteers developed symptomatic disease if infected 1 year later with the same strain of HCoV-229E.[356]

SARS-CoV Infections

In contrast to the mild illness usually associated with human coronavirus infections, SARS-CoV nearly always resulted in a serious lower respiratory tract illness that required hospitalization, often in an intensive care unit (up to 20% of infections)[332] (Fig. 10.17). In the 2002–2003 epidemic, approximately 8,000 individuals were infected, with an overall mortality rate of 10%. Disease severity increased proportionally to age. Thus, no mortality occurred in patients less than 24 years old, but about 50% of infected individuals greater than 60 years succumbed to the infection. Mortality was also greater in patients with underlying disease. No clinical manifestations distinguished SARS from other severe respiratory diseases.[42,334] Illness usually had an onset of 4 to 7 days, although occasionally an incubation period of 10 to 14 days was observed. Disease was characterized by systemic symptoms such as fever, malaise, and myalgias. Unlike many other respiratory tract infections, URT signs and symptoms were not common. The first lower respiratory tract symptoms (usually a nonproductive cough and shortness of breath) and concomitant abnormalities on radiological examination developed several days after onset of systemic symptoms.[331] Respiratory symptoms were often accompanied by evidence of involvement of other organ systems. Virus particles and RNA were detected in several organs including the gastrointestinal tract, kidneys, and brain.[158] Thus, while diarrhea occurred at disease onset in less than 25% of patients, up to 70% developed gastrointestinal disease during the course of the illness. Most patients developed abnormal liver function tests and lymphopenia with a substantial drop in both CD4 and CD8 T-cell numbers.[102] Patients, generally those greater than 50 years of age or who had underlying disease, often had progressive respiratory failure leading to ARDS and death.[334,354] In these patients, lymphocyte and platelet counts remained abnormally low, while neutrophilia, presence of infectious virus or viral RNA in clinical specimens, and elevated proinflammatory cytokines for prolonged periods of time were common features. Asymptomatic or mild illness was uncommon.[171] Most survivors of SARS-CoV infection achieved full recovery, although pulmonary function abnormalities sometimes took months to subside,[464] and some had persistently abnormal pulmonary function.

MERS-CoV Infections

Like SARS-CoV, MERS-CoV initiates infection via the respiratory tract. The spectrum of human disease caused by MERS-CoV ranges from asymptomatic to severe, with an overall mortality of approximately 36%.[183] Older individuals and those with underlying conditions develop the most severe disease. Patients with severe disease develop respiratory failure and multiorgan dysfunction.[19] No specific clinical or laboratory signs distinguish MERS from other respiratory disease so that laboratory-based diagnosis is critical.[20] Health care workers generally develop mild disease in large part because most do not have underlying conditions. As was the case with SARS patients, MERS patients usually seek medical attention for nonspecific signs including fever, cough, difficult breathing, and diarrhea. As in SARS patients,[331] peak virus loads occur in the 2nd week of illness.[317] Renal damage is common in MERS patients.[19,63] Kidney damage may result from direct infection, possibly because levels of renal DPP4 are high: coronavirus-like particles were observed on autopsy of a patient with MERS.[12] Patients develop laboratory abnormalities similar to those described for SARS.[489] MERS is relatively uncommon in pediatric patients, and those that become infected generally develop mild disease.[6]

DIAGNOSIS

Most human coronavirus infections, other than SARS and MERS, are not diagnosed because they cause mild, self-limited upper respiratory disease, and no specific therapy is available. Diagnosis is laboratory-based because coronavirus infections cannot be distinguished clinically from other causes of URT infections, such as rhinoviruses. However, in some clinical settings, such as in hospitalized patients with pneumonia and in epidemiological studies, specific diagnosis is important. Coronavirus infections in animals and humans were initially diagnosed by isolation of infectious virus, by electron microscopy and using serologic assays, with the caveat that some coronaviruses, especially those in the stool, are not easily cultured. HCoV-229E, HCoV-OC43, and HCoV-NL63 can now be grown in tissue culture cells, but HCoV-HKU1 has been grown only in primary human airway epithelial cells.[351] As is now true for many virus infections, reverse transcription (RT)-PCR–based methods and immunofluorescence assays (IFAs) for virus antigen are the gold standards for diagnosis of respiratory coronavirus infections. PCR primers can be designed to be broadly reactive or strain specific, based on primer location and design. Use of these primers in multiplex assays provides a convenient and rapid method of diagnosis.[145,440] With a sensitive system to detect the PCR amplicon (e.g., a real-time assay), less than five RNA copies in the reaction mixture can be consistently detected.[134] While EM examination of clinical material contributed to the identification and characterization of many coronaviruses, including SARS-CoV,[127,222,284,333] its use at present is confined to the identification of coronaviruses in patients with enteritis,[206] recognizing that such findings are suggestive but not diagnostic.

A variety of serologic assays have been used to detect URT-associated coronavirus infections, including complement fixation, hemagglutination inhibition (HI) for viruses with an HE protein (i.e., some betacoronaviruses), neutralization and immunofluorescence (IFA) assays, and ELISAs (enzyme-linked immunosorbent assays). These assays use virus lysates, inactivated whole virus, cloned expressed proteins, synthesized peptides, and pseudoviruses (e.g., references[39,439]).

SARS and MERS present a different diagnostic situation. A specific diagnosis is critical to guide clinical management, and the diagnosis of MERS or SARS has public health implications. However, testing should only be considered when, based on the likelihood of an exposure and clinical features of the illness, infection is plausible. SARS-CoV was initially isolated in tissue culture cells, but during the 2002–2003 epidemic, a combination of serologic and RT-PCR assays, not

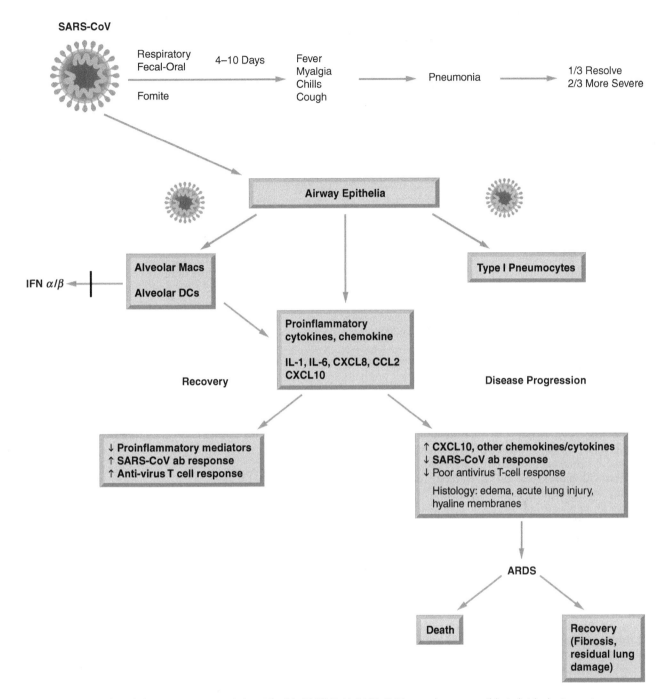

FIGURE 10.17 Clinical disease in patients infected with SARS-CoV. SARS-CoV spread to susceptible individuals via respiratory and fecal–oral routes and, less commonly, if at all, via fomites. Virus replication was initiated in the upper airway epithelial cells, based primarily on animal studies and *in vitro* studies using primary cultures of airway epithelial cells. Virus subsequently spread to the lower respiratory tract, with infection of type 1 pneumocytes and macrophages and dendritic cells most prominent. The infection of the latter two cell types was abortive, resulting in production of proinflammatory cytokines and chemokines such as CXCL10 and CXCL8 but not type I IFN. In patients who recovered, expression of proinflammatory cytokines diminished, and robust antivirus antibody responses were detected. In patients who developed progressively more severe disease, cytokine production continued, and patients remained lymphopenic without developing an effective anti–SARS-CoV antibody response. Some of these patients died and significant long-term morbidity was found in many of the survivors.

virus culture, was used to detect and confirm SARS-CoV infection.[332] With very sensitive PCR assays (e.g., a nested or real-time PCR assay) and RNA extraction procedures that increased the amount of specimen available for the assay, the positivity rate in respiratory specimens obtained during the 2nd and 3rd

days of illness increased from less than 40% to more than 80% as the epidemic progressed.[346] SARS-CoV N protein ELISAs were positive in 50% to 80% of serum specimens collected during the 1st week of illness and in more than 50% of respiratory and stool specimens collected during the 2nd and 3rd weeks of illness.[239] SARS-CoV–specific antibodies were usually detected by 14 days into the illness, but sometimes not until 4 weeks after infection.[177,181] Whereas RT-PCR provided the best way to make an early diagnosis, serologic assays were important in confirming or ruling out SARS-CoV as the cause of infection. Because serum specimens from persons not infected with SARS during the 2002–2003 outbreak have rarely tested positive for SARS-CoV antibodies,[247] a single serum specimen positive for SARS-CoV antibodies was usually considered diagnostic; a negative test on a serum specimen collected late in the illness (28 days or later after onset of illness) was used to rule out SARS-CoV infection. SARS-CoV–specific antibodies were relatively transient, because they could not be detected 6 years after the epidemic ended.[410]

MERS, like SARS, must be diagnosed rapidly and accurately because its clinical features are indistinguishable from those of other acute respiratory infections.[65] Guidelines for MERS testing and diagnosis have been published.[60,207,448] Only patients with a high suspicion for MERS should be tested, to avoid false-positive results. During the acute phase of the illness, a two-step quantitative RT-PCR assay is used for diagnosis, with confirmation by sequencing of PCR products if only a single RT-PCR assay is positive. Isolation of infectious MERS-CoV requires a BSL3 laboratory, so virus isolation is not generally attempted. Measurements of MERS-CoV–specific antibodies are not used for diagnosis during the acute phase since they are generally not detected until 2 to 3 weeks after infection onset.[128] Antibody measurements are useful for studies of disease prevalence, but MERS-CoV–specific antibodies are not detected or are transient in some patients with mild or subclinical disease,[13,217] making them insensitive for this purpose. Even in patients with more severe disease, antibody responses appear to rapidly wane. Initially, screening is generally performed by ELISA, with confirmation by IFA and neutralizing antibody measurements. Patients with detectable neutralization titers may be ELISA negative or borderline, indicating that a combination of ELISA and neutralization assays should be considered in high-risk patients.[14] Virus-specific T cells can be detected during the acute phase in patients with severe disease[383] as well as at 6 to 24 months in all survivors of severe MERS and in some with mild disease. Most of the latter were seronegative.[477] Additionally, SARS-CoV–specific T-cell responses were detected for up to 11 years after the epidemic ended,[312] again suggesting that the T-cell response may be a better measure of prior infection. Detection of virus-specific T-cell responses is technically difficult, but their measurement will be useful in some epidemiological studies. Antibody and T-cell measurements must be carefully controlled and standardized to minimize nonspecific responses mediated by cross-reaction with community-acquired coronavirus infections. Serological cross-reactivity has been reported for SARS-CoV, but not for other coronaviruses.[64]

TREATMENT

At present, there are no approved antiviral drugs for human coronavirus infections and therapy is supportive. During the SARS epidemic, most patients were treated with ribavirin and high-dose steroids, based on the belief that the virus would be susceptible to ribavirin and steroids might diminish immune-mediated bystander damage. However, meta-analyses of outcomes showed that neither drug was efficacious and steroid use was associated with worse outcomes.[400] Late in the epidemic, IFN-α, SARS convalescent phase immunoglobulin, and lopinavir plus ritonavir, two proteases licensed for the treatment of HIV, were used to treat patients. Review of all of these therapies concluded that while some showed efficacy in inhibiting SARS-CoV replication in tissue culture cells, none showed a beneficial effect in patients.[400] Similarly, convalescent sera and various combinations of ribavirin, IFN-α, corticosteroids, and lopinavir–ritonavir did not improve outcomes in MERS patients, although corticosteroid use delayed virus clearance.[21,488] The mechanism of coronavirus replication involves several proteins that are potential targets for antiviral drugs, including the viral RdRp, virus-encoded proteases, host cell receptors used by the virus for entry, and the viral S glycoprotein. Consequently, several antiviral drugs targeting these viral proteins or processes have been developed and evaluated for their ability to inhibit SARS-CoV and MERS-CoV replication *in vitro* and in experimentally infected animals.[65,488] These include protease inhibitors,[18] monoclonal antibodies that inhibit binding to cells, peptides from the heptad repeat regions of the S protein that inhibit receptor binding or fusion, small interfering RNAs, and polymerase and helicase inhibitors.[65,382,488] A second promising category of drug is a set of 3CLpro inhibitors with broad activity against coronaviruses. One drug, GC376, is most active against feline coronaviruses, although it also has activity against other coronaviruses. Remarkably, it was shown to effect recovery of cats with clinical FIPV, a uniformly fatal disease.[211]

PREVENTION

No vaccines are available to prevent human coronavirus infection, but vaccines against domestic animal coronaviruses, such as IBV, PEDV, TGEV, and BCoV, are routinely used to prevent serious disease in young animals. Efforts are ongoing to improve these vaccines and to enhance safety and efficacy while minimizing the likelihood of reversion to a virulent strain and recombination with circulating strains.[367] In addition, several SARS-CoV vaccines have been developed, including inactivated whole virus, live virus vectors expressing single viral proteins, and recombinant proteins and DNA vaccines.[156] Nearly all of these vaccines express the surface glycoprotein and are designed to induce SARS-CoV neutralizing antibodies. For some of these vaccines, efficacy has been demonstrated in animal models. Large stocks of anti–SARS-CoV neutralizing antibody have been prepared and are available for passive immunization of health care workers and other high-risk personnel if SARS recurs.

MERS was identified in 2018 by the WHO and Coalition for Epidemic Preparedness Innovations (CEPI) as a key target for vaccine development, because it may evolve to pose an epidemic threat. Similar to SARS-CoV, several MERS-CoV–specific vaccines are under development, including subunit, measles, adenovirus, and vaccinia vaccines expressing the S glycoprotein, recombinant proteins, nanoparticles, VLPs, and DNA vaccines.[318] Some of these vaccines are presently in phase I clinical trials. Additionally, several potently neutralizing antibodies have been detected,[65,488] which will be useful for passively immunizing health care workers and other exposed individuals in outbreak settings. Given the small number of MERS patients, it is unlikely that active vaccination will ever be used widely in human populations, unless the virus mutates so that human-to-human transmission is greatly increased. As an alternative strategy, vaccination of camels is considered a more feasible approach. Vaccination with a camel poxvirus expressing the MERS S glycoprotein conferred immunity against both MERS-CoV and camelpox, representing a vaccine candidate with dual efficacy.[163] Use of a poxvirus has the advantage of inducing potent antivirus T-cell as well as antibody responses.

In general, live attenuated vaccines are most effective in inducing protective immune responses against coronaviruses. This has been illustrated elegantly in the case of transmissible gastroenteritis virus (TGEV), an important cause of neonatal diarrhea and death in swine. In the mid-1980s, a naturally occurring, attenuated variant of TGEV, porcine respiratory coronavirus (PRCoV), was identified in pig populations. This virus, which causes mild disease and no enteritis, induces an immune response in pigs that is protective against TGEV and largely eliminated it from infected populations.[241] Live attenuated vaccines induce not only neutralizing antibodies but also antivirus T-cell responses, which are required for virus clearance from infected cells in SARS, MERS, and other coronavirus infections.[71] However, the development of live coronavirus vaccines is challenging.[367] First, in many instances, natural infection does not prevent subsequent infection or disease, so an effective vaccine would need to be superior to immunity induced naturally. Second, the genetic and antigenic variability of coronaviruses and their ability to readily recombine hinder vaccine development. Thus, a vaccine may not provide equal protection to all antigenic variants, and subsequent recombination with vaccine strains could increase the number of different strains circulating in the wild. As an example, recombinants of IBV vaccine and wild-type strains have caused disease outbreaks in chicken flocks.[194] In addition, the finding that immunization with an S protein–expressing FIPV vaccine led to more severe disease after subsequent natural infection raises the concern that other coronavirus vaccines might also enhance rather than protect from disease.[431] Several strategies to minimize the likelihood of recombination and to attenuate candidate vaccines without compromising efficacy have been recently described. These include engineering viruses with deletions or mutations in nsp1, important for immune evasion[492]; nsp14, critical for RNA genome fidelity; or E protein, important for virus assembly.[156] In other approaches to minimizing recombination of vaccine viruses, the coronavirus genome has been reconstructed, modifying the leader and body TRSs (see *Viral RNA Synthesis*) to eliminate homology with naturally occurring virus sequences.[472]

In the absence of effective vaccines and antiviral drugs, the most important ways to prevent human coronavirus infections are a highly active public health surveillance system and good infection control practices. This was demonstrated unequivocally during the SARS outbreak in 2002–2003, in which sharing of information by national public health agencies and governments and involvement of international agencies such as the World Health Organization resulted in the rapid identification of a coronavirus as the cause of SARS and implementation of measures that minimized spread. At the local level, strict attention to good isolation and infection control practices and identification and management of exposed persons (contacts) minimized human-to-human spread of the virus within a few months of its global spread. The low risk of SARS-CoV transmission before hospitalization and the low rate of asymptomatic infection facilitated the efficacy of these public health measures.[78] The identification of cases of laboratory-acquired SARS-CoV, with subsequent transmission to others after one of these cases,[260,261] reinforces the importance of strict attention to safe laboratory practices. These practices include handling the virus in the appropriate type of facility, using standardized operating procedures and providing appropriate training and medical surveillance programs for staff. Similarly, stringent use of infection control measures and careful screening of patients has diminished nosocomial transmission of MERS-CoV and helped end the Korean outbreak.[183,325]

PERSPECTIVES

Many important problems remain to be resolved in future studies. One critical task will be to develop a detailed understanding of how coronaviruses cross species. Are cross species viral trafficking events rare or common, and what features facilitate or inhibit cross species transmission? While there has been a recent expansion of our knowledge of spike protein interactions with receptors and associated proteases, we cannot yet fully gauge the likelihood of productive adaptation by a spike protein to new receptors and proteases. Such information will be directly relevant to forestalling or coping with the emergence or reemergence of pathogenic HCoVs from ubiquitous bat reservoirs. A second area of crucial importance will be to increase our understanding of the immunopathogenesis of the more severe human and animal coronaviruses and to more precisely define the correlates of immune protection. This will involve delineating the relationship between coronaviruses and their host immune response. Understanding the intricacies in this relationship will inform the effective design and evaluation of vaccines for control of these agents. Third, one of the most exciting areas of future research continues to be addressing the many gaps in our basic knowledge of the intricacies of the coronavirus RTC, the largest and most complicated machinery of RNA synthesis found in any RNA virus. The past few years have seen tremendous advances resulting from structural and biochemical studies, and it is likely that progress will continue apace. A long-term goal is the total *in vitro* reconstitution of coronavirus RNA synthesis, which would definitively identify or confirm the roles of the many viral replicase subunits as well as of putative host factors. It can be expected that studies of this type will reveal fundamental principles common to all RNA-dependent RNA synthesis, in addition to mechanisms unique to the order *Nidovirales*. Knowledge derived from this enterprise will be critical for the design of antiviral drugs to combat diseases caused by existing and emerging coronaviruses.

REFERENCES

1. Abdul-Rasool S, Fielding BC. Understanding human coronavirus HCoV-NL63. *Open Virol J* 2010;4:76–84.
2. Adney DR, van Doremalen N, Brown VR, et al. Replication and shedding of MERS-CoV in upper respiratory tract of inoculated dromedary camels. *Emerg Infect Dis* 2014;20:1999–2005.
3. Afzelius BA. Ultrastructure of human nasal epithelium during an episode of coronavirus infection. *Virchows Arch* 1994;424:295–300.
4. Agrawal AS, Garron T, Tao X, et al. Generation of a transgenic mouse model of Middle East respiratory syndrome coronavirus infection and disease. *J Virol* 2015;89:3659–3670.

5. Alekseev KP, Vlasova AN, Jung K, et al. Bovine-like coronaviruses isolated from four species of captive wild ruminants are homologous to bovine coronaviruses based on complete genomic sequences. *J Virol* 2008;82:12422–12431.

6. Alfaraj SH, Al-Tawfiq JA, Altuwaijri TA, et al. Middle East respiratory syndrome coronavirus in pediatrics; a report of seven cases from Saudi Arabia. *Front Med* 2018. doi: 10.1007/s11684-017-0603-y.

7. Almazán F, DeDiego ML, Sola I, et al. Engineering a replication-competent, propagation-defective Middle East respiratory syndrome coronavirus as a vaccine candidate. *MBio* 2013;4:e00650-13.

8. Almazán F, González JM, Pénzes Z, et al. Engineering the largest RNA virus genome as an infectious bacterial artificial chromosome. *Proc Natl Acad Sci U S A* 2000;97:5516–5521.

9. Almazán F, Sola I, Zuñiga S, et al. Coronavirus reverse genetic systems: infectious clones and replicons. *Virus Res* 2014;189:262–270.

10. Almeida JD, Tyrrell DA. The morphology of three previously uncharacterized human respiratory viruses that grow in organ culture. *J Gen Virol* 1967;1:175–178.

11. Alraddadi BM, Al-Salmi HS, Jacobs-Slifka K, et al. Risk factors for Middle East Respiratory Syndrome coronavirus infection among healthcare personnel. *Emerg Infect Dis* 2016;22:1915–1920.

12. Alsaad KO, Hajeer AH, Al Balwi M, et al. Histopathology of Middle East respiratory syndrome coronavirus (MERS-CoV) infection—clinicopathological and ultrastructural study. *Histopathology* 2017;72:516–524.

13. Alshukairi AN, Khalid I, Ahmed WA, et al. Antibody response and disease severity in healthcare worker MERS survivors. *Emerg Infect Dis* 2016;22:1113–1115.

14. Alshukairi AN, Zheng J, Zhao J, et al. High prevalence of MERS-CoV infection in camel workers in Saudi Arabia. *MBio* 2018;9:e01985-18.

15. Anand K, Palm GJ, Mesters JR, et al. Structure of coronavirus main proteinase reveals combination of a chymotrypsin fold with an extra alpha-helical domain. *EMBO J* 2002;21:3213–3224.

16. Angelini MM, Akhlaghpour M, Neuman BW, et al. Severe acute respiratory syndrome coronavirus nonstructural proteins 3, 4, and 6 induce double-membrane vesicles. *MBio* 2013;4:e00524-13.

17. Anghelina D, Pewe L, Perlman S. Pathogenic role for virus-specific CD4 T cells in mice with coronavirus-induced acute encephalitis. *Am J Pathol* 2006;169:209–222.

18. Arabi YM, Alothman A, Balkhy HH, et al. Treatment of Middle East respiratory syndrome with a combination of lopinavir-ritonavir and interferon-beta1b (MIRACLE trial): study protocol for a randomized controlled trial. *Trials* 2018;19:81.

19. Arabi YM, Arifi AA, Balkhy HH, et al. Clinical course and outcomes of critically ill patients with Middle East respiratory syndrome coronavirus infection. *Ann Intern Med* 2014;160:389–397.

20. Arabi YM, Balkhy HH, Hayden FG, et al. Middle East respiratory syndrome. *N Engl J Med* 2017;376:584–594.

21. Arabi YM, Mandourah Y, Al-Hameed F, et al. Corticosteroid therapy for critically ill patients with Middle East Respiratory Syndrome. *Am J Respir Crit Care Med* 2018;197:757–767.

22. Arbour N, Day R, Newcombe J, et al. Neuroinvasion by human respiratory coronaviruses. *J Virol* 2000;74:8913–8921.

23. Arndt AL, Larson BJ, Hogue BG. A conserved domain in the coronavirus membrane protein tail is important for virus assembly. *J Virol* 2010;84:11418–11428.

24. Athmer J, Fehr AR, Grunewald ME, et al. Selective packaging in murine coronavirus promotes virulence by limiting type I interferon responses. *MBio* 2018;9:e00272-18.

25. Bailey O, Pappenheimer AM, Cheever FS, et al. A murine virus (JHM) causing disseminated encephalomyelitis with extensive destruction of myelin. *J Exp Med* 1949;90:195–212.

26. Bakkers MJ, Lang Y, Feitsma LJ, et al. Betacoronavirus adaptation to humans involved progressive loss of hemagglutinin-esterase lectin activity. *Cell Host Microbe* 2017;21:356–366.

27. Banner LR, Lai MM. Random nature of coronavirus RNA recombination in the absence of selection pressure. *Virology* 1991;185:441–445.

28. Bárcena M, Oostergetel GT, Bartelink W, et al. Cryo-electron tomography of mouse hepatitis virus: insights into the structure of the coronavirion. *Proc Natl Acad Sci U S A* 2009;106:582–587.

29. Baric RS, Fu K, Schaad MC, et al. Establishing a genetic recombination map for murine coronavirus strain A59 complementation groups. *Virology* 1990;177:646–656.

30. Baric RS, Sullivan E, Hensley L, et al. Persistent infection promotes cross-species transmissibility of mouse hepatitis virus. *J Virol* 1999;73:638–649.

31. Baric RS, Yount B. Subgenomic negative-strand RNA function during mouse hepatitis virus infection. *J Virol* 2000;74:4039–4046.

32. Becares M, Pascual-Iglesias A, Nogales A, et al. Mutagenesis of coronavirus nsp14 reveals Its potential role in modulation of the innate immune response. *J Virol* 2016;90:5399–5414.

33. Becker MM, Graham RL, Donaldson EF, et al. Synthetic recombinant bat SARS-like coronavirus is infectious in cultured cells and in mice. *Proc Natl Acad Sci U S A* 2008;105:19944–19949.

34. Belouzard S, Chu VC, Whittaker GR. Activation of the SARS coronavirus spike protein via sequential proteolytic cleavage at two distinct sites. *Proc Natl Acad Sci U S A* 2009;106:5871–5876.

35. Benbacer L, Kut E, Besnardeau L, et al. Interspecies aminopeptidase-N chimeras reveal species-specific receptor recognition by canine coronavirus, feline infectious peritonitis virus, and transmissible gastroenteritis virus. *J Virol* 1997;71:734–737.

36. Beniac DR, Andonov A, Grudeski E, et al. Architecture of the SARS coronavirus prefusion spike. *Nat Struct Mol Biol* 2006;13:751–752.

37. Bergmann CC, Lane TE, Stohlman SA. Coronavirus infection of the central nervous system: host-virus stand-off. *Nat Rev Microbiol* 2006;4:121–132.

38. Bin SY, Heo JY, Song MS, et al. Environmental contamination and viral shedding in MERS patients during MERS-CoV outbreak in South Korea. *Clin Infect Dis* 2016;62:755–760.

39. Blanchard EG, Miao C, Haupt TE, et al. Development of a recombinant truncated nucleocapsid protein based immunoassay for detection of antibodies against human coronavirus OC43. *J Virol Methods* 2011;177:100–106.

40. Bonavia A, Zelus BD, Wentworth DE, et al. Identification of a receptor-binding domain of the spike glycoprotein of human coronavirus HCoV-229E. *J Virol* 2003;77:2530–2538.

41. Bonny TS, Yezli S, Lednicky JA. Isolation and identification of human coronavirus 229E from frequently touched environmental surfaces of a university classroom that is cleaned daily. *Am J Infect Control* 2018;46:105–107.

42. Booth CM, Matukas LM, Tomlinson GA, et al. Clinical features and short-term outcomes of 144 patients with SARS in the greater Toronto area. *JAMA* 2003;289:2801–2809.

43. Bos EC, Luytjes W, van der Meulen HV, et al. The production of recombinant infectious DI-particles of a murine coronavirus in the absence of helper virus. *Virology* 1996;218:52–60.

44. Boscarino JA, Logan HL, Lacny JJ, et al. Envelope protein palmitoylations are crucial for murine coronavirus assembly. *J Virol* 2008;82:2989–2999.

45. Bosch BJ, de Haan CA, Smits SL, et al. Spike protein assembly into the coronavirion: exploring the limits of its sequence requirements. *Virology* 2005;334:306–318.

46. Bosch BJ, Rottier PJM. Nidovirus entry into cells. In: Perlman S, Gallagher T, Snijder EJ, eds. *Nidoviruses*. Washington: ASM Press; 2008:361–377.

47. Bosch BJ, van der Zee R, de Haan CA, et al. The coronavirus spike protein is a class I virus fusion protein: structural and functional characterization of the fusion core complex. *J Virol* 2003;77:8801–8811.

48. Bouvet M, Imbert I, Subissi L, et al. RNA 3′-end mismatch excision by the severe acute respiratory syndrome coronavirus nonstructural protein nsp10/nsp14 exoribonuclease complex. *Proc Natl Acad Sci U S A* 2012;109:9372–9377.

49. Brierley I, Digard P, Inglis SC. Characterization of an efficient coronavirus ribosomal frameshifting signal: requirement for an RNA pseudoknot. *Cell* 1989;57:537–547.

50. Brierley I, Rolley NJ, Jenner AJ, et al. Mutational analysis of the RNA pseudoknot component of a coronavirus ribosomal frameshifting signal. *J Mol Biol* 1991;220:889–902.

51. Calvo E, Escors D, López JA, et al. Phosphorylation and subcellular localization of transmissible gastroenteritis virus nucleocapsid protein in infected cells. *J Gen Virol* 2005;86:2255–2267.

52. Cameron MJ, Ran L, Xu L, et al. Interferon-mediated immunopathological events are associated with atypical innate and adaptive immune responses in patients with severe acute respiratory syndrome. *J Virol* 2007;81:8692–8706.

53. Canton J, Fehr AR, Fernandez-Delgado R, et al. MERS-CoV 4b protein interferes with the NF-kappaB-dependent innate immune response during infection. *PLoS Pathog* 2018;14:e1006838.

54. Casais R, Thiel V, Siddell SG, et al. Reverse genetics system for the avian coronavirus infectious bronchitis virus. *J Virol* 2001;75:12359–12369.

55. Case JB, Li Y, Elliott R, et al. Murine hepatitis virus nsp14 exoribonuclease activity is required for resistance to innate immunity. *J Virol* 2018;92:e01531-17.

56. Cauchemez S, Nouvellet P, Cori A, et al. Unraveling the drivers of MERS-CoV transmission. *Proc Natl Acad Sci U S A* 2016;113:9081–9086.

57. Caul EO, Ashley CR, Ferguson M, et al. Preliminary studies on the isolation of coronavirus 229E nucleocapsids. *FEMS Microbiol Lett* 1979;5:101–105.

58. Cavanagh D, Davis PJ, Pappin DJ. Coronavirus IBV glycopolypeptides: locational studies using proteases and saponin, a membrane permeabilizer. *Virus Res* 1986;4:145–156.

59. Cavanagh D, Davis PJ, Pappin DJ, et al. Coronavirus IBV: partial amino terminal sequencing of spike polypeptide S2 identifies the sequence Arg-Arg-Phe-Arg-Arg at the cleavage site of the spike precursor propolypeptide of IBV strains Beaudette and M41. *Virus Res* 1986;4:133–143.

60. CDC. Middle East respiratory syndrome (MERS): case definitions. 2014. Available at: http://www.cdc.gov/coronavirus/mers/case-def.html

61. Cervantes-Barragan L, Kalinke U, Zust R, et al. Type I IFN-mediated protection of macrophages and dendritic cells secures control of murine coronavirus infection. *J Immunol* 2009;182:1099–1106.

62. Cervantes-Barragan L, Zust R, Weber F, et al. Control of coronavirus infection through plasmacytoid dendritic cell-derived type I interferon. *Blood* 2006;109:1131–1137.

63. Cha RH, Joh JS, Jeong I, et al. Renal complications and their prognosis in Korean patients with Middle East Respiratory Syndrome-Coronavirus from the central MERS-CoV designated hospital. *J Korean Med Sci* 2015;30:1807–1814.

64. Chan KH, Chan JF, Tse H, et al. Cross-reactive antibodies in convalescent SARS patients' sera against the emerging novel human coronavirus EMC (2012) by both immunofluorescent and neutralizing antibody tests. *J Infect* 2013;67:130–140.

65. Chan JF, Lau SK, To KK, et al. Middle East respiratory syndrome coronavirus: another zoonotic betacoronavirus causing SARS-like disease. *Clin Microbiol Rev* 2015;28:465–522.

66. Chan KH, Poon LL, Cheng VC, et al. Detection of SARS coronavirus in patients with suspected SARS. *Emerg Infect Dis* 2004;10:294–299.

67. Chang CK, Chen CM, Chiang MH, et al. Transient oligomerization of the SARS-CoV N protein–implication for virus ribonucleoprotein packaging. *PLoS One* 2013;8:e65045.

68. Chang CK, Hou MH, Chang CF, et al. The SARS coronavirus nucleocapsid protein–forms and functions. *Antiviral Res* 2014;103:39–50.

69. Chang CK, Hsu YL, Chang YH, et al. Multiple nucleic acid binding sites and intrinsic disorder of severe acute respiratory syndrome coronavirus nucleocapsid protein: implications for ribonucleocapsid protein packaging. *J Virol* 2009;83:2255–2264.

70. Channappanavar R, Fehr AR, Vijay R, et al. Dysregulated type I interferon and inflammatory monocyte-macrophage responses cause lethal pneumonia in SARS-CoV-infected mice. *Cell Host Microbe* 2016;19:181–193.

71. Channappanavar R, Zhao J, Perlman S. T cell-mediated immune response to respiratory coronaviruses. *Immunol Res* 2014;59:118–128.

72. Chen Y, Cai H, Pan J, et al. Functional screen reveals SARS coronavirus nonstructural protein nsp14 as a novel cap N7 methyltransferase. *Proc Natl Acad Sci U S A* 2009;106:3484–3489.

73. Chen CY, Chang CK, Chang YW, et al. Structure of the SARS coronavirus nucleocapsid protein RNA-binding dimerization domain suggests a mechanism for helical packaging of viral RNA. *J Mol Biol* 2007;368:1075–1086.

74. Chen H, Gill A, Dove BK, et al. Mass spectroscopic characterization of the coronavirus infectious bronchitis virus nucleoprotein and elucidation of the role of phosphorylation in RNA binding by using surface plasmon resonance. *J Virol* 2005;79:1164–1179.

75. Chen H, Hou J, Jiang X, et al. Response of memory CD8+ T cells to severe acute respiratory syndrome (SARS) coronavirus in recovered SARS patients and healthy individuals. *J Immunol* 2005;175:591–598.

76. Chen J, Subbarao K. The immunobiology of SARS. *Annu Rev Immunol* 2007;25:443–472.

77. Chen SC, van den Born E, van den Worm SH, et al. New structure model for the packaging signal in the genome of group IIa coronaviruses. *J Virol* 2007;81:6771–6774.

78. Cheng VC, Chan JF, To KK, et al. Clinical management and infection control of SARS: lessons learned. *Antiviral Res* 2013;100:407–419.

79. Chibo D, Birch C. Analysis of human coronavirus 229E spike and nucleoprotein genes demonstrates genetic drift between chronologically distinct strains. *J Gen Virol* 2006;87:1203–1208.

80. Chinese SMEC. Molecular evolution of the SARS coronavirus during the course of the SARS epidemic in China. *Science* 2004;303:1666–1669.

81. Cho SY, Kang JM, Ha YE, et al. MERS-CoV outbreak following a single patient exposure in an emergency room in South Korea: an epidemiological outbreak study. *Lancet* 2016;388:994–1001.

82. Choi S, Jung E, Choi BY, et al. High reproduction number of Middle East respiratory syndrome coronavirus in nosocomial outbreaks: mathematical modelling in Saudi Arabia and South Korea. *J Hosp Infect* 2018;99:162–168.

83. Chu DKW, Hui KPY, Perera R, et al. MERS coronaviruses from camels in Africa exhibit region-dependent genetic diversity. *Proc Natl Acad Sci U S A* 2018;115:3144–3149.

84. Chu H, Zhou J, Wong BH, et al. Middle East Respiratory Syndrome coronavirus efficiently infects human primary T lymphocytes and activates the extrinsic and intrinsic apoptosis pathways. *J Infect Dis* 2016;213:904–914.

85. Cockrell AS, Yount BL, Scobey T, et al. A mouse model for MERS coronavirus-induced acute respiratory distress syndrome. *Nat Microbiol* 2016;2:16226.

86. Collins AR, Knobler RL, Powell H, et al. Monoclonal antibodies to murine hepatitis virus-4 (strain JHM) define the viral glycoprotein responsible for attachment and cell-cell fusion. *Virology* 1982;119:358–371.

87. Cologna R, Spagnolo JF, Hogue BG. Identification of nucleocapsid binding sites within coronavirus-defective genomes. *Virology* 2000;277:235–249.

88. Compton SR, Barthold SW, Smith AL. The cell and molecular pathogenesis of coronaviruses. *Lab Anim Sci* 1993;43:15–28.

89. Cong Y, Kriegenburg F, de Haan CAM, et al. Coronavirus nucleocapsid proteins assemble constitutively in high molecular oligomers. *Sci Rep* 2017;7:5740.

90. Cong Y, Ren X. Coronavirus entry and release in polarized epithelial cells: a review. *Rev Med Virol* 2014;24:308–315.

91. Conzade R, Grant R, Malik MR, et al. Reported direct and indirect contact with dromedary camels among laboratory-confirmed MERS-CoV cases. *Viruses* 2018;10:425.

92. Corman VM, Baldwin HJ, Tateno AF, et al. Evidence for an ancestral association of human coronavirus 229E with bats. *J Virol* 2015;89:11858–11870.

93. Corman VM, Eckerle I, Memish ZA, et al. Link of a ubiquitous human coronavirus to dromedary camels. *Proc Natl Acad Sci U S A* 2016;113:9864–9869.

94. Corman VM, Ithete NL, Richards LR, et al. Rooting the phylogenetic tree of middle East respiratory syndrome coronavirus by characterization of a conspecific virus from an African bat. *J Virol* 2014;88:11297–11303.

95. Cornelissen LA, Wierda CM, van der Meer FJ, et al. Hemagglutinin-esterase, a novel structural protein of torovirus. *J Virol* 1997;71:5277–5286.

96. Corse E, Machamer CE. Infectious bronchitis virus E protein is targeted to the Golgi complex and directs release of virus-like particles. *J Virol* 2000;74:4319–4326.

97. Corse E, Machamer CE. The cytoplasmic tail of infectious bronchitis virus E protein directs Golgi targeting. *J Virol* 2002;76:1273–1284.

98. Cotten M, Watson SJ, Zumla AI, et al. Spread, circulation, and evolution of the Middle East respiratory syndrome coronavirus. *MBio* 2014;5:e01062-13.

99. Cowley JA, Walker PJ. Molecular biology and pathogenesis of roniviruses. In: Perlman S, Gallagher T, Snijder EJ, eds. *Nidoviruses*. Washington: ASM Press; 2008:361–377.

100. Cruz JL, Becares M, Sola I, et al. Alphacoronavirus protein 7 modulates host innate immune response. *J Virol* 2013;87:9754–9767.

101. Cruz JL, Sola I, Becares M, et al. Coronavirus gene 7 counteracts host defenses and modulates virus virulence. *PLoS Pathog* 2011;7:e1002090.

102. Cui W, Fan Y, Wu W, et al. Expression of lymphocytes and lymphocyte subsets in patients with severe acute respiratory syndrome. *Clin Infect Dis* 2003;37:857–859.

103. Daffis S, Szretter KJ, Schriewer J, et al. 2'-O methylation of the viral mRNA cap evades host restriction by IFIT family members. *Nature* 2010;468:452–456.

104. Davies HA, Dourmashkin RR, Macnaughton MR. Ribonucleoprotein of avian infectious bronchitis virus. *J Gen Virol* 1981;53:67–74.

105. de Groot RJ. Structure, function and evolution of the hemagglutinin-esterase proteins of corona- and toroviruses. *Glycoconj J* 2006;23:59–72.

106. de Groot RJ, Baker SC, Baric R, et al. Family–Coronaviridae. In: King AMQ, Adams MJ, Carstens EB, et al. eds. *Virus Taxonomy Classification and Nomenclature of Viruses Ninth Report of the International Committee on Taxonomy of Viruses*. San Diego: Elsevier; 2012:806–828.

107. de Groot RJ, Luytjes W, Horzinek MC, et al. Evidence for a coiled-coil structure in the spike proteins of coronaviruses. *J Mol Biol* 1987;196:963–966.

108. de Groot-Mijnes JD, van Dun JM, van der Most RG, et al. Natural history of a recurrent feline coronavirus infection and the role of cellular immunity in survival and disease. *J Virol* 2005;79:1036–1044.

109. de Haan CA, de Wit M, Kuo L, et al. The glycosylation status of the murine hepatitis coronavirus M protein affects the interferogenic capacity of the virus in vitro and its ability to replicate in the liver but not the brain. *Virology* 2003;312:395–406.

110. de Haan CA, Masters PS, Shen X, et al. The group-specific murine coronavirus genes are not essential, but their deletion, by reverse genetics, is attenuating in the natural host. *Virology* 2002;296:177–189.

111. de Haan CA, Roestenberg P, de Wit M, et al. Structural requirements for O-glycosylation of the mouse hepatitis virus membrane protein. *J Biol Chem* 1998;273:29905–29914.

112. de Haan CA, Rottier PJ. Molecular interactions in the assembly of coronaviruses. *Adv Virus Res* 2005;64:165–230.

113. de Haan CA, Volders H, Koetzner CA, et al. Coronaviruses maintain viability despite dramatic rearrangements of the strictly conserved genome organization. *J Virol* 2002;76:12491–12502.

114. Decroly E, Imbert I, Coutard B, et al. Coronavirus nonstructural protein 16 is a cap-0 binding enzyme possessing (nucleoside-2'O)-methyltransferase activity. *J Virol* 2008;82:8071–8084.

115. DeDiego ML, Alvarez E, Almazán F, et al. A severe acute respiratory syndrome coronavirus that lacks the E gene is attenuated in vitro and in vivo. *J Virol* 2007;81:1701–1713.

116. Delmas B, Gelfi J, Kut E, et al. Determinants essential for the transmissible gastroenteritis virus-receptor interaction reside within a domain of aminopeptidase-N that is distinct from the enzymatic site. *J Virol* 1994;68:5216–5224.

117. Delmas B, Gelfi J, L'Haridon R, et al. Aminopeptidase N is a major receptor for the enteropathogenic coronavirus TGEV. *Nature* 1992;357:417–420.

118. Delmas B, Gelfi J, Sjöström H, et al. Further characterization of aminopeptidase-N as a receptor for coronaviruses. *Adv Exp Med Biol* 1993;342:293–298.

119. Delmas B, Laude H. Assembly of coronavirus spike protein into trimers and its role in epitope expression. *J Virol* 1990;64:5367–5375.

120. Deming DJ, Baric RS. Genetics and reverse genetics of nidoviruses. In: Perlman S, Gallagher T, Snijder EJ, eds. *Nidoviruses*. Washington: ASM Press; 2008:47–64.

121. Deming DJ, Graham RL, Denison MR, et al. Processing of open reading frame 1a replicase proteins nsp7 to nsp10 in murine hepatitis virus strain A59 replication. *J Virol* 2007;81:10280–10291.

122. Deng X, Baker SC. An "old" protein with a new story: Coronavirus endoribonuclease is important for evading host antiviral defenses. *Virology* 2018;517:157–163.

123. Deng X, Hackbart M, Mettelman RC, et al. Coronavirus nonstructural protein 15 mediates evasion of dsRNA sensors and limits apoptosis in macrophages. *Proc Natl Acad Sci U S A* 2017;114:E4251–E4260.

124. Devaraj SG, Wang N, Chen Z, et al. Regulation of IRF-3-dependent innate immunity by the papain-like protease domain of the severe acute respiratory syndrome coronavirus. *J Biol Chem* 2007;282:32208–32221.

125. Ding Z, Fang L, Yuan S, et al. The nucleocapsid proteins of mouse hepatitis virus and severe acute respiratory syndrome coronavirus share the same IFN-beta antagonizing mechanism: attenuation of PACT-mediated RIG-I/MDA5 activation. *Oncotarget* 2017;8:49655–49670.

126. Donnelly CA, Ghani AC, Leung GM, et al. Epidemiological determinants of spread of causal agent of severe acute respiratory syndrome in Hong Kong. *Lancet* 2003;361:1761–1766.

127. Drosten C, Günther S, Preiser W, et al. Identification of a novel coronavirus in patients with severe acute respiratory syndrome. *N Engl J Med* 2003;348:1967–1976.

128. Drosten C, Meyer B, Muller MA, et al. Transmission of MERS-coronavirus in household contacts. *N Engl J Med* 2014;371:828–835.

129. Dveksler GS, Dieffenbach CW, Cardellichio CB, et al. Several members of the mouse carcinoembryonic antigen-related glycoprotein family are functional receptors for the coronavirus mouse hepatitis virus-A59. *J Virol* 1993;67:1–8.

130. Dveksler GS, Pensiero MN, Cardellichio CB, et al. Cloning of the mouse hepatitis virus (MHV) receptor: expression in human and hamster cell lines confers susceptibility to MHV *J Virol* 1991;65:6881–6891.

131. Dye C, Temperton N, Siddell SG. Type I feline coronavirus spike glycoprotein fails to recognize aminopeptidase N as a functional receptor on feline cell lines. *J Gen Virol* 2007;88:1753–1760.

132. Earnest JT, Hantak MP, Li K, et al. The tetraspanin CD9 facilitates MERS-coronavirus entry by scaffolding host cell receptors and proteases. *PLoS Pathog* 2017;13:e1006546.

133. Eckerle LD, Becker MM, Halpin RA, et al. Infidelity of SARS-CoV Nsp14-exonuclease mutant virus replication is revealed by complete genome sequencing. *PLoS Pathog* 2010;6:e1000896.

134. Emery SL, Erdman DD, Bowen MD, et al. Real-time reverse transcription-polymerase chain reaction assay for SARS-associated coronavirus. *Emerg Infect Dis* 2004;10: 311–316.

135. Escors D, Izeta A, Capiscol C, et al. Transmissible gastroenteritis coronavirus packaging signal is located at the 5' end of the virus genome. *J Virol* 2003;77:7890–7902.

136. Escors D, Ortego J, Laude H, et al. The membrane M protein carboxy terminus binds to transmissible gastroenteritis coronavirus core and contributes to core stability. *J Virol* 2001;75:1312–1324.

137. Fan H, Ooi A, Tan YW, et al. The nucleocapsid protein of coronavirus infectious bronchitis virus: crystal structure of its N-terminal domain and multimerization properties. *Structure* 2005;13:1859–1868.

138. Fang P, Fang L, Ren J, et al. Porcine deltacoronavirus accessory protein NS6 antagonizes interferon beta production by interfering with the binding of RIG-I/MDA5 to double-stranded RNA. *J Virol* 2018;92:e00712–e00718.

139. FAO-OIE-WHO MERS Technical Working Group. MERS: Progress on the global response, remaining challenges and the way forward. *Antiviral Res* 2018;159:35–44.

140. Fehr AR, Athmer J, Channappanavar R, et al. The nsp3 macrodomain promotes virulence in mice with coronavirus-induced encephalitis. *J Virol* 2015;89:1523–1536.

141. Fehr AR, Jankevicius G, Ahel I, et al. Viral macrodomains: unique mediators of viral replication and pathogenesis. *Trends Microbiol* 2018;26:598–610.

142. Frieman M, Ratia K, Johnston RE, et al. Severe acute respiratory syndrome coronavirus papain-like protease ubiquitin-like domain and catalytic domain regulate antagonism of IRF3 and NF-kappaB signaling. *J Virol* 2009;83:6689–6705.

143. Frieman M, Yount B, Heise M, et al. Severe acute respiratory syndrome coronavirus ORF6 antagonizes STAT1 function by sequestering nuclear import factors on the rough endoplasmic reticulum/Golgi membrane. *J Virol* 2007;81:9812–9824.

144. Garwes DJ, Pocock DH, Pike BV. Isolation of subviral components from transmissible gastroenteritis virus. *J Gen Virol* 1976;32:283–294.

145. Gaunt ER, Hardie A, Claas EC, et al. Epidemiology and clinical presentations of the four human coronaviruses 229E, HKU1, NL63, and OC43 detected over 3 years using a novel multiplex real-time PCR method. *J Clin Microbiol* 2010;48:2940–2947.

146. Ge XY, Li JL, Yang XL, et al. Isolation and characterization of a bat SARS-like coronavirus that uses the ACE2 receptor. *Nature* 2013;503:535–538.

147. Godet M, Grosclaude J, Delmas B, et al. Major receptor-binding and neutralization determinants are located within the same domain of the transmissible gastroenteritis virus (coronavirus) spike protein. *J Virol* 1994;68:8008–8016.

148. Goebel SJ, Hsue B, Dombrowski TF, et al. Characterization of the RNA components of a putative molecular switch in the 3′ untranslated region of the murine coronavirus genome. *J Virol* 2004;78:669–682.

149. Goebel SJ, Miller TB, Bennett CJ, et al. A hypervariable region within the 3′ cis-acting element of the murine coronavirus genome is nonessential for RNA synthesis but affects pathogenesis. *J Virol* 2007;81:1274–1287.

150. Goebel SJ, Taylor J, Masters PS. The 3′ cis-acting genomic replication element of the severe acute respiratory syndrome coronavirus can function in the murine coronavirus genome. *J Virol* 2004;78:7846–7851.

151. Goldstein SA, Thornbrough JM, Zhang R, et al. Lineage A betacoronavirus NS2 proteins and the homologous torovirus Berne pp1a carboxy-terminal domain are phosphodiesterases that antagonize activation of RNase L. *J Virol* 2017;91:e02201–e02216.

152. Gorbalenya AE. Genomics and evolution of the *Nidovirales*. In: Perlman S, Gallagher T, Snijder EJ, eds. *Nidoviruses*. Washington, DC: ASM Press; 2008:15–28.

153. Gorbalenya AE, Enjuanes L, Ziebuhr J, et al. Nidovirales: evolving the largest RNA virus genome. *Virus Res* 2006;117:17–37.

154. Gorbalenya AE, Koonin EV, Donchenko AP, et al. Coronavirus genome: prediction of putative functional domains in the non-structural polyprotein by comparative amino acid sequence analysis. *Nucleic Acids Res* 1989;17:4847–4861.

155. Gorse GJ, O'Connor TZ, Hall SL, et al. Human coronavirus and acute respiratory illness in older adults with chronic obstructive pulmonary disease. *J Infect Dis* 2009;199:847–857.

156. Graham RL, Donaldson EF, Baric RS. A decade after SARS: strategies for controlling emerging coronaviruses. *Nat Rev Microbiol* 2013;11:836–848.

157. Grossoehme NE, Li L, Keane SC, et al. Coronavirus N protein N-terminal domain (NTD) specifically binds the transcriptional regulatory sequence (TRS) and melts TRS-cTRS RNA duplexes. *J Mol Biol* 2009;394:544–557.

158. Gu J, Gong E, Zhang B, et al. Multiple organ infection and the pathogenesis of SARS. *J Exp Med* 2005;202:415–424.

159. Guan BJ, Su YP, Wu HY, et al. Genetic evidence of a long-range RNA-RNA interaction between the genomic 5′ untranslated region and the nonstructural protein 1 coding region in murine and bovine coronaviruses. *J Virol* 2012;86:4631–4643.

160. Guan BJ, Wu HY, Brian DA. An optimal cis-replication stem-loop IV in the 5′ untranslated region of the mouse coronavirus genome extends 16 nucleotides into open reading frame 1. *J Virol* 2011;85:5593–5605.

161. Guan Y, Zheng BJ, He YQ, et al. Isolation and characterization of viruses related to the SARS coronavirus from animals in southern China. *Science* 2003;302:276–278.

162. Guy JS, Breslin JJ, Breuhaus B, et al. Characterization of a coronavirus isolated from a diarrheic foal. *J Clin Microbiol* 2000;38:4523–4526.

163. Haagmans BL, van den Brand JM, Raj VS, et al. An orthopoxvirus-based vaccine reduces virus excretion after MERS-CoV infection in dromedary camels. *Science* 2016;351(6268):77–81.

164. Hagemeijer MC, Monastyrska I, Griffith J, et al. Membrane rearrangements mediated by coronavirus nonstructural proteins 3 and 4. *Virology* 2014;458–459:125–135.

165. Haijema BJ, Volders H, Rottier PJ. Switching species tropism: an effective way to manipulate the feline coronavirus genome. *J Virol* 2003;77:4528–4538.

166. Hand J, Rose EB, Salinas A, et al. Severe respiratory illness outbreak associated with human coronavirus NL63 in a long-term care facility. *Emerg Infect Dis* 2018;24:1964–1966.

167. Hao W, Wojdyla JA, Zhao R, et al. Crystal structure of Middle East respiratory syndrome coronavirus helicase. *PLoS Pathog* 2017;13:e1006474.

168. Harrison SC. Viral membrane fusion. *Nat Struct Mol Biol* 2008;15:690–698.

169. Heald-Sargent T, Gallagher T. Ready, set, fuse! The coronavirus spike protein and acquisition of fusion competence. *Viruses* 2012;4:557–580

170. Hemmila E, Turbide C, Olson M, et al. Ceacam1a-/- mice are completely resistant to infection by murine coronavirus mouse hepatitis virus A59. *J Virol* 2004;78:10156–10165.

171. Ho KY, Singh KS, Habib AG, et al. Mild illness associated with severe acute respiratory syndrome coronavirus infection: lessons from a prospective seroepidemiologic study of health-care workers in a teaching hospital in Singapore. *J Infect Dis* 2004;189:642–647.

172. Hofmann H, Pyrc K, van der Hoek L, et al. Human coronavirus NL63 employs the severe acute respiratory syndrome coronavirus receptor for cellular entry. *Proc Natl Acad Sci U S A* 2005;102:7988–7993.

173. Hogue BG, Kienzle TE, Brian DA. Synthesis and processing of the bovine enteric coronavirus haemagglutinin protein. *J Gen Virol* 1989;70:345–352.

174. Hogue BG, Machamer CE. Coronavirus structural proteins and virus assembly. In: Perlman S, Gallagher T, Snijder EJ, eds. *Nidoviruses*. Washington: ASM Press; 2008:179–200.

175. Holmes KV, Doller EW, Sturman LS. Tunicamycin resistant glycosylation of coronavirus glycoprotein: demonstration of a novel type of viral glycoprotein. *Virology* 1981;115:334–344.

176. Hoskins JD. Coronavirus infection in cats. *Vet Clin North Am Small Anim Pract* 1993;23:1–16.

177. Hsueh PR, Huang LM, Chen PJ, et al. Chronological evolution of IgM, IgA, IgG and neutralisation antibodies after infection with SARS-associated coronavirus. *Clin Microbiol Infect* 2004;10:1062–1066.

178. Hu Y, Li W, Gao T, et al. The severe acute respiratory syndrome coronavirus nucleocapsid inhibits Type I interferon production by interfering with TRIM25-mediated RIG-I ubiquitination. *J Virol* 2017;91:e02143-16.

179. Hu B, Zeng LP, Yang XL, et al. Discovery of a rich gene pool of bat SARS-related coronaviruses provides new insights into the origin of SARS coronavirus. *PLoS Pathog* 2017;13:e1006698.

180. Huang IC, Bosch BJ, Li F, et al. SARS coronavirus, but not human coronavirus NL63, utilizes cathepsin L to infect ACE2-expressing cells. *J Biol Chem* 2006;281:3198–3203.

181. Huang LR, Chiu CM, Yeh SH, et al. Evaluation of antibody responses against SARS coronaviral nucleocapsid or spike proteins by immunoblotting or ELISA. *J Med Virol* 2004;73:338–346.

182. Huang C, Liu WJ, Xu W, et al. A bat-derived putative cross-family recombinant coronavirus with a reovirus gene. *PLoS Pathog* 2016;12:e1005883.

183. Hui DS, Azhar EI, Kim YJ, et al. Middle East respiratory syndrome coronavirus: risk factors and determinants of primary, household, and nosocomial transmission. *Lancet Infect Dis* 2018;18:e217–e227.

184. Hurst KR, Koetzner CA, Masters PS. Identification of in vivo-interacting domains of the murine coronavirus nucleocapsid protein. *J Virol* 2009;83:7221–7234.

185. Hurst KR, Koetzner CA, Masters PS. Characterization of a critical interaction between the coronavirus nucleocapsid protein and nonstructural protein 3 of the viral replicase-transcriptase complex. *J Virol* 2013;87:9159–9172.

186. Hurst KR, Kuo L, Koetzner CA, et al. A major determinant for membrane protein interaction localizes to the carboxy-terminal domain of the mouse coronavirus nucleocapsid protein. *J Virol* 2005;79:13285–13297.

187. Hurst KR, Ye R, Goebel SJ, et al. An interaction between the nucleocapsid protein and a component of the replicase-transcriptase complex is crucial for the infectivity of coronavirus genomic RNA. *J Virol* 2010;84:10276–10288.

188. International Committee on Taxonomy of Viruses (ICTV). Virus Taxonomy: 2017 Release. Available at: https://talk.ictvonline.org/taxonomy/

189. Ireland DD, Stohlman SA, Hinton DR, et al. Type I interferons are essential in controlling neurotropic coronavirus infection irrespective of functional CD8 T cells. *J Virol* 2008;82:300–310.

190. Irigoyen N, Firth AE, Jones JD, et al. High-resolution analysis of coronavirus gene expression by RNA sequencing and ribosome profiling. *PLoS Pathog* 2016;12:e1005473.

191. Isaacs D, Flowers D, Clarke JR, et al. Epidemiology of coronavirus respiratory infections. *Arch Dis Child* 1983;58:500–503.

192. Ivanov KA, Hertzig T, Rozanov M, et al. Major genetic marker of nidoviruses encodes a replicative endoribonuclease. *Proc Natl Acad Sci U S A* 2004;101:12694–12699.

193. Ivanov KA, Thiel V, Dobbe JC, et al. Multiple enzymatic activities associated with severe acute respiratory syndrome coronavirus helicase. *J Virol* 2004;78:5619–5632.

194. Jackwood MW, Boynton TO, Hilt DA, et al. Emergence of a group 3 coronavirus through recombination. *Virology* 2010;398:98–108.

195. Jacobs L, van der Zeijst BA, Horzinek MC. Characterization and translation of transmissible gastroenteritis virus mRNAs. *J Virol* 1986;57:1010–1015.

196. Jacobse-Geels HE, Daha MR, Horzinek MC. Antibody, immune complexes, and complement activity fluctuations in kittens with experimentally induced feline infectious peritonitis. *Am J Vet Res* 1982;43:666–670.

197. Jeffers SA, Tusell SM, Gillim-Ross L, et al. CD209L (L-SIGN) is a receptor for severe acute respiratory syndrome coronavirus. *Proc Natl Acad Sci U S A* 2004;101:15748–15753.

198. Jung K, Hu H, Saif LJ. Porcine deltacoronavirus infection: etiology, cell culture for virus isolation and propagation, molecular epidemiology and pathogenesis. *Virus Res* 2016;226:50–59.

199. Kang H, Feng M, Schroeder ME, et al. Putative cis-acting stem-loops in the 5′ untranslated region of the severe acute respiratory syndrome coronavirus can substitute for their mouse hepatitis virus counterparts. *J Virol* 2006;80:10600–10614.

200. Kanjanahaluethai A, Chen Z, Jukneliene D, et al. Membrane topology of murine coronavirus replicase nonstructural protein 3. *Virology* 2007;361:391–401.

201. Kapke PA, Tung FY, Hogue BG, et al. The amino-terminal signal peptide on the porcine transmissible gastroenteritis coronavirus matrix protein is not an absolute requirement for membrane translocation and glycosylation. *Virology* 1988;165:367–376.

202. Kaye HS, Dowdle WR. Seroepidemiologic survey of coronavirus (strain 229E) infections in a population of children. *Am J Epidemiol* 1975;101:238–244.

203. Kazi L, Lissenberg A, Watson R, et al. Expression of hemagglutinin esterase protein from recombinant mouse hepatitis virus enhances neurovirulence. *J Virol* 2005;79:15064–15073.

204. Keane SC, Giedroc DP. Solution structure of mouse hepatitis virus (MHV) nsp3a and determinants of the interaction with MHV nucleocapsid (N) protein. *J Virol* 2013;87:3502–3515.

205. Kennedy DA, Johnson-Lussenburg CM. Isolation and morphology of the internal component of human coronavirus, strain 229E. *Intervirology* 1975–1976;6:197–206.

206. Kheyami AM, Nakagomi T, Nakagomi O, et al. Detection of coronaviruses in children with acute gastroenteritis in Maddina, Saudi Arabia. *Ann Trop Paediatr* 2010;30:45–50.

207. Ki CS, Lee H, Sung H, et al. Korean Society for Laboratory Medicine practice guidelines for the molecular diagnosis of Middle East respiratory syndrome during an outbreak in Korea in 2015. *Ann Lab Med* 2016;36:203–208.

208. Killerby ME, Biggs HM, Haynes A, et al. Human coronavirus circulation in the United States 2014-2017. *J Clin Virol* 2018;101:52–56.

209. Kim SH, Chang SY, Sung M, et al. Extensive viable Middle East respiratory syndrome (MERS) coronavirus contamination in air and surrounding environment in MERS isolation wards. *Clin Infect Dis* 2016;63:363–369.

210. Kim Y, Cheon S, Min CK, et al. Spread of mutant Middle East respiratory syndrome coronavirus with reduced affinity to human CD26 during the South Korean outbreak. *MBio* 2016;7:e00019.

211. Kim Y, Liu H, Galasiti Kankanamalage AC, et al. Reversal of the progression of fatal coronavirus infection in cats by a broad-spectrum coronavirus protease inhibitor. *PLoS Pathog* 2016;12:e1005531.

212. Kindler E, Gil-Cruz C, Spanier J, et al. Early endonuclease-mediated evasion of RNA sensing ensures efficient coronavirus replication. *PLoS Pathog* 2017;13:e1006195.

213. Kindler E, Thiel V, Weber F. Interaction of SARS and MERS coronaviruses with the antiviral interferon response. *Adv Virus Res* 2016;96:219–243.

214. Kirchdoerfer RN, Cottrell CA, Wang N, et al. Pre-fusion structure of a human coronavirus spike protein. *Nature* 2016;531:118–121.

215. Kirchdoerfer RN, Ward AB. Structure of the SARS-CoV nsp12 polymerase bound to nsp7 and nsp8 co-factors. *Nat Commun* 2019;10:2342.

216. Knoops K, Kikkert M, Worm SH, et al. SARS-coronavirus replication is supported by a reticulovesicular network of modified endoplasmic reticulum. *PLoS Biol* 2008;6:e226.

217. Ko JH, Muller MA, Seok H, et al. Serologic responses of 42 MERS-coronavirus-infected patients according to the disease severity. *Diagn Microbiol Infect Dis* 2017;89:106–111.

218. Koetzner CA, Kuo L, Goebel SJ, et al. Accessory protein 5a is a major antagonist of the antiviral action of interferon against murine coronavirus. *J Virol* 2010;84:8262–8274.

219. Koetzner CA, Parker MM, Ricard CS, et al. Repair and mutagenesis of the genome of a deletion mutant of the coronavirus mouse hepatitis virus by targeted RNA recombination. *J Virol* 1992;66:1841–1848.

220. Kopecky-Bromberg SA, Martinez-Sobrido L, Frieman M, et al. SARS coronavirus proteins Orf 3b, Orf 6, and nucleocapsid function as interferon antagonists. *J Virol* 2006;81:548–557.

221. Kottier SA, Cavanagh D, Britton P. Experimental evidence of recombination in coronavirus infectious bronchitis virus. *Virology* 1995;213:569–580.

222. Ksiazek TG, Erdman D, Goldsmith CS, et al. A novel coronavirus associated with severe acute respiratory syndrome. *N Engl J Med* 2003;348:1953–1966.

223. Kuba K, Imai Y, Rao S, et al. A crucial role of angiotensin converting enzyme 2 (ACE2) in SARS coronavirus-induced lung injury. *Nat Med* 2005;11:875–879.

224. Kubo H, Yamada YK, Taguchi F. Localization of neutralizing epitopes and the receptor-binding site within the amino-terminal 330 amino acids of the murine coronavirus spike protein. *J Virol* 1994;68:5403–5410.

225. Kuhn JH, Lauck M, Bailey AL, et al. Reorganization and expansion of the nidoviral family Arteriviridae. *Arch Virol* 2016;161:755–768.

226. Künkel F, Herrler G. Structural and functional analysis of the surface protein of human coronavirus OC43. *Virology* 1993;195:195–202.

227. Kuo L, Godeke GJ, Raamsman MJ, et al. Retargeting of coronavirus by substitution of the spike glycoprotein ectodomain: crossing the host cell species barrier. *J Virol* 2000;74:1393–1406.

228. Kuo L, Hurst KR, Masters PS. Exceptional flexibility in the sequence requirements for coronavirus small envelope protein function. *J Virol* 2007;81:2249–2262.

229. Kuo L, Koetzner CA, Hurst KR, et al. Recognition of the murine coronavirus genomic RNA packaging signal depends on the second RNA-binding domain of the nucleocapsid protein. *J Virol* 2014;88:4451–4465.

230. Kuo L, Koetzner CA, Masters PS. A key role for the carboxy-terminal tail of the murine coronavirus nucleocapsid protein in coordination of genome packaging. *Virology* 2016;494:100–107.

231. Kuo L, Masters PS. Genetic evidence for a structural interaction between the carboxy termini of the membrane and nucleocapsid proteins of mouse hepatitis virus. *J Virol* 2002;76:4987–4999.

232. Kuo L, Masters PS. The small envelope protein E is not essential for murine coronavirus replication. *J Virol* 2003;77:4597–4608.

233. Kuo L, Masters PS. Evolved variants of the membrane protein can partially replace the envelope protein in murine coronavirus assembly. *J Virol* 2010;84:12872–12885.

234. Kuo L, Masters PS. Functional analysis of the murine coronavirus genomic RNA packaging signal. *J Virol* 2013;87:5182–5192.

235. Lai MM, Cavanagh D. The molecular biology of coronaviruses. *Adv Virus Res* 1997;48:1–100.

236. Lassnig C, Sanchez CM, Egerbacher M, et al. Development of a transgenic mouse model susceptible to human coronavirus 229E. *Proc Natl Acad Sci U S A* 2005;102:8275–8280.

237. Lau SK, Lee P, Tsang AK, et al. Molecular epidemiology of human coronavirus OC43 reveals evolution of different genotypes over time and recent emergence of a novel genotype due to natural recombination. *J Virol* 2011;85:11325–11337.

238. Lau SKP, Wong EYM, Tsang CC, et al. Discovery and sequence analysis of four deltacoronaviruses from birds in the Middle East suggest interspecies jumping and recombination as potential mechanism for avian-to-avian and avian-to-mammalian transmission. *J Virol* 2018;92:e00265-18.

239. Lau SK, Woo PC, Wong BH, et al. Detection of severe acute respiratory syndrome (SARS) coronavirus nucleocapsid protein in sars patients by enzyme-linked immunosorbent assay. *J Clin Microbiol* 2004;42:2884–2889.

240. Laude H, Gelfi J, Lavenant L, et al. Single amino acid changes in the viral glycoprotein M affect induction of alpha interferon by the coronavirus transmissible gastroenteritis virus. *J Virol* 1992;66:743–749.

241. Laude H, Van Reeth K, Pensaert M. Porcine respiratory coronavirus: molecular features and virus-host interactions. *Vet Res* 1993;24:125–150.

242. Law HK, Cheung CY, Ng HY, et al. Chemokine upregulation in SARS coronavirus infected human monocyte derived dendritic cells. *Blood* 2005;106:2366–2376.

243. Lee C. Porcine epidemic diarrhea virus: an emerging and re-emerging epizootic swine virus. *Virol J* 2015;12:193.

244. Lehmann KC, Gulyaeva A, Zevenhoven-Dobbe JC, et al. Discovery of an essential nucleotidylating activity associated with a newly delineated conserved domain in the RNA polymerase-containing protein of all nidoviruses. *Nucleic Acids Res* 2015;43:8416–8434.

245. Lehmann KC, Snijder EJ, Posthuma CC, et al. What we know but do not understand about nidovirus helicases. *Virus Res* 2015;202:12–32.

246. Lei J, Kusov Y, Hilgenfeld R. Nsp3 of coronaviruses: structures and functions of a large multi-domain protein. *Antiviral Res* 2018;149:58–74.

247. Leung DT, van Maren WW, Chan FK, et al. Extremely low exposure of a community to Severe Acute Respiratory Syndrome coronavirus: false seropositivity due to use of bacterially derived antigens. *J Virol* 2006;80:8920–8928.

248. Li F. Receptor recognition mechanisms of coronaviruses: a decade of structural studies. *J Virol* 2015;89:1954–1964. doi: 10.1128/JVI.02615-14.

249. Li F. Structure, function, and evolution of coronavirus spike proteins. *Annu Rev Virol* 2016;3:237–261.

250. Li F, Berardi M, Li W, et al. Conformational states of the severe acute respiratory syndrome coronavirus spike protein ectodomain. *J Virol* 2006;80:6794–6800.

251. Li C, Debing Y, Jankevicius G, et al. Viral macro domains reverse protein ADP-ribosylation. *J Virol* 2016;90:8478–8486.

252. Li Z, He W, Lan Y, et al. The evidence of porcine hemagglutinating encephalomyelitis virus induced nonsuppurative encephalitis as the cause of death in piglets. *PeerJ* 2016;4:e2443.

253. Li W, Hulswit RJG, Kenney SP, et al. Broad receptor engagement of an emerging global coronavirus may potentiate its diverse cross-species transmissibility. *Proc Natl Acad Sci U S A* 2018;115:E5135–E5143.

254. Li L, Kang H, Liu P, et al. Structural lability in stem-loop 1 drives a 5' UTR-3' UTR interaction in coronavirus replication. *J Mol Biol* 2008;377:790–803.

255. Li F, Li W, Farzan M, et al. Structure of SARS coronavirus spike receptor-binding domain complexed with receptor. *Science* 2005;309:1864–1868.

256. Li J, Liu Y, Zhang X. Murine coronavirus Induces Type I interferon in oligodendrocytes through recognition by RIG-I and MDA5. *J Virol* 2010;84:6472–6482.

257. Li W, Luo R, He Q, et al. Aminopeptidase N is not required for porcine epidemic diarrhea virus cell entry. *Virus Res* 2017;235:6–13.

258. Li W, Moore MJ, Vasilieva N, et al. Angiotensin-converting enzyme 2 is a functional receptor for the SARS coronavirus. *Nature* 2003;426:450–454.

259. Li K, Wohlford-Lenane CL, Channappanavar R, et al. Mouse-adapted MERS coronavirus causes lethal lung disease in human DPP4 knockin mice. *Proc Natl Acad Sci U S A* 2017;114:E3119–E3128.

260. Liang G, Chen Q, Xu J, et al. Laboratory diagnosis of four recent sporadic cases of community-acquired SARS, Guangdong Province, China. *Emerg Infect Dis* 2004;10:1774–1781.

261. Lim PL, Kurup A, Gopalakrishna G, et al. Laboratory-acquired severe acute respiratory syndrome. *N Engl J Med* 2004;350:1740–1745.

262. Lin HX, Feng Y, Wong G, et al. Identification of residues in the receptor-binding domain (RBD) of the spike protein of human coronavirus NL63 that are critical for the RBD-ACE2 receptor interaction. *J Gen Virol* 2008;89:1015–1024.

263. Lin MT, Hinton DR, Marten NW, et al. Antibody prevents virus reactivation within the central nervous system. *J Immunol* 1999;162:7358–7368.

264. Lin MT, Stohlman SA, Hinton DR. Mouse hepatitis virus is cleared from the central nervous systems of mice lacking perforin-mediated cytolysis. *J Virol* 1997;71:383–391.

265. Lipsitch M, Cohen T, Cooper B, et al. Transmission dynamics and control of severe acute respiratory syndrome. *Science* 2003;300:1966–1970.

266. Liu J, Sun Y, Qi J, et al. The membrane protein of severe acute respiratory syndrome coronavirus acts as a dominant immunogen revealed by a clustering region of novel functionally and structurally defined cytotoxic T-lymphocyte epitopes. *J Infect Dis* 2010;202:1171–1180.

267. Locker JK, Rose JK, Horzinek MC, et al. Membrane assembly of the triple-spanning coronavirus M protein. Individual transmembrane domains show preferred orientation. *J Biol Chem* 1992;267:21911–21918.

268. Lopez LA, Riffle AJ, Pike SL, et al. Importance of conserved cysteine residues in the coronavirus envelope protein. *J Virol* 2008;82:3000–3010.

269. Lorusso A, Decaro N, Schellen P, et al. Gain, preservation, and loss of a group 1a coronavirus accessory glycoprotein. *J Virol* 2008;82:10312–10317.

270. Lu G, Hu Y, Wang Q, et al. Molecular basis of binding between novel human coronavirus MERS-CoV and its receptor CD26. *Nature* 2013;500:227–331.

271. Lui PY, Wong LY, Fung CL, et al. Middle East respiratory syndrome coronavirus M protein suppresses type I interferon expression through the inhibition of TBK1-dependent phosphorylation of IRF3. *Emerg Microbes Infect* 2016;5:e39.

272. Luo CM, Wang N, Yang XL, et al. Discovery of novel bat coronaviruses in south China that use the same receptor as MERS coronavirus. *J Virol* 2018;92:e00116–e00118.

273. Luytjes W, Bredenbeek PJ, Noten AF, et al. Sequence of mouse hepatitis virus A59 mRNA 2: indications for RNA recombination between coronaviruses and influenza C virus. *Virology* 1988;166:415–422.

274. Luytjes W, Gerritsma H, Bos E, et al. Characterization of two temperature-sensitive mutants of coronavirus mouse hepatitis virus strain A59 with maturation defects in the spike protein. *J Virol* 1997;71:949–955.

275. Luytjes W, Sturman LS, Bredenbeek PJ, et al. Primary structure of the glycoprotein E2 of coronavirus MHV-A59 and identification of the trypsin cleavage site. *Virology* 1987;161:479–487.

276. Machamer CE, Rose JK. A specific transmembrane domain of a coronavirus E1 glycoprotein is required for its retention in the Golgi region. *J Cell Biol* 1987;105:1205–1214.

277. Macnaughton MR, Davies HA, Nermut MV. Ribonucleoprotein-like structures from coronavirus particles. *J Gen Virol* 1978;39:545–549.

278. Madhugiri R, Fricke M, Marz M, et al. Coronavirus cis-acting RNA elements. *Adv Virus Res* 2016;96:127–163.

279. Madhugiri R, Karl N, Petersen D, et al. Structural and functional conservation of cis-acting RNA elements in coronavirus 5'-terminal genome regions. *Virology* 2018;517:44–55.

280. Marsden PA, Ning Q, Fung LS, et al. The Fgl2/fibroleukin prothrombinase contributes to immunologically mediated thrombosis in experimental and human viral hepatitis. *J Clin Invest* 2003;112:58–66.

281. Masters PS. The molecular biology of coronaviruses. *Adv Virus Res* 2006;66:193–292.

282. Masters PS, Koetzner CA, Kerr CA, et al. Optimization of targeted RNA recombination and mapping of a novel nucleocapsid gene mutation in the coronavirus mouse hepatitis virus. *J Virol* 1994;68:328–337.

283. Masters PS, Rottier PJ. Coronavirus reverse genetics by targeted RNA recombination. *Curr Top Microbiol Immunol* 2005;287:133–159.

284. McIntosh K. Coronaviruses: a comparative review. *Curr Top Microbiol Immunol* 1974;63:85–129.

285. McIntosh K, Dees JH, Becker WB, et al. Recovery in tracheal organ cultures of novel viruses from patients with respiratory disease. *Proc Natl Acad Sci U S A* 1967;57:933–940.

286. Menachery VD, Mitchell HD, Cockrell AS, et al. MERS-CoV accessory ORFs play key role for infection and pathogenesis. *MBio* 2017;8:e00665-17.

287. Menachery VD, Yount BL Jr, Sims AC, et al. SARS-like WIV1-CoV poised for human emergence. *Proc Natl Acad Sci U S A* 2016;113:3048–3053.

288. Mielech AM, Chen Y, Mesecar AD, et al. Nidovirus papain-like proteases: multifunctional enzymes with protease, deubiquitinating and deISGylating activities. *Virus Res* 2014;194:184–190.

289. Mihindukulasuriya KA, Wu G, St Leger J, et al. Identification of a novel coronavirus from a beluga whale by using a panviral microarray. *J Virol* 2008;82:5084–5088.

290. Millet JK, Whittaker GR. Host cell proteases: critical determinants of coronavirus tropism and pathogenesis. *Virus Res* 2015;202:120–134.

291. Millet JK, Whittaker GR. Physiological and molecular triggers for SARS-CoV membrane fusion and entry into host cells. *Virology* 2018;517:3–8.

292. Minskaia E, Hertzig T, Gorbalenya AE, et al. Discovery of an RNA virus 3′->5′ exoribonuclease that is critically involved in coronavirus RNA synthesis. *Proc Natl Acad Sci U S A* 2006;103:5108–5113.

293. Molenkamp R, Spaan WJ. Identification of a specific interaction between the coronavirus mouse hepatitis virus A59 nucleocapsid protein and packaging signal. *Virology* 1997;239:78–86.

294. Monto AS. Medical reviews. Coronaviruses. *Yale J Biol Med* 1974;47:234–251.

295. Morales L, Mateos-Gomez PA, Capiscol C, et al. Transmissible gastroenteritis coronavirus genome packaging signal is located at the 5′ end of the genome and promotes viral RNA incorporation into virions in a replication-independent process. *J Virol* 2013;87:11579–11590.

296. Morfopoulou S, Brown JR, Davies EG, et al. Human coronavirus OC43 associated with fatal encephalitis. *N Engl J Med* 2016;375:497–498.

297. Muller MA, Meyer B, Corman VM, et al. Presence of Middle East respiratory syndrome coronavirus antibodies in Saudi Arabia: a nationwide, cross-sectional, serological study. *Lancet Infect Dis* 2015;15:559–564.

298. Nakagawa K, Narayanan K, Wada M, et al. The endonucleolytic RNA cleavage function of nsp1 of Middle East Respiratory Syndrome Coronavirus promotes the production of infectious virus particles in specific human cell lines. *J Virol* 2018;92:e01157-18.

299. Nakagawa K, Narayanan K, Wada M, et al. Inhibition of stress granule formation by Middle East Respiratory Syndrome Coronavirus 4a accessory protein facilitates viral translation, leading to efficient virus replication. *J Virol* 2018;92:e00902-e00918.

300. Nal B, Chan C, Kien F, et al. Differential maturation and subcellular localization of severe acute respiratory syndrome coronavirus surface proteins S, M and E. *J Gen Virol* 2005;86:1423–1434.

301. Namy O, Moran SJ, Stuart DI, et al. A mechanical explanation of RNA pseudoknot function in programmed ribosomal frameshifting. *Nature* 2006;441:244–247.

302. Narayanan K, Chen CJ, Maeda J, et al. Nucleocapsid-independent specific viral RNA packaging via viral envelope protein and viral RNA signal. *J Virol* 2003;77:2922–2927.

303. Narayanan K, Huang C, Makino S. Coronavirus accessory proteins. In: Perlman S, Gallagher T, Snijder EJ, eds. *Nidoviruses*. Washington, DC: ASM Press; 2008:235–244.

304. Narayanan K, Kim KH, Makino S. Characterization of N protein self-association in coronavirus ribonucleoprotein complexes. *Virus Res* 2003;98:131–140.

305. Narayanan K, Ramirez SI, Lokugamage KG, et al. Coronavirus nonstructural protein 1: Common and distinct functions in the regulation of host and viral gene expression. *Virus Res* 2015;202:89–100.

306. Neuman BW. Bioinformatics and functional analyses of coronavirus nonstructural proteins involved in the formation of replicative organelles. *Antiviral Res* 2016;135:97–107.

307. Neuman BW, Adair BD, Yoshioka C, et al. Supramolecular architecture of severe acute respiratory syndrome coronavirus revealed by electron cryomicroscopy. *J Virol* 2006;80:7918–7928.

308. Neuman BW, Chamberlain P, Bowden F, et al. Atlas of coronavirus replicase structure. *Virus Res* 2014;194:49–66.

309. Neuman BW, Joseph JS, Saikatendu KS, et al. Proteomics analysis unravels the functional repertoire of coronavirus nonstructural protein 3. *J Virol* 2008;82:5279–5294.

310. Neuman BW, Kiss G, Kunding AH, et al. A structural analysis of M protein in coronavirus assembly and morphology. *J Struct Biol* 2011;174:11–22.

311. Ng DL, Al Hosani F, Keating MK, et al. Clinicopathologic, immunohistochemical, and ultrastructural findings of a fatal case of Middle East Respiratory syndrome coronavirus infection in the United Arab Emirates, April 2014. *Am J Pathol* 2016;186:652–658.

312. Ng OW, Chia A, Tan AT, et al. Memory T cell responses targeting the SARS coronavirus persist up to 11 years post-infection. *Vaccine* 2016;34:2008–2014.

313. Nga PT, Parquet MdC, Lauber C, et al. Discovery of the first insect nidovirus, a missing evolutionary link in the emergence of the largest RNA virus genomes. *PLoS Pathog* 2011;7:e1002215.

314. Nicholls JM, Butany J, Poon LL, et al. Time course and cellular localization of SARS-CoV nucleoprotein and RNA in lungs from fatal cases of SARS. *PLoS Med* 2006;3:e27.

315. Nieto-Torres JL, Dediego ML, Alvarez E, et al. Subcellular location and topology of severe acute respiratory syndrome coronavirus envelope protein. *Virology* 2011;415:69–82.

316. Nikiforuk AM, Leung A, Cook BWM, et al. Rapid one-step construction of a Middle East Respiratory Syndrome (MERS-CoV) infectious clone system by homologous recombination. *J Virol Methods* 2016;236:178–183.

317. Oh MD, Park WB, Choe PG, et al. Viral load kinetics of MERS coronavirus infection. *N Engl J Med* 2016;375:1303–1305.

318. Okba NM, Raj VS, Haagmans BL. Middle East respiratory syndrome coronavirus vaccines: current status and novel approaches. *Curr Opin Virol* 2017;23:49–58.

319. Omrani AS, Al-Tawfiq JA, Memish ZA. Middle East respiratory syndrome coronavirus (MERS-CoV): animal to human interaction. *Pathog Glob Health* 2015;109:354–362.

320. Oostra M, Hagemeijer MC, van Gent M, et al. Topology and membrane anchoring of the coronavirus replication complex: not all hydrophobic domains of nsp3 and nsp6 are membrane spanning. *J Virol* 2008;82:12392–12405.

321. Opstelten DJ, de Groote P, Horzinek MC, et al. Disulfide bonds in folding and transport of mouse hepatitis coronavirus glycoproteins. *J Virol* 1993;67:7394–7401.

322. Ortego J, Escors D, Laude H, et al. Generation of a replication-competent, propagation-deficient virus vector based on the transmissible gastroenteritis coronavirus genome. *J Virol* 2002;76:11518–11529.

323. Ou X, Zheng W, Shan Y, et al. Identification of the fusion peptide-containing region in Betacoronavirus spike glycoproteins. *J Virol* 2016;90:5586–5600.

324. Oudshoorn D, Rijs K, Limpens RWAL, et al. Expression and cleavage of Middle East respiratory syndrome coronavirus nsp3-4 polyprotein induce the formation of double-membrane vesicles that mimic those associated with coronaviral RNA replication. *MBio* 2017;8:e01658-17.

325. Park GE, Ko JH, Peck KR, et al. Control of an outbreak of Middle East Respiratory Syndrome in a tertiary hospital in Korea. *Ann Intern Med* 2016;165:87–93.

326. Parker SE, Gallagher TM, Buchmeier MJ. Sequence analysis reveals extensive polymorphism and evidence of deletions within the E2 glycoprotein gene of several strains of murine hepatitis virus. *Virology* 1989;173:664–673.

327. Parra B, Hinton D, Marten N, et al. IFN-gamma is required for viral clearance from central nervous system oligodendroglia. *J Immunol* 1999;162:1641–1647.

328. Pascal KE, Coleman CM, Mujica AO, et al. Pre- and postexposure efficacy of fully human antibodies against Spike protein in a novel humanized mouse model of MERS-CoV infection. *Proc Natl Acad Sci U S A* 2015;112:8738–8743.

329. Pasternak AO, van den Born E, Spaan WJ, et al. Sequence requirements for RNA strand transfer during nidovirus discontinuous subgenomic RNA synthesis. *EMBO J* 2001;20:7220–7228.

330. Payne DC, Biggs HM, Al-Abdallat MM, et al. Multihospital outbreak of a Middle East Respiratory syndrome coronavirus deletion variant, Jordan: a molecular, serologic, and epidemiologic investigation. *Open Forum Infect Dis* 2018;5:ofy095.

331. Peiris JS, Chu CM, Cheng VC, et al. Clinical progression and viral load in a community outbreak of coronavirus-associated SARS pneumonia: a prospective study. *Lancet* 2003;361:1767–1772.

332. Peiris JS, Guan Y, Yuen KY. Severe acute respiratory syndrome. *Nat Med* 2004;10:S88–S97.

333. Peiris JS, Lai ST, Poon LL, et al. Coronavirus as a possible cause of severe acute respiratory syndrome. *Lancet* 2003;361:1319–1325.

334. Peiris JS, Yuen KY, Osterhaus AD, et al. The severe acute respiratory syndrome. *N Engl J Med* 2003;349:2431–2341.

335. Peng G, Xu L, Lin YL, et al. Crystal structure of bovine coronavirus spike protein lectin domain. *J Biol Chem* 2012;287:41931–41938.

336. Peng H, Yang LT, Wang LY, et al. Long-lived memory T lymphocyte responses against SARS coronavirus nucleocapsid protein in SARS-recovered patients. *Virology* 2006;351:466–475.

337. Percy DH, Williams KL. Experimental Parker's coronavirus infection in Wistar rats. *Lab Anim Sci* 1990;40:603–607.

338. Perlman S. Pathogenesis of coronavirus-induced infections: review of pathological and immunological aspects. *Adv Exp Med Biol* 1998;440:503–513.

339. Pervushin K, Tan E, Parthasarathy K, et al. Structure and inhibition of the SARS coronavirus envelope protein ion channel. *PLoS Pathog* 2009;5:e1000511.

340. Pewe L, Wu G, Barnett EM, et al. Cytotoxic T cell-resistant variants are selected in a virus-induced demyelinating disease. *Immunity* 1996;5:253–262.

341. Phillips JJ, Chua MM, Lavi E, et al. Pathogenesis of chimeric MHV4/MHV-A59 recombinant viruses: the murine coronavirus spike protein is a major determinant of neurovirulence. *J Virol* 1999;73:7752–7760.

342. Pitkaranta A, Virolainen A, Jero J, et al. Detection of rhinovirus, respiratory syncytial virus, and coronavirus infections in acute otitis media by reverse transcriptase polymerase chain reaction. *Pediatrics* 1998;102:291–295.

343. Plant EP, Pérez-Alvarado GC, Jacobs JL, et al. A three-stemmed mRNA pseudoknot in the SARS coronavirus frameshift signal. *PLoS Biol* 2005;3:e172.

344. Plant EP, Rakauskaite R, Taylor DR, et al. Achieving a golden mean: mechanisms by which coronaviruses ensure synthesis of the correct stoichiometric ratios of viral proteins. *J Virol* 2010;84:4330–4340.

345. Pohl-Koppe A, Raabe T, Siddell SG, et al. Detection of human coronavirus 229E-specific antibodies using recombinant fusion proteins. *J Virol Methods* 1995;55:175–183.

346. Poon LL, Chan KH, Wong OK, et al. Early diagnosis of SARS coronavirus infection by real time RT-PCR. *J Clin Virol* 2003;28:233–238.

347. Posthuma CC, Te Velthuis AJW, Snijder EJ. Nidovirus RNA polymerases: complex enzymes handling exceptional RNA genomes. *Virus Res* 2017;234:58–73.

348. Promkuntod N, van Eijndhoven RE, de Vrieze G, et al. Mapping of the receptor-binding domain and amino acids critical for attachment in the spike protein of avian coronavirus infectious bronchitis virus. *Virology* 2014;448:26–32.

349. Pyrc K, Berkhout B, van der Hoek L. The novel human coronaviruses NL63 and HKU1. *J Virol* 2007;81:3051–3057.

350. Pyrc K, Dijkman R, Deng L, et al. Mosaic structure of human coronavirus NL63, one thousand years of evolution. *J Mol Biol* 2006;364:964–973.

351. Pyrc K, Sims AC, Dijkman R, et al. Culturing the unculturable: human coronavirus HKU1 infects, replicates, and produces progeny virions in human ciliated airway epithelial cell cultures. *J Virol* 2010;84:11255–11263.

352. Qian Z, Ou X, Góes LG, et al. Identification of the receptor-binding domain of the spike glycoprotein of human betacoronavirus HKU1. *J Virol* 2015;89:8816–8827.

353. Rabouw HH, Langereis MA, Knaap RC, et al. Middle East respiratory coronavirus accessory protein 4a inhibits PKR-mediated antiviral stress responses. *PLoS Pathog* 2016;12:e1005982.

354. Rainer TH, Chan PK, Ip M, et al. The spectrum of severe acute respiratory syndrome-associated coronavirus infection. *Ann Intern Med* 2004;140:614–619.

355. Raj VS, Mou H, Smits SL, et al. Dipeptidyl peptidase 4 is a functional receptor for the emerging human coronavirus-EMC. *Nature* 2013;495:251–254.

356. Reed SE. The behaviour of recent isolates of human respiratory coronavirus in vitro and in volunteers: evidence of heterogeneity among 229E-related strains. *J Med Virol* 1984;13:179–192.

357. Reguera J, Santiago C, Mudgal G, et al. Structural bases of coronavirus attachment to host aminopeptidase N and its inhibition by neutralizing antibodies. *PLoS Pathog* 2012;8:e1002859.

358. Riley S, Fraser C, Donnelly CA, et al. Transmission dynamics of the etiological agent of SARS in Hong Kong: impact of public health interventions. *Science* 2003;300:1961–1966.

359. Roberts A, Deming D, Paddock CD, et al. A mouse-adapted SARS-coronavirus causes disease and mortality in BALB/c mice. *PLoS Pathog* 2007;3:e5.

360. Roberts A, Paddock C, Vogel L, et al. Aged BALB/c mice as a model for increased severity of severe acute respiratory syndrome in elderly humans. *J Virol* 2005;79:5833–5838.

361. Roth-Cross JK, Bender SJ, Weiss SR. Murine coronavirus mouse hepatitis virus is recognized by MDA5 and induces type I interferon in brain macrophages/microglia. *J Virol* 2008;82:9829–9838.

362. Rottier P, Brandenburg D, Armstrong J, et al. Assembly in vitro of a spanning membrane protein of the endoplasmic reticulum: the E1 glycoprotein of coronavirus mouse hepatitis virus A59. *Proc Natl Acad Sci U S A* 1984;81:1421–1425.

363. Rottier PJ, Horzinek MC, van der Zeijst BA. Viral protein synthesis in mouse hepatitis virus strain A59-infected cells: effect of tunicamycin. *J Virol* 1981;40:350–357.

364. Ruch TR, Machamer CE. A single polar residue and distinct membrane topologies impact the function of the infectious bronchitis coronavirus E protein. *PLoS Pathog* 2012;8:e1002674.

365. Ruch TR, Machamer CE. The coronavirus E protein: assembly and beyond. *Viruses* 2012;4:363–382.

366. Sabir JS, Lam TT, Ahmed MM, et al. Co-circulation of three camel coronavirus species and recombination of MERS-CoVs in Saudi Arabia. *Science* 2016;351:81–84.

367. Saif LJ. Animal coronavirus vaccines: lessons for SARS. *Dev Biol* 2004;119:129–140.

368. Sánchez CM, Izeta A, Sánchez-Morgado JM, et al. Targeted recombination demonstrates that the spike gene of transmissible gastroenteritis coronavirus is a determinant of its enteric tropism and virulence. *J Virol* 1999;73:7607–7618.

369. Sawicki SG, Sawicki DL. Coronavirus transcription: subgenomic mouse hepatitis virus replicative intermediates function in RNA synthesis. *J Virol* 1990;64:1050–1056.

370. Sawicki SG, Sawicki DL, Siddell SG. A contemporary view of coronavirus transcription. *J Virol* 2007;81:20–29.

371. Sawicki SG, Sawicki DL, Younker D, et al. Functional and genetic analysis of coronavirus replicase-transcriptase proteins. *PLoS Pathog* 2005;1(4):e39.

372. Sawicki DL, Wang T, Sawicki SG. The RNA structures engaged in replication and transcription of the A59 strain of mouse hepatitis virus. *J Gen Virol* 2001;82:385–396.

373. Scheuplein VA, Seifried J, Malczyk AH, et al. High secretion of interferons by human plasmacytoid dendritic cells upon recognition of Middle East respiratory syndrome coronavirus. *J Virol* 2015;89:3859–3869.

374. Schultze B, Herrler G. Bovine coronavirus uses N-acetyl-9-O-acetylneuraminic acid as a receptor determinant to initiate the infection of cultured cells. *J Gen Virol* 1992;73:901–906.

375. Schütze H, Ulferts R, Schelle B, et al. Characterization of white bream virus reveals a novel genetic cluster of nidoviruses. *J Virol* 2006;80:11598–11609.

376. Sethna PB, Hofmann MA, Brian DA. Minus-strand copies of replicating coronavirus mRNAs contain antileaders. *J Virol* 1991;65:320–325.

377. Sethna PB, Hung SL, Brian DA. Coronavirus subgenomic minus-strand RNAs and the potential for mRNA replicons. *Proc Natl Acad Sci U S A* 1989;86:5626–5630.

378. Sevajol M, Subissi L, Decroly E, et al. Insights into RNA synthesis, capping, and proofreading mechanisms of SARS-coronavirus. *Virus Res* 2014;194:90–99.

379. Shang J, Zheng Y, Yang Y, et al. Cryo-EM structure of porcine delta coronavirus spike protein in the pre-fusion state. *J Virol* 2017;92:e01556-17.

380. Shang J, Zheng Y, Yang Y, et al. Cryo-EM structure of infectious bronchitis coronavirus spike protein reveals structural and functional evolution of coronavirus spike proteins. *PLoS Pathog* 2018;14:e1007009.

381. Sheahan T, Morrison TE, Funkhouser W, et al. MyD88 is required for protection from lethal infection with a mouse-adapted SARS-CoV. *PLoS Pathog* 2008;4:e1000240.

382. Sheahan TP, Sims AC, Graham RL, et al. Broad-spectrum antiviral GS-5734 inhibits both epidemic and zoonotic coronaviruses. *Sci Transl Med* 2017;9:eaal3653.

383. Shin HS, Kim Y, Kim G, et al. Immune responses to MERS coronavirus during the acute and convalescent phases of human infection. *Clin Infect Dis* 2019;68(6):984–992.

384. Shirato K, Kanou K, Kawase M, et al. Clinical isolates of human coronavirus 229E bypass the endosome for cell entry. *J Virol* 2017;91:e01387-16.

385. Shirato K, Kawase M, Matsuyama S. Wild-type human coronaviruses prefer cell-surface TMPRSS2 to endosomal cathepsins for cell entry. *Virology* 2018;517:9–15.

386. Shirato K, Maejima M, Islam MT, et al. Porcine aminopeptidase N is not a cellular receptor of porcine epidemic diarrhea virus, but promotes its infectivity via aminopeptidase activity. *J Gen Virol* 2016;97:2528–2539.

387. Shulla A, Heald-Sargent T, Subramanya G, et al. A transmembrane serine protease is linked to the severe acute respiratory syndrome coronavirus receptor and activates virus entry. *J Virol* 2011;85:873–882.

388. Simmons G, Reeves JD, Rennekamp AJ, et al. Characterization of severe acute respiratory syndrome-associated coronavirus (SARS-CoV) spike glycoprotein-mediated viral entry. *Proc Natl Acad Sci U S A* 2004;101:4240–4245.

389. Siu KL, Kok KH, Ng MH, et al. Severe acute respiratory syndrome coronavirus M protein inhibits type I interferon production by impeding the formation of TRAF3.TANK.TBK1/IKKepsilon complex. *J Biol Chem* 2009;284:16202–16209.

390. Siu YL, Teoh KT, Lo J, et al. The M, E, and N structural proteins of the severe acute respiratory syndrome coronavirus are required for efficient assembly, trafficking, and release of virus-like particles. *J Virol* 2008;82:11318–11330.

391. Siu KL, Yeung ML, Kok KH, et al. Middle east respiratory syndrome coronavirus 4a protein is a double-stranded RNA-binding protein that suppresses PACT-induced activation of RIG-I and MDA5 in the innate antiviral response. *J Virol* 2014;88:4866–4876.

392. Snijder EJ, Bredenbeek PJ, Dobbe JC, et al. Unique and conserved features of genome and proteome of SARS-coronavirus, an early split-off from the coronavirus group 2 lineage. *J Mol Biol* 2003;331:991–1004.

393. Snijder EJ, Decroly E, Ziebuhr J. The nonstructural proteins directing coronavirus RNA synthesis and processing. *Adv Virus Res* 2016;96:59–126.

394. Snijder EJ, den Boon JA, Horzinek MC, et al. Comparison of the genome organization of toro- and coronaviruses: evidence for two nonhomologous RNA recombination events during Berne virus evolution. *Virology* 1991;180:448–452.

395. Sola I, Almazán F, Zúñiga S, et al. Continuous and discontinuous RNA synthesis in coronaviruses. *Annu Rev Virol* 2015;2:265–288.

396. Song W, Gui M, Wang X, et al. Cryo-EM structure of the SARS coronavirus spike glycoprotein in complex with its host cell receptor ACE2. *PLoS Pathog* 2018;14:e1007236.

397. Spiegel M, Schneider K, Weber F, et al. Interaction of severe acute respiratory syndrome-associated coronavirus with dendritic cells. *J Gen Virol* 2006;87:1953–1960.

398. Stewart H, Brown K, Dinan AM, et al. The transcriptional and translational landscape of equine torovirus. *J Virol* 2018;92:e00589-18.

399. Stobart CC, Lee AS, Lu X, et al. Temperature-sensitive mutants and revertants in the coronavirus nonstructural protein 5 protease (3CLpro) define residues involved in longdistance communication and regulation of protease activity. *J Virol* 2012;86:4801–4810.

400. Stockman LJ, Bellamy R, Garner P. SARS: systematic review of treatment effects. *PLoS Med* 2006;3:e343.

401. Stohlman SA, Bergmann CC, Perlman S. Mouse hepatitis virus. In: Ahmed R, Chen I, eds. *Persistent Viral Infections*. New York: John Wiley & Sons, Ltd.; 1998:537–557.

402. Stohlman SA, Fleming JO, Patton CD, et al. Synthesis and subcellular localization of the murine coronavirus nucleocapsid protein. *Virology* 1983;130:527–532.

403. Stokes HL, Baliji S, Hui CG, et al. A new cistron in the murine hepatitis virus replicase gene. *J Virol* 2010;84:10148–10158.

404. Sturman LS, Holmes KV. The molecular biology of coronaviruses. *Adv Virus Res* 1983;28:35–111.

405. Sturman LS, Holmes KV, Behnke J. Isolation of coronavirus envelope glycoproteins and interaction with the viral nucleocapsid. *J Virol* 1980;33:449–462.

406. Subbarao K, Roberts A. Is there an ideal animal model for SARS? *Trends Microbiol* 2006;14:299–303.

407. Subissi L, Posthuma CC, Collet A, et al. One severe acute respiratory syndrome coronavirus protein complex integrates processive RNA polymerase and exonuclease activities. *Proc Natl Acad Sci U S A* 2014;111:E3900–E3909.

408. Taguchi F, Hirai-Yuki A. Mouse hepatitis virus receptor as a determinant of the mouse susceptibility to MHV infection. *Front Microbiol* 2012;3:68.

409. Talbot HK, Crowe JE Jr, Edwards KM, et al. Coronavirus infection and hospitalizations for acute respiratory illness in young children. *J Med Virol* 2009;81:853–856.

410. Tang F, Quan Y, Xin ZT, et al. Lack of peripheral memory B cell responses in recovered patients with severe acute respiratory syndrome: a six-year follow-up study. *J Immunol* 2011;186:7264–7268.

411. Tangudu C, Olivares H, Netland J, et al. Severe acute respiratory syndrome coronavirus protein 6 accelerates murine coronavirus infections. *J Virol* 2007;81:1220–1229.

412. Tao X, Hill TE, Morimoto C, et al. Bilateral entry and release of Middle East respiratory syndrome coronavirus induces profound apoptosis of human bronchial epithelial cells. *J Virol* 2013;87:9953–9958.

413. Tao Y, Shi M, Chommanard C, et al. Surveillance of bat coronaviruses in Kenya identifies relatives of human coronaviruses NL63 and 229E and their recombination history. *J Virol* 2017;91.

414. Tekes G, Thiel HJ. Feline coronaviruses: pathogenesis of feline infectious peritonitis. *Adv Virus Res* 2016;96:193–218.

415. Thiel V, Herold J, Schelle B, et al. Infectious RNA transcribed in vitro from a cDNA copy of the human coronavirus genome cloned in vaccinia virus. *J Gen Virol* 2001;82:1273–1281.

416. Thornbrough JM, Jha BK, Yount B, et al. Middle East respiratory syndrome coronavirus NS4b protein inhibits host RNase L activation. *MBio*. 2016;7(2):e00258.

417. To J, Surya W, Fung TS, et al. Channel-inactivating mutations and their revertant mutants in the envelope protein of infectious bronchitis virus. *J Virol* 2017;91:e02158-16.

418. Trandem K, Anghelina D, Zhao J, et al. Regulatory T cells inhibit T cell proliferation and decrease demyelination in mice chronically infected with a coronavirus. *J Immunol* 2010;184:4391–4400.

419. Trandem K, Zhao J, Fleming E, et al. Highly activated cytotoxic CD8 T cells express protective IL-10 at the peak of coronavirus-Induced encephalitis. *J Immunol* 2011;186:3642–3652.

420. Tresnan DB, Levis R, Holmes KV. Feline aminopeptidase N serves as a receptor for feline, canine, porcine, and human coronaviruses in serogroup I. *J Virol* 1996;70:8669–8674.

421. Tsai TL, Lin CH, Lin CN, et al. Interplay between the poly(A) tail, poly(A)-binding protein, and coronavirus nucleocapsid protein regulates gene expression of coronavirus and the host cell. *J Virol* 2018;92:e01162-18.

422. Tynell J, Westenius V, Ronkko E, et al. Middle East respiratory syndrome coronavirus shows poor replication but significant induction of antiviral responses in human monocyte-derived macrophages and dendritic cells. *J Gen Virol* 2016;97:344–355.

423. Ujike M, Taguchi F. Incorporation of spike and membrane glycoproteins into coronavirus virions. *Viruses* 2015;7:1700–1725.

424. van Beurden SJ, Berends AJ, Krämer-Kühl A, et al. A reverse genetics system for avian coronavirus infectious bronchitis virus based on targeted RNA recombination. *Virol J* 2017;14:109.

425. van der Hoek L, Pyrc K, Jebbink MF, et al. Identification of a new human coronavirus. *Nat Med* 2004;10:368–373.

426. van der Hoek L, Sure K, Ihorst G, et al. Croup is associated with the novel coronavirus NL63. *PLoS Med* 2005;2:e240.

427. van Hemert MJ, van den Worm SH, Knoops K, et al. SARS-coronavirus replication/transcription complexes are membrane-protected and need a host factor for activity in vitro. *PLoS Pathog* 2008;4:e1000054.

428. van Marle G, Dobbe JC, Gultyaev AP, et al. Arterivirus discontinuous mRNA transcription is guided by base pairing between sense and antisense transcription-regulating sequences. *Proc Natl Acad Sci U S A* 1999;96:12056–12061.

429. Varghese L, Zachariah P, Vargas C, et al. Epidemiology and clinical features of human coronaviruses in the pediatric population. *J Pediatric Infect Dis Soc* 2018;7:151–158.

430. Venkatagopalan P, Daskalova SM, Lopez LA, et al. Coronavirus envelope (E) protein remains at the site of assembly. *Virology* 2015;478:75–85.

431. Vennema H, de Groot RJ, Harbour DA, et al. Early death after feline infectious peritonitis virus challenge due to recombinant vaccinia virus immunization. *J Virol* 1990;64:1407–1409.

432. Vennema H, Godeke GJ, Rossen JW, et al. Nucleocapsid-independent assembly of coronavirus-like particles by co-expression of viral envelope protein genes. *EMBO J* 1996;15:2020–2028.

433. Verma S, Bednar V, Blount A, et al. Identification of functionally important negatively charged residues in the carboxy end of mouse hepatitis coronavirus A59 nucleocapsid protein. *J Virol* 2006;80:4344–4355.

434. Versteeg GA, Bredenbeek PJ, van den Worm SH, et al. Group 2 coronaviruses prevent immediate early interferon induction by protection of viral RNA from host cell recognition. *Virology* 2007;361:18–26.

435. Vijgen L, Keyaerts E, Lemey P, et al. Evolutionary history of the closely related group 2 coronaviruses: porcine hemagglutinating encephalomyelitis virus, bovine coronavirus, and human coronavirus OC43. *J Virol* 2006;80:7270–7274.

436. Walls AC, Tortorici MA, Bosch BJ, et al. Cryo-electron microscopy structure of a coronavirus spike glycoprotein trimer. *Nature* 2016;531:114–117.

437. Walls AC, Tortorici MA, Frenz B, et al. Glycan shield and epitope masking of a coronavirus spike protein observed by cryo-electron microscopy. *Nat Struct Mol Biol* 2016;23:899–905.

438. Walls AC, Tortorici MA, Snijder J, et al. Tectonic conformational changes of a coronavirus spike glycoprotein promote membrane fusion. *Proc Natl Acad Sci U S A* 2017;114:11157–11162.

439. Walsh EE, Shin JH, Falsey AR. Clinical impact of human coronaviruses 229E and OC43 infection in diverse adult populations. *J Infect Dis* 2013;208:1634–1642.

440. Wan Z, Zhang Y, He Z, et al. A melting curve-based multiplex RT-qPCR assay for simultaneous detection of four human coronaviruses. *Int J Mol Sci* 2016;17.

441. Wang L, Junker D, Hock L, et al. Evolutionary implications of genetic variations in the S1 gene of infectious bronchitis virus. *Virus Res* 1994;34:327–338.

442. Wang B, Liu Y, Ji CM, et al. Porcine deltacoronavirus engages the transmissible gastroenteritis virus functional receptor porcine aminopeptidase N for infectious cellular entry. *J Virol* 2018;92:e00318-18.

443. Wang N, Shi X, Jiang L, et al. Structure of MERS-CoV spike receptor-binding domain complexed with human receptor DPP4. *Cell Res* 2013;23:986–993.

444. Wang F, Stohlman SA, Fleming JO. Demyelination induced by murine hepatitis virus JHM strain (MHV-4) is immunologically mediated. *J Neuroimmunol* 1990;30:31–41.

445. Weiner LP. Pathogenesis of demyelination induced by a mouse hepatitis virus (JHM virus). *Arch Neurol* 1973;28:298–303.

446. Westerbeck JW, Machamer CE. A coronavirus E protein is present in two distinct pools with different effects on assembly and the secretory pathway. *J Virol* 2015;89:9313–9323.

447. White TC, Yi Z, Hogue BG. Identification of mouse hepatitis coronavirus A59 nucleocapsid protein phosphorylation sites. *Virus Res* 2007;126:139–148.

448. WHO. Laboratory testing for Middle East respiratory syndrome coronavirus. 2013. Available at: http://www.who.int/csr/disease/coronavirus_infections/MERS_Lab_recos_16_Sept_2013.pdf

449. Williams GD, Chang RY, Brian DA. A phylogenetically conserved hairpin-type 3' untranslated region pseudoknot functions in coronavirus RNA replication. *J Virol* 1999;73:8349–8355.

450. Williams RK, Jiang G, Holmes KV. Receptor for mouse hepatitis virus is a member of the carcinoembryonic antigen family of glycoproteins. *Proc Natl Acad Sci U S A* 1991;88:5533–5536.

451. Williams RK, Jiang GS, Snyder SW, et al. Purification of the 110-kilodalton glycoprotein receptor for mouse hepatitis virus (MHV)-A59 from mouse liver and identification of a nonfunctional, homologous protein in MHV-resistant SJL/J mice. *J Virol* 1990;64:3817–3823.

452. Wilson L, McKinlay C, Gage P, et al. SARS coronavirus E protein forms cation-selective ion channels. *Virology* 2004;330:322–331.

453. Wong SK, Li W, Moore MJ, et al. A 193-amino acid fragment of the SARS coronavirus S protein efficiently binds angiotensin-converting enzyme 2. *J Biol Chem* 2004;279:3197–3201.

454. Wong AHM, Tomlinson ACA, Zhou D, et al. Receptor-binding loops in alphacoronavirus adaptation and evolution. *Nat Commun* 2017;8:1735.

455. Woo PC, Lau SK, Chu CM, et al. Characterization and complete genome sequence of a novel coronavirus, coronavirus HKU1, from patients with pneumonia. *J Virol* 2005;79:884–895.

456. Woo PCW, Lau SKP, Huang Y, et al. Coronavirus diversity, phylogeny and interspecies jumping. *Exp Biol Med* 2009;234:1117–1127.

457. Woo PC, Lau SK, Lam CS, et al. Discovery of seven novel mammalian and avian coronaviruses in the genus deltacoronavirus supports bat coronaviruses as the gene source of alphacoronavirus and betacoronavirus and avian coronaviruses as the gene source of gammacoronavirus and deltacoronavirus. *J Virol* 2012;86:3995–4008.

458. Woo PC, Lau SK, Tsoi HW, et al. Clinical and molecular epidemiological features of coronavirus HKU1-associated community-acquired pneumonia. *J Infect Dis* 2005;192:1898–1907.

459. Woo PC, Wang M, Lau SK, et al. Comparative analysis of twelve genomes of three novel group 2c and group 2d coronaviruses reveals unique group and subgroup features. *J Virol* 2007;81:1574–1585.

460. Wu CH, Chen PJ, Yeh SH. Nucleocapsid phosphorylation and RNA helicase DDX1 recruitment enables coronavirus transition from discontinuous to continuous transcription. *Cell Host Microbe* 2014;16:462–472.

461. Wu GF, Dandekar AA, Pewe L, et al. CD4 and CD8 T cells have redundant but not identical roles in virus-induced demyelination. *J Immunol* 2000;165:2278–2286.

462. Wu HY, Ke TY, Liao WY, et al. Regulation of coronaviral poly(A) tail length during infection. *PLoS One* 2013;8:e70548.

463. Xie Q, Cao Y, Su J, et al. Two deletion variants of Middle East respiratory syndrome coronavirus found in a patient with characteristic symptoms. *Arch Virol* 2017;162:2445–2449.

464. Xie L, Liu Y, Fan B, et al. Dynamic changes of serum SARS-coronavirus IgG, pulmonary function and radiography in patients recovering from SARS after hospital discharge. *Respir Res* 2005;6:5.

465. Xiong X, Tortorici MA, Snijder J, et al. Glycan shield and fusion activation of a deltacoronavirus spike glycoprotein fine-tuned for enteric infections. *J Virol* 2017;92:e01628-17.

466. Yang D, Leibowitz JL. The structure and functions of coronavirus genomic 3' and 5' ends. *Virus Res* 2015;206:120–133.

467. Yang H, Xie W, Xue X, et al. Design of wide-spectrum inhibitors targeting coronavirus main proteases. *PLoS Biol* 2005;3:e324.

468. Yang Y, Ye F, Zhu N, et al. Middle East respiratory syndrome coronavirus ORF4b protein inhibits type I interferon production through both cytoplasmic and nuclear targets. *Sci Rep* 2015;5:17554.

469. Ye R, Montalto-Morrison C, Masters PS. Genetic analysis of determinants for spike glycoprotein assembly into murine coronavirus virions: distinct roles for charge-rich and cysteine-rich regions of the endodomain. *J Virol* 2004;78:9904–9917.

470. Yeager CL, Ashmun RA, Williams RK, et al. Human aminopeptidase N is a receptor for human coronavirus 229E. *Nature* 1992;357:420–422.

471. Yount B, Curtis KM, Baric RS. Strategy for systematic assembly of large RNA and DNA genomes: transmissible gastroenteritis virus model. *J Virol* 2000;74:10600–10611.

472. Yount B, Roberts RS, Lindesmith L, et al. Rewiring the severe acute respiratory syndrome coronavirus (SARS-CoV) transcription circuit: Engineering a recombination-resistant genome. *Proc Natl Acad Sci U S A* 2006;103:12546–12551.

473. Yuan Y, Cao D, Zhang Y, et al. Cryo-EM structures of MERS-CoV and SARS-CoV spike glycoproteins reveal the dynamic receptor binding domains. *Nat Commun* 2017;8:15092.

474. Zaki AM, van Boheemen S, Bestebroer TM, et al. Isolation of a novel coronavirus from a man with pneumonia in Saudi Arabia. *N Engl J Med* 2012;367:1814–1820.

475. Zeng LP, Gao YT, Ge XY, et al. Bat severe acute respiratory syndrome-like coronavirus WIV1 encodes an extra accessory protein, ORFX, involved in modulation of the host immune response. *J Virol* 2016;90:6573–6582.

476. Zeng Q, Langereis MA, van Vliet AL, et al. Structure of coronavirus hemagglutinin-esterase offers insight into corona and influenza virus evolution. *Proc Natl Acad Sci U S A* 2008;105:9065–9069.

477. Zhao J, Alshukairi AN, Baharoon SA, et al. Recovery from the Middle East respiratory syndrome is associated with antibody and T-cell responses. *Sci Immunol* 2017;2:eaan5393.

478. Zhao L, Jha BK, Wu A, et al. Antagonism of the interferon-induced OAS-RNase L pathway by murine coronavirus ns2 protein is required for virus replication and liver pathology. *Cell Host Microbe* 2012;11:607–616.

479. Zhao J, Li K, Wohlford-Lenane C, et al. Rapid generation of a mouse model for Middle East respiratory syndrome. *Proc Natl Acad Sci U S A* 2014;111:4970–4975.

480. Zhao J, Zhao J, Legge K, et al. Age-related increases in PGD(2) expression impair respiratory DC migration, resulting in diminished T cell responses upon respiratory virus infection in mice. *J Clin Invest* 2011;121:4921–4930.

481. Zhao J, Zhao J, Van Rooijen N, et al. Evasion by stealth: inefficient immune activation underlies poor T cell response and severe disease in SARS-CoV-infected mice. *PLoS Pathog* 2009;5:e1000636.

482. Zhou J, Chu H, Li C, et al. Active replication of Middle East respiratory syndrome coronavirus and aberrant induction of inflammatory cytokines and chemokines in human macrophages: implications for pathogenesis. *J Infect Dis* 2014;209:1331–1342.

483. Zhou P, Fan H, Lan T, et al. Fatal swine acute diarrhoea syndrome caused by an HKU2-related coronavirus of bat origin. *Nature* 2018;556:255–258.

484. Zhou H, Perlman S. Mouse hepatitis virus does not induce Beta interferon synthesis and does not inhibit its induction by double-stranded RNA. *J Virol* 2007;81:568–574.

485. Zhu X, Fang L, Wang D, et al. Porcine deltacoronavirus nsp5 inhibits interferon-beta production through the cleavage of NEMO. *Virology* 2017;502:33–38.

486. Ziebuhr J. The coronavirus replicase. *Curr Top Microbiol Immunol* 2005;287:57–94.

487. Ziebuhr J, Thiel V, Gorbalenya AE. The autocatalytic release of a putative RNA virus transcription factor from its polyprotein precursor involves two paralogous papain-like proteases that cleave the same peptide bond. *J Biol Chem* 2001;276:33220–33232.

488. Zumla A, Chan JF, Azhar EI, et al. Coronaviruses—drug discovery and therapeutic options. *Nat Rev Drug Discov* 2016;15:327–347.

489. Zumla A, Hui DS, Perlman S. Middle East respiratory syndrome. *Lancet* 2015;386:995–1007.

490. Zúñiga S, Sola I, Alonso S, et al. Sequence motifs involved in the regulation of discontinuous coronavirus subgenomic RNA synthesis. *J Virol* 2004;78:980–994.

491. Zust R, Cervantes-Barragan L, Habjan M, et al. Ribose 2'-O-methylation provides a molecular signature for the distinction of self and non-self mRNA dependent on the RNA sensor Mda5. *Nat Immunol* 2011;12:137–143.

492. Zust R, Cervantes-Barragan L, Kuri T, et al. Coronavirus non-structural protein 1 is a major pathogenicity factor: implications for the rational design of coronavirus vaccines. *PLoS Pathog* 2007;3:e109.

493. Züst R, Miller TB, Goebel SJ, et al. Genetic interactions between an essential 3' cis-acting RNA pseudoknot, replicase gene products, and the extreme 3' end of the mouse coronavirus genome. *J Virol* 2008;82:1214–1228.

Jens H. Kuhn • Gaya K. Amarasinghe • Donna L. Perry

HISTORY

The known history of filovirus infections spans five decades. Since the first discovery of a filovirus in 1967,[684] 43 natural human filovirus disease (FVD) outbreaks and at least five laboratory-acquired infections (LAIs) have been recorded (Figs. 11.1 and 11.2). Limited clusters of human filovirus infections were likely overlooked in the past.[425] However, improved surveillance and reporting systems together with progress in diagnostic methodologies still support the notion that human filovirus spillover events are extremely rare. Almost all FVD outbreaks have occurred in Equatorial (Western, Middle, and Eastern) Africa,[425] suggesting that filoviruses pathogenic to humans are endemic primarily on the African continent. The majority of FVD outbreaks has been caused by single introductions of a filovirus from an unknown source into the affected human populations with subsequent amplification by direct person-to-person transmission. FVD outbreaks have most commonly occurred in isolated rural areas, rarely involving more than a few hundred people.[425] However, some outbreaks have occurred in urban areas. One outbreak affected almost 29,000 people,[106] demonstrating that filoviruses have the potential for pandemic spread associated with significant socioeconomic impacts.[340]

Marburgviruses

Marburg Virus

The first recorded filovirus, Marburg virus (MARV), was discovered in 1967. Three nearly simultaneous case clusters of severe and frequently lethal human disease occurred among laboratory personnel working in poliomyelitis vaccine–manufacturing institutes in Marburg an der Lahn and Frankfurt am Main, Hesse, West Germany (today Germany) and Belgrade, Yugoslavia (today Serbia).[294,486,684] The initial West German infections happened during routine tissue harvesting from infected grivets (Primates: Cercopithecidae: *Chlorocebus aethiops* Linnaeus, 1758) imported from Uganda, with subsequent secondary transmission among colleagues and nosocomial transmissions during clinical treatment of patients.[294,486,684] In Yugoslavia, a veterinarian became infected during the necropsy of a grivet that had died from unknown causes. His wife attended to him during his illness and, thereby, became infected herself.[871] These grivets had been imported from the same Ugandan nonhuman primate (NHP) exporter that supplied the West German facilities. Thus, all three case clusters were epidemiologically connected through grivets that likely became infected in Eastern Africa.[320,694] However, the true source of MARV that caused this outbreak, which ultimately affected 31 people and killed 7, was never identified, and this outbreak was the only recorded natural occurrence of MARV infection involving grivets.

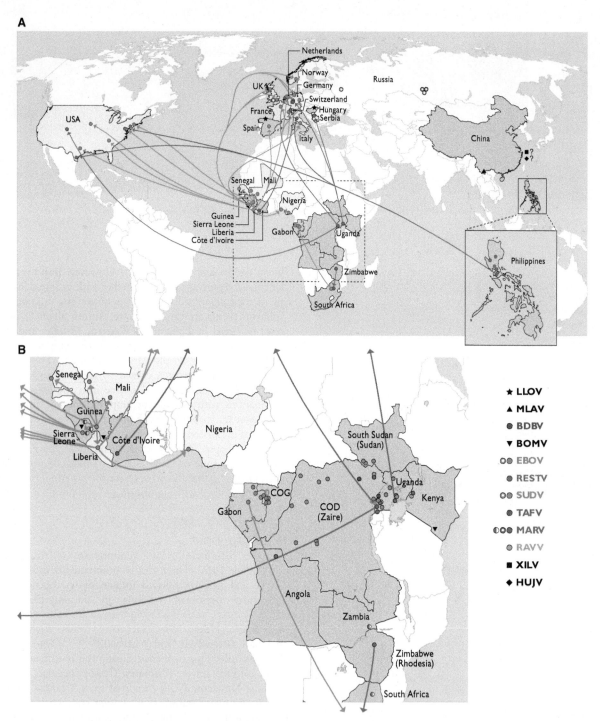

FIGURE 11.1 Global filovirus distribution. A: Human filovirus infections are indicated on a global map by colored dots indicating different filoviruses. Countries where filoviruses are suspected to be endemic are colored pink. Countries affected by imported cases are colored yellow, with arrows indicating origin and destination of cases. Hollow dots indicate locations of laboratory-acquired infections (LAIs; in this text defined as filovirus infections acquired in nonclinical laboratories during activities known to involve filoviruses). Half-colored dots indicate unambiguous human filovirus detection in nonhuman animals. *Asterisks, triangles, squares,* and *diamonds* indicate discovery locations of filoviruses, thus far, not associated with human infections. Question marks indicate uncertain origins. Only current country names are shown. **B:** Magnification of *central insert* indicated by *dashed lines* in **(A)**. Former country names are listed in parenthesis under current names. BDBV, Bundibugyo virus; BOMV, Bombali virus; COD, Democratic Republic of the Congo; COG, Republic of the Congo; EBOV, Ebola virus; HUJV, Huángjiāo virus; LLOV, Lloviu virus; MARV, Marburg virus; MLAV, Měnglà virus; RAVV, Ravn virus; RESTV, Reston virus; SUDV, Sudan virus; TAFV, Taï Forest virus; USA, United States of America; XILV, Xīlǎng virus. (Adapted from Kuhn JH. Ebolavirus and marburgvirus infections. In: Jameson JL, Fauci AS, Kasper DL, et al., eds. *Harrison's Principles of Internal Medicine,* Vol. 2. 20th ed. Columbus: McGraw-Hill Education; 2018: 1509–1515; Radoshitzky SR, Bavari S, Jahrling PB, et al. Filoviruses. In: Bozue J, Cote CK, Glass PJ, eds. *Medical Aspects of Biological Warfare.* Fort Sam Houston: Borden Institute, US Army Medical Department Center and School, Health Readiness Center of Excellence; 2018:569–614, Refs.[426,615] Figure courtesy of Jiro Wada, IRF-Frederick, Fort Detrick, MD, USA.)

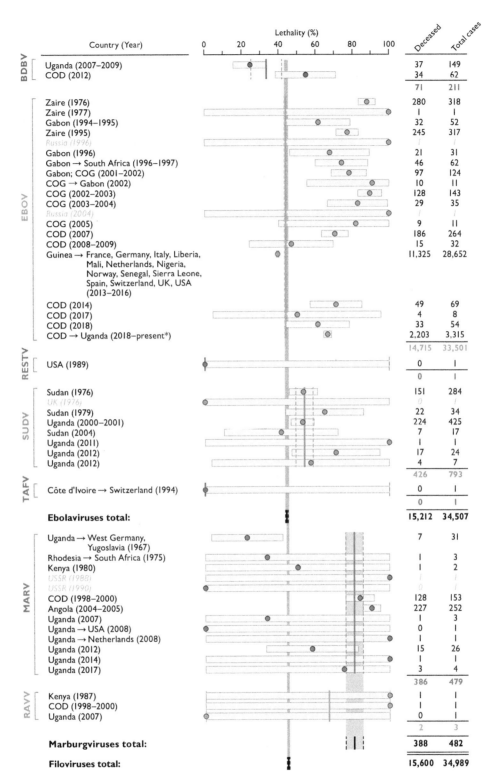

FIGURE 11.2 Global human filovirus infections. Occurrences are listed by year and etiologic agent. Laboratory-acquired infections are indicated by gray italics; international case exportations are indicated using arrows (*left column*). Case numbers and deaths for each filovirus, all filoviruses of a particular genus, and all filoviruses together are listed for each outbreak in the utmost right columns. Lethality/case-fatality rates for each individual outbreak are indicated by dots plotted in the middle column on a 0% to 100% scale along with 99% confidence intervals (*gray horizontal bars*). Average lethalities over all outbreaks caused by an individual filovirus, filoviruses of a particular genus, or all filoviruses are indicated by vertical lines with 99% confidence intervals shown by dashed lines (*partially overlapping*). Countries are listed according to their official names at the time of filovirus detection. BDBV, Bundibugyo virus; COD, Democratic Republic of the Congo; COG, Republic of the Congo; EBOV, Ebola virus; MARV, Marburg virus; RAVV, Ravn virus; RESTV, Reston virus; SUDV, Sudan virus; TAFV, Taï Forest virus; UK, United Kingdom; USA; United States of America; USSR, Union of Soviet Socialist Republics. *, case numbers as of December 1, 2019. (Inspired by Kuhn JH. Ebolavirus and marburgvirus infections. In: Jameson JL, Fauci AS, Kasper DL, et al., eds. *Harrison's Principles of Internal Medicine*, Vol. 2. 20th ed. Columbus: McGraw-Hill Education; 2018:1509–1515. Figure courtesy of Jiro Wada, IRF-Frederick, Fort Detrick, MD, USA.)

Over the subsequent five decades, MARV has caused only a few sporadic infections. In 1975, a student became infected with the virus from an unknown source in Rhodesia (now Zimbabwe). Prior to his death, the student transmitted the virus to his companion and later to a medical professional during treatment in Johannesburg, South Africa.[142,254,256] In 1980, MARV, again acquired from an unknown source and at an unknown location, killed a French citizen in Kenya and led to the infection of one of his doctors.[695]

Further cases of MARV infection occurred in Uganda from 2007 to 2017. In 2007, an outbreak occurred in Ibanda District among three visitors of a Kamwenge District gold mine (Kitaka Cave) inhabited by (cavernicolous and frugivorous) Egyptian rousettes (Chiroptera: Pteropodidae: *Rousettus aegyptiacus* E. Geoffroy, 1810).[2] These bats are now known to be natural hosts of the virus.[21–23,585,737] In 2008, in Bushenyi District, two tourists who had independently visited Python Cave inhabited by Egyptian rousettes became infected and inadvertently exported MARV to Colorado, the United States,[118] and South Holland, the Netherlands,[731] respectively. In 2012, an outbreak in the Ibanda, Kabale, and Kamwenge Districts affected 26 people (15 deaths). Though suspected, none of these infections could be associated with Egyptian rousette exposure.[402] In 2014, MARV killed a health care worker in Kampala, Uganda.[565] In 2017, the last recorded outbreak occurred in Uganda's Kween District. Four family members became infected, two of them died.[566] Direct exposure to bats did not appear to play a role in these latter outbreaks and the route of MARV introduction into human populations remains unclear.

Thus far, MARV has caused only two large disease outbreaks. From 1998 to 2000, numerous independent introductions of MARV into a population of illegal gold miners caused an outbreak consisting of multiple short transmission chains (at least 153 cases and 128 deaths) in Orientale Province (today Haut-Uele Province), Democratic Republic of the Congo (COD). The outbreak ended after the underground mine was flooded, suggesting that exposures occurred within the mine, likely involving Egyptian rousettes.[52,53,66] In 2004, MARV infected a single individual in northern Angola by unknown means and urban person-to-person transmission ultimately led to a total of 252 infected individuals and 227 deaths.[335,692,738]

In addition to natural outbreaks, MARV has been implicated in at least two additional LAIs. These infections occurred at the same Soviet (today Russian) institute in Novosibirsk Oblast in 1988 and 1990 during research involving the injection of MARV into domesticated guinea pigs (Rodentia: Caviidae: *Cavia porcellus* Linnaeus, 1758).[447,870]

MARV has rarely been detected in the wild in the absence of human infections. Next-generation sequencing (NGS) detected MARV in Egyptian rousette samples collected in 2013–2014 in Limpopo Province, South Africa.[585] Interestingly, the sequenced genome was found to be very closely related to the MARV isolate that caused the 1975 Rhodesia infections.[585] In 2018, MARV was discovered by NGS in Egyptian rousettes sampled in three locations in Sierra Leone (unpublished,[290]) and in Lusaka Province, Zambia.[381]

Ravn Virus

In 1987, a close relative of MARV, Ravn virus (RAVV), was discovered after a 15-year-old Danish boy succumbed to infection in Kenya during a vacation trip.[372] The source of infection was never identified. Since then, RAVV caused at least two additional human infections. One infection occurred during the 1998–2000 disease outbreak among gold miners caused predominantly by MARV in COD.[53] The other affected an individual who, in 2007, visited the same gold mine (Kitaka Cave) in Uganda that was pinpointed as the origin of three human MARV infections that year.[2] In addition, RAVV was repeatedly detected in or isolated from Egyptian rousettes from Kitaka Cave and from nearby Python Cave from 2007 to 2012.[21,23,737]

Ebolaviruses

Ebola Virus

Ebola virus (EBOV) was discovered in 1976 during a large outbreak that killed 280 of 318 infected people from 55 villages in Équateur Province (today Mongala Province) in Zaire (today COD). In addition to direct person-to-person contact, transmission was associated with the reuse of contaminated needles within health care facilities.[86,373,582,583,821]

Over the past five decades, EBOV has caused at least 17 additional disease outbreaks. One outbreak was a single infection in a 9-year-old girl in Équateur Province (today Sud-Ubangi Province), Zaire in 1977.[327] In 1994–1995, another cluster of at least 52 cases occurred after five independent virus introductions into populations working in three Gabonese gold mining camps in Woleu-Ntem Province.[277] In 1995, an outbreak involved at least 317 urban infections, many of them nosocomial, in and around Kikwit, Bandundu Province (today Kwilu Province), Zaire.[393] Seven smaller outbreaks occurred in the Ogooué-Ivindo and Ogooué-Lolo Provinces of Gabon and/or the Cuvette-Ouest Department of the Republic of the Congo (COG) from 1996 to 2005. Among these, a 1996 outbreak was noteworthy because it began with 18 infected children, whereas a 1996–1997 outbreak occurred among adults in a logging camp. The remainder of the outbreaks were all traced back to hunters who had been in contact with various NHPs or other animals destined for consumption.[85,239,241,275–277,450,510,556,557,602]

After these outbreaks, with one notable exception, EBOV infections were only recorded in COD. These outbreaks occurred in 2007 and 2008–2009 in Kasaï Occidental Province (today Kasaï Province),[289] in 2014 and 2018 in Équateur Province,[471,500] in 2017 in Bas-Uele Province,[564] and from 2018 to time of writing (December 2019) in the Ituri and Nord-Kivu Provinces.[351,499] The exception is the largest EVD outbreak ever recorded. This outbreak likely began in 2013 in Guinea with the typical single index case,[32] followed by substantial direct person-to-person transmission that ultimately involved 28,652 infections and 11,325 deaths distributed over 15 countries (predominantly Guinea, Liberia, and Sierra Leone).[106,115,188,280,735] True to historical precedent, the source of initial human infection in Guinea remains unclear. Indeed, EBOV has yet to be unambiguously detected and/or isolated from a wild animal.

EBOV has also caused at least two lethal LAIs in Russia. The first infection occurred in 1996 within a classified research program at a military institute in Moscow Oblast.[447,867] The second infection occurred in 2004 at the same institute in Novosibirsk Oblast that experienced previous laboratory-acquired MARV infections.[865]

Sudan Virus

Sudan virus (SUDV) was discovered almost simultaneously with EBOV in 1976. While EBOV spread through the population in Zaire, SUDV affected neighboring Sudan (today South Sudan). The three index cases worked in a cotton factory in Nzara, Western Equatoria State (today Gbudwe State). After their admission to Maridi City Hospital, SUDV spread within the hospital and then, via person-to-person transmission, into Maridi and neighboring towns. In total, 151 of 284 people died.[33,86,173,197,244,387,582,822] SUDV reemerged in 1979 in an employee from the same cotton factory implicated in the 1976 outbreak. As before, nosocomial transmission of SUDV contributed to the outbreaks, which ultimately claimed 22 lives.[40]

SUDV was not reencountered until the end of August 2000, when the virus emerged by unknown means in Gulu District, Uganda. Nosocomial transmission amplified the outbreak into Masindi and Mbarara Districts, ultimately affecting 425 people and killing 224.[73,117,572] After the Gulu outbreak, SUDV caused at least four more outbreaks. In 2004, the virus infection killed 7 of 17 people in South Sudan in the same area that experienced outbreaks in 1976 and 1979.[575,728] In 2011, SUDV infection killed a 12-year-old girl in Luweero District, Uganda.[681] Then, SUDV reappeared twice in Uganda in 2012, in Kibaale District (24 cases, 17 deaths) and Luweero District (7 cases, 4 deaths).[9]

Thus far, a single, nonlethal, laboratory-acquired SUDV infection is on record. In 1976, shortly after the discovery of SUDV in Sudan, a British investigator stuck himself with a contaminated needle at a military laboratory in South West England, United Kingdom, and became ill several days later.[87,205]

Reston Virus

Reston virus (RESTV) infection was identified in 1989 and 1990 in severely ill crab-eating macaques (Primates: Cercopithecidae: *Macaca fascicularis* Raffles, 1821) in U.S. NHP facilities located in Pennsylvania, Texas, and Virginia shortly after arrival from a NHP export facility in Laguna, Luzon, Philippines. The macaques presented with clinical signs typical of simian hemorrhagic fever (SHF); indeed, further studies revealed coinfection of some of the macaques with SHF-causing simarteriviruses (*Arteriviridae*: *Simarterivirinae*).[268,315,357,513] Despite increased surveillance and quarantine measures, RESTV was again exported in crab-eating macaques from the same Filipino primate supplier to Tuscany, Italy, in 1992 and to Texas, United States, in 1996. Simarterivirus coinfections were found only in the macaques euthanized in Texas.[134,512–514,636]

In 2008–2009, RESTV cocirculated together with porcine reproductive and respiratory syndrome virus 2 (PRRSV-2; *Arteriviridae*: *Variarterivirinae*) and porcine circovirus 2 (PCV-2; *Circoviridae*: *Circovirus*) in severely sick domestic pigs (Artiodactyla: Suidae: *Sus scrofa domesticus* Erxleben, 1777) bred in two piggeries on Luzon, Philippines.[42] The contribution of RESTV to the observed disease is unclear. In 2015, RESTV once again emerged in the Philippines, this time again in crab-eating macaques, some coinfected with measles virus, in a NHP facility close to Manila.[166] Finally, short RESTV gene-like fragments were detected in molossid, pteropodid, and vespertilionid bats trapped in the Philippines[364] and in samples

from PRRSV-2–coinfected domestic pigs in China,[580] suggesting widespread RESTV distribution in Asia.

Thus far, a single asymptomatic human infection with RESTV has been proven unambiguously,[12] but seroconversions have been reported several times in individuals in contact with RESTV-infected animals.[42,116,513,824]

Taï Forest Virus

Taï Forest virus (TAFV) was discovered in 1994 during an investigation into the cause of unusual deaths in a troop of western chimpanzees (Primates: Hominidae: *Pan troglodytes verus* Schwartz, 1934) in Taï National Park, western Côte d'Ivoire. A Swiss ethologist, who had performed a field necropsy on one of the apes, fell sick with a dengue fever–like disease. She fully recovered after medical evacuation from Abidjan to Switzerland.[238,442] Histopathological examination of the tissues from the necropsied western chimpanzee suggested that the troop indeed had been infected with, and decimated by, TAFV.[833]

Bundibugyo Virus

Bundibugyo virus (BDBV) was first discovered in Bundibugyo District, Uganda, during a human disease outbreak that lasted from 2007 to 2008, resulting in at least 149 cases and 37 deaths.[470,740,779] BDBV has since been encountered during a smaller outbreak in 2012 in Orientale Province, COD (62 cases, 34 deaths). As in all previous disease outbreaks caused by ebolaviruses, these two outbreaks began with single BDBV introductions into the human population from unknown sources.[9,414] Thus far, BDBV infections have not been associated with human exposure to a particular animal or geographic or ecologic feature or associated with a certain socioeconomic background.

Bombali Virus

Bombali virus (BOMV), which has yet to be isolated, was discovered by NGS in oral and rectal swabs taken from apparently healthy insectivorous little free-tailed bats (Chiroptera: Molossidae: *Chaerephon pumilus* Cretzschmar, 1826) and Angolan free-tailed bats (Chiroptera: Molossidae: *Mops condylurus* A. Smith, 1933) sampled in Sierra Leone in 2016. Although the sampled bats have roosted inside occupied homes, no human BOMV infections have been recorded,[285] and BOMV's pathogenic potential remains to be determined. BOMV RNA has also been found in various organs of Angolan free-tailed bats sampled in Taita-Taveta County, Kenya, in 2018 and Nzérékoré Region, Guinea, in 2018–2019.[237,386]

Cuevaviruses

Lloviu virus (LLOV) was discovered in dead Schreiber's long-fingered bats (Chiroptera: Vespertilionidae: *Miniopterus schreibersii* Kuhl, 1817) by NGS performed on samples collected in Cueva del Lloviu, Asturias Principality, Spain, in 2002.[550] LLOV was also detected by NGS in dead Schreiber's long-fingered bats found in caves in North Hungarian Mountains, Hungary, in 2016.[391] Thus far, LLOV has not been isolated. Whether LLOV caused the deaths of the bats it was sequenced from remains as unclear as is the potential of LLOV to cause human disease.

Striaviruses

Xīlǎng virus (XILV) was discovered by NGS in a striated frog-fish (Lophiiformes: Antennariidae: *Antennarius striatus* Shaw, 1794) captured by a fishing trawler in the East China Sea in 2011.[679] XILV has not yet been isolated.

Thamnoviruses

Huángjiāo virus (HUJV) was discovered by NGS in a greenfin horse-faced filefish (Tetraodontiformes: Monacanthidae: *Thamnaconus septentrionalis* Günther, 1874) captured by a fishing trawler in the East China Sea in 2011.[679] HUJV has not yet been isolated.

Dianloviruses

Měnglǎ virus (MLAV), first described in 2019, was discovered by NGS in a liver sample collected from an apparently healthy *Rousettus* sp. sampled in 2015 in Yúnnán Province, China. Thus far, MLAV has not been isolated and its pathogenic potential is currently unclear.[841,842]

Other Filoviruses

The recent discovery of BOMV, HUJV, LLOV, MLAV, and XILV in highly diverse animals (e.g., actinopterygid fish, frugivorous and insectivorous bats) in geographically separated areas (e.g., Africa, Asia, Europe) suggests that filovirus diversity and distribution are much broader than previously appreciated. Indeed, filovirus gene-like sequences were discovered in 2009 and 2015 by NGS in samples taken from apparently healthy frugivorous lesser dawn bats (Chiroptera: Pteropodidae: *Eonycteris spelaea* Dobson, 1871) and unspecified rousettes in Yúnnán Province, China. Additional sequences were detected by NGS in frugivorous Leschenault's rousettes (*Rousettus leschenaultii* Desmarest, 1820) sampled in 2013 in the same area.[316,842] In addition, endogenous filovirus-like sequences were found in the genomes of various afrosoricids, bats, eulipotyphla, and rodents, as well as in marsupials, indicating that filoviruses have a long evolutionary history.[62,195,388,721,722]

CLASSIFICATION

Filoviruses are the members of the family *Filoviridae*, which is one of the 11 families in the haploviricotine order *Mononegavirales*.[20] Filoviruses are most closely related to viruses of the mononegaviral families *Paramyxoviridae*, *Pneumoviridae*, and *Sunviridae* and are assigned to six official genera (Table 11.1). Filovirus genus assignment is based on nine determinants: (a) pairwise genome sequence similarities,[39,428] (b) phylogenetic distance of coding-complete genomes, (c) large protein gene (*L*) sequences (Fig. 11.3), (d) RNA-directed RNA polymerase (RdRp) core domain amino acid sequences,[428,814] (e) number and location of open reading frames (ORFs) in genomes, (f) the presence or absence of cotranscriptional editing sites, (g) geographic distribution, (h) host tropism, and (i) pathogenic potential.[428]

Only the genera *Ebolavirus* and *Marburgvirus* contain viruses known to infect humans. The World Health Organization (WHO) consequently recognizes two major FVD subcategories, Ebola disease (EBOD; caused by BDBV, EBOV, SUDV, or TAFV) and Marburg disease (MARD; caused by MARV and RAVV) along with several secondary subcategories.[427,827]

TABLE 11.1 Filovirus classification and nomenclature as of 2019

Realm *Riboviria*
Kingdom *Orthornavirae**
Phylum *Negarnaviricota*
Subphylum *Haploviricotina*
Class *Monjiviricetes*
Order *Mononegavirales*
Family *Filoviridae*
Genus *Cuevavirus*
Species *Lloviu cuevavirus*[a]
Virus: Lloviu virus (LLOV)
Genus *Dianlovirus**
Species *Mengla dianlovirus**,[a]
Virus: Měnglǎ virus (MLAV)
Genus *Ebolavirus*
Species *Bombali ebolavirus**
Virus: Bombali virus (BOMV)
Species *Bundibugyo ebolavirus*
Virus: Bundibugyo virus (BDBV)
Species *Zaire ebolavirus*
Virus: Ebola virus (EBOV)[a]
Species *Reston ebolavirus*
Virus: Reston virus (RESTV)
Species *Sudan ebolavirus*
Virus: Sudan virus (SUDV)
Species *Tai Forest ebolavirus*
Virus: Taï Forest virus (TAFV)
Genus *Marburgvirus*
Species *Marburg marburgvirus*[a]
Virus 1: Marburg virus (MARV)
Virus 2: Ravn virus (RAVV)
Genus *Striavirus*
Species *Xilang striavirus*[a]
Virus: Xīlǎng virus (XILV)
Genus *Thamnovirus*
Species *Huangjiao thamnovirus*[a]
Virus: Huángjiāo virus (HUJV)

Asterisks mark taxa that have been approved by the International Committee on Taxonomy of Viruses (ICTV) Executive Committee in December of 2019 but still await ratification by the entire ICTV in 2020. Colors indicate filoviruses associated with human infections. Virus name abbreviations are shown in parentheses.
[a]Type species.
From Kuhn JH, Amarasinghe GK, Basler CF, et al. ICTV virus taxonomy profile: *Filoviridae*. *J Gen Virol* 2019;100:911–912.

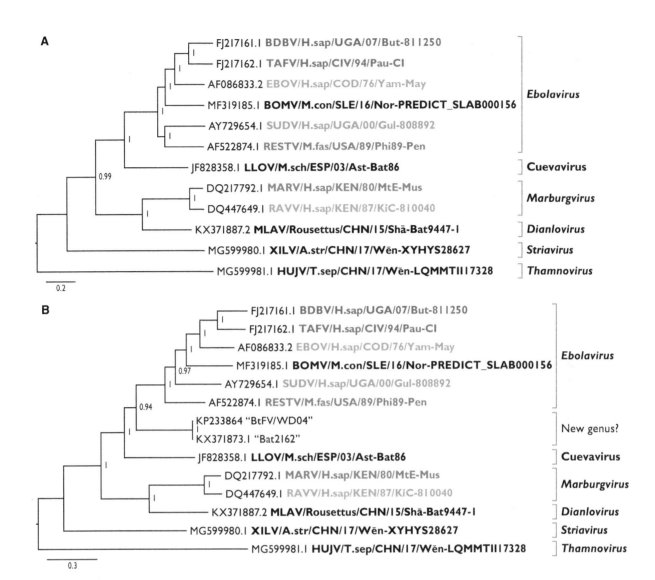

FIGURE 11.3 Phylogenetic relationships of filoviruses. Maximum-likelihood tree (midpoint-rooted) inferred by using **(A)** coding-complete or complete filovirus genome sequences and **(B)** filovirus RNA-directed RNA polymerase gene (*L*) sequences. Sequences were aligned using Clustal-Omega version 1.2.1 (http://www.clustal.org/omega/) and were manually curated in Geneious version R9 (http://www.geneious.com). Trees were inferred in FastTree version 2.1 (http://www.microbesonline.org/fasttree/) using a general time reversible (GTR) model with 20 gamma-rate categories, 5,000 bootstrap replicates, and exhaustive search parameters (-slow) and pseudocounts (-pseudo). Numbers near nodes on the trees indicate bootstrap values in decimal form. Tree branches are scaled to nucleotide substitutions per site (scale bars). Tips of branches indicate GenBank accession numbers and the medium-length abbreviation[429] of each filovirus isolate used for the analyses in the form of <virus name abbreviation>/<isolation host species name abbreviation>/<UN Geoscheme country name abbreviation>/<year of isolation>/<variant name>-<isolate name>. BDBV, Bundibugyo virus; BOMV, Bombali virus; EBOV, Ebola virus; HUJV, Huángjiāo virus; LLOV, Lloviu virus; MARV, Marburg virus; MLAV, Měnglà virus; RAVV, Ravn virus; RESTV, Reston virus; SUDV, Sudan virus; TAFV, Taï Forest virus; XILV, Xīlǎng virus. (Adapted and expanded from Kuhn JH, Amarasinghe GK, Basler CF, et al. ICTV virus taxonomy profile: *Filoviridae*. *J Gen Virol* 2019;100:911–912. Analysis courtesy of Dr. Nicholas Di Paola, PhD, USAMRIID, Fort Detrick, MD, USA. Figure courtesy of Jiro Wada, IRF-Frederick, Fort Detrick, MD, USA.)

Due to the extraordinarily high case-fatality rates of most human filovirus infections (Fig. 11.2), the ability of certain filoviruses to spread from one individual to another by direct contact, and the absence of efficacious licensed medical countermeasures (MCMs), filovirus research is prioritized within public health preparedness and biodefense efforts.[121,549] WHO considers all filoviruses that are known to infect humans to be Risk Group 4 (RG-4) pathogens.[823] In the United States, any research involving viable forms or ebolaviruses and marburg-

viruses requires biosafety level 4 (BSL-4) or animal biosafety level 4 (ABSL-4) containment and adherence to associated standard operating procedures to protect laboratory workers and the public.[750] In addition, most filoviruses are classified as Select Agents under U.S. Federal Law for regulation and oversight of filovirus research activities and/or possession[749] (Table 11.2). Similar classification systems used by other countries also list filoviruses at the top of their risk, safety, or priority categories.

TABLE 11.2 Major filovirus biosafety and biosecurity risk classifications

Filovirus (Abbreviation)	Biocontainment Requirement[750]	CDC Bioterrorism Agent/Disease[121]	NIAID Priority Pathogen[549]	HHS Select Agent[749]	Australia Group Human Pathogen for Export Control[725]
Bombali virus (BOMV)	(A)BSL-4[a]	No	No[c]	Yes (Tier 1)[d]	Yes
Bundibugyo virus (BDBV)	(A)BSL-4[a]	Yes (Category A)[b]	Yes (Category A)[c]	Yes (Tier 1)[d]	Yes
Ebola virus (EBOV)	(A)BSL-4	Yes (Category A)	Yes (Category A)	Yes (Tier 1)	Yes
Huángjiāo virus (HUJV)	?	No	No	No	No
Lloviu virus (LLOV)	(A)BSL-4[a]	No	No	No	No
Marburg virus (MARV)	(A)BSL-4	Yes (Category A)	Yes (Category A)	Yes (Tier 1)	Yes
Měnglà virus (MLAV)	(A)BSL-4[a]	No	No	No	No
Ravn virus (RAVV)	(A)BSL-4[a]	Yes (Category A)[b]	Yes (Category A)[c]	Yes (Tier 1)[d]	Yes
Reston virus (RESTV)	(A)BSL-4	No	No	Yes (Tier 1)[d]	Yes
Sudan virus (SUDV)	(A)BSL-4[a]	Yes (Category A)[b]	Yes (Category A)[c]	Yes (Tier 1)[d]	Yes
Taï Forest virus (TAFV)	(A)BSL-4[a]	Yes (Category A)[b]	Yes (Category A)[c]	Yes (Tier 1)[d]	Yes
Xīlǎng virus (XILV)	?	No	No	No	No

(A)BSL, US (animal) biosafety level; CDC, U.S. Centers for Disease Control and Prevention; HHS, U.S. Department of Health and Human Services; NIAID, U.S. National Institute of Allergy and Infectious Diseases.
[a]Reference[750] lists "Ebola (including Reston)" and "Marburg" as requiring (A)BSL-4 biocontainment. Here, it is assumed that these terms include all ebolaviruses/marburgviruses with significant genomic similarities.
[b]Reference[121] assigns "Viral hemorrhagic fevers, including … [f]iloviruses (Ebola, Marburg)" to Category A. Because the terms "Ebola" and "Marburg" are ambiguous, all human disease-causing ebolaviruses and marburgviruses (rather than just Ebola virus and Marburg virus) are listed here in Category A.
[c]Interpreted here to be included in the ambiguous list phrases "Ebola" or "Marburg."
[d]Interpreted here to be included in the ambiguous list phrases "Ebola virus" or "Marburg virus."

VIRION STRUCTURE

Filovirion morphology data are only available for ebolaviruses and marburgviruses because cuevaviruses, dianloviruses, striaviruses, and thamnoviruses have not yet been isolated. The hallmark of ebolavirus and marburgvirus particles is their predominantly filamentous appearance that is easily identifiable in electron micrographs (Fig. 11.4). Depending on culture conditions and cell or tissue types, particles also can assume branched, toroid, U-shaped, or 6-shaped ("shepherd's crook") forms. Filamentous and other particles are typically less than 1 μm long, but in cell culture, these particles can reach lengths of greater than 20 μm. Their diameters are more uniform, ranging from ≈91 to 98 nm.[63,68,69,202,203,269,644] An initial study using recombinantly expressed proteins suggests that cuevavirions may also form predominantly filamentous particles.[490]

Ebolavirions and marburgvirions possess a central core, the helically-arranged ribonucleoprotein (RNP) complex. This RNP is ≈30 to 41 nm in diameter with a pitch of ≈7 to 7.5 nm. The RNP is embedded in a matrix layer surrounded by a lipid envelope obtained during particle budding from host cell membranes. The lipid envelope is decorated with globular peplomers (≈7 nm in diameter and ≈13 nm in length) at intervals of ≈15 ± 4 nm (1 peplomer per 250 nm²).[63,68,69,202,203,269,644,802] These peplomers largely determine the antigenicity of filovirions.

Filovirions are sensitive to desiccation, heat, pressure, UV light, γ-irradiation, detergents (e.g., diethyl ether, phenolic compounds, sodium deoxycholate), formaldehyde, and commercial oxidizing agents (e.g., sodium hypochlorite/bleach), but inactivation/disinfection efficiency is dependent on disinfectant type, concentration, and contact time and varies based on the volume, titer, and type of contaminated material.[17,88,126,224,229,301,433,522,604,696,805,869]

GENOME STRUCTURE AND ORGANIZATION

Filovirus Genomic Organization

Filovirus genomes are components of filovirion RNPs and are organized like those of most mononegaviruses,[576] consisting of linear, nonsegmented, negative-sense RNAs with the general gene order 3'-N-P-M-G-L-5' (filovirus terminology: 3'-NP-VP35-VP40-GP-L-5'). Filovirus-specific genes are inserted at various locations throughout the genome depending on genus affiliation. For instance, dianlovirus, ebolavirus, and marburgvirus genomes have the gene order 3'-NP-VP35-VP40-GP-VP30-VP24-L-5' (Fig. 11.5). However, cuevaviruses appear to synthesize VP24 and L expression products from a single gene using a bicistronic transcript. Striavirus genomes appear to contain at least 10 genes with only 9 (NP, VP35, VP40, GP, VP30, and L) that are obvious homologs to those of ebolaviruses and marburgviruses.[343,679] Finally, thamnoviruses are classified as filoviruses primarily because of their NP, GP, and L genes, whereas their four other genes do not have obvious filovirus homologs.[343,679] In addition to gene content, filovirus genomes differ in length (≈15 kb [thamnoviruses] to ≈19 kb [cuevaviruses, ebolaviruses, and marburgviruses]), number and location of gene overlaps (0–9), and absence (dianloviruses, marburgviruses, striaviruses, thamnoviruses) or presence (cuevaviruses, ebolaviruses) of overlapping reading frames in the GP gene that can be accessed via cotranscriptional editing[222,349,550,649,652,679,765,841] (Fig. 11.5).

Complete genome information has only been obtained for five ebolaviruses (BDBV, BOMV, EBOV, RESTV, and SUDV) and one marburgvirus (MARV). The 3' ends of these genomes are not polyadenylated, and the 5' ends are neither

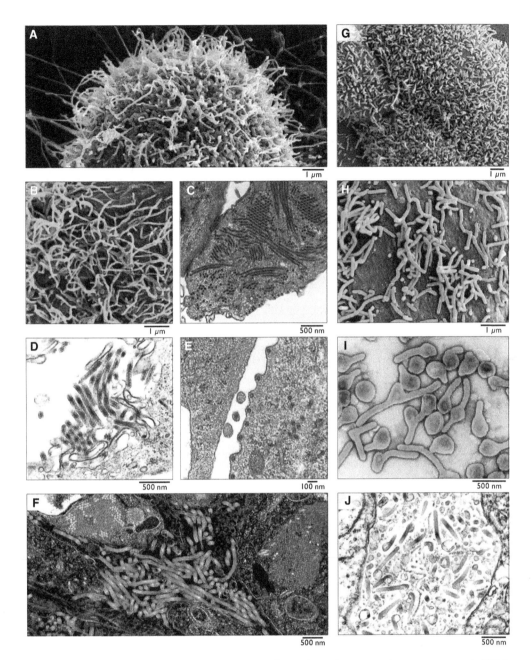

FIGURE 11.4 Mammalian filovirion structure. A and B: Colorized scanning electron microscopic (SEM) images of Ebola virus (EBOV) particles budding from Vero E6 cells. Virions are *blue* in **(A)** and *green* in **(B)**. **C–E:** Transmission electron microscopic (TEM) images of EBOV nucleocapsids forming in an intracytoplasmic inclusion body **(C)**, mature virus particles (*colored green*) **(D)**, and budding virus particles **(E)** in Vero E6 cells. **F:** TEM image of intracytoplasmic inclusion bodies forming EBOV nucleocapsid structures (*stippled red and white*) and intercellular, filamentous, mature virion particles (*red*) from the ovary of a crab-eating macaque. **G and H:** SEM images of Marburg virus (MARV) particles on the surface of Vero E6 cells (**H** *colored blue*). **I:** Negative-stain TEM image of mature filamentous MARV particles (*colored blue*) forming characteristic shepherd's crook structures collected from infected Vero E6 cell culture supernatants. **J:** TEM image of mature filamentous MARV particles (*colored blue*) from the liver of a rhesus monkey. (Figure courtesy of John G. Bernbaum and Jiro Wada, IRF-Frederick, Fort Detrick, MD, USA.)

capped nor covalently linked to any protein. The 3′ leader and 5′ trailer sequences of the genomes are conserved (particularly within genera) and, in part, complementary. They contain *cis*-acting signals for mRNA transcription and genome replication, including promoters.[79,148,222,396,624,768]

Mammalian filovirus (cuevavirus, dianlovirus, ebolavirus, and marburgvirus) genes are identifiable through their genus-/species-specific conserved gene start and end/polyadenylation signals within relatively long noncoding regions.[104,222,349,649,651,740] These regions may be separated from each other by intergenic

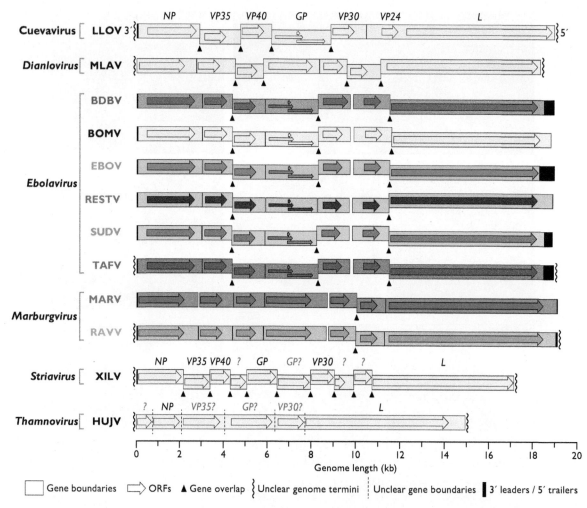

FIGURE 11.5 Filovirus genome organization. Genomes are drawn to scale. BDBV, Bundibugyo virus; BOMV, Bombali virus; EBOV, Ebola virus; HUJV, Huángjiāo virus; LLOV, Lloviu virus; MARV, Marburg virus; MLAV, Měnglà virus; ORF, open reading frame; RAVV, Ravn virus; RESTV, Reston virus; SUDV, Sudan virus; TAFV, Taï Forest virus; XILV, Xīlǎng virus. (Adapted and expanded from Kuhn JH, Amarasinghe GK, Basler CF, et al. ICTV virus taxonomy profile: *Filoviridae. J Gen Virol* 2019;100:911–912. Figure courtesy of Jiro Wada, IRF-Frederick, Fort Detrick, MD, USA.)

regions or overlaps, which influence transcription reinitiation and/or virus growth in manners that need to be better defined.[93]

Filovirus Genome Expression Products

Filovirus genomes encode 6 to 10 proteins, some of which are further processed by proteolytic cleavage. Most of the main proteins are expressed from single genes, although cotranscriptional editing (cuevaviruses, ebolaviruses) and possibly bicistronic transcripts (cuevaviruses) are also used to access ORFs.[550,652,765] The mammalian filovirus *NP, VP35, VP40, VP30, VP24,* and *L* genes encode nucleoprotein (NP), polymerase cofactor (VP35), matrix protein (VP40), transcriptional activator (VP30), RNA complex–associated protein (VP24), and large protein (L), respectively. Dianlovirus and marburgvirus *GP* genes encode only the glycoprotein ($GP_{1,2}$) and a cleavage product thereof (shed glycoprotein [$GP_{1,2\Delta}$]), whereas cuevaviruses and ebolaviruses express six products from these genes: secreted glycoprotein (sGP), Δ-peptide, $GP_{1,2}$, $GP_{1,2\Delta}$, sGP–GP_2, and secondary secreted glycoprotein (ssGP).[198,199,222,395,649] NP, VP35, VP40,

$GP_{1,2}$, and L are the functional analogs (and NP and L are also functional homologs[41,814]) (Fig. 11.5) of core proteins encoded by all mononegaviruses (typically designated N, P, M, G, and L, respectively).[41,605,814] The expression products of piscine filoviruses (striaviruses and thamnoviruses) have yet to be characterized. However, these viruses encode some obvious homologs to proteins expressed by other filoviruses (striaviruses, NP, VP40, VP30, L; thamnoviruses, NP and L) (Fig. 11.5; Table 11.3).

Filovirus Ribonucleoprotein Complex Components

NP, VP35, VP30, VP24, L, and the viral genome form the mammalian filovirus RNP complex, which is embedded in the virion matrix composed of VP40 surrounded by the envelope containing $GP_{1,2}$ peplomers[38,60,63,401,534,709,802] (Fig. 11.6). Mammalian filovirions may be polyploid, containing up to 22 individual RNPs. Extremely long particles, typically seen in tissue culture, are likely highly polyploid.[63] The RNPs of piscine filoviruses remain to be defined.

TABLE 11.3 Characterized mammalian filovirus proteins

Protein Designation (Abbreviation)	Characteristics	Function
Nucleoprotein (NP)	• RNP complex and cellular inclusion body component. Homo-oligomerizes to form helical polymers • Binds to ssRNA, VP35, VP40, VP30, and VP24 • Phosphorylated and, in ebolaviruses, also *O*-glycosylated and possibly sialylated • Marburgviruses: contain a late-budding (PSAP) motif	• RNP formation through encapsidation of filovirus genomic or antigenomic RNA • Genome replication and transcription • Marburgviruses: RNP transport and budding • Determinant in filovirus rodent adaptation
Polymerase cofactor (VP35)	• RNP complex and cellular inclusion body component • Homo-oligomerizes and binds to dsRNA, NP, and L; phosphorylated • Absent from striaviruses and thamnoviruses • Interacts with DYNLL1 • EBOV: ubiquitinylated by TRIM6	• Polymerase cofactor in the filovirus polymerase holoenzyme (L+VP35) • Cuevaviruses: inhibits IRF3 phosphorylation, IFNA1/B1 production, and protein kinase R phosphorylation • Ebolaviruses: inhibits innate immune response by interfering with IRF3, IRF7, IFIH1, DDX58, and RNAi pathways; inhibits stress granule formation • Marburgviruses: inhibits innate immune response by interfering with IRF3, IRF7, and DDX58 pathways and inhibits EIF2AK2 activity • Ebolaviruses: RNA silencing suppressor; prevents stress granule formation
Matrix protein (VP40)	• Consists of two distinct functional domains that drive homo-oligomerization to form dimers, linear hexamers, and circular octamers. Dimers bind to cellular membranes; hexamers polymerize to matrix filaments; octamers bind ssRNA. Binds NP • Dianloviruses and marburgviruses: contains PPXY late-budding motif that interacts with NEDD4 and TSG101 • Cuevaviruses and ebolaviruses: contains PPXY and P(T/S)AP late-budding motifs that interact with NEDD4 and TSG101; binds to α-tubulin and are ubiquitinylated • Absent from thamnoviruses	• Matrix component • Negative regulator of genome transcription and replication • Regulator of virion morphogenesis and egress • Ebolaviruses: RNAi silencing suppressor • Marburgviruses: inhibits JAK1/TYK2 STAT pathway
Glycoprotein (GP$_{1,2}$)	• Trimeric type I transmembrane and class I fusion protein consisting of disulfide-linked GP$_1$–GP$_2$ heterodimers; heavily *N*- and *O*-glycosylated, phosphorylated, acylated. Sialylation extent different depending on the virus • Absent from striaviruses and thamnoviruses	• Virion adsorption to filovirus-susceptible cells via cellular attachment factors; induction of virus–cell membrane fusion subsequent to endolysosomal binding to NPC1 • Determines filovirus cell and tissue tropism • Inhibits intrinsic immune response by interfering with BST2
Shed glycoprotein (GP$_{1,2\Delta}$)	• Secreted GP$_{1,2}$ trimer produced by ADAM17-mediated cleavage of membrane-bound GP$_{1,2}$ • Absent from striaviruses and thamnoviruses	Hypothesized to be an anti-GP$_{1,2}$ antibody decoy
Secreted glycoprotein (sGP)	• Secreted disulfide-linked parallel homodimeric nonstructural protein that is C-mannosylated and *N*-glycosylated • Not encoded by marburgviruses, dianloviruses, striaviruses, and thamnoviruses	Hypothesized to be an anti-GP$_{1,2}$ antibody decoy and an anti-inflammatory agent
Secondary secreted glycoprotein (ssGP)	• Secreted disulfide-linked homodimeric nonstructural protein that is *N*-glycosylated • Not encoded by marburgviruses, dianloviruses, striaviruses, and thamnoviruses	Unknown
Δ-peptide	• Secreted nonstructural protein that is *O*-glycosylated and sialylated. Assembles as a pentameric chloride-selective viroporin • Not encoded by marburgviruses, dianloviruses, striaviruses, and thamnoviruses	Hypothesized to suppress filovirus superinfection of infected host cells

(continued)

TABLE 11.3 Characterized mammalian filovirus proteins (*Continued*)

Protein Designation (Abbreviation)	Characteristics	Function
Transcriptional activator (VP30)	• RNP complex and cellular inclusion body component • Homo-oligomerizes; Cys$_3$-His zinc finger; binds ssRNA, NP, and L; phosphorylated • Absent from thamnoviruses	• Transcription initiation, reinitiaition, enhancement, and antitermination • Cuevaviruses and ebolaviruses: *GP* gene editing regulator • Ebolaviruses: RNAi silencing suppressor
RNP complex–associated protein (VP24)	• RNP complex and cellular inclusion body component • Associates with membranes • Absent from striaviruses and thamnoviruses	• Negative regulator of genome transcription and replication; regulator of virion morphogenesis and egress; determinant in filovirus rodent adaptation • Cuevaviruses: inhibits tyrosine phosphorylated STAT1 binding to KPNA5, STAT1 nuclear accumulation, and IFN-induced gene expression • Ebolaviruses: inhibits phosphorylation of MAPK14 and prevent karyopherin shuttling from the cytoplasm into the nucleus; inhibits host cell signaling downstream of IFNA1/B1/G • Marburgviruses: targets KEAP1 to activate NFE2L2-induced cytoprotective responses
Large protein (L)	• RNP complex and cellular inclusion body component and catalytic center of the filovirus polymerase holo-enzyme (VP35+L) • Binds to filovirus genomic and antigenomic RNA and recognizes specific promoters and gene start and end signals • Binds directly to VP35 and VP30	• Genome replication via antigenomic intermediates • mRNA synthesis, capping, methylation, and polyadenylation • Determinant in filovirus rodent adaptation • Cuevaviruses and ebolaviruses; cotranscriptional editing of *GP* mRNAs

ADAM metallopeptidase domain 17 (ADAM17, formerly TACE); DDX58, DExD/H-box helicase 58 (formerly RIG-I); IFIH1, interferon induced with helicase C domain 1 (formerly MDA5); IFN, interferon; IRF, interferon regulatory factor; KEAP1, Kelch-like ECH-associated protein 1; MAPK, mitogen-activated protein kinase; NPC1, NPC intracellular cholesterol transporter 1; RNAi, RNA interference; RNP, ribonucleoprotein; STAT1, signal transducer and activator of transcription 1.

Nucleoprotein

Ebolavirus and marburgvirus NPs are phosphorylated or dephosphorylated by cellular kinases and phosphatases at C-terminal threonine and serine residues at various stages of the filovirus life cycle.[58,198,465] Partially phosphorylated NP monomers associate via their two-lobed N-terminal domains (NTDs) to form long, left-handed helical polymers that encapsidate filovirus genomes or antigenomes[58,63,68,69,400,498,558,560,706] (Fig. 11.7). These complexes serve as the templates for transcription and replication performed by L and VP35 and also for underlying structures of an array of morphologically distinct inclusion bodies. These inclusion bodies take the shape of lamellae, threads, or sponges (likely representing different RNP maturation forms) in the cytoplasm of filovirus-infected cells.[269,339,408,787,872] NP, via its NTD, binds directly to viral single-stranded (ss) RNA, VP35, and VP30,[58,60,292] all of which also interact directly with L and are recruited into inclusion bodies.[74,292,526] The EBOV NP NTD recruits PP2A-B56 phosphatase through an LxxIxE motif. This interaction dephosphorylates VP30, thereby triggering its transcriptional activation function.[419] The NP NTD also binds directly to VP24[38] and to VP40, which forms a matrix around RNPs.[562] Marburgvirus, but not ebolavirus, NP C-terminal domain (CTD) contains a late-budding (PSAP) motif that likely regulates RNP transport and particle budding. In ebolaviruses, such a motif (PTAP) is located in VP40.[178] The function of the ebolavirus NP CTD, which is tethered to the NTD through an unstructured sequence, is currently unclear.

Polymerase Cofactor (VP35)

VP35 consists of two distinct domains. The VP35 N-terminal oligomerization domain mediates VP35 homo-oligomerization and, thereby, filoviral replication and RNP complex formation. Binding of this domain via an SQTQT motif to host dynein light chain LC8-type 1 (DYNLL1) stabilizes the domain and increases viral RNA synthesis. The VP35 C-terminal interferon inhibitory domain (IID) binds double-stranded (ds) RNA at a distinct central basic patch. The region between the N-terminal and the C-terminal regions is likely unstructured in the absence of binding partners. VP35 IID's N-terminal NP-binding peptide (NPBP) binds to the NP NTD, and phosphorylation of IID may regulate this interaction[49,111,311,421,451,453,454,467,528,860] (Fig. 11.8). Interleukin enhancer-binding factor 3 (ILF3) binds to VP35 IID and, thereby, inhibits filovirus VP35–NP interaction and transcription/replication.[675] Ubiquitinylation of IID, promoted by host cell TRIM6, promotes EBOV replication.[67] A recent study has revealed that EBOV VP35 can hydrolyze all types of NTPs and unwind RNA helices in 5′→3′ direction in an ATP-dependent manner.[682] In addition, filovirus VP35 is an immunomodulator that antagonizes infected host cell antiviral responses via its IID.[49,50,111,124,194,218,226,342,606,669]

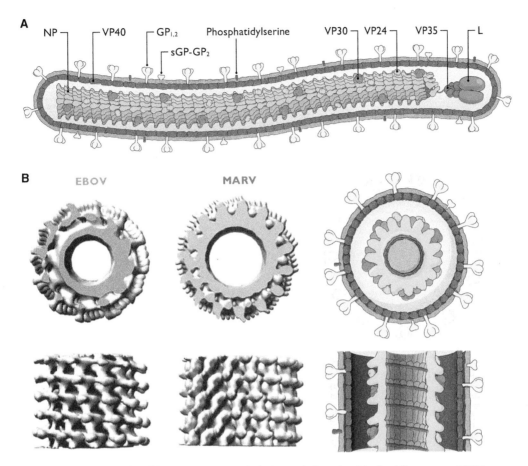

FIGURE 11.6 Mammalian filovirion structure. A: Artist rendering of an idealized filamentous EBOV particle. A ribonucleoprotein (RNP) complex, consists of the filovirus genome bound to helically polymerized nucleoprotein (NP) monomers in association with VP35, VP30, VP24, and L. The complex is embedded in the virion matrix composed of VP40 polymers surrounded by a cellular membrane–derived envelope containing $GP_{1,2}$ peplomers, sGP–GP_2, and, among other components, phosphatidylserine. (Cartoon inspired by Hoenen T, Brandt J, Caì Y, et al. Reverse genetics of filoviruses. *Curr Top Microbiol Immunol* 2017;411:421–445, Ref.[329]) **B:** Reconstruction of the EBOV RNP (*left, top*, viewed along the helical axis; *bottom*, side view) and MARV (*middle, top*, viewed along the helical axis; *bottom*, side view) from cryoelectron tomography and subtomogram averaging.[69] Right: Artist rendering of RNP in combination with matrix and envelope using the same color scheme as in **(A)**. (Figure courtesy of Jiro Wada, IRF-Frederick, Fort Detrick, MD, USA.)

Transcriptional Activator (VP30)

Ebolavirus VP30 is a Cys_3–His zinc finger that acts as a transcriptional activator and regulator of ebolavirus RNA synthesis. VP30 facilitates L to read through an RNA hairpin in the 5′-untranslated region (UTR).[369,797,836] In addition, ebolavirus VP30 is speculated to promote L transcription reinitiation during the sequential transcription of all ebolavirus genes[482] and to regulate cotranscriptional *GP* gene editing.[507] VP30's activity is regulated via phosphorylation (resulting in transcriptional repression) and dephosphorylation (transcriptional activation) by cellular kinases and phosphatases[72,419,525,526,730] and by Zn^{2+}.[369,524] VP30 oligomerization is required for activation of ebolavirus transcription but not for NP binding.[307,308] In addition, ebolavirus VP30 antagonizes the cellular RNA interference (RNAi) pathway.[214] The VP30 CTD binds a PPXPXY motif located in the NP CTD (Fig. 11.8B). The cellular ubiquitin ligase RB binding protein 6 (RBBP6) mimics ebolavirus NP and binds to ebolavirus VP30 using a similar motif, thereby down-regulating ebolavirus transcription and replication.[51]

The role of marburgvirus (and likely dianlovirus) VP30 is not as clear as that of ebolavirus VP30. Although marburgvirus VP30 is structurally very similar to ebolavirus VP30, Marburgvirus VP30 enhances transcription only minimally but is essential for the marburgvirus life cycle. Akin to ebolavirus VP30, marburgvirus VP30 phosphorylation regulates its activity.[10,207,399,531,730,803]

RNP Complex–Associated Protein (VP24)

VP24, which adopts single-domain α/β-structure with the overall shape resembling a pyramid[855,856] (Fig. 11.8C), is a RNP assembly factor. VP24 acts through a direct interaction with NP, thereby condensing RNP complexes. This interaction inhibits transcription and replication and facilitates RNP transport to budding sites and packaging into virions.[38,330,561,719,790,791] In addition, cuevavirus and ebolavirus VP24s counter the innate host cell antiviral response by binding to nuclear transporter karyopherins (KPNA1, 5, and 6) that transport STAT proteins to the nucleus to activate interferon-stimulated gene expression.[193,374,495,578,626,627,671,834]

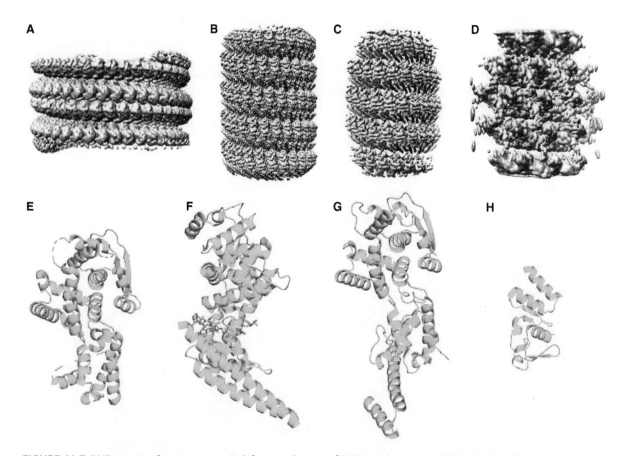

FIGURE 11.7 RNP structural components. Multifunctional states of EBOV nucleoprotein (NP). **A–D:** Cryoelectron micros-copy reconstruction of EBOV nucleocapsid-like and nucleocapsid cores containing **(A)** NP residues 25-457 (Protein Data Bank [PDB] 6C54),[706] **(B)** NP residues 1-450 (PDB 5Z9W),[709] **(C)** NP residues 1-450 (PDB 6EHL[780]), and **(D)** full-length NP (residues 1-739) from virions (PDB 6EHM).[780] **E–H:** X-ray crystal structures of EBOV NP. **(E)** N-terminal domain alone (*green*; PDB 4Z9P), **(F)** N-terminal domain (*green*) in complex with ssRNA (*gray*; PDB 5Z9W), **(G)** N-terminal domain (*green*) in complex with EBOV VP35 NP-binding peptide (NPBP; *blue*; PDB 4YPI), and **(H)** C-terminal domain (*green*; PDB 4QAZ).

Large Protein (L)

Filovirus L is the catalytic part of the filovirus polymerase holoenzymes (VP35+L).[79,532,534,723,768] Filovirus Ls contain six highly conserved regions (CRs) mediating nucleotide triphos-phate binding (CRI), RNA template recognition (CRII), RNA polymerization (CRIII), polyadenylation (CRIII), mRNA capping/polyribonucleotidyl transfer (CRIV and CRV), and methylation (CRVI). These regions are organized in four dis-tinct domains: (a) RdRp and polyribonucleotidyltransferase (PRNTase), (b) a connector domain, (c) methyltransferase (MTase), and (d) a CTD. Structurally, all mononegavirus RdRps resemble right hands with clearly discernible finger, palm, and thumb structural domains. Since efforts to obtain structural information on filovirus L have not been successful thus far, structural considerations currently rely on computa-tional modeling[227,360,457,458,479,532,658,745] (Fig. 11.8D). Analogous to other mononegaviruses, filoviral genomes and antigenomes likely possess a single L entry site (promoter) at the 3′ ends of the encapsidated genomes and antigenomes, respectively. After binding to the promoter region, L either replicates the genome or antigenomes over their entire lengths (replication) or scans the genome (but not the antigenome) for gene start and gene end signals to transcribe the individual genes (transcription). Transcription includes viral mRNA G capping, N^7 methylation

of the G cap and 2′-*O*-methylation (capI structure), cap-inde-pendent methylation, and polyadenylation. Cuevavirus and ebolavirus polymerases additionally mediate cotranscriptional mRNA editing.[479,652,765] Adaptation of MARV to domesticated guinea pigs results in mutations in the L sequence, thereby up-regulating L's activity.[404]

Matrix Protein (VP40)

Mammalian filovirus VP40 is a multifunctional protein that can assume multiple structural states.[81,618,789] The basis for these structural states is the VP40 protomer, which con-sists of a distinct NTD and a distinct CTD[168] (Fig. 11.9A). Within the protomer, the position of NTD and CTD rela-tive to each other[81,168,286,672] drives at least three types of VP40 polymerization. One type is a symmetric NTD–NTD VP40 dimer in which the CTDs are tightly bound to the NTDs, resulting in a structure resembling a butterfly[81,168,732] (Fig. 11.9B). Butterfly dimers traffic through the cell and ulti-mately localize at cell membranes. Through VP40's ability to directly bind to NP and VP35, VP40 recruits RNPs to cell membranes.[3,68,69,78,81,198,328,333,370,546,559,561,581,734] The second type of VP40 polymerization originates in CTD interaction with membrane phosphatidylserine, resulting in VP40 hexamer-ization with hexamers consisting of three linearly arranged

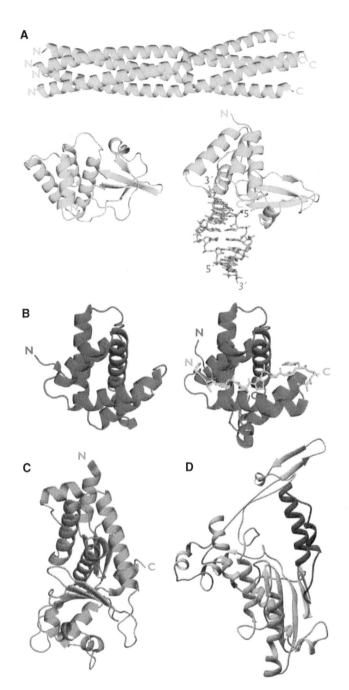

FIGURE 11.8 RNP structural components. A: EBOV polymerase cofactor (VP35) contains an N-terminal oligomerization domain (*blue, top*; PDB 6GBO) and a C-terminal interferon inhibitory domain (IID; PDB 3FKE; *blue, bottom left*), which binds to dsRNA (*gray, bottom right*; PDB 4GHL).[860] **B:** EBOV transcriptional activator (VP30) has a C-terminal domain (*purple, left*; PDB 2I8B) that binds to NP's PPXPXY motif (*right*; PDB 5VAO).[836] **C:** EBOV RNP complex–associated protein (VP24) adopts a pyramid-like structure (*orange*) that is important for binding to a subset of importin molecules that transport STAT1 into the nucleus (PDB 4U2X).[856] **D:** Prediction structural model of EBOV large protein (L). Monomers resemble right hands with fingers (*chartreuse*), palms (*green*), and thumbs (*rust*) structural domains. (**D** from Jácome R, Becerra A, Ponce de León S, et al. Structural analysis of monomeric RNA-dependent polymerases: evolutionary and therapeutic implications. PLoS One 2015;10(9):e0139001.)

VP40 dimers that are structurally distinct from butterfly dimers[3–5,81,672,699] (Fig. 11.9C). CTD–CTD interactions at ends of hexamers then polymerize the hexamers, resulting in virion matrix filaments that cylindrically engulf RNPs[3,5,81,584] (Fig. 11.9D) and facilitate budding.[4,5,168,312,363,581,641,672,700] Finally, VP40 can form octameric rings via NTD–NTD interactions used for hexamerization and additional, distinct NTD–NTD interfaces not available in either butterfly or hexamer dimers[81,286,641,732] (Fig. 11.9E). The VP40 octamer is a nonstructural protein that does not localize to cell membranes but instead binds RNA in its lumen, thereby likely negatively regulating filovirus transcription.[81,286,328,330,333,581,734]

The N-terminus of VP40 contains late-budding motifs that are important for budding. Filoviruses differ in type and number of these motifs. For instance, ebolavirus VP40s have overlapping P(T/S)AP and PPXY motifs, whereas marburgvirus VP40s only contain PPXY motifs.[313,459,704] Finally, marburgvirus and likely dianlovirus, but not ebolavirus VP40 counter the cellular innate antiviral response.[568,757,758]

Filovirus *GP* Gene Expression Products

The cuevavirus and ebolavirus *GP* genes contain three ORFs located in the three possible reading frames (Fig. 11.10). The 0 frame is preceded by a Kozak sequence and contains a stretch of seven consecutive uridine residues (7U editing site) within a predicted hairpin loop. Transcription of this ORF by the filovirus polymerase (L+VP35) and subsequent translation yield a nonstructural protein precursor (pre-sGP). The two other ORFs begin in the −1 and +1 reading frames at the 7U editing site, respectively. Cotranscriptional polymerase stuttering (editing) at the 7U site results in mRNA transcripts that contain more or less than the expected seven cognate adenosine residues, thereby transcribing the −1 and +1 ORFs.[550,652,674,765,771]

Expression of these mRNAs, therefore, yields two distinct proteins, the major glycoprotein ($GP_{1,2}$) precursor (preGP; −1 frame editing) and the secondary secreted glycoprotein precursor (pre-ssGP; +1 frame editing). The N-termini of the three *GP* gene-encoded proteins are identical (i.e., the amino acid residues encoded in the 0 reading frame up to the editing site; EBOV: 295 N-terminal amino acid residues), but the proteins differ in their C-termini.[652,765] Because multiple adenosine residues can be inserted or skipped during cotranscriptional editing, all three proteins are expressed in various isoforms. For instance, insertion of three adenosine residues into the nascent mRNA still yields pre-sGP because the 0 frame is maintained, but this sGP now contains one additional amino acid residue compared to unedited mRNA.[14,674] Cotranscriptional editing is regulated by *cis*-acting sequences located nine nucleotides upstream and downstream of the editing site in synergy with VP30 as a *trans*-acting factor.[507] The expression ratio of pre-sGP:preGP:pre-ssGP is roughly 61% to 72%:19% to 28%:1% to 5% depending on cell type and virus in the 7U context.[11,506,674]

Cell culture passaging or animal inoculation of ebolaviruses can result in uridine additions or deletions in the *GP* editing site within the genome, thereby shifting the pre-sGP:preGP:pre-ssGP expression ratio at the genomic level.[766] For instance, passaging of 7U EBOV or 7U SUDV in Vero E6 cells results in the selection of 8U viruses. However, injection of a domesticated guinea pig–adapted 8U EBOV into domesticated guinea pigs or crab-eating macaques results in evolution of predominantly 7U EBOV. Likewise, injection of 9U

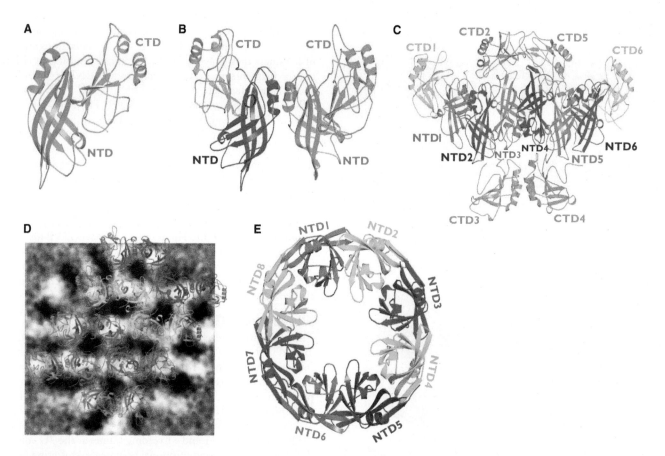

FIGURE 11.9 Structure of EBOV matrix protein (VP40). A: VP40 protomer showing the characteristic N-terminal domain (NTD, *blue*) and C-terminal domain (CTD, *orange*). **B:** Butterfly dimer consisting of two VP40 monomers that interact via their NTDs with sprung CTDs. **C:** Hexamer. **D:** Octamer. **E:** Model of the cylindrical VP40 matrix showing four VP40 hexamers side by side superimposed on 2D averages of virion tomograms. (From Pavadai E, Gerstman BS, Chapagain PP. Pavadai E, Gerstman BS, Chapagain PP. A cylindrical assembly model and dynamics of the Ebola virus VP40 structural matrix. *Sci Rep* 2018;8(1):9776. Figure arrangement courtesy of Jiro Wada, IRF-Frederick, Fort Detrick, MD, USA.)

SUDV into crab-eating macaques results in partial reversion to 7U SUDV. On the other hand, injected 7U SUDV does not convert to 8U SUDV.[14,425,770] The significance of these selections remains to be clarified. Differences in disease progression were not observed in domesticated guinea pigs or crab-eating macaques injected with either 7U or 8U EBOV[743,766] or in crab-eating macaques injected with either 7U or 8U SUDV at high inoculation doses.[14] However, at extremely low inoculation doses (0.01 plaque-forming units [PFU]), both 8U EBOV and 8U SUDV can be less lethal to crab-eating macaques than 7U control viruses.[15]

Dianlovirus and marburgvirus GP genes contain single ORFs without editing sites. The only deduced or known expression product from these genes is preGP.[807,841]

Secreted Glycoprotein

Cuevavirus and ebolavirus pre-sGP is synthetized into the endoplasmic reticulum (ER). Proteolytic cleavage of pre-sGP by furin-like endoproteases at a conserved C-terminal R-X-R-R↓ motif and further maturation in the ER yield mature sGP and Δ-peptide. sGP is a nonstructural protein that is C-mannosylated at a conserved W̲-X-X-W motif, *N*-glycosylated, and is secreted through the Golgi apparatus in high amounts by infected cells as a disulfide-linked parallel homodimer.[43,44,216,579,772,773] In EBOD patients, this secretion leads to high sGP concentrations

in the blood. Because sGP, $GP_{1,2}$, and ssGP have identical N-terminal amino acid sequences (including one of the two cysteine residues responsible for sGP homodimerization), each sGP monomer contains the residues that correspond to the GP_1 head, glycan cap, and base (see below). Therefore, this monomer is partially cross-reactive with several anti-GP_1 antibodies.[336,520,538,579,741,857] The observed serologic cross-reactivity with anti-$GP_{1,2}$ antibodies suggests an antibody decoy function for circulating sGP in infected animals.[354,527] However, the function of sGP is still unknown. *In vitro*, sGP restores the endothelial barrier destroyed by exposure to Ebola virion–like particles and tumor necrosis factor (TNF), suggesting an anti-inflammatory role of sGP.[774] However, recombinant domesticated guinea pig–adapted EBOV engineered not to produce sGP is not attenuated in infected domesticated guinea pigs compared to wild-type EBOV,[331] and marburgviruses are as virulent as ebolaviruses without producing sGP.

Δ-peptide

Δ-peptide, the C-terminal cleavage product of cuevavirus and ebolavirus pre-sGP, is an *O*-glycosylated and sialylated peptide of ≈40 amino acid residues that is secreted from infected cells.[773] Exogenous BDBV, EBOV, SUDV, and TAFV (but not LLOV or RESTV) Δ-peptides inhibit EBOV and MARV replication in cell culture, suggesting that these peptides may

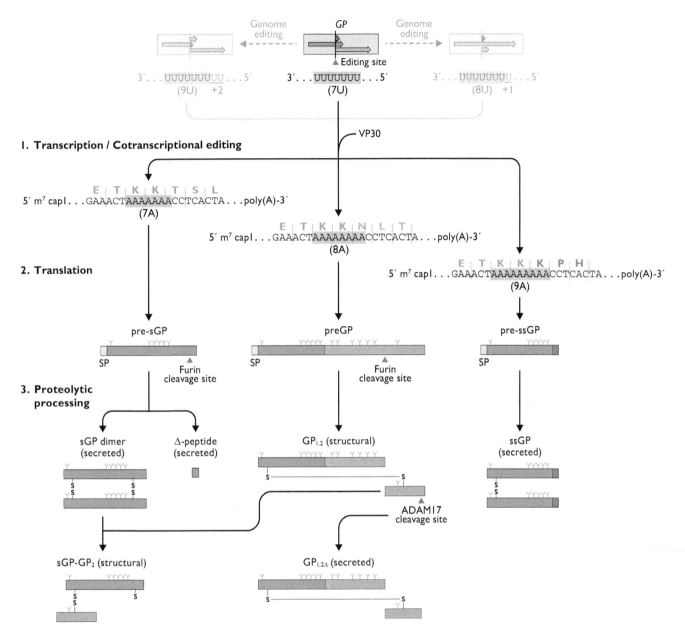

FIGURE 11.10 EBOV *GP* gene expression. The *GP* of most wild-type ("7U") EBOV isolates contains a single open reading frame (ORF) preceded by a proper Kozak sequence (*blue arrow*, emphasized middle *GP* gene, top) and a 7U editing site (*vertical black bar*). Transcription of this ORF, regulated by VP30, results in a capped and polyadenylated 7A mRNA, which is translated into pre-sGP (*left pathway*). Pre-sGP's signal peptide (SP) is removed by a signalase, and the protein is further proteolytically processed by furin into secreted sGP and Δ-peptide. At top middle of figure: cotranscriptional mRNA editing by the EBOV polymerase holoenzyme (L+VP35) under VP30 regulation leads to frameshifts, thereby accessing novel ORFs (*orange and red arrows*, emphasized middle *GP* gene, top). Addition of a single nontemplated A results in mRNAs that are translated into preGP, which is further processed by a signalase (SP removal) and furin to the EBOV GP$_{1,2}$ peplomer, which can be shed from membranes after ADAM metallopeptidase domain 17 (ADAM17, formerly TACE) cleavage (*middle pathway*). Disulfide bond switching between the sGP homodimer and the GP$_{1,2}$ heterodimer can connect sGP monomers to GP$_2$ monomers to form virion-structural sGP–GP$_2$ heterodimers. Addition of two nontemplated As results in mRNAs that are translated into pre-ssGP, which is further processed by a signalase and matures to secreted ssGP (*right pathway*). Genome editing can result in alternative *GP* editing sites (top, deemphasized *left and right* GP genes). Cotranscriptional mRNA editing results in the same expression products but with altered expression frequencies. (Figure courtesy of Jiro Wada, IRF-Frederick, Fort Detrick, MD, USA.)

control filovirus superinfection of host cells.[617] Recent studies indicate that Δ-peptide is a chloride-selective viroporin that forms pentameric pores in host cell plasma membranes.[317,601] The actual function of the peptide during *in vivo* infection remains to be determined.

Glycoprotein (GP$_{1,2}$)

Mammalian filovirus preGP contains a signal peptide at the N-terminus that targets the protein into the ER and a C-terminal type I transmembrane domain that tethers the protein to the ER membrane. In the ER, the protein acquires oligomannosidic *N*-glycans. After translocation to the Golgi, hybrid and complex *N*-glycan modifications are finalized, and the protein becomes *O*-glycosylated. Ebolavirus preGPs are typically also highly sialylated, whereas sialylation is weaker or absent in marburgvirus preGPs, dependent on cell type. The overall glycan content constitutes at least one-third of the molecular mass of the preGP. The majority of glycosylations occurs in a highly variable, so-called mucin-like subdomain at the center of preGP.[59,139,223,225,278,629,767,769] Glycosylated preGP dimerizes via a disulfide bond and is then cleaved in the *trans*-Golgi apparatus by furin-like endoproteases at a conserved R-X-R-R↓ motif into GP_1 and GP_2 subunits. The role of this highly conserved cleavage event is unclear, as recombinant EBOV engineered to forgo preGP cleavage is fully functional and equally virulent in rhesus monkeys (Primates: Cercopithecidae:

Macaca mulatta Zimmermann, 1780) as wild-type control virus.[553] These subunits remain attached to each other through a disulfide bond ($GP_{1,2}$ heterodimer). Prior to transport to the cell membrane, which is independent from any other filovirus proteins, these heterodimers trimerize to form the mature $GP_{1,2}$ peplomer that is incorporated into virions.[546,653,767,769,820]

GP_1 is the virion surface-exposed $GP_{1,2}$ moiety that mediates cell-surface attachment via a distinct filovirus receptor-binding site.[34,171,365,431,445,476,477] GP_1 is structured into base, head, glycan cap, and mucin-like subdomains (Fig. 11.11A). The receptor-binding site is situated in the head of each GP_1 monomer in the trimer, but the sites are masked by the glycan caps consisting of *N*-glycans. The mucin-like subdomains are located upward and outward from these caps and shield $GP_{1,2}$ from host antibodies.[63,314,742] Marburgvirus GP_1 is

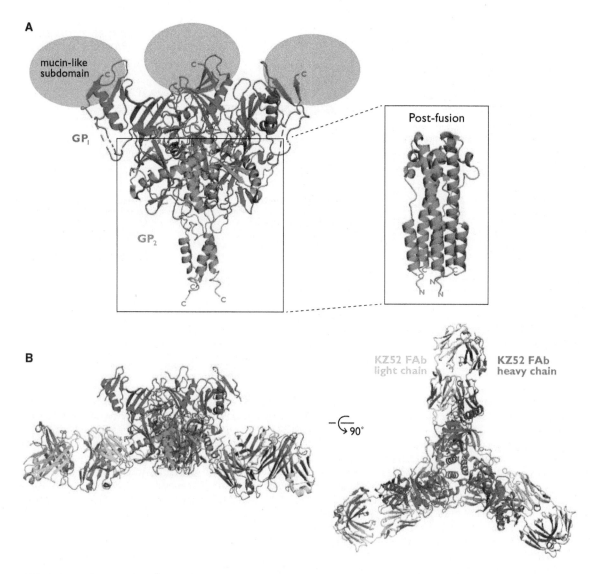

FIGURE 11.11 Glycoprotein ($GP_{1,2}$) structure. A: Side view of the mature prefusion EBOV $GP_{1,2}$ peplomer consisting of three GP_1 (*red*)-GP_2 (*pink*) heterodimers ("chalice"-like structure with the three GP_2s pointing toward the envelope and the three mucin-like subdomains decorating the bowl; PDB 5JQ3). Low pH and cathepsin cleavage lead to glycan cap and mucin-like subdomain removal, insertion of the fusion peptide into the cellular target membrane, membrane–envelope fusion, and a characteristic "six-helix bundle" $GP_{1,2}$ postfusion structure (*inset box*; PDB 2EBO). **B:** Prefusion EBOV $GP_{1,2}$ in complex with EBOV-neutralizing mAb KZ52's antigen-binding fragment (Fab light chain, *light brown*; heavy chain, *dark brown*), which binds at the GP_1–GP_2 interface (PDB 1CSY).

phosphorylated, but the role of this posttranslational modification is unclear.[654]

GP$_2$ is a typical class I fusion protein containing helical heptad-repeat regions that flank a CX$_6$CC motif, a conserved fusion loop defined by a disulfide bridge between two cysteine residues and the transmembrane domain that tethers GP$_{1,2}$ to the virion membrane.[103,250,251,445] Similar to retrovirus transmembrane proteins, filovirus GP$_2$ also contains a short immunosuppressive motif.[103,838] In addition, GP$_2$s are acylated at their cytoplasmic domains.[247] GP$_2$ drives fusion of the viral envelope with host cell membranes through GP$_{1,2}$ conformational changes induced by GP$_1$ receptor binding.

Virion GP$_{1,2}$ trimers assume the shape of a chalice, with the three GP$_1$ subunits angling outward but bound together at their bases where they connect to the stalk-like GP$_2$ trimer (Fig. 11.11A). The GP$_2$ fusion loops wrap around the outside of the GP$_2$ trimer into the neighboring GP$_1$s.[34,171,445]

Filovirion antigenicity is primarily determined by GP$_{1,2}$. Cuevavirions, ebolavirions, and marburgvirions are antigenically distinct, and individual species members can be differentiated with certain anti-GP$_{1,2}$ antibodies. Monoclonal antibodies that neutralize filovirus infection *in vitro* do not necessarily protect experimentally infected animals *in vivo*. Vice versa, nonneutralizing antibodies have been described that play important parts in disease protection.[91,171,234,235,246,314,398,445,490,493,516,655,656,794,804] Filovirus-neutralizing monoclonal antibodies, such as EBOV-specific KZ52, EBOV-specific 2G4, EBOV-specific 4G7, and EBOV-specific mAb114 and SUDV-specific 16F6, often bind to a GP$_1$–GP$_2$ epitope at the base of the GP$_{1,2}$ trimer, thereby mechanically preventing the GP$_{1,2}$ conformational changes required for fusion[171,445,520,538,579,741] (Fig. 11.11B). Other antibodies target the fusion loop or the GP$_2$ stalk[82,236,248,389] or the mucin-like subdomain.[446,809]

Shed Glycoprotein (GP$_{1,2\Delta}$)

Luminal proteolytic cleavage of EBOV and MARV GP$_{1,2}$ near the GP$_2$'s transmembrane anchor by ADAM metallopeptidase domain 17 (ADAM17, formerly TACE) produces a soluble, trimeric GP$_{1,2}$ variant (GP$_{1,2\Delta}$).[181] ADAM17 expression is up-regulated at days 4 to 6 postexposure in EBOV-infected crab-eating macaques, and GP$_{1,2\Delta}$ can be detected at high concentrations at that time.[639] *In vitro*, GP$_{1,2\Delta}$ activates noninfected dendritic cells and macrophages to secrete pro- and anti-inflammatory cytokines (TNF, CXCL8, interleukin [IL] 1B, IL1R1, IL6, IL10, IL12B) that increase endothelial cell permeability.[210] Because the structure of GP$_{1,2\Delta}$ is highly similar to that of GP$_{1,2}$, GP$_{1,2\Delta}$ could also serve as an antibody decoy in the circulation.

sGP–GP$_2$

Under yet-to-be-defined conditions, sGP monomers can connect to GP$_2$ monomers via a disulfide bridge between cysteine residues most often used for sGP dimerization and the GP$_1$–GP$_2$ connection. The resulting sGP–GP$_2$ heterodimer is anchored to the ER and, later, to the plasma membrane via the GP$_2$ transmembrane domain and may become incorporated into the envelope of budding virions. Due to the significant sequence similarity between sGP and GP$_1$, sGP–GP$_2$ could function as an anti-GP$_{1,2}$ antibody decoy directly on the virion, thereby protecting GP$_{1,2}$ peplomers from host recognition.[160,355]

Secondary Secreted Glycoprotein

Pre-ssGP is produced at low frequency by cuevaviruses and ebolaviruses via cotranscriptional editing from the *GP* gene.[11,506,674] During maturation in the ER, pre-ssGP becomes *N*-glycosylated and is subsequently secreted from infected cells as a disulfide-linked homodimer (mature sGP). The function of the protein is unclear, but similarly to sGP and sGP–GP$_2$, ssGP could be an antibody decoy.[506,772]

STAGES OF REPLICATION

The filovirus life cycle can be divided into virion attachment/entry, replication/transcription/translation, and assembly/budding (Fig. 11.12).

Filovirion Cell-Surface Attachment and Host Cell Entry

Mammalian filoviruses infect a wide variety of vertebrate cell types from a broad range of species.[425,644,848] The cell types and host tropisms of all mammalian filoviruses are almost identical *in vitro*. However, some filovirus genus- or species-specific tropism differences have been uncovered.[220,555] Filovirus *in vitro* species and cell-type specificity are not necessarily predictive of *in vivo* tropism, as, thus far, only mammals of a few species have been infected successfully with mammalian filoviruses (Table 11.4).

Filovirion attachment to host cells is mediated, likely at neutral pH, by the GP$_{1,2}$ peplomer[476,477,717,819] or by filovirion outer leaflet envelope components such as phosphatidylserine. The glycans on GP$_{1,2}$ bind directly to a broad range of C-type lectins (CLECs), such as asialoglycoprotein receptor 1 (ASGR1), CD209 (formerly DC-SIGN), C-type lectin domain family 4 member M (CLEC4M, formerly DC-SIGNR), C-type lectin domain containing 10A (CLEC10A, formerly MGL), C-type lectin domain family 4 member G (CLEC4G, formerly LSECTin), and mannose-binding lectin 2 (MBL2).[18,61,288,367,490,492,685,716,754] Filovirion attachment can also be mediated by hepatitis A virus cellular receptor 1 (HAVCR1, formerly TIM-1) and T-cell immunoglobulin and mucin domain containing 4 (TIMD4, formerly TIM-4), which bind phosphatidylserine at the outer leaflet of the filovirion envelope.[186,409,434,628,849] In addition, other cell-surface factors, such TAM family receptor tyrosine kinases (i.e., AXL, MERTK, TYRO3), facilitate filovirion attachment in an unknown manner.[99,680]

Importantly, filovirion attachment factors are not bona fide virion receptors, because individual factors are not necessary or sufficient for filovirion entry. Instead, they appear to function in a complementary manner to adsorb virions at the target cell surface—if a particular factor is absent, another will take over this function.[496,853] For instance, deletion of the GP$_{1,2}$ mucin-like subdomain, and thereby deletion of most GP$_{1,2}$ glycans, does not diminish but rather increases EBOV GP$_{1,2}$–mediated particle entry *in vitro*,[365] indicating that factors such as HAVCR1 could substitute for lectins. Likewise, absence of HAVCR1 (for instance, on primary filovirus targets such as macrophages) does not abrogate filovirion entry—possibly TIMD4 or other, yet-to-be-identified, attachment factors could take over. In addition, within-species HAVCR1 polymorphism influences host cell susceptibility to filovirus infection,[435] suggesting that the temporal progression of filovirus infection from

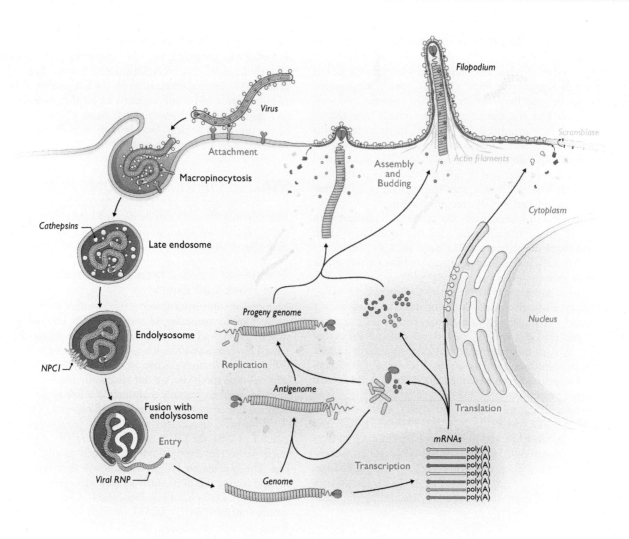

Filopodium

Virus

Attachment

Macropinocytosis

Cathepsins

Late endosome

Endolysosome

NPC1

Fusion with
endolysosome

Entry

Viral RNP

Progeny genome

Replication

Antigenome

Genome

Transcription

Translation

mRNAs

poly(A)
poly(A)
poly(A)
poly(A)
poly(A)
poly(A)
poly(A)

Assembly
and
Budding

Actin filaments

Scramblase

Cytoplasm

Nucleus

FIGURE 11.12 Mammalian filovirus life cycle. Filovirion GP$_{1,2}$ peplomers and/or phosphatidylserine in the filovirion envelope mediates binding to host cell-surface attachment factor (*orange*), resulting in virion endocytosis (predominantly macropinocytosis). Low pH and cathepsin-mediated cleavage of GP$_{1,2}$ in the late endosome lead to engagement of the filovirus receptor, NPC intracellular cholesterol transporter 1 (NPC1; *light blue*) and, thereby, fusion of the virion envelope with the endolysosomal membrane. The virion ribonucleoprotein (RNP) core is released into the cytosol, where filovirus gene transcription and genome replication take place. Replication occurs by synthesis of encapsidated antigenomes that serve as templates for progeny genome synthesis. Following translation, mature progeny RNPs are transported to the GP$_{1,2}$-containing plasma membrane of filopodia for matrix embedding and envelopment. Budding occurs at the plasma membrane via a VP40-mediated process. (Figure courtesy of Jiro Wada, IRF-Frederick, Fort Detrick, MD, USA.)

initial to late target cells may be influenced by multiple factors at the cell-attachment step.

Subsequent to attachment, filoviruses enter host cells by endocytosis, generally, but likely not exclusively, by macropinocytosis.[13,70,345,536,543,646,648] In the low pH environment of the endolysosome, the GP$_1$ subunit is cleaved by cathepsins B and L,[123,284,287,483,490,519,656,663] thereby releasing the mucin-like subdomains and glycan caps to expose the receptor-binding site.[82,187,334,383,782] β1 integrins are thought to regulate these cathepsins, explaining why β1 integrin–deficient cells are refractory to filovirus infection.[664,718] Once exposed, the GP$_1$ receptor-binding site engages the second luminal domain C of the universal mammalian filovirus receptor, the lysosomal NPC intracellular cholesterol transporter 1 (NPC1),[112,144,285,324,417,555,782,841] which also interacts directly with HAVCR1.[434] The GP$_1$–NPC1 interaction results in extensive conformational changes in the metastable prefusion GP$_{1,2}$ molecule. These changes involve unwinding GP$_2$ from GP$_1$ (and possibly release of GP$_1$) and unwinding of GP$_2$'s fusion loop containing a fusion peptide from the GP$_2$ trimer and penetrating the fusion loop into the endolysosomal membrane. While assuming a so-called six-helix bundle structure (Fig. 11.11A), GP$_2$ pulls the endolysosomal membrane into proximity of the filovirion envelope, thereby triggering membrane–membrane fusion and release of the filovirion RNP into the cytosol of the host cell.[405,445,473,799,800] These last steps are controlled by host two pore segment channels 1 and 2 (TPCN1 and TPCN2), but their exact mechanism of action remains to be determined.[647]

TABLE 11.4   Overview of animal models of mammalian filovirus infections

Experimental Animal (Species)	Exposure Filovirus	Outcomes
Artiodactyla		
Domestic pigs/wild boars (*Sus scrofa domesticus* Erxleben, 1777)	EBOV, RESTV	Viremia in the absence of overt clinical signs[403,478,554,798]
Carnivora		
Domestic ferrets (*Mustela putorius furo* Linnaeus, 1758)	BDBV, EBOV, RESTV, SUDV	Uniformly lethal disease[149,398,404,819]; partially lethal transmission model[159]
	MARV, RAVV	Absence of viremia and clinical signs[150,818]
Chiroptera		
Egyptian rousettes (*Rousettus aegyptiacus* E. Geoffroy, 1810)	BDBV, EBOV, RESTV, SUDV, TAFV	Absence of viremia and clinical signs[377,587]
	MARV, RAVV	Viremia in the absence of overt clinical signs[22,376,377,586]
Lagomorpha		
European rabbits (*Oryctolagus cuniculus* Linnaeus, 1758)	Domesticated guinea pig–adapted EBOV	Variably lethal disease[643]
Primates		
Common marmosets (*Callithrix jacchus* Linnaeus, 1758)	EBOV, MARV	Uniformly lethal disease[113,697,698]
Common squirrel monkeys (*Saimiri sciureus* Linnaeus, 1758)	MARV	Uniformly lethal disease[687,688]
Crab-eating macaques (*Macaca fascicularis* Raffles, 1821)	EBOV, MARV, RAVV	Uniformly lethal disease[16,19,153,245,266,272,273,321]
	BDBV, RESTV, SUDV, TAFV	Variably lethal disease[215,230,263,322,361,517,864]
Grivets (*Chlorocebus aethiops* Linnaeus, 1758)	EBOV, RESTV, SUDV, MARV	Variably lethal disease[47,155,230,298,623,642,687,688,864,866]
Hamadryas baboons (*Papio hamadryas* Linnaeus, 1758)	EBOV, MARV	Uniformly lethal disease[642,644,868]
Rhesus monkeys (*Macaca mulatta* Zimmermann, 1780)	EBOV, SUDV, MARV, RAVV	Uniformly lethal disease[47,154,200,232,259,356,358,371,439,623,687,688,864]
Rodentia		
Domesticated guinea pigs (*Cavia porcellus* Linnaeus, 1758)	Domesticated guinea pig–adapted EBOV, SUDV, MARV, and RAVV	Uniformly lethal disease[57,140,149,265,410,462,645,707,714,748,816]; partially lethal transmission model[817]
	RESTV	Viremia in absence of overt clinical signs[162]
Golden hamsters (*Mesocricetus auratus* Waterhouse, 1839)	Laboratory mouse–adapted EBOV, domesticated guinea pig- and golden hamster-adapted MARV	Uniformly lethal disease[191,686,775,862]
	RESTV	Viremia in the absence of overt clinical signs[162]
Laboratory mice (immunocompetent)	Laboratory mouse–adapted EBOV, MARV, RAVV	Uniformly lethal disease[96,98,296,611,620,785,795,863]
	RESTV	Viremia in the absence of overt clinical signs[162]
Laboratory mice (immunodeficient)	BDBV	Nonlethal disease[92]
	EBOV, RESTV, SUDV	Partially to uniformly lethal disease[92,98,162,455,621,863]
	TAFV	Viremia in the absence of overt clinical signs[92,621]
	MARV, RAVV	Uniformly lethal disease[95,455,621,783]

Filovirus Genome Replication and Transcription

Filovirus replication occurs exclusively in the cytosol and begins with mRNA transcription from incoming genomic RNPs. The filovirus replication promoter is bipartite, consisting of a first promoter element (PEI) located in the 3′ genomic leader region and a second promoter element (PEII) located in the UTR of the *NP* gene, downstream of the *NP* gene start signal (Fig. 11.13A). The antigenomic promoter, likely also bipartite, is located at the 3′ end of the antigenome. Ebolavirus and marburgvirus promoters are similarly organized but differ in length and secondary structure.[206,796] Importantly, in contrast to most other mononegavirus genomes that have complementary 3′ and 5′ terminal nucleotides, filovirus genome termini are heterogenous, and the terminal nucleotides are not completely complementary.[164] The 3′ ends of ebolavirus genomes and antigenomes have a single nucleotide overhang compared to the complementary sequence at the 5′ ends. Ebolavirus genome replication begins with the polymerase initiating RNA opposite of a highly conserved 3′-CCUGU motif with the first C residue located at position 2 of the genome. In contrast, MARV genomes lack a 3′ overhang, and the conserved motif

has the sequence 3′-UCUGU. The polymerase commences the synthesis of full-length antigenomes that are encapsidated by NP as the antigenome chain elongates. Using the antigenomic promoter, these antigenomic RNPs then serve as templates for the synthesis of progeny genomic RNPs.[164,531,534] Synthesized genomic and antigenomic RNPs accumulate in cytoplasmic perinuclear inclusion bodies, which are readily visible in filovirus-infected cells.[180,332,339,546]

The mechanism regulating the switch from transcription to replication is still unclear, but analagous to other mononegaviruses, the concentration of NP might play a role. Ebolavirus VP30 serves as a transcriptional activator and replication inhibitor in a phosphorylation-dependent manner. The transcription-activating function of VP30 depends on an RNA hairpin structure that is formed at the gene start signal of the first gene, the *NP* gene.[72,419,525,526,730] Marburgvirus VP30 functions like ebolavirus VP30 but is a much less potent transcriptional activator.[72,307,308,419,482,524–526,730] Binding of a small stem–loop structure in the genomic trailer by heat shock protein family A (Hsp70) member 8 (HSPA8) is essential for replication.[715] In addition, VP40 and VP24 are both involved in regulation of transcription and replication in ways that remain

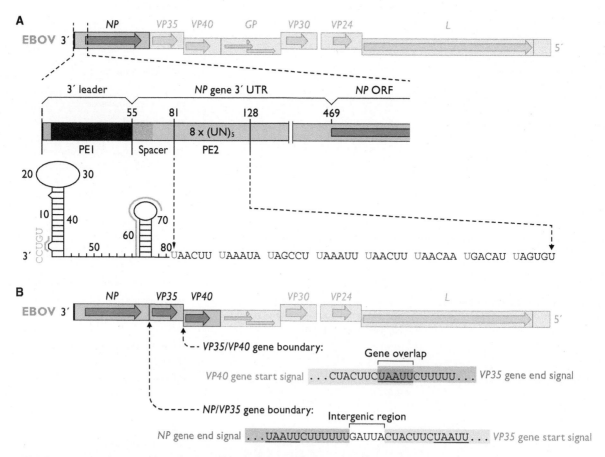

FIGURE 11.13 Mammalian filovirus genomic regulatory signals. A: Organization of the bipartite EBOV promoter, which consists of two promoter elements (PE1 and PE2) separated by a spacer containing the *NP* gene start signal (*orange*). PEII consists of an EBOV-characteristic 8x(UN)₅ sequence. The EBOV polymerase initiates RNA synthesis opposite of a highly conserved 3′-CCUGU motif (*green*) at position 2 of the genome. This motif is located within a putative hairpin structure. **B:** Examples for EBOV gene overlaps and intergenic regions. ORF, open reading frame; UTR, untranslated region. (Figure inspired by Mühlberger E. Filovirus replication and transcription. *Future Virol* 2007;2(2):205–215, Ref.[530] and courtesy of Jiro Wada, IRF-Frederick, Fort Detrick, MD, USA.)

to be defined,[330] but in the case of VP24, it most likely involves nucleocapsid condensation.[38]

The typically monocistronic, cotranscriptionally capped and polyadenylated mRNAs are synthesized by the viral polymerase from the viral genome (Fig. 11.5) with polar attenuation. mRNAs produced from the utmost 3′ gene (typically *NP*) are synthesized in high abundance, whereas mRNAs produced from the utmost 5′ gene (*L*) are synthesized in the lowest concentrations. Each filovirus gene is flanked by filovirus species/genus-conserved gene start ($\approx$12–14 nt) and gene end ($\approx$11–12 nt) signals (frequently containing the sequence pentamer 3′-UAAUU-5′; Fig. 11.13B). The gene-specific mRNA concentration gradient likely results because the polymerase complex enters the genome at the 3′ end and then moves along the template until it recognizes a gene end signal, which contains a short stretch of uridines. Here, the polymerase stutters, leading to the addition of a poly(A) tail to the nascent mRNA strand. Concomitantly, the polymerase occasionally falls off the template. Since only a single polymerase entry site is at the 3′ end of the genome, the more 5′-located genes are less likely to be transcribed by the polymerase.[79,293,531,533,534]

Filovirion Assembly and Budding

Mammalian filovirion morphogenesis is regulated by NP, VP35, VP40, and VP24, which initiate and regulate RNP transport, RNP envelopment, and virion budding. Mature genomic progeny RNPs move from their perinuclear location to the plasma membrane or, in particular cell types, to the membranes of endosomal multivesicular bodies (MVBs) in an actin-dependent manner.[69,180,406,407,546,665,719] RNP transport is mediated at least in part by late-budding motifs contained in VP40 of ebolaviruses or in NP and VP40 of marburgviruses. These motifs interact with cellular proteins that contain WW domains, such as components of the endosomal sorting complexes required for transport (ESCRT) and MVB trafficking pathways (e.g., programmed cell death 6 interacting protein [PDCD6IP; formerly Alix], itchy E3 ubiquitin protein ligase [ITCH], NEDD4 E3 ubiquitin protein ligase [NEDD4], tumor susceptibility 101 [TSG101], WW domain containing E3 ubiquitin protein ligase 1 [WWP1]),[178,179,304–306,459,489,552,733,751,752,843] and are dependent on numerous other proteins, such as vacuolar protein sorting 4 homolog A (VPS4A), RAB9A, and RAB11A.[541,545]

ESCRT-dependent filovirion budding at the plasma membrane occurs at VP40 layer–associated lipid rafts and/or filopodia, which also accumulate $GP_{1,2}$ trimers in a tubulin-dependent manner.[55,523,581,665] Consequently, budding filovirions not only contain part of the plasma membrane (including phosphatidylserine) but also the membrane-incorporated $GP_{1,2}$ as progeny peplomers.[4,165,406,700,802] Phosphatidylserine, the substrate for filovirion attachment factors such as HAVCR1, is flipped from the inner leaflet of the plasma membrane to the outer leaflet of the filovirion envelope by cellular scramblases (e.g., XK-related family [XKR], anoctamin 6 [ANO6]).[544,847]

PATHOGENESIS AND PATHOLOGY

The understanding of FVD pathogenesis has been limited by the very low number of autopsies that have been performed in affected individuals.[174,201,256,257,267,384,539,683,694,695,850,852] This low number is explained by opposition to these procedures among particular FVD-affected populations, by a lack of appropriate facilities and staff that could perform these procedures in outbreak areas, and by biosafety risk assessments (exposure to even a very low filovirion numbers can result in lethal FVD).

As a result, the current understanding of FVD pathogenesis (Fig. 11.14) is an amalgam gathered from experimental exposures of mammals belonging to different species using different filoviruses, filovirus variants, and variable exposure doses and inoculation routes (Table 11.4). In the past, animal models that achieved face validity (phenotypic similarity of the disease induced in an animal compared to that observed with human infections) were favored. Face validity was relatively easily achieved because little was known about FVD pathogenesis in humans. Consequently, any "gold-standard" animal model only needs to mimic a few salient characteristics of human FVD to be considered valid. Ethical, financial, logistical, and regulatory (e.g., Food and Drug Administration [FDA] Animal Efficacy Rule) arguments further influence the debate on which of these animal models ought to be used for a particular experiment.[411]

Rodent models of FVD have the advantage of being less expensive than primates, but clinically evident infection in immunocompetent laboratory mice requires exposure to relatively high doses of species-adapted filoviruses. However, infection of rodents with serially passaged or adapted virus in most immunocompetent rodent FVD models still fails to reproduce hallmark features of FVD including cutaneous rashes, coagulopathies, and lymphocyte death.[96,140,191,686,783,785] Nonetheless, because of the genetic homogeneity of rodent strains and small size, sufficiently powered, highly standardized experiments can be performed using rodents with reduced sampling error attributable to population variance. Similar studies would be difficult to replicate using a genetically diverse study population due to the sample sizes required. In addition, some strains of laboratory mice are very well characterized immunologically, making them advantageous for studies of the host immune response against filoviruses. The increasing ability to create novel laboratory mice (e.g., creation of knockout mice, collaborative cross mice, or humanized mice susceptible to wild-type filoviruses) expands the spectrum of possible pathogenesis studies.[98,441,620,701]

The domestic ferret (*Mustela putorius furo* Linnaeus, 1758) is a recently characterized and promising model of EBOD (but not MARD). Intramuscular or intranasal exposure of domestic ferrets to wild-type ebolaviruses results in a rapid onset of uniformly lethal clinical disease with the development of a cutaneous rash, lymphopenia, a consumptive coagulopathy, and necrotizing lesions in both the liver and spleen.[150,151,159,412,418,818,839] These are all features seen in NHP FVD models. Whereas NHPs are sometimes considered to be the best available or "gold-standard" FVD models,[271] studies using NHPs can typically be performed with only small numbers of animals at high financial cost. These restrictions make the verification of research findings or validation through reproducibility difficult. These issues are compounded by the challenges associated with working in maximum containment and ethical considerations, as NHP experimentation is controversial.

Experimental infection of NHPs is typically achieved via parenteral injection or small particle aerosol exposure (i.e., exposure routes that do not mimic the direct person-to-person transmission route in naturally acquired infection).[411] Injection or inhalation of large doses of virus leads to rapid, fulminating disease that is typically uniformly fatal 6 to 9 days later. The hallmark features of human FVD including cutaneous rashes,

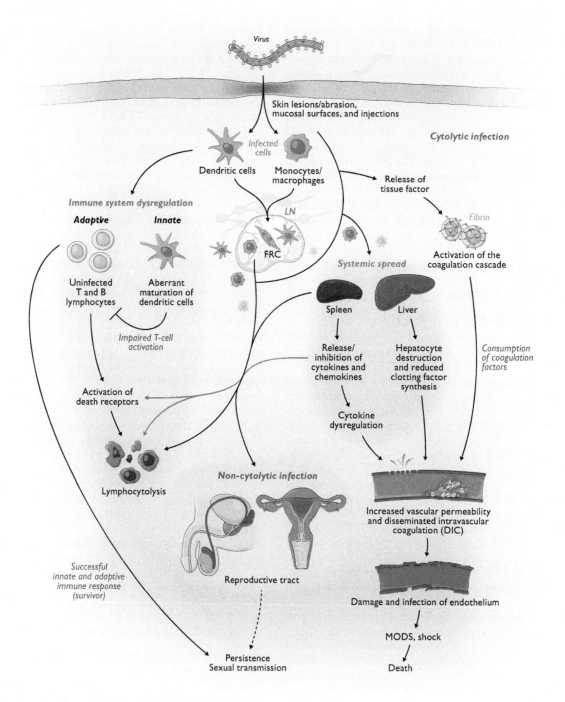

FIGURE 11.14 Overview of pathogenesis of filovirus disease (FVD). Following exposure to virions through skin lesions, contact with mucosal surfaces, or injection, filoviruses infect dermal dendritic cells and/or monocytes/macrophages and begin replicating. The infected cells transport virus via the lymphatics to regional lymph nodes (LNs). In the LN, the virus spreads to follicular dendritic cells, to monocyte/macrophage populations, and to resident fibroblastic reticular cells (FRCs) that create the three-dimensional network in LNs on which leukocytes compartmentalize and migrate. Filovirus VP35 inhibition of DDX58 inhibits dendritic cell maturation, impairing antigen presentation to T cells and B cells. Infected mononuclear phagocytic cells release a variety of cytokines CXCL8, IL1B, IL6, TNF and express coagulation factor III, increasing vascular permeability and inducing a proinflammatory and procoagulable state. A dysregulated immune response leads to largely unimpeded viral replication. From lymph nodes near the exposure site, the virus spreads systemically, infecting resident macrophages throughout the body, including those in the lungs, spleen, and liver. Lymphocytolysis occurs by unknown mechanisms thought to be associated with cytokine dysregulation and paracrine signaling from infected fibroblastic reticular cells (FRCs), resulting in severe lymphopenia. Hepatocyte infection leads to widespread hepatocellular degeneration and necrosis with a concomitant decrease in the production hepatocyte-synthesized clotting factors and albumin. A consumptive coagulopathy or disseminated intravascular coagulation results in thrombosis, shock, and multiple organ dysfunction syndrome (MODS). Alternatively, in individuals that mount a successful immune response and survive infection, rare cases of sexual transmission have been reported. (Inspired by Schmidt KM, Mühlberger E. Marburg virus reverse genetics systems. *Viruses* 2016;8(6):178, Ref.[659] and figure courtesy of Jiro Wada, IRF-Frederick, Fort Detrick, MD, USA.)

coagulopathies, and lymphocyte death[96,140,191,686,783,785] are consistently observed in NHP models following intramuscular exposure to even low doses of wild-type virus.[15,515] Whereas humans with FVD commonly develop massive gastrointestinal fluid losses,[413] gastrointestinal signs are typically absent in the NHP models. Uniform mortality, or a lack of heterogeneity in disease severity, in the high-dose NHP FVD models is appropriate for stringent studies of vaccine protection or MCMs. However, with a uniform mortality model, questions of the natural correlates of protection leading to survival, subclinical infection, viral persistence and sexual transmission, or clinical sequelae seen in convalescent human survivors (including disease relapse) cannot be answered. Although perfect animal disease models do not exist, refinement of existing models based on the most current data may result in models with construct validity in the near future (i.e., animal models in which pathogenic processes are homologous to those in humans with FVD).

The pathologic characterization of filoviruses in their natural reservoir hosts or accidental hosts other than humans has barely started and is thus far restricted to individual studies of EBOV and RESTV in subclinically infected domestic pigs,[403,478,554,798] a histopathological examination of TAFV in a western chimpanzee,[833] and the characterization of MARV and RAVV in subclinically infected Egyptian rousettes.[22,376,377,586]

Pathogenesis Following Filovirus Host Entry

Human-to-human filovirus transmission occurs through direct contact via microabrasions, cuts, or scratches in the skin or mucous membranes. Fomite-to-human transmission can occur through contact with contaminated biological or nonbiological materials, accidental needlesticks, or contact with deceased FVD victims during preparation of bodies for burial.[185,353,393,577,821,822,852]

The filovirion $GP_{1,2}$ peplomer, the host cell–specific expression of $GP_{1,2}$ attachment factors, and NPC1 are the major factors that determine filovirus *in vivo* cell and tissue tropism and the sequence in which susceptible cells and tissues become infected. At the exposure site, filoviruses target resident tissue (typically dermal or submucosal) dendritic cells and macrophages and begin replicating. These infected mononuclear cells migrate to the lymphatics and enter regional lymph nodes. Virus replication continues in dendritic cells, monocytes, and fibroblastic reticular cells within the regional lymph nodes. Then, both mature virions and infected monocytes spread the virus systemically.[155,747] Filoviruses exhibit a wide tissue tropism, infecting resident tissue macrophages throughout the body; mesenchymal connective tissue cells, including those in lymphoid organs and the reproductive tract; and epithelial cells. The liver is a major target organ of infection[48,97,143,221,266,270,588,644,852] (Fig. 11.15).

Most infected cells produce copious amounts of progeny virions, resulting in tissue and blood titers reaching 10^6 to 10^8 PFU/mL in humans and up to 10^9 PFU/mL in certain animal models.[158,273,321,420,738,852] The relationship between inoculum/exposure dose and route has been impossible to characterize in humans, but limited data from animal models suggest a very low median lethal dose in EBOV-infected laboratory mice ($LD_{50} \approx 1$ PFU).[96] In crab-eating macaques infected with EBOV or SUDV, a target dose of 0.01 PFU of EBOV or SUDV still suffices to cause fatalities.[15] Extrapolating from animal data, human-to-human filovirus transmission via microabrasions is, not surprisingly, highly efficient.

Filovirus Intrahost Distribution and Pathologic Consequences

Viremia has been detected in the NHP model as soon as 2 days following intramuscular EBOV exposure, often coinciding with the onset of fever,[189] but the temporal development of infection varies with the dose and route of exposure.[16] Whereas few studies with a limited number of animals have evaluated coagulation abnormalities, detectable derangements in hemostasis, such as increases in coagulation factor III (F3, tissue factor) expression and fibrinogen concentrations, have been seen as early as 2 days postexposure. Increases in laboratory-measured clotting times, activated partial thromboplastin time, and prothrombin time occur as early as 3 to 4 days postexposure, and elevations in fibrin degradation products are detected at 5 days postexposure.[189,273,321,488] A similar consumptive coagulopathy has been reported in humans with EVD shortly after the onset of clinical signs.[810] A maculopapular rash of varying severity can be seen as early as day 2 postexposure[266] but typically manifests later, by 5 days postexposure[189] (Fig. 11.16).

Hematologic findings include changes in total leukocyte, monocyte, and platelet numbers. A neutrophilic leukocytosis typically increases the white blood cell count with a concomitant lymphopenia and a decrease in platelet numbers, while monocyte numbers vary. Lymphopenia and decreased platelet numbers are consistent clinicopathologic findings by 4 days postexposure in most NHPs infected with 1,000 PFU of EBOV by the intramuscular exposure route. Platelet numbers typically continue to decrease with disease progression. A terminal thrombocytopenia is one of the clinicopathologic hallmarks of FVD, and thrombocytopenia and clinically significant increases in laboratory measurements of clotting time and fibrin degradation products are diagnostic for disseminated intravascular coagulation (DIC).[189,266,488] Normal megakaryocyte numbers in the bone marrow have been reported in the few human patients examined with FVD.[481] However, a systematic assessment of the presence or absence of megakaryocyte infection by filoviruses and study of the effect of FVD on megakaryopoiesis or megakaryocyte and platelet function have not been undertaken in any animal model of FVD.

Systemic filovirus spread results in the infection of hepatocytes and Kupffer cells causing acute degeneration with marked (>10 times the upper limit of normal range) increases in alanine transaminase (ALT) and aspartate transaminase (AST) activities. As the disease progresses, hepatocellular necrosis occurs (Fig. 11.15A-C), further increasing both ALT and AST activities. ALT, a cytosolic enzyme, is the most specific marker of hepatocyte damage commonly measured in FVD, though lower activity of this enzyme is present in the kidneys, myocardium, skeletal muscle, pancreas, spleen, lungs, and red blood cells. AST, a cytosolic and mitochondrial enzyme, is present in the cardiac muscle, skeletal muscle, the kidneys, pancreas, spleen, lungs, and red blood cells, in addition to the liver. Terminally, increases in AST activity could be associated with ischemic damage and/or hemorrhage in any of these organs, but the abrupt, marked increases in AST activity seen typically by 4 days postexposure are thought to be derived from hepatocytes. Whereas cholestasis is not a feature in the NHP FVD model, marked increases in gamma-glutamyltransferase (GGT) activity are also typical. Although GGT is present in cells of several organs, including intestine, kidneys, pancreas, and prostate gland, the enzyme is interpreted to be a specific marker for hepatocellular and biliary epithelial cell damage. Increases in alkaline

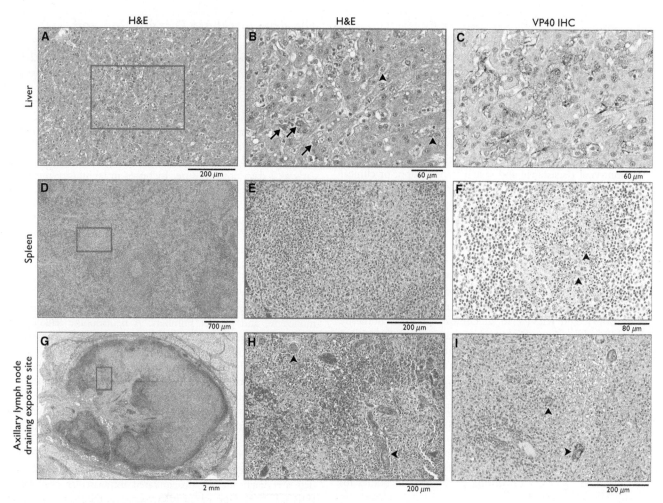

FIGURE 11.15 Histopathology of experimental filovirus infection in rhesus monkeys. A: Hepatocellular degeneration and necrosis in the liver 8 days after EBOV exposure (magnification bar 200 μm). **B:** *Insert* of **(A)**. Hepatocellular swelling is diffuse, apart from individual and small clusters of hepatocytes that are hypereosinophilic and irregularly shrunken (necrotic hepatocytes, *black arrows*). Kupffer cells are enlarged with vacuolated cytoplasm (*black arrow head*) (magnification bar 60 μm). **C:** EBOV VP40 staining (DAB, *brown*) identifies individual hepatocytes and Kupffer cells within the sinusoids in addition to positive serum staining (magnification bar 60 μm). **D:** Severe fibrinoid necrosis and lymphoid depletion in the spleen 7 days after MARV exposure (magnification bar 700 μm). Fibrin deposits expand and replace the pre-existing sinusoidal splenic architecture. **E:** *Insert* of **(D)**. A splenic lymphoid follicle with severe lymphoid depletion and lympho-cytolysis (magnification bar 200 μm). **F:** EBOV VP40 staining (DAB, *brown*, IHC) reveals infection in the few degenerate follicular dendritic cells remaining (*black arrowheads*), whereas the surrounding lymphocytes are uninfected (magnification bar 80 μm). **G:** Axillary lymph node draining an intramuscular EBOV exposure site 8 days after EBOV exposure (magnification bar 2 mm). **H:** *Insert* of **(G)**. Diffuse necrosis effaces the normal architecture of the lymph node with hemorrhage extending into the perinodal connective tissues. Diffuse congestion and hemorrhage with multifocal vascular thrombosis (*black arrowheads*) are present within the subcapsular sinuses and extend into the underlying cortex. The normal cortical lymphoid tissue has been replaced by fibrin admixed with hemorrhage and cellular debris (magnification bar 200 μm). **I:** EBOV VP40 staining (DAB, *brown*, IHC) reveals infection of the few intact macrophages, fibroblastic reticular cells, and virions in the serum (*black arrow heads*; magnification bar 200 μm). DAB, 3,3'-diaminobenzidine; H&E, hematoxylin and eosin stain; IHC, immunohistochemical stain. (Figure courtesy of Reed F. Johnson, NIH/NIAID/DIR/EVPS, and Matthias J. Schnell, Thomas Jefferson University.)

phosphatase (ALP) activity are also observed, but the multiple isoforms of this enzyme in different tissue types have typically not been measured individually. ALP is therefore not as specific as other markers of hepatic damage commonly measured in FVD models. As the disease progresses, ongoing hepatocellular damage is thought to decrease the production of albumin and hepatocellular-synthesized coagulation factors, potentiating the coagulopathy.[189] Similar changes have been documented in human disease, albeit in small numbers of patients.

Fibrin accumulation in the spleen is a consistent histopathologic feature in NHPs, regardless of exposure route, as is severe lymphoid depletion and destruction in both the splenic white

pulp and lymph nodes[16,747] (Fig. 11.15D–I). Currently no evidence is available that lymphocytes are infected with filoviruses in vivo. However, in vitro, abortive infection of lymphocytes by EBOV appears to occur. The lymphopenia observed in FVD had previously been thought to be a result of paracrine signaling, possibly stemming from infected fibroblastic reticular cells in lymphoid tissues. However, the molecular mechanisms underlying FVD-associated lymphocyte death are not clear.[155,702,848]

Prerenal azotemia (secondary to dehydration) occurs later in the disease course, typically from days 5 to 8 postexposure. The kidneys are likely not initial targets in FVD, though terminal DIC often results in thrombosis of vasa recta and, occasionally, the

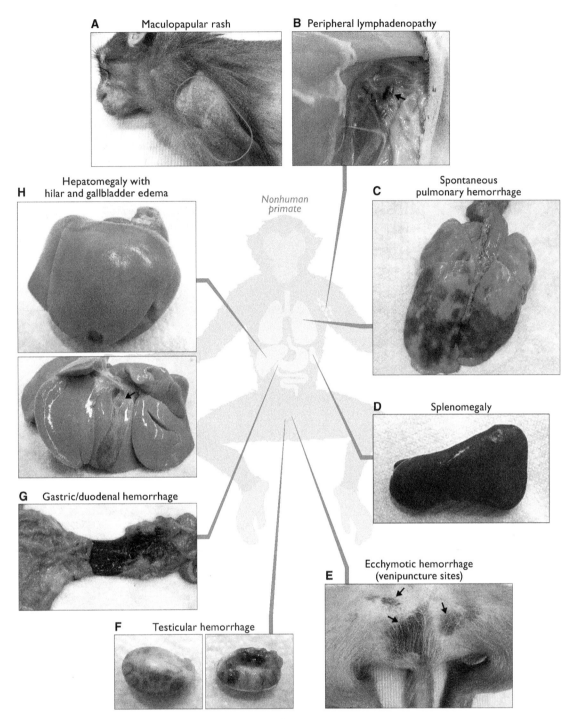

FIGURE 11.16 Gross pathology of experimental filovirus infection in rhesus monkeys. A: The left lateral face, thorax, and arm of a macaque 8 days after exposure to Marburg virus (MARV) showing a locally extensive, maculo-papular rash. **B:** The left axilla with exposed axillary lymph nodes *in situ* showing diffuse axillary lymphadenopathy with moderate edema in the surrounding connective tissues from a macaque 7 days after exposure to Ebola virus (EBOV). **C:** The dorsal surface of the lungs with multifocal to locally extensive, acute pulmonary hemorrhage in a macaque 9 days after MARV exposure. **D:** Severe diffuse splenomegaly in a macaque 9 days after MARV exposure. **E:** Inguinal skin with multifocal ecchymotic hemorrhages at venipuncture sites in a macaque 6 days after MARV expo-sure. **F:** Testicles (the testis on the right is cross-sectioned) with multifocal, acute-to-subacute testicular hemorrhage in a macaque 7 days after EBOV exposure. **G:** The stomach and proximal duodenum with acute-to-subacute, locally extensive, proximal duodenal hemorrhage in a macaque 8 days after EBOV exposure. **H:** Diaphragmatic (top image) and visceral (bottom image) surfaces of the liver. Severe, diffuse hepatomegaly and pallor with edema of the hilar con-nective tissue and gallbladder wall in a macaque 9 days after MARV exposure. (Figure courtesy of Reed F. Johnson, NIH/NIAID/DIR/EVPS, and Matthias J. Schnell, Thomas Jefferson University.)

glomeruli in affected animals. Multifocal acute tubular necrosis, thought to be secondary to reduced perfusion or ischemia associated with multiple organ dysfunction syndrome (MODS), is sometimes seen in macaque models histopathologically.[266,321,481]

Adrenal cortical cells are also often infected.[642] This observation has led to widespread speculation that filovirus infection decreases both mineralocorticoid and glucocorticoid production leading to reductions in blood volume and vascular tone. However, concentrations of these hormones in animal models of FVD and in humans with FVD have not been reported. A progressive hypoproteinemia, perhaps secondary to both reduced hepatic production of albumin and protein loss resulting from increased vascular permeability, reduces oncotic pressure. This hypoproteinemia is occasionally severe enough to result in third spacing or edema. Quantitative assessments of protein loss via renal and gastrointestinal routes have not been reported. The coagulopathy associated with FVD can lead to spontaneous hemorrhage, but more frequently, DIC with thrombosis occurs in the NHP model. Thrombosis can be seen in almost any organ, but in the NHP model, thrombosis is predominantly seen in lymph nodes near the exposure site (Fig. 11.15G, H), renal vasa recta, the submucosal vessels supplying the proximal duodenum (Fig. 11.16G), lungs, ciliary pars plicata, renal glomeruli, testes, hepatic sinusoids, and choroid plexus of the brain. Death occurs as a result of MODS.[19,47,48,97,98,155,189,230–232,256,259,266,267,270–273, 321,353,356,540,635,642–645,660,717,851,861]

Immune Response to Filovirus Infection

Filoviruses have evolved to overcome elements of the intrinsic, innate (Fig. 11.17), and adaptive arms of the host immune system. The result is almost unrestricted replication and ultimately cytolysis in the absence of a significant influx of inflammatory cells

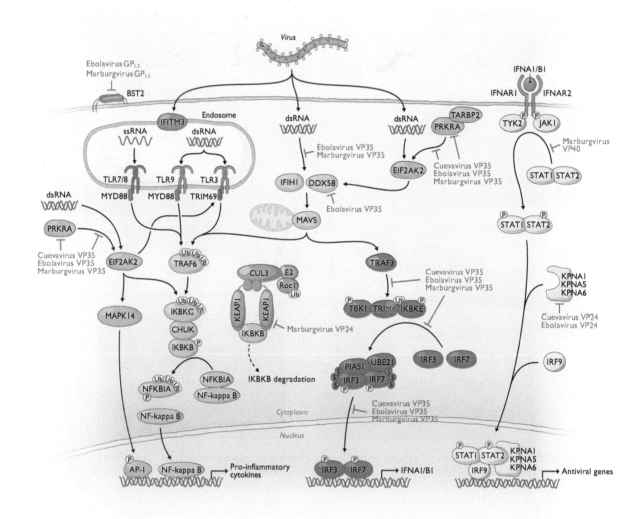

FIGURE 11.17 Mammalian filovirus escape from host intrinsic and innate immune responses. Simplified cartoon showing major intrinsic and innate immune pathways and sites of putative inhibition by filovirus proteins. BST2, bone marrow stromal cell antigen 2 (formerly also tetherin); DDX58, DExD/H-box helicase 58 (formerly RIG-I); EIF2AK2, eukaryotic translation initiation factor 2 alpha kinase 2 (formerly PKR); IKBKB, inhibitor of nuclear factor kappa B kinase subunit beta (formerly IKK-β); IKBKE, inhibitor of nuclear factor kappa B kinase subunit epsilon (formerly IKKε); PRKRA, protein activator of interferon-induced protein kinase EIF2AK2 (formerly PACT). For meaning of other protein abbreviations, see https://www.genenames.org/. (Inspired by Olejnik J, Hume AJ, Leung DW, et al. Filovirus strategies to escape antiviral responses. *Curr Top Microbiol Immunol* 2017;411:293–322, Ref.[574] and figure courtesy of Jiro Wada and Laura Bollinger, IRF-Frederick, Fort Detrick, MD, USA.)

in infected tissues.[481,521] Key filoviral proteins facilitating evasion of the host immune response include VP35, VP40, VP24, and GP$_{1,2}$.

Filovirus VP35 IID cloaks dsRNA intermediates, thereby preventing dsRNA detection by host pathogen-associated molecular pattern (PAMP) receptors such as interferon induced with helicase C domain 1 (IFIH1, formerly MDA5) and DExD/H-box helicase 58 (DDX58, formerly RIG-I).[35,36,397,454] For instance, EBOV VP35 binds protein activator of interferon-induced protein kinase EIF2AK2 (PRKRA, formerly PACT), thereby blocking PRKRA-induced DDX58 signaling and preventing DDX58-triggered IFNA1/B1 production. VP35 also prevents IFNA1/B1 production in two ways by (a) binding kinases that otherwise would activate interferon regulatory factors 3 and 7 (IRF3/IRF7), inhibitor of nuclear factor kappa B kinase subunit epsilon (IKBKE, formerly IKKε), and TANK-binding kinase 1 (TBK1) via phosphorylation[49,50,111,194,218,309,311,453,468,475,606,619] and (b) forming a complex with IRF7 and protein inhibitor of activated STAT 1 (PIAS1, a small ubiquitin modifier [SUMO] E3 ligase), promoting sumoylation and therefore inactivation of IRF7.[124] VP35 also associates noncovalently with polyubiquitin chains and thereby inhibits TRIM6-mediated type I IFN induction.[67] In addition, filovirus VP35 inhibits the cellular response to IFNA1 expression and induction of apoptosis by inhibiting EIF2AK2 (formerly PKR).[218,226,342,669] Ebolavirus VP35 also acts as a host cell RNAi silencing suppressor (RSS) by interaction with PRKRA and TARBP2 subunit of RISC-loading complex, two components of the RNA-induced silencing complex (RISC), independent of the presence of small interfering RNA (siRNA).[214,299] In addition, PRKRA interaction with ebolavirus VP35 impairs the association between VP35 and L and downstream viral RNA synthesis.[468]

Through EBOV VP35 inhibition of DDX58 signaling, virus-induced maturation of dendritic cells is blocked.[350,368,452,466,844,845] Exposure of cells to mutant EBOV encoding altered VP35 resulted in a strong IFN immune response.[310] *In vivo* administration of mutant EBOV that impairs VP35 suppression of DDX58 signaling to laboratory mice and guinea pigs resulted in severely attenuated EBOV infection.[607]

Marburgvirus and likely dianlovirus, but not cuevavirus and ebolavirus, VP40 synergistically supports VP35 by inhibiting Janus kinase1 (JAK1)-dependent tyrosine phosphorylation of signal transducer and activator of transcription (STAT) proteins, thereby disrupting JAK-STAT signaling in response to type I and II IFN.[568,757,758]

Cuevavirus and ebolavirus, but not marburgvirus, VP24 synergistically supports VP35 and inhibits IFN signaling by binding to karyopherin subunit alpha 1, 5, and 6 (KPNA1, KPNA5, KPNA6) proteins in the cytoplasm, preventing karyopherin-directed shuttling of tyrosine-phosphorylated STAT1 from the cytoplasm into the nucleus.[218,495,626,627,671,834] Although structurally similar to ebolavirus VP24, marburgvirus VP24 does not bind karyopherin directly. Instead, dimerized cytosolic marburgvirus VP24 binds to cellular oxidative stress pathway–related ubiquitin E3 ligase Kelch-like ECH-associated protein 1 (KEAP1), a repressor of antioxidant transcriptional signaling. KEAP1 up-regulates transcription factor nuclear factor (erythroid-derived 2)-like 2 (NFE2L2) for ubiquitinylation and degradation, which leads to an oxidative stress response.[193,374,578] In absence of the marburgviruses, KEAP1 interacts with inhibitor of nuclear factor kappa B kinase subunit beta (IKBKB), and IKBKB subsequently degrades and prevents the response of

nuclear factor-kappa beta (NF-κB) to activating stimuli. Upon binding to KEAP1, marburgvirus VP24 disrupts the interaction of IKBKB with KEAP1, and IKBKB is free to respond to NF-κB-activating stimuli with subsequent gene expression.[192]

Finally, filovirus GP$_{1,2}$ antagonizes the cellular viral restriction factor bone marrow stromal cell antigen 2 (BST2, formerly also tetherin), which is a type I interferon-inducible factor that restricts release of virions from infected cells.[100,378,382,424,464,616] Host cell IFN-inducible transmembrane proteins 1 to 3 (IFITM-1–IFITM3) restrict mammalian filovirus infection at an unknown step during virion cell entry,[338,830] but not sufficiently to prevent entry.

The effects of the various filoviral immunomodulating factors are likely dependent on the host. For instance, adaptation of EBOV to laboratory mice by serial passaging results in selection of mutations in the EBOV *NP* and *VP24* genes, and these mutations increase the ability of adapted EBOV to evade the IFN response.[190] Adaptation of MARV to laboratory mice or domesticated guinea pigs consistently leads to accumulation of mutations in the VP40 ORF.[795] MARV and RAVV VP40 from the parental viruses do not inhibit IFN signaling in murine cells, but laboratory mouse-adapted VP40s acquire the capacity to function in murine cells. These results suggest that inhibition of IFN signaling may be important for virulence.[219,757] Interestingly, laboratory mouse-adapted RAVV VP40 has impaired capacity to bud from human cells in the absence of GP$_{1,2}$.[217]

Productively infected macrophages are activated and release proinflammatory cytokines (CXCL8, IL1B, IL6, TNF) that recruit further infection-susceptible macrophages to the area. These cytokines alter cell adhesion protein expression and remodel intercellular adherens junction composition that increase vascular endothelial permeability. Increased F3 expression promotes a procoagulative state. EBOV GP$_{1,2}$ plays a crucial role in macrophage activation. EBOV GP$_{1,2}$ and GP$_{1,2Δ}$ activate toll-like receptor 4 (TLR4) on macrophages, which leads to the induction of the observed proinflammatory response. However, the extent of macrophage activation is species-specific, with EBOV and RESTV inducing profound and weak inflammatory responses, respectively.[94,97,221,272,371,481,573,639,642,660–662,705,774] Interestingly, *in vitro* macrophage activation with subsequent expression of proinflammatory and proapoptotic mediators occurs at the GP$_{1,2}$-cell binding stage, that is, prior to filovirus gene expression.[776]

General measurements of cytokine and reactive oxygen species (ROS) and nitric oxide responses as filovirus disease progresses suggest extensive immune dysregulation that is directly associated with MODS.[30,31,189,266,272,273,295,321,323,346,347,650,764,792] In infected dendritic cells, major histocompatibility complex (MHC) class II expression is suppressed by VP35, inhibiting antigen-presenting cell activity and the development of an adaptive immune response.[350] However, expression of F3 and TNF superfamily member 10 (TNFSF10, formerly TRAIL) increases. The latter factor may contribute to massive death of uninfected (in particular, T cell and natural killer [NK]) lymphocytes and to general immunosuppression and consequent secondary infections. Bystander lymphocyte death is thought to be provoked by numerous pathways. For instance, VP40-containing exosomes cause apoptosis in recipient T cells. VP40 in parental cells or in exosomes delivered to naïve cells result in the down-regulation of RNAi machinery components argonaute, DICER1, and

DROSHA, which therefore may play a role in the induction of cell death in recipient immune cells.[598]

Histopathologically, severe lymphoid depletion occurs in all lymphatic organs and is measurable clinically in the peripheral blood as lymphopenia.[19,31,83,84,189,231,232,245,257,264,266,267,272,273, 321,323,356,472,540,622,650,792,861] B cells and NK cells are thought to remain functional, whereas T-cell function is likely disrupted. In addition, filovirus infection ultimately greatly influences the numbers of all three cell types (concomitant with diminished T-cell–derived IL2 and IL4 in blood) and, hence, the ability to mount an effective host humoral and cytotoxic immune response. Retrospective analysis of limited numbers of human patients suggests that the presence or absence of a robust cell-mediated (CD8+ and CD4+) and humoral immune response may determine survival in patients with FVD,[7,90,133,474,501,640] though true mechanistic correlates of protection from infection, disease, or death remain to be identified.

In EVD survivors, cytokines peak only briefly and return to normal concentrations during convalescence. In lethal cases, cytokine concentrations remain uncontrolled, leading to systemic inflammation resembling sepsis.[30,318,792] Survivors typically develop high titers of IgM and IgG antibodies, whereas nonsurvivors do not mount IgG responses and have very low IgM titers.[31,712]

Virulence

From the currently available data detailing FVD case numbers and associated deaths, one cannot determine the most virulent filovirus, although the absolute case numbers and case-fatality rates suggest that marburgviruses may be more lethal than ebolaviruses (Fig. 11.2). However, all case numbers need to be regarded with caution. Case definitions and diagnostic criteria changed considerably since 1967 and were applied differently during different outbreaks. In addition, lethality differences among different outbreak areas are likely influenced by overall population health status, host genetics, and the specific availability and quality of clinical health care. Experimentally, true side-by-side comparisons of similarly grown and characterized filoviruses in the same animal model are extremely challenging to perform, and statistically significant comparisons can rarely be determined.[430] However, some studies indicate that particular isolates of individual filoviruses may be more virulent than others.[76]

Persistence

Clinical observation of human FVD survivors reveals that mammalian filoviruses may persist for extended periods of time in fluids from immune-privileged compartments (e.g., semen and aqueous humor) in the absence of viremia. This persistence leads to rare but documented recrudescent organ-specific inflammatory disease relapses (meningoencephalitis, uveitis) and sexual (or other undefined) transmission events.[71,75,167,170,177,337,359,390,394,432,485,494,632,760,870] These events have not yet been studied systematically, as current animal models of FVD do not result in significant numbers of survivors. However, widespread, noncytolytic infection of the supporting mesenchymal connective tissues, including the endothelium, throughout the male and female reproductive tract occurs in the NHP model as early as 6 days postexposure (Figs. 11.18–11.20).[588] Retrospective analyses of tissues from a few NHPs that did survive experimental EBOV or MARV infection (and treatment with candidate MCMs) have demonstrated filovirus persistence

in tissues such as the eyes, testes, and brain.[137,854] Despite localization of the virus in immune-privileged sites in macaque models, the molecular mechanisms underlying persistence and sexual transmission in the host remain unclear. Experiments with laboratory mice indicate that filovirus persistence can be established through depletion of B cells, suggesting that persistence in humans may be due to certain types of acquired or inherited immunodeficiencies.[297]

EPIDEMIOLOGY

Filoviruses associated with human disease have been encountered in Western Africa (EBOV, MARV, TAFV), Middle Africa (BDBV, EBOV, MARV), Eastern Africa (BDBV, SUDV, MARV, RAVV), and Southern Africa (MARV) (Figs. 11.1 and 11.2). The definite distribution of pathogenic filoviruses is further substantiated by the proven infection of western chimpanzees with TAFV (Western Africa)[833] and of Egyptian rousettes with MARV and RAVV (Western, Eastern, and Southern Africa).[21–23,290,381,585,737] Classical epidemiological investigations, but also environmental niche modeling, indicate that ebolaviruses are endemic in humid rain forests and that marburgviruses occur in caves located in arid woodlands. Ebolavirus emergence appears to be correlated with unusually heavy rainfall subsequent to extended dry periods. These predictions suggest that some filovirus reservoir hosts might react to climate anomalies in ways that further their interaction with humans.[440,589,590,592–596,746] Finally, serological surveys indicate that humans are exposed to filoviruses in numerous countries that, thus far, have not reported disease outbreaks (e.g., certain African countries, Belarus, Ukraine). However, the results of most of these surveys are considered controversial because of the applied methodologies and the likelihood of serological cross-reactions.[89,425,668]

The discovery of Egyptian rousettes as marburgvirus hosts[21–23,585,737] and the presence of BOMV and MLAV in insectivorous and frugivorous bats, respectively,[237,285,841,842] tempt one to hypothesize a chiropteran connection for all mammalian filoviruses. Indeed, numerous studies have either detected anti-ebolavirus antibodies in bats of various species or found short viral genomic fragments. However, the definitive reservoir host(s) of pathogenic ebolaviruses remain(s) unknown, and the means of human transmission of marburgviruses from Egyptian rousettes are unclear. As a result, the origins of all FVD outbreaks remain murky.[24,107,777]

Indeed, the majority of the few recorded FVD outbreaks began with single human infections through contact with unknown reservoir hosts. These rare events indicate that host–human transmissions are likely not as simplistic as exposure of a human to an infected bat or its excreta or secreta. For instance, MARV and RAVV transmission occurs at low levels among Egyptian rousettes throughout the year with peaks of infection occurring only in older (male and female) juveniles. Such juveniles shed marburgviruses orally and rectally.[21,22,377,737] In experimental settings, this shedding is sufficient for bat-to-bat transmission,[666] but infected bats clear the virus and develop long-term protective immunity against reinfection.[667] These results suggest that contact with particular subpopulations of bats, such as juveniles, at certain times of the year may increase the risk for bat-to-human marburgvirus transmission.

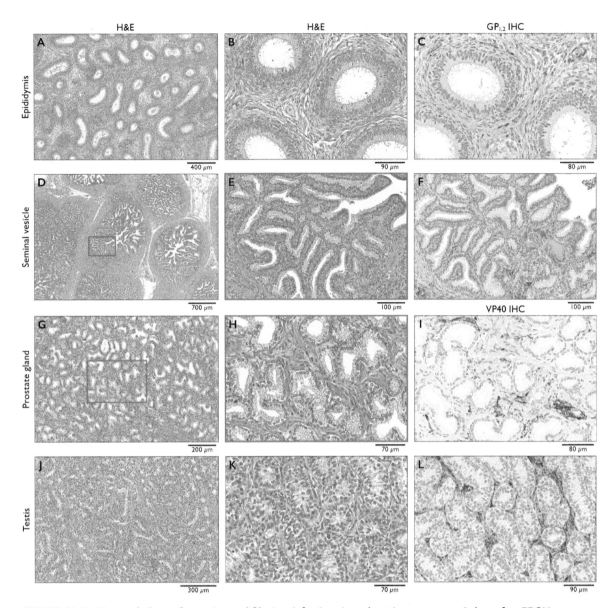

FIGURE 11.18 Histopathology of experimental filovirus infections in crab-eating macaques 6 days after EBOV exposure. A–C: Slight interstitial edema is present multifocally between epididymal tubules 6 days postexposure (magnification bars **(A)** 400 μm and **(B)** 90 μm). **C:** EBOV GP$_{1,2}$ staining (DAB, *brown*, IHC) is multifocally positive within the stroma despite a lack of significant histopathologic lesions at the light microscopic level (magnification bar 80 μm). **D and E:** (*insert* of **D**) No significant lesions are present of the seminal vesicle at the light microscopic level (magnification bars **(D)** 700 μm and **(E)** 100 μm). **F:** EBOV GP$_{1,2}$ staining (DAB, *brown*, IHC) shows multifocal positivity within the stroma and rare epithelial cells (magnification bar 100 μm). **(G and H)** (*insert* of **G**) No significant lesions are present within the prostate gland of a macaque at the light microscopic level (magnification bars **(G)** 200 μm and **(H)** 70 μm). **I:** EBOV VP40 staining (DAB, *brown*, IHC) shows multifocal positivity within the stromal connective tissue supporting the prostatic acini (magnification bar 80 μm). **J and K:** No significant lesions are present within the testis at the light microscopic level (magnification bar **(J)** 300 μm and **(K)** 70 μm). **L:** EBOV VP40 staining (DAB, *brown*, IHC) shows positive staining within the interstitial stromal cells supporting the seminiferous tubules (magnification bar 90 μm). DAB, 3,3′-diaminobenzidine; H&E, hematoxylin and eosin stain; IHC, immunohistochemical stain. (Figure courtesy of Reed F. Johnson, NIH/NIAID/DIR/EVPS, and Matthias J. Schnell, Thomas Jefferson University.)

Numerous outbreaks have occurred that were not even anecdotally associated with bat exposure but instead associated with exposure of the index cases to various mammals, including NHPs.[379,425] Past EVD outbreaks were temporally associated with significant declines of central chimpanzee (*Pan troglodytes troglodytes* Blumenbach, 1775), western lowland gorilla (*Gorilla gorilla gorilla* Savage, 1847), and

arteriodactyl duiker (*Cephalophus* spp.) populations in Gabon and COG, and EBOV antigen and short genomic fragments were detected in a few of these animals.[65,341,449,638,778,812] These data indicate that apes, and likely other primates, and duikers are occasionally exposed to filoviruses and that human infection could begin through human contact with such accidental hosts.

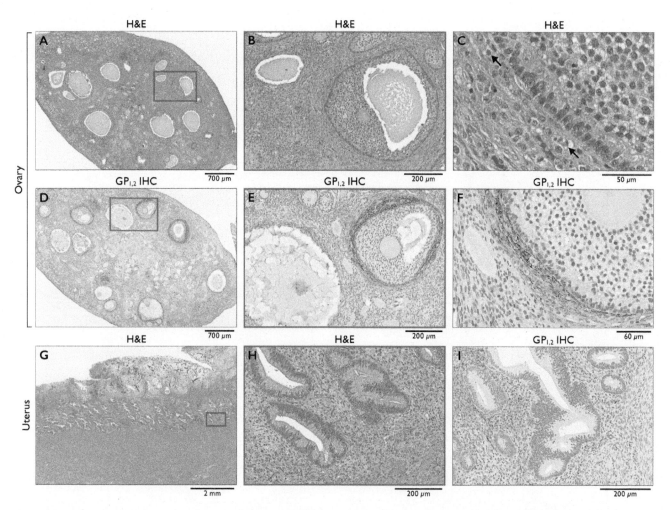

FIGURE 11.19 Histopathology of experimental EBOV infections. A–C: (**B**, *insert* of **A**) Ovary from a crab-macaque 7 days after EBOV exposure. At the light microscopic level, no significant lesions can be seen within the ovary except for mild, multifocal degeneration and eosinophilic intracytoplasmic inclusion bodies (**C**, *black arrow*) within the thecal cells surrounding maturing ovarian follicles (magnification bars (**A**) 700 μm, (**B**) 200 μm, (**C**) 50 μm). **D and E:** (*insert* of **D, F**) (*insert* of **E**) EBOV GP$_{1,2}$ staining (DAB, *brown*, IHC) shows positive staining within the theca cell layers of maturing ovarian follicles and multifocally within ovarian stromal cells (magnification bars (**D**) 700 μm, (**E**) 200 μm, (**F**) 60 μm). **G and H:** (*insert* of **G, I**) The uterus from a menstruating crab-eating macaque 7 days postexposure. (**G and H**) At the light microscopic level, no significant lesions can be seen (magnification bars (**G**) 2 mm and (**H**) 200 μm). **I:** EBOV GP$_{1,2}$ staining (DAB, *brown*, IHC) shows multifocal positive staining within the endometrial stroma and underlying myometrium (magnification bar 200 μm). DAB, 3,3'-diaminobenzidine; H&E, hematoxylin and eosin stain; IHC, immunohistochemical stain. (Figure courtesy of Reed F. Johnson, NIH/NIAID/DIR/EVPS, and Matthias J. Schnell, Thomas Jefferson University.)

Once a host–human transmission has occurred, filoviruses spread by direct, human-to-human contact (in particular, within the family unit and among patients and health care workers) or contact with contaminated bodily fluids (e.g., amniotic fluid, blood/plasma/serum, breast milk, feces, saliva, semen, skin swabs, tears, urine) or fomites contaminated with infectious material derived from patients or cadavers. Importantly, asymptomatic individuals only rarely transmit virus to another human. Airborne transmission does not contribute to FVD outbreaks except in hospital or laboratory environments, where centrifugation of samples, intubation of patients, or suction during surgical procedures can potentially lead to aerosolization of large numbers of virions.[25,54,185,249,379,380,529,563,633,678] Nosocomial spread by means of contaminated and reused equipment, in particular needles and syringes, was a major contributor to past FVD outbreaks.[185,274,380,633,678,821,822]

In regard to host susceptibility to infection or severe outcome, filovirus infections do not have a sex or ethnicity predilection, and individuals of all ages can become infected. Differences in sex, ethnicity, and age distribution between outbreaks can be largely explained by local demographics. For instance, in countries where women traditionally care for the sick, women become infected in higher numbers compared to men. Fewer children are typically affected by FVD than adults during an outbreak, but this finding may be due to children having less direct contact to potentially infected people than adults. However, children less than 5 years old with EVD typically have a shorter incubation period, shorter disease duration, and increased lethality.[8,27,127,184,282,385,693] Infected pregnant women often miscarry or deliver stillbirths due to transplacental filovirus transmission. Neonates of infected mothers rarely survive, and maternal lethality is very high.[28,56,300,537,551,569–571,670] Only two studies have evaluated the influence of host genetics on FVD outcome. Expression of killer immunoglobulin-like receptor proteins KIR2DS1 and KIR2DS3 was associated with

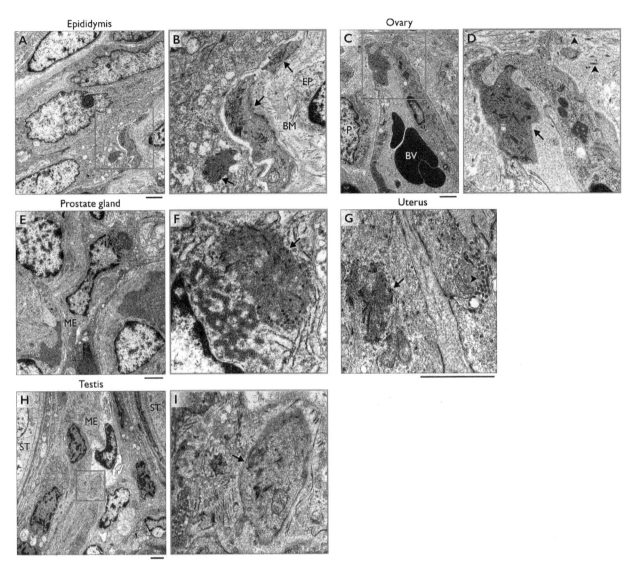

FIGURE 11.20 Transmission electron micrographs from reproductive organs following experimental EBOV infections. A and B: (*insert of* **A**) Epididymis (crab-eating macaque 6 days after EBOV exposure): three intracytoplasmic inclusion bodies are present within the mesenchymal cells (*red-boxed area*) adjacent to the basement membrane (*BM*) of the epididymal epithelium (*Ep*). Higher magnification shows filamentous nucleocapsid structures forming within the inclusion bodies (*black arrows*). **C and D:** (*insert of* **C**) Ovary (crab-eating macaque 7 days after EBOV exposure): intracytoplasmic inclusion bodies (*red boxed area*) are present in the endothelium lining a blood vessel (*BV*) and in an adjacent pericyte (*P, left*). Higher magnification shows a large intracytoplasmic inclusion body (*black arrow*) containing nucleocapsid proteins forming filamentous nucleocapsid structures within the endothelial cell. Adjacent to the vessel, a few mature EBOV particles are free within the interstitium (*black arrowheads*). **E and F:** (*insert of* **E**) Prostate gland: an intracytoplasmic EBOV inclusion body (*red boxed area*) is present within a mesenchymal cell (*Me*) of the prostate gland. Higher magnification shows filamentous EBOV nucleocapsid structures forming within the inclusion body (*black arrow*). **G:** Uterus (crab-eating macaque 7 days after EBOV exposure): an intracytoplasmic inclusion body (*black arrow*) is present in a smooth muscle cell of the myometrium. Adjacent to the smooth muscle cells, mature filamentous EBOV particles are free within the interstitial spaces (*black arrow head*). **H and I:** (*insert of* **H**) Testis: two intracytoplasmic EBOV inclusion bodies (*red boxed area*) are present within mesenchymal cells (Me) of the testis adjacent to the seminiferous tubules (ST). Higher magnification shows filamentous EBOV nucleocapsid structures forming within one of these inclusion bodies (*black arrow*). (Figure courtesy of Reed F. Johnson, NIH/NIAID/DIR/EVPS, and Matthias J. Schnell, Thomas Jefferson University.)

fatal EVD outcome in a Gabonese population.[793] HLA-B alleles B*67 and B*15 were associated with fatal outcomes, and alleles B*07 and B*14 were associated with nonfatal SVD outcomes in a Ugandan population.[635]

The evolution of filoviruses during human-to-human transmission has only been analyzed during the 2013–2016 Western African EVD outbreak. Interestingly, genomic mutations leading to at least three amino acid mutations rose to high frequency early in the outbreak and became fixed over time: mutation R111C in the homo-oligomerization domain of NP, A82V in GP$_1$'s receptor-binding site, and D759G in the active center of L. *In vitro*, GP$_1$ A82V increased GP$_{1,2}$-mediated cell entry into primate cells but decreased cell entry into bat cells, whereas NP R111C and L D759G decreased and increased viral replication and transcription depending on cell type.[172,176,491,753,781] The selective pressure leading to these mutations is unclear, as are their effects on EBOV transmissibility and virulence. Initial experiments in immunocompromised laboratory mice and rhesus monkeys did not reveal phenotypic disease associated with these mutations, but the viruses used differed by additional nucleotide changes beyond these three mutations, thereby preventing direct comparison.[491] Results from a second study indicated that L D759G may increase survival of EBOV-infected laboratory mice and delay death in infected domestic ferrets.[815]

CLINICAL FEATURES

Since the discovery of the first filovirus, MARV, in West Germany and Yugoslavia in 1967[684] until the large disease outbreak caused by EBOV in Western Africa in 2013–2016,[32,106,115,188,280,735,826] filoviruses have caused only 36 known FVD outbreaks (2,882 infections/1,968 deaths) (Fig. 11.2). The majority of these outbreaks has occurred in resource-limited and often remote African settings without efficient epidemiological surveillance programs, modern health care facilities, and well-trained and capacitated health care workers. Consequently, the clinical presentation and evolution of FVD in humans have not been well characterized by systematic study. Instead, clinical descriptions have been based on an accumulation of case or case cluster observations summarized by different individuals or expert groups in different locations, often focusing on different clinical parameters.[53,108,353,387,470,572,597,630] These descriptions were further complemented by more detailed clinical observations made from a few patients cared for in modern health care settings in 1967, 1975, and 1994[196,240,256,484,703] and from three individuals with filovirus LAIs.[205,865,870]

A lack of systematic data collection and country- and region-specific differences in overall patient health status has led clinicians to conclude that FVD caused by distinct filoviruses follow a common path. FVD infections were correctly described to begin with a nonspecific influenza-like phase followed by either recovery or progression to critical illness leading to MODS, shock, and death. However, experimental laboratory infections of mammals (Table 11.4) and the increased molecular–biological characterization of distinct filoviruses indicated that pathogenic ebolaviruses (BDBV, EBOV, SUDV, TAFV) and marburgviruses (MARV, RAVV) may cause infections with distinct clinical phenotypes. Infections by distinct ebolaviruses likely are more similar to each other than to those of marburgviruses and vice versa. This hypothesis is now reflected in WHO's International Classification of Diseases revision 11, which divides FVD into diseases caused by ebolaviruses (EBOD) and marburgviruses (MARD). These subcategories are further subdivided according to the specific filoviruses: Bundibugyo virus disease (BDV), Ebola virus disease (EVD), Sudan virus disease (SVD), and Marburg virus disease (MVD), respectively (Table 11.5).[427,827]

The 2013–2016 Western African EVD outbreak (28,652 cases and 11,325 deaths)[32,106,115,280,735] was the first opportunity to systematically characterize a FVD using increased patient cohorts that achieved statistical significance. In August of 2014, WHO formally declared the outbreak a Public Health Emergency of International Concern (PHEIC). This declaration further supported an already steadily growing international response, which resulted in the establishment of local, sometimes modern, Ebola [virus disease] Treatment Units (ETUs) staffed with national health care workers and international health care providers, occasionally including specialist infectious disease and critical care physicians.[1,110,242,281,362,436,461,463,788]

The international concern about the outbreak, combined with growing local and international support capacities for identification, isolation, treatment, and longitudinal follow-up of patients, resulted in a much more sophisticated definition of EVD than was used prior to 2013. This definition was further defined by data collected during subsequent outbreaks.[547]

Though presentation is variable from patient to patient, EVD can generally be characterized after an incubation period into typical clinical phases: a nonspecific prodrome, a gastrointestinal phase progressing to peak illness, and subsequent death or slow recovery (Fig. 11.21). Classically bounded from 2 to 21 days and only mildly influenced by EBOV exposure route and dose,[761] the incubation period is 6 to 10 days, after which patients develop an influenza-like illness that usually includes fever, anorexia, severe fatigue/asthenia, myalgia/arthralgia, and headache. Around day 5 of illness, patients often develop gastrointestinal symptoms (diarrhea, nausea/vomiting, abdominal pain) that may result in dramatic gastrointestinal fluid losses (stool volumes of 5–10 L/day) with concomitant hypotension, third-spacing due to increased vascular permeability with edema (often apparent in the face), and rhabdomyolysis. Patients with milder initial prodrome or gastrointestinal symptoms may begin to improve. Other less common signs include conjunctival injection or hemorrhage, hiccups, dyspnea, and cough. Infrequently, patients may develop hemorrhagic manifestations (ecchymoses, epistaxis, hematemesis, melena, oozing from injection sites, and petechial rashes) likely due to clotting factor deficiency, thrombocytopenia, or DIC. As illness progresses, severely ill patients develop signs of hypovolemic or septic shock (often with metabolic acidosis and severe electrolyte abnormalities) progressing to MODS, including acute kidney and liver injury, respiratory failure, and encephalopathy or seizures. Often presenting with altered mental status or seizures, the etiology of CNS manifestations may include meningoencephalitis (associated with EBOV detection in cerebrospinal fluid), metabolic causes (hypoglycemia, hyponatremia), and CNS hypoperfusion associated with hypovolemia or septic shock.[45,128,129,146,156,175,243,413,469,505,610,810,813,835]

Although the underlying mechanistic correlates have yet to be defined, accumulated clinical experience has identified a number of host and illness-specific predictors of fatal FVD outcomes. The most consistent factor across multiple outbreaks and filoviruses is the admission or peak viral load (or nadir cycle threshold value in RT-qPCR). The most ominous clinical factors include signs of organ dysfunction, most significantly acute kidney injury (AKI; signaled by elevated creatinine levels), CNS manifestations (altered mental status, coma, seizures), and severe liver injury (indicated by AST and ALT activity increases).[156,420,502,505,563,835] Only recently, retrospective analyses of EVD and SVD outbreak data have identified biomarkers that predict human disease outcome. Of interest, these biomarkers may be different in adult and pediatric disease. For instance, in adults with EVD, hemorrhage and death have been associated with increased serum thrombomodulin and ferritin concentrations. In addition, increased serum concentrations of soluble vascular cell adhesion molecule 1 (VCAM-1) and von Willebrand factor (VWF) have been associated with hemorrhage, and elevated concentrations of F3 and tissue plasminogen correlate with viremia. Increased concentrations of sCD40LG have been associated with survival. Increased serum concentrations of soluble intracellular adhesion molecule and VWF are also characteristic in fatal pediatric cases, but increased serum C–C motif chemokine ligand 5 (CCL5, formerly RANTES) and decreased serpin family E member 1 (SERPINE1,

TABLE 11.5 Human filovirus disease classification as of 2018

ICD-11 Code/Disease Name (Abbreviation)	ICD-11 Description
1D60 Filovirus disease (FVD)	A severe disease with high lethality caused by filovirus infection. Filovirus disease is typically characterized by acute onset of fever with nonspecific symptoms/signs (e.g., abdominal pain, anorexia, fatigue, malaise, myalgia, sore throat) usually followed several days later by nausea, vomiting, diarrhea, and occasionally a variable rash. Hiccups may occur. Severe illness may include hemorrhagic manifestations (e.g., bleeding from puncture sites, ecchymoses, petechiae, visceral effusions), encephalopathy, shock/hypotension, multiorgan failure, and spontaneous abortion in infected pregnant women. Common laboratory findings include thrombocytopenia, elevated transaminase concentrations, electrolyte abnormalities, and signs of renal dysfunction. Individuals who recover may experience prolonged sequelae (e.g., arthralgia, neurocognitive dysfunction, uveitis sometimes followed by cataract formation), and clinical and subclinical persistent infection may occur in immune-privileged compartments (e.g., CNS, eyes, testes). Person-to-person transmission occurs by direct contact with blood, other bodily fluids, organs, or contaminated surfaces and materials with risk beginning at the onset of clinical signs and increasing with disease severity. Family members, sexual contacts, health care providers, and participants in burial ceremonies with direct contact with the deceased are at particular risk. The incubation period typically is 7–11 days (range ≈2–21 days).
1D60.0 Ebola disease (EBOD)	A severe disease with high case fatality caused by infection with Ebola virus or a closely related virus. Ebola disease is typically characterized by acute onset of fever with nonspecific symptoms/signs (e.g., abdominal pain, anorexia, fatigue, malaise, myalgia, sore throat) usually followed several days later by nausea, vomiting, diarrhea, and occasionally a variable rash. Hiccups may occur. Severe illness may include hemorrhagic manifestations (e.g., bleeding from puncture sites, ecchymoses, petechiae, visceral effusions), encephalopathy, shock/hypotension, multiorgan failure, and spontaneous abortion in infected pregnant women. Common laboratory findings include thrombocytopenia, elevated transaminase concentrations, electrolyte abnormalities, and signs of renal dysfunction. Individuals who recover may experience prolonged sequelae (e.g., arthralgia, neurocognitive dysfunction, uveitis sometimes followed by cataract formation), and clinical and subclinical persistent infection may occur in immune-privileged compartments (e.g., CNS, eyes, testes). Person-to-person transmission occurs by direct contact with blood, other bodily fluids, organs, or contaminated surfaces and materials with risk beginning at the onset of clinical signs and increasing with disease severity. Family members, sexual contacts, health care providers, and participants in burial ceremonies with direct contact with the deceased are at particular risk. The incubation period typically is 7–11 days (range ≈2–21 days).
1D60.00 Bundibugyo virus disease (BVD)	EBOD caused by BDBV
1D60.01 Ebola virus disease (EVD)	EBOD caused by EBOV
1D60.02 Sudan virus disease (SVD)	EBOD caused by SUDV
1D60.03 Atypical Ebola disease	To be used in conjunction with codes that identify the causative virus. Unusual manifestations of disease include organ-specific (e.g., meningoencephalitis) or systemic inflammatory syndromes associated with viral recrudescence occurring after clinical recovery from acute disease. These manifestations may occur several months following infection. Additionally, this code may be used for unusual presentations of acute disease not included in the general description of Ebola disease.
1D60.0Y Other specified Ebola disease	EBOD known to be caused by a virus closely related to EBOV that is not BDBV, EBOV, or SUDV.
1D60.0Z Ebola disease, virus unspecified	EBOD caused by a novel, unidentified virus closely related to EBOV and its relatives.
1D60.1 Marburg disease (MARD)	A severe disease with high case fatality caused by infection with Marburg virus or a closely related virus. Marburg disease is typically characterized by acute onset of fever with nonspecific symptoms/signs (e.g., abdominal pain, anorexia, fatigue, malaise, myalgia, sore throat) usually followed several days later by nausea, vomiting, and occasionally a variable rash. Severe illness may include hemorrhagic manifestations (e.g., bleeding from puncture sites, ecchymoses, petechiae, visceral effusions), encephalopathy, shock/hypotension, and multiorgan failure. Common laboratory findings include thrombocytopenia, elevated transaminase concentrations, electrolyte abnormalities, and signs of renal dysfunction. Individuals who recover may experience prolonged sequelae (e.g., arthralgia, neurocognitive dysfunction, uveitis), and clinical and subclinical persistent infection may occur in immune-privileged compartments (e.g., CNS, eyes, testes). Person-to-person transmission occurs by direct contact with blood, other bodily fluids, organs, or contaminated surfaces and materials with risk beginning at the onset of clinical signs and increasing with disease severity. Family members, sexual contacts, health care providers, and participants in burial ceremonies with direct contact with the deceased are at particular risk. The incubation period typically is 7–11 days (range ≈2–21 days).

(continued)

TABLE 11.5 Human filovirus disease classification as of 2018 (*Continued*)

ICD-11 Code/Disease Name (Abbreviation)	ICD-11 Description
1D60.10 Marburg virus disease (MVD)	MARD caused by MARV or RAVV.
1D60.11 Atypical Marburg disease	To be used in conjunction with codes that identify the causative virus. Unusual manifestations of disease include organ-specific (e.g., orchitis, uveitis) or systemic inflammatory syndromes associated with viral recrudescence occurring after clinical recovery from acute disease. These manifestations may occur several months following infection. Additionally, this code may be used for unusual presentations of acute disease not included in the general description of Marburg disease.
1D60.1Y Other specified Marburg disease	MARD known to be caused by a virus closely related to MARV that is not MARV or RAVV.
1D60.1Z Marburg disease, virus unspecified	MARD caused by a novel, unidentified virus closely related to MARV and its relatives.
1D60.Y Other specified filovirus disease	FVD known to be caused by an identified filovirus that is not closely related to EBOV, MARV, and their immediate relatives.
1D60.Z Filovirus disease, virus unspecified	FVD suspected through incomplete diagnostic testing in the absence of known viral etiology.

BDBV, Bundibugyo virus; CNS, central nervous system; EBOV, Ebola virus; ICD-11, International [Statistical] Classification of Diseases [and Related Health Problems] (ICD) version 11; MARV, Marburg virus; RAVV, Ravn virus; SUDV, Sudan virus.
From World Health Organization. ICD-11 for mortality and morbidity statistics. December 2018. Available at: https://icd.who.int/browse11/l-m/en; Kuhn JH, Adachi T, Adhikari NKJ, et al. New filovirus disease classification and nomenclature. *Nat Rev Microbiol* 2019;17(5):261–263.

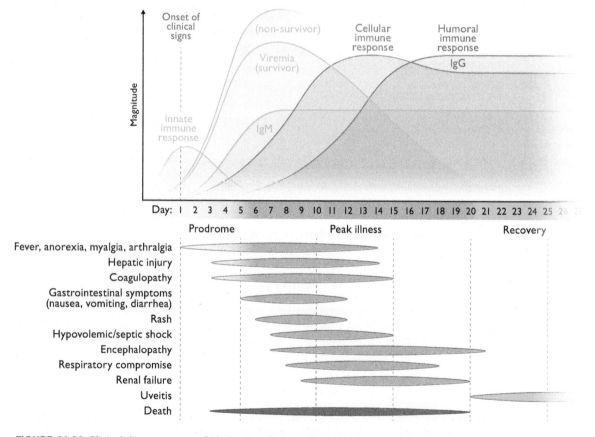

FIGURE 11.21 Clinical disease course of Ebola virus disease (EVD). Idealized progression of key parameters and clinical signs. (Inspired by Baseler L, Chertow DS, Johnson KM, et al. The pathogenesis of Ebola virus disease. *Annu Rev Pathol* 2017;12:387–418; Ploquin A, Zhou Y, Sullivan NJ. Ebola immunity: gaining a winning position in lightning chess. *J Immunol* 2018;201(3):833–842; Chertow DS, Nath A, Suffredini AF, et al. Severe meningoencephalitis in a case of Ebola virus disease: a case report. *Ann Intern Med* 2016;165(4):301–304. Refs.[46,599] and figure courtesy of Jiro Wada, IRF-Frederick, Fort Detrick, MD, USA.)

formerly plasminogen activator inhibitor 1) and VCAM-1 concentrations correlate with survival.[502–504] In both EVD and SVD, viral load is inversely associated with patient survival.[152,233,650,739]

The impact of co- or secondary infections that complicate and/or confuse the clinical presentation (e.g., gram-negative sepsis due to bacterial translocation from the gastrointestinal tract, HIV-1, plasmodium infections)[114,138,415,416,591,637,763] on prognosis remains an important question that requires systematic investigation. The observation of disseminated *Pseudomonas aeruginosa* superinfection in a child with RAVV infection[372] and the development of mucormycosis in an acute EVD patient[384] indicate that secondary infections may be common complications of FVD.

Prolonged sequelae (2 years and longer) in some FVD survivors and occasional filovirus persistence associated with disease relapse or sexual transmission were observed prior to the 2013–2016 EVD outbreak[29,37,108,394,432,485,632,870] and also during a BVD outbreak.[135] However, longitudinal follow-up of EVD survivors of the 2013–2016 EVD outbreak clarified that sequelae such

as abdominal pain, symmetric polyarticular arthralgia, fatigue, headaches, myalgia, and insomnia are common complaints (Fig. 11.22). Alopecia, confusion, hearing loss or tinnitus, seizures, and uveitis and other ocular sequelae (e.g., blurry vision, cataracts, light sensitivity) have been relatively frequent events that could be confirmed clinically.[208,212,497,548,612,673,676,677,727,729]

Thus far, substantiation of whether EBOV causes these symptoms or clinical signs has been difficult. Currently, no animal EVD survivor models are available in which causal relationships between infection and sequelae can be established. However, individual case reports indicate that some of the reported sequelae could be due directly to persistent (nonlatent) EBOV infection. For instance, EBOV was detected in the cerebrospinal fluid of two nonviremic EVD survivors with encephalopathy[337,359] and in the aqueous humor of a nonviremic survivor with uveitis.[760] Additionally, EBOV RNA could be detected in breast milk and vaginal swabs and up to 2 years or longer in the seminal fluid of numerous EVD survivors.[54,163,229,460,690,755] Both

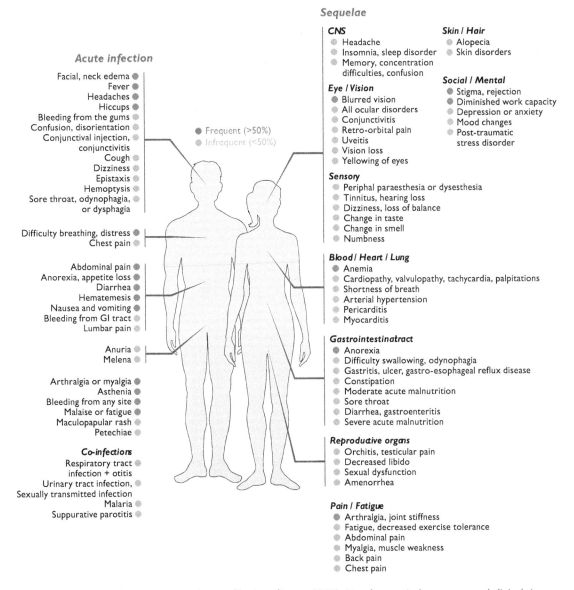

FIGURE 11.22 Clinical presentation of acute filovirus disease (FVD). Listed are typical symptoms and clinical signs of adults in acute infections and reported or observed sequelae among survivors.[53,64,108,470] (Figure courtesy of Jiro Wada, IRF-Frederick, Fort Detrick, MD, USA.)

genomic and antigenomic EBOV RNAs, indicating ongoing replication, could be detected in the aqueous humor, semen, and urine of EVD survivors.[806] In at least some instances, EBOV persistence led to sexual or undefined EBOV transmission from survivors to naïve contacts, thereby causing new EVD cases and transmission chains.[167,170,177,228,494]

DIAGNOSIS

Differential Diagnosis

No pathognomonic features exist to establish an unequivocal diagnosis of FVD at the bedside. Instead, FVD needs to be considered a possibility in any patient (febrile or not) with a recent travel history to or in Africa, particularly if the patient traveled to areas with known prior or ongoing outbreaks and/or

had contact with wildlife (bats, duikers, or primates) or visited rain forests or caves/mines. The differential diagnosis includes numerous other infectious and noninfectious diseases that present similarly with a much higher prevalence and incidence than FVD[80,567] (Table 11.6). Any suspicion of FVD should be reported to the responsible public health authorities, and special operating procedures should be implemented to ensure safety of hospital staff and prevention of further filovirus transmission.

Laboratory Diagnosis

Today, filoviruses can be detected safely and in a straightforward fashion in mobile, field, and international reference laboratories using a variety of complementary methods and samples (Table 11.7). Several methods, in particular commercial PCR-based assays and handheld lateral flow immunoassays, are recommended for field use (Table 11.8). The choice of assay

TABLE 11.6 Filovirus disease (FVD) differential diagnosis

Bacterial Disease	Etiological Bacterium
Cholera	*Vibrio cholerae*
Enterohemorrhagic *Escherichia coli* infection	Enterohemorrhagic *Escherichia coli* (EHEC)
Gram-negative bacterial septicemia	Gram-negative bacterium
Intestinal infections due to *Shigella*	*Shigella* spp.
Leptospirosis	*Leptospira* spp.
Rickettsioses	*Rickettsia prowazekii, Rickettsia typhi*
Typhoid fever	*Salmonella* Typhi
Fungal Disease	**Etiological Fungus**
Histoplasmosis	*Histoplasma capsulatum*
Protozoan Disease	**Etiological Protozoan**
Malaria due to *Plasmodium falciparum*	*Plasmodium falciparum*
Viral Disease	**Etiological Virus**
Acute or subacute hepatic failure due to hepatitis virus (fulminant hepatitis)	Hepatitis A virus (HAV), hepatitis B virus (HBV), hepatitis C virus (HCV), hepatitis D virus (HDV)
Crimean-Congo hemorrhagic fever (CCHF)	Crimean-Congo hemorrhagic fever virus (CCHFV)
Lassa fever (LF)	Lassa virus (LASV)
Measles	Measles virus (MeV)
Rift Valley fever (RFV)	Rift Valley fever virus (RVFV)
Rubella	Rubella virus (RuV)
Yellow fever (YF)	Yellow fever virus (YFV)
Other	**Cause**
Acute promyelocytic leukemia	White blood cell cancer
Dermatoses resulting from anticoagulant therapy	Warfarin
Factor VII, IX, and X deficiencies	
Hemolytic uremic syndrome	Genetic disorder
Hereditary hemorrhagic telangiectasia	Genetic disorder
Mucocutaneous lymph node syndrome	Idiopathic
Snake envenomation	Snake bites
Thrombotic thrombocytopenic purpura	Idiopathic

Adapted from Kuhn JH. Filoviruses. A compendium of 40 years of epidemiological, clinical, and laboratory studies. *Arch Virol Suppl* 2008;20:13–360; Radoshitzky SR, Bavari S, Jahrling PB, et al. Filoviruses. In: Bozue J, Cote CK, Glass PJ, eds. *Medical Aspects of Biological Warfare*. Fort Sam Houston: Borden Institute, US Army Medical Department Center and School, Health Readiness Center of Excellence; 2018:569–614; Gear JHS. The diagnosis of hemorrhagic fever. In: Gear JHS, ed. *CRC Handbook of Viral and Rickettsial Hemorrhagic Fevers*. Boca Raton: CRC Press; 1988:231–239; Grolla A, Lucht A, Dick D, et al. Laboratory diagnosis of Ebola and Marburg hemorrhagic fever. *Bull Soc Pathol Exot* 2005;98(3):205–209. Refs.[255,291]

TABLE 11.7 Advantages and disadvantages of common filovirus laboratory detection methods

Test	Target	Source Material	Advantages	Disadvantages
Primary methods				
Antigen enzyme-linked immunosorbent assay (ELISA)	Filovirus antigen/proteins	Blood, serum, tissues	Rapid (faster than RT-qPCR) and highly sensitive; can be performed on inactivated samples	Requires special equipment, but capable of high-throughput; less specific than RT-qPCR; low sensitivity in early infection
IgG or IgM enzyme-linked immunosorbent assay (ELISA)	Antifiloviral antibodies	Serum	Rapid (faster than RT-qPCR) and highly sensitive; useful for seroprevalence studies in nonviremic populations; can be performed on inactivated samples	Requires special equipment, but capable of high-throughput; less specific than RT-qPCR; relatively high rate of false positives or within-genus cross-reactions; need to consider time point of appearance of IgG and IgM antibodies in response to infection (of limited use early in infection); some patients do not seroconvert
Reverse transcription quantitative polymerase chain reaction (RT-qPCR)	Filovirus genomic or antigenomic nucleic acids	Blood, serum, tissues	Most sensitive detection method; rapid and easy to adapt to any known or new filovirus; relatively simple to perform (in particular when commercialized); can be multiplexed; can be performed on inactivated samples	Requires expensive equipment sensitive to environmental factors and dependent on electricity; reagents may be temperature-sensitive; cannot be used for detection after viral clearance; number and types of fluorescent dyes limit multiplexing; release of RT-PCR inhibitors from tissue can lead to false-negative results
Reverse transcription polymerase chain reaction (RT-PCR)	Filovirus genomic or antigenomic nucleic acids	Blood, serum, tissues	Most straightforward nucleic acid detection method; minimal training requires (in particular when commercialized); more rapid than RT-qPCR; can be performed on inactivated samples	Requires expensive equipment sensitive to environmental factors and dependent on electricity; reagents may be temperature sensitive; cannot be used for detection after viral clearance; less sensitive than RT-qPCR; release of RT-PCR inhibitors from tissue can lead to false-negative results
Confirmatory methods				
Electron microscopy (EM)	Filoviral particles or cellular inclusion bodies	Blood, serum, tissues	Unique morphology enables family-specific diagnosis; immunostaining is possible for confirmation and species-specific differentiation	Insensitive; requires expensive equipment
Indirect fluorescent assay (IFA)	Antifiloviral antibodies	Serum	Rapid and simple; useful for seroprevalence studies in nonviremic populations	Subjective interpretation; high rate of false positives; low sensitivity; some patients do not seroconvert
Immunohistochemistry (IHC)	Filovirus antigen/proteins	Tissues	Detection of filovirus antigen in the absence of viremia	Slow; for use outside of BSL-4 containment, material needs to be inactivated but works well in fixed tissues
In situ hybridization (ISH)	Filovirus genomic or antigenomic nucleic acids	Tissues	Highly sensitive if used with amplification (e.g., RNAscope); useful for detection of persistent infection in the absence of viremia	Slow; material needs to be inactivated but works well in fixed tissues
Fluorescence assay (FA)	Filovirus antigen/proteins	Tissues	Rapid and simple	Subjective interpretation; high rate of false positives; low sensitivity
Next-generation sequencing (NGS)	Filovirus genomic or antigenomic nucleic acids	Blood, serum, tissues	Unequivocal identification of filovirus; discovery of novel filoviruses; enables monitoring of genetic drift and MCM escape; can be performed on inactivated material	Expensive; slow; requires special equipment and highly trained staff for *in silico* interpretation of data

(continued)

TABLE 11.7 Advantages and disadvantages of common filovirus laboratory detection methods (Continued)

Test	Target	Source Material	Advantages	Disadvantages
Virus isolation	Filovirus	Blood, bodily fluids, tissues	Definite diagnosis; availability of virus isolates for experiments, including validation of novel detection methods	Requires transport of potentially infectious material to facilities with BSL-4 containment laboratories; need for filovirus-susceptible cells and secondary filovirus detection methods to confirm isolation; increased risk to laboratory workers due to work with live virus; cannot be applied for batch testing
Western blot	Antifiloviral antibodies	Serum	Specific	Interpretation sometimes difficult; dependent on availability of filovirus-specific antibodies

MCM, medical countermeasure.

Adapted from Broadhurst MJ, Brooks TJG, Pollock NR. Diagnosis of Ebola virus disease: past, present, and future. *Clin Microbiol Rev* 2016;29(4):773–793; de la Vega M-A, Bello A, Chaillet P, et al. Diagnosis and management of Ebola samples in the laboratory. *Expert Rev Anti Infect Ther* 2016;14(6):557–567; Grolla A, Lucht A, Dick D, et al. Laboratory diagnosis of Ebola and Marburg hemorrhagic fever. *Bull Soc Pathol Exot* 2005;98(3):205–209; Kuhn JH. Ebolavirus and marburgvirus infections. In: Jameson JL, Fauci AS, Kasper DL, et al., eds. *Harrison's Principles of Internal Medicine*, Vol. 2. 20th ed. Columbus: McGraw-Hill Education; 2018:1509–1515; Radoshitzky SR, Bavari S, Jahrling PB, et al. Filoviruses. In: Bozue J, Cote CK, Glass PJ, eds. *Medical Aspects of Biological Warfare*. Fort Sam Houston: Borden Institute, US Army Medical Department Center and School, Health Readiness Center of Excellence; 2018:569–614; Tembo J, Simulundu E, Changula K, et al. Recent advances in the development and evaluation of molecular diagnostics for Ebola virus disease. *Expert Rev Mol Diagn* 2019;19:325–340. Refs.[101,157,724]

TABLE 11.8 Field filovirus rapid diagnostic tests (RTDs) and next-generation diagnostic tests (NGDSs)

Test Name	Test Manufacturer	Test Type (Protein/Gene Target)	Targeted Filovirus[684]	Approval Type and Authority
Filovirus antigen detections tests				
Dual Path Platform (DPP) Ebola Antigen System	Chembio	LFI (VP40)	EBOV	EUA (FDA)
One-step Ebola test	Intec	LFI (not disclosed)	EBOV	EUAL (WHO)
OraQuick Ebola Rapid Antigen Test	OraSure Technologies	LFI (VP40)	BDBV, EBOV, SUDV	Approved by FDA, EUAL (WHO)
ReEBOV Antigen test kit	Corgenix	LFI (VP40)	BDBV, EBOV, SUDV	EUA (FDA), EUAL (WHO)
SD Q Line Ebola Zaire Ag test	SD Biosensor	LFI (NP, GP$_{1,2}$, VP40)	EBOV	EUAL (WHO)
Filovirus nucleic acid detection tests				
Ebola Virus (EBOV) Real-Time RT-PCR Kit	Liferiver Bio-Tech	RT-qPCR (*NP*)	BDBV, EBOV, MARV, RAVV, SUDV	EUAL (WHO)
Ebola Virus NP Real-Time RT-PCR Assay	CDC	RT-qPCR (*NP*)	EBOV	EUA (FDA)
Ebola Virus VP40 Real-Time RT-PCR Assay	CDC	RT-qPCR (*VP40*)	EBOV	EUA (FDA)
Ebola Zaire (EZ1) rRT-PCR Assay	U.S. Naval Medical Research Center	RT-qPCR (*GP*)	EBOV	EUA (FDA)
FilmArray BioThreat-E Test	BioFire Defense	RT-PCR (*L*)	EBOV	EUA (FDA), EUAL (WHO)
FilmArray BT-E Assay	BioFire Defense	RT-PCR (*L*)	EBOV	EUA (FDA)
FilmArray Warrior Control Panel M290	Maine Molecular Quality Controls	RT-PCR (not disclosed)	BDBV, EBOV, MARV, RAVV, RESTV, SUDV, TAFV	Approved by FDA
Idylla Ebola Virus Triage Test	Biocartis	RT-qPCR (*GP*)	EBOV, SUDV	EUA (FDA)
LightMix Ebola Zaire rRT-PCR Test	TIB Molbiol	RT-qPCR (*L*)	EBOV	EUA (FDA)
RealStar Ebolavirus RT-PCR Kit 1.0	altona Diagnostics	RT-qPCR (*L*)	BDBV, EBOV, RESTV, SUDV, TAFV	EUA (FDA), EUAL (WHO)
Xpert Ebola Assay	Cepheid	RT-PCR (*NP, GP*)	EBOV	EUA (FDA), EUAL (WHO)

Although some assays listed in this table target multiple filoviruses, EUA and EULA approval is not necessarily given to all of them. CDC, U.S. Centers for Disease Control and Prevention; ELISA, enzyme-linked immunosorbent assay; EUA, Emergency Use Authorization; EUAL, Emergency Use Assessment and Listing; FDA, U.S. Food and Drug Administration; LFI, lateral flow immunoassay; RT-qPCR, reverse transcription quantitative polymerase chain reaction; RT-PCR, reverse transcription polymerase chain reaction; WHO, World Health Organization.

Adapted from Broadhurst MJ, Brooks TJG, Pollock NR. Diagnosis of Ebola virus disease: past, present, and future. *Clin Microbiol Rev* 2016;29(4):773–793; Cnops L, de Smet B, Mbala-Kingebeni P, et al. Where are the Ebola diagnostics from last time? *Nature* 2019;565(7740):419–421. Refs.[101,136]

may depend on the filovirus and filovirus variant, stage of illness, available sample type, laboratory capacity, and training of the diagnostician. For the first time, in COD in 2018 to time of writing, a single diagnostic field-deployable platform (Cepheid GeneXpert) and a single set of protocols are used across all laboratory sites, making systematic comparison of viral titers at the time of diagnosis and during disease progression possible. Even in this setting, diagnostic challenges include test interpretation in the setting of large-scale preventive vaccination of close contacts as vaccinated individuals may test positive as a result of vaccination. Also, infected asymptomatic or paucisymptomatic people (including acutely infected as well as survivors with ongoing filovirus replication in immune-privileged compartments) pose a challenge because of the absence of viremia and the time lag between infection and development of detectable IgM and IgG antibodies.[54,132,169,209,283,448,563,689,690]

PREVENTION AND CONTROL

Prevention

Prevention of initial filovirus introductions into human populations is currently impossible due to the lack of understanding of filovirus reservoir hosts, host-to-human transmission dynamics, and the likely existence of inapparent human infections outside of the context of an ongoing FVD outbreak. However, the risk of filovirus infection can be mitigated through behavioral education. Avoidance of direct contact with wildlife (in particular, apes, bats, and duikers), caution during preparation of freshly hunted bushmeat, rejection of undercooked or uncooked meat, sexual abstinence or sexual intercourse using appropriate protection, and elimination of direct person-to-person contact with apparently sick individuals will decrease the risk of filovirus transmission. During ongoing FVD outbreaks, such behavioral education should be emphasized via local media and community outreach. Locals and anthropologists should be consulted to help modify cultural practices that are associated with increased filovirus transmission risk (e.g., embalming of bodies, handshaking) in community-acceptable ways. Health care personnel should always wear appropriate personal protective equipment, apply strict barrier nursing procedures, avoid reuse of any medical equipment in the absence of appropriate disinfection, and wear powered air-purifying respirators (PAPRs) or fit-tested N95 respirators during procedures that may generate virus-contaminated aerosols.[54,119,122,352,366,380,613,614,631,634] Patient isolation until resolution of clinical signs for greater than 3 days and/or negative RT-qPCR testing, ideally in local ETUs staffed with experienced infectious disease experts, greatly diminishes further filovirus transmission.[422,825] Cadavers of FVD patients ought to be buried as soon as possible because they may contain viable filoviruses for up to 7 days after death.[604] Any potentially contaminated, disposable material in the surrounding area of a patient or body should be autoclaved, irradiated, or burned as filoviruses can stay viable in drying blood for up to 5 days.[229] For dried blood, 5% peracetic acid can be used to inactivate filovirions.[696]

FDA has recently approved single vaccine for EVD prevention. Numerous candidate vaccines have been developed and shown promise in animal models of FVD. These candidates include adenovirus,[131,258,322,603,710,711,713] alphavirus,[325,326,608,609,808] lyssavirus,[77,78] orthopoxvirus,[279] paramyxovirus,[102,105,509,840,846] and vesiculovirus[154,252,260–262,517] platforms that encode filovirus proteins, naked DNA vaccines that encode filovirus proteins,[322,480,508,759,837] and filovirion-like particles created by coexpression of recombinant filovirus NP, VP40, and $GP_{1,2}$.[487,714,784,786] A few promising candidate vaccines for the prevention of EVD are in various phases of clinical trials (Table 11.9). A few promising candidate vaccines for the prevention of EVD are in various phases of clinical trials (Table 11.9) with one of them, rVSVΔG-ZEBOV-GP, now FDA-approved.[319] The same candidate vaccine has been administered to more than 255,000 people at risk of EBOV infection during the currently still ongoing EVD outbreak in the Ituri and Nord-Kivu Provinces of COD. Preliminary evaluation indicates that the vaccine may be efficacious.[801,828] and the vaccine has recently been granted conditional marketing authorization by the European Medicines Agency. A second candidate vaccine, hAd26-ZEBOV-GP/MVA-BN-Filo, is currently administered in COD.

Treatment

Currently, no FDA-approved filovirus-specific antivirals are available for the treatment of FVD. Regardless, FVD patients should receive aggressive supportive care to mitigate homeostatic imbalances. Pillars of supportive care include the standardized assessment, triage, and monitoring of vital signs, recognition and appropriate administration of oral or intravenous fluids to prevent and treat hypovolemic or septic shock, supplemental oxygen, laboratory monitoring and appropriate treatment of hypoglycemia and common electrolyte imbalance, the prevention and treatment of co- or secondary infections (with antimalarials and broad-spectrum antibiotics), and the relief of symptoms (acetaminophen for fever and pain, antiemetics, sedation as needed).[130,145,344,437,469,657,756,825] Though not always the case, the will and capacity to routinely provide optimized supportive or standard of care (oSOC) are increasingly emphasized in African outbreak settings.

Care of FVD patients who progress to MODS is extremely challenging in outbreak areas. Thus far, the utmost critical care (e.g., renal replacement therapy, mechanical ventilation) has been delivered routinely only in well-resourced US or European settings, though such care has been administered in extraordinary circumstances in Western Africa.[26,141,243,303,375,438,542,708,736,756,813,829] Likewise, management of high-risk obstetric cases and children less than 5 years old with EVD remains a significant challenge, but population-specific care is being similarly emphasized and optimized to improve patient outcomes.[109,120,183,744]

Numerous promising filovirus-specific candidate therapeutics have been evaluated *in vitro* and in animal models *in vivo*.[831] Some of them have been administered to EVD patients under compassionate care protocols, but their safety and efficacy could not be established in these anecdotal settings. During the Western African outbreak, a number of clinical trials of varying design were initiated. Unfortunately, the only one that was designed to truly determine safety and efficacy (PREVAIL II randomized controlled trial [RCT]) failed to enroll the target number of patients to provide a definitive result. This trial did however, suggest that the monoclonal antibody cocktail ZMapp was superior to standard-of-care alone. Accordingly, ZMapp was chosen as the control arm for the PALM study, an RCT comparing the nucleotide analogue remdesivir, the single

TABLE 11.9   Examples for candidate vaccines for prevention of Ebola virus disease evaluated in clinical trials

Candidate Vaccine	Vaccine Type	Clinical Trial Stage	Advantages and Disadvantages	References
• rVSVΔG-ZEBOV-GP • rVSVN4CT1-EBOVGP1	Replication-competent recombinant vesicular stomatitis Indiana viruses (rVSIVs) expressing EBOV GP$_{1,2}$ instead of VSIV glycoprotein (G)	I–III in numerous studies performed in at least 10 countries with and without homotypic boosts; rVSVΔG-ZEBOV-GP received conditional marketing authorization by the European Medicines Agency and FDA approval in the USA in December 2019	• Antibody titers resulting from single injection last ≥2 years • rVSVΔG-ZEBOV-GP submitted for WHO EUAL • rVSVΔG-ZEBOV-GP used to vaccinate >255,000 people during the 2018–present EVD outbreak in COD • Mild adverse effects such as arthralgia, fever, headaches, myalgia pain at injection site, vector viremia	6,204,252,302,319,348,392,518,600,625,828
• GamEvac-Combi • GamEvac-Lyo	Replication-competent recombinant vesicular stomatitis Indiana virus (rVSIV) and human adenovirus 5 (hAd5) vectors expressing EBOV GP$_{1,2}$	I–II	Pain at injection site	182
• hAd5-ZEBOV-GP • hAd26 ZEBOV-GP • hAd35 ZEBOV-GP • ChAd3-EBO Z GP	Replication-defective chimpanzee or human adenovirus vectors expressing EBOV GP$_{1,2}$	I–III with and without homotypic boosts and with modified vaccinia virus Ankara (MVA) expressing EBOV GP$_{1,2}$ (MVA-BN-Filo or MVA-EBO-Z) boosts; hAd26-ZEBOV-GP/MVA-BN-Filo currently in use in COD.	• Pain at injection site (human vectors); fatigue, headaches, malaise, pain at injection site (chimpanzee vector) • Preexisting immunity to used human adenovirus vector is a common issue	161,213,392,443,444,456,511,720,762,811,832,858,859

monoclonal antibody mAb114, and the monoclonal antibody cocktail REGN-EB3 to ZMapp. This study was prematurely stopped when the mAb114 and REGN-EB3 arms were shown to be superior to ZMapp.[535] These two investigational products are now the treatments of choice for patients with EVD. Only a handful of candidate therapeutics have been or currently are evaluated in clinical trials, thus far, with unclear results (Table 11.10). Of note, an ongoing randomized clinical trial of four candidate therapeutics is enrolling patients in the EVD outbreak that at the time of writing was still ongoing in COD.

PERSPECTIVE

Since the discovery of MARV in 1967 until 2012, filoviruses were largely considered exotic tropical pathogens with little overall public health impact. This view changed dramatically during the 2013–2016 Western African EVD outbreak, which demonstrated that filoviruses can infect tens of thousands of individuals and be inadvertently exported globally. Results from recent studies, performed with international urgency, illuminated many forgotten or novel aspects of filovirus infection (e.g., filovirus persistence in immune-privileged sites, frequent sequelae in survivors, sexual transmission). In addition, these results greatly advanced the repertoire of potential MCMs (e.g., EUA-/EULA-approved diagnostic tests, two candidate vaccines in the field, and two standard-of-care therapeutics). Nevertheless, true control of FVD, let alone complete FVD pre-

vention, remains a remote prospect. The still very fragmented understanding of filovirus ecology, including the lack of identified viral host(s) and potential vectors, makes prediction of hot spots of filovirus–human interfaces difficult. The socioeconomic, logistic, and infrastructural shortcomings in potentially filovirus-endemic or filovirus-epidemic areas continue to pose immense challenges to outbreak responders and to hinder performance of clinical trials. In some FVD outbreaks, ongoing strife within epidemic regions can foster mistrust of existing institutions. As foreign responders align themselves with the host government to contain the outbreak, mistrust of government may morph into mistrust of the offered foreign assistance. Cultural norms, linguistic diversity, and differences in disease concepts held by traditional healers and western medicine create cognitive dissonance in the community that also contributes to resistance of foreign assistance. A combination of scientific advances, investment in infrastructure, and social anthropology will hopefully be brought to bear in future outbreaks.

FOOTNOTE

Country and geographic region nomenclature (including country abbreviations) was standardized throughout according to the United Nations geoscheme (https://unstats.un.org/unsd/methodology/m49/). Gene and protein names were standardized throughout according to the most recent nomenclature of the HUGO Gene Nomenclature Committee

TABLE 11.10 Candidate therapeutics in clinical trials for treatment of Ebola virus disease

Investigational Agent	Drug Class	Efficacy	Advantages	Disadvantages
mAb114	Monoclonal antibody against EBOV GP$_{1,2}$	• Phase II randomized study comparing drug with remdesivir, REGN-EB3, and ZMapp prematurely terminated. mAb114 and REGN-EB3 are now the treatments of choice for EVD.[535]	• Antibody isolated by from a COD survivor[253] • Single rapid infusion (30 minutes) • Currently, no dose-limiting toxicity[147]	• Associated with myalgia, headache, chills, nausea, arthralgia, fever, shaking, nausea, vomiting, pain, dizziness, dyspnea, hypo- or hypertension, pruritus, rash, facial edema, diarrhea, tachycardia, or chest pain
REGN3470, REGN3471, REGN3479 (REGN-EB3)	Monoclonal antibody cocktail against EBOV GP$_{1,2}$	• Phase II-III randomized study comparing drug with remdesivir, mAb114, and ZMapp prematurely terminated. REGN-EB3 and mAb114 are now considered treatments of choice for EVD.[147,535,691] • Available through extension phase of study	• Single intravenous infusion • Antibodies were isolated from humanized mice • Generally well tolerated[147]	• Associated with headache, myalgia, dyspnea, chills, shaking, dizziness, fainting, cough, hypotension, rash, hives, or swelling around the mouth, throat, or eyes
Remdesivir (GS-5734)	Prodrug of adenosine nucleoside analog	• Phase II randomized study comparing drug with REGN-EB3, mAb114, and ZMapp prematurely terminated. REGN-EB3 and mAb114 are now considered treatments of choice for EVD.[535]	Does not require refrigeration[125]	• Requires monitoring of ALT/AST; may not be available in limited resource settings • Associated with transient constipation, heartburn, pruritus, dizziness, loss of appetite, nausea, vomiting, shaking, headache, loose stools, or upset stomach
ZMapp	Monoclonal antibody cocktail (c2G4, c4G7, c13C6) against EBOV GP$_{1,2}$	• Trend in efficacy from phase I trial in Western Africa[726] • Phases II–III randomized study comparing drug with REGN-EB3, mAb114, and remdesivir prematurely terminated. REGN-EB3 and mAb 114 now considered treatments of choice for EVD.[147,535]	Showed the potential for mAb cocktails like REGN-EB3 to be effective against EVD.[211]	• Long IV infusion duration under supervision[147] • Requires cold chain[125] • Antibodies were isolated from immunized mice[253] • Erythema, tachycardia, chills, hypo- or hypertension, pruritus

COD, Democratic Republic of the Congo; mAb, monoclonal antibody.

(https://www.genenames.org/). Mammal and mammal species names were standardized throughout following recommendations in Wilson and Reeder's *Mammal Species of the World*, third edition (https://www.departments.bucknell.edu/biology/resources/msw3/).

ACKNOWLEDGMENTS

We thank Laura Bollinger, John G. Bernbaum, and Jiro Wada (IRF-Frederick, MD, USA) for critically editing the manuscript (L.B.) and for figure preparation (J.G.B., J.W.), respectively. We are also thankful for critical review of the manuscript by IRF-Frederick staff Richard S. Bennett, Timothy K. Cooper, Ian Crozier, Lisa E. Hensley, Michael R. Holbrook, Louis M. Huzella, Reed F. Johnson, James Logue, and Gabriella Worwa. In addition, Christopher F. Basler (Georgia State University, Atlanta, GA, USA), Alexander Bukreyev (UTMB, Galveston, TX, USA), Olga Dolnik (Philipps University of Marburg, Marburg an der Lahn, Germany), Thomas Hoenen (FLI, Greifswald, Germany), St. Patrick Reid (University of Nebraska Medical Center, Omaha, NE, USA), Elke Mühlberger (NEIDL, Boston University, MA, USA), Jonathan S. Towner (CDC, Atlanta, GA, USA), and Victoria Wahl (NBACC, Frederick, MD, USA) provided highly appreciated feedback.

DISCLAIMER

This work was supported in part through Battelle Memorial Institute's prime contract with the U.S. National Institute of Allergy and Infectious Diseases (NIAID) under Contract No. HHSN272200700016I (J.H.K.). D.L.P. performed this work as an employee of Charles River Laboratories, a subcontractor of Battelle Memorial Institute under Contract No. HHSN272200700016I. The views and conclusions contained in this document are those of the authors and should not be interpreted as necessarily representing the official policies, either expressed or implied, of the U.S. Department of Health and Human Services or of the institutions and companies affiliated with the authors. In no event shall any of these entities have any responsibility or liability for any use, misuse, inability to use, or reliance upon the information contained herein. The U.S. Department of Health and Human Services does not endorse any products or commercial services mentioned in this publication.

REFERENCES

1. Abramowitz SA, McLean KE, McKune SL, et al. Community-centered responses to Ebola in urban Liberia: the view from below. *PLoS Negl Trop Dis* 2015;9(4):e0003706.
2. Adjemian J, Farnon EC, Tschioko F, et al. Outbreak of Marburg hemorrhagic fever among miners in Kamwenge and Ibanda Districts, Uganda, 2007. *J Infect Dis* 2011;204(Suppl 3):S796–S799.
3. Adu-Gyamfi E, Digman MA, Gratton E, et al. Investigation of Ebola VP40 assembly and oligomerization in live cells using number and brightness analysis. *Biophys J* 2012;102(11):2517–2525.
4. Adu-Gyamfi E, Johnson KA, Fraser ME, et al. Host cell plasma membrane phosphatidylserine regulates the assembly and budding of Ebola virus. *J Virol* 2015;89(18):9440–9453.
5. Adu-Gyamfi E, Soni SP, Xue Y, et al. The Ebola virus matrix protein penetrates into the plasma membrane: a key step in viral protein 40 (VP40) oligomerization and viral egress. *J Biol Chem* 2013;288(8):5779–5789.
6. Agnandji ST, Huttner A, Zinser ME, et al. Phase 1 trials of rVSV Ebola vaccine in Africa and Europe. *N Engl J Med* 2016;374(17):1647–1660.
7. Agrati C, Castilletti C, Casetti R, et al. Longitudinal characterization of dysfunctional T cell-activation during human acute Ebola infection. *Cell Death Dis* 2016;7:e2164.
8. Agua-Agum J, Ariyarajah A, Blake IM, et al. Ebola virus disease among children in West Africa. *N Engl J Med* 2015;372(13):1274–1277.
9. Albariño CG, Shoemaker T, Khristova ML, et al. Genomic analysis of filoviruses associated with four viral hemorrhagic fever outbreaks in Uganda and the Democratic Republic of the Congo in 2012. *Virology* 2013;442(2):97–100.
10. Albariño CG, Uebelhoer LS, Vincent JP, et al. Development of a reverse genetics system to generate recombinant Marburg virus derived from a bat isolate. *Virology* 2013;446(1–2):230–237.
11. Albariño CG, Wiggleton Guerrero L, Chakrabarti AK, et al. Transcriptional analysis of viral mRNAs reveals common transcription patterns in cells infected by five different filoviruses. *PLoS One* 2018;13(8):e0201827.
12. Albariño CG, Wiggleton Guerrero L, Jenks HM, et al. Insights into Reston virus spillovers and adaption from virus whole genome sequences. *PLoS One* 2017;12(5):e0178224.
13. Aleksandrowicz P, Marzi A, Biedenkopf N, et al. Ebola virus enters host cells by macropinocytosis and clathrin-mediated endocytosis. *J Infect Dis* 2011;204(Suppl 3):S957–S967.
14. Alfson KJ, Avena LE, Beadles MW, et al. Genetic changes at the glycoprotein editing site associated with serial passage of Sudan virus. *J Infect Dis* 2015;212(Suppl 2):S295–S304.
15. Alfson KJ, Avena LE, Beadles MW, et al. Intramuscular exposure of Macaca fascicularis to low doses of low passage- or cell culture-adapted Sudan virus or Ebola virus. *Viruses* 2018;10(11):642.
16. Alfson KJ, Avena LE, Worwa G, et al. Development of a lethal intranasal exposure model of Ebola virus in the cynomolgus macaque. *Viruses* 2017;9(11):319.
17. Alfson KJ, Griffiths A. Development and testing of a method for validating chemical inactivation of Ebola virus. *Viruses* 2018;10(3):126.
18. Alvarez CP, Lasala F, Carrillo J, et al. C-type lectins DC-SIGN and L-SIGN mediate cellular entry by Ebola virus in cis and in trans. *J Virol* 2002;76(13):6841–6844.
19. Alves DA, Glynn AR, Steele KE, et al. Aerosol exposure to the Angola strain of Marburg virus causes lethal viral hemorrhagic fever in cynomolgus macaques. *Vet Pathol* 2010;47(5):831–851.
20. Amarasinghe GK, Ayllón MA, Bào Y, et al. Taxonomy of the order Mononegavirales: update 2019. *Arch Virol* 2019;164:1967–1980.
21. Amman BR, Carroll SA, Reed ZD, et al. Seasonal pulses of Marburg virus circulation in juvenile Rousettus aegyptiacus bats coincide with periods of increased risk of human infection. *PLoS Pathog* 2012;8(10):e1002877.
22. Amman BR, Jones MEB, Sealy TK, et al. Oral shedding of Marburg virus in experimentally infected Egyptian fruit bats (Rousettus aegyptiacus). *J Wildl Dis* 2015;51(1):113–124.
23. Amman BR, Nyakarahuka L, McElroy AK, et al. Marburgvirus resurgence in Kitaka Mine bat population after extermination attempts, Uganda. *Emerg Infect Dis* 2014;20(10):1761–1764.
24. Amman BR, Swanepoel R, Nichol ST, et al. Ecology of filoviruses. *Curr Top Microbiol Immunol* 2017;411:23–61.
25. Arias A, Watson SJ, Asogun D, et al. Rapid outbreak sequencing of Ebola virus in Sierra Leone identifies transmission chains linked to sporadic cases. *Virus Evol* 2016;2(1):vew016.
26. Auffermann WF, Kraft CS, Vanairsdale S, et al. Radiographic imaging for patients with contagious infectious diseases: how to acquire chest radiographs of patients infected with the Ebola virus. *AJR Am J Roentgenol* 2015;204(1):44–48.
27. Aylward B, Barboza P, Bawo L, et al. Ebola virus disease in West Africa - the first 9 months of the epidemic and forward projections. *N Engl J Med* 2014;371(16):1481–1495.
28. Baggi FM, Taybi A, Kurth A, et al. Management of pregnant women infected with Ebola virus in a treatment centre in Guinea, June 2014. *Euro Surveill* 2014;19(49):20983.
29. Bah EI, Lamah M-C, Fletcher T, et al. Clinical presentation of patients with Ebola virus disease in Conakry, Guinea. *N Engl J Med* 2015;372(1):40–47.
30. Baize S, Leroy EM, Georges AJ, et al. Inflammatory responses in Ebola virus-infected patients. *Clin Exp Immunol* 2002;128(1):163–168.
31. Baize S, Leroy EM, Georges-Courbot M-C, et al. Defective humoral responses and extensive intravascular apoptosis are associated with fatal outcome in Ebola virus-infected patients. *Nat Med* 1999;5(4):423–426.
32. Baize S, Pannetier D, Oestereich L, et al. Emergence of Zaire Ebola virus disease in Guinea. *N Engl J Med* 2014;371(15):1418–1425.
33. Bakri AG. Fighting the first Ebola virus epidemic in the World in 1976: memoirs of a young doctor. *Sudan J Paediatr* 2014;14(2):94–100.
34. Bale S, Dias JM, Fusco ML, et al. Structural basis for differential neutralization of ebolaviruses. *Viruses* 2012;4(4):447–470.
35. Bale S, Julien J-P, Bornholdt ZA, et al. Marburg virus VP35 can both fully coat the backbone and cap the ends of dsRNA for interferon antagonism. *PLoS Pathog* 2012;8(9):e1002916.
36. Bale S, Julien J-P, Bornholdt ZA, et al. Ebolavirus VP35 coats the backbone of double-stranded RNA for interferon antagonism. *J Virol* 2013;87(18):10385–10388.
37. Baltzer G, Slenczka W, Stöppler L, et al. Marburg-Virus-Krankheit. Verlaufsbeobachtungen über 12 Jahre (1967-1979). *Verh Dtsch Ges Inn Med* 1979;83:1203–1206.
38. Banadyga L, Hoenen T, Ambroggio X, et al. Ebola virus VP24 interacts with NP to facilitate nucleocapsid assembly and genome packaging. *Sci Rep* 2017;7(1):7698.
39. Bào Y, Amarasinghe GK, Basler CF, et al. Implementation of objective PASC-derived taxon demarcation criteria for official classification of filoviruses. *Viruses* 2017;9(5):106.
40. Baron RC, McCormick JB, Zubeir OA. Ebola virus disease in southern Sudan: hospital dissemination and intrafamilial spread. *Bull World Health Organ* 1983;61(6):997–1003.
41. Barr J, Chambers P, Pringle CR, et al. Sequence of the major nucleocapsid protein gene of pneumonia virus of mice: sequence comparisons suggest structural homology between nucleocapsid proteins of pneumoviruses, paramyxoviruses, rhabdoviruses and filoviruses. *J Gen Virol* 1991;72(Pt. 3):677–685.
42. Barrette RW, Metwally SA, Rowland JM, et al. Discovery of swine as a host for the Reston ebolavirus. *Science* 2009;325(5937):204–206.
43. Barrientos LG, Martin AM, Rollin PE, et al. Disulfide bond assignment of the Ebola virus secreted glycoprotein sGP. *Biochem Biophys Res Commun* 2004;323(2):696–702.
44. Barrientos LG, Martin AM, Wohlhueter RM, et al. Secreted glycoprotein from Live Zaire ebolavirus-infected cultures: preparation, structural and biophysical characterization, and thermodynamic stability. *J Infect Dis* 2007;196(Suppl 2):S220–S231.
45. Barry M, Touré A, Traoré FA, et al. Clinical predictors of mortality in patients with Ebola virus disease. *Clin Infect Dis* 2015;60(12):1821–1824.
46. Baseler L, Chertow DS, Johnson KM, et al. The pathogenesis of Ebola virus disease. *Annu Rev Pathol* 2017;12:387–418.
47. Baskerville A, Bowen ETW, Platt GS, et al. The pathology of experimental Ebola virus infection in monkeys. *J Pathol* 1978;125(3):131–138.
48. Baskerville A, Fisher-Hoch SP, Neild GH, et al. Ultrastructural pathology of experimental Ebola haemorrhagic fever virus infection. *J Pathol* 1985;147(3):199–209.
49. Basler CF, Mikulasova A, Martinez-Sobrido L, et al. The Ebola virus VP35 protein inhibits activation of interferon regulatory factor 3. *J Virol* 2003;77(14):7945–7956.
50. Basler CF, Wang X, Mühlberger E, et al. The Ebola virus VP35 protein functions as a type I IFN antagonist. *Proc Natl Acad Sci U S A* 2000;97(22):12289–12294.
51. Batra J, Hultquist JF, Liu D, et al. Protein interaction mapping identifies RBBP6 as a negative regulator of Ebola virus replication. *Cell* 2018;175(7):1917.e1913–1930.e1913.
52. Bausch DG, Borchert M, Grein T, et al. Risk factors for Marburg hemorrhagic fever, Democratic Republic of the Congo. *Emerg Infect Dis* 2003;9(12):1531–1537.
53. Bausch DG, Nichol ST, Muyembe-Tamfum J-J, et al. Marburg hemorrhagic fever associated with multiple genetic lineages of virus. *N Engl J Med* 2006;355(9):909–919.
54. Bausch DG, Towner JS, Dowell SF, et al. Assessment of the risk of Ebola virus transmission from bodily fluids and fomites. *J Infect Dis* 2007;196(Suppl 2):S142–S147.
55. Bavari S, Bosio CM, Wiegand E, et al. Lipid raft microdomains: a gateway for compartmentalized trafficking of Ebola and Marburg viruses. *J Exp Med* 2002;195(5):593–602.
56. Bebell LM, Oduyebo T, Riley LE. Ebola virus disease and pregnancy: a review of the current knowledge of Ebola virus pathogenesis, maternal, and neonatal outcomes. *Birth Defects Res* 2017;109(5):353–362.
57. Bechtelsheimer H, Korb G, Gedigk P. Die "Marburg-Virus"-Hepatitis—Untersuchungen bei Menschen und Meerschweinchen. *Virchows Arch A Pathol Pathol Anat* 1970;351(4):273–290.
58. Becker S, Huppertz S, Klenk H-D, et al. The nucleoprotein of Marburg virus is phosphorylated. *J Gen Virol* 1994;75(Pt. 4):809–818.
59. Becker S, Klenk H-D, Mühlberger E. Intracellular transport and processing of the Marburg virus surface protein in vertebrate and insect cells. *Virology* 1996;225(1):145–155.
60. Becker S, Rinne C, Hofsäß U, et al. Interactions of Marburg virus nucleocapsid proteins. *Virology* 1998;249(2):406–417.
61. Becker S, Spiess M, Klenk H-D. The asialoglycoprotein receptor is a potential liver-specific receptor for Marburg virus. *J Gen Virol* 1995;76(Pt. 2):393–399.
62. Belyi VA, Levine AJ, Skalka AM. Unexpected inheritance: multiple integrations of ancient bornavirus and ebolavirus/marburgvirus sequences in vertebrate genomes. *PLoS Pathog* 2010;6(7):e1001030.
63. Beniac DR, Melito PL, Devarennes SL, et al. The organisation of Ebola virus reveals a capacity for extensive, modular polyploidy. *PLoS One* 2012;7(1):e29608.
64. Bennett RS, Huzella LM, Jahrling PB, et al. Nonhuman primate models of Ebola virus disease. *Curr Top Microbiol Immunol* 2017;411:171–193.
65. Bermejo M, Rodríguez-Teijeiro JD, Illera G, et al. Ebola outbreak killed 5000 gorillas. *Science* 2006;314(5805):1564.
66. Bertherat E, Talarmin A, Zeller H; Comité international de coordination technique et scientifique de l'épidémie de Durba. République Démocratique du Congo: entre guerre civile et virus Marburg. *Méd Trop (Mars)* 1999;59(2):201–204.
67. Bharaj P, Atkins C, Luthra P, et al. The host E3-ubiquitin ligase TRIM6 ubiquitinates the Ebola virus VP35 protein and promotes virus replication. *J Virol* 2017;91(18):e00833-e00817.
68. Bharat TAM, Noda T, Riches JD, et al. Structural dissection of Ebola virus and its assembly determinants using cryo-electron tomography. *Proc Natl Acad Sci U S A* 2012;109(11):4275–4280.
69. Bharat TAM, Riches JD, Kolesnikova L, et al. Cryo-electron tomography of Marburg virus particles and their morphogenesis within infected cells. *PLoS Biol* 2011;9(11):e1001196.
70. Bhattacharyya S, Hope TJ, Young JAT. Differential requirements for clathrin endocytic pathway components in cellular entry by Ebola and Marburg glycoprotein pseudovirions. *Virology* 2011;419(1):1–9.
71. Biava M, Caglioti C, Bordi L, et al. Detection of viral RNA in tissues following plasma clearance from an Ebola virus infected patient. *PLoS Pathog* 2017;13(1):e1006065.
72. Biedenkopf N, Hartlieb B, Hoenen T, et al. Phosphorylation of Ebola virus VP30 influences the composition of the viral nucleocapsid complex: impact on viral transcription and replication. *J Biol Chem* 2013;288(16):11165–11174.
73. Bitekyerezo M, Kyobutungi C, Kizza R, et al. The outbreak and control of Ebola viral haemorrhagic fever in a Ugandan medical school. *Trop Doct* 2002;32(1):10–15.
74. Björndal AS, Szekely L, Elgh F. Ebola virus infection inversely correlates with the overall expression levels of promyelocytic leukaemia (PML) protein in cultured cells. *BMC Microbiol* 2003;3(1):6.

This chapter represents a revised and updated version of the chapter from the Sixth Edition of Fields Virology written by Heinz Feldman, Anthony Sanchez, and Thomas Gilbert. Some of the figures and tables, as well as portions of the text have been carried forward from previous editions.

75. Blackley D, Wiley MR, Ladner JT, et al. Reduced evolutionary rate in reemerged Ebola virus transmission chains. *Sci Adv* 2016;2(4):e1600378.
76. Blair PW, Keshtkar-Jahromi M, Psoter KJ, et al. Virulence of Marburg virus Angola compared to Mt. Elgon (Musoke) in macaques: a pooled survival analysis. *Viruses* 2018; 10(11):658.
77. Blaney JE, Marzi A, Willet M, et al. Antibody quality and protection from lethal Ebola virus challenge in nonhuman primates immunized with rabies virus based bivalent vaccine. *PLoS Pathog* 2013;9(5):e1003389.
78. Blaney JE, Wirblich C, Papaneri AB, et al. Inactivated or live-attenuated bivalent vaccines that confer protection against rabies and Ebola viruses. *J Virol* 2011;85(20):10605–10616.
79. Boehmann Y, Enterlein S, Randolf A, et al. A reconstituted replication and transcription system for Ebola virus Reston and comparison with Ebola virus Zaire. *Virology* 2005;332(1):406–417.
80. Boggild AK, Esposito DH, Kozarsky PE, et al. Differential diagnosis of illness in travelers arriving from Sierra Leone, Liberia, or Guinea: a cross-sectional study from the GeoSentinel Surveillance Network. *Ann Intern Med* 2015;162(11):757–764.
81. Bornholdt ZA, Noda T, Abelson DM, et al. Structural rearrangement of Ebola virus VP40 begets multiple functions in the virus life cycle. *Cell* 2013;154(4):763–774.
82. Bornholdt ZA, Turner HL, Murin CD, et al. Isolation of potent neutralizing antibodies from a survivor of the 2014 Ebola virus outbreak. *Science* 2016;351(6277):1078–1083.
83. Bosio CM, Aman MJ, Grogan C, et al. Ebola and Marburg viruses replicate in monocyte-derived dendritic cells without inducing the production of cytokines and full maturation. *J Infect Dis* 2003;188(11):1630–1638.
84. Bosio CM, Moore BD, Warfield KL, et al. Ebola and Marburg virus-like particles activate human myeloid dendritic cells. *Virology* 2004;326(2):280–287.
85. Boumandouki P, Formenty P, Epelboin A, et al. Prise en charge des malades et des défunts lors de l'épidémie de fièvre hémorragique due au virus Ebola d'octobre à décembre 2003 au Congo. *Bull Soc Pathol Exot* 2005;98(3):218–223.
86. Bowen ETW, Lloyd G, Harris WJ, et al. Viral haemorrhagic fever in southern Sudan and northern Zaire. Preliminary studies on the aetiological agent. Lancet 1977;1(8011 Part 1):571–573.
87. Bowen ETW, Lloyd G, Platt G, et al. Virological studies on a case of Ebola virus infection in man and in monkeys. In: Pattyn SR, ed. *Ebola Virus Haemorrhagic Fever*. Amsterdam: Elsevier/North-Holland Biomedical Press; 1978:95–102.
88. Bowen ETW, Simpson DIH, Bright WF, et al. Vervet monkey disease: studies on some physical and chemical properties of the causative agent. *Br J Exp Pathol* 1969;50(4):400–407.
89. Bower H, Glynn JR. A systematic review and meta-analysis of seroprevalence surveys of ebolavirus infection. *Sci Data* 2017;4:160133.
90. Bradfute SB, Warfield KL, Bavari S. Functional CD8+ T cell responses in lethal Ebola virus infection. *J Immunol* 2008;180(6):4058–4066.
91. Bramble MS, Hoff N, Gilchuk P, et al. Pan-filovirus serum neutralizing antibodies in a subset of Congolese ebolavirus infection survivors. *J Infect Dis* 2018;218(12):1929–1936.
92. Brannan JM, Froude JW, Prugar LI, et al. Interferon α/β receptor-deficient mice as a model for Ebola virus disease. *J Infect Dis* 2015;212(Suppl 2):S282–S294.
93. Brauburger K, Boehmann Y, Tsuda Y, et al. Analysis of the highly diverse gene borders in Ebola virus reveals a distinct mechanism of transcriptional regulation. *J Virol* 2014;88(21):12558–12571.
94. Brauburger K, Deflubé LR, Mühlberger E. Filovirus transcription and replication. In: Pattnaik AK, Whitt MA, eds. *Biology and Pathogenesis of Rhabdo- and Filoviruses*. Singapore: World Scientific Publishing; 2015:515–555.
95. Bray M. The role of the type I interferon response in the resistance of mice to filovirus infection. *J Gen Virol* 2001;82(Pt. 6):1365–1373.
96. Bray M, Davis K, Geisbert T, et al. A mouse model for evaluation of prophylaxis and therapy of Ebola hemorrhagic fever. *J Infect Dis* 1998;178(3):651–661.
97. Bray M, Geisbert TW. Ebola virus: the role of macrophages and dendritic cells in the pathogenesis of Ebola hemorrhagic fever. *Int J Biochem Cell Biol* 2005;37(8):1560–1566.
98. Bray M, Hatfill S, Hensley L, et al. Haematological, biochemical and coagulation changes in mice, guinea-pigs and monkeys infected with a mouse-adapted variant of Ebola Zaire virus. *J Comp Pathol* 2001;125(4):243–253.
99. Brindley MA, Hunt CL, Kondratowicz AS, et al. Tyrosine kinase receptor Axl enhances entry of Zaire ebolavirus without direct interactions with the viral glycoprotein. *Virology* 2011;415(2):83–94.
100. Brinkmann C, Nehlmeier I, Walendy-Gnirß K, et al. The tetherin antagonism of the Ebola virus glycoprotein requires an intact receptor-binding domain and can be blocked by GP1-specific antibodies. *J Virol* 2016;90(24):11075–11086.
101. Broadhurst MJ, Brooks TJG, Pollock NR. Diagnosis of Ebola virus disease: past, present, and future. *Clin Microbiol Rev* 2016;29(4):773–793.
102. Bukreyev A, Rollin PE, Tate MK, et al. Successful topical respiratory tract immunization of primates against Ebola virus. *J Virol* 2007;81(12):6379–6388.
103. Bukreyev A, Volchkov VE, Blinov VM, et al. The GP-protein of Marburg virus contains the region similar to the "immunosuppressive domain" of oncogenic retrovirus P15E proteins. *FEBS Lett* 1993;323(1–2):183–187.
104. Bukreyev AA, Volchkov VE, Blinov VM, et al. The complete nucleotide sequence of the Popp (1967) strain of Marburg virus: a comparison with the Musoke (1980) strain. *Arch Virol* 1995;140(9):1589–1600.
105. Bukreyev A, Yang L, Zaki SR, et al. A single intranasal inoculation with a paramyxovirus-vectored vaccine protects guinea pigs against a lethal-dose Ebola virus challenge. *J Virol* 2006;80(5):2267–2279.
106. Bullard SG. *A Day-by-Day Chronicle of the 2013-2016 Ebola Outbreak*. Cham: Springer; 2018.
107. Burk R, Bollinger L, Johnson JC, et al. Neglected filoviruses. *FEMS Microbiol Rev* 2016;40(4):494–519.
108. Bwaka MA, Bonnet M-J, Calain P, et al. Ebola hemorrhagic fever in Kikwit, Democratic Republic of the Congo: clinical observations in 103 patients. *J Infect Dis* 1999;179(Suppl 1):S1–S7.
109. Caluwaerts S, Fautsch T, Lagrou D, et al. Dilemmas in managing pregnant women with Ebola: 2 case reports. *Clin Infect Dis* 2016;62(7):903–905.
110. Cao J, Zhang L, Xi H, et al. Providing nursing care to Ebola virus disease patients: China Ebola Treatment Unit experience. *J Glob Health* 2015;5(2):020301.
111. Cárdenas WB, Loo Y-M, Gale M Jr, et al. Ebola virus VP35 protein binds double-stranded RNA and inhibits alpha/beta interferon production induced by RIG-I signaling. *J Virol* 2006;80(11):5168–5178.
112. Carette JE, Raaben M, Wong AC, et al. Ebola virus entry requires the cholesterol transporter Niemann-Pick C1. *Nature* 2011;477(7364):340–343.
113. Carrion R Jr, Ro Y, Hoosien K, et al. A small nonhuman primate model for filovirus-induced disease. *Virology* 2011;420(2):117–124.
114. Carroll MW, Haldenby S, Rickett NY, et al. Deep sequencing of RNA from blood and oral swab samples reveals the presence of nucleic acid from a number of pathogens in patients with acute Ebola virus disease and is consistent with bacterial translocation across the gut. mSphere 2017;2(4):e00325.
115. Carroll MW, Matthews DA, Hiscox JA, et al. Temporal and spatial analysis of the 2014-2015 Ebola virus outbreak in West Africa. *Nature* 2015;524(7563):97–101.
116. Centers for Disease Control. Update: filovirus infection in animal handlers. *MMWR Morb Mortal Wkly Rep* 1990;39(13):221.
117. Centers for Disease Control and Prevention. Outbreak of Ebola hemorrhagic fever Uganda, August 2000-January 2001. *MMWR Morb Mortal Wkly Rep* 2001;50(5):73–77.
118. Centers for Disease Control and Prevention. Imported case of Marburg hemorrhagic fever—Colorado, 2008. *MMWR Morb Mortal Wkly Rep* 2009;58(49):1377–1381.
119. Centers for Disease Control and Prevention. Infection prevention and control recommendations for hospitalized patients under investigation (PUIs) for Ebola virus disease (EVD) in U.S. hospitals. 2015. Available at: http://www.cdc.gov/vhf/ebola/hcp/infection-prevention-and-control-recommendations.html
120. Centers for Disease Control and Prevention. Interim guidance for U.S. hospitals on the care of a neonate born to a mother who is confirmed to have Ebola, is a person under investigation (PUI), or has been exposed to Ebola. 2016. Available at: http://www.cdc.gov/vhf/ebola/healthcare-us/hospitals/neonatal-care.html
121. Centers for Disease Control and Prevention. Bioterrorism agents/diseases. 2018. Available at: https://emergency.cdc.gov/agent/agentlist-category.asp
122. Centers for Disease Control and Prevention, World Health Organization. Teaching and prevention materials "Infection control for viral haemorrhagic fevers in the African health care setting". WHO Document. 1999. WHO/EMC/ESR/98-2.
123. Chandran K, Sullivan NJ, Felbor U, et al. Endosomal proteolysis of the Ebola virus glycoprotein is necessary for infection. *Science* 2005;308(5728):1643–1645.
124. Chang T-H, Kubota T, Matsuoka M, et al. Ebola Zaire virus blocks type I interferon production by exploiting the host SUMO modification machinery. *PLoS Pathog* 2009;5(6):e1000493.
125. Check Hayden E. Experimental drugs poised for use in Ebola outbreak. *Nature* 2018;557(7706):475–476.
126. Chepurnov AA, Bakulina LF, Dadaeva AA, et al. Inactivation of Ebola virus with a surfactant nanoemulsion. *Acta Trop* 2003;87(3):315–320.
127. Chérif MS, Koonrungsesomboon N, Kassé D, et al. Ebola virus disease in children during the 2014-2015 epidemic in Guinea: a nationwide cohort study. *Eur J Pediatr* 2017; 176(6):791–796.
128. Chertow DS, Kleine C, Edwards JK, et al. Ebola virus disease in West Africa—clinical manifestations and management. *N Engl J Med* 2014;371(22):2054–2057.
129. Chertow DS, Nath A, Suffredini AF, et al. Severe meningoencephalitis in a case of Ebola virus disease: a case report. *Ann Intern Med* 2016;165(4):301–304.
130. Chertow DS, Uyeki TM, DuPont HL. Loperamide therapy for voluminous diarrhea in Ebola virus disease. *J Infect Dis* 2015;211(7):1036–1037.
131. Choi JH, Jonsson-Schmunk K, Qiu X, et al. A single dose respiratory recombinant adenovirus-based vaccine provides long-term protection for non-human primates from lethal Ebola infection. *Mol Pharm* 2015;12(8):2712–2731.
132. Chughtai AA, Barnes M, Macintyre CR. Persistence of Ebola virus in various body fluids during convalescence: evidence and implications for disease transmission and control. *Epidemiol Infect* 2016;144(8):1652–1660.
133. Cimini E, Viola D, Cabeza-Cabrerizo M, et al. Different features of Cδ2 T and NK cells in fatal and non-fatal human Ebola infections. *PLoS Negl Trop Dis* 2017;11(5):e0005645.
134. Ciorba A, Matteucci G, Perini L, et al. Infezione da virus Ebola nella scimmia: reperti clinici et anatomoistopatologici. Osservati nel corso del primo episidio verificatosi in Europa. *Veterinaria* 1997;11(3):109–112.
135. Clark DV, Kibuuka H, Millard M, et al. Long-term sequelae after Ebola virus disease in Bundibugyo, Uganda: a retrospective cohort study. *Lancet Infect Dis* 2015;15(8):905–912.
136. Cnops L, de Smet B, Mbala-Kingebeni P, et al. Where are the Ebola diagnostics from last time? *Nature* 2019;565(7740):419–421.
137. Coffin KM, Liu J, Warren TK, et al. Persistent Marburg virus infection in the testes of nonhuman primate survivors. *Cell Host Microbe* 2018;24(3):405.e403–416.e403.
138. Colebunders RL. Is Plasmodium species parasitemia really associated with increased survival in Ebola virus-infected patients? *Clin Infect Dis* 2017;64(2):231–232.
139. Collar AL, Clarke EC, Anaya E, et al. Comparison of N- and O-linked glycosylation patterns of ebolavirus glycoproteins. *Virology* 2017;502:39–47.
140. Connolly BM, Steele KE, Davis KJ, et al. Pathogenesis of experimental Ebola virus infection in guinea pigs. *J Infect Dis* 1999;179(Suppl 1):S203–S217.
141. Connor MJ Jr, Kraft C, Mehta AK, et al. Successful delivery of RRT in Ebola virus disease. *J Am Soc Nephrol* 2015;26(1):31–37.
142. Conrad JL, Isaacson M, Smith EB, et al. Epidemiologic investigation of Marburg virus disease, Southern Africa, 1975. *Am J Trop Med Hyg* 1978;27(6):1210–1215.
143. Cooper TK, Huzella L, Johnson JC, et al. Histology, immunohistochemistry, and in situ hybridization reveal overlooked Ebola virus target tissues in the Ebola virus disease guinea pig model. *Sci Rep* 2018;8(1):1250.
144. Côté M, Misasi J, Ren T, et al. Small molecule inhibitors reveal Niemann-Pick C1 is essential for Ebola virus infection. *Nature* 2011;477(7364):344–348.
145. Cotte J, Cordier P-Y, Bordes J, et al. Fluid resuscitation in Ebola virus disease: aA comparison of peripheral and central venous accesses. *Anaesth Crit Care Pain Med* 2015;34(6):317–320.

146. Cournac JM, Karkowski L, Bordes J, et al. Rhabdomyolysis in Ebola virus disease. Results of an observational study in a treatment center in Guinea. *Clin Infect Dis* 2016;62(1):19–23.

147. Cox E, Antierens A, Bavari S, et al. Notes on the rRecord: cConsultation on mMonitored eEmergency use of uUnregistered and iInvestigational iInterventions for Ebola vVirus dDisease (EVD). Geneva: World Health Organization; 2018. Available at: https://www.who.int/emergencies/ebola/MEURI-Ebola.pdf

148. Crary SM, Towner JS, Honig JE, et al. Analysis of the role of predicted RNA secondary structures in Ebola virus replication. *Virology* 2003;306(2):210–218.

149. Cross RW, Fenton KA, Geisbert JB, et al. Comparison of the pathogenesis of the Angola and Ravn strains of Marburg virus in the outbred guinea pig model. *J Infect Dis* 2015;212(Suppl 2):S258–S270.

150. Cross RW, Mire CE, Agans KN, et al. Marburg and Ravn viruses fail to cause disease in the domestic ferret (Mustela putorius furo). *J Infect Dis* 2018;218(Suppl 5):S448–S452.

151. Cross RW, Mire CE, Borisevich V, et al. The domestic ferret (Mustela putorius furo) as a lethal infection model for 3 species of Ebolavirus. *J Infect Dis* 2016;214(4):565–569.

152. Crowe SJ, Maenner MJ, Kuah S, et al. Prognostic indicators for Ebola patient survival. *Emerg Infect Dis* 2016;22(2):217–223.

153. Daddario-DiCaprio KM, Geisbert TW, Geisbert JB, et al. Cross-protection against Marburg virus strains by using a live, attenuated recombinant vaccine. *J Virol* 2006;80(19):9659–9666.

154. Daddario-DiCaprio KM, Geisbert TW, Stroher U, et al. Postexposure protection against Marburg haemorrhagic fever with recombinant vesicular stomatitis virus vectors in non-human primates: an efficacy assessment. *Lancet* 2006;367(9520):1399–1404.

155. Davis KJ, Anderson AO, Geisbert TW, et al. Pathology of experimental Ebola virus infection in African green monkeys. Involvement of fibroblastic reticular cells. *Arch Pathol Lab Med* 1997;121(8):805–819.

156. de Greslan T, Billhot M, Rousseau C, et al. Ebola virus-related encephalitis. *Clin Infect Dis* 2016;63(8):1076–1078.

157. de la Vega M-A, Bello A, Chaillet P, et al. Diagnosis and management of Ebola samples in the laboratory. *Expert Rev Anti Infect Ther* 2016;14(6):557–567.

158. de la Vega M-A, Caleo G, Audet J, et al. Ebola viral load at diagnosis associates with patient outcome and outbreak evolution. *J Clin Invest* 2015;125(12):4421–4428.

159. de la Vega M-A, Soule G, Tran KN, et al. Modeling Ebola virus transmission using ferrets mSphere 2018;3(5):e00309–e00318.

160. de la Vega M-A, Wong G, Kobinger GP, et al. The multiple roles of sGP in Ebola pathogenesis. *Viral Immunol* 2015;28(1):3–9.

161. de Santis O, Audran R, Pothin E, et al. Safety and immunogenicity of a chimpanzee adenovirus-vectored Ebola vaccine in healthy adults: a randomised, double-blind, placebo-controlled, dose-finding, phase 1/2a study. *Lancet Infect Dis* 2016;16(3):311–320.

162. de Wit E, Munster VJ, Metwally SA, et al. Assessment of rodents as animal models for Reston ebolavirus. *J Infect Dis* 2011;204(Suppl 3):S968–S972.

163. Deen GF, Broutet N, Xu W, et al. Ebola RNA persistence in semen of Ebola virus disease survivors—final report. *N Engl J Med* 2017;377(15):1428–1437.

164. Deflubé LR, Cressey TN, Hume AJ, et al. Ebolavirus polymerase uses an unconventional genome replication mechanism. *Proc Natl Acad Sci U S A* 2019;116(17):8535–8543.

165. del Vecchio K, Frick CT, Gc JB, et al. A cationic, C-terminal patch and structural rearrangements in Ebola virus matrix VP40 protein control its interactions with phosphatidylserine. *J Biol Chem* 2018;293(9):3335–3349.

166. Demetria C, Smith I, Tan T, et al. Reemergence of Reston ebolavirus in cynomolgus monkeys, the Philippines, 2015. *Emerg Infect Dis* 2018;24(7):1285–1291.

167. den Boon S, Marston BJ, Nyenswah TG, et al. Ebola virus infection associated with transmission from survivors. *Emerg Infect Dis* 2019;25(2):249–255.

168. Dessen A, Volchkov V, Dolnik O, et al. Crystal structure of the matrix protein VP40 from Ebola virus. *EMBO J* 2000;19(16):4228–4236.

169. Diallo MSK, Rabilloud M, Ayouba A, et al. Prevalence of infection among asymptomatic and paucisymptomatic contact persons exposed to Ebola virus in Guinea: a retrospective, cross-sectional observational study. *Lancet Infect Dis* 2019;19(3):308–316.

170. Diallo B, Sissoko D, Loman NJ, et al. Resurgence of Ebola virus disease in Guinea linked to a survivor with virus persistence in seminal fluid for more than 500 days. *Clin Infect Dis* 2016;63(10):1353–1356.

171. Dias JM, Kuehne AI, Abelson DM, et al. A shared structural solution for neutralizing ebolaviruses. *Nat Struct Mol Biol* 2011;18(12):1424–1427.

172. Diehl WE, Lin AE, Grubaugh ND, et al. Ebola virus glycoprotein with increased infectivity dominated the 2013-2016 epidemic. *Cell* 2016;167(4):1088–1098.e1086.

173. Dietrich M, Knobloch J. Maridi-hämorrhagisches Fieber; die Bedeutung einer neuen Viruskrankheit. *Verh Dtsch Ges Inn Med* 1978;84:931–933.

174. Dietrich M, Schumacher HH, Peters D, et al. Human pathology of Ebola (Maridi) virus infection in the Sudan. In: Pattyn SR, ed. *Ebola Virus Haemorrhagic Fever*. Amsterdam: Elsevier/North-Holland Biomedical Press; 1978:37–41.

175. Dietz PM, Jambai A, Paweska JT, et al. Epidemiology and risk factors for Ebola virus disease in Sierra Leone-23 May 2014 to 31 January 2015. *Clin Infect Dis* 2015;61(11):1648–1654.

176. Dietzel E, Schudt G, Krähling V, et al. Functional characterization of adaptive mutations during the West African Ebola virus outbreak. *J Virol* 2017;91(2):e01913–e01916.

177. Dokubo EK, Wendland A, Mate SE, et al. Persistence of Ebola virus after the end of widespread transmission in Liberia: an outbreak report. *Lancet Infect Dis* 2018;18(9):1015–1024.

178. Dolnik O, Kolesnikova L, Stevermann L, et al. Tsg101 is recruited by a late domain of the nucleocapsid protein to support budding of Marburg virus-like particles. *J Virol* 2010;84(15):7847–7856.

179. Dolnik O, Kolesnikova L, Welsch S, et al. Interaction with Tsg101 is necessary for the efficient transport and release of nucleocapsids in Mmarburg virus-infected cells. *PLoS Pathog* 2014;10(10):e1004463.

180. Dolnik O, Stevermann L, Kolesnikova L, et al. Marburg virus inclusions: a virus-induced microcompartment and interface to multivesicular bodies and the late endosomal compartment. *Eur J Cell Biol* 2015;94(7-9):323–331.

181. Dolnik O, Volchkova V, Garten W, et al. Ectodomain shedding of the glycoprotein GP of Ebola virus. *EMBO J* 2004;23(10):2175–2184.

182. Dolzhikova IV, Zubkova OV, Tukhvatulin AI, et al. Safety and immunogenicity of GamEvac-Combi, a heterologous VSV- and Ad5-vectored Ebola vaccine: an open phase I/II trial in healthy adults in Russia. *Hum Vaccin Immunother* 2017;13(3):613–620.

183. Dörnemann J, Burzio C, Ronsse A, et al. First newborn baby to receive experimental therapies survives Ebola virus disease. *J Infect Dis* 2017;215(2):171–174.

184. Dowell SF. Ebola hemorrhagic fever: why were children spared? *Pediatr Infect Dis J* 1996;15(3):189–191.

185. Dowell SF, Mukunu R, Ksiazek TG, et al. Transmission of Ebola hemorrhagic fever: a study of risk factors in family members, Kikwit, Democratic Republic of the Congo, 1995. Commission de Lutte contre les Epidemies a Kikwit. *J Infect Dis* 1999;179(Suppl 1):S87–S91.

186. Dragovich MA, Fortoul N, Jagota A, et al. Biomechanical characterization of TIM protein-mediated Ebola virus-host cell adhesion. *Sci Rep* 2019;9(1):267.

187. Dube D, Brecher MB, Delos SE, et al. The primed ebolavirus glycoprotein (19-kilodalton GP$_{1,2}$): sequence and residues critical for host cell binding. *J Virol* 2009;83(7):2883–2891.

188. Dudas G, Carvalho LM, Bedford T, et al. Virus genomes reveal factors that spread and sustained the Ebola epidemic. *Nature* 2017;544(7650):309–315.

189. Ebihara H, Rockx B, Marzi A, et al. Host response dynamics following lethal infection of rhesus macaques with Zaire ebolavirus. *J Infect Dis* 2011;204(Suppl 3):S991–S999.

190. Ebihara H, Takada A, Kobasa D, et al. Molecular determinants of Ebola virus virulence in mice. *PLoS Pathog* 2006;2(7):e73.

191. Ebihara H, Zivcec M, Gardner D, et al. A Syrian golden hamster model recapitulating Ebola hemorrhagic fever. *J Infect Dis* 2013;207(2):306–318.

192. Edwards MR, Basler CF. Marburg virus VP24 protein relieves suppression of the NF-κB pathway through interaction with Kelch-like ECH-associated protein 1. *J Infect Dis.* 2015;212(Suppl 2):S154–159.

193. Edwards MR, Johnson B, Mire CE, et al. The Marburg virus VP24 protein interacts with Keap1 to activate the cytoprotective antioxidant response pathway. *Cell Rep* 2014;6(6):1017–1025.

194. Edwards MR, Liu G, Mire CE, et al. Differential regulation of interferon responses by Ebola and Marburg virus VP35 proteins. *Cell Rep* 2016;14(7):1632–1640.

195. Edwards MR, Liu H, Shabman RS, et al. Conservation of structure and immune antagonist functions of filoviral VP35 homologs present in microbat genomes. *Cell Rep* 2018;24(4):861.e866–872.e866.

196. Egbring R, Slenczka W, Baltzer G. Clinical manifestations and mechanism of the haemorrhagic diathesis in Marburg virus disease. In: Martini GA, Siegert R, eds. *Marburg Virus Disease*. Berlin: Springer-Verlag; 1971:41–49.

197. el Tahir BM. The haemorrhagic fever outbreak in Maridi, Western Equatoria, southern Sudan. In: Pattyn SR, ed. *Ebola Virus Haemorrhagic Fever*. Amsterdam: Elsevier/North-Holland Biomedical Press; 1978:125–127.

198. Elliott LH, Kiley MP, McCormick JB. Descriptive analysis of Ebola virus proteins. *Virology* 1985;147(1):169–176.

199. Elliott LH, Sanchez A, Holloway BP, et al. Ebola protein analyses for the determination of genetic organization. *Arch Virol* 1993;133(3–4):423–436.

200. Ellis DS, Bowen ETW, Simpson DIH, et al. Ebola virus: a comparison, at ultrastructural level, of the behaviour of the Sudan and Zaire strains in monkeys. *Br J Exp Pathol* 1978;59(6):584–593.

201. Ellis DS, Simpson DIH, Francis DP, et al. Ultrastructure of Ebola virus particles in human liver. *J Clin Pathol* 1978;31(3):201–208.

202. Ellis DS, Stamford S, Lloyd G, et al. Ebola and Marburg viruses: I. Some ultrastructural differences between strains when grown in Vero cells. *J Med Virol* 1979;4(3):201–211.

203. Ellis DS, Stamford S, Tvoey DG, et al. Ebola and Marburg viruses: II. Their development within Vero cells and the extra-cellular formation of branched and torus forms. *J Med Virol* 1979;4(3):213–225.

204. ElSherif MS, Brown C, MacKinnon-Cameron D, et al. Assessing the safety and immunogenicity of recombinant vesicular stomatitis virus Ebola vaccine in healthy adults: a randomized clinical trial. *CMAJ* 2017;189(24):E819–E827.

205. Emond RT, Evans B, Bowen ET, et al. A case of Ebola virus infection. *Br Med J* 1977;2(6086):541–544.

206. Enterlein S, Schmidt KM, Schümann M, et al. The Marburg virus 3′ noncoding region structurally and functionally differs from that of Ebola virus. *J Virol* 2009;83(9):4508–4519.

207. Enterlein S, Volchkov V, Weik M, et al. Rescue of recombinant Marburg virus from cDNA is dependent on nucleocapsid protein VP30. *J Virol* 2006;80(2):1038–1043.

208. Epstein L, Wong KK, Kallen AJ, et al. Post-Ebola signs and symptoms in U.S. survivors. *N Engl J Med* 2015;373(25):2484–2486.

209. Erickson BR, Sealy TK, Flietstra T, et al. Ebola virus disease diagnostics, Sierra Leone: analysis of real-time reverse transcription-polymerase chain reaction values for clinical blood and oral swab specimens. *J Infect Dis* 2016;214(Suppl 3):S258–S262.

210. Escudero-Pérez B, Volchkova VA, Dolnik O, et al. Shed GP of Ebola virus triggers immune activation and increased vascular permeability. *PLoS Pathog* 2014;10(11):e1004509.

211. Espeland EM, Tsai C-W, Larsen J, et al. Safeguarding against Ebola: vaccines and therapeutics to be stockpiled for future outbreaks. *PLoS Negl Trop Dis* 2018;12(4):e0006275.

212. Etard J-F, Sow MS, Leroy S, et al. Multidisciplinary assessment of post-Ebola sequelae in Guinea (Postebogui): an observational cohort study. *Lancet Infect Dis* 2017;17(5):545–552.

213. Ewer K, Rampling T, Venkatraman N, et al. A monovalent chimpanzee adenovirus Ebola vaccine boosted with MVA. *N Engl J Med* 2016;374(17):1635–1646.

214. Fabozzi G, Nabel CS, Dolan MA, et al. Ebolavirus proteins suppress the effects of small interfering RNA by direct interaction with the mammalian RNA interference pathway. *J Virol* 2011;85(6):2512–2523.

215. Falzarano D, Feldmann F, Grolla A, et al. Single immunization with a monovalent vesicular stomatitis virus-based vaccine protects nonhuman primates against heterologous challenge with Bundibugyo ebolavirus. *J Infect Dis* 2011;204(Suppl 3):S1082–S1089.

216. Falzarano D, Krokhin O, Wahl-Jensen V, et al. Structure-function analysis of the soluble glycoprotein, sGP, of Ebola virus. *Chembiochem* 2006;7(10):1605–1611.

217. Feagins AR, Basler CF. The VP40 protein of Marburg virus exhibits impaired budding and increased sensitivity to human tetherin following mouse adaptation. *J Virol* 2014;88(24):14440–14450.

218. Feagins AR, Basler CF. Lloviu virus VP24 and VP35 proteins function as innate immune antagonists in human and bat cells. *Virology* 2015;485:145–152.
219. Feagins AR, Basler CF. Amino acid residue at position 79 of Marburg virus VP40 confers interferon antagonism in mouse cells. *J Infect Dis* 2015;212(Suppl 2):S219–225.
220. Fedewa G, Radoshitzky SR, Chī X, et al. Ebola virus, but not Marburg virus, replicates efficiently and without required adaptation in snake cells. *Virus Evol* 2018;4(2):vey034.
221. Feldmann H, Bugany H, Mahner F, et al. Filovirus-induced endothelial leakage triggered by infected monocytes/macrophages. *J Virol* 1996;70(4):2208–2214.
222. Feldmann H, Mühlberger E, Randolf A, et al. Marburg virus, a filovirus: messenger RNAs, gene order, and regulatory elements of the replication cycle. *Virus Res* 1992;24(1):1–19.
223. Feldmann H, Nichol ST, Klenk H-D, et al. Characterization of filoviruses based on differences in structure and antigenicity of the virion glycoprotein. *Virology* 1994; 199(2):469–473.
224. Feldmann F, Shupert WL, Haddock E, et al. Gamma irradiation as an effective method for inactivation of emerging viral pathogens. *Am J Trop Med Hyg* 2019;100(5):1275–1277.
225. Feldmann H, Will C, Schikore M, et al. Glycosylation and oligomerization of the spike protein of Marburg virus. *Virology* 1991;182(1):353–356.
226. Feng Z, Cerveny M, Yan Z, et al. The VP35 protein of Ebola virus inhibits the antiviral effect mediated by double-stranded RNA-dependent protein kinase PKR. *J Virol* 2007;81(1):182–192.
227. Ferron F, Longhi S, Henrissat B, et al. Viral RNA-polymerases—a predicted 2′-O-ribose methyltransferase domain shared by all Mononegavirales. *Trends Biochem Sci* 2002;27(5):222–224.
228. Fischer WA, Brown J, Wohl DA, et al. Ebola virus ribonucleic acid detection in semen more than two years after resolution of acute Ebola virus infection. *Open Forum Infect Dis* 2017;4(3):ofx155.
229. Fischer R, Judson S, Miazgowicz K, et al. Ebola virus stability on surfaces and in fluids in simulated outbreak environments. *Emerg Infect Dis* 2015;21(7):1243–1246.
230. Fisher-Hoch SP, Brammer TL, Trappier SG, et al. Pathogenic potential of filoviruses: role of geographic origin of primate host and virus strain. *J Infect Dis* 1992;166(4):753–763.
231. Fisher-Hoch SP, Platt GS, Lloyd G, et al. Haematological and biochemical monitoring of Ebola infection in rhesus monkeys: implications for patient management. *Lancet* 1983;2(8358):1055–1058.
232. Fisher-Hoch SP, Platt GS, Neild GH, et al. Pathophysiology of shock and hemorrhage in a fulminating viral infection (Ebola). *J Infect Dis* 1985;152(5):887–894.
233. Fitzpatrick G, Vogt F, Moi Gbabai OBM, et al. The contribution of Ebola viral load at admission and other patient characteristics to mortality in a Médecins Sans Frontières Ebola case management centre, Kailahun, Sierra Leone, June-October 2014. *J Infect Dis* 2015;212(11):1752–1758.
234. Flyak AI, Ilinykh PA, Murin CD, et al. Mechanism of human antibody-mediated neutralization of Marburg virus. *Cell* 2015;160(5):893–903.
235. Flyak AI, Kuzmina N, Murin CD, et al. Broadly neutralizing antibodies from human survivors target a conserved site in the Ebola virus glycoprotein HR2-MPER region. *Nat Microbiol* 2018;3(6):670–677.
236. Flyak AI, Shen X, Murin CD, et al. Cross-reactive and potent neutralizing antibody responses in human survivors of natural ebolavirus infection. *Cell* 2016;164(3):392–405.
237. Forbes KM, Webala PW, Jääskeläinen AJ, et al. Bombali virus in Mops condylurus Bat, Kenya, *Emerg Infect Dis* 2019;25(5):955–957.
238. Formenty P, Boesch C, Wyers M, et al. Ebola virus outbreak among wild chimpanzees living in a rain forest of Côte d'Ivoire. *J Infect Dis* 1999;179(Suppl 1):S120–S126.
239. Formenty P, Epelboin A, Allarangar Y, et al. Séminaire de formation des formateurs et d'analyse des épidémies de fièvre hémorragique due au virus Ebola en Afrique centrale de 2001 à 2004. Brazzaville, République du Congo, 6-8 avril 2004. *Bull Soc Pathol Exot* 2005;98(3):244–254.
240. Formenty P, Hatz C, Le Guenno B, et al. Human infection due to Ebola virus, subtype Côte d'Ivoire: clinical and biologic presentation. *J Infect Dis* 1999;179(Suppl 1):S48–S53.
241. Formenty P, Libama F, Epelboin A, et al. L'épidémie de fièvre hémorragique à virus Ebola en république du Congo, 2003: une nouvelle stratégie? *Méd Trop (Mars)* 2003;63(3):291–295.
242. Forrester JD, Hunter JC, Pillai SK, et al. Cluster of Ebola cases among Liberian and U.S. health care workers in an Ebola treatment unit and adjacent hospital—Liberia, 2014. *MMWR Morb Mortal Wkly Rep* 2014;63(41):925–929.
243. Fowler RA, Fletcher T, Fischer WA, II, et al. Caring for critically ill patients with Ebola virus disease. Perspectives from West Africa. *Am J Respir Crit Care Med* 2014;190(7):733–737.
244. Francis DP, Smith DH, Highton RB, et al. Ebola fever in the Sudan, 1976: epidemiological aspects of the disease. In: Pattyn SR, ed. *Ebola Virus Haemorrhagic Fever*. Amsterdam: Elsevier/North-Holland Biomedical Press; 1978:129–135.
245. Fritz EA, Geisbert JB, Geisbert TW, et al. Cellular immune response to Marburg virus infection in cynomolgus macaques. *Viral Immunol* 2008;21(3):355–363.
246. Froude JW, Pelat T, Miethe S, et al. Generation and characterization of protective antibodies to Marburg virus. *MAbs* 2017;9(4):696–703.
247. Funke C, Becker S, Dartsch H, et al. Acylation of the Marburg virus glycoprotein. *Virology* 1995;208(1):289–297.
248. Furuyama W, Marzi A, Nanbo A, et al. Discovery of an antibody for pan-ebolavirus therapy. *Sci Rep* 2016;6:20514.
249. Gałaś A. The determinants of spread of Ebola virus disease—an evidence from the past outbreak experiences. *Folia Med Cracov* 2014;54(3):17–25.
250. Gallaher WR. Similar structural models of the transmembrane proteins of Ebola and avian sarcoma viruses. *Cell* 1996;85(4):477–478.
251. Gallaher WR, DiSimone C, Buchmeier MJ. The viral transmembrane superfamily: possible divergence of Arenavirus and Filovirus glycoproteins from a common RNA virus ancestor. *BMC Microbiol* 2001;1(1):1.
252. Garbutt M, Liebscher R, Wahl-Jensen V, et al. Properties of replication-competent vesicular stomatitis virus vectors expressing glycoproteins of filoviruses and arenaviruses. *J Virol* 2004;78(10):5458–5465.
253. Gaudinski MR, Coates EE, Novik L, et al. Safety, tolerability, pharmacokinetics, and immunogenicity of the therapeutic monoclonal antibody mAb114 targeting Ebola virus glycoprotein (VRC 608): an open-label phase 1 study. *Lancet* 2019;393(10174):889–898.
254. Gear JHS. Marburg fever in the Johannesburg General Hospital—a personal account of the outbreak. *Bacteria* 1975;(1):7–14.
255. Gear JHS. The diagnosis of hemorrhagic fever. In: Gear JHS, ed. *CRC Handbook of Viral and Rickettsial Hemorrhagic Fevers*. Boca Raton: CRC Press; 1988:231–239.
256. Gear JSS, Cassel GA, Gear AJ, et al. Outbreak of Marburg virus disease in Johannesburg. *Br Med J* 1975;4(5995):489–493.
257. Gedigk P, Bechtelsheimer H, Korb G. Die pathologische Anatomie der "Marburg-Virus"-Krankheit (sog. "Marburger Affenkrankheit"). *Dtsch Med Wochenschr* 1968;93(12):590–601.
258. Geisbert TW, Bailey M, Hensley L, et al. Recombinant adenovirus serotype 26 (Ad26) and Ad35 vaccine vectors bypass immunity to Ad5 and protect nonhuman primates against ebolavirus challenge. *J Virol* 2011;85(9):4222–4233.
259. Geisbert TW, Daddario-DiCaprio KM, Geisbert JB, et al. Marburg virus Angola infection of rhesus macaques: pathogenesis and treatment with recombinant nematode anticoagulant protein c2. *J Infect Dis* 2007;196(Suppl 2):S372–S381.
260. Geisbert TW, Daddario-Dicaprio KM, Geisbert JB, et al. Vesicular stomatitis virus-based vaccines protect nonhuman primates against aerosol challenge with Ebola and Marburg viruses. *Vaccine* 2008;26(52):6894–6900.
261. Geisbert TW, Daddario-Dicaprio KM, Lewis MG, et al. Vesicular stomatitis virus-based Ebola vaccine is well-tolerated and protects immunocompromised nonhuman primates. *PLoS Pathog* 2008;4(11):e1000225.
262. Geisbert TW, Daddario-DiCaprio KM, Williams KJN, et al. Recombinant vesicular stomatitis virus vector mediates postexposure protection against Sudan Ebola hemorrhagic fever in nonhuman primates. *J Virol* 2008;82(11):5664–5668.
263. Geisbert TW, Geisbert JB, Leung A, et al. Single-injection vaccine protects nonhuman primates against infection with Marburg virus and three species of Ebola virus. *J Virol* 2009;83(14):7296–7304.
264. Geisbert TW, Hensley LE, Gibb TR, et al. Apoptosis induced in vitro and in vivo during infection by Ebola and Marburg viruses. *Lab Invest* 2000;80(2):171–186.
265. Geisbert TW, Hensley LE, Kagan E, et al. Postexposure protection of guinea pigs against a lethal ebola virus challenge is conferred by RNA interference. *J Infect Dis* 2006;193(12):1650–1657.
266. Geisbert TW, Hensley LE, Larsen T, et al. Pathogenesis of Ebola hemorrhagic fever in cynomolgus macaques: evidence that dendritic cells are early and sustained targets of infection. *Am J Pathol* 2003;163(6):2347–2370.
267. Geisbert TW, Jaax NK. Marburg hemorrhagic fever: report of a case studied by immunohistochemistry and electron microscopy. *Ultrastruct Pathol* 1998;22(1):3–17.
268. Geisbert TW, Jahrling PB. Use of immunoelectron microscopy to show Ebola virus during the 1989 United States epizootic. *J Clin Pathol* 1990;43(10):813–816.
269. Geisbert TW, Jahrling PB. Differentiation of filoviruses by electron microscopy. *Virus Res* 1995;39(2-3):129–150.
270. Geisbert TW, Jahrling PB, Hanes MA, et al. Association of Ebola-related Reston virus particles and antigen with tissue lesions of monkeys imported to the United States. *J Comp Pathol* 1992;106(2):137–152.
271. Geisbert TW, Strong JE, Feldmann H. Considerations in the use of nonhuman primate models of Ebola virus and Marburg virus infection. *J Infect Dis* 2015;212(Suppl 2):S91–S97.
272. Geisbert TW, Young HA, Jahrling PB, et al. Mechanisms underlying coagulation abnormalities in Ebola hemorrhagic fever: overexpression of tissue factor in primate monocytes/macrophages is a key event. *J Infect Dis* 2003;188(11):1618–1629.
273. Geisbert TW, Young HA, Jahrling PB, et al. Pathogenesis of Ebola hemorrhagic fever in primate models: evidence that hemorrhage is not a direct effect of virus-induced cytolysis of endothelial cells. *Am J Pathol* 2003;163(6):2371–2382.
274. Georges AJ, Baize S, Leroy EM, et al. Virus Ebola: l'essentiel pour le praticien. *Méd Trop (Mars)* 1998;58(2):177–186.
275. Georges A-J, Leroy EM, Renaut AA, et al. Ebola hemorrhagic fever outbreaks in Gabon, 1994-1997: epidemiologic and health control issues. *J Infect Dis* 1999;179(Suppl 1):S65–S75.
276. Georges-Courbot MC, Lu CY, Lansoud-Soukate J, et al. Isolation and partial molecular characterisation of a strain of Ebola virus during a recent epidemic of viral haemorrhagic fever in Gabon. *Lancet* 1997;349(9046):181.
277. Georges-Courbot M-C, Sanchez A, Lu C-Y, et al. Isolation and phylogenetic characterization of Ebola viruses causing different outbreaks in Gabon. *Emerg Infect Dis* 1997;3(1):59–62.
278. Geyer H, Will C, Feldmann H, et al. Carbohydrate structure of Marburg virus glycoprotein. *Glycobiology* 1992;2(4):299–312.
279. Gilligan KJ, Geisbert JB, Jahrling PB, et al. Assessment of protective immunity conferred by recombinant vaccinia viruses to guinea pigs challenged with Ebola virus. In: Brown F, Burton D, Doherty P, et al., eds. *Vaccines97: Modern Approaches to New Vaccines, Including Prevention of AIDS*. New York: Cold Spring Harbor Laboratory Press; 1997:87–92.
280. Gire SK, Goba A, Andersen KG, et al. Genomic surveillance elucidates Ebola virus origin and transmission during the 2014 outbreak. *Science* 2014;345(6202):1369–1372.
281. Gleason B, Redd J, Kilmarx P, et al. Establishment of an Ebola treatment unit and laboratory—Bombali District, Sierra Leone, July 2014-January 2015. *MMWR Morb Mortal Wkly Rep* 2015;64(39):1108–1111.
282. Glynn JR. Age-specific incidence of Ebola virus disease. *Lancet* 2015;386(9992):432.
283. Glynn JR, Bower H, Johnson S, et al. Asymptomatic infection and unrecognised Ebola virus disease in Ebola-affected households in Sierra Leone: a cross-sectional study using a new non-invasive assay for antibodies to Ebola virus. *Lancet Infect Dis* 2017;17(6):645–653.
284. Gnirß K, Kühl A, Karsten C, et al. Cathepsins B and L activate Ebola but not Marburg virus glycoproteins for efficient entry into cell lines and macrophages independent of TMPRSS2 expression. *Virology* 2012;424(1):3–10.
285. Goldstein T, Anthony SJ, Gbakima A, et al. The discovery of Bombali virus adds further support for bats as hosts of ebolaviruses. *Nat Microbiol* 2018;3(10):1084–1089.
286. Gomis-Rüth FX, Dessen A, Timmins J, et al. The matrix protein VP40 from Ebola virus octamerizes into pore-like structures with specific RNA binding properties. *Structure* 2003;11(4):423–433.

287. González-Hernández M, Müller A, Hoenen T, et al. Calu-3 cells are largely resistant to entry driven by filovirus glycoproteins and the entry defect can be rescued by directed expression of DC-SIGN or cathepsin L. *Virology* 2019;532:22–29.
288. Gramberg T, Hofmann H, Möller P, et al. LSECtin interacts with filovirus glycoproteins and the spike protein of SARS coronavirus. *Virology* 2005;340(2):224–236.
289. Grard G, Biek R, Tamfum J-J, et al. Emergence of divergent Zaire Ebola virus strains in Democratic Republic of the Congo in 2007 and 2008. *J Infect Dis* 2011;204(Suppl 3):S776–S784.
290. Grens K. Bats in Sierra Leone carry Marburg virus. *Scientist.* 2018. Available at: https://wwwthe-scientistcom/news-opinion/bats-in-sierra-leone-carry-marburg-virus-65271
291. Grolla A, Lucht A, Dick D, et al. Laboratory diagnosis of Ebola and Marburg hemorrhagic fever. *Bull Soc Pathol Exot* 2005;98(3):205–209.
292. Groseth A, Charton JE, Sauerborn M, et al. The Ebola virus ribonucleoprotein complex: a novel VP30-L interaction identified. *Virus Res* 2009;140(1-2):8–14.
293. Groseth A, Feldmann H, Theriault S, et al. RNA polymerase I-driven minigenome system for Ebola viruses. *J Virol* 2005;79(7):4425–4433.
294. Grosse-Brockhoff F, Krauss H, Rosie RH, et al. Eine bisher unbekannte Infektionskrankheit durch Kontakt mit Affen—Zusammenfassender Bericht. *Dtsch Med Wochenschr* 1968;93(12a).
295. Gupta M, MacNeil A, Reed ZD, et al. Serology and cytokine profiles in patients infected with the newly discovered Bundibugyo ebolavirus. *Virology* 2012;423(2):119–124.
296. Gupta M, Mahanty S, Bray M, et al. Passive transfer of antibodies protects immunocompetent and immunodeficient mice against lethal Ebola virus infection without complete inhibition of viral replication. *J Virol* 2001;75(10):4649–4654.
297. Gupta M, Mahanty S, Greer P, et al. Persistent infection with Ebola virus under conditions of partial immunity. *J Virol* 2004;78(2):958–967.
298. Haas R, Maass G, Müller J, et al. Experimentelle Infektionen von Cercopithecus aethiops mit dem Erreger des Frankfurt-Marburg-Syndroms (FMS). *Z Med Mikrobiol Immunol* 1968;154(3):210–220.
299. Haasnoot J, de Vries W, Geutjes E-J, et al. The Ebola virus VP35 protein is a suppressor of RNA silencing. *PLoS Pathog* 2007;3(6):e86.
300. Haddad LB, Jamieson DJ, Rasmussen SA. Pregnant women and the Ebola crisis. *N Engl J Med* 2018;379(26):2492–2493.
301. Haddock E, Feldmann F, Feldmann H. Effective chemical inactivation of Ebola virus. *Emerg Infect Dis* 2016;22(7):1292–1294.
302. Halperin SA, Arribas JR, Rupp R, et al. Six-month safety data of recombinant vesicular stomatitis virus-Zaire Ebola virus envelope glycoprotein vaccine in a phase 3 double-blind, placebo-controlled randomized study in healthy adults. *J Infect Dis* 2017;215(12):1789–1798.
303. Halpern SD, Emanuel EJ. Use of life-sustaining therapies for patients with Ebola virus disease. *Ann Intern Med* 2015;163(1):70.
304. Han Z, Madara JJ, Liu Y, et al. ALIX rescues budding of a double PTAP/PPEY L-domain deletion mutant of Ebola VP40: a role for ALIX in Ebola virus egress. *J Infect Dis* 2015;212(Suppl 2):S138–S145.
305. Han Z, Sagum CA, Bedford MT, et al. ITCH E3 ubiquitin ligase interacts with Ebola virus VP40 to regulate budding. *J Virol* 2016;90(20):9163–9171.
306. Han Z, Sagum CA, Takizawa F, et al. Ubiquitin ligase WWP1 interacts with Ebola virus VP40 to regulate egress. *J Virol* 2017;91(20):e00812–e00817.
307. Hartlieb B, Modrof J, Mühlberger E, et al. Oligomerization of Ebola virus VP30 is essential for viral transcription and can be inhibited by a synthetic peptide. *J Biol Chem* 2003;278(43):41830–41836.
308. Hartlieb B, Muziol T, Weissenhorn W, et al. Crystal structure of the C-terminal domain of Ebola virus VP30 reveals a role in transcription and nucleocapsid association. *Proc Natl Acad Sci U S A* 2007;104(2):624–629.
309. Hartman AL, Bird BH, Towner JS, et al. Inhibition of IRF-3 activation by VP35 is critical for the high level of virulence of Ebola virus. *J Virol* 2008;82(6):2699–2704.
310. Hartman AL, Ling L, Nichol ST, Hibberd ML. Whole-genome expression profiling reveals that inhibition of host innate immune response pathways by Ebola virus can be reversed by a single amino acid change in the VP35 protein. *J Virol* 2008;82(11):5348–5358.
311. Hartman AL, Towner JS, Nichol ST. A C-terminal basic amino acid motif of Zaire ebolavirus VP35 is essential for type I interferon antagonism and displays high identity with the RNA-binding domain of another interferon antagonist, the NS1 protein of influenza A virus. *Virology* 2004;328(2):177–184.
312. Harty RN. No exit: targeting the budding process to inhibit filovirus replication. *Antiviral Res* 2009;81(3):189–197.
313. Harty RN, Brown ME, Wang G, et al. A PPxY motif within the VP40 protein of Ebola virus interacts physically and functionally with a ubiquitin ligase: implications for filovirus budding. *Proc Natl Acad Sci U S A* 2000;97(25):13871–13876.
314. Hashiguchi T, Fusco ML, Bornholdt ZA, et al. Structural basis for Marburg virus neutralization by a cross-reactive human antibody. *Cell* 2015;160(5):904–912.
315. Hayes CG, Burans JP, Ksiazek TG, et al. Outbreak of fatal illness among captive macaques in the Philippines caused by an Ebola-related filovirus. *Am J Trop Med Hyg* 1992;46(6):664–671.
316. He B, Feng Y, Zhang H, et al. Filovirus RNA in fruit bats, China. *Emerg Infect Dis* 2015;21(9):1675–1677.
317. He J, Melnik LI, Komin A, et al. Ebola virus delta peptide is a viroporin. *J Virol* 2017;91(16):e00438–e00417.
318. Hellman J. Addressing the complications of Ebola and other viral hemorrhagic fever infections: using insights from bacterial and fungal sepsis. *PLoS Pathog* 2015;11(10):e1005088.
319. Henao-Restrepo AM, Camacho A, Longini IM, et al. Efficacy and effectiveness of an rVSV-vectored vaccine in preventing Ebola virus disease: final results from the Guinea ring vaccination, open-label, cluster-randomised trial (Ebola Ça Suffit!). *Lancet* 2017;389(10068):505–518.
320. Hennessen W. Epidemiology of "Marburg virus" disease. In: Martini GA, Siegert R, eds. *Marburg Virus Disease.* Berlin: Springer-Verlag; 1971:161–165.
321. Hensley LE, Alves DA, Geisbert JB, et al. Pathogenesis of Marburg hemorrhagic fever in cynomolgus macaques. *J Infect Dis* 2011;204(Suppl 3):S1021–S1031.
322. Hensley LE, Mulangu S, Asiedu C, et al. Demonstration of cross-protective vaccine immunity against an emerging pathogenic Ebolavirus Species. *PLoS Pathog* 2010;6(5):e1000904.
323. Hensley LE, Young HA, Jahrling PB, et al. Proinflammatory response during Ebola virus infection of primate models: possible involvement of the tumor necrosis factor receptor superfamily. *Immunol Lett* 2002;80(3):169–179.
324. Herbert AS, Davidson C, Kuehne AI, et al. Niemann-Pick C1 is essential for ebolavirus replication and pathogenesis in vivo. *MBio* 2015;6(3):e00565.
325. Herbert AS, Kuehne AI, Barth JF, et al. Venezuelan equine encephalitis virus replicon particle vaccine protects nonhuman primates from intramuscular and aerosol challenge with ebolavirus. *J Virol* 2013;87(9):4952–4964.
326. Hevey M, Negley D, Pushko P, et al. Marburg virus vaccines based upon alphavirus replicons protect guinea pigs and nonhuman primates. *Virology* 1998;251(1):28–37.
327. Heymann DL, Weisfeld JS, Webb PA, et al. Ebola hemorrhagic fever: Tandala, Zaire, 1977-1978. *J Infect Dis* 1980;142(3):372–376.
328. Hoenen T, Biedenkopf N, Zielecki F, et al. Oligomerization of Ebola virus VP40 is essential for particle morphogenesis and regulation of viral transcription. *J Virol* 2010;84(14):7053–7063.
329. Hoenen T, Brandt J, Caì Y, et al. Reverse genetics of filoviruses. *Curr Top Microbiol Immunol* 2017;411:421–445.
330. Hoenen T, Jung S, Herwig A, et al. Both matrix proteins of Ebola virus contribute to the regulation of viral genome replication and transcription. *Virology* 2010;403(1):56–66.
331. Hoenen T, Marzi A, Scott DP, et al. Soluble glycoprotein is not required for Ebola virus virulence in guinea pigs. *J Infect Dis* 2015;212(Suppl 2):S242–S246.
332. Hoenen T, Shabman RS, Groseth A, et al. Inclusion bodies are a site of ebolavirus replication. *J Virol* 2012;86(21):11779–11788.
333. Hoenen T, Volchkov V, Kolesnikova L, et al. VP40 octamers are essential for Ebola virus replication. *J Virol* 2005;79(3):1898–1905.
334. Hood CL, Abraham J, Boyington JC, et al. Biochemical and structural characterization of cathepsin L-processed Ebola virus glycoprotein: implications for viral entry and immunogenicity. *J Virol* 2010;84(6):2972–2982.
335. Hovette P. Epidémie de fièvre hémorragique à virus Marburg en Angola. *Méd Trop (Mars)* 2005;65(2):127–128.
336. Howell KA, Qiu X, Brannan JM, et al. Antibody treatment of Ebola and Sudan virus infection via a uniquely exposed epitope within the glycoprotein receptor-binding site. *Cell Rep* 2016;15(7):1514–1526.
337. Howlett P, Brown C, Helderman T, et al. Ebola virus disease complicated by late-onset encephalitis and polyarthritis, Sierra Leone., *Emerg Infect Dis* 2016;22(1):150–152.
338. Huang I-C, Bailey CC, Weyer JL, et al. Distinct patterns of IFITM-mediated restriction of filoviruses, SARS coronavirus, and influenza A virus. *PLoS Pathog* 2011;7(1):e1001258.
339. Huang Y, Xu L, Sun Y, et al. The assembly of Ebola virus nucleocapsid requires virion-associated proteins 35 and 24 and posttranslational modification of nucleoprotein. *Mol Cell* 2002;10(2):307–316.
340. Huber C, Finelli L, Stevens W. The economic and social burden of the 2014 Ebola outbreak in West Africa. *J Infect Dis* 2018;218(Suppl 5):S698–S704.
341. Huijbregts B, de Wachter P, Obiang LSN, et al. Ebola and the decline of gorilla Gorilla gorilla and chimpanzee Pan troglodytes populations in Minkebe Forest, north-eastern Gabon. *Oryx* 2003;37(4):437–443.
342. Hume A, Mühlberger E. Marburg virus viral protein 35 inhibits protein kinase R activation in a cell type-specific manner. *J Infect Dis* 2018;218(Suppl 5):S403–S408.
343. Hume AJ, Mühlberger E. Distinct genome replication and transcription strategies within the growing filovirus family. *J Mol Biol* 2019;431(21):4290–4320.
344. Hunt L, Gupta-Wright A, Simms V, et al. Clinical presentation, biochemical, and haematological parameters and their association with outcome in patients with Ebola virus disease: an observational cohort study. *Lancet Infect Dis* 2015;15(11):1292–1299.
345. Hunt CL, Kolokoltsov AA, Davey RA, et al. The Tyro3 receptor kinase Axl enhances macropinocytosis of Zaire ebolavirus. *J Virol* 2011;85(1):334–347.
346. Hutchinson KL, Rollin PE. Cytokine and chemokine expression in humans infected with Sudan Ebola virus. *J Infect Dis* 2007;196(Suppl 2):S357–S363.
347. Hutchinson KL, Villinger F, Miranda ME, et al. Multiplex analysis of cytokines in the blood of cynomolgus macaques naturally infected with Ebola virus (Reston serotype). *J Med Virol* 2001;65(3):561–566.
348. Huttner A, Agnandji ST, Combescure C, et al. Determinants of antibody persistence across doses and continents after single-dose rVSV-ZEBOV vaccination for Ebola virus disease: an observational cohort study. *Lancet Infect Dis* 2018;18(7):738–748.
349. Ikegami T, Calaor AB, Miranda ME, et al. Genome structure of Ebola virus subtype Reston: differences among Ebola subtypes. *Arch Virol* 2001;146(10):2021–2027.
350. Ilinykh PA, Lubaki NM, Widen SG, et al. Different temporal effects of Ebola virus VP35 and VP24 proteins on global gene expression in human dendritic cells. *J Virol* 2015;89(15):7567–7583.
351. Ilunga Kalenga O, Moeti M, Sparrow A, et al. The ongoing Ebola epidemic in the Democratic Republic of Congo, 2018-2019. *N Engl J Med* 2019;381(4):373–383.
352. Isaäcson M. Prevention and control of viral hemorrhagic fevers. In: Gear JHS, ed. *CRC Handbook of Viral and Rickettsial Hemorrhagic Fevers.* Boca Raton: CRC Press; 1988:253–261.
353. Isaacson M, Sureau P, Courteille G, et al. Clinical aspects of Ebola virus disease at the Ngaliema Hospital, Kinshasa, Zaire, 1976. In: Pattyn SR, ed. *Ebola Virus Haemorrhagic Fever.* Amsterdam: Elsevier/North-Holland Biomedical Press; 1978:22–26.
354. Ito H, Watanabe S, Takada A, et al. Ebola virus glycoprotein: proteolytic processing, acylation, cell tropism, and detection of neutralizing antibodies. *J Virol* 2001;75(3):1576–1580.
355. Iwasa A, Shimojima M, Kawaoka Y. sGP serves as a structural protein in Ebola virus infection. *J Infect Dis* 2011;204(Suppl 3):S897–S903.
356. Jaax NK, Davis KJ, Geisbert TJ, et al. Lethal experimental infection of rhesus monkeys with Ebola-Zaire (Mayinga) virus by the oral and conjunctival route of exposure. *Arch Pathol Lab Med* 1996;120(2):140–155.
357. Jaax J, Jaax NK. An Ebola filovirus is discovered in the USA: Reston, Virginia, USA, 1989. *Vet Herit* 2016;39(1):16–19.

358. Jaax N, Jahrling P, Geisbert T, et al. Transmission of Ebola virus (Zaire strain) to uninfected control monkeys in a biocontainment laboratory. *Lancet* 1995;346(8991-8992):1669–1671.
359. Jacobs M, Rodger A, Bell DJ, et al. Late Ebola virus relapse causing meningoencephalitis: a case report. *Lancet* 2016;388(10043):498–503.
360. Jácome R, Becerra A, Ponce de León S, et al. Structural analysis of monomeric RNA-dependent polymerases: evolutionary and therapeutic implications. PLoS One 2015;10(9):e0139001.
361. Jahrling PB, Geisbert TW, Jaax NK, et al. Experimental infection of cynomolgus macaques with Ebola-Reston filoviruses from the 1989-1990 U.S. epizootic. *Arch Virol Suppl* 1996;11:115–134.
362. Janke C, Heim KM, Steiner F, et al. Beyond Ebola treatment units: severe infection temporary treatment units as an essential element of Ebola case management during an outbreak. *BMC Infect Dis* 2017;17(1):124.
363. Jasenosky LD, Neumann G, Lukashevich I, et al. Ebola virus VP40-induced particle formation and association with the lipid bilayer. *J Virol* 2001;75(11):5205–5214.
364. Jayme SI, Field HE, de Jong C, et al. Molecular evidence of Ebola Reston virus infection in Philippine bats. *Virol J* 2015;12:107.
365. Jeffers SA, Sanders DA, Sanchez A. Covalent modifications of the Ebola virus glycoprotein. *J Virol* 2002;76(24):12463–12472.
366. Jeffs B, Roddy P, Weatherill D, et al. The Médecins Sans Frontières intervention in the Marburg hemorrhagic fever epidemic, Uíge, Angola, 2005. I. Lessons learned in the hospital. *J Infect Dis* 2007;196(Suppl 2):S154—S161.
367. Ji X, Olinger GG, Aris S, et al. Mannose-binding lectin binds to Ebola and Marburg envelope glycoproteins, resulting in blocking of virus interaction with DC-SIGN and complement-mediated virus neutralization. *J Gen Virol* 2005;86(Pt. 9):2535–2542.
368. Jin H, Yan Z, Prabhakar BS, et al. The VP35 protein of Ebola virus impairs dendritic cell maturation induced by virus and lipopolysaccharide. *J Gen Virol* 2010;91(Pt. 2):352–361.
369. John SP, Wang T, Steffen S, et al. Ebola virus VP30 is an RNA binding protein. *J Virol* 2007;81(17):8967–8976.
370. Johnson RF, Bell P, Harty RN. Effect of Ebola virus proteins GP, NP and VP35 on VP40 VLP morphology. *Virol J* 2006;3(1):31.
371. Johnson E, Jaax N, White J, et al. Lethal experimental infections of rhesus monkeys by aerosolized Ebola virus. *Int J Exp Pathol* 1995;76(4):227–236.
372. Johnson ED, Johnson BK, Silverstein D, et al. Characterization of a new Marburg virus isolated from a 1987 fatal case in Kenya. *Arch Virol Suppl* 1996;11:101–114.
373. Johnson KM, Lange JV, Webb PA, et al. Isolation and partial characterisation of a new virus causing acute haemorrhagic fever in Zaire. *Lancet* 1977;1(8011):569–571.
374. Johnson B, Li J, Adhikari J, et al. Dimerization controls Marburg virus VP24-dependent modulation of host antioxidative stress responses. *J Mol Biol* 2016;428(17):3483–3494.
375. Johnson DW, Sullivan JN, Piquette CA, et al. Lessons learned: critical care management of patients with Ebola in the United States. *Crit Care Med* 2015;43(6):1157–1164.
376. Jones MEB, Amman BR, Sealy TK, et al. Clinical, histopathologic, and immunohistochemical characterization of experimental Marburg virus infection in a natural reservoir host, the Egyptian rousette bat (Rousettus aegyptiacus). *Viruses* 2019;11(3):214.
377. Jones MEB, Schuh AJ, Amman BR, et al. Experimental inoculation of Egyptian rousette bats (Rousettus aegyptiacus) with viruses of the Ebolavirus and Marburgvirus genera. *Viruses* 2015;7(7):3420–3442.
378. Jouvenet N, Neil SJ, Zhadina M, et al. Broad-spectrum inhibition of retroviral and filoviral particle release by tetherin. *J Virol* 2009;83(4):1837–1844.
379. Judson SD, Fischer R, Judson A, et al. Ecological contexts of index cases and spillover events of different ebolaviruses. *PLoS Pathog* 2016;12(8):e1005780.
380. Judson S, Prescott J, Munster V. Understanding Ebola virus transmission. *Viruses* 2015;7(2):511–521.
381. Kajihara M, Hang'ombe BM, Changula K, et al. Marburgvirus in Egyptian fruit bats, Zambia. *Emerg Infect Dis* 2019;25(8):1577–1580.
382. Kaletsky RL, Francica JR, Agrawal-Gamse C, et al. Tetherin-mediated restriction of filovirus budding is antagonized by the Ebola glycoprotein. *Proc Natl Acad Sci U S A* 2009;106(8):2886–2891.
383. Kaletsky RL, Simmons G, Bates P. Proteolysis of the Ebola virus glycoproteins enhances virus binding and infectivity. *J Virol* 2007;81(24):13378–13384.
384. Kalongi Y, Mwanza K, Tshisuaka M, et al. Isolated case of Ebola hemorrhagic fever with mucormycosis complications, Kinshasa, Democratic Republic of the Congo. *J Infect Dis* 1999;179(Suppl 1):S15–S17.
385. Kangbai JB, Heumann C, Hoelscher M, et al. Epidemiological characteristics, clinical manifestations, and treatment outcome of 139 paediatric Ebola patients treated at a Sierra Leone Ebola treatment center. *BMC Infect Dis* 2019;19(1):81.
386. Karan LS, Makenov MT, Korneev MG, et al. Bombali virus in Mops condylurus Bats, Guinea. *Emerg Infect Dis* 2019;25(9):1174–1175.
387. Karrar MO, Mahdi AO. Maridi virus disease. A clinical report of the outbreak of the haemorrhagic fever which occurred in Maridi area, Equatoria provinces, in the southern region of the Sudan. *Sudan J Paediatr* 2014;14(2):103–111.
388. Katzourakis A, Gifford RJ. Endogenous viral elements in animal genomes. *PLoS Genet* 2010;6(11):e1001191.
389. Keck Z-Y, Enterlein SG, Howell KA, et al. Macaque monoclonal antibodies targeting novel conserved epitopes within filovirus glycoprotein. *J Virol* 2016;90(1):279–291.
390. Keita M, Duraffour S, Loman NJ, et al. Unusual Ebola virus chain of transmission, Conakry, Guinea, 2014-2015. *Emerg Infect Dis* 2016;22(12):2149–2152.
391. Kemenesi G, Kurucz K, Dallos B, et al. Re-emergence of Lloviu virus in Miniopterus schreibersii bats, Hungary, 2016. *Emerg Microbes Infect* 2018;7(1):66.
392. Kennedy SB, Bolay F, Kieh M, et al. Phase 2 placebo-controlled trial of two vaccines to prevent Ebola in Liberia. *N Engl J Med* 2017;377(15):1438–1447.
393. Khan AS, Tshioko FK, Heymann DL, et al. The reemergence of Ebola hemorrhagic fever, Democratic Republic of the Congo, 1995. *J Infect Dis* 1999;179(Suppl 1):S76–S86.
394. Kibadi K, Mupapa K, Kuvula K, et al. Late ophthalmologic manifestations in survivors of the 1995 Ebola virus epidemic in Kikwit, Democratic Republic of the Congo. *J Infect Dis* 1999;179(Suppl 1):S13–S14.
395. Kiley MP, Cox NJ, Elliott LH, et al. Physicochemical properties of Marburg virus: evidence for three distinct virus strains and their relationship to Ebola virus. *J Gen Virol* 1988;69(Pt. 8):1957–1967.
396. Kiley MP, Wilusz J, McCormick JB, et al. Conservation of the 3′ terminal nucleotide sequences of Ebola and Marburg virus. *Virology* 1986;149(2):251–254.
397. Kimberlin CR, Bornholdt ZA, Li S, et al. Ebolavirus VP35 uses a bimodal strategy to bind dsRNA for innate immune suppression. *Proc Natl Acad Sci U S A* 2010;107(1):314–319.
398. King LB, Fusco ML, Flyak AI, et al. The marburgvirus-neutralizing human monoclonal antibody MR191 targets a conserved site to block virus receptor binding. Cell Host Microbe 2018;23(1):101.e104–109.e104.
399. Kirchdoerfer RN, Moyer CL, Abelson DM, et al. The Ebola virus VP30-NP interaction is a regulator of viral RNA synthesis. *PLoS Pathog* 2016;12(10):e1005937.
400. Kirchdoerfer RN, Saphire EO, Ward AB. Cryo-EM structure of the Ebola virus nucleoprotein-RNA complex. *Acta Crystallogr F Struct Biol Commun* 2019;75(Pt 5):340–347.
401. Kirchdoerfer RN, Wasserman H, Amarasinghe GK, et al. Filovirus structural biology: the molecules in the machine. *Curr Top Microbiol Immunol* 2017;411:381–417.
402. Knust B, Schafer IJ, Wamala J, et al. Multidistrict outbreak of Marburg virus disease—Uganda, 2012. *J Infect Dis* 2015;212(Suppl 2):S119–S128.
403. Kobinger GP, Leung A, Neufeld J, et al. Replication, pathogenicity, shedding, and transmission of Zaire ebolavirus in pigs. *J Infect Dis* 2011;204(2):200–208.
404. Koehler A, Kolesnikova L, Becker S. An active site mutation increases the polymerase activity of the guinea pig-lethal Marburg virus. *J Gen Virol* 2016;97(Pt. 10):2494–2500.
405. Koellhoffer JF, Malashkevich VN, Harrison JS, et al. Crystal structure of the Marburg virus GP2 core domain in its postfusion conformation. *Biochemistry* 2012;51(39):7665–7675.
406. Kolesnikova L, Berghöfer B, Bamberg S, et al. Multivesicular bodies as a platform for formation of the Marburg virus envelope. *J Virol* 2004;78(22):12277–12287.
407. Kolesnikova L, Bugany H, Klenk H-D, et al. VP40, the matrix protein of Marburg virus, is associated with membranes of the late endosomal compartment. *J Virol* 2002;76(4):1825–1838.
408. Kolesnikova L, Mühlberger E, Ryabchikova E, et al. Ultrastructural organization of recombinant Marburg virus nucleoprotein: comparison with Marburg virus inclusions. *J Virol* 2000;74(8):3899–3904.
409. Kondratowicz AS, Lennemann NJ, Sinn PL, et al. T-cell immunoglobulin and mucin domain 1 (TIM-1) is a receptor for Zaire Ebolavirus and Lake Victoria Marburgvirus. *Proc Natl Acad Sci U S A* 2011;108(20):8426–8431.
410. Korb G, Slenczka W, Bechtelsheimer H, et al. Die "Marburg-Virus"-Hepatitis im Tierexperiment. Versuche an Meerschweinchen. *Virchows Arch A Pathol Pathol Anat* 1971;353(2):169–184.
411. Korch GW Jr, Niemi SM, Bergman NH, et al. *Animal Models for Assessing Countermeasures to Bioterrorism Agents.* Washington: Institute for Laboratory Animal Research (ILAR), Division on Earth and Life Studies, The National Academies of Sciences (NAS); 2011.
412. Kozak R, He S, Kroeker A, et al. Ferrets infected with Bundibugyo virus or Ebola virus recapitulate important aspects of human filovirus disease. *J Virol* 2016;90(20):9209–9223.
413. Kraft CS, Hewlett AL, Koepsell S, et al. The use of TKM-100802 and convalescent plasma in 2 patients with Ebola virus disease in the United States. *Clin Infect Dis* 2015;61(4):496–502.
414. Kratz T, Roddy P, Tshomba Oloma A, et al. Ebola virus disease outbreak in Isiro, Democratic Republic of the Congo, 2012: signs and symptoms, management and outcomes. *PLoS One* 2015;10(6):e0129333.
415. Kreuels B, Addo MM, Schmiedel S. Severe Ebola virus infection complicated by gram-negative septicemia. *N Engl J Med* 2015;372(14):1377.
416. Kreuels B, Wichmann D, Emmerich P, et al. A case of severe Ebola virus infection complicated by gram-negative septicemia. *N Engl J Med* 2014;371(25):2394–2401.
417. Krishnan A, Miller EH, Herbert AS, et al. Niemann-Pick C1 (NPC1)/NPC1-like1 chimeras define sequences critical for NPC1's function as a filovirus entry receptor. *Viruses* 2012;4(11):2471–2484.
418. Kroeker A, He S, de La Vega M-A, et al. Characterization of Sudan ebolavirus infection in ferrets. *Oncotarget* 2017;8(28):46262–46272.
419. Kruse T, Biedenkopf N, Hertz EPT, et al. The Ebola virus nucleoprotein recruits the host PP2A-B56 phosphatase to activate transcriptional support activity of VP30. *Mol Cell* 2018;69(1):136.e136–145.e136.
420. Ksiazek TG, Rollin PE, Williams AJ, et al. Clinical virology of Ebola hemorrhagic fever (EHF): virus, virus antigen, and IgG and IgM antibody findings among EHF patients in Kikwit, Democratic Republic of the Congo, 1995. *J Infect Dis* 1999;179(Suppl 1):S177–S187.
421. Kubota T, Matsuoka M, Chang T-H, et al. Ebolavirus VP35 interacts with the cytoplasmic dynein light chain 8. *J Virol* 2009;83(13):6952–6956.
422. Kucharski AJ, Camacho A, Flasche S, et al. Measuring the impact of Ebola control measures in Sierra Leone. *Proc Natl Acad Sci U S A* 2015;112(46):14366–14371.
423. Kugelman JR, Lee MS, Rossi CA, et al. Ebola virus genome plasticity as a marker of its passaging history: a comparison of in vitro passaging to non-human primate infection. *PLoS One* 2012;7(11):e50316.
424. Kühl A, Banning C, Marzi A, et al. The Ebola virus glycoprotein and HIV-1 Vpu employ different strategies to counteract the antiviral factor tetherin. *J Infect Dis* 2011;204(Suppl 3):S850–S860.
425. Kuhn JH. Filoviruses. A compendium of 40 years of epidemiological, clinical, and laboratory studies. *Arch Virol Suppl* 2008;20:13–360.
426. Kuhn JH. Ebolavirus and marburgvirus infections. In: Jameson JL, Fauci AS, Kasper DL, et al., eds. *Harrison's Principles of Internal Medicine, Vol. 2.* 20th ed. Columbus: McGraw-Hill Education; 2018:1509–1515.
427. Kuhn JH, Adachi T, Adhikari NKJ, et al. New filovirus disease classification and nomenclature. *Nat Rev Microbiol* 2019;17(5):261–263.
428. Kuhn JH, Amarasinghe GK, Basler CF, et al. ICTV virus taxonomy profile: Filoviridae. *J Gen Virol* 2019;100:911–912.
429. Kuhn JH, Bao Y, Bavari S, et al. Virus nomenclature below the species level: a standardized nomenclature for natural variants of viruses assigned to the family Filoviridae. *Arch Virol* 2013;158(1):301–311.

430. Kuhn JH, Dodd LE, Wahl-Jensen V, et al. Evaluation of perceived threat differences posed by filovirus variants. *Biosecur Bioterror* 2011;9(4):361–371.
431. Kuhn JH, Radoshitzky SR, Guth AC, et al. Conserved receptor-binding domains of Lake Victoria marburgvirus and Zaire ebolavirus bind a common receptor. *J Biol Chem* 2006;281(23):15951–15958.
432. Kuming BS, Kokoris N. Uveal involvement in Marburg virus disease. *Br J Ophthalmol* 1977;61(4):265–266.
433. Kunz C, Hofmann H. Some characteristics of the Marburg virus. In: Martini GA, Siegert R, eds. *Marburg Virus Disease.* Berlin: Springer-Verlag; 1971:109–111.
434. Kuroda M, Fujikura D, Nanbo A, et al. Interaction between TIM-1 and NPC1 is important for cellular entry of Ebola virus. *J Virol* 2015;89(12):6481–6493.
435. Kuroda M, Fujikura D, Noyori O, et al. A polymorphism of the TIM-1 IgV domain: implications for the susceptibility to filovirus infection. *Biochem Biophys Res Commun* 2014;455(3-4):223–228.
436. Lamb LE, Cox AT, Fletcher T, et al. Formulating and improving care while mitigating risk in a military Ebola virus disease treatment unit. *J R Army Med Corps* 2017;163(1):2–6.
437. Lamontagne F, Fowler RA, Adhikari NK, et al. Evidence-based guidelines for supportive care of patients with Ebola virus disease. *Lancet* 2018;391(10121):700–708.
438. Langer M, Portella G, Finazzi S, et al. Intensive care support and clinical outcomes of patients with Ebola virus disease (EVD) in West Africa. *Intensive Care Med* 2018;44(8):1266–1275.
439. Larsen T, Stevens EL, Davis KJ, et al. Pathologic findings associated with delayed death in nonhuman primates experimentally infected with Zaire Ebola virus. *J Infect Dis* 2007;196(Suppl 2):S323–S328.
440. Lash RR, Brunsell NA, Peterson AT. Spatiotemporal environmental triggers of Ebola and Marburg virus transmission. *Geocarto Int* 2008;23(6):451–466.
441. Lavender KJ, Williamson BN, Saturday G, et al. Pathogenicity of Ebola and Marburg viruses is associated with differential activation of the myeloid compartment in humanized triple knockout-bone marrow, liver, and thymus mice. *J Infect Dis* 2018;218(Suppl 5):S409–S417.
442. Le Guenno B, Formenty P, Wyers M, et al. Isolation and partial characterisation of a new strain of Ebola virus. *Lancet* 1995;345(8960):1271–1274.
443. Ledgerwood JE, Costner P, Desai N, et al. A replication defective recombinant Ad5 vaccine expressing Ebola virus GP is safe and immunogenic in healthy adults. *Vaccine* 2010;29(2):304–313.
444. Ledgerwood JE, DeZure AD, Stanley DA, et al. Chimpanzee adenovirus vector Ebola vaccine. *N Engl J Med* 2017;376(10):928–938.
445. Lee JE, Fusco ML, Hessell AJ, et al. Structure of the Ebola virus glycoprotein bound to an antibody from a human survivor. *Nature* 2008;454(7201):177–182.
446. Lee JE, Kuehne A, Abelson DM, et al. Complex of a protective antibody with its Ebola virus GP peptide epitope: unusual features of a $V\lambda_x$ light chain. *J Mol Biol* 2008;375(1):202–216.
447. Leitenberg M, Zilinskas RA, Kuhn JH. *The Soviet Biological Weapons Program—A History.* Cambridge: Harvard University Press; 2012.
448. Leroy EM, Baize S, Volchkov VE, et al. Human asymptomatic Ebola infection and strong inflammatory response. *Lancet* 2000;355(9222):2210–2215.
449. Leroy EM, Rouquet P, Formenty P, et al. Multiple Ebola virus transmission events and rapid decline of central African wildlife. *Science* 2004;303(5656):387–390.
450. Leroy EM, Souquière S, Rouquet P, et al. Re-emergence of Ebola haemorrhagic fever in Gabon. *Lancet* 2002;359(9307):712.
451. Leung DW, Ginder ND, Fulton DB, et al. Structure of the Ebola VP35 interferon inhibitory domain. *Proc Natl Acad Sci U S A* 2009;106(2):411–416.
452. Leung LW, Park M-S, Martinez O, et al. Ebolavirus VP35 suppresses IFN production from conventional but not plasmacytoid dendritic cells. *Immunol Cell Biol* 2011;89(7):792–802.
453. Leung DW, Prins KC, Borek DM, et al. Structural basis for dsRNA recognition and interferon antagonism by Ebola VP35. *Nat Struct Mol Biol* 2010;17(2):165–172.
454. Leung DW, Shabman RS, Farahbakhsh M, et al. Structural and functional characterization of Reston Ebola virus VP35 interferon inhibitory domain. *J Mol Biol* 2010;399(3):347–357.
455. Lever MS, Piercy TJ, Steward JA, et al. Lethality and pathogenesis of airborne infection with filoviruses in A129 α/β -/- interferon receptor-deficient mice. *J Med Microbiol* 2012;61:8–15.
456. Li J-X, Hou L-H, Meng F-Y, et al. Immunity duration of a recombinant adenovirus type-5 vector-based Ebola vaccine and a homologous prime-boost immunisation in healthy adults in China: final report of a randomised, double-blind, placebo-controlled, phase 1 trial. *Lancet Glob Health* 2017;5(3):e324–e334.
457. Li J, Rahmeh A, Morelli M, et al. A conserved motif in region v of the large polymerase proteins of nonsegmented negative-sense RNA viruses that is essential for mRNA capping. *J Virol* 2008;82(2):775–784.
458. Liang B, Li Z, Jenni S, et al. Structure of the L protein of vesicular stomatitis virus from electron cryomicroscopy. *Cell* 2015;162(2):314–327.
459. Licata JM, Simpson-Holley M, Wright NT, et al. Overlapping motifs (PTAP and PPEY) within the Ebola virus VP40 protein function independently as late budding domains: involvement of host proteins TSG101 and VPS-4. *J Virol* 2003;77(3):1812–1819.
460. Liu WJ, Sesay FR, Coursier A, et al. Comprehensive clinical and laboratory follow-up of a female patient with Ebola virus disease: Sierra Leone Ebola virus persistence study. Open Forum Infect Dis 2019;6(3):ofz068.
461. Liu L, Yin H, Liu D. Zero health worker infection: experiences from the China Ebola Treatment Unit during the Ebola epidemic in Liberia. *Disaster Med Public Health Prep* 2017;11(2):262–266.
462. Lofts LL, Ibrahim MS, Negley DL, et al. Genomic differences between guinea pig lethal and nonlethal Marburg virus variants. *J Infect Dis* 2007;196(Suppl 2):S305–S312.
463. Logan G, Vora NM, Nyensuah TG, et al. Establishment of a community care center for isolation and management of Ebola patients—Bomi County, Liberia, October 2014. *MMWR Morb Mortal Wkly Rep* 2014;63(44):1010–1012.
464. Lopez LA, Yang SJ, Hauser H, et al. Ebola virus glycoprotein counteracts BST-2/Tetherin restriction in a sequence-independent manner that does not require tetherin surface removal. *J Virol* 2010;84(14):7243–7255.
465. Lötfering B, Mühlberger E, Tamura T, et al. The nucleoprotein of Marburg virus is target for multiple cellular kinases. *Virology* 1999;255(1):50–62.
466. Lubaki NM, Younan P, Santos RI, et al. The Ebola interferon inhibiting domains attenuate and dysregulate cell-mediated immune responses. *PLoS Pathog* 2016;12(12):e1006031.
467. Luthra P, Jordan DS, Leung DW, et al. Ebola virus VP35 interaction with dynein LC8 regulates viral RNA synthesis. *J Virol* 2015;89(9):5148–5153.
468. Luthra P, Ramanan P, Mire CE, et al. Mutual antagonism between the Ebola virus VP35 protein and the RIG-I activator PACT determines infection outcome. *Cell Host Microbe* 2013;14(1):74–84.
469. Lyon GM, Mehta AK, Varkey JB, et al. Clinical care of two patients with Ebola virus disease in the United States. *N Engl J Med* 2014;371(25):2402–2409.
470. MacNeil A, Farnon EC, Wamala J, et al. Proportion of deaths and clinical features in Bundibugyo Ebola virus infection, Uganda. *Emerg Infect Dis* 2010;16(12):1969–1972.
471. Maganga GD, Kapetshi J, Berthet N, et al. Ebola virus disease in the Democratic Republic of Congo. *N Engl J Med* 2014;371(22):2083–2091.
472. Mahanty S, Hutchinson K, Agarwal S, et al. Impairment of dendritic cells and adaptive immunity by Ebola and Lassa viruses. *J Immunol* 2003;170(6):2797–2801.
473. Malashkevich VN, Schneider BJ, McNally ML, et al. Core structure of the envelope glycoprotein GP2 from Ebola virus at 1.9-Å resolution. *Proc Natl Acad Sci U S A* 1999;96(6):2662–2667.
474. Mandl JN, Feinberg MB. Robust and sustained immune activation in human Ebola virus infection. *Proc Natl Acad Sci U S A* 2015;112(15):4518–4519.
475. Manhart WA, Pacheco JR, Hume AJ, et al. A chimeric Lloviu virus minigenome system reveals that the bat-derived filovirus replicates more similarly to ebolaviruses than marburgviruses. Cell Rep 2018;24(10):2573.e2574–2580.e2574.
476. Manicassamy B, Wang J, Jiang H, et al. Comprehensive analysis of Ebola virus GP1 in viral entry. *J Virol* 2005;79(8):4793–4805.
477. Manicassamy B, Wang J, Rumschlag E, et al. Characterization of Marburg virus glycoprotein in viral entry. *Virology* 2007;358(1):79–88.
478. Marsh GA, Haining J, Robinson R, et al. Ebola Reston virus infection of pigs: clinical significance and transmission potential. *J Infect Dis* 2011;204(Suppl 3):S804–S809.
479. Martin B, Coutard B, Guez T, et al. The methyltransferase domain of the Sudan ebolavirus L protein specifically targets internal adenosines of RNA substrates, in addition to the cap structure. *Nucleic Acids Res* 2018;46(15):7902–7912.
480. Martin JE, Sullivan NJ, Enama ME, et al. A DNA vaccine for Ebola virus is safe and immunogenic in a phase I clinical trial. *Clin Vaccine Immunol* 2006;13(11):1267–1277.
481. Martines RB, Ng DL, Greer PW, et al. Tissue and cellular tropism, pathology and pathogenesis of Ebola and Marburg viruses. *J Pathol* 2015;235(2):153–174.
482. Martínez MJ, Biedenkopf N, Volchkova V, et al. Role of Ebola virus VP30 in transcription reinitiation. *J Virol* 2008;82(24):12569–12573.
483. Martinez O, Johnson J, Manicassamy B, et al. Zaire Ebola virus entry into human dendritic cells is insensitive to cathepsin L inhibition. *Cell Microbiol* 2010;12(2):148–157.
484. Martini GA. Marburg virus disease. Clinical syndrome. In: Martini GA, Siegert R, eds. *Marburg Virus Disease.* Berlin: Springer-Verlag; 1971:1–9.
485. Martini GA, Schmidt HA. Spermatogene Übertragung des "Virus Marburg" (Erreger der "Marburger Affenkrankheit"). *Klin Wochenschr* 1968;46(7):398–400.
486. Martini GA, Siegert R. *Marburg Virus Disease.* Berlin: Springer-Verlag; 1971.
487. Martins K, Carra JH, Cooper CL, et al. Cross-protection conferred by filovirus virus-like particles containing trimeric hybrid glycoprotein. *Viral Immunol* 2015;28(1):62–70.
488. Martins K, Cooper C, Warren T, et al. Characterization of clinical and immunological parameters during Ebola virus infection of rhesus macaques. *Viral Immunol* 2015;28(1):32–41.
489. Martin-Serrano J, Zang T, Bieniasz PD. HIV-1 and Ebola virus encode small peptide motifs that recruit Tsg101 to sites of particle assembly to facilitate egress. *Nat Med* 2001;7(12):1313–1319.
490. Maruyama J, Miyamoto H, Kajihara M, et al. Characterization of the envelope glycoprotein of a novel filovirus, Lloviu virus. *J Virol* 2014;88(1):99–109.
491. Marzi A, Chadinah S, Haddock E, et al. Recently identified mutations in the Ebola virus-Makona genome do not alter pathogenicity in animal models. *Cell Rep* 2018;23(6):1806–1816.
492. Marzi A, Gramberg T, Simmons G, et al. DC-SIGN and DC-SIGNR interact with the glycoprotein of Marburg virus and the S protein of severe acute respiratory syndrome coronavirus. *J Virol* 2004;78(21):12090–12095.
493. Marzi A, Haddock E, Kajihara M, et al. Monoclonal antibody cocktail protects hamsters from lethal Marburg virus infection. *J Infect Dis* 2018;218(Suppl 5):S662–S665.
494. Mate SE, Kugelman JR, Nyenswah TG, et al. Molecular evidence of sexual transmission of Ebola virus. *N Engl J Med* 2015;373(25):2448–2454.
495. Mateo M, Reid SP, Leung LW, et al. Ebolavirus VP24 binding to karyopherins is required for inhibition of interferon signaling. *J Virol* 2010;84(2):1169–1175.
496. Matsuno K, Nakayama E, Noyori O, et al. C-type lectins do not act as functional receptors for filovirus entry into cells. *Biochem Biophys Res Commun* 2010;403(1):144–148.
497. Mattia JG, Vandy MJ, Chang JC, et al. Early clinical sequelae of Ebola virus disease in Sierra Leone: a cross-sectional study. *Lancet Infect Dis* 2016;16(3):331–338.
498. Mavrakis M, Kolesnikova L, Schoehn G, et al. Morphology of Marburg virus NP-RNA. *Virology* 2002;296(2):300–307.
499. Mbala-Kingebeni P, Aziza A, di Paola N, et al. Medical countermeasures during the 2018 Ebola virus disease outbreak in the North Kivu and Ituri Provinces of the Democratic Republic of the Congo: a rapid genomic assessment. *Lancet Infect Dis* 2019;19:648–657.
500. Mbala-Kingebeni P, Pratt CB, Wiley MR, et al. 2018 Ebola virus disease outbreak in Équateur Province, Democratic Republic of the Congo: a retrospective genomic characterisation. *Lancet Infect Dis* 2019;19:641–647.
501. McElroy AK, Akondy RS, Davis CW, et al. Human Ebola virus infection results in substantial immune activation. *Proc Natl Acad Sci U S A* 2015;112(15):4719–4724.
502. McElroy AK, Erickson BR, Flietstra TD, et al. Ebola hemorrhagic fever: novel biomarker correlates of clinical outcome. *J Infect Dis* 2014;210(4):558–566.
503. McElroy AK, Erickson BR, Flietstra TD, et al. Biomarker correlates of survival in pediatric patients with Ebola virus disease. *Emerg Infect Dis* 2014;20(10):1683–1690.

504. McElroy AK, Erickson BR, Flietstra TD, et al. Von Willebrand factor is elevated in individuals infected with Sudan virus and is associated with adverse clinical outcomes. *Viral Immunol* 2015;28(1):71–73.

505. McElroy AK, Harmon JR, Flietstra TD, et al. Kinetic analysis of biomarkers in a cohort of US patients with Ebola virus disease. *Clin Infect Dis* 2016;63(4):460–467.

506. Mehedi M, Falzarano D, Seebach J, et al. A new Ebola virus nonstructural glycoprotein expressed through RNA editing. *J Virol* 2011;85(11):5406–5414.

507. Mehedi M, Hoenen T, Robertson S, et al. Ebola virus RNA editing depends on the primary editing site sequence and an upstream secondary structure. *PLoS Pathog* 2013;9(10):e1003677.

508. Mellquist-Riemenschneider JL, Garrison AR, Geisbert JB, et al. Comparison of the protective efficacy of DNA and baculovirus-derived protein vaccines for EBOLA virus in guinea pigs. *Virus Res* 2003;92(2):187–193.

509. Meyer M, Garron T, Lubaki NM, et al. Aerosolized Ebola vaccine protects primates and elicits lung-resident T cell responses. *J Clin Invest* 2015;125(8):3241–3255.

510. Milleliri J-M, Tévi-Benissan C, Baize S, et al. Les épidémies de fièvre hémorragique due au virus Ebola au Gabon (1994–2002): aspects épidémiologiques et réflexions sur les mesures de contrôle. *Bull Soc Pathol Exot* 2004;97(3):199–205.

511. Milligan ID, Gibani MM, Sewell R, et al. Safety and immunogenicity of novel adenovirus type 26- and modified vaccinia Ankara-vectored Ebola vaccines: a randomized clinical trial. *JAMA* 2016;315(15):1610–1623.

512. Miranda ME, Ksiazek TG, Retuya TJ, et al. Epidemiology of Ebola (subtype Reston) virus in the Philippines, 1996. *J Infect Dis* 1999;179(Suppl 1):S115–S119.

513. Miranda MEG, Miranda NLJ. Reston ebolavirus in humans and animals in the Philippines: a review. *J Infect Dis* 2011;204(Suppl 3):S757–S760.

514. Miranda ME, Yoshikawa Y, Manalo DL, et al. Chronological and spatial analysis of the 1996 Ebola Reston virus outbreak in a monkey breeding facility in the Philippines. *Exp Anim* 2002;51(2):173–179.

515. Mire CE, Geisbert JB, Agans KN, et al. Oral and conjunctival exposure of nonhuman primates to low doses of Ebola Makona virus. *J Infect Dis* 2016;214(Suppl 3):S263–S267.

516. Mire CE, Geisbert JB, Borisevich V, et al. Therapeutic treatment of Marburg and Ravn virus infection in nonhuman primates with a human monoclonal antibody. *Sci Transl Med* 2017;9(384):eaai8711.

517. Mire CE, Geisbert JB, Marzi A, et al. Vesicular stomatitis virus-based vaccines protect nonhuman primates against Bundibugyo ebolavirus. *PLoS Negl Trop Dis* 2013;7(12):e2600.

518. Mire CE, Matassov D, Geisbert JB, et al. Single-dose attenuated Vesiculovax vaccines protect primates against Ebola Makona virus. *Nature* 2015;520(7549):688–691.

519. Misasi J, Chandran K, Yang J-Y, et al. Filoviruses require endosomal cysteine proteases for entry but exhibit distinct protease preferences. *J Virol* 2012;86(6):3284–3292.

520. Misasi J, Gilman MSA, Kanekiyo M, et al. Structural and molecular basis for Ebola virus neutralization by protective human antibodies. *Science* 2016;351(6279):1343–1346.

521. Misasi J, Sullivan NJ. Camouflage and misdirection: the full-on assault of Ebola virus disease. *Cell* 2014;159(3):477–486.

522. Mitchell SW, McCormick JB. Physicochemical inactivation of Lassa, Ebola, and Marburg viruses and effect on clinical laboratory analyses. *J Clin Microbiol* 1984;20(3):486–489.

523. Mittler E, Schudt G, Halwe S, et al. A fluorescently labeled Marburg virus glycoprotein as a new tool to study viral transport and assembly. *J Infect Dis* 2018;218(Suppl 5):S318–S326.

524. Modrof J, Becker S, Mühlberger E. Ebola virus transcription activator VP30 is a zinc-binding protein. *J Virol* 2003;77(5):3334–3338.

525. Modrof J, Möritz C, Kolesnikova L, et al. Phosphorylation of Marburg virus VP30 at serines 40 and 42 is critical for its interaction with NP inclusions. *Virology* 2001;287(1):171–182.

526. Modrof J, Mühlberger E, Klenk HD, et al. Phosphorylation of VP30 impairs Ebola virus transcription. *J Biol Chem* 2002;277(36):33099–33104.

527. Mohan GS, Li W, Ye L, et al. Antigenic subversion: a novel mechanism of host immune evasion by Ebola virus. *PLoS Pathog* 2012;8(12):e1003065.

528. Möller P, Pariente N, Klenk H-D, et al. Homo-oligomerization of Marburgvirus VP35 is essential for its function in replication and transcription. *J Virol* 2005;79(23):14876–14886.

529. Moreau M, Spencer C, Gozalbes JG, et al. Lactating mothers infected with Ebola virus: EBOV RT-PCR of blood only may be insufficient. *Euro Surveill* 2015;20(3):21017.

530. Mühlberger E. Filovirus replication and transcription. *Future Virol* 2007;2(2):205–215.

531. Mühlberger E, Lötfering B, Klenk H-D, et al. Three of the four nucleocapsid proteins of Marburg virus, NP, VP35, and L, are sufficient to mediate replication and transcription of Marburg virus-specific monocistronic minigenomes. *J Virol* 1998;72(11):8756–8764.

532. Mühlberger E, Sanchez A, Randolf A, et al. The nucleotide sequence of the L gene of Marburg virus, a filovirus: homologies with paramyxoviruses and rhabdoviruses. *Virology* 1992;187(2):534–547.

533. Mühlberger E, Trommer S, Funke C, et al. Termini of all mRNA species of Marburg virus: sequence and secondary structure. *Virology* 1996;223(2):376–380.

534. Mühlberger E, Weik M, Volchov VE, et al. Comparison of the transcription and replication strategies of Marburg virus and Ebola virus by using artificial replication systems. *J Virol* 1999;73(3):2333–2342.

535. Mulangu S, Dodd LE, Davey RT Jr, et al. A randomized, controlled trial of Ebola virus disease therapeutics. *N Engl J Med* 2019.

536. Mulherkar N, Raaben M, de la Torre JC, et al. The Ebola virus glycoprotein mediates entry via a non-classical dynamin-dependent macropinocytic pathway. *Virology* 2011;419(2):72–83.

537. Mupapa K, Mukundu W, Bwaka MA, et al. Ebola hemorrhagic fever and pregnancy. *J Infect Dis* 1999;179(Suppl 1):S11–S12.

538. Murin CD, Fusco ML, Bornholdt ZA, et al. Structures of protective antibodies reveal sites of vulnerability on Ebola virus. *Proc Natl Acad Sci U S A* 2014;111(48):17182–17187.

539. Murphy FA. Pathology of Ebola virus infection. In: Pattyn SR, ed. *Ebola Virus Haemorrhagic Fever*. Amsterdam: Elsevier/North-Holland Biomedical Press; 1978:43–59.

540. Murphy FA, Simpson DIH, Whitfield SG, et al. Marburg virus infection in monkeys. Ultrastructural studies. *Lab Invest* 1971;24(4):279–291.

541. Murray JL, Mavrakis M, McDonald NJ, et al. Rab9 GTPase is required for replication of human immunodeficiency virus type 1, filoviruses, and measles virus. *J Virol* 2005;79(18):11742–11751.

542. Murthy S; Ebola Clinical Care authors group. Ebola and provision of critical care. *Lancet* 2015;385(9976):1392–1393.

543. Nanbo A, Imai M, Watanabe S, et al. Ebolavirus is internalized into host cells via macropinocytosis in a viral glycoprotein-dependent manner. *PLoS Pathog* 2010;6(9):e1001121.

544. Nanbo A, Maruyama J, Imai M, et al. Ebola virus requires a host scramblase for externalization of phosphatidylserine on the surface of viral particles. *PLoS Pathog* 2018;14(1):e1006848.

545. Nanbo A, Ohba Y. Budding of Ebola virus particles requires the Rab11-dependent endocytic recycling pathway. *J Infect Dis* 2018;218(Suppl 5):S388–S396.

546. Nanbo A, Watanabe S, Halfmann P, et al. The spatio-temporal distribution dynamics of Ebola virus proteins and RNA in infected cells. *Sci Rep* 2013;3:1206.

547. Nanclares C, Kapetshi J, Lionetto F, et al. Ebola virus disease, Democratic Republic of the Congo, 2014. *Emerg Infect Dis* 2016;22(9):1579–1586.

548. Nanyonga M, Saidu J, Ramsay A, et al. Sequelae of Ebola virus disease, Kenema District, Sierra Leone. *Clin Infect Dis* 2016;62(1):125–126.

549. National Institute of Allergy and Infectious Diseases. NIAID emerging infectious diseases/pathogens. 2018. Available at: https://www.niaid.nih.gov/research/emerging-infectious-diseases-pathogens

550. Negredo A, Palacios G, Vázquez-Morón S, et al. Discovery of an ebolavirus-like filovirus in Europe. *PLoS Pathog* 2011;7(10):e1002304.

551. Nelson JM, Griese SE, Goodman AB, et al. Live neonates born to mothers with Ebola virus disease: a review of the literature. *J Perinatol* 2016;36(6):411–414.

552. Neumann G, Ebihara H, Takada A, et al. Ebola virus VP40 late domains are not essential for viral replication in cell culture. *J Virol* 2005;79(16):10300–10307.

553. Neumann G, Geisbert TW, Ebihara H, et al. Proteolytic processing of the Ebola virus glycoprotein is not critical for Ebola virus replication in nonhuman primates. *J Virol* 2007;81(6):2995–2998.

554. Nfon CK, Leung A, Smith G, et al. Immunopathogenesis of severe acute respiratory disease in Zaire ebolavirus-infected pigs. *PLoS One* 2013;8(4):e61904.

555. Ng M, Ndungo E, Kaczmarek ME, et al. Filovirus receptor NPC1 contributes to species-specific patterns of ebolavirus susceptibility in bats. *Elife* 2015;4:e11785.

556. Nkoghe D, Formenty P, Leroy ÉM, et al. Plusieurs épidémies de fièvre hémorragique à virus Ebola au Gabon, d'octobre 2001 à avril 2002. *Bull Soc Pathol Exot* 2005;98(3):224–229.

557. Nkoghe D, Kone ML, Yada A, et al. A limited outbreak of Ebola haemorrhagic fever in Etoumbi, Republic of Congo, 2005. *Trans R Soc Trop Med Hyg* 2011;105(8):466–472.

558. Noda T, Aoyama K, Sagara H, et al. Nucleocapsid-like structures of Ebola virus reconstructed using electron tomography. *J Vet Med Sci* 2005;67(3):325–328.

559. Noda T, Ebihara H, Muramoto Y, et al. Assembly and budding of Ebolavirus. *PLoS Pathog* 2006;2(9):e99.

560. Noda T, Hagiwara K, Sagara H, et al. Characterization of the Ebola virus nucleoprotein-RNA complex. *J Gen Virol* 2010;91(Pt. 6):1478–1483.

561. Noda T, Halfmann P, Sagara H, et al. Regions in Ebola virus VP24 that are important for nucleocapsid formation. *J Infect Dis* 2007;196(Suppl 2):S247–S250.

562. Noda T, Watanabe S, Sagara H, et al. Mapping of the VP40-binding regions of the nucleoprotein of Ebola virus. *J Virol* 2007;81(7):3554–3562.

563. Nordenstedt H, Bah EI, de la Vega M-A, et al. Ebola virus in breast milk in an Ebola virus-positive mother with twin babies, Guinea, 2015. *Emerg Infect Dis* 2016;22(4):759–760.

564. Nsio J, Kapetshi J, Makiala S, et al. 2017 outbreak of Ebola virus disease in northern Democratic Republic of Congo. *J Infect Dis* 2019. doi: 10.1093/infdis/jiz107. Available at: https://academic.oup.com/jid/advance-article/doi/10.1093/infdis/jiz107/5426903

565. Nyakarahuka L, Ojwang J, Tumusiime A, et al. Isolated case of Marburg virus disease, Kampala, Uganda, 2014. *Emerg Infect Dis* 2017;23(6):1001–1004.

566. Nyakarahuka L, Shoemaker TR, Balinandi S, et al. Marburg virus disease outbreak in Kween District Uganda, 2017: epidemiological and laboratory findings. *PLoS Negl Trop Dis* 2019;13(3):e0007257.

567. O'Shea MK, Clay KA, Craig DG, et al. Diagnosis of febrile illnesses other than Ebola virus disease at an Ebola Treatment Unit in Sierra Leone. *Clin Infect Dis* 2015;61(5):795–798.

568. Oda S-I, Noda T, Wijesinghe KJ, et al. Crystal structure of Marburg virus VP40 reveals a broad, basic patch for matrix assembly and a requirement of the N-terminal domain for immunosuppression. *J Virol* 2016;90(4):1839–1848.

569. Oduyebo T, Bennett SD, Nallo AS, et al. Stillbirths and neonatal deaths surveillance during the 2014-2015 Ebola virus disease outbreak in Sierra Leone. *Int J Gynaecol Obstet* 2019;144(2):225–231.

570. Oduyebo T, Pineda D, Lamin M, et al. A pregnant patient with Ebola virus disease. *Obstet Gynecol* 2015;126(6):1273–1275.

571. Okoror L, Kamara A, Kargbo B, et al. Transplacental transmission: aA rare case of Ebola virus transmission. *Infect Dis Rep* 2018;10(3):7725.

572. Okware SI, Omaswa FG, Zaramba S, et al. An outbreak of Ebola in Uganda. *Trop Med Int Health* 2002;7(12):1068–1075.

573. Olejnik J, Forero A, Deflubé LR, et al. Ebolaviruses associated with differential pathogenicity induce distinct host responses in human macrophages. *J Virol* 2017;91(11):e00179.

574. Olejnik J, Hume AJ, Leung DW, et al. Filovirus strategies to escape antiviral responses. *Curr Top Microbiol Immunol* 2017;411:293–322.

575. Onyango CO, Opoka ML, Ksiazek TG, et al. Laboratory diagnosis of Ebola hemorrhagic fever during an outbreak in Yambio, Sudan, 2004. *J Infect Dis* 2007;196(Suppl 2):S193–S198.

576. Ortín J, Martín-Benito J. The RNA synthesis machinery of negative-stranded RNA viruses. *Virology* 2015;479-480:532–544.

577. Osterholm MT, Moore KA, Kelley NS, et al. Transmission of Ebola viruses: what we know and what we do not know. *MBio* 2015;6(2):e00137.

578. Page A, Volchkova VA, Reid SP, et al. Marburgvirus hijacks nrf2-dependent pathway by targeting nrf2-negative regulator keap1. *Cell Rep* 2014;6(6):1026–1036.

579. Pallesen J, Murin CD, de Val N, et al. Structures of Ebola virus GP and sGP in complex with therapeutic antibodies. *Nat Microbiol* 2016;1(9):16128.

580. Pan Y, Zhang W, Cui L, et al. Reston virus in domestic pigs in China. *Arch Virol* 2014;159(5):1129–1132.

581. Panchal RG, Ruthel G, Kenny TA, et al. In vivo oligomerization and raft localization of Ebola virus protein VP40 during vesicular budding. *Proc Natl Acad Sci U S A* 2003;100(26):15936–15941.

582. Pattyn SR. *Ebola Virus Haemorrhagic Fever*. Amsterdam: Elsevier/North-Holland Biomedical Press; 1978.
583. Pattyn S, van der Groen G, Jacob W, et al. Isolation of Marburg-like virus from a case of haemorrhagic fever in Zaire. *Lancet* 1977;1(8011):573–574.
584. Pavadai E, Gerstman BS, Chapagain PP. A cylindrical assembly model and dynamics of the Ebola virus VP40 structural matrix. *Sci Rep* 2018;8(1):9776.
585. Pawęska JT, Jansen van Vuren P, Kemp A, et al. Marburg virus infection in Egyptian rousette bats, South Africa, 2013-2014. *Emerg Infect Dis* 2018;24(6):1134–1137.
586. Paweska JT, Jansen van Vuren P, Masumu J, et al. Virological and serological findings in Rousettus aegyptiacus experimentally inoculated with Vero cells-adapted Hogan strain of Marburg virus. *PLoS One* 2012;7(9):e45479.
587. Paweska JT, Storm N, Grobbelaar AA, et al. Experimental inoculation of Egyptian fruit bats (Rousettus aegyptiacus) with Ebola virus. *Viruses* 2016;8(2):29.
588. Perry DL, Huzella LM, Bernbaum JG, et al. Ebola virus localization in the macaque reproductive tract during acute Ebola virus disease. *Am J Pathol* 2018;188(3):550–558.
589. Peterson AT, Bauer JT, Mills JN. Ecologic and geographic distribution of filovirus disease. *Emerg Infect Dis* 2004;10(1):40–47.
590. Peterson AT, Lash RR, Carroll DS, et al. Geographic potential for outbreaks of Marburg hemorrhagic fever. *Am J Trop Med Hyg* 2006;75(1):9–15.
591. Petrosillo N, Nicastri E, Lanini S, et al. Ebola virus disease complicated with viral interstitial pneumonia: a case report. *BMC Infect Dis* 2015;15(1):432.
592. Pigott DM, Deshpande A, Letourneau I, et al. Local, national, and regional viral haemorrhagic fever pandemic potential in Africa: a multistage analysis. *Lancet* 2017;390(10113):2662–2672.
593. Pigott DM, Golding N, Mylne A, et al. Mapping the zoonotic niche of Ebola virus disease in Africa. *Elife* 2014;3:e04395.
594. Pigott DM, Golding N, Mylne A, et al. Mapping the zoonotic niche of Marburg virus disease in Africa. *Trans R Soc Trop Med Hyg* 2015;109(6):366–378.
595. Pigott DM, Millear AI, Earl L, et al. Updates to the zoonotic niche map of Ebola virus disease in Africa. *Elife* 2016;5:e16412.
596. Pinzon JE, Wilson JM, Tucker CJ, et al. Trigger events: enviroclimatic coupling of Ebola hemorrhagic fever outbreaks. *Am J Trop Med Hyg* 2004;71(5):664–674.
597. Piot P, Bureau P, Breman G, et al. Clinical aspects of Ebola virus infection in Yambuku area, Zaire, 1976. In: Pattyn SR, ed. *Ebola Virus Haemorrhagic Fever*. Amsterdam: Elsevier/North-Holland Biomedical Press; 1978:7–14.
598. Pleet ML, Mathiesen A, DeMarino C, et al. Ebola VP40 in exosomes can cause immune cell dysfunction. *Front Microbiol* 2016;7:1765.
599. Ploquin A, Zhou Y, Sullivan NJ. Ebola immunity: gaining a winning position in lightning chess. *J Immunol* 2018;201(3):833–842.
600. Poetsch JH, Dahlke C, Zinser ME, et al. Detectable vesicular stomatitis virus (VSV)-specific humoral and cellular immune responses following VSV-Ebola virus vaccination in humans. *J Infect Dis* 2019;219(4):556–561.
601. Pokhrel R, Pavadai E, Gerstman BS, et al. Membrane pore formation and ion selectivity of the Ebola virus delta peptide. *Phys Chem Chem Phys* 2019;21(10):5578–5585.
602. Pourrut X, Kumulungui B, Wittmann T, et al. The natural history of Ebola virus in Africa. *Microbes Infect* 2005;7(7-8):1005–1014.
603. Pratt WD, Wang D, Nichols DK, et al. Protection of nonhuman primates against two species of Ebola virus infection with a single complex adenovirus vector. *Clin Vaccine Immunol* 2010;17(4):572–581.
604. Prescott J, Bushmaker T, Fischer R, et al. Postmortem stability of Ebola virus. *Emerg Infect Dis* 2015;21(5):856–859.
605. Pringle CR, Easton AJ. Monopartite negative strand RNA genomes. *Semin Virol* 1997;8(1):49–57.
606. Prins KC, Cárdenas WB, Basler CF. Ebola virus protein VP35 impairs the function of interferon regulatory factor-activating kinases IKKε and TBK-1. *J Virol* 2009;83(7):3069–3077.
607. Prins KC, Delpeut S, Leung DW, et al. Mutations abrogating VP35 interaction with double-stranded RNA render Ebola virus avirulent in guinea pigs. *J Virol* 2010;84(6):3004–3015.
608. Pushko P, Bray M, Ludwig GV, et al. Recombinant RNA replicons derived from attenuated Venezuelan equine encephalitis virus protect guinea pigs and mice from Ebola hemorrhagic fever virus. *Vaccine* 2000;19(1):142–153.
609. Pushko P, Geisbert J, Parker M, et al. Individual and bivalent vaccines based on alphavirus replicons protect guinea pigs against infection with Lassa and Ebola viruses. *J Virol* 2001;75(23):11677–11685.
610. Qin E, Bi J, Zhao M, et al. Clinical features of patients with Ebola virus disease in Sierra Leone. *Clin Infect Dis* 2015;61(4):491–495.
611. Qiu X, Wong G, Audet J, et al. Establishment and characterization of a lethal mouse model for the Angola strain of Marburg virus. *J Virol* 2014;88(21):12703–12714.
612. Qureshi AI, Chughtai M, Loua TO, et al. Study of Ebola virus disease survivors in Guinea. *Clin Infect Dis* 2015;61(7):1035–1042.
613. Raabe VN, Borcherta M. Infection control during filoviral hemorrhagic fever outbreaks. *J Glob Infect Dis* 2012;4(1):69–74.
614. Raabe VN, Mutyaba I, Roddy P, et al. Infection control during filoviral hemorrhagic fever outbreaks: preferences of community members and health workers in Masindi, Uganda. *Trans R Soc Trop Med Hyg* 2010;104(1):48–50.
615. Radoshitzky SR, Bavari S, Jahrling PB, et al. Filoviruses. In: Bozue J, Cote CK, Glass PJ, eds. *Medical Aspects of Biological Warfare*. Fort Sam Houston: Borden Institute, US Army Medical Department Center and School, Health Readiness Center of Excellence; 2018:569–614.
616. Radoshitzky SR, Dong L, Chi X, et al. Infectious Lassa virus, but not filoviruses, is restricted by BST-2/tetherin. *J Virol* 2010;84(20):10569–10580.
617. Radoshitzky SR, Warfield KL, Chi X, et al. Ebolavirus Δ-peptide immunoadhesins inhibit marburgvirus and ebolavirus cell entry. *J Virol* 2011;85(17):8502–8513.
618. Radzimanowski J, Effantin G, Weissenhorn W. Conformational plasticity of the Ebola virus matrix protein. *Protein Sci* 2014;23(11):1519–1527.
619. Ramanan P, Edwards MR, Shabman RS, et al. Structural basis for Marburg virus VP35-mediated immune evasion mechanisms. *Proc Natl Acad Sci U S A* 2012;109(50):20661–20666.
620. Rasmussen AL, Okumura A, Ferris MT, et al. Host genetic diversity enables Ebola hemorrhagic fever pathogenesis and resistance. *Science* 2014;346(6212):987–991.
621. Raymond J, Bradfute S, Bray M. Filovirus infection of STAT-1 knockout mice. *J Infect Dis* 2011;204(Suppl 3):S986–S990.
622. Reed DS, Hensley LE, Geisbert JB, et al. Depletion of peripheral blood T lymphocytes and NK cells during the course of Ebola hemorrhagic Fever in cynomolgus macaques. *Viral Immunol* 2004;17(3):390–400.
623. Reed DS, Lackemeyer MG, Garza NL, et al. Aerosol exposure to Zaire ebolavirus in three nonhuman primate species: differences in disease course and clinical pathology. *Microbes Infect* 2011;13(11):930–936.
624. Regnery RL, Johnson KM, Kiley MP. Virion nucleic acid of Ebola virus. *J Virol* 1980;36(2):465–469.
625. Regules JA, Beigel JH, Paolino KM, et al. A recombinant vesicular stomatitis virus Ebola vaccine. *N Engl J Med* 2017;376(4):330–341.
626. Reid SP, Leung LW, Hartman AL, et al. Ebola virus VP24 binds karyopherin α1 and blocks STAT1 nuclear accumulation. *J Virol* 2006;80(11):5156–5167.
627. Reid SP, Valmas C, Martinez O, et al. Ebola virus VP24 proteins inhibit the interaction of NPI-1 subfamily karyopherin α proteins with activated STAT1. *J Virol* 2007;81(24):13469–13477.
628. Rhein BA, Brouillette RB, Schaack GA, et al. Characterization of human and murine T-cell immunoglobulin mucin domain 4 (TIM-4) IgV domain residues critical for Ebola virus entry. *J Virol* 2016;90(13):6097–6111.
629. Ritchie G, Harvey DJ, Stroeher U, et al. Identification of N-glycans from Ebola virus glycoproteins by matrix-assisted laser desorption/ionisation time-of-flight and negative ion electrospray tandem mass spectrometry. *Rapid Commun Mass Spectrom* 2010;24(5):571–585.
630. Roddy P, Howard N, van Kerkhove MD, et al. Clinical manifestations and case management of Ebola haemorrhagic fever caused by a newly identified virus strain, Bundibugyo, Uganda, 2007-2008. *PLoS One* 2012;7(12):e52986.
631. Roddy P, Weatherill D, Jeffs B, et al. The Médecins Sans Frontières intervention in the Marburg hemorrhagic fever epidemic, Uige, Angola, 2005. II. Lessons learned in the community. *J Infect Dis* 2007;196(Suppl 2):S162–S167.
632. Rodriguez LL, de Roo A, Guimard Y, et al. Persistence and genetic stability of Ebola virus during the outbreak in Kikwit, Democratic Republic of the Congo, 1995. *J Infect Dis* 1999;179(Suppl 1):S170–S176.
633. Roels TH, Bloom AS, Buffington J, et al. Ebola hemorrhagic fever, Kikwit, Democratic Republic of the Congo, 1995: risk factors for patients without a reported exposure. *J Infect Dis* 1999;179(Suppl 1):S92–S97.
634. Rogstad KE, Tunbridge A. Ebola virus as a sexually transmitted infection. *Curr Opin Infect Dis* 2015;28(1):83–85.
635. Rollin PE, Bausch DG, Sanchez A. Blood chemistry measurements and D-Dimer levels associated with fatal and nonfatal outcomes in humans infected with Sudan Ebola virus. *J Infect Dis* 2007;196(Suppl 2):S364–S371.
636. Rollin PE, Williams RJ, Bressler DS, et al. Ebola (subtype Reston) virus among quarantined nonhuman primates recently imported from the Philippines to the United States. *J Infect Dis* 1999;179(Suppl 1):S108–S114.
637. Rosenke K, Adjemian J, Munster VJ, et al. Plasmodium parasitemia associated with increased survival in Ebola virus-infected patients. *Clin Infect Dis* 2016;63(8):1026–1033.
638. Rouquet P, Froment J-M, Bermejo M, et al. Wild animal mortality monitoring and human Ebola outbreaks, Gabon and Republic of Congo, 2001-2003. *Emerg Infect Dis* 2005;11(2):283–290.
639. Rubins KH, Hensley LE, Wahl-Jensen V, et al. The temporal program of peripheral blood gene expression in the response of nonhuman primates to Ebola hemorrhagic fever. *Genome Biol* 2007;8(8):R174.
640. Ruibal P, Oestereich L, Lüdtke A, et al. Unique human immune signature of Ebola virus disease in Guinea. *Nature* 2016;533(7601):100–104.
641. Ruigrok RWH, Schoehn G, Dessen A, et al. Structural characterization and membrane binding properties of the matrix protein VP40 of Ebola virus. *J Mol Biol* 2000;300(1):103–112.
642. Ryabchikova EI, Kolesnikova LV, Luchko SV. An analysis of features of pathogenesis in two animal models of Ebola virus infection. *J Infect Dis* 1999;179(Suppl 1):S199–S202.
643. Ryabchikova E, Kolesnikova L, Smolina M, et al. Ebola virus infection in guinea pigs: presumable role of granulomatous inflammation in pathogenesis. *Arch Virol* 1996;141(5):909–921.
644. Ryabchikova EI, Price BBS. *Ebola and Marburg Viruses. A View of Infection Using Electron Microscopy*. Columbus: Battelle Press; 2004.
645. Ryabchikova E, Strelets L, Kolesnikova L, et al. Respiratory Marburg virus infection in guinea pigs. *Arch Virol* 1996;141(11):2177–2190.
646. Saeed MF, Kolokoltsov AA, Albrecht T, et al. Cellular entry of Ebola virus involves uptake by a macropinocytosis-like mechanism and subsequent trafficking through early and late endosomes. *PLoS Pathog* 2010;6(9):e1001110.
647. Sakurai Y, Kolokoltsov AA, Chen C-C, et al. Two-pore channels control Ebola virus host cell entry and are drug targets for disease treatment. *Science* 2015;347(6225):995–998.
648. Sanchez A. Analysis of filovirus entry into Vero e6 cells, using inhibitors of endocytosis, endosomal acidification, structural integrity, and cathepsin (B and L) activity. *J Infect Dis* 2007;196(Suppl 2):S251–S258.
649. Sanchez A, Kiley MP, Holloway BP, et al. Sequence analysis of the Ebola virus genome: organization, genetic elements, and comparison with the genome of Marburg virus. *Virus Res* 1993;29(3):215–240.
650. Sanchez A, Lukwiya M, Bausch D, et al. Analysis of human peripheral blood samples from fatal and nonfatal cases of Ebola (Sudan) hemorrhagic fever: cellular responses, virus load, and nitric oxide levels. *J Virol* 2004;78(19):10370–10377.
651. Sanchez A, Rollin PE. Complete genome sequence of an Ebola virus (Sudan species) responsible for a 2000 outbreak of human disease in Uganda. *Virus Res* 2005;113(1):16–25.
652. Sanchez A, Trappier SG, Mahy BWJ, et al. The virion glycoproteins of Ebola viruses are encoded in two reading frames and are expressed through transcriptional editing. *Proc Natl Acad Sci U S A* 1996;93(8):3602–3607.
653. Sanchez A, Yang Z-Y, Xu L, et al. Biochemical analysis of the secreted and virion glycoproteins of Ebola virus. *J Virol* 1998;72(8):6442–6447.
654. Sänger C, Mühlberger E, Lötfering B, et al. The Marburg virus surface protein GP is phosphorylated at its ectodomain. *Virology* 2002;295(1):20–29.
655. Sangha AK, Dong J, Williamson L, et al. Role of non-local interactions between CDR loops in binding affinity of MR78 antibody to Marburg virus glycoprotein. *Structure* 2017;25(12):1820.e1822–1828.e1822.

656. Saphire EO, Schendel SL, Fusco ML, et al. Systematic analysis of monoclonal antibodies against Ebola virus GP defines features that contribute to protection. *Cell* 2018;174(4):938.e913–952.e913.
657. Schieffelin JS, Shaffer JG, Goba A, et al. Clinical illness and outcomes in patients with Ebola in Sierra Leone. *N Engl J Med* 2014;371(22):2092–2100.
658. Schmidt ML, Hoenen T. Characterization of the catalytic center of the Ebola virus L polymerase. *PLoS Negl Trop Dis* 2017;11(10):e0005996.
659. Schmidt KM, Mühlberger E. Marburg virus reverse genetics systems. *Viruses* 2016;8(6):178.
660. Schnittler H-J, Feldmann H. Marburg and Ebola hemorrhagic fevers: does the primary course of infection depend on the accessibility of organ-specific macrophages? *Clin Infect Dis* 1998;27(2):404–406.
661. Schnittler H-J, Feldmann H. Molecular pathogenesis of filovirus infections: role of macrophages and endothelial cells. *Curr Top Microbiol Immunol* 1999;235:175–204.
662. Schnittler H-J, Feldmann H. Viral hemorrhagic fever—a vascular disease? *Thromb Haemost* 2003;89(6):967–972.
663. Schornberg K, Matsuyama S, Kabsch K, et al. Role of endosomal cathepsins in entry mediated by the Ebola virus glycoprotein. *J Virol* 2006;80(8):4174–4178.
664. Schornberg KL, Shoemaker CJ, Dube D, et al. $\alpha_5\beta_1$-Integrin controls ebolavirus entry by regulating endosomal cathepsins. *Proc Natl Acad Sci U S A* 2009;106(19):8003–8008.
665. Schudt G, Kolesnikova L, Dolnik O, et al. Live-cell imaging of Marburg virus-infected cells uncovers actin-dependent transport of nucleocapsids over long distances. *Proc Natl Acad Sci U S A* 2013;110(35):14402–14407.
666. Schuh AJ, Amman BR, Jones MEB, et al. Modelling filovirus maintenance in nature by experimental transmission of Marburg virus between Egyptian rousette bats. *Nat Commun* 2017;8:14446.
667. Schuh AJ, Amman BR, Sealy TK, et al. Egyptian rousette bats maintain long-term protective immunity against Marburg virus infection despite diminished antibody levels. *Sci Rep* 2017;7(1):8763.
668. Schuh AJ, Amman BR, Sealy TS, et al. Comparative analysis of serologic cross-reactivity using convalescent sera from filovirus-experimentally infected fruit bats. *Sci Rep* 2019;9(1):6707.
669. Schümann M, Gantke T, Mühlberger E. Ebola virus VP35 antagonizes PKR activity through its C-terminal interferon inhibitory domain. *J Virol* 2009;83(17):8993–8997.
670. Schwartz DA, Anoko JN, Abramowitz SA. *Pregnant in the Time of Ebola*. Cham: Springer International Publishing; 2019.
671. Schwarz TM, Edwards MR, Diederichs A, et al. VP24-karyopherin alpha binding affinities differ between Ebolavirus species, influencing interferon inhibition and VP24 stability. *J Virol* 2017;91(4):e01715–e01716.
672. Scianimanico S, Schoehn G, Timmins J, et al. Membrane association induces a conformational change in the Ebola virus matrix protein. *EMBO J* 2000;19(24):6732–6741.
673. Scott JT, Sesay FR, Massaquoi TA, et al. Post-Ebola syndrome, Sierra Leone. *Emerg Infect Dis* 2016;22(4):641–646.
674. Shabman RS, Jabado OJ, Mire CE, et al. Deep sequencing identifies noncanonical editing of Ebola and Marburg virus RNAs in infected cells. *MBio* 2014;5(6):e02011.
675. Shabman RS, Leung DW, Johnson J, et al. DRBP76 associates with Ebola virus VP35 and suppresses viral polymerase function. *J Infect Dis* 2011;204(Suppl 3):S911–S918.
676. Shantha JG, Crozier I, Varkey JB, et al. Long-term management of panuveitis and iris heterochromia in an Ebola survivor. *Ophthalmology* 2016;123(12):2626.e2622–2628.e2622.
677. Shantha JG, Mattia JG, Goba A, et al. Ebola virus persistence in ocular tissues and fluids (EVICT) study: reverse transcription-polymerase chain reaction and cataract surgery outcomes of Ebola survivors in Sierra Leone. *EBioMedicine* 2018;30:217–224.
678. Shears P, O'Dempsey TJD. Ebola virus disease in Africa: epidemiology and nosocomial transmission. *J Hosp Infect* 2015;90(1):1–9.
679. Shi M, Lin X-D, Chen X, et al. The evolutionary history of vertebrate RNA viruses. *Nature* 2018;556(7700):197–202.
680. Shimojima M, Takada A, Ebihara H, et al. Tyro3 family-mediated cell entry of Ebola and Marburg viruses. *J Virol* 2006;80(20):10109–10116.
681. Shoemaker T, MacNeil A, Balinandi S, et al. Reemerging Sudan Ebola virus disease in Uganda, 2011. *Emerg Infect Dis* 2012;18(9):1480–1483.
682. Shu T, Gan T, Bai P, et al. Ebola virus VP35 has novel NTPase and helicase-like activities. *Nucleic Acids Res* 2019;47:5837–5851.
683. Siegert R, Shu H-L, Slenczka W. Nachweis des "Marburg-Virus" beim Patienten. *Dtsch Med Wochenschr* 1968;93(12):616–619.
684. Siegert R, Shu H-L, Slenczka W, et al. Zur Ätiologie einer unbekannten, von Affen ausgegangenen menschlichen Infektionskrankheit. *Dtsch Med Wochenschr* 1967;92(51):2341–2343.
685. Simmons G, Reeves JD, Grogan CC, et al. DC-SIGN and DC-SIGNR bind ebola glycoproteins and enhance infection of macrophages and endothelial cells. *Virology* 2003;305(1):115–123.
686. Simpson DIH. Vervent monkey disease. Transmission to the hamster. *Br J Exp Pathol* 1969;50(4):389–392.
687. Simpson DIH. Marburg agent disease: in monkeys. *Trans R Soc Trop Med Hyg* 1969;63(3):303–309.
688. Simpson DIH. Marburg virus disease: experimental infection in monkeys. *Lab Anim Handb* 1969;4:149–154.
689. Sissoko D, Duraffour S, Kerber R, et al. Persistence and clearance of Ebola virus RNA from seminal fluid of Ebola virus disease survivors: a longitudinal analysis and modelling study. *Lancet Glob Health* 2017;5(1):e80–e88.
690. Sissoko D, Keïta M, Diallo B, et al. Ebola virus persistence in breast milk after no reported illness: a likely source of virus transmission from mother to child. *Clin Infect Dis* 2017;64(4):513–516.
691. Sivapalasingam S, Kamal M, Slim R, et al. Safety, pharmacokinetics, and immunogenicity of a co-formulated cocktail of three human monoclonal antibodies targeting Ebola virus glycoprotein in healthy adults: a randomised, first-in-human phase 1 study. *Lancet Infect Dis* 2018;18(8):884–893.
692. Smetana J, Chlíbek R, Vacková M. Marburgská hemoragická horečka—epidemie v Angole. *Epidemiol Mikrobiol Imunol* 2006;55(2):63–67.
693. Smit MA, Michelow IC, Glavis-Bloom J, et al. Characteristics and outcomes of pediatric patients with Ebola virus disease admitted to treatment units in Liberia and Sierra Leone: a retrospective cohort study. *Clin Infect Dis* 2017;64(3):243–249.
694. Smith MW. Field aspects of the Marburg virus outbreak: 1967. *Primate Supply* 1982;7(1):11–15.
695. Smith DH, Johnson BK, Isaacson M, et al. Marburg-virus disease in Kenya. *Lancet* 1982;1(8276):816–820.
696. Smither SJ, Eastaugh L, Filone CM, et al. Two-center evaluation of disinfectant efficacy against Ebola virus in clinical and laboratory matrices. *Emerg Infect Dis* 2018;24(1):135–139.
697. Smither SJ, Nelson M, Eastaugh L, et al. Experimental respiratory Marburg virus haemorrhagic fever infection in the common marmoset (*Callithrix jacchus*). *Int J Exp Pathol* 2013;94(2):156–168.
698. Smither SJ, Nelson M, Eastaugh L, et al. Experimental respiratory infection of marmosets (*Callithrix jacchus*) with Ebola virus Kikwit. *J Infect Dis* 2015;212(Suppl 2):S336–S345.
699. Soni SP, Adu-Gyamfi E, Yong SS, et al. The Ebola virus matrix protein deeply penetrates the plasma membrane: an important step in viral egress. *Biophys J* 2013;104(9):1940–1949.
700. Soni SP, Stahelin RV. The Ebola virus matrix protein VP40 selectively induces vesiculation from phosphatidylserine-enriched membranes. *J Biol Chem* 2014;289(48):33590–33597.
701. Spengler JR, Saturday G, Lavender KJ, et al. Severity of disease in humanized mice infected with Ebola virus or Reston virus is associated with magnitude of early viral replication in liver. *J Infect Dis* 2017;217(1):58–63.
702. Steele KE, Anderson AO, Mohamadzadeh M. Fibroblastic reticular cell infection by hemorrhagic fever viruses. *Immunotherapy* 2009;1(2):187–197.
703. Stille W, Böhle E. Clinical course and prognosis of Marburg virus ("green-monkey") disease. In: Martini GA, Siegert R, eds. *Marburg Virus Disease*. Berlin: Springer-Verlag; 1971:10–18.
704. Strack B, Calistri A, Göttlinger HG. Late assembly domain function can exhibit context dependence and involves ubiquitin residues implicated in endocytosis. *J Virol* 2002;76(11):5472–5479.
705. Ströher U, West E, Bugany H, et al. Infection and activation of monocytes by Marburg and Ebola viruses. *J Virol* 2001;75(22):11025–11033.
706. Su Z, Wu C, Shi L, et al. Electron cryo-microscopy structure of Ebola virus nucleoprotein reveals a mechanism for nucleocapsid-like assembly. *Cell* 2018;172(5):966.e912–978.e912.
707. Subbotina E, Dadaeva A, Kachko A, et al. Genetic factors of Ebola virus virulence in guinea pigs. *Virus Res* 2010;153(1):121–133.
708. Sueblinvong V, Johnson DW, Weinstein GL, et al. Critical care for multiple organ failure secondary to Ebola virus disease in the United States. *Crit Care Med* 2015;43(10):2066–2075.
709. Sugita Y, Matsunami H, Kawaoka Y, et al. Cryo-EM structure of the Ebola virus nucleoprotein-RNA complex at 3.6 Å resolution. *Nature* 2018;563(7729):137–140.
710. Sullivan NJ, Geisbert TW, Geisbert JB, et al. Accelerated vaccination for Ebola virus haemorrhagic fever in non-human primates. *Nature* 2003;424(6949):681–684.
711. Sullivan NJ, Geisbert TW, Geisbert JB, et al. Immune protection of nonhuman primates against Ebola virus with single low-dose adenovirus vectors encoding modified GPs. *PLoS Med* 2006;3(6):e177.
712. Sullivan NJ, Martin JE, Graham BS, et al. Correlates of protective immunity for Ebola vaccines: implications for regulatory approval by the animal rule. *Nat Rev Microbiol* 2009;7(5):393–400.
713. Swenson DL, Wang D, Luo M, et al. Vaccine to confer to nonhuman primates complete protection against multistrain Ebola and Marburg virus infections. *Clin Vaccine Immunol* 2008;15(3):460–467.
714. Swenson DL, Warfield KL, Larsen T, et al. Monovalent virus-like particle vaccine protects guinea pigs and nonhuman primates against infection with multiple Marburg viruses. *Expert Rev Vaccines* 2008;7(4):417–429.
715. Sztuba-Solinska J, Diaz L, Kumar MR, et al. A small stem-loop structure of the Ebola virus trailer is essential for replication and interacts with heat-shock protein A8. *Nucleic Acids Res* 2016;44(20):9831–9846.
716. Takada A, Fujioka K, Tsuiji M, et al. Human macrophage C-type lectin specific for galactose and N-acetylgalactosamine promotes filovirus entry. *J Virol* 2004;78(6):2943–2947.
717. Takada A, Robison C, Goto H, et al. A system for functional analysis of Ebola virus glycoprotein. *Proc Natl Acad Sci U S A* 1997;94(26):14764–14769.
718. Takada A, Watanabe S, Ito H, et al. Downregulation of β1 integrins by Ebola virus glycoprotein: implication for virus entry. *Virology* 2000;278(1):20–26.
719. Takamatsu Y, Kolesnikova L, Becker S. Ebola virus proteins NP, VP35, and VP24 are essential and sufficient to mediate nucleocapsid transport. *Proc Natl Acad Sci U S A* 2018;115(5):1075–1080.
720. Tapia MD, Sow SO, Lyke KE, et al. Use of ChAd3-EBO-Z Ebola virus vaccine in Malian and US adults, and boosting of Malian adults with MVA-BN-Filo: a phase 1, single-blind, randomised trial, a phase 1b, open-label and double-blind, dose-escalation trial, and a nested, randomised, double-blind, placebo-controlled trial. *Lancet Infect Dis* 2016;16(1):31–42.
721. Taylor DJ, Dittmar K, Ballinger MJ, et al. Evolutionary maintenance of filovirus-like genes in bat genomes. *BMC Evol Biol* 2011;11(1):336.
722. Taylor DJ, Leach RW, Bruenn J. Filoviruses are ancient and integrated into mammalian genomes. *BMC Evol Biol* 2010;10:193.
723. Tchesnokov EP, Raeisimakiani P, Ngure M, et al. Recombinant RNA-dependent RNA polymerase complex of Ebola virus. *Sci Rep* 2018;8(1):3970.
724. Tembo J, Simulundu E, Changula K, et al. Recent advances in the development and evaluation of molecular diagnostics for Ebola virus disease. *Expert Rev Mol Diagn* 2019;19:325–340.
725. The Australia Group. List of human and animal pathogens and toxins for export control. 2017. Available at: http://www.australiagroup.net/en/human_animal_pathogens.html
726. The PREVAIL II Writing Group. A randomized, controlled trial of ZMapp for Ebola virus infection. *N Engl J Med* 2016;375(15):1448–1456.
727. The PREVAIL III Study Group. A longitudinal study of Ebola sequelae in Liberia. *N Engl J Med* 2019;380(10):924–934.
728. Thill M, Tolou H. Fièvre hémorragique à virus Ebola: nouvel opus meurtrier au Soudan. *Méd Trop (Mars)* 2004;64(4):331–333.
729. Tiffany A, Vetter P, Mattia J, et al. Ebola virus disease complications as experienced by survivors in Sierra Leone. *Clin Infect Dis* 2016;62(11):1360–1366.

730. Tigabu B, Ramanathan P, Ivanov A, et al. Phosphorylated VP30 of Marburg virus is a repressor of transcription. *J Virol* 2018;92(21):e00426.
731. Timen A, Koopmans MPG, Vossen ACTM, et al. Response to imported case of Marburg hemorrhagic fever, the Netherlands. *Emerg Infect Dis* 2009;15(8):1171–1175.
732. Timmins J, Schoehn G, Kohlhaas C, et al. Oligomerization and polymerization of the filovirus matrix protein VP40. *Virology* 2003;312(2):359–368.
733. Timmins J, Schoehn G, Ricard-Blum S, et al. Ebola virus matrix protein VP40 interaction with human cellular factors Tsg101 and Nedd4. *J Mol Biol* 2003;326(2):493–502.
734. Timmins J, Scianimanico S, Schoehn G, et al. Vesicular release of Ebola virus matrix protein VP40. *Virology* 2001;283(1):1–6.
735. Tong Y-G, Shi W-F, Liu D, et al. Genetic diversity and evolutionary dynamics of Ebola virus in Sierra Leone. *Nature* 2015;524(7563):93–96.
736. Torabi-Parizi P, Davey RT Jr, Suffredini AF, et al. Ethical and practical considerations in providing critical care to patients with Ebola virus disease. *Chest* 2015;147(6):1460–1466.
737. Towner JS, Amman BR, Sealy TK, et al. Isolation of genetically diverse Marburg viruses from Egyptian fruit bats. *PLoS Pathog* 2009;5(7):e1000536.
738. Towner JS, Khristova ML, Sealy TK, et al. Marburgvirus genomics and association with a large hemorrhagic fever outbreak in Angola. *J Virol* 2006;80(13):6497–6516.
739. Towner JS, Rollin PE, Bausch DG, et al. Rapid diagnosis of Ebola hemorrhagic fever by reverse transcription-PCR in an outbreak setting and assessment of patient viral load as a predictor of outcome. *J Virol* 2004;78(8):4330–4341.
740. Towner JS, Sealy TK, Khristova ML, et al. Newly discovered Ebola virus associated with hemorrhagic fever outbreak in Uganda. *PLoS Pathog* 2008;4(11):e1000212.
741. Tran EEH, Nelson EA, Bonagiri P, et al. Mapping of ebolavirus neutralization by monoclonal antibodies in the ZMapp cocktail using cryo-electron tomography and studies of cellular entry. *J Virol* 2016;90(17):7618–7627.
742. Tran EEH, Simmons JA, Bartesaghi A, et al. Spatial localization of the Ebola virus glycoprotein mucin-like domain determined by cryo-electron tomography. *J Virol* 2014;88(18):10958–10962.
743. Trefry JC, Wollen SE, Nasar F, et al. Ebola virus infections in nonhuman primates are temporally influenced by glycoprotein poly-U editing site populations in the exposure material. *Viruses* 2015;7(12):6739–6754.
744. Trehan I, Kelly T, Marsh RH, et al. Moving towards a more aggressive and comprehensive model of care for children with Ebola. *J Pediatr* 2016;170:28.e21–33.e27.
745. Trunschke M, Conrad D, Enterlein S, et al. The L-VP35 and L-L interaction domains reside in the amino terminus of the Ebola virus L protein and are potential targets for antivirals. *Virology* 2013;441(2):135–145.
746. Tucker CJ, Wilson JM, Mahoney R, et al. Climatic and ecological context of the 1994-1996 Ebola outbreaks. *Photogrammetric Eng Remote Sensing* 2002;68(2):147–152.
747. Twenhafel NA, Mattix ME, Johnson JC, et al. Pathology of experimental aerosol Zaire ebolavirus infection in rhesus macaques. *Vet Pathol* 2013;50(3):514–529.
748. Twenhafel NA, Shaia CI, Bunton TE, et al. Experimental aerosolized guinea pig-adapted Zaire ebolavirus (variant: Mayinga) causes lethal pneumonia in guinea pigs. *Vet Pathol* 2015;52(1):21–25.
749. U.S. Department of Health and Human Services, U.S. Centers for Disease Control and Prevention, U.S. Department of Agriculture. Select Agents and Toxins List. 2017. Available at: https://www.selectagents.gov/selectagentsandtoxinslist.html
750. U.S. Department of Health and Human Services, U.S. Centers for Disease Control and Prevention, U.S. National Institutes of Health. *Biosafety in Microbiological and Biomedical Laboratories (BMBL)*. Revised 5th ed. Washington: U.S. Government Printing Office; 2009. Available at: https://www.cdc.gov/labs/BMBL.html. HHS Publication No. (CDC) 93-8395.
751. Urata S, Noda T, Kawaoka Y, et al. Interaction of Tsg101 with Marburg virus VP40 depends on the PPPY motif, but not the PT/SAP motif as in the case of Ebola virus, and Tsg101 plays a critical role in the budding of Marburg virus-like particles induced by VP40, NP, and GP. *J Virol* 2007;81(9):4895–4899.
752. Urata S, Yasuda J. Regulation of Marburg virus (MARV) budding by Nedd4.1: a different WW domain of Nedd4.1 is critical for binding to MARV and Ebola virus VP40. *J Gen Virol* 2010;91(Pt. 1):228–234.
753. Urbanowicz RA, McClure CP, Sakuntabhai A, et al. Human adaptation of Ebola virus during the West African outbreak. Cell 2016;167(4):1079.e1075–1087.e1075.
754. Usami K, Matsuno K, Igarashi M, et al. Involvement of viral envelope GP2 in Ebola virus entry into cells expressing the macrophage galactose-type C-type lectin. *Biochem Biophys Res Commun* 2011;407(1):74–78.
755. Uyeki TM, Erickson BR, Brown S, et al. Ebola virus persistence in semen of male survivors. *Clin Infect Dis* 2016;62(12):1552–1555.
756. Uyeki TM, Mehta AK, Davey RT Jr, et al. Clinical management of Ebola virus disease in the United States and Europe. *N Engl J Med* 2016;374(7):636–646.
757. Valmas C, Basler CF. Marburg virus VP40 antagonizes interferon signaling in a species-specific manner. *J Virol* 2011;85(9):4309–4317.
758. Valmas C, Grosch MN, Schümann M, et al. Marburg virus evades interferon responses by a mechanism distinct from Ebola virus. *PLoS Pathog* 2010;6(1):e1000721.
759. Vanderzanden L, Bray M, Fuller D, et al. DNA vaccines expressing either the GP or NP genes of Ebola virus protect mice from lethal challenge. *Virology* 1998;246(1):134–144.
760. Varkey JB, Shantha JG, Crozier I, et al. Persistence of Ebola virus in ocular fluid during convalescence. *N Engl J Med* 2015;372(25):2423–2427.
761. Velásquez GE, Aibana O, Ling EJ, et al. Time from infection to disease and infectiousness for Ebola virus disease, a systematic review. *Clin Infect Dis* 2015;61(7):1135–1140.
762. Venkatraman N, Ndiaye BP, Bowyer G, et al. Safety and immunogenicity of a heterologous prime-boost Ebola virus vaccine regimen in healthy adults in the United Kingdom and Senegal. *J Infect Dis* 2019;219(8):1187–1197.
763. Vernet M-A, Reynard S, Fizet A, et al. Clinical, virological, and biological parameters associated with outcomes of Ebola virus infection in Macenta, Guinea. *JCI Insight* 2017;2(6):e88864.
764. Villinger F, Rollin PE, Brar SS, et al. Markedly elevated levels of interferon (IFN)-γ, IFN-α, interleukin (IL)-2, IL-10, and tumor necrosis factor-α associated with fatal Ebola virus infection. *J Infect Dis* 1999;179(Suppl 1):S188–S191.
765. Volchkov VE, Becker S, Volchkova VA, et al. GP mRNA of Ebola virus is edited by the Ebola virus polymerase and by T7 and vaccinia virus polymerases. *Virology* 1995;214(2):421–430.
766. Volchkov VE, Chepurnov AA, Volchkova VA, et al. Molecular characterization of guinea pig-adapted variants of Ebola virus. *Virology* 2000;277(1):147–155.
767. Volchkov VE, Feldmann H, Volchkova VA, et al. Processing of the Ebola virus glycoprotein by the proprotein convertase furin. *Proc Natl Acad Sci U S A* 1998;95(10):5762–5767.
768. Volchkov VE, Volchkova VA, Chepurnov AA, et al. Characterization of the L gene and 5′ trailer region of Ebola virus. *J Gen Virol* 1999;80(Pt. 2):355–362.
769. Volchkov VE, Volchkova VA, Ströher U, et al. Proteolytic processing of Marburg virus glycoprotein. *Virology* 2000;268(1):1–6.
770. Volchkova VA, Dolnik O, Martinez MJ, et al. Genomic RNA editing and its impact on Ebola virus adaptation during serial passages in cell culture and infection of guinea pigs. *J Infect Dis* 2011;204(Suppl 3):S941–S946.
771. Volchkova VA, Dolnik O, Martinez MJ, et al. RNA editing of the GP gene of Ebola virus is an important pathogenicity factor. *J Infect Dis* 2015;212(Suppl 2):S226–S233.
772. Volchkova VA, Feldmann H, Klenk H-D, et al. The nonstructural small glycoprotein sGP of Ebola virus is secreted as an antiparallel-orientated homodimer. *Virology* 1998;250(2):408–414.
773. Volchkova VA, Klenk H-D, Volchkov VE. Delta-peptide is the carboxy-terminal cleavage fragment of the nonstructural small glycoprotein sGP of Ebola virus. *Virology* 1999;265(1):164–171.
774. Wahl-Jensen VM, Afanasieva TA, Seebach J, et al. Effects of Ebola virus glycoproteins on endothelial cell activation and barrier function. *J Virol* 2005;79(16):10442–10450.
775. Wahl-Jensen V, Bollinger L, Safronetz D, et al. Use of the Syrian hamster as a new model of Ebola virus disease and other viral hemorrhagic fevers. *Viruses* 2012;4(12):3754–3784.
776. Wahl-Jensen V, Kurz S, Feldmann F, et al. Ebola virion attachment and entry into human macrophages profoundly effects early cellular gene expression. *PLoS Negl Trop Dis* 2011;5(10):e1359.
777. Wahl-Jensen V, Radoshitzky SR, de Kok-Mercado F, et al. Role of rodents and bats in human viral hemorrhagic fevers. In: Singh SK, Ruzek D, eds. Viral Hemorrhagic Fevers. Boca Raton: Taylor & Francis/CRC Press; 2013:99–127.
778. Walsh PD, Abernethy KA, Bermejo M, et al. Catastrophic ape decline in western equatorial Africa. *Nature* 2003;422(6932):611–614.
779. Wamala JF, Lukwago L, Malimbo M, et al. Ebola hemorrhagic fever associated with novel virus strain, Uganda, 2007-2008. *Emerg Infect Dis* 2010;16(7):1087–1092.
780. Wan W, Kolesnikova L, Clarke M, et al. Structure and assembly of the Ebola virus nucleocapsid. *Nature* 2017;551(7680):394–397.
781. Wang MK, Lim S-Y, Lee SM, et al. Biochemical basis for increased activity of Ebola glycoprotein in the 2013-16 Epidemic. *Cell Host Microbe* 2017;21(3):367–375.
782. Wang H, Shi Y, Song J, et al. Ebola viral glycoprotein bound to its endosomal receptor Niemann-Pick C1. *Cell* 2016;164(1-2):258–268.
783. Warfield KL, Alves DA, Bradfute SB, et al. Development of a model for marburgvirus based on severe-combined immunodeficiency mice. *Virol J* 2007;4:108.
784. Warfield KL, Bosio CM, Welcher BC, et al. Ebola virus-like particles protect from lethal Ebola virus infection. *Proc Natl Acad Sci U S A* 2003;100(26):15889–15894.
785. Warfield KL, Bradfute SB, Wells J, et al. Development and characterization of a mouse model for Marburg hemorrhagic fever. *J Virol* 2009;83(13):6404–6415.
786. Warfield KL, Swenson DL, Olinger GG, et al. Ebola virus-like particle-based vaccine protects nonhuman primates against lethal Ebola virus challenge. *J Infect Dis* 2007;196(Suppl 2):S430–S437.
787. Warren TK, Jordan R, Lo MK, et al. Therapeutic efficacy of the small molecule GS-5734 against Ebola virus in rhesus monkeys. *Nature* 2016;531(7594):381–385.
788. Washington ML, Meltzer ML; Centers for Disease Control and Prevention. Effectiveness of Ebola treatment units and community care centers—Liberia, September 23-October 31, 2014. *MMWR Morb Mortal Wkly Rep* 2015;64(3):67–69.
789. Wasserman H, Saphire EO. More than meets the eye: hidden structures in the proteome. *Annu Rev Virol* 2016;3(1):373–386.
790. Watanabe S, Noda T, Halfmann P, et al. Ebola virus (EBOV) VP24 inhibits transcription and replication of the EBOV genome. *J Infect Dis* 2007;196(Suppl 2):S284–S290.
791. Watt A, Moukambi F, Banadyga L, et al. A novel life cycle modeling system for Ebola virus shows a genome length-dependent role of VP24 in virus infectivity. *J Virol* 2014;88(18):10511–10524.
792. Wauquier N, Becquart P, Padilla C, et al. Human fatal Zaire Ebola virus infection is associated with an aberrant innate immunity and with massive lymphocyte apoptosis. *PLoS Negl Trop Dis* 2010;4(10):e837.
793. Wauquier N, Padilla C, Becquart P, et al. Association of KIR2DS1 and KIR2DS3 with fatal outcome in Ebola virus infection. *Immunogenetics* 2010;62(11-12):767–771.
794. Wec AZ, Herbert AS, Murin CD, et al. Antibodies from a human survivor define sites of vulnerability for broad protection against ebolaviruses. *Cell* 2017;169(5):878.e815–890.e815.
795. Wei H, Audet J, Wong G, et al. Deep-sequencing of Marburg virus genome during sequential mouse passaging and cell-culture adaptation reveals extensive changes over time. *Sci Rep* 2017;7(1):3390.
796. Weik M, Enterlein S, Schlenz K, et al. The Ebola virus genomic replication promoter is bipartite and follows the rule of six. *J Virol* 2005;79(16):10660–10671.
797. Weik M, Modrof J, Klenk H-D, et al. Ebola virus VP30-mediated transcription is regulated by RNA secondary structure formation. *J Virol* 2002;76(17):8532–8539.
798. Weingartl HM, Embury-Hyatt C, Nfon C, et al. Transmission of Ebola virus from pigs to non-human primates. *Sci Rep* 2012;2:811.
799. Weissenhorn W, Calder LJ, Wharton SA, et al. The central structural feature of the membrane fusion protein subunit from the Ebola virus glycoprotein is a long triple-stranded coiled coil. *Proc Natl Acad Sci U S A* 1998;95(11):6032–6036.
800. Weissenhorn W, Carfi A, Lee K-H, et al. Crystal structure of the Ebola virus membrane fusion subunit, GP2, from the envelope glycoprotein ectodomain. *Mol Cell* 1998;2(5):605–616.
801. Wells CR, Pandey A, Parpia AS, et al. Ebola vaccination in the Democratic Republic of the Congo. *Proc Natl Acad Sci U S A* 2019;116:10178–10183.
802. Welsch S, Kolesnikova L, Krähling V, et al. Electron tomography reveals the steps in filovirus budding. *PLoS Pathog* 2010;6(4):e1000875.

803. Wenigenrath J, Kolesnikova L, Hoenen T, et al. Establishment and application of an infectious virus-like particle system for Marburg virus. *J Gen Virol* 2010;91(Pt 5):1325–1334.
804. West BR, Moyer CL, King LB, et al. Structural basis of pan-ebolavirus neutralization by a human antibody against a conserved, yet cryptic epitope. *MBio* 2018;9(5):e01674.
805. Westhoff Smith D, Hill-Batorski L, N'Jai A, et al. Ebola virus stability under hospital and environmental conditions. *J Infect Dis* 2016;214(Suppl 3):S142–S144.
806. Whitmer SLM, Ladner JT, Wiley MR, et al. Active Ebola virus replication and heterogeneous evolutionary rates in EVD survivors. *Cell Rep* 2018;22(5):1159–1168.
807. Will C, Mühlberger E, Linder D, et al. Marburg virus gene 4 encodes the virion membrane protein, a type I transmembrane glycoprotein. *J Virol* 1993;67(3):1203–1210.
808. Wilson JA, Bray M, Bakken R, et al. Vaccine potential of Ebola virus VP24, VP30, VP35, and VP40 proteins. *Virology* 2001;286(2):384–390.
809. Wilson JA, Hevey M, Bakken R, et al. Epitopes involved in antibody-mediated protection from Ebola virus. *Science* 2000;287(5458):1664–1666.
810. Wilson AJ, Martin DS, Maddox V, et al. Thromboelastography in the management of coagulopathy associated with Ebola virus disease. *Clin Infect Dis* 2016;62(5):610–612.
811. Winslow RL, Milligan ID, Voysey M, et al. Immune responses to novel adenovirus type 26 and modified vaccinia virus Ankara-vectored Ebola vaccines at 1 year. *JAMA* 2017;317(10):1075–1077.
812. Wittmann TJ, Biek R, Hassanin A, et al. Isolates of Zaire ebolavirus from wild apes reveal genetic lineage and recombinants. *Proc Natl Acad Sci U S A* 2007;104(43):17123–17127.
813. Wolf T, Kann G, Becker S, et al. Severe Ebola virus disease with vascular leakage and multiorgan failure: treatment of a patient in intensive care. *Lancet* 2015;385(9976):1428–1435.
814. Wolf YI, Kazlauskas D, Iranzo J, et al. Origins and evolution of the global RNA virome. *MBio* 2018;9(6):e02329.
815. Wong G, He S, Leung A, et al. Naturally occurring single mutations in Ebola virus observably impact infectivity. *J Virol* 2019;93(1):e01098.
816. Wong G, He S, Wei H, et al. Development and characterization of a Guinea pig-adapted Sudan virus. *J Virol* 2016;90(1):392–399.
817. Wong G, Qiu X, Richardson JS, et al. Ebola virus transmission in guinea pigs. *J Virol* 2015;89(2):1314–1323.
818. Wong G, Zhang Z, He S, et al. Marburg and Ravn virus infections do not cause observable disease in ferrets. *J Infect Dis* 2018;218(Suppl 5):S471–S474.
819. Wool-Lewis RJ, Bates P. Characterization of Ebola virus entry by using pseudotyped viruses: identification of receptor-deficient cell lines. *J Virol* 1998;72(4):3155–3160.
820. Wool-Lewis RJ, Bates P. Endoproteolytic processing of the ebola virus envelope glycoprotein: cleavage is not required for function. *J Virol* 1999;73(2):1419–1426.
821. World Health Organization. Ebola haemorrhagic fever in Zaire, 1976. Report of an International Commission. Bull World Health Organ 1978;56(2):271–293.
822. World Health Organization. Ebola haemorrhagic fever in Sudan, 1976. Report of a WHO/International Study Team. *Bull World Health Organ* 1978;56(2):247–270.
823. World Health Organization. *Laboratory Biosafety Manual.* 3rd ed. Geneva: World Health Organization; 2004.
824. World Health Organization. Ebola Reston in pigs and humans, Philippines. *Wkly Epidemiol Rec* 2009;84(7):49–50.
825. World Health Organization. Clinical management of patients with viral haemorrhagic fever: a pocket guide for the front-line health worker. 2016. Available at: http://apps.who.int/iris/bitstream/10665/205570/1/9789241549608_eng.pdf?ua=1
826. World Health Organization. Ebola outbreak 2014-2015. 2017. Available at: http://www.who.int/csr/disease/ebola/en/
827. World Health Organization. ICD-11 for mortality and morbidity statistics. December 2018. Available at: https://icd.who.int/browse11/l-m/en
828. World Health Organization. Preliminary results on the efficacy of rVSV-ZEBOV-GP Ebola vaccine using the ring vaccination strategy in the control of an Ebola outbreak in the Democratic Republic of the Congo: an example of integration of research into epidemic response. 2019. Available at: https://www.who.int/csr/resources/publications/ebola/ebola-ring-vaccination-results-12-april-2019.pdf
829. Wren SM, Kushner AL, Hoyt DB. Operation Ebola. Surgical Care During the West African Outbreak. Baltimore: Johns Hopkins University Press; 2017.
830. Wrensch F, Karsten CB, Gnirß K, et al. Interferon-induced transmembrane protein-mediated inhibition of host cell entry of ebolaviruses. *J Infect Dis* 2015;212(Suppl 2):S210–S218.
831. Wu W, Liu S. The drug targets and antiviral molecules for treatment of Ebola virus infection. *Curr Top Med Chem* 2017;17(3):361–370.
832. Wu L, Zhang Z, Gao H, et al. Open-label phase I clinical trial of Ad5-EBOV in Africans in China. *Hum Vaccin Immunother* 2017;13(9):2078–2085.
833. Wyers M, Formenty P, Cherel Y, et al. Histopathological and immunohistochemical studies of lesions associated with Ebola virus in a naturally infected chimpanzee. *J Infect Dis* 1999;179(Suppl 1):S54–S59.
834. Xu W, Edwards MR, Borek DM, et al. Ebola virus VP24 targets a unique NLS binding site on karyopherin alpha 5 to selectively compete with nuclear import of phosphorylated STAT1. *Cell Host Microbe* 2014;16(2):187–200.
835. Xu Z, Jin B, Teng G, et al. Epidemiologic characteristics, clinical manifestations, and risk factors of 139 patients with Ebola virus disease in western Sierra Leone. *Am J Infect Control* 2016;44(11):1285–1290.
836. Xu W, Luthra P, Wu C, et al. Ebola virus VP30 and nucleoprotein interactions modulate viral RNA synthesis. *Nat Commun* 2017;8:15576.
837. Xu L, Sanchez A, Yang Z-Y, et al. Immunization for Ebola virus infection. *Nat Med* 1998;4(1):37–42.
838. Yaddanapudi K, Palacios G, Towner JS, et al. Implication of a retrovirus-like glycoprotein peptide in the immunopathogenesis of Ebola and Marburg viruses. *FASEB J* 2006;20(14):2519–2530.
839. Yan F, He S, Banadyga L, et al. Characterization of Reston virus infection in ferrets. *Antiviral Res* 2019;165:1–10.
840. Yang L, Sanchez A, Ward JM, et al. A paramyxovirus-vectored intranasal vaccine against Ebola virus is immunogenic in vector-immune animals. *Virology* 2008;377(2):255–264.
841. Yang X-L, Tan CW, Anderson DE, et al. Characterization of a filovirus (Měnglà virus) from Rousettus bats in China. *Nat Microbiol* 2019;4(3):390–395.
842. Yang X-L, Zhang Y-Z, Jiang R-D, et al. Genetically diverse filoviruses in Rousettus and Eonycteris spp. bats, China, 2009 and 2015. *Emerg Infect Dis* 2017;23(3):482–486.
843. Yasuda J, Nakao M, Kawaoka Y, et al. Nedd4 regulates egress of Ebola virus-like particles from host cells. *J Virol* 2003;77(18):9987–9992.
844. Yen BC, Basler CF. Effects of filovirus interferon antagonists on responses of human monocyte-derived dendritic cells to RNA virus infection. *J Virol* 2016;90(10):5108–5118.
845. Yen B, Mulder LCF, Martinez O, Basler CF. Molecular basis for ebolavirus VP35 suppression of human dendritic cell maturation. *J Virol* 2014;88(21):12500–12510.
846. Yoshida A, Kim S-H, Manoharan VK, et al. Novel avian paramyxovirus-based vaccine vectors expressing the Ebola virus glycoprotein elicit mucosal and humoral immune responses in guinea pigs. *Sci Rep* 2019;9(1):5520.
847. Younan P, Iampietro M, Santos RI, et al. Role of transmembrane protein 16F in the incorporation of phosphatidylserine into budding Ebola virus virions. *J Infect Dis* 2018;218(Suppl 5):S335–S345.
848. Younan P, Santos RI, Ramanathan P, et al. Ebola virus-mediated T-lymphocyte depletion is the result of an abortive infection. *PLoS Pathog* 2019;15(10):e1008068.
849. Yuan S, Cao L, Ling H, et al. TIM-1 acts a dual-attachment receptor for Ebolavirus by interacting directly with viral GP and the PS on the viral envelope. *Protein Cell* 2015;6(11):814–824.
850. Zaki SR, Goldsmith CS. Pathologic features of filovirus infections in humans. *Curr Top Microbiol Immunol* 1999;235:97–116.
851. Zaki SR, Peters CJ. Viral hemorrhagic fevers. In: Connor DH, Chandler FW, Schwartz DA, et al., eds. *The Pathology of Infectious Diseases.* Norwalk: Appleton and Lange; 1997:347–364.
852. Zaki SR, Shieh W-J, Greer PW, et al. A novel immunohistochemical assay for the detection of Ebola virus in skin: implications for diagnosis, spread, and surveillance of Ebola hemorrhagic fever. *J Infect Dis* 1999;179(Suppl 1):S36–S47.
853. Zapatero-Belinchon FJ, Dietzel E, Dolnik O, et al. Characterization of the filovirus-resistant cell line SH-SY5Y reveals redundant role of cell surface entry factors. *Viruses* 2019;11(3):275.
854. Zeng X, Blancett CD, Koistinen KA, et al. Identification and pathological characterization of persistent asymptomatic Ebola virus infection in rhesus monkeys. *Nat Microbiol* 2017;2:17113.
855. Zhang APP, Bornholdt ZA, Abelson DM, et al. Crystal structure of Marburg virus VP24. *J Virol* 2014;88(10):5859–5863.
856. Zhang APP, Bornholdt ZA, Liu T, et al. The Ebola virus interferon antagonist VP24 directly binds STAT1 and has a novel, pyramidal fold. *PLoS Pathog* 2012;8(2):e1002550.
857. Zhang Q, Gui M, Niu X, et al. Potent neutralizing monoclonal antibodies against Ebola virus infection. *Sci Rep* 2016;6:25856.
858. Zhu F-C, Hou L-H, Li JX, et al. Safety and immunogenicity of a novel recombinant adenovirus type-5 vector-based Ebola vaccine in healthy adults in China: preliminary report of a randomised, double-blind, placebo-controlled, phase 1 trial. *Lancet* 2015;385(9984):2272–2279.
859. Zhu F-C, Wurie AH, Hou L-H, et al. Safety and immunogenicity of a recombinant adenovirus type-5 vector-based Ebola vaccine in healthy adults in Sierra Leone: a single-centre, randomised, double-blind, placebo-controlled, phase 2 trial. *Lancet* 2017;389(10069):621–628.
860. Zinzula L, Nagy I, Orsini M, et al. Structures of Ebola and Reston virus VP35 oligomerization domains and comparative biophysical characterization in all ebolavirus species. Structure 2019;27(1):39.e36–54.e36.
861. Zlotnik I. Marburg agent disease: pathology. *Trans R Soc Trop Med Hyg* 1969;63(3):310–327.
862. Zlotnik I, Simpson DIH. The pathology of experimental vervet monkey disease in hamsters. *Br J Exp Pathol* 1969;50(4):393–399.
863. Zumbrun EE, Abdeltawab NF, Bloomfield HA, et al. Development of a murine model for aerosolized ebolavirus infection using a panel of recombinant inbred mice. *Viruses* 2012;4(12):3468–3493.
864. Zumbrun EE, Bloomfield HA, Dye JM, et al. A characterization of aerosolized Sudan virus infection in African green monkeys, cynomolgus macaques, and rhesus macaques. *Viruses* 2012;4(10):2115–2136.
865. Акинфеева ЛА, Аксёнова ОИ, Василевич ИВ, et al. Случай вирусной геморрагической лихорадки Эбола. *Инфекционные Болезни.* 2005;3(1):85–88.
866. Бажутин НБ, Беланов ЕФ, Спиридонов ВА, et al. Влияние способов экспериментального заражения вирусом Марбург на особенности протекания болезни у зеленых мартышек. *Вопр Вирусол.* 1992;37(3):153–156.
867. Борисевич ИВ, Маркин ВА, Фирсова ИВ, et al. Эпидемиология, профилактика, клиника и лечение геморрагических лихорадок (Марбург, Эбола, Ласса и Боливийской). *Вопр Вирусол.* 2006;51(5):8–16.
868. Михайлов ВВ, Борисевич ИВ, Черникова НК, et al. Оценка на павианах гамадрилах возможности специфической профилактики лихорадки Эбола. *Вопр Вирусол.* 1994;39(2):82–84.
869. Мунтянов ВП, Крюк ВД, Беланов ЕФ. Дезинфицирующее действие хлорамина Б на вирус Марбург. *Вопр Вирусол.* 1996;41(1):42–43.
870. Никифоров ВВ, Туровский ЮИ, Калинин ПП, et al. Случай лабораторного заражения лихорадкой Марбург. Ж Микробиол Эпидемиол Иммунобиол. 1994(3):104–106.
871. Тодоровић К, Моцић М, Клашња Р, et al. Непознато вирусно обољење пренето са инфицираних-оболелих мајмуна на човека. *Глас Срп Акад Наука Мед.* 1969;CCLXXV(22):91–101.
872. Чеусова ТБ, Becker S, Muehlberger E, Рябчикова ЕИ. Субмикроскопические особенности репликации вируса Марбург и его минигеномного аналога в культурах клеток. *Мол Ген Микробиол Вирусол.* 2002(2):27–30.

Paramyxoviridae: The Viruses and Their Replication

Richard K. Plemper • Robert A. Lamb

INTRODUCTION

The *Paramyxoviridae* are important and ubiquitous disease-causing viruses of humans and animals, including one of the most infectious viruses known (measles virus [MeV]); some of the most prevalent viruses known (MeV, parainfluenza viruses, and mumps virus [MuV]); a virus that has been targeted by the World Health Organization for eradication (MeV) and the second virus successfully eradicated (rinderpest virus [RPV]); viruses that have a major agricultural impact (Newcastle disease virus [NDV] and Nipah virus [NiV]); and many recently identified viruses (Hendra virus [HeV], NiV, J virus, and Belong virus), some of which cause deadly diseases (HeV and NiV). The *Paramyxoviridae* are enveloped negative-strand RNA viruses that have special relationships with three other families of negative-strand RNA viruses, namely, the *Orthomyxoviridae* (for the biological properties of the envelope glycoproteins) and the *Pneumoviridae* and *Rhabdoviridae* (for the similarity of organization of the nonsegmented genome and its expression).

Both the *Paramyxoviridae* and the *Pneumoviridae* are defined by having a fusion (F) protein that causes merger of viral and cell membranes at neutral pH. The genomic RNA of all negative-strand RNA viruses has to serve two functions: (a) as a template for synthesis of mRNAs and (b) as a template for synthesis of the antigenome (+) strand. Negative-strand RNA viruses encode and package their own RNA-dependent RNA polymerase (RdRP), but mRNAs are only synthesized once the virion has been uncoated in the infected cell. Viral replication occurs only after the synthesis of viral mRNAs and proteins has been initiated and requires the continuous synthesis of viral proteins. Newly synthesized antigenome (+) strands serve as the template for further copies of the (−) strand genomic RNA.

CLASSIFICATION

According to the February 2019 classification accepted by the International Committee on the Taxonomy of Viruses, the family *Paramyxoviridae* is grouped into seven genera: *Morbillivirus, Henipavirus, Respirovirus, Rubulavirus, Avulavirus, Aquaparamyxovirus,* and *Ferlavirus* (Table 12.1). This organization was originally developed based on historic classification criteria such as morphologic features, genome organization, and biological activities of individual proteins and further refined based on sequence relationships after an increasing number of genome sequences became available. However, the recent discovery of numerous new paramyxoviruses has prompted a proposal for taxonomic reorganization driven by novel, sequence-based demarcation criteria including RdRP sequence motifs and pairwise amino acid sequence comparison to negotiate inconsistencies that arose from the historical classification approach.[487] This initiative organizes the *Paramyxoviridae* into four subfamilies, the *Avulavirinae, Rubulavirinae, Orthoparamyxovirinae,* and *Metaparamyxovirinae* (Table 12.2), that contain a combined total of 14 different genera with 69 classified and 3 unassigned species. The future discovery of additional new paramyxoviruses is highly likely.[595]

The distinguishing morphologic feature among enveloped viruses for the family *Paramyxoviridae* is the size and shape of the nucleocapsids (variable among different family members; approximate length is 1 μm, diameter and pitch range from 18–20 nm and 4.7–8.3 nm, respectively), which have a left-handed helical symmetry. Historic biological organization

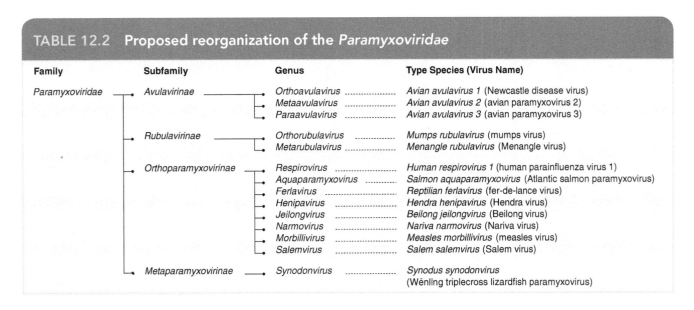

TABLE 12.1 Classification of the *Paramyxoviridae* family, ICTV 2018

Family	Genus	Type Species (Virus Name)
Paramyxoviridae	*Aquaparamyxovirus*	*Salmon aquaparamyxovirus* (Atlantic salmon paramyxovirus)
	Avulavirus	*Avian avulavirus 1* (Newcastle disease virus)
	Ferlavirus	*Reptilian ferlavirus* (fer-de-lance virus)
	Henipavirus	*Hendra henipavirus* (Hendra virus)
	Morbillivirus	*Measles morbillivirus* (measles virus)
	Respirovirus	*Murine respirovirus* (Sendai virus)
	Rubulavirus	*Mumps rubulavirus* (mumps virus)

criteria are (a) antigenic cross-reactivity between members of a genus and (b) the presence or absence of neuraminidase (NA) activity. In addition, the differing coding potentials of the *P* genes were considered—members of the *Avulavirinae*, *Rubulavirinae*, and *Metaparamyxovirinae* and the genus *Ferlavirus* do not encode a C protein—and some *Rubulavirinae* and *Jeilongviruses* contain an extra *SH* gene. Most closely related to the *Paramyxoviridae* are the *Pneumoviridae*, which until recently were jointly classified in a single family. Pneumoviruses (respiratory syncytial viruses [RSVs] and the metapneumoviruses) can be distinguished from the *Paramyxoviridae* based on their narrower nucleocapsids, a greater number of open reading frames (ORFs) in the genomes, and a different structural organization and functional role of their attachment proteins.

THE STRUCTURE AND REPLICATION STRATEGY OF THE *PARAMYXOVIRIDAE*

Paramyxoviruses contain nonsegmented single-stranded RNA genomes of negative polarity and replicate entirely in the cytoplasm. Their genomes are 14,296 to 21,523 bp in length and harbor six (*Avulavirinae*, most *Orthoparamyxovirinae*, *Metarubulavirus* genus) to eight (*Jeilongvirus* genus) tandemly linked genes. By the convention used for paramyxoviruses, the term "gene" refers to the genome sequence encoding a single mRNA, even if that mRNA contains more than one ORF and encodes more than one protein. A lipid envelope containing two surface glycoproteins (F and the attachment glycoprotein variously called hemagglutinin-neuraminidase (HN), hemagglutinin (H), or glycoprotein (G)) surrounds the virions. Inside the envelope lies a helical nucleocapsid core containing the RNA genome and the nucleocapsid (N), phosphoprotein (P), and large (L) proteins, which initiate intracellular transcription and replication. Residing between the envelope and the core is the viral matrix (M) protein that serves as a virion assembly organizer and is released from the core during virus entry. In addition to the genes encoding structural proteins, paramyxoviruses express "accessory" proteins that are encoded in alternative reading frames overlapping with the *P* gene.

Intracellular replication of paramyxoviruses begins with the viral RdRP (minimally, a hetero-oligomeric complex consisting of a P homotetramer and a single L protein) transcribing the N-encapsidated genomic RNA (N–RNA) into 5′-capped and 3′-polyadenylated mRNAs. In transcriptase mode, the viral RdRP initiates RNA synthesis at the 3′ end of the genome and transcribes the genes into mRNAs in a sequential (and polar) manner by terminating and reinitiating at each gene junction. The junctions consist of a gene-end (GE) sequence, at which polyadenylation occurs by the reiterative copying of four to seven uridines (followed by release of the mRNA), a short nontranscribed intergenic (IG) region,

TABLE 12.2 Proposed reorganization of the *Paramyxoviridae*

Family	Subfamily	Genus	Type Species (Virus Name)
Paramyxoviridae	*Avulavirinae*	*Orthoavulavirus*	*Avian avulavirus 1* (Newcastle disease virus)
		Metaavulavirus	*Avian avulavirus 2* (avian paramyxovirus 2)
		Paraavulavirus	*Avian avulavirus 3* (avian paramyxovirus 3)
	Rubulavirinae	*Orthorubulavirus*	*Mumps rubulavirus* (mumps virus)
		Metarubulavirus	*Menangle rubulavirus* (Menangle virus)
	Orthoparamyxovirinae	*Respirovirus*	*Human respirovirus 1* (human parainfluenza virus 1)
		Aquaparamyxovirus	*Salmon aquaparamyxovirus* (Atlantic salmon paramyxovirus)
		Ferlavirus	*Reptilian ferlavirus* (fer-de-lance virus)
		Henipavirus	*Hendra henipavirus* (Hendra virus)
		Jeilongvirus	*Beilong jeilongvirus* (Beilong virus)
		Narmovirus	*Nariva narmovirus* (Nariva virus)
		Morbillivirus	*Measles morbillivirus* (measles virus)
		Salemvirus	*Salem salemvirus* (Salem virus)
	Metaparamyxovirinae	*Synodonvirus*	*Synodus synodonvirus* (Wēnlíng triplecross lizardfish paramyxovirus)

and a gene-start sequence that specifies mRNA initiation and, presumably, by analogy with rhabdovirus gene expression, capping. While RdRP generates predominantly monocistronic viral mRNAs, it occasionally misses GE sequences resulting in the synthesis of polycistronic mRNAs, of which only the first gene is translated. In addition, the RdRP sometimes fails to reinitiate transcription at a gene-start sequence and/or detaches from the template N–RNA prematurely, resulting in the creation of an mRNA transcription gradient that is inversely proportional to the distance of the gene from the 3′ end of the genome. After primary transcription and translation, when sufficient amounts of unassembled N protein have accumulated in the infected cell, the RdRP can switch into replicase mode, becoming highly processive and concomitantly N-encapsidating the nascent RNA chain while ignoring all IG junctions and editing sites. The resulting product is an exact complementary antigenomic [+] RNA chain of the viral genome in a fully assembled nucleocapsid.

VIRION STRUCTURE

The *Paramyxoviridae* contain a lipid bilayer envelope that is derived from the plasma membrane of the host cell in which the virus is grown (reviewed in Ref.[93]). *Paramyxoviridae* are generally spherical, 150 to 350 nm in diameter, but can be pleiomorphic in shape, and filamentous forms exceeding one micron in length have been observed.[266] Inserted into the envelope are glycoprotein spikes that extend approximately 8 to 12 nm from the surface of the membrane and can be readily visualized by electron microscopy (EM). Inside the viral membrane is the ribonucleoprotein (RNP) core that contains the 14,296 to 21,523 (depending on paramyxovirus species) nucleotide single-stranded RNA genome. Figure 12.1 shows a stylized schematic diagram of the virion by example of the *Morbillivirus* genus. The pleiomorphic nature of virion particles is illustrated in the negative-stain electron micrographs and cryoelectron

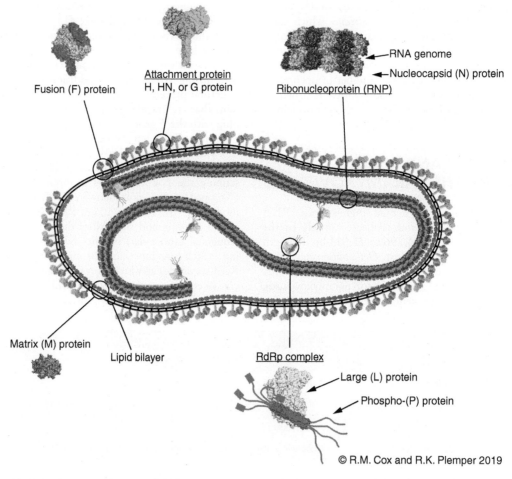

© R.M. Cox and R.K. Plemper 2019

FIGURE 12.1 Schematic diagram of a paramyxovirus (not drawn to scale). Shown are the lipid envelope and the underlying viral M protein array. Inserted into the envelope are the attachment protein (hemagglutinin [H], hemagglutinin-neuraminidase [HN], or glycoprotein [G] depending on virus species) and the F protein. The relative abundance of attachment and F proteins is not accurately illustrated by the diagram. The attachment proteins form tetrameric structures composed of a stalk region and a globular head. The F proteins exist as trimers. The ribonucleoprotein (RNP) complex is composed of the negative-strand viral RNA genome encapsidated by the N protein. Associated with the RNP are RNA-dependent RNA polymerase (RdRP) complexes, consisting of the L and P proteins. (Images copyright © 2019 by Richard K. Plemper and Robert M. Cox.)

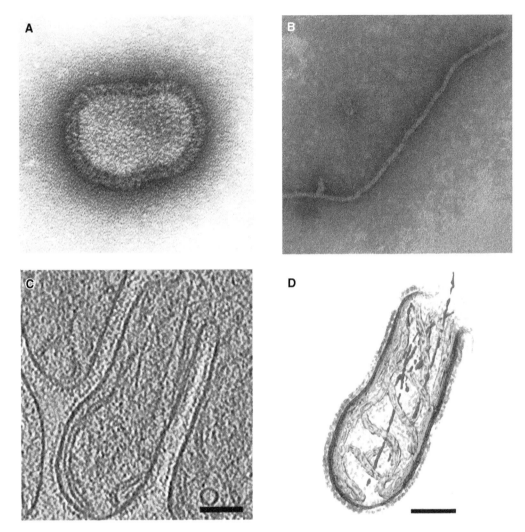

FIGURE 12.2 Electron microscopy images of paramyxoviruses. A: Ultrastructure of PIV-5 virions revealed by negative staining. The glycoprotein spikes on intact 150- to 300-nm virus particles can be observed (226,280×). **B:** Negatively stained PIV-5 nucleocapsid (74,570×). **C and D:** Cryoelectron tomography (cryo-ET) **(C)** and 3D segmentation of the cryo-ET data **(D)** provided detailed insights into the organization of a MeV virion budding from infected cells.[266] Scale bars represent 100 nm. (Images of budding MeV and corresponding 3D segmentation were modified from Ke Z, Strauss JD, Hampton CM, et al. Promotion of virus assembly and organization by the measles virus matrix protein. *Nat Commun* 2018;9(1):1736, CC BY 4.0; the original image was cropped, scale bars were relocated, and *arrows* were removed; http://creativecommons.org/licenses/by/4.0/.)

microscopy (cryo-EM)–derived tomograms shown in Figure 12.2, and a comparison of the RNPs of influenza virus, rabies virus, and Sendai virus (SeV) is shown in Figure 12.3.

The helical nucleocapsid, rather than free genome RNA, serves as the template for all RNA synthesis. For SeV, each nucleocapsid is composed of approximately 2,600 N, 300 P, and 50 L proteins.[291] The N protein and genomic RNA together form a core structure, to which the P-L complexes are attached. This nucleocapsid core is remarkably stable because it withstands the high salt and gravity forces of CsCl density gradient centrifugation. In the EM of nucleocapsids and more recent cryoelectron tomography (cryo-ET) reconstructions, the P and L proteins are not observed, and they have only been visualized through immunostaining.[467] Holonucleocapsids (N–RNA plus P-L) have the capacity to transcribe mRNAs *in vitro*,

presumably mimicking primary transcription in infected cells, and they are believed to be the minimum unit of infectivity.

SeV nucleocapsids were shown to exist in several distinct morphologic states at normal salt concentration.[150,210] The most prevalent form in negatively stained preparations is the most tightly coiled one, with a helical pitch of 5.3 nm. Two other forms, one with a slightly larger pitch of 6.8 nm and another with a much larger pitch of 37.5 nm, have also been noted. The fact that no structures of intermediate pitch have been found indicates that these are distinct states. It is believed that the template is copied without dissociation of N protein from the nucleocapsid, routing the interlocking N protein chain over the surface of the P-L complex as the polymerase advances. Local uncoiling of the nucleocapsid may be necessary for the polymerase to gain access to the RNA bases. It is possible that the viral polymerase

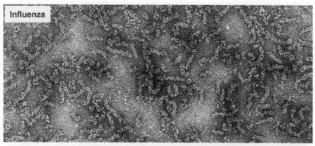

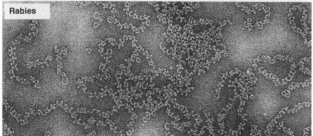

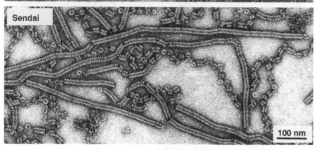

FIGURE 12.3 Nucleocapsids of negative-strand RNA viruses.
Negative-stain electron micrographs of the nucleocapsids of three
negative-strand RNA viruses. **Top:** Ribonucleoprotein particles
of influenza virus (*Orthomyxoviridae*) with a stoichiometry of 24
nucleotides per NP monomer. **Middle:** Nucleocapsids of rabies virus
(*Rhabdoviridae*) with a stoichiometry of 9 nucleotides per N monomer. **Bottom:** Nucleocapsids of SeV (*Paramyxoviridae*) with a stoichiometry of 6 nucleotides per N monomer. All micrographs have the
same magnification; scale bar is 100 nm. (Micrographs courtesy of
Rob Ruigrok, EMBL, Grenoble, France.)

traverses the nucleocapsid template by uncoiling the helix in
front of it and recoiling it once the polymerase has passed a
given position, much the same as cellular RNA polymerase generates its template "bubble" in traversing dsDNA.

As expected, the diameter of the nucleocapsid decreases as
the pitch increases and the nucleocapsid lengthens. For SeV,
the diameter is 3.5 nm less for the 6.8-nm form than for the
5.3-nm pitch form. These latter values are similar to those of
Pneumoviridae nucleocapsids, which also have a pitch of 7 nm.
As discussed previously, these differences in nucleocapsid morphology can be used to distinguish between the *Paramyxoviridae*
and *Pneumoviridae*, but they may relate simply to which form
predominates in negatively stained preparations.

THE *PARAMYXOVIRIDAE* GENOMES AND THEIR ENCODED PROTEINS

The complete genome sequences for all known members
of the *Paramyxoviridae* have been obtained and are available

online. The genomic RNAs contain a 3′ extracistronic region
of approximately 50 nucleotides known as the leader and a 5′
extracistronic region of 50 to 161 nucleotides known as the
trailer (or [−] leader). These control regions are essential for
transcription and replication and flank the six to eight genes.
The coding capacity of the genomes is extended by the use of
overlapping ORFs in the *P* gene. The gene order of representative paramyxoviruses is shown in Figure 12.4. At the beginning and end of each gene are conserved transcriptional control
sequences that are copied into mRNA. Between the gene
boundaries are IG regions. These are precisely three nucleotides
long for the respiroviruses and morbilliviruses but are quite
variable in length for the *Rubulavirinae* (1–47 nucleotides)
(Table 12.3).

The Nucleocapsid Protein

The nucleocapsid (N) protein is present as the first transcribed
gene in the viral genome of all paramyxoviruses and ranges in
size from 489 to 553 amino acids (molecular weight ~53–57
kDa). N is an RNA-binding protein that coats full-length viral
(−) sense genomic and (+) sense antigenomic RNAs to form
the helical nucleocapsid template, which is the only biologically
active form of these viral RNAs. EM and three-dimensional
image reconstruction for MeV, parainfluenza virus 5 (PIV-5),
and SeV nucleocapsids reveals that N binds precisely 6 consecutive nucleotides and 13 N subunits constitute each turn of
the nucleocapsid helix.[6,150,193] In general, these parameters also
apply to other paramyxovirus nucleocapsids, although there
can be slight differences in the number of N subunits per helix
turn and in the pitch of the helix.[27] The binding of N to RNA
to form a helical structure is believed to serve several functions,
including protection from nuclease digestion, alignment of distal RNA segments to create a functional 3′-end promoter, and
providing interaction sites for assembly of progeny nucleocapsids into budding virions.

Expression of paramyxovirus N proteins in the absence of
other viral components results in the formation of nucleocapsid-like structures, suggesting that N has inherent self-assembly properties and that N–N interactions drive nucleocapsid
assembly.[163,386,387,403,529,557] Biochemical and mutational studies
have shown that the N protein can be generally divided into
two main structural regions: (a) Ncore, an N-terminal domain
representing approximately three-fourths of the protein that
is conserved in sequence among related viruses, and (b) Ntail,
a C-terminal nonconserved acidic domain. The N-terminal
approximately 400 residues of the SeV and MeV Ncore are
essential for self-assembly and RNA binding.[55,111,271]

A cryo-EM–based reconstruction of purified MeV nucleocapsids after removal of the Ntail domain has revealed an
organization of Ncore into two distinct globular domains, the
N-terminal NTD (residues 37–265) and C-terminal CTD
(residues 266–372), which are preceded and followed by short
NT-arm (residues 1–36) and CT-arm (residues 373–391)
extensions, respectively (Fig. 12.5A–C).[193] In the nucleocapsid
assembly, the NT-arms interlock with the CTD of the subsequent N protomer, and CT-arms interact with the preceding protomer, creating a stable chain link–like arrangement.
Although Ntails were removed prior to reconstruction, the
position of the CT-arm suggests that Ntails protrude to the
outside of the nucleocapsid between adjacent rungs of the
helix. The RNA populates a cleft between NTD and CTD,

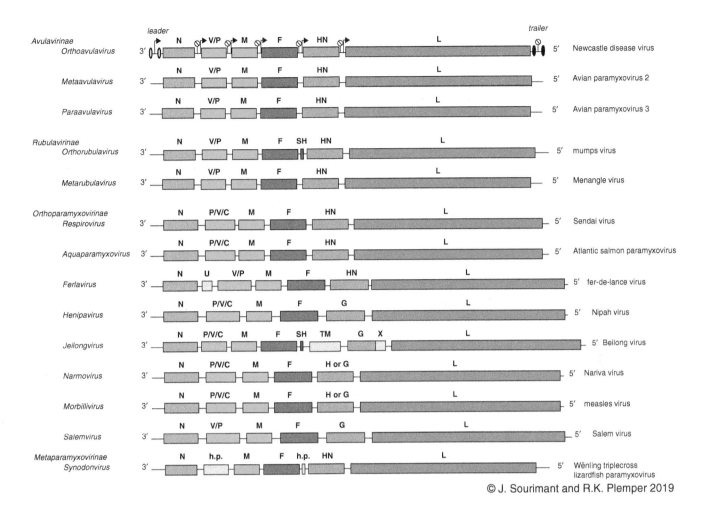

FIGURE 12.4 Schematic diagram of the genomes of selected viruses representing each genus of the *Paramyxoviridae*. Intergenic junctions are shown as single *black lines*; transcribed sections are depicted as *boxes* drawn to approximate gene length scale and color-coded by encoded protein type: N proteins (*orange*), P proteins (*green*), M proteins (*light blue*), F proteins (*red*), attachment proteins (*pink*), and L proteins (*dark blue*). When present, SH proteins are shown in *red*. Uncharacterized proteins are colored in *gray*. For *Jeilongvirus* genus, X denotes an internal ORF in the G gene of unknown function. Hypothetical proteins (h.p.) predicted based on the complete genome of the newly discovered *Synodonvirus* genus are indicated. Bipartite promoters (*oval circle*) and transcriptional gene end (*crossed circle*) and transcription gene start (*black arrow*) sequence are shown for NDV only. (Images copyright © 2019 by Richard K. Plemper and Julien Sourimant.)

winding around the outside of the RNP helix (Figs. 12.5D, E and 12.6A).[193] However, paramyxovirus N proteins do not contain conventional RNA-binding motifs that are typically found on cellular RNA-binding proteins. Biophysical properties are furthermore unusual for RNA-binding proteins, since

they feature an overall acidic charge (net charge of −7 to −12, with the exception of MuV [+2]). A central region of Ncore that is highly conserved among all members of the family (residues 258–369 for SeV) contains an F-X4-Y-X3-ϕ–S–ϕ-A-M motif (where X is any residue and ϕ is an aromatic amino acid).

TABLE 12.3 Gene-end, Gene-start, and intergenic sequences in representative members of the *Paramyxoviridae*

Gene-End	Intergenic	Gene-Start	
NAUUCU$_5$	Gaa	UCCCaNUUU	Sendai virus
AuuuuU$_4$	Gaa	UCCcnggU	Measles virus
AAuUcU$_{5-6}$	GAA	UCCUngGU	Nipah virus
aauuCU$_{4-7}$	1–22	UcCgggCa	Parainfluenza virus 5
AauucU$_{4-6}$	8–70	CuCgGgcU	Tioman virus

Consensus sequences are listed as (−) sense genomic RNA. Strictly conserved nucleotides are shown as upper case letters; nucleotides that are mostly conserved (≥3 junctions per genome) are shown in lowercase letters.

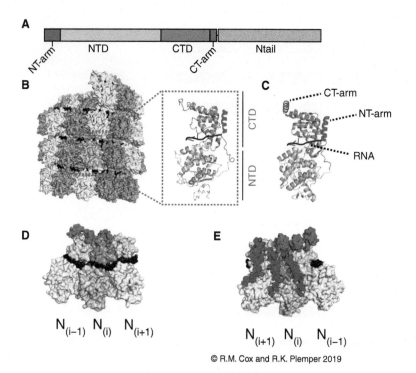

FIGURE 12.5 Structure of the paramyxovirus N protein and RNP assembly. A: Schematic of the domain organization of the N protein. NT-arm (*blue*) and CT-arm (*red*) are responsible for N–N homo-oligomerization. RNA is encapsidated between NTD (*light blue*) and CTD (*pink*). The C-terminal Ntail domain is flexible and disordered. **B:** Cryoelectron microscopy structure of the MeV nucleocapsid (PDB ID: 4UFT).[193] The structure is based on a truncated N protein (residues 1–391) and lacks Ntail. *Insert*: Single N protomer. The NTD (*light blue*) and CTD (*pink*) domains and viral RNA (*black*) are highlighted. **C:** Crystal structure of the PIV-5 N protein lacking the Ntail domain. The domain architecture is similar to MeV N, color-coding as in (**B**). **D and E:** Enlarged views of three neighboring protomers, taken from outside (**D**) or inside (**E**) the helical RNP. NT-arm of $N_{(i)}$ interacts with an adjacent $N_{(N+1)}$, while CT-arm interacts with the other neighboring $N_{(N-1)}$ monomer. Color-coding of the arms as in (**C**). (Images copyright © 2019 by Richard K. Plemper and Robert M. Cox.)

© R.M. Cox and R.K. Plemper 2019

This region is essential for self-assembly of N with RNA[385] and important for N–RNA interactions.[6,193,349]

The approximately 125–amino acid C-terminal Ntail region is intrinsically structurally disordered[40] and poorly conserved among different paramyxoviruses. It is dispensable for RNA binding and the assembly of N–RNA complexes.[111] While Ncores are resistant to trypsin proteolysis, treatment of purified nucleocapsids with trypsin removes most of Ntail, resulting in bioinactive, rigidified RNP helixes with a shortened pitch of 5 nm compared to the native 6.4-nm form detected in infected cells.[27,28,111,209,377,529] This apparent link between the physical presence of Ntail and flexibility of the native nucleocapsid is consistent with Ntail being routed between adjacent turns of the helix. Supported by the high degree of structural disorder, a role of Ntail in a diverse array of protein–protein interactions was proposed. For instance, three short conserved sequence elements (Boxes 1–3) are embedded in *Morbillivirus* Ntails, spanning residues 400 to 420, 489 to 506, and 517 to 525 (Fig. 12.6A).[130] The second of these elements, termed a molecular recognition element (MoRE), has been shown to interact with a C-terminal X domain of the P protein (P-XD), undergoing an induced conversion into a short alpha helical structure upon contact.[40,197,252,620] A crystal structure of a recombinant MeV P-XD fused to a MoRE-derived peptide was solved, revealing a stable four-helix arrangement.[273] This interaction with P appeared to support a proposed role of Ntail in recruiting P-L to the nucleocapsid, since a C-terminal truncation of residues 495 to 525 had been shown to abolish RdRP activity in MeV minireplicon reporter assays.[659] However, further truncation of the MeV Ntail by up to 40 additional residues has been unexpectedly shown to progressively restore polymerase activity, indicating that initial loading of the RdRP complex onto the template occurs independent of interaction between Ntail and P-L.[282] Rather, recruitment of the RdRP complex to the RNP is thought to depend on direct interactions between P-L and Ncore.[555] While specific microdomains involved in this interaction are unknown, binding of MuV P to Ncore was demonstrated.[101,271]

Once the polymerase complex is loaded onto the template, iterative cycles of MoRE to P-XD binding and release contribute to preventing premature termination of the advancing RdRP.[57,271,325] These productive interaction cycles are independent of spatial flexibility provided by Ntail-embedded MoRE and cis-acting elements in Ntail, since recombinant MeVs expressing engineered N proteins in which MoRE was relocated from Ntail into Ncore replicated efficiently.[102] However, these engineered MeVs and likewise recombinant canine distemper viruses (CDVs) containing N proteins lacking up to 55 of the structurally disordered central Ntail residues showed altered RdRP transcriptase function, implicating Ntail in regulating proper viral protein expression.[594] A nonessential role of the structurally disordered Ntail section was also confirmed for the related henipaviruses,[594] although the relative positioning of N–P interaction regions within Ntail differs between the henipaviruses and morbilliviruses (Fig. 12.6A).[194]

In the case of MeV, two serine-phosphorylation sites (S479 and S510) located before and after MoREs have been mapped that, when mutated to alanines, affect RdRP bioactivity.[195] Both the second and third conserved elements at the Ntail C-terminus were furthermore proposed to bind the cellular chaperone HSP72 and its cofactor HSP40,[100,659] opening an additional path to regulate RdRP activity by modulating the stability of the Ntail P-XD interaction. Residues in the third conserved element in addition interact with the viral matrix (M) protein, outlining a role of Ntail in virion assembly through creation of a link between RNP and viral envelope.[245,485]

The interactions of paramyxovirus N proteins with RNA are remarkably stable, and nucleocapsid-associated RNA is protected from nucleases even at very high salt concentrations or after proteolytic removal of the Ntail domain.[209,377,529]

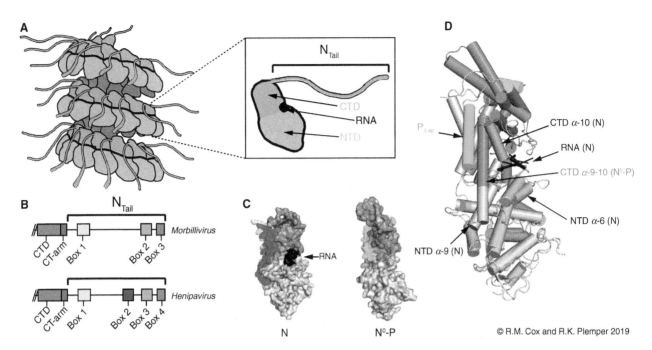

FIGURE 12.6 N–RNA binding and N⁰–P interaction. The N-terminus of the P protein is responsible for chaperoning newly synthesized N proteins to the nascent RNA strand during replication. Crystal structures of these N⁰–P complexes have been solved.[4,192,641] **A:** Cartoon of an assembled helical nucleocapsid with intact Ntails (not drawn to scale). The Ntail domain is proposed to extend from the helical nucleocapsid into the surrounding environment.[251] *Insert:* Enlargement of a single N protomer; major folding domains, the tail domain, and the RNA are highlighted. **B:** Three conserved sections exist in the Ntail of a *Morbillivirus*, termed Boxes 1 to 3. The function of Box 1 is still unclear, but Box 2 contains a molecular recognition element (MoRE) responsible for interaction with the C-terminal XD domain in the homotypic P protein,[273] and Box 3 contains an M binding site that is required for efficient assembly of virions.[485] The Ntail of henipaviruses contains four patches of partially conserved residues that were termed Boxes 1 to 4 and predicted to be MoREs.[30] Binding of Box 3 to the henipavirus P-XD was demonstrated, but the role of Boxes 1, 2, and 4 remains still unclear. **C:** *Left,* surface representation of an MeV N protomer in the RNP assembly with the NT-arm of the neighboring N protomer shown in *blue; top,* surface representation of an MeV N⁰–P crystal structure (complex [PDB ID: 5E4V][192]). **D:** Cartoon representation of overlays of MeV N⁰–P (NTD, *light blue*; CTD, *pink*; P, *green*) and NC model (*light gray*). The N-terminus of P (P_{1-48}) interacts specifically with the first and second helices of the CTD of N (α-9 and α-10; *arrow*). This interaction blocks NT-arm interactions from neighboring N subunits, preventing premature N–N oligomerization. In addition, binding of P_{1-48} induces a conformational change in the α-6 helix of the NTD, blocking RNA encapsidation. (Images copyright © 2019 by Richard K. Plemper and Robert M. Cox.)

N binding to RNA is believed to be independent of nucleotide sequence and thought to occur through interactions with the phosphodiester backbone.[242] However, the MeV RNP reconstructions have revealed that of the six nucleotides interacting with a single N protomer, only the first, fifth, and sixth bases are orientated outward and therefore accessible to viral RdRP, while the second to fourth bases face inward.[64,193,259] Encapsidation therefore imprints a hexamer phase on the viral RNA that is consistent with the earlier finding that SeV RNPs are hyperreactive to chemical treatment of cytidine residues predicted to be located at positions one and six of a hexamer of nucleotides.[242] Correct imprinting is ensured by the bipartite organization of the paramyxovirus promoter, which allows formation of a functional promoter only when nucleotides of the distinct promoter elements are properly juxtaposed next to each other in consecutive turns of the RNP helix.[126,365,587,618]

N protein exists in at least two forms in infected cells, one stably associated with RNA in a nucleocapsid structure and a second unassembled soluble form termed N⁰, which has been found associated with P in N⁰–P complexes for a number of viruses, including SeV,[222] PIV-5 (SV5),[472] HPIV-2 and HPIV-3,[403,661] and MeV.[231,557] N⁰ is believed to be the RNA-free func-

tional form of N that allows accumulation of a large pool of RNA-free N in an infected cell before the viral RdRP switches to replicase mode.[114,223] N-terminal regions of Ncore are important for formation of the N⁰–P complex,[220] and these domains are distinct from those involved in binding of P to N in the assembled nucleocapsid. A crystal structure of a MeV Ncore fragment (residues 21–408) fused to the first 48 amino acids of P supports comparison of RNA-bound and RNA-free N proteins.[192] In this structure, the P residues directly interact with the first alpha helix in the CTD of the N protein, partially occupying space claimed by the NT- and CT-arms of Ni−1 and Ni+1 of an Ni protomer in RNP assembly (Fig. 12.6C, D). Conceivably, steric hindrance mediated by P residues 1 to 48 prevents spontaneous N homo-oligomerization when in N⁰–P complexes.

The *P* Gene and Its Encoded Proteins

The *Paramyxoviridae P* gene is a remarkable example of expanding the coding capacity within a viral gene. The SeV P/V/C gene is the most diverse of the paramyxovirus *P* genes, directing the expression of at least seven polypeptides, including the P, V, W, C′, C, Y1, and Y2 proteins (Fig. 12.7). Although

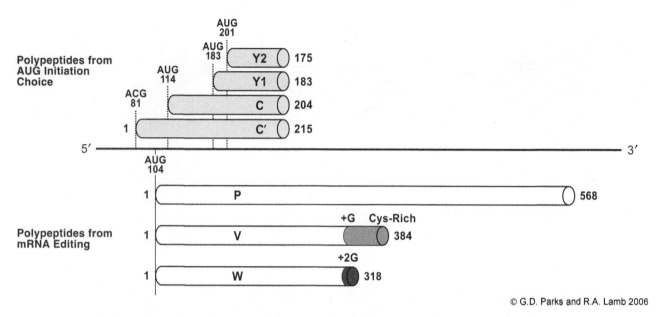

© G.D. Parks and R.A. Lamb 2006

FIGURE 12.7 Representation of the Sendai virus P mRNA to illustrate the mechanisms of producing P, V, and C proteins. The positions of four unique initiation codons for the C', C, Y1, and Y2 ORFs are shown above the *horizontal black line* representing the *P* gene mRNA. The position of the common initiation codon for the P, V, and W ORFs at base 104 is shown below the mRNA. The *gray cylinder* indicates the V protein Cys-rich C-terminal domain that is fused to the shared P N-terminal domain by addition of a G residue during viral transcription; the *black cylinder* indicates the short W domain, which is accessed by insertion of 2G residues. Numbers denote the amino acids contained within each polypeptide chain. Note that the initiation codon for C' is ACG. (Images copyright © 2006 by G.D. Parks and R.A. Lamb.)

other paramyxoviruses express fewer proteins from the *P/V/C* gene than SeV, the *P* gene always produces more than one polypeptide species (Table 12.4). Expression of P/V/C proteins can involve two main mechanisms, with members of a paramyxovirus genus having a characteristic combination of

Paramyxovirus		mRNA Insertion			
		0	+1G	+2G	Alternative ORFs
Rubulavirus	PIV-5	V	W/I	P	
	MuV; HPIV-2				
	HPIV-4				
Avulavirus	NDV	P	V	I	
Respirovirus	SeV	P	V	W	C' C Y1 Y2
	BPIV-3	P	V	D	C
	HPIV-3	P	V	D	C
	HPIV-1	P			C' C
Henipavirus	NiV; HeV	P	V	W	C
Morbillivirus	MeV; CDV	P	V	W	C
Unclassified	J virus; TPMV	P	V	W	C
	MoV				
	MenV; TiV	V	W	P	
	FDLV	V	W	P	

TABLE 12.4 Examples of distinct ORFs identified in the paramyxovirus P genes

these expression strategies. The first expression mechanism that produces the P, V, and W/I/D proteins has been termed "RNA editing" or pseudotemplated addition of nucleotides.[70,204,438,596,608] This mechanism involves the production of mRNAs whose ORFs are altered by insertion of G residues at a specific position in the mRNA. As described below, the second expression mechanism involves ribosome initiation at alternative translation codons and produces the family of C proteins.

The P and V proteins, as well as virus-specific proteins variously called W, I, and D, are produced as a nested set of proteins sharing identical N-terminal sections. These polypeptides are translation products from distinct mRNAs that differ only by inserted G nucleotides that shift the translational reading frame at the site of insertion, the editing site. As shown in Figure 12.7, the *P* gene of the *Avulavirinae* and members of the *Respirovirus*, *Morbillivirus*, and *Henipavirus* genus codes for a long N-terminal ORF shared by all three proteins and three shorter ORFs starting at approximately base 400 in the mRNA. During transcription of the nucleocapsid template, the viral RdRP is directed to make an accurate copy of the *P* gene template or to insert one or two G residues at the editing site in the nascent mRNA. The result is that the accurate transcription product encodes the full-length P ORF, while the mRNAs with insertions of +1G and +2G have a shift in the translational ORF such that the 5'-end P ORF is fused at the site of insertion in the mRNA coding sequence to a more 3' ORF encoding V (+1G) or W (+2G). Thus, the P, V, and W/I/D proteins that are produced as a result of RNA editing share a common N-terminal region but differ in their C-terminal regions, starting at the site of G insertion.

All paramyxoviruses except Cedar virus and HPIV-1[350] encode a characteristic editing site in the *P* gene, and the

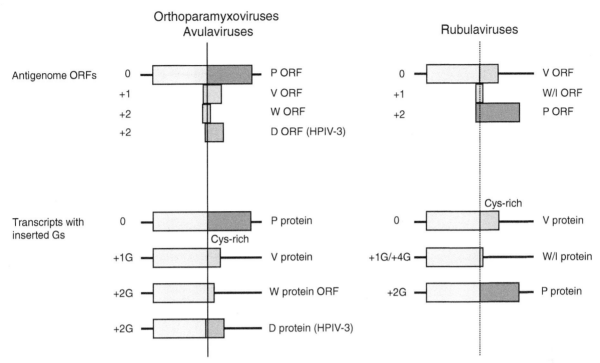

adapted from G.D. Parks and R.A. Lamb 2006, with permission ©

FIGURE 12.8 Schematic diagram of *P* gene ORFs accessed through RNA editing by different paramyxoviruses. The shared N-terminal ORF is shown as a *light green box*. The RNA editing site, at which nontemplated nucleotides are added to the mRNA, is indicated by the *vertical line*. At the bottom, RNA transcripts are shown to contain insertions of up to two additional G residues at the editing site, with *colored boxes* indicating unique C-terminal ORFs fused to the common N-terminal ORF. For the *Orthoparamyxovirinae* and *Avulavirinae*, the mRNA for the P protein is transcribed faithfully (unedited) from the viral genome and is shown as a *light green box* fused to a *dark green box*. Transcriptional RNA editing with the addition of one G nucleotide at the editing site produces an mRNA that encodes the V protein, in which the common N-terminal domain is fused to a different C-terminal frame, represented in *yellow box*. Addition of two G nucleotides at the editing site produces an mRNA that encodes the W (*blue box*) or D (*pink box*) or I proteins (depending on paramyxovirus species). For the *Rubulavirinae*, the unedited mRNA encodes the V protein, the addition of either one or four G nucleotides produces mRNA encoding the W or I protein, and the addition of two G nucleotides produces the mRNA encoding the P protein. (Adapted from G.D. Parks and R.A. Lamb, 2006, with permission ©)

number of inserted G residues, as well as the frequency of inserting G nucleotides, is thought to be determined by both sequences surrounding and within the editing site[204] and the position of the editing site relative to the hexamer phase of the encapsidated genome.[277,300] For example, Sendai and MeV encode the P protein as the translation product from the unedited mRNA (+0G; Fig. 12.8). The V protein is produced from a transcript containing a single G residue at the insertion site (+1G), which fuses the common N-terminal ORF to the V-specific ORF, whereas two inserted G nucleotides code for the W protein (+2G). As depicted in Figure 12.8, *Rubulavirinae* differ from other paramyxoviruses in that V protein is produced by translation of the unedited mRNA (+0G) and P is produced by translation of an mRNA containing a two G insertion (+2G).

Insertion of G residues into *P* gene mRNA transcripts is a cotranscriptional event catalyzed by the viral RdRP[608,609] and is usually limited to insertions of between zero and two nucleotides, depending on the virus. Relative abundance of the different *P* gene mRNA species often rapidly declines with the number of nucleotides inserted,[102,277] but NiV and human and

bovine PIV3 are exceptions to these rules, since the different mRNA species were found to be equally abundant and transcripts with multiple G insertion were detected.[168,284]

The Phosphoprotein

The P protein is the only *P/V/C* gene product that is essential for viral RNA synthesis.[114,115] Paramyxovirus P proteins are generally 400 to 600 amino acids long and heavily phosphorylated at serine and threonine residues, predominantly within the N-terminal region. The major sites of P phosphorylation and the respective kinases have been identified for several viruses.[117,232] The P protein features a modular organization of ordered and intrinsically highly disordered domains,[40,41,257,258] consistent with the requirement for interacting with multiple partners during the viral replication cycle. While lacking inherent enzymatic activity, P is an essential component of both the viral RdRP[196] and the N⁰ nascent chain assembly complex that functions to encapsidate RNA during replication.[222] Structural information has been obtained for distinct modular N- and C-terminal domains of P proteins derived from different paramyxoviruses (Fig. 12.9). These domains are instrumental for

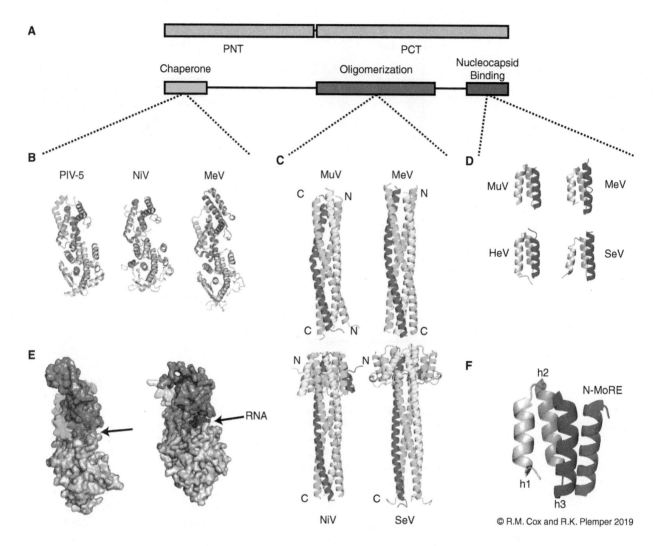

FIGURE 12.9 Structures of paramyxovirus P protein domains. A: Schematic of the P protein organization. P proteins are divided into an N-terminal domain (PNT) and a C-terminal domain (PCT). Known functional domains involved in chaperoning, oligomerization, and nucleocapsid binding are highlighted. **B and E:** The chaperone domain prevents premature N multimerization and RNA binding. Three crystal structures have been solved for paramyxovirus N⁰–P complexes (PIV-5, PDB ID: 5WKN; NiV, 4CO6; MeV, 5E4V).[4,192,641] **C:** Crystal structures of the P oligomerization domains of MuV (PDB ID: 4EIJ), MeV (PDB ID: 4BHV), NiV (PDB ID: 4N5B), and SeV (PDB ID: 1EZJ).[54,91,101,589] P tetramers form a coiled coil of four parallel helices, except for MuV, which emerged as a tetramer of parallel and antiparallel helices. **D:** Structures of the nucleocapsid binding X domain (XD) that have been solved for MuV (PDB ID: 3BBZ), MeV (PDB ID: 1OKS), HeV (PDB ID: 4HEO), and SeV (PDB ID: 1R4G).[29,92,252,272] XD structures are highly conserved, all featuring three-helix bundle arrangements. **F:** Crystal structure of MeV P-XD in complex with a C-terminal fragment of MeV N (PDB ID: 1T6O).[273] XD interacts directly with a molecular recognition element (MoRE) located in Box 2 of MeV Ntail. (Images copyright © 2019 by Richard K. Plemper and Robert M. Cox.)

P activity as an essential polymerase cofactor, mediator of P-L complex loading onto the RNP template, and inhibitor of premature termination of the advancing polymerase complex during transcription and replication.

The C-terminal half of the paramyxovirus P protein (termed PCT, residues 304–507 in the case of MeV P) is relatively well conserved in predicted secondary structure across the family. P proteins function as multimers, with an oligomerization domain (P_{OD}) located in the central region of P near the beginning of the PCT. However, P_{OD} sequences and the organization of the assembly may vary considerably between different Ps. While crystal structures of SeV, MeV, and NiV P_{ODS} have been shown to form tetrameric alpha helical coiled coils

in parallel arrangements,[54,91,588] a crystal structure of MuV P_{OD} (residues 213–277) suggested a tetramer organization consisting of two parallel pairs of alpha helices, arranged in opposite orientation to each other[101] (Fig. 12.9C).

SeV PCT (residues 325–568) is sufficient for catalyzing viral RNA synthesis because this fragment alone can substitute for intact P protein in all aspects of mRNA transcription.[115] Although the L protein contains all RdRP catalytic activities, L binds to the nucleocapsid template via the P protein.[222] In addition to establishing physical contact between the RNP and L, P proteins are required as cochaperones for proper L protein folding. Transient expression of MeV L protein in the absence of the P protein resulted in low L protein steady-state levels,[225] and MeV P proteins have furthermore been suggested to recruit the host cell chaperone Hsp90 to the L protein.[32] While the exact nature of the interface between P and L proteins is still unknown, residues located at the C-terminal end of the P_{OD} and in the following domains were consistently found to contribute to facilitating proper interactions in SeV,[45,115] MeV,[91,252] RPV,[78] and human parainfluenza viruses type 2 and 3 (HPIV-2 and HPIV-3)[85,402] P-L complexes. Located at the end of the PCT, the P-XD as discussed above establishes an interaction between P-L and the MoRE residues located in Box 2 of the Ntail.[45,115,506] Structural data obtained for MeV indicate that P-XD induces partial folding of resides in the MoRE, establishing a four-helix bundle arrangement consisting of three XD-derived helices and one formed by the MoRE residues (Fig. 12.9F).[40,197,252,326,620] These interactions with Ntail appear to be predominantly required for preventing premature termination of the polymerase complex at IG junctions,[282] and a correlation between binding strength and transcriptase reinitiation efficiency after IG regions was proposed for MeV RdRP.[31] The ability of P-XD and Ntail to form interactions between intrinsically disordered domains may be important to allow movement of the P-L complex along the RNP template,[29,40,271] although it is unclear at present how separation of P-XD from Ntail, once the induced-fit interface has been established, is initiated and coordinated. So far only for MuV P, the N-terminal PNT has been implicated in RNA de-encapsidation and the local uncoiling of the RNP in front of the approaching RdRP, indicating a direct interaction of MuV PNT with the RNP.[103]

In contrast to viral transcription, genome replication depends on the availability of unassembled N^0 (in N^0–P complexes)

facilitating concomitant encapsidation of the nascent strand. The residues located at the N-terminus of the PNT (residues 33–41 for SeV[114,222] and 1–48 for MeV P[192]) have been implicated in preventing premature N aggregation and ensuring productive assembly of the RNP. The remainder of the SeV PNT appears to be dispensable for RNA synthesis and assembly, since a P protein in which residues 78 to 324 have been deleted is still active for minigenome replication in transfected cells.[114] However, phosphorylation of RPV P protein at serine residue 88 prevented the initiation of polymerization,[476] and the phosphorylation status of RPV P appears to modulate transcriptase versus replicase activity,[507] suggesting a major regulatory role of PNT in controlling RdRP activity. Consistent with this theme, the phosphorylation status of MeV P protein residues S86 and S151 likewise alters RdRP transcriptase activity.[569]

The V Protein

The V protein is an approximately 25- to 30-kDa polypeptide that shares an N-terminal domain with the P protein but has a unique C-terminal domain as a result of RNA editing.[70,203,438,439,596,608] The C-terminal V-specific domain is highly conserved among related paramyxoviruses, with invariantly spaced histidine and cysteine residues forming a novel domain that binds two zinc molecules per V protein[167,307,317,441] (Fig. 12.10). In the case of PIV-5 and MuV, this cysteine-rich domain of V protein directs spontaneous self-assembly into spherical high molecular weight particles that can be visualized by EM.[604] Despite the high level of intracellular synthesis, paramyxovirus particles typically incorporate little V protein into virions,[441] although there can be some variation.[110,626]

Avulavirinae	*Orthoavulavirus*	NDV	175...	PG**H**RREHSISWTMGGVTTISW**C**NPS**C**SPIRAEPRQYS**C**TCGS**C**PAT**C**RL**C**AS...226
Rubulavirinae	*Orthorubulavirus*	PIV-5	169...	GF**H**RREYSIGWVGDEVKVTEW**C**NPS**C**SPITAAARRFE**C**TCHQ**C**PVT**C**SE**C**ER...220
	Orthorubulavirus	HPIV-2	172...	GN**H**RREWSIAWVGDQVKVFEW**C**NPR**C**APVTASARKFT**C**TCGS**C**PSI**C**GE**C**EG...223
	Orthorubulavirus	MuV	168...	GG**H**RREWSLSWVQGEVRVFEW**C**NPI**C**SPITAAARFHS**C**KCGN**C**PAK**C**DQ**C**ER...219
	Metarubulavirus	MenaV	164...	GG**H**RREIAIDWIGGRPRVTEW**C**NPI**C**HPISQSTFRGS**C**RCGN**C**PGI**C**SL**C**ER...215
	Metarubulavirus	TioV	162...	GG**H**RREIAISWATGTPRVTEW**C**NPI**C**HPISQFTYRGT**C**RCGC**C**PDV**C**SL**C**ER...213
Orthoparamyxovirinae	*Respirovirus*	SeV	312...	KG**H**RREHIIYERDGYIVDESW**C**NPV**C**SRIRIIPRREL**C**VCKT**C**PKV**C**KL**C**RD...367
	Respirovirus	BPIV-3	346...	RG**H**RREHSIYREGDYIITESW**C**NPI**C**SKIRPVPRQES**C**VCGE**C**PKQ**C**GY**C**IE...397
	Henipavirus	HeV	404...	KG**H**RREVSICWDGRRAWVEEW**C**NPV**C**SRITPQPRKQE**C**YCGE**C**PTE**C**SQ**C**CH...455
	Henipavirus	NiV	404...	KG**H**RREISICWDGKRAWVEEW**C**NPA**C**SRITPLPRRQE**C**QCGE**C**PTE**C**FH**C**G....456
	Jeilongvirus	JV	234...	KG**H**RREFCIDNFGGKTYIREW**C**NPQ**C**APITVTPTQSR**C**TCGE**C**PKV**C**AR**C**IK...285
	Narmovirus	TupV	228...	KG**H**RREYSMVWSNDGVFIESW**C**NPM**C**ARIRPLPIREI**C**VCGR**C**PLK**C**SK**C**LL...279
	Morbillivirus	MeV	230...	KG**H**RREISLIWDGDRVFIDRW**C**NPM**C**SKVTLGTIRAR**C**TCGE**C**PRV**C**EQ**C**RT...281
	Morbillivirus	CDV	230...	KG**H**RREVSLTWNGDSCWIDKW**C**NPI**C**TQVNWGIIRAK**C**FCGE**C**PPT**C**NE**C**KD...281
	Morbillivirus	RPV	230...	KG**H**RREIDLIWNDGRVFIDRW**C**NPT**C**SKVTVGTVRAK**C**ICGE**C**PRV**C**EQ**C**IT...281
	Salemvirus	SalV	250...	SR**H**RREYSIIWDSEGIQIESW**C**NPV**C**SKVRSTPRREK**C**RCGK**C**PAR**C**SE**C**GD...301

FIGURE 12.10 Amino acid sequence alignment of the conserved cysteine-rich C-terminal region of selected paramyxovirus V proteins. Numbers indicate the amino acid position within the respective proteins. Positions of the conserved histidine and seven conserved cysteine residues that are involved in coordinating Zn are indicated by *asterisks*. Additional areas of sequence identity are shaded in *red*. New abbreviations: MenaV, Menangle virus; TioV, Tioman virus; BPIV-3, bovine parainfluenza virus 3; JV, J virus; TupV, Tupaia paramyxovirus; CDV, canine distemper virus; SalV, Salem virus.

Paramyxovirus V proteins are the primary viral countermeasure against the host innate antiviral immune response, interfering with type I interferon (IFN) expression and signaling (reviewed in Ref.[433]) and thus ultimately blocking the activation of hundreds of IFN-stimulated genes (ISGs) and the induction of an antiviral state. Accordingly, V proteins are important pathogenesis factors and play a central role in the virus replication cycle, as evidenced by a range of different recombinant paramyxoviruses that have been engineered to disrupt expression of the V protein cysteine-rich domain.[22,120,127,143,207,261,265,527,600,614,650] In many cases, these mutant viruses display an elevated RNA synthesis phenotype, but they generally grow well in many tissue culture cell lines.[121,261,527] However, severely attenuated growth *in vivo* is common, and/or the mutant viruses are cleared more rapidly than the corresponding parental forms from lungs of infected animals.[143,262,446,572,606]

Several paramyxovirus V proteins interact in the cytoplasm with the cellular damage-specific DNA-binding protein 1 (DDB1),[11,316] and a crystal structure of PIV-5 V protein complexed with DDB1 has been solved.[307] This structure reveals a bipartite organization, consisting of a core domain built around a central seven-stranded β sheet, which is in turn sandwiched between one alpha helix and two long loops (Fig. 12.11). The unique C-terminal domain forms the middle two β sheets and part of the central core, and this structure is anchored through the cys-rich zinc-binding region. Thus, despite sharing a 164–amino acid N-terminal domain, the PIV-5 P and V proteins can adopt very different structures due to the unique properties of the C-terminal cys-rich region.

Through distinct, genus-specific strategies, the paramyxovirus V proteins interfere with type I IFN expression and signaling, antagonizing the innate host cell antiviral response (discussed in the section Paramyxovirus Accessory Genes and their Interference with the Cellular Antiviral Response). In addition to this primary function, V proteins have been shown to regulate viral RNA synthesis in transfection experiments involving model RNA genomes,[114,226,315,645] and recombinant

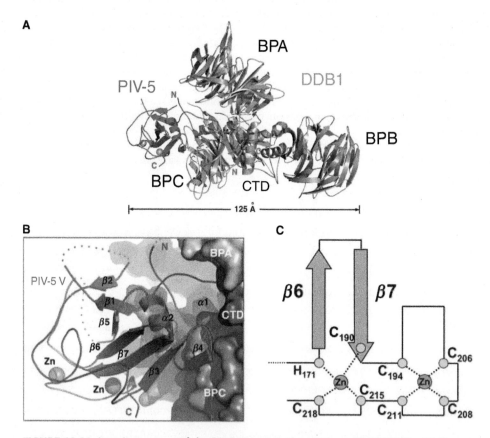

FIGURE 12.11 Atomic structure of the PIV-5 V protein in complex with DDB1. The PIV-5 V protein binds to DDB1, which adopts a four-domain structure consisting of a three-propeller cluster and a helical C-terminal domain. **A:** Overall view of the DDB1-PIV-5-V complex with DDB1 in *blue* and the V protein in *red*. The zinc ions in PIV-5-V are shown as *orange spheres*. The four DDB1 domains are labeled BPA, BPB, BPC, and CTD. The longest dimension of the complex is indicated. **B:** The PIV-5 V protein adopts a bipartite structure upon interacting with the DDB1 BPC domain. DDB1 and PIV-5-V are shown in surface and ribbon representation, respectively. The N-terminal part of the V protein, which is also found in the viral P protein, is colored *red*. The rest of the V protein, including the zinc-binding sequence, is colored in *gray*. **C:** A novel zinc-finger fold found in the PIV-5-V protein. (Adapted from Li T, Chen X, Garbutt KC, et al. Structure of DDB1 in complex with a paramyxovirus V protein: viral hijack of a propeller cluster in ubiquitin ligase. *Cell* 2006;124(1):105–117, with permission.)

viruses that are engineered with V protein mutations often show increased viral RNA synthesis.[22,120,143,261,265,527,600,625] The shared N-terminal domain of P/V is responsible for the assembly of N[0]–P complexes, and V proteins from PIV-5, SeV, and MeV have been found in equivalent N[0]–V interactions that, however, are incapable of mediating RNA encapsidation during viral genome replication.[114,226,472,600] A model has been proposed in which V-mediated inhibition of viral RNA synthesis may be a result of V and P competition for soluble N[0].[114,226,645] The cysteine-rich C-terminal domain of MeV and PIV-5 V proteins were likewise implicated in inhibiting viral RNA synthesis.[435,636,645] While mechanistically unclear at present, it is speculated that this inhibitory effect may be mediated through interaction with a host cell factor.[645] Lastly, the V protein is also capable of binding RNA,[316] and in the case of MeV V protein, it has been proposed that this interaction may contribute to inhibiting RNA synthesis.[435]

The W/D/I Proteins

The W and D ORFs of respiroviruses, morbilliviruses, and henipaviruses are expressed from mRNAs with two inserted G residues (Fig. 12.8). Since the W ORF is typically closed by a stop codon shortly after the editing site, the W protein is essentially a truncated P protein containing the N-terminal N[0] assembly module of the P protein and a very short C-terminal extension. The W protein is abundantly expressed during infection[109,321] and, in the case of SeV, has been found to interact with unassembled N[0].[226] Accordingly, W proteins are thought to function as regulators of viral RNA synthesis. In contrast to the predominant presence of P and V in the cytoplasm, however, *Henipavirus* W proteins are transported to the nucleus through specific interaction of an NLS located in the unique C-terminus with cellular importin-α3.[15,537,553] Different subcellular localizations suggested a distinct immunomodulatory strategy for NiV W and V. Consistent with this notion, binding to NiV W is thought to trap STAT1 in the nucleus, blocking IFN signaling through the formation of nonfunctional complexes containing STAT1.

In the case of bovine and human PIV-3, the +2 ORF extends for 131 residues from the editing site, resulting in the synthesis of a unique D protein that is a chimera of the common N-terminal domain of P and this ORF downstream of the editing site.[168] *Rubulavirinae* I protein is generated when the upstream N-terminal P region is fused to a downstream ORF by the insertion of either one or four G residues during RNA editing.[438,596]

The C Proteins

In addition to RNA editing, some paramyxoviruses use a second mechanism to express *P* gene polypeptides that involves the use of alternative translation initiation codons to yield the C proteins (Fig. 12.7). The SeV C', C, Y1, and Y2 proteins constitute a nested set of carboxy-coterminal polypeptides that range in size from 175 to 215 residues. These proteins are expressed independently from a P/V mRNA through the use of alternative start codons (Fig. 12.7), with the C protein ORF being in the +1 reading frame relative to the P ORF. Consequently, all ORFs of the C protein set terminate at the same stop codon, and the C proteins thus share a common C-terminus. The C' and C proteins are translated by a leaky scanning mechanism, being initiated at an unconventional ACG triplet at base 81

and AUG at base 114, respectively.[112] In contrast, translation of the Y1 and Y2 proteins occurs through a scanning-independent ribosome-shunting mechanism that is directed by a 5′ noncoding RNA segment, resulting in ribosomes initiating at AUG codons at bases 183 and 201, respectively. The C protein is abundantly expressed in infected cells at levels higher than C', Y1, and Y2, but virions contain only very low levels of these polypeptides.[296] morbilliviruses and henipaviruses express only one C protein,[26,198,621,623] whereas respiroviruses such as SeV and HPIV-1 express all four C', C, Y1, and Y2 polypeptides.[176] *Rubulavirinae* and *Avulavirinae* do not express C proteins (Table 12.4).

C proteins are small basic polypeptides that like the V proteins play important roles in regulating the host IFN response. They are involved in controlling viral RdRP transcription versus replication activity,[19,263,296,335,393,586] enhancing polymerase fidelity,[35,453,577] and facilitating the release of virus from infected cells.[238,431,508,568] The regulatory effect of C proteins on RNA synthesis correlates with their ability to bind to the L subunit of the viral polymerase,[223] and, in the case of SeV, naturally occurring variant C proteins can have differential effects on inhibition of virus RNA synthesis.[19]

Although nonessential for infectivity, SeV mutants engineered to express only a subset of C proteins or lacking expression of all four proteins show defects in virus growth[238,286] and in the absence of all C proteins were entirely unable to suppress the expression of ISGs.[184] Recombinant HPIV-3, SeV, NiV, and MeV with disrupted C protein expression are growth attenuated in mice, hamsters, and nonhuman primates, respectively.[127,143,170,348,650] An additional role for C proteins in the release of some paramyxovirus particles was proposed based on enhanced budding of SeV-like particles (VLPs) when SeV C was coexpressed with the viral M protein.[568] The effect was dependent on the host endosomal sorting complex required for transport (ESCRT) pathway (discussed below), possibly through interactions with the ESCRT factor Alix.[238,508] A similar ESCRT-dependent budding enhancing effect was described for NiV C, in this case through recruiting the ESCRT-I component TSG101.[431]

The Large Protein

The large (L) protein is an essential subunit of the paramyxovirus RdRP. Originally named after its high molecular weight of approximately 220 to 250 kDa, the L protein is invariably encoded as the most promoter-distal gene in the paramyxovirus genome (Fig. 12.4). L proteins are generally present in only very low amounts in infected cells or virions,[291] where they are found on the nucleocapsid in P-L clusters.[468] L is believed to possess all the enzymatic activities needed for viral RNA synthesis, including phosphodiester bond formation, 5′-end mRNA capping and methylation, and 3′-end mRNA polyadenylation.[90,188,213,416,575] In the presence of amounts of N[0]–P complexes sufficient to allow the encapsidation of nascent full-length viral RNAs, the L protein also mediates synthesis of viral genomes and antigenomes.[190,222]

Paramyxovirus L proteins are generally approximately 2,200 amino acids in length. Although the primary L protein amino acid sequences are diverse, the proteins share a similar overall organization and conserved functional motifs. Sequence alignments have identified two short hinge regions of high variability (approximately located at residues 600 and 1,700) in

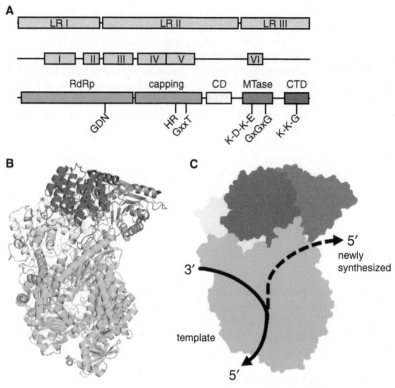

© R.M. Cox and R.K. Plemper 2019

FIGURE 12.12 Structural overview of the L polymerase protein. A: Domain organization of the paramyxovirus L protein. **A, top:** The paramyxovirus L proteins can be divided into three large regions (LR I-III), determined by insertion analysis. LR I-II and LR III represent independent folding domains that can form a functional polymerase when expressed separately.[135] **A, middle:** Sequence alignments have revealed six conserved regions (CR I–VI) in the L polymerase proteins. **A, bottom; B:** A cryo-EM–based reconstruction of the VSV L structure shows five main structural domains: polymerase (*cyan*), capping (*green*), connector domain (*yellow*), methyltransferase (*orange*), and C-terminal domain (*red*).[311] The locations of active site residues are shown for each domain in the cartoon. **C:** Approximate locations of the RNA template and exit channels within the VSV L protein are shown in *black*. Template RNA (*solid line*) is proposed to enter and exit the polymerase complex from the one side, while the newly synthesized strand (*dashed line*) exits on the opposite side. This position of the proposed exit channel places the 5' end of the nascent mRNA strand in close proximity to the capping and MTase domains. (Images copyright © 2019 by Richard K. Plemper and Robert M. Cox.)

L proteins of SeV, NiV, and morbilliviruses such as RPV and MeV that connect three large regions[53,135,141,354] (Fig. 12.12A). Insertion of green fluorescent protein (GFP) into the downstream hinge region maintained substantial RdRP activity and allowed recovery of viable recombinant viruses encoding these L-GFP hybrid proteins, while insertion into the upstream junction abolished bioactivity.[53,141] It was unclear, however, whether the L regions before and after the downstream hinge region represent fully independent folding domains or assume a native conformation only when synthesized as a single polypeptide, since L proteins of the related rhabdovirus vesicular stomatitis virus (VSV) likewise tolerated large insertions in an interdomain region between subunits,[499] but these subunits were unable to reconstitute a functional polymerase when expressed separately.[478] By contrast, individually expressed NiV and MeV have been found able to restore bioactivity through homotypic

transcomplementation when dimerization tags were fused to the fragments, indicating that paramyxovirus L proteins are composed of at least two independent folding domains.[135]

Sequence alignments have identified six conserved regions (CRs I–VI) that were originally proposed to be individually responsible for each of the distinct L functions[461,542,571] (Fig. 12.12A). Residues in regions overlapping with CR I were found to be involved in the essential L interaction with the P protein that is required for the formation of functional P-L complexes.[32,74,79,196,219,222,225,432] CRs II and III contain subdomains common to all L polymerases.[461] Based on a high net positive charge, CR II is considered to be an RNA-binding domain, whereas a GDN tripeptide motif in CR III is extremely conserved and, based on mutational analyses, thought to form part of the catalytic center for nucleotide polymerization.[78,79,246,334] In a cryo-EM structure of the VSV L protein, CRs IV and V mapped to an mRNA capping domain.[462] VSV is a member of the rhabdovirus family that like the paramyxoviruses belongs to the mononegavirales, which are thought to share a comparable overall L organization. CR VI and the L C-terminal domain are required for viral mRNA methylation.

Expression and purification of native L proteins is challenging, reflected by a current lack of high-resolution structural information of the spatial organization of any paramyxovirus L protein. However, recent negative-stain EM images of copurified NiV P-L complexes showed two particle classes, globular 5- to 8-nm particles with even density, and larger 8- to 11-nm ring-like structures.[253] The latter class resembles previous negative-stain EM images of VSV L proteins that showed a doughnut-like architecture with a globular appendage covering the center of the doughnut and three smaller globular appendages.[478] A cryo-EM reconstruction of VSV L to near-atomic resolution mapped CRs I to III to the polymerase domain, CRs IV and V, the single appendage covering the doughnut, to the capping domain, and the smaller appendages to a connector, CR VI, and C-terminal domain, respectively[462] (Fig. 12.12B, C). A crystal structure of a C-terminal L fragment of human metapneumovirus, a member of the closely related pneumovirus family, revealed that CR VI and the C-terminal domain build a functional MTase.[422] Although small globular attachments comparable to those seen in VSV L were not detectable in the EM images of NiV L, the preserved outline of the CRs and reoccurrence of key features of the low-resolution negative-stain EM images suggest that the molecular organization of the different L proteins may be similar.

mRNA cap formation and cap methylation are crucial processes to form stable mRNA, and viruses have adapted different strategies to form those structures.[119] In mammalian cells, RNA triphosphatase (RTPase) activity first removes the 5′ phosphate of pre-mRNA. Guanylyltransferase (GTase) then transfers a guanylyl monophosphate (GMP) from a guanosine 5′ triphosphate (GTP) molecule on the pre-mRNA, followed by successive methylation of a new cap through guanine-N7-methyltransferase (GN7-MTase) (cap 0 structure) on the cap and 2′O methyltransferase (2′O MTase) (cap-1 structure) activity on the first nucleotide. GN7-MTase activity for cap methylation was attributed to a C-terminal L protein fragment (residues 717–2,183), and sequence alignments revealed K-D-K-E and GxGxG motifs characteristic for 2′O MTases.[161,181,310,416,461,473]

Among mononegaviruses, cap formation strategies are most extensively characterized for rhabdoviruses, which follow an unconventional pathway[411,413,415]: (a) GTP is hydrolyzed to guanosine 5′ diphosphate (GDP) through a nucleotide triphosphatase (NTPase) activity,[411,412] and (b) the nascent 5′ triphosphorylated RNA strand (pppA-RNA) is covalently ligated as a 5′ monophosphate RNA (p-A-RNA) and transferred to GDP to form the capped Gppp-N-RNA through a polyribonucleotidyltransferase [PRNTase] activity.[411,413] The cap is methylated successively at the 2′-O-position of the first nucleotide (Gppp-Am-RNA) and at the cap N7 position (m7Gppp-Am-RNA).[477] Interestingly, PRNTase motifs are conserved across the mononegaviruses suggesting that all viruses in this order could implement an unconventional capping mechanism.[397] Support for this notion comes from the finding that mutation of critical residues in the HR motif of the PRNTase resulted in the loss of the capping activities in HPIV-2[397] and pneu-

moviruses (RSV[47]). Use of GDP instead of GMP to form the cap structure and NTPase activity has also been described for pneumoviruses.[20,422]

Despite conservation of PRNTase motifs, however, the paramyxovirus mRNA cap formation mechanism is not yet fully understood mechanistically, and PRNTase activity has so far only been confirmed for rhabdovirus L proteins.[411,413,415] Surprisingly, also a C-terminal "K-K-G motif" located downstream of CR VI is well conserved among para-, filo-, and pneumovirus L proteins. This motif appears reminiscent of eukaryotic cell–style GTase activity[397] and is absent from rhabdovirus L proteins but has been shown to be essential for HPIV2 mRNA synthesis.[397] Also, GTase[180] and RTPase[13,546,547] activities have been proposed for RPV L proteins, but a direct structural comparison of the C-terminal domains of HMPV and VSV L reveals that the structural organization of the K-K-G motif in HMPV is distinct from that in eukaryotic GTases, arguing against guanylyltransferase activity as a universal mechanism for paramyxovirus cap formation.

L protein activity in RNA synthesis is highly dependent on protein–protein interactions. Based on biochemical evidence and genetic complementation studies with Sendai and MeV L proteins, the possibility of L-L self-assembly through an N-terminal domain was raised.[74,550,552] The resolution of the NiV L protein EM data is not high enough to extract quaternary structure information, but potential spatial organization and physiological relevance of L-L assembly are not immediately evident from the high-resolution VSV L structure. In contrast, L protein interaction with P is essential for proper folding, and interaction sites were consistently mapped to N-terminal domains of different paramyxovirus L proteins.[74,219,432] A physical interaction of RPV and SeV L proteins with the viral C protein was furthermore demonstrated, in the case of SeV involving the polymerase domain (CRs I–III[223,573]). Paramyxoviruses spontaneously produce some amount of dsRNAs during replication. Infection of cells with engineered SeV, HPIV-1, and MeV lacking functional C proteins, however, resulted in greatly elevated dsRNA levels, which is consistent with C reducing the formation of defective interfering (DI) genomes by enhancing polymerase fidelity. Other proteins encoded in the SeV *P/V/C* gene (C′, Y1, and Y2) also interact with L and inhibit defective interfering (DI)-RNA synthesis *in vitro*[189] and *in vivo*.[263]

In addition to interaction with viral proteins, an association of paramyxovirus L proteins with host cell proteins has been proposed. In the case of MeV and SeV, L interactions with tubulin are believed to promote L activity.[378,379] Other cellular proteins have also been suggested to promote viral RNA synthesis (e.g., β-catenin for HPIV-3[36]), but the precise role that these proteins play in RdRP function has not been determined.

The Matrix Protein

The paramyxovirus matrix (M) protein is the most abundant protein in the virion. The M proteins contain 341 to 375 residues (Mr ~38,500–41,500), are quite basic in nature (net charge at neutral pH of +14 to +17), and are somewhat hydrophobic. Three major roles have been proposed for the M proteins in the paramyxovirus replication cycle: organization of virions assembly, promotion of particle budding, and sequestering of inhibitory host proteins from the cytoplasm.

Early fractionation studies of infected cells and virions indicated that the M proteins can peripherally associate with membranes, but they are not integral membrane proteins.[155,289,390,513] A temperature-sensitive SeV first suggested a link between changes in M and virus budding efficiency.[651] Purified SeV M proteins have furthermore been shown to self-associate and form two-dimensional paracrystalline arrays (sheets and tubes) in low-salt conditions,[16,211] and M proteins of several paramyxoviruses including SeV and the henipaviruses

expressed in isolation are sufficient to drive virus-like particle (VLP) formation.[436,581]

At present, high-resolution structures have only been solved for the NDV and HeV M proteins,[23,318] but the overall organization of M proteins from different mononegavirales is considered to be well conserved.[295] The NDV M crystal structure (Fig. 12.13A–D) showed the protein in a homodimer

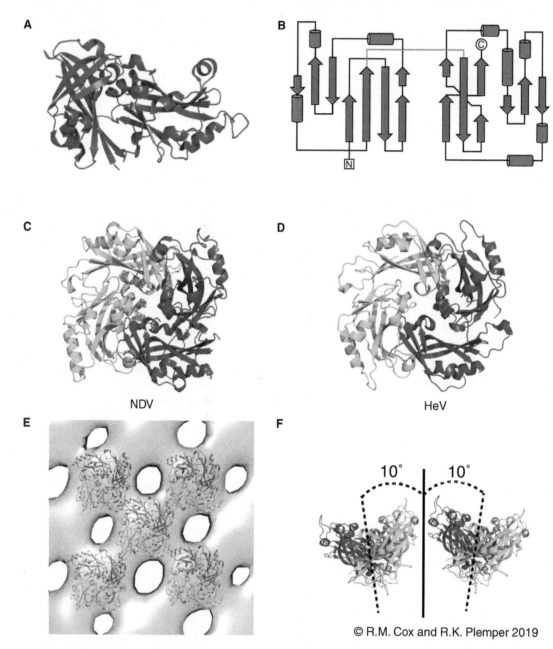

NDV

HeV

10°   10°

© R.M. Cox and R.K. Plemper 2019

FIGURE 12.13 Structure of the paramyxovirus matrix protein. A: Ribbon drawing of the monomeric NDV M crystal structure (PDB ID: 4G1G).[23] **B:** Schematic of the secondary structure of the NDV M monomer. Each NDV M monomer is composed of two β-sandwich domains (*red*) that are lined by several α-helices (*cyan*). **C and D:** Structures of the NDV and HeV (PDB ID: 6BK6) matrix proteins,[23,318] showing similar features and folds. **E:** The M protein forms 2D paracrystalline arrays in cells. A subtomographic average of the NDV M protein is shown with the crystal structure docked into place. **F:** Crystal contacts in matrix dimers are similar to those made between adjacent dimers in the virus. The M dimer in the crystal structure forms contacts with adjacent dimers with a 20-degree angle between dimers. Similar contacts are made between adjacent M dimers in NDV virions, but with a smaller 6-degree angle between dimers. This arrangement is thought to allow the M protein to induce membrane curvature to facilitate budding of virions from infected cells. (Images copyright © 2019 by Richard K. Plemper and Robert M. Cox.)

assembly.[23] Each monomer features two β-sheet sandwiches with approximately orthogonal orientation of the opposing β strands, which are connected by a 16-residue linker and surrounded by several short α-helices. A high density of positive charge of the nearly square-shaped face of the dimer oriented toward the membrane supports membrane association of M proteins through electrostatic interactions. Cryo-ET reconstructions of purified NDV particles showed a grid-like arrangement of the matrix layer with approximately square-shaped appearance of the repeating protein units, into which the dimer assembly could be fitted.[23] Electrostatic interactions and hydrogen bonding between pairs of two α-helices in each dimer are proposed to mediate dimer-to-dimer contacts, introducing an approximately 20-degree angle between the symmetry axes of neighboring dimers that results in an overall curvature of the assembled matrix array similar to the membrane curvature in a budding virus (Fig. 12.13E, F).

Discussed in detail in the *Virus Particle Formation* section, biochemical data and the reconstruction of cryopreserved paramyxovirus particles have indicated specific interactions between the M protein layer and the cytoplasmic tails of the envelope glycoproteins that are instrumental for efficient particle assembly.[69,266,513,514,521,574] In addition to contacts with the glycoproteins, M specifically associates with the viral RNP, creating a bridge between viral envelope and genome. For instance, SeV M has been shown to associate with nucleocapsids[567]; MuV M, fusion, and N proteins together promote efficient VLP production[309]; and a specific interaction between MeV M and the C-terminal, third conserved element in Ntail was demonstrated in yeast two-hybrid studies and biochemically.[245]

While M lattice-mediated induction of membrane curvature emerged as an important step of the paramyxovirus budding process, several paramyxovirus M proteins appear to engage the actin cytoskeleton,[33,156,177,560] possibly for efficient membrane targeting. Likely, M proteins recruit the cellular vesicle budding machinery for fission of the viral envelope and cellular membranes, although paramyxovirus M proteins lack canonical "late domains" that mediate interaction with components of the host cell ESCRT machinery. Budding of PIV-5, NDV, MuV, and NiV has been shown to depend on vacuolar protein sorting–associated protein 4 (VPS4) ATPase activity.[140,309,431,523] Together with ESCRT-III proteins, VPS4 catalyzes membrane fission. A noncanonical late domain, however, has been suggested for PIV-5, NDV, and MuV protein,[140,309,522,523] while the nonstructural C proteins of SeV and NiV have been implicated in recruiting ESCRT components Alix and TSG101, respectively.[238,431]

Suggesting a possible role of the paramyxovirus M protein distinct from its function in virion assembly and budding, transient nuclear localization of SeV, NDV, and NiV M has been described.[448,622,651] Best characterized for Nipah M, nuclear import was shown to be dependent on the integrity of a putative bipartite nuclear localization signal (NLS) in M that was conserved in SeV and MuV also.[451,622] Following nuclear import, both NDV and NiV M proteins associate with the nucleolar compartment.[139,451] A lysine residue in the NiV M NLS that was found to be subject to monoubiquitination is proposed to regulate subcellular localization of the protein. When ubiquitinated, a likewise conserved nuclear export sequence located in one of the α-helix pairs forming the M dimer–dimer interface redirects M to the cytoplasm.[451,622] While the functional importance of transient M localization to the nucleolus is not yet understood, a recent study proposed that *Henipavirus* M specifically targets Treacle protein–enriched regions of the nucleolus, potentially modulating the host DNA damage response–Treacle pathway to optimize the cellular environment for efficient virus replication.[484]

Envelope Glycoproteins

All *Paramyxoviridae* possess two integral membrane proteins, some *Rubulavirinae* encode a third integral membrane protein, and members of *Jeilongvirus* genus feature two additional membrane proteins. One major glycoprotein (HN, H, or G) is involved in cell attachment and the other major glycoprotein (F) in mediating pH-independent fusion of the viral envelope with the plasma membrane of the host cell (Fig. 12.14). The *Rubulavirinae* third integral membrane protein is called SH, and for PIV-5, this 44–amino acid integral membrane protein is believed to block virus-induced apoptosis. *Jeilongvirus* (i.e., J virus, Tioman virus, and Beilong virus) encode a fourth integral membrane protein between SH and G, designated TM.[247] The assignment of specific biological activities of F and HN was originally made on the basis of purification and reconstitution studies, mainly for SeV and PIV-5 proteins.[517,518] The attachment proteins (HN, H, or G) are all type II integral membrane proteins, and bioinformatics and structural predictions indicate the proteins all exhibit a related propellerlike fold despite having different receptors and the presence or absence of NA activity.

For the respiroviruses and *Rubulavirinae*, the attachment glycoprotein binds to cellular sialic acid–containing receptors, which can be glycoproteins or glycolipids. The binding is probably of fairly low affinity but of sufficiently high avidity that these viruses agglutinate erythrocytes (hemagglutination). The attachment proteins of respiroviruses and *Rubulavirinae* also have NA (receptor-destroying) activity, and the proteins have been designated HN. However, a possible role of a specific protein–protein involvement in infection of host cells has not been ruled out.

The *Morbillivirus* attachment protein (H) can cause agglutination of primate erythrocytes but lacks detectable NA or esterase activity. The restricted host range of MeV for primate cells made it unlikely that sialic acid was the primary receptor for MeV. In 1993, human CD46 was identified as a cellular receptor for Edmonston and Halle strains of MeV.[137,395] Edmonston and Vero cell–adapted strains of MeV are capable of infecting any CD46+ primate cell. However, viruses isolated from B-cell and T-cell lines do not grow in CD46+ cells. To identify the receptor in B cells, a VSV recombinant virus was used that expressed GFP as a marker of infection and MeV H (from a virus isolate propagated on B cells) in place of VSV G. Nonsusceptible 293T cells were transfected with a cDNA library from B95a cells (marmoset B cells) and then infected with VSV-GFP-H. From cells expressing GFP, a cDNA was identified that supported MeV replication in 293T cells. This cDNA encoded the equivalent of human CD150 (also known as signaling lymphocyte activation molecule [SLAM]), a membrane glycoprotein involved in lymphocyte activation.[591,644] All MeV isolates can productively interact with hSLAM, and its predominant expression on activated lymphocytes, dendritic cells, and macrophages is consistent with the strong lymphotropism of the virus.[418] SLAM-dependent infection therefore outlined a

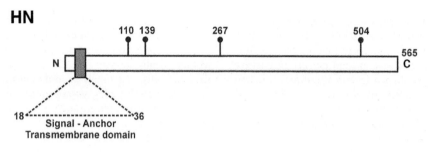

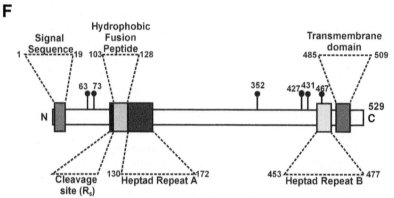

© G.D. Parks and R.A. Lamb 2006

FIGURE 12.14 Schematic diagram showing the orientation and domains of paramyxovirus integral membrane proteins. **Top:** Hemagglutinin-neuraminidase attachment protein (based on the predicted sequence of the PIV-5 HN gene).[214] The signal anchor transmembrane domain and the sites used for addition of N-linked carbohydrate (lollipops)[399] are indicated. **Bottom:** Fusion protein (based on the predicted sequence of the PIV-5 F gene). The position of the signal sequence, the transmembrane domain, the cleavage site, the hydrophobic fusion peptide, and the heptad repeats A and B are indicated. The sites used for addition of N-linked carbohydrate (lollipops)[17] are indicated. R_5 indicates the five arginine residues site for cleavage activation. (Images copyright © 2006 by G.D. Parks and R.A. Lamb.)

path toward the observed initial virus replication in mediastinal lymph nodes followed by PBMC-associated viremia. However, SLAM tissue distribution was incompatible with basolateral MeV re-entry into the respiratory tract and subsequent dissemination, since the receptor is not expressed on respiratory epithelial cells. The mystery was solved by identifying the adherence junction protein nectin-4 as the missing epithelial cell receptor based on microarray profiling of epithelial cells differentially permissive for CD46 and hSLAM-independent MeV infection.[408] A subsequent report confirmed MeV infection of epithelial cells through nectin-4.[380]

In addition to the morbilliviruses, members of the *Henipavirus* genus also gain cell entry through proteinaceous receptors. Ephrin B2 has been identified as a cognate receptor for both HeV and NiV G glycoprotein. In one approach, direct binding of Nipah G to receptor was obtained, and the identity of the receptor was determined by protein sequencing and bioinformatics.[396] In another approach, microarray analysis was used to identify mRNAs that were expressed in *Henipavirus*-susceptible cells and not in cells refractory to *Henipavirus* infection.[34] Ephrin B2 is a member of a family of cell surface glycoprotein ligands that bind to ephrin (Eph) receptors, a large family of tyrosine kinases. The identification of ephrin B2 as the cellular receptor for both HeV and NiV and the widespread occurrence of ephrin B2 in vertebrates, particularly in arterial endothelial cells and in neurons, provides an explana-

tion for the wide host range of the zoonotic henipaviruses and their ability to cause systemic infections.[147]

Paramyxovirus Attachment Protein Organization

The paramyxovirus attachment glycoproteins are both multifunctional proteins and the major antigenic determinant for the humoral immune response. They are responsible for the adsorption of the virus to target cells, either through contact with sialic acid–containing cell surface molecules (*Respirovirus* and *Rubulavirinae* HN) or specific interaction with proteinaceous receptors (*Morbillivirus* H and *Henipavirus* G). Independent of the chemical nature of the host cell receptor, subsequent to particle binding, the attachment proteins trigger fusion between viral envelope and target cell membranes, mediated through the F glycoprotein (see below). In addition, HN proteins mediate enzymatic cleavage of sialic acid (NA activity) from the surface of virions and the surface of infected cells. By analogy with the role of influenza virus NA, it seems likely that the role of this NA activity is to prevent self-aggregation of viral particles during budding at the plasma membrane. These dual activities of HN can be modulated by halide ion concentration and pH.[361] Whereas chemical properties of the extracellular environment are optimal for hemagglutination activity, paramyxovirus NAs have acidic pH optima (pH 4.8–5.5), suggesting that NA acts in the acidic trans-Golgi network to remove sialic acid from the HN carbohydrate chains and from the F protein carbohydrate chains.

The attachment protein polypeptide chain ranges from 420 (NiV) to an exceptional 1,052 residues (Tailam virus) but, in most cases, is approximately 600 residues in length. HN proteins of some NDV strains are synthesized as biologically inactive precursors (HN_o) that are activated through proteolytic removal of 90 residues from the C-terminus.[388,389,654] All paramyxovirus attachment proteins are type II integral membrane proteins that span the membrane once and contain an N-terminal cytoplasmic tail, a single N-terminal transmembrane (TM) domain, a membrane-proximal stalk domain, and a large C-terminal globular head domain.[214] The globular head domain harbors the receptor binding and, in the case of HN proteins, enzymatic activity.[434,517,597] The protein is glycosylated and contains from four to six potential sites for the addition of N-linked carbohydrate chains. For PIV-5 and NDV HN and for MeV H, four sites are used.[229,351,400] The attachment proteins are noncovalently associated to form a tetramer, based on biochemical, cross-linking, EM, and structural studies, which, depending on the paramyxovirus, can be composed of two disulfide-linked dimers.[50,106,297,330,352,399,400,457,598,656] The covalent linkage occurs through cysteine residues at the C-terminal end of the stalk domain, adjacent to the beginning of the head domain. The stalk domain is instrumental in tetramerization,[51,656] while the head domains expressed in isolation remain monomeric.[106,297,656]

The structure of the enzymatically active head domain of the attachment protein has been predicted to be similar to that of other NAs or sialidases, such as influenza NA,[152] with the globular head composed of identical subunits arranged with fourfold symmetry. Each NA domain was expected to exhibit the six-blade propeller fold typical of neuraminidase/sialidase structures from viral, protozoan, or bacterial origin.[58,59,294,592] The predicted structure of the attachment protein head domain was confirmed by the x-ray structures of soluble NDV, HPIV-3, and PIV-5 HN,[106,297,656,658] soluble MeV H,[202,515,660] and soluble NiV G[44,640] globular regions, and it shows the typical sialidase fold consisting of six antiparallel β strands organized as a super barrel with a centrally located active site (Fig. 12.15). The sialidase fold was conserved even in MeV and NiV attachment proteins that bind to proteinaceous receptors and have accu-

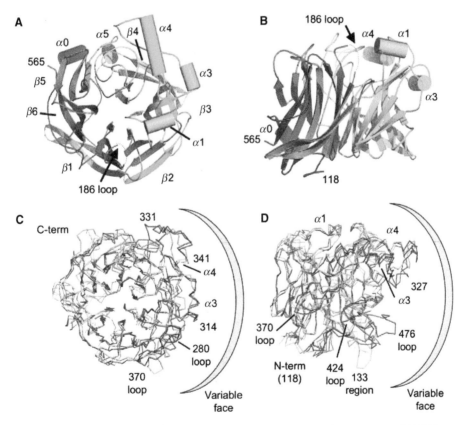

FIGURE 12.15 PIV-5 HN monomer structure and comparison with NDV HN and HPIV-3 HN. A and B: Schematic cartoon diagrams showing top and side views of PIV-5 HN. Helices are shown in *cylinders*, and β strands are shown in *arrowed belts*. The N-terminus is shown in *blue*, and the C-terminus is shown in *red*. The missing loop from residues 186 to 190 is indicated as a *dashed blue line*. **C and D:** Ribbon diagram of the superposition of PIV-5 HN with NDV and HPIV-3 HN, shown in top and side views. Major differences in the PIV-5, NDV, and HPIV HN structures are colored *red, blue,* and *green,* respectively. Areas of major structural differences are labeled, and the highly variable face of the HN monomer is highlighted. (Adapted from Yuan P, Thompson T, Wurzburg BA, et al. Structural studies of the parainfluenza virus 5 hemagglutinin-neuraminidase tetramer in complex with its receptor, sialyllactose. *Structure* 2005;13:803–815, with permission.)

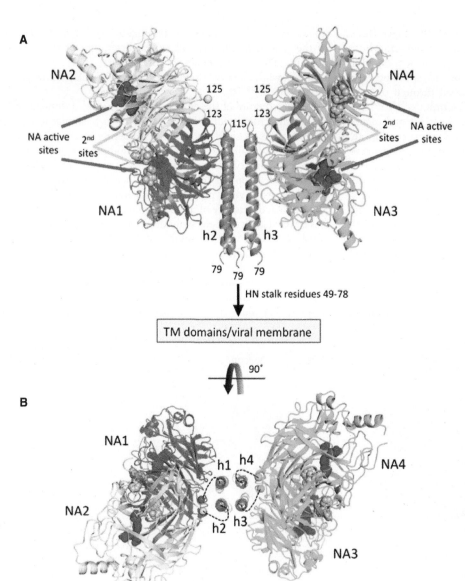

FIGURE 12.16 PIV-5 HN tetramers. Active sites are marked by space-filling representations of the ligand sialyllactose. The four subunits are shown in different colors. **A:** Top view of the PIV-5 HN tetramer arrangement. **B:** Side view of the PIV-5 HN tetramer arrangement, with a 60-degree packing angle between dimers. (Adapted from Yuan P, Thompson T, Wurzburg BA, et al. Structural studies of the parainfluenza virus 5 hemagglutinin-neuraminidase tetramer in complex with its receptor, sialyllactose. *Structure* 2005;13:803–815, with permission.)

mulated mutations eliminating NA catalytic activity. For PIV-5, the HN structure was determined with a bound uncleaved receptor sialyllactose[656] (Fig. 12.16). The seven highly conserved active site residues found in NA and sialidases are found in the paramyxovirus HN structures. Superimposition of the NDV, HPIV-3, and PIV-5 HN monomer structures indicated a high degree of conservation on one face of the molecule with the other face containing more variability and additional protein loops.[656]

It has long been debated whether the hemagglutinin and NA activities of the HN-type attachment proteins involve one or two separate sialic acid–binding sites.[106,469,598,658] The disparate theories of one site with dual function or of two distinct sites that are intimately related are both consistent with the observation that sialic acid–derived NA inhibitors interfere with receptor binding.[235,384,518] A single site can provide both hemagglutinin and NA activities by binding sialic acid tightly and hydrolyzing the molecules slowly.[518] For NDV HN, two sialic acid sites have been observed in the x-ray structures: one is the active site and the second site is located at the dimer

interface.[658] Strong biological evidence supports the notion of a second sialic acid–binding site in NDV.[43,465] Mutagenesis of a key residue involved in the dimer interface sialic acid–binding site abolishes sialic acid binding to the second site.[43] However, virus containing this key residue mutation is only marginally affected in growth properties.[43] For HPIV-3 and PIV-5 HN, not only was a second sialic acid molecule not observed, but the PIV-5 HN molecule is also unable to form the second sialic acid–binding site between two monomers due to changes in sequence and conformation.[297,656] Thus, the biological importance of the second sialic acid–binding site in NDV HN is unclear.

From the structural studies of NDV HN, it was also suggested that the NA domain could form two distinct dimeric assemblies that were ligand dependent.[106] One of the dimers, observed after cocrystallization with ligand, formed an extensive buried interface, while the second dimer, crystallized in the absence of ligand and at low pH, formed a much smaller interface. Conformational changes were observed in the paramyxovirus attachment protein upon ligand binding, but the dimer of HN that is observed in the HPIV-3 and PIV-5 structures occurs in the absence of ligand binding, and there is no crystallographic or biochemical evidence that ligand binding influences the oligomeric status of the attachment protein tetramer itself.[52,297,319,656]

The attachment protein tetrameric arrangement[656,658] is unusual because, rather than having fourfold rotational symmetry as might be anticipated, it is arranged with two twofold symmetry axes that are orientated at 60 degrees to each other and in the crystal lattice, allowing neighboring dimers and tetramers to associate in infinitely long oligomers. The calculated buried surface area for each monomer in the PIV-5 HN dimer is 1,818 Å.[595] In contrast to the dimer interaction, the dimer-of-dimers interface is much smaller, involving only 10 residues and burying only 657 Å.[595] The small surface of interaction suggests that the arrangement is not very strong and that the head domain dimers may dissociate.

Upon being transported to the cell surface, the PIV-5 HN protein is rapidly internalized by the clathrin-mediated endocytosis pathway.[305] The signal for internalization is unusual because it is not located in the cytoplasmic tail but rather at the boundary of the TM domain and the ectodomain.[306] The reason for the internalization of PIV-5 HN, a process seemingly in conflict with virus assembly, is not known.

Paramyxovirus Fusion Protein Organization

The paramyxovirus fusion (F) proteins mediate viral penetration by fusion between the viral envelope and the host cell membranes at neutral pH. The consequence of the fusion reaction is that the nucleocapsid is delivered to the cytoplasm. Later in infection, coexpression of the F proteins and the homotypic attachment proteins at the plasma membrane of infected cells can mediate fusion of the infected cell with uninfected neighboring cells to form multinucleated giant cells (syncytia), the hallmark cytopathic effect associated with paramyxovirus infection in cell culture that can lead to tissue necrosis *in vivo* and might be a mechanism of virus spread.

The F proteins are type I integral membrane proteins with a single TM domain and short C-terminal cytosolic tails. The physiological oligomer is a noncovalently associated homotrimer.[80,201,505,637,647,648] First synthesized as inactive precursor proteins (F0), F proteins must be cleaved by a host cell protease at a specific cleavage activation site located in the ectodomain to be biologically active. This proteolytic maturation step generates a larger, membrane-integral F1 subunit and shorter F2 ectodomain subunit that remains connected to F1 through an intra–monomeric disulfide link.[221,519] A short hydrophobic membrane attack domain, the fusion peptide, is located at the newly liberated N-terminus of the F1 subunit. The paramyxovirus F genes encode 540 to 580 residues. The F0 protein carries at the N-terminus a cleavable signal sequence that targets the nascent polypeptide chain to the membrane of the endoplasmic reticulum (ER) for cotranslational ER import. Located near the C-termini, a hydrophobic stop-transfer TM domain anchors the protein in the membrane leaving a short cytoplasmic tail of approximately 20 to 40 residues. Sequences adjacent to the fusion peptide and the TM anchor domain typically reveal a 4–3 (heptad) pattern of hydrophobic repeats and are designated HRA and HRB, respectively. Approximately 250 residues separate the HRA and HRB domains (Fig. 12.17A).

Like other viral and cellular fusogenic proteins, the paramyxovirus F proteins are believed to be membrane-bending machineries that drive membrane fusion by coupling irreversible protein refolding to the localized introduction of extreme negative curvature into juxtapositioned donor and target membranes.[82,455] Initially folding into a metastable prefusion form, they undergo a series of discrete/stepwise conformational changes to a lower energy state, the postfusion form, when triggered.[248,288] Cleavage of F0 primes the protein for productive membrane fusion by liberating the internal N-terminus of the fusion peptide, but uncleaved soluble F0 complexes are capable of refolding into a postfusion-like conformation (discussed below).[647] The varying nature of the residues found at the cleavage site, the enzymes involved in cleavage, and the role of cleavage in pathogenesis are discussed later in this chapter.

Comparison of the amino acid sequences of paramyxovirus F proteins (reviewed in Ref.[374]) does not show major regions of sequence identity overall, with the exception of the fusion peptide, which has a conserved sequence (up to 90% identity). However, the overall placement of cysteine, glycine, and proline residues suggests a similar structure for all F proteins and a conserved intramonomeric disulfide bond scaffold of the F ectodomain. The *Respirovirus* and *Rubulavirus* F2 and F1 subunits are glycosylated, and there are a total of three to six potential sites for the addition of N-linked carbohydrate. For PIV-5 F protein, it is known that all four potential sites for addition of N-linked carbohydrate are used.[17] The MeV F protein contains three sites in the F2 subunit for N-linked carbohydrate addition, and all three sites are used; there are no sites in F1 for N-linked carbohydrate addition.[8]

Class I viral fusion proteins

The paramyxovirus F proteins belong to the class I viral fusion protein type, of which the longest-standing and structurally first characterized member is the influenza virus hemagglutinin (HA). In addition to the ortho- and paramyxoviruses, major human and animal viral pathogens feature class I fusion proteins including the retroviruses (i.e., HIV-1 Env/gp160), coronaviruses (i.e., SARS coronavirus S), filoviruses (i.e., Ebola virus G), and pneumoviruses (i.e., RSV F).[89,145,146,248,455] Models for class I viral fusion protein-mediated membrane merger have been developed, until recently, primarily based on the structural studies of HA.[548] The general mechanism for class I viral fusion proteins comprises initial folding of the uncleaved protein into a metastable prefusion state, which can be activated through distinct, virus family–characteristic stimuli to undergo large structural reorganizations into a thermodynamically more stable postfusion conformation. The attainment of the prefusion state, its regulation, and its relative free energy as compared to the postfusion form are all key to the process by which class I viral fusion proteins function.

Class I viral fusion proteins and the helical hairpin (core trimer)

Biophysical data indicated that HRA and HRB form a complex, and crystallographic studies have shown that HRA and HRB associate into a helical hairpin or six-helix bundle (6HB) structure (core trimer) that is reminiscent of the low-pH–induced proteolytic fragment of influenza virus HA (TBHA2). The core trimers of PIV-5 and hRSV F,[18,254,661] HIV gp41,[62,76,583,629] Moloney murine leukemia virus envelope

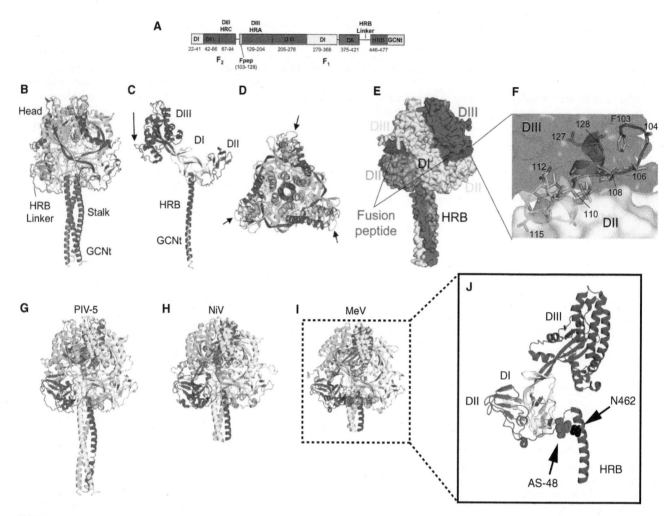

FIGURE 12.17 The F protein prefusion structure. A: Schematic diagram of the F-GCNt domains. Important domains are colored, and their corresponding residue ranges indicated. **B:** Ribbon diagram of the F trimer, with each chain colored by residue number in a gradient from *blue* (N-terminus) to *red* (C-terminus). The head and stalk regions are indicated. HRB linker residues 429 to 432 could not be modeled in one subunit and had high temperature factors in the other two. **C:** Ribbon diagram of one subunit of the F trimer colored by domain. The domains are labeled and the colors correspond to those used in **(A)**. The cleavage/activation site is marked by an *arrow*. **D:** Top view of the trimer colored as in **(A)**. Cleavage/activation sites are indicated by *arrows*. **E:** Surface representation of the F trimer colored by subunit. The fusion peptide exposed surface is shown in *blue*. **F:** Close-up view of the fusion peptide (residues 103–128). The peptide is folded back on itself with a small hydrophobic core and contains a mixture of extended chain, 1 β strand, and a C-terminal α-helix. The fusion peptide is sandwiched between two subunits of the trimer, between DII and DIII domains. (Adapted from Yin HS, Wen X, Paterson RG, et al. Structure of the parainfluenza virus 5 F protein in its metastable, prefusion conformation. *Nature* 2006;439:38–44, with permission.) **G–I:** Crystal structures of the prefusion forms of HPIV-5 (PDB ID: 4WSG),[464] NiV (PDB ID: 5EVM),[638] and MeV F (PDB ID: 5YZC)[201] proteins displaying the similar overall structure and domain architecture of paramyxovirus F proteins. **J:** Close-up of the MeV F monomer, showing the docking pose of the small-molecule MeV entry inhibitor AS-48 (*red spheres*) that was identified in cocrystals.[201] The compound binds at the intersection of the top of the prefusion F stalk with the head domain. The location of the N462 resistance hot spot to AS-48[138] is shown as *black spheres*.

protein,[158] Ebola GP2,[332,630] and HTLV-1[276] fusion proteins all share this similarity in structure (Fig. 12.18A). Although the structural details vary, all reveal a trimeric coiled coil beginning near the C-terminal end of the hydrophobic fusion peptide. The C-terminal segment abutting the TM domain is also often helical and packs in an antiparallel direction along the outside of the N-terminal coiled coil, placing the fusion peptides and TM anchors at the same end of a rod-like structure (for PIV-5 6HB, see Fig. 12.18A). These 6HBs typically represent a relatively small fraction of the intact fusion protein, yet their structures are generally extremely thermostable, with

melting temperatures near 100°C. Intermediates along the pathway of membrane fusion can be trapped by the addition of peptides derived from either the N-terminal (HRA) or the C-terminal (HRB) heptad repeat regions for many class I fusion proteins,[146,149,157,503,653] indicating that the intact protein undergoes multistep conformational changes that consecutively expose both HR regions, prior to assembly of the final 6HB. While structurally not yet characterized, these intermediates are believed to represent partially refolded forms of the fusion protein, with the hydrophobic fusion peptide anchored in the target cell membrane and the TM domains integrated

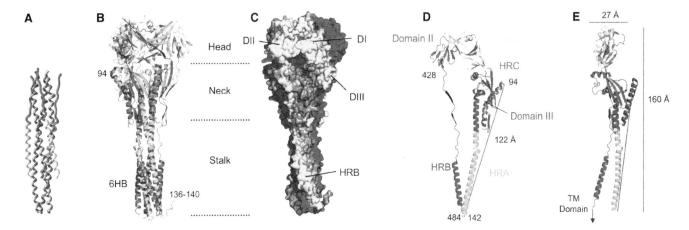

FIGURE 12.18 The F protein postfusion structure. A: The complete PIV-5 F1 core trimer is shown with the N1 helix colored *gray* and the C1 peptide colored *blue*, except for the extended chain N-terminal residues of C1 that are colored *red*. **B:** Ribbon diagram of the HPIV-3 solF0 trimer. The three chains are colored similarly from *blue* (N-terminus) to *red* (C-terminus). Residues 95 to 135 are disordered in all chains. Residue 94 is labeled in one chain, and residues 136 to 140 at the base of the stalk are ordered in one chain due to crystal packing interactions. **C:** Surface representation of the solF0 trimer. Each chain is a different color, and domains I to III and HRB for one chain (*yellow*) are indicated by the DI, DII, DIII, and HRB labels. One radial channel is readily apparent below domains I and II of the *yellow* chain and above domain III of the *red* chain. **D:** Ribbon diagram of the solF0 protein monomer colored by domain. The direct distance within one monomer between residue 94 at the end of HRC and residue 142 at the base of the stalk region is 122 Å. **E:** Ribbon diagram of the monomer rotated by 90 degrees, indicating the width and height of the solF0 monomer. An *arrow* at the C-terminus of the HRB segment points toward the likely position of the transmembrane anchor domain that would be present in the full-length protein. (Adapted from Yin HS, Paterson RG, Wen X, et al. Structure of the uncleaved ectodomain of the paramyxovirus (hPIV3) fusion protein. *Proc Natl Acad Sci USA* 2005;102:9288–9293, with permission.)

in the viral envelope. The formation of the 6HB is linked to the merger of lipid bilayers and is believed to couple the free energy released on protein refolding to membrane fusion.[359,503] Resembling the requirements for HIV gp41–mediated fusion pore opening,[360] however, transition of paramyxovirus F into a 6HB causes fusion without full closure of the bundle configuration.[49]

Atomic structures of the paramyxovirus F protein
Structure of the prefusion F protein
The crystal structures of the PIV-5 F protein ectodomain, and subsequently of NiV, HeV, and MeV F, have been determined in their metastable prefusion forms.[201,637,638,648] To solve the atomic structures, the secreted PIV-5 and HeV F proteins were stabilized by the addition of a soluble trimeric TM domain (GCNt) that supplants the hydrophobic TM domain, or in the case of MeV F through engineered disulfide bonds added to the membrane-proximal F stalk domain. In all cases, the F trimer was found to have a large globular head attached to a three-helix coiled-coil stalk formed by HRB (Fig. 12.17B–E), orienting the head away from the viral membrane. The F head contains three domains (DI–DIII) per subunit that extend around the trimer axis, making extensive intersubunit contacts. A large cavity is present at the base of the head, with the bottom and sides formed by DI and DII. DIII (residues 42–278) covers the top of the cavity, HRA, and the fusion peptide (Fig. 12.17B–F). At the C-terminus of DII, an extended linker to HRB wraps around the outside of the trimer and into the center of the base of the head where the stalk begins. The structure has three lateral vertices projecting from the trimer axis, exposing the cleavage/activation sites adjacent to the fusion peptides (Fig. 12.17C, D). Helices line the central threefold axis at the top and bottom

of the trimer. In DIII, two sets of six helices form rings sealing the top of the head, while the HRB three-helix bundle seals the bottom (Fig. 12.17D). The network of noncovalent interactions between the top of the stalk and base of the head domain is considered to contribute to conformational stability of the prefusion F trimer, and a cocrystal structure of MeV F with a small-molecule MeV entry inhibitor stabilizing an F prefusion conformation[138,456] demonstrated specific targeting of this intersection by the compound[201] (Fig. 12.17G–J).

Illustrated by example of prefusion PIV-5 F, the hydrophobic fusion peptide (residues 103–128) is wedged between two subunits of the trimer (Fig. 12.17E). The N-terminal end of the fusion peptide is exposed at the F surface and then proceeds inward, becoming increasingly buried from solvent. The fusion peptide adopts a partly extended, partly β sheet, and partly α-helical conformation and is sandwiched between DIII of its own subunit and DII of another. Residues 107 to 117 pack against the hydrophobic edge of the neighboring DII domain. The fusion peptide folds back on itself, forming a small hydrophobic core between its N- and C-terminal ends, making less extensive contacts with DIII (Fig. 12.17E, F). Proteolytic maturation of F0 might allow the N-terminus of the fusion peptide to make additional contacts with DII and to affect intersubunit interactions, but the transition of prefusion paramyxovirus F from the uncleaved to cleaved form does not entail a major relocation of the fusion peptides, as has been described, for instance, for influenza virus HA fusion peptides.[561] The crystal structure of soluble NiV F, expressed at high concentration, revealed a unique high molecular weight supercomplex that was interpreted as a hexameric ring of F protein trimers.[638] The physiological significance of this higher-order F organization is not known, and analogous supercomplex structures have not been noted in crystals of PIV-5, MeV, or HeV F. It is furthermore challenging to reconcile a ring-like F arrangement with the regular F layer, arranged in sync with the M protein array, that was revealed by reconstruction of cryopreserved near-native MeV virions (Ref.[266] discussed below).

Structure of the postfusion form of the F protein

The atomic structure of intact uncleaved F protein in its postfusion form[647] has also been determined. The structure of the HPIV-3 F protein was solved by molecular replacement using as a model a fragment of the NDV F structure that had been obtained earlier.[80] The NDV F structure had revealed a trimer, with distinct head, neck, and stalk regions.

The HPIV-3 F also forms a trimer, with distinct head, neck, and stalk regions (Fig. 12.18A–D). The only part of the structure lacking electron density is the fusion peptide and cleavage site, but these residues would be draped flexibly on the exterior of the stalk region. Given that the uncleaved F ectodomain was secreted from cells by removal of the TM domain, it was initially unexpected that the structure contained a 6HB (Fig. 12.18A–D) that represents the postfusion conformation of the protein. It had been widely anticipated that cleavage of F at the cleavage site was a requirement for conversion to the postfusion form. Nonetheless, many lines of evidence suggested that the observed HPIV-3 conformation represented the postfusion form, although the polypeptide chains were intact in the crystal and the fusion peptide was not located at the appropriate end of the 6HB: (a) the 6HB was well formed and undistorted, similar to the previously determined PIV-5 and hRSV F 6HB structures[18,662]; (b) the HPIV-3 structure appeared to be inconsistent with peptide inhibition data that show, at least for PIV-5 F, that the HRA and HRB peptides are exposed at distinct steps of the membrane fusion reaction[503]; (c) the HPIV-3 structure does not provide a simple mechanism for how membrane fusion could be achieved. Cleavage of the HPIV-3 solF0

protein would appear to simply allow repositioning of the fusion peptide to the N-terminus of the HRA coiled-coil and concomitant insertion into the anchoring membrane for the TM domain; and, (d) the HPIV-3 structure did not explain the behavior of F protein mutants that destabilize the prefusion conformation of F and significantly enhance its membrane fusion activity.[89,138,292,442,504,647]

The observation that the soluble, secreted HPIV-3 and NDV F proteins were in the postfusion conformation was unexpected, and there are at least two possible explanations for this finding. First, the TM anchor (and potentially the cytoplasmic tail[624]) could be an important determinant of the stability of the prefusion conformation, providing a significant fraction of the energy barrier that traps the protein in a metastable state. In this case, the secreted protein may fold into the prefusion form transiently but then refold to the postfusion conformation. A second possible explanation for the structural results is that the TM domain is important for the protein to attain the prefusion metastable state and that, in the absence of this region, the soluble F protein folds directly to the final, most stable postfusion conformation. In either case, it appears that the amino acids constituting the intact F protein ectodomain are not sufficient for the protein to fold to and maintain a metastable conformation. Hence, to preserve a soluble form of a paramyxovirus F protein in its metastable form, the prefusion stalk domain had to be stabilized either through in-frame addition of a trimeric GCNt or bacterial fold on domain as mimetics of the hydrophobic TM domain[48,637,648] or a scaffold of engineered disulfide bonds.[201]

Comparison of the pre- and postfusion F structures

The available prefusion F structures and the HPIV-3 postfusion F structure are in strikingly different conformations (Fig. 12.19), consistent with a transition from pre- to postfusion forms. None of the intersubunit contacts are conserved in the pre- and postfusion

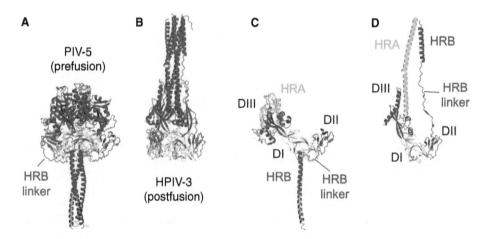

FIGURE 12.19 Structural changes between the pre- and postfusion F protein conformations.
A: Ribbon diagram of the PIV-5 F-GCNt trimer. DI is colored *yellow*, DII is colored *red*, DIII is colored *magenta*, HRB is colored *blue*, and GCNt is colored *gray*. **B:** Ribbon diagram of the HPIV-3 (postfusion) trimer, colored as in **(A)**. **C:** Ribbon diagram of a single subunit of the PIV-5 F-GCNt trimer, colored as in **(A)**, except for HRA residues, which are colored *green*. **D:** Ribbon diagram of a single subunit of the HPIV-3 F trimer, colored as in **(C)**. (Adapted from Yin HS, Wen X, Paterson RG, et al. Structure of the parainfluenza virus 5 F protein in its metastable, prefusion conformation. *Nature* 2006;439:38–44, with permission.)

forms. The two F conformations are related by flipping the stalk and TM domains relative to the F head. Substantial compacting of the head is observed in HPIV-3 postfusion F compared to the prefusion F structures. DI domains pivot slightly inward, shearing intersubunit contacts, and DII domains swing across, contacting neighboring subunits. Individual DI and DII domains in the two conformations remain similar. Closely related forms of the paramyxovirus F proteins have been observed in electron micrographs and crystal structures of RSV F of the pneumovirus family.[65,179,355,356,500,501]

DIII undergoes major refolding between the two structures, projecting a newly assembled coiled coil (HRA) upward and away from DI, the prefusion stalk and the viral membrane. The fusion peptides, located at the top of this HRA triple helix coiled coil, move approximately 115 Å from their initial position between subunits in the prefusion conformation, allowing DII domains to reposition. None of the postfusion HRA intersubunit coiled-coil contacts are observed in the stabilized F structures. Instead, they are replaced by two sets of six-helix rings at the DIII interfaces (Fig. 12.17D). To assemble the HRA coiled coil to form, DIII must rotate and collapse inward, further compacting the head. In the prefusion conformation, HRA is broken up into four helices, two β strands, and five loop, kink, or turn segments. Thus, the conformational changes in HRA involve the refolding of 11 distinct segments into a single, extended α-helical conformation (Fig. 12.20).

The conformational change also requires the opening and translocation of the HRB stalk (Fig. 12.19). In the prefusion form, HRB is located at the base of the head region. During the conversion to the postfusion conformation, HRB segments must separate and swing around the base of the head to pack against the HRA coiled coil (hairpin formation). Since the C-terminal residues of HRB are neighboring the TM domains

anchored in the viral envelope, hairpin formation most likely entails asymmetric refolding of individual monomers constituting the F trimer.

The mechanism of paramyxovirus-mediated membrane fusion

The pre- and postfusion F structures suggest how discrete refolding intermediates are coupled to the activation and progression of F-mediated membrane fusion. Although proteolytic cleavage of the paramyxovirus F protein is required for membrane fusion activity, it is not necessary for the formation of the postfusion conformation. In a current model of membrane fusion, the HRB helices melt in a first step (open-stalk form, Fig. 12.21), breaking interactions at the base of the head but leaving HRA in the prefusion conformation. This intermediate is consistent with effects of mutations of PIV-5 F residues 443, 447, and 449, peptide inhibition data, and inter–monomeric disulfide bonds engineered to link the top of prefusion MeV F stalk to the base of the head domain.[303,442,503,504] These disulfide bonds covalently stabilized prefusion F but allowed fusion to proceed when exposed to reducing conditions. HRA-derived peptides, which likely bind to the endogenous HRB segment, inhibited an early intermediate along the fusion pathway, while HRB-derived peptides inhibited a later intermediate by binding the endogenous HRA coiled coil. Opening of the HRB stalk could initiate further changes in F by affecting the packing of DII and the fusion peptide (through the HRB linker) and by affecting the stability of the head intersubunit contacts, which shift during the conformational transition. It seems possible that transient dissociation of the F trimer could occur, analogous to dimer-to-trimer transition characterized in alpha- and flavivirus fusion proteins. The open-stalk intermediate is then likely followed by refolding of DIII, the assembly of the HRA

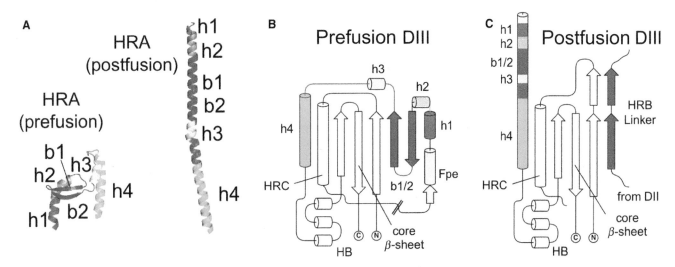

FIGURE 12.20 F protein refolding: the role of DIII in HRA folding and transformation. A: HRA refolds from 11 distinct segments (h1, h2, b1, b2, h3, h4, and the intervening residues) in the prefusion conformation into a single approximately 120-Å–long helix in the postfusion form. **B:** Secondary structure diagram for DIII in the prefusion (PIV-5) conformation. The "DIII core" includes three antiparallel strands, HRC, a helical bundle (HB), and h4 of HRA. HRA segments are colored as in **(A)**, and the cleavage site (//) and fusion peptide are indicated. The DIII core sheet is extended by the b1 and b2 strands from HRA. **C:** Secondary structure diagram for DIII in the postfusion (HPIV-3) conformation colored as in **(B)**. The DIII core sheet is extended by one strand from HRB linker from a neighboring subunit (*dark violet*). (Adapted from Yin HS, Wen X, Paterson RG, et al. Structure of the parainfluenza virus 5 F protein in its metastable, prefusion conformation. *Nature* 2006;439:38–44, with permission.)

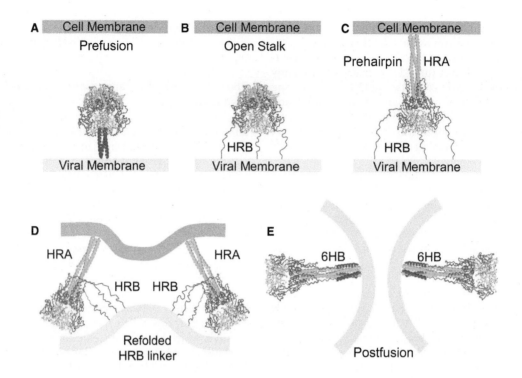

FIGURE 12.21 A model for F-mediated membrane fusion. A: Structure of the prefusion conformation. HRB is colored *blue*, HRA is colored *green*, and domains I, II, and III are colored *yellow*, *red*, and *magenta*, respectively. **B:** An "open-stalk" conformation, in which the HRB stalk melts and separates from the prefusion head region. HRB is shown as three extended chains because the individual segments are unlikely to be helical. This conformation is consistent with a low-temperature intermediate that is inhibited by HRA peptides, but not HRB peptides. Mutations of the switch peptide residues 443, 447, and 449 would influence the formation of this intermediate by affecting stabilizing interactions between the prefusion stalk and head domains. **C:** A prehairpin intermediate can form by refolding of DIII, allowing the formation of the HRA coiled coil and insertion of the fusion peptide into the target cell membrane. This intermediate can be inhibited by peptides derived from both HRA and HRB regions. **D:** Prior to forming the final 6HB, the close approach of viral and cellular membranes may be trapped by folding of the HRB linker onto the newly exposed DIII core, with the formation of two β strands. **E:** The formation of the postfusion 6HB is tightly linked to membrane fusion and pore formation, juxtaposing the membrane-interacting fusion peptide and TM domains. (Adapted from Yin HS, Wen X, Paterson RG, et al. Structure of the parainfluenza virus 5 F protein in its metastable, prefusion conformation. *Nature* 2006;439:38–44, with permission.)

coiled coil, and the translocation of the fusion peptide toward the target cell membrane (Fig. 12.21). This prehairpin intermediate has been trapped and coprecipitated with HRB peptides.[503] Removal of the fusion peptide from the intersubunit interfaces is believed to enable an inward swing of DII and the formation of new contacts with DI of a neighboring subunit, compacting the head. The refolding of DIII HRA would also expose its core β sheet and, together with the inward movement of DII, allow the HRB linker (at the C-terminus of DII) to form parallel β strands with the DIII core, likely preceding and initiating the final positioning of HRB (Fig. 12.21). The assembly of the final 6HB completes the conformational change and membrane merger.

The attachment protein activates the F protein for membrane fusion

The exact molecular triggering mechanism that regulates F protein refolding such that it occurs when a target cell is within reach is still unknown, although most paramyxovirus F proteins require the presence of the receptor-binding protein (HN, H, or G) for activation of cell-to-cell fusion (reviewed in Refs.[292,372,455]) and engineered paramyxoviruses lacking the attachment protein have not been recovered. The precise role of the HN, H, or G protein in stimulating the F conformational change remains to be understood, but the emerging picture indicates a highly controlled, complex biological machine.

For all paramyxoviruses, coexpression of F and HN, H, or G is required to mediate viral entry.[73,148,227,230,373,509,634,646] Furthermore, typically the homotypic attachment protein (i.e., of the same virus), and not a heterotypic protein derived from a different member of the family, has to be coexpressed in the same cell as the F protein to promote fusion,[227,230,533] although cases of heterotypic fusion activation between glycoproteins derived from different viruses within the same paramyxovirus genus (i.e., for the morbilliviruses) have been described.[302] However, expression of the F of PIV-5 alone causes some syncytium formation in transient cell-to-cell fusion assays,[8,227,255,419,440,443] and point mutations within NDV F render the protein somewhat

HN-independent for fusion.[534] It therefore appears likely that the different paramyxovirus F proteins have different activation energy thresholds for fusion activation and that HN, H, or G enable the F protein to cross this activation energy barrier in a receptor binding–dependent manner.

It was hypothesized that a type-specific interaction would occur between the attachment and F protein.[230,288,535] Immunoprecipitation assays show that F and attachment proteins coprecipitate specifically,[5,125,358,459,564,646] native MeV F and H proteins were found to first interact intracellularly in the ER of the infected cells,[458] and HPIV-3 F and HN have been shown to undergo antibody-induced cocapping,[646] indicating the formation of a protein complex. A lot of effort has been spent on mapping the regions of F and the attachment protein that interact. Mutations have been identified in the globular attachment protein head domain,[123,366] the helix repeat–like domains of the attachment protein stalk region,[52,124,302,358,421,466,535,565,584,657] and TM anchor[42,352] that decrease or abolish fusogenic activity with no or little effect on receptor recognition. Analysis of the fusion promoting activity of chimeric or engineered paramyxovirus attachment proteins largely suggests that the stalk domain and, in some cases, parts of the globular head impart productive interaction with F.[124,421,584,602] Crystal structures of the NDV HN ectodomain and the PIV-5 HN stalk[38,655] have revealed a parallel 4-helix bundle arrangement of the stalks, in which 11-mer and 7-mer helical repeat sections are separated by a central kink. In the NDV HN structure, the dimeric head domains flank the 4-helix bundles with one of the head monomers of each dimer directly associating with the stalk (Fig. 12.22). This conformation, termed a "heads-down" arrangement, is considered to represent the prereceptor-bound arrangement.[249] By contrast, the PIV-5 HN crystal structure posited the globular head domains oriented away from the stalk and receptor-binding sites facing toward the target membrane, which was hypothesized to resemble a postreceptor-bound "heads-up" organization[632] (Fig. 12.22C). Biochemical assessment of native MeV H tetramers revealed

conformational changes upon receptor binding, suggesting that the HN-based observations likely extend to paramyxoviruses binding to proteinaceous receptors.[52] Extension of the helical MeV H stalk domain by 41 amino acids in α-helical arrangement, corresponding to approximately 7.5 nm in pitch or an elongation of the stalk by an additional half of its original length, was furthermore compatible with efficient fusion promotion in transient expression assays and engineered recombinant virions, provided the extension was placed downstream of stalk residue 118,[51,421] indicating that MeV H stalk residues membrane-proximal of position 118 interact with prefusion F. The structural and biochemical data suggest a modular organization of the attachment protein, organized in a receptor-binding (head domains) regulatory module and an F-triggering (stalk domain) effector module. First demonstrated for PIV-5 HN and confirmed for MeV H, NiV G, and MuV and NDV HN, engineered "headless" attachment protein stalk domains are sufficient to specifically trigger homotypic F trimers in transient cell-to-cell fusion assays.[37,39,51,319] Presumably due to premature constitutive F activation, however, these isolated effector modules are unable to support efficient replication of engineered recombinant viruses.[51]

Initial mechanistic models of the fusion process considered that the paramyxovirus attachment proteins may stabilize associated F protein trimers in prefusion conformation, thus acting like a molecular clamp that prevents F refolding until receptor-binding–induced separation of the attachment and F protein oligomers. An implication of this model is that F protein trimers expressed in the absence of the attachment proteins should spontaneously assume a postfusion-like conformation, potentially immediately after insertion into the ER membrane but latest after proteolytic maturation. Through use of monoclonal antibodies that selectively recognize conformation-dependent epitopes present only in the prefusion forms of the PIV-5, MeV, CDV, or NiV F trimers, however, it was demonstrated that these F proteins remained in prefusion conformation when expressed on their own and did not convert to the

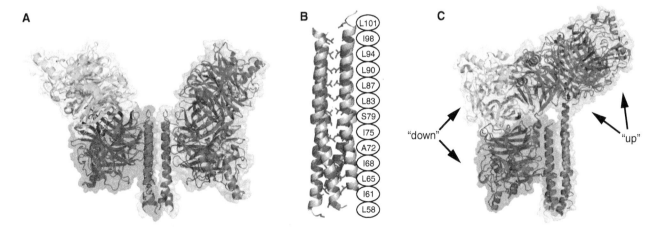

FIGURE 12.22 Crystal structures of the PIV-5 and NDV HN proteins. A: The NDV HN structure (PDB ID: 3T1E) possesses four ectodomains in a "heads-down" orientation.[655] The receptor-binding sites (E400, R415, and Y525) are shown as *yellow spheres*. **B:** Structure of the HPIV-5 HN stalk (amino acids of 56–108) (PDB ID: 3TSI) forms a four-helix bundle.[38] Residues that form the hydrophobic core of the four-helix bundle are labeled. **C:** A crystal structure of the PIV-5 ectodomain (PDB ID: 4JF7) revealed an alternative conformation.[632] In this structure, one head domain dimer is in "heads-down" orientation and the other dimer in "heads-up" orientation (*black arrows*).

postfusion form unless subjected to a trigger such as heat.[2,52,77,94] These observations and the constitutive fusion promotion activity of headless attachment protein effector domains called for an alternative triggering mechanism.

Rather than attachment proteins acting as a molecular clamp, the current model of paramyxovirus fusion promotion proposes that in the case of paramyxoviruses with HN-type attachment proteins featuring relatively short stalk domains, the prereceptor-bound heads-down conformation sterically prevents premature contact of prefusion F with the HN stalk (Fig. 12.23A). Receptor binding rotates HN head domains into the heads-up configuration, giving F access to the now exposed stalk effector module. Subsequent rearrangements in the HN stalk-F contact zone may alter the interface with F, activating the F trimer for membrane fusion.[249] Variations of this triggering mechanism appear to have evolved in the binding of paramyxoviruses, such as members of the *Morbillivirus* genus, to proteinaceous receptors (Fig. 12.23B). A seemingly counterintuitive inverse correlation between fusion promotion activity and strength of F-attachment protein interaction has been demonstrated for H-type and G-type attachment proteins of the *Morbillivirus* and *Henipavirus* genus, respectively,[96,367,459] and MeV F-H complexes are tightly associated in early secretory compartments of the host cell prior to proteolytic maturation

of F and receptor binding of H.[458] Through use of headless MeV H stalks and F mutants stabilized in prefusion conformation, it has been shown that the MeV H head domains do not block F access to the stalk domain prior to receptor binding.[48] Rather, uncleaved MeV F0s tightly preassemble with H stalks in the ER, and subsequent F maturation in the Golgi partially destabilizes this assembly, preparing for F activation. However, H head domains in prereceptor-bound configuration appear to suppress H stalk rearrangements required for F triggering until receptor binding. Receptor-induced rotation of the H head domains into a heads-up configuration may then be directly linked to stalk rearrangements at the H–F interface, triggering F.[3] The intracellular preassembly of the fusion complexes has been shown to affect MeV fusion profiles[48] and may account for the extremely high cell-to-cell fusion activity characteristic of the *Morbillivirus* genus.

Cleavage activation

As discussed previously, the precursor F0 molecule is biologically inactive, and cleavage of F0 to the disulfide-linked chains F1 and F2 activates the protein, rendering the molecule fusion-active and permitting viral infectivity. It is important to remember, however, that F2 and F1 are not separate domains in the atomic structure of F and thus are not individual parts

Model of *Respirovirus* (i.e., PIV-5) fusion activation

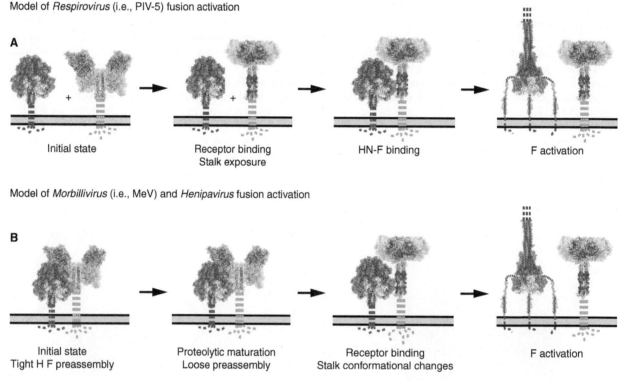

A

Initial state   Receptor binding Stalk exposure   HN-F binding   F activation

Model of *Morbillivirus* (i.e., MeV) and *Henipavirus* fusion activation

B

Initial state Tight H F preassembly   Proteolytic maturation Loose preassembly   Receptor binding Stalk conformational changes   F activation

© R.M.Cox, R.K. Plemper and R.A. Lamb 2019

FIGURE 12.23 Models for paramyxovirus fusion activation. Presenting variations of common elements, two F activation models are favored for paramyxoviruses entering through carbohydrate (i.e., PIV-5) **(A)** or proteinaceous (i.e., MeV) **(B)** receptors. In **(A)**, the F binding site in the attachment protein stalk is masked by the head dimers in heads-down configuration until receptor binding. Then, the F binding domain in the stalk is exposed and glycoprotein hetero-oligomers associated, triggering F refolding. In **(B)**, a longer stalk domain allows tight intracellular preassociation of envelope glycoprotein hetero-oligomers. Proteolytic maturation of F late in the secretory system relaxes the interaction, and receptor binding by the attachment protein head domains induces conformational changes in the tetrameric stalk that trigger F refolding. (Images copyright © 2019 by Richard K. Plemper, Robert A. Lamb, and Robert M. Cox.)

of the protein. Cleavage of F0 is a candidate to be a key determinant for infectivity and pathogenicity, and for certain viruses, this appears to be the case. Proteolytic activation of F0 involves the sequential action of two enzymes, the host protease that cleaves at the carboxyl side of an arginine residue, and a host carboxypeptidase that removes the basic residues. The *Paramyxoviridae* can be divided into two groups: those that have F proteins with multibasic residues at the cleavage site and those with F proteins that have a single basic residue at the cleavage site (Table 12.5). Cleavage of F proteins containing multibasic residues at the cleavage site occurs intracellularly during transport of the protein through the *trans*-Golgi network.

Furin is a cellular protease localized to the *trans*-Golgi network, and its sequence specificity for cleavage is R-X-K/R-R. The available evidence suggests that furin, a subtilisin-like endoprotease, is the (or one of the) protease(s) that cleaves most F proteins intracellularly (Ref.[420]; reviewed in Ref.[275]).

Paramyxoviruses that have F proteins with single basic residues in the cleavage site (e.g., SeV) are not usually cleaved when grown in tissue culture, and, thus, only a single cycle of growth is obtained. However, the F0 precursor that is expressed at the cell surface and incorporated into released virions can be cleavage activated by the addition of exogenous protease,[519] leading to multiple rounds of replication. Purification of a protease from the allantoic fluid of embryonated chicken eggs has indicated that the endoprotease responsible for SeV activation is homologous to the blood clotting factor Xa, a member of the prothrombin family.[183,186] A protease with similar substrate specificity is secreted from Clara cells of the bronchial epithelium in rats and mice, and this enzyme is probably responsible for activating paramyxoviruses in the respiratory tract. For NDV, the nature of the cleavage site correlates with virulence of the virus. Those strains with multibasic residues in the F0 cleavage site are virulent strains and readily disseminate through the host, whereas strains with F0 molecules having single basic residues are avirulent and tend to be restricted to the respiratory tracts where the necessary secreted protease can be found.[388]

A variation on the cleavage theme is found with HeV because its F protein does not contain a multibasic cleavage site. HeV F is cleaved in expressing cells at the sequence HDLVDGVK ,[105] but the K residue is not essential for cleavage.[368] In the search for the cleavage enzyme, it was found that inhibition of cathepsin L blocks cleavage,[423] suggesting cleavage occurs in the endocytic pathway.[133,363]

Other Envelope Proteins

The *Rubulavirinae* such as PIV-5 and MuV and the Jeilongvirus paramyxoviruses contain a small gene located between F and HN designated SH.[1,214,215,308] The PIV-5 SH protein is a 44-residue, type II integral membrane protein that is expressed at the plasma membrane and is packaged in virions. The MuV SH protein is a 57-residue integral membrane protein orientated in the opposite direction from the PIV-5 SH protein with a C-terminal cytoplasmic domain.[151,580] Due to the variability in sequence among different strains of MuV, the *SH* gene sequence has been used as marker to identify MuV isolates.[579] PIV-5 lacking SH (rSV5deltaSH) grows as well as wild-type in tissue culture cells, but the virus is attenuated *in vivo*.[205] rSV5deltaSH induces apoptosis in L929 and MDCK cells (but not in HeLa cells) through a tumor necrosis factor alpha (TNFα)-mediated extrinsic apoptotic pathway.[206,314] *In vivo* virus attenuation and a comparable TNFα-mediated effect on pathogenesis were more recently reported for Jeilongviruses engineered to lack SH.[1] While the *SH* gene has been found in all strains of MuV, expression of the SH protein is also not required for MuV replication in tissue culture,[580] and in the Enders strain of MuV, a monocistronic mRNA encoding SH is not found. MuV SH may have a similar role as PIV-5 and *Jeilongvirus* SH.[635]

TM protein, the fourth integral membrane protein of members of the *Jeilongvirus* genus, has been found in association with F and G in biochemical assays and was shown to stimulate cell-to-cell fusion activity in cell culture. However, TM was dispensable for growth of recombinant viruses in tissue culture.[308]

STAGES OF REPLICATION

General Aspects

Transient nuclear localization of the matrix protein has emerged as a recurring theme that may apply to all *Paramyxoviridae*, but all aspects of paramyxovirus genome transcription, replication, and virion assembly occur in the cytoplasm. A schematic overview of the paramyxovirus life cycle is provided in Figure 12.24, and an overview of transcription and replication is shown in Figure 12.25. In contrast to, for instance, the *Orthomyxoviridae*, paramyxovirus mRNA synthesis is insensitive to DNA-intercalating drugs such as actinomycin D (reviewed in Ref.[84]), and the *Paramyxoviridae* can replicate in enucleated cells.[450] In cell culture, single cycle growth curves are generally of 14 to 30 hours' duration, but virulent strains of NDV can complete a replication cycle in as little as 10 hours. The effect of viral replication on host macromolecular synthesis is quite variable, ranging from almost complete shutoff late in infection for NDV to no obvious effect in PIV-5–infected cells.

TABLE 12.5 Amino acid sequences upstream of the F protein cleavage site of some *Paramyxoviridae*	
SeV	G-V-*P*-Q-S–R↓
HPIV-1	D-N-P-Q-S–R↓
HPIV-3	D-P-**R**-T-**K**-**R**↓
PIV-5	T-R-**R**-R-**R**-**R**↓
MuV	S-**R**-**R**-H-**K**-**R**↓
NDV (virulent strain)	G-R-**R**-Q-**R**↓ **K**
NDV (avirulent strain)	G-K-G G-Q-R↓ E-R-S
MeV	S-**R**-**R**-H-**K**-**R**↓
HeV	H-D-L-V-D-G-V-K↓

Consensus sequence for furin protease cleavage is R-X—R↓.[228]

(with superscript R above and subscript K below the X)

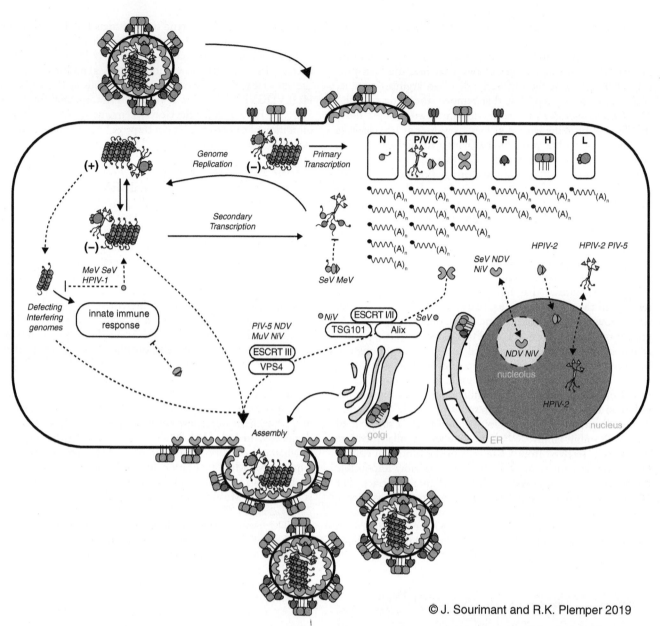

© J. Sourimant and R.K. Plemper 2019

FIGURE 12.24 Schematic representation of the paramyxovirus life cycle. Incoming virions (*top*) fuse with the plasma membrane to release the (−) sense nucleocapsid into the cytoplasm. Viral mRNAs are represented by *zigzag lines*; 5′ mRNA caps are shown as filled *black circles* and 3′ poly-A tails by (A)$_n$. The transcription gradient is symbolized. The relative abundance of genomic and antigenomic RNPs is not shown. Primary and secondary transcription, stages of genome replication, and the role of P proteins in forming P-L polymerase and RNA-free N^0–P complexes are shown. The V protein has been observed to be able to bind the nucleoprotein for MeV and SeV, although the N^0–V complex seems unable to form nucleocapsids. The newly synthesized RNPs are assembled into budding virions through interactions with the M protein. The polymerase can prematurely abort replication and release dsRNA structures that can trigger innate immune responses. The C proteins limit these phenomena by increasing polymerase fidelity, likely through direct binding to L. Nuclear transport of some M proteins and nucleolar localization are represented by a *dashed arrow*. Nuclear shuttling observed for some P proteins is represented by a *dashed arrow*. Integral envelope proteins are transported through the host cell secretory system. The proposed interactions of some M proteins with host cell ESCRT including TSG101 and Alix are represented by *dotted lines*, and recruitment of ESCRT-III and VPS4 to the budding site (*bottom*) proposed for some paramyxoviruses is shown. Release of progeny virions is thought to occur from the plasma membrane. (Images copyright © 2019 by Richard K. Plemper and Julien Sourimant.)

Virus Adsorption and Entry

It has long been accepted that molecules containing sialic acid (sialoglycoconjugates) serve as cell surface receptors for the respiroviruses and *Rubulavirinae*. This was originally based on the finding that sialidase of *Vibrio cholerae* acted as a "receptor-destroying enzyme" and protected the host cell from infection (reviewed in Ref.[340]). Sialic acid, the acyl derivative of neuraminic acid, is found on both glycoproteins and lipids (sialoglycolipids or gangliosides). For SeV, gangliosides function as both the attachment factor and the viral receptor.[341–343]

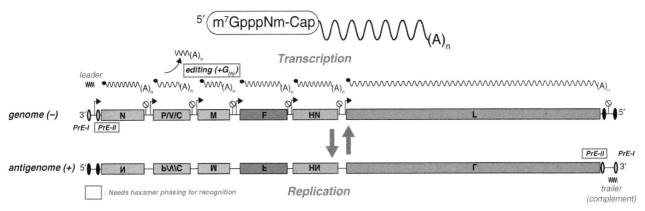

FIGURE 12.25 Schematic of the paramyxovirus negative-sense genomic and positive-sense antigenomic RNA. The locations of the 3′-end promoter element I (PrE-I) and internal promoter element II (PrE-II) are indicated by *blue oval circles*; color-coded areas refer to transcribed sections. The 5′ end of the antigenome contains sequences that are the compliment to the genomic RNA promoter and are partially complimentary to the 3′ region of the antigenomic RNA. Transcription products are represented with *black zigzag lines* above the schematic genome, mRNAs are represented with a 5′ cap (*black dot*) and a poly-A tail: (A)n. The 5′ cap of paramyxoviruses has a cap-1 structure typical of eukaryotic mRNAs. Guanine-7-methylation activity has been shown to be carried by the L protein of SeV, RPV and PPRV, and conserved motifs among mononegaviruses and MTases suggest that the L may also mediate ribose-2′O-methylation. PrE-II function and the P/V mRNA editing site are optimized for most paramyxoviruses based on their position relative to the RNP phase. (Images copyright © 2019 by Richard K. Plemper and Julien Sourimant.)

As described above, the morbilliviruses and henipaviruses bind to proteinaceous receptors displayed on the target cell surface; cognate receptors for the morbilliviruses are the host species–specific homologues of human SLAM and nectin-4, while the zoonotic henipaviruses use highly conserved ephrin-B2 and ephrin-B3 for cell entry. Upon adsorption of the virus to the cellular receptor, the viral envelope fuses with the target membrane at neutral pH conditions, ultimately resulting in release of the helical nucleocapsids into the cytoplasm.

Cryo-ET–based reconstructions of paramyxovirus particles have revealed numerous contacts between the M protein arrays and the nucleocapsid, necessitating the existence of a specific uncoating mechanism that allows separation of the nucleocapsid from the membrane-associated viral proteins after fusion of the envelope with cellular membranes. Unlike influenza virus, for instance, that encounters different environmental conditions at the assembly site (plasma membrane) and acidic uncoating compartment (endosomes), paramyxovirus self-assembly and disassembly are believed to both occur at the plasma membrane. Components of the host cell ESCRT machinery have been implicated in participating in the assembly and budding process, but the driving force for paramyxovirus uncoating is not known.

Viral RNA Synthesis

Paramyxoviruses control both the level and type of viral RNA that is synthesized at different stages of the infection cycle through the use of cis-acting RNA sequences and trans-acting proteins. The relationship between RNA sequences and the RdRP functions that they control is particularly complex because these cis-acting signals are only properly recognized when they are in the context of the nucleocapsid structure. Overlaying these RNA-encoded control elements are regulatory protein–protein interactions between components of the P-L polymerase and the RNP and trans-acting accessory

proteins that govern specific activities of the RdRP. Because all RdRP functionalities are essential for completion of the viral replication cycle, synthetic minigenome systems using cDNA-derived viral components that allow the targeted assessment of individual activities of the viral polymerase machinery have been instrumental for the functional analysis of both cis-acting sequences and regulatory protein interactions.

The paramyxovirus genome expression and replication cycle can be divided into three major phases. Early after infection, before the synthesis of appreciable amounts of viral proteins (or in the presence of inhibitors such as cycloheximide that block protein synthesis), the RdRP, in the primary transcription phase, transcribes viral mRNAs from the incoming virus genome (Fig. 12.24). When a sufficiently large N protein pool has been synthesized to ensure encapsidation of full-length RNA genome copies, the RdRP in processive replicase mode generates (+)-sense antigenomes, which serve as templates to synthesize (−)-sense progeny genomes. Both antigenomic and genomic RNAs must be encapsidated cotranscriptionally. The accumulating progeny genomes then serve as additional templates for viral mRNA synthesis in a secondary transcription phase, which yields the message required to produce the bulk of the viral proteins. Because of the increasing number of template genomes transcribed, viral mRNA copies present in the infected cell expand exponentially during secondary transcription, compared to linear accumulation during primary transcription.[460]

Paramyxovirus Promoter Organization

The paramyxovirus RdRP gains access to the viral genome and antigenome through single entry sites located at the 3′ ends. While the promoter present on antigenomes (hence termed the antigenomic promoter) only directs the synthesis of full-length genomic RNA, the promoter on genome RNA (termed the genomic promoter) is responsible for the generation of both mRNAs and antigenomes. Genomic RNA is present in higher copy numbers than antigenomic RNA in infected cells,[299] which was originally thought to reflect greater strength of the antigenomic than the genomic promoter. Using C protein–deficient recombinant SeV, however, it has more recently been demonstrated that the genomic promoter is in fact stronger than the antigenomic.[240] The greater relative abundance of genomic RNA is attributed rather to the C protein, which can interact with the L protein and regulate polymerase activity at the promoter.[189,223,239,240] The promoters of all paramyxoviruses have a bipartite organization, in which the first of two discontinuous promoter elements (PrE-I) is located at the 3′ end of the RNA strand and the second (PrE-II) between positions 73 and 96, depending on the virus,[217,339,365,381,587,618,619] placing the PrE-II sequence within the *N* or *L* gene for the genomic and antigenomic promoter, respectively (Fig. 12.26A). PrE-I sequences are highly conserved within the family, while the PrE-IIs feature three-time repetitions of one of two simple motifs, either (CNNNNN)$_3$ or (NNNNGC)$_3$.[217,339,365,381,587,618,619] Additional elements located between antigenomic PrE-I and PrE-II in PIV-5 (bases 51–66) and HPIV-3 (bases 13–55) are believed to act as nonessential enhancer of replication.[217,267]

As discussed above, precisely six nucleotides interact with each N protein protomer, and the phase of interaction determines the orientation of each base toward the outside or the nucleocapsid core.[64,193] Furthermore, each turn of the helical nucleocapsid assembly comprises on average approximately 12 to 13 N protein protomers. Mapping of the promoter elements onto the nucleocapsid structure has revealed that bases forming key sequence motifs are placed in phase positions facing outward and that the relative distance of the two PrEs relative to each other posits them on the same face of the helix in immediate proximity of each other (Fig. 12.26A).[126,365,381,587,617,618] It is believed that the RdRP complex recognizes both promoter elements in conjunction, initiating loading onto the template RNA and allowing identification of the transcription start site. The correct initial positioning of the paramyxovirus polymerase appears to be independent of the 3′ end of the RNA itself, since relocation of the SeV bipartite promoter to an internal position did not abolish bioactivity, provided relative phase of the PrEs and distance to each other remained intact.[617] Experimental support for this promoter model comes from the observations that paramyxovirus promoter activity is governed by three factors: (a) the RNA sequence of promoter motifs, (b) the relative distance between the PrEs, and (c) the position of promoter motifs relative to the hexamer phase imprinted by N encapsidation of the RNA.

Specifically, mutational analyses of the PIV-5 and SeV antigenomic promoters have demonstrated that deletions or insertions in the RNA segment located between the promoter elements prevented RNA replication.[381,587] Furthermore, it was demonstrated that the overall length of a paramyxovirus N–RNA complex can affect the efficiency of RNA replication.[64] This RNA chain-length requirement was termed the "rule of six," which entails that efficient replication of a paramyxovirus genomic or antigenomic RNA will only occur when the total number of nucleotides in the RNA is an even multiple of six. However, there is large variability in the stringency to which various groups of paramyxoviruses adhere to the rule of six requirements. RNA replication of SeV, all morbilliviruses, and the henipaviruses is strictly dependent on adherence to the rule of six. In contrast, the efficiency of PIV-5, NDV, and HPIV-3

RNA replication is boosted if genome lengths adhere to the rule of six, but this is not a stringent requirement.[144,339,383] It is currently believed that the rule of six reflects less a need for precise genome encapsidation without overhanging terminal nucleotides[617] but rather arises from imprinting the correct hexamer phase on the RNA,[449] orienting key bases of the promoter sequence outward and thereby recognizable by the polymerase complex (Fig. 12.26B).[277,300] Correct phase positioning is considered to be a prerequisite for efficient RNA editing in the *P* gene.[277,300] For HPIV-2, it has been demonstrated that a glutamine residue at position 202 of the N protein functions as a gatekeeper for PrE-II–dependent RdRP initiation.[349] Gln202 is the only residue in the RNA-binding groove that directly contacts a nucleotide base and not the backbone in the N–RNA assembly and apparently ensures that only genomes imprinted with the correct hexameric phase of the mRNA editing site are replicated.

It should be noted that RNA synthesis can be promoted *in vitro* from an unencapsidated PrE-I,[253] suggesting that successful RdRP initiation on encapsidated template relies on (a) recognition of the promoter elements on the nucleocapsid and (b) direct contact of the unencapsidated PrE-I element by the polymerase. Since *in vivo* only N-encapsidated viral RNA can serve as template for paramyxovirus RNA synthesis, promoter binding by the incoming P-L polymerase complex must be followed by displacing of the N capsid and threading of the locally exposed RNA strand into the template channel of the RdRP complex. As discussed before, the viral RNA is positioned in the RNP assembly in the groove that is created by the parallel alignment of the NTD and CTD folding domains of neighboring N protomers. Comparison of PIV-5 N assemblies[6] with free NiV N[641] and direct comparisons of PIV-5[4] and MeV[192] N with N[0] drove the hypothesis that RNA release may result from deep-seated local conformational changes upon P-L binding that entail opening of the RNA groove through an outward rotation of the CTD.[6] Alternatively, it was suggested based on the overlay of a cryo-EM reconstruction of MuV nucleocapsids with the PIV-5 N crystal structure that P-L contacts with a loop–helix domain located adjacent to the central groove may be sufficient to unveil the sequestered RNA through a local conformational change, bypassing the need for major rearrangements of the tightly assembled N protein core.[536] While the precise molecular mechanism of local RNA release from the nucleocapsid remains unknown, the N protein core—stabilized by extensive side-to-side interactions between the protomers—is considered to be routed over the surface of the RdRP while the locally unveiled RNA passes through the RdRP complex, followed by re-encapsidation as the template RNA emerges from the template channel.[277]

RdRP Initiation

Different initiation mechanisms of RNA synthesis have been identified for paramyxoviruses compared to the pneumoviruses. Two distinct initiation sites, +3 for transcription and +1 for replication, have been proposed for RSV, the archetype of the pneumovirus family,[406,601] although initiation at +3 likely represents the default and +1 may result from nontemplated preloading of the polymerase with a dinucleotide.[107,404,405] Paramyxovirus polymerase initiation sites have not been fully mapped yet, but several lines of evidence support templated initiation at +1 position[159]: (a) RdRPs preferentially initiate

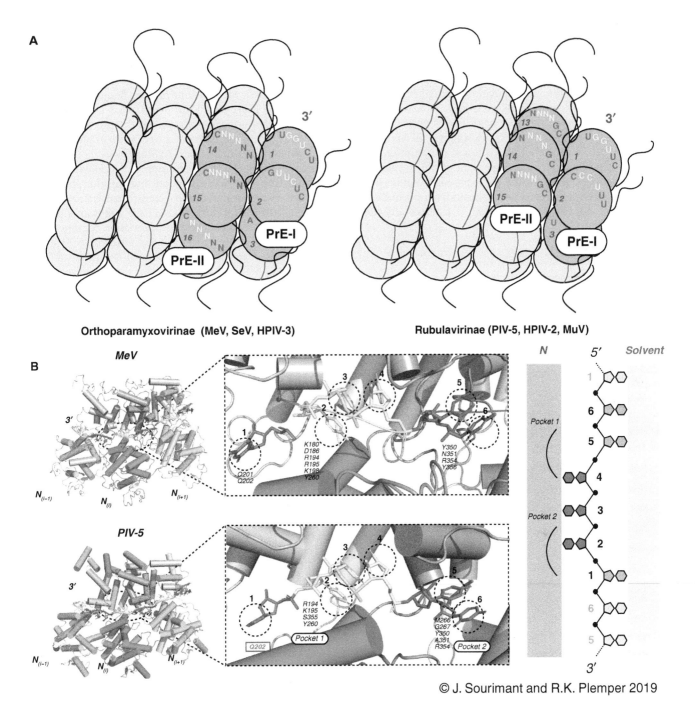

© J. Sourimant and R.K. Plemper 2019

FIGURE 12.26 Nucleocapsid structure, hexamer phasing of nucleotide sequences, and the bipartite replication promoters of the ***Paramyxoviridae***. **A:** Left-handed helix models of the SeV (*left*) and PIV-5 (*right*) nucleocapsid assemblies. Single N protein protomers (*gray spheres with black tail*) bind precisely six nucleotides, 13 N subunits per helix turn. Numbers refer to the position of each N subunit from the RNA 3′ end. The N protomers bound to the PrE-I and PrE-II elements are colored in *blue*. Both PrE-I and PrE-II of the bipartite replication promoter are found on the same face of the helix. Bases oriented toward the solvent are colored in *yellow*, while bases oriented toward the nucleoprotein are represented in *red*. Note that for the internal PrE-II element, essential C residues are located in the first position of each hexamer for SeV, whereas GC residues are located in the fifth and sixth positions in the case of PIV-5. **B:** Cartoon representations of the structure of three successive protomers of the RNA-bound Ncore structures of MeV (*top left*) (PDB ID: 4UFT) and PIV-5 (*bottom left*) (PDBank ID: 4XJN). N-terminal domains are shown in *blue*, C-terminal domains in salmon. The central protomers (N$_i$) are colored with increased saturation; RNAs are shown as stick representations. Bases oriented toward the solvent are colored in *yellow*, while bases oriented toward the nucleoprotein are shown in *red*. *Center*: Magnification of the N–RNA interaction, circling and numbering the six bases defining a hexamer phase from 3′ to 5′. N residues defining the two RNA-binding pockets in PIV-5 RNPs and equivalents in MeV RNPs are marked. The residue Q202 of the *Orthorubulavirus* genus is the only residue demonstrated to directly interact with an RNA base. *Right*: 2D representation of the relative base orientation in a hexamer phase. The six bases bound to each protomer are numbered 3′ to 5′. The nucleoprotein surface is represented in *purple*; solvent is shown in *blue*. *Gray* bases are encapsidated by a preceding or subsequent N protomer. (Images copyright © 2019 by Richard K. Plemper and Julien Sourimant.)

with purine (thus opposite a pyrimidine base),[409] but paramyxovirus promoters contain purines (G residues) at positions +2, +3, and in some cases—for instance, the *Ferlaviruses*—+4 (Fig. 12.27); (b) extension of primers representing SeV promoters did not reveal product populations derived from internal initiation sites[610]; and (c) unlike the experience with RSV polymerase, for instance, the amount of free N protein available is inversely correlated to transcription activity of MeV and SeV RdRP,[113,460] consistent with initiation of transcription and replication at position +1 by a single pool of polymerases. A current model of paramyxovirus RNA synthesis initiation proposes that polymerase alignment with the uridine tract in PrE-I drives initiation opposite the +1 position,[159] in all cases starting with pppApC.[406]

A *Paramyxoviridae 3′ genomic nucleotides*

Avulavirinae
Orthoavulavirus   NDV   3′   UGGUUUGUCUCUUAG

Metaavulavirus   APMV-2   3′   UGGUUUUGUUCCUUAU

Paraavulavirus   APMV-3   3′   UGAUUUGUCUUUUAA

Rubulavirinae
Orthorubulavirus   MuV   3′   UGGUUCCCCUUUUAC

Metarubulavirus   MenV   3′   UGGUUCCCCUUUUAG

Orthoparamyxovirinae
Respirovirus   HPIV-1   3′   UGGUUUGUUCUCCUU

Aquaparamyxovirus   ASPMV   3′   UGGUUUGUUCUUCCU

Ferlavirus   FdLV   3′   UGGGUUGUUCCCCUU

Henipavirus   HeV   3′   UGGCUUGUUCCCCUU

Jeilongvirus   BeiV   3′   UGGUUUGUUUCUACA

Narmovirus   NarV   3′   UGGUGUGUUUCCACC

Morbillivirus   MeV   3′   UGGUUUGUUUCAACC

Salemvirus   SalV   3′   UGGUUUGUUCUGUUA

Metaparamyxovirinae
Synodonvirus   WTLPV   3′   UAUCCCAUAUUAUAA

B *Pneumoviridae 3′ genomic nucleotides*

Orthopneumovirus   HRSV   3′   UGCGCUUUUUUACGC

Metapneumovirus   HMPV   3′   UGCGCUUUUUUUGCG

▨ : pyrimidine   ▨ : purine

FIGURE 12.27 Selected 3′ termini sequences (nucleotides 1–15) of the *Paramyxoviridae* and related *Pneumoviridae*.
A: Representative sequences from each genus of the *Paramyxoviridae*. The first three nucleotides are overlayed with *blue* for pyrimidines or *green* for purines; uracil bases are shown in *red*. Viruses of most *Paramyxoviridae* subfamilies but the *Synodonvirus* genus initiate with UGG (predominant) or UGA (pyrimidine–purine–pyrimidine), followed by uracil repeats. The newly proposed *Synodonvirus* WTLPV does not follow this pattern, but its first three nucleotides UAU (pyrimidine–purine–pyrimidine) are reminiscent of the *Pneumoviridae* 3′ termini, and the uracil-rich region is less defined. **B:** 3′ termini sequences (nucleotides 1–15) of selected viruses from members of the *Pneumoviridae* family. Color-coding as in **(A)**. Characteristic are 3′ UGCGC (pyrimidine–purine–pyrimidine–purine–pyrimidine) initiation sequences, followed by uracil repeats.

Initiation of *de novo* RNA synthesis typically involves an aromatic residue in a priming loop that interacts with the incoming first ribonucleotide.[14,60,593] While the paramyxovirus priming loop is not yet fully defined due to lack of high-resolution native structural information, homology models of paramyxovirus L proteins based on the VSV L reconstruction have highlighted aromatic residues on the predicted priming loop[159] that, albeit not fully conserved in all paramyxoviruses, appear homologous to a critical tryptophan in the VSV priming loop[311,414] (Fig. 12.28). Transition of the polymerase complex from RNA synthesis initiation to elongation must entail significant reorganization of the reconstructed L structure, creating exit channels for both the template and transcript RNA strands. Support for a structural reorganization of mononegavirales polymerases at the transition from initiation to elongation comes from mechanistic studies with small-molecule inhibitors of the related RSV RNA polymerase that did not prevent initiation and extension by up to two nucleotides but blocked subsequent RNA elongation.[104,407] Resistance sites for one of these compounds were mapped to the L connector domain linking the polymerase subunit to the methyltransferase (MTase) and C-terminal domains. Mutations in the SeV L capping and MTase domains have furthermore been identified that are distant from the catalytic site for phosphodiester bond formation and do not affect L protein steady-state levels but prevent RNA synthesis.[99,160,382] Although not experimentally validated yet, these data suggest that capping, MTase, and C-terminal domains relocate relative to the RdRP core domain of the polymerase complex, allowing egress of the nascent strand.

mRNA Synthesis

Following initiation of RNA synthesis at the 3′ promoter, the paramyxovirus polymerase generates a nontranslated short RNA copy of the leader (*le*) region of the viral genome. It is believed that encapsidation of this leader RNA, which depends on availability of free N⁰–P complexes, serves as an important determinant for the switch of the paramyxovirus RdRP into replicase mode. If left unencapsidated, the leader RNA is typically released before the polymerase complex has reached the end of the *le* region[175,224,285,304,601,610] and the RdRP scans the template for the first gene-start (GS) signal, which in all paramyxoviruses is that of the *N* gene. Once the GS is located, RNA synthesis is reinitiated *de novo*.[601,610] All GS sequences in the genome resemble the genomic promoter, and initiation of mRNA synthesis is consistently with a purine (ATP),[406] suggesting a conserved underlying principle governing polymerase contact with the promoter and the GS and incoming ATP. In contrast to original initiation at +1 position, however, the scanning polymerase complex is preloaded with template RNA, requiring the presence of a fully formed exit channel and thus reducing the scope of conformational rearrangements at the switch from initiation to elongation. Nascent mRNA strands are expected to be released from the exit channel in proximity to the capping domain, enabling efficient capping and methylation (Fig. 12.29). Lack of capping results in the release of abortive RNA transcripts from VSV and RSV RdRPs of less than 40 or 50 nucleotides in length, respectively,[320,410,562] and a similar mechanism may prevent efficient elongation of uncapped paramyxovirus pre-mRNAs. SeV MTase expressed in isolation has been demonstrated to be able to methylate capped mRNAs in trans,[416] which is consistent with successful

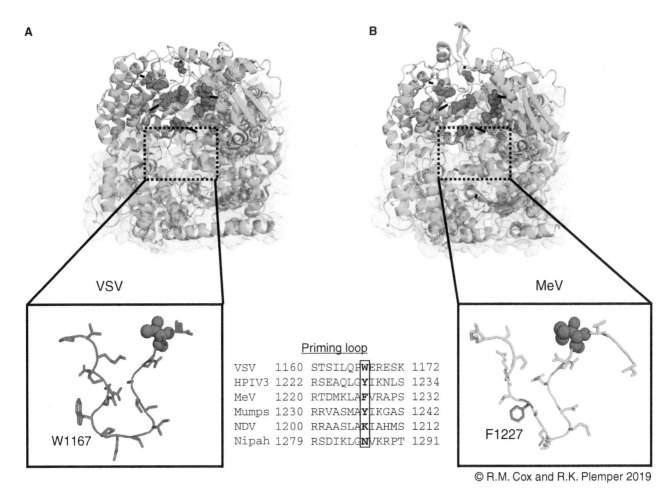

FIGURE 12.28 VSV and MeV RdRP priming loops. *Top*: 3D structural model of the RdRP (*cyan*) and PRNTase (*green*) domains of VSV L (PDB ID: 5A22)[311] **(A)**. Conserved motifs in the PRNTase domain are highlighted by *red spheres*. **B**: Corresponding domains in an MeV L homology model are shown in equivalent orientation. *Bottom inserts*: VSV L residue W1167 located in a priming loop facing the polymerase catalytic center is instrumental for RNA synthesis.[397,414] A homologous aromatic residue (F1227) in the predicted MeV L priming loop is highlighted. Sequence alignments of selected priming loop structures are shown, but presence of an aromatic residue is not fully conserved. Sequence alignments were performed using Clustal Omega,[543] the MeV homology model was generated using the PHYRE2 homology modeling server.[268] (Images copyright © 2019 by Richard K. Plemper and Robert M. Cox.)

transcomplementation of distinct mutations in the N-terminal and C-terminal domains of SeV L, respectively,[550] and suggests that MTase recognizes a specific RNA sequence for activity.

Starting with the intersection between the *N* and *P* gene, all paramyxovirus gene junctions comprise three distinct segments: a GE region at the 3′ end of the upstream gene, an IG region between the two genes that is normally not transcribed, and a gene-start (GS) region signaling reinitiation of transcription of the subsequent gene (Table 12.3). Located downstream of the stop codon of each viral gene, the GE sections are 10 to 13 nucleotides long and signal the advancing transcriptase complex to terminate RNA synthesis and add a poly-A tail at a stretch of four to seven uridine residues, the U tract. The resulting approximately 300- to 400-nucleotide–long poly-A tails are nontemplated, however, and are considered to be generated through reiterative backsliding of the polymerase complex in the U tract region,[277] followed by release of the newly synthesized *bona fide* mRNA molecule through an unknown trigger. Backsliding entails slippage of the nascent strand relative to the template RNA within the RdRP active site, although the

molecular mechanism enabling this movement has not yet been elucidated. Shortening the length of the unstructured C-terminal Ntail domains or relocation of the P-binding MoRE domain from Ntail into Ncore has lowered the efficiency of GE signal recognition and instead caused the synthesis of multicistronic mRNAs with increased frequency.[102,594] These results suggest that the unstructured Ntail sections located upstream of the MoRE may allow structural flexibility between the P-L complex and the RNP template that enables efficient backsliding. In addition to protein–protein interactions between P-L and the N protein chain, GE sequences determine the frequency of readthrough transcription. Although generally infrequent, polymerases of HPIV-1 types 1 to 3, MeV, and PIV-5 generate bicistronic mRNAs most often at the M-F junction, where approximately 50% to 80% of the mRNA can be locked into M-F readthrough products.[42,71,481,559] This high readthrough frequency is a consequence of insertions[559] or substitutions[481] at the M GE, which modify termination efficiency. Conceivably, some paramyxoviruses experience a heightened selective pressure to increase transcriptase access to the more 3′ distal genes

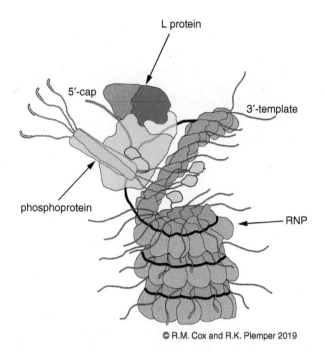

L protein

5'-cap

3'-template

phosphoprotein

RNP

© R.M. Cox and R.K. Plemper 2019

FIGURE 12.29 Model of the paramyxovirus transcriptase complex. The encapsidated viral genome serves as the template for the RdRP. The P protein acts as a bridge between the L polymerase and the RNP template, harboring binding sites for both the N and L proteins. The polymerase engages the template from the 3′ end of the viral genome, routing the N protein chain over the surface of the RdRP after local release of the encapsidated RNA. Nascent mRNAs emerge from a proposed exit channel, located in close proximity to the capping domain. (Images copyright © 2019 by Richard K. Plemper and Robert M. Cox.)

(e.g., attachment protein and L), or frequent M-F readthrough may present a mechanism to selectively reduce F protein expression, since polycistronic paramyxovirus mRNAs do not contain internal ribosomal entry sites and the F ORF locked into a bicistronic M-F transcript would presumably not be translated.[260,481] F protein down-regulation has been demonstrated to be critically linked to virulence of some paramyxoviruses.[9]

After termination of transcription, the RdRP complex advances through the IG region, scanning for the next downstream GS site.[454] Paramyxovirus IG regions minimally consist of a conserved trinucleotide segment, but many are highly variable in length and sequence (Table 12.3).[290] In fact, paramyxoviruses can be divided based on the degree of variability of the GE and IG sequences. For instance, these regions are highly conserved in SeV, HPIV-1, and HPIV-3.[279] Each SeV GE sequence consists of a 3′-AUUCU$_5$-5′ motif, and the IG region is 3′-GAA-5′ (except the HN-L junction, which is 3′-GGG-5′). In contrast, the GE and IG regions of HPIV-2, MuV, and PIV-5 are highly diverse, providing an additional level of transcriptional control of individual viral genes.[199,482] Since the viral polymerase complex initiates exclusively at the 3′ leader promoter and is unable to mount the RNA template at internal GS sites, the template RNA must remain threaded through the template channel as the transcriptase scans the IG, displacing the N protein scaffold as the complexes advance. Despite this local separation of template RNA and N protein chain, some paramyxoviruses require correct positioning of the GS site

relative to the encapsidation phase, suggesting that reinitiation of mRNA synthesis of at least some paramyxovirus transcriptases appears to be governed by both the RNA sequence and signals from the N protein.[277] Once the next downstream GS has been identified, mRNA synthesis reinitiates as described for the *N* gene GS, and this sequential "stop–start" mechanism of mRNA synthesis continues across the viral genome in a 3′ to 5′ direction. However, the frequency of reinitiation is not perfect, some RdRP complexes may advance along the template nonproductively or prematurely detach from the template RNA while negotiating an IG region, and the occasional readthrough transcription renders downstream ORFs locked in polycistronic mRNAs inaccessible to translation, resulting in a gradient of functional mRNA abundance that is inversely correlated to distance from the genome 3′ end, with functional N mRNAs being found in far higher abundance than L mRNAs.[72]

P Gene mRNA Editing

mRNA editing, the pseudotemplated addition of nucleotides altering the ORF, is a mechanism to expand the coding capacity of a gene that for paramyxoviruses was first identified for PIV-5.[444,596] It is now known that most paramyxovirus *P* genes contain a functional editing site within the coding region of the *P* gene (Fig. 12.8). As described above, in addition to a faithful (unedited) mRNA, transcription across the *P/V/C* gene yields edited versions that contain variable numbers of inserted G residues. The number of G insertions can differ for each virus group and mirrors their requirements for mRNAs that encode the individual P/V/W/I/D proteins (Fig. 12.8). Mechanistically, mRNA editing is believed to be achieved through controlled cotranscriptional polymerase stuttering and backsliding relative to the RNA template[203,608] that is triggered by the sequence of the editing site and in principle is reminiscent of the stuttering and backsliding employed to generate poly-A tails. The efficiency of G insertion by the stuttering polymerase is furthermore influenced by the position of the editing site relative to the N-bound hexameric phase,[242] providing another example for control of RdRP activity by a combination of RNA sequence and N protein phase imprinted on the template.

Genome Replication

Replication of the paramyxovirus genetic information occurs through generation of single-stranded, N-encapsidated antigenome copies that serve as template for the synthesis of progeny genomic RNA. Antigenomes do not code for any known functional ORF or template mRNAs. However, the synthesis and release of a short SeV trailer complement have been shown to antagonize stress granule formation and apoptosis through specific interaction with cellular TIAR.[243] If protein biosynthesis is pharmaceutically blocked in infected cells, viral mRNA synthesis continues normally, but antigenome and genome synthesis are both aborted rapidly. This observation underscores that active protein synthesis is essential to sustain RdRP in replicase mode, in which the polymerase ignores all GE regions, polyadenylation signals, and editing sites and generates exact, full-length copies of the viral genomic or antigenomic RNA, respectively.[190,353,610] Nascent transcripts of the replicase complex must be encapsidated cotranscriptionally[190] to generate bioactive antigenomes and genomes, mandating a continued supply of unassembled N proteins that are provided in the form of N⁰–P complexes (approximately 2,600 N monomers are required per full-length RNA copy).[40] This coupling of genome assembly and synthesis establishes a self-regulatory system for controlling the relative levels of viral transcription and replication. As encapsidation of the leader RNA is critical for the switch of the RdRP complex into replicase mode, early during the growth cycle, when N⁰–P complexes are limiting, leader RNA remains unencapsidated. The RdRP then acts predominantly in transcriptase mode, increasing the intracellular level of viral proteins until a sufficiently deep N⁰–P pool has been generated. Similarly, the 3′ promoter of the antigenome directs synthesis of a short trailer RNA (also called [−] leader). Cotranscriptional encapsidation of this trailer RNA again serves as trigger for commitment of the polymerase to become fully processive and synthesize encapsidated minus-strand genomes. As shown in Figure 12.24, the progeny genomes can serve three distinct functions: they template the bulk of viral mRNA that is generated during secondary transcription; they can serve as template for additional antigenomes; and they can be incorporated into progeny virus particles during virion budding.

In vitro assembly of six-nucleotide RNA molecules with purified MeV N⁰–P complexes resulted in spontaneous release of P and encapsidation of the discrete RNAs into a nucleocapsid, provided the RNA sequence corresponded to the 5′ end of the viral genome.[364] This study indicated that the initiation of the encapsidation process is sequence-dependent and that formation of helical RNP assemblies is a function solely of the N protein chain, not of a continuous RNA strand. However, the subsequent efficient cotranscriptional encapsidation of nascent genomic and antigenomic RNA transcripts is sequence independent, suggesting an interaction between the free N⁰–P complexes and the P-L polymerase. Because there is no evidence for a direct interaction between L and N, the P protein presumably serves as a bridge facilitating both the P-L interaction with the RNP and, in case of P-L in replicase mode, the incoming N⁰–P molecules. Substitutions have been described that specifically inhibit SeV L-mediated replication but not transcription.[160,551] Mapped onto the VSV L structure, the majority of these mutations are located on the same face of L, potentially outlining residues that are involved in guiding the transfer of free N protein to the newly synthesized RNA for efficient encapsidation.[159] The paramyxovirus nonstructural proteins provide a second avenue to control replicase versus transcriptase function of the viral RdRP. SeV V is believed to sequester N protein in N⁰–V complexes, inhibiting RNA replication by reducing the pool of bioactive unassembled N.[226] As discussed above, engineered paramyxoviruses unable to express the nonstructural C protein are viable in cell culture but produce abortive dsRNA transcripts in high frequency, highlighting a role of the C protein in controlling, among others, replicase fidelity.

Virion Assembly and Release

Paramyxovirus virions are generated through a budding process that entails the formation of buds from sites on the plasma membrane where viral components have assembled, followed by pinching off of progeny particles. This assembly is believed to require coordinated localization of multiple but distinct virus components, including viral glycoproteins, which are transported to the plasma membrane through the secretory system, and soluble viral components such as the RNP. This coordination appears to be accomplished through a series of

protein–protein and protein–lipid interactions, many of which involve the viral matrix protein array that can interact with lipids, with the glycoproteins via their cytoplasmic tails, and with N proteins assembled in the RNPs. It furthermore appears to involve interactions between viral components and the host exocytotic machinery that allows bud formation and membrane fission. Paramyxoviruses with HN-type attachment proteins contain glycoproteins that lack sialic modification of their carbohydrate chains, and it is believed that the HN NA activity serves the same purpose as NA of influenza virus, to prevent self-binding and to prevent reattachment to the infected cell.

Assembly of the Nucleocapsid

Nucleocapsids assemble in the cytoplasm concomitant to RNA synthesis, through continuous encapsidation of the nascent genomic and antigenomic RNA copies by newly synthesized N proteins as the replicase complex advances. As discussed above, it is believed that specific interactions between the L protein and free N⁰–P complexes guide encapsidation. While this process ensures that only viral RNAs are efficiently encapsidated in infected cells, transient expression of N proteins in the absence of other viral components results in the spontaneous and random encapsidation of host RNAs into short nucleocapsid-like structures, suggesting that encapsidation can occur independent of specific RNA sequence elements,[97,153,524,558,568] although as discussed above RNA sequence can greatly influence efficiency of the process.[364] However, encapsidation is only initiated *de novo* during synthesis of the terminal 3′ leader RNA (and 3′ trailer RNA for antigenome templates), since once in transcriptase mode, reinitiation of RNA synthesis by the polymerase at downstream GS regions does not randomly prompt unproductive encapsidation of nascent mRNAs. To ensure that a new replication cycle can be started after infection, paramyxoviruses must package copies of the P-L polymerase complex, which are thought to associate with the helical RNP prior to particle assembly.[270] Packaging of one complete copy of the viral genome is sufficient for infectivity, but biochemical studies and particle reconstructions have revealed that paramyxoviruses can—in low frequency—incorporate multiple RNP copies in a single virion.[178,266,324,475] The RNP packaging efficiency is determined by RNP polarity, genome length,[98,278,375] and compatibility of the N and M proteins.

Virus Particle Assembly

Due to its ability to engage in multiple interprotein and protein–lipid contacts, the paramyxovirus M protein serves as the central virion assembly organizer. Matrix proteins are found stably attached to RNPs when purified from virions, they bind to lipid membranes both *in vitro* and in living cells, and they self-assemble into ordered structures as purified proteins *in vitro* and in virus-infected cells. As discussed above, specific, homotypic N and M interactions have been demonstrated for a range of paramyxoviruses spanning different subfamilies, and these interactions are thought to guide the RNP to the assembly sites at the plasma membrane where M arrays form.[98,245,266,525] However, live cell imaging studies with SeV and MeV outlined an active role also of the host cytoskeleton in RNP trafficking to the plasma membrane. Both SeV and MeV RNPs were found moving along microtubules in Rab11A transport vesicles.[75,392] In the case of MeV, virus budding from polarized cells specifically appears to require Rab11A-dependent transport, whereas this association is important for efficient SeV assembly independent of whether or not host cells are polarized. Both SeV and NDV M proteins have furthermore been shown to interact with actin,[177] and a candidate actin binding site was located in SeV M that, when mutated, affected particle production, suggesting a requirement for SeV M interaction with the cytoskeleton for efficient particle assembly.[581] Consistent with this observation, major actin cytoskeleton reorganizations have been described after infection of cells with MeV, MuV, or NDV,[156] and MeV budding in particular requires uninhibited actin cytoskeleton dynamics.[560] NiV M has been found in proteomics studies in complex with AP3B1,[451,570] the beta subunit of the host cell AP-3 complex that facilitates vesicular budding from Golgi membranes and protein sorting in the late Golgi and endosomes. Disruption of NiV and HeV M interaction with AP3B1 blocked efficient virion production, suggesting that *Henipavirus* M relies on AP-3–directed vesicular trafficking for sorting from internal host membranes to the plasma membrane.[570]

Reconstructions of cryopreserved paramyxovirus particles have revealed that, once located at the assembly sites, the viral RNPs are arranged with the membrane-associated M lattice in high order. In NDV particles, the RNP helix was found in sync with the M protein dimers, placing the 7-nm pitch of the helical RNP along the diagonal 7-nm repeat of the matrix array.[23] Similarly, tomograms of both budding and cell-free MeV virions showed the viral RNP in register with the matrix array, the average 7.8-nm pitch of the RNP helix matching the 7.8 nm subunit spacing of the MeV M lattice.[266] Alternatively reported wrapping of MeV RNP into membrane-detached helical M tubes[313] was rare and restricted to structurally compromised virions.[266] Rather than representing a *bona fide* MeV assembly intermediate, coating of the viral RNP by an M-derived external helical structure may therefore likely result from M lattice reorganization during particle purification for imaging.

Driving efficient assembly of the viral envelope, multiple lines of evidence support specific interactions between the M protein layer and the cytoplasmic tails of the paramyxovirus envelope glycoproteins: (a) the M protein of SeV has been shown to specifically engage membranes individually expressing the F and HN glycoproteins, which implies an interaction.[513,514] Engineered recombinant PIV-5 and MeV that lack glycoprotein cytoplasmic tails show a subcellular redistribution of the matrix protein,[69,521] and colocalization and mutational studies revealed an interaction between the NDV and MeV attachment and M proteins.[424,574] A recombinant SeV carrying an F protein mutant with altered cytoplasmic tail furthermore showed defects in particle assembly and viral subunit clustering at assembly sites, underscoring the importance of glycoprotein tail interactions with the M layer for coordinated virion formation.[154,563] (b) Coexpression of MeV or NiV M and envelope glycoproteins in polarized cells redirected intracellular sorting. While envelope glycoproteins expressed in isolation are targeted to basolateral membranes, the presence of apically sorted M proteins directed glycoproteins to the apical side,[293,331] consistent with apical budding of these viruses. (c) Cryo-ET reconstructions of budding MeV virions showed a coordinated two-layered fusion-M protein lattice at the budding site and in released particles (Fig. 12.30). In contrast, tomograms of NDV,[23] SeV,[324] and HPIV-3[191] particles did not reveal any appreciable organization of the fusion glycoprotein ectodomains,

although the MeV matrix array itself resembled that of NDV. The co-organized arrangement of the fusion glycoprotein in a 2D array with a subunit spacing of approximately 11 nm provided structural evidence that the viral M protein drives particle assembly. Despite the biochemical evidence supporting an interaction between MeV M and H protein cytoplasmic tail, however, no obvious organization of the viral attachment protein was appreciable in the tomograms of MeV,[266] even when recombinant MeV particles were analyzed that expressed elongated attachment proteins, harboring an extension of the helical stalk domain by 41 residues[48] to reduce local electron density in the envelope glycoprotein layer.

Additional experimental confirmation for the instrumental role of matrix in proper virion assembly came from the analysis of paramyxoviruses with defective M proteins. A temperature-sensitive SeV strain has been isolated that is defective in proper virion assembly at the nonpermissive temperature due to mutations in its *M* gene.[651] This M protein variant is unstable at the nonpermissive temperature, indicating that low abundance of M prevents efficient virion assembly. In subsequent studies, engineered MeV and NiV mutants were recovered through reverse genetics techniques that lacked a functional *M* gene entirely.[68,134] These engineered viruses showed a dramatic reduction in progeny titers, infectivity remained essentially cell-associated, and virions were less stable, all consistent with a severe virion assembly and budding defect in the absence of the M protein. Moreover, in model systems of persistent SeV infection in culture in which the normally lytic infection is converted to a persistent one using DI particles, this change from lytic to persistent infection correlates mainly with M protein instability and an absence of virion assembly.[498]

Paramyxovirus Budding

While particle assembly entails the induction of local membrane curvature and the concentration of virus components in the nascent vesicular structures, budding—the release of cell-free progeny virions—requires an energy-demanding membrane fission event to pinch off the particle from the host cell membrane. An extensive list of enveloped viruses has been demonstrated to recruit components of the host cell vesicularization pathways to complete this final step in the replication cycle, and many others are thought to also follow this strategy.[81] Major experimental insight into the budding process was gained from the analysis of VLP systems. VLPs are nonreplication competent membrane-wrapped vesicles that contain only a subset of the viral structural proteins expressed from cloned cDNAs but lack genetic information. This section will assess minimal protein composition and protein–protein interaction requirements for paramyxovirus budding based on VLPs and recombinant virions, followed by a discussion of a role of the host vesicularization machinery in paramyxovirus particle fission and the contribution of the lipid composition to bud zone selection.

VLP systems to identify viral proteins essential for budding

VLP systems have been established for a number of different paramyxoviruses and have revealed diverse, virus-specific protein requirements for budding. In the most basic scenario, expression of M proteins in isolation is sufficient for VLP formation, as has been described, for instance, for NDV and several

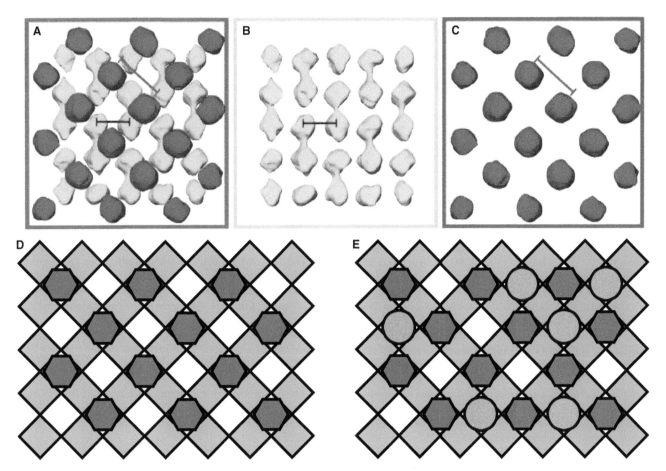

FIGURE 12.30 Symmetric arrangements of the F and M arrays observed in MeV particles. Cryoelectron tomography studies revealed a two-layered F–M lattice (EMDB entry: EMD-7591),[266] suggesting that M and F interact to facilitate efficient MeV assembly. **A–C:** Subtomogram averages of the MeV F–M lattice. The top layer of the averages reveals a regular array of F proteins (*dark blue*) **(A)**. The distance between F trimers is shown. Underlying the F layer, the M proteins (*cyan*) form a 2D array **(B)**. Distances between individual M dimers are shown. Overlay of the M and F lattices suggests coordination between the M and F protein arrangements **(C)**. **D:** Schematic of the F–M lattice displaying the organization of M (*blue*) and F (*red*) proteins above and below the viral envelope. **E:** The MeV H (*orange*) protein did not form regular arrays with the M or F proteins. However, the positions of the M and F proteins allow for variable distribution of H proteins above the M lattices. (Modified from Ke Z, Strauss JD, Hampton CM, et al. Promotion of virus assembly and organization by the measles virus matrix protein. *Nat Commun* 2018;9(1):1736, CC BY 4.0; http://creativecommons.org/licenses/by/4.0/)

Orthoparamyxovirinae such as SeV, HPIV-1, MeV, and NiV.[86,97,424,436,463,502,568,581] These studies confirmed that the M proteins of these viruses are inherently sufficient to interact with lipids, assemble into larger membrane-associated arrays that introduce local lipid curvature, and promote membrane fission. In contrast, PIV-5 M protein alone is unable to trigger efficient VLP formation, but coexpression with the N protein and either one of the viral glycoproteins induces budding with an efficiency approaching that observed in virus-infected cells.[524] M proteins of MuV, another member of the *Rubulavirinae* subfamily, also require coexpression with a viral glycoprotein for efficient budding, but a stimulatory effect is only observed when M is combined with the F and not the HN protein.[309,520,524] While the envelope glycoproteins of a number of *Orthoparamyxovirinae* subfamily members specifically engage the M protein layer as discussed above, these interactions do not impact virus budding in most cases. Accordingly, the ability to facilitate induction of local membrane curvature is a discrete function of some glycoproteins, rather than merely a consequence of M-mediated

local glycoprotein concentration in discrete plasma membrane regions. However, VLP budding after expression of the M protein alone, for instance, becomes more efficient when SeV M is coexpressed with the F glycoprotein.[581] Efficient transport of the F–M complexes to the cell surface for budding depends on the integrity of a five-residue TYTLE motif in the SeV F cytoplasmic tail.[154] F mutants lacking this motif remained capable of interacting with SeV M but were retained in the ER, thus preventing transport of F–M complexes to particle assembly sites at the plasma membrane.

The VLP-based insight into particle assembly requirements has been largely corroborated by studies with engineered viruses. Recombinant MeV expressing F proteins with truncated or modified cytoplasmic tails showed an increased cell-to-cell fusion rate of infected and uninfected, neighboring cells, indicating a redistribution of the envelope glycoproteins from bud sites to other plasma membrane regions.[69,370] Increased cell fusion activity is consistent with a shift of these recombinant viruses to a mode of virus propagation that is independent of budding. Recombinant PIV-5 was budding-impaired when the cytoplasmic tail was removed from the HN protein.[520] However, engineered PIV-5 similarly expressing tail-truncated F glycoprotein mutants remained capable of efficient replication and particle formation in cell culture.[624] Recombinant SeVs with F or HN cytoplasmic tail truncations reportedly showed an approximately 20- to 50-fold reduction in particle production,[164] and a follow-up study specifically confirmed the importance of the TYTLE motif in the F cytosolic tail for efficient production of progeny virions.[154]

Role of the host vesicularization machinery in membrane scission

Enveloped viruses of many different families are known to contain specific protein motifs that, when disrupted, cause defects late during budding, typically at the final stage of membrane fission.[81,122,173,187,250] These late (L) domains have been shown to engage host proteins of the cellular vacuolar protein sorting (VPS) pathway that is responsible for biogenesis of the multivesicular body (MVB). MVB formation is a key function of the cellular ESCRT machinery, a large network of cytoplasmic proteins that in its core consists of the ESCRT complexes I, II, and III, Alix and the VPS4 ATPase (reviews in Ref.[233,401,531,554]). Consistent with its central role in MVB formation, the hallmark of ESCRT activity is reverse-topology membrane scission, vesicularization away from the cytosol as opposed to, for instance, vesicle formation for intracellular vesicular transport or endocytotic pathways. Representing two distinct branches leading toward membrane fission, ESCRT-I, which forms a supercomplex with ESCRT-II when activated, and Alix recognize various protein interaction signals, triggering recruitment to cellular membranes and the induction of initial membrane curvature. Membrane-associated ESCRT-I–II or Alix then activates ESCRT-III polymerization in the nascent bud neck to high-energy dome-shaped spiral structures that cause membrane scission when VPS4 dependently resolved.[531] Because the unique reverse-topology of ESCRT-mediated vesicularization is equivalent to that of virus budding into internal cellular compartments or the extracellular environment, ESCRT pathway components are likely candidates for exploitation by enveloped viruses. Viral L domains serve as the molecular adapters required to engage the ESCRT machinery, and at least one of three types of canonical L domain motifs can be found in, for instance, retroviruses, filoviruses, flaviviruses, rhabdoviruses, and herpesviruses: P(T/S)AP, YP(x)$_n$L, and PPxY.[616] Each of these sequences resembles a host cell protein interaction motif. For instance, P(T/S)AP-type L domains mediate binding to TSG101,[173,347] an ESCRT-I subunit, YP(x)$_n$L recruits Alix[346,566,612,615] and the PPxY motif engages the WW domains of NEDD4 and similar HECT domain–containing E3 ubiquitin ligases.[200,269,599] Ubiquitin has been identified as the main pathway-specific signal in MVB biogenesis, and HIV Gag protein ubiquitination, for instance, promoting binding by TSG101 and Alix may be a major recruitment pathway for ESCRT components to bind Gag proteins.[539]

Although paramyxoviruses do not contain any of the canonical viral late domains, overexpression of a dominant-negative VPS4A ATPase mutant suppressed efficient budding of PIV-5,[523] NDV,[524] and MuV,[309] implicating the ESCRT machinery in particle release. Consistent with this observation, M proteins of these three paramyxoviruses contain a conserved, noncanonical FP(I/V)(I/V) motif that distantly resembles known viral L domains. In PIV-5, the core sequence of this motif is FPIV, which has been demonstrated to functionally compensate for lack of a PTAP L domain in budding HIV-1 VLPs.[523] The proline residue in this noncanonical motif emerged as critically important for bioactivity, since substitution in PIV-5 M protein resulted in poor VLP formation and failure of a corresponding recombinant PIV-5 to replicate normally. In addition, a screen for host factors interacting with PIV-5 M proteins identified AMOTL1, which itself contains three L/PPxY motifs and may in a novel host factor recruitment strategy serve as a bridge between a paramyxovirus M protein and NEDD4 ubiquitin ligases and the ESCRT machinery.[486] Consistent with a role of ubiquitination in engaging the PIV-5 budding machinery, formation of PIV-5 VLPs and virions was reduced by treatment of cells with the proteasome inhibitor MG-132,[523] which depletes the free ubiquitin pool in the cell by preventing recycling of ubiquitin after delivery of proteins marked for degradation to the proteasome.[613] Similar effects of proteasome inhibitor treatment on virus budding have been observed for retroviruses such as HIV-1[532] and Rous sarcoma virus,[445] which contain PTAP and PPxY late domains for budding.[523]

Despite this experimental support for a possible role of the ESCRT machinery in paramyxovirus budding, the evidence is mixed, and it remains unclear whether paramyxoviruses in general rely on ESCRT components for virion release. The noncanonical paramyxovirus L domain candidate is not universally conserved in the family, no physical interaction between paramyxovirus M proteins and the ESCRT machinery has been demonstrated, and NiV VLP formation, SeV virion budding,[182] and both MeV VLP and progeny virion formation are apparently unaffected by dominant-negative VPS4A.[437,510] Although deletion of candidate L domains in NiV M abrogated VLP budding, this effect appeared to be due to unexpected relocation of the mutated M proteins to the nucleus.[86,437] Since nuclear localization is naturally incompatible with budding from the plasma membrane, these studies did not provide clear evidence that the budding arrest was due to impaired interaction with ESCRT components. In contrast to the indifference of NiV VLP formation to dominant-negative VPS4A, however, budding of NiV virions from infected cells has subsequently been demonstrated to depend on VPS4 activity,[431] indicating that VLP and virion budding can be mechanistically distinct. Apparently, this discrepancy is due to the presence of the nonstructural NiV C protein in infected cells, which can act as a molecular bridge between NiV M and the ESCRT-I component Tsg101. While *Henipavirus* C proteins lack L domains, they show homology to the Vps28 subunit of the ESCRT-I complex, suggesting that all members of this genus may employ a molecular mimicry strategy to engage the ESCRT pathway for virion release.[627]

This probudding effect of the NiV C protein through recruitment of ESCRT components is reminiscent of the demonstrated ability of SeV C to engage ESCRT-III/VPS4 through the Alix branch of the pathway.[238,568] In addition, a putative L domain, YLDL, was identified in SeV M that was attributed to engage Alix independent of the C protein.[241] Despite these links to the ESCRT pathway, neither suppression of Alix nor expression of dominant-negative VPS4A abrogated budding of SeV virions.[182] Also, VLP formation and virion budding by all members of the *Morbillivirus* genus appear to be independent of ESCRT, but it remains unclear whether these viruses achieve membrane scission through noncanonical engagement of selected ESCRT components or through alternative fission mechanisms. As a structure-independent alternative strategy, local crowding of membrane-bound proteins at nascent fission sites has been proposed to generate sufficient steric pressure through lateral collisions to drive membrane vesiculation.[554]

Contribution of membrane subcompartments to paramyxovirus budding

Lipid molecules within the plasma membrane are not distributed homogenously in each leaflet of the bilayer but rather participate in lateral associations to form subcompartments within the membrane. These fluctuating nanoscale assemblies are enriched in sphingolipids, cholesterol, and a distinct set of membrane-bound proteins and can be stabilized into raft platforms by oligomerization.[544] Rafts were originally identified based on a simple assay, resistance to solubilization by some nonionic detergents such TX-100 at low temperature,[545] although these detergent-resistant membrane (DRM) extracts are unlikely to reflect the reality of a live cell.[67,131] Rafts are now recognized as highly dynamic structures that are involved, for instance, in cell signaling, assembly of many viruses,[24,66,495,576] and membrane trafficking. Rafts mediate lipid-based secretory sorting from the Golgi to the plasma membrane and in polarized cells locate predominantly to the apical site.[67,131] With the caveat of unclear physiological relevance of DRM extracts, a number of paramyxovirus proteins have been found enriched in detergent-insoluble membrane domains. For instance, MeV M, N, and F proteins[61,337,463,611]; SeV N, F, and HN proteins[182,512]; and NDV N, F, and HN proteins[136,287] are all selectively targeted to DRMs. MeV F targeting into rafts is apparently achieved through palmitoylation of two cysteine residues in the transmembrane domain of the protein.[24,61,66,495,576] Because functional MeV F and H protein complexes preassemble in the ER,[48,458] sorting of F into DRMs will pull H into the same subcompartment.[337] For some paramyxoviruses, lipid-mediated sorting may facilitate the local accumulation of envelope glycoproteins and matrix proteins, potentially resulting in the formation of viral assembly platforms.[329] However, engineered targeting of NiV M proteins into raft or nonraft domains did not affect VLP formation,[622] suggesting that NiV particle budding does not depend on a specific lipid environment.

Polarized budding from epithelial cells

Association of viral envelope components with raft microdomains could provide an attractive mechanistic explanation for preferential virion budding from the apical side in polarized epithelial cells, which has been reported for a number of paramyxoviruses including SeV, MeV, PIV-5, and NiV.[293,331,492] Quite counterintuitively, however, the glycoproteins of MeV and NiV are trafficked to basolateral membranes when expressed on their own, which is determined by tyrosine-dependent sorting signals[331,369,628] and in the case of MeV F appears to override F targeting into DRM domains. These observations underscore that intrinsic trafficking signals of the envelope glycoproteins do not control the location of virion budding for these viruses. Rather, coexpression of the M protein as experienced in infected cells induces rerouting of the glycoproteins to the apical bud zones,[293,391,628] although no direct intracellular

contacts between these M proteins and glycoproteins have been demonstrated yet.

Despite this mechanistic ambiguity, preferential apical virion budding and basolateral glycoprotein targeting are considered to be important contributors to viral pathogenesis. Budding from the apical surface could favor restriction of the infection to the epithelial cell layer, whereas budding from the basolateral surface allows viral access to underlying tissue and could favor development of a systemic infection. Consistent with this view, standard SeV and PIV-5 both produce localized infections of the respiratory tract *in vivo*, whereas a SeV mutant strain (F1-R) was described that is released bidirectionally and causes systemic infection.[590] In the case of MeV, redirecting the envelope glycoproteins away from basolateral membranes resulted in virus attenuation, coinciding with reduced lateral spread through cell-to-cell fusion in the respiratory epithelium.[371] The identification of SLAM and nectin-4 as cellular receptors for MeV has provided a solution to the conundrum of preferred apical release and efficient systemic dissemination of MeV. Mediated through SLAM-dependent cell entry, incoming MeV is considered to most likely initially infect respiratory macrophages and dendritic cells, using them as vehicle for homing to draining mediastinal lymph nodes where first centers of virus replication are established.[118,362] Subsequently, primary viremia ensues that is carried by circulating, SLAM-positive lymphocytes. Infected lymphocytes and dendritic cells in the epithelial submucosa are considered to then transmit the virus late during infection to epithelial cells displaying nectin-4 on the basolateral side.[166,328] This infection of nectin-4–positive respiratory epithelial cells sets the stage for apical release into the mucus layer lining the lumen of the respiratory tract, enabling airborne viral transmission in aerosols through coughing and sneezing.

PARAMYXOVIRUS ACCESSORY GENES AND THEIR INTERFERENCE WITH THE CELLULAR ANTIVIRAL RESPONSE

Type I IFNs form a group of the most important antiviral cytokines that can be major determinants of tropism, pathogenesis, and viral dissemination.[108] As shown in Figure 12.31, the cellular IFN response involves two general phases: the induction of IFN synthesis in a primary transcriptional phase and signaling through IFN signaling pathways to activate in a positive feedback loop a secondary transcriptional phase of IFNs and greater than 300 ISGs, at least 51 of which directly contribute to host defense.[301,357] A large body of work has emerged on the role of paramyxovirus accessory proteins in counteracting the host cell IFN pathways at the level of both the induction of IFN synthesis and IFN-mediated signaling.[95,218,433] Albeit through different specific interactions, predominantly the paramyxovirus V/W proteins interfere with the cellular sensing pathways that trigger type I IFN transcription and IFN signaling, while C proteins can modulate the antiviral response by reducing the production of virus-specific signals that are recognized by these host cell sensors.

Antagonists of Interferon Synthesis

Providing the first line of defense against viruses and other microbial pathogens, the type I IFN response is triggered by

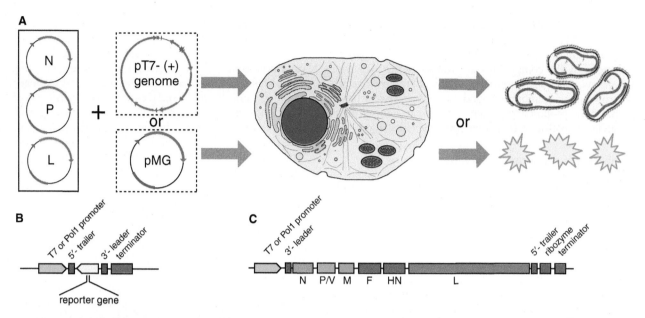

FIGURE 12.31 Minigenome reporter systems and recovery of recombinant paramyxoviruses from cloned cDNA. A and B: Paramyxovirus reverse genetics requires N, P, and L proteins provided *in trans* (plasmid-encoded or stable cell lines) and expression of viral genomic (minigenome) or antigenomic (minigenome, virus recovery) RNA, in most cases under the control of the T7 polymerase promoter. Ribozyme elements flanking the viral RNA ensure the generation of precise 3′ and 5′ ends. Minigenome reporter systems allow for quantitative assessment (i.e., luciferase reporter) of RdRP activity in the absence of viral replication. **C:** Schematic of a full-length viral genome expression cassette. Minigenomic or full-length viral RNAs are spontaneously encapsidated by the viral N protein, following RdRP-mediated transcription and amplification. (Images copyright © 2019 by Richard K. Plemper and Julien Sourimant.)

pattern recognition receptors (PRRs) that detect pathogen-associated molecular patterns (PAMPs). PAMPs can be by-products of virus infection, for instance, cytosolic dsRNA, other unique viral replication products, or capsid proteins, which all contain distinct features not normally present in the cell.[244] Major PRRs sensing RNA virus infections include the Toll-like receptor (TLR) family and the RIG-I–like receptor (RLR) RNA helicases. Sensing microbial RNAs, TLR3, TLR7, and TLR8 are associated with endosomal compartments,[7,212] while the RLR prototype retinoic acid–inducible gene I (RIG-I) and melanoma differentiation–associated gene 5 (MDA-5) represent the main cytosolic receptors responsible for the recognition of RNA.[234,516] Different downstream pathways and adapter proteins transduce the signal when these PRRs are triggered (Fig. 12.32), but most converge on activation of IFN regulatory factor (IRF) transcription factor family members IRF3 and IRF7 as the primary inducers of IFN-α and IFN-β expression.[582]

Results from transient transfection–based studies and the analysis of viruses that have been engineered to encode altered or deleted nonstructural protein genes have elucidated paramyxovirus antagonists of the cellular innate immune response. Most of these studies focused on pathogens of the *Morbillivirus*, *Respirovirus*, *Henipavirus*, and *Rubulavirus* genera. Common to all paramyxoviruses examined, the V proteins are instrumental for the suppression of type I IFN expression. Experimentally confirmed for many paramyxoviruses including, for instance, PIV-5, MeV, NiV, HPIV-2, and SeV,[10,83,116,336,376,425,479] the unique C-terminal zinc-finger domain of the V proteins associates with MDA-5 and also LGP2, the third member of the RLR family that lacks caspase recruitment domains (CARDs). Binding of paramyxovirus V to the helicase domain of MDA-5 has been shown to block association of MDA-5 with dsRNA, inhibiting MDA-5 association and signaling.[83] Originally, it

was thought that paramyxovirus V proteins are incapable of interacting with the RLR prototype, RIG-I, itself. Subsequent reports were mixed, however, and recent work has suggested binding of a number of different paramyxovirus V proteins including those derived from NiV, MeV, SeV, and parainfluenza viruses to the RIG-I regulatory protein TRIM25 and to RIG-I as a novel mechanism to block type I IFN expression.[511] Although LGP2 lacks CARDs, LGP2 overexpression has been shown to impair both MDA-5 and RIG-I signaling,[281,496] mice deficient in LGP2 were more susceptible to viral infection, and coexpression of MDA-5 and LGP2 led to synergistic signal transduction.[516,607] Consistent with the notion that LGP2 facilitates MDA-5 and RIG-I mediated recognition of viral RNAs, binding of MeV and PIV-5 V proteins to LGP2 blocked LGP2-dependent promotion of MDA5 signaling.[489,490]

In addition to directly blocking RLR sensing, paramyxoviruses interrupt the downstream signaling cascade to prevent IFN expression. Rubulavirus V proteins have been proposed to compete with IRF3 for phosphorylation by TBK1/IKKε kinase, preventing phosphorylation and nuclear translocation of the IRF3 transcription factor.[327] Similarly, MeV V protein has been shown to bind as a decoy substrate to IKKα kinase, competing with IRF7 for IKKα-mediated phosphorylation and thus blocking TLR7/9 signaling.[452] V proteins of MeV, HPIV-2, SeV, and NiV have furthermore been suggested to directly interact with IRF7, preventing its transcriptional activity.[274,452] MeV, SeV, and NDV V proteins have also been shown to directly associate with IRF3—in the case of SeV, V association takes place in the cytosol and prevents IRF3 nuclear translocation, while MeV V was proposed to associate with IRF3 after translocation—and block IRF3 transcription activation activity.[236] Likewise in the nucleus, NiV W but not V blocks IRF3-mediated IFN expression.[236,537]

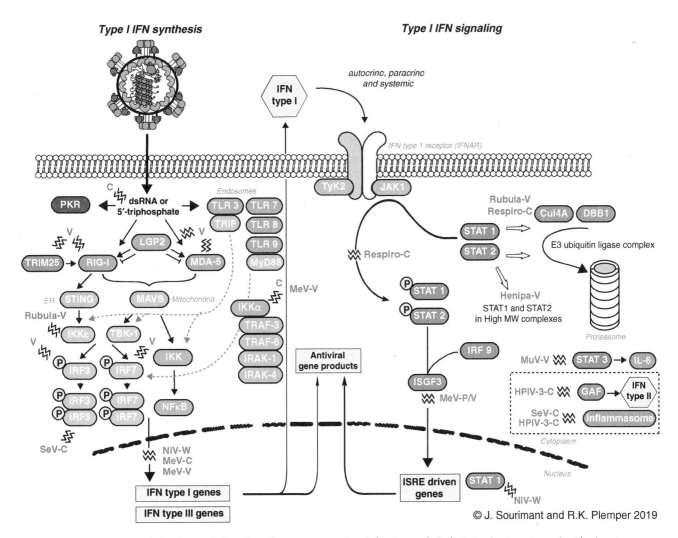

FIGURE 12.32 Type I IFN induction and signaling after paramyxovirus infection and viral strategies to antagonize the innate antiviral response. Schematic overview of induction of IFN synthesis (*left*) and autocrine or paracrine IFN signaling (*right*) after infection. Currently known broad and paramyxovirus genus- or subfamily-specific interference pathways are specified. (Images copyright © 2019 by Richard K. Plemper and Julien Sourimant.)

Rather than interfering with the PAMP sensing pathways, several paramyxovirus C proteins appear to lower signal intensity through a regulatory effect on polymerase fidelity. For instance, cells infected with C-deficient recombinant SeV, HPIV-1, or MeV strains accumulated increased amounts of dsRNAs,[35,453,577] which triggered the RLR and protein kinase R (PKR)-mediated response pathways, stimulating type I IFN expression.[35,577] In the case of MeV, short virus-derived DI-RNAs with duplex structures were found in cells infected with a C protein–defective, but not standard, MeV, confirming a dsRNA-mediated effect.[453] *Henipavirus* C proteins likewise regulate viral RNA synthesis, lowering the impetus for type I IFN expression.[322,323,348,549] Constituting a second mechanism by which *Morbillivirus* C proteins inhibit IFN induction, a NLS was identified in MeV C, and the presence of *Morbillivirus* C in the nucleus was found to be associated with a block in IFN-β expression downstream of IRF3 activation.[46,556] Also *Respirovirus* C has been found to directly inhibit type I IFN expression, in this case by targeting IRF3 translocation into the nucleus.[237] One study in addition suggested a C-mediated suppression of IRF7 phosphorylation and consequently TLR7/9

signaling through direct binding to, and inhibition of, IKKα by C proteins of SeV, MeV, and NiV.[642]

Antagonists of Interferon Signaling Pathways

Once virus-sensing host cell PRRs are triggered, the ensuing first wave of type I IFN can result in autocrine, paracrine, or systemic stimulation, activating multiple downstream signaling pathways through binding to the type I IFN receptor (IFNAR). The canonical response pathway involves formation of the signal transducer and activator of transcription 1 (STAT1)–STAT2–IRF9 signaling complex, also known as the IFN-stimulated gene factor 3 (ISGF3), which translocates to the nucleus and induces ISG expression through activation of IFN-stimulated response elements (ISREs) in gene promoters (Fig. 12.32).[357] ISGF3 formation is initiated by phosphorylation of STAT1 and STAT2 by the JAK kinases Tyk2 and Jak1. Major ISGs with effector activity against some or all negative-sense RNA viruses include, for instance, the myxovirus resistance (Mx) proteins, the IFN-induced protein with tetratricopeptide (IFIT) repeats and the IFN-inducible transmembrane (IFITM) families, members of the TRIM superfamily and the poly(ADP-ribose) polymerase (PARP) family, and the OAS/RNase L system.[108,526]

In addition to suppressing type I IFN synthesis, paramyxoviruses have developed a diverse range of strategies to interrupt IFN signaling that include the degradation of signaling pathway components and the sequestration of signaling complexes, and the V proteins again assume a central role in this activity. First demonstrated for PIV-5, rubulavirus V proteins directly induce the degradation of STAT proteins. PIV-5[12,132] and MuV V[283] both target STAT1 for degradation, while HPIV-2 V induces breakdown of STAT2.[427] Although STAT-specific, degradation requires the presence of both STAT1 and STAT2[428] and involves both the cysteine-rich C-terminal domain of V and residues located in the N-terminal section shared by P/V.[11,207,625] MuV V has furthermore been demonstrated to also induce STAT3 turnover, which results in an additional block in proinflammatory IL-6–mediated signaling.[605] Virulent MuV strains were found to bind STATs efficiently and limit the production of IL-6.[494,639] Mechanistically, these *Rubulavirinae* V proteins are thought to form a cytoplasmic V–dependent degradation complex that comprises STAT1, STAT2 and two components of a host cell E3 ubiquitin ligase, the UV-damaged DNA-binding protein DDB1, and the Cullin family of ubiquitin ligase subunit member Cullin 4A (Cul4A).[470,471,603] Assembly of this complex triggers polyubiquitination of the target protein, inducing its proteasomal degradation. PIV-5 V protein degradation of STAT1 occurs in human cells but not mouse cells, and PIV-5 growth in mouse cells is restricted.[132] However, efficient STAT1 degradation and higher PIV-5 replication levels can be restored in mouse cells engineered to express human STAT2.[426] Likewise, a single amino acid substitution in the PIV-5 V protein N-terminal domain is sufficient to allow targeted degradation of mouse STAT1 and block IFN signaling.[652] Thus, the ability to assemble specific STAT degradation complexes and disrupt IFN signaling may be a factor determining the host range of some paramyxoviruses such as PIV-5 and NDV,[426,429] which are restricted for growth in cells from particular species.

Rather than inducing breakdown of IFN signaling proteins, V proteins of a number of viruses of the *Orthoparamyxovirinae* subfamily have been shown to bind and sequester STATs in the cytosol, preventing shuttling into the nucleus and transcription activation. For instance, P/V proteins of MeV of the *Morbillivirus* genus target STAT1 through a tyrosine-based motif in the shared N-terminal domain[129,417,497] and STAT2 through nonconserved residues in the V protein C-terminal domain.[63,480,497] Binding prevents STAT protein nuclear import, and a recombinant MeV unable to target STAT1 specifically due to three point mutations in the shared N-terminal region of P/V was found to less efficiently control the proinflammatory response and experience reduced viremia titers in a rhesus monkey model of infection.[128] *Henipavirus* V proteins form high molecular weight aggregates with nonphosphorylated STAT1 and STAT2,[491] and a nuclear export signal in NiV V ensures localization in the cytosol.[488] In contrast, NiV W harbors a nuclear import signal in its short C-terminal unique region and forms nonfunctional complexes containing STAT1 in the nucleus.[87,538] Underscoring the importance of *Henipavirus* V and W for viral pathogenesis, the more recently identified low-pathogenic Cedar virus of the *Henipavirus* genus[344] does not express V or W, and Cedar virus P is unable to efficiently target STAT1 or STAT2 and therefore cannot effectively inhibit IFN signaling.[312]

C proteins of the respiroviruses, morbilliviruses, and henipaviruses have been proposed to interfere with IFN signaling, but in the case of *Morbillivirus* and *Henipavirus* C, these antisignaling effects were subsequently found to be minor.[162,322,323,348,394] In contrast, a number of studies have indicated that *Respirovirus* C proteins can interfere with IFN signaling pathways. HPIV-1 C proteins have been shown to bind STATs, prevent phosphorylation of STAT1 and STAT2, and retain STAT1 in perinuclear aggregates, preventing nuclear translocation.[530] SeV and HPIV-3 C proteins have been found to alter STAT phosphorylation patterns,[185] were detected as interacting partners with STAT1,[169,333,578] and could induce ubiquitination and degradation of STAT1 in some mouse cells.[171] HPIV-3 C protein has also been shown to inhibit type II IFN signaling by blocking the formation of the gamma interferon activation factor (GAF) complex, and an N-terminal region of 25 amino acids was found to be involved in mediating both STAT1- and GAF-dependent antisignaling effects.[338] A recent study furthermore implicated HPIV-3 C in counteracting inflammasome activation in macrophages following HPIV-3 infection.[540] Inflammasomes are cytosolic multiprotein complexes that combat microbial infections by regulating production of proinflammatory IL-1β and IL-18, controlling the immune response and pathogen clearance.[165,483] They can be activated by a number of different viruses including SeV.[256,280,430,541] While the SeV V protein was suggested to antagonize inflammasome activity,[280] in the case of HPIV-3, the C protein was found to specifically block assembly of the NLRP3/ASC inflammasome by interaction with, and promotion of proteasomal degradation of, the NLRP3 protein.[540] These observations underscore that the mechanisms by which the paramyxovirus C proteins interfere with the host antiviral response depend on both host cell type and virus species.

ENGINEERED PARAMYXOVIRUS MINIGENOMES AND RECOMBINANT VIRUSES: REVERSE GENETICS

The study of viruses has benefited greatly from the ability to specifically modify viral genomes and recover the corresponding recombinant viruses, a technique known as reverse genetics.[631] For RNA viruses, the first recovery of a virus from a cloned cDNA copy has been described for the positive-sense RNA bacteriophage Qβ,[585] and many more positive polarity RNA viruses were recovered subsequently following this strategy. Adaptation of this approach to negative-strand RNA viruses was challenging, however, since synthetic genomic RNA copies are noninfectious. Only protein-encapsidated negative-strand RNA virus genomes and antigenomes are biologically active, and exclusively, the viral polymerase machinery can productively interact with the RNPs. Instrumental for the development of *Mononegavirales* reverse genetics technology were shortened minigenome reporter systems, which minimally consist of a single reporter gene flanked by cDNA copies of the untranslated terminal regions of the viral genome (Fig. 12.32). Expressed under the control of a T7 RNA polymerase promoter and fused to a hepatitis delta virus–derived ribozyme to create precise 5′ and 3′ ends equivalent to those of genomic viral RNA, proof of concept was first established through successful replication of synthetic VSV-derived RNAs when plasmid-encoded VSV N, P, and L proteins were expressed in trans.[447]

Building on this strategy, rabies virus was the first infectious *Mononegavirales* to be recovered entirely from cloned cDNA,[528] followed several months later by VSV[298,633] and, as the first paramyxoviruses recovered, MeV and SeV.[172,474] In contrast to the first-generation minigenome reporter technology, which produced negative-strand RNAs, all of these initial full-length reverse genetics systems were engineered to express antigenomic, positive polarity RNA molecules (Fig. 12.32). Attempts to directly recover virions from direct expression of genomic RNAs were either unsuccessful or highly ineffective,[264] supposedly because simultaneous expression of negative polarity genomic RNA and positive polarity mRNAs in the same cell sets the stage for dsRNA formation through hybridization, triggering IFN-1 response pathways and preventing encapsidation.[528]

Although progress has been made to optimize the technology and many more paramyxoviruses have successfully been generated from cloned cDNAs (i.e., NDV,[493] NiV,[649] HeV,[345] CDV,[174] RPV,[21] MuV,[88] HPIV-1,[398] HPIV-2,[265] HPIV-3,[142,216] and PIV-5[208]), the frequency of virus recovery remains relatively low. Rate limiting remains the initial formation of bioactive antigenomes through inefficient, spontaneous encapsidation of the antigenomic RNA molecules expressed from the cloned full-length cDNAs by N protein provided in trans. Process improvements included the use of engineered cell lines stably expressing T7 polymerase[56] rather than the original superinfection of transfected cells with a recombinant vaccinia virus encoding T7 polymerase,[528] the use of helper plasmids encoding mammalian-cell codon-optimized versions of N, P, and L under the control of strong constitutive mammalian promoters, and the combination of a self-cleaving hammerhead ribozyme sequence preceding the viral antigenome RNA in combination with overexpression of plasmid-encoded codon-optimized T7 polymerase.[25] In particular, the production of RNA transcripts with precise 3' and 5' ends of the viral genomes through inclusion of ribozyme elements has increased rescue efficiency dramatically, advancing from approximately 1 per 10^6 to 10^7 to 1 per 10^2 to 10^3 transfected cells. Based on the design of T7 polymerase–independent reverse genetics systems for influenza virus, *Mononegavirales* minigenome technology has also been developed that employs the cellular RNA polymerase I (Pol I) promoter.[643] Naturally responsible for the synthesis of ribosomal RNAs in higher eukaryotes, Pol I–driven systems, when combined with helper plasmids under the control of constitutive mammalian RNA polymerase II promoters, provide superior flexibility in the choice of host cell type while bypassing the need for transforming an additional, T7 polymerase–encoding plasmid or superinfecting with a T7 polymerase–expressing helper virus. However, Pol I–mediated RNA synthesis in the nucleus is less suitable for the synthesis of full-length viral RNAs and may require codon optimization of viral coding regions, making this technology most useful for minigenome reporter systems.

As discussed throughout this chapter, recombinant paramyxovirus viruses have been instrumental in elucidating the role of individual viral proteins and protein subdomains in the viral life cycle, better understanding the molecular interplay between the replicating virus and the host cell, and identifying determinants of viral pathogenesis. Reporter paramyxoviruses expressing,

for instance, luciferases or fluorescent proteins from additional transcription units have elucidated host invasion pathways, increasingly in combination with noninvasive *in vivo* imaging technology. Reporter viruses have furthermore been game-changing for the identification and development of novel antiviral drug candidates through automated drug screening campaigns and the targeted engineering of next-generation vaccine candidates.

REFERENCES

1. Abraham M, Arroyo-Diaz NM, Li Z, et al. Role of small hydrophobic protein of J paramyxovirus in virulence. *J Virol* 2018;92(20).
2. Ader N, Brindley M, Avila M, et al. Mechanism for active membrane fusion triggering by morbillivirus attachment protein. *J Virol* 2013;87:314–326.
3. Ader-Ebert N, Khosravi M, Herren M, et al. Sequential conformational changes in the morbillivirus attachment protein initiate the membrane fusion process. *PLoS Pathog* 2015;11(5):e1004880.
4. Aggarwal M, Leser GP, Kors CA, et al. Structure of the paramyxovirus parainfluenza virus 5 nucleoprotein in complex with an amino-terminal peptide of the phosphoprotein. *J Virol* 2018;92(5).
5. Aguilar HC, Ataman ZA, Aspericueta V, et al. A novel receptor-induced activation site in the Nipah virus attachment glycoprotein (G) involved in triggering the fusion glycoprotein (F). *J Biol Chem* 2009;284:1628–1635.
6. Alayyoubi M, Leser GP, Kors CA, et al. Structure of the paramyxovirus parainfluenza virus 5 nucleoprotein-RNA complex. *Proc Natl Acad Sci U S A* 2015;112(14):E1792–E1799.
7. Alexopoulou L, Holt AC, Medzhitov R, et al. Recognition of double-stranded RNA and activation of NF-kappaB by Toll-like receptor 3. *Nature* 2001;413(6857):732–738.
8. Alkhatib G, Richardson C, Shen SH. Intracellular processing, glycosylation, and cell-surface expression of the measles virus fusion protein (F) encoded by a recombinant adenovirus. *Virology* 1990;175:262–270.
9. Anderson DE, von Messling V. Region between the canine distemper virus M and F genes modulates virulence by controlling fusion protein expression. *J Virol* 2008;82(21):10510–10518.
10. Andrejeva J, Childs KS, Young DF, et al. The V proteins of paramyxoviruses bind the IFN-inducible RNA helicase, mda-5, and inhibit its activation of the IFN-beta promoter. *Proc Natl Acad Sci U S A* 2004;101(49):17264–17269.
11. Andrejeva J, Poole E, Young DF, et al. The p127 subunit (DDB1) of the UV-DNA damage repair binding protein is essential for the targeted degradation of STAT1 by the V protein of the paramyxovirus simian virus 5. *J Virol* 2002;76:11379–11386.
12. Andrejeva J, Young DF, Goodbourn S, et al. Degradation of STAT1 and STAT2 by the V proteins of simian virus 5 and human parainfluenza virus type 2, respectively: consequences for virus replication in the presence of alpha/beta and gamma interferons. *J Virol* 2002;76:2159–2167.
13. Ansari MY, Singh PK, Rajagopalan D, et al. The large protein 'L' of Peste-des-petits-ruminants virus exhibits RNA triphosphatase activity, the first enzyme in mRNA capping pathway. *Virus Genes* 2019;55(1):68–75.
14. Appleby TC, Perry JK, Murakami E, et al. Viral replication. Structural basis for RNA replication by the hepatitis C virus polymerase. *Science* 2015;347(6223):771–775.
15. Audsley MD, Jans DA, Moseley GW. Nucleocytoplasmic trafficking of Nipah virus W protein involves multiple discrete interactions with the nuclear import and export machinery. *Biochem Biophys Res Commun* 2016;479(3):429–433.
16. Bachi T. Intramembrane structural differentiation in Sendai virus maturation. *Virology* 1980;106:41–49.
17. Bagai S, Lamb RA. Individual roles of N-linked oligosaccharide chains in intracellular transport of the paramyxovirus SV5 fusion protein. *Virology* 1995;209:250–256.
18. Baker KA, Dutch RE, Lamb RA, et al. Structural basis for paramyxovirus-mediated membrane fusion. *Mol Cell* 1999;3:309–319.
19. Bankamp B, Wilson J, Bellini WJ, et al. Identification of naturally occurring amino acid variations that affect the ability of the measles virus C protein to regulate genome replication and transcription. *Virology* 2005;336:120–129.
20. Barik S. The structure of the 5' terminal cap of the respiratory syncytial virus mRNA. *J Gen Virol* 1993;74(Pt 3):485–490.
21. Baron MD, Barrett T. Rescue of rinderpest virus from cloned cDNA. *J Virol* 1997;71:1265–1271.
22. Baron MD, Barrett T. Rinderpest viruses lacking the C and V proteins show specific defects in growth and transcription of viral RNAs. *J Virol* 2000;74:2603–2611.
23. Battisti AJ, Meng G, Winkler DC, et al. Structure and assembly of a paramyxovirus matrix protein. *Proc Natl Acad Sci U S A* 2012;109(35):13996–14000.
24. Bavari S, Bosio CM, Wiegand E, et al. Lipid raft microdomains: a gateway for compartmentalized trafficking of Ebola and Marburg viruses. *J Exp Med* 2002;195:593–602.
25. Beaty SM, Park A, Won ST, et al. Efficient and robust *Paramyxoviridae* reverse genetics systems. *mSphere* 2017;2(2).
26. Bellini WJ, Englund G, Rozenblatt S, et al. Measles virus P gene codes for two proteins. *J Virol* 1985;53:908–919.
27. Bhella D, Ralph A, Murphy LB, et al. Significant differences in nucleocapsid morphology within the *Paramyxoviridae*. *J Gen Virol* 2002;83:1831–1839.
28. Bhella D, Ralph A, Yeo RP. Conformational flexibility in recombinant measles virus nucleocapsids visualised by cryo-negative stain electron microscopy and real-space helical reconstruction. *J Mol Biol* 2004;340(2):319–331.
29. Blanchard L, Tarbouriech N, Blackledge M, et al. Structure and dynamics of the nucleocapsid-binding domain of the Sendai virus phosphoprotein in solution. *Virology* 2004;319:201–211.

30. Blocquel D, Habchi J, Gruet A, et al. Compaction and binding properties of the intrinsically disordered C-terminal domain of Henipavirus nucleoprotein as unveiled by deletion studies. *Mol Biosyst* 2012;8(1):392–410.
31. Bloyet LM, Brunel J, Dosnon M, et al. Modulation of re-initiation of measles virus transcription at intergenic regions by PXD to NTAIL binding strength. *PLoS Pathog* 2016;12(12):e1006058.
32. Bloyet LM, Welsch J, Enchery F, et al. HSP90 chaperoning in addition to phosphoprotein required for folding but not for supporting enzymatic activities of measles and Nipah virus L polymerases. *J Virol* 2016;90(15):6642–6656.
33. Bohn W, Rutter G, Hohenberg H, et al. Involvement of actin filaments in budding of measles virus: studies on cytoskeletons of infected cells. *Virology* 1986;149:91–106.
34. Bonaparte MI, Dimitrov AS, Bossart KN, et al. Ephrin-B2 ligand is a functional receptor for Hendra virus and Nipah virus. *Proc Natl Acad Sci U S A* 2005;102:10652–10657.
35. Boonyaratanakornkit J, Bartlett E, Schomacker H, et al. The C proteins of human parainfluenza virus type 1 limit double-stranded RNA accumulation that would otherwise trigger activation of MDA5 and protein kinase R. *J Virol* 2011;85:1495–1506.
36. Bose S, Banerjee AK. Beta-catenin associates with human parainfluenza virus type 3 ribonucleoprotein complex and activates transcription of viral genome RNA in vitro. *Gene Expr* 2004;11:241–249.
37. Bose S, Song AS, Jardetzky TS, et al. Fusion activation through attachment protein stalk domains indicates a conserved core mechanism of paramyxovirus entry into cells. *J Virol* 2014;88(8):3925–3941.
38. Bose S, Welch BD, Kors CA, et al. Structure and mutagenesis of the parainfluenza virus 5 hemagglutinin-neuraminidase stalk domain reveals a four-helix bundle and the role of the stalk in fusion promotion. *J Virol* 2011;85:12855–12866.
39. Bose S, Zokarkar A, Welch BD, et al. Fusion activation by a headless parainfluenza virus 5 hemagglutinin-neuraminidase stalk suggests a modular mechanism for triggering. *Proc Natl Acad Sci U S A* 2012;109:E2625–E2634.
40. Bourhis JM, Canard B, Longhi S. Structural disorder within the replicative complex of measles virus: functional implications. *Virology* 2006;344(1):94–110.
41. Bourhis JM, Receveur-Brechot V, Oglesbee M, et al. The intrinsically disordered C-terminal domain of the measles virus nucleoprotein interacts with the C-terminal domain of the phosphoprotein via two distinct sites and remains predominantly unfolded. *Protein Sci* 2005;14(8):1975–1992.
42. Bousse T, Matrosovich T, Portner A, et al. The long noncoding region of the human parainfluenza virus type 1 F gene contributes to the read-through transcription at the M-F gene junction. *J Virol* 2002;76:8244–8251.
43. Bousse TL, Taylor G, Krishnamurthy S, et al. Biological significance of the second receptor binding site of Newcastle disease virus hemagglutinin-neuraminidase protein. *J Virol* 2004;78:13351–13355.
44. Bowden TA, Crispin M, Harvey DJ, et al. Crystal structure and carbohydrate analysis of Nipah virus attachment glycoprotein: a template for antiviral and vaccine design. *J Virol* 2008;82:11628–11636.
45. Bowman MC, Smallwood S, Moyer SA. Dissection of individual functions of the Sendai virus phosphoprotein in transcription. *J Virol* 1999;73:6474–6483.
46. Boxer EL, Nanda SK, Baron MD. The rinderpest virus non-structural C protein blocks the induction of type 1 interferon. *Virology* 2009;385(1):134–142.
47. Braun MR, Deflube LR, Noton SL, et al. RNA elongation by respiratory syncytial virus polymerase is calibrated by conserved region V. *PLoS Pathog* 2017;13(12):e1006803.
48. Brindley MA, Chaudhury S, Plemper RK. Measles virus glycoprotein complexes preassemble intracellularly and relax during transport to the cell surface in preparation for fusion. *J Virol* 2015;89:1230–1241.
49. Brindley MA, Plattet P, Plemper RK. Efficient replication of a paramyxovirus independent of full zippering of the fusion protein six-helix bundle domain. *Proc Natl Acad Sci U S A* 2014,111(36).E3795–E3804.
50. Brindley MA, Plemper RK. Blue native PAGE and biomolecular complementation reveal a tetrameric or higher-order oligomer organization of the physiological measles virus attachment protein H. *J Virol* 2010;84:12174–12184.
51. Brindley MA, Suter R, Schestak I, et al. A stabilized headless measles virus attachment protein stalk efficiently triggers membrane fusion. *J Virol* 2013;87:11693–11703.
52. Brindley MA, Takeda M, Plattet P, et al. Triggering the measles virus membrane fusion machinery. *Proc Natl Acad Sci U S A* 2012;109:E3018–E3027.
53. Brown DD, Rima BK, Allen IV, et al. Rational attenuation of a morbillivirus by modulating the activity of the RNA-dependent RNA polymerase. *J Virol* 2005;79:14330–14338.
54. Bruhn JF, Barnett KC, Bibby J, et al. Crystal structure of the nipah virus phosphoprotein tetramerization domain. *J Virol* 2014;88(1):758–762.
55. Buchholz UJ, Biacchesi S, Pham QN, et al. Deletion of M2 gene open reading frames 1 and 2 of human metapneumovirus: effects on RNA synthesis, attenuation, and immunogenicity. *J Virol* 2005;79:6588–6597.
56. Buchholz UJ, Finke S, Conzelmann KK. Generation of bovine respiratory syncytial virus (BRSV) from cDNA: BRSV NS2 is not essential for virus replication in tissue culture, and the human RSV leader region acts as a functional BRSV genome promoter. *J Virol* 1999;73:251–259.
57. Buchholz CJ, Retzler C, Homann HE, et al. The carboxy-terminal domain of Sendai virus nucleocapsid protein is involved in complex formation between phosphoprotein and nucleocapsid-like particles. *Virology* 1994;204:770–776.
58. Buschiazzo A, Amaya MF, Cremona ML, et al. The crystal structure and mode of action of trans-sialidase, a key enzyme in Trypanosoma cruzi pathogenesis. *Mol Cell* 2002;10:757–768.
59. Buschiazzo A, Tavares GA, Campetella O, et al. Structural basis of sialyltransferase activity in trypanosomal sialidases. *EMBO J* 2000;19:16–24.
60. Butcher SJ, Grimes JM, Makeyev EV, et al. A mechanism for initiating RNA-dependent RNA polymerization. *Nature* 2001;410(6825):235–240.
61. Caballero M, Carabana J, Ortego J, et al. Measles virus fusion protein is palmitoylated on transmembrane-intracytoplasmic cysteine residues which participate in cell fusion. *J Virol* 1998;72(10):8198–8204.
62. Caffrey M, Cai M, Kaufman J, et al. Three-dimensional solution structure of the 44 kDa ectodomain of SIV gp41. *EMBO J* 1998;17:4572–4584.
63. Caignard G, Bourai M, Jacob Y; Infection MpIMAP, et al. Inhibition of IFN-alpha/beta signaling by two discrete peptides within measles virus V protein that specifically bind STAT1 and STAT2. *Virology* 2009;383(1):112–120.
64. Calain P, Roux L. The rule of six, a basic feature for efficient replication of Sendai virus defective interfering RNA. *J Virol* 1993;67:4822–4830.
65. Calder LJ, Gonzalez-Reyes L, Garcia-Barreno B, et al. Electron microscopy of the human respiratory syncytial virus fusion protein and complexes that it forms with monoclonal antibodies. *Virology* 2000;271:122–131.
66. Campbell SM, Crowe SM, Mak J. Lipid rafts and HIV-1: from viral entry to assembly of progeny virions. *J Clin Virol* 2001;22:217–227.
67. Cao X, Surma MA, Simons K. Polarized sorting and trafficking in epithelial cells. *Cell Res* 2012;22(5):793–805.
68. Cathomen T, Mrkic B, Spehner D, et al. A matrix-less measles virus is infectious and elicits extensive cell fusion: consequences for propagation in the brain. *EMBO J* 1998;17:3899–3908.
69. Cathomen T, Naim HY, Cattaneo R. Measles viruses with altered envelope protein cytoplasmic tails gain cell fusion competence. *J Virol* 1998;72:1224–1234.
70. Cattaneo R, Kaelin K, Baezko K, et al. Measles virus editing provides an additional cysteine-rich protein. *Cell* 1989;56:759–764.
71. Cattaneo R, Rebmann G, Baczko K, et al. Altered ratios of measles virus transcripts in diseased human brains. *Virology* 1987;160:523–526.
72. Cattaneo R, Rebmann G, Schmid A, et al. Altered transcription of a defective measles virus genome derived from a diseased human brain. *EMBO J* 1987;6:681–688.
73. Cattaneo R, Rose JK. Cell fusion by the envelope glycoproteins of persistent measles viruses which caused lethal human brain disease. *J Virol* 1993;67:1493–1502.
74. Cevik B, Holmes DE, Vrotsos E, et al. The phosphoprotein (P) and L binding sites reside in the N-terminus of the L subunit of the measles virus RNA polymerase. *Virology* 2004;327:297–306.
75. Chambers R, Takimoto T. Trafficking of Sendai virus nucleocapsids is mediated by intracellular vesicles. *PLoS One* 2010;5(6):e10994.
76. Chan DC, Fass D, Berger JM, et al. Core structure of gp41 from the HIV envelope glycoprotein. *Cell* 1997;89:263–273.
77. Chan YP, Lu M, Dutta S, et al. Biochemical, conformational and immunogenic analysis of soluble trimeric forms of henipavirus fusion glycoproteins. *J Virol* 2012;86:11457–11471.
78. Chattopadhyay A, Shaila MS. Rinderpest virus RNA polymerase subunits: mapping of mutual interacting domains on the large protein L and phosphoprotein P. *Virus Genes* 2004;28:169–178.
79. Chen M, Cortay JC, Gerlier D. Measles virus protein interactions in yeast: new findings and caveats. *Virus Res* 2003;98(2):123–129.
80. Chen L, Gorman JJ, McKimm-Breschkin J, et al. The structure of the fusion glycoprotein of Newcastle disease virus suggests a novel paradigm for the molecular mechanism of membrane fusion. *Structure* 2001;9:255–266.
81. Chen BJ, Lamb RA. Mechanisms for enveloped virus budding: can some viruses do without an ESCRT? *Virology* 2008;372:221–232.
82. Chernomordik LV, Kozlov MM. Protein-lipid interplay in fusion and fission of biological membranes. *Annu Rev Biochem* 2003;72:175–207.
83. Childs KS, Andrejeva J, Randall RE, et al. Mechanism of mda-5 inhibition by paramyxovirus V proteins. *J Virol* 2009;83:1465–1473.
84. Choppin PW, Compans RW. Reproduction of paramyxoviruses. In: Fraenkel-Conrat H, Wagner RR, eds. *Comprehensive Virology*. Vol. 4. New York: Plenum Press; 1975:95–178.
85. Choudhary SK, Malur AG, Huo Y, et al. Characterization of the oligomerization domain of the phosphoprotein of human parainfluenza virus type 3. *Virology* 2002;302(2):373–382.
86. Ciancanelli MJ, Basler CF. Mutation of YMYL in the Nipah virus matrix protein abrogates budding and alters subcellular localization. *J Virol* 2006;80(24):12070–12078.
87. Ciancanelli MJ, Volchkova VA, Shaw ML, et al. Nipah virus sequesters inactive STAT1 in the nucleus via a P gene-encoded mechanism. *J Virol* 2009;83(16):7828–7841.
88. Clarke DK, Sidhu MS, Johnson JE, et al. Rescue of mumps virus from cDNA. *J Virol* 2000;74:4831–4838.
89. Colman PM, Lawrence MC. The structural biology of type I viral membrane fusion. *Nat Rev Mol Cell Biol* 2003;4:309–319.
90. Colonno RJ, Stone HO. Newcastle disease virus mRNA lacks 2′-O-methylated nucleotides. *Nature* 1976;261(5561):611–614.
91. Communie G, Crepin T, Maurin D, et al. Structure of the tetramerization domain of measles virus phosphoprotein. *J Virol* 2013;87(12):7166–7169.
92. Communie G, Habchi J, Yabukarski F, et al. Atomic resolution description of the interaction between the nucleoprotein and phosphoprotein of Hendra virus. *PLoS Pathog* 2013;9(9):e1003631.
93. Compans RW, Choppin PW. Reproduction of myxoviruses. In: Fraenkel-Conrat H, Wagner RR, eds. *Comprehensive Virology*. Vol. IV New York: Plenum Press; 1975:179–252.
94. Connolly SA, Leser GP, Jardetzky TS, et al. Bimolecular complementation of paramyxovirus fusion and hemagglutinin-neuraminidase proteins enhances fusion: implications for the mechanism of fusion triggering. *J Virol* 2009;83:10857–10868.
95. Conzelmann KK. Transcriptional activation of alpha/beta interferon genes: interference by nonsegmented negative-strand RNA viruses. *J Virol* 2005;79:5241–5248.
96. Corey EA, Iorio RM. Mutations in the stalk of the measles virus hemagglutinin protein decrease fusion but do not interfere with virus-specific interaction with the homologous fusion protein. *J Virol* 2007;81:9900–9910.
97. Coronel EC, Murti KG, Takimoto T, et al. Human parainfluenza virus type 1 matrix and nucleoprotein genes transiently expressed in mammalian cells induce the release of virus-like particles containing nucleocapsid-like structures. *J Virol* 1999;73:7035–7038.
98. Coronel EC, Takimoto T, Murti KG, et al. Nucleocapsid incorporation into parainfluenza virus is regulated by specific interaction with matrix protein. *J Virol* 2001;75:1117–1123.
99. Cortese CK, Feller JA, Moyer SA. Mutations in domain V of the Sendai virus L polymerase protein uncouple transcription and replication and differentially affect replication in vitro and in vivo. *Virology* 2000;277(2):387–396.

100. Couturier M, Buccellato M, Costanzo S, et al. High affinity binding between Hsp70 and the C-terminal domain of the measles virus nucleoprotein requires an Hsp40 co-chaperone. *J Mol Recognit* 2010;23(3):301–315.

101. Cox R, Green TJ, Purushotham S, et al. Structural and functional characterization of the mumps virus phosphoprotein. *J Virol* 2013;87(13):7558–7568.

102. Cox RM, Krumm SA, Thakkar VD, et al. The structurally disordered paramyxovirus nucleocapsid protein tail domain is a regulator of the mRNA transcription gradient. *Sci Adv* 2017;3(2):e1602350.

103. Cox R, Pickar A, Qiu S, et al. Structural studies on the authentic mumps virus nucleocapsid showing uncoiling by the phosphoprotein. *Proc Natl Acad Sci U S A* 2014;111(42):15208–15213.

104. Cox RM, Toots M, Yoon JJ, et al. Development of an allosteric inhibitor class blocking RNA elongation by the respiratory syncytial virus polymerase complex. *J Biol Chem* 2018;293(43):16761–16777.

105. Craft WW Jr, Dutch RE. Sequence motif upstream of the Hendra virus fusion protein cleavage site is not sufficient to promote efficient proteolytic processing. *Virology* 2005;341:130–140.

106. Crennell S, Takimoto T, Portner A, et al. Crystal structure of the multifunctional paramyxovirus hemagglutinin-neuraminidase. *Nat Struct Biol* 2000;7:1068–1074.

107. Cressey TN, Noton SL, Nagendra K, et al. Mechanism for de novo initiation at two sites in the respiratory syncytial virus promoter. *Nucleic Acids Res* 2018;46(13):6785–6796.

108. Crosse KM, Monson EA, Beard MR, et al. Interferon-stimulated genes as enhancers of antiviral innate immune signaling. *J Innate Immun* 2018;10(2):85–93.

109. Curran J, Boeck R, Kolakofsky D. The Sendai virus P gene expresses both an essential protein and an inhibitor of RNA synthesis by shuffling modules via mRNA editing. *EMBO J* 1991;10:3079–3085.

110. Curran J, de Melo M, Moyer S, et al. Characterization of the Sendai virus V protein with an anti-peptide antiserum. *Virology* 1991;184:108–116.

111. Curran J, Homann H, Buchholz C, et al. The hypervariable C-terminal tail of the Sendai paramyxovirus nucleocapsid protein is required for template function but not for RNA encapsidation. *J Virol* 1993;67:4358–4364.

112. Curran J, Kolakofsky D. Ribosomal initiation from an ACG codon in the Sendai virus P/C mRNA. *EMBO J* 1988;7:245–251.

113. Curran J, Kolakofsky D. Nonsegmented negative-strand RNA virus RNA synthesis in vivo. *Virology* 2008;371(2):227–230.

114. Curran J, Marq JB, Kolakofsky D. An N-terminal domain of the Sendai paramyxovirus P protein acts as a chaperone for the NP protein during the nascent chain assembly step of genome replication. *J Virol* 1995;69:849–855.

115. Curran J, Pelet T, Kolakofsky D. An acidic activation-like domain of the Sendai virus P protein is required for RNA synthesis and encapsidation. *Virology* 1994;202:875–884.

116. Davis ME, Wang MK, Rennick LJ, et al. Antagonism of the phosphatase PP1 by the measles virus V protein is required for innate immune escape of MDA5. *Cell Host Microbe* 2014;16(1):19–30.

117. De BP, Gupta S, Banerjee AK. Cellular protein kinase C isoform zeta regulates human parainfluenza virus type 3 replication. *Proc Natl Acad Sci U S A* 1995;92:5204–5208.

118. de Swart RL, Ludlow M, de Witte L, et al. Predominant infection of CD150+ lymphocytes and dendritic cells during measles virus infection of macaques. *PLoS Pathog* 2007;3(11):e178.

119. Decroly E, Ferron F, Lescar J, et al. Conventional and unconventional mechanisms for capping viral mRNA. *Nat Rev Microbiol* 2011;10(1):51–65.

120. Delenda C, Hausmann S, Garcin D, et al. Normal cellular replication of Sendai virus without the trans-frame, nonstructural V protein. *Virology* 1997;228:55–62.

121. Delenda C, Taylor G, Hausmann S, et al. Sendai viruses with altered P, V, and W protein expression. *Virology* 1998;242:327–337.

122. Demirov DG, Ono A, Orenstein JM, et al. Overexpression of the N-terminal domain of TSG101 inhibits HIV-1 budding by blocking late domain function. *Proc Natl Acad Sci U S A* 2002;99:955–960.

123. Deng R, Wang Z, Glickman RL, et al. Glycosylation within an antigenic site on the HN glycoprotein of Newcastle disease virus interferes with its role in the promotion of membrane function. *Virology* 1994;204:17–26.

124. Deng R, Wang Z, Mahon PJ, et al. Mutations in the Newcastle disease virus hemagglutinin-neuraminidase protein that interfere with its ability to interact with the homologous F protein in the promotion of fusion. *Virology* 1999;253:43–54.

125. Deng R, Wang Z, Mirza AM, et al. Localization of a domain on the paramyxovirus attachment protein required for the promotion of cellular fusion by its homologous fusion protein spike. *Virology* 1995;209:457–469.

126. Desfosses A, Goret G, Farias Estrozi L, et al. Nucleoprotein-RNA orientation in the measles virus nucleocapsid by three-dimensional electron microscopy. *J Virol* 2011;85(3):1391–1395.

127. Devaux P, Hodge G, McChesney MB, et al. Attenuation of V- or C-defective measles viruses: infection control by the inflammatory and interferon responses of rhesus monkeys. *J Virol* 2008;82(11):5359–5367.

128. Devaux P, Hudacek AW, Hodge G, et al. A recombinant measles virus unable to antagonize STAT1 function cannot control inflammation and is attenuated in rhesus monkeys. *J Virol* 2011;85(1):348–356.

129. Devaux P, von Messling V, Songsungthong W, et al. Tyrosine 110 in the measles virus phosphoprotein is required to block STAT1 phosphorylation. *Virology* 2007;360:72–83.

130. Diallo A, Barrett T, Barbron M, et al. Cloning of the nucleocapsid protein gene of peste-des-petits-ruminants virus: relationship to other morbilliviruses. *J Gen Virol* 1994;75(Pt 1):233–237.

131. Diaz-Rohrer B, Levental KR, Levental I. Rafting through traffic: membrane domains in cellular logistics. *Biochim Biophys Acta* 2014;1838(12):3003–3013.

132. Didcock L, Young DF, Goodbourn S, et al. The V protein of simian virus 5 inhibits interferon signalling by targeting STAT1 for proteasome-mediated degradation. *J Virol* 1999;73:9928–9933.

133. Diederich S, Moll M, Klenk HD, et al. The Nipah virus fusion protein is cleaved within the endosomal compartment. *J Biol Chem* 2005;280:29899–29903.

134. Dietzel E, Kolesnikova L, Sawatsky B, et al. Nipah virus matrix protein influences fusogenicity and is essential for particle infectivity and stability. *J Virol* 2015;90(5):2514–2522.

135. Dochow M, Krumm SA, Crowe JE Jr, et al. Independent structural domains in paramyxovirus polymerase protein. *J Biol Chem* 2012;287(9):6878–6891.

136. Dolganiuc V, McGinnes L, Luna EJ, et al. Role of the cytoplasmic domain of the Newcastle disease virus fusion protein in association with lipid rafts. *J Virol* 2003;77:12968–12979.

137. Dorig RE, Marcil A, Chopra A, et al. The human CD46 molecule is a receptor for measles virus (Edmonston strain). *Cell* 1993;75:295–305.

138. Doyle J, Prussia A, White LK, et al. Two domains that control prefusion stability and transport competence of the measles virus fusion protein. *J Virol* 2006;80(3):1524–1536.

139. Duan Z, Chen J, Xu H, et al. The nucleolar phosphoprotein B23 targets Newcastle disease virus matrix protein to the nucleoli and facilitates viral replication. *Virology* 2014;452–453:212–222.

140. Duan Z, Hu Z, Zhu J, et al. Mutations in the FPIV motif of Newcastle disease virus matrix protein attenuate virus replication and reduce virus budding. *Arch Virol* 2014;159(7):1813–1819.

141. Duprex WP, Collins FM, Rima BK. Modulating the function of the measles virus RNA-dependent RNA polymerase by insertion of green fluorescent protein into the open reading frame. *J Virol* 2002;76:7322–7328.

142. Durbin AP, Hall SL, Siew JW, et al. Recovery of infectious human parainfluenza virus type 3 from cDNA. *Virology* 1997;235:323–332.

143. Durbin AP, McAuliffe JM, Collins PL, et al. Mutations in the C, D, and V open reading frames of human parainfluenza virus type 3 attenuate replication in rodents and primates. *Virology* 1999;261:319–330.

144. Durbin AP, Siew JW, Murphy BR, et al. Minimum protein requirements for transcription and RNA replication of a minigenome of human parainfluenza virus type 3 and evaluation of the rule of six. *Virology* 1997;234:74–83.

145. Dutch RE, Jardetzky TS, Lamb RA. Virus membrane fusion proteins: biological machines that undergo a metamorphosis. *Biosci Rep* 2000;20:597–612.

146. Earp LJ, Delos SE, Park HE, et al. The many mechanisms of viral membrane fusion proteins. *Curr Top Microbiol Immunol* 2005;285:25–66.

147. Eaton BT, Broder CC, Middleton D, et al. Hendra and Nipah viruses: different and dangerous. *Nat Rev Microbiol* 2006;4:23–35.

148. Ebata SN, Cote MJ, Kang CY, et al. The fusion and hemagglutinin-neuraminidase glycoproteins of human parainfluenza virus 3 are both required for fusion. *Virology* 1991;183:437–441.

149. Eckert DM, Kim PS. Mechanisms of viral membrane fusion and its inhibition. *Annu Rev Biochem* 2001;70:777–810.

150. Egelman EH, Wu SS, Amrein M, et al. The Sendai virus nucleocapsid exists in at least four different helical states. *J Virol* 1989;63:2233–2243.

151. Elango N, Kovamees J, Varsanyi TM, et al. mRNA sequence and deduced amino acid sequence of the mumps virus small hydrophobic protein gene. *J Virol* 1989;63:1413–1415.

152. Epa VC. Modeling the paramyxovirus hemagglutinin-neuraminidase protein. *Proteins* 1997;29:264–281.

153. Errington W, Emmerson PT. Assembly of recombinant Newcastle disease virus nucleocapsid protein into nucleocapsid-like structures is inhibited by the phosphoprotein. *J Gen Virol* 1997;78:2335–2339.

154. Essaidi-Laziosi M, Shevtsova A, Gerlier D, et al. Mutation of the TYTLE motif in the cytoplasmic tail of the sendai virus fusion protein deeply affects viral assembly and particle production. *PLoS One* 2013;8(12):e78074.

155. Faaberg KS, Peeples ME. Association of soluble matrix protein of Newcastle disease virus with liposomes is independent of ionic conditions. *Virology* 1988;166:123–132.

156. Fagraeus A, Tyrrell DL, Norberg R, et al. Actin filaments in paramyxovirus-infected human fibroblasts studied by indirect immunofluorescence. *Arch Virol* 1978;57(4):291–296.

157. Fass D. Conformational changes in enveloped virus surface proteins during cell entry. *Adv Protein Chem* 2003;64:325–362.

158. Fass D, Harrison SC, Kim PS. Retrovirus envelope domain at 1.7 Å resolution. *Nat Struct Biol* 1996;3:465–469.

159. Fearns R, Plemper RK. Polymerases of paramyxoviruses and pneumoviruses. *Virus Res* 2017;234:87–102.

160. Feller JA, Smallwood S, Horikami SM, et al. Mutations in conserved domains IV and VI of the large (L) subunit of the sendai virus RNA polymerase give a spectrum of defective RNA synthesis phenotypes. *Virology* 2000;269(2):426–439.

161. Ferron F, Longhi S, Henrissat B, et al. Viral RNA-polymerases—a predicted 2'-O-ribose methyltransferase domain shared by all Mononegavirales. *Trends Biochem Sci* 2002;27:222–224.

162. Fontana JM, Bankamp B, Bellini WJ, et al. Regulation of interferon signaling by the C and V proteins from attenuated and wild-type strains of measles virus. *Virology* 2008;374(1):71–81.

163. Fooks AR, Stephenson JR, Warnes A, et al. Measles virus nucleocapsid protein expressed in insect cells assembles into nucleocapsid-like structures. *J Gen Virol* 1993;74(Pt 7):1439–1444.

164. Fouillot-Coriou N, Roux L. Structure-function analysis of the Sendai virus F and HN cytoplasmic domain: different role for the two proteins in the production of virus particle. *Virology* 2000;270:464–475.

165. Franchi L, Munoz-Planillo R, Reimer T, et al. Inflammasomes as microbial sensors. *Eur J Immunol* 2010;40(3):611–615.

166. Frenzke M, Sawatsky B, Wong XX, et al. Nectin-4-dependent measles virus spread to the cynomolgus monkey tracheal epithelium: role of infected immune cells infiltrating the lamina propria. *J Virol* 2013;87(5):2526–2534.

167. Fukuhara N, Huang C, Kiyotani K, et al. Mutational analysis of the Sendai virus V protein: importance of the conserved residues for Zn binding, virus pathogenesis, and efficient RNA editing. *Virology* 2002;299:172–181.

168. Galinski MS, Troy RM, Banerjee AK. RNA editing in the phosphoprotein gene of the human parainfluenza virus type 3. *Virology* 1992;186:543–550.

169. Garcin D, Curran J, Itoh M, et al. Longer and shorter forms of Sendai virus C proteins play different roles in modulating the cellular antiviral response. *J Virol* 2001;75(15):6800–6807.

170. Garcin D, Itoh M, Kolakofsky D. A point mutation in the Sendai virus accessory C proteins attenuated virulence for mice, but not virus growth in cell culture. *Virology* 1997;238:424–431.
171. Garcin D, Marq JB, Strahle L, et al. All four Sendai virus C proteins bind STAT1, but only the larger forms also induce its mono-ubiquitination and degradation. *Virology* 2002;295(2):256–265.
172. Garcin D, Pelet T, Calain P, et al. A highly recombinogenic system for the recovery of infectious Sendai paramyxovirus from cDNA: generation of a novel copy-back nondefective interfering virus. *EMBO J* 1995;14:6087–6094.
173. Garrus JE, von Schwedler UK, Pornillos OW, et al. Tsg101 and the vacuolar protein sorting pathway are essential for HIV-1 budding. *Cell* 2001;107(1):55–65.
174. Gassen U, Collins FM, Duprex WP, et al. Establishment of a rescue system for canine distemper virus. *J Virol* 2000;74(22):10737–10744.
175. Ghosh A, Nayak R, Shaila MS. Synthesis of leader RNA and editing of P mRNA during transcription by rinderpest virus. *Virus Res* 1996;41(1):69–76.
176. Giorgi C, Blumberg BM, Kolakofsky D. Sendai virus contains overlapping genes expressed from a single mRNA. *Cell* 1983;35:829–836.
177. Giuffre RM, Tovell DR, Kay CM, et al. Evidence for an interaction between the membrane protein of a paramyxovirus and actin. *J Virol* 1982;42(3):963–968.
178. Goff PH, Gao Q, Palese P. A majority of infectious Newcastle disease virus particles contain a single genome, while a minority contain multiple genomes. *J Virol* 2012;86(19):10852–10856.
179. Gonzâlez-Reyes L, Ruiz-Argèuello MB, Garcâia-Barreno B, et al. Cleavage of the human respiratory syncytial virus fusion protein at two distinct sites is required for activation of membrane fusion. *Proc Natl Acad Sci U S A* 2001;98:9859–9864.
180. Gopinath M, Shaila MS. RNA triphosphatase and guanylyl transferase activities are associated with the RNA polymerase protein L of rinderpest virus. *J Gen Virol* 2009;90(Pt 7):1748–1756.
181. Gopinath M, Shaila MS. Evidence for N(7) guanine methyl transferase activity encoded within the modular domain of RNA-dependent RNA polymerase L of a Morbillivirus. *Virus Genes* 2015;51(3):356–360.
182. Gosselin-Grenet AS, Marq JB, Abrami L, et al. Sendai virus budding in the course of an infection does not require Alix and VPS4A host factors. *Virology* 2007;365(1):101–112.
183. Gotoh B, Ogasawara T, Toyoda T, et al. An endoprotease homologous to the blood clotting factor X as a determinant of viral tropism in chick embryo. *EMBO J* 1990;9:4189–4195.
184. Gotoh B, Takeuchi K, Komatsu T, et al. Knockout of the Sendai virus C gene eliminates the viral ability to prevent the interferon-alpha/beta-mediated responses. *FEBS Lett* 1999;459(2):205–210.
185. Gotoh B, Takeuchi K, Komatsu T, et al. The STAT2 activation process is a crucial target of Sendai virus C protein for the blockade of alpha interferon signaling. *J Virol* 2003;77(6):3360–3370.
186. Gotoh B, Yamauchi F, Ogasawara T, et al. Isolation of factor Xa from chick embryo as the amniotic endoprotease responsible for paramyxovirus activation. *FEBS Lett* 1992;296:274–278.
187. Gottlinger HG, Dorfman T, Sodroski JG, et al. Effect of mutations affecting the p6 gag protein on human immunodeficiency virus particle release. *Proc Natl Acad Sci U S A* 1991;88(8):3195–3199.
188. Grdzelishvili VZ, Smallwood S, Tower D, et al. A single amino acid change in the L-polymerase protein of vesicular stomatitis virus completely abolishes viral mRNA cap methylation. *J Virol* 2005;79:7327–7337.
189. Grogan CC, Moyer SA. Sendai virus wild-type and mutant C proteins show a direct correlation between L polymerase binding and inhibition of viral RNA synthesis. *Virology* 2001;288:96–108.
190. Gubbay O, Curran J, Kolakofsky D. Sendai virus genome synthesis and assembly are coupled: a possible mechanism to promote viral RNA polymerase processivity. *J Gen Virol* 2001;82:2895–2903.
191. Gui L, Jurgens EM, Ebner JL, et al. Electron tomography imaging of surface glycoproteins on human parainfluenza virus 3: association of receptor binding and fusion proteins before receptor engagement. *MBio* 2015;6:e02393–e02414.
192. Guryanov SG, Liljeroos L, Kasaragod P, et al. Crystal structure of the measles virus nucleoprotein core in complex with an N-terminal region of phosphoprotein. *J Virol* 2015;90(6):2849–2857.
193. Gutsche I, Desfosses A, Effantin G, et al. Structural virology. Near-atomic cryo-EM structure of the helical measles virus nucleocapsid. *Science* 2015;348(6235):704–707.
194. Habchi J, Blangy S, Mamelli L, et al. Characterization of the interactions between the nucleoprotein and the phosphoprotein of Henipavirus. *J Biol Chem* 2011;286(15):13583–13602.
195. Hagiwara K, Sato H, Inoue Y, et al. Phosphorylation of measles virus nucleoprotein upregulates the transcriptional activity of minigenomic RNA. *Proteomics* 2008;8(9):1871–1879.
196. Hamaguchi M, Yoshida T, Nishikawa K, et al. Transcriptive complex of Newcastle disease virus. I. Both L and P proteins are required to constitute an active complex. *Virology* 1983;128:105–117.
197. Han M, Xu J, Ren Y, et al. Simulation of coupled folding and binding of an intrinsically disordered protein in explicit solvent with metadynamics. *J Mol Graph Model* 2016;68:114–127.
198. Harcourt BH, Tamin A, Ksiazek TG, et al. Molecular characterization of Nipah virus, a newly emergent paramyxovirus. *Virology* 2000;271:334–349.
199. Harmon SB, Wertz GW. Transcriptional termination modulated by nucleotides outside the characterized gene end sequence of respiratory syncytial virus. *Virology* 2002;300:304–315.
200. Harty RN, Paragas J, Sudol M, et al. A proline-rich motif within the matrix protein of vesicular stomatitis virus and rabies virus interacts with WW domains of cellular proteins: implications for viral budding. *J Virol* 1999;73:2921–2929.
201. Hashiguchi T, Fukuda Y, Matsuoka R, et al. Structures of the prefusion form of measles virus fusion protein in complex with inhibitors. *Proc Natl Acad Sci U S A* 2018;115(10):2496–2501.
202. Hashiguchi T, Ose T, Kubota M, et al. Structure of the measles virus hemagglutinin bound to its cellular receptor SLAM. *Nat Struct Biol* 2011;18:135–141.
203. Hausmann S, Garcin D, Delenda C, et al. The versatility of paramyxovirus RNA polymerase stuttering. *J Virol* 1999;73:5568–5576.
204. Hausmann S, Gardin D, Morel AS, et al. Two nucleotides immediately upstream of the essential A6G3 slippery sequence modulate the pattern of G insertions during Sendai virus mRNA editing. *J Virol* 1999;73:343–351.
205. He B, Leser GP, Paterson RG, et al. The paramyxovirus SV5 small hydrophobic (SH) protein is not essential for virus growth in tissue culture cells. *Virology* 1998;250:30–40.
206. He B, Lin GY, Durbin JE, et al. The SH integral membrane protein of the paramyxovirus simian virus 5 is required to block apoptosis in MDBK cells. *J Virol* 2001;75:4068–4079.
207. He B, Paterson RG, Stock N, et al. Recovery of paramyxovirus simian virus 5 with a V protein lacking the conserved cysteine-rich domain: the multifunctional V protein blocks both interferon-beta induction and interferon signaling. *Virology* 2002;303:15–32.
208. He B, Paterson RG, Ward CD, et al. Recovery of infectious SV5 from cloned DNA and expression of a foreign gene. *Virology* 1997;237:249–260.
209. Heggeness MH, Scheid A, Choppin PW. Conformation of the helical nucleocapsids of paramyxoviruses and vesicular stomatitis virus: reversible coiling and uncoiling induced by changes in salt concentration. *Proc Natl Acad Sci U S A* 1980;77:2631–2635.
210. Heggeness MH, Scheid A, Choppin PW. The relationship of conformational changes in the Sendai virus nucleocapsid to proteolytic cleavage of the NP polypeptide. *Virology* 1981;114:555–562.
211. Heggeness MH, Smith PR, Choppin PW. In vitro assembly of the nonglycosylated membrane protein (M) of Sendai virus. *Proc Natl Acad Sci U S A* 1982;79(20):6232–6236.
212. Heil F, Hemmi H, Hochrein H, et al. Species-specific recognition of single-stranded RNA via toll-like receptor 7 and 8. *Science* 2004;303(5663):1526–1529.
213. Hercyk N, Horikami SM, Moyer SA. The vesicular stomatitis virus L protein possesses the mRNA methyltransferase activities. *Virology* 1988;163:222–225.
214. Hiebert SW, Paterson RG, Lamb RA. Hemagglutinin-neuraminidase protein of the paramyxovirus simian virus 5: nucleotide sequence of the mRNA predicts an N-terminal membrane anchor. *J Virol* 1985;54:1–6.
215. Hiebert SW, Richardson CD, Lamb RA. Cell surface expression and orientation in membranes of the 44-amino-acid SH protein of simian virus 5. *J Virol* 1988;62:2347–2357.
216. Hoffman MA, Banerjee AK. An infectious clone of human parainfluenza virus type 3. *J Virol* 1997;71:4272–4277.
217. Hoffman MA, Banerjee AK. Precise mapping of the replication and transcription promoters of human parainfluenza virus type 3. *Virology* 2000;269:201–211.
218. Hoffmann HH, Schneider WM, Rice CM. Interferons and viruses: an evolutionary arms race of molecular interactions. *Trends Immunol* 2015;36(3):124–138.
219. Holmes DE, Moyer SA. The phosphoprotein (P) binding site resides in the N terminus of the L polymerase subunit of sendai virus. *J Virol* 2002;76:3078–3083.
220. Homann HE, Willenbrink W, Buchholz CJ, et al. Sendai virus protein-protein interactions studied by a protein-blotting protein-overlay technique: mapping of domains on NP protein required for binding to P protein. *J Virol* 1991;65:1304–1309.
221. Homma M, Ohuchi M. Trypsin action on the growth of Sendai virus in tissue culture cells. III. Structural differences of Sendai viruses grown in eggs and tissue culture cells. *J Virol* 1973;12:1457–1465.
222. Horikami SM, Curran J, Kolakofsky D, et al. Complexes of Sendai virus NP-P and P-L proteins are required for defective interfering particle genome replication in vitro. *J Virol* 1992;66:4901–4908.
223. Horikami SM, Hector RC, Smallwood S, et al. The Sendai virus C protein binds the L polymerase protein to inhibit viral RNA synthesis. *Virology* 1997;235:261–270.
224. Horikami SM, Moyer SA. Synthesis of leader RNA and editing of the P mRNA during transcription by purified measles virus. *J Virol* 1991;65(10):5342–5347.
225. Horikami SM, Smallwood S, Bankamp B, et al. An amino-proximal domain of the L protein binds to the P protein in the measles virus RNA polymerase complex. *Virology* 1994;205(2):540–545.
226. Horikami S, Smallwood S, Moyer SA. The Sendai virus V protein interacts with the NP protein to regulate viral genome RNA replication. *Virology* 1996;222:383–390.
227. Horvath CM, Paterson RG, Shaughnessy MA, et al. Biological activity of paramyxovirus fusion proteins: factors influencing formation of syncytia. *J Virol* 1992;66:4564–4569.
228. Hosaka M, Nagahama M, Kim W-S, et al. Arg-X-Lys/Arg-Arg motif as a signal for precursor cleavage catalyzed by furin within the constitutive secretory pathway. *J Biol Chem* 1991;266:12127–12130.
229. Hu A, Cattaneo R, Schwartz S, et al. Role of N-linked oligosaccharide chains in the processing and antigenicity of measles virus haemagglutinin protein. *J Gen Virol* 1994;75:1043–1052.
230. Hu X, Ray R, Compans RW. Functional interactions between the fusion protein and hemagglutinin-neuraminidase of human parainfluenza viruses. *J Virol* 1992;66:1528–1534.
231. Huber M, Cattaneo R, Spielhofer P, et al. Measles virus phosphoprotein retains the nucleocapsid protein in the cytoplasm. *Virology* 1991;185:299–308.
232. Huntley CC, De BP, Banerjee AK. Phosphorylation of Sendai virus phosphoprotein by cellular protein kinase C zeta. *J Biol Chem* 1997;272(26):16578–16584.
233. Hurley JH, Emr SD. The ESCRT complexes: structure and mechanism of a membrane-trafficking network. *Annu Rev Biophys Biomol Struct* 2006;35:277–298.
234. Ikegame S, Takeda M, Ohno S, et al. Both RIG-I and MDA5 RNA helicases contribute to the induction of alpha/beta interferon in measles virus-infected human cells. *J Virol* 2010;84(1):372–379.
235. Iorio RM, Field GM, Sauvron JM, et al. Structural and functional relationship between the receptor recognition and neuraminidase activities of the Newcastle disease virus hemagglutinin-neuraminidase protein: receptor recognition is dependent on neuraminidase activity. *J Virol* 2001;75:1918–1927.
236. Irie T, Kiyotani K, Igarashi T, et al. Inhibition of interferon regulatory factor 3 activation by paramyxovirus V protein. *J Virol* 2012;86(13):7136–7145.
237. Irie T, Nagata N, Igarashi T, et al. Conserved charged amino acids within Sendai virus C protein play multiple roles in the evasion of innate immune responses. *PLoS One* 2010;5(5):e10719.

238. Irie T, Nagata N, Yoshida T, et al. Recruitment of Alix/AIP1 to the plasma membrane by Sendai virus C protein facilitates budding of virus-like particles. *Virology* 2008;371(1):108–120.
239. Irie T, Nagata N, Yoshida T, et al. Paramyxovirus Sendai virus C proteins are essential for maintenance of negative-sense RNA genome in virus particles. *Virology* 2008;374(2): 495–505.
240. Irie T, Okamoto I, Yoshida A, et al. Sendai virus C proteins regulate viral genome and antigenome synthesis to dictate the negative genome polarity. *J Virol* 2014;88(1):690–698.
241. Irie T, Shimazu Y, Yoshida T, et al. The YLDL sequence within Sendai virus M protein is critical for budding of virus-like particles and interacts with Alix/AIP1 independently of C protein. *J Virol* 2007;81(5):2263–2273.
242. Iseni F, Baudin F, Garcin D, et al. Chemical modification of nucleotide bases and mRNA editing depend on hexamer or nucleoprotein phase in Sendai virus nucleocapsids. *RNA* 2002;8:1056–1067.
243. Iseni F, Garcin D, Nishio M, et al. Sendai virus trailer RNA binds TIAR, a cellular protein involved in virus-induced apoptosis. *EMBO J* 2002;21(19):5141–5150.
244. Iwasaki A. A virological view of innate immune recognition. *Annu Rev Microbiol* 2012;66:177–196.
245. Iwasaki M, Takeda M, Shirogane Y, et al. The matrix protein of measles virus regulates viral RNA synthesis and assembly by interacting with the nucleocapsid protein. *J Virol* 2009;83(20):10374–10383.
246. Jablonski SA, Luo M, Morrow CD. Enzymatic activity of poliovirus RNA polymerase mutants with single amino acid changes in the conserved YGDD amino acid motif. *J Virol* 1991;65(9):4565–4572.
247. Jack PJ, Boyle DB, Eaton BT, et al. The complete genome sequence of J virus reveals a unique genome structure in the family *Paramyxoviridae*. *J Virol* 2005;79(16):10690–10700.
248. Jardetzky TS, Lamb RA. Virology: a class act. *Nature* 2004;427:307–308.
249. Jardetzky TS, Lamb RA. Activation of paramyxovirus membrane fusion and virus entry. *Curr Opin Virol* 2014;5:24–33.
250. Jayakar HR, Murti KG, Whitt MA. Mutations in the PPPY motif of vesicular stomatitis virus matrix protein reduce virus budding by inhibiting a late step in virion release. *J Virol* 2000;74:9818–9827.
251. Jensen MB, Bhatia VK, Jao CC, et al. Membrane curvature sensing by amphipathic helices: a single liposome study using alpha-synuclein and annexin B12. *J Biol Chem* 2011;286:42603–42614.
252. Johansson K, Bourhis JM, Campanacci V, et al. Crystal structure of the measles virus phosphoprotein domain responsible for the induced folding of the C-terminal domain of the nucleoprotein. *J Biol Chem* 2003;278:44567–44573.
253. Jordan PC, Liu C, Raynaud P, et al. Initiation, extension, and termination of RNA synthesis by a paramyxovirus polymerase. *PLoS Pathog* 2018;14(2):e1006889.
254. Joshi SB, Dutch RE, Lamb RA. A core trimer of the paramyxovirus fusion protein: parallels to influenza virus hemagglutinin and HIV-1 gp41. *Virology* 1998;248:20–34.
255. Kahn JS, Schnell MJ, Buonocore L, et al. Recombinant vesicular stomatitis virus expressing respiratory syncytial virus (RSV) glycoproteins: RSV fusion protein can mediate infection and cell fusion. *Virology* 1999;254:81–91.
256. Kanneganti TD, Body-Malapel M, Amer A, et al. Critical role for Cryopyrin/Nalp3 in activation of caspase-1 in response to viral infection and double-stranded RNA. *J Biol Chem* 2006;281(48):36560–36568.
257. Karlin D, Ferron F, Canard B, et al. Structural disorder and modular organization in Paramyxovirinae N and P. *J Gen Virol* 2003;84(Pt 12):3239–3252.
258. Karlin D, Longhi S, Receveur V, et al. The N-terminal domain of the phosphoprotein of morbilliviruses belongs to the natively unfolded class of proteins. *Virology* 2002;296: 251–262.
259. Katayama H, Hori M, Sato K, et al. Role of actin microfilaments in canine distemper virus replication in vero cells. *J Vet Med Sci* 2004;66(4):409–415.
260. Kato A, Kiyotani K, Hasan MK, et al. Sendai virus gene start signals are not equivalent in reinitiation capacity: moderation at the fusion protein gene. *J Virol* 1999;73:9237–9246.
261. Kato A, Kiyotani K, Sakai Y, et al. Importance of the cysteine-rich carboxyl-terminal half of V protein for Sendai virus pathogenesis. *J Virol* 1997;71:7266–7272.
262. Kato A, Kiyotani K, Sakai Y, et al. The paramyxovirus, Sendai virus, V protein encodes a luxury function required for viral pathogenesis. *EMBO J* 1997;16:578–587.
263. Kato A, Ohnishi Y, Kohase M, et al. Y2, the smallest of the Sendai virus C proteins, is fully capable of both counteracting the antiviral action of interferons and inhibiting viral RNA synthesis. *J Virol* 2001;75:3802–3810.
264. Kato A, Sakai Y, Shioda T, et al. Initiation of Sendai virus multiplication from transfected cDNA or RNA with negative or positive sense. *Genes Cells* 1996;1:569–579.
265. Kawano M, Kaito M, Kozuka Y, et al. Recovery of infectious human parainfluenza type 2 virus from cDNA clones and properties of the defective virus without V-specific cysteine-rich domain. *Virology* 2001;284:99–112.
266. Ke Z, Strauss JD, Hampton CM, et al. Promotion of virus assembly and organization by the measles virus matrix protein. *Nat Commun* 2018;9(1):1736.
267. Keller MA, Parks GD. Positive- and negative-acting signals combine to determine differential RNA replication from the paramyxovirus simian virus 5 genomic and antigenomic promoters. *Virology* 2003;306:347–358.
268. Kelley LA, Mezulis S, Yates CM, et al. The Phyre2 web portal for protein modeling, prediction and analysis. *Nat Protoc* 2015;10(6):845–858.
269. Kikonyogo A, Bouamr F, Vana ML, et al. Proteins related to the Nedd4 family of ubiquitin protein ligases interact with the L domain of Rous sarcoma virus and are required for gag budding from cells. *Proc Natl Acad Sci U S A* 2001;98(20):11199–11204.
270. Kingsbury DW, Hsu CH, Murti KG. Intracellular metabolism of Sendai virus nucleocapsids. *Virology* 1978;91:86–94.
271. Kingston RL, Baase WA, Gay LS. Characterization of nucleocapsid binding by the measles virus and mumps virus phosphoproteins. *J Virol* 2004;78:8630–8640.
272. Kingston RL, Gay LS, Baase WS, et al. Structure of the nucleocapsid-binding domain from the mumps virus polymerase; an example of protein folding induced by crystallization. *J Mol Biol* 2008;379(4):719–731.
273. Kingston RL, Hamel DJ, Gay LS, et al. Structural basis for the attachment of a paramyxoviral polymerase to its template. *Proc Natl Acad Sci U S A* 2004;101(22):8301–8306.
274. Kitagawa Y, Yamaguchi M, Zhou M, et al. A tryptophan-rich motif in the human parainfluenza virus type 2 V protein is critical for the blockade of toll-like receptor 7 (TLR7)- and TLR9-dependent signaling. *J Virol* 2011;85(9):4606–4611.
275. Klenk HD, Garten W. Host cell proteases controlling virus pathogenicity. *Trends Microbiol* 1994;2:39–43.
276. Kobe B, Center RJ, Kemp BE, et al. Crystal structure of human T cell leukemia virus type 1 gp21 ectodomain crystallized as a maltose-binding protein chimera reveals structural evolution of retroviral transmembrane proteins. *Proc Natl Acad Sci U S A* 1999;96:4319–4324.
277. Kolakofsky D. Paramyxovirus RNA synthesis, mRNA editing, and genome hexamer phase: a review. *Virology* 2016;498:94–98.
278. Kolakofsky D, Bruschi A. Antigenomes in Sendai virions and Sendai virus-infected cells. *Virology* 1975;66:185–191.
279. Kolakofsky D, Pelet T, Garin D, et al. Paramyxovirus RNA synthesis and the requirement for hexamer genome length: The rule of six revisited. *J Virol* 1998;72:891–899.
280. Komatsu T, Tanaka Y, Kitagawa Y, et al. Sendai virus V protein inhibits the secretion of interleukin-1β by preventing NLRP3 inflammasome assembly. *J Virol* 2018;92(19).
281. Komuro A, Bamming D, Horvath CM. Negative regulation of cytoplasmic RNA-mediated antiviral signaling. *Cytokine* 2008;43(3):350–358.
282. Krumm SA, Takeda M, Plemper RK. The measles virus nucleocapsid protein tail domain is dispensable for viral polymerase recruitment and activity. *J Biol Chem* 2013;288(41):29943–29953.
283. Kubota T, Yokosawa N, Yokota S, et al. C terminal CYS-RICH region of mumps virus structural V protein correlates with block of interferon alpha and gamma signal transduction pathway through decrease of STAT 1-alpha. *Biochem Biophys Res Commun* 2001;283:255–259.
284. Kulkarni S, Volchkova V, Basler CF, et al. Nipah virus edits its P gene at high frequency to express the V and W proteins. *J Virol* 2009;83(8):3982–3987.
285. Kurilla MG, Stone HO, Keene JD. RNA sequence and transcriptional properties of the 3′ end of the Newcastle disease virus genome. *Virology* 1985;145(2):203–212.
286. Kurotani A, Kiyotani K, Kato A, et al. Sendai virus C proteins are categorically nonessential gene products but silencing their expression severely impairs viral replication and pathogenesis. *Genes Cells* 1998;3:111–124.
287. Laliberte JP, McGinnes LW, Morrison TG. Incorporation of functional HN-F glycoprotein-containing complexes into newcastle disease virus is dependent on cholesterol and membrane lipid raft integrity. *J Virol* 2007;81(19):10636–10648.
288. Lamb RA. Paramyxovirus fusion: a hypothesis for changes. *Virology* 1993;197:1–11.
289. Lamb RA, Choppin PW. The synthesis of Sendai virus polypeptides in infected cells. II Intracellular distribution of polypeptides. *Virology* 1977;81:371–381.
290. Lamb RA, Kolakofsky D. *Paramyxoviridae*: the viruses and their replication. In: Knipe DM, Howley PM, eds. *Fields Virology*. 4th ed. Philadelphia: Lippincott, Williams and Wilkins; 2001:1305–1340.
291. Lamb RA, Mahy BW, Choppin PW. The synthesis of Sendai virus polypeptides in infected cells. *Virology* 1976;69:116–131.
292. Lamb RA, Paterson RG, Jardetzky TS. Paramyxovirus membrane fusion: lessons from the F and HN atomic structures. *Virology* 2006;344:30–37.
293. Lamp B, Dietzel E, Kolesnikova L, et al. Nipah virus entry and egress from polarized epithelial cells. *J Virol* 2013;87(6):3143–3154.
294. Langedijk JPM, Daus FJ, van Oirschot JT. Sequence and structure alignment of *Paramyxoviridae* attachment proteins and discovery of enzymatic activity for a morbillivirus hemagglutinin. *J Virol* 1997;71:6155–6167.
295. Latiff K, Meanger J, Mills J, et al. Sequence and structure relatedness of matrix protein of human respiratory syncytial virus with matrix proteins of other negative-sense RNA viruses. *Clin Microbiol Infect* 2004;10(10):945–948.
296. Latorre P, Cadd T, Itoh M, et al. The various Sendai virus C proteins are not functionally equivalent and exert both positive and negative effects on viral RNA accumulation during the course of infection. *J Virol* 1998;72:5984–5993.
297. Lawrence MC, Borg NA, Streltsov VA, et al. Structure of the haemagglutinin-neuraminidase from human parainfluenza virus type III. *J Mol Biol* 2004;335:1343–1357.
298. Lawson ND, Stillman EA, Whitt MA, et al. Recombinant vesicular stomatitis viruses from DNA. *Proc Natl Acad Sci U S A* 1995;92(10):4477–4481.
299. Le Mercier P, Garcin D, Hausmann S, et al. Ambisense Sendai viruses are inherently unstable but are useful to study viral RNA synthesis. *J Virol* 2002;76:5492–5502.
300. le Mercier P, Kolakofsky D. Bipartite promoters and RNA editing of paramyxoviruses and filoviruses. *RNA* 2019;25(3):279–285.
301. Lee AJ, Ashkar AA. The dual nature of type I and type II interferons. *Front Immunol* 2018;9:2061.
302. Lee JK, Prussia A, Paal T, et al. Functional interaction between paramyxovirus fusion and attachment proteins. *J Biol Chem* 2008;283:16561–16572.
303. Lee JK, Prussia A, Snyder JP, et al. Reversible inhibition of the fusion activity of measles virus F protein by an engineered intersubunit disulfide bridge. *J Virol* 2007;81:8821–8826.
304. Leppert M, Rittenhouse L, Perrault J, et al. Plus and minus strand leader RNAs in negative strand virus-infected cells. *Cell* 1979;18(3):735–747.
305. Leser GP, Ector KJ, Ng DT, et al. The signal for clathrin-mediated endocytosis of the paramyxovirus SV5 HN protein resides at the transmembrane domain-ectodomain boundary region. *Virology* 1999;262:79–92.
306. Leser GP, Lamb RA. Influenza virus assembly and budding in raft-derived microdomains: a quantitative analysis of the surface distribution of HA, NA and M2 proteins. *Virology* 2005;342:215–227.
307. Li T, Chen X, Garbutt KC, et al. Structure of DDB1 in complex with a paramyxovirus V protein: viral hijack of a propeller cluster in ubiquitin ligase. *Cell* 2006;124(1):105–117.
308. Li Z, Hung C, Paterson RG, et al. Type II integral membrane protein, TM of J paramyxovirus promotes cell-to-cell fusion. *Proc Natl Acad Sci U S A* 2015;112:12504–12509.
309. Li M, Schmitt PT, Li Z, et al. Mumps virus matrix, fusion, and nucleocapsid proteins cooperate for efficient production of virus-like particles. *J Virol* 2009;83(14):7261–7272.

310. Li J, Wang JT, Whelan SP. A unique strategy for mRNA cap methylation used by vesicular stomatitis virus. *Proc Natl Acad Sci U S A* 2006;103(22):8493–8498.

311. Liang B, Li Z, Jenni S, et al. Structure of the L protein of vesicular stomatitis virus from electron cryomicroscopy. *Cell* 2015;162:314–327.

312. Lieu KG, Marsh GA, Wang LF, et al. The non-pathogenic Henipavirus Cedar paramyxovirus phosphoprotein has a compromised ability to target STAT1 and STAT2. *Antiviral Res* 2015;124:69–76.

313. Liljeroos L, Huiskonen JT, Ora A, et al. Electron cryotomography of measles virus reveals how matrix protein coats the ribonucleocapsid within intact virions. *Proc Natl Acad Sci U S A* 2011;108(44):18085–18090.

314. Lin Y, Bright AC, Rothermel TA, et al. Induction of apoptosis by paramyxovirus simian virus 5 lacking a small hydrophobic gene. *J Virol* 2003;77:3371–3383.

315. Lin Y, Horvath F, Aligo JA, et al. The role of simian virus 5 V protein on viral RNA synthesis. *Virology* 2005;338:270–280.

316. Lin GY, Paterson RG, Richardson CD, et al. The V protein of the paramyxovirus SV5 interacts with damage-specific DNA binding protein. *Virology* 1998;249:189–200.

317. Liston P, Briedis DJ. Measles virus V protein binds zinc. *Virology* 1994;198:399–404.

318. Liu YC, Grusovin J, Adams TE. Electrostatic interactions between Hendra virus matrix proteins are required for efficient virus-like-particle assembly. *J Virol* 2018;92(13).

319. Liu Q, Stone JA, Bradel-Tretheway B, et al. Unraveling a three-step spatiotemporal mechanism of triggering of receptor-induced Nipah virus fusion and cell entry. *PLoS Pathog* 2013;9:e1003770.

320. Liuzzi M, Mason SW, Cartier M, et al. Inhibitors of respiratory syncytial virus replication target cotranscriptional mRNA guanylylation by viral RNA-dependent RNA polymerase. *J Virol* 2005;79(20):13105–13115.

321. Lo MK, Harcourt BH, Mungall BA, et al. Determination of the henipavirus phosphoprotein gene mRNA editing frequencies and detection of the C, V and W proteins of Nipah virus in virus-infected cells. *J Gen Virol* 2009;90(Pt 2):398–404.

322. Lo MK, Peeples ME, Bellini WJ, et al. Distinct and overlapping roles of Nipah virus P gene products in modulating the human endothelial cell antiviral response. *PLoS One* 2012;7(10):e47790.

323. Lo MK, Sogaard TM, Karlin DG. Evolution and structural organization of the C proteins of paramyxovirinae. *PLoS One* 2014;9(2):e90003.

324. Loney C, Mottet-Osman G, Roux L, et al. Paramyxovirus ultrastructure and genome packaging: cryo-electron tomography of sendai virus. *J Virol* 2009;83(16):8191–8197.

325. Longhi S, Bloyet LM, Gianni S, et al. How order and disorder within paramyxoviral nucleoproteins and phosphoproteins orchestrate the molecular interplay of transcription and replication. *Cell Mol Life Sci* 2017;74(17):3091–3118.

326. Longhi S, Receveur-Brechot V, Karlin D, et al. The C-terminal domain of the measles virus nucleoprotein is intrinsically disordered and folds upon binding to the C-terminal moiety of the phosphoprotein. *J Biol Chem* 2003;278:18638–18648.

327. Lu LL, Puri M, Horvath CM, et al. Select paramyxoviral V proteins inhibit IRF3 activation by acting as alternative substrates for inhibitor of kappaB kinase epsilon (IKKe)/TBK1. *J Biol Chem* 2008;283:14269–14276.

328. Ludlow M, Lemon K, de Vries RD, et al. Measles virus infection of epithelial cells in the macaque upper respiratory tract is mediated by subepithelial immune cells. *J Virol* 2013;87(7):4033–4042.

329. Lyles DS. Assembly and budding of negative-strand RNA viruses. *Adv Virus Res* 2013;85:57–90.

330. Maar D, Harmon B, Chu D, et al. Cysteines in the stalk of the nipah virus g glycoprotein are located in a distinct subdomain critical for fusion activation. *J Virol* 2012;86:6632–6642.

331. Maisner A, Klenk H, Herrler G. Polarized budding of measles virus is not determined by viral surface glycoproteins. *J Virol* 1998;72(6):5276–5278.

332. Malashkevich VN, Schneider BJ, McNally ML, et al. Core structure of the envelope glycoprotein GP2 from Ebola virus at 1.9-A resolution. *Proc Natl Acad Sci U S A* 1999;96:2662–2667.

333. Malur AG, Chattopadhyay S, Maitra RK, et al. Inhibition of STAT 1 phosphorylation by human parainfluenza virus type 3 C protein. *J Virol* 2005;79(12):7877–7882.

334. Malur AG, Gupta NK, De Bishnu P, et al. Analysis of the mutations in the active site of the RNA-dependent RNA polymerase of human parainfluenza virus type 3 (HPIV3). *Gene Expr* 2002;10:93–100.

335. Malur AG, Hoffman MA, Banerjee AK. The human parainfluenza virus type 3 (hPIV 3) C protein inhibits viral transcription. *Virus Res* 2004;99:199–204.

336. Mandhana R, Qian LK, Horvath CM. Constitutively active MDA5 proteins are inhibited by paramyxovirus V proteins. *J Interferon Cytokine Res* 2018;38(8):319–332.

337. Manie SN, Debreyne S, Vincent S, et al. Measles virus structural components are enriched into lipid raft microdomains: a potential cellular location for virus assembly. *J Virol* 2000;74:305–311.

338. Mao H, Chattopadhyay S, Banerjee AK. Domain within the C protein of human parainfluenza virus type 3 that regulates interferon signaling. *Gene Expr* 2010;15(1):43–50.

339. Marcos F, Ferreira L, Cros J, et al. Mapping of the RNA promoter of Newcastle disease virus. *Virology* 2005;331:396–406.

340. Markwell MAK. New frontiers opened by the exploration of host cell receptors. In: Kingsbury DW, ed. *The Paramyxoviruses*. New York: Plenum Press; 1991:407–425.

341. Markwell MAK, Fredman P, Svennerholm L. Specific gangliosides are receptors for Sendai virus. *Adv Exp Med Biol* 1984;174:369–379.

342. Markwell MAK, Moss J, Hom BE, et al. Expression of gangliosides as receptors at the cell surface controls infection of NCTC 2071 cells by Sendai virus. *Virology* 1986;155:356–364.

343. Markwell MA, Portner A, Schwartz AL. An alternative route of infection for viruses: entry by means of the asialoglycoprotein receptor of a Sendai virus mutant lacking its attachment protein. *Proc Natl Acad Sci U S A* 1985;82:978–982.

344. Marsh GA, de Jong C, Barr JA, et al. Cedar virus: a novel henipavirus isolated from Australian bats. *PLoS Pathog* 2012;8:e1002836.

345. Marsh GA, Virtue ER, Smith I, et al. Recombinant Hendra viruses expressing a reporter gene retain pathogenicity in ferrets. *Virol J* 2013;10:95.

346. Martin-Serrano J, Yarovoy A, Perez-Caballero D, et al. Divergent retroviral late-budding domains recruit vacuolar protein sorting factors by using alternative adaptor proteins. *Proc Natl Acad Sci U S A* 2003;100:12414–12419.

347. Martin-Serrano J, Zang T, Bieniasz PD. HIV-1 and Ebola virus encode small peptide motifs that recruit Tsg101 to sites of particle assembly to facilitate egress. *Nat Med* 2001;7:1313–1319.

348. Mathieu C, Guillaume V, Volchkova VA, et al. Nonstructural Nipah virus C protein regulates both the early host proinflammatory response and viral virulence. *J Virol* 2012;86(19):10766–10775.

349. Matsumoto Y, Ohta K, Kolakofsky D, et al. The control of paramyxovirus genome hexamer length and mRNA editing. *RNA* 2018;24(4):461–467.

350. Matsuoka Y, Curran J, Pelet T, et al. The P gene of human parainfluenza virus type 1 encodes P and C proteins but not a cysteine-rich V protein. *J Virol* 1991;65:3406–3410.

351. McGinnes LW, Morrison TG. The role of individual oligosaccharide chains in the activities of the HN glycoprotein of Newcastle disease virus. *Virology* 1995;212:398–410.

352. McGinnes L, Sergel T, Morrison T. Mutations in the transmembrane domain of the HN protein of Newcastle disease virus affect the structure and activity of the protein. *Virology* 1993;196:101–110.

353. McGivern DR, Collins PL, Fearns R. Identification of internal sequences in the 3′ leader region of human respiratory syncytial virus that enhance transcription and confer replication processivity. *J Virol* 2005;79(4):2449–2460.

354. McIlhatton MA, Curran MD, Rima BK. Nucleotide sequence analysis of the large (L) genes of phocine distemper virus and canine distemper virus (corrected sequence). *J Gen Virol* 1997;78:571–576.

355. McLellan JS, Chen M, Leung S, et al. Structure of RSV fusion glycoprotein trimer bound to a prefusion-specific neutralizing antibody. *Science* 2013;340:1113–1117.

356. McLellan JS, Yang Y, Graham BS, et al. Structure of respiratory syncytial virus fusion glycoprotein in the postfusion conformation reveals preservation of neutralizing epitopes. *J Virol* 2011;85:7788–7796.

357. McNab F, Mayer-Barber K, Sher A, et al. Type I interferons in infectious disease. *Nat Rev Immunol* 2015;15(2):87–103.

358. Melanson VR, Iorio RM. Addition of N-glycans in the stalk of the Newcastle disease virus HN protein blocks its interaction with the F protein and prevents fusion. *J Virol* 2006;80:623–633.

359. Melikyan GB, Grener SA, Ok DC, et al. Inner but not outer membrane leaflets control the transition from glycosylphosphatidylinositol-anchored influenza hemagglutinin-induced hemifusion to full fusion. *J Cell Biol* 1997;136:995–1005.

360. Melikyan GB, Markosyan RM, Hemmati H, et al. Evidence that the transition of HIV-1 gp41 into a six-helix bundle, not the bundle configuration, induces membrane fusion. *J Cell Biol* 2000;151:413–423.

361. Merz DC, Prehm P, Scheid A, et al. Inhibition of the neuraminidase of paramyxoviruses by halide ions: a possible means of modulating the two activities of the HN protein. *Virology* 1981;112:296–305.

362. Mesman AW, de Vries RD, McQuaid S, et al. A prominent role for DC-SIGN+ dendritic cells in initiation and dissemination of measles virus infection in non-human primates. *PLoS One* 2012;7(12):e49573.

363. Meulendyke KA, Wurth MA, McCann RO, et al. Endocytosis plays a critical role in proteolytic processing of the Hendra virus fusion protein. *J Virol* 2005;79:12643–12649.

364. Milles S, Jensen MR, Communie G, et al. Self-assembly of measles virus nucleocapsid-like particles: kinetics and RNA sequence dependence. *Angew Chem Int Ed Engl* 2016;55(32):9356–9360.

365. Mioulet V, Barrett T, Baron MD. Scanning mutagenesis identifies critical residues in the rinderpest virus genome promoter. *J Gen Virol* 2001;82(Pt 12):2905–2911.

366. Mirza AM, Deng R, Iorio RM. Site-directed mutagenesis of a conserved hexapeptide in the paramyxovirus hemagglutinin-neuraminidase glycoprotein: effects on antigenic structure and function. *J Virol* 1994;68:5093–5099.

367. Mirza AM, Iorio RM. A mutation in the stalk of the newcastle disease virus hemagglutinin-neuraminidase (HN) protein prevents triggering of the F protein despite allowing efficient HN-F complex formation. *J Virol* 2013;87(15):8813–8815.

368. Moll M, Diederich S, Klenk HD, et al. Ubiquitous activation of the Nipah virus fusion protein does not require a basic amino acid at the cleavage site. *J Virol* 2004;78:9705–9712.

369. Moll M, Klenk HD, Herrler G, et al. A single amino acid change in the cytoplasmic domains of measles virus glycoproteins H and F alters targeting, endocytosis, and cell fusion in polarized Madin-Darby canine kidney cells. *J Biol Chem* 2001;276(21):17887–17894.

370. Moll M, Klenk HD, Maisner A. Importance of the cytoplasmic tails of the measles virus glycoproteins for fusogenic activity and the generation of recombinant measles viruses. *J Virol* 2002;76:7174–7186.

371. Moll M, Pfeuffer J, Klenk HD, et al. Polarized glycoprotein targeting affects the spread of measles virus in vitro and in vivo. *J Gen Virol* 2004;85(Pt 4):1019–1027.

372. Morrison TG. Structure and function of a paramyxovirus fusion protein. *Biochim Biophys Acta* 2003;1614:73–84.

373. Morrison T, McQuain C, McGinnes L. Complementation between avirulent Newcastle disease virus and a fusion protein gene expressed from a retrovirus vector: requirements for membrane fusion. *J Virol* 1991;65:813–822.

374. Morrison T, Portner A. Structure, function, and intracellular processing of the glycoproteins of *Paramyxoviridae*. In: Kingsbury DW, ed. *The Paramyxoviruses*. New York: Plenum Press; 1991:347–382.

375. Mottet G, Roux L. Budding efficiency of Sendai virus nucleocapsids: influence of size and ends of the RNA. *Virus Res* 1989;14:175–187.

376. Motz C, Schuhmann KM, Kirchhofer A, et al. Paramyxovirus V proteins disrupt the fold of the RNA sensor MDA5 to inhibit antiviral signaling. *Science* 2013;339(6120):690–693.

377. Mountcastle WE, Compans RW, Lackland H, et al. Proteolytic cleavage of subunits of the nucleocapsid of the paramyxovirus simian virus 5. *J Virol* 1974;14:1253–1261.

378. Moyer SA, Baker SC, Horikami SM. Host cell proteins required for measles virus reproduction. *J Gen Virol* 1990;71:775–783.

379. Moyer SA, Baker SC, Lessard JL. Tubulin: a factor necessary for the synthesis of both Sendai virus and vesicular stomatitis virus RNAs. *Proc Natl Acad Sci U S A* 1986;83:5405–5409.

380. Muhlebach MD, Mateo M, Sinn PL, et al. Adherens junction protein nectin-4 is the epithelial receptor for measles virus. *Nature* 2011;480:530–533.

381. Murphy SK, Ito Y, Parks GD. A functional antigenomic promoter for the paramyxovirus simian virus 5 requires proper spacing between an essential internal segment and the 3′ terminus. *J Virol* 1998;72:10–19.
382. Murphy AM, Moerdyk-Schauwecker M, Mushegian A, et al. Sequence-function analysis of the Sendai virus L protein domain VI. *Virology* 2010;405(2):370–382.
383. Murphy SK, Parks GD. Genome nucleotide lengths that are divisible by six are not essential but enhance replication of defective interfering RNAs of the paramyxovirus simian virus 5. *Virology* 1997;232:145–157.
384. Murrell MT, Porotto M, Greengard O, et al. A single amino acid alteration in the human parainfluenza virus type 3 hemagglutinin-neuraminidase glycoprotein confers resistance to the inhibitory effects of zanamivir on receptor binding and neuraminidase activity. *J Virol* 2001;75(14):6310–6320.
385. Myers TM, Moyer SA. An amino-terminal domain of the Sendai virus nucleocapsid protein is required for template function in viral RNA synthesis. *J Virol* 1997;71:918–924.
386. Myers TM, Pieters A, Moyer SA. A highly conserved region of the Sendai virus nucleocapsid protein contributes to the NP-NP binding domain. *Virology* 1997;229:322–335.
387. Myers TM, Smallwood S, Moyer SA. Identification of nucleocapsid protein residues required for Sendai virus nucleocapsid formation and genome replication. *J Gen Virol* 1999;80:1383–1391.
388. Nagai Y, Klenk HD. Activation of precursors to both glycoproteins of Newcastle disease virus by proteolytic cleavage. *Virology* 1977;77:125–134.
389. Nagai Y, Klenk HD, Rott R. Proteolytic cleavage of the viral glycoproteins and its significance for the virulence of Newcastle disease virus. *Virology* 1976;72(2):494–508.
390. Nagai Y, Ogura H, Klenk HD. Studies on the assembly of the envelope of Newcastle disease virus. *Virology* 1976;69:523–538.
391. Naim HY, Ehler E, Billeter MA. Measles virus matrix protein specifies apical virus release and glycoprotein sorting in epithelial cells. *EMBO J* 2000;19:3576–3585.
392. Nakatsu Y, Ma X, Seki F, et al. Intracellular transport of the measles virus ribonucleoprotein complex is mediated by Rab11A-positive recycling endosomes and drives virus release from the apical membrane of polarized epithelial cells. *J Virol* 2013;87(8):4683–4693.
393. Nakatsu Y, Takeda M, Ohno S, et al. Translational inhibition and increased interferon induction in cells infected with C protein-deficient measles virus. *J Virol* 2006;80(23):11861–11867.
394. Nakatsu Y, Takeda M, Ohno S, et al. Measles virus circumvents the host interferon response by different actions of the C and V proteins. *J Virol* 2008;82(17):8296–8306.
395. Naniche D, Varior-Krishnan G, Cervoni F, et al. Human membrane cofactor protein (CD46) acts as a cellular receptor for measles virus. *J Virol* 1993;67:6025–6032.
396. Negrete OA, Levroney EL, Aguilar HC, et al. EphrinB2 is the entry receptor for Nipah virus, an emergent deadly paramyxovirus. *Nature* 2005;436:401–405.
397. Neubauer J, Ogino M, Green TJ, et al. Signature motifs of GDP polyribonucleotidyltransferase, a non-segmented negative strand RNA viral mRNA capping enzyme, domain in the L protein are required for covalent enzyme-pRNA intermediate formation. *Nucleic Acids Res* 2016;44(1):330–341.
398. Newman JT, Surman SR, Riggs JM, et al. Sequence analysis of the Washington/1964 strain of human parainfluenza virus type 1 (HPIV1) and recovery and characterization of wild-type recombinant HPIV1 produced by reverse genetics. *Virus Genes* 2002;24(1):77–92.
399. Ng DT, Hiebert SW, Lamb RA. Different roles of individual N-linked oligosaccharide chains in folding, assembly, and transport of the simian virus 5 hemagglutinin-neuraminidase. *Mol Cell Biol* 1990;10:1989–2001.
400. Ng DT, Randall RE, Lamb RA. Intracellular maturation and transport of the SV5 type II glycoprotein hemagglutinin-neuraminidase: specific and transient association with GRP78-BiP in the endoplasmic reticulum and extensive internalization from the cell surface. *J Cell Biol* 1989;109:3273–3289.
401. Nickerson DP, Russell MR, Odorizzi G. A concentric circle model of multivesicular body cargo sorting. *EMBO Rep* 2007;8(7):644–650.
402. Nishio M, Tsurudome M, Ito M, et al. Human parainfluenza virus type 2 phosphoprotein: mapping of monoclonal antibody epitopes and location of the multimerization domain. *J Gen Virol* 1997;78(Pt 6):1303–1308.
403. Nishio M, Tsurudome M, Ito M, et al. Mapping of domains on the human parainfluenza virus type 2 nucleocapsid protein (NP) required for NP-phosphoprotein or NP-NP interaction. *J Gen Virol* 1999;80:2017–2022.
404. Noton SL, Cowton VM, Zack CR, et al. Evidence that the polymerase of respiratory syncytial virus initiates RNA replication in a nontemplated fashion. *Proc Natl Acad Sci U S A* 2010;107(22):10226–10231.
405. Noton SL, Fearns R. The first two nucleotides of the respiratory syncytial virus antigenome RNA replication product can be selected independently of the promoter terminus. *RNA* 2011;17(10):1895–1906.
406. Noton SL, Fearns R. Initiation and regulation of paramyxovirus transcription and replication. *Virology* 2015;479–480:545–554.
407. Noton SL, Nagendra K, Dunn EF, et al. Respiratory syncytial virus inhibitor AZ-27 differentially inhibits different polymerase activities at the promoter. *J Virol* 2015;89(15): 7786–7798.
408. Noyce RS, Bondre DG, Ha MN, et al. Tumor cell marker PVRL4 (nectin 4) is an epithelial cell receptor for measles virus. *PLoS Pathog* 2011;7:e1002240.
409. O'Reilly EK, Kao CC. Analysis of RNA-dependent RNA polymerase structure and function as guided by known polymerase structures and computer predictions of secondary structure. *Virology* 1998;252(2):287–303.
410. Ogino T. Capping of vesicular stomatitis virus pre-mRNA is required for accurate selection of transcription stop-start sites and virus propagation. *Nucleic Acids Res* 2014;42(19): 12112–12125.
411. Ogino T, Banerjee AK. Unconventional mechanism of mRNA capping by the RNA-dependent RNA polymerase of vesicular stomatitis virus. *Mol Cell* 2007;25(1):85–97.
412. Ogino T, Banerjee AK. Formation of guanosine(5′)tetraphospho(5′)adenosine cap structure by an unconventional mRNA capping enzyme of vesicular stomatitis virus. *J Virol* 2008;82(15):7729–7734.
413. Ogino T, Banerjee AK. The HR motif in the RNA-dependent RNA polymerase L protein of Chandipura virus is required for unconventional mRNA-capping activity. *J Gen Virol* 2010;91(Pt 5):1311–1314.
414. Ogino M, Gupta N, Green TJ, et al. A dual-functional priming-capping loop of rhabdoviral RNA polymerases directs terminal de novo initiation and capping intermediate formation. *Nucleic Acids Res* 2019;47(1):299–309.
415. Ogino M, Ito N, Sugiyama M, et al. The rabies virus L protein catalyzes mRNA capping with GDP polyribonucleotidyltransferase activity. *Viruses* 2016;8(5).
416. Ogino T, Kobayashi M, Iwama M, et al. Sendai virus RNA-dependent RNA polymerase L protein catalyzes cap methylation of virus-specific mRNA. *J Biol Chem* 2005;280:4429–4435.
417. Ohno S, Ono N, Takeda M, et al. Dissection of measles virus V protein in relation to its ability to block alpha/beta interferon signal transduction. *J Gen Virol* 2004;85:2991–2999.
418. Oldstone MBA, Homann D, Lewicki H, et al. One, two, or three step: measles virus receptor dance. *Virology* 2002;299:162-163.
419. Olmsted RA, Elango N, Prince GA, et al. Expression of the F glycoprotein of respiratory syncytial virus by a recombinant vaccinia virus: comparison of the individual contributions of the F and G glycoproteins to host immunity. *Proc Natl Acad Sci U S A* 1986;83:7462–7466.
420. Ortmann D, Ohuchi M, Angliker H, et al. Proteolytic cleavage of wild type and mutants of the F protein of human parainfluenza virus type 3 by two subtilisin-like endoproteases, furin and KEX2. *J Virol* 1994;68:2772–2776.
421. Paal T, Brindley MA, St Clair C, et al. Probing the spatial organization of measles virus fusion complexes. *J Virol* 2009;83:10480–10493.
422. Paesen GC, Collet A, Sallamand C, et al. X-ray structure and activities of an essential Mononegavirales L-protein domain. *Nat Commun* 2015;6:8749.
423. Pager CT, Dutch RE. Cathepsin L is involved in proteolytic processing of the Hendra virus fusion protein. *J Virol* 2005;79:12714–12720.
424. Pantua HD, McGinnes LW, Peeples ME, et al. Requirements for the assembly and release of Newcastle disease virus-like particles. *J Virol* 2006;80(22):11062–11073.
425. Parisien JP, Bamming D, Komuro A, et al. A shared interface mediates paramyxovirus interference with antiviral RNA helicases MDA5 and LGP2. *J Virol* 2009;83(14):7252–7260.
426. Parisien JP, Lau JF, Horvath CM. STAT2 acts as a host range determinant for species-specific paramyxovirus interferon antagonism and simian virus 5 replication. *J Virol* 2002;76:6435–6441.
427. Parisien JP, Lau JF, Rodriguez JJ, et al. The V protein of human parainfluenza virus 2 antagonizes type I interferon responses by destabilizing signal transducer and activator of transcription 2. *Virology* 2001;283:230–239.
428. Parisien JP, Lau JF, Rodriguez JJ, et al. Selective STAT protein degradation induced by paramyxoviruses requires both STAT1 and STAT2 but is independent of alpha/beta interferon signal transduction. *J Virol* 2002;76:4190–4198.
429. Park MS, Garcia-Sastre A, Cros JF, et al. Newcastle disease virus V protein is a determinant of host range restriction. *J Virol* 2003;77:9522–9532.
430. Park S, Juliana C, Hong S, et al. The mitochondrial antiviral protein MAVS associates with NLRP3 and regulates its inflammasome activity. *J Immunol* 2013;191(8):4358–4366.
431. Park A, Yun T, Vigant F, et al. Nipah virus C protein recruits Tsg101 to promote the efficient release of virus in an ESCRT-dependent pathway. *PLoS Pathog* 2016;12(5):e1005659.
432. Parks GD. Mapping of a region of the paramyxovirus L protein required for the formation of a stable complex with the viral phosphoprotein P. *J Virol* 1994;68:4862–4872.
433. Parks GD, Alexander-Miller MA. Paramyxovirus activation and inhibition of innate immune responses. *J Mol Biol* 2013;425(24):4872–4892.
434. Parks GD, Lamb RA. Folding and oligomerization properties of a soluble and secreted form of the paramyxovirus hemagglutinin-neuraminidase glycoprotein. *Virology* 1990;178:498–508.
435. Parks CL, Witko SE, Kotash C, et al. Role of V protein RNA binding in inhibition of measles virus minigenome replication. *Virology* 2006;348(1):96–106.
436. Patch JR, Crameri G, Wang LF, et al. Quantitative analysis of Nipah virus proteins released as virus-like particles reveals central role for the matrix protein. *Virol J* 2007;4:1.
437. Patch JR, Han Z, McCarthy SE, et al. The YPLGVG sequence of the Nipah virus matrix protein is required for budding. *Virol J* 2008;5:137.
438. Paterson RG, Lamb RA. RNA editing by G-nucleotide insertion in mumps virus P-gene mRNA transcripts. *J Virol* 1990;64:4137–4145.
439. Paterson RG, Harris TJR, Lamb RA. Analysis and gene assignment of mRNAs of a paramyxovirus, simian virus 5. *Virology* 1984;138:310–323.
440. Paterson RG, Hiebert SW, Lamb RA. Expression at the cell surface of biologically active fusion and hemagglutinin-neuraminidase proteins of the paramyxovirus simian virus 5 from cloned cDNA. *Proc Natl Acad Sci U S A* 1985;82:7520–7524.
441. Paterson RG, Leser GP, Shaughnessy MA, et al. The paramyxovirus SV5 V protein binds two atoms of zinc and is a structural component of virions. *Virology* 1995;208:121–131.
442. Paterson RG, Russell CJ, Lamb RA. Fusion protein of the paramyxovirus SV5: destabilizing and stabilizing mutants of fusion activation. *Virology* 2000;270:17–30.
443. Paterson RG, Shaughnessy MA, Lamb RA. Analysis of the relationship between cleavability of a paramyxovirus fusion protein and length of the connecting peptide. *J Virol* 1989;63:1293–1301.
444. Paterson RG, Thomas SM, Lamb RA. Specific nontemplated nucleotide addition to a simian virus 5 mRNA: prediction of a common mechanism by which unrecognized hybrid P-cysteine-rich proteins are encoded by paramyxovirus "P" genes. In: Kolakofsky D, Mahy BWJ, eds. *Genetics and Pathogenicity of Negative Strand Viruses*. London: Elsevier; 1989:232–245.
445. Patnaik A, Chau V, Wills JW. Ubiquitin is part of the retrovirus budding machinery. *Proc Natl Acad Sci U S A* 2000;97(24):13069–13074.
446. Patterson JB, Thomas D, Lewicki H, et al. V and C proteins of measles virus function as virulence factors in vivo. *Virology* 2000;267:80–89.
447. Pattnaik AK, Ball LA, LeGrone AW, et al. Infectious defective interfering particles of VSV from transcripts of a cDNA clone. *Cell* 1992;69:1011–1020.
448. Peeples ME, Wang C, Gupta KC, et al. Nuclear entry and nucleolar localization of the Newcastle disease virus (NDV) matrix protein occur early in infection and do not require other NDV proteins. *J Virol* 1992;66:3263–3269.
449. Pelet T, Delenda C, Gubbay O, et al. Partial characterization of a Sendai virus replication promoter and the rule of six. *Virology* 1996;224:405–414.

450. Pennington TH, Pringle CR. Negative strand viruses in enucleate cells. In: Mahy BWJ, Barry RD, eds. *Negative Strand Viruses and the Host Cell*. New York: Academic Press, Inc.; 1978:457–464.
451. Pentecost M, Vashisht AA, Lester T, et al. Evidence for ubiquitin-regulated nuclear and subnuclear trafficking among Paramyxovirinae matrix proteins. *PLoS Pathog* 2015;11(3): e1004739.
452. Pfaller CK, Conzelmann KK. Measles virus V protein is a decoy substrate for IkappaB kinase alpha and prevents Toll-like receptor 7/9-mediated interferon induction. *J Virol* 2008;82:12365–12373.
453. Pfaller CK, Radeke MJ, Cattaneo R, et al. Measles virus C protein impairs production of defective copyback double-stranded viral RNA and activation of protein kinase R. *J Virol* 2014;88(1):456–468.
454. Plattet P, Strahle L, le Mercier P, et al. Sendai virus RNA polymerase scanning for mRNA start sites at gene junctions. *Virology* 2007;362(2):411–420.
455. Plemper RK. Cell entry of enveloped viruses. *Curr Opin Virol* 2011;1(2):92–100.
456. Plemper RK, Erlandson KJ, Lakdawala AS, et al. A target site for template-based design of measles virus entry inhibitors. *Proc Natl Acad Sci U S A* 2004;101(15):5628–5633.
457. Plemper RK, Hammond AL, Cattaneo R. Characterization of a region of the measles virus hemagglutinin sufficient for its dimerization. *J Virol* 2000;74:6485–6493.
458. Plemper RK, Hammond AL, Cattaneo R. Measles virus envelope glycoproteins hetero-oligomerize in the endoplasmic reticulum. *J Biol Chem* 2001;276:44239–44246.
459. Plemper RK, Hammond AL, Gerlier D, et al. Strength of envelope protein interaction modulates cytopathicity of measles virus. *J Virol* 2002;76:5051–5061.
460. Plumet S, Duprex WP, Gerlier D. Dynamics of viral RNA synthesis during measles virus infection. *J Virol* 2005;79(11):6900–6908.
461. Poch O, Blumberg BM, Bougueleret L, et al. Sequence comparison of five polymerases (L proteins) of unsegmented negative-strand RNA viruses: theoretical assignment of functional domains. *J Gen Virol* 1990;71:1153–1162.
462. Poch O, Sauvaget I, Delarue M, et al. Identification of four conserved motifs among the RNA-dependent polymerase encoding elements. *EMBO J* 1989;8:3867–3874.
463. Pohl C, Duprex WP, Krohne G, et al. Measles virus M and F proteins associate with detergent-resistant membrane fractions and promote formation of virus-like particles. *J Gen Virol* 2007;88(Pt 4):1243–1250.
464. Poor TA, Song AS, Welch BD, et al. On the stability of parainfluenza virus 5 F proteins. *J Virol* 2015;89(6):3438–3441.
465. Porotto M, Fornabaio M, Greengard O, et al. Paramyxovirus receptor-binding molecules: engagement of one site on the hemagglutinin-neuraminidase protein modulates activity at the second site. *J Virol* 2006;80:1204–1213.
466. Porotto M, Murrell M, Greengard O, et al. Triggering of human parainfluenza virus 3 fusion protein (F) by the hemagglutinin-neuraminidase (HN) protein: an HN mutation diminishes the rate of F activation and fusion. *J Virol* 2003;77:3647–3654.
467. Portner A, Marx PA, Kingsbury DW. Isolation and characterization of Sendai virus temperature-sensitive mutants. *J Virol* 1974;13:298–304.
468. Portner A, Murti KG, Morgan EM, et al. Antibodies against Sendai virus L protein: distribution of the protein in nucleocapsids revealed by immunoelectron microscopy. *Virology* 1988;163:236–239.
469. Portner A, Scroggs RA, Metzger DW. Distinct functions of antigenic sites of the HN glycoprotein of Sendai virus. *Virology* 1987;158:61–68.
470. Precious BL, Carlos TS, Goodbourn S, et al. Catalytic turnover of STAT1 allows PIV5 to dismantle the interferon-induced anti-viral state of cells. *Virology* 2007;368:114–121.
471. Precious B, Childs K, Fitzpatrick-Swallow V, et al. Simian virus 5 V protein acts as an adaptor, linking DDB1 to STAT2, to facilitate the ubiquitination of STAT1. *J Virol* 2005;79: 13434–13441.
472. Precious B, Young DF, Bermingham A, et al. Inducible expression of the P, V, and NP genes of the paramyxovirus simian virus 5 in cell lines and an examination of NP-P and NP-V interactions. *J Virol* 1995;69:8001–8010.
473. Qiu S, Ogino M, Luo M, et al. Structure and function of the N-terminal domain of the vesicular stomatitis virus RNA polymerase. *J Virol* 2016;90(2):715–724.
474. Radecke F, Spielhofer P, Schneider H, et al. Rescue of measles viruses from cloned DNA. *EMBO J* 1995;14:5773–5784.
475. Rager M, Vongpunsawad S, Duprex WP, et al. Polyploid measles virus with hexameric genome length. *EMBO J* 2002;21(10):2364–2372.
476. Raha T, Kaushik R, Shaila MS. Phosphoprotein P of rinderpest virus binds to plus sense leader RNA: regulation by phosphorylation. *Virus Res* 2004;104(2):191–200.
477. Rahmeh AA, Li J, Kranzusch PJ, et al. Ribose 2′-O methylation of the vesicular stomatitis virus mRNA cap precedes and facilitates subsequent guanine-N-7 methylation by the large polymerase protein. *J Virol* 2009;83(21):11043–11050.
478. Rahmeh AA, Schenk AD, Danek EI, et al. Molecular architecture of the vesicular stomatitis virus RNA polymerase. *Proc Natl Acad Sci U S A* 2010;107(46):20075–20080.
479. Ramachandran A, Horvath CM. Dissociation of paramyxovirus interferon evasion activities: universal and virus-specific requirements for conserved V protein amino acids in MDA5 interference. *J Virol* 2010;84(21):11152–11163.
480. Ramachandran A, Parisien JP, Horvath CM. STAT2 is a primary target for measles virus V protein-mediated alpha/beta interferon signaling inhibition. *J Virol* 2008;82(17): 8330–8338.
481. Rassa JC, Parks GD. Molecular basis for naturally occurring elevated readthrough transcription across the M-F junction of the paramyxovirus SV5. *Virology* 1998;247:274–286.
482. Rassa JC, Parks GD. Highly diverse intergenic regions of the paramyxovirus simian virus 5 cooperate with the gene end U tract in viral transcription termination and can influence reinitiation at a downstream gene. *J Virol* 1999;73:3904–3912.
483. Rathinam VA, Vanaja SK, Fitzgerald KA. Regulation of inflammasome signaling. *Nat Immunol* 2012;13(4):333–342.
484. Rawlinson SM, Zhao T, Rozario AM, et al. Viral regulation of host cell biology by hijacking of the nucleolar DNA-damage response. *Nat Commun* 2018;9(1):3057.
485. Ray G, Schmitt PT, Schmitt AP. C-terminal DxD-containing sequences within paramyxovirus nucleocapsid proteins determine matrix protein compatibility and can direct foreign proteins into budding particles. *J Virol* 2016;90(7):3650–3660.
486. Ray G, Schmitt PT, Schmitt AP. Angiomotin-like 1 links paramyxovirus M proteins to NEDD4 family ubiquitin ligases. *Viruses* 2019;11(2).
487. Rima B, Collins P, Easton A, et al. Problems of classification in the family *Paramyxoviridae*. *Arch Virol* 2018;163(5):1395–1404.
488. Rodriguez JJ, Cruz CD, Horvath CM. Identification of the nuclear export signal and STAT-binding domains of the Nipah virus V protein reveals mechanisms underlying interferon evasion. *J Virol* 2004;78:5358–5367.
489. Rodriguez KR, Horvath CM. Amino acid requirements for MDA5 and LGP2 recognition by paramyxovirus V proteins: a single arginine distinguishes MDA5 from RIG-I. *J Virol* 2013;87(5):2974–2978.
490. Rodriguez KR, Horvath CM. Paramyxovirus V protein interaction with the antiviral sensor LGP2 disrupts MDA5 signaling enhancement but is not relevant to LGP2-mediated RLR signaling inhibition. *J Virol* 2014;88(14):8180–8188.
491. Rodriguez JJ, Wang LF, Horvath CM. Hendra virus V protein inhibits interferon signaling by preventing STAT1 and STAT2 nuclear accumulation. *J Virol* 2003;77: 11842–11845.
492. Rodriguez-Boulan E, Sabatini DD. Asymmetric budding of viruses in epithelial monolayers; a model system for study of epithelial polarity. *Proc Natl Acad Sci U S A* 1978;75:5071–5075.
493. Romer-Oberdorfer A, Mundt E, Mebatsion T, et al. Generation of recombinant lentogenic Newcastle disease virus from cDNA. *J Gen Virol* 1999;80(Pt 11):2987–2995.
494. Rosas-Murrieta NH, Herrera-Camacho I, Palma-Ocampo H, et al. Interaction of mumps virus V protein variants with STAT1-STAT2 heterodimer: experimental and theoretical studies. *Virol J* 2010;7:263.
495. Rossman JS, Lamb RA. Influenza virus assembly and budding. *Virology* 2011;411:229–236.
496. Rothenfusser S, Goutagny N, DiPerna G, et al. The RNA helicase Lgp2 inhibits TLR-independent sensing of viral replication by retinoic acid-inducible gene-I. *J Immunol* 2005;175(8):5260–5268.
497. Rothlisberger A, Wiener D, Schweizer M, et al. Two domains of the V protein of virulent canine distemper virus selectively inhibit STAT1 and STAT2 nuclear import. *J Virol* 2010;84(13):6328–6343.
498. Roux L, Waldvogel FA. Instability of the viral M protein in BHK-21 cells persistently infected with Sendai virus. *Cell* 1982;28:293–302.
499. Ruedas JB, Perrault J. Insertion of enhanced green fluorescent protein in a hinge region of vesicular stomatitis virus L polymerase protein creates a temperature-sensitive virus that displays no virion-associated polymerase activity in vitro. *J Virol* 2009;83(23):12241–12252.
500. Ruiz-Arguello MB, Gonzalez-Reyes L, Calder LJ, et al. Effect of proteolytic processing at two distinct sites on shape and aggregation of an anchorless fusion protein of human respiratory syncytial virus and fate of the intervening segment. *Virology* 2002;298:317–326.
501. Ruiz-Arguello MB, Martin D, Wharton SA, et al. Thermostability of the human respiratory syncytial virus fusion protein before and after activation: implications for the membrane-fusion mechanism. *J Gen Virol* 2004;85:3677–3687.
502. Runkler N, Pohl C, Schneider-Schaulies S, et al. Measles virus nucleocapsid transport to the plasma membrane requires stable expression and surface accumulation of the viral matrix protein. *Cell Microbiol* 2007;9(5):1203–1214.
503. Russell CJ, Jardetzky TS, Lamb RA. Membrane fusion machines of paramyxoviruses: capture of intermediates of fusion. *EMBO J* 2001;20:4024–4034.
504. Russell CJ, Kantor KL, Jardetzky TS, et al. A dual-functional paramyxovirus F protein regulatory switch segment: activation and membrane fusion. *J Cell Biol* 2003;163: 363–374.
505. Russell R, Paterson RG, Lamb RA. Studies with cross-linking reagents on the oligomeric form of the paramyxovirus fusion protein. *Virology* 1994;199:160–168.
506. Ryan KW, Morgan EM, Portner A. Two noncontiguous regions of Sendai virus P protein combine to form a single nucleocapsid binding domain. *Virology* 1991;180:126–134.
507. Saikia P, Gopinath M, Shaila MS. Phosphorylation status of the phosphoprotein P of rinderpest virus modulates transcription and replication of the genome. *Arch Virol* 2008;153(4):615–626.
508. Sakaguchi T, Kato A, Sugahara F, et al. AIP1/Alix is a binding partner of Sendai virus C protein and facilitates virus budding. *J Virol* 2005;79:8933–8941.
509. Sakai Y, Shibuta H. Syncytium formation by recombinant vaccinia viruses carrying bovine parainfluenza 3 virus envelope protein genes. *J Virol* 1989;63:3661–3668.
510. Salditt A, Koethe S, Pohl C, et al. Measles virus M protein-driven particle production does not involve the endosomal sorting complex required for transport (ESCRT) system. *J Gen Virol* 2010;91(Pt 6):1464–1472.
511. Sanchez-Aparicio MT, Feinman LJ, Garcia-Sastre A, et al. Paramyxovirus V proteins interact with the RIG-I/TRIM25 regulatory complex and inhibit RIG-I signaling. *J Virol* 2018;92(6).
512. Sanderson CM, Avalos R, Kundu A, et al. Interaction of Sendai viral F, HN, and M proteins with host cytoskeletal and lipid components in Sendai virus-infected BHK cells. *Virology* 1995;209:701–707.
513. Sanderson CM, McQueen NL, Nayak DP. Sendai virus assembly: M protein binds to viral glycoproteins in transit through the secretory pathway. *J Virol* 1993;67:651–663.
514. Sanderson CM, Wu HH, Nayak DP. Sendai virus M protein binds independently to either the F or the HN glycoprotein in vivo. *J Virol* 1993;68:69–76.
515. Santiago C, Celma ML, Stehle T, et al. Structure of the measles virus hemagglutinin bound to the CD46 receptor. *Nat Struct Mol Biol* 2010;17:124–129.
516. Satoh T, Kato H, Kumagai Y, et al. LGP2 is a positive regulator of RIG-I- and MDA5-mediated antiviral responses. *Proc Natl Acad Sci U S A* 2010;107(4):1512–1517.
517. Scheid A, Caliguiri LA, Compans RW, et al. Isolation of paramyxovirus glycoproteins. Association of both hemagglutinating and neuraminidase activities with the larger SV5 glycoprotein. *Virology* 1972;50:640–652.
518. Scheid A, Choppin PW. The hemagglutinating and neuraminidase protein of a paramyxovirus: interaction with neuraminic acid in affinity chromatography. *Virology* 1974;62:125–133.
519. Scheid A, Choppin PW. Identification of biological activities of paramyxovirus glycoproteins. Activation of cell fusion, hemolysis, and infectivity of proteolytic cleavage of an inactive precursor protein of Sendai virus. *Virology* 1974;57:475–490.

520. Schmitt AP, He B, Lamb RA. Involvement of the cytoplasmic domain of the hemagglutinin-neuraminidase protein in assembly of the paramyxovirus simian virus 5. *J Virol* 1999;73:8703–8712.
521. Schmitt AP, Lamb RA. Escaping from the cell: assembly and budding of negative-strand RNA viruses. *Curr Top Microbiol Immunol* 2004;283:145–196.
522. Schmitt AP, Lamb RA. Influenza virus assembly and budding at the viral budozone. *Adv Virus Res* 2005;64:383–416.
523. Schmitt AP, Leser GP, Morita E, et al. Evidence for a new viral late-domain core sequence, FPIV, necessary for budding of a paramyxovirus. *J Virol* 2005;79:2988–2997.
524. Schmitt AP, Leser GP, Waning DL, et al. Requirements for budding of paramyxovirus simian virus 5 virus-like particles. *J Virol* 2002;76:3952–3964.
525. Schmitt PT, Ray G, Schmitt AP. The C-terminal end of parainfluenza virus 5 NP protein is important for virus-like particle production and M-NP protein interaction. *J Virol* 2010;84(24):12810–12823.
526. Schneider WM, Chevillotte MD, Rice CM. Interferon-stimulated genes: a complex web of host defenses. *Annu Rev Immunol* 2014;32:513–545.
527. Schneider H, Kaelin K, Billeter MA. Recombinant measles viruses defective for RNA editing and V protein synthesis are viable in cultured cells. *Virology* 1997;227:314–322.
528. Schnell MJ, Mebatsion T, Conzelmann KK. Infectious rabies viruses from cloned cDNA. *EMBO J* 1994;13(18):4195–4203.
529. Schoehn G, Mavrakis M, Albertini A, et al. The 12 A structure of trypsin-treated measles virus N-RNA. *J Mol Biol* 2004;339:301–312.
530. Schomacker H, Hebner RM, Boonyaratanakornkit J, et al. The C proteins of human parainfluenza virus type 1 block IFN signaling by binding and retaining STAT1 in perinuclear aggregates at the late endosome. *PLoS One* 2012;7(2):e28382.
531. Schoneberg J, Lee IH, Iwasa JH, et al. Reverse-topology membrane scission by the ESCRT proteins. *Nat Rev Mol Cell Biol* 2017;18(1):5–17.
532. Schubert U, Ott DE, Chertova EN, et al. Proteasome inhibition interferes with gag polyprotein processing, release, and maturation of HIV-1 and HIV-2. *Proc Natl Acad Sci U S A* 2000;97(24):13057–13062.
533. Sergel R, McGinnes LW, Morrison TG. The fusion promotion activity of the NDV HN protein does not correlate with neuraminidase activity. *Virology* 1993;196:831–834.
534. Sergel TA, McGinnes LW, Morrison TG. A single amino acid change in the Newcastle disease virus fusion protein alters the requirement for HN protein in fusion. *J Virol* 2000;74:5101–5107.
535. Sergel T, McGinnes LW, Peeples ME, et al. The attachment function of the Newcastle disease virus hemagglutinin-neuraminidase protein can be separated from fusion promotion by mutation. *Virology* 1993;193:717–726.
536. Severin C, Terrell JR, Zengel JR, et al. Releasing the genomic RNA sequestered in the mumps virus nucleocapsid. *J Virol* 2016;90(22):10113–10119.
537. Shaw ML, Cardenas WB, Zamarin D, et al. Nuclear localization of the Nipah virus W protein allows for inhibition of both virus- and toll-like receptor 3-triggered signaling pathways. *J Virol* 2005;79:6078–6088.
538. Shaw ML, Garcia-Sastre A, Palese P, et al. Nipah virus V and W proteins have a common STAT1-binding domain yet inhibit STAT1 activation from the cytoplasmic and nuclear compartments, respectively. *J Virol* 2004;78:5633–5641.
539. Shields SB, Piper RC. How ubiquitin functions with ESCRTs. *Traffic* 2011;12(10):1306–1317.
540. Shil NK, Pokharel SM, Banerjee AK, et al. Inflammasome antagonism by human parainfluenza virus type 3 C protein. *J Virol* 2018;92(4).
541. Shrivastava G, Leon-Juarez M, Garcia-Cordero J, et al. Inflammasomes and its importance in viral infections. *Immunol Res* 2016;64(5–6):1101–1117.
542. Sidhu MS, Menonna JP, Cook SD, et al. Canine distemper virus L gene: sequence and comparison with related viruses. *Virology* 1993;193:50–65.
543. Sievers F, Higgins DG. Clustal omega. *Curr Protoc Bioinformatics* 2014;48:3. 13 11-16.
544. Simons K, Gerl MJ. Revitalizing membrane rafts: new tools and insights. *Nat Rev Mol Cell Biol* 2010;11(10):688–699.
545. Simons K, Ikonen E. Functional rafts in cell membranes. *Nature* 1997;387:569–572.
546. Singh PK, Ratnam N, Narayanarao KB, et al. A carboxy terminal domain of the L protein of rinderpest virus possesses RNA triphosphatase activity—The first enzyme in the viral mRNA capping pathway. *Biochem Biophys Res Commun* 2015;464(2):629–634.
547. Singh PK, Subbarao SM. The RNA triphosphatase domain of L protein of Rinderpest virus exhibits pyrophosphatase and tripolyphosphatase activities. *Virus Genes* 2016;52(5):743–747.
548. Skehel JJ, Wiley DC. Receptor binding and membrane fusion in virus entry: the influenza hemagglutinin. *Annu Rev Biochem* 2000;69:531–569.
549. Sleeman K, Bankamp B, Hummel KB, et al. The C, V and W proteins of Nipah virus inhibit minigenome replication. *J Gen Virol* 2008;89(Pt 5):1300–1308.
550. Smallwood S, Cevik B, Moyer SA. Intragenic complementation and oligomerization of the L subunit of the sendai virus RNA polymerase. *Virology* 2002;304:235–245.
551. Smallwood S, Easson CD, Feller JA, et al. Mutations in conserved domain II of the large (L) subunit of the Sendai virus RNA polymerase abolish RNA synthesis. *Virology* 1999;262:375–383.
552. Smallwood S, Moyer SA. The L polymerase protein of parainfluenza virus 3 forms an oligomer and can interact with the heterologous Sendai virus L, P and C proteins. *Virology* 2004;318:439–450.
553. Smith KM, Tsimbalyuk S, Edwards MR, et al. Structural basis for importin alpha 3 specificity of W proteins in Hendra and Nipah viruses. *Nat Commun* 2018;9(1):3703.
554. Snead WT, Stachowiak JC. Structure versus stochasticity-the role of molecular crowding and intrinsic disorder in membrane fission. *J Mol Biol* 2018;430(16):2293–2308.
555. Sourimant J, Plemper RK. Organization, function, and therapeutic targeting of the morbillivirus RNA-dependent RNA polymerase complex. *Viruses* 2016;8(9).
556. Sparrer KM, Pfaller CK, Conzelmann KK. Measles virus C protein interferes with Beta interferon transcription in the nucleus. *J Virol* 2012;86:796–805.
557. Spehner D, Drillien R, Howley PM. The assembly of the measles virus nucleoprotein into nucleocapsid-like particles is modulated by the phosphoprotein. *Virology* 1997;232:260–268.
558. Spehner D, Kirn A, Drillien R. Assembly of nucleocapsidlike structures in animal cells infected with a vaccinia virus recombinant encoding the measles virus nucleoprotein. *J Virol* 1991;65:6296–6300.
559. Spriggs MK, Collins PL. Human parainfluenza virus type 3: messenger RNAs, polypeptide coding assignments, intergenic sequences, and genetic map. *J Virol* 1986;59:646–654.
560. Stallcup KC, Raine CS, Fields BN. Cytochalasin B inhibits the maturation of measles virus. *Virology* 1983;124(1):59–74.
561. Steinhauer DA, Plemper RK. Structure of the primed paramyxovirus fusion protein. *Proc Natl Acad Sci U S A* 2012;109(41):16404–16405.
562. Stillman EA, Whitt MA. Transcript initiation and 5′-end modifications are separable events during vesicular stomatitis virus transcription. *J Virol* 1999;73(9):7199–7209.
563. Stone R, Takimoto T. Critical role of the fusion protein cytoplasmic tail sequence in parainfluenza virus assembly. *PLoS One* 2013;8(4):e61281.
564. Stone-Hulslander J, Morrison TG. Detection of an interaction between the HN and F proteins in Newcastle disease virus-infected cells. *J Virol* 1997;71:6287–6295.
565. Stone-Hulslander J, Morrison TG. Mutational analysis of heptad repeats in the membrane-proximal region of Newcastle disease virus HN protein. *J Virol* 1999;73:3630–3637.
566. Strack B, Calistri A, Accola MA, et al. A role for ubiquitin ligase recruitment in retrovirus release. *Proc Natl Acad Sci U S A* 2000;97(24):13063–13068.
567. Stricker R, Mottet G, Roux L. The Sendai virus matrix protein appears to be recruited in the cytoplasm by the viral nucleocapsid to function in viral assembly and budding. *J Gen Virol* 1994;75:1031–1042.
568. Sugahara F, Uchiyama T, Watanabe H, et al. Paramyxovirus Sendai virus-like particle formation by expression of multiple viral proteins and acceleration of its release by C protein. *Virology* 2004;325:1–10.
569. Sugai A, Sato H, Yoneda M, et al. Phosphorylation of measles virus phosphoprotein at S86 and/or S151 downregulates viral transcriptional activity. *FEBS Lett* 2012;586(21):3900–3907.
570. Sun W, McCrory TS, Khaw WY, et al. Matrix proteins of Nipah and Hendra viruses interact with beta subunits of AP-3 complexes. *J Virol* 2014;88(22):13099–13110.
571. Svenda M, Berg M, Moreno-Lopez J, et al. Analysis of the large (L) protein gene of the porcine rubulavirus LPMV: identification of possible functional domains. *Virus Res* 1997;48:57–70.
572. Svitek N, Gerhauser I, Goncalves C, et al. Morbillivirus control of the interferon response: relevance of STAT2 and mda5 but not STAT1 for canine distemper virus virulence in ferrets. *J Virol* 2014;88(5):2941–2950.
573. Sweetman DA, Miskin J, Baron MD. Rinderpest virus C and V proteins interact with the major (L) component of the viral polymerase. *Virology* 2001;281:193–204.
574. Tahara M, Takeda M, Yanagi Y. Altered interaction of the matrix protein with the cytoplasmic tail of hemagglutinin modulates measles virus growth by affecting virus assembly and cell-cell fusion. *J Virol* 2007;81(13):6827–6836.
575. Takagi T, Muroya K, Iwama M, et al. In vitro mRNA synthesis by Sendai virus: isolation and characterization of the transcription initiation complex. *J Biochem* 1995;118(2):390–396.
576. Takahashi T, Suzuki T. Function of membrane rafts in viral lifecycles and host cellular response. *Biochem Res Int* 2011;2011:245090.
577. Takeuchi K, Komatsu T, Kitagawa Y, et al. Sendai virus C protein plays a role in restricting PKR activation by limiting the generation of intracellular double-stranded RNA. *J Virol* 2008;82:10102–10110.
578. Takeuchi K, Komatsu T, Yokoo J, et al. Sendai virus C protein physically associates with STAT1. *Genes Cells* 2001;6(6):545–557.
579. Takeuchi K, Tanabayashi K, Hishiyama M, et al. Variation of nucleotide sequences and transcription of the SH gene among mumps virus strains. *Virology* 1991;181:364–366.
580. Takeuchi K, Tanabayashi K, Hishiyama M, et al. The mumps virus SH protein is a membrane protein and not essential for virus growth. *Virology* 1996;225:156–162.
581. Takimoto T, Murti KG, Bousse T, et al. Role of matrix and fusion proteins in budding of Sendai virus. *J Virol* 2001;75:11384–11391.
582. Tamura T, Yanai H, Savitsky D, et al. The IRF family transcription factors in immunity and oncogenesis. *Annu Rev Immunol* 2008;26:535–584.
583. Tan K, Liu JH, Wang JH, et al. Atomic structure of a thermostable subdomain of HIV-1 gp41. *Proc Natl Acad Sci U S A* 1997;94:12303–12308.
584. Tanabayashi K, Compans RW. Functional interaction of paramyxovirus glycoproteins: identification of a domain in Sendai virus HN which promotes cell fusion. *J Virol* 1996;70:6112–6118.
585. Taniguchi T, Palmieri M, Weissmann C. Qb DNA-containing hybrid plasmids giving rise to Qb phage formation in the bacterial host. *Nature* 1978;274:223–228.
586. Tapparel C, Hausmann S, Pelet T, et al. Inhibition of Sendai virus genome replication due to promoter-increased selectivity: a possible role for the accessory C proteins. *J Virol* 1997;71:9588–9599.
587. Tapparel C, Maurice D, Roux L. The activity of Sendai virus genomic and antigenomic promoters requires a second element past the leader template regions: a motif (GNNNNN)3 is essential for replication. *J Virol* 1998;72(4):3117–3128.
588. Tarbouriech N, Curran J, Ebel C, et al. On the domain structure and the polymerization state of the sendai virus P protein. *Virology* 2000;266:99–109.
589. Tarbouriech N, Curran J, Ruigrok RW, et al. Tetrameric coiled coil domain of Sendai virus phosphoprotein. *Nat Struct Biol* 2000;7:777–781.
590. Tashiro M, Yamakawa M, Tobita K, et al. Altered budding site of a pantropic mutant of Sendai virus, F1-R, in polarized epithelial cells. *J Virol* 1990;64(10):4672–4677.
591. Tatsuo H, Ono N, Tanaka K, et al. SLAM (CDw150) is a cellular receptor for measles virus. *Nature* 2000;406(6798):893–897.
592. Taylor G. Sialidases: structures, biological significance and therapeutic potential. *Curr Opin Struct Biol* 1996;6:830–837.
593. Te Velthuis AJ, Robb NC, Kapanidis AN, et al. The role of the priming loop in influenza A virus RNA synthesis. *Nat Microbiol* 2016;1:16029.
594. Thakkar VD, Cox RM, Sawatsky B, et al. The unstructured paramyxovirus nucleocapsid protein tail domain modulates viral pathogenesis through regulation of transcriptase activity. *J Virol* 2018;92(8).

595. Thibault PA, Watkinson RE, Moreira-Soto A, et al. Zoonotic potential of emerging Paramyxoviruses: knowns and unknowns. *Adv Virus Res* 2017;98:1–55.

596. Thomas SM, Lamb RA, Paterson RG. Two mRNAs that differ by two nontemplated nucleotides encode the amino coterminal proteins P and V of the paramyxovirus SV5. *Cell* 1988;54:891–902.

597. Thompson SD, Laver WG, Murti KG, et al. Isolation of a biologically active soluble form of the hemagglutinin-neuraminidase protein of Sendai virus. *J Virol* 1988;62: 4653–4660.

598. Thompson SD, Portner A. Localization of functional sites on the hemagglutinin-neuraminidase glycoprotein of Sendai virus by sequence analysis of antigenic and temperature-sensitive mutants. *Virology* 1987;160:1–8.

599. Timmins J, Schoehn G, Ricard-Blum S, et al. Ebola virus matrix protein VP40 interaction with human cellular factors Tsg101 and Nedd4. *J Mol Biol* 2003;326:493–502.

600. Tober C, Seufert M, Schneider H, et al. Expression of measles virus V protein is associated with pathogenicity and control of viral RNA synthesis. *J Virol* 1998;72:8124–8132.

601. Tremaglio CZ, Noton SL, Deflube LR, et al. Respiratory syncytial virus polymerase can initiate transcription from position 3 of the leader promoter. *J Virol* 2013;87(6):3196–3207.

602. Tsurudome M, Bando H, Kawano M, et al. Transcripts of simian virus 41 (SV41) matrix gene are exclusively dicistronic with the fusion gene which is also transcribed as a monocistron. *Virology* 1991;184:93–100.

603. Ulane CM, Horvath CM. Paramyxoviruses SV5 and HPIV2 assemble STAT protein ubiquitin ligase complexes from cellular components. *Virology* 2002;304:160–166.

604. Ulane CM, Kentsis A, Cruz CD, et al. Composition and assembly of STAT-targeting ubiquitin ligase complexes: paramyxovirus V protein carboxyl terminus is an oligomerization domain. *J Virol* 2005;79:10180–10189.

605. Ulane CM, Rodriguez JJ, Parisien JP, et al. STAT3 ubiquitylation and degradation by mumps virus suppress cytokine and oncogene signaling. *J Virol* 2003;77:6385–6393.

606. Valsamakis A, Schneider H, Auwaerter PG, et al. Recombinant measles viruses with mutations in the C, V, or F gene have altered growth phenotypes in vivo. *J Virol* 1998;72:7754–7761.

607. Venkataraman T, Valdes M, Elsby R, et al. Loss of DExD/H box RNA helicase LGP2 manifests disparate antiviral responses. *J Immunol* 2007;178(10):6444–6455.

608. Vidal S, Curran J, Kolakofsky D. Editing of the Sendai virus P/C mRNA by G insertion occurs during mRNA synthesis via a virus-encoded activity. *J Virol* 1990;64:239–246.

609. Vidal S, Curran J, Kolakofsky D. A stuttering model for paramyxovirus P mRNA editing. *EMBO J* 1990;9:2017–2022.

610. Vidal S, Kolakofsky D. Modified model for the switch from Sendai virus transcription to replication. *J Virol* 1989;63:1951–1958.

611. Vincent S, Gerlier D, Manie SN. Measles virus assembly within membrane rafts. *J Virol* 2000;74:9911–9915.

612. Vincent O, Rainbow L, Tilburn J, et al. YPXL/I is a protein interaction motif recognized by aspergillus PalA and its human homologue, AIP1/Alix. *Mol Cell Biol* 2003;23: 1647–1655.

613. Vogt VM. Ubiquitin in retrovirus assembly: actor or bystander? *Proc Natl Acad Sci U S A* 2000;97(24):12945–12947.

614. von Messling V, Svitek N, Cattaneo R. Receptor (SLAM [CD150]) recognition and the V protein sustain swift lymphocyte-based invasion of mucosal tissue and lymphatic organs by a morbillivirus. *J Virol* 2006;80(12):6084–6092.

615. von Schwedler UK, Stuchell M, Muller B, et al. The protein network of HIV budding. *Cell* 2003;114:701–713.

616. Votteler J, Sundquist WI. Virus budding and the ESCRT pathway. *Cell Host Microbe* 2013;14(3):232–241.

617. Vulliemoz D, Roux L. "Rule of six": how does the Sendai virus RNA polymerase keep count? *J Virol* 2001;75:4506–4518.

618. Walpita P. An internal element of the measles virus antigenome promoter modulates replication efficiency. *Virus Res* 2004;100:199–211.

619. Walpita P, Peters CJ. Cis-acting elements in the antigenomic promoter of Nipah virus. *J Gen Virol* 2007;88(Pt 9):2542–2551.

620. Wang Y, Chu X, Longhi S, et al. Multiscaled exploration of coupled folding and binding of an intrinsically disordered molecular recognition element in measles virus nucleoprotein. *Proc Natl Acad Sci U S A* 2013;110(40):E3743–E3752.

621. Wang LF, Michalski WP, Yu M, et al. A novel P/V/C gene in a new member of the *Paramyxoviridae* family, which causes lethal infection in humans, horses, and other animals. *J Virol* 1998;72:1482–1490.

622. Wang YE, Park A, Lake M, et al. Ubiquitin-regulated nuclear-cytoplasmic trafficking of the Nipah virus matrix protein is important for viral budding. *PLoS Pathog* 2010;6(11):e1001186.

623. Wang LF, Yu M, Hansson E, et al. The exceptionally large genome of Hendra virus: support for creation of a new genus within the family *Paramyxoviridae*. *J Virol* 2000;74:9972–9979.

624. Waning DL, Schmitt AP, Leser GP, et al. Roles for the cytoplasmic tails of the fusion and hemagglutinin-neuraminidase proteins in budding of the paramyxovirus simian virus 5. *J Virol* 2002;76:9284–9297.

625. Wansley EK, Parks GD. Naturally occurring substitutions in the P/V gene convert the noncytopathic paramyxovirus simian virus 5 into a virus that induces alpha/beta interferon synthesis and cell death. *J Virol* 2002;76:10109–10121.

626. Wardrop EA, Briedis DJ. Characterization of V protein in measles virus-infected cells. *J Virol* 1991;65:3421–3428.

627. Watkinson RE, Lee B. Nipah virus matrix protein: expert hacker of cellular machines. *FEBS Lett* 2016;590(15):2494–2511.

628. Weise C, Erbar S, Lamp B, et al. Tyrosine residues in the cytoplasmic domains affect sorting and fusion activity of the Nipah virus glycoproteins in polarized epithelial cells. *J Virol* 2010;84(15):7634–7641.

629. Weissenhorn W, Calder LJ, Dessen A, et al. Assembly of a rod-shaped chimera of a trimeric GCN4 zipper and the HIV-1 gp41 ectodomain expressed in *Escherichia coli*. *Proc Natl Acad Sci U S A* 1997;94:6065–6069.

630. Weissenhorn W, Carfi A, Lee KH, et al. Crystal structure of the Ebola virus membrane fusion subunit, GP2, from the envelope glycoprotein ectodomain. *Mol Cell* 1998;2:605–616.

631. Weissmann C. Reversed genetics. A new approach to the elucidation of structure-function relationships. *Trends Biochem Sci* 1978;3:N109–N111.

632. Welch BD, Yuan P, Bose S, et al. Structure of the parainfluenza virus 5 (PIV5) hemagglutinin-neuraminidase (HN) ectodomain. *PLoS Pathog* 2013;9:e1003534.

633. Whelan SP, Ball LA, Barr JN, et al. Efficient recovery of infectious vesicular stomatitis virus entirely from cDNA clones. *Proc Natl Acad Sci U S A* 1995;92:8388–8392.

634. Wild TF, Malvoisin E, Buckland R. Measles virus: both the haemagglutinin and fusion glycoproteins are required for fusion. *J Gen Virol* 1991;72:439–442.

635. Wilson RL, Fuentes SM, Wang P, et al. Function of small hydrophobic proteins of paramyxovirus. *J Virol* 2006;80:1700–1709.

636. Witko SE, Kotash C, Sidhu MS, et al. Inhibition of measles virus minireplicon-encoded reporter gene expression by V protein. *Virology* 2006;348(1):107–119.

637. Wong JJ, Paterson RG, Lamb RA, et al. Structure and stabilization of the Hendra virus F glycoprotein in its prefusion form. *Proc Natl Acad Sci U S A* 2016;113:1056–1061.

638. Xu K, Chan YP, Bradel-Tretheway B, et al. Crystal structure of the pre-fusion Nipah virus fusion glycoprotein reveals a novel hexamer-of-trimers assembly. *PLoS Pathog* 2015;11(12):e1005322.

639. Xu P, Luthra P, Li Z, et al. The V protein of mumps virus plays a critical role in pathogenesis. *J Virol* 2012;86(3):1768–1776.

640. Xu K, Rajashankar KR, Chan YP, et al. Host cell recognition by the henipaviruses: crystal structures of the Nipah G attachment glycoprotein and its complex with ephrin-B3. *Proc Natl Acad Sci U S A* 2008;105:9953–9958.

641. Yabukarski F, Lawrence P, Tarbouriech N, et al. Structure of Nipah virus unassembled nucleoprotein in complex with its viral chaperone. *Nat Struct Mol Biol* 2014;21(9):754–759.

642. Yamaguchi M, Kitagawa Y, Zhou M, et al. An anti-interferon activity shared by paramyxovirus C proteins: inhibition of Toll-like receptor 7/9-dependent alpha interferon induction. *FEBS Lett* 2014;588(1):28–34.

643. Yan D, Lee S, Thakkar VD, et al. Cross-resistance mechanism of respiratory syncytial virus against structurally diverse entry inhibitors. *Proc Natl Acad Sci U S A* 2014;111(33):E3441–E3449.

644. Yanagi Y, Ono N, Tatsuo H, et al. Measles virus receptor SLAM (CD150). *Virology* 2002;299:155–161.

645. Yang Y, Zengel J, Sun M, et al. Regulation of viral RNA synthesis by the V protein of parainfluenza virus 5. *J Virol* 2015;89(23):11845–11857.

646. Yao Q, Hu X, Compans RW. Association of the parainfluenza virus fusion and hemagglutinin-neuraminidase glycoproteins on cell surfaces. *J Virol* 1997;71:650–656.

647. Yin HS, Paterson RG, Wen X, et al. Structure of the uncleaved ectodomain of the paramyxovirus (hPIV3) fusion protein. *Proc Natl Acad Sci U S A* 2005;102:9288–9293.

648. Yin HS, Wen X, Paterson RG, et al. Structure of the parainfluenza virus 5 F protein in its metastable, prefusion conformation. *Nature* 2006;439:38–44.

649. Yoneda M, Guillaume V, Ikeda F, et al. Establishment of a Nipah virus rescue system. *Proc Natl Acad Sci U S A* 2006;103(44):16508–16513.

650. Yoneda M, Guillaume V, Sato H, et al. The nonstructural proteins of Nipah virus play a key role in pathogenicity in experimentally infected animals. *PLoS One* 2010;5(9):e12709.

651. Yoshida T, Nagai Y, Maeno K, et al. Studies on the role of M protein in virus assembly using a ts mutant of HVJ (Sendai virus). *Virology* 1979;92(1):139–154.

652. Young DF, Chatziandreou N, He B, et al. Single amino acid substitution in the V protein of simian virus 5 differentiates its ability to block interferon signaling in human and murine cells. *J Virol* 2001;75:3363–3370.

653. Young JK, Hicks RP, Wright GE, et al. Analysis of a peptide inhibitor of paramyxovirus (NDV) fusion using biological assays, NMR, and molecular modeling. *Virology* 1997;238:291–304.

654. Yuan P, Paterson RG, Leser GP, et al. Structure of the Ulster strain Newcastle disease virus hemagglutinin-neuraminidase reveals auto-inhibitory interactions associated with low virulence. *PLoS Pathog* 2012;8:e1002855.

655. Yuan P, Swanson KA, Leser GP, et al. Structure of the Newcastle disease virus hemagglutinin-neuraminidase (HN) ectodomain reveals a four-helix bundle stalk. *Proc Natl Acad Sci U S A* 2011;108:14920–14925.

656. Yuan P, Thompson TB, Wurzburg BA, et al. Structural studies of the parainfluenza virus 5 hemagglutinin-neuraminidase tetramer in complex with its receptor, sialyllactose. *Structure* 2005;13:803–815.

657. Yuasa T, Kawano M, Tabata N, et al. A cell fusion-inhibiting monoclonal antibody binds to the presumed stalk domain of the human parainfluenza type 2 virus hemagglutinin-neuraminidase protein. *Virology* 1995;206:1117–1125.

658. Zaitsev V, Von Itzstein M, Groves D, et al. Second sialic acid binding site in Newcastle disease virus hemagglutinin-neuraminidase: implications in fusion. *J Virol* 2004;78:3733–3741.

659. Zhang X, Glendening C, Linke H, et al. Identification and characterization of a regulatory domain on the carboxyl terminus of the measles virus nucleocapsid protein. *J Virol* 2002;76(17):8737–8746.

660. Zhang X, Lu G, Qi J, et al. Structure of measles virus hemagglutinin bound to its epithelial receptor nectin-4. *Nat Struct Mol Biol* 2013;20(1):67–72.

661. Zhao H, Banerjee AK. Interaction between the nucleocapsid protein and the phosphoprotein of human parainfluenza virus 3. *J Biol Chem* 1995;270:12485–12490.

662. Zhao X, Singh M, Malashkevich VN, et al. Structural characterization of the human respiratory syncytial virus fusion protein core. *Proc Natl Acad Sci U S A* 2000;97:14172–14177.

Henipaviruses: Hendra and Nipah Viruses

Benhur Lee • Christopher C. Broder • Lin-Fa Wang

HISTORY

Hendra virus (HeV), the first known member of the genus *Henipavirus* in the family *Paramyxoviridae*, came to light in September 1994 as the causative agent of a sudden outbreak of acute respiratory disease in thoroughbred horses at a stable in Brisbane, Australia. A total of 21 horses and 2 humans (a horse trainer and a stable hand) became infected. The horse trainer and 14 horses died.[1,2] A virus was isolated, initially called *equine morbillivirus* but later renamed *Hendra virus* after

the Brisbane suburb where the outbreak occurred. A second person died from HeV infection 13 months after the Brisbane outbreak, a farmer from Mackay, nearly 1,000 km north of Brisbane. Unlike the first case, however, the man succumbed to encephalitis caused by HeV infection 14 months after his initial mild meningitic illness.[3,4] After initial serologic evidence suggested that fruit bats (flying foxes) of the genus *Pteropus* in the suborder Yinpterochiroptera were the reservoir hosts,[5] HeV was isolated from two species of flying fox.[6] In total, there have been 60 recognized occurrences of HeV in Australia between 1994 and 2018, with at least 1 occurrence per year since 2006 (Table 13.1A).[7] Every occurrence of HeV has involved horses as the initial infected host, causing lethal respiratory disease and/or encephalitis, along with a total of seven human cases arising from exposure to infected horses, among which four have been fatal and the most recent in 2009 (Table 13.1B).[8]

Nipah virus (NiV), the second known member of the genus *Henipavirus*, emerged as the cause of an outbreak of disease in pigs and humans in Peninsular Malaysia in 1998 through 1999. The epidemic started in Perak State as clusters of cases of encephalitis among pig farmers. It was initially believed to be caused by Japanese encephalitis virus; however, various features of the outbreak, including a high proportion of cases in direct contact with pigs and illness and deaths in pigs, differed from those expected with Japanese encephalitis.[9] Indeed, respiratory illness and encephalitis in pigs preceded human cases in the same district.[10] The epidemic spread south to the intensive pig farming areas of Negeri Sembilan in December 1998 and subsequently peaked between February and April 1999. More than 1 million pigs were destroyed to halt the spread of the epidemic, and by late May, 265 human cases of acute encephalitis with 105 deaths were recorded.[9,11] A cluster of 11 cases with 1 death occurred among abattoir workers in Singapore.[12] In early March 1999, a virus was isolated from the cerebrospinal fluid (CSF) of a patient with encephalitis and identified as the etiologic agent.[9,11] Named *Nipah virus* after the village from which the patient had come, it was shown to be closely related to HeV. NiV was subsequently isolated from the urine of Malaysian flying foxes.[13] A highly related NiV emerged in Bangladesh in 2001,[14] and outbreaks of NiV-related encephalitis have occurred in people from that country almost every year since, along with three reports of NiV encephalitis in India,[15,16] albeit in Bangladesh adjacent regions.

TABLE 13.1A Summary of Hendra virus outbreaks in horses in Australia

Year	Month	State[a]	Location	Total Cases[b]
1994	Aug	QLD	Mackay	2
1994	Sep	QLD	Hendra	20
1999	Jan	QLD	Cairns	1
2004	Oct	QLD	Cairns	1
	Dec	QLD	Townsville	1
2006	Jun	QLD	Peachester	1
	Oct	NSW	Murwillumbah	1
2007	Jun	QLD	Peachester	1
	Jul	QLD	Cairns	1
2008	Jun	QLD	Redlands	8
	Jul	QLD	Proserpine	4
2009	Jul	QLD	Cawarral	4
	Sep	QLD	Bowen	2
2010	May	QLD	Tewantin	1
2011	Jun	QLD	Beaudesert	1
		QLD	Boonah	3
		QLD	Logan	1
		NSW	Wollongbar	2
	Jul	QLD	Park Ridge	1
		NSW	Macksville	1
		QLD	Kuranda	1
		NSW	Lismore	1
		QLD	Hervey Bay	1
		QLD	Boondall	1
		QLD	Chinchilla	1
		NSW	Mullumbimby	1
	Aug	NSW	South Ballina	1
		NSW	South Ballina	2
		NSW	Mullumbimby	1
		QLD	Gold Coast Hinterland	1
		NSW	North Ballina	1
	Oct	QLD	Beachmere	3
2012	Jan	QLD	Townsville	1
	May	QLD	Rockhampton	1
		QLD	Ingham	1
	Jun	QLD	Mackay	1
	Jul	QLD	Rockhampton	3
		QLD	Cairns	1
	Sep	QLD	Port Douglas	1
	Oct	QLD	Ingham	1

(continued)

TABLE 13.1A   Summary of Hendra virus outbreaks in horses in Australia *(Continued)*

Year	Month	State[a]	Location	Total Cases[b]
2013	Jan	QLD	Mackay	1
	Feb	QLD	Atherton Tablelands	1
	Jun	NSW	Macksville	1
		QLD	Brisbane Valley	1
	Jul	QLD	Gold Coast Hinterland	1
		NSW	Macksville	1
		NSW	Kempsey	2
2014	Mar	QLD	Bundaberg	1
	Jun	QLD	Beenleigh	1
		NSW	Murwillumbah	1
	Jul	QLD	Gladstone	1
2015	Jun	NSW	Murwillumbah	1
	Jul	QLD	Atherton Tablelands	1
	Sep	NSW	Lismore	1
2016	Dec	NSW	Casino	1
2017	May	QLD	Gold Cost Hinterland	1
	Jun	NSW	Lismore	1
	Aug	NSW	Murwillumbah	1
		NSW	Lismore	1
2018	Sep	NSW	Tween Heads	1
Total				**103**

[a]QLD, Queensland; NSW, New South Wales.
[b]All cases were deceased.

However, the most recent outbreak of NiV occurred in 2018 in Kerala (India), more than 2,500 km southwest of NiV-endemic Bangladesh counties. This outbreak claimed 21 lives out of 23 infected human cases.[17] In 2014, an NiV outbreak occurred in the Province of Sultan Kudarat, the Philippines, which resulted in the death of 9 humans from 11, which showed an acute encephalitis syndrome.[18] The human case fatality rate of these NiV outbreaks averages around 60% (Table 13.1C). So far human NiV outbreaks have been documented in a total of five countries: Malaysia, Singapore, Bangladesh, India, and the Philippines. Seroepidemiological evidence for henipavirus spillover events from bats into high-risk human populations have also been reported in Cameroon.[19]

INFECTIOUS AGENT

Classification
When HeV was first isolated in 1994, partial sequencing of the matrix gene (M) revealed that it most closely resembled members of the genus *Morbillivirus* in the subfamily *Paramyxovirinae*.[2]

TABLE 13.1B   Summary of Hendra virus outbreaks in humans

Year	Month	Country	Location	No. of Cases	No. of Deaths	Case Fatality Rate
1994	Aug	Australia	Mackay	1	1	100%
1994	Sep		Hendra	2	1	50%
2004	Oct		Cairns	1	0	0%
2008	Jul		Redlands	2	1	50%
2009	Aug		Carrara	1	1	10%
Total				**7**	**4**	**57%**

TABLE 13.1C   Summary of Nipah virus outbreaks in humans

Year	Month	Country	Location	No. of Cases	No. of Deaths	NiV Clade (M/B)		Case Fatality Rate
1998	Sep–Apr 1999	Malaysia	Started from Nipah near Ipoh	265	105	M		40%
1999	Mar	Singapore	Singapore	11	1	M		9%
2001	Feb	India	Siliguri	66	45		B	68%
2001	Apr–May	Bangladesh	Meherpur	13	9		B	69%
2003	Jan		Naogaon	12	8		B	67%
2004	Jan		Raibari	31	23		B	74%
	Apr		Faridpur	36	27		B	75%
2005	Jan–Mar		Tangail	12	11		B	92%
2007	Jan–Feb		Thakurgaon	7	3		B	43%
	Mar		Kushtia	8	5		B	63%
	Apr		Pabna, Natore, Naogaon	3	1		B	33%
	Apr	India	Nadia	5	5		B	100%
2008	Feb	Bangladesh	Manikganj	4	4		B	100%
	Apr		Rajbari	7	5		B	71%
2009	Jan		Gaibandha, Rangpur, Nilphamari	3	0		B	0%
			Rajbari	1	1		B	100%
2010	Feb–Mar		Faridpur, Rajbari, Gopalganj, Kurigram	17	15		B	88%
2011	Jan–Feb		Lalmonirhat, Dinajpur, Comilla, Nilphamari, Faridpur, Rajbari	44	40		B	91%
2012	Jan		Joypurhat	12	10		B	83%
2013	Jan–Apr		Pabna, Natore, Naogaon, Gaibandha, Manikganj	24	21			88%
2014	Jan–Feb		13 districts	18	9		B	50%
2014	Mar–May	The Philippines	Senator Ninoy Aquino	17	9	M		53%
2015	Jan–Feb	Bangladesh	Nilphamari, Panchagarh, Faridpur, Magura, Naogaon, Rajbari	9	6			67%
2018	May	India	Kerala	23	21		B	94%
				293	*115*	*M*		*39%*
				355	*269*		*B*	*76%*
Total				**648**	**384**	***M***	***B***	**59%**

Subsequent characterization of the full-length genome, however, revealed that many of the genetic features of HeV were unique among paramyxoviruses and that the virus did not fit within any of the existing genera at that time.[20,21] After the isolation of NiV in 1999, it was shown that sera raised against HeV were able to neutralize NiV and vice versa and that both viruses shared a high degree of similarity in genome organization and protein size and sequence.[11,22–24] In 2002, the genus *Henipavirus* was created to accommodate these novel paramyxoviruses, and HeV was designated the type species.[25] Since 1994, there have been 38 isolations of HeV or NiV from humans, bats, horses, and pigs over a wide geographic area and spanning a period of approximately 20 years (Table 13.2). The susceptibility of humans, the virulence of the viruses, and absence of therapeutics and vaccines led to classification of HeV and NiV as biosafety level 4 (BSL4) pathogens. In the latest report from the paramyxovirus study group under the order Mononegavirales, the genus *Henipavirus* has been expanded to include three new species[26,27]; they are *Cedar henipavirus* (Cedar virus [CedV]) isolated from bats in Australia,[28] *Ghanaian bat henipavirus* (Ghana virus [GhV]) detected in bats from Ghana,[29] and *Mojiang henipavirus* (Mòjiāng [MojV]) detected in rats in China.[30] These three new species are highly divergent from NiV and HeV, and only CedV has been isolated. GhV and MojV are only known from sequence information. *Henipavirus* is now classified as one of the fourteen ICTV-approved genera in the family *Paramyxoviridae*.

Propagation in Cell Culture and Cytopathic Effect

The ultrastructural characteristics of henipavirus-infected cells resemble those found in cells infected by other members of the *Paramyxoviridae*. Shared features include generation of large

TABLE 13.2 **Summary of Henipaviruses isolated from different species and geographic locations**

| Virus | Isolate Name and Number | Isolation Details | | | References |
		Year	Country	Host Species/Tissue	
Hendra	Horse-1	1994	Australia	Horse/spleen, lung	2
	VR-1			Human/lung, liver, kidney, spleen	
	Bat-1-1	1996	Australia	Gray-headed flying fox (*Pteropus poliocephalus*)/ uterine fluid	6
	Bat-1-2			Gray-headed flying fox (*P. poliocephalus*)/fetus	
	Bat-2			Black flying fox (*Pteropus alecto*)/fetal lung	
	Murwillumbah	2006	Australia	Horse/lung	219
	Clifton Beach	2007		Horse/lung	
	Peachester	2008		Horse/blood	
	Redlands			Horse/lung	
	Proserpine			Horse/lung	
Nipah	PKL	1999	Malaysia	Human/cerebrospinal fluid	9,11
	EKK			Human/cerebrospinal fluid	
	WWS			Human/cerebrospinal fluid	
	UMMC1	1999	Malaysia	Human/cerebrospinal fluid	220
	UMMC2			Human/throat secretion	
	UM-0128	1999	Malaysia	Human	303
	VRI-0626			Pig/lung	
	VRI-1413			Pig/lung	
	VRI-2794			Pig/lung	
	B13/6-18	2000	Malaysia	Bat/pooled urine	13
	B13/6-43			Bat/pooled urine	
	JA13/6-4			Bat/partially eaten jambu air fruit	
	Rajbari-1	2004	Bangladesh	Human/oropharyngeal	33
	Rajbari-2			Human/cerebrospinal fluid	
	Faridpur			Human/urine	
	Rajshahi			Human/urine	
	CSUR381	2004	Cambodia	Flying fox (*Pteropus lylei*)/urine	89
	CSUR382			Flying fox (*Pteropus lylei*)/urine	
	Raypur-31	2013	Bangladesh	Flying fox (*Pteropus medius*)/urine	206
	Raypur-36			Flying fox (*Pteropus medius*)/urine	
	Raypur-38			Flying fox (*Pteropus medius*)/urine	
	Raypur-40			Flying fox (*Pteropus medius*)/urine	
	Raypur-41			Flying fox (*Pteropus medius*)/urine	
	Raypur-42			Flying fox (*Pteropus medius*)/urine	
	Raypur-43			Flying fox (*Pteropus medius*)/urine	
	Raypur-46			Flying fox (*Pteropus medius*)/urine	
	Raypur-47			Flying fox (*Pteropus medius*)/urine	
	Sylhet-47			Flying fox (*Pteropus medius*)/urine	

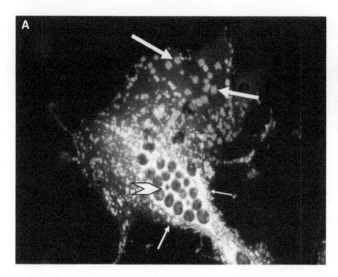
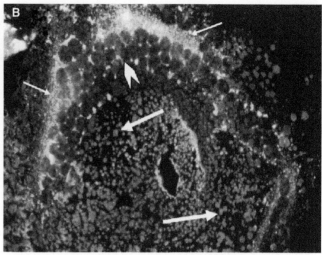

FIGURE 13.1 Syncytia induced in Vero cells 24 hours after infection by Hendra virus (HeV) (A) and Nipah virus (NiV) (B). Methanol-fixed infected cells were labeled with rabbit monospecific antiserum to the HeV P protein and fluorescein-conjugated goat antirabbit immunoglobulin G. P protein is detected in extensive perinuclear ribonucleoprotein complexes (*small arrow*) and in discrete regularly shaped arrays (*large arrow*) distributed throughout the cytoplasm and believed to be sites of virus egress from the cell. Nuclei are indicated by *chevrons*.

syncytia and the presence of viral nucleocapsids in cytoplasmic inclusion bodies and underlying electron-dense areas of the plasma membrane.[31,32] In Vero cells, NiV-induced syncytia are significantly larger than those generated by HeV, and nuclei and nucleocapsids are frequently located at the cell periphery, compared with HeV-induced syncytia, where they tend to be more centrally located or distributed randomly throughout the cytoplasm (Fig. 13.1). Henipavirus-infected cells also contain structures that are not seen with other paramyxoviruses—specifically a network of membrane-like reticular structures in the cytoplasm and long tubules that appear to be continuous with the plasma membrane in NiV-infected cells. Tubules can

also be observed in NiV virions (Fig. 13.2A). *In situ* hybridization suggests that these reticular structures contain viral RNA and may play a role in viral transcription.[31]

Virus Morphology

Henipavirus particles are pleomorphic, varying from spherical to filamentous and ranging in size from 40 to 1,900 nm.[2,31,32] Nucleocapsids have a diameter of 18 to 19 nm with an average pitch of 5 nm. When examined by electron microscopy (EM), HeV has a unique double-fringed appearance, caused by the presence of surface projections 15 ± 1 nm and 8 ± 1 nm in length (see Fig. 13.2B). Approximately 95% of virions

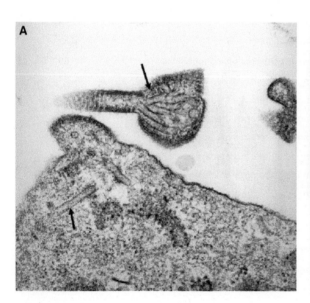
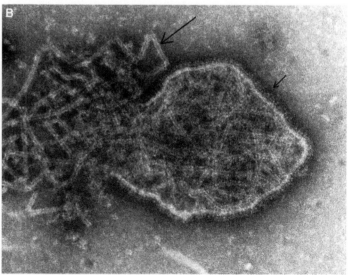

FIGURE 13.2 A: Electron micrograph of Nipah virus (NiV)–infected Vero cells showing tubule-like structures, both in the cytoplasm and in a maturing virus particle (*arrows*). **B:** Electron micrograph of negatively stained Hendra virus (HeV) displaying the double fringe at the virus envelope (*small arrow*) and the herringbone nucleocapsids (*large arrow*). (Courtesy of Dr. Alex Hyatt, CSIRO Australian Animal Health Laboratory.)

contain the double fringe, and the remaining 5% display a uniform fringe length of 15 ± 1 nm. Unlike HeV, NiV possesses a single layer of surface projections with an average length of 17 ± 1 nm, and NiV particles released into the culture medium are difficult to image because they are routinely penetrated by negative stains. This suggests that the viruses may differ in the physical nature of their envelope.[32]

Genome Length and Organization

In the family *Paramyxoviridae*, the genome length of all characterized viruses is divisible by 6, an observation caused by the requirement of each N protein in the viral ribonucleoprotein to bind 6 nucleotide (nt) residues (see Chapter 12). This is also true for HeV and NiV despite their much larger genome sizes.[24] The genomes of the Malaysian (MY) and Bangladesh (BD) strains of NiV differ by 6 nt because of a 6-nt increase in the 3'-untranslated region of the *F* gene in NiV-BD.[33]

A minigenome replicon study confirms that NiV complies with the rule of six.[34] When the complete genome sequence of HeV was determined, its length (18,234 nt) was more than 2,700 nt or 15% longer than the genomes of all other paramyxoviruses known at that time.[21] The size of NiV genomes at 18,246 nt to 18,252 nt is slightly larger than that of HeV.[22,23,33] These large genome sizes of greater than 18 kb are a conserved feature of henipaviruses as even the recently discovered and more divergent CedV, GhV, and MojV all have genomes between 18,162 nt (CedV) and approximately 18,430 nt (GhV). Given the caveat that there is wide variation among individual species of the other paramyxovirus genera, the extra length of the henipavirus genome is primarily due to the longer 3' untranslated regions (3' UTRs) at the end of several of its six genes and a larger *P* gene relative to the other paramyxovirus genera. A comparison of genome length and gene organization of representative members of the *Paramyxoviridae* is shown in Figure 13.3A.

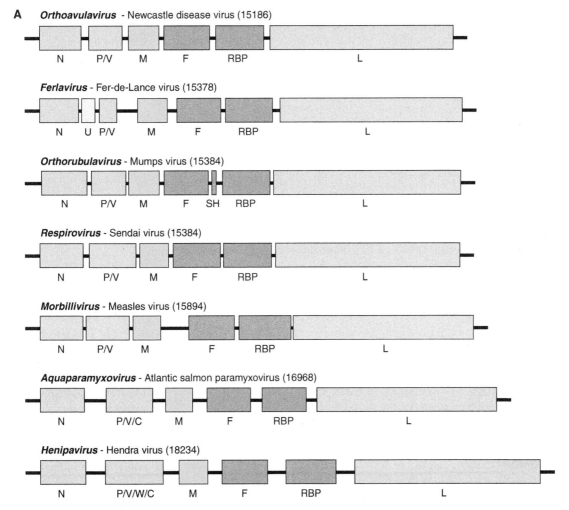

FIGURE 13.3 Genome size and organization of Hendra virus in comparison with the type species from representative genera genera in the family Paramyxoviridae. A: Genome length (in nucleotides) are given in brackets after each virus. Color coding: *blue*, N, P and L genes nucleocapsid responsible for replication and transcription; *orange*, M (Matrix); *purple*, envelope (F and RBP). **B:** 3' UTR of certain genes in henipaviruses (N, P, and G) are longer than their counterparts from representative members of paramyxovirus genera that infect mammals. The 3' UTR length (number of nucleotides) of each gene from representative members of the indicated genera is compared separately in box-and-whisker plots (N, P, M, F, RBP, and L). P values are calculated based on one-tailed t-test (*Henipavirus* vs. all other genera); five virus species from *Henipavirus* (HeV, NC_001906; NiV, NC_002728; CedV, NC_025351.1; GhV, NC_025256.1; MojV, NC_025352.1) and three each from *Morbillivirus* (MeV, NC_001498.1; CDV, NC_001921.1; FeMV, NC_039196.1), *Rubulavirus* (MuV, NC_002200.1; HPIV-2, NC_003443.1; PIV-5, NC_006430.1), and *Respirovirus* (SeV, NC_001552; HPIV-1, NC_003461; HPIV-3, NC_001796.2). (Courtesy of Satoshi Ikegame and Christian Stevens, Icahn School of Medicine at Mount Sinai, New York.)

B

Length of 3′ UTR

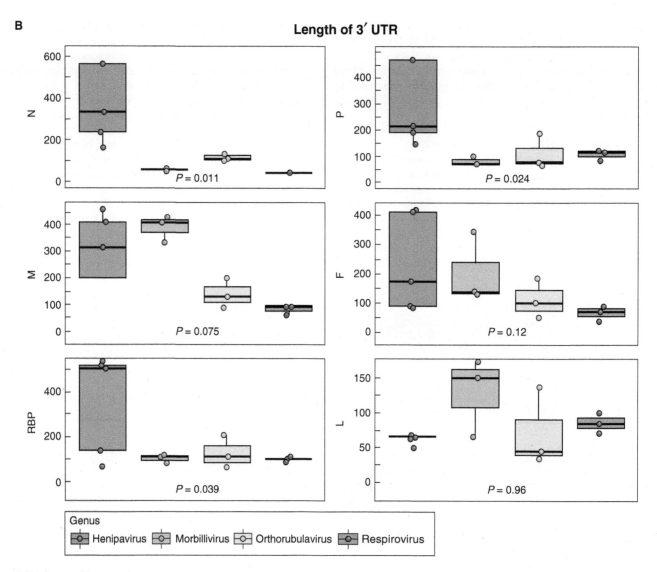

FIGURE 13.3 (Continued)

The nomenclature of each of the six major genes common to all paramyxoviruses has been updated to reflect the latest ICTV convention.[35] An analysis of the 3′ UTR lengths between extant henipaviruses and representative species from each paramyxovirus genera that infects mammals is presented in Figure 13.3B. The most significant differences are in the 3′ UTRs of *N*, *P*, and *RBP* genes even given the wide variance seen within each genus. The significance of long 3′ UTRs, especially in HeV and NiV, is generally unknown. However, the N gene 3′ UTR of NiV appears to play a role in the down-regulation of N mRNAs via specific interactions with hnRNP-D.[36]

The genome organization of henipaviruses resembles that in the genera *Respirovirus* and *Morbillivirus*, in that the first 12 nt of the 3′ and 5′ genomic terminal sequences of paramyxoviruses are highly conserved and complementary, containing promoter elements for replication and transcription (see Chapter 12). The first 3 nt of the henipavirus genome termini are 5′-ACC-3′—a sequence that is absolutely conserved in members of the family *Paramyxoviridae* and different from that found in the family *Pneumoviridae*.

Virus Proteins and Their Properties

Analysis of purified viruses by polyacrylamide gel electrophoresis reveals L, P, RBP (G), F_0, N, F_1, M, and F_2 proteins[20,24] where F_0 is the uncleaved and F_1 and F_2 are the cleaved products of the *F* gene (Fig. 13.4A). Interestingly, F_0 is more readily detected in HeV compared with other paramyxoviruses, including NiV,[24,37] which may suggest that HeV F is less efficiently cleaved. Overall, the proteins of henipaviruses are typical of those of *Paramyxoviridae*, with the exception of the P protein, which is significantly larger than cognate proteins in this virus family.[26] The P protein is translated from messenger RNA (mRNA) that is colinear with genomic RNA. For most henipaviruses, the *P* gene also encodes V and W proteins, produced from mRNA in which one and two nontemplated G residues, respectively, are inserted at the RNA editing site during transcription. The P, V, and W proteins, therefore, are identical for the first 405 amino acid residues of NiV and HeV. A C protein is encoded by the 5′ end of the gene in an overlapping reading frame and is produced by an internal translational initiation mechanism, which is common to other

FIGURE 13.4 The major proteins of Hendra virus and Nipah virus and their roles in the henipavirus life cycle. A: Viruses were purified and analyzed as described in Wang et al.[20] Major virus proteins and the molecular weights of standard marker proteins are shown on the *right* and *left*, respectively. (Reproduced with permission from Wang LF, et al. Molecular biology of Hendra and Nipah viruses. *Microbes Infect* 2001;3:279–287.) **B:** Henipavirus replication cycle is depicted. The virus receptor–binding protein (RBP, *gold lollipops*) attaches the virus to the cell via its cognate receptor, typically ephrin-B2/ephrin-B3 (*1*) and triggers virus–cell membrane fusion mediated by the viral fusion protein (F, filled *orange trapezoids*) (*2*). Fusion delivers the nucleoprotein (N)–encapsidated negative-sense virus RNA genome (vRNA[–], *red*) to the cytosol (*3*). The vRNA(–) serves as template for viral transcripts made by the transcriptase complex comprised of the phosphoprotein (P) and the large RNA-dependent RNA polymerase (L) (P-L, *transparent hexagons*) (*4*). Viral transcripts are made following a 3′ to 5′ attenuation gradient. The vRNA(–) is also the template for making full-length antigenomic cRNA(+) (*5*), which in turn is a template for vRNA(–) synthesis during virus genome replication (*6*). Henipavirus genome replication mediated by the N-P-L replicase complex is similar to the details described for the *Paramyxoviridae* in Chapter 12. However, some aspects of henipavirus assembly are relatively unique. The matrix protein (M, *purple octagons*) needs to transit through the nucleus (*7*) in a ubiquitin-regulated manner (*8*), in order to traffic properly to the plasma membrane. This nuclear sojourn involves shuttling through subnuclear compartments such as nucleoli (*9*). Proper trafficking is required for M to orchestrate the assembly of the viral RNPs with the viral envelope glycoproteins into budding infectious virions bearing the vRNA(–) (*10*). Matrix also has nonstructural functions such as antagonizing type I IFN responses (*11*); see Figure 13.9 and text for details. Additionally, in order for the henipavirus F protein to be cleaved and become fusion competent, it needs to access cathepsins L/B in the endosomal compartment. To do this, F first reaches the plasma membrane via the secretory pathway in an uncleaved form (*open beige trapezoids*) (*12*). Subsequent endocytosis and recycling back to the plasma membrane (*12a*) is required to form infectious virions where cleaved fusion-competent F (*filled orange trapezoids*) (*12b*) is complexed with the RBP in its proper oligomeric state. Where this occurs along the vesicular trafficking pathway and/or the plasma membrane is unresolved (*13*). F protein cleavage is seldom complete, and uncleaved F can be detected in budded virions (*14*). (Adapted from Aguilar HC, Lee B. Emerging paramyxoviruses: molecular mechanisms and antiviral strategies. *Expert Rev Mol Med* 2011;13:e6.)

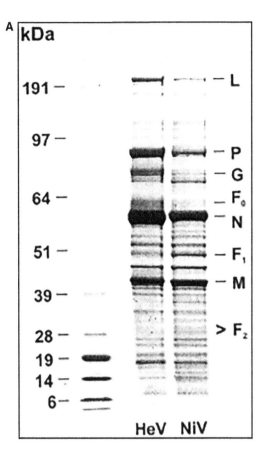

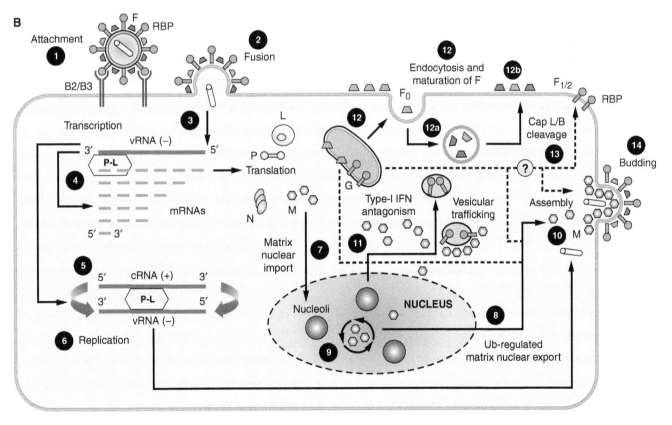

members of *Paramyxoviridae*, except for rubulaviruses (see Chapter 12). The *P*-derived V, W, and C proteins are present in HeV-infected and/or NiV-infected cells.[24,38] It is worth noting that CedV lacks both the RNA editing and expression of the V protein.[28] Similar to other paramyxoviruses, P itself and its derived proteins (V, W, and C in the case of most henipaviruses), all antagonize innate immune responses via a diverse set of mechanisms.[39,40] The C protein also interacts with the host cell ESCRT machinery and the virus matrix (M) protein itself to facilitate virus budding (see Pathogenesis section for details on the function of these *P*-derived proteins).[41]

Paramyxovirus N, P, and L proteins are necessary and sufficient for replication of viral RNA both *in vitro* and *in vivo* as discussed in Chapter 12. This has been confirmed for henipaviruses by reverse genetics using a minigenome replicon containing leader and trailer sequences of the NiV genome with its entire coding region replaced with a reporter gene.[34,42] NiV N, P, and L proteins were also able to rescue an HeV minigenome, demonstrating the close genetic relationship between the viruses. Full-length recombinant NiV bearing the matrix (M), fusion (F), and receptor-binding protein (RBP) genes from HeV, singly or in combination, can also be functionally rescued. These chimeric but isogenic rNiVs replicate well in primary human endothelial and neuronal cells, further underscoring the genetic relatedness of NiV and HeV that allows for heterotypic complementation between their major structural proteins.[43] These henipavirus structural proteins contribute to unique aspects of the henipavirus life cycle (Fig. 13.4B) and play different roles in the spread and virulence of henipaviruses. Indeed, multiple groups have developed recombinant virus systems for NiV, HeV, and CedV bearing various reporters and/or relevant mutations.[43–53] These additional tools have facilitated work toward understanding the virological and pathogenic similarities and differences among the henipaviruses (see Pathogenesis section for details).

The L protein of nonsegmented, negative-strand RNA (NNR) viruses in the order *Mononegavirales* contains a highly conserved GDNQ motif, believed to be important for polymerase activity.[54] Henipaviruses were the first NNR viruses in which GDNQ was replaced by GDNE. It was speculated that this motif might be unique to paramyxoviruses with relatively large genomes[21,24]; however, the GDNE motif has since been found in the L protein of Mossman virus that has a genome length of 16,650 nt.[55] Conversely, other henipaviruses of both Asiatic (CedV) and African lineages (GhV) also have the GDNQ motif that is common to most other NNR viruses. High-resolution cryo-EM structures of VSV-L (another NNR virus, family *Rhabdoviridae*) suggest that GDN is the truly conserved catalytic motif essential for the polymerase function of L.[56]

The receptor-binding proteins (RBPs) of the *Paramyxoviridae* display hemagglutination (H) and neuraminidase (N) activities in a predominantly genus-specific manner. Viruses in the genera *Respirovirus*, *Avulavirus*, and *Rubulavirus* possess both activities; hence their RBPs were formerly termed HN proteins,[57] whereas viruses in the genus *Morbillivirus* do not behave uniformly and only some possess hemagglutination activity, but nonetheless their RBPs were formerly termed H.[58] This is an unfortunate misnomer. Paramyxoviruses with RBPs bearing HN activity genuinely use sialic acid–based receptors

for entry, whereas "H" activity of some morbilliviruses arise from the ability of their RBPs to bind CD46 expressed on some nonhuman primate (NHP) red blood cells.[59] In contrast, henipavirus RBPs have neither of these activities[24,60]; rather, they utilize at least ephrin-B2, and in many cases, also ephrin-B3 expressed on host cell surfaces as attachment and entry receptors.[28,61–65] The exception is MojV, which does not appear to use any known paramyxovirus receptors.[66] Recent solution structures of various henipavirus RBPs alone and in complex with the ephrin-B2 and/or ephrin-B3 receptors have revealed the details of the virus–host cell binding process, distinguishing it from other paramyxoviruses' receptor-binding strategies[59,65–69] (Fig. 13.5).

Proteolytic processing of paramyxovirus F proteins is essential for the generation of a fusogenic form of the protein. For most paramyxoviruses that generate systemic infections, furin-like proteases in the secretory pathway cleave their F proteins at a multibasic cleavage site.[70] Surprisingly, henipavirus F proteins are cleaved without the involvement of furin and, although cleavage occurs at a single basic residue—lysine for HeV and arginine for NiV[37]—activation of the NiV F protein does not require a basic amino acid at the cleavage site.[71] Instead, endosomal/lysosomal cysteine proteases such as cathepsins L and B are responsible for the cleavage of henipavirus F proteins.[72–75] To access cathepsins L/B, henipavirus F proteins are endocytosed upon initially reaching the cell surface in an uncleaved form and subsequently have to traffic back to the cell surface once they are cleaved into a fusion-competent form (Fig. 13.4B).[55,57] Classical endocytic YXXØ motifs[76,77] in the cytoplasmic tails of henipavirus F proteins and specific residues in the transmembrane domain of at least HeV F regulate this trafficking behavior through the early/sorting (S490) and recycling endosomal (Y498) compartments.[78] Henipavirus F proteins also have the ability to bud by themselves, forming F-only particles in the absence of M.[79,80]

The matrix protein (M) plays a major role in the efficient assembly and budding of infectious paramyxoviruses.[81,82] M interacts specifically with N, the cytoplasmic tail of F, as well as cognate lipid ligands along the vesicular trafficking pathway. These orchestrated interactions help to coordinate the envelopment of encapsidated viral genomes (RNPs) and the budding of infectious virions bearing a relatively high density of viral envelope glycoprotein spikes. General details on the role that matrix plays in paramyxovirus assembly and budding are given in Chapter 12.

Henipavirus M exhibits some relatively unique behaviors and functions. For example, NiV and HeV M have classical nuclear localization and export sequences (NLS, NES) that when mutated give the relevant nuclear exclusion and nuclear retention phenotypes, respectively.[83] Time-course monitoring of M trafficking during live NiV and HeV infection indicates that M first appears in the nucleus and localizes to subnuclear compartments, including the nucleolus, before exiting into the cytoplasm and trafficking to the plasma membrane to coordinate virus assembly and budding (Fig. 13.4B).[83,84] This nuclear transit is regulated by ubiquitination and is critical for M to acquire its budding functionality.[83,85] Henipavirus M is multimono- and polyubiquitinated; a lysine to arginine mutation of a key residue in its bipartite NLS is sufficient to dysregulate ubiquitination of M and abrogate its budding function.[83,85]

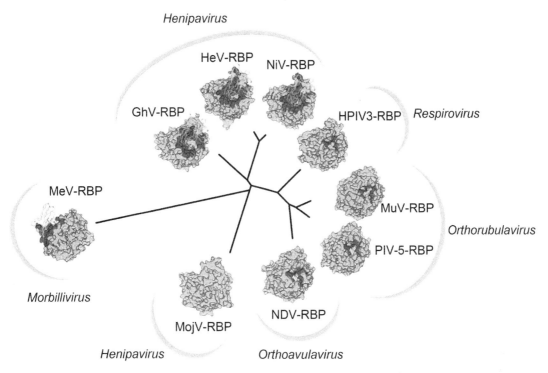

FIGURE 13.5 A structure-based phylogeny of paramyxoviral receptor-binding proteins. Structure-based phylogenetic analysis on extant structures of henipavirus RBPs and representative RBPs from at least one virus in other paramyxovirus genera for which structural data are available. RBPs are shown besides the tree and are rendered as surface representation (*gray*). All receptor-binding proteins, with the exception of the MojV-G, are shown in complex with their respective receptor molecules (*yellow*), with the receptor-binding interface colored *red*. Analysis was performed and produced as described in Rissanen et al.[66] Paramyxoviral RBPs generally cluster according to their respective genera and cellular receptor usage with the exception MojV-RBP, which is almost equidistant to all structurally studied genera. (Courtesy of Dr. Thomas Bowden, University of Oxford, UK.)

The latter is true not only in HeV and NiV but also in divergent henipaviruses (GhV, CedV, MojV), albeit to varying degrees.[86] Matrix interactome studies have identified many nuclear interacting factors, including importins and exportins, consistent with the nucleocytoplasmic trafficking phenotype of M.[85,87]

Host Range
For most paramyxoviruses, host range is limited and interspecies transmission is rare. In contrast, henipaviruses display a broad species tropism. In addition to a large number of bat hosts at various geographic locations (see more detail in Epidemiology section), NiV has naturally infected pigs, humans, dogs, horses, and cats,[10,11,88–90] whereas HeV infects all four Australian flying fox species and has naturally infected humans, horses, and dogs.[2,91–93] Confirmation of the wide host range of these henipaviruses and the identical cell tropism of HeV and NiV were obtained early using an *in vitro* cell fusion system that relies on vaccinia virus–mediated cell surface expression of G and F glycoproteins.[94–96] Bats, guinea pigs, hamsters, ferrets, squirrel monkeys, and African green monkeys (AGMs) are also susceptible to experimental NiV infection.[97–101] Laboratory studies have added cats, guinea pigs, hamsters, ferrets, dogs, and AGMs to the list of HeV-susceptible species.[93,102–106] CedV, isolated from flying foxes (*Pteropus* sp.) in Cedar Grove, Australia, can establish transient but nonpathogenic infections

in laboratory-challenged guinea pigs and ferrets.[28] GhV and MojV, known only from sequence information, were identified from bats[29] and rats,[30] respectively.

PATHOGENESIS AND PATHOLOGY

Entry Into the Host
Epidemiologic and experimental studies generally support an oronasal[8,107,108] or oropharyngeal[109–111] route of entry. This occurs directly or indirectly via saliva, urine, or oronasal secretions that are contaminated with relatively high levels of HeV or NiV.[93,105,107,112–123] Figure 13.6 summarizes what is known about how NiV is transmitted to humans either directly from their pteropid reservoir hosts—fruit bats or flying foxes—or indirectly via a secondary amplifying host such as pigs, horses, and humans. Direct bat-to-human transmission has been associated with consuming contaminated fruit or liquid (e.g., date palm sap).[109–111] Human-to-human transmission of NiV has been well documented, especially in Bangladesh[117,124–126] and the most recent outbreak in Kerala (India).[17] However, all seven known cases of HeV infections in humans have resulted from contact with sick horses already exhibiting symptoms of respiratory distress,[127] likely after being exposed to food

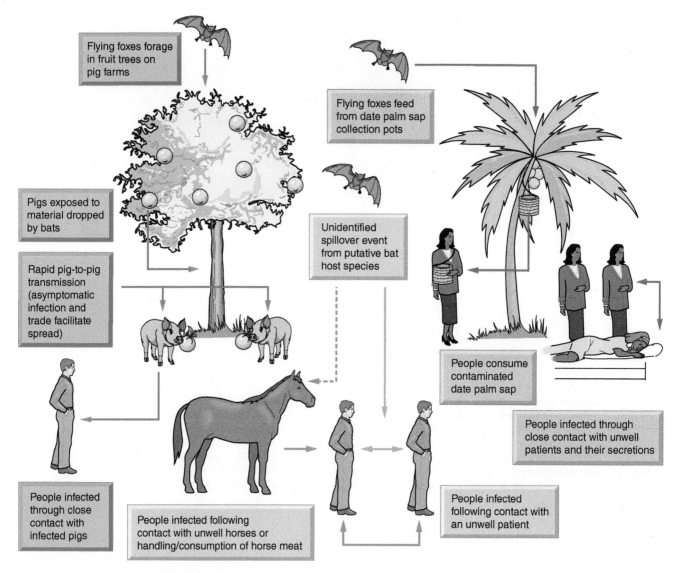

FIGURE 13.6 Nipah virus transmission. Major pathways of human Nipah virus infection are summarized for Malaysia (*blue arrows*), Bangladesh (*red arrows*), the Philippines (*green arrows*), and the latest outbreak in Kerala, India (*orange arrows*). (Adapted from Clayton BA. Nipah virus: transmission of a zoonotic paramyxovirus. *Curr Opin Virol* 2017;22:97–104.)

or water contaminated with saliva and urine/droppings from HeV-infected flying foxes.[128] While patients that succumb to henipavirus infections eventually die from encephalitic complications that often involve brainstem neuronal dysfunction,[108,129] there is diversity of clinical presentations.[130] For example, NiV-MY–infected patients in Malaysia present less often with respiratory involvement (~40%) than the vast majority of NiV-BD–infected patients in Bangladesh and India. A handful of HeV-infected humans have also presented with encephalitic illness with or without a respiratory component (see Clinical Features section). To better understand the pathogenesis and pathology associated with henipavirus disease in humans, many relevant animal models have been developed that either represent natural amplifying hosts (pigs and horses) or reproduce well the respiratory and encephalitic disease seen in humans (hamsters, ferrets, and AGMs).[131,132] Despite the broad host range mentioned in the prior section, other animal challenge models (guinea pigs, cats, dogs) either do not represent the full

spectrum of disease seen in humans or are relatively asymptomatic when challenged with NiV and/or HeV.[93,131]

Site of Primary Replication, Virus Spread, and Cell and Tissue Tropism

The clinical and pathological data from humans (see Clinical Features section), relevant animal models, and cell tropism studies (Table 13.3) indicate that the initial site of replication is within the respiratory system, likely involving cells lining the oro-/nasopharyngeal epithelium as well as bronchiolar epithelial cells, type I pneumocytes, alveolar macrophages, or pulmonary airway dendritic cells (DCs).[40,132–135] The distribution and time of appearance of lesions throughout the vasculature and in the brain and lung in NiV encephalitis suggest that secondary infection probably arises via hematogenous spread of the virus, with secondary replication occurring in vascular endothelium.[136] Inflammation of blood vessels (vasculitis) occurs in

TABLE 13.3 Henipavirus cell tropism and receptor expression

Cell Line/Primary Cells	Species/Cell Type	Virus	EFNB2[a]	EFNB3[a]	Infection Permissive[b]	References[c]
Human						
HeLa-CCL2	Human cervical cancer	NiV HeV	+	−	+	44,62
HeLa-USU	Human cervical cancer	NiV HeV	−	−	−	62
HeLa-USU-EFNB2	HeLa-USU stably expressing EFNB2	HeV CedV	+ +	− −	+ +	28,53
HeLa-USU-EFNB3	HeLa-USU stably expressing EFNB3	HeV CedV	− −	+ +	+ −	28,53
Vero (various subclones)	African green monkey kidney epithelial	NiV HeV CedV GhV	++	+	+	2,11,28,62,304,305
293T	Human embryonic kidney fibroblast		+	+	+	306–309
A549	Human lung adenocarcinoma	NiV HeV	+	+	+	49,87,310
PCI 13	Human head and neck carcinoma	NiV HeV	+	+	+	62,267
U373-MG	Human astroglioma	NiV	+	++	+	62,150,267
U87-MG	Human glioblastoma	NiV GhV	+	+	+	65,305,311,312
HBMEC (primary)	Human brain microvascular endothelial	NiV	+	−	+	136,304
HUVEC (primary)	Human umbilical cord endothelial	NiV HeV	+	+	+	43,313
HuNSC neurons/ astrocytes (Primary)	Human neural stem cell–derived neurons and astrocytes	NiV HeV	+	+	+	43,314
NHBE (primary)	(Normal) human bronchial epithelial	NiV HeV	+	+	+	315,316
SAEC (primary)	Human small airway epithelial	NiV HeV	+	+	+	315,316
Hu PBL (primary)	Human peripheral blood lymphocytes	NiV	(+/−)[d]	(+/−)[d]	−	150
HuMono/Mac/DCs (primary)	Human monocytes, macrophages, dendritic cells	NiV	Mono/Mac (+/−)[d] DC (+/−)[d]	Mono/Mac (+/−)[d] DC (−)	Mono (−) Mac (−) DC (+/−)	150,182
HuOE (primary)	Human olfactory epithelial	NiV HeV	(?)	+	+	142,317
Nonhuman						
BHK-21	Baby hamster kidney fibroblast	NiV	+	(?)	+	44,310
CHO	Chinese hamster ovary	NiV HeV	−	−	−	44,63,64
CHO-B2	CHO stably expressing ephrin-B2	NiV HeV	+	−	+	63,64
CHO-B3	CHO stably expressing ephrin-B3	NiV HeV	−	+	+	63,64
CRFK	Cat (feline) kidney epithelial	NiV HeV	+	+	+	308

(continued)

TABLE 13.3   Henipavirus cell tropism and receptor expression *(Continued)*

Cell Line/Primary Cells	Species/Cell Type	Virus	EFNB2[a]	EFNB3[a]	Infection Permissive[b]	References[c]
PBMEC (primary)	Porcine brain microvascular endothelial	NiV	+	+	+	304,318
PAEC (primary)	Pig aorta endothelial	NiV	−	−	−	304
PK13	Pig kidney fibroblast	NiV	−	−	−	63,319
Rat cortical neurons	Rat cortical neurons (Primary)	NiV	+	+	+	63,307
4/4RM4	Rat pleural mesothelial	NiV	+	ND	+	44,320
L2	Rat lung epithelial	NiV	+	ND	+	44,321
208f	Rat embryonic fibroblast	NiV	+	ND	−	44,321
P815	Mouse mast cell	NiV	+	ND	−	44,321
MyEnd	Mouse myocardial endothelial	NiV	(?)	(?)	−	304
PaLuT02	Immortalized *P. alecto* (fruit bat) lung cells	NiV HeV	+	+	+	175,322
PaKi	Primary *P. alecto* (fruit bat) kidney cells	HeV	+	+	+	175,322
PaBrH04	Immortalized *P. alecto* (fruit bat) brain cells	NiV HeV	+	+	+	322,323
MMEC	Mouse microvascular endothelium	NiV HeV	(?)	(?)	(+/−)[d]	310

[a]Expression inferred from (1) transcriptional data (microarray, next-generation sequencing, RT-PCR, etc.) provided in the cited references, or (2) independently verified through the Gene Expression Omnibus (GEO) database (https://www.ncbi.nlm.nih.gov/geo/), or (3) competition with soluble ephrin-B ligands or interference with cognate henipavirus receptor–binding proteins.
[b]For clarity and uniformity, only infection-permissive (not fusion-permissive) data are indicated; infection includes use of live virus and/or pseudotyped virus.
[c]References cited support expression, infection data, or cell-type origin where relevant and are representative, not comprehensive.
[d]Indicates greater than 10–100-fold below positive control when quantitative data are available. ND, not determined; (?), not specifically mentioned.

most organs but is particularly prominent in the brain, lung, heart, kidney, and spleen.[9,136,137] Vasculitis is limited to small arteries, arterioles, and capillaries where NiV antigen is found in both endothelial cells and the smooth muscle of the tunica media. The pattern and time of appearance of vasculitis and viral antigen distribution are consistent with endothelial cell infection occurring before infection of the smooth muscle. The 5-day interval between maximal vasculitis in the brain and parenchymal infection in acute NiV encephalitis suggests that virus replication occurs first in endothelial cells, with infection of neurons occurring as a result of vascular damage and break-down of the blood–brain barrier (BBB). In humans as well as in pigs and hamsters, viral antigen–positive brain microvascular endothelial cells can be observed in areas of compromised BBB integrity.[136,138,139] The presence of inclusion bodies and viral antigen in neurons, along with widespread histologic and radiologic lesions, suggests that neurologic impairment in NiV (and HeV) encephalitis may be caused by both the effects of ischemia and infarction and viral infection of neurons.[12,107,136]

In addition to the systemic vasculitis, NiV antigen is clearly present in the parenchyma of multiple organs mentioned above. The same pathology has been reported for a fatal case of acute HeV encephalitis.[140] Similar widespread infection and multiorgan vasculopathy has been demonstrated in relevant animal models with the highest viral antigen load consistently

seen in the lung and brain (Fig. 13.7).[131,132] Interestingly, intra-nasal inoculation in pigs, hamsters, and ferrets suggests that NiV can also directly invade the central nervous system (CNS) through the olfactory epithelium (OE). NiV antigen–positive neurons or olfactory nerves can be found extending through the cribriform plate or in the nasal turbinate into the olfactory bulb.[133,139,141] While primary human OE cells are susceptible to henipavirus infection,[142] the olfactory route is unlikely to be the major mode of CNS invasion in humans (and the AGM model). Primates have a relatively smaller area of OE compared to hamsters, pigs, or ferrets where the majority of evidence regarding the olfactory route of entry has been gathered.[97,139,141] In addition, NiV antigen was not detected in the olfactory bulbs of at least nine infected patients from the autopsy series reported from the Malaysian outbreak.[136]

The widespread cell and tissue tropism of NiV and HeV seen in humans and the various animal models is determined by the expression pattern of the henipavirus receptors, ephrin-B2 and ephrin-B3.[61–64] The ephrin-B ligands and their cognate EphB receptors are both receptor tyrosine kinases that mediate bidirectional cell–cell signaling events upon engaging each other. They are critical modulators of cell remodeling events, especially within the nervous and vascular systems.[143,144] They are also highly conserved among vertebrates, which explains, at least in part, the unusually broad species tropism of

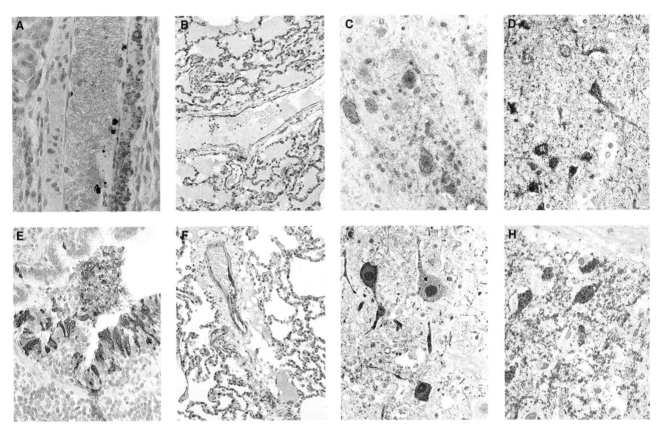

FIGURE 13.7 Immunohistochemistry detection of Nipah virus (NiV) and Hendra virus (HeV) antigen in henipavirus-infected tissues.
A–D: Hendra virus–infected tissues. **A:** Staining of HeV antigen (N protein–specific rabbit antibody) within the wall of superficial arteriole in the submucosa of the nasal cavity in an HeV-infected horse. **B:** Immunolabeling (N protein–specific rabbit antibody) of the endothelium of medium-caliber vessels and alveolar septa in the lung of an HeV-infected African green monkey (AGM) (10×). **C:** Immunolabeling of HeV antigen (N protein–specific rabbit antibody) within neurons in the brainstem of an HeV-infected AGM (40×). **D:** Immunolabeling of HeV antigens (mouse anti-HeV polyclonal antibody) in neurons of acute HeV-infected human case (40×). **E:** Positive immunolabeling (using anti–Nipah virus rabbit serum) within the lung of an NiV-infected pig. Involvement of bronchial epithelium and airway debris is noted. **F:** Immunolabeling (N protein–specific antibody) of the endothelium of medium-caliber vessels and alveolar septa in the lung of an NiV-infected AGM (20×). **G:** Immunolabeling of NiV antigen (N protein–specific antibody) within neurons in the brainstem of an NiV-infected AGM (40×). **H:** Immunolabeling of NiV antigens (hyperimmune anti-NiV mouse ascitic fluid) in the cytoplasm and nuclei of neurons and neuronal processes in the brain of acute NiV-infected human case (158×). (**A and E:** Courtesy of Dr. Deborah Middleton, CSIRO Australian Animal Health Laboratory. **B, C, F and G**: Courtesy of Dr. Karla Fenton, University of Texas Medical Branch at Galveston, Texas. **D:** Courtesy of Dr. Kum Thong Wong, University of Malaya. **H:** From Wong KT, Shieh WJ, Kumar S, et al. Nipah virus infection: pathology and pathogenesis of an emerging paramyxoviral zoonosis. *Am J Pathol* 2002;161(6):2153–2167.)

henipaviruses. Ephrin-B2 is found in arteries, arterioles, and capillaries in multiple organs and is more broadly distributed across multiple tissues and cell types (Fig. 13.8), including neurons, arterial smooth muscle, and human bronchiolar epithelial cells,[143,145–147] but is absent from venous components of the vasculature.[148,149] In contrast, ephrin-B3 is essentially restricted to the brain[144] where it is expressed higher than ephrin-B2 (Fig. 13.8). Its relative absence from organs such as the lung, kidney, and spleen, as well as from arterial endothelium, suggests that the systemic vasculitis, respiratory distress, and other end-organ pathologies seen in henipavirus infections are largely a consequence of ephrin-B2–mediated entry. Conversely, ephrin-B3–mediated entry may play a larger role in the spread of HeV and NiV within the CNS.

Human lymphocytes (mainly T and B cells), and monocytes, despite being nonpermissive for NiV infection[150] or HeV F/RBP–induced fusion,[94] can bind and transfer NiV to permissive microvascular endothelial cells *in vitro*.[150] This transinfection phenotype, thought to be mediated by heparan sulfates,[151] may be an efficient form of hematogenous spread in addition to the free form viruses that make up the plasma viremia seen in acute NiV and HeV infections in humans. This acute but transient viremia appears about 4 to 7 days post onset of illness (POI) and, in survivors, is usually undetectable within 2 to 4 weeks POI depending on severity of the disease course.[17,152–154] A similar course of plasma viremia can also be detected in AGMs challenged intratracheally and orally with NiV.[98] The next section on the Immune Response will discuss possible mechanisms by which viremia is cleared in survivors.

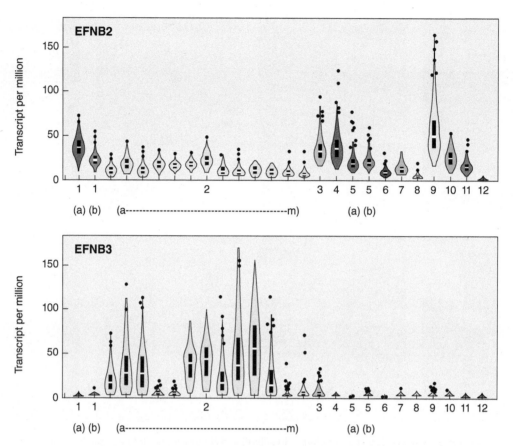

FIGURE 13.8 Ephrin-B2 and ephrin-B3 RNA-seq expression data across representative human nondisease tissues. Shown here are ephrin-B2 (*upper*) and ephrin-B3 (*lower*) expression data obtained from the Genotype-Tissue Expression (GTEx) Portal. The GTEx project is a public resource where up to 53 nondisease tissue sites obtained from nearly 1,000 individuals are subjected to RNA-seq by next-generation sequencing among other assays. Details on datasets can be found on https://gtexportal.org. Data from all available brain regions are shown. The nonbrain tissues are chosen for illustrative purposes based on their relevance to henipavirus pathogenesis. Expression data in transcripts per million are plotted as *violin plots* with the medians and 25th and 75th percentiles shown; points are displayed as outliers if they are above or below 1.5 times the interquartile range. 1a Artery, aorta; 1b artery, coronary; 2a brain, amygdala; 2b brain, anterior cingulate cortex (BA24); 2c brain, caudate (basal ganglia); 2d brain, cerebellar hemisphere; 2e brain, cerebellum; 2f brain, cortex; 2g brain, frontal cortex (BA9); 2h brain, hippocampus; 2i brain, hypothalamus; 2j brain, nucleus accumbens (basal ganglia); 2k brain, putamen (basal ganglia); 2l brain, spinal cord (cervical c-1); 2m brain, substantia nigra; 3 breast, mammary tissue; 4 colon, transverse; 5 esophagus, gastroesophageal junction; esophagus, mucosa; 6 heart, left ventricle; 7 kidney, cortex; 8 liver; 9 lung; 10 minor salivary gland; 11 spleen; 12 whole blood.

Immune Response

Viral Antagonism of Innate Immune Responses

HeV and NiV have a broad host range that is uncommon in paramyxoviruses. This ability to replicate, spread, and cause acutely lethal disease among multiple species suggests that these viruses have evolved effective means to antagonize or evade innate antiviral responses that might otherwise keep them in check until adaptive immune responses develop. In henipaviruses, as in other paramyxoviruses,[40] the major anti-interferon (IFN) activities are encoded by the *P* gene, and *in vitro* studies indicate that *P* gene products inhibit both IFN induction and signaling (Fig. 13.9).[39] In IFN induction, various forms of viral double-stranded RNA (dsRNA) are detected by cytoplasmic RNA helicases[155–157] such as RIG-I and MDA5 and by toll-like receptor-3 (TLR3).[157,158] Both of these dsRNA signaling pathways, via a cascade of signaling events depicted in Figure 13.9 (left), lead to activation and nuclear translocation of interferon regulatory factor (IRF) 3, or if present, IRF7, and nuclear factor kappa B (NF-κB), transcription factors that induce the expression of IFN-α/β proteins. HeV and NiV inhibit dsRNA signaling via its V protein, which binds to MDA5 and prevents downstream signaling[155,159,160] but does not abrogate dsRNA signaling through TLR3.[161] Recent evidence suggests that NiV V also binds RIG-I and its regulator (TRIM25), disrupting downstream signaling.[162] In an additional strategy unique to henipaviruses, the W protein, by virtue of an NLS located in the unique carboxy-terminal, inhibits induction of IFN-α/β expression in the nucleus by targeting a process that is part of both helicase-dependent and TLR3-dependent signaling pathways.[163] Unexpectedly, the NiV M protein can also inhibit

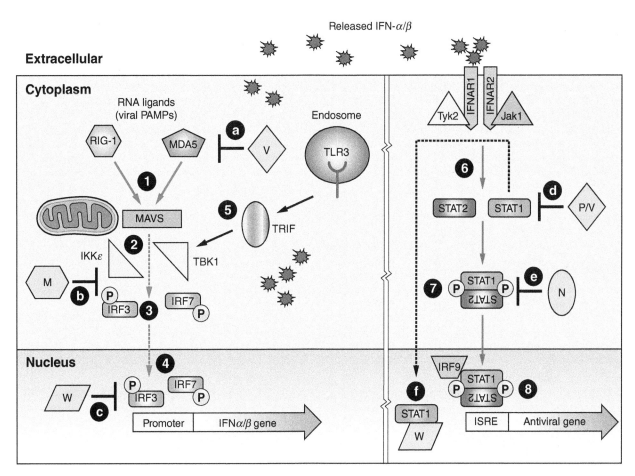

FIGURE 13.9 Innate immune evasion mechanisms of the Nipah virus N, P, V, W, and M proteins. Left: The V and W proteins (*green diamonds and trapezoids, respectively*) block IFN-α/β expression by different mechanisms. Depicted are simplified versions of the RIG-I–like receptor (RLR) signaling (*blue arrows*) and TLR3 signaling (*black arrows*) pathways. Both lead to activation of interferon regulatory factors 3 and 7 (IRF3 and IRF7) (*blue dashed arrow*). RIG-I, MDA5, and TLR3 can sense RNAs produced during viral infection. Activation of RIG-I or MDA5 leads to their interaction with the mitochondria-associated adapter protein MAVS (*1*). This leads to activation of the kinases IKKε and/or TBK-1 (*2*), which phosphorylate and activate IRF3 and, when present, IRF7 (*3*). For clarity, MAVS activation of NF-κB is not shown. Activated IRF3 and IRF7 translocate into and accumulate in the nucleus; both contribute to IFN-α/β gene transcription (*4*). TLR3 signals through adaptor protein TRIF to activate IKKε/TBK-1 (*5*). The cytoplasmic NiV and HeV V proteins interact with and inhibit MDA5, thereby inhibiting the induction of IFN-α/β expression early on in the pathway (*a*); however NiV V does not appear to inhibit TLR3 signaling. The nucleocytoplasmic shuttling NiV M protein (*green hexagon*), while it is in the cytoplasm, antagonizes induction of type I IFNs by blocking IKKε activation (*b*). This prevents downstream phosphorylation and nuclear translocation of IRF3, which also leads to a failure of IFN-α/β induction. The nuclear W protein (*green trapezoid*) effectively blocks RLR and TLR3 activation of the IFN-β promoter by preventing the accumulation of phosphorylated IRF3 (*c*). This function requires the nuclear localization of W. **Right:** The Nipah virus N, P, V, and W proteins each block IFN signaling pathways at distinct steps (*red arrows*), ultimately leading to reduced expression of interferon- stimulated (antiviral) genes (ISGs). The P, V, and W proteins can each inhibit the phosphorylation and activation of STAT1 and STAT2 in response to IFN-α/β (*6*) and block the phosphorylation and activation of STAT1 in response to IFNγ. The inhibition of the IFN-α/β signaling pathway is depicted. The cytoplasmic P and V proteins interact with and inhibit STAT1 (*d*). The V protein also interacts with STAT2, in a STAT1-dependent manner. P and V prevent nuclear accumulation of pSTAT1/pSTAT2 following IFN-α/β addition to cells and cause the STAT proteins to accumulate in a high molecular weight complex. The NiV and HeV N proteins (*green oval*) were recently reported to disrupt phospho-STAT1 complex formation (*7*), though not phosphorylation of STAT1 itself (*e*). Nonetheless, this N-mediated disruption of STAT complexes reduces nuclear accumulation of the activated STAT complexes required to stimulate ISG expression (*8*). The nuclear W protein relocalizes nonphosphorylated STAT1 from its typically cytoplasmic localization to the nucleus (*f*). STAT1 relocalized to the nucleus by W remains unphosphorylated and does not activate transcription of ISGs in response to IFN-α/β addition. (Adapted from Basler CF. Nipah and Hendra virus interactions with the innate immune system. *Curr Top Microbiol Immunol* 2012;359:123–152.)

IFN-α/β induction by indirectly antagonizing the activity of IKKε, the kinase responsible for IRF3 activation.[51]

In the IFN signaling pathway (Fig. 13.9, right), IFN binds to the IFN-α/β receptor (IFNAR) on cells and initiates a signaling sequence that leads to activation of members of a family of proteins called *signal transducers and activators of transcription* (STAT).[164,165] Henipaviruses inhibit IFN signaling by sequestering STAT proteins in high molecular weight complexes and preventing their phosphoactivation.[166,167] The anti-IFN signaling activity is a property of the V protein, as has been observed for other paramyxoviruses, but also of the W and P proteins.[45,161,166,167] The P, V, and W proteins of henipaviruses have an N-terminal extension of 100 to 200 amino acids compared with cognate proteins in the subfamily,[20,23] and the STAT-binding domain of NiV V maps to this region.[161,168,169] The V and P proteins bind STAT in the cytoplasm, whereas the W protein, which is imported into the nucleus via specific interactions of its NLS with importin α-3,[170] likely sequesters unactivated STAT1 in the nucleus.[161,163] Recently, NiV and HeV N proteins were also found to antagonize IFN signaling by interfering with formation of activated phospho (p)-STAT1 complexes. This NiV N–mediated antagonism of pSTAT1 nuclear accumulation does *not* rely on direct binding to or inhibiting phosphorylation of STAT1 itself.[171] NiV C has also been demonstrated to interfere with IFN signaling.[47,172] However, its mechanism and true function remain unclear. Antagonizing IFN signaling is unlikely to be the main function of the C protein since recombinant C-deficient NiVs have an attenuated replication phenotype even in Vero cells,[41,45,46] which are genetically deficient in IFN production.

There is little doubt that inhibition of IFN-α/β production is one major contributor to the acute virulence of HeV and NiV *in vivo*. Daily administration of poly(I)–poly(C[12]U), a potent IFN inducer, results in greater than 80% survival in a lethal challenge hamster model for NiV infections.[173] Most of the studies described previously were carried out *in vitro* using single-gene transfection expression systems. Understanding the true function(s) of these proteins requires assessing their impact in the context of a live virus infection or the phenotype of viruses deficient in the cognate protein(s). For example, IFN signaling apparently remains functional during live HeV and NiV infection of human cell lines, whereas IFN production was inhibited.[174] However, henipaviruses also clearly antagonize both IFN production and signaling in bat cells derived from *Pteropus* sp. that serve as their natural hosts.[175]

The diverse phenotypes observed in the various animal models when challenged with recombinant viruses deficient in the various *P*-derived accessory proteins make interpretation difficult. The clearest phenotype comes from rNiVs engineered to be V-deficient. rNiV-ΔV are extremely attenuated in both hamster and ferret challenge models.[46,50] Each model recapitulates the respiratory and neurological disease seen in human infections when infected with wt NiV, albeit in different ways and in a dose-dependent fashion.[103,131,176] However, challenge with V-deficient rNiV under conditions where their wt counterparts effectuate 100% mortality always results in 100% survival, and almost never results in any overt respiratory or neurological signs.[46,50] On the other hand, C-deficient rNiVs give a variety of phenotypes that range from strong attenuation in the hamster model[177] to 100% mortality in the ferret model, albeit with less severe histological lesions in the lung.[52] Similarly, W-deficient rNiVs did not show significant attenuation compared to their wild-type counterparts in both the hamster[46] and ferret models, although the disease symptomology appeared to be more neurologic in the latter.[50,52] Interestingly, an rNiV lacking both C and W still resulted in 60% mortality with reduced respiratory disease but markedly increased neurological disease.[52]

Adaptive Immune Responses

In patients with encephalitis, anti-NiV antibodies were observed more frequently in the serum than the CSF. Immunoglobulin M (IgM) antibodies occurred more frequently than immunoglobulin G (IgG) antibodies in both locations.[9,12,136] The appearance of specific IgM antibodies in serum preceded their appearance in the CSF, a sequence consistent with viremia preceding central nervous system (CNS) infection. Anti-NiV antibodies were present in most patients with clinical NiV encephalitis; however, no difference was observed in clinical features, laboratory results, or mortality between seropositive and seronegative patients.[108,178] Seroconversion of IgG against HeV was seen in two human cases of HeV infection in 2008, with one progressing to fatal encephalitis.[8] From these cases, seroconversion in acute henipavirus disease may have diagnostic but no apparent prognostic value. Conversely, in the most recent NiV outbreak in Kerala involving 23 cases, careful monitoring of humoral and cellular immune responses in the 2 survivors revealed that there was a dramatic increase in activated (Ki67+) CD8+ T cells with an acute effector phenotype (CD38+/HLA-DR+/Granzyme B+/PD1+), suggesting that virus-specific naïve T cells were actively proliferating in response to the virus. Interestingly, clearance of viremia coincided with the peak of proliferating Ki67+ CD8+ T cells and occurred before peak IgG titers.[152] Increases in activated CD8+ T cells in lethal (NHP)[179] and nonlethal (swine) animal models of NiV infection have also been observed[180]; in the latter, prevention of virus shedding appears correlated with such T-cell responses. However, most animal studies do not monitor adaptive immune responses with the requisite precision and sophistication in order to make definitive statements regarding the relative importance of T- or B-cell responses in protective immunity against acute henipavirus infections.[181]

The high CFR associated with the acute nature of henipavirus infections already suggests that the virus interferes with the timely generation of effective T- or B-cell responses during the *natural* history of the disease in the majority of infected individuals. Indeed, although NiV replicates poorly in DCs (Table 13.3),[150,182] *in vitro* NiV-infected DCs induce an inflammatory proapoptotic milieu (TNF-α, IL-1β, IL-8) that leads not only to defective T-cell priming but apoptosis of cognate T cells and DCs.[182] This *in vitro* phenomenon, if recapitulated *in vivo* by NiV-infected DCs that traffic to lymph nodes, may account for the lymphoid depletion and lymphoid necrotic lesions seen in humans[136] and various relevant animal models.[50,183,184]

Release from Host and Transmission

Transmission is generally accepted to occur via the oronasal route[8,107,108] or liquid/food (palm sap/fruit),[109–111] with transmissibility of HeV (horse–human or human-to-human)[185,186] being much less efficient than that of NiV transmission (pig-to-human or human-to-human).[9,15,17,108,115,117,126,187,188] Infectious NiV can be recovered from urine and the tracheal and nasopharyngeal secretions of infected patients in the early phase of their illness in the original Malaysian outbreak.[3,107,108] Nonetheless, human-to-human transmission in the Malaysian outbreak was extremely rare,[189] although it has been reported in the more recent outbreak in the Philippines. In contrast, person-to-person transmission in Bangladesh has been well documented and typically occurs during the final stages of disease in the index patient when not only symptoms of respiratory involvement are most prominent but also more frequent and closer contact with familial caretakers occurs.[125,187,188]

Replication in the respiratory epithelium and shedding in oronasal secretions is most likely responsible for virus release and transmission. Ferrets have been used to model the respiratory transmission of henipaviruses[112,184] as their respiratory symptoms (cough, serous nasal discharge, dyspnea) mimic the human disease.[97] Despite shedding relatively large amounts of virus in their oronasal secretions (4–5 log10 $TCID_{50}$ equivalents/mL at peak titers), passively cohoused naïve ferrets never got infected, regardless of whether the index ferrets were infected with HeV, NiV-MY, or NiV-BD.[112,184] However, following assisted or direct exposure to infectious oronasal fluids from the index ferrets, all the naïve ferrets developed acute infections, regardless of virus strain used.[112] Thus, the efficiency of NiV transmission appears low and likely requires direct and repeated oro- or nasomucosal exposure to infectious oronasal secretions. This is consistent with epidemiological investigations into the many recurrent outbreaks in Bangladesh where despite chains of person-to-person transmission, the estimated basic reproductive number R_0 of NiV-BD strains that have spilled over in Bangladesh have averaged 0.48.[187]

Virulence

Infection with HeV appears more severe than infection with NiV-MY and NiV-BD in the hamster[138,190] and AGM model.[191] The dose-dependent disease symptomology in the hamster model[138,192] makes it difficult to make generalized statements about any intrinsic pathogenic difference between these three genetically distinct henipaviruses. However, the intratracheal and intranasal AGM challenge model appears to recapitulate the clinical pathologies seen in human patients more robustly.[98,103] Interestingly, it is also in this model that NiV-BD is shown to be more pathogenic than NiV-MY,[191] which reflects the observed differences in pathogenicity between NiV-MY and NiV-BD. Previous studies comparing NiV-MY and NiV-BD in hamsters[190] and in ferrets[112] gave conflicting and confusing results. But more careful comparisons of fully sequenced NiV-MY and NiV-BD strains in the AGM model provide support that NiV-BD is more pathogenic than NiV-MY,[191] consistent with the higher mortality rates associated with NiV-BD (see Table 13.1C). Under identical experimental conditions, not only is NiV-BD shown to be more pathogenic in terms of viral load in the lungs, spleen, and blood, but also the therapeutic window for postexposure prophylaxis using human monoclonal antibody (m102.4) is significantly shorter in NiV-BD–infected AGMs.[191] m102.4 is a potent neutralizing mAb previously shown to rescue NiV-MY– and HeV-infected AGMs even when administered up to 7 days postinfection.[193,194]

CedV lacks the editing site in the *P* gene and does not make the V protein,[28] a potent type I IFN antagonist required for henipavirus virulence *in vivo*.[39] Not surprisingly, CedV, which is naturally V-deficient, also does not induce any overt disease in ferrets and guinea pigs.[28] Reactive hyperplasia of oropharyngeal lymphoid tissues and detection of viral RNA in select bronchial associated lymphoid tissue (BALT) accompanied by increasing neutralizing Ab titers suggests that CedV likely replicates transiently in the upper and lower respiratory tracts of the challenged animals.[28] While recent evidence suggests that the CedV P protein itself is also a less efficient antagonizer of IFN-α signaling compared to HeV P,[195] whether CedV is truly nonpathogenic in humans or horses remains to be seen. Given the fact that CedV does not appear to use ephrin-B3 as receptor, one might also predict CedV to be less encephalopathic even in more susceptible animals.

Persistence

A small percentage of NiV-infected patients (3%–7%) experience late-onset or relapse encephalitis months to years after the initial NiV infection; the former describes patients with initially mild or asymptomatic NiV infections, while the latter are survivors of acute NiV encephalitis.[108,129,196,197] One case of fatal late-onset HeV encephalitis has also been reported.[3,140] These cases suggest that NiV and HeV can persist in sanctuary sites like the brain especially since virus has never been isolated from oronasal secretions of relapsed encephalitis cases[9,107,136,196–198] (see Clinical Features section for details). There is one report of NiV RNA being detected in the semen of an NiV survivor 4 weeks POI, but this was gone 2 weeks later. Longitudinal studies on two HeV survivors show no evidence of viral shedding by RT-qPCR, up to 6 years postsymptom onset.[154] It is unlikely that NiV and HeV in humans can persist in infectious forms. Thus, relapse henipavirus encephalitis might resemble measles virus–associated subacute sclerosing panencephalitis, which can occur years after recovery from measles virus infection.[199,200]

EPIDEMIOLOGY

Age

The age of patients with encephalitis in the Malaysian outbreak ranged from 9 to 76 years, with almost 50% of cases occurring in those 40 to 44 years.[108,136,153,178,201] The male-to-female ratio was approximately 3:1, and more than 80% of the patients were Chinese, with statistics reflecting the increased risk to those working with infected pigs.[108,201] In Bangladesh, the age of patients ranged from 4 to 60 years, and males constituted 47% and 67% of the cases in the 2001 and 2003 outbreaks, respectively.[14,202] The outbreak in early 2011 in Bangladesh claimed at least 35 lives, including many children and infants, with ages ranging from 2 to 56 years.[127,203] Among the 18 suspected patients in the 2014 outbreak in the Philippines, the age distribution is between 21 and 60 years old.[18] In the most recent NiV outbreak in Kerala, India, the age distribution ranged from a 17-year-old male to a 75-year-old female among a total of 23 human cases.[17]

Morbidity and Mortality

In Malaysia, between September 1998 and June 1999, 256 patients who developed acute NiV encephalitis were admitted to Malaysian hospitals, and 105 died, a mortality rate of approximately 40%.[9,201] The rate of subclinical infection in households and farms where cases of NiV encephalitis occurred was calculated to be 8% and 11%, respectively.[196,201] In Singapore, where 11 patients were confirmed to have acute NiV encephalitis, a further 2 asymptomatic abattoir workers were serologically positive, representing a rate of subclinical infection of 15%.[204] Subsequently, 89 individuals were identified on the basis of positive serology as having experienced either an asymptomatic or mildly symptomatic NiV infection.[129] This increases the number of people infected with NiV to 345 and decreases the mortality rate to approximately 30%.[137] In Bangladesh, 98 of 135 patients died in 8 outbreaks from 2001 to 2008, giving a combined case fatality rate of 73%.[117,188,202] In the Philippines outbreak, the case mortality is 53% out of all the suspected cases or 81% for those with encephalitic clinical signs.[18] The case mortality is 94% for the 2018 Kerala outbreak in India.[17] There have only been seven known human cases of HeV infection in Australia in the past 16 years, four of which have been fatal (three acute and one case of relapsed encephalitis).[2,3,8]

Origin and Spread of Epidemics

Fruit bats (flying foxes) in the genus *Pteropus*, family Pteropodidae, and suborder Megachiroptera are main reservoir hosts of HeV and NiV.[5,6,13,89,205] In Australia, HeV has been shown to occur in all four flying fox species, with the crude seroprevalence of 47%, indicating an endemic pattern of infection throughout Australia.[91] Serologic tests show that NiV or NiV-related virus is widely dispersed in bats from Indonesia to the west border of Africa (Fig. 13.10). NiV was first isolated from the urine of island flying foxes and from the saliva on partially eaten fruit[13] and has since been isolated from Lyle's flying foxes (*Pteropus lylei*) in Cambodia[89] and *Pteropus medius* in Bangladesh.[206] The Indian flying fox (*Pteropus giganteus*) is the main pteropid species throughout Bangladesh and the

Indian subcontinent with a high seroprevalence of henipavirus-specific antibody.[14,110,187,207] Additional serologic and limited nucleic acid evidence has suggested that related henipaviruses are circulating in other regions, including Thailand, Indonesia, Vietnam, China, Madagascar, and several countries and regions in Africa (Fig. 13.10 and Table 13.4).

Neither HeV nor NiV appear to cause clinical disease in naturally infected bats.[91,202,205,208] Experimental infection with doses of HeV that are lethal in horses generates sporadic vasculitis in the lung, spleen, meninges, kidney, and gastrointestinal tract and, even then, only in a proportion of infected bats.[105] Viral antigen is detected in the tunica media rather than endothelial cells, a fact that may spare these bats from the clinical effects associated with vasculitis.[209] In infected pregnant fruit bats, antigen was observed in similar locations and in the placenta.[210] The mode of transmission between fruit bats is unknown. Transplacental transmission has also been observed experimentally without apparent harm to the fetus.[210] Experimental infection of fruit bats with NiV produced a subclinical infection with a transient presence of virus within selected viscera along with periodic viral excretion in bat urine and seroconversion with neutralizing antibody present.[100]

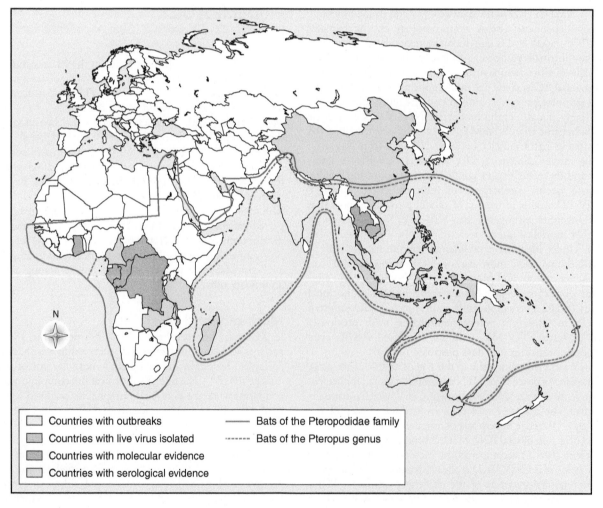

FIGURE 13.10 Distribution of frugivorous bats belonging to various genera in the Pteropodidae family where evidence of henipavirus presence have been detected. The presence of henipavirus is graded into four levels with known outbreak (*yellow*), virus isolation (*blue*), molecular detection (*brown*), and antibody detection (*green*).

TABLE 13.4 Detection of nipah or nipah-related virus infection in bats (geographic surveillance studies)

Bat Species	Method and Country of Detection			References
	Serology	PCR	Isolation	
Suborder: Yinpterochiroptera				
Cynopterus brachyotis	Malaysia			205
Cynopterus sphinx	Vietnam			292
Eidolon dupreanum	Madagascar			324
Eidolon helvum	Ghana, Zambia, Malawi, Tanzania, Uganda, Rio Muni, Bioko, Príncipe, São Tomé, Annobón, Cameroon	Ghana, Gabon, Democratic Republic of the Congo, Central African Republic		19,29,222,296,325
Eonycteris spelaea	Malaysia			205
Epomophorus gambianus	Ghana	Democratic Republic of the Congo, Gabon, Republic of the Congo		29,296
Hipposideros armiger	China			287
Hipposideros larvatus	Thailand	Thailand		286
Hipposideros pomona	China			287
Hypsignathus monstrosus	Ghana	Republic of the Congo, Central African Republic,		29,296
Myonycteris torquata		Democratic Republic of the Congo, Gabon, Republic of the Congo		29
Rhinolophus affinis	China			287
Rhinolophus sinicus	China			287
Rousettus leschenaulti	China, Vietnam			287,292
Rousettus aegyptiacus		Gabon		29
Pteropus giganteus	Bangladesh, India			207
Pteropus hypomelanus	Malaysia, Thailand	Thailand	Malaysia	205,221,326
Pteropus lylei	Cambodia, Thailand	Thailand	Cambodia	89,290,327
Pteropus medius		Bangladesh, India	Bangladesh	206,328,329
Pteropus rufus	Madagascar			324
Pteropus vampyrus	Malaysia, Thailand			205,286
Suborder: Yangochiroptera				
Carollia perspicillata		Costa Rica		29
Miniopterus spp.	China			287
Myotis daubentonii	China			287
Myotis ricketti	China			287
Pteronotus parnellii		Costa Rica		29
Scotophilus kuhlii	Malaysia			205

The spillover and epidemic hosts of HeV and NiV were horses in Australia and the Philippines and pigs in Malaysia. All human infections with HeV in Australia and NiV in Malaysia have only occurred through transmission from these domestic animal hosts.[9,201] No evidence exists of direct transmission from pteropid bats to humans in Australia or Malaysia, despite many opportunities in Australia for transmission to bat carers.[196,211] In contrast, fruit bats apparently play a direct role in the transmission of NiV to humans in the many recent outbreaks of disease in Bangladesh, where epidemiologic evidence in support of a role for an intermediate host was lacking.[14,202] Three pathways

of NiV transmission from bats to people have been identified based on epidemiologic investigations in Bangladesh.[117] Consumption of fresh date palm sap appears to be the predominant risk factor, and infrared camera studies have confirmed that *P. giganteus* bats frequently visit date palm sap trees and consume sap during collection.[212] In the 2005 NiV outbreak in Tangail District, Bangladesh, drinking raw date palm sap was the only activity significantly associated with illness (64% among cases vs. 18% among controls).[110] Another route of transmission for NiV from bats to people in Bangladesh could be via domestic animals. Contact with a sick cow in Meherpur,

Bangladesh, in 2001 was strongly associated with NiV infection,[14] and contact with pigs and diseased goats has also been implicated in other occurrences of NiV in Bangladesh.[117] Although NiV has never been isolated in domestic livestock animals, serological evidence was reported for antibodies to NiV or NiV-related viruses in cattle, goats, and pigs in Bangladesh.[213] Transmission via direct contact with NiV-infected bat secretions also appears possible from evidence in the Goalando outbreak in 2004, where individuals who climbed trees were more likely to develop NiV infection than controls.[214]

The mode of transmission from bats to spillover hosts in Australia and Malaysia remains to be determined. Three principal hypotheses exist. One is that masticated pellets of virus-contaminated, residual fruit pulp spat out by flying foxes are ingested by horses or pigs.[205] The second is that urine from infected animals contaminates pastures or pigsties. The third is that infected fetal tissues or fluids contaminate pastures or sties and are ingested. The latter is based largely on the fact that the HeV outbreaks have occurred during the birthing period of some species of flying fox and is supported by the isolation of virus from a pregnant flying fox and its fetus.[6]

HeV has been transmitted from horse to man on seven occasions from 1994 to 2009, twice during the initial outbreak in Brisbane,[1,2] twice during necropsy of horses that died in the field,[1,4] twice during either daily nasal cavity lavage or participating in a necropsy,[8] and once from performing an endoscopy on an infected horse.[8,215] HeV is rarely found in the bronchi or bronchioles of infected horses, which suggests that aerosol transmission to either man or horses is less likely[216] and horse-to-horse transmission of HeV has not been demonstrated.[105] The presence of HeV in equine saliva, however, suggests that close contact with infected horses, such as might occur during manual feeding of the animals, may facilitate horse-to-human transmission.[1] The presence of virus in a wide range of tissues and in the nasal discharge commonly found at the terminal stage of infection offers a range of sources for virus transmission during necropsy.[2,217] As shown in Figure 13.7, high level of viral antigen can be detected in the nasal cavity of HeV-infected horses.

In the Malaysian NiV outbreak, contact with pigs or fresh pig products was required for transmission of the virus to humans, with greater likelihood of transfer to those in direct contact with sick or dying pigs on farms or in abattoirs.[9,201] The presence of NiV in the respiratory epithelium of naturally and experimentally infected pigs (Fig. 13.7) indicated that virus probably spread to humans and within the pig population by aerosol or by direct contact with oropharyngeal or nasal secretions.[10,121,139] The presence of the virus in a wide range of organs indicates that humans may also have been infected during processes such as slaughtering or farrowing. In Bangladesh, pigs were excluded as potential sources of NiV on epidemiological grounds, and human-to-human transmission was observed.[126,188] The virus may have been transmitted to human index cases directly through contact with fruit bat secretions in contaminated fruit or date palm sap before circulation in the human population (Fig. 13.6).[13,14,117,202] Nosocomial transmission has been detected in some of the Bangladesh and India outbreaks.[15,117,218] In the Philippine NiV outbreak, of the 17 case patients, a total of 7 (41%) had participated in horse slaughtering and horse meat consumption; 3 (18%) had only consumed horse meat but had no history of slaughtering or

meat preparation; and 5 (29%) case patients had been exposed to other human case patients but not to any horses. So it is possible that both horse-to-human and human-to-human transmission might have occurred (Fig. 13.6).[18] For the Kerala NiV outbreak, while it remains undefined how the index case was exposed to NiV, it was evident that human-to-human transmission was the main driver for the spread of the virus in both family/community and hospital settings (Fig. 13.6).[17]

Genetic Diversity

Genome sequencing revealed that HeV isolated from equine and human sources during the outbreak in Brisbane appears identical and differs little from HeV isolated from flying foxes 2 years later.[2,6] Sequencing of five additional horse isolates from five different locations from the 2006 to 2008 HeV occurrences has also demonstrated a very high genetic similarity.[219] Similar observations were made in Malaysia, where it was demonstrated that NiV isolated from pigs at the height of the outbreak and at its geographic focus was essentially identical to human isolates made at that time and isolates obtained from flying foxes several years later.[13,22,23,220]

In Bangladesh, four human isolates obtained in 2004 demonstrate significant genetic heterogeneity, which might suggest multiple spillovers of NiV from flying foxes into the human population.[33] The NiV sequences detected from human patients in India from 2001 to 2018 were more related to NiV from Bangladesh than NiV from Malaysia.[15,17,218] A recently whole genome sequencing study of 10 NiV isolates obtained from bats in 2013 in Bangladesh at two different geographic locations revealed that the isolated viruses were very similar in sequences. This suggests that multiple strains were not cocirculating in the bat population at the time.[206] Furthermore, none of the bat NiV isolate sequences was identical with any previously detected human NiV isolate sequences, suggesting that NiV spillover into humans is a rare event and more intensive surveillance is required to appreciate the full genetic diversity of NiV in bats in an area with frequent spillover events into human populations.[206] NiV isolated from the flying fox *Pteropus lylei* in Cambodia[89] represents an evolutionary lineage that is separated from the Malaysia or Bangladesh/India cluster. Partial *N* gene sequences detected in *Pteropus lylei* in Thailand indicate the circulation of at least two lineages of NiV—one related to the Bangladesh NiV and the other more related to the Malaysian NiV.[119] On the other hand, NiV sequences detected in *Pteropus hypomelanus* in Southern Thailand are clearly more related to the Malaysian NiV.[221] As the RNA-dependent RNA polymerase (RdRP), designated as the L protein, is the most highly conserved protein for paramyxoviruses, it has been used as a more reliable indicator of evolutionary relationship among different paramyxoviruses. Figure 13.11 shows an L-based phylogenetic tree of henipavirus species and strains, selected to represent major species origin, geographic location, and time of isolation. Prototype species from other genera in the family *Paramyxoviridae* are also shown for context and comparison.

The presence of henipavirus-reactive (but not neutralizing) antibodies and viral RNA in bats from other regions of the world (Fig. 13.10 and Table 13.4) indicates that a much greater genetic diversity of henipaviruses exists in different bat populations.[29,222,223] These divergent but yet to be characterized henipaviruses likely have different transmissibility, pathogenicity, and receptor usage patterns, as has already been shown for

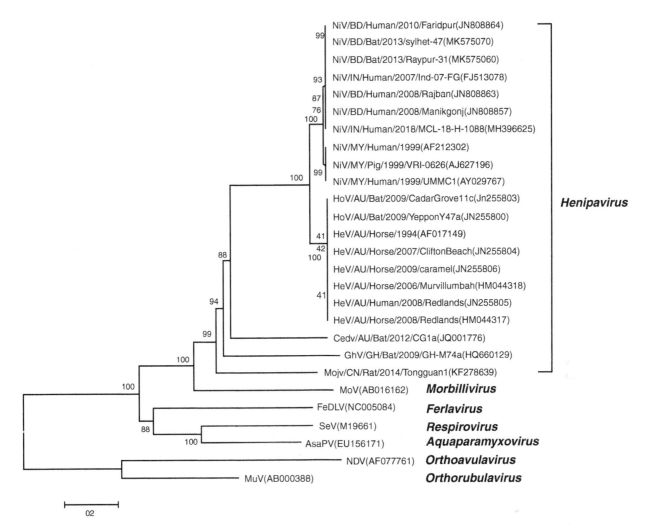

FIGURE 13.11 Phylogenetic tree based on RdRP proteins of selected henipaviruses and prototype species of the other genera in the family *Paramyxoviridae*. Tree was constructed by using neighbor-joining approach with 1,000 bootstrap replicates. Numbers at the nodes represent bootstrap values. Scale bar indicates amino acid substitutions per site. Sequences are labeled with the following ordination when all relative information is available for any given genome sequence: Virus/Country/Host/Year/Strain (GenBank accession number). For example, NiV/BD/Human/2010/Faridpur(JN808864) represents a Nipah virus isolated in Bangladesh from humans in 2010 with Faridpur as its isolate name and JN808864 as its GenBank accession number.

CedV,[28,53,195] GhV,[65,224,225] and MojV.[66] The latter is an outlier in many ways[41,66,86] and is currently the only henipavirus identified in rodents rather than bats.[30]

CLINICAL FEATURES

Incubation Period

Based on the time interval between the last exposure to pigs and onset of disease, the incubation period for NiV ranged from 2 to 45 days; however, for 90% of patients, it was 2 weeks or less.[108,153,178] An estimate of 2 to 3 weeks was made based on the time interval between importation of pigs from NiV-affected areas of Malaysia and development of human disease at a Singaporean abattoir.[204] A mean incubation period of 9.4 days was calculated for four patients who had a fixed period of exposure.[178] The NiV outbreak in Kerala, India, 2018, revealed a median incubation period was 9.5 days among 23 cases, 22 of

which were nosocomial.[17] In the occurrence of HeV in Australia in 2008, a detailed examination of exposure histories from two infected patients (one fatal) suggested a likely incubation period of 9 to 16 days, with exposure occurring some 3 days before the onset of symptoms of HeV infection in the horse.[8]

Acute Clinical Features

The first two patients infected with HeV presented with fever, myalgia, headaches, lethargy, and vertigo. One patient recovered; however, the other developed pneumonitis, respiratory failure, renal failure, and arterial thrombosis and died of cardiac arrest 7 days after admission to the hospital. Findings at autopsy were consistent with a viral infection; both lungs were congested, hemorrhagic, and filled with serous fluid, and the histology revealed focal necrotizing alveolitis with many giant cells, some syncytial formation, and viral inclusions.[1] Although the predominant clinical features of NiV encephalitis derived from CNS involvement in the initial Malaysian outbreak, a proportion (40%) of patients displayed pulmonary involvement, which presented as an atypical pneumonia with fever, cough, and headache.[12,108,136,178] In the Kerala, India, NiV outbreak, 19 cases (83%) presented with acute respiratory distress syndrome (ARDS) and shortness of breath, and 20 cases (87%) had respiratory symptoms.[17] The clinical presentation of NiV infections in Bangladesh also shows severe respiratory disease involvement.[226] A chest x-ray of an acute NiV-infected human case showing diffuse bilateral opacities of the lung fields consistent with ARDS (Fig. 13.12A) and a similar presentation were reported in the first fatal human HeV case.[1] Chest x-ray images of NiV- and HeV-infected AGMs have also demonstrated severe respiratory disease (Fig. 13.12B). Case definitions for suspected NiV infection in Bangladesh[226] and India[15,17] generally included individuals residing in an outbreak area who presented with fever, headache, vomiting, or altered mental status or with history of cough or shortness of breath and fever.

With NiV in Malaysia, most patients presented with acute encephalitis characterized by fever, headache, drowsiness, dizziness, myalgia, and vomiting, and more than 50% had a reduced level of consciousness.[9,12,108,178] The major clinical signs included drowsiness, areflexia, segmental myoclonus, tachycardia, hypertension, pinpoint pupils, and an abnormal doll's eye reflex. Such clinical features as these suggested involvement of the brainstem and upper cervical spinal cord and were observed more frequently in patients with a reduced level of consciousness.[108] In Kerala, India, 2018, NiV-infected patients presented with altered sensorium (74%), along with myalgia, headache, vomiting, and seizures.[17] Patients in the NiV-Malaysian outbreak who retained normal levels of consciousness throughout their illness recovered fully; however, only 15% with reduced levels of consciousness survived. Figure 13.13 shows magnetic resonance imaging (MRI) images of human cases of acute NiV encephalitis. Such neurological manifestations are consistent with vasculitis-induced thrombosis in the brain and the direct infection of neurons.[9,11,12,136] The multiple discrete lesions 1 to 5 mm in diameter in the cerebral white matter detected by MRI may be the site of such microinfarctions and are distinct from lesions

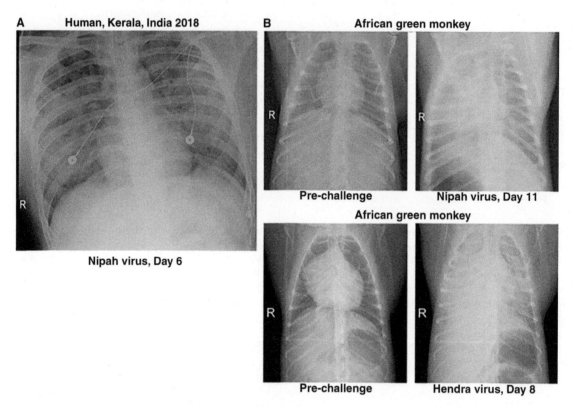

FIGURE 13.12 Chest radiographs of a Nipah virus (NiV)–infected patient and Nipah virus (NiV)– and Hendra virus (HeV)–infected African green monkeys. A: Chest x-ray of patient infected with Nipah virus (Nipah-Bangladesh clade) from Kerala, India, 2018, at 6 days following onset of symptoms showing diffuse bilateral opacities covering the majority of the lung fields, consistent with acute respiratory distress syndrome (ARDS). **B:** *Top*, comparison of prechallenge to Nipah virus (Nipah-Malaysia clade)–infected African green monkey at 11 days postchallenge showing congestion and pneumonia with infiltrates on the lung fields. *Bottom*, comparison of prechallenge to Hendra virus–infected African green monkey at 8 days postchallenge showing diffuse interstitial infiltrates and pulmonary consolidation and severe respiratory distress. (**Panel A:** Courtesy of Prof. Govindakarnavar Arunkumar, Manipal Centre for Virus Research, Manipal Academy of Higher Education (deemed to be University), Karnataka State, India, and Dr. Suresh Kumar E.K., Malabar Institute of Medical Sciences, Kerala State, India. **Panel B**, *top:* From Geisbert TW, Daddario-DiCaprio KM, Hickey AC, et al. Development of an acute and highly pathogenic nonhuman primate model of Nipah virus infection. *PLoS One* 2010;5(5):e10690; *bottom:* From Rockx B, Bossart KN, Feldmann F, et al. A novel model of lethal Hendra virus infection in African green monkeys and the effectiveness of ribavirin treatment. *J Virol* 2010;84(19):9831–9839, reproduced with permission.)

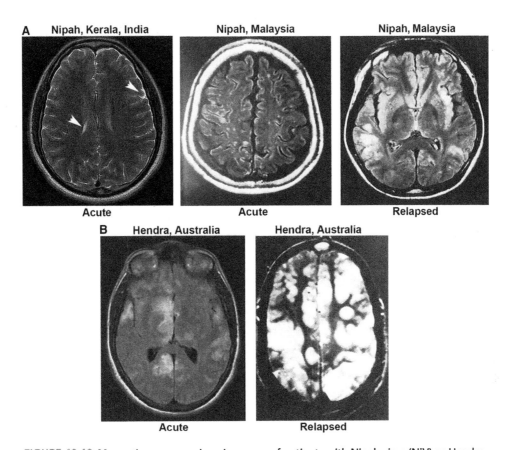

FIGURE 13.13 Magnetic resonance imaging scans of patients with Nipah virus (NiV) or Hendra virus (HeV) encephalitis. A: *Left*, patient with NiV encephalitis (Nipah-Bangladesh clade) from Kerala, India, 2018, at 6 days following onset of symptoms showing cortical and subcortical hyperintense foci (*arrow heads*). *Middle*, patient with acute NiV encephalitis (Nipah-Malaysia clade) from Malaysia, 1999, showing multiple discrete hyperintense lesions in the gray and white matter. *Right*, patient with relapsed NiV encephalitis from Malaysia, 1999, showing confluent lesions involving primarily the cortical gray matter. **B:** *Left*, acute HeV encephalitis in a patient on day 18 of illness, showing cortical and subcortical hyperintense foci. *Right*, relapsed HeV encephalitis in a patient on day 14 following symptoms onset showing widespread multifocal neocortical involvement. (**Panel A,** *left* (India): Courtesy of Prof. Govindakarnavar Arunkumar, Manipal Centre for Virus Research, Manipal Academy of Higher Education (deemed to be University), Karnataka State, India, and Dr. Suresh Kumar. E.K, Malabar Institute of Medical Sciences, Kerala State, India. **A,** *middle and right* (Malaysia): From Goh KJ, Tan CT, Chew NK, et al. Clinical features of Nipah virus encephalitis among pig farmers in Malaysia. *N Engl J Med* 2000;342(17):1229–1235. Copyright © 2000 Massachusetts Medical Society. Reprinted with permission from Massachusetts Medical Society. **B,** *left*: From Playford EG, McCall B, Smith G, et al. Human Hendra virus encephalitis associated with equine outbreak, Australia, 2008. *Emerg Infect Dis* 2010;16(2):219–223. **B,** *right*: From O'Sullivan JD, Allworth AM, Paterson DL, et al. Fatal encephalitis due to novel paramyxovirus transmitted from horses. *Lancet* 1997;349(9045):93–95, reproduced with permission.)

caused by other viruses.[9,12,140,196,228] A third case of HeV infection presented first with meningitis and a 12-day history of sore throat, headache, drowsiness, vomiting, and neck stiffness. After an apparent full recovery, this patient developed fatal encephalitis 13 months later and was admitted to the hospital with a generalized tonic–clonic seizure after 2 weeks of irritable mood and low-back pain. Recurrent focal motor seizures occurred over the next 7 days, as did secondarily generalized seizures and low-grade fever, followed by dense right hemiplegia, signs of brainstem involvement, and depressed consciousness requiring intubation. The patient remained comatose and died 25 days after admission.[3] Two patients in 2008[8] presented with initial influenza-like

illness, although soon after apparent clinical improvement and an absence of fever, encephalitis developed in both. MRI revealed widespread cortical, subcortical, and deep white matter involvement, similar to the previous late-onset case of HeV encephalitis[3] and to NiV encephalitis cases (Fig. 13.13B).[108,196,229]

Outcome of Infection

Most patients who survived acute NiV encephalitis in Malaysia made a full recovery; however, approximately 20% had residual neurologic deficits.[108,178,230] Neurologic sequelae included cognitive difficulties, tetraparesis, cerebellar signs, nerve palsies, and clinical depression. A few patients remained in a vegetative state.

In patients with encephalitis who recovered, most brain lesions revealed by MRI disappeared or became smaller over a period of 12 to 18 months, although some remained unchanged.[230] Approximately 7.5% of patients who recovered from acute encephalitis and 3.4% of those who experienced nonencephalitic or asymptomatic infection developed late neurologic disease (Fig. 13.13).[108,129,196,197] Relapse encephalitis and late-onset encephalitis presented several months to 4 years after the initial infection, with the longest reported case 11 years after an initial acute infection.[231] Relapsed cases had elevated IgG, but not IgM, and no vasculitis, and unlike the situation in acute encephalitis, virus was not isolated from throat and nasal secretions.[9,107,136,196–198]

The clinical features associated with relapse and late-onset encephalitis resembled those found with acute NiV encephalitis, although decreased incidence was seen of fever, coma, segmental myoclonus, and meningism and an increased occurrence of seizures and focal cortical signs compared with the acute manifestation of the disease.[129] The clinical, radiologic, and pathological features of relapse NiV encephalitis resembled those of the patient who became infected with HeV; suffered mild, transient aseptic meningitis; and recovered but died of a fatal meningoencephalitis 13 months later.[3,140] Most patients with relapse and late-onset encephalitis had only one neurologic episode, although some patients experienced two episodes separated by a mean of 7.6 months (6 weeks–1 year).[129] The mortality rate associated with relapse and late-onset encephalitis at 18% was lower than that associated with acute encephalitis, at 30% to 40%. However, 61% of patients with relapse and late onset had further neurologic sequelae compared with 22% after acute encephalitis. Among NiV survivors in Bangladesh, some 30% have moderate to severe persistent neurologic dysfunction for years following acute infection.[196]

The demographics, clinical features, serology, and MRI of patients with relapsed and late-onset encephalitis were similar, suggesting that the two diseases have identical pathogenesis[129] and that the initial infection in late-onset encephalitis patients may not have been sufficiently severe to cause neurologic symptoms. MRI abnormalities similar to those observed in patients with acute encephalitis were also seen in 16% of asymptomatic patients, although the lesions were fewer in number.[227] The involvement of the cortex in relapse and late-onset encephalitis suggests a different pathologic mechanism compared with acute encephalitis. Relapse and late-onset encephalitis are considered to be caused by the recrudescence and rapid replication of virus that had persisted following acute or asymptomatic NiV infection.[129] NiV, however, was not isolated from CSF and brain tissue of patients with relapse and late-onset encephalitis.[129]

The generalized understanding of the infection process along with the clinical features of human NiV and HeV infection is diagrammed in Figure 13.14. Transmission is likely via the oronasal route as described above (Pathogenesis section). The initial site of replication in humans is likely within the respiratory system, and disease onset is characterized by fever, myalgia, shortness of breath, and cough, which may progress to ARDS. Possible invasion into the CNS via the olfactory bulb has been demonstrated in nonprimate animal models.[133,139,141] Virus replication and hematogenous systemic spread occurs (cell-free or cell-associated viremia), and established infection is characterized by a widespread vasculitis with endothelial and smooth muscle cell tropism resulting in multinucleated syncytial cells.[136] CNS infection and encephalitis results in altered sensorium, headache, vomiting, and seizures along with fever and other systemic symptoms. Infection of other organs in addition to the lung and brain in human cases occurs and has been reported in the kidney, heart, spleen, and lymphoid tissues,[136] and similar widespread infection has been demonstrated in multiple animal models.[131]

DIAGNOSIS

Virus isolation, EM, immuno-EM, immunohistochemistry (IHC), serology, and polymerase chain reaction (PCR) played key roles in the initial discovery of HeV[2] and NiV.[11] They remain essential elements in the repertoire of procedures for the rapid and specific diagnosis of henipavirus infections in humans and animals.

During investigation of a suspected disease outbreak, attempts to grow henipaviruses may be initiated in a BSL3 laboratory. However, if a cytopathic effect (CPE) is observed and the growth of henipavirus is confirmed by PCR or immunostaining, infected cultures need to be handled under BSL4 conditions and subsequent work with live virus restricted to BSL4. Both HeV and NiV replicate in various cell lines—a feature that contributed to the efficiency with which they were isolated during the initial disease outbreak investigations.[2,11] Vero cells are commonly used, generating titers of virus as high as 10^8 infectious virions per milliliter.[153,232] In fatal cases, attempts should be made to isolate virus from the brain, lung, kidney, and spleen.[232] For tissue specimens containing a high virus load, direct examination by immuno-EM and IHC can be very useful in providing early diagnosis. Various antibody reagents have been developed for this purpose, including polyclonal antisera, monospecific antibodies raised against recombinant antigens,[20] and monoclonal antibodies (mAb) raised against whole virions or vaccinia virus–expressed viral proteins.[233–236] Using HeV- or NiV-specific mAb, it is possible to differentiate between the two viruses.[235,236] Quantitative real-time PCR (TaqMan assay) has been the method of choice to detect viral materials in infected tissues because of its speed, specificity, and sensitivity. The first-generation henipavirus TaqMan assays are either HeV specific[237] or NiV specific.[238] Since then, several consensus henipavirus real-time PCR assays have been developed that target different conserved regions of the viral genome.[239] It should be cautioned that the current PCR tests may not work with new henipaviruses yet to be discovered, especially those from African bats, owing to expected greater genetic divergence than those detected in Australia and Asia.

For henipaviruses, serologic tests are important both during outbreak investigation and for disease surveillance. The virus neutralization test (VNT) is accepted as the reference standard.[232] Few laboratories, however, can conduct neutralization tests because of the requirement to handle live virus at BSL4. For surveillance and diagnostic purposes, three types of tests that do not require BSL4 containment have been developed:

1. *Enzyme-linked immunosorbent assay (ELISA):* Several ELISA-based tests have been reported for the detection of henipavirus antibodies.[232,240,241] For diagnosis of human infections, two different ELISA tests have been applied: an IgM capture ELISA for early diagnosis of infection and an indirect ELISA for detection of IgG antibodies.[232]

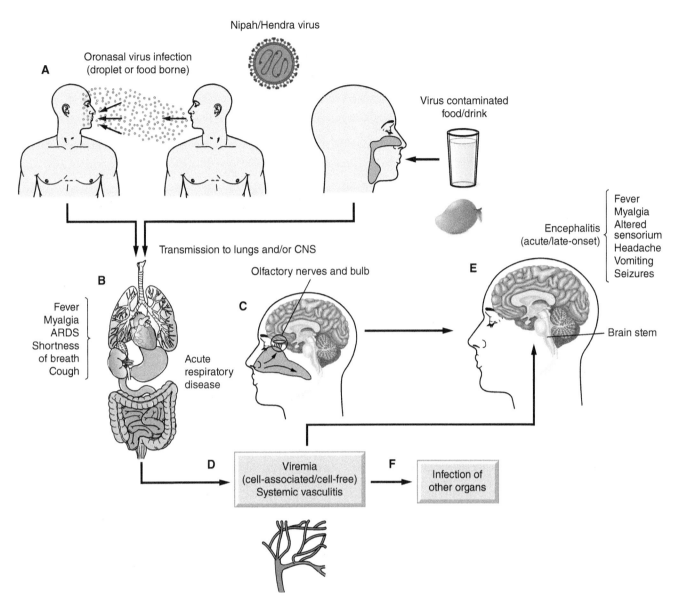

FIGURE 13.14 Generalized understanding of infection and clinical features of human Nipah virus (NiV) and Hendra virus (HeV) infection. A: Transmission is generally accepted to occur via the oronasal route presumably by virus-contaminated respiratory secretions or droplets from infected animals or people or liquid/food (palm sap/fruit). **B:** The initial site of replication in humans is ill-defined but is thought to occur within the respiratory system, and disease onset is characterized by fever, myalgia, shortness of breath, and cough, which may progress to an acute respiratory distress syndrome (ARDS). **C:** Possible invasion into the central nervous system (CNS) via the olfactory bulb has also been suggested and has been demonstrated in animal models. **D:** Virus replication and hematogenous systemic spread occurs (cell-free or cell-associated viremia), and established infection is characterized by a widespread vasculitis with endothelial and smooth muscle cell tropism resulting in multinucleated syncytial cells. **E:** CNS infection and encephalitis results in altered sensorium, headache, vomiting, and seizures along with fever and other systemic symptoms. **F:** Infection of other organs in addition to lung and brain in human cases occurs and has been reported in kidney, heart, spleen, and lymphoid tissues, and similar widespread infection has been demonstrated in multiple animal models.

2. *Liquid protein array multiplex test:* A Luminex-based test based on recombinant soluble G proteins of HeV and NiV was developed that is capable of mimicking VNT with great sensitivity and differentiating between antibody responses of HeV and NiV infection.[242]

3. *Pseudotype virus:* Different pseudotype systems carrying the henipavirus F and G proteins have been developed as a surrogate VNT for detecting henipavirus-specific antibodies.[18,243–245] Incorporation of reporter genes in these systems resulted in greater sensitivity and reproducibility.

PREVENTION AND CONTROL

Drugs and Small Molecules

Ribavirin, which inhibits replication of HeV *in vitro*,[246] was used during the NiV outbreak in Malaysia in an open-label study in which 140 patients with encephalitis were given the drug and 54 patients who presented before ribavirin became available or who refused treatment acted as controls.[247] Mortality in the treated group was 32% compared with 54% in the control group, representing a 35% reduction (P = 0.011). Duration of ventilation and that of total hospital stay were both significantly shorter in the ribavirin group (P = 0.0002 and P < 0.0001, respectively). In the absence of other therapies, ribavirin may be an option for treatment of henipavirus infections. However, two HeV-infected patients in 2008[8] were given a high-dose intravenous regimen of ribavirin, although basal concentrations appeared inadequate given the results of *in vitro* susceptibility testing of HeV, and the efficacy of ribavirin as therapy or prophylaxis in people remains at best uncertain. Chloroquine, an antimalarial drug, was first demonstrated to block the critical proteolytic processing needed for HeV F maturation and function.[248] Not surprisingly, the drug was later shown to inhibit NiV and HeV infection in cell culture experiments.[249] Chloroquine was administered along with ribavirin to one HeV-infected individual in 2009[250] with no apparent clinical benefit. Remdesivir (GS-5734) is a nucleotide analog prodrug that showed therapeutic efficacy in a NHP model of Ebola virus infection.[251] GS-5734 has been administered under compassionate use to Ebola virus–infected patients and is currently in phase II clinical development for treatment of Ebola virus disease. The antiviral activities of GS-5734 have been demonstrated to be broad showing *in vitro* activity against viruses in the *Coronaviridae*, *Filoviridae*, and *Paramyxoviridae* including NiV and HeV.[252]

In vivo, ribavirin only delayed but did not prevent deaths caused by NiV and had no effect on HeV infection in a hamster model.[173,253] Ribavirin treatment also only delayed disease onset by 1 to 2 days in AGMs challenged with HeV with no significant benefit for disease progression or outcome.[103] Chloroquine administration, either alone or in combination with ribavirin, had no therapeutic benefit in ferrets challenged with NiV or hamsters challenged with either NiV or HeV.[253,254] Poly(I)–poly(C12U), which induces IFN-α and IFN-β production and can completely block NiV replication *in vitro*, displayed approximately 80% protective efficacy in the hamster model of lethal NiV infection.[173]

Peptide Fusion Inhibitors

The first potential henipavirus-specific therapeutic was shown to be a heptad peptide–based fusion inhibitor,[95] analogous to HIV-1–specific peptide, enfuvirtide (Fuzeon) approved by the Food and Drug Administration (FDA) in March 2003. The henipavirus F_1 glycoprotein resembles other fusion glycoproteins in having α-helical heptad repeat (HR) domains proximal to both the fusion peptide at the amino (N) terminus and the transmembrane domain near the carboxy (C) terminus of the protein. The HR domains are involved in the formation of a trimer-of-hairpins structure during the membrane fusion and virus infection process. Addition of exogenous peptide from either HR domain blocks formation of the trimer-of-hairpins and abrogates membrane fusion and virus infection.[94,95,255] These observations were followed up with testing cholesterol tagged HR-derived peptides in the hamster model of NiV infection providing the first evidence of *in vivo* effectiveness of a fusion inhibiting peptide against NiV.[256]

Vaccines

A wide variety of immunization strategies have been developed for NiV and HeV prevention and include live-recombinant virus platforms, protein subunit, virus-like particles, and DNA vaccines; however, many of these approaches have only been examined for HeV- or NiV-specific neutralizing antibody induction.[257] A more limited number of vaccine candidates have been examined for both immune response and efficacy using a variety of animal challenge models (Table 13.5). Attenuated vaccinia virus strain NYVAC recombinants encoding either the NiV F or G glycoproteins used to immunize hamsters provided complete protection from NiV-mediated disease following challenge and demonstrated that an immune response to the viral envelope glycoproteins was an important immunogen in protection.[258] A second poxvirus-based approach was developed as a potential livestock vaccine using recombinant canarypox virus with the NiV F and G genes inserted into ALVAC vectors (Table 13.5). ALVAC vectors expressing either NiV F or NiV G were tested individually and in combination by vaccination of piglets, and animals were challenged intranasally with NiV. Piglets were protected from NiV-mediated illness by either ALVAC vector alone or in combination, and immunized animals shed only low levels of nucleic acid detectable virus, and no recoverable virus was evident.[259] Three other viral vector-based NiV vaccines have been examined in animal challenge studies (Table 13.5). An adeno-associated virus (AAV) platform using the NiV G glycoprotein was tested in the hamster model using NiV challenge, showing complete protection against NiV, but only low level cross-protection (three of six animals) against an HeV challenge.[260] A recombinant measles virus vector encoding the NiV G glycoprotein was examined using two different vectors; the HL (rMV-HL-G) and Edmonston (rMV-Ed-G) measles virus strains[261] (Table 13.5). Here, complete protection from NiV disease was achievable in the hamster challenge model following vaccination with either rMV-HL-G or rMV-Ed-G, and the rMV-Ed-G was tested in the NHP model demonstrating two of two AGMs were protected against NiV challenge. Several groups have tested the vesicular stomatitis virus (VSV)–based platform using the NiV F or G glycoproteins (Table 13.5). In the ferret model, a single immunization with VSV encoding either NiV F or NiV G could afford complete protection from NiV challenge.[262] Similarly, NiV G or F glycoproteins in VSV vectors were successful in protection from NiV challenge in the hamster model,[263,264] and a single immunization of NiV G encoding VSV was protective in the AGM model.[265,266]

The most extensively tested vaccine against NiV and HeV has been a recombinant protein subunit strategy because of the inherent safety of such an approach. Soluble, secreted, oligomeric forms of the G glycoprotein (sG) from both NiV and HeV were developed and tested as possible vaccine candidates, and the HeV-sG was shown capable of eliciting a more potent cross-reactive polyclonal antibody response and also a better cross-protective response[267,268] (Table 13.5). HeV-sG is a soluble and secreted version of the molecule with a genetically deleted transmembrane and cytoplasmic tail that is produced in mammalian cell culture systems and is properly N-linked glycosylated[269] (Fig. 13.15). HeV-sG has been shown to retain many native characteristics including oligomerization and ability to bind ephrin receptors[62,267] and is capable of eliciting potent cross-reactive (HeV and NiV) neutralizing antibody responses in a variety of animals including mice, rabbits, cats, ferrets, monkeys, and horses.[257] The HeV-sG vaccine in the cat model provided complete protection against a lethal NiV challenge[268] and suggested a single subunit vaccine (HeV-sG) could be effective against both HeV and NiV. Further studies in the cat model revealed that antibody titers as low as 1:32 could protect

TABLE 13.5 Summary of advanced henipavirus vaccination development initiatives evaluated in animal challenge models

Platform	Viral Antigen Target or Immunogen	Animal Challenge Model
Active vaccination		
Recombinant vaccinia virus	Nipah F and/or G glycoprotein	Hamster[a] (NiV)
Recombinant canarypox virus	Nipah F and/or G glycoprotein	Pig[b] (NiV)
Recombinant VSV	Nipah F and/or G glycoprotein	Ferret[c] (NiV), hamster[d] (NiV), nonhuman primate[e] (NiV)
Recombinant AAV	Nipah G glycoprotein	Hamster[f] (NiV, HeV)
Recombinant measles virus	Nipah G glycoprotein	Hamster[g], nonhuman primate (NiV, HeV)
Recombinant subunit	Hendra virus soluble G glycoprotein	Cat[h] (NiV), Ferret[i] (HeV, NiV), nonhuman primate[j] (HeV, NiV), horse[k] (HeV)
VLP based	Purified virus-like particles made from NiV M, F, and G proteins	Hamster (NiV)[n]
Passive immunization		
Human monoclonal antibody m102.4	Hendra/Nipah G glycoprotein	Ferret[l] (NiV) Nonhuman primate[m] (HeV, NiV)

[a]Hamsters immunized with NiV F and/or G glycoprotein encoding recombinant vaccinia viruses were protected against disease following intraperitoneal challenge with 10^3 PFU of NiV.[258]

[b]Pigs immunized with NiV F and/or G glycoprotein encoding recombinant canarypox viruses were protected against intranasal challenge with 2.5×10^5 PFU of NiV.[259]

[c]Ferrets immunized with NiV F and/or G glycoprotein encoding recombinant vesicular stomatitis virus (VSV) vectors were protected against lethal intranasal challenge with 5×10^3 PFU of NiV.[262]

[d]Hamsters immunized with NiV F and/or G glycoprotein encoding recombinant vesicular stomatitis virus (VSV) vectors were protected against lethal intraperitoneal challenge with 10^5 TCID$_{50}$ of NiV[264] or 6.8×10^4 TCID$_{50}$ of NiV.[263]

[e]African green monkeys immunized with an NiV G encoding recombinant VSV vector were protected against lethal intratracheal challenge with 10^5 TCID$_{50}$ of NiV.[265,266]

[f]Hamsters immunized with an NiV G encoding recombinant adeno-associated virus (AAV) vector were protected against lethal intraperitoneal with 10^4 PFU of NiV.[260]

[g]Hamsters and African green monkeys immunized with an NiV G encoding recombinant measles virus vector were protected against lethal intraperitoneal challenge with 10^3 TCID$_{50}$ of NiV (hamsters) or 10^5 TCID$_{50}$ of NiV (AGMs).[261]

[h]Hendra virus soluble G glycoprotein (HeV-sG) used to immunize cats protects against lethal subcutaneous (500 TCID$_{50}$)[268] or oronasal (5×10^4 TCID$_{50}$) NiV challenge.[270]

[i]HeV-sG used to immunize ferrets protects against lethal oronasal challenge with 5×10^3 TCID$_{50}$ of HeV[106] or 5×10^3 TCID$_{50}$ of NiV challenge.[271]

[j]HeV-sG used to immunize African green monkeys protects against lethal intratracheal challenge with 10^5 TCID$_{50}$ of NiV[272] or 5×10^5 PFU of HeV.[273]

[k]HeV-sG used to immunize horses protects against lethal oronasal challenge with 2×10^6 TCID$_{50}$ of HeV.[274]

[l]An NiV and HeV cross-reactive G glycoprotein–specific neutralizing human mAb (m102.4) protects ferrets against lethal oronasal challenge with 5×10^3 TCID$_{50}$ of NiV[97] or 5×10^3 TCID$_{50}$ of HeV (J. Pallister and C. Broder, unpublished) by postexposure infusion.

[m]Human mAb m102.4 protects African green monkeys by postexposure infusion following lethal intratracheal challenge with 4×10^5 TCID$_{50}$ of HeV[193] or lethal intratracheal challenge with 5×10^5 PFU of NiV.[191,194]

[n]Hamsters immunized with VLPs (either one dose or three doses) composed of Nipah virus M, F, and G (RBP) proteins were completely protected against lethal intraperitoneal challenge with 1.6×10^4 pfu of NiV.[330]

against NiV-Malaysia challenge[270] (Table 13.5). Studies in the ferret model with low vaccine doses of HeV-sG formulated in CpG and Alhydrogel™ could completely protect against high-dose HeV challenge.[106] Immunization and challenge studies in ferrets with the NiV-Bangladesh strain also demonstrated complete protection.[271] In addition, good durable immunity was shown in other ferrets challenged 434 days postvaccination.[271] However, preliminary studies with HeV-sG as a vaccine in the pig model was less effective against HeV and unprotective against NiV, and both humoral and cellular immune responses were required for protection of swine against henipaviruses in that challenge model.[180]

The HeV-sG vaccine has also been extensively evaluated in nonhuman primates (AGMs). Monkeys immunized with HeV-sG formulated in Alhydrogel™ and CpG were completely protected against intratracheal challenge with NiV-Malaysia, some with prechallenge neutralizing titers as low as 1:28, and no evidence of clinical disease, virus replication, or pathology was observed in any vaccinated monkeys.[272] Similarly, HeV-sG vaccination and protection from an HeV challenge in AGMs have also been shown, including HeV-sG formulated in Alhydrogel™ alone.[273] The inherent safety and effectiveness of

the HeV-sG vaccine led to its development as an equine vaccine to prevent not only HeV infection of horses but also as the means to reduce the risk of HeV transmission to people (Fig. 13.16A). HeV-sG was licensed by Zoetis™ Inc., (formerly Pfizer Animal Health) and developed as an equine vaccine for use in Australia. Horse HeV-sG vaccination and HeV challenge studies were conducted at the BSL4 facilities of the Australian Animal Health Laboratory (AAHL) in Geelong[274] (Table 13.5). HeV-sG was formulated in an approved equine adjuvant (Zoetis, Inc.), and two initial efficacy studies in horses tested 50-μg and 100-μg doses of the same HeV-sG used in published animal studies were used to immunize horses. Additional studies used a 100-μg dose of HeV-sG produced in CHO cells (Zoetis, Inc.). Immunizations were two doses given intramuscularly 3 weeks apart. All horses in these efficacy studies were challenged oronasally with 2×10^6 TCID$_{50}$ of HeV. Seven horses were challenged at 28 days, and three horses were challenged 194 days, after the second immunization. All vaccinated horses remained clinically healthy following challenge, demonstrating protection with prechallenge HeV neutralizing titers as low as 1:16.[274] There was no gross or histologic evidence of HeV infection in any of the vaccinated horses at study

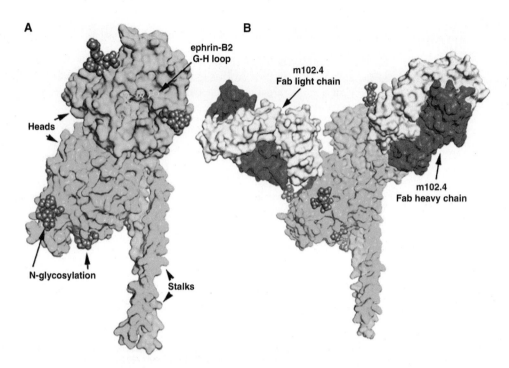

FIGURE 13.15 Model of the Hendra virus soluble G glycoprotein subunit vaccine (HeV-sG) and its complex with the Hendra and Nipah virus–neutralizing human monoclonal antibody m102.4. A: The HeV-sG glycoprotein subunit vaccine is composed of the entire ectodomain (amino acids 76–604) of the HeV G glycoprotein. HeV-sG is shown as dimer with one monomer colored *green* and the other *cyan*. The secondary structure elements of the two globular head domains are derived from the crystal structure of the HeV G head domain, the stalk regions of each G monomer (residues 77–136) are modeled, and N-linked glycosylation sites are shown as *gray spheres*. The ephrin-binding face of the *cyan* globular head is facing forward with an overlay of the interacting ephrin-B2 G-H loop residues in *yellow*. **B:** The HeV-sG dimer is modeled in complex with two m102.4 Fab antibody fragments. The two HeV-sG monomers are colored *green* and *cyan* as in **panel A** and rotated slightly to the right, and the two Fab molecules are shown with their heavy chains colored in *magenta* and light chain in *yellow*, each binding one globular head domains of G. (Modified from Broder CC, Xu K, Nikolov DB, et al. A treatment for and vaccine against the deadly Hendra and Nipah viruses. *Antiviral Res* 2013;100(1):8–13A.)

completion, and all tissues examined were negative for HeV antigen by IHC, with no viral genome detected in any tissue. In 9 of 10 vaccinated horses, HeV nucleic acid was not detected in daily nasal, oral, or rectal swab specimens or from blood, urine, or fecal samples collected before euthanasia, and no recoverable virus was present.[274]

Equivac® HeV was launched in November 2012 on a Minor Use Permit by the regulatory authority, the Australian Pesticides and Veterinary Medicines Authority (APVMA), and is the first commercially developed and deployed vaccine against a BSL4 agent and is currently the only licensed antiviral approach for henipavirus infection. All vaccinated horses receive a microchip, and database is maintained, and in August 2015, Equivac® HeV received full registration by the APVMA. To date, more than 640,000 doses of Equivac® HeV vaccine have been administered to more than 153,000 unique horses (Fig. 13.16B). Since vaccine release, laboratory-confirmed HeV infections in horses ($n = 21$) have only occurred in unvaccinated horses. The HeV-sG recombinant subunit vaccine for NiV and HeV is now in clinical development with support from the Coalition for Epidemic Preparedness Innovations (CEPI),[275] and phase I clinical trials set to commence in 2019. Recent vaccination and challenge studies in NHPs have shown that a

single immunizing dose of HeV-sG in Alhydrogel™ can protect against HeV and NiV-Bangladesh challenge (Geisbert and Broder, unpublished), and together with the results of recombinant VSV-based NiV vaccines, these findings highlight their potential usefulness in an emergency use or outbreak scenario.

Passive Immunization

Initial passive immunization studies using either NiV G– and F–specific polyclonal antiserums or mouse monoclonal antibodies (mAbs) specific for the NiV or HeV G or F glycoproteins were shown to be protective in the hamster model.[102,258,276] HeV- and NiV-neutralizing human mAbs reactive to the G glycoproteins of both HeV and NiV have been developed using recombinant antibody technology.[277] One mAb, m102.4, possessed strong cross-reactive neutralizing activity against HeV and NiV and was later produced in an IgG1 format in a CHO-K1 cell line.[278] The m102.4 mAb epitope maps to the receptor-binding site of G and engages G in a similar fashion as the ephrin receptors[279,302] (Fig. 13.5). The m102.4 mAb can neutralize all HeV and NiV isolates tested, including HeV-1994, HeV-Redlands, NiV-Malaysia, and NiV-Bangladesh.[97,280] NiV challenge experiments in the ferret demonstrated that complete protection was possible by a single dose of m102.4 mAb administered

A

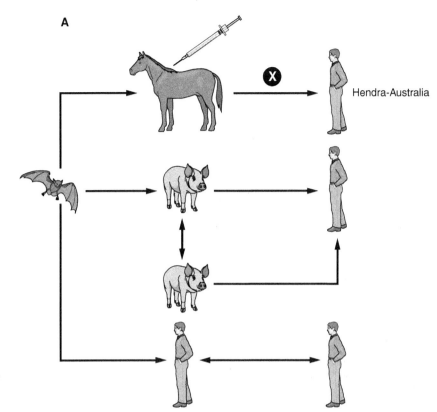

FIGURE 13.16 One Health vaccine strategy.
A: The known modes of henipavirus transmission in different countries. In Australia, all seven human cases were infected via contacting infected horses. A One Health vaccine strategy was developed for immunization of horses with the dual purposes of saving horses from lethal Hendra virus infection and prevention of transmission from bats to humans via horses. **B:** Location densities of Equivac® HeV vaccine administered to horses around Australia. As of 2018, more than 700,000 doses of Equivac® HeV have been administered to horses around Australia, equating to more than 168,000 unique horses vaccinated. (Courtesy of Dr. Richard L'Estrange, Zoetis Inc.)

B

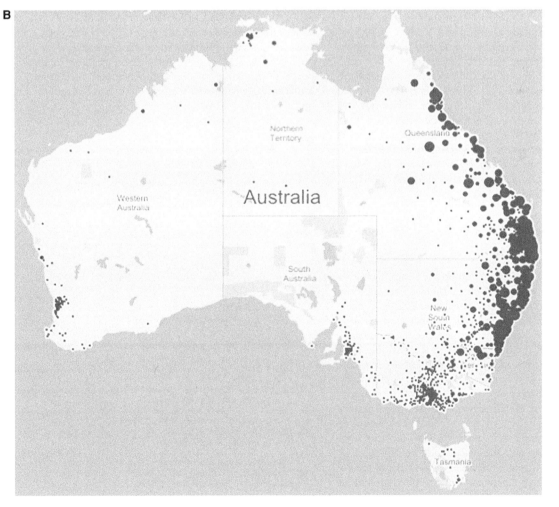

by intravenous infusion 10 hours following a lethal virus challenge.[97] The therapeutic efficacy of mAb m102.4 has also been examined in NHPs against both NiV and HeV challenge as a postexposure therapeutic reflective of a potential real-life virus exposure scenario[193,194] (Table 13.5). In one study, AGMs were challenged intratracheally with HeV, and following virus administration, they were infused twice with m102.4 (~15 mg/kg) beginning at 10 hours, 24 hours, or 72 hours postinfection followed by a the second infusion approximately 48 hours after the first. In this study, all subjects became infected following challenge, and all animals that received m102.4 survived, whereas all controls succumbed to severe systemic disease 8 days following virus challenge. Animals in a 72 hours treatment group did exhibit neurologic signs, but all recovered by day 16, but there was no evidence of HeV-specific pathology in any of the m102.4–treated animals, and no infectious HeV could be recovered from any tissues from any m102.4–treated subjects. A later study evaluated the efficacy of m102.4 against NiV-Malaysia challenge in AGMs, at several time points after virus exposure by intratracheal challenge including as late as the onset of clinical illness.[194] Here, animals were infused twice with m102.4 (15 mg/kg) beginning at either 1, 3, or 5 days following NiV-Malaysia challenge and again 48 hours after the first dose. All animals became infected following virus exposure, and again all subjects that received m102.4 therapy survived the infection, whereas the untreated control subjects succumbed to disease between days 8 and 10 following virus challenge. The m102.4 mAb was also shown to be effective in the NHP model against NiV-Bangladesh infection, although its therapeutic window was much shorter as compared to NiV-Malaysia–infected subjects.[191] Taken together, these studies have shown that m102.4 mAb therapy can prevent HeV or NiV lethal disease in exposed subjects is the only effective postexposure therapeutic tested *in vivo* in NHPs. The mAb m102.4 has since been used by emergency protocol in 13 people in Australia and one in the United States because of significant risk of HeV or NiV infection.[257] The m102.4 antibody has completed a phase I clinical trial in Australia and has recently been supplied to Government of India and included in an international Nipah treatment protocol sponsored by the Indian Council of Medical Research (ICMR) with support from the NIAID, NIH, USA.

PERSPECTIVE

Nipah and henipaviral diseases remain on the latest WHO list of Blueprint priority diseases (February 2018).[281] This acknowledges that NiV (or related virulent henipaviruses) is a major threat to global public health and calls for increased research and development into henipaviruses and their countermeasures, including surveillance and diagnostics. In addition, both NiV and HeV emergence and reemergence remain continuous infectious disease transboundary threats to economically important livestock throughout South Asia and Australia.[282] NiV is also one of the top three viral agents prioritized for vaccine development by the CEPI.[275,283] The high virulence of the henipaviruses and the requirement for BSL4 facilities have hampered investigations into the biology and pathogenesis of these novel paramyxoviruses. Nonetheless, the advent of reverse genetics for henipaviruses, coupled with the development of

animal models that recapitulate the clinical features and pathology seen in virus-infected humans, has provided insights into the functions of many henipavirus proteins and the role they play in the pathogenesis of henipavirus disease. While the virulence of henipaviruses necessitates the initial functional characterization of henipavirus proteins from cloned genes, it is imperative that these functional characteristics be examined in the context of a live virus infection. Even then, it appears increasingly important to investigate why henipaviruses appear so much more virulent in many of their terrestrial hosts versus their chiropteran counterparts.[284]

Despite our expanded understanding of the henipaviruses, many questions relating to the ecology and biology of henipaviruses remain unanswered. *Pteropus* species of fruit bats are clearly the major reservoir host of these viruses,[202,207,208] but new studies have suggested that an even wider group of chiropteran species host not only the known henipaviruses but also multiple divergent clades of new henipavirus species.[29,222,285] Molecular or serologic evidence of henipaviruses can now be found in frugivorous and insectivorous bats that range from Australia and Austronesia to China, Southeast Asia, countries of the Indian subcontinent, Madagascar, sub-Saharan Africa, and even into the New World (Costa Rica and Brazil).[19,29,207,286–297] The emergence of these and related viruses is probably associated with the destruction of the flying fox native habitats, driving the animals to seek food from orchards and ornamental trees in urban and peri-urban areas. Continued deforestation and amplification of factors that drive zoonotic spillover from reservoir hosts will undoubtedly lead to further outbreaks of HeV, NiV, and novel related members of the genus.[298–301] Continued surveillance coupled with identification and characterization of these putative new species of henipavirus is required to provide a proper assessment as to the countermeasures, such as the CEPI initiatives, that would be necessary to control or prevent future outbreaks and spillovers.

REFERENCES

1. Selvey LA, Wells RM, McCormack JG, et al. Infection of humans and horses by a newly described morbillivirus. *Med J Aust* 1995;162(12):642–645.
2. Murray K, Selleck P, Hooper P, et al. A morbillivirus that caused fatal disease in horses and humans. *Science* 1995;268(5207):94–97.
3. O'Sullivan JD, Allworth AM, Paterson DL, et al. Fatal encephalitis due to novel paramyxovirus transmitted from horses. *Lancet* 1997;349(9045):93–95.
4. Rogers RJ, Douglas IC, Baldock FC, et al. Investigation of a second focus of equine morbillivirus infection in coastal Queensland. *Aust Vet J* 1996;74(3):243–244.
5. Young PL, Halpin K, Selleck PW, et al. Serologic evidence for the presence in Pteropus bats of a paramyxovirus related to equine morbillivirus. *Emerg Infect Dis* 1996;2(3):239–240.
6. Halpin K, Young PL, Field HE, et al. Isolation of Hendra virus from pteropid bats: a natural reservoir of Hendra virus. *J Gen Virol* 2000;81(Pt 8):1927–1932.
7. Summary of Hendra virus incidents in horses. Queensland Government; 2018. Business Queensland Web site. Available at: https://www.business.qld.gov.au/industries/service-industries-professionals/service-industries/veterinary-surgeons/guidelines-hendra/incident-summary. Accessed September 20, 2018.
8. Playford EG, McCall B, Smith G, et al. Human Hendra virus encephalitis associated with equine outbreak, Australia, 2008. *Emerg Infect Dis* 2010;16(2):219–223.
9. Chua KB, Goh KJ, Wong KT, et al. Fatal encephalitis due to Nipah virus among pig-farmers in Malaysia. *Lancet* 1999;354(9186):1257–1259.
10. Mohd Nor MN, Gan CH, Ong BL. Nipah virus infection of pigs in peninsular Malaysia. *Rev Sci Tech* 2000;19(1):160–165.
11. Chua KB, Bellini WJ, Rota PA, et al. Nipah virus: a recently emergent deadly paramyxovirus. *Science* 2000;288(5470):1432–1435.
12. Paton NI, Leo YS, Zaki SR, et al. Outbreak of Nipah-virus infection among abattoir workers in Singapore. *Lancet* 1999;354(9186):1253–1256.
13. Chua KB, Koh CL, Hooi PS, et al. Isolation of Nipah virus from Malaysian Island flying-foxes. *Microbes Infect* 2002;4(2):145–151.
14. Hsu VP, Hossain MJ, Parashar UD, et al. Nipah virus encephalitis reemergence, Bangladesh. *Emerg Infect Dis* 2004;10(12):2082–2087.
15. Chadha MS, Comer JA, Lowe L, et al. Nipah virus-associated encephalitis outbreak, Siliguri, India. *Emerg Infect Dis* 2006;12(2):235–240.

16. Harit AK, Ichhpujani RL, Gupta S, et al. Nipah/Hendra virus outbreak in Siliguri, West Bengal, India in 2001. *Indian J Med Res* 2006;123(4):553–560.
17. Arunkumar G, Chandni R, Mourya DT, et al. Outbreak investigation of Nipah Virus Disease in Kerala, India, 2018. *J Infect Dis* 2019;219(12):1867–1878.
18. Ching PK, de los Reyes VC, Sucaldito MN, et al. Outbreak of henipavirus infection, Philippines, 2014. *Emerg Infect Dis* 2015;21(2):328–331.
19. Pernet O, Schneider BS, Beaty SM, et al. Evidence for henipavirus spillover into human populations in Africa. *Nat Commun* 2014;5:5342.
20. Wang LF, Michalski WP, Yu M, et al. A novel P/V/C gene in a new member of the Paramyxoviridae family, which causes lethal infection in humans, horses, and other animals. *J Virol* 1998;72(2):1482–1490.
21. Wang LF, Yu M, Hansson E, et al. The exceptionally large genome of Hendra virus: support for creation of a new genus within the family Paramyxoviridae. *J Virol* 2000;74(21):9972–9979.
22. Harcourt BH, Tamin A, Halpin K, et al. Molecular characterization of the polymerase gene and genomic termini of Nipah virus. *Virology* 2001;287(1):192–201.
23. Harcourt BH, Tamin A, Ksiazek TG, et al. Molecular characterization of Nipah virus, a newly emergent paramyxovirus. *Virology* 2000;271(2):334–349.
24. Wang L, Harcourt BH, Yu M, et al. Molecular biology of Hendra and Nipah viruses. *Microbes Infect* 2001;3(4):279–287.
25. Lamb RA, Collins PL, Kolakofsky D, et al. Family Paramyxoviridae. In: Fauquet CM, Mayo J, Maniloff J, Desselberger U, Ball LA, eds. *Virus Taxonomy: 8th Report of the International Committee on Taxonomy of Viruses.* San Diego: Elsevier Academic Press; 2005:655–668.
26. Amarasinghe GK, Arechiga Ceballos NG, Banyard AC, et al. Taxonomy of the order Mononegavirales: update 2018. *Arch Virol* 2018;163(8):2283–2294.
27. Maes P, Amarasinghe GK, Ayllon MA, et al. Taxonomy of the order Mononegavirales: second update 2018. *Arch Virol* 2019;164(4):1233–1244.
28. Marsh GA, de Jong C, Barr JA, et al. Cedar virus: a novel Henipavirus isolated from Australian bats. *PLoS Pathog* 2012;8(8):e1002836.
29. Drexler JF, Corman VM, Muller MA, et al. Bats host major mammalian paramyxoviruses. *Nat Commun* 2012;3:796.
30. Wu Z, Yang L, Yang F, et al. Novel Henipa-like virus, Mojiang Paramyxovirus, in rats, China, 2012. *Emerg Infect Dis* 2014;20(6):1064–1066.
31. Goldsmith CS, Whistler T, Rollin PE, et al. Elucidation of Nipah virus morphogenesis and replication using ultrastructural and molecular approaches. *Virus Res* 2003;92(1):89–98.
32. Hyatt AD, Zaki SR, Goldsmith CS, et al. Ultrastructure of Hendra virus and Nipah virus within cultured cells and host animals. *Microbes Infect* 2001;3(4):297–306.
33. Harcourt BH, Lowe L, Tamin A, et al. Genetic characterization of Nipah virus, Bangladesh, 2004. *Emerg Infect Dis* 2005;11(10):1594–1597.
34. Halpin K, Bankamp B, Harcourt BH, et al. Nipah virus conforms to the rule of six in a minigenome replication assay. *J Gen Virol* 2004;85(Pt 3):701–707.
35. Rima BK, Balkema-Buschmann A, Dundon WG, et al. ICTV Virus Taxonomy Profile: Paramyxoviridae. *J Gen Virol* 2019 Oct 14. doi: 10.1099/jgv.0.001328. [Epub ahead of print]
36. Hino K, Sato H, Sugai A, et al. Downregulation of Nipah virus N mRNA occurs through interaction between its 3′ untranslated region and hnRNP D. *J Virol* 2013;87(12):6582–6588.
37. Michalski WP, Crameri G, Wang L, et al. The cleavage activation and sites of glycosylation in the fusion protein of Hendra virus. *Virus Res* 2000;69(2):83–93.
38. Lo MK, Harcourt BH, Mungall BA, et al. Determination of the henipavirus phosphoprotein gene mRNA editing frequencies and detection of the C, V and W proteins of Nipah virus in virus-infected cells. *J Gen Virol* 2009;90(Pt 2):398–404.
39. Basler CF. Nipah and hendra virus interactions with the innate immune system. *Curr Top Microbiol Immunol* 2012;359:123–152.
40. Parks GD, Alexander-Miller MA. Paramyxovirus activation and inhibition of innate immune responses. *J Mol Biol* 2013;425(24):4872–4892.
41. Park A, Yun T, Vigant F, et al. Nipah virus C protein recruits Tsg101 to promote the efficient release of virus in an ESCRT-dependent pathway. *PLoS Pathog* 2016;12(5):e1005659.
42. Freiberg A, Dolores LK, Enterlein S, et al. Establishment and characterization of plasmid-driven minigenome rescue systems for Nipah virus: RNA polymerase I- and T7-catalyzed generation of functional paramyxoviral RNA. *Virology* 2008;370(1):33–44.
43. Yun T, Park A, Hill TE, et al. Efficient reverse genetics reveals genetic determinants of budding and fusogenic differences between Nipah and Hendra viruses and enables real-time monitoring of viral spread in small animal models of henipavirus infection. *J Virol* 2015;89(2):1242–1253.
44. Yoneda M, Guillaume V, Ikeda F, et al. Establishment of a Nipah virus rescue system. *Proc Natl Acad Sci U S A* 2006;103(44):16508–16513.
45. Ciancanelli MJ, Volchkova VA, Shaw ML, et al. Nipah virus sequesters inactive STAT1 in the nucleus via a P gene-encoded mechanism. *J Virol* 2009;83(16):7828–7841.
46. Yoneda M, Guillaume V, Sato H, et al. The nonstructural proteins of Nipah virus play a key role in pathogenicity in experimentally infected animals. *PLoS One* 2010;5(9):e12709.
47. Lo MK, Peeples ME, Bellini WJ, et al. Distinct and overlapping roles of Nipah virus P gene products in modulating the human endothelial cell antiviral response. *PLoS One* 2012;7(10):e47790.
48. Marsh GA, Virtue ER, Smith I, et al. Recombinant Hendra viruses expressing a reporter gene retain pathogenicity in ferrets. *Virol J* 2013;10:95.
49. Dietzel E, Kolesnikova L, Sawatsky B, et al. Nipah virus matrix protein influences fusogenicity and is essential for particle infectivity and stability. *J Virol* 2015;90(5):2514–2522.
50. Satterfield BA, Cross RW, Fenton KA, et al. The immunomodulating V and W proteins of Nipah virus determine disease course. *Nat Commun* 2015;6:7483.
51. Bharaj P, Wang YE, Dawes BE, et al. The matrix protein of Nipah virus targets the E3-Ubiquitin Ligase TRIM6 to inhibit the IKKepsilon kinase-mediated type-I IFN antiviral response. *PLoS Pathog* 2016;12(9):e1005880.
52. Satterfield BA, Cross RW, Fenton KA, et al. Nipah virus C and W proteins contribute to respiratory disease in ferrets. *J Virol* 2016;90(14):6326–6343.
53. Laing ED, Amaya M, Navaratnarajah CK, et al. Rescue and characterization of recombinant cedar virus, a non-pathogenic Henipavirus species. *Virol J* 2018;15(1):56.
54. Poch O, Blumberg BM, Bougueleret L, et al. Sequence comparison of five polymerases (L proteins) of unsegmented negative-strand RNA viruses: theoretical assignment of functional domains. *J Gen Virol* 1990;71(Pt 5):1153–1162.
55. Miller PJ, Boyle DB, Eaton BT, et al. Full-length genome sequence of Mossman virus, a novel paramyxovirus isolated from rodents in Australia. *Virology* 2003;317(2):330–344.
56. Liang B, Li Z, Jenni S, et al. Structure of the L protein of vesicular stomatitis virus from electron cryomicroscopy. *Cell* 2015;162(2):314–327.
57. Lamb RA, Parks GD. *Paramyxoviridae*: the viruses and their replication. In: Fields BN, Knipe DM, Howley PM, eds. *Fields Virology*. 6th ed. Philadelphia: Lippincott Williams & Wilkins; 2013:957–995.
58. Langedijk JP, Daus FJ, van Oirschot JT. Sequence and structure alignment of Paramyxoviridae attachment proteins and discovery of enzymatic activity for a morbillivirus hemagglutinin. *J Virol* 1997;71(8):6155–6167.
59. Lee B, Ataman ZA. Modes of paramyxovirus fusion: a Henipavirus perspective. *Trends Microbiol* 2011;19(8):389–399.
60. Yu M, Hansson E, Langedijk JP, et al. The attachment protein of Hendra virus has high structural similarity but limited primary sequence homology compared with viruses in the genus Paramyxovirus. *Virology* 1998;251(2):227–233.
61. Bishop KA, Stantchev TS, Hickey AC, et al. Identification of Hendra virus G glycoprotein residues that are critical for receptor binding. *J Virol* 2007;81(11):5893–5901.
62. Bonaparte MI, Dimitrov AS, Bossart KN, et al. Ephrin-B2 ligand is a functional receptor for Hendra virus and Nipah virus. *Proc Natl Acad Sci U S A* 2005;102(30):10652–10657.
63. Negrete OA, Levroney EL, Aguilar HC, et al. EphrinB2 is the entry receptor for Nipah virus, an emergent deadly paramyxovirus. *Nature* 2005;436(7049):401–405.
64. Negrete OA, Wolf MC, Aguilar HC, et al. Two key residues in ephrinB3 are critical for its use as an alternative receptor for Nipah virus. *PLoS Pathog* 2006;2(2):e7.
65. Lee B, Pernet O, Ahmed AA, et al. Molecular recognition of human ephrinB2 cell surface receptor by an emergent African henipavirus. *Proc Natl Acad Sci U S A* 2015;112(17):E2156–E2165.
66. Rissanen I, Ahmed AA, Azarm K, et al. Idiosyncratic Mojiang virus attachment glycoprotein directs a host-cell entry pathway distinct from genetically related henipaviruses. *Nat Commun* 2017;8:16060.
67. Bowden TA, Aricescu AR, Gilbert RJ, et al. Structural basis of Nipah and Hendra virus attachment to their cell-surface receptor ephrin-B2. *Nat Struct Mol Biol* 2008;15(6):567–572.
68. Bowden TA, Crispin M, Harvey DJ, et al. Dimeric architecture of the Hendra virus attachment glycoprotein: evidence for a conserved mode of assembly. *J Virol* 2010;84(12):6208–6217.
69. Xu K, Rajashankar KR, Chan YP, et al. Host cell recognition by the henipaviruses: crystal structures of the Nipah G attachment glycoprotein and its complex with ephrin-B3. *Proc Natl Acad Sci U S A* 2008;105(29):9953–9958.
70. Bose S, Jardetzky TS, Lamb RA. Timing is everything: Fine-tuned molecular machines orchestrate paramyxovirus entry. *Virology* 2015;479–480:518–531.
71. Moll M, Diederich S, Klenk HD, et al. Ubiquitous activation of the Nipah virus fusion protein does not require a basic amino acid at the cleavage site. *J Virol* 2004;78(18):9705–9712.
72. Pager CT, Dutch RE. Cathepsin L is involved in proteolytic processing of the Hendra virus fusion protein. *J Virol* 2005;79(20):12714–12720.
73. Diederich S, Sauerhering L, Weis M, et al. Activation of the Nipah virus fusion protein in MDCK cells is mediated by cathepsin B within the endosome-recycling compartment. *J Virol* 2012;86(7):3736–3745.
74. Kruger N, Hoffmann M, Weis M, et al. Surface glycoproteins of an African henipavirus induce syncytium formation in a cell line derived from an African fruit bat, Hypsignathus monstrosus. *J Virol* 2013;87(24):13889–13891.
75. Pager CT, Craft WW Jr, Patch J, et al. A mature and fusogenic form of the Nipah virus fusion protein requires proteolytic processing by cathepsin L. *Virology* 2006;346(2):251–257.
76. Meulendyke KA, Wurth MA, McCann RO, et al. Endocytosis plays a critical role in proteolytic processing of the Hendra virus fusion protein. *J Virol* 2005;79(20):12643–12649.
77. Vogt C, Eickmann M, Diederich S, et al. Endocytosis of the Nipah virus glycoproteins. *J Virol* 2005;79(6):3865–3872.
78. Popa A, Carter JR, Smith SE, et al. Residues in the hendra virus fusion protein transmembrane domain are critical for endocytic recycling. *J Virol* 2012;86(6):3014–3026.
79. Cifuentes-Munoz N, Sun W, Ray G, et al. Mutations in the transmembrane domain and cytoplasmic tail of Hendra virus fusion protein disrupt virus-like-particle assembly. *J Virol* 2017;91(14).
80. Johnston GP, Contreras EM, Dabundo J, et al. Cytoplasmic motifs in the Nipah virus fusion protein modulate virus particle assembly and egress. *J Virol* 2017;91(10).
81. El Najjar F, Schmitt AP, Dutch RE. Paramyxovirus glycoprotein incorporation, assembly and budding: a three way dance for infectious particle production. *Viruses* 2014;6(8):3019–3054.
82. Harrison MS, Sakaguchi T, Schmitt AP. Paramyxovirus assembly and budding: building particles that transmit infections. *Int J Biochem Cell Biol* 2010;42(9):1416–1429.
83. Wang YE, Park A, Lake M, et al. Ubiquitin-regulated nuclear-cytoplasmic trafficking of the Nipah virus matrix protein is important for viral budding. *PLoS Pathog* 2010;6(11):e1001186.
84. Monaghan P, Green D, Pallister J, et al. Detailed morphological characterisation of Hendra virus infection of different cell types using super-resolution and conventional imaging. *Virol J* 2014;11:200.
85. Pentecost M, Vashisht AA, Lester T, et al. Evidence for ubiquitin-regulated nuclear and subnuclear trafficking among Paramyxovirinae matrix proteins. *PLoS Pathog* 2015;11(3):e1004739.
86. McLinton EC, Wagstaff KM, Lee A, et al. Nuclear localization and secretion competence are conserved among henipavirus matrix proteins. *J Gen Virol* 2017;98(4):563–576.
87. Bauer A, Neumann S, Karger A, et al. ANP32B is a nuclear target of henipavirus M proteins. *PLoS One* 2014;9(5):e97233.
88. Hooper P, Zaki S, Daniels P, et al. Comparative pathology of the diseases caused by Hendra and Nipah viruses. *Microbes Infect* 2001;3(4):315–322.
89. Reynes JM, Counor D, Ong S, et al. Nipah virus in Lyle's flying foxes, Cambodia. *Emerg Infect Dis* 2005;11(7):1042–1047.

90. Mills JN, Alim AN, Bunning ML, et al. Nipah virus infection in dogs, Malaysia, 1999. *Emerg Infect Dis* 2009;15(6):950–952.
91. Field H, Young P, Yob JM, et al. The natural history of Hendra and Nipah viruses. *Microbes Infect* 2001;3(4):307–314.
92. Kirkland PD, Gabor M, Poe I, et al. Hendra virus infection in dog, Australia, 2013. *Emerg Infect Dis* 2015;21(12):2182–2185.
93. Middleton DJ, Riddell S, Klein R, et al. Experimental Hendra virus infection of dogs: virus replication, shedding and potential for transmission. *Aust Vet J* 2017;95(1–2):10–18.
94. Bossart KN, Wang LF, Eaton BT, et al. Functional expression and membrane fusion tropism of the envelope glycoproteins of Hendra virus. *Virology* 2001;290(1):121–135.
95. Bossart KN, Wang LF, Flora MN, et al. Membrane fusion tropism and heterotypic functional activities of the Nipah virus and Hendra virus envelope glycoproteins. *J Virol* 2002;76(22):11186–11198.
96. Tamin A, Harcourt BH, Ksiazek TG, et al. Functional properties of the fusion and attachment glycoproteins of Nipah virus. *Virology* 2002;296(1):190–200.
97. Bossart KN, Zhu Z, Middleton D, et al. A neutralizing human monoclonal antibody protects against lethal disease in a new ferret model of acute nipah virus infection. *PLoS Pathog* 2009;5(10):e1000642.
98. Geisbert TW, Daddario-DiCaprio KM, Hickey AC, et al. Development of an acute and highly pathogenic nonhuman primate model of Nipah virus infection. *PLoS One* 2010;5(5):e10690.
99. Marianneau P, Guillaume V, Wong T, et al. Experimental infection of squirrel monkeys with nipah virus. *Emerg Infect Dis* 2010;16(3):507–510.
100. Middleton DJ, Morrissy CJ, van der Heide BM, et al. Experimental Nipah virus infection in pteropid bats (Pteropus poliocephalus). *J Comp Pathol* 2007;136(4):266–272.
101. Wong KT, Grosjean I, Brisson C, et al. A golden hamster model for human acute Nipah virus infection. *Am J Pathol* 2003;163(5):2127–2137.
102. Guillaume V, Wong KT, Looi RY, et al. Acute Hendra virus infection: analysis of the pathogenesis and passive antibody protection in the hamster model. *Virology* 2009;387(2):459–465.
103. Rockx B, Bossart KN, Feldmann F, et al. A novel model of lethal Hendra virus infection in African green monkeys and the effectiveness of ribavirin treatment. *J Virol* 2010;84(19): 9831–9839.
104. Williamson MM, Hooper PT, Selleck PW, et al. A guinea-pig model of Hendra virus encephalitis. *J Comp Pathol* 2001;124(4):273–279.
105. Williamson MM, Hooper PT, Selleck PW, et al. Transmission studies of Hendra virus (equine morbillivirus) in fruit bats, horses and cats. *Aust Vet J* 1998;76(12):813–818.
106. Pallister J, Middleton D, Wang LF, et al. A recombinant Hendra virus G glycoprotein-based subunit vaccine protects ferrets from lethal Hendra virus challenge. *Vaccine* 2011;29(34): 5623–5630.
107. Chua KB, Lam SK, Goh KJ, et al. The presence of Nipah virus in respiratory secretions and urine of patients during an outbreak of Nipah virus encephalitis in Malaysia. *J Infect* 2001;42(1):40–43.
108. Goh KJ, Tan CT, Chew NK, et al. Clinical features of Nipah virus encephalitis among pig farmers in Malaysia. *N Engl J Med* 2000;342(17):1229–1235.
109. Islam MS, Sazzad HM, Satter SM, et al. Nipah virus transmission from bats to humans associated with drinking traditional liquor made from date palm sap, Bangladesh, 2011-2014. *Emerg Infect Dis* 2016;22(4):664–670.
110. Luby SP, Rahman M, Hossain MJ, et al. Foodborne transmission of Nipah virus, Bangladesh. *Emerg Infect Dis* 2006;12(12):1888–1894.
111. Rahman MA, Hossain MJ, Sultana S, et al. Date palm sap linked to Nipah virus outbreak in Bangladesh, 2008. *Vector Borne Zoonotic Dis* 2012;12(1):65–72.
112. Clayton BA, Middleton D, Arkinstall R, et al. The nature of exposure drives transmission of Nipah viruses from Malaysia and Bangladesh in ferrets. *PLoS Negl Trop Dis* 2016; 10(6):e0004775.
113. Edson D, Field H, McMichael L, et al. Routes of Hendra virus excretion in naturally-infected flying-foxes: implications for viral transmission and spillover risk. *PLoS One* 2015;10(10):e0140670.
114. Middleton DJ, Weingartl HM. Henipaviruses in their natural animal hosts. *Curr Top Microbiol Immunol* 2012;359:105–121.
115. Homaira N, Rahman M, Hossain MJ, et al. Cluster of Nipah virus infection, Kushtia District, Bangladesh, 2007. *PLoS One* 2010;5(10):e13570.
116. Chua KB. Epidemiology, surveillance and control of Nipah virus infections in Malaysia. *Malays J Pathol* 2010;32(2):69–73.
117. Luby SP, Gurley ES, Hossain MJ. Transmission of human infection with Nipah virus. *Clin Infect Dis* 2009;49(11):1743–1748.
118. Fogarty R, Halpin K, Hyatt AD, et al. Henipavirus susceptibility to environmental variables. *Virus Res* 2008;132(1–2):140–144.
119. Wacharapluesadee S, Hemachudha T. Duplex nested RT-PCR for detection of Nipah virus RNA from urine specimens of bats. *J Virol Methods* 2007;141(1):97–101.
120. Looi LM, Chua KB. Lessons from the Nipah virus outbreak in Malaysia. *Malays J Pathol* 2007;29(2):63–67.
121. Middleton DJ, Westbury HA, Morrissy CJ, et al. Experimental Nipah virus infection in pigs and cats. *J Comp Pathol* 2002;126(2–3):124–136.
122. Chakraborty A, Sazzad HM, Hossain MJ, et al. Evolving epidemiology of Nipah virus infection in Bangladesh: evidence from outbreaks during 2010-2011. *Epidemiol Infect* 2016;144(2):371–380.
123. Hegde ST, Sazzad HM, Hossain MJ, et al. Investigating rare risk factors for Nipah virus in Bangladesh: 2001-2012. *Ecohealth* 2016;13(4):720–728.
124. Blum LS, Khan R, Nahar N, et al. In-depth assessment of an outbreak of Nipah encephalitis with person-to-person transmission in Bangladesh: implications for prevention and control strategies. *Am J Trop Med Hyg* 2009;80(1):96–102.
125. Sazzad HM, Hossain MJ, Gurley ES, et al. Nipah virus infection outbreak with nosocomial and corpse-to-human transmission, Bangladesh. *Emerg Infect Dis* 2013;19(2):210–217.
126. Gurley ES, Montgomery JM, Hossain MJ, et al. Person-to-person transmission of Nipah virus in a Bangladeshi community. *Emerg Infect Dis* 2007;13(7):1031–1037.
127. Luby SP, Gurley ES. Epidemiology of henipavirus disease in humans. *Curr Top Microbiol Immunol* 2012;359:25–40.
128. Field HE. Hendra virus ecology and transmission. *Curr Opin Virol* 2016;16:120–125.
129. Tan CT, Goh KJ, Wong KT, et al. Relapsed and late-onset Nipah encephalitis. *Ann Neurol* 2002;51(6):703–708.
130. Wong KT, Tan CT. Clinical and pathological manifestations of human henipavirus infection. *Curr Top Microbiol Immunol* 2012;359:95–104.
131. Geisbert TW, Feldmann H, Broder CC. Animal challenge models of henipavirus infection and pathogenesis. *Curr Top Microbiol Immunol* 2012;359:153–177.
132. de Wit E, Munster VJ. Animal models of disease shed light on Nipah virus pathogenesis and transmission. *J Pathol* 2015;235(2):196–205.
133. Baseler L, Scott DP, Saturday G, et al. Identifying early target cells of Nipah virus infection in Syrian Hamsters. *PLoS Negl Trop Dis* 2016;10(11):e0005120.
134. Hammoud DA, Lentz MR, Lara A, et al. Aerosol exposure to intermediate size Nipah virus particles induces neurological disease in African green monkeys. *PLoS Negl Trop Dis* 2018;12(11):e0006978.
135. Lambrecht BN, Hammad H. Lung dendritic cells in respiratory viral infection and asthma: from protection to immunopathology. *Annu Rev Immunol* 2012;30:243–270.
136. Wong KT, Shieh WJ, Kumar S, et al. Nipah virus infection: pathology and pathogenesis of an emerging paramyxoviral zoonosis. *Am J Pathol* 2002;161(6):2153–2167.
137. Wong KT, Shieh WJ, Zaki SR, et al. Nipah virus infection, an emerging paramyxoviral zoonosis. *Springer Semin Immunopathol* 2002;24(2):215–228.
138. Rockx B, Brining D, Kramer J, et al. Clinical outcome of henipavirus infection in hamsters is determined by the route and dose of infection. *J Virol* 2011;85(15):7658–7671.
139. Weingartl H, Czub S, Copps J, et al. Invasion of the central nervous system in a porcine host by nipah virus. *J Virol* 2005;79(12):7528–7534.
140. Wong KT, Robertson T, Ong BB, et al. Human Hendra virus infection causes acute and relapsing encephalitis. *Neuropathol Appl Neurobiol* 2009;35(3):296–305.
141. Munster VJ, Prescott JB, Bushmaker T, et al. Rapid Nipah virus entry into the central nervous system of hamsters via the olfactory route. *Sci Rep* 2012;2:736.
142. Borisevich V, Ozdener MH, Malik B, et al. Hendra and Nipah virus infection in cultured human olfactory epithelial cells. *mSphere* 2017;2(3).
143. Miao H, Wang B. Eph/ephrin signaling in epithelial development and homeostasis. *Int J Biochem Cell Biol* 2009;41(4):762–770.
144. Pasquale EB. Eph-ephrin bidirectional signaling in physiology and disease. *Cell* 2008;133(1):38–52.
145. Barquilla A, Pasquale EB. Eph receptors and ephrins: therapeutic opportunities. *Annu Rev Pharmacol Toxicol* 2015;55:465–487.
146. Bennett KM, Afanador MD, Lal CV, et al. Ephrin-B2 reverse signaling increases $\alpha 5\beta 1$ integrin-mediated fibronectin deposition and reduces distal lung compliance. *Am J Respir Cell Mol Biol* 2013;49(4):680–687.
147. Genotype-Tissue Expression (GTEx) Portal: dbGaP Accession phs000424.v7.p2. The Broad Institute of MIT and Harvard; 2019. Available at: https://gtexportal.org/home/. Accessed January 31, 2019.
148. Gale NW, Baluk P, Pan L, et al. Ephrin-B2 selectively marks arterial vessels and neovascularization sites in the adult, with expression in both endothelial and smooth-muscle cells. *Dev Biol* 2001;230(2):151–160.
149. Shin D, Garcia-Cardena G, Hayashi S, et al. Expression of ephrinB2 identifies a stable genetic difference between arterial and venous vascular smooth muscle as well as endothelial cells, and marks subsets of microvessels at sites of adult neovascularization. *Dev Biol* 2001;230(2):139–150.
150. Mathieu C, Pohl C, Szecsi J, et al. Nipah virus uses leukocytes for efficient dissemination within a host. *J Virol* 2011;85(15):7863–7871.
151. Mathieu C, Dhondt KP, Chalons M, et al. Heparan sulfate-dependent enhancement of henipavirus infection. *MBio* 2015;6(2):e02427.
152. Arunkumar G, Devadiga S, McElroy AK, et al. Adaptive immune responses in humans during Nipah virus acute and convalescent phases of infection. *Clin Infect Dis* 2019. doi: 10.1093/cid/ciz010.
153. Chua KB. Nipah virus outbreak in Malaysia. *J Clin Virol* 2003;26(3):265–275.
154. Taylor C, Playford EG, McBride WJ, et al. No evidence of prolonged Hendra virus shedding by 2 patients, Australia. *Emerg Infect Dis* 2012;18(12):2025–2027.
155. Andrejeva J, Childs KS, Young DF, et al. The V proteins of paramyxoviruses bind the IFN-inducible RNA helicase, mda-5, and inhibit its activation of the IFN-beta promoter. *Proc Natl Acad Sci U S A* 2004;101(49):17264–17269.
156. Levy DE, Marie IJ. RIGging an antiviral defense—it's in the CARDs. *Nat Immunol* 2004;5(7):699–701.
157. Jensen S, Thomsen AR. Sensing of RNA viruses: a review of innate immune receptors involved in recognizing RNA virus invasion. *J Virol* 2012;86(6):2900–2910.
158. Matsumoto M, Oshiumi H, Seya T. Antiviral responses induced by the TLR3 pathway. *Rev Med Virol* 2011;21(2):67–77.
159. Parisien JP, Bamming D, Komuro A, et al. A shared interface mediates paramyxovirus interference with antiviral RNA helicases MDA5 and LGP2. *J Virol* 2009;83(14):7252–7260.
160. Childs KS, Andrejeva J, Randall RE, et al. Mechanism of mda-5 Inhibition by paramyxovirus V proteins. *J Virol* 2009;83(3):1465–1473.
161. Shaw ML, Garcia-Sastre A, Palese P, et al. Nipah virus V and W proteins have a common STAT1-binding domain yet inhibit STAT1 activation from the cytoplasmic and nuclear compartments, respectively. *J Virol* 2004;78(11):5633–5641.
162. Sanchez-Aparicio MT, Feinman LJ, Garcia-Sastre A, et al. Paramyxovirus V proteins interact with the RIG-I/TRIM25 regulatory complex and inhibit RIG-I signaling. *J Virol* 2018;92(6).
163. Shaw ML, Cardenas WB, Zamarin D, et al. Nuclear localization of the Nipah virus W protein allows for inhibition of both virus- and toll-like receptor 3-triggered signaling pathways. *J Virol* 2005;79(10):6078–6088.
164. Aaronson DS, Horvath CM. A road map for those who don't know JAK-STAT. *Science* 2002;296(5573):1653–1655.
165. Platanias LC. Mechanisms of type-I- and type-II-interferon-mediated signalling. *Nat Rev Immunol* 2005;5(5):375–386.
166. Rodriguez JJ, Wang LF, Horvath CM. Hendra virus V protein inhibits interferon signaling by preventing STAT1 and STAT2 nuclear accumulation. *J Virol* 2003;77(21):11842–11845.

167. Rodriguez JJ, Parisien JP, Horvath CM. Nipah virus V protein evades alpha and gamma interferons by preventing STAT1 and STAT2 activation and nuclear accumulation. *J Virol* 2002;76(22):11476–11483.
168. Rodriguez JJ, Cruz CD, Horvath CM. Identification of the nuclear export signal and STAT-binding domains of the Nipah virus V protein reveals mechanisms underlying interferon evasion. *J Virol* 2004;78(10):5358 5367.
169. Ludlow LE, Lo MK, Rodriguez JJ, et al. Henipavirus V protein association with Polo-like kinase reveals functional overlap with STAT1 binding and interferon evasion. *J Virol* 2008;82(13):6259–6271.
170. Smith KM, Tsimbalyuk S, Edwards MR, et al. Structural basis for importin alpha 3 specificity of W proteins in Hendra and Nipah viruses. *Nat Commun* 2018;9(1):3703.
171. Sugai A, Sato H, Takayama I, et al. Nipah and Hendra Virus nucleoproteins inhibit nuclear accumulation of signal transducer and activator of transcription 1 (STAT1) and STAT2 by interfering with their complex formation. *J Virol* 2017;91(21).
172. Park MS, Shaw ML, Munoz-Jordan J, et al. Newcastle disease virus (NDV)-based assay demonstrates interferon-antagonist activity for the NDV V protein and the Nipah virus V, W, and C proteins. *J Virol* 2003;77(2):1501–1511.
173. Georges-Courbot MC, Contamin H, Faure C, et al. Poly(I)-poly(C12U) but not ribavirin prevents death in a hamster model of Nipah virus infection. *Antimicrob Agents Chemother* 2006;50(5):1768–1772.
174. Virtue ER, Marsh GA, Wang LF. Interferon signaling remains functional during henipavirus infection of human cell lines. *J Virol* 2011;85(8):4031–4034.
175. Virtue ER, Marsh GA, Baker ML, et al. Interferon production and signaling pathways are antagonized during henipavirus infection of fruit bat cell lines. *PLoS One* 2011;6(7):e22488.
176. Rockx B. Recent developments in experimental animal models of Henipavirus infection. *Pathog Dis* 2014;71(2):199–206.
177. Mathieu C, Guillaume V, Volchkova VA, et al. Nonstructural Nipah virus C protein regulates both the early host proinflammatory response and viral virulence. *J Virol* 2012;86(19):10766–10775.
178. Chong HT, Kunjapan SR, Thayaparan T, et al. Nipah encephalitis outbreak in Malaysia, clinical features in patients from Seremban. *Can J Neurol Sci* 2002;29(1):83–87.
179. Cong Y, Lentz MR, Lara A, et al. Loss in lung volume and changes in the immune response demonstrate disease progression in African green monkeys infected by small-particle aerosol and intratracheal exposure to Nipah virus. *PLoS Negl Trop Dis* 2017;11(4):e0005532.
180. Pickering BS, Hardham JM, Smith G, et al. Protection against henipaviruses in swine requires both, cell-mediated and humoral immune response. *Vaccine* 2016;34(40):4777–4786.
181. Satterfield BA, Dawes BE, Milligan GN. Status of vaccine research and development of vaccines for Nipah virus. *Vaccine* 2016;34(26):2971–2975.
182. Gupta M, Lo MK, Spiropoulou CF. Activation and cell death in human dendritic cells infected with Nipah virus. *Virology* 2013;441(1):49–56.
183. Berhane Y, Weingartl HM, Lopez J, et al. Bacterial infections in pigs experimentally infected with Nipah virus. *Transbound Emerg Dis* 2008;55(3–4):165–174.
184. Leon AJ, Borisevich V, Boroumand N, et al. Host gene expression profiles in ferrets infected with genetically distinct henipavirus strains. *PLoS Negl Trop Dis* 2018;12(3):e0006343.
185. Barclay AJ, Paton DJ. Hendra (equine morbillivirus). *Vet J* 2000;160(3):169–176.
186. McCormack JG, Allworth AM, Selvey LA, et al. Transmissibility from horses to humans of a novel paramyxovirus, equine morbillivirus (EMV). *J Infect* 1999;38(1):22–23.
187. Luby SP, Hossain MJ, Gurley ES, et al. Recurrent zoonotic transmission of Nipah virus into humans, Bangladesh, 2001-2007. *Emerg Infect Dis* 2009;15(8):1229–1235.
188. Homaira N, Rahman M, Hossain MJ, et al. Nipah virus outbreak with person-to-person transmission in a district of Bangladesh, 2007. *Epidemiol Infect* 2010;138(11):1630–1636.
189. Mounts AW, Kaur H, Parashar UD, et al. A cohort study of health care workers to assess nosocomial transmissibility of Nipah virus, Malaysia, 1999. *J Infect Dis* 2001;183(5):810–813.
190. DeBuysscher BL, de Wit E, Munster VJ, et al. Comparison of the pathogenicity of Nipah virus isolates from Bangladesh and Malaysia in the Syrian hamster. *PLoS Negl Trop Dis* 2013;7(1):e2024.
191. Mire CE, Satterfield BA, Geisbert JB, et al. Pathogenic differences between Nipah virus Bangladesh and Malaysia Strains in Primates: implications for antibody therapy. *Sci Rep* 2016;6:30916.
192. Rockx B, Winegar R, Freiberg AN. Recent progress in henipavirus research: molecular biology, genetic diversity, animal models. *Antiviral Res* 2012;95(2):135–149.
193. Bossart KN, Geisbert TW, Feldmann H, et al. A neutralizing human monoclonal antibody protects african green monkeys from hendra virus challenge. *Sci Transl Med* 2011;3(105):105ra103.
194. Geisbert TW, Mire CE, Geisbert JB, et al. Therapeutic treatment of Nipah virus infection in nonhuman primates with a neutralizing human monoclonal antibody. *Sci Transl Med* 2014;6(242):242ra282.
195. Lieu KG, Marsh GA, Wang LF, et al. The non-pathogenic Henipavirus Cedar paramyxovirus phosphoprotein has a compromised ability to target STAT1 and STAT2. *Antiviral Res* 2015;124:69–76.
196. Sejvar JJ, Hossain J, Saha SK. et al. Long-term neurological and functional outcome in Nipah virus infection. *Ann Neurol* 2007;62(3):235–242.
197. Wong SC, Ooi MH, Wong MN, et al. Late presentation of Nipah virus encephalitis and kinetics of the humoral immune response. *J Neurol Neurosurg Psychiatry* 2001;71(4):552–554.
198. Chua KB, Lam SK, Tan CT, et al. High mortality in Nipah encephalitis is associated with presence of virus in cerebrospinal fluid. *Ann Neurol* 2000;48(5):802–805.
199. Griffin DE, Lin WW, Nelson AN. Understanding the causes and consequences of measles virus persistence. *F1000Res* 2018;7:237.
200. Watanabe S, Shirogane Y, Sato Y, et al. New insights into Measles virus brain infections. *Trends Microbiol* 2019;27(2):164–175.
201. Parashar UD, Sunn LM, Ong F, et al. Case-control study of risk factors for human infection with a new zoonotic paramyxovirus, Nipah virus, during a 1998-1999 outbreak of severe encephalitis in Malaysia. *J Infect Dis* 2000;181(5):1755–1759.
202. Field HE, Mackenzie JS, Daszak P. Henipaviruses: emerging paramyxoviruses associated with fruit bats. *Curr Top Microbiol Immunol* 2007;315:133–159.
203. Luby SP. The pandemic potential of Nipah virus. *Antiviral Res* 2013;100(1):38–43.
204. Chew MH, Arguin PM, Shay DK, et al. Risk factors for Nipah virus infection among abattoir workers in Singapore. *J Infect Dis* 2000;181(5):1760–1763.
205. Yob JM, Field H, Rashdi AM, et al. Nipah virus infection in bats (order Chiroptera) in peninsular Malaysia. *Emerg Infect Dis* 2001;7(3):439–441.
206. Anderson DE, Islam A, Crameri G, et al. Isolation and full-genome characterization of Nipah viruses from Bats, Bangladesh. *Emerg Infect Dis* 2019;25(1):166–170.
207. Epstein JH, Prakash V, Smith CS, et al. Henipavirus infection in fruit bats (Pteropus giganteus), India. *Emerg Infect Dis* 2008;14(8):1309–1311.
208. Rahman SA, Hassan SS, Olival KJ, et al. Characterization of Nipah virus from naturally infected Pteropus vampyrus bats, Malaysia. *Emerg Infect Dis* 2010;16(12):1990–1993.
209. Eaton BT, Broder CC, Middleton D, et al. Hendra and Nipah viruses: different and dangerous. *Nat Rev Microbiol* 2006;4(1):23–35.
210. Williamson MM, Hooper PT, Selleck PW, et al. Experimental hendra virus infection in pregnant guinea-pigs and fruit Bats (Pteropus poliocephalus). *J Comp Pathol* 2000;122(2-3):201-207.
211. Selvey L, Taylor R, Arklay A, et al. Screening of bat carers for antibodies to equine morbillivirus. *Commun Dis Intell* 1996;20:477–478.
212. Khan MS, Hossain J, Gurley ES, et al. Use of infrared camera to understand bats' access to date palm sap: implications for preventing Nipah virus transmission. *Ecohealth* 2010;7(4):517–525.
213. Chowdhury S, Khan SU, Crameri G, et al. Serological evidence of henipavirus exposure in cattle, goats and pigs in Bangladesh. *PLoS Negl Trop Dis* 2014;8(11):e3302.
214. Montgomery JM, Hossain MJ, Gurley E, et al. Risk factors for Nipah virus encephalitis in Bangladesh. *Emerg Infect Dis* 2008;14(10):1526–1532.
215. Mahalingam S, Herrero LJ, Playford EG, et al. Hendra virus: an emerging paramyxovirus in Australia. *Lancet Infect Dis* 2012;12(10):799–807.
216. Hooper PT, Westbury HA, Russell GM. The lesions of experimental equine morbillivirus disease in cats and guinea pigs. *Vet Pathol* 1997;34(4):323–329.
217. Murray K, Rogers R, Selvey L, et al. A novel morbillivirus pneumonia of horses and its transmission to humans. *Emerg Infect Dis* 1995;1(1):31–33.
218. Arankalle VA, Bandyopadhyay BT, Ramdasi AY, et al. Genomic characterization of Nipah virus, West Bengal, India. *Emerg Infect Dis* 2011;17(5):907–909.
219. Marsh GA, Todd S, Foord A, et al. Genome sequence conservation of Hendra virus isolates during spillover to horses, Australia. *Emerg Infect Dis* 2010;16(11):1767–1769.
220. Chan YP, Chua KB, Koh CL, et al. Complete nucleotide sequences of Nipah virus isolates from Malaysia. *J Gen Virol* 2001;82(Pt 9):2151–2155.
221. Wacharapluesadee S, Samseeneam P, Phermpool M, et al. Molecular characterization of Nipah virus from Pteropus hypomelanus in Southern Thailand. *Virol J* 2016;13:53.
222. Peel AJ, Sargan DR, Baker KS, et al. Continent-wide panmixia of an African fruit bat facilitates transmission of potentially zoonotic viruses. *Nat Commun* 2013;4:2770.
223. Weiss S, Nowak K, Fahr J, et al. Henipavirus-related sequences in fruit bat bushmeat, Republic of Congo. *Emerg Infect Dis* 2012;18(9):1536–1537.
224. Kruger N, Hoffmann M, Drexler JF, et al. Attachment protein G of an African bat henipavirus is differentially restricted in chiropteran and nonchiropteran cells. *J Virol* 2014;88(20):11973–11980.
225. Weis M, Behner L, Hoffmann M, et al. Characterization of African bat henipavirus GH-M74a glycoproteins. *J Gen Virol* 2014;95(Pt 3):539–548.
226. Hossain MJ, Gurley ES, Montgomery JM, et al. Clinical presentation of nipah virus infection in Bangladesh. *Clin Infect Dis* 2008;46(7):977–984.
227. Tan KS, Sarji SA, Tan CT, et al. Patients with asymptomatic Nipah virus infection may have abnormal cerebral MR imaging. *Neurol J Southeast Asia* 2000;5:69–73.
228. Lim CC, Lee KE, Lee WL, et al. Nipah virus encephalitis: serial MR study of an emerging disease. *Radiology* 2002;222(1):219–226.
229. Lee KE, Umapathi T, Tan CB, et al. The neurological manifestations of Nipah virus encephalitis, a novel paramyxovirus. *Ann Neurol* 1999;46(3):428–432.
230. Lim CC, Lee WL, Leo YS, et al. Late clinical and magnetic resonance imaging follow up of Nipah virus infection. *J Neurol Neurosurg Psychiatry* 2003;74(1):131–133.
231. Abdullah S, Chang LY, Rahmat K, et al. Late-onset Nipah virus encephalitis 11 years after the initial outbreak: a case report. *Neurol Asia* 2012;17(1):71–74.
232. Wang LF, Daniels P. Diagnosis of henipavirus infection: current capabilities and future directions. *Curr Top Microbiol Immunol* 2012;359:179–196.
233. Imada T, Abdul Rahman MA, Kashiwazaki Y, et al. Production and characterization of monoclonal antibodies against formalin-inactivated Nipah virus isolated from the lungs of a pig. *J Vet Med Sci* 2004;66(1):81–83.
234. Tanimura N, Imada T, Kashiwazaki Y, et al. Monoclonal antibody-based immunohistochemical diagnosis of Malaysian Nipah virus infection in pigs. *J Comp Pathol* 2004;131(2–3):199–206.
235. Tanimura N, Imada T, Kashiwazaki Y, et al. Reactivity of anti-Nipah virus monoclonal antibodies to formalin-fixed, paraffin-embedded lung tissues from experimental Nipah and Hendra virus infections. *J Vet Med Sci* 2004;66(10):1263–1266.
236. White JR, Boyd V, Crameri GS, et al. Location of, immunogenicity of and relationships between neutralization epitopes on the attachment protein (G) of Hendra virus. *J Gen Virol* 2005;86(Pt 10):2839–2848.
237. Smith IL, Halpin K, Warrilow D, et al. Development of a fluorogenic RT-PCR assay (TaqMan) for the detection of Hendra virus. *J Virol Methods* 2001;98(1):33–40.
238. Guillaume V, Lefeuvre A, Faure C, et al. Specific detection of Nipah virus using real-time RT-PCR (TaqMan). *J Virol Methods* 2004;120(2):229–237.
239. Feldman KS, Foord A, Heine HG, et al. Design and evaluation of consensus PCR assays for henipaviruses. *J Virol Methods* 2009;161(1):52–57.
240. Eshaghi M, Tan WS, Mohidin TB, et al. Nipah virus glycoprotein: production in baculovirus and application in diagnosis. *Virus Res* 2004;106(1):71–76.
241. Kashiwazaki Y, Na YN, Tanimura N, et al. A solid-phase blocking ELISA for detection of antibodies to Nipah virus. *J Virol Methods* 2004;121(2):259–261.

242. Bossart KN, McEachern JA, Hickey AC, et al. Neutralization assays for differential henipavirus serology using Bio-Plex protein array systems. *J Virol Methods* 2007;142(1–2):29–40.
243. Kaku Y, Noguchi A, Marsh GA, et al. A neutralization test for specific detection of Nipah virus antibodies using pseudotyped vesicular stomatitis virus expressing green fluorescent protein. *J Virol Methods* 2009;160(1–2):7–13.
244. Kaku Y, Noguchi A, Marsh GA, et al. Second generation of pseudotype-based serum neutralization assay for Nipah virus antibodies: sensitive and high-throughput analysis utilizing secreted alkaline phosphatase. *J Virol Methods* 2012;179(1):226–232.
245. Tamin A, Harcourt BH, Lo MK, et al. Development of a neutralization assay for Nipah virus using pseudotype particles. *J Virol Methods* 2009;160(1–2):1–6.
246. Wright PJ, Crameri G, Eaton BT. RNA synthesis during infection by Hendra virus: an examination by quantitative real-time PCR of RNA accumulation, the effect of ribavirin and the attenuation of transcription. *Arch Virol* 2005;150(3):521–532.
247. Chong HT, Kamarulzaman A, Tan CT, et al. Treatment of acute Nipah encephalitis with ribavirin. *Ann Neurol* 2001;49(6):810–813.
248. Pager CT, Wurth MA, Dutch RE. Subcellular localization and calcium and pH requirements for proteolytic processing of the Hendra virus fusion protein. *J Virol* 2004; 78(17):9154–9163.
249. Porotto M, Orefice G, Yokoyama CC, et al. Simulating henipavirus multicycle replication in a screening assay leads to identification of a promising candidate for therapy. *J Virol* 2009;83(10):5148–5155.
250. International Society for Infectious Diseases. *Hendra virus, human, equine—Australia (05): Queensland*. Brookline, MA: Pro-med; 2009. Archive no. 20090910.3189. Available at: www.promedmail.org
251. Warren TK, Jordan R, Lo MK, et al. Therapeutic efficacy of the small molecule GS-5734 against Ebola virus in rhesus monkeys. *Nature* 2016;531(7594):381–385.
252. Lo MK, Jordan R, Arvey A, et al. GS-5734 and its parent nucleoside analog inhibit Filo-, Pneumo-, and Paramyxoviruses. *Sci Rep* 2017;7:43395.
253. Freiberg AN, Worthy MN, Lee B, et al. Combined chloroquine and ribavirin treatment does not prevent death in a hamster model of Nipah and Hendra virus infection. *J Gen Virol* 2010;91(Pt 3):765–772.
254. Pallister J, Middleton D, Crameri G, et al. Chloroquine administration does not prevent Nipah virus infection and disease in ferrets. *J Virol* 2009;83(22):11979–11982.
255. Eaton BT, Broder CC, Wang LF. Hendra and Nipah viruses: pathogenesis and therapeutics. *Curr Mol Med* 2005;5(8):805–816.
256. Porotto M, Rockx B, Yokoyama CC, et al. Inhibition of Nipah virus infection in vivo: targeting an early stage of paramyxovirus fusion activation during viral entry. *PLoS Pathog* 2010;6(10):e1001168.
257. Broder CC, Weir DL, Reid PA. Hendra virus and Nipah virus animal vaccines. *Vaccine* 2016;34(30):3525–3534.
258. Guillaume V, Contamin H, Loth P, et al. Nipah virus: vaccination and passive protection studies in a hamster model. *J Virol* 2004;78(2):834–840.
259. Weingartl HM, Berhane Y, Caswell JL, et al. Recombinant nipah virus vaccines protect pigs against challenge. *J Virol* 2006;80(16):7929–7938.
260. Ploquin A, Szecsi J, Mathieu C, et al. Protection against henipavirus infection by use of recombinant adeno-associated virus-vector vaccines. *J Infect Dis* 2013;207(3):469–478.
261. Yoneda M, Georges-Courbot MC, Ikeda F, et al. Recombinant measles virus vaccine expressing the Nipah virus glycoprotein protects against lethal Nipah virus challenge. *PLoS One* 2013;8(3):e58414.
262. Mire CE, Versteeg KM, Cross RW, et al. Single injection recombinant vesicular stomatitis virus vaccines protect ferrets against lethal Nipah virus disease. *Virol J* 2013;10:353.
263. DeBuysscher BL, Scott D, Marzi A, et al. Single-dose live-attenuated Nipah virus vaccines confer complete protection by eliciting antibodies directed against surface glycoproteins. *Vaccine* 2014;32(22):2637–2644.
264. Lo MK, Bird BH, Chattopadhyay A, et al. Single-dose replication-defective VSV-based Nipah virus vaccines provide protection from lethal challenge in Syrian hamsters. *Antiviral Res* 2014;101:26–29.
265. Prescott J, DeBuysscher BL, Feldmann F, et al. Single-dose live-attenuated vesicular stomatitis virus-based vaccine protects African green monkeys from Nipah virus disease. *Vaccine* 2015;33(24):2823–2829.
266. DeBuysscher BL, Scott D, Thomas T, et al. Peri-exposure protection against Nipah virus disease using a single-dose recombinant vesicular stomatitis virus-based vaccine. *NPJ Vaccines* 2016;1.
267. Bossart KN, Crameri G, Dimitrov AS, et al. Receptor binding, fusion inhibition, and induction of cross-reactive neutralizing antibodies by a soluble G glycoprotein of Hendra virus. *J Virol* 2005;79(11):6690–6702.
268. Mungall BA, Middleton D, Crameri G, et al. Feline model of acute nipah virus infection and protection with a soluble glycoprotein-based subunit vaccine. *J Virol* 2006; 80(24):12293–12302.
269. Colgrave ML, Snelling HJ, Shiell BJ, et al. Site occupancy and glycan compositional analysis of two soluble recombinant forms of the attachment glycoprotein of Hendra virus. *Glycobiology* 2012;22(4):572–584.
270. McEachern JA, Bingham J, Crameri G, et al. A recombinant subunit vaccine formulation protects against lethal Nipah virus challenge in cats. *Vaccine* 2008;26(31):3842–3852.
271. Pallister JA, Klein R, Arkinstall R, et al. Vaccination of ferrets with a recombinant G glycoprotein subunit vaccine provides protection against Nipah virus disease for over 12 months. *Virol J* 2013;10:237.
272. Bossart KN, Rockx B, Feldmann F, et al. A Hendra virus G glycoprotein subunit vaccine protects African green monkeys from Nipah virus challenge. *Sci Transl Med* 2012;4(146):146ra107.
273. Mire CE, Geisbert JB, Agans KN, et al. A recombinant Hendra virus G glycoprotein subunit vaccine protects nonhuman primates against Hendra virus challenge. *J Virol* 2014;88(9):4624–4631.
274. Middleton D, Pallister J, Klein R, et al. Hendra virus vaccine, a one health approach to protecting horse, human, and environmental health. *Emerg Infect Dis* 2014;20(3):372–379.
275. Plotkin SA. Vaccines for epidemic infections and the role of CEPI. *Hum Vaccin Immunother* 2017;13(12):2755–2762.
276. Guillaume V, Contamin H, Loth P, et al. Antibody prophylaxis and therapy against Nipah virus infection in hamsters. *J Virol* 2006;80(4):1972–1978.
277. Zhu Z, Dimitrov AS, Bossart KN, et al. Potent neutralization of Hendra and Nipah viruses by human monoclonal antibodies. *J Virol* 2006;80(2):891–899.
278. Zhu Z, Bossart KN, Bishop KA, et al. Exceptionally potent cross-reactive neutralization of Nipah and Hendra viruses by a human monoclonal antibody. *J Infect Dis* 2008;197(6):846–853.
279. Xu K, Rockx B, Xie Y, et al. Crystal structure of the Hendra virus attachment G glycoprotein bound to a potent cross-reactive neutralizing human monoclonal antibody. *PLoS Pathog* 2013;9(10):e1003684.
280. Broder CC. Henipavirus outbreaks to antivirals: the current status of potential therapeutics. *Curr Opin Virol* 2012;2(2):176–187.
281. WHO. 2018 annual review of the Blueprint list of priority diseases. WHO; 2018. Available at: https://www.who.int/blueprint/priority-diseases/en/
282. USDA. Henipavirus Gap Analysis Workshop Report. U.S. Department of Agriculture, Agricultural Research Service. Available at: http://go.usa.gov/xnHgR. Published 2018. Accessed.
283. CEPI. Coalition of Epidemic Preparedness Innovations: Vaccine Portfolio. 2019. Available at: https://cepi.net/research_dev/our-portfolio/
284. Schountz T, Baker ML, Butler J, et al. Immunological control of viral infections in bats and the emergence of viruses highly pathogenic to humans. *Front Immunol* 2017;8:1098.
285. Breed AC, Meers J, Sendow I, et al. The distribution of henipaviruses in Southeast Asia and Australasia: is Wallace's line a barrier to Nipah virus? *PLoS One* 2013;8(4):e61316.
286. Wacharapluesadee S, Lumlertdacha B, Boongird K, et al. Bat Nipah virus, Thailand. *Emerg Infect Dis* 2005;11(12):1949–1951.
287. Li Y, Wang J, Hickey AC, et al. Antibodies to Nipah or Nipah-like viruses in bats, China. *Emerg Infect Dis* 2008;14(12):1974–1976.
288. Breed AC, Yu M, Barr JA, et al. Prevalence of henipavirus and rubulavirus antibodies in pteropid bats, Papua New Guinea. *Emerg Infect Dis* 2010;16(12):1997–1999.
289. Sendow I, Field HE, Adjid A, et al. Screening for Nipah virus infection in West Kalimantan Province, Indonesia. *Zoonoses Public Health* 2010;57(7–8):499–503.
290. Wacharapluesadee S, Boongird K, Wanghongsa S, et al. A longitudinal study of the prevalence of Nipah virus in Pteropus lylei bats in Thailand: evidence for seasonal preference in disease transmission. *Vector Borne Zoonotic Dis* 2010;10(2):183–190.
291. Plowright RK, Foley P, Field HE, et al. Urban habituation, ecological connectivity and epidemic dampening: the emergence of Hendra virus from flying foxes (Pteropus spp.). *Proc Biol Sci* 2011;278(1725):3703–3712.
292. Hasebe F, Thuy NT, Inoue S, et al. Serologic evidence of nipah virus infection in bats, Vietnam. *Emerg Infect Dis* 2012;18(3):536–537.
293. Yadav PD, Raut CG, Shete AM, et al. Detection of Nipah virus RNA in fruit bat (Pteropus giganteus) from India. *Am J Trop Med Hyg* 2012;87(3):576–578.
294. Field H, de Jong CE, Halpin K, et al. Henipaviruses and fruit bats, Papua New Guinea. *Emerg Infect Dis* 2013;19(4):670–671.
295. de Araujo J, Lo MK, Tamin A, et al. Antibodies against Henipa-Like viruses in Brazilian bats. *Vector Borne Zoonotic Dis* 2017;17(4):271–274.
296. Hayman DT, Suu-Ire R, Breed AC, et al. Evidence of henipavirus infection in West African fruit bats. *PLoS One* 2008;3(7):e2739.
297. Peel AJ, Baker KS, Crameri G, et al. Henipavirus neutralising antibodies in an isolated island population of African fruit bats. *PLoS One* 2012;7(1):e30346.
298. Kessler MK, Becker DJ, Peel AJ, et al. Changing resource landscapes and spillover of henipaviruses. *Ann N Y Acad Sci* 2018;1429(1):78–99.
299. Giles JR, Eby P, Parry H, et al. Environmental drivers of spatiotemporal foraging intensity in fruit bats and implications for Hendra virus ecology. *Sci Rep* 2018;8(1):9555.
300. Plowright RK, Peel AJ, Streicker DG, et al. Transmission or within-host dynamics driving pulses of zoonotic viruses in reservoir-host populations. *PLoS Negl Trop Dis* 2016;10(8):e0004796.
301. Wood JL, Leach M, Waldman L, et al. A framework for the study of zoonotic disease emergence and its drivers: spillover of bat pathogens as a case study. *Philos Trans R Soc Lond B Biol Sci* 2012;367(1604):2881–2892.
302. Broder CC, Xu K, Nikolov DB, et al. A treatment for and vaccine against the deadly Hendra and Nipah viruses. *Antiviral Res* 2013;100(1):8–13.
303. AbuBakar S, Chang LY, Ali AR, et al. Isolation and molecular identification of Nipah virus from pigs. *Emerg Infect Dis* 2004;10(12):2228–2230.
304. Erbar S, Diederich S, Maisner A. Selective receptor expression restricts Nipah virus infection of endothelial cells. *Virol J* 2008;5:142.
305. Pernet O, Wang YE, Lee B. Henipavirus receptor usage and tropism. *Curr Top Microbiol Immunol* 2012;359:59–78.
306. Yoneda M. Nipah and Hendra virus infectious diseases. *Nihon Rinsho* 2016;74(12):1973–1978.
307. Talekar A, Pessi A, Porotto M. Infection of primary neurons mediated by nipah virus envelope proteins: role of host target cells in antiviral action. *J Virol* 2011;85(16):8422–8426.
308. Sawatsky B, Grolla A, Kuzenko N, et al. Inhibition of henipavirus infection by Nipah virus attachment glycoprotein occurs without cell-surface downregulation of ephrin-B2 or ephrin-B3. *J Gen Virol* 2007;88(Pt 2):582–591.
309. Martinez-Gil L, Vera-Velasco NM, Mingarro I. Exploring the Human-Nipah virus Protein-Protein interactome. *J Virol* 2017;91(23).
310. Aljofan M, Porotto M, Moscona A, et al. Development and validation of a chemiluminescent immunodetection assay amenable to high throughput screening of antiviral drugs for Nipah and Hendra virus. *J Virol Methods* 2008;149(1):12–19.
311. Bender RR, Muth A, Schneider IC, et al. Receptor-targeted Nipah virus glycoproteins improve cell-type selective gene delivery and reveal a preference for membrane-proximal cell attachment. *PLoS Pathog* 2016;12(6):e1005641.
312. Khetawat D, Broder CC. A functional henipavirus envelope glycoprotein pseudotyped lentivirus assay system. *Virol J* 2010;7:312.
313. Mathieu C, Guillaume V, Sabine A, et al. Lethal Nipah virus infection induces rapid overexpression of CXCL10. *PLoS One* 2012;7(2):e32157.
314. Palomares K, Vigant F, Van Handel B, et al. Nipah virus envelope-pseudotyped lentiviruses efficiently target ephrinB2-positive stem cell populations in vitro and bypass the liver sink when administered in vivo. *J Virol* 2013;87(4):2094–2108.
315. Escaffre O, Borisevich V, Carmical JR, et al. Henipavirus pathogenesis in human respiratory epithelial cells. *J Virol* 2013;87(6):3284–3294.
316. Escaffre O, Borisevich V, Vergara LA, et al. Characterization of Nipah virus infection in a model of human airway epithelial cells cultured at an air-liquid interface. *J Gen Virol* 2016;97(5):1077–1086.

317. Tanos T, Saibene AM, Pipolo C, et al. Isolation of putative stem cells present in human adult olfactory mucosa. *PLoS One* 2017;12(7):e0181151.
318. Erbar S, Maisner A. Nipah virus infection and glycoprotein targeting in endothelial cells. *Virol J* 2010;7:305.
319. Chua KB, Wong EM, Cropp BC, et al. Role of electron microscopy in Nipah virus outbreak investigation and control. *Med J Malaysia* 2007;62(2):139–142.
320. Hudson AL, Weir C, Moon E, et al. Establishing a panel of chemo-resistant mesothelioma models for investigating chemo-resistance and identifying new treatments for mesothelioma. *Sci Rep* 2014;4:6152.
321. Yoneda M, Fujita K, Sato H, et al. Reverse genetics of Nipah virus to probe viral pathogenicity. *Methods Mol Biol* 2009;515:329–337.
322. Bossart KN, Tachedjian M, McEachern JA, et al. Functional studies of host-specific ephrin-B ligands as Henipavirus receptors. *Virology* 2008;372(2):357–371.
323. Crameri G, Todd S, Grimley S, et al. Establishment, immortalisation and characterisation of pteropid bat cell lines. *PLoS One* 2009;4(12):e8266.
324. Iehle C, Razafitrimo G, Razainirina J, et al. Henipavirus and Tioman virus antibodies in pteropodid bats, Madagascar. *Emerg Infect Dis* 2007;13(1):159–161.
325. Drexler JF, Corman VM, Gloza-Rausch F, et al. Henipavirus RNA in African bats. *PLoS One* 2009;4(7):e6367.
326. Chua KB. A novel approach for collecting samples from fruit bats for isolation of infectious agents. *Microbes Infect* 2003;5(6):487–490.
327. Olson JG, Rupprecht C, Rollin PE, et al. Antibodies to Nipah-like virus in bats (Pteropus lylei), Cambodia. *Emerg Infect Dis* 2002;8(9):987–988.
328. Epstein JH, Anthony SJ, Islam A, et al. Nipah virus ecology and infection dynamics in its bat reservoir, *Pteropus medius*, in Bangladesh. *Int J Infect Dis* 2016;53:20–21.
329. Mourya DT, Yadav P, Sudeep AB, et al. Spatial association between a Nipah virus outbreak in India and Nipah virus infection in Pteropus bats. *Clin Infect Dis* 2019;69(2):378–379.
330. Walpita P, Cong Y, Jahrling PB, et al. A VLP-based vaccine provides complete protection against Nipah virus challenge following multiple-dose or single-dose vaccination schedules in a hamster model. *NPJ Vaccines* 2017;2:21.

Orthomyxoviridae: The Viruses and Their Replication

Florian Krammer • Peter Palese

INTRODUCTION

Influenza viruses were possibly responsible for an epidemic disease in Athens in the in 5th century BC,[52] and thus they would have been with us for a long, long time. Influenza remains a major cause of morbidity and mortality worldwide, and large segments of the human population are affected every year. In addition, many animal species can be infected by influenza viruses, and some of these viruses may give rise to pandemic strains in humans, as in the case of the 2009 H1N1 pandemic. Most threatening is the possibility of another pandemic similar to that experienced in 1918, which is estimated to have caused on the order of 50 million deaths worldwide.[438]

CLASSIFICATION

The family of *Orthomyxoviridae* is defined by viruses that have a negative-sense, single-stranded, and segmented RNA genome. The definition of negative-sense RNA viruses came from work by David Baltimore, who showed that the packaged genome of this class of viruses is complementary to the messenger RNA (mRNA), which is defined as positive.[32] There are seven different genera in the family of *Orthomyxoviridae*: the *Thogotovirus*; *Alpha-, Beta-, Gamma-,* and *Deltainfluenzavirus* (or *Influenzavirus A, B, C, and D*); *Quaranjavirus; and Isavirus* (Fig. 14.1) (http://www.ictvonline.org/). Members belonging to any of the four different genera of influenza viruses can undergo genetic reassortment within the genus (see below) and thus readily exchange genetic information. However, reassortment between members of different genera (types) has never been reported. This absence of genetic exchange between viruses of different genera (types) is one manifestation of speciation as a result of evolutionary divergence. It is likely that many more members of the family *Orthomyxoviridae* will be discovered as more and more species and their viruses will be sequenced in the future.

Different influenza virus strains are named according to their genus (type), the species from which the virus was isolated (omitted if human), the location of the isolate, the number of the isolate, the year of isolation, and, in the case of the influenza A viruses, the hemagglutinin (H) and neuraminidase (N) subtypes. For example, the 220th isolate of an influenza virus isolated from a chicken in Hong Kong in 1997 is designated as influenza A/chicken/Hong Kong/220/97(H5N1) virus. There are now 18 different hemagglutinin (H1–H16 and hemagglutinin-like proteins H17 and H18) subtypes and 11 different neuraminidase (N1–N9 and neuraminidase-like proteins N10 and N11) subtypes for influenza A viruses, while there are no influenza B virus hemagglutinin and neuraminidase subtypes (Fig. 14.2).

VIRION STRUCTURE

Influenza A viruses have a complex structure and possess a lipid membrane derived from the host cell (Fig. 14.3A). This envelope harbors the hemagglutinin (HA) and the neuraminidase (NA) that project from the surface of the virus and the membrane integral M2 ion channel. The matrix (M1) protein lies just beneath the envelope, and the core of the virus particle is made up of the RNP (**ribo**nucleo**p**rotein) complex, consisting of the viral RNA (vRNA) segments, the polymerase proteins

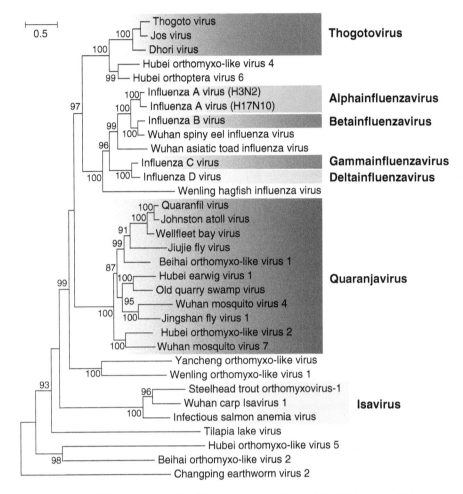

FIGURE 14.1 *Phylogenetic relationships among members of the Orthomyxoviridae.* Amino acid sequences of the polymerase basic 1 (PB1) protein were aligned using the MAFFT program,[456] with the phylogeny then inferred using the maximum likelihood algorithm implemented in PhyML.[328] The tree was midpoint rooted for clarity only and the support for individual nodes was assessed using an approximate likelihood ratio test (aLRT). The scale bar represents the number of amino acid substitutions per site. (Figure was kindly provided by Edward C. Holmes and Mang Shi.)

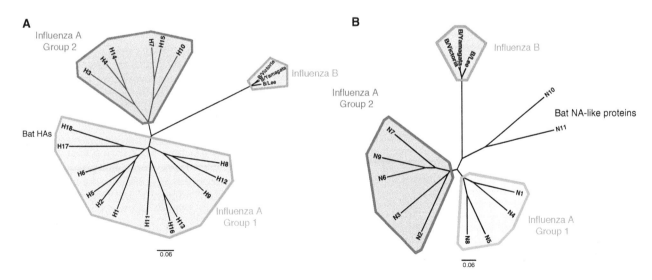

FIGURE 14.2 Phylogeny of influenza A and B virus hemagglutinins (HAs) and neuraminidases (NAs). Unrooted, radial phylogenetic trees based on amino acid sequences of the HA **(A)** and NA **(B)** proteins from representative influenza A and B viruses. Representative viruses were selected from the Global Initiative on Sharing All Influenza Data (GISAID) and aligned using ClustalW. Phylogenetic trees were visualized using FigTree (v1.4.3). The scale bars represent an amino acid change of 6%. (Courtesy of Ericka Kirkpatrick.)

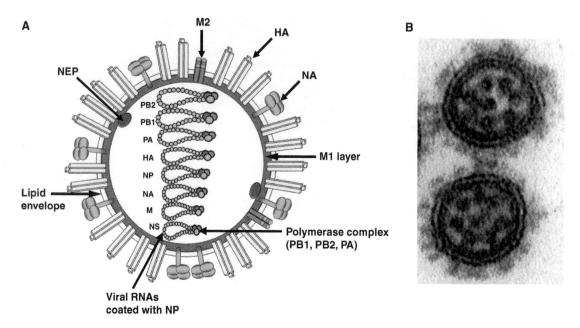

FIGURE 14.3 Schematic diagram and electron micrograph of influenza virus particles. A: The hemagglutinin (HA), neuraminidase (NA), and M2 proteins are inserted into the host-derived lipid envelope. HA is found as a trimer and NA and M2 both as tetramers. The matrix (M1) protein underlies the lipid envelope. A nuclear export protein (NEP) is also associated with the virus. The viral RNA segments are coated with nucleoprotein and are bound by the polymerase complex. Of note, this is a schematic representation and does not represent the actual architecture of the different viral components. **B:** Electron micrograph thin-section image of influenza virus particles (diameter ~100 nm) with the HA and NA spikes visible on the surface and the eight ribonucleoprotein (RNP) segments visible in the interior of each particle. (Courtesy of Yi-ying Chou.)

(PB1 [**p**olymerase **b**asic 1], PB2 [**p**olymerase **b**asic 2], and PA [**p**olymerase **a**cid]), and the nucleoprotein (NP).[486] The NEP (**n**uclear **e**xport **p**rotein) protein is also present in purified viral preparations.[747] The overall composition of virus particles is about 1% RNA, 5% to 8% carbohydrate, 20% lipid, and approximately 70% protein.[3,162,265] Specifically, it is important to get quantitative data on the presence of individual viral components as well as cellular components that are packaged into the virus.[414,808] Excellent analyses have already been performed using electron microscopy (EM) of negatively stained or frozen-hydrated (cryoelectron microscopy) particles and tomographic reconstructions.[20,106,270,352,354,664,905,946] The morphology of influenza A virus particles is characterized by distinctive spikes that are readily observable in electron micrographs of negatively stained virus particles (Fig. 14.3B). These spikes, made up of HA and NA, have lengths of approximately 10 to 14 nm, with an approximate ratio of four HA trimers to one NA tetramer. Influenza viruses are pleomorphic. The spherical particles have a diameter of about 100 nm, but filamentous particles with elongated viral structures (more than 300 nm) have frequently been observed, particularly in fresh clinical isolates[176] and in preparations of viruses with specific M1, M2, or NP proteins (Fig. 14.4).[54,73,100,107,176,226,227,768]

Less is known about the internal structures of influenza viruses. However, the underlying M1 layer can be visualized and reveals a helical superstructure.[106,774,776] The RNP complexes were first separated by Duesberg[207] on sucrose gradients and were visualized by EM using positive staining with uranyl acetate.[161] These RNP structures appear to consist of a strand that is folded back on itself to form a double-helical arrangement covered by NP and affixed to a trimeric polymerase with one open end and a loop on the other end.[161,632,723] Most recently, RNPs or individual RNA segments have been visualized by EM of thin-section virus particles and cryotomography.[20,606,664,665,858]

Influenza B viruses are mostly indistinguishable from the A viruses by EM. They have four proteins inserted in their lipid envelopes: the HA, NA, NB, and BM2.[53,81,671,1021] The M1 and the RNP complexes make up the interior of the particle. It has also been shown that the influenza B virus NEP is associated with purified virus preparations.[420]

Influenza C and D viruses have been found to possess hexagonal reticular (net-like) structures on the surface[15,642] and to form unusually long (500 μm) cord-like structures on the surface of infected cells (which seem to be more prevalent in influenza C than influenza D viruses).[628,642,659] Influenza C and D viruses also contain a core of three polymerase proteins and the NP, which are associated with seven RNA segments. The influenza C and D virus M1 appears to have a similar role to those of influenza A and B viruses. The major glycoprotein, HEF (**h**emagglutinin-**e**sterase **f**usion), combines the functions of the HA and NA (and thus influenza C and D viruses contain one less RNA segment than do the A and B viruses).[379] The HEF of influenza C and D viruses is inserted into the lipid membrane, as are the glycosylated CM2 and DM2, which are analogous to the M2 of influenza A viruses and the BM2 of influenza B viruses.[460,636,704,834]

WSN   Udorn   WSN-Mud

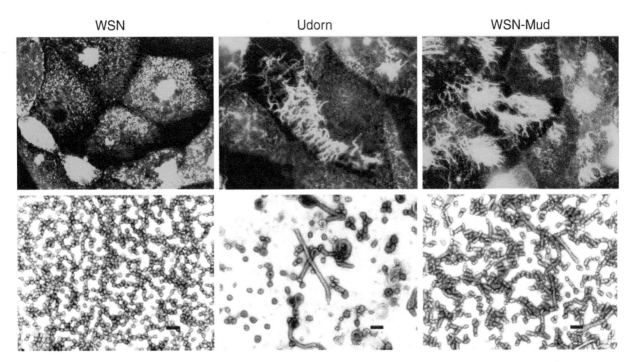

FIGURE 14.4 The filamentous phenotype depends on the M segment. Indirect immunofluorescence of viral antigens on the surfaces of infected cells (*top panels*) and electron microscopy images of negatively stained virus preparations (*bottom panels*). Particles of influenza A/WSN/33 virus are spherical, whereas those of influenza A/Udorn/72 virus are filamentous. Substitution of the WSN M segment with that of Udorn (WSN-Mud) results in a recombinant/reassortant virus with a filamentous phenotype. Calibration bar represents 300 nm. For details, see Ref.[73] (Courtesy of Adolfo García-Sastre and Svetlana Bourmakina.)

GENOME STRUCTURE AND ORGANIZATION

Influenza Viruses

All A- and B-type influenza viruses possess eight RNA segments, whereas influenza C and D viruses only have seven different RNAs (Figs. 14.5–14.7). This genome assignment for influenza A viruses was first shown by using polyacrylamide gel electrophoresis of isolated RNAs from two parent influenza A virus strains and their reassortants. Identifying the derivation of an RNA segment (by gel electrophoresis) in a reassortant and simultaneous protein analysis (by serologic or gel analysis) allowed the assignment of individual RNAs to specific viral proteins[687] (Figs. 14.5–14.7). Interestingly, influenza A viruses increase the coding capacity of their genomes via both splicing and use of alternative open reading frames (ORFs). The M and NS genes each give rise to a spliced mRNA encoding the M2 and the NEP (formerly NEP/NS2) proteins, respectively.[501,502] The PB1-F2 is expressed from an alternative ORF within the *PB1* gene, while PB1-N40 is an N-terminal truncation produced by the use of a downstream AUG and leaky scanning[122,970] (Fig. 14.5), although not all influenza A virus strains encode these proteins, making them true accessory proteins. Recently, a frameshift product, termed PA-X, was identified comprising the endonuclease domain of the viral PA protein with a C-terminal domain encoded by the X-ORF[433] (Fig. 14.5). PA-X can function to repress cellular gene expression,[433] and mutations in the PA-X gene have the potential to improve the hemagglutinin yield of vaccine viruses.[413] The PA-X protein, like the NS1 protein, is multifunctional and has

effects on the innate immune response of the host.[668] Each viral segment contains noncoding regions at both the 5′ and 3′ ends. The extreme ends are highly conserved among all segments of influenza A viruses, and they are followed by less conserved segment-specific noncoding regions.

The influenza B virus genome is similar to that of influenza A virus (Fig. 14.6A). Again, eight RNA segments code for one or more viral proteins with the three largest RNAs coding for the polymerase proteins, the fourth RNA for the HA, and the fifth and sixth RNAs for the NP and NA, respectively.[738] The NA gene codes for the NB protein as well as for the NA. The NB protein is encoded by a −1 ORF seven nucleotides upstream (…AUGAACA<u>AUG</u>…) of the NA coding frame.[806] The seventh RNA codes for the M1 protein (248 amino acids in length). Its termination codon (…U<u>AAUG</u>) overlaps with the initiation codon (U<u>AAUG</u>…) for the BM2 (109 amino acids in length), which allows for a "stop–start" translation mechanism.[400] The eighth RNA codes for the NS1 as well as for the NEP protein, the latter via a spliced mRNA. Cognate PB1-F2, PB1-N40, and PA-X proteins have not yet been identified in influenza B viruses. The noncoding regions of the influenza B virus genome are longer than those in influenza A virus.

The genome of influenza C viruses has only seven RNA segments, with the three largest RNAs each coding for one of the polymerase proteins (Fig. 14.6B). The PB1 and PB2 proteins are homologous to the corresponding influenza A and B virus proteins. The third influenza C virus polymerase protein is named P3 because it does not display acid charge features at neutral pH, as do the corresponding PA proteins of influenza A and B viruses.[995] The fourth RNA codes for the HEF protein,[379] combining the hemagglutinin, receptor-destroying, and

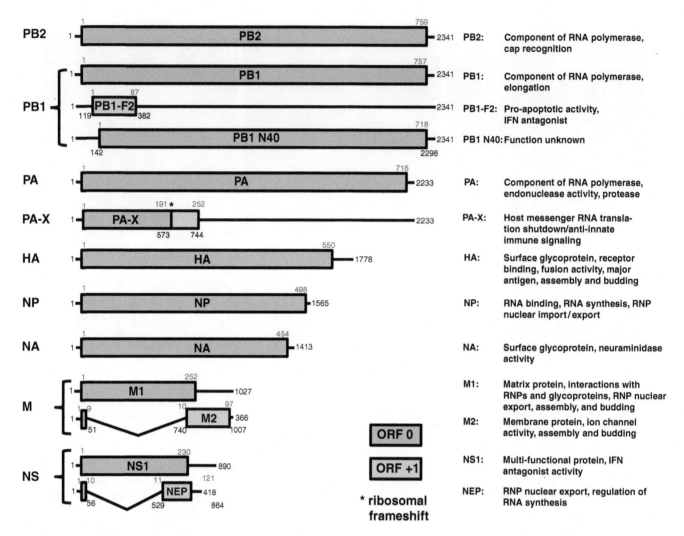

FIGURE 14.5 Genome structure of influenza A/Puerto Rico/8/34 virus. RNA segments (nucleotides in *black*) shown in positive sense and their encoded proteins (amino acids in *red*). The *lines* at the 5' and 3' termini represent the noncoding regions. The polymerase basic 1 (PB1) protein segment contains a second open reading frame (ORF) in the +1 frame resulting in the PB1-F2 protein and a third ORF in the 0 frame resulting in the PB1-N40 protein. The PA segment contains codes for a second protein that consist of the N-terminus of PA and a novel C-terminal sequence that is added after a frameshift to +1 at the codon for amino acid 191. The M2 and nuclear export protein (NEP) proteins are encoded by spliced messenger RNAs (mRNAs) (the introns are indicated by the *V-shaped lines*). Additional accessory proteins are not shown but discussed in the main text. (Courtesy of Heinrich Hoffmann.)

fusion activities. The NP is encoded by the fifth RNA. The sixth RNA codes for the M protein, which is expressed from a spliced mRNA, and from the unspliced mRNA a long precursor is translated (p42), which is then processed by signal peptide cleavage into CM2. This 115–amino acid (aa)-long protein consists of an amino-terminal extracellular domain (with a carbohydrate chain), a hydrophobic transmembrane domain (TMD), and an intracellular cytoplasmic tail.[703,704,995] Finally, RNA 7 codes for the NS1 protein (246 amino acids)[637] and, via a spliced mRNA, for the NEP protein (182 amino acids).[5,394] The genome structure of influenza D virus seems to be very similar to that of influenza C virus.[855]

Evolutionarily, influenza A, B, C, and D viruses have a common precursor, and it is also likely that influenza A and B viruses diverged from each other more recently than did influenza C and D viruses. Based on comparative sequencing studies using the hemagglutinin molecules, it has been postulated that the influenza A viruses diverged about 2,000 years ago and the influenza B and C viruses about 4,000 and 8,000 years ago, respectively.[867] Clearly, these numbers are based on a series of unprovable assumptions, including a steady rate of evolution over time, and therefore must be taken *cum grano salis*. Interestingly, influenza C[152,359,646] viruses have only seven distinct RNA segments, but scanning transmission electron microscopic tomography suggests that the majority of their virus particles package 7+1 viral RNPs,[642] similar to what is observed with influenza A and B viruses (the latter each having eight different RNA segments).

Thogoto Virus

The genomes of Thogoto viruses, including Bourbon virus, possess only six single-stranded RNA segments of negative polarity, with a total coding capacity for seven proteins.[220,508] As with the influenza viruses, three proteins make up the RNA-dependent RNA polymerase complex. The NP, the glycoprotein (G), the matrix protein (M), and one nonessential accessory

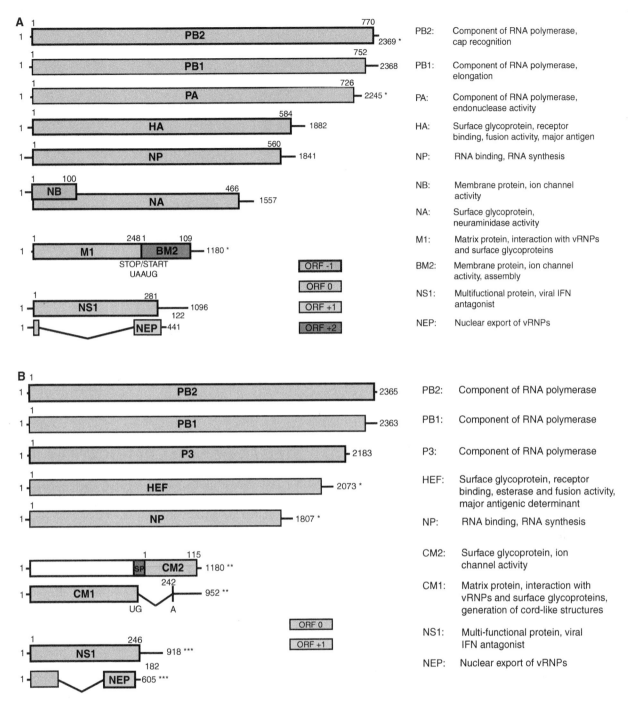

FIGURE 14.6 A: Genome structure of influenza B/Lee/40 virus. RNA segments (in nucleotides) shown in positive sense and their encoded proteins (in amino acids). The *lines* at the 5′ and 3′ termini represent the noncoding regions. The NA segment contains an additional open reading frame (ORF) in the −1 frame starting four nucleotides upstream of the NA start codon, resulting in the NB protein. The M segment encodes the M1 and the BM2 protein. The M1 termination codon UAA overlaps with the BM2 initiation codon AUG in a translational stop-and-start pentanucleotide UAAUG (shown in *capital letters*). The NS segment codes for NS1 and NEP. NS1 is a translation product of a colinear messenger RNA (mRNA), whereas NEP is a product of spliced mRNA (intron is shown by the *V-shaped line*). Asterisks indicate that RNA segments are from influenza B/Memphis/97/12 virus. **B:** Genome structure of influenza C virus. RNA segments (in nucleotides) shown in positive sense and their encoded proteins (in amino acids). The lines at the 5′ and 3′ termini represent the noncoding regions. The M segment encodes the CM1 and CM2 proteins. The CM2 protein is derived from a colinear messenger RNA (mRNA). The p42 precursor contains a signal peptide (SP) that becomes cleaved and releases CM2. CM1 is the product of a spliced mRNA in which the stop codon UGA (shown in *capital letters*) is introduced by mRNA splicing. The NS segment codes for NS1 by a colinear mRNA and for NEP by a spliced mRNA (intron is shown by the *V-shaped line*). (PB2, PB1, and P3 are derived from C/JJ/50 virus; HEF* is derived from C/JHB/1/66 virus; NP** and M** are derived from C/AnnArbor/1/50 virus; and NS*** is derived from C/Yamagata/1/88 virus.) (Courtesy of Heinrich Hoffmann.)

A

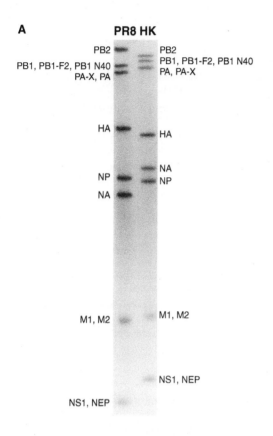

B

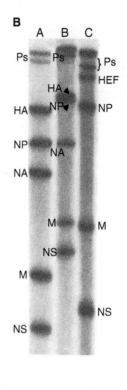

FIGURE 14.7 A: RNA segments of influenza A/Puerto Rico/8/34 (H1N1) and A/Hong Kong/8/68 (H3N2) viruses. The viral RNAs are separated on a polyacrylamide gel and the proteins encoded by the RNAs are indicated. (Adapted from Palese P. The genes of influenza virus. *Cell* 1977;10(1):1–10.) **B:** Separation of RNAs from influenza A, B, and C viruses on a polyacrylamide gel. The ^{32}P-labeled RNAs of influenza A/PR/8/34 virus (*lane 1*), influenza B/Lee/40 virus (*lane 2*), and influenza C/JHB/1/66 virus (*lane 3*) were isolated from purified virus preparations. The RNAs were treated with glyoxal for complete denaturation and separated by polyacrylamide gel electrophoresis. (Adapted from Palese P, Racaniello VR, Desselberger U, et al. Genetic structure and genetic variation of influenza viruses [and Discussion]. *Philos Trans R Soc Lond Ser B Biol Sci* 1980;288(1029):299–305, Ref. [691])

protein (ML) are coded for by the remaining three RNAs. The M and ML proteins are both encoded by the shortest RNA, with the M protein being derived from a spliced mRNA.[336,474] The 304-aa-long ML protein has been shown to possess interferon antagonist activity[92,333,336,434] and is virion associated.[336]

Quaranjavirus

The genomes of viruses in the *Quaranjavirus* genus consist of six or seven negative-sense, single-stranded RNA segments.[7,708] The ends of each segment are conserved and partially complementary. Segments 1, 2, and 3 encode the PB2, PA, and PB1 polymerase subunits, respectively, while segment 5 codes for a protein that is distantly related to the Thogoto virus glycoprotein and the gp64 surface glycoprotein of baculoviruses and thus is likely the attachment protein.[7,731]

Isavirus (Infectious Salmon Anemia Virus)

The genome of infectious salmon anemia virus consists of eight negative-sense, single-stranded RNA segments similar to those of influenza A and B viruses,[167,604] and an important reverse genetics system has been established.[893,894] Segment 6 encodes the hemagglutinin-esterase (HE) protein, which is also present on the viral surface and whose function is to bind sialic acid residues of the cellular receptor.[372] The HE protein also presents receptor-destroying enzyme (RDE) activity that favors the release of new viral particles that emerge from the cellular membrane.[623] This activity is similar to the binding and RDE activities previously observed for the HEF protein of influenza C viruses and the HE glycoprotein of coronaviruses.[372,379,918,919] Segment 8 encodes two proteins of 27.6 and 22 kD, the larger of which has interferon antagonist activity.[167,295]

STAGES OF VIRAL REPLICATION

An overview of the influenza virus life cycle is illustrated in Figure 14.8, and in the following pages, we will discuss each stage of this life cycle in order.

Mechanism of Attachment

Influenza viruses bind to neuraminic acids (sialic acids) on the surface of cells to initiate infection and replication. The interaction of influenza viruses with a ubiquitous molecule such as sialic acid is constrained by the fact that the HAs (Fig. 14.9) of viruses that replicate in different species show specificity toward sialic acids with different linkages.

Human viruses preferentially bind to *N*-acetylneuraminic acid attached to the penultimate galactose sugar by an α2,6 linkage (SAα2,6Gal), whereas avian viruses mostly bind to sialic acid with an α2,3 linkage[165,765,957] (Fig. 14.10). In agreement with this finding is the fact that human tracheal epithelial cells contain mostly SAα2,6Gal, while the gut epithelium from ducks possesses mostly SAα2,3Gal sugar moieties.[168,424] It should be noted, however, that this viral specificity is not absolute and that avian and human cells can contain both neuraminic acid linkages (2,3 as well as 2,6). Studies have shown that sialylated proteins with α2,3 linkages are present on cells in the human airways and that these cells can be infected with avian influenza viruses.[582,819,931] Furthermore, the relevant glycan structure consists of more than just the terminal sialic acid linkage, and evidence suggests that factors such as the type of backbone, chain length, and branching pattern as well as sulfation and fucosylation may also influence the interactions with HA.[137,837,846,931] In fact, studies have shown that recent human H3N2 viruses have evolved to bind to

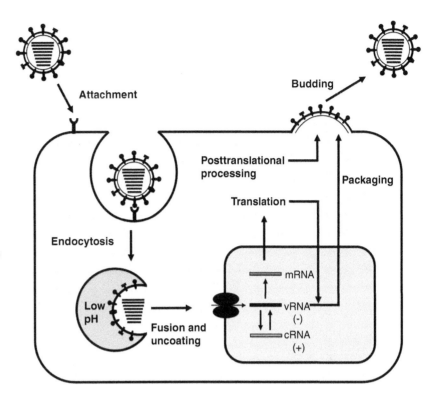

FIGURE 14.8 Illustration of the influenza virus replication cycle. Upon binding at the cell surface, the virus is internalized by receptor-mediated endocytosis. The low pH in the endosome triggers fusion of the viral and endosomal membranes, releasing the viral ribonucleoproteins (vRNPs) into the cytoplasm. vRNPs are imported into the nucleus where they serve as the template for transcription. New proteins are synthesized from viral mRNA. The viral genome (vRNA) is replicated through a positive-sense intermediate (complementary RNA [cRNA]). Newly synthesized viral RNPs are exported from the nucleus to the assembly site at the apical plasma membrane, where virus particles bud and are released.

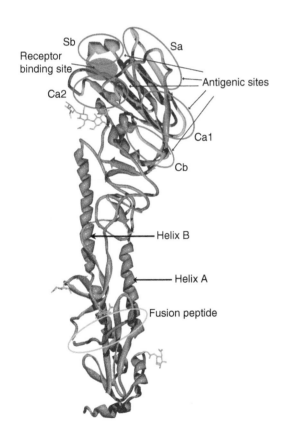

FIGURE 14.9 Ribbon representation of the uncleaved hemagglutinin monomer from the 1918 influenza virus based on x-ray diffraction analysis. The five predicted antigenic sites (Ca2, Sb, Sa, Ca1, and Cb) surround the sialic acid receptor–binding site. Toward the membrane-proximal end (*bottom*) is the fusion peptide and helices A and B are indicated. For details, see Ref.[847] (Courtesy of James Stevens and Ian A. Wilson.)

branched human-type receptors with extended poly-*N*-acetyl-lactosamine chains.[706] Glycan microarrays that contain a wide spectrum of glycan structures are now being used as tools to better understand the specificity of receptor binding.[845] Also, when viruses are passaged in a particular host, they can adapt to that host by mutating the receptor-binding site in the viral HA.[284,605] In a study of the A/New York/1/1918 virus HA, it was shown that the binding specificity can be changed by a single amino acid mutation (D190E) to a preference for α2,3-linked sialic acids. It is thus hypothesized that the HA gene of the 1918 influenza virus has its origin in avian influenza viruses and that a single amino acid change (E190D) allowed the hemagglutinin to recognize the α2,6-linked sialic acids prevalent in human cells.[307,844] Similar changes in binding phenotype based on a small number of mutations have now been shown for many virus subtypes.[182] The interactions between HA and sialic acid are relatively well understood, but it is less clear if influenza viruses bind to N-linked glycans attached to specific surface proteins or if there is no specificity in terms of the protein carrying the glycan. Interestingly, it has been shown that the HA-like proteins of the H17N10 and H18N11 subtypes do not bind to sialic acid but can use MHC II as receptor.[450,865,892,1048]

Mechanism of Entry

While some viruses (e.g., paramyxoviruses and herpes viruses) can enter cells directly through the plasma membrane by a pH-independent fusion process, influenza viruses require a low pH to initiate fusion and are therefore internalized by endocytic compartments. There are several internalization mechanisms including clathrin-coated pits, via caveolae, through macropinocytosis and through alternative mechanisms.[211,371,600,997] Clathrin-mediated endocytosis has traditionally been the model for influenza virus entry.[581] However, a nonclathrin, non–caveolae-mediated internalization mechanism has also been described for influenza viruses.[821] The latter pathway is dependent on low pH

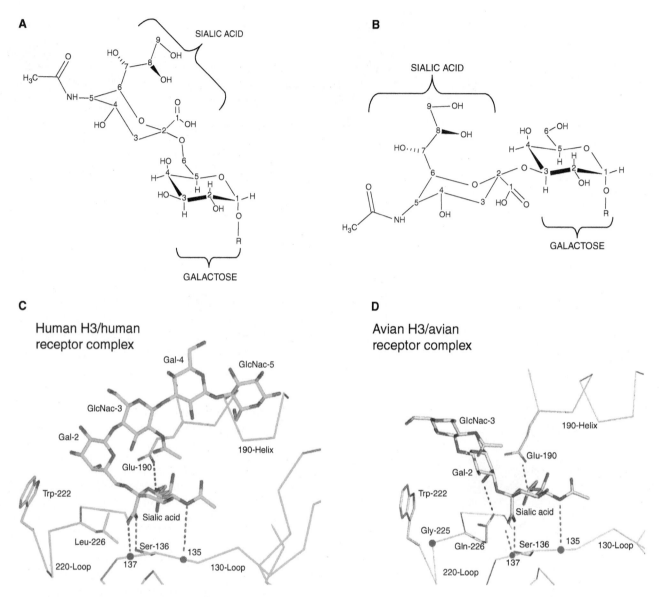

FIGURE 14.10 Sialic acid linkages preferred by human or avian influenza viruses. A: $\alpha2,6$-linkage (human): The sialic acid is bound to C atom 6 of the galactose molecule via its C atom 2. **B:** $\alpha2,3$-linkage (avian): The sialic acid is attached by its C atom 2 to the three positions (C atom 3) of the penultimate sugar, galactose. These different linkages result in receptor molecules with different steric configurations. (Courtesy of Laurel Glaser.) Conformational differences in the receptor-binding sites of the H3 avian and H3 human hemagglutinins (HAs). Interactions of human subtype 3 HA with a human receptor analog **(C)** and avian H3 HA with an avian receptor analog **(D)**. The three secondary structure components (190-helix, 130-loop, 220-loop) of the binding site are labeled in this backbone representation together with some of the most relevant side chains. The broken lines indicate potential hydrogen bond interactions between the HA and the receptor. Residues making interactions via main chain carbonyl groups are shown as red spheres, while those interacting via main chain nitrogens are shown as blue spheres. In the pentasaccharide ligand model, the galactose molecule is bound to sialic acid in an $\alpha2,6$ or an $\alpha2,3$ linkage **(C** and **D**, respectively). The human HA is from A/Aichi/68 (H3) virus and the avian HA is from A/duck/Ukraine/63 (H3) virus. For details, see Ref.[332] (Courtesy of John Skehel.)

and trafficking to late endosomes, as it requires protein kinase C, Rab5, and Rab7 functions.[820] More recently, through the use of specific inhibitors and RNA interference (RNAi), it has been shown that in addition to entering via a dynamin-dependent, clathrin-driven pathway, influenza viruses can also enter via a dynamin-independent pathway that is characteristic of macropinocytosis.[184] This mechanism has specifically been implicated for entry of filamentous influenza virions.[771] Potential differences in the entry pathways defined in polarized versus nonpolarized cells should also be appreciated, as, for example, the actin cytoskeleton appears to be critical for uptake of influenza viruses into polarized cells but not nonpolarized cells.[866] Of note, it is still unclear if binding of virus particles to sialylated glycans is sufficient or if additional interactions are needed to trigger/initiate efficient entry. A number of proteins have been identified to be of importance in influenza virus entry. Epsin 1 has been shown to be specifically required for clathrin-mediated uptake of influenza virus.[131] The epidermal growth factor receptor (EGFR) has also been demonstrated to play a role during influenza virus entry,[217] and it is thought that virus attachment to the cell stimulates EGFR, which leads to activation of signaling cascades such as phosphatidylinositol 3-kinase (PI3K) signaling, which is known to promote influenza virus entry.[214] Additional proteins including phospholipase D, the sialylated voltage-dependent Ca^{2+} channel $Ca_v 1.2$, cell-surface nucleolin, prolidase, and fibronectin have been identified as factors important for influenza virus entry.[115,269,527,672,722] There are also questions over whether sialic acid is the only attachment molecule. Lec-1 cells, which are deficient in N-linked glycosylation (but still contain sialylated proteins), are unable to internalize influenza viruses.[143] Similarly, cells deficient in sialic acid can be made to support influenza virus entry if they express one of the C-type lectins, DC-SIGN or L-SIGN.[382,549,655]

Mechanism of Fusion and Uncoating

Influenza viruses and other enveloped viruses (including rhabdo-, flavi-, bunya-, and filoviruses) require low pH to fuse with endosomal membranes. After binding to the target cell surface and endocytosis, the low pH of the endosome activates fusion of the viral membrane with that of the endosome. This fusion activity is induced by a structural change in the HA of influenza viruses (Fig. 14.11), but in order for this to occur, the HA0 precursor must first be cleaved into two subunits, HA1 and HA2 (which typically occurs after release of new virions/before attachment; for details, see the following section on Hemagglutinin). Once in the acidic environment of the endosome, the cleaved HA molecule undergoes a conformational change, and this exposes the fusion peptide at the N-terminus of the HA2 subunit, enabling it to interact with the membrane of the endosome[66,355,963,980] (for details, see the following section on Hemagglutinin). The transmembrane domain (TMD) of the HA2 (inserted into the viral membrane) and the fusion peptide (inserted into the endosomal membrane) are in juxtaposition in the low pH–induced HA structure. The concerted structural change of several hemagglutinin molecules then opens up a pore, which releases the contents of the virion (i.e., viral RNPs) into the cytoplasm of the cell (Fig. 14.12). The precise timing and the location of uncoating depend on the pH-mediated transition of the specific HA molecule involved.[282]

The uncoating of influenza viruses is blocked by changes in pH caused by weak bases (e.g., ammonium chloride or chloroquine) or ionophores (e.g., monensin).[573] Effective uncoating is also dependent on the presence of the M2 protein, which has ion channel activity.[567,716] Early on, it was recognized that

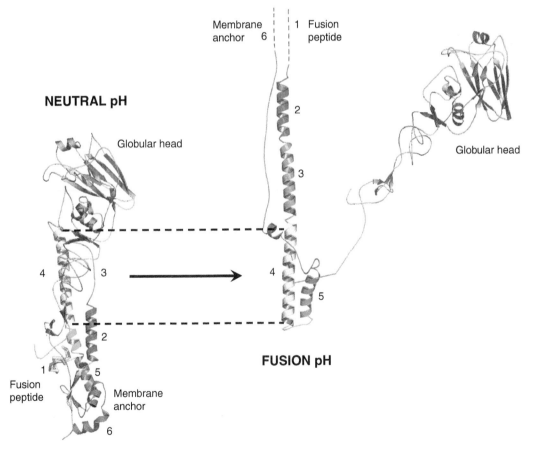

FIGURE 14.11 Ribbon representation of the structural changes that occur in hemagglutinin (HA) at low pH. Bromelain-treated HA monomer with regions of HA2 undergoing conformational changes at low pH as indicated by numbered domains (*left*). The domains, starting at the fusion peptide (domain 1), are numbered sequentially until the membrane anchor is reached (domain 6). The structure and the position of the region comprising residues 75 to 106 (domain 4) are the same before and after the conformational change (denoted by the *dotted lines*). The globular head domains retain their structures but detrimerize (falling to the right, away from the HA2 portion). For details, see Refs.[127,825] (Courtesy of John Skehel and Rupert Russell.)

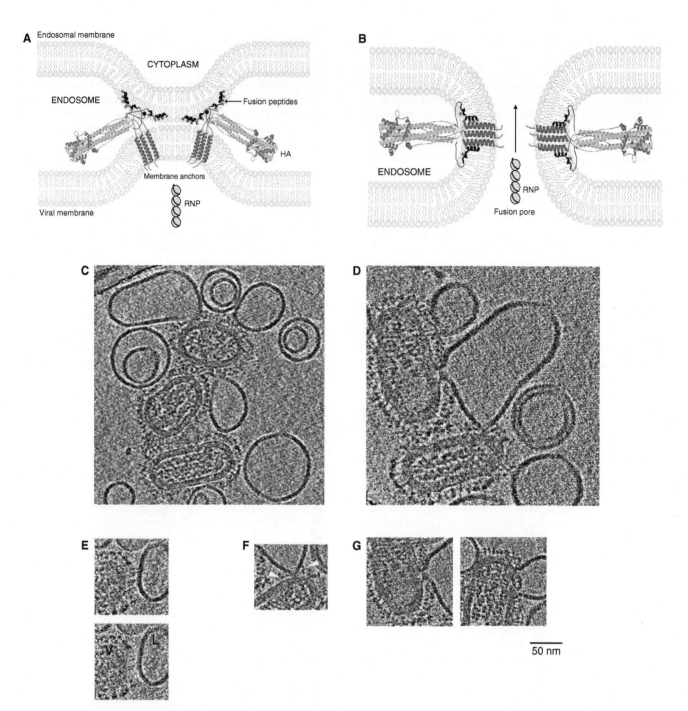

FIGURE 14.12 Model for juxtaposition of viral and endosomal membranes resulting in formation of a fusion pore and release of ribonucleoproteins (RNPs). Structures of influenza virus hemagglutinins in their postfusion state modeled into a possible fusion inter-mediate **(A)** and into a fusion pore **(B)**. The fusion peptides are shown inserted into the endosomal membrane, while the transmembrane domains remain anchored in the viral membrane. Note the large conformational changes of the ecto- and fusion domains when compared to their prefusion structures (see Figs. 14.9 and 14.11). The small spheres (*pink*) on the fusion peptide denote glycines that may mediate helix interactions, and the small squares (*blue*) denote glutamates that may be responsible for the pH dependence of the fusion peptide penetration into lipid bilayers. Following the formation of a pore, the RNPs are released from the interior of the virus particle into the cyto-plasm, completing the uncoating process. (Courtesy of Lukas Tamm.) Influenza virus membrane fusion with liposomes **(C-G)**. **C:** Sections of an electron cryotomogram of A/Udorn/72 virus and liposomes after incubation at pH 4.9. **D:** HA glycoprotein–mediated interaction and perturbation of liposomes. **E:** Fusion pores between liposomes and virus with tomogram section showing thin densities (*green*) extending between virus (V) and liposome (L) membranes (*red*) as indicated in the annotated image below. **F:** Protein densities (*yellow arrow heads*) surrounding a point contact between liposome and membrane. **G:** Tomogram sections showing fusion pores (*red arrow heads*) between virus and liposomes. (Adapted from Calder LJ, Rosenthal PB. Cryomicroscopy provides structural snapshots of influenza virus membrane fusion. *Nat Struct Mol Biol* 2016;23(9):853–858; courtesy of Peter Rosenthal.)

amantadine and rimantadine inhibit replication immediately following virus infection.[826] Later, it was found that the virus-associated M2 protein allows the influx of H+ ions from the endosome into the virus particle, which disrupts protein–protein interactions and results in the release of RNP free of the M1 protein.[567,581,1037] Amantadine and rimantadine have been shown to block the ion channel activity of the M2 protein and thus uncoating.[138,391,716,862,942] The HA-mediated fusion of the viral membrane with the endosomal membrane and the M2-mediated release of the RNP result in the appearance of free RNP complexes in the cytoplasm. This completes the uncoating process.[575] Cellular factors like Itch, transportin 1, and the cellular aggresome have been shown to play important roles in this process.[34,603,736,853] The time frame for the uncoating process was examined by inhibiting virus penetration with ammonium chloride. The majority of virus particles showed a half-time for penetration of about 25 minutes (after adsorption). Barely 10 minutes later (half-time of 34 minutes after adsorption), RNP complexes are found in the nucleus.[575] The following uptake of RNP molecules through nuclear pores is an active process, involving the nucleocytoplasmic trafficking machinery of the host cell (for details, see Nuclear Import of RNPs).

Much less is known about the uptake and uncoating of influenza B, C, and D viruses. Influenza B viruses are more like influenza A viruses as both recognize *N*-acetylneuraminic acid as receptors, while influenza C and D viruses bind to 9-*O*-acetylated neuraminic acid derivatives.[380,834] Like influenza A viruses, the B- and C-type viruses go through an endosome-mediated uncoating process, which requires proteolytic activation (cleavage) of the HA or HEF proteins and subsequent fusion of the viral and endosomal membranes. Although the viral glycoproteins of both HA and HEF are dependent on a low pH–triggered fusion process, the influenza C virus HEF-mediated fusion/uncoating may occur at a higher pH in early endosomes.[257,1037] The opposite seems to be true for the HEF protein of influenza D virus, which has been shown to be relatively acid stable leaving a question mark about its specific entry mechanism.[1014] At this point, the role of CM2 and DM2 in uncoating of influenza C and D viruses is less well established than that of the BM2 protein of influenza B viruses, which is the homolog of the influenza A virus M2 protein.[273,358,393,460,620,940,945] The NB ion channel of influenza B viruses does not seem to be required for virus infectivity *in vitro* and *in vivo*.[225,358]

The Hemagglutinin

Structural features

Much is known about the HA molecule, and excellent reviews are available.[66,286,355,777,984,985] In fact, the influenza virus HA has become a model for studies of protein folding and trafficking, protein quality control, membrane fusion, protein–receptor interactions, and antigen–antibody complexes and, last but not least, for investigating how the immune system reacts to a foreign protein. The major functions of the HA are the receptor-binding and fusion activities, but there may also be a structural role for the HA in budding and particle formation. The HA is a trimeric rod-shaped molecule with the carboxy-terminus inserted into the viral membrane and the hydrophilic end projecting as a spike away from the viral surface (i.e., a type I integral membrane protein). Early on, it was shown that (a) posttranslational modifications of the precursor molecule (i.e., glycosylation and palmitoylation), (b) cleavage of the signal peptide in the endoplasmic reticulum (ER), and (c) cleavage of the HA0 precursor into HA1 and HA2 subunits are required for the full activity of the molecule.[469,513,727] During human infections, HA is cleaved when expressed on the cell surface or virus surface by airway proteases potentially including matriptase, transmembrane protease, serine 2 (TMPRSS2), and human airway trypsin-like protease (HAT).[46,70,282,347] HAs with a polybasic cleavage site, for example from specific H5 and H7 strains, can also be cleaved in the Golgi apparatus by furin/furin-like proteases.[849] In cell culture, tosyl phenylalanyl chloromethyl ketone (TPCK)-treated trypsin is usually added to culture medium to facilitate cleavage. The attachment of N-linked glycans is also a very important posttranslational modification for the viral HA. N-linked glycosylation sites in the stalk domain are conserved within groups/subtypes and contribute to protein folding and stability. Glycosylation of the head domain is more variable between strains and subtypes and plays an important role in immune evasion and pathogenicity.[592]

The first x-ray crystallographic structure of an HA (the ectodomain released from the virus by bromelain treatment) was resolved in 1981 by Wilson et al.[969] At that time, the HA (from A/Aichi/68 [H3N2] virus) was the largest biological molecule for which a structure had been resolved, and it started an unprecedented drive to study the structure/function relationships of biologically important molecules, which continues unabated to this day. The structures of numerous HAs have now been resolved, including the subtype 1 HA molecules of the 1918 and 2009 pandemic influenza viruses[285,847,989] and that of an H2 subtype HA (Fig. 14.9).[990] Remarkably, even though the overall amino acid sequence identity can be less than 50%, the structure and functions of these HAs are highly conserved. This represents a case of evolution and sequence variation proceeding to an extreme level while structure and function have remained conserved. Even more surprising is that the structure of the influenza B virus HA is similar to that of influenza A virus HA despite sharing only approximately 25% sequence identity.[934,944]

The crystallographic structure of the uncleaved influenza A virus HA is superimposable onto that of the cleaved HA1 and HA2, with the exception of the amino acids adjacent to the cleavage site. The major features of the structure are (a) a long fibrous stem, which is made up of a triple-stranded coiled coil of α-helices derived from the ectodomain of the three HA2 parts of the molecule (helix A and helix B; Fig. 14.9) and the N-terminal and C-terminal portions of HA1, and (b) the globular head, which is also made up of three identical domains whose sequences are derived from the central region (C52–C277 in H3 numbering) of the HA1 of the three monomers.

A major function of HA is binding to receptors and the receptor-binding site lies within the globular head of the molecule. This site has been defined through crystallization and structure analysis of HA–receptor complexes, as well as by mutational analysis. In the H3-subtype viruses, it appears that within the receptor-binding pocket of an avian HA, a glutamine in position 226 and a glycine in position 228 preferentially accommodate the 2,3-linked sialic acid, whereas leucine and serine in these positions in human H3 HAs preferentially accommodate the 2,6-linked sialic acid (Fig. 14.10).[165,332] (See the previous section on Attachment for more details.) Similar receptor-specificity defining amino acids have been characterized for many influenza A HA subtypes.

The second major function of the HA is acid pH–triggered fusion, which is required for the uncoating process. Low pH treatment changes the structure of the HA dramatically.

The molecule becomes susceptible to protease digestion, and the disulfide bond linking the HA1 and HA2 subunits becomes susceptible to mercaptoethanol.[320,824] However, the important feature of the acid pH–mediated change is that the fusion peptide becomes aligned antiparallel to the membrane anchor of the HA2 (Fig. 14.11). The end result is that the fusion peptide brings the endosomal membrane into juxtaposition with the viral membrane, leading to fusion. The presence of more than one hemagglutinin then leads to the formation of a fusion pore through which the RNPs can enter the cytoplasm (Fig. 14.12). Structures of the postfusion HA as well as an early fusion intermediate have helped to reveal the molecular details of the changes that occur during the transition from pre- to postfusion state.[98,991] The dynamics of the fusion process have recently been further elucidated using cryoelectronmicroscopy, cryotomography, and single-molecule FRET.[105,178] Structures of the fusion peptide in lipid environments have been resolved by nuclear magnetic resonance (NMR) and show that the peptide forms a tight helical hairpin structure that angles back on itself.[348,497,551,980] This hook structure may help to pull the endosomal membrane close to the viral membrane, resulting in the initiation of the actual fusion process.

Another important structural element (c) of the HA is the TMD, which is relatively conserved and consists of a trimeric helical bundle. The TMD is connected to the ectodomain by a short, flexible linker, which allows the HA ectodomain to tilt more than 25 degrees, which is likely needed to facilitate structural rearrangements during fusion.[51]

The last major structural element of the HA, the cytoplasmic tail (d), is highly conserved among all subtypes. There are three cysteines that are palmitoylated (with one of them located in the TMD). The role of this cytoplasmic tail (and the palmitates attached to the cysteines) is not entirely clear due to subtype- and cell/host-specific differences.[128,437,928,1049]

Antigenic determinants

In addition to having an important role in receptor binding, fusion, and assembly, the influenza virus HA is also the *major determinant* recognized by the adaptive immune system of the host. Following infection and replication, a vigorous immune response is induced, which usually results in the formation of neutralizing antibodies.[483] These antibodies then lead to the selection of "antibody escape" variants. The amino acids undergoing change are almost exclusively on the globular head domain (and on the outside of the molecule). Many of these changes get fixed (accumulate over time), defining the antigenic drift of influenza viruses. Using insertion and mutagenesis libraries as well as evolutionary analysis, it has also been shown that the head domain of influenza A virus HA is highly plastic as compared to the conserved stalk domain and tolerates drastic changes enabling fast antigenic drift (Fig. 14.13).[202,369,465] Using the same methods, the influenza B virus HA head domain was shown to be less tolerant to changes than its A counterpart.[272,465]

Fab antibody fragments have been shown to bind to different regions of the HA head (Fig. 14.14) and, interestingly, not in all cases do three Fabs bind to one trimeric spike (3:1 ratio). Examples have been found where only one Fab molecule binds to one HA spike (1:1 ratio) or where just two Fab molecules bind to a trimeric spike (2:1 ratio) (Fig. 14.14).[471] In the latter case, the two Fab fragments cross-link two monomers so that the HA molecule cannot undergo an acid pH–induced conformational change.[471] Attempts have also been made to measure antigenic evolution of influenza virus strains by pairwise comparison of hemagglutination inhibition assay titers.[256,259]

Unexpectedly, broadly cross-reactive monoclonal antibodies have been identified, which do not bind to the tip of the HA molecules but also have neutralizing activity. These antibodies are directed against the conserved stalk region of the HA spike and recognize the membrane-proximal part of HA1 in combination with HA2 or the HA2 alone (Fig. 14.14). In

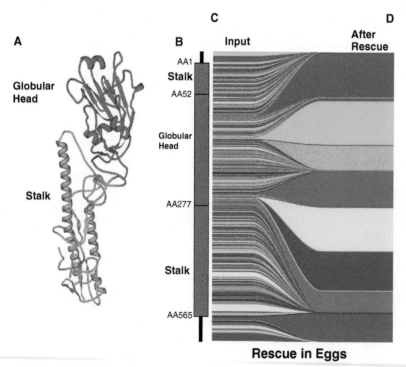

FIGURE 14.13 Relative tolerance to insertions in the head (*red*) of the influenza A virus hemagglutinin versus the stalk (*green*) **(A and B)**. Plots represent individual insertion sites. Individual insertions in the input **(C)** and after rescue **(D)** of viruses are represented by different colors; the thickness of the lines is representative of the proportion in the population. (The figure was kindly provided by Drs. Nicholas Heaton and Peter Palese.) For details, see Ref.[369]

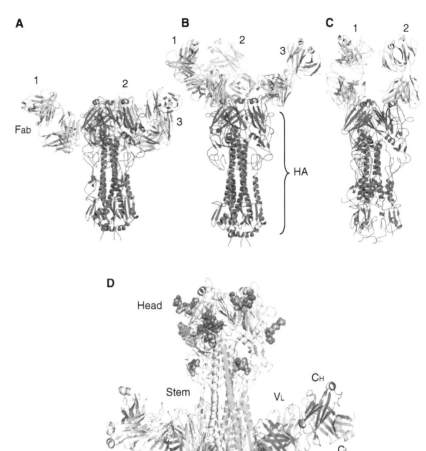

FIGURE 14.14 Ribbon diagram of H3 hemagglutinin (HA) in complex with Fab molecules. A and B: The first two complexes are examples where three Fab molecules (shown in *green*) are bound per HA trimer (i.e., one per HA monomer). **C:** The third complex has only two Fab molecules bound as the third is blocked by steric hindrance. For details, see Ref.[471] (Courtesy of John Skehel and Rupert Russell.) **D:** Crystal structure of antibody CR8020 bound to the H3 hemagglutinin. CR8020 binds an epitope on the hemagglutinin (HA) stem and has broad neutralizing activity against multiple group 2 influenza A viruses, including H3, H7, and H10. One monomer from the HA trimer is depicted in yellow and green (HA1 and HA2 subunits, respectively) and CR8020 is colored *blue* and *cyan* (heavy chain and light chain, respectively). N-linked carbohydrates are represented as pink van der Waals spheres. See for details Ref.[222] (Courtesy of Damian Ekiert and Ian A. Wilson.)

general, these antibodies recognize HAs within either group 1[221,455,678,863,873,885] or group 2.[223,264,943] However, very rare cross-group monoclonal antibodies[14,166,376,444,982] and one monoclonal antibody that binds to influenza A and B virus HA have also been isolated.[203] These cross-reactive antistalk antibodies protect from influenza virus infection via several mechanisms including by blocking conformational rearrangements associated with membrane fusion (antifusion vs. hemagglutination inhibition activity), by blocking viral egress, by blocking the function of the viral NA via steric hindrance, and by inhibiting the cleavage of HA0 and, importantly, via Fc–Fc receptor–mediated effector functions.[79,193,874,972] A number of antibodies that broadly bind to the head domain of HA have been isolated as well. These antibodies target the conserved sialic acid–binding site or a conserved area at the trimer interface of the head domain.[223,517,985] Antihead cross-reactive antibodies seem to be more prevalent for influenza B HA than for A HA, likely due to the higher conservation of influenza B virus HA.[872] Universal influenza virus vaccine approaches that target conserved epitopes in the stalk and/or head domain are currently being tested in preclinical and early clinical trials.[485,634,635]

The HEF of Influenza C and D Viruses

In contrast to the HA of influenza A and B viruses, the major glycoprotein of the C and D viruses has receptor-destroying activity. This is mediated by HEF's esterase activity, which cleaves off an acetyl group at position 9 of the neuraminic (sialic) acid receptor, eliminating the ligand.[851] This activity is important for entry of

the virus, implying a role in releasing the incoming virus from the receptor so that the uncoating process can begin.[834,920] Thus, in addition to receptor-binding (**h**emagglutination) and **f**usion activities, the molecule also has **e**sterase activity, hence the name HEF.[380] Although there is only about a 12% sequence identity between HAs and HEF, the overall structure of the molecule is similar, as was shown by x-ray crystallographic analysis.[766,834] Even more surprising are structural and sequence similarities between influenza virus HEF and some coronavirus esterases.[1022]

The M2 Protein

The M2 protein of influenza A viruses is a tetrameric type III (lacking a signal peptide sequence) integral membrane protein. It has a short ectodomain, a TMD, and a cytoplasmic domain with palmitate and phosphate modifications.[567,717,794] M2 has been shown to possess ion channel activity, and its major role is thought to be that of conducting protons from the acidified endosomes into the interior of the virus to dissociate the RNP complexes from the rest of the viral components, thus facilitating the uncoating process (see earlier section on Fusion and Uncoating). The structural and genetic analyses of the M2 protein have revealed that the ion channel is acid gated (but not voltage gated) and highly selective for H^+ and K^+ ions.[121,138,618,619,660,840] The structures of the transmembrane regions of M2 and of those that include the cytoplasmic sequences reveal a good understanding of the mechanism of proton conductance, which is controlled by the histidine-37 and tryptophan-41 cluster.[1,104,405,657,790,803,850,883] The transmembrane

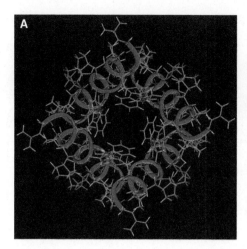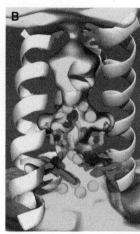

FIGURE 14.15 Structure of the tetrameric M2 ion channel. A: As seen from the top, four helices sit at an angle in the lipid membrane forming a pore. The backbone structure was determined by solid-state nuclear magnetic resonance (NMR) spectroscopy of the aligned bilayers. The histidine-37 and the tryptophan-41 side chains form the bottom of the pore in the closed state at neutral pH. For details, see Ref.[660] (Courtesy of Tim Cross.) **B:** X-ray structure of the transmembrane section of the M2 proton channel. The protein backbone is shown as a cartoon, viewed from across the viral membrane (lipid molecules and one of the monomers are not shown). Cyan spheres represent crystallographically resolved water molecules, which are stepping stones in possible proton conduction pathways. The three most important groups of side chains (the Val27-valve [*blue*], the His37-box [*orange*], and the Trp41-basket [*magenta*]) are shown in sticks. The three-dimensional density of water at 37°C, calculated from molecular dynamics simulations, is drawn as a gray contour. See Ref.[1] for details. (Courtesy of Giacomo Fiorin.)

region, when viewed from the top, shows four helices that sit at an angle in the lipid bilayer, forming a pore (Fig. 14.15). Structural studies on M2 in complex with adamantine drugs indicate two potential sites of interaction. In the x-ray structure, a single drug molecule binds to the core of the pore.[850] In contrast, the NMR structure shows four drug molecules binding to the lipid-exposed surface of the channel close to the cytoplasmic ends of the helices.[790] More recent data confirm the existence of these two interaction sites and propose that both drug-binding mechanisms may have physiologic significance.[104,482] The structure and the precise function of the extracellular portion of the M2 protein remain to be resolved. This external portion of M2 has been considered as the basis of a universal influenza virus vaccine approach because the M2 protein maintains a relatively conserved sequence over long periods of time.[786]

The ion channel activity of M2 has also been implicated in stabilizing HAs from premature low pH transitions in the trans-Golgi network, but this second function may only come into play for viruses carrying highly acid-sensitive HAs.[146] This is the case for some strains of H5 and H7 HAs, which have a multibasic cleavage site that can be cleaved by ubiquitous proteases and are therefore more susceptible to a premature low pH–induced conformational change. Further functions attributed to the M2 protein include roles in particle morphology,[319,427,756,757,768] genome packaging,[319,427,587] membrane scission[579,757,769] (see Assembly and Release), and inhibition of autophagy.[287] M2 expression also activates the inflammasome via the NLRP3 pathway.[244,418]

Influenza Virus Transcription and Replication
Overview

After uncoating, the viral ribonucleoproteins (vRNPs) are transported into the nucleus, and the incoming negative-sense vRNAs are transcribed into mRNA by a primer-dependent mechanism. These mRNA products are incomplete copies of the vRNA templates and are capped and polyadenylated, unlike vRNA. Replication occurs via a two-step process. A full-length, positive-sense copy of the vRNA is first made, which is referred to as complementary RNA (cRNA), and is in turn used as a template to produce more vRNA.

Nuclear Import of Ribonucleoproteins

One of the characteristics of the influenza virus life cycle is its dependence on nuclear functions. All vRNA synthesis occurs in the nucleus, and the trafficking of the viral genome into and out of the nucleus is a tightly regulated process.[72,173] The eight influenza virus genome segments never exist as naked RNAs but are associated with four viral proteins to form vRNP complexes. The major viral protein in the RNP complex is the nucleoprotein (NP), which coats the RNA. The remaining proteins are the three polymerase proteins (PB1, PB2, and PA), which bind to the partially complementary ends of the vRNA. RNPs (10–20 nm wide)[577] are considered too large to allow for passive diffusion into the nucleus, and therefore they must rely on an active nuclear import mechanism. All proteins in the RNP complex possess nuclear localization signals (NLSs), which mediate their interaction with the nuclear import machinery.[440,622,644,830,939,956] However, the signals on NP have been shown to be both sufficient and necessary for the import of vRNA.[96,172,639,669,682]

NP interactions with importin-α

The transport of proteins across the nuclear membrane is an energy-driven process that is initiated upon recognition of an NLS-containing cargo protein by members of the importin-α (also called karyopherin-α) family. Importin-α binds directly to the NLS and then recruits importin-β into a trimeric complex, which docks at the nuclear pore (Fig. 14.16A). Interestingly, the NP NLS-binding site on importin-α is distinct from that of classical NLS-containing proteins and relies on a low affinity–high avidity interaction with the nuclear import machinery.[172,595,639,890] One could postulate that this serves to avoid competition for importin-α binding with host proteins and may explain the use of an unconventional NLS. There is also evidence that differential interactions with human versus avian importin-α proteins may determine species specificity of influenza viruses.[278,279]

The Viral Ribonucleoprotein Template

Each vRNA segment exists as an RNP complex in which the RNA is coated with NP and forms a helical hairpin that is bound on one end by the heterotrimeric polymerase complex.[713,745] NP is an arginine-rich protein and has a net positive charge (at pH 6.5), which reflects its RNA-binding activity and its primary role in encapsidation.[726] The RNA/NP interaction is thought to be mediated by the positively charged residues on NP and the negatively charged phosphate backbone of the RNA, and thus there is no apparent sequence specificity to the interaction.[40,228] The RNA within the influenza virus RNP also remains sensitive to digestion with RNase and chemical

modifications,[207,470] supporting the model that the bases are exposed so that they can be accessed by the polymerase without disrupting the RNP structure.[40] Approximately 24 nucleotides of RNA are bound by each NP monomer,[681] and NP also has homo-oligomerization properties,[734] which adds structure to the RNP complex. This is maintained even in the absence of RNA[207,723,775] and has been shown to be crucial for maintaining the RNP in a transcriptionally active form.[116,229] Crystal structures of NP show that it is composed of a head domain and body domain and that a flexible tail loop mediates oligomerization.[656,1005] A potential RNA-binding groove, which is highly positively charged, has been identified between the head and body domains.[1005] Structural data based on EM also provide evidence that NP makes direct contact with the bound polymerase complex on the RNP,[19,159,577] which may reflect the previously reported interaction of free NP with both PB1 and PB2.[57] Mutagenesis and mapping of conserved residues in NP indicate the regions that are involved in genome replication/transcription and also genome packaging.[23,521,539,615,967]

The RNA Polymerase Complex

The influenza virus RNA-dependent RNA polymerase is a 270-kD complex of three proteins: PB1, PB2, and PA.[77] Three-dimensional images of the complex obtained by EM and x-ray analyses indicate that the three subunits are tightly associated to form a compact structure (Fig. 14.17).[19,374,712,713,743,895]

The PB1 protein

The PB1 protein catalyzes the sequential addition of nucleotides during RNA chain elongation[77] and contains the conserved motifs characteristic of RNA-dependent RNA polymerases.[58] The active site for the polymerization activity is an S–D–D

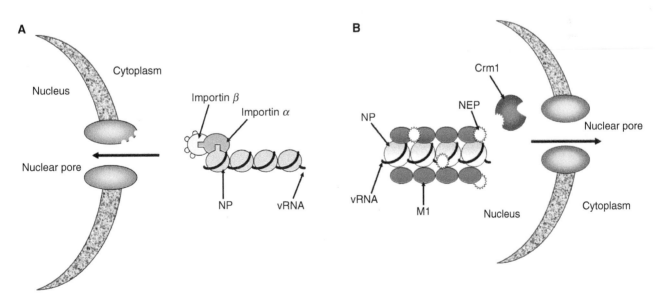

FIGURE 14.16 A: Illustration of influenza viral ribonucleoprotein (RNP) nuclear import. Viral RNPs (shown as viral RNA [vRNA] wrapped around nucleoprotein [NP]) are imported into the nucleus by an energy-dependent process, requiring interactions with soluble host factors. NP interacts with importin-α via its nuclear localization signals. Importin-α binds to importin-β, which mediates the interaction with proteins of the nuclear pore. For details, see Ref.[173] **B:** Illustration of influenza viral ribonucleoprotein (RNP) nuclear export. The nuclear export of newly synthesized viral RNP complexes is mediated by the viral nuclear export protein (NEP). NEP interacts with a cellular export factor, Crm1, and with the viral RNPs via the M1 protein. This interaction with the cellular export machinery facilitates the transport of the viral genome through the nuclear pore and into the cytoplasm.

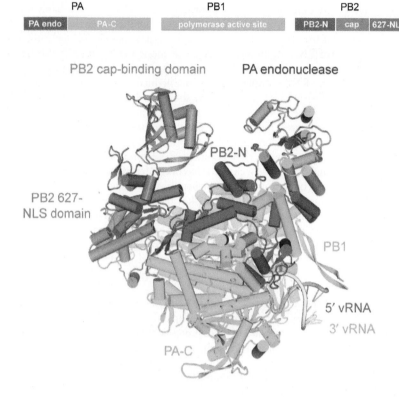

PA   PB1   PB2

| PA endo | PA-C | polymerase active site | PB2-N | cap | 627-NLS |

PB2 cap-binding domain   PA endonuclease

PB2-N

PB2 627-NLS domain

PB1

5′ vRNA
3′ vRNA

PA-C

FIGURE 14.17 Structure of the heterotrimeric influenza polymerase, bound to the viral RNA promotor (ribbon representation, color-coded according to the scheme above). The 3′ end of the promotor is in *yellow* and the 5′ end in *pink*. The domain organization of the subunits is shown above. (Courtesy of Maria Lukarska and Stephen Cusack, European Molecular Biology Laboratory.)

motif at positions 444 to 446.[58] The PB1, or more precisely the polymerase core, consisting of the PB1, the C-terminal domain of PA (PA-C), and the N-terminal domain of PB2 (PB2-N), is also responsible for binding to the terminal ends of both vRNA[312,537] and cRNA[313] for initiation of transcription and replication (Fig. 14.18).[712,743]

The PB2 protein

The PB2 protein plays a critical role in the initiation of transcription as it is responsible for binding the cap on host pre-mRNA molecules (Figs. 14.17 and 14.18).[60,713,904] Despite earlier discrepancy in the position of the binding site, it has now been shown that a domain encompassing PB2 residues 318 to 483 is sufficient for cap binding[327] and confirms the findings of a mutagenesis study that identified two aromatic residues (F363 and F404) as being important for the interaction.[240] PB2 has also been shown to localize to mitochondria, and this is determined by an N-terminal mitochondrial-targeting signal.[112] However, avian influenza viruses have a polymorphism in this signal, so it appears that mitochondrial localization of PB2 is unique to human influenza viruses.[317] Finally, as well as interacting with PB1 via its N-terminus,[860] the PB2 is also reported to interact with PA.[373] The PB2 also participates in genome replication as mutations affecting this activity but not transcription have been reported.[299]

The PA protein

Until several years ago, the specific function of PA was unknown, but crystal structures of the N-terminal domain revealed that the endonuclease activity of the polymerase, which is required to generate the capped primer, resides in the PA protein (Figs. 14.17 and 14.18).[191,712,1017] Previous work had mistakenly attributed this function to the PB1 protein. In the structure, the fold and position of the active site identify the PA endo-

nuclease as a member of the PD-(D/E)XK family of nucleases. The catalytic site involves residues His 41, Glu 80, Asp 108, Glu 119, and Lys 134 and harbors two $Mn^{(2+)}$ ions.[170,191] Mutation of these residues abolishes the transcriptional activity of the trimeric polymerase, but replication activity is unaffected, confirming the specific role of the endonuclease in viral transcription.[170,1017] PA does, however, participate in genome replication as mutations affecting this process have been described.[252,410] In addition to encoding nuclease function, the N-terminus of PA (aa 1–100) is also involved in an interaction with PB2,[373] while the C-terminus makes contact with PB1.[713]

The vRNA Promoter

All influenza virus RNA segments contain noncoding sequences at their 5′ and 3′ ends, which flank the coding region. Some of this sequence is segment specific,[1036] but the terminal ends are highly conserved between all segments in all influenza viruses. These conserved 13 nucleotides at the 5′ end and 12 nucleotides at the 3′ end display partial and inverted complementarity, which led to the proposal of a panhandle structure created by base pairing of the 5′ and 3′ ends.[189,758] This is supported by cross-linking experiments that demonstrated a circular configuration for virion RNAs[402] as well as by more recent structural analyses.[29,577] The panhandle model was refined to incorporate a fork model and a corkscrew style conformation.[249] Studies using *in vitro* transcription of model RNA templates or reporter gene expression *in vivo* have shown that both 5′- and 3′-terminal ends are necessary for promoter activity and that base pairing is required.[250,649] Furthermore, it has been demonstrated that the polymerase can interact with both 5′ and 3′ ends and that the binding affinity decreases when the duplex is disrupted.[254,312,334,520,887] A full understanding of the promoter has

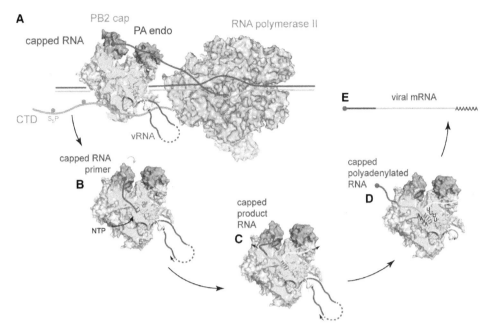

FIGURE 14.18 Schematic representation of the transcription cycle of influenza polymerase. **A: Cap snatching:** association with the Ser5-phosphorylated C-terminal domain of RNA polymerase II brings the influenza virus polymerase in proximity to the nascent capped transcript, which is recognized by the PB2 cap-binding site and cleaved by the endonuclease activity around 10 to 15 nucleotides after the cap. The conserved ends of the viral RNA are bound to the polymerase (*pink* and *yellow* for 5′ and 3′ end, respectively). **B: Transcription initiation:** the cap-binding domain rotates by about 70 degrees to direct the capped RNA primer into the active site of the polymerase, where it serves to initiate transcription of the vRNA segment at the 3′ end of the template (*yellow*). **C: Elongation:** incorporation of NTPs leads to elongation of the capped transcript and translocation of the template. **D: Termination/polyadenylation:** near the end of the template, the polymerase stutters over a oligouridine stretch, while the 5′ hook remains tightly bound to the polymerase, producing a poly(A) tail. **E:** The product of the transcription cycle is a hybrid RNA, containing a cap and a host-derived sequence at its 5′ end (*red*), the coding sequence of the viral segment (*blue*) and poly(A) tail. (Courtesy of Maria Lukarska and Stephen Cusack, European Molecular Biology Laboratory.)

been obtained following the successful x-ray analysis of the bat influenza virus polymerase complex by S. Cusack and his group (Fig. 14.19).[693,743,753,891] These data define the vRNA promoter as an element that features a double-stranded region created by pairing between 5′ and 3′ ends, forking of ssRNA for the 5′ end and a hairpin on the 5′ end making a partial corkscrew.[662,712,743]

While the need for base pairing of the 5′ and 3′ ends is clear, the stem–loop structures are also involved in binding and stabilizing the polymerase complex.[85]

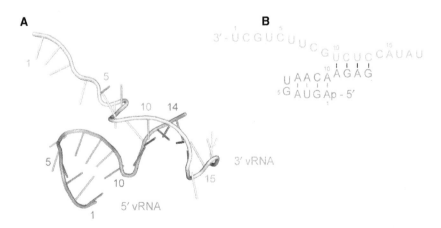

FIGURE 14.19 A: Structure of the vRNA promotor, bound to the polymerase, showing the 5′ hook and the distal base-pairing region between the 5′ and 3′ ends. **B:** Schematic diagram of the 5′ and 3′ end of the vRNA promotor, with base pairing indicated with lines. (Courtesy of Maria Lukarska and Stephen Cusack, European Molecular Biology Laboratory.)

Initiation of Messenger RNA Synthesis

Influenza virus mRNA synthesis is dependent on cellular RNA polymerase II activity. This is because it requires a 5′-capped primer, which it steals from host pre-mRNA transcripts, to initiate its own mRNA synthesis.[721] This process is known as cap snatching and involves the cap-binding function of the PB2 protein and endonuclease function of the PA protein. The initiation of transcription commences with binding of the 5′ end of the vRNA to the PB1 subunit (Fig. 14.18). This induces an allosteric change in the polymerase, which allows the PB2 protein to recognize and bind the cap structure on host pre-mRNAs.[148,239,537,713] This structural change in the polymerase also increases its affinity for the 3′ vRNA end, which is bound by PB1. Endonuclease activation leads to cleavage of the bound mRNAs and small nuclear RNAs.[322,479] This occurs approximately 10 to 14 nucleotides from their 5′ caps, usually after a purine residue.[44,721] Transcription is then initiated by the addition of a "G" residue to the primer, directed by the penultimate "C" nucleotide at the 3′ end of the vRNA template,[44] although in some instances the incorporation of a "C" that is directed by the "G" at position 3 in the vRNA has also been observed.[255] Unlike influenza viruses, Thogoto viruses lack host-derived sequences at the 5′ end of their capped mRNAs.[955] RNA chain elongation is catalyzed by the polymerase function of PB1 and continues until a stretch of uridine residues is encountered approximately 16 nucleotides before the 5′ end of the vRNA.[535,557,759] This is the signal for polyadenylation (Fig. 14.18).[713]

Polyadenylation

Unlike host cells, which use a specific poly(A) polymerase for generating the poly(A) tail on mRNA transcripts, polyadenylation of influenza virus mRNAs is catalyzed by the same polymerase that is used for transcription. This activity is dependent on an uninterrupted stretch of five to seven "U" residues and the adjacent double-stranded region of the vRNA promoter.[535,557,759] The current model proposes that the 5′ end of the vRNA remains bound to the polymerase during elongation while the template is threaded through in a 3′ to 5′ direction (Fig. 14.18).[713] In support of this model, mutations introduced into the 5′ end of the vRNA that prevent or weaken polymerase binding have been shown to also inhibit polyadenylation.[253,725,732,733] The polyadenylation signal is vital for gene expression as replacement of the uridines with adenosines has been shown to result in transcripts with poly(U) tails, which fail to be properly exported from the nucleus.[724]

Splicing

Members of the *Orthomyxovirus* family can extend the coding capacity of their genomes by producing two proteins from one gene via an alternative splicing mechanism. *Orthomyxovirus* genome segments that encode proteins from both spliced and unspliced mRNA transcripts include segments 7 and 8 of influenza A virus,[504,507] segment 8 of influenza B virus,[82] segments 6 and 7 of influenza C virus,[638,994] segment 6 of Thogoto virus,[474] and segment 7 of isavirus[56] (see Genome Structure and Organization section). The primary transcripts from these segments have 5′ and 3′ splice sites, which (more or less) fit the consensus sequence for the exon/intron boundaries of cellular

transcripts. This, combined with the fact that splicing can be demonstrated in the absence of any viral proteins,[505,506] indicates that the virus is using the cellular splicing machinery. However, unlike cellular splicing, which is extremely efficient, splicing of viral mRNA has to be relatively inefficient because proteins must be expressed from both spliced and unspliced mRNAs. In influenza virus–infected cells, splicing is tightly regulated such that the steady-state level of spliced viral transcripts is only 10% that of the unspliced viral transcripts.[503,507] These control mechanisms may act on several different levels. The rate of nuclear export of the unspliced transcript is certainly crucial as this determines its availability for splicing. It has been proposed that the NS1 protein inhibits both the splicing and nuclear export of NS1 transcripts via negative feedback,[9,293] but contradictory reports[751] suggest that alternative mechanisms may exist for regulating splicing of viral transcripts. Potentially, these may involve *cis*-acting sequences in the NS1 transcript that negatively control the rate of splicing.[8,648] Strangely, the influenza C virus NS1 protein (C/NS1) has been reported to up-regulate viral mRNA splicing.[625] Splicing of the influenza A virus M1 transcript is controlled by the aforementioned rate of nuclear export[906] as well as by the viral polymerase and a cellular splicing factor, SF2/ASF. The polymerase determines the time at which splicing (and hence production of M2) occurs and SF2/ASF is required to activate splicing.[811,813] Other host proteins have also been shown to modulate splicing of influenza virus RNAs.[260,884,899]

Replication Products: cRNA and vRNA

Full-length copies of the incoming vRNAs have to be made, and these positive-sense cRNAs serve as templates for the synthesis of new negative-sense genomic vRNAs. The cRNA promoter is complementary to the vRNA promoter and has also been reported to assume a corkscrew configuration, albeit with subtle differences.[28,174,697,753,1036] This variation has been implicated in determining whether or not the endonuclease function of the polymerase is activated and therefore may play an important regulatory role.[515]

The Switch from Transcription to Replication

The vRNA serves as a template for both mRNA and cRNA synthesis, and yet the means of initiation and termination for the generation of these two molecules are quite different. In contrast to the primer-dependent mechanism of initiation of mRNA synthesis, initiation of cRNA synthesis occurs without a capped primer, and cRNA molecules are full-length copies of the vRNA and thus are not prematurely terminated and polyadenylated as are mRNAs. The different initiation and termination reactions therefore have to be coordinated, but exactly how the polymerase switches between these two modes is still not well understood. It has been proposed that the transcription-competent polymerase is structurally different from the replication-competent polymerase. Support comes from evidence that different domains of PB1 are involved in binding vRNA versus cRNA and that PA is more critical for binding the cRNA than the vRNA promoter.[313,374,564,877,882] One obvious difference is that the cap-binding and endonuclease functions of PB2 and PA, respectively, are not required when the polymerase is in replication mode.

In contrast to mRNAs, newly synthesized cRNAs and vRNAs are encapsidated. It has been proposed that the availability of soluble NP (i.e., not associated with RNPs) controls the switch between mRNA and cRNA synthesis. This hypothesis arose from the observation that replication is dependent on *de novo* protein synthesis, which means that the incoming RNPs are only capable of transcription.[360] Indeed, free NP has been shown to be required for production of full-length cRNA (antitermination),[45] and this is consistent with data from temperature-sensitive (ts) NP mutants,[489,591,802] which show that cRNA but not mRNA synthesis is affected at the nonpermissive temperature. However, this model has been challenged by a report demonstrating that overexpressed NP does not promote replication.[624] Another study disputes the existence of a switch, instead suggesting a stabilization role for NP and the polymerase.[926] This model claims that the incoming polymerase is able to synthesize both mRNA and cRNA,[922] but until there is a sufficient pool of polymerase and NP to encapsidate the cRNA, it is degraded and therefore at early times postinfection there is a bias toward mRNA accumulation. Also, requirements for higher nucleotide concentrations to initiate cRNA synthesis may determine the timing of transcription versus replication.[925] Furthermore, the accumulation of NEP is associated with a decrease in transcription and an increase in replication, suggesting a regulatory role.[97,752] Interestingly, NEP is also required for the generation of small viral RNAs (svRNAs), which have been implicated in the initiation of vRNA synthesis.[709] The svRNAs are 22 to 27 nt in length and correspond to the 5′ end of each vRNA segment. These segment-specific svRNAs are needed for vRNA but not cRNA synthesis, so according to this model the polymerase is in replication mode when these svRNAs are present. It has also been proposed that the switch from transcription to replication is the result of accumulation of a newly synthesized free polymerase complex, which enhances cRNA to vRNA synthesis (and vice versa) over mRNA synthesis.[441] The role of host factors in regulating influenza virus replication, including posttranslational modification of viral proteins, should also be considered.[69,132,442,542,584,607,609,611,612]

Regulation of Viral Gene Expression

Early studies have provided evidence for temporal regulation of viral gene expression,[360,829] but the mechanism(s) is (are) still unresolved. Disproportionate accumulation of mRNAs from the different segments has been observed, but whether this represents specific up-regulation of transcription for these segments[232,357] or reflects different rates of vRNA synthesis[801,829] or RNA stability is unclear. Regardless, the synthesis of NP and NS1 mRNAs and protein is favored at early stages, whereas the synthesis of HA, NA, and particularly M1 mRNAs and proteins is delayed.[357,360,801,829] This differential expression is mirrored by the roles these proteins play at different points in the virus life cycle. As discussed earlier, NP is required for replication and NS1 plays a crucial role in combating the host immune response; thus, both of these proteins are needed early in the virus life cycle. M1 has been found to inhibit viral transcription,[707,947] which demands its delayed expression, and at later stages, M1 accumulation probably dictates the arrest of viral mRNA synthesis. M1 is also involved in the export of RNPs from the nucleus,[576] which must only occur once replication is complete.

Another control mechanism for differential gene expression resides in the vRNA promoter. A natural variation is found at position 4 from the 3′ vRNA end in an otherwise totally conserved region. The PB1, PB2, and PA RNA segments have a "C" at this position, while the remaining segments usually have a "U." The C4-containing promoter is associated with a down-regulation in transcription and an up-regulation in replication compared to the U4 promoter,[523] which correlates with the lower amounts of polymerase mRNAs and proteins found in infected cells.[360,829] A structural analysis of the C4 and U4 promoters has revealed differences that may alter their interaction with the polymerase and thereby regulate gene expression.[516]

As observed with many other viruses, influenza virus gene expression is also controlled at the level of translation. This is achieved via numerous mechanisms and results in the selective translation of viral genes and suppression of host protein synthesis.[281,924,1003] These mechanisms include (a) degradation of host pre-mRNAs following cleavage (due to cap snatching), (b) inhibition of host mRNA processing, (c) degradation of cellular RNA polymerase II, and (d) preferential translation of viral mRNA transcripts. Several of these processes involve the influenza virus NS1 and PA-X proteins. The NS1-mediated and PA-X–mediated effects on mRNA processing are discussed in a later section (see below). NS1 is also involved in the specific translational enhancement of viral mRNAs through its association with the 5′ noncoding region of viral mRNA transcripts and with cellular proteins involved in translation initiation.[16,99,698] These include the translation initiation factor eIF4GI and poly(A)-binding protein 1, and it has been proposed that this protein complex acts to specifically recruit ribosomes to the 5′ end of viral mRNA transcript. Another cellular protein that may play a role is GRSF-1, an RNA-binding protein that has been reported to interact with the 5′ end of the NP transcript and to stimulate the specific translation of a template driven by the NP 5′ noncoding region in a cell-free translation system.[454,699] Whether this interaction is relevant *in vivo* remains to be determined.

An interesting model explaining the selective translation of viral mRNAs has been proposed suggesting that the viral polymerase complex remains associated with the viral mRNA transcript in the cytoplasm. It is thought that this interaction eliminates the need for complex formation with eIF4E. Since eIF4E is inactivated in influenza virus–infected cells,[241] this would explain the selective translation of viral transcripts over cellular transcripts. Other components of the translation machinery, such as eIF4A and eIF4G, are required for influenza viral protein translation.[1001] Although this model is compelling in its simplicity, this mechanism is questioned by the finding that viral mRNAs in the cytoplasm are devoid of viral polymerase but are associated with cellular cap-binding proteins, including eIF4E.[55] Clearly, further investigation is required to explain the selective translation of viral transcripts in infected cells.

An additional host shutoff mechanism is controlled by the viral polymerase at the level of host transcription. It has been shown that the influenza virus polymerase interacts with the C-terminal domain of the large subunit of cellular RNA polymerase II[235] and that this interaction mediates the degradation of RNA polymerase II at late times postinfection.[763,923] This shutoff mechanism may play a role in viral pathogenicity because attenuated influenza viruses have been shown not to induce RNA polymerase II degradation.[762] Another mechanism involves the reduction of free RNA polymerase II due termination defects.[42,1034]

Virus Assembly and Release
Nuclear Export of Ribonucleoproteins
Association of RNP complexes with M1

Following virus replication, newly formed RNP complexes are assembled in the nucleus from which they are then exported into the cytoplasm. Two viral proteins, the matrix (M1) protein and the NEP, are involved in directing the nuclear export of RNPs[72,173,416,499] in a proposed daisy chain model in which M1 binds to the RNP complexes and NEP then binds to M1.[499] Our present understanding of this process indicates that M1 associates with RNPs in the nucleus, a process potentially facilitated by the host protein clustered mitochondria homolog (CLUH).[13] This association may actually promote the formation of RNP complexes.[409] M1 makes contact with both the vRNA and NP,[41,173,645,1006] and evidence that M1 also binds to nucleosomes[294,1039] has led to the hypothesis that M1 interactions cause the dissociation of RNP from the nuclear matrix. This agrees with the significant finding that nuclear import of M1 is required for subsequent export of RNP complexes.[96,576] Furthermore, at high temperatures, heat shock protein 70 is found bound to RNP, which prevents association with M1 and results in a block in RNP export.[384,780] It has been reported that sumoylation of M1 is essential for its nuclear export function.[983] An alternative to the daisy chain model has also recently been proposed in which the C-terminal part of NEP interacts with both PB2 and PB1 and facilitates binding of M1 to NP and vRNA.[88] In this model, the N-terminal part of NEP then interacts with Crm1. This model is attractive since it has recently been shown that the polymerase complex can assume different conformations when bound to cRNPs and vRNPs.[499] Selective binding of NEP to the vRNP polymerase conformation in this model might regulate the export of vRNP versus cRNPs.

NEP interacts with the cellular export machinery

Initial data suggested that M1 alone could control RNP export, but as is the case for import, nuclear export of large molecules involves direct interactions with the cellular export machinery and no such interactions with M1 had initially been demonstrated. However, NEP has been found to interact with the export receptor Crm1[651] and several nucleoporins.[123,670] NEP also associates with M1,[4,816,1004] so the current model proposes that an RNP–M1–NEP complex is formed in the nucleus and that NEP is responsible for recruiting the export machinery and directing export of the complex (Fig. 14.16B). In support of this role, it has been shown that injection of anti-NEP antibodies into the nucleus of infected cells inhibits RNP export,[670] which is also seen in a system using recombinant virus-like particles (VLPs) lacking NEP.[651] A methionine/leucine-rich and a leucine-rich nuclear export signal (NES), NES1 and NES2, respectively, have been identified in the N-terminus of NEP[407,670] and shown to be critical for RNP export and virus growth.[407,426,651] NES2 potentially interacts directly with Crm1, while NES1's contribution might be indirect by involving host factor chromodomain–helicase–DNA-binding protein 3 (CHD3) since it does not interact with Crm1.[403,407,651] Treatment with leptomycin B, a Crm1 inhibitor, completely inhibits RNP export in infected cells, which indicates that export does occur in a Crm1-dependent manner.[230,426,952] Interactions between Crm1 and the RNP–M1–NEP complex have been shown to occur at chromatin structures rich in Ran nucleotide exchange factor Rcc1, a protein that generates Ran-GTP, which in turn activates Crm1.[119,878]

Another viral protein, NP, has also been shown to bind to Crm1 and to the NTF2-related export protein 1 (NXT1)[145,230] and therefore is proposed to play a role in export as well as import. Both this study and another also revealed that RNPs are localized to the periphery of the nucleus after leptomycin B treatment but that M1 and NEP retain diffuse nuclear staining.[230,561] The RNPs were shown to colocalize with nuclear lamins just beneath the nuclear pore complex, which may represent an intermediate step prior to export through the pore.[561] The roles of M1 and NEP are obviously called into question by their differing staining pattern compared to RNPs,[230,561] but this could be explained if only a fraction of the total M1 and NEP pool was used for export. In addition to potential involvement of NP in nuclear export of vRNPs, an NES on M1 has been identified recently as well. Removal of this NES impaired export of RNPs and suggests that M1 might have a more active role in nuclear export than previously thought.[109] These findings raise the possibility that redundant export mechanisms may exist. Already in the nucleus, the RNP–M1–NEP complexes associate with Y-box–binding protein 1 (YB-1), which is coexported from the nucleus and likely facilitates interactions with microtubules at microtubule-organizing centers (MTOCs). There, the RNPs are thought to be delivered to Rab11a-positive recycling endosomes.[457]

Regulation of RNP export

As discussed earlier, the late expression of M1 determines that export takes place only after a full round of replication has occurred, therefore preventing premature exit of RNPs from the nucleus. The process is also controlled by a number of other mechanisms including the enlargement of nuclear pores by caspases induced by virus replication and the slow accumulation of NEP in the nucleus due to inefficient splicing.[144,621] Similarly, control mechanisms must also exist to stop the re-entry of RNPs into the nucleus following export. Studies with a temperature-sensitive virus (ts51) showed that when grown at the nonpermissive temperature, this virus is unable to retain its RNPs in the cytoplasm following export.[965] This defect mapped to M1,[966] once again demonstrating the vital role of this protein in regulating the nucleocytoplasmic transport of RNPs. It is interesting to note that the canonical NEP-binding site on M1 maps to the M1 NLS,[4] which suggests that NEP may act to mask the NLS on M1 and therefore prevent the complex from re-entering the nucleus. NP is also proposed to cause the cytoplasmic retention of RNPs by binding to filamentous actin and thereby anchoring the RNPs in the cytoplasm.[192] All these processes are likely to be regulated at some level, and protein modification by phosphorylation is probably involved as several studies have reported alterations in M1, NEP, and NP trafficking in the presence of kinase inhibitors.[93–95,594,720,744,966]

RNP export in influenza B and C viruses

Few studies concerning export in influenza B and C viruses have been performed, but it has been shown that as with influenza A viruses, the NEP proteins possess nuclear export activities.[696] They both have been shown to interact with Crm1 (and a subset of nucleoporins), and NES motifs have been defined for each protein. Similar to that of influenza A viruses, the influenza C virus NES is composed of two separate leucine-rich domains, both of which are required for full activity.[696]

In contrast to influenza A virus where M1 acts as a bridge between NEP and the RNP complex, the influenza B NEP has been proposed to bind directly to the RNP as well as to M1,[420] which suggests that the model for export of influenza B virus RNPs may be slightly different than the canonical model for influenza A virus. Interestingly, the influenza B virus M1 protein also contains two NES motifs that could be involved in export of RNPs.[108] Not much information is available for RNP export of influenza D virus, but it can be assumed—based on the genome structure and the presence of an M1 and NEP protein—that the mechanisms are likely similar to those for influenza C virus.[855]

The Site of Virus Assembly and Budding

Influenza viruses assemble and bud from the apical plasma membrane of polarized cells (e.g., lung epithelial cells of the infected host)[477,761,770] (Fig. 14.20). This asymmetrical process (i.e., apical vs. basolateral) is thought to have an important role in viral pathogenesis and tissue tropism. Viruses that bud from the internal cell surface (e.g., Marburg virus) tend to cause systemic disease, whereas viruses, such as influenza virus, that bud from the external cell surface generally have a more restricted tissue tropism.[242] The influenza virus HA, NA, and M2 have all been shown to localize to the apical surface of polarized cells when expressed alone,[411,439,772] and apical sorting signals have been identified within the TMDs of HA and NA. The vRNPs are thought to arrive at the site of virus assembly and budding in a Rab11-dependent manner although the exact mechanism is still unclear.[499]

The M1 protein

M1 is the most abundant virion protein and lies just beneath the lipid envelope where it is believed to make contact with the cytoplasmic tails of the glycoproteins and with the RNPs, thereby forming a bridge between the inner core components and the membrane proteins.[770] Structural analyses indicate that the M1 protein consists of two globular helical domains that are linked by a protease-sensitive region.[21,353,799] Rods (6 nm in length) corresponding to M1 monomers have been observed by negative-stain EM of virions with one end in contact with the membrane and the other end pointing toward the interior of the particle.[4] These rods form an ordered structure consistent with the homo-oligomerization properties of M1[106,1030,1032] and are arranged such that the positive and negatively charged residues are on opposite sides of the oligomer.[21,353] Several reports have documented the ability of M1 to associate with lipid membranes,[231,383,774,1026]

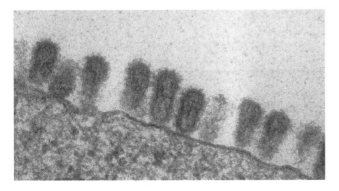

FIGURE 14.20 Budding influenza virus particles. Electron micrograph thin-section image of influenza virus particles budding from the apical surface of an infected cell. (Courtesy of Yi-ying Chou.)

and as mentioned previously (see section on Nuclear Export of Ribonucleoproteins), M1 interacts with both RNPs and NEP. M1 also interacts with the cytoplasmic tail of M2.[124] Therefore, it is proposed that M1 plays a vital role in assembly by recruiting the viral components to the site of assembly at the plasma membrane.

Assembly of Viral Components

Following synthesis on membrane-bound ribosomes, the three integral membrane proteins, HA, NA, and M2, enter the ER where they are folded and HA and NA are glycosylated. There, it is traditionally believed that the HA is assembled into a trimer, assisted by membrane protein translocator SEC61, and NA and M2 are assembled into tetramers.[196,368] However, it has recently also been shown that trimer assembly for HA might occur at a later stage in the Golgi network.[563] Of note, M2 associates with the E3 ubiquitin–protein ligase UBR4 in the ER. UBR4 has been shown to be required for effective shuttling of M2 to the plasma membrane as is ubiquitination of M2 (but not by UBR4).[857,898] Lack of UBR4 or ubiquitination leads to transport of M2 to the autophagosome.[857,898] HA, NA, and M2 are subsequently transported to the Golgi apparatus where cysteine residues on HA and M2 are palmitoylated in the *cis*-Golgi network and M2 is acetylated.[842,861,913–915] For those HAs that have a multibasic cleavage site (e.g., some H5 and H7 subtypes), furin cleavage of HA into HA1 and HA2 subunits may occur in the *trans*-Golgi network.[849] From here, HA, NA, and M2 are all directed to the virus assembly site on the apical plasma membrane via their apical sorting signals. The signals for HA and NA have been described to reside in their TMDs.[36,495,544,976] The TMDs of HA and NA also contain the determinants for association with lipid rafts.[35,36,544] Lipid rafts are proposed to be nonionic detergent-resistant lipid microdomains within the plasma membrane that are rich in sphingolipids and cholesterol. The significance of lipid rafts/transient lipid nanodomains for virus budding is still controversial and an area of ongoing research.[311,528,798,835] However, the lipid raft model is helpful in explaining influenza virus assembly and budding, and examination of the lipid content of purified virus particles indicates that influenza virus might bud preferentially from these domains.[784,1028] HA and NA individually also selectively accumulate at and are incorporated into rafts.[495,785] Also, it has been shown that reduction of cholesterol levels in the plasma membrane impacts negatively on titers of progeny virus, while increases in cholesterol levels positively affect titers.[633] The signals for apical sorting and raft association both lie within the TMD and are not mutually exclusive.[35,183,645] Raft association of HA has been shown to be essential for efficient virus replication.[869] This is thought to be because of a requirement for concentrated "patches" of HA at the plasma membrane, which governs the level of HA incorporation into budding particles and subsequently affects fusion. A similar scenario holds for raft association of NA, as an optimal amount of NA must be incorporated to allow for efficient virus release.[35] Coexpression of HA and NA seems to induce raft clustering leading to acceleration of their apical transport.[673] It is important to mention that a recent study using high-resolution secondary ion mass spectroscopy in fibroblasts found that there was no enrichment of cholesterol or sphingolipids in HA clusters on the cell membrane, which questions the significance of lipid rafts for influenza virus assembly and budding.[968] While not mutually exclusive with lipid raft–based mechanisms, clustering of HA has recently also been associated with actin-rich membrane regions (ARMRs) that lacked cofilin providing an alternative mechanism for the formation of HA nanoclusters.[326] In contrast to HA and NA, the majority of M2 protein is excluded from lipid rafts,[1028] which may reflect its low abundance in virus particles. M2 has been shown to bind cholesterol, and this property is suggested to target M2 to the raft periphery where it may act to bridge several raft domains.[791] Mutation of the cholesterol recognition/interaction amino acid consensus (CRAC) motif in M2 is reported to affect membrane targeting but not raft association,[879–881] and in the context of infection, it is shown to attenuate the virus *in vivo* but not in tissue culture.[848] There is also evidence that M2 is involved in capturing the RNPs at the assembly site. Experimental evidence for this mechanism was first demonstrated with an influenza B virus that lacked BM2 expression and produced particles devoid of RNPs.[419] Subsequently, mutation or truncation of the influenza A virus M2 cytoplasmic tail has been shown to correspond with decreased incorporation of genome segments into virions.[319,427,587,588,857]

In comparison to the integral membrane proteins, less is known about how the remaining viral components reach the assembly site. A long-standing hypothesis is that M1 acts as the master recruiter dictated by its position between the viral envelope and the RNP core. This is supported by evidence that the availability of M1 affects the timing of assembly and maturation, as seen with a virus engineered to express reduced levels of protein from the M segment.[74] This virus showed no defects in virion protein composition but displayed delayed growth kinetics, suggesting that a minimum amount of M1 protein must accumulate before assembly can begin. The association of M1 with the RNP–NEP complex is well described (see section on Nuclear Export of Ribonucleoproteins), but the specific interaction of M1 with the membrane-bound glycoproteins has been difficult to prove because of M1's intrinsic membrane-binding properties, which has resulted in some conflicting reports.[231,487,1026] However, it was noted that in influenza virus–infected cells, M1 becomes resistant to extraction with Triton X-100 (a marker for lipid raft association), whereas M1 expressed alone remains soluble.[6,1026] This suggested a role for other viral proteins, and indeed, coexpression of HA and NA together with M1 has been shown to promote raft association of M1.[6] This requires the TMDs and cytoplasmic tails of HA and NA,[6,1028] and in the absence of the cytoplasmic tails of these two proteins, virus particles have been found to be grossly distorted, which perhaps indicates reduced M1 association.[436] A recent study using EM, electron tomography, and cryoelectron tomography also showed that, while expression of HA, NA, or HA and NA led to the formation of particles, only coexpression of the M proteins clustered the glycoproteins together into filamentous membrane protrusions and led to the formation of particles with characteristics similar to authentic budding virus.[139]

The hypothetical model for transport of M1 to the plasma membrane proposes that M1 becomes associated with the glycoproteins during their passage through the exocytic pathway and "hitches a ride" to raft domains in the apical membrane. The initial model also proposed that M1 was taking the RNP–NEP complex with it. However, the current working hypothesis is that the vRNPs use the cytoskeleton to reach the virus assembly site. This is based on the finding that RNPs can interact with cytoskeletal components and Rab11.[12,25,86,141,218,610]

In this model, vRNP–M1–NEP complexes delivered to microtubules at MTOCs by YB-1 (as described above) lead to an interaction between PB2 and Rab11.[12,26,457] Interactions between human immunodeficiency virus Rev-binding protein (HRB) and potentially between NP and actin might also play a role early in this process.[25,192,219] It is unclear if M1 and NEP disassemble from the RNPs at this point or if they stay attached. While costaining of RNPs and Rab11 has been observed, interactions with M1 have not been detected in the cytoplasm, although M1 can interact with cytoskeletal components.[12,25,610] Rab11 proteins are small GTPases that are involved in transport of recycling endosomes. These Rab11a-containing recycling endosomes can be transported along microtubules or along actin filaments.[907] This might provide an explanation why inhibition of microtubules[12,608] or actin filaments[18,492,755,823] on their own does not drastically impact influenza virus replication. It remains controversial if Rab11-based RNP transport is mainly microtubule-[12,26,608] or actin filament–dependent.[18,492] However, an intact cytoskeleton has only been found to be necessary for the production of filamentous virus particles,[755,823] so a specific role in assembly remains to be confirmed. Interestingly, a recent report suggested that the RNPs are transported in a Rab11a-dependent manner on infection-induced irregular coated vesicles associated with a reorganized tubulated endoplasmatic reticulum that stretches throughout the cell to the plasma membrane.[181] Independent of the transport mechanism, it has been observed using fluorescent *in situ* hybridization that different RNPs start to colocalize in the cytoplasm. This colocalization is associated with Rab11 and suggests that Rab11-positive vesicles facilitate association of different RNPs.[141,500] It was recently suggested that RNPs could then be transferred from Rab11-positive vesicles to the plasma membrane by interaction of NP with phosphatidylinositol 4,5-bisphosphate, a component of lipid rafts.[447] Finally, there is evidence that NP alone is intrinsically targeted to the apical plasma membrane and associates with lipid rafts in a cholesterol-dependent manner, which suggests that RNPs could reach the assembly site independently of the cytoskeleton.[113] How exactly the RNPs reach the plasma membrane is an ongoing area of research and future studies will bring more clarity.[11]

Packaging of Eight RNA Segments

Correct assembly and packaging of a full complement of RNA genome segments is a requirement for a fully infectious virion. The precise mechanism of packaging of the eight vRNA segments is still not well understood, although different models have been proposed. The first model, *the random incorporation model*, assumes that a common structural feature is present on all vRNAs (vRNPs), which enables them to be randomly incorporated into budding virions. This model is supported by evidence that virions may possess more than eight vRNPs, ensuring the presence of a full complement of eight vRNPs in a significant percentage of virus particles.[33,234,290] Mathematical analysis of packaging suggests that if eight RNA segments were randomly packaged into budding virions, only 0.24% of released virus particles would be infectious.[234] However, if a greater number of RNA segments were randomly packaged, then the percentage of infectious particles increases.[84,160,197]

The second model, *the selective incorporation model*, suggests that each vRNA segment acts independently, allowing each segment to be packaged selectively. A similar model has been reported for the packaging of the 3 double-stranded RNA (dsRNA) segments of bacteriophage-ϕ6[602] and for the packaging of the 11 dsRNA segments of rotavirus (RV).[589] This model suggests that each vRNA segment contains a unique "packaging signal" and predicts that every virion possesses a full complement of the eight vRNP segments. There is increasing evidence to support this model. The precise number of vRNPs packaged in a single virion has been determined by imaging of serially sectioned budding virions using EM and electron tomography.[261,262,643,663,664] The vast majority of virions from influenza A and B viruses appear to contain exactly eight vRNPs organized in a distinct pattern: one in the center and seven in the surrounding positions (1+7 configuration).[663] The eight vRNPs are oriented perpendicular to the budding tip. These findings were also corroborated by multicolor single-molecule fluorescent *in situ* hybridization.[142] In addition, the existence of packaging signals within the noncoding and coding regions at both the 5′ and 3′ ends of the genomic RNAs has been confirmed (Fig. 14.21).[574] Coding regions of the NA[267]; HA[954]; NS[266]; PB2, PB1, and PA[150,540,630]; NP[682]; and M[684] segments have all been demonstrated to increase the ability of a reporter sequence

to be incorporated within assembling virions. Similar sequence features have been shown to govern packaging in influenza B viruses.[809] Goto and colleagues proposed that the 5′ and 3′ noncoding regions act as virus incorporation signals, while the sequences in the coding regions act as bundling signals bringing the eight segments together.[315] Both the coding and noncoding regions of the packaging signals are relatively conserved compared to other parts of the sequences.[275,309] Mutations introduced into the packaging signal region of one segment can result in a decrease in packaging efficiency of the segment itself and of other segments,[415,417,541,572,574] suggesting the existence of specific interactions among genomic segments. Interestingly, data also show that efficient packaging of the NA or NS segment does not absolutely require the original sequences of the packaging signal, while this is required for efficient HA segment packaging.[268,962] In addition, it has been shown that certain segments are preferentially interacting with each other, a mechanism that might play a role in governing the position of each segment in the 1+7 configuration.[150,289,306] Segment-specific packaging is hypothesized to occur via specific RNA–RNA or protein–RNA interactions, but exactly how the packaging signals

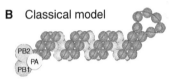

B Classical model

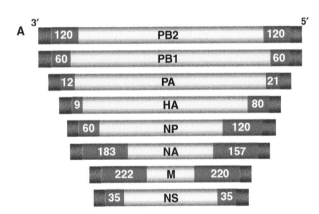

A

C Revised model

NP binds viral RNA in a non-uniform, non-random manner

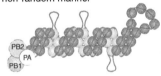

D Proposed model of vRNA-vRNA interaction

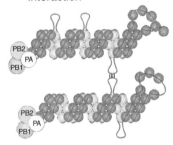

FIGURE 14.21 A: Schematic diagram of the packaging signals on each RNA segment. Each influenza virus RNA segment is depicted with the conserved noncoding regions on both 3′ and 5′ ends. The adjacent numbered domains indicate the number of nucleotides in the coding regions required for effective incorporation of viral RNA (vRNA) into virions. For details, see Refs.[266,267,540,630,682,684,954] (Courtesy of Yoshihiro Kawaoka and updated by Qinshan Gao.) **B:** Model of vRNP structure. The classical model of vRNP is a uniform association of NP to viral RNA. **C:** Recent work[514,521,967] supports a revised model where NP binds viral RNA in a nonuniform manner unique to each viral RNA segment. The nonuniform binding produces regions of viral RNA free of NP and accessible for putative RNA–RNA interactions. **D:** Proposed strategy for intersegmental viral RNA interactions, which likely occur at NP-free sites. (Courtesy of Seema Lakdawala; adapted from Lee N, Le Sage V, Nanni AV, et al. Genome-wide analysis of influenza viral RNA and nucleoprotein association. *Nucleic Acids Res* 2017;45(15):8968–8977.)

participate during the genome packaging process is yet to be determined. Another piece of evidence supporting the specific packaging model is the generation of a rewired influenza virus carrying the HA packaging signal on the NS segment and the NS packaging signal on the HA segment.[291] The modified virus grew well; however, it lost its ability to independently reassort its rewired HA or NS segment with a wild-type (WT) virus, indicating that only viruses containing a full complement of all eight packaging signals will grow to high yields. This model is also supported by data showing specific interference of deleted RNA segments with packaging of the corresponding WT RNA segment but not with any other genome segment.[208,209] Furthermore, segments carrying two different reporter genes but the same packaging signals compete with each other for incorporation into virions and produce viruses that express only one or the other reporter but not both.[421] It has now also been demonstrated that packaging signals, specifically the portions in coding regions, can have a strain-specific component that can limit reassortment and can impact on viral fitness of reassortant viruses.[236,961,962] Recently, a novel hypothesis regarding the concerted packaging of eight distinct genomic segments has emerged. While it was thought that the vRNA interacts uniformly with NP in a beads-on-a-string manner, it has recently been shown using high-throughput sequencing techniques that this binding is relatively heterogeneous leaving loops of RNA free of NP.[521,967] These loops are vulnerable to RNAse digestion in an experimental setting, and loops from different RNPs can freely interact with each other. Sequence-specific interactions between these loops from different RNPs (kissing loops) have been proposed to govern the packaging of eight distinct genomic segments (Fig. 14.21).[300,521,967] These regions include some of the previously identified more canonical packaging sequences.[967] However, since these loops include regions of low genetic conservation, this hypothesis might provide an explanation for reassortment incompatibility between viruses or fitness loss after reassortment.[521,961,967] This model also leaves room for a more active role of NP in determining packaging specificity and may explain why specific NP sequences or mutations may affect reassortment and packaging.[63,83,615] It will be interesting to define the precise sequences, structures, and mechanisms that determine the specific packaging of each segment. Such conserved features must also be compatible with the divergent sequences observed among influenza viruses. Taken together, there is now good evidence for selective packaging of eight distinct genomic segments per virion mediated by packaging/bundling sequences in the 5′ and 3′ noncoding regions as well as the coding regions of the genomic segments.

The Budding Process

Initiation of bud formation requires outward curvature of the plasma membrane (Fig. 14.20). The virus bud is then extruded until the inner core is enveloped. The budding process is completed when the membranes fuse at the base of the bud and the enveloped virus particle is released following fission from the cell membrane.[770,787] It is likely that several of the influenza virus structural proteins contribute to the budding process. HA, NA, and M2, when expressed alone in transfected cells, are all capable of forming VLPs[125,496,1012] although only in the presence of M proteins are HA and NA brought together in filamentous membrane protrusions that resemble budding virus.[139] Although M1 obviously participates in the formation of virus

particles from infected cells, unlike other viral matrix proteins, it does not appear to possess a late domain sequence that mediates interaction with the cellular ESCRT pathway.[87,769,949] It has initially been demonstrated that in the absence of other viral proteins, M1 does not associate with membranes.[935] More recent data suggest that M1 does associate with membranes on its own.[383,526] It is likely a concerted action of all structural components of the virus as well as host factors that brings the components together and initiates budding of authentic virus particles.[526] The extent to which the membrane is extruded before pinching off occurs will affect the size and shape of the virus particle. Generally, influenza virus particles are either spherical or filamentous, and this characteristic morphology is genetically linked to the M segment (Fig. 14.4).[73,226,756,828] It has been further shown that the determinants for a particular filamentous isolate (A/Udorn/72[H3N2]) map to two residues (R95 and E204) in the M1 protein,[73] although other residues in M1 as well as in the cytoplasmic tail of M2 are also involved in regulating morphology.[319,756,757,768,900] Host factors such as polarization and an intact actin cytoskeleton also play a critical role in determining the morphology of virus particles.[492,755,823] The final step of the budding process is membrane scission, which may be facilitated by both viral and cellular factors. The amphipathic helix in the cytoplasmic tail of M2 has been demonstrated to mediate membrane curvature and scission.[579,757,769] Also, the small guanosine triphosphate (GTP)-binding protein, Rab11, has been implicated in this process.[86]

Release

Influenza virus particles have to be actively released after the viral envelope has separated from the cell membrane during the completion of budding. This is because the HA anchors the virus to the cell by binding to sialic acid–containing receptors on the cell surface. The enzymatic activity of the NA protein is required to remove the sialic acid and thereby releases the virus from its host cell. NA activity is also required to remove sialic acid from the carbohydrates present on the viral glycoproteins themselves so that the individual virus particles do not aggregate. The essential function of NA in particle release has been demonstrated through the use of NA inhibitors,[558,688] temperature-sensitive (ts) NA mutant viruses,[688] and NA-deficient viruses.[546] In all cases, the absence of NA enzymatic activity was seen to cause viral particles to amass in clumps at the cell surface (Fig. 14.22), resulting in a loss in infectivity that could be restored by addition of exogenous sialidase. Virions released from infected cells can, as described above, be spherical or filamentous, but often have a pleomorphic character. Recently, it was proposed that morphologically different particles released during infection might be a strategy to survive different environments that fluctuate over different replication cycles.[905]

Due to the fact that both HA and NA recognize the same molecule (sialic acid) but have opposing effects (receptor binding vs. receptor destroying), a delicate balance exists between the HA and NA functions.[929] This is optimized for individual viruses but if disturbed can result in attenuation.[103,301,1008]

The neuraminidase

The NA is the second major glycoprotein of influenza A and B viruses and is a type II integral membrane protein with its N-terminus oriented toward the interior of the virus

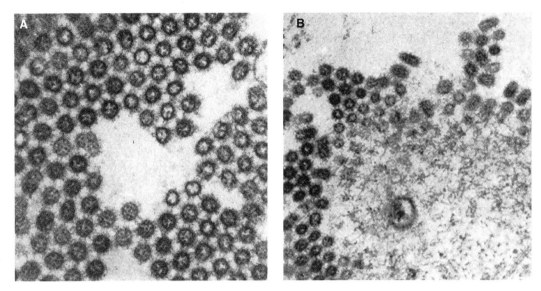

FIGURE 14.22 Aggregate formation of influenza virus particles in the absence of neuraminidase activity. Electron micrograph thin-section images showing aggregates of temperature-sensitive neuraminidase (NA) mutant influenza virus grown at nonpermissive temperature **(A)** or grown in the presence of the neuraminidase inhibitor FANA **(B)**. For details, see Refs.[688,693]

(Fig. 14.23).[154,512,973] The nine subtypes of the A virus NA fall into two major groups (N1, N4, N5, N8 and N2, N3, N6, N7, N9) based on sequence comparisons (Fig. 14.2).[973] In addition, the NA-like proteins from H17N10 and H18N11 viruses do not possess NA activity despite their structural similarity with authentic NAs.[263,892,1047] No subtypes have been found for the NAs of B viruses, possibly because these viruses do not have an animal reservoir. The influenza A virus NAs have a highly conserved short cytoplasmic tail and a hydrophobic transmembrane region, which provides the anchor for the stalk and the head domains. The purified head domain of an N2 NA (obtained by pronase treatment of whole virus) was first crystallized by Graeme Laver, and its x-ray crystallographic structure was solved by Peter Colman.[158] The structure of the N1 NA from the 1918 pandemic virus and of several other NA subtypes has also been determined.[992] The head of the NA is a homotetramer, each monomer of which is composed of six topologically identical β-sheets arranged in a propeller formation. The structure of the influenza B virus neuraminidase, similar to that of the A virus, is characterized by the interaction of the sialic acid ligand with nine conserved active site residues.[101] The enzymatic activity of NA was first recognized by George Hirst, who found that red blood cells treated with virus were refractory to reagglutination by another virus preparation.[385] The enzyme was also found to cleave ketosidically bound sugars of alcohols (at position 2 of neuraminic acid).[90] Neuraminidases from different subtypes are described to have different substrate specificities.[531,728] Transition state inhibitors such as 2-deoxy-2,3-dehydro-*N*-trifluoroacetylneuraminic acid, which mimic the enzymatic substrate, were shown early on to inhibit influenza virus replication,[692] and compounds with the same mechanism of action were later developed for use as highly effective antivirals in humans.[43,195,430,658] Early work had

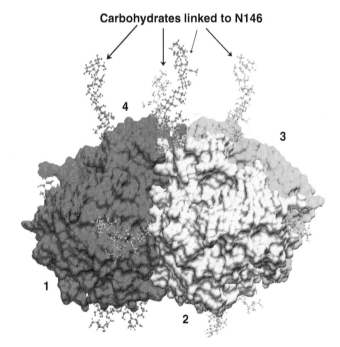

FIGURE 14.23 Molecular surface drawing of the x-ray structure of an N2 neuraminidase head. The neuraminidase is a tetramer made up of a bulky head attached to a slender stalk. A side-on view of the head only is shown consisting of four identical monomers (from this perspective, the two rear monomers, *blue and green*, are mostly hidden). The carbohydrates attached to asparagine residue 146 of each monomer are shown in ball-and-stick model and form antennae-like structures rising from the top of the molecule. For details, see Ref.[911] (Courtesy of Peter Colman.)

also elucidated the function of the NA in virus replication. Cells infected by temperature-sensitive mutants with defects in the NA were shown by EM to have large aggregates of intact virus particles accumulating near the cell surface (Fig. 14.22). This finding was interpreted to mean that the viral NA must remove the sialic/neuraminic acid receptor from the surface of the cell as well as from the virus particles to prevent recognition by the HA of the virus. The NA thus has a role in releasing the virus from the infected cell and in cleansing the environment (e.g., mucus and cell surfaces in the respiratory tract) of sialic acid receptors to allow for virus spread.[688,693] In addition, it has been shown that the viral NA may also play a role early in infection, possibly facilitating entry of the virus[151,583,674,1000] and/or modulating late endosome/lysosome trafficking.[445,868] A role in immunomodulation by interaction with TGF-β has also been proposed.[111,484,793] As described earlier (see Budding Process), the NA can also mediate virus budding[496,1012] and the cellular restriction factor, tetherin, can influence this step.[950,1012] Another function for at least one NA subtype has also been reported. In the case of an N9 NA, a hemadsorption activity was found to be associated with the purified molecule, and x-ray structure analysis revealed a second independent binding site for sialic acid.[910] A similar site has been described for N1 as well,[205] but its relevance in human influenza virus strains remains unclear[903] Of note, mutations in the regular enzymatic site of NA can lead to receptor-binding activity as well, which in some instances can completely replace the receptor-binding activity of HA (but not its fusion mechanism).[395,396,1046]

It is assumed that the function of the influenza B virus NA is similar, if not identical, to that of the A virus NA.[304,559,739] Additionally, the active sites of influenza A and B virus NAs are conserved, which allows for broad-spectrum activity of NA inhibitors. In influenza C and D viruses, the receptor-destroying role of the NA is played by the esterase activity of the viral HEF. By removing the acetyl group from 9-O-acetylneuraminic acid, the HEF facilitates the release and spread of virus from infected cells. In addition, it appears that the enzyme is needed for virus entry, suggesting release of the HEF from cell receptors during the endosomal uptake and fusion/uncoating process.[920]

Like the HA, NA molecules are antigenic and variants are selected in nature.[782] Antibodies directed against the NA are usually not neutralizing, but can be broadly protective in animals and humans.[130,169,216,484,614,975] Immunization with NA preparations has been proposed as an infection-permissive, disease-preventing vaccine approach against influenza, and NA has recently re-emerged as an attractive vaccine antigen.[216,463,484,973,974]

Interactions of Influenza Virus with the Host Cell

Cellular Functions Required for Influenza Virus Replication

A virus with a small coding capacity, such as influenza virus, relies on numerous host cell functions in order to complete its replication cycle. In comparison to our understanding of the role of each viral protein in the influenza virus life cycle, we know relatively little about the contribution of host cell proteins. Some well-characterized interactions between viral and host proteins are noted in the sections covering specific viral proteins (e.g., NP and importin-α, NEP and Crm1, NS1 and CPSF30), but these probably represent only a small fraction of the molecular interactions that occur between influenza virus and its host cell during the viral life cycle. Initial efforts to expand our knowledge of these cellular binding partners have involved a yeast two-hybrid analysis of 10 influenza virus proteins (all except PB1-F2 and PA-X), which identified interactions with 87 human proteins.[800] These interactions exist in a tightly connected network, as 24 of the human proteins interact with two or more viral proteins and there are 51 known interactions occurring between the 87 human proteins. Other studies have examined interacting partners of viral protein complexes rather than individual proteins and particularly those that retain functionality such as the RNP or trimeric polymerase complexes. Forty-one human proteins were reported to interact with the viral RNP complex of influenza A/WSN/33 (H1N1) virus, and 10 interacting proteins were identified in another study using the polymerase complex.[442,584] A large-scale proteomic analysis of an H5N1 influenza virus polymerase complex has revealed an astonishing 859 human proteins that are associated with either the full polymerase complex or PA-containing subcomponents thereof.[78] In their analyses, the authors also distinguished between those interactions that are dependent on RNA and those that are not. In summary, 166 PA interacting proteins, 23 that bind to the PB1-PA dimer and 10 that associate with the full polymerase, were identified irrespective of the presence of RNA. Using RNAi, 31 proteins known for interacting with the vRNP or polymerase complex were assessed for their role in polymerase activity.[69] Eighteen were shown to facilitate the activities of both H1N1 and H5N1 polymerases, while two antagonized both polymerases, supporting the idea that interacting proteins are likely to play functional roles. Recent large-scale studies queried additional interactions between individual viral proteins and the host.[368,746,948]

Completion of the analysis of the human genome and the discovery of RNAi have made it possible to query the participation of each human gene product in functional assays using genome-wide small interfering ribonucleic acid (siRNA) libraries. Using this powerful tool, genome-wide RNAi screens have been performed on influenza virus–infected cells to identify those genes that are required for efficient virus growth.[843,953] These five studies[80,350,451,478,800] identified a total of 1,077 unique genes that when targeted by siRNAs lead to decreased influenza virus replication. Each study employed different assay conditions, and this likely contributes to the finding that only 85 genes were common to two or more of the screens. However, a greater degree of concordance is seen when one analyzes the results at the level of cellular function rather than gene name.[804,843,953] Following these initial studies, many different screens using different technologies including RNAi screens,[49,133,194,201,853] CRISPR screens,[349,366] transcriptomics profiling,[377,788] proteomic screening,[368,543,746,948,1013] kinase profiling,[24,611,832,1002] radiation hybrid mapping,[550] and meta-analysis/network analysis of existing screening data[2,120,898] have been performed. These and many other studies have identified a large number of host and restriction factors that play significant roles in influenza virus interactions with the host cell. Host factors involved in attachment and internalization,[131,184,217,224,269,349,773,1045] endosome trafficking,[321,498,722,749,820,822,996] fusion, uncoating and nuclear import,[34,39,70,212,329,365,519,568,603,669,710,853,1002] transcription and replication,[110,194,235,260,451,509,571,764,812,856,859,899,916,1027] protein synthesis, nuclear export[13,22,145,274,292,403,651,720,730,797,878,951,986] and transport to the bud zone,[12,219,368,457,864,898,937] and packaging, assembling, and budding[187,314,365] have been described above and/or are depicted in Figure 14.24. In addition, important restriction factors including interferon-inducible transmembrane (IFITM) proteins were identified in this manner.[80,237,729,741,1044]

Future progress in this area will depend on integrating the data obtained from these global approaches (e.g., proteomics, RNAi, microarray, CRISPR, etc.) to build a clearer picture of the cellular networks that govern efficient influenza virus

growth. Such information may address questions concerning species specificity and also provide new avenues to explore for drug discovery (see section on Inhibition of Cellular Factors).

The Actions of the NS1 Protein

When a virus infects a cell, it has to contend with the rapid onset of the host innate immune response, whose mission it is to establish an antiviral state within the cell and prevent

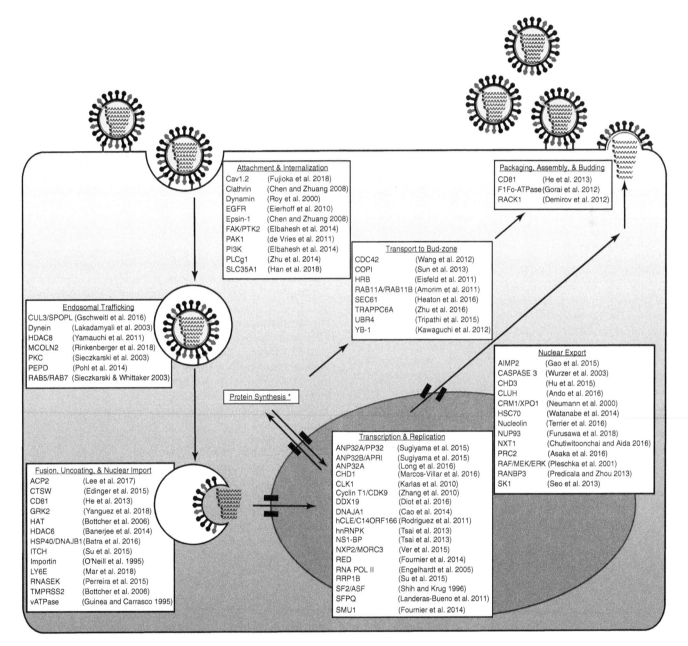

FIGURE 14.24 Host factors of influenza A virus. Shown are a subset of identified host factors required by influenza A virus during different stages of the viral life cycle. Of the depicted cellular proteins, experimental evidence exists indicating that influenza A virus is dependent on the expression/function of the respective protein for productive infection. The listed host factors are categorized based on individual stages of the influenza A virus life cycle during which they exhibit their proviral function: (1) attachment and internalization; (2) endosomal trafficking, fusion, uncoating, and nuclear import; (3) transcription and replication; (4) protein synthesis*; (5) nuclear export; (6) transport to bud zone; and (7) packaging, assembly, and budding. See Ref.[807] for more details. *Influenza A virus depends on a large variety of cellular proteins during viral protein synthesis. However, current screening methodologies for the identification of host factors of IAV involve manipulation of host gene expression. Therefore, proteins crucial for host cell viability, such as proteins involved in translation and protein expression, are usually not identified in such screening efforts. (Courtesy of Silke Stertz, Marie Pohl, and Eva Spieler.)

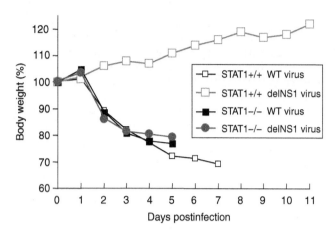

FIGURE 14.25 Pathogenicity of influenza A virus lacking NS1 expression in STAT1−/− mice. Wild-type (STAT1+/+) or STAT1−/− mice were infected with either wild-type (WT) or delNS1 viruses as indicated. DelNS1 virus is apathogenic in STAT1+/+ mice; however, the weight loss (shown in percentage) of delNS1 virus–infected STAT1−/− mice is comparable to that of WT virus–infected mice. DelNS1 and WT virus are equally lethal in STAT1−/− mice. (For details, see Ref.[297]; courtesy of Adolfo García-Sastre.)

virus replication. A critical component of this response is type I interferon (IFN-α/β), which is secreted from virus-infected cells. A characteristic feature of all orthomyxoviruses is their sensitivity to the inhibitory effect of IFN-inducible Mx GTPases.[346] In fact, IFN was first described as a factor induced by heat-inactivated influenza virus,[422] although interestingly, live influenza virus was found to inhibit the induction of IFN by inactivated virus.[545] The reason for this observation did not become clear until almost 40 years later when, with the benefit of reverse genetics technology, it was possible to engineer an influenza A virus that lacked the *NS1* gene (delNS1).[297] This virus displayed unusual growth properties as it was severely attenuated in IFN-competent systems but grew well in IFN-deficient systems such as Vero cells and 6-day-old embryonated eggs and was lethal in STAT1$^{-/-}$ mice (Fig. 14.25).[297,871] Thus, in the absence of an IFN response, NS1 appears to be dispensable, whereas in the context of an immunocompetent host, it is essential. Microarray analysis has demonstrated that infection with delNS1 virus leads to enhanced expression of IFN and IFN-regulated genes compared to WT influenza virus infection,[303] and NS1 is therefore termed an *IFN antagonist* because it acts to suppress the virus-induced host IFN response.[340,977] These findings have given rise to a new concept for the design of live attenuated vaccines based on mutations in the NS1 gene.[689,690,748,871] Studies on viruses expressing truncated forms of NS1 have shown that the level of attenuation is determined by the amount of IFN induced by the virus (i.e., highly attenuated viruses induce larger quantities of IFN)[37,243,737,833,871] and immunization with these mutant viruses produced protective immunity in mice, chickens, swine, horses, and macaques.[667,748]

Structural features of the NS1 protein
NS1 is a nuclear, dimeric protein that is highly expressed in infected cells and has a dsRNA-binding domain, an effector domain, and a disordered tail.[345,668] The RNA-binding domain lies within the N-terminal 73 amino acids,[735] for which both

NMR and crystal structures have been obtained.[134,135,548,1009] These data indicate that the NS1 RNA-binding domain forms a symmetric homodimer with a six-helical fold and that conserved tracks consisting of basic and hydrophilic residues on each monomer mediate interactions with dsRNA. Mutational analysis has further demonstrated that dimer formation is crucial for RNA binding as are residues R38, R35, and R46.[134,941] Residue K41 strongly enhances the binding affinity[941] and residues S42 and T49 also participate in dsRNA binding.[134] It is suggested that the basic residues make contact with the phosphate backbone of the RNA via electrostatic interactions,[136,941,1009] which is consistent with the observed lack of sequence specificity.[356,735] Structural data indicate that the NS1 dimer spans the major groove of canonical A-form dsRNA in a length-independent mode.[134] Structures of the influenza B virus NS1 RNA-binding domain indicate a similar binding mode.[1009]

The remaining portion of NS1 has been termed the effector domain and includes binding sites for several host factors (Fig. 14.26).[345] Crystallographic structures of the NS1 effector domain have been determined for several influenza A virus strains. While the monomer conformation is very similar, different dimer interfaces have been determined, specifically one that is mediated by a helix–helix interaction[17,341,458,987] and another mediated by a strand–strand interaction.[67,459] The helix–helix interaction is dependent on residue W187 in each monomer,[341,988] and it has been proposed that the monomer interface can twist and therefore the dimer can exist in both open and closed conformations.[458] Finally, one structure of a full-length NS1 protein has been reported.[68] Strikingly, instead of individual dimers, NS1 is shown to form a chain with alternating interactions occurring via the dsRNA-binding and effector domains. Moreover, three of these chains are shown to interact with one another to form a tubular structure that can accommodate dsRNA in its center. This chain-like structure opens up questions regarding how interactions between NS1 and its cellular partners can be accommodated, but models for how this may occur in the context of an individual NS1 dimer have been proposed.[458]

Inhibition of the interferon synthesis
WT influenza virus infection induces far less IFN than does delNS1 virus, and this difference lies at the level of mRNA molecules.[303,870,938] This implies that NS1 either acts to prevent the synthesis of IFN mRNA or destabilizes IFN mRNA (Figs. 14.25 and 14.26). The transcriptional activation of IFN-β in response to virus infection is regulated by transcription factors including interferon-regulatory factor-3 (IRF3), nuclear factor-κB (NF-κB), and activator protein-1 (AP-1).[668] Each one of these transcription factors has been shown to be activated in delNS1 virus–infected cells but not in WT virus–infected cells,[554,870,938] which corresponds with the differential induction of IFN-β by these viruses. Moreover, expression of NS1 alone inhibits the activation of the IFN-β promoter in response to infection with a heterologous virus or even delNS1 virus.[554,938] Substantial progress has been made to understand the precise mechanism by which NS1 suppresses IFN synthesis[340,345] (Fig. 14.26). First, dsRNA binding is important as expression of the RNA-binding domain alone is sufficient to block virus induction of IFN.[938] However, a virus expressing only the first 73 residues is still attenuated in mice (with a phenotype intermediate to that of delNS1 and WT virus), pointing to a role for

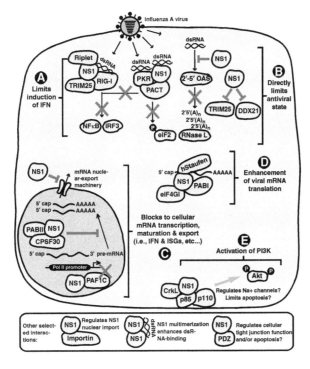

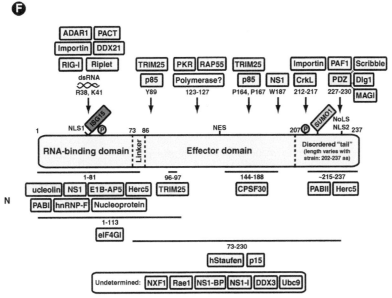

FIGURE 14.26 Schematic diagram of the multiple functions of NS1 within infected cells. A: Pretranscriptional limitation of interferon-β (IFN-β) induction. **B:** Inhibition of the antiviral properties of protein kinase R (PKR) and 2′-5′-oligoadenylate synthetase (OAS)/RNase L. **C:** Posttranscriptional block to processing and nuclear export of all cellular messenger RNAs (mRNAs). **D:** Enhancement of viral mRNA translation. **E:** Activation of phosphatidylinositol 3-kinase (PI3K). Some other interactions that have been characterized are detailed in the *lower box.* See Refs.[27,345,468,570,668] for details (Adapted from Hale BG, Randall RE, Ortin J, et al. The multifunctional NS1 protein of influenza A viruses. *J Gen Virol* 2008;89(Pt 10):2359–2376; courtesy of Ben Hale.). **F:** Schematic representation of the influenza A virus NS1 protein, together with its known interactors. The influenza A virus NS1 protein (*yellow*) is 202 to 237 amino acids long depending on the strain. The N-terminal 73 amino acids form a functional RNA-binding domain, while the effector domain predominantly mediates interactions with host cell proteins. The final C-terminal approximately 20 amino acids appear to be natively unstructured. NS1 contains two nuclear localization sequences (NLS1 and NLS2) and a nuclear export signal (NES). A nucleolar localization sequence (NoLS) has been reported for some strains and is concomitant with NLS2. The interaction of NS1 with itself to form homomultimers via both the RNA-binding domain and effector domain (W187) is important for function. Residues involved in RNA binding (Arg-38 [R38] and Lys-41 [K41]) are implicated in the inhibition of 2′-5′-oligoadenylate synthetase/RNase L, Jun N-terminal kinase, and RIG-I/TRIM25. Additionally, NS1 contains binding sites for poly(A)-binding protein I (PABPI), p85β, importin-α, nucleolin, NS1-BP, eIF4GI, hStaufen, NS1-I, PKR, PACT, hnRNP-F, Ubc9, CPSF30, poly(A)-binding protein II (PABPII), Crk/CrkL, PDZ domain–containing proteins (e.g., Scribble, Dlg-1, PDlim2, and the MAGIs), the viral polymerase/nucleoprotein, and components of the cellular messenger RNA (mRNA) nuclear export machinery (E1B-AP5, p15, NXF1, and Rae1). Several posttranslational modifications to NS1 have also been described: ISG15 modification (*red*) by the interferon (IFN)-inducible Herc5 protein mediates negative effects on NS1 function, while phosphorylation and sumoylation (*green*) appear to enhance NS1 function. See Refs.[27,345,468,570,668] for details. (Adapted from Hale BG, Randall RE, Ortin J, et al. The multifunctional NS1 protein of influenza A viruses. *J Gen Virol* 2008;89(Pt 10):2359–2376; courtesy of Ben Hale.)

the effector domain *in vivo*.[243,871,932] Alanine substitution of the residues involved in RNA binding (R38 and K41) was found to significantly reduce the ability of NS1 to inhibit IRF3 and NF-κB activation[870,938] and, hence, IFN-β synthesis.[198] In the context of a virus, lack of NS1 resulted in increased IFN-β production and, therefore, an attenuated phenotype in mice (Fig. 14.25).[198] Second, NS1 is found in complex with the cytoplasmic sensor RIG-I and acts to prevent RIG-I signaling and IFN-β production.[330,601,680,715] This interaction appears to depend on the same residues implicated in dsRNA binding, indicating that it is potentially mediated by RNA.[715] Third, NS1 interacts with TRIM25 via residues E96 and E97.[280] TRIM25 is responsible for ubiquitinating and activating RIG-I and the presence of NS1 blocks this activity (Fig. 14.26). However, *in vivo*, different influenza viruses show different patterns of interferon inhibition,[740] which are difficult to reconcile based on the known mechanism of action in tissue culture.[488] Dozens of different host factors involved in the suppression of the IFN response by NS1 have been identified.[668]

Inhibition of host mRNA processing

Influenza virus–infected cells harbor pre-mRNAs in their nuclei that do not undergo efficient 3′-end processing and therefore cannot be exported.[126,815] This is thought to be an NS1-mediated effect that occurs via interaction of the NS1 effector domain with two components of the 3′-end processing machinery: the 30-kD subunit of the cleavage and polyadenylation specificity factor (CPSF)[179,473,647] and the poly(A)-binding protein II (PABII).[126,340,345,490] The NS1 interaction effectively inhibits these processing factors and results in pre-mRNAs that either remain uncleaved[647,815] or only acquire short poly(A) tails.[126] NS1 also inhibits splicing of pre-mRNAs, which also results in their retention in the nucleus,[258,552] and evidence for the requirement of CPSF in splicing suggests that both of these mRNA-processing defects in influenza virus–infected cells may be related to the inhibition of CPSF (Fig. 14.26).[532] NS1 also interferes with mRNA export via complex formation with several components of the nuclear export machinery.[783] As the induction of the host antiviral response relies so heavily on transcriptional up-regulation of genes, this global posttranscriptional inhibition may aid in aborting or at least delaying the onset of this response. This is reflected in data from a CPSF-binding mutant virus, which is attenuated in tissue culture and which causes an earlier induction of antiviral gene products compared to WT virus.[661] It should be noted, however, that the delNS1 virus shows shutoff of host protein synthesis at levels similar to that of WT virus in an A/PR/8/34 background (which cannot bind to CPSF40).[781] This suggests that other (or additional) factors may be responsible for inhibition of general gene expression.[675,930]

Additional NS1 interactions with host cell factors

The influenza A virus NS1 protein binds directly to the p85β regulatory subunit of PI3K via its C-terminal effector domain, and NS1 expression is sufficient to activate PI3K signaling.[215,343,818] Specifically, residues Y89, M93, P164, P167, L141, and E142 in the NS1 protein, which are located in predicted src homology 2 (SH2)- and SH3-binding motifs, have been implicated in the interaction with p85β.[343,530,817,818] The NS1-binding site on p85β is located in an inter-SH2 domain,[342] and a cocrystal of the NS1 effector domain in complex with this

region of p85β shows that residues Y89 and P167 of NS1 are at the binding interface.[344] Furthermore, a model of a heterotrimeric complex consisting of NS1–p85β–p110 predicts that the presence of NS1 would disrupt the inhibitory contact between p85β and p110.[344] This explains the PI3K-activating properties of NS1, which theoretically serve to delay apoptosis at late stages of infection.[213] However, recombinant viruses expressing NS1 proteins that fail to activate PI3K were not seen to induce any more apoptosis than WT virus, so the biological significance of NS1-mediated PI3K activation remains unclear.[432] It also should be noted that a proapoptotic activity of NS1 has been reported.[792]

NS1 has also been reported to interact with several other host factors (Fig. 14.26), including the eukaryotic translation initiation factor 4GI, poly(A)-binding protein I, Staufen, NS1-I and NS1-BP, nucleolin, hnRNP-F, E1B-AP5, Herc5, PABII, importin-α, CrkL, Scribble, Dlg1, PDLim2, p15, NXF1, Rae1, PACT, Ubc9, and others.[16,99,126,238,310,370,401,547,596,631,783,789,875,978,979,1015,1029,1033] It has been shown that disruption of the Staufen-1/NS1 interaction inhibits influenza virus replication, indicating that this virus–host interaction is required for optimal virus growth.[522] Furthermore, it has been shown that NS1 can act like a histone mimic.[569]

Anti-interferon proteins of influenza B, C, and D viruses; thogoto virus; and isavirus

Like its A virus counterpart, the NS1 protein of influenza B virus (B/NS1) exists as a dimer and has RNA-binding activity in its N-terminal domain (residues 1–93).[199,936,1016] A virus lacking B/NS1 has also been demonstrated to induce larger amounts of IFN than WT virus,[180] and the B/NS1 protein can complement the growth of influenza A delNS1 virus,[199] indicating that A/NS1 and B/NS1 are functional equivalents. Therefore, as described for influenza A virus, recombinant influenza B viruses either lacking NS1 or expressing truncated NS1 proteins have been proposed as vaccine candidates.[338,981] Expression of B/NS1 has been shown to inhibit virus activation of the IFN-β promoter,[180,199] but interestingly, both N- and C-terminal domains of the protein encode this inhibitory activity, and hence RNA binding was found not to be essential for inhibition of IFN-β synthesis.[199] However, in the context of expression of the N-terminal domain alone, RNA binding was required. Similarly, both portions of B/NS1 were shown to independently inhibit virus activation of the transcription factor, IRF3.[199] B/NS1 is also an inhibitor of PKR, but unlike A/NS1, it does not interfere with mRNA processing.[936] B/NS1 does possess the unique ability to bind to *ISG15* (an IFN-inducible gene) and prevent its conjugation to target proteins,[1018] which it does through its N-terminal domain independently of RNA binding.[435,1016,1035] Structural analysis shows that a dimer of the B/NS1 N-terminal domain interacts with two ISG15 molecules, with each ISG15 molecule binding distinct regions of each NS1 monomer.[323] ISG15 conjugation or ISGylation has been shown to regulate the IFN signaling pathway and to be critical for host antiviral defense.[565,750,1031] Interestingly, B/NS1 inhibits ISGylation in a species-specific manner, binding only to human and nonhuman primate ISG15 proteins.[836,917] This likely contributes to the fact that influenza B infections are restricted to humans. The influenza B virus NS1 protein may also have a role in virus replication as the virus lacking B/NS1 grows to lower titers, even in IFN-deficient cells.[180] It has also been shown that B/NS1 associates with nuclear speckles and that this is linked to residues in its N-terminal region.[789]

The C/NS1 has been shown to inhibit RIG-I–mediated activation of the IFN-β promoter through a region located in its C-terminus.[686] C/NS1 has also been shown to up-regulate splicing of viral mRNAs.[625] While no data are available, similar mechanisms are probably used by influenza D virus since it expresses a D/NS1 protein.[855]

Unlike the influenza viruses, Thogoto virus has no NS segment and instead, its anti-IFN activity is encoded by the M segment.[336] The M segment produces the M protein from a spliced transcript and the ML protein from an unspliced transcript, of which the latter has been shown to be an IFN antagonist protein.[336,474] As seen with the delNS1 influenza virus, a recombinant Thogoto virus lacking the ML protein was shown to induce far greater levels of IFN in infected cells than WT virus[336] and was remarkably attenuated in mice expressing functional Mx1 (an IFN-inducible protein that protects against orthomyxovirus infection).[714] ML has also been demonstrated to inhibit virus-induced activation of IRF3 but in a manner distinct from that of NS1.[434] Another striking difference between ML and NS1 is that ML is a structural protein.[335] Because expression of ML is controlled by the same promoter as that of the M protein (which is expressed late in infection), this strategy ensures that ML is present (as part of the incoming virion) at the initial stages of virus infection when it can most effectively exert its effect on the host immune response.[335]

The isavirus IFN antagonist proteins are expressed from the unspliced transcript of RNA segment 7 and the larger ORF of RNA segment 8.[167,295,886]

The Actions of the PB1-F2 Protein

Influenza A viruses can express an 11th protein, PB1-F2, which is encoded by the +1 alternate ORF in the *PB1* gene.[122,448,480] PB1-F2 is 87 to 90 aa long, depending on the virus strain, and is expressed by most human H3N2 viruses, while a large number of human H1N1 isolates have a premature stop codon in the PB1-F2 ORF. Of note, the pandemics that occurred in 1918, 1957, and 1968 were all caused by influenza viruses that express full-length PB1-F2 and so do many zoonotic influenza viruses.[10] The protein has been shown to contribute to influenza virus pathogenicity through several mechanisms. Initially, a proapoptotic function was described for PB1-F2. It was found to localize to the mitochondria and disturb the mitochondrial membrane potential, leading to the efflux of cytochrome c into the cytoplasm.[122,305] The induction of apoptosis by PB1-F2 is thought to occur specifically in immune cells in a strain-dependent manner and, thus, contribute to immune evasion by influenza viruses.[91,122,585,1020] It was demonstrated that PB1-F2 triggers an apoptotic response by interacting with the mitochondrial adenine nucleotide translocase 3 (ANT3) and voltage-dependent anion channel 1 (VDAC1) proteins[1019] and/or forms pores via self-oligomerization (Fig. 14.27).[89,117,375]

In addition to its proapoptotic activity, PB1-F2 was reported to have proinflammatory properties. Specifically, it was observed that PB1-F2–expressing viruses increase the levels of several cytokines and chemokines, enhance cell infiltration, and exacerbate lung injury in infected mice.[163,164,585,586] Notably, it was found that a serine (S) at position 66 in the PB1-F2 protein dramatically increases immunopathology and mortality caused by the 1918 pandemic strain and by highly

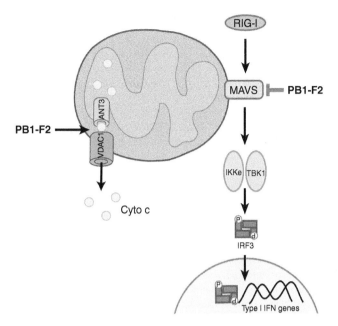

FIGURE 14.27 The proapoptotic and anti-interferon activities of the influenza A virus protein PB1-F2. The protein promotes apoptosis by interacting with the mitochondrial VDAC1 and ANT3 proteins and interferes with the induction of interferon at the level of the MAVS adaptor protein. Cyto c, cytochrome c. (Courtesy of Zsuzsanna T. Varga.)

pathogenic H5N1 viruses.[164] Transcriptional profiling of mice infected with a PB1-F2 N66S-expressing virus revealed an early suppression of interferon-stimulated genes (ISGs),[163] and *in vitro* studies demonstrated an anti-interferon activity of PB1-F2 at the level of the MAVS adaptor protein (Fig. 14.27).[909] Interestingly, PB1-F2 N66S, which is associated with increased pathogenicity, inhibited the induction of IFN more efficiently than a WT PB1-F2 protein.[909] It is hypothesized that there may be a possible link between the proapoptotic and anti-interferon functions of PB1-F2 through the MAVS protein.[908]

The Actions of the PA-X Protein

Recently, a novel protein translated from the PA segment has been discovered and named PA-X.[433] This protein consists of the N-terminal 191 amino acids of PA plus additional amino acids that are added from an alternative reading frame. At the codon for amino acid 191, a +1 ribosomal frameshift occurs resulting in attachment of 41 or 61 novel amino acids to the N-terminus of PA.[246,810] The N-terminus of PA, which is retained in PA-X, hosts the endonuclease domain of the protein.[188] It has been shown that PA-X has cap-snatching activity, which induces degradation of host mRNA and leads to shutoff of the host protein expression.[188] The first 15 amino acids of the C-terminus of PA-X are also actively involved in this activity.[361,675] It is assumed that the main activity of PA-X takes place in the nucleus, but mRNA degradation in the cytoplasm by this protein has also been demonstrated.[361,668,676] Importantly, the shutoff of host mRNA translation leads to suppression of the antiviral response and disables antiviral stress-induced arrest.[362,461] NS1 also has mRNA translation shutoff activity and it was recently reported that there is an interplay between NS1 and PA-X that modulates pathogenesis and suppression of the innate immune response.[114,668] While NS1 shutoff activity seems to be more targeted toward antiviral gene expression, the PA-X activity has been described as relatively unspecific but with a preference for RNA polymerase II–transcribed mRNA in the nucleus.[114,462] Strong activity of both proteins can decrease viral fitness and pathogenesis suggesting that the effect of PA-X activity on virulence might be strain specific and dependent on NS1.[668]

The Role of Other Accessory Proteins

Several additional accessory proteins or putative ORFs have been described for influenza A viruses including PB2-S1, PB1-N40, PA-N155, PA-N182, M42, NS3, and ORF NEG8.[912] A hallmark of accessory proteins is that they are not required for virus replication and might not be expressed by all strains. PB2-S1 is a splice variant that includes the 462 N-terminal of PB2 plus 46 additional amino acids from a +1 ORF. It is found in pandemic H1N1 viruses but not seasonal H3N2 or prepandemic seasonal H1N1 viruses, and its biological function is unclear.[998] PB1-N40 is a truncated version of PB1 that lacks the N-terminal 39 amino acids and starts at PB1 methionine 40.[970] The lack of the N-terminus ablates its ability to interact with PA and its proposed role is in regulation of PB1 and PB1-F2 expression.[876] PA-N155 and PA-N182 are proteins expressed from the PA segment, lack the N-terminal endonuclease domain of PA, and start at methionines 155 and 182 of PA, respectively.[876] Their deletion has been shown to have a slightly negative impact on virus replication and pathogenicity, but no specific function has been assigned to them.[629] In addition to the M segment splice variant that forms the M2 mRNA, two more splice variants, M mRNA3 and M mRNA4, have been detected.[814,971] M mRNA3 does not encode a protein, but mRNA4 has been predicted to encode a protein named M4.[814] A variant of this predicted protein, M42, was indeed found in a mutated virus lacking M2 (through deletion of the M mRNA2 splice donor site) and functionally replaced M2. This is not surprising since M42 is basically M2 with a variant ectodomain.[971] Similarly, a splice variant of the NS segment has been detected that translates into the NS3 protein, which is a NS1 protein isoform with a large deletion in its effector domain.[796] Again, the function of this protein is unknown and it is only encoded by a very small number of natural viral isolates. Finally, the enigmatic NEG8 ORF is a highly conserved antisense direction ORF of the NS segment. The putative approximately 25-kDa protein it might encode was termed NSP and is predicted to have a signal peptide, two TMDs, and an N-linked glycosylation motif.[778] However, despite significant efforts, this protein has never been detected in infected cells except for a T-cell response.[30,381,912] It remains unclear if influenza viruses express additional accessory proteins with significant functionality. Especially for influenza B, C, and D viruses, this area is not well explored.

Reverse Genetics

Because the *Orthomyxoviridae* are negative-strand RNA viruses, introduction of the genomic RNAs into cells does not result in the formation of infectious virus (as it does in the case of positive-strand RNA viruses). Initial experiments eventually leading to the genetic engineering of influenza viruses involved the reconstitution of functional RNP complexes *in vitro*[392,700] and transfection of functional RNPs into cells. In these experiments, cDNA-derived RNA for a specific segment was mixed with purified virion NP and polymerase proteins and transfected into cells before or after infection with a helper influenza virus

in order to provide the remaining vRNP segments.[560] Initially, rescue of infectious virus containing the cDNA-derived RNA required selection of the novel virus against the helper virus.[233] Instead of using cDNA-derived RNA, cells can be transfected with a plasmid construct containing the gene of interest flanked by an RNA polymerase I promoter and terminator sequences. Cellular RNA polymerase I normally transcribes rRNA (which lacks a 5′ cap and 3′ poly[A] tail), and therefore the RNA synthesized from the plasmid construct is an exact replica of the vRNA. The viral polymerase proteins were supplied by transfection with polymerase II–driven expression plasmids, and the remaining genomic segments were provided by infection with a helper influenza virus.[654,719] A disadvantage of these early systems was the need for helper virus, which must be selected against in order to isolate the rescued virus.

In 1999, a decade after the initial influenza reverse genetics system had been described, Fodor et al.[251] and Neumann et al.[653] reported the generation of influenza viruses entirely from cloned cDNAs. In the system reported by Fodor et al., cDNA from each of the eight genome segments was cloned in negative orientation between a truncated human RNA polymerase I promoter and the hepatitis delta virus ribozyme.[251] Transfection of the eight vRNA-encoding plasmids into Vero cells along with four polymerase II–driven plasmids expressing NP and the polymerase complex (PB1, PB2, PA) resulted in recovery of infectious virus (Fig. 14.28). As helper virus is not required for the generation of recombinant virus, the cumbersome selection process was unnecessary. Improvements to this system now include the transfection of cocultured 293T cells (necessary due to the human RNA polymerase I promoter) and Madin-Darby Canine Kidney (MDCK) cells, which support high levels of virus replication.[652]

Further improvements to these systems were reported in which only eight plasmids were required.[389,390] The plasmids contained cDNAs of genomic segments cloned in negative orientation with a human RNA polymerase I promoter at the 5′ end and the mouse RNA polymerase I terminator at the 3′ end. The cellular RNA polymerase I was responsible for copying the cDNA into vRNA. Downstream of the RNA polymerase I terminator was a CMV immediate-early promoter. A polyadenylation sequence was inserted at the other end, giving rise to a polymerase II–driven mRNA transcript from the opposite DNA strand. Expressed viral proteins and vRNAs then assembled in the transfected cells and resulted in the formation of infectious virus derived entirely from only eight plasmids. A single plasmid containing the cDNAs of all eight RNAs resulted in the generation of infectious virus when transfected into human cells.[650] Most likely, transcription of mRNA-like molecules occurred from this plasmid, which then gave rise to the formation of the complementing viral polymerase proteins. These proteins, together with the full-length vRNA segments (also transcribed from the plasmid), allowed rescue of fully infectious virus. Another one-plasmid system was developed for the rescue of influenza A viruses in chicken cells.[1025] Other modifications of the rescue system involve the use of uncloned PCR-amplified products, which obviates possible problems in cloning toxic sequences,[200,1042,1043] and the use of adenovirus as a vector to deliver the required plasmid constructs.[683] In past studies, others have demonstrated that reducing the number of required plasmids for rescue could greatly increase virus recovery.[650,1025] Therefore, two plasmids, termed pRS A/PR8 7 segment and pRS B/Mal04

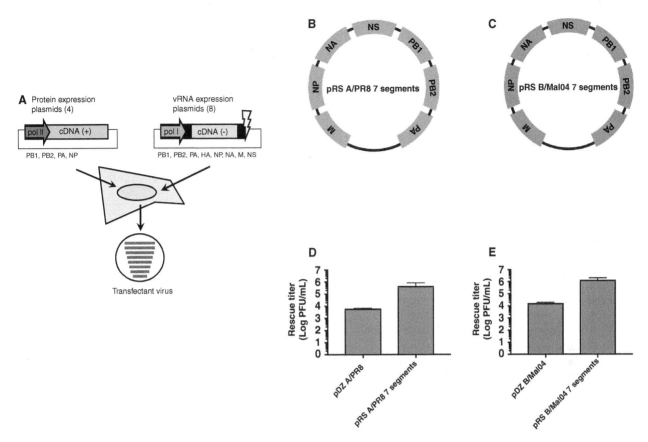

FIGURE 14.28 A: Schematic representation of the plasmid-based rescue system for influenza A virus. The negative-sense complementary DNA (cDNA) for each viral segment is cloned between a polymerase I promoter and the hepatitis delta virus ribozyme or polymerase I terminator. These eight plasmids are transfected into mammalian cells along with four expression plasmids for the polymerase proteins and nucleoprotein (NP). The resulting transfectant virus is then passaged on fresh cells. For details, see Ref.[251] (Courtesy of Adolfo García-Sastre.) The plasmid-based rescue system can be optimized by combining bidirectional (including Pol I and Pol II promoters) transcription cassettes for multiple genomic segments onto one plasmid. Examples include pRS A/PR8 7 for influenza A virus **(B)** and pRS B/Mal04 for influenza B virus **(C)**, which contain seven genomic segments (PB2, PB1, PA, NP, NA, M, NS) and can be combined with a second plasmid encoding the HA of choice. These optimized rescue systems result in increased rescue efficiency as compared to the eight-plasmid pDZ system **(D and E**, respectively).[272] Segments are not to scale but show their order within the plasmid backbone. (Courtesy of Weina Sun.)

7 segment, were generated for the A/PR8 (H1N1) and B/Mal04 (Vic/87) viruses, respectively (Fig. 14.28B, C). The plasmids contain all of the segments of the influenza viral genome except HA. Viral rescue with this system requires only two plasmids: the pRS 7 segment plasmid and an additional plasmid encoding the HA segment. Transfection of the pRS rescue system results in an approximately 2-log increase in rescue titer over the conventional methodology (Fig. 14.28D, E).[272] De Wit et al.[185] designed a rescue system built on transcription by the T7 polymerase, which allows the rescue of influenza viruses in practically all cells independent of the species origin.

Influenza viruses expressing foreign genes have also been generated, demonstrating the use of influenza virus as a vector to deliver foreign antigens to the immune system. Numerous approaches have been successful for the expression of foreign antigens by influenza viruses. These include (a) replacement of the antigenic domains of either the influenza HA or NA glycoproteins with epitopes from foreign proteins[536,538] and (b) modification of existing viral genomic segments to express influenza viral proteins fused to other foreign proteins. These polyproteins can then be subsequently cleaved into two separate proteins. Also reported was the rescue of an influenza virus that expresses an uncleaved chimeric HA with a 140–amino acid insertion of the receptor-binding domain of the *Bacillus anthracis*–protective antigen (PA),[534] (c) replacement of ectodomains of surface glycoproteins with those of foreign glycoproteins,[247] and (d) preparation of viruses with foreign antigens encoded by a ninth RNA segment.[296,351,652,705]

Advantages of influenza viruses over other viruses for the expression of foreign proteins include the fact that influenza viruses are extremely safe as a nonintegrating and nononcogenic virus. Infection with influenza viruses also elicit a strong and long-lasting immune response, and thus recombinant influenza viruses may be useful as vaccine vectors in the future. The limitations related to the use of influenza viruses for the expression of foreign antigens include the limited (but not yet well-defined) capacity of influenza viruses to express foreign sequences and the requirement for packaging signals on both the 5′ and 3′ ends of the vRNA, which may interfere with the expression of foreign genes.

The advances in reverse genetics technology have been of great benefit to the study of structure/function of different influenza virus genes and their proteins. In many cases, the definitive role of a gene or of a domain (or even of a single amino acid) can only be explored by introducing appropriate mutations into the genome of the virus and then analyzing the phenotype of the rescued virus. As discussed, rescue systems have been described for influenza A viruses[296,524,578] and B viruses.[388,429,431] Also, rescue systems have now been developed for influenza C viruses.[171,626,627,685] Influenza viruses have been generated that express chimeric (type A/B) HAs and NAs. For example, such viruses may express, in a type A genetic background, the extracellular portion (ectodomain) of an influenza B HA and/or NA.[247,397,399] These findings show that the HA and NA of an influenza A virus can be functionally replaced with the corresponding protein from an influenza B virus. In turn, viruses have been made in the influenza B virus background expressing proteins derived from influenza A viruses.[337] By taking advantage of the knowledge about packaging sequences, influenza A viruses have been made to contain nine segments expressing an H1 and an H3 HA[290] or only seven segments.[288] In the latter virus, the HA and the NA have been replaced by the HEF protein of an influenza C virus. Whole-organ imaging and analysis of infected cells are now facilitated by chimeric influenza viruses that express a green fluorescent protein (GFP) molecule for visualization of influenza virus–infected cells.[175,271,367,452,453,566,694,896,897] Reverse genetics has also been successfully used to rescue an influenza virus expressing all eight genes of the "extinct" 1918 pandemic virus, which has allowed its extraordinary virulence to be studied.[695,901]

Reverse genetics has also helped in designing improved influenza virus vaccines.[666] The live attenuated pH1N1 2009 vaccine was made from a plasmid-generated strain, into which HA gene mutations were introduced to give high yields without changing the antigenicity of the strain.[129] Also, killed and live pandemic H5N1 virus vaccines were prepared using reverse genetics, allowing the removal of the basic peptide from the HA cleavage site, to make the strains used for manufacturing less virulent.[398]

Thogoto virus, which has six negative-strand RNA segments, has also been rescued by a reverse genetics system.[472,927] The vRNAs were transcribed from the plasmids under the control of a polymerase I promoter, and the structural proteins were expressed from six plasmids driven by a T7 polymerase promoter in the presence of a T7 vaccinia recombinant.

Inhibitors of Influenza Viruses

Because influenza viruses remain a constant health threat, major efforts have been directed at discovering effective antivirals over the past several decades. Presently, there are seven drugs available for use in humans: amantadine, rimantadine, oseltamivir, zanamivir, peramivir, laninamivir (in Japan), and baloxavir marboxil (Fig. 14.29). Past and current approaches to antiviral therapy are briefly discussed here (according to the steps in the viral replication cycle targeted by each drug). Extensive reviews cover the vast literature on this subject.[38,50,64,157,190,302,363,430,481,754,805]

Inhibition of Attachment and Uncoating

While vaccination, in essence, targets the HA so that specific antibodies are generated that block attachment of the virus to the receptor, drugs that interfere with the HA–sialic acid interaction have not been successfully developed.[1023] This is perhaps

surprising because the x-ray crystallographic structures of the HA and of HA–ligand complexes have now been known for decades. In principle, such an approach could work,[140,308] but this strategy, using sialic acid analogs (or polymers bearing sialic acids), has not led to an FDA-approved drug. Whether removal of receptor molecules from the respiratory tract by administration of exogenous sialidase/neuraminidase is a viable antiviral approach remains to be seen. A sialidase fusion protein, DAS181, has been shown to be an effective antiviral strategy in tissue culture and animal models.[48,510] Ongoing clinical trials with this drug will demonstrate if it is effective in humans.[1024]

Quinone derivatives that prevent the first stage of the conformational change of the HA and thus inhibit infection were discovered in 1993,[62] and other compounds with a similar mechanism showed inhibition for some strains but not for others.[177,839] Additional examples include Arbidol (umifenovir) and S20.[59,446,960] Compounds have also been identified that appear to push the HA into an inactive state[386] or that associate with the N-terminal heptad-repeat trimer, thus interfering with the *trimer of hairpin* (helix bundle) formation.[147] This latter approach would be similar to that successfully applied for human immunodeficiency virus (HIV) using the fusion inhibitor T-20.[464] In addition, several other approaches aimed at preventing virus attachment have been reported.[283,331,525,617,779,827,838] Nitazoxanide (a thiazolide) is thought to prevent terminal glycosylation of HA and thereby impair HA maturation and trafficking to the cell surface.[481,767] Of these approaches, Arbidol is currently used in humans in Russia and China and nitazoxanide is in late-stage clinical trials.

Monoclonal antibodies that broadly bind to the HA and block attachment to sialic acid receptors or fusion between viral and endosomal membranes and/or work via effector functions have recently been discovered and might also serve as therapeutics. A number of these antibodies are currently in clinical development.[634,985] Insights from these monoclonal antibodies have also been used to design and engineer small proteins that block attachment or fusion.[248,475,852,964] In addition, multidomain camelid antibody constructs capable of blocking both fusion and attachment have been developed as well.[511] Polyclonal antibodies in the form of influenza-specific human intravenous immunoglobulin (IVIG) are currently tested in clinical trials as well.[760]

Another approach concerns the inhibition of the posttranslational cleavage of the HA, which results in a molecule unable to undergo the conformational change required for fusion/uncoating. Several exogenous protease inhibitors have been investigated,[47,71,518,1040,1041] of which aprotinin has been found to be effective in humans.[1038] Drugs belonging to this general class have been successful against HIV but have not been further developed for widespread therapeutic or prophylactic use against influenza virus in humans.

Amantadine, which has been known for many decades to inhibit most influenza A viruses, has been found to target the M2 ion channel (for details, see M2 Protein and Fig. 14.28A). During uptake, virus enters endosomes where the acid pH activates the ion channel, resulting in the transport of protons into the viral interior. This process, which is required for the dissociation of the RNP complex from the M1 protein and subsequent release of the RNP into the cytoplasm, is blocked by amantadine and its derivatives (including rimantadine;

Fig. 14.28B).[718,958] In addition, amantadine can affect the pH regulation of vesicles involved in the transport of viral glycoproteins to the cell surface during assembly.[841] Thus, there are two possible steps at which amantadine can exert an antiviral effect: uncoating and HA stability (in some strains) during transport in vesicles. Unfortunately, resistance to amantadine and to its 10-fold more active derivative, rimantadine, develops with increased use in humans and animals.[613] In fact, according to Centers for Disease Control and Prevention (CDC) guidelines, adamantanes are not recommended for clinical use as of 2018/2019.

Inhibitors of the Viral Replication Complex

The vRNA-dependent RNA polymerase is a good antiviral target as it possesses unique features not found in the cell. In recent years, rapid progress has been made in the development of inhibitors of the influenza virus polymerase complex. Increases in structural and functional knowledge of the influenza virus polymerases are expected to even further catalyze the development of drugs interfering with this molecular machine.[555,712,743,930]

Already in the 1990s, Tomassini et al.[888,889] reported that 2,4-dioxobutanoic acid and 2,6-diketopiperazine derivatives selectively inhibit the endonuclease activity (PA) of the influenza virus polymerase. Since then, rapid progress has been made with the first inhibitor against this activity of both the influenza A and B PA, baloxavir marboxil (S-033188), which is already in the market in the United States (Fig. 14.28G, H).[364,999] Of note, resistant mutants have already been detected during clinical trials and at low frequency within the population.[364] Additional endonuclease inhibitors including AL-974 are also in development.[1011]

Capped- and uncapped-RNA fragments that can interfere with cap binding, capped-RNA primed transcription, or panhandle formation have been reported,[556] but these compounds would have pharmacologic limitations because of difficulties in getting charged molecules into cells. A small molecule inhibitor of the cap-snatching activity of PB2, pimodivir, is currently being tested in late-stage clinical trials.[245] Other compounds with similar activity are in earlier stages of development.[149,562,702,711]

Ribavirin (which is approved for treatment of hepatitis C) and several other nucleotide analogs are known to inhibit influenza virus replication in humans, but toxicity remains a problem.[443,529,556] For RNA viruses, most of the antiviral effects of ribavirin are likely due to its incorporation as a purine analog during viral replication, resulting in lethal mutations. Favipiravir (T-705) inhibits influenza virus RNA polymerase activity also by acting as a purine analog and has been shown to be effective against several RNA viruses.[186,276,277,467] Favipiravir is approved for use in Japan as treatment for influenza virus infections in a pandemic setting. Screens of small molecules have also uncovered novel inhibitors of influenza virus replication that target the NP and PB1 proteins.[406,408,449,854,959]

Neuraminidase Inhibitors

The study of temperature-sensitive influenza virus mutants with defects in the NA has shown that the function of this enzyme is to release the newly formed virus from the cell surface.[693] Additional studies showed that neuraminic acid analogs inhibit influenza virus replication in tissue culture and that aggregates of virus are formed at the cell surface in the presence of these drugs (Fig. 14.22).[688,692] von Itzstein et al.[921] designed a derivative of neuraminic acid that had a guanidino group at C atom 4 instead of the OH group of the previously studied neuraminidase inhibitor, 2,3-didchydro-2-deoxy-*N*-acetylneuraminic acid (DANA).[593] This compound, zanamivir (Fig. 14.29), is not orally bioavailable and is FDA approved for administration by inhalation or by nasal spray. Most recently, intravenous administration has been investigated.[742] In numerous studies, this compound has been shown to be a potent anti-influenza drug, both prophylactically and therapeutically.[155,298,430,590,658] Peramivir is another approved neuraminidase inhibitor that can be administered intravenously.[476,641] A long-acting neuraminidase inhibitor (laninamivir) that requires only a single administration for the entire course of treatment was recently developed and is currently approved for use in Japan.[993] The search for compounds with oral bioavailability led to the development of oseltamivir.[533] Its prodrug is an ethyl ester of a compound that has the three OH groups of C atoms 7, 8, and 9 of sialic acid replaced by a hydrophobic side chain, which allows the drug to pass through the gut and into the bloodstream (Fig. 14.29). Oseltamivir has been shown to be highly effective against both influenza A and B viruses, including strains containing the NA gene of the 1918 pandemic virus.[423,430,590,658,902] Although neuraminidase inhibitor–resistant variants had been described with escape mutations in the HA as well as the NA,[31,156,324,428,466] it was still unexpected that such widespread resistance would be seen among the seasonal H1N1 viruses by the 2009 season.[412,679] Prior to 2007, the presence of the NA H274Y (H275Y in N1 numbering) mutation was associated with a cost to viral fitness.[378,425] By 2008/2009, this mutation had a fitness advantage even in the absence of oseltamivir, and these resistant viruses were shown to be highly transmissible in a guinea pig model.[76] It has been proposed that compensating mutations in the NA resulted in a more stable molecule with enhanced expression at the cell surface than was observed for a mutant with only the H274Y mutation.[61] Interestingly, for the H3N2 viruses, oseltamivir resistance is associated with a loss of fitness and is detrimental to transmissibility of these viruses.[75,1007] Resistant H3N2 viruses have been isolated particularly from immunocompromised patients undergoing therapy.[598,677] Similarly, oseltamivir-resistant isolates of the 2009 pandemic virus have been observed in these patient populations but not in the community.[318,599] Based on experiments in animal models, it is predicted that an H274Y change in the NA of the 2009 pandemic virus would not be associated with any substantial loss in fitness or transmissibility.[206,597,795] With this virus already being resistant to the adamantanes, acquisition of oseltamivir resistance would make it a multi–drug-resistant virus and a significant threat. Oseltamivir-resistant influenza B viruses have also been detected, although at a relatively low frequency.[102,428,701] Of note, avian and zoonotic influenza viruses can also carry resistance mutations.[210,316,339,404] For H7N9, it has been shown that these mutations do not impact on viral fitness.[339] Fortunately, mutations associated with oseltamivir resistance do not generally confer zanamivir resistance, and reports of zanamivir resistance in patients are rare.[325] Structures of oseltamivir-resistant NAs that remain sensitive to zanamivir show that this is due to an altered hydrophobic pocket in the active site that affects oseltamivir but not zanamivir binding.[153]

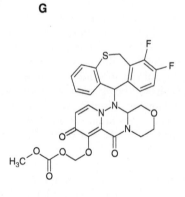
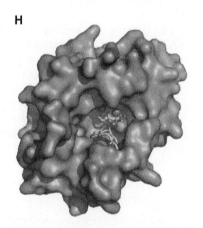

FIGURE 14.29 Anti-influenza virus compounds. The chemical structures of **(A)** amantadine, **(B)** rimantadine, **(C)** oseltamivir, **(D)** zanamivir, **(E)** peramivir, **(F)** laninamivir, and **(G)** baloxavir marboxil are shown. (Courtesy of Kris White.) **H:** Endonuclease domain of PA (surface representation), bound to inhibitor baloxavir marboxil (sticks). (Courtesy of Maria Lukarska and Stephen Cusack, European Molecular Biology Laboratory.)

As an alternative to small molecule inhibitors, broadly protective monoclonal antibodies that inhibit the NA have recently been isolated. Like antibodies to HA, they are being considered for development into future therapeutics.[130,975]

Inhibition of Cellular Factors

The identification of host factors that are required for optimal influenza virus replication (see section Cellular Functions Required for Influenza Virus Replication) provides additional targets that can be explored for potential antiviral development.[211,368,553,742,804,807,1010] There are distinct advantages and disadvantages to this approach. The obvious disadvantage is that inhibition of a cellular activity that is essential for cell survival or growth may be detrimental to the host, so such proteins may not be suitable as antiviral targets. However, particularly with acute infections like influenza, the short duration of therapy may allow for temporary loss or down-regulation of a cellular function without harming the host. The major advantage of targeting a host factor over a viral factor is that resistance is much less likely to develop. There is also greater opportunity for host-directed compounds to have broad-spectrum activity as many viruses may rely on the same host function. For example, HSP90 inhibitors have been shown to inhibit influenza virus[118] and other viruses including hepatitis C virus and Ebola virus.[640,831] Several inhibitors of enzymes in the *de novo* pyrimidine synthesis pathway have been shown to inhibit the replication of a wide range of viruses, including influenza virus,[65,387,933] presumably because viral replication is particularly dependent on large pyrimidine pools. Inhibitors of receptor tyrosine kinases have also been shown to inhibit influenza virus replication as well as other viruses.[493,494] Identification of the target of a novel compound can be difficult, but a cellular target is strongly suggested if the compound can inhibit viruses belonging to different families and/or shows species-specific activity. This is the case with a compound shown to block replication of both influenza viruses and several paramyxoviruses,[491] and future identification of the target may reveal an important virus–host interaction. Likewise, known inhibitors of host factors or signaling pathways identified as critical for influenza virus replication could be repurposed as antivirals or at least chemical probes for investigating the function of specific virus–host interactions. Inhibitors of the following cellular factors have all been shown to inhibit influenza virus growth: MEK, CAMK2B, vATPase, and CLK1.[204,451,478,720] Rather than inhibiting the activity of a required host protein, it is also feasible for an antiviral compound to function by activating a cellular factor with antiviral activity, as shown by chemical activation of REDD1 expression, which decreases growth of both influenza and vesicular stomatitis viruses.[580]

PERSPECTIVES

Human influenza viruses were first isolated in 1933, and since that time, they have been studied extensively. Extraordinary progress has been made in elucidating the components of the virus and in understanding the medical consequences of an influenza virus infection. Many of these discoveries have had implications far beyond the influenza virus field and have sparked new developments in disciplines such as immunology

and protein structure as well as furthering our basic understanding of viruses in general. For example, the ability of virus to agglutinate red blood cells (hemagglutination) was first recognized as a property associated with influenza virus, hence the name of its major surface glycoprotein. With the discovery that this phenomenon extends to other viruses (e.g., measles virus, rubella virus), this property became the basis for viral diagnostic tests, allowing for easy detection of virus or of protective antibody (hemagglutination inhibition) in patient sera. The influenza virus neuraminidase was also the first enzyme found to be associated with an animal virus, even before it was recognized that viruses encode their own polymerases, including those with reverse transcriptase activity. The discovery of interferon by Isaacs and Lindenmann in 1957 was the result of studying infection with heat-inactivated influenza virus (the anti-interferon activity of the NS1 protein was inhibited by the heat inactivation of the virus).

Structural analyses of the HA and NA proteins helped to lay the foundation for the exploration of structure/function relationships of large, biologically active proteins. Today, the intensity of influenza research has not diminished, and a PubMed search yields more than 100,000 entries at the time this chapter was revised.

Many approaches that served us well in the past have now been superseded by newer techniques, but the contribution of these earlier techniques to our current knowledge should not be overlooked. The superb collections of temperature-sensitive mutants obtained and characterized by Akira Sugiura in Japan and by Christoph Scholtissek and Rudolf Rott in Germany made it possible to study the genetics of the virus on a gene-by-gene level and allowed the field to take giant steps forward. The early sequencing of the influenza virus proteins and RNAs was an effort of months, if not years. Now, this can be done in a matter of hours, and since the last edition of this book, there has been an enormous increase in the number of influenza virus sequences submitted to GenBank and GISAID. We also have exciting new molecular technologies (including reverse genetics) that have allowed us to obtain an excellent understanding of the virus on a molecular level and to learn how it has changed over the years. Using this technology, we have even been able to resurrect the 1918 pandemic influenza virus from sequenced RNA fragments and to study its pathogenicity in animal models. Reverse genetics is also a technique that allows us to develop influenza virus constructs, which can induce long-lasting and broadly protective antibody responses in humans and animals bringing us closer to a universal influenza virus vaccine.

What are the challenges for the future? With the threat of yet another pandemic influenza virus emerging, a detailed molecular understanding of virus–host interactions is needed in order to know how best to disable the virus. Perhaps, one of the most pressing questions is, what makes an influenza virus transmissible from human to human and from animal to animal? This aspect has been notoriously difficult to study and will require the use of complex animal models. On a molecular level, it will be important to learn more about the cell's signaling pathways and how they are modulated during influenza virus replication. What makes the virus a pathogen in one species and not in another? How does the virus affect the host immune response, and—in turn—how is the virus globally affected by the immune system in humans and animals? What role does the age of a person (child, adult, elderly), the sex of a person,[616] and conditions/diseases (pregnancy, obesity, diabetes) play in influenza virus replication? What are the complicating factors (coinfection with other viral/bacterial agents, environmental changes) in an influenza virus infection? And last but not least, we need to address the question of host genetics in influenza virus infection and in virus infections in general. Which genetic makeup (polymorphisms and gene expression profiles) determines susceptibility to (and recovery from) influenza virus infection in humans and animals?

These efforts will need to be accompanied by the development of reliable rapid diagnostic tests and safe, broadly effective antivirals. As we begin to obtain a better understanding of the host factors involved in influenza virus replication, we have the opportunity to start using these host factors as new antiviral drug targets. Potentially, this approach can lead to the development of broad-spectrum antivirals that can be used to treat influenza and other viral diseases. Since the isolation and characterization of broadly protective monoclonal antibodies directed against conserved portions of the HA, it is now possible to design novel immunogens that may serve as vaccine constructs. Such universal influenza vaccines may eliminate the need for annual revaccinations against influenza and provide protection against intrasubtype variants (antigenic drift) and against strains belonging to different subtypes (antigenic shift). In a new pandemic outbreak, the availability of such tools will be imperative. We might even consider eradicating influenza B with an effective universal influenza B virus vaccine since humans are the only reservoir for the virus. It is likely that answers to these challenges will come from a vigorous basic science enterprise, which has brought us a long way in the past several decades of influenza virus research.

ACKNOWLEDGMENTS

We want to apologize to all our colleagues whose work we could not reference due to space limitations. We would also like to acknowledge the work of Megan Shaw, Ph.D., coauthor of this chapter in the fifth and sixth editions of *Fields Virology*. Finally, we want to thank Jordan Bragg and Molly Deroy for their help with editing as well as Fatima Amanat, Guha Asthagiri-Arunkumar, Mark Bailey, James Duehr, Alec Freyn, Ericka Kirkpatrick, Andrea Parsons, Daniel Stadlbauer, Gayathri Vijayakumar, and Allen Zheng for their help proofreading this chapter.

REFERENCES

1. Acharya R, Carnevale V, Fiorin G, et al. Structure and mechanism of proton transport through the transmembrane tetrameric M2 protein bundle of the influenza A virus. *Proc Natl Acad Sci U S A* 2010;107(34):15075–15080.
2. Ackerman EE, Kawakami J, Katoh M, et al. Network-guided discovery of influenza virus replication host factors. *MBio* 2018;9(6).
3. Ada GL, Perry BT. The nucleic acid content of influenza virus. *Aust J Exp Biol Med Sci* 1954;32(4):453–468.
4. Akarsu H, Burmeister WP, Petosa C, et al. Crystal structure of the M1 protein-binding domain of the influenza A virus nuclear export protein (NEP/NS2). *EMBO J* 2003;22(18):4646–4655.
5. Alamgir AS, Matsuzaki Y, Hongo S, et al. Phylogenetic analysis of influenza C virus nonstructural (NS) protein genes and identification of the NS2 protein. *J Gen Virol* 2000;81:1933–1940.
6. Ali A, Avalos RT, Ponimaskin E, et al. Influenza virus assembly: effect of influenza virus glycoproteins on the membrane association of M1 protein. *J Virol* 2000;74(18):8709–8719.
7. Allison AB, Ballard JR, Tesh RB, et al. Cyclic avian mass mortality in the northeastern United States is associated with a novel orthomyxovirus. *J Virol* 2015;89(2):1389–1403.
8. Alonso-Caplen FV, Krug RM. Regulation of the extent of splicing of influenza virus NS1 mRNA: role of the rates of splicing and of the nucleocytoplasmic transport of NS1 mRNA. *Mol Cell Biol* 1991;11(2):1092–1098.
9. Alonso-Caplen FV, Nemeroff ME, Qiu Y, et al. Nucleocytoplasmic transport: the influenza virus NS1 protein regulates the transport of spliced NS2 mRNA and its precursor NS1 mRNA. *Genes Dev* 1992;6(2):255–267.
10. Alymova IV, McCullers JA, Kamal RP, et al. Virulent PB1-F2 residues: effects on fitness of H1N1 influenza A virus in mice and changes during evolution of human influenza A viruses. *Sci Rep* 2018;8(1):7474.
11. Amorim MJ. A comprehensive review on the interaction between the host GTPase Rab11 and influenza A virus. *Front Cell Dev Biol* 2018;6:176.
12. Amorim MJ, Bruce EA, Read EK, et al. A Rab11- and microtubule-dependent mechanism for cytoplasmic transport of influenza A virus viral RNA. *J Virol* 2011;85(9):4143–4156.
13. Ando T, Yamayoshi S, Tomita Y, et al. The host protein CLUH participates in the subnuclear transport of influenza virus ribonucleoprotein complexes. *Nat Microbiol* 2016;1(8):16062.
14. Andrews SF, Joyce MG, Chambers MJ, et al. Preferential induction of cross-group influenza A hemagglutinin stem-specific memory B cells after H7N9 immunization in humans. *Sci Immunol* 2017;2(13).
15. Apostolov K, Flewett TH. Further observations on the structure of influenza viruses A and C. *J Gen Virol* 1969;4(3):365–370.
16. Aragon T, de la Luna S, Novoa I, et al. Eukaryotic translation initiation factor 4GI is a cellular target for NS1 protein, a translational activator of influenza virus. *Mol Cell Biol* 2000;20(17):6259–6268.
17. Aramini JM, Ma LC, Zhou L, et al. Dimer interface of the effector domain of non-structural protein 1 from influenza A virus: an interface with multiple functions. *J Biol Chem* 2011;286(29):26050–26060.
18. Arcangeletti MC, De Conto F, Ferraglia F, et al. Host-cell-dependent role of actin cytoskeleton during the replication of a human strain of influenza A virus. *Arch Virol* 2008;153(7):1209–1221.
19. Area E, Martín-Benito J, Gastaminza P, et al. 3D structure of the influenza virus polymerase complex: localization of subunit domains. *Proc Natl Acad Sci U S A* 2004;101(1):308–313.
20. Arranz R, Coloma R, Chichón FJ, et al. The structure of native influenza virion ribonucleoproteins. *Science* 2012;338(6114):1634–1637.
21. Arzt S, Baudin F, Barge A, et al. Combined results from solution studies on intact influenza virus M1 protein and from a new crystal form of its N-terminal domain show that M1 is an elongated monomer. *Virology* 2001;279(2):439–446.
22. Asaka MN, Kawaguchi A, Sakai Y, et al. Polycomb repressive complex 2 facilitates the nuclear export of the influenza viral genome through the interaction with M1. *Sci Rep* 2016;6:33608.
23. Ashenberg O, Padmakumar J, Doud MB, et al. Deep mutational scanning identifies sites in influenza nucleoprotein that affect viral inhibition by MxA. *PLoS Pathog* 2017;13(3):e1006288.
24. Atkins C, Evans CW, Nordin B, et al. Global human-kinase screening identifies therapeutic host targets against influenza. *J Biomol Screen* 2014;19(6):936–946.
25. Avalos RT, Yu Z, Nayak DP. Association of influenza virus NP and M1 proteins with cellular cytoskeletal elements in influenza virus-infected cells. *J Virol* 1997;71(4):2947–2958.
26. Avilov SV, Moisy D, Naffakh N, et al. Influenza A virus progeny vRNP trafficking in live infected cells studied with the virus-encoded fluorescently tagged PB2 protein. *Vaccine* 2012;30(51):7411–7417.
27. Ayllon J, García-Sastre A. The NS1 protein: a multitasking virulence factor. *Curr Top Microbiol Immunol* 2015;386:73–107.
28. Azzeh M, Flick R, Hobom G. Functional analysis of the influenza A virus cRNA promoter and construction of an ambisense transcription system. *Virology* 2001;289(2):400–410.
29. Bae S-H, Cheong H-K, Lee J-H, et al. Structural features of an influenza virus promoter and their implications for viral RNA synthesis. *Proc Natl Acad Sci U S A* 2001;98(19):10602–10607.
30. Baez M, Taussig R, Zazra JJ, et al. Complete nucleotide sequence of the influenza A/PR/8/34 virus NS gene and comparison with the NS genes of the A/Udorn/72 and A/FPV/Rostock/34 strains. *Nucleic Acids Res* 1980;8(23):5845–5858.
31. Baigent SJ, Bethell RC, McCauley JW. Genetic analysis reveals that both haemagglutinin and neuraminidase determine the sensitivity of naturally occurring avian influenza viruses to zanamivir in vitro. *Virology* 1999;263(2):323–338.
32. Baltimore D. Expression of animal virus genomes. *Bacteriol Rev* 1971;35(3):235–241.
33. Bancroft CT, Parslow TG. Evidence for segment-nonspecific packaging of the influenza a virus genome. *J Virol* 2002;76(14):7133–7139.
34. Banerjee I, Miyake Y, Nobs SP, et al. Influenza A virus uses the aggresome processing machinery for host cell entry. *Science* 2014;346(6208):473–477.
35. Barman S, Ali A, Hui EK, et al. Transport of viral proteins to the apical membranes and interaction of matrix protein with glycoproteins in the assembly of influenza viruses. *Virus Res* 2001;77(1):61–69.
36. Barman S, Nayak DP. Analysis of the transmembrane domain of influenza virus neuraminidase, a type II transmembrane glycoprotein, for apical sorting and raft association. *J Virol* 2000;74(14):6538–6545.
37. Baskin CR, Bielefeldt-Ohmann H, Garcia-Sastre A, et al. Functional genomic and serological analysis of the protective immune response resulting from vaccination of macaques with an NS1-truncated influenza virus. *J Virol* 2007;81(21):11817–11827.
38. Basler CF. Influenza viruses: basic biology and potential drug targets. *Infect Disord Drug Targets* 2007;7(4):282–293.
39. Batra J, Tripathi S, Kumar A, et al. Human heat shock protein 40 (Hsp40/DnaJB1) promotes influenza A virus replication by assisting nuclear import of viral ribonucleoproteins. *Sci Rep* 2016;6:19063.
40. Baudin F, Bach C, Cusack S, et al. Structure of influenza virus RNP. I. Influenza virus nucleoprotein melts secondary structure in panhandle RNA and exposes the bases to the solvent. *EMBO J* 1994;13(13):3158–3165.
41. Baudin F, Petit I, Weissenhorn W, et al. In vitro dissection of the membrane and RNP binding activities of influenza virus M1 protein. *Virology* 2001;281(1):102–108.

42. Bauer DLV, Tellier M, Martínez-Alonso M, et al. Influenza virus mounts a two-pronged attack on host RNA polymerase II transcription. *Cell Rep* 2018;23(7):2119–2129.e2113.

43. Beard KR, Brendish NJ, Clark TW. Treatment of influenza with neuraminidase inhibitors. *Curr Opin Infect Dis* 2018;31(6):514–519.

44. Beaton AR, Krug RM. Selected host cell capped RNA fragments prime influenza viral RNA transcription in vivo. *Nucleic Acids Res* 1981;9(17):4423–4436.

45. Beaton AR, Krug RM. Transcription antitermination during influenza viral template RNA synthesis requires the nucleocapsid protein and the absence of a 5′ capped end. *Proc Natl Acad Sci U S A* 1986;83(17):6282–6286.

46. Beaulieu A, Gravel É, Cloutier A, et al. Matriptase proteolytically activates influenza virus and promotes multicycle replication in the human airway epithelium. *J Virol* 2013;87(8):4237–4251.

47. Becker GL, Sielaff F, Than ME, et al. Potent inhibitors of furin and furin-like proprotein convertases containing decarboxylated P1 arginine mimetics. *J Med Chem* 2010;53(3):1067–1075.

48. Belser JA, Lu X, Szretter KJ, et al. DAS181, a novel sialidase fusion protein, protects mice from lethal avian influenza H5N1 virus infection. *J Infect Dis* 2007;196(10):1493–1499.

49. Benitez AA, Panis M, Xue J, et al. In Vivo RNAi screening identifies MDA5 as a significant contributor to the cellular defense against influenza A virus. *Cell Rep* 2015;11(11):1714–1726.

50. Bennink JR, Palmore TN. The promise of siRNAs for the treatment of influenza. *Trends Mol Med* 2004;10(12):571–574.

51. Benton DJ, Nans A, Calder LJ, et al. Influenza hemagglutinin membrane anchor. *Proc Natl Acad Sci U S A* 2018;115(40):10112–10117.

52. Berger MJ. Influenza, not Ebola, more likely the cause of 430 bce Athenian Outbreak. *Clin Infect Dis* 2015;61(9):1492–1493.

53. Betakova T, Nermut MV, Hay AJ. The NB protein is an integral component of the membrane of influenza B virus. *J Gen Virol* 1996;77(Pt 11):2689–2694.

54. Bialas KM, Bussey KA, Stone RL, et al. Specific nucleoprotein residues affect influenza virus morphology. *J Virol* 2014;88(4):2227–2234.

55. Bier K, York A, Fodor E. Cellular cap-binding proteins associate with influenza virus mRNAs. *J Gen Virol* 2011;92(Pt 7):1627–1634.

56. Bierin E, Falk K, Hoel E, et al. Segment 8 encodes a structural protein of infectious salmon anaemia virus (ISAV); the co-linear transcript from segment 7 probably encodes a nonstructural or minor structural protein. *Dis Aquat Organ* 2002;49(2):117–122.

57. Biswas SK, Boutz PL, Nayak DP. Influenza virus nucleoprotein interacts with influenza virus polymerase proteins. *J Virol* 1998;72(7):5493–5501.

58. Biswas SK, Nayak DP. Mutational analysis of the conserved motifs of influenza A virus polymerase basic protein 1. *J Virol* 1994;68(3):1819–1826.

59. Blaising J, Polyak SJ, Pécheur EI. Arbidol as a broad-spectrum antiviral: an update. *Antiviral Res* 2014;107:84–94.

60. Blass D, Patzelt E, Kuechler E. Identification of the cap binding protein of influenza virus. *Nucleic Acids Res* 1982;10(15):4803–4812.

61. Bloom JD, Gong LI, Baltimore D. Permissive secondary mutations enable the evolution of influenza oseltamivir resistance. *Science* 2010;328(5983):1272–1275.

62. Bodian DL, Yamasaki RB, Buswell RL, et al. Inhibition of the fusion-inducing conformational change of influenza hemagglutinin by benzoquinones and hydroquinones. *Biochemistry* 1993;32(12):2967–2978.

63. Bolte H, Rosu ME, Hagelauer E, et al. Packaging of the influenza A virus genome is governed by a plastic network of RNA/protein interactions. *J Virol* 2019;93(4).

64. Boltz DA, Aldridge JR, Webster RG, et al. Drugs in development for influenza. *Drugs* 2010;70(11):1349–1362.

65. Bonavia A, Franti M, Pusateri Keaney E, et al. Identification of broad-spectrum antiviral compounds and assessment of the druggability of their target for efficacy against respiratory syncytial virus (RSV). *Proc Natl Acad Sci U S A* 2011;108(17):6739–6744.

66. Boonstra S, Blijleven JS, Roos WH, et al. Hemagglutinin-mediated membrane fusion: a biophysical perspective. *Annu Rev Biophys* 2018;47:153–173.

67. Bornholdt ZA, Prasad BV. X-ray structure of influenza virus NS1 effector domain. *Nat Struct Mol Biol* 2006;13(6):559–560.

68. Bornholdt ZA, Prasad BV. X-ray structure of NS1 from a highly pathogenic H5N1 influenza virus. *Nature* 2008;456(7224):985–988.

69. Bortz E, Westera L, Maamary J, et al. Host- and strain-specific regulation of influenza virus polymerase activity by interacting cellular proteins. *MBio* 2011;2(4).

70. Böttcher E, Matrosovich T, Beyerle M, et al. Proteolytic activation of influenza viruses by serine proteases TMPRSS2 and HAT from human airway epithelium. *J Virol* 2006;80(19):9896–9898.

71. Böttcher-Friebertshäuser E, Stein DA, Klenk HD, et al. Inhibition of influenza virus infection in human airway cell cultures by an antisense peptide-conjugated morpholino oligomer targeting the hemagglutinin-activating protease TMPRSS2. *J Virol* 2011;85(4):1554–1562.

72. Boulo S, Akarsu H, Ruigrok RW, et al. Nuclear traffic of influenza virus proteins and ribonucleoprotein complexes. *Virus Res* 2007;124(1–2):12–21.

73. Bourmakina S, García-Sastre A. Reverse genetics studies on the filamentous morphology of influenza A virus. *J Gen Virol* 2003;84(Pt 3):517–527.

74. Bourmakina S, García-Sastre A. The morphology and composition of influenza A virus particles are not affected by low levels of M1 and M2 proteins in infected cells. *J Virol* 2005;79(12):7926–7932.

75. Bouvier NM, Lowen AC, Palese P. Oseltamivir-resistant influenza A viruses are transmitted efficiently among guinea pigs by direct contact but not by aerosol. *J Virol* 2008;82(20):10052–10058.

76. Bouvier NM, Rahmat S, Pica N. Enhanced mammalian transmissibility of seasonal influenza A/H1N1 viruses encoding an oseltamivir-resistant neuraminidase. *J Virol* 2012;86(13):7268–7279.

77. Braam J, Ulmanen I, Krug RM. Molecular model of a eucaryotic transcription complex: functions and movements of influenza P proteins during capped RNA-primed transcription. *Cell* 1983;34(2):609–618.

78. Bradel-Tretheway BG, Mattiacio JL, Krasnoselsky A, et al. Comprehensive proteomic analysis of influenza virus polymerase complex reveals a novel association with mitochondrial proteins and RNA polymerase accessory factors. *J Virol* 2011;85(17):8569–8581.

79. Brandenburg B, Koudstaal W, Goudsmit J, et al. Mechanisms of hemagglutinin targeted influenza virus neutralization. *PLoS One* 2013;8(12):e80034.

80. Brass AL, Huang IC, Benita Y, et al. The IFITM proteins mediate cellular resistance to influenza A H1N1 virus, West Nile virus, and dengue virus. *Cell* 2009;139(7):1243–1254.

81. Brassard DL, Leser GP, Lamb RA. Influenza B virus NB glycoprotein is a component of the virion. *Virology* 1996;220(2):350–360.

82. Briedis DJ, Lamb RA. Influenza B virus genome: sequences and structural organization of RNA segment 8 and the mRNAs coding for the NS1 and NS2 proteins. *J Virol* 1982;42(1):186–193.

83. Brooke CB, Ince WL, Wei J, et al. Influenza A virus nucleoprotein selectively decreases neuraminidase gene-segment packaging while enhancing viral fitness and transmissibility. *Proc Natl Acad Sci U S A* 2014;111(47):16854–16859.

84. Brooke CB, Ince WL, Wrammert J, et al. Most influenza a virions fail to express at least one essential viral protein. *J Virol* 2013;87(6):3155–3162.

85. Brownlee GG, Sharps JL. The RNA polymerase of influenza A virus is stabilized by interaction with its viral RNA promoter. *J Virol* 2002;76(14):7103–7113.

86. Bruce EA, Digard P, Stuart AD. The Rab11 pathway is required for influenza A virus budding and filament formation. *J Virol* 2010;84(12):5848–5859.

87. Bruce E, Medcalf L, Crump C, et al. Budding of filamentous and non-filamentous influenza A virus occurs via a VPS4 and VPS28-independent pathway. *Virology* 2009;390(2):268–278.

88. Brunotte L, Flies J, Bolte H, et al. The nuclear export protein of H5N1 influenza A viruses recruits Matrix 1 (M1) protein to the viral ribonucleoprotein to mediate nuclear export. *J Biol Chem* 2014;289(29):20067–20077.

89. Bruns K, Studtrucker N, Sharma A, et al. Structural characterization and oligomerization of PB1-F2, a proapoptotic influenza A virus protein. *J Biol Chem* 2007;282(1):353–363.

90. Bucher D, Palese P. The biologically active proteins of influenza virus: neuraminidase. In: Kilbourne ED, ed. *The Influenza Viruses and Influenza*. New York: Academic Press; 1975.

91. Buehler J, Navi D, Lorusso A, et al. Influenza A virus PB1-F2 protein expression is regulated in a strain-specific manner by sequences located downstream of the PB1-F2 initiation codon. *J Virol* 2013;87(19):10687–10699.

92. Buettner N, Vogt C, Martinez-Sobrido L, et al. Thogoto virus ML protein is a potent inhibitor of the interferon regulatory factor-7 transcription factor. *J Gen Virol* 2010;91(Pt 1):220–227.

93. Bui M, Myers JE, Whittaker GR. Nucleo-cytoplasmic localization of influenza virus nucleoprotein depends on cell density and phosphorylation. *Virus Res* 2002;84(1–2):37–44.

94. Bui M, Whittaker G, Helenius A. Effect of M1 protein and low pH on nuclear transport of influenza virus ribonucleoproteins. *J Virol* 1996;70(12):8391–8401.

95. Bui M, Wills EG, Helenius A, et al. Role of the influenza virus M1 protein in nuclear export of viral ribonucleoproteins. *J Virol* 2000;74(4):1781–1786.

96. Bullido R, Gómez-Puertas P, Albo C, et al. Several protein regions contribute to determine the nuclear and cytoplasmic localization of the influenza A virus nucleoprotein. *J Gen Virol* 2000;81(Pt 1):135–142.

97. Bullido R, Gomez-Puertas P, Saiz MJ, et al. Influenza A virus NEP (NS2 protein) downregulates RNA synthesis of model template RNAs. *J Virol* 2001;75(10):4912–4917.

98. Bullough PA, Hughson FM, Skehel JJ, et al. Structure of influenza haemagglutinin at the pH of membrane fusion. *Nature* 1994;371(6492):37–43.

99. Burgui I, Aragon T, Ortin J, et al. PABP1 and eIF4GI associate with influenza virus NS1 protein in viral mRNA translation initiation complexes. *J Gen Virol* 2003;84:3263–3274.

100. Burleigh LM, Calder LJ, Skehel JJ, et al. Influenza a viruses with mutations in the m1 helix six domain display a wide variety of morphological phenotypes. *J Virol* 2005;79(2):1262–1270.

101. Burmeister WP, Ruigrok RW, Cusack S. The 2.2 A resolution crystal structure of influenza B neuraminidase and its complex with sialic acid. *EMBO J* 1992;11(1):49–56.

102. Burnham AJ, Armstrong J, Lowen AC, et al. Competitive fitness of influenza B viruses with neuraminidase inhibitor-resistant substitutions in a coinfection model of the human airway epithelium. *J Virol* 2015;89(8):4575–4587.

103. Byrd-Leotis L, Cummings RD, Steinhauer DA. The interplay between the host receptor and influenza virus hemagglutinin and neuraminidase. *Int J Mol Sci* 2017;18(7).

104. Cady SD, Schmidt-Rohr K, Wang J, et al. Structure of the amantadine binding site of influenza M2 proton channels in lipid bilayers. *Nature* 2010;463(7281):689–692.

105. Calder LJ, Rosenthal PB. Cryomicroscopy provides structural snapshots of influenza virus membrane fusion. *Nat Struct Mol Biol* 2016;23(9):853–858.

106. Calder LJ, Wasilewski S, Berriman JA, et al. Structural organization of a filamentous influenza A virus. *Proc Natl Acad Sci U S A* 2010;107(23):10685–10690.

107. Campbell PJ, Kyriakis CS, Marshall N, et al. Residue 41 of the Eurasian avian-like swine influenza a virus matrix protein modulates virion filament length and efficiency of contact transmission. *J Virol* 2014;88(13):7569–7577.

108. Cao S, Jiang J, Li J, et al. Characterization of the nucleocytoplasmic shuttle of the matrix protein of influenza B virus. *J Virol* 2014;88(13):7464–7473.

109. Cao S, Liu X, Yu M, et al. A nuclear export signal in the matrix protein of influenza A virus is required for efficient virus replication. *J Virol* 2012;86(9):4883–4891.

110. Cao M, Wei C, Zhao L, et al. DnaJA1/Hsp40 is co-opted by influenza A virus to enhance its viral RNA polymerase activity. *J Virol* 2014;88(24):14078–14089.

111. Carlson CM, Turpin EA, Moser LA, et al. Transforming growth factor-β: activation by neuraminidase and role in highly pathogenic H5N1 influenza pathogenesis. *PLoS Pathog* 2010;6(10):e1001136.

112. Carr SM, Carnero E, García-Sastre A, et al. Characterization of a mitochondrial-targeting signal in the PB2 protein of influenza viruses. *Virology* 2006;344(2):492–508.

113. Carrasco M, Amorim MJ, Digard P. Lipid raft-dependent targeting of the influenza A virus nucleoprotein to the apical plasma membrane. *Traffic* 2004;5(12):979–992.

114. Chaimayo C, Dunagan M, Hayashi T, et al. Specificity and functional interplay between influenza virus PA-X and NS1 shutoff activity. *PLoS Pathog* 2018;14(11):e1007465.

115. Chan CM, Chu H, Zhang AJ, et al. Hemagglutinin of influenza A virus binds specifically to cell surface nucleolin and plays a role in virus internalization. *Virology* 2016;494:78–88.
116. Chan W-H, Ng AK-L, Robb NC, et al. Functional analysis of the influenza virus H5N1 nucleoprotein tail loop reveals amino acids that are crucial for oligomerization and ribonucleoprotein activities. *J Virol* 2010;84(14):7337–7345.
117. Chanturiya AN, Basanez G, Schubert U, et al. PB1-F2, an influenza A virus-encoded proapoptotic mitochondrial protein, creates variably sized pores in planar lipid membranes. *J Virol* 2004;78(12):6304–6312.
118. Chase G, Deng T, Fodor E, et al. Hsp90 inhibitors reduce influenza virus replication in cell culture. *Virology* 2008;377(2):431–439.
119. Chase GP, Rameix-Welti MA, Zvirbliene A, et al. Influenza virus ribonucleoprotein complexes gain preferential access to cellular export machinery through chromatin targeting. *PLoS Pathog* 2011;7(9):e1002187.
120. Chasman D, Walters KB, Lopes TJ, et al. Integrating transcriptomic and proteomic data using predictive regulatory network models of host response to pathogens. *PLoS Comput Biol* 2016;12(7):e1005013.
121. Chekmenev EY, Hu J, Gor'kov PL, et al. 15N and 31P solid-state NMR study of transmembrane domain alignment of M2 protein of influenza A virus in hydrated cylindrical lipid bilayers confined to anodic aluminum oxide nanopores. *J Magn Reson* 2005;173(2):322–327.
122. Chen W, Calvo PA, Malide D, et al. A novel influenza A virus mitochondrial protein that induces cell death. *Nat Med* 2001;7(12):1306–1312.
123. Chen J, Huang S, Chen Z. Human cellular protein nucleoporin hNup98 interacts with influenza A virus NS2/nuclear export protein and overexpression of its GLFG repeat domain can inhibit virus propagation. *J Gen Virol* 2010;91(Pt 10):2474–2484.
124. Chen BJ, Leser GP, Jackson D, et al. The influenza virus M2 protein cytoplasmic tail interacts with the M1 protein and influences virus assembly at the site of virus budding. *J Virol* 2008;82(20):10059–10070.
125. Chen B, Leser G, Morita E, et al. Influenza virus hemagglutinin and neuraminidase, but not the matrix protein, are required for assembly and budding of plasmid-derived virus-like particles. *J Virol* 2007;81(13):7111–7123.
126. Chen Z, Li Y, Krug RM. Influenza A virus NS1 protein targets poly(A)-binding protein II of the cellular 3′-end processing machinery. *EMBO J* 1999;18(8):2273–2283.
127. Chen J, Skehel JJ, Wiley DC. N- and C-terminal residues combine in the fusion-pH influenza hemagglutinin HA(2) subunit to form an N cap that terminates the triple-stranded coiled coil. *Proc Natl Acad Sci U S A* 1999;96(16):8967–8972.
128. Chen BJ, Takeda M, Lamb RA. Influenza virus hemagglutinin (H3 subtype) requires palmitoylation of its cytoplasmic tail for assembly: M1 proteins of two subtypes differ in their ability to support assembly. *J Virol* 2005;79(21):13673–13684.
129. Chen Z, Wang W, Zhou H, et al. Generation of live attenuated novel influenza virus A/California/7/09 (H1N1) vaccines with high yield in embryonated chicken eggs. *J Virol* 2010;84(1):44–51.
130. Chen YQ, Wohlbold TJ, Zheng NY, et al. Influenza infection in humans induces broadly cross-reactive and protective neuraminidase-reactive antibodies. *Cell* 2018;173(2):417–429.e410.
131. Chen C, Zhuang X. Epsin 1 is a cargo-specific adaptor for the clathrin-mediated endocytosis of the influenza virus. *Proc Natl Acad Sci U S A* 2008;105(33):11790–11795.
132. Chenavas S, Estrozi LF, Slama-Schwok A, et al. Monomeric nucleoprotein of influenza A virus. *PLoS Pathog* 2013;9(3):e1003275.
133. Cheng H, Koning K, O'Hearn A, et al. A parallel genome-wide RNAi screening strategy to identify host proteins important for entry of Marburg virus and H5N1 influenza virus. *Virol J* 2015;12:194.
134. Cheng A, Wong SM, Yuan YA. Structural basis for dsRNA recognition by NS1 protein of influenza A virus. *Cell Res* 2009;19(2):187–195.
135. Chien CY, Tejero R, Huang Y, et al. A novel RNA-binding motif in influenza A virus nonstructural protein 1. *Nat Struct Biol* 1997;4(11):891–895.
136. Chien CY, Xu Y, Xiao R, et al. Biophysical characterization of the complex between double-stranded RNA and the N-terminal domain of the NS1 protein from influenza A virus: evidence for a novel RNA-binding mode. *Biochemistry* 2004;43(7):1950–1962.
137. Childs RA, Palma AS, Wharton S, et al. Receptor-binding specificity of pandemic influenza A (H1N1) 2009 virus determined by carbohydrate microarray. *Nat Biotechnol* 2009;27(9):797–799.
138. Chizhmakov IV, Geraghty FM, Ogden DC, et al. Selective proton permeability and pH regulation of the influenza virus M2 channel expressed in mouse erythroleukaemia cells. *J Physiol* 1996;494(Pt 2):329–336.
139. Chlanda P, Schraidt O, Kummer S, et al. Structural analysis of the roles of influenza a virus membrane-associated proteins in assembly and morphology. *J Virol* 2015;89(17):8957–8966.
140. Choi SK, Mammen M, Whitesides GM. Monomeric inhibitors of influenza neuraminidase enhance the hemagglutination inhibition activities of polyacrylamides presenting multiple C-sialoside groups. *Chem Biol* 1996;3(2):97–104.
141. Chou YY, Heaton NS, Gao Q, et al. Colocalization of different influenza viral RNA segments in the cytoplasm before viral budding as shown by single-molecule sensitivity FISH analysis. *PLoS Pathog* 2013;9(5):e1003358.
142. Chou YY, Vafabakhsh R, Doğanay S, et al. One influenza virus particle packages eight unique viral RNAs as shown by FISH analysis. *Proc Natl Acad Sci U S A* 2012;109(23):9101–9106.
143. Chu VC, Whittaker GR. Influenza virus entry and infection require host cell N-linked glycoprotein. *Proc Natl Acad Sci U S A* 2004;101(52):18153–18158.
144. Chua MA, Schmid S, Perez JT, et al. Influenza A virus utilizes suboptimal splicing to coordinate the timing of infection. *Cell Rep* 2013;3(1):23–29.
145. Chutiwitoonchai N, Aida Y. NXT1, a novel influenza A NP binding protein, promotes the nuclear export of NP via a CRM1-dependent pathway. *Viruses* 2016;8(8).
146. Ciampor F, Bayley PM, Nermut MV, et al. Evidence that the amantadine-induced, M2-mediated conversion of influenza A virus hemagglutinin to the low pH conformation occurs in an acidic trans Golgi compartment. *Virology* 1992;188(1):14–24.
147. Cianci C, Langley DR, Dischino DD, et al. Targeting a binding pocket within the trimer-of-hairpins: small-molecule inhibition of viral fusion. *Proc Natl Acad Sci U S A* 2004;101(42):15046–15051.
148. Cianci C, Tiley L, Krystal M. Differential activation of the influenza virus polymerase via template RNA binding. *J Virol* 1995;69(7):3995–3999.
149. Clark MP, Ledeboer MW, Davies I, et al. Discovery of a novel, first-in-class, orally bioavailable azaindole inhibitor (VX-787) of influenza PB2. *J Med Chem* 2014;57(15):6668–6678.
150. Cobbin JC, Ong C, Verity E, et al. Influenza virus PB1 and neuraminidase gene segments can cosegregate during vaccine reassortment driven by interactions in the PB1 coding region. *J Virol* 2014;88(16):8971–8980.
151. Cohen M, Zhang XQ, Senaati HP, et al. Influenza A penetrates host mucus by cleaving sialic acids with neuraminidase. *Virol J* 2013;10:321.
152. Collin EA, Sheng Z, Lang Y, et al. Cocirculation of two distinct genetic and antigenic lineages of proposed influenza D virus in cattle. *J Virol* 2015;89(2):1036–1042.
153. Collins PJ, Haire LF, Lin YP, et al. Crystal structures of oseltamivir-resistant influenza virus neuraminidase mutants. *Nature* 2008;453(7199):1258–1261.
154. Colman PM. Influenza virus neuraminidase: structure, antibodies, and inhibitors. *Protein Sci* 1994;3(10):1687–1696.
155. Colman PM. A novel approach to antiviral therapy for influenza. *J Antimicrob Chemother* 1999;44(Suppl B):17–22.
156. Colman PM. Zanamivir: an influenza virus neuraminidase inhibitor. *Expert Rev Anti Infect Ther* 2005;3(2):191–199.
157. Colman PM. New antivirals and drug resistance. *Annu Rev Biochem* 2009;78:95–118.
158. Colman PM, Varghese JN, Laver WG. Structure of the catalytic and antigenic sites in influenza virus neuraminidase. *Nature* 1983;303(5912):41–44.
159. Coloma R, Valpuesta JM, Arranz R, et al. The structure of a biologically active influenza virus ribonucleoprotein complex. *PLoS Pathog* 2009;5(6):e1000491.
160. Compans R, Choppin P. Reproduction of myxoviruses. In: Fraenkel-Conrat H, Wagner RR, eds. *Comprehensive Virology: Reproduction of Large RNA Viruses*, vol. 4. New York: Plenum Publishing Corp.; 1975:179–252.
161. Compans RW, Content J, Duesberg PH. Structure of the ribonucleoprotein of influenza virus. *J Virol* 1972;10(4):795–800.
162. Compans RW, Meier-Ewert H, Palese P. Assembly of lipid-containing viruses. *J Supramol Struct* 1974;2(2–4):496–511.
163. Conenello GM, Tisoncik JR, Rosenzweig E, et al. A single N66S mutation in the PB1-F2 protein of influenza A virus increases virulence by inhibiting the early interferon response in vivo. *J Virol* 2011;85(2):652–662.
164. Conenello GM, Zamarin D, Perrone LA, et al. A single mutation in the PB1-F2 of H5N1 (HK/97) and 1918 influenza A viruses contributes to increased virulence. *PLoS Pathog* 2007;3(10):1414–1421.
165. Connor RJ, Kawaoka Y, Webster RG, et al. Receptor specificity in human, avian, and equine H2 and H3 influenza virus isolates. *Virology* 1994;205(1):17–23.
166. Corti D, Voss J, Gamblin SJ, et al. A neutralizing antibody selected from plasma cells that binds to group 1 and group 2 influenza A hemagglutinins. *Science* 2011;333(6044):850–856.
167. Cottet L, Rivas-Aravena A, Cortez-San Martin M, et al. Infectious salmon anemia virus—genetics and pathogenesis. *Virus Res* 2011;155(1):10–19.
168. Couceiro JN, Paulson JC, Baum LG. Influenza virus strains selectively recognize sialyloligosaccharides on human respiratory epithelium; the role of the host cell in selection of hemagglutinin receptor specificity. *Virus Res* 1993;29(2):155–165.
169. Couch RB, Atmar RL, Franco LM, et al. Antibody correlates and predictors of immunity to naturally occurring influenza in humans and the importance of antibody to the neuraminidase. *J Infect Dis* 2013;207(6):974–981.
170. Crépin T, Dias A, Palencia A, et al. Mutational and metal binding analysis of the endonuclease domain of the influenza virus polymerase PA subunit. *J Virol* 2010;84(18):9096–9104.
171. Crescenzo-Chaigne B, van der Werf S. Rescue of influenza C virus from recombinant DNA. *J Virol* 2007;81(20):11282–11289.
172. Cros JF, Garcia-Sastre A, Palese P. An unconventional NLS is critical for the nuclear import of the influenza A virus nucleoprotein and ribonucleoprotein. *Traffic* 2005;6(3):205–213.
173. Cros JF, Palese P. Trafficking of viral genomic RNA into and out of the nucleus: influenza, Thogoto and Borna disease viruses. *Virus Res* 2003;95(1–2):3–12.
174. Crow M, Deng T, Addley M, et al. Mutational analysis of the influenza virus cRNA promoter and identification of nucleotides critical for replication. *J Virol* 2004;78(12):6263–6270.
175. Czakó R, Vogel L, Lamirande EW, et al. In vivo imaging of influenza virus infection in immunized mice. *MBio* 2017;8(3):e00714–e00717.
176. Dadonaite B, Vijayakrishnan S, Fodor E, et al. Filamentous influenza viruses. *J Gen Virol* 2016;97(8):1755–1764.
177. Dang Z, Jung K, Zhu L, et al. Phenolic diterpenoid derivatives as anti-influenza a virus agents. *ACS Med Chem Lett* 2015;6(3):355–358.
178. Das DK, Govindan R, Nikić-Spiegel I, et al. Direct visualization of the conformational dynamics of single influenza hemagglutinin trimers. *Cell* 2018;174(4):926–937.e912.
179. Das K, Ma LC, Xiao R, et al. Structural basis for suppression of a host antiviral response by influenza A virus. *Proc Natl Acad Sci U S A* 2008;105(35):13093–13098.
180. Dauber B, Heins G, Wolff T. The influenza B virus nonstructural NS1 protein is essential for efficient viral growth and antagonizes beta interferon induction. *J Virol* 2004;78(4):1865–1872.
181. de Castro Martin IF, Fournier G, Sachse M, et al. Influenza virus genome reaches the plasma membrane via a modified endoplasmic reticulum and Rab11-dependent vesicles. *Nat Commun* 2017;8(1):1396.
182. de Graaf M, Fouchier RA. Role of receptor binding specificity in influenza A virus transmission and pathogenesis. *EMBO J* 2014;33(8):823–841.
183. de Vries M, Herrmann A, Veit M. A cholesterol consensus motif is required for efficient intracellular transport and raft association of a group 2 HA from influenza virus. *Biochem J* 2015;465(2):305–314.

184. de Vries E, Tscherne DM, Wienholts MJ, et al. Dissection of the influenza A virus endocytic routes reveals macropinocytosis as an alternative entry pathway. *PLoS Pathog* 2011;7(3):e1001329.
185. de Wit E, Spronken MI, Vervaet G, et al. A reverse-genetics system for Influenza A virus using T7 RNA polymerase. *J Gen Virol* 2007;88(Pt 4):1281–1287.
186. Delang L, Abdelnabi R, Neyts J. Favipiravir as a potential countermeasure against neglected and emerging RNA viruses. *Antiviral Res* 2018;153:85–94.
187. Demirov D, Gabriel G, Schneider C, et al. Interaction of influenza A virus matrix protein with RACK1 is required for virus release. *Cell Microbiol* 2012;14(5):774–789.
188. Desmet EA, Bussey KA, Stone R, et al. Identification of the N-terminal domain of the influenza virus PA responsible for the suppression of host protein synthesis. *J Virol* 2013;87(6):3108–3118.
189. Desselberger U, Racaniello VR, Zazra JJ, et al. The 3′ and 5′-terminal sequences of influenza A, B and C virus RNA segments are highly conserved and show partial inverted complementarity. *Gene* 1980;8(3):315–328.
190. DeVincenzo JP. The promise, pitfalls and progress of RNA-interference-based antiviral therapy for respiratory viruses. *Antivir Ther* 2012;17(1 Pt B):213–225.
191. Dias A, Bouvier D, Crépin T, et al. The cap-snatching endonuclease of influenza virus polymerase resides in the PA subunit. *Nature* 2009;458(7240):914.
192. Digard P, Elton D, Bishop K, et al. Modulation of nuclear localization of the influenza virus nucleoprotein through interaction with actin filaments. *J Virol* 1999;73(3):2222–2231.
193. Dilillo DJ, Tan GS, Palese P, et al. Broadly neutralizing hemagglutinin stalk-specific antibodies require FcγR interactions for protection against influenza virus in vivo. *Nat Med* 2014;20(2):143–151.
194. Diot C, Fournier G, Dos Santos M, et al. Influenza A virus polymerase recruits the RNA helicase DDX19 to promote the nuclear export of viral mRNAs. *Sci Rep* 2016;6:33763.
195. Dobson J, Whitley RJ, Pocock S, et al. Oseltamivir treatment for influenza in adults: a meta-analysis of randomised controlled trials. *Lancet* 2015;385(9979):1729–1737.
196. Doms RW, Lamb RA, Rose JK, et al. Folding and assembly of viral membrane proteins. *Virology* 1993;193(2):545–562.
197. Donald HB, Isaacs A. Counts of influenza virus particles. *J Gen Microbiol* 1954;10(3):457–464.
198. Donelan NR, Basler CF, Garcia-Sastre A. A recombinant influenza A virus expressing an RNA-binding-defective NS1 protein induces high levels of beta interferon and is attenuated in mice. *J Virol* 2003;77(24):13257–13266.
199. Donelan NR, Dauber B, Wang X, et al. The N- and C-terminal domains of the NS1 protein of influenza B virus can independently inhibit IRF-3 and beta interferon promoter activation. *J Virol* 2004;78(21):11574–11582.
200. Dormitzer PR, Suphaphiphat P, Gibson DG, et al. Synthetic generation of influenza vaccine viruses for rapid response to pandemics. *Sci Transl Med* 2013;5(185):185ra168.
201. Dornfeld D, Dudek AH, Vausselin T, et al. SMARCA2-regulated host cell factors are required for MxA restriction of influenza A viruses. *Sci Rep* 2018;8(1):2092.
202. Doud MB, Bloom JD. Accurate measurement of the effects of all amino-acid mutations on influenza hemagglutinin. *Viruses* 2016;8(6).
203. Dreyfus C, Laursen NS, Kwaks T, et al. Highly conserved protective epitopes on influenza B viruses. *Science* 2012;337(6100):1343–1348.
204. Droebner K, Pleschka S, Ludwig S, et al. Antiviral activity of the MEK-inhibitor U0126 against pandemic H1N1v and highly pathogenic avian influenza virus in vitro and in vivo. *Antiviral Res* 2011;92(2):195–203.
205. Du W, Dai M, Li Z, et al. Substrate binding by the second sialic acid-binding site of influenza A virus N1 neuraminidase contributes to enzymatic activity. *J Virol* 2018;92(20).
206. Duan S, Boltz DA, Seiler P, et al. Oseltamivir-resistant pandemic H1N1/2009 influenza virus possesses lower transmissibility and fitness in ferrets. *PLoS Pathog* 2010;6(7):e1001022.
207. Duesberg PH. Distinct subunits of the ribonucleoprotein of influenza virus. *J Mol Biol* 1969;42(3):485–499.
208. Duhaut SD, Dimmock NJ. Defective segment 1 RNAs that interfere with production of infectious influenza A virus require at least 150 nucleotides of 5′ sequence: evidence from a plasmid-driven system. *J Gen Virol* 2002;83(Pt 2):403–411.
209. Duhaut SD, McCauley JW. Defective RNAs inhibit the assembly of influenza virus genome segments in a segment-specific manner. *Virology* 1996;216(2):326–337.
210. Earhart KC, Elsayed NM, Saad MD, et al. Oseltamivir resistance mutation N294S in human influenza A(H5N1) virus in Egypt. *J Infect Public Health* 2009;2(2):74–80.
211. Edinger TO, Pohl MO, Stertz S. Entry of influenza A virus: host factors and antiviral targets. *J Gen Virol* 2014;95(Pt 2):263–277.
212. Edinger TO, Pohl MO, Yángüez E, et al. Cathepsin W is required for escape of influenza A virus from late endosomes. *MBio* 2015;6(3):e00297.
213. Ehrhardt C, Ludwig S. A new player in a deadly game: influenza viruses and the PI3K/Akt signalling pathway. *Cell Microbiol* 2009;11(6):863–871.
214. Ehrhardt C, Marjuki H, Wolff T, et al. Bivalent role of the phosphatidylinositol-3-kinase (PI3K) during influenza virus infection and host cell defence. *Cell Microbiol* 2006;8(8):1336–1348.
215. Ehrhardt C, Wolff T, Pleschka S, et al. Influenza A virus NS1 protein activates the PI3K/Akt pathway to mediate antiapoptotic signaling responses. *J Virol* 2007;81(7):3058–3067.
216. Eichelberger MC, Morens DM, Taubenberger JK. Neuraminidase as an influenza vaccine antigen: a low hanging fruit, ready for picking to improve vaccine effectiveness. *Curr Opin Immunol* 2018;53:38–44.
217. Eierhoff T, Hrincius ER, Rescher U, et al. The epidermal growth factor receptor (EGFR) promotes uptake of influenza A viruses (IAV) into host cells. *PLoS Pathog* 2010;6(9):e1001099.
218. Eisfeld AJ, Kawakami E, Watanabe T, et al. RAB11A is essential for transport of the influenza virus genome to the plasma membrane. *J Virol* 2011;85(13):6117–6126.
219. Eisfeld AJ, Neumann G, Kawaoka Y. Human immunodeficiency virus rev-binding protein is essential for influenza a virus replication and promotes genome trafficking in late-stage infection. *J Virol* 2011;85(18):9588–9598.
220. Ejiri H, Lim C-K, Isawa H, et al. Characterization of a novel thogotovirus isolated from Amblyomma testudinarium ticks in Ehime, Japan: a significant phylogenetic relationship to Bourbon virus. *Virus Res* 2018;249:57–65.
221. Ekiert DC, Bhabha G, Elsliger MA, et al. Antibody recognition of a highly conserved influenza virus epitope. *Science* 2009;324(5924):246–251.
222. Ekiert DC, Friesen RH, Bhabha G, et al. A highly conserved neutralizing epitope on group 2 influenza A viruses. *Science* 2011;333(6044):843–850.
223. Ekiert DC, Kashyap AK, Steel J, et al. Cross-neutralization of influenza A viruses mediated by a single antibody loop. *Nature* 2012;489(7417):526–532.
224. Elbahesh H, Cline T, Baranovich T, et al. Novel roles of focal adhesion kinase in cytoplasmic entry and replication of influenza A viruses. *J Virol* 2014;88(12):6714–6728.
225. Elderfield RA, Koutsakos M, Frise R, et al. NB protein does not affect influenza B virus replication in vitro and is not required for replication in or transmission between ferrets. *J Gen Virol* 2016;97(3):593–601.
226. Elleman CJ, Barclay WS. The M1 matrix protein controls the filamentous phenotype of influenza A virus. *Virology* 2004;321(1):144–153.
227. Elton D, Bruce EA, Bryant N, et al. The genetics of virus particle shape in equine influenza A virus. *Influenza Other Respir Viruses* 2013;7(Suppl 4):81–89.
228. Elton D, Medcalf L, Bishop K, et al. Identification of amino acid residues of influenza virus nucleoprotein essential for RNA binding. *J Virol* 1999;73(9):7357–7367.
229. Elton D, Medcalf E, Bishop K, et al. Oligomerization of the influenza virus nucleoprotein: identification of positive and negative sequence elements. *Virology* 1999;260(1):190–200.
230. Elton D, Simpson-Holley M, Archer K, et al. Interaction of the influenza virus nucleoprotein with the cellular CRM1-mediated nuclear export pathway. *J Virol* 2001;75(1):408–419.
231. Enami M, Enami K. Influenza virus hemagglutinin and neuraminidase glycoproteins stimulate the membrane association of the matrix protein. *J Virol* 1996;70(10):6653–6657.
232. Enami M, Fukuda R, Ishihama A. Transcription and replication of eight RNA segments of influenza virus. *Virology* 1985;142(1):68–77.
233. Enami M, Luytjes W, Krystal M, et al. Introduction of site-specific mutations into the genome of influenza virus. *Proc Natl Acad Sci U S A* 1990;87(10):3802–3805.
234. Enami M, Sharma G, Benham C, et al. An influenza virus containing nine different RNA segments. *Virology* 1991;185(1):291–298.
235. Engelhardt OG, Smith M, Fodor E. Association of the influenza A virus RNA-dependent RNA polymerase with cellular RNA polymerase II. *J Virol* 2005;79(9):5812–5818.
236. Essere B, Yver M, Gavazzi C, et al. Critical role of segment-specific packaging signals in genetic reassortment of influenza A viruses. *Proc Natl Acad Sci U S A* 2013;110(40):E38 40–E3848.
237. Everitt AR, Clare S, Pertel T, et al. IFITM3 restricts the morbidity and mortality associated with influenza. *Nature* 2012;484(7395):519–523.
238. Falcon AM, Fortes P, Marion RM, et al. Interaction of influenza virus NS1 protein and the human homologue of Staufen in vivo and in vitro. *Nucleic Acids Res* 1999;27(11):2241–2247.
239. Fechter P, Brownlee GG. Recognition of mRNA cap structures by viral and cellular proteins. *J Gen Virol* 2005;86(5):1239–1249.
240. Fechter P, Mingay L, Sharps J, et al. Two aromatic residues in the PB2 subunit of influenza A RNA polymerase are crucial for cap binding. *J Biol Chem* 2003;278(22):20381–20388.
241. Feigenblum D, Schneider RJ. Modification of eukaryotic initiation factor 4F during infection by influenza virus. *J Virol* 1993;67(6):3027–3035.
242. Feldmann A, Schäfer MK, Garten W, et al. Targeted infection of endothelial cells by avian influenza virus A/FPV/Rostock/34 (H7N1) in chicken embryos. *J Virol* 2000;74(17):8018–8027.
243. Ferko B, Stasakova J, Romanova J, et al. Immunogenicity and protection efficacy of replication-deficient influenza A viruses with altered NS1 genes. *J Virol* 2004;78(23):13037–13045.
244. Fernandez MV, Miller E, Krammer F, et al. Ion efflux and influenza infection trigger NLRP3 inflammasome signaling in human dendritic cells. *J Leukoc Biol* 2016;99(5):723–734.
245. Finberg RW, Lanno R, Anderson D, et al. Phase 2b study of pimodivir (JNJ-63623872) as monotherapy or in combination with oseltamivir for treatment of acute uncomplicated seasonal influenza A: TOPAZ trial. *J Infect Dis* 2019;219(7):1026–1034.
246. Firth AE, Jagger BW, Wise HM, et al. Ribosomal frameshifting used in influenza A virus expression occurs within the sequence UCC_UUU_CGU and is in the +1 direction. *Open Biol* 2012;2(10):120109.
247. Flandorfer A, Garcia-Sastre A, Basler CF, et al. Chimeric influenza A viruses with a functional influenza B virus neuraminidase or hemagglutinin. *J Virol* 2003;77(17):9116–9123.
248. Fleishman SJ, Whitehead TA, Ekiert DC, et al. Computational design of proteins targeting the conserved stem region of influenza hemagglutinin. *Science* 2011;332(6031):816–821.
249. Flick R, Neumann G, Hoffmann E, et al. Promoter elements in the influenza vRNA terminal structure. *RNA* 1996;2(10):1046–1057.
250. Fodor E, Brownlee GG. Influenza virus replication. In: Potter CW, ed. *Perspectives in Medical Virology*, vol. 7. Amsterdam: Elsevier B.V.; 2002:1–29.
251. Fodor E, Devenish L, Engelhardt OG, et al. Rescue of influenza A virus from recombinant DNA. *J Virol* 1999;73(11):9679–9682.
252. Fodor E, Mingay LJ, Crow M, et al. A single amino acid mutation in the PA subunit of the influenza virus RNA polymerase promotes the generation of defective interfering RNAs. *J Virol* 2003;77(8):5017–5020.
253. Fodor E, Palese P, Brownlee GG, et al. Attenuation of influenza A virus mRNA levels by promoter mutations. *J Virol* 1998;72(8):6283–6290.
254. Fodor E, Pritlove DC, Brownlee GG. The influenza virus panhandle is involved in the initiation of transcription. *J Virol* 1994;68(6):4092–4096.
255. Fodor E, Pritlove DC, Brownlee GG. Characterization of the RNA-fork model of virion RNA in the initiation of transcription in influenza A virus. *J Virol* 1995;69(7):4012–4019.
256. Fonville JM, Wilks SH, James SL, et al. Antibody landscapes after influenza virus infection or vaccination. *Science* 2014;346(6212):996–1000.
257. Formanowski F, Wharton SA, Calder LJ, et al. Fusion characteristics of influenza C viruses. *J Gen Virol* 1990;71(Pt 5):1181–1188.
258. Fortes P, Beloso A, Ortin J. Influenza virus NS1 protein inhibits pre-mRNA splicing and blocks mRNA nucleocytoplasmic transport. *EMBO J* 1994;13(3):704–712.
259. Fouchier RA, Smith DJ. Use of antigenic cartography in vaccine seed strain selection. *Avian Dis* 2010;54(1 Suppl):220–223.

260. Fournier G, Chiang C, Munier S, et al. Recruitment of RED-SMU1 complex by influenza A virus RNA polymerase to control viral mRNA splicing. *PLoS Pathog* 2014;10(6):e1004164.
261. Fournier E, Moules V, Essere B, et al. Interaction network linking the human H3N2 influenza A virus genomic RNA segments. *Vaccine* 2012;30(51):7359–7367.
262. Fournier E, Moules V, Essere B, et al. A supramolecular assembly formed by influenza A virus genomic RNA segments. *Nucleic Acids Res* 2012;40(5):2197–2209.
263. Freidl GS, Binger T, Müller MA, et al. Serological evidence of influenza A viruses in frugivorous bats from Africa. *PLoS One* 2015;10(5):e0127035.
264. Friesen RH, Lee PS, Stoop EJ, et al. A common solution to group 2 influenza virus neutralization. *Proc Natl Acad Sci U S A* 2014;111(1):445–450.
265. Frommhagen LH, Knight CA, Freeman NK. The ribonucleic acid, lipid, and polysaccharide constituents of influenza virus preparations. *Virology* 1959;8(2):176–197.
266. Fujii K, Fujii Y, Noda T, et al. Importance of both the coding and the segment-specific noncoding regions of the influenza A virus NS segment for its efficient incorporation into virions. *J Virol* 2005;79(6):3766–3774.
267. Fujii Y, Goto H, Watanabe T, et al. Selective incorporation of influenza virus RNA segments into virions. *Proc Natl Acad Sci U S A* 2003;100(4):2002–2007.
268. Fujii K, Ozawa M, Iwatsuki-Horimoto K, et al. Incorporation of influenza A virus genome segments does not absolutely require wild-type sequences. *J Gen Virol* 2009;90(Pt 7):1734–1740.
269. Fujioka Y, Nishide S, Ose T, et al. A sialylated voltage-dependent Ca^{2+} channel binds hemagglutinin and mediates influenza A virus entry into mammalian cells. *Cell Host Microbe* 2018;23(6):809–818.e805.
270. Fujiyoshi Y, Kume NP, Sakata K, et al. Fine structure of influenza A virus observed by electron cryo-microscopy. *EMBO J* 1994;13(2):318–326.
271. Fulton BO, Palese P, Heaton NS. Replication-competent influenza B reporter viruses as tools for screening antivirals and antibodies. *J Virol* 2015;89(23):12226–12231.
272. Fulton BO, Sun W, Heaton NS, et al. The Influenza B virus hemagglutinin head domain is less tolerant to transposon mutagenesis than that of the influenza A virus. *J Virol* 2018;92(16).
273. Furukawa T, Muraki Y, Noda T, et al. Role of the CM2 protein in the influenza C virus replication cycle. *J Virol* 2011;85(3):1322–1329.
274. Furusawa Y, Yamada S, Kawaoka Y. Host factor nucleoporin 93 is involved in the nuclear export of influenza virus RNA. *Front Microbiol* 2018;9:1675.
275. Furuse Y, Oshitani H. Evolution of the influenza A virus untranslated regions. *Infect Genet Evol* 2011;11(5):1150–1154.
276. Furuta Y, Takahashi K, Kuno-Maekawa M, et al. Mechanism of action of T-705 against influenza virus. *Antimicrob Agents Chemother* 2005;49(3):981–986.
277. Furuta Y, Takahashi K, Shiraki K, et al. T-705 (favipiravir) and related compounds: novel broad-spectrum inhibitors of RNA viral infections. *Antiviral Res* 2009;82(3):95–102.
278. Gabriel G, Herwig A, Klenk HD. Interaction of polymerase subunit PB2 and NP with importin alpha1 is a determinant of host range of influenza A virus. *PLoS Pathog* 2008;4(2):e11.
279. Gabriel G, Klingel K, Otte A, et al. Differential use of importin-alpha isoforms governs cell tropism and host adaptation of influenza virus. *Nat Commun* 2011;2:156.
280. Gack MU, Albrecht RA, Urano T, et al. Influenza A virus NS1 targets the ubiquitin ligase TRIM25 to evade recognition by the host viral RNA sensor RIG-I. *Cell Host Microbe* 2009;5(5):439–449.
281. Gale M, Jr., Tan SL, Katze MG. Translational control of viral gene expression in eukaryotes. *Microbiol Mol Biol Rev* 2000;64(2):239–280.
282. Galloway SE, Reed ML, Russell CJ, et al. Influenza HA subtypes demonstrate divergent phenotypes for cleavage activation and pH of fusion: implications for host range and adaptation. *PLoS Pathog* 2013;9(2):e1003151.
283. Gambaryan AS, Boravleva EY, Matrosovich TY, et al. Polymer-bound 6′ sialyl-N-acetyllactosamine protects mice infected by influenza virus. *Antiviral Res* 2005;68(3):116–123.
284. Gambaryan AS, Robertson JS, Matrosovich MN. Effects of egg-adaptation on the receptor-binding properties of human influenza A and B viruses. *Virology* 1999;258(2):232–239.
285. Gamblin S, Haire L, Russell R, et al. The structure and receptor binding properties of the 1918 influenza hemagglutinin. *Science* 2004;303(5665):1838–1842.
286. Gamblin SJ, Skehel JJ. Influenza hemagglutinin and neuraminidase membrane glycoproteins. *J Biol Chem* 2010;285(37):28403–28409.
287. Gannagé M, Dormann D, Albrecht R, et al. Matrix protein 2 of influenza A virus blocks autophagosome fusion with lysosomes. *Cell Host Microbe* 2009;6(4):367–380.
288. Gao Q, Brydon EW, Palese P. A seven-segmented influenza A virus expressing the influenza C virus glycoprotein HEF. *J Virol* 2008;82(13):6419–6426.
289. Gao Q, Chou YY, Doğanay S, et al. The influenza A virus PB2, PA, NP, and M segments play a pivotal role during genome packaging. *J Virol* 2012;86(13):7043–7051.
290. Gao Q, Lowen AC, Wang TT, et al. A nine-segment influenza a virus carrying subtype H1 and H3 hemagglutinins. *J Virol* 2010;84(16):8062–8071.
291. Gao Q, Palese P. Rewiring the RNAs of influenza virus to prevent reassortment. *Proc Natl Acad Sci U S A* 2009;106(37):15891–15896.
292. Gao S, Wu J, Liu RY, et al. Interaction of NS2 with AIMP2 facilitates the switch from ubiquitination to SUMOylation of M1 in influenza A virus-infected cells. *J Virol* 2015;89(1):300–311.
293. Garaigorta U, Ortin J. Mutation analysis of a recombinant NS replicon shows that influenza virus NS1 protein blocks the splicing and nucleo-cytoplasmic transport of its own viral mRNA. *Nucleic Acids Res* 2007;35(14):4573–4582.
294. Garcia-Robles I, Akarsu H, Müller CW, et al. Interaction of influenza virus proteins with nucleosomes. *Virology* 2005;332(1):329–336.
295. Garcia-Rosado E, Markussen T, Kileng O, et al. Molecular and functional characterization of two infectious salmon anaemia virus (ISAV) proteins with type I interferon antagonizing activity. *Virus Res* 2008;133(2):228–238.
296. Garcia-Sastre A. Transfectant influenza viruses as antigen delivery vectors. *Adv Virus Res* 2000;55:579–597.
297. Garcia-Sastre A, Egorov A, Matassov D, et al. Influenza A virus lacking the NS1 gene replicates in interferon-deficient systems. *Virology* 1998;252(2):324–330.
298. Garman E, Laver G. Controlling influenza by inhibiting the virus's neuraminidase. *Curr Drug Targets* 2004;5(2):119–136.
299. Gastaminza P, Perales B, Falcón AM, et al. Mutations in the N-terminal region of influenza virus PB2 protein affect virus RNA replication but not transcription. *J Virol* 2003;77(9):5098–5108.
300. Gavazzi C, Yver M, Isel C, et al. A functional sequence-specific interaction between influenza A virus genomic RNA segments. *Proc Natl Acad Sci U S A* 2013;110(41):16604–16609.
301. Gaymard A, Le Briand N, Frobert E, et al. Functional balance between neuraminidase and haemagglutinin in influenza viruses. *Clin Microbiol Infect* 2016;22(12):975–983.
302. Ge Q, Eisen HN, Chen J. Use of siRNAs to prevent and treat influenza virus infection. *Virus Res* 2004;102(1):37–42.
303. Geiss GK, Salvatore M, Tumpey TM, et al. Cellular transcriptional profiling in influenza A virus-infected lung epithelial cells: the role of the nonstructural NS1 protein in the evasion of the host innate defense and its potential contribution to pandemic influenza. *Proc Natl Acad Sci U S A* 2002;99(16):10736–10741.
304. Ghate AA, Air GM. Influenza type B neuraminidase can replace the function of type A neuraminidase. *Virology* 1999;264(2):265–277.
305. Gibbs JS, Malide D, Hornung F, et al. The influenza A virus PB1-F2 protein targets the inner mitochondrial membrane via a predicted basic amphipathic helix that disrupts mitochondrial function. *J Virol* 2003;77(13):7214–7224.
306. Gilbertson B, Zheng T, Gerber M, et al. Influenza NA and PB1 gene segments interact during the formation of viral progeny: localization of the binding region within the PB1 gene. *Viruses* 2016;8(8).
307. Glaser L, Stevens J, Zamarin D, et al. A single amino acid substitution in 1918 influenza virus hemagglutinin changes receptor binding specificity. *J Virol* 2005;79(17):11533–11536.
308. Glick GD, Toogood PL, Wiley DC, et al. Ligand recognition by influenza virus. The binding of bivalent sialosides. *J Biol Chem* 1991;266(35):23660–23669.
309. Gog JR, Afonso Edos S, Dalton RM, et al. Codon conservation in the influenza A virus genome defines RNA packaging signals. *Nucleic Acids Res* 2007;35(6):1897–1907.
310. Golebiewski L, Liu H, Javier RT, et al. The avian influenza virus NS1 ESEV PDZ binding motif associates with Dlg1 and Scribble to disrupt cellular tight junctions. *J Virol* 2011;85(20):10639–10648.
311. Goñi FM. "Rafts": a nickname for putative transient nanodomains. *Chem Phys Lipids* 2019;218:34–39.
312. Gonzalez S, Ortín J. Characterization of influenza virus PB1 protein binding to viral RNA: two separate regions of the protein contribute to the interaction domain. *J Virol* 1999;73(1):631–637.
313. González S, Ortín J. Distinct regions of influenza virus PB1 polymerase subunit recognize vRNA and cRNA templates. *EMBO J* 1999;18(13):3767–3775.
314. Gorai T, Goto H, Noda T, et al. F1Fo-ATPase, F-type proton-translocating ATPase, at the plasma membrane is critical for efficient influenza virus budding. *Proc Natl Acad Sci U S A* 2012;109(12):4615–4620.
315. Goto H, Muramoto Y, Noda T, et al. The genome-packaging signal of the influenza A virus genome comprises a genome incorporation signal and a genome-bundling signal. *J Virol* 2013;87(21):11316–11322.
316. Govorkova EA, Baranovich T, Seiler P, et al. Antiviral resistance among highly pathogenic influenza A (H5N1) viruses isolated worldwide in 2002–2012 shows need for continued monitoring. *Antiviral Res* 2013;98(2):297–304.
317. Graef KM, Vreede FT, Lau Y-F, et al. The PB2 subunit of the influenza virus RNA polymerase affects virulence by interacting with the mitochondrial antiviral signaling protein and inhibiting expression of beta interferon. *J Virol* 2010;84(17):8433–8445.
318. Graitcer SB, Gubareva L, Kamimoto L, et al. Characteristics of patients with oseltamivir-resistant pandemic (H1N1) 2009, United States. *Emerg Infect Dis* 2011;17(2):255–257.
319. Grantham ML, Stewart SM, Lalime EN, et al. Tyrosines in the influenza A virus M2 protein cytoplasmic tail are critical for production of infectious virus particles. *J Virol* 2010;84(17):8765–8776.
320. Graves PN, Schulman JL, Young JF, et al. Preparation of influenza virus subviral particles lacking the HA1 subunit of hemagglutinin: unmasking of cross-reactive HA2 determinants. *Virology* 1983;126(1):106–116.
321. Gschweitl M, Ulbricht A, Barnes CA, et al. A SPOPL/Cullin-3 ubiquitin ligase complex regulates endocytic trafficking by targeting EPS15 at endosomes. *Elife* 2016;5:e13841.
322. Gu W, Gallagher GR, Dai W, et al. Influenza A virus preferentially snatches noncoding RNA caps. *RNA* 2015;21(12):2067–2075.
323. Guan R, Ma LC, Leonard PG, et al. Structural basis for the sequence-specific recognition of human ISG15 by the NS1 protein of influenza B virus. *Proc Natl Acad Sci U S A* 2011;108(33):13468–13473.
324. Gubareva LV, Bethell R, Hart GJ, et al. Characterization of mutants of influenza A virus selected with the neuraminidase inhibitor 4-guanidino-Neu5Ac2en. *J Virol* 1996;70(3):1818–1827.
325. Gubareva LV, Trujillo AA, Okomo-Adhiambo M, et al. Comprehensive assessment of 2009 pandemic influenza A (H1N1) virus drug susceptibility in vitro. *Antivir Ther* 2010;15(8):1151–1159.
326. Gudheti MV, Curthoys NM, Gould TJ, et al. Actin mediates the nanoscale membrane organization of the clustered membrane protein influenza hemagglutinin. *Biophys J* 2013;104(10):2182–2192.
327. Guilligay D, Tarendeau F, Resa-Infante P, et al. The structural basis for cap binding by influenza virus polymerase subunit PB2. *Nat Struct Mol Biol* 2008;15(5):500.
328. Guindon S, Dufayard JF, Lefort V, et al. New algorithms and methods to estimate maximum-likelihood phylogenies: assessing the performance of PhyML 3.0. *Syst Biol* 2010;59(3):307–321.
329. Guinea R, Carrasco L. Requirement for vacuolar proton-ATPase activity during entry of influenza virus into cells. *J Virol* 1995;69(4):2306–2312.
330. Guo Z, Chen LM, Zeng H, et al. NS1 protein of influenza A virus inhibits the function of intracytoplasmic pathogen sensor, RIG-I. *Am J Respir Cell Mol Biol* 2007;36(3):263–269.
331. Guo CT, Ohta S, Yoshimoto A, et al. A unique phosphatidylinositol bearing a novel branched-chain fatty acid from *Rhodococcus equi* binds to influenza virus hemagglutinin and inhibits the infection of cells. *J Biochem* 2001;130(3):377–384.

332. Ha Y, Stevens DJ, Skehel JJ, et al. X-ray structure of the hemagglutinin of a potential H3 avian progenitor of the 1968 Hong Kong pandemic influenza virus. *Virology* 2003;309(2):209–218.

333. Haas DA, Meiler A, Geiger K, et al. Viral targeting of TFIIB impairs de novo polymerase II recruitment and affects antiviral immunity. *PLoS Pathog* 2018;14(4):e1006980.

334. Hagen M, Chung T, Butcher JA, et al. Recombinant influenza virus polymerase: requirement of both 5′ and 3′ viral ends for endonuclease activity. *J Virol* 1994;68(3):1509–1515.

335. Hagmaier K, Gelderblom HR, Kochs G. Functional comparison of the two gene products of Thogoto virus segment 6. *J Gen Virol* 2004;85:3699–3708.

336. Hagmaier K, Jennings S, Buse J, et al. Novel gene product of Thogoto virus segment 6 codes for an interferon antagonist. *J Virol* 2003;77(4):2747–2752.

337. Hai R, Garcia-Sastre A, Swayne DE, et al. A reassortment-incompetent live attenuated influenza virus vaccine for protection against pandemic virus strains. *J Virol* 2011;85(14):6832–6843.

338. Hai R, Martinez-Sobrido L, Fraser KA, et al. Influenza B virus NS1-truncated mutants: live-attenuated vaccine approach. *J Virol* 2008;82(21):10580–10590.

339. Hai R, Schmolke M, Leyva-Grado VH, et al. Influenza A(H7N9) virus gains neuraminidase inhibitor resistance without loss of in vivo virulence or transmissibility. *Nat Commun* 2013;4:2854.

340. Hale BG, Albrecht RA, Garcia-Sastre A. Innate immune evasion strategies of influenza viruses. *Future Microbiol* 2010;5(1):23–41.

341. Hale BG, Barclay WS, Randall RE, et al. Structure of an avian influenza A virus NS1 protein effector domain. *Virology* 2008;378(1):1–5.

342. Hale BG, Batty IH, Downes CP, et al. Binding of influenza A virus NS1 protein to the inter-SH2 domain of p85 suggests a novel mechanism for phosphoinositide 3-kinase activation. *J Biol Chem* 2008;283(3):1372–1380.

343. Hale BG, Jackson D, Chen YH, et al. Influenza A virus NS1 protein binds p85beta and activates phosphatidylinositol-3-kinase signaling. *Proc Natl Acad Sci U S A* 2006;103(38):14194–14199.

344. Hale BG, Kerry PS, Jackson D, et al. Structural insights into phosphoinositide 3-kinase activation by the influenza A virus NS1 protein. *Proc Natl Acad Sci U S A* 2010;107(5):1954–1959.

345. Hale BG, Randall RE, Ortin J, et al. The multifunctional NS1 protein of influenza A viruses. *J Gen Virol* 2008;89(Pt 10):2359–2376.

346. Haller O, Staeheli P, Kochs G. Protective role of interferon-induced Mx GTPases against influenza viruses. *Rev Sci Tech* 2009;28(1):219–231.

347. Hamilton BS, Gludish DW, Whittaker GR. Cleavage activation of the human-adapted influenza virus subtypes by matriptase reveals both subtype and strain specificities. *J Virol* 2012;86(19):10579–10586.

348. Han X, Bushweller JH, Cafiso DS, et al. Membrane structure and fusion-triggering conformational change of the fusion domain from influenza hemagglutinin. *Nat Struct Biol* 2001;8(8):715–720.

349. Han J, Perez JT, Chen C, et al. Genome-wide CRISPR/Cas9 screen identifies host factors essential for influenza virus replication. *Cell Rep* 2018;23(2):596–607.

350. Hao L, Sakurai A, Watanabe T, et al. Drosophila RNAi screen identifies host genes important for influenza virus replication. *Nature* 2008;454(7206):890–893.

351. Harding AT, Heaton BE, Dumm RE, et al. Rationally designed influenza virus vaccines that are antigenically stable during growth in eggs. *MBio* 2017;8(3):e00669.

352. Harris A, Cardone G, Winkler D, et al. Influenza virus pleiomorphy characterized by cryo-electron tomography. *Proc Natl Acad Sci U S A* 2006;103(50):19123–19127.

353. Harris A, Forouhar F, Qiu S, et al. The crystal structure of the influenza matrix protein M1 at neutral pH: M1-M1 protein interfaces can rotate in the oligomeric structures of M1. *Virology* 2001;289(1):34–44.

354. Harris AK, Meyerson JR, Matsuoka Y, et al. Structure and accessibility of HA trimers on intact 2009 H1N1 pandemic influenza virus to stem region-specific neutralizing antibodies. *Proc Natl Acad Sci U S A* 2013;110(12):4592–4597.

355. Harrison SC. Viral membrane fusion. *Virology* 2015;479–480:498–507.

356. Hatada E, Fukuda R. Binding of influenza A virus NS1 protein to dsRNA in vitro. *J Gen Virol* 1992;73:3325–3329.

357. Hatada E, Hasegawa M, Mukaigawa J, et al. Control of influenza virus gene expression: quantitative analysis of each viral RNA species in infected cells. *J Biochem (Tokyo)* 1989;105(4):537–546.

358. Hatta M, Kawaoka Y. The NB protein of influenza B virus is not necessary for virus replication in vitro. *J Virol* 2003;77(10):6050–6054.

359. Hause BM, Ducatez M, Collin EA, et al. Isolation of a novel swine influenza virus from Oklahoma in 2011 which is distantly related to human influenza C viruses. *PLoS Pathog* 2013;9(2):e1003176.

360. Hay AJ, Lomniczi B, Bellamy AR, et al. Transcription of the influenza virus genome. *Virology* 1977;83(2):337–355.

361. Hayashi T, Chaimayo C, McGuinness J, et al. Critical role of the PA-X C-terminal domain of influenza A virus in its subcellular localization and shutoff activity. *J Virol* 2016;90(16):7131–7141.

362. Hayashi T, MacDonald LA, Takimoto T. Influenza A virus protein PA-X contributes to viral growth and suppression of the host antiviral and immune responses. *J Virol* 2015;89(12):6442–6452.

363. Hayden F. Developing new antiviral agents for influenza treatment: what does the future hold? *Clin Infect Dis* 2009;48(Suppl 1):S3–S13.

364. Hayden FG, Sugaya N, Hirotsu N, et al. Baloxavir marboxil for uncomplicated influenza in adults and adolescents. *N Engl J Med* 2018;379(10):913–923.

365. He J, Sun E, Bujny MV, et al. Dual function of CD81 in influenza virus uncoating and budding. *PLoS Pathog* 2013;9(10):e1003701.

366. Heaton BE, Kennedy EM, Dumm RE, et al. A CRISPR activation screen identifies a pan-avian influenza virus inhibitory host factor. *Cell Rep* 2017;20(7):1503–1512.

367. Heaton NS, Leyva-Grado VH, Tan GS, et al. In vivo bioluminescent imaging of influenza a virus infection and characterization of novel cross-protective monoclonal antibodies. *J Virol* 2013;87(15):8272–8281.

368. Heaton NS, Moshkina N, Fenouil R, et al. Targeting viral proteostasis limits influenza virus, HIV, and dengue virus infection. *Immunity* 2016;44(1):46–58.

369. Heaton NS, Sachs D, Chen CJ, et al. Genome-wide mutagenesis of influenza virus reveals unique plasticity of the hemagglutinin and NS1 proteins. *Proc Natl Acad Sci U S A* 2013;110(50):20248–20253.

370. Heikkinen LS, Kazlauskas A, Melen K, et al. Avian and 1918 Spanish influenza a virus NS1 proteins bind to Crk/CrkL Src homology 3 domains to activate host cell signaling. *J Biol Chem* 2008;283(9):5719–5727.

371. Helenius A. Virus entry: looking back and moving forward. *J Mol Biol* 2018;430(13):1853–1862.

372. Hellebo A, Vilas U, Falk K, et al. Infectious salmon anemia virus specifically binds to and hydrolyzes 4-O-acetylated sialic acids. *J Virol* 2004;78(6):3055–3062.

373. Hemerka JN, Wang D, Weng Y, et al. Detection and characterization of influenza A virus PA-PB2 interaction through a bimolecular fluorescence complementation assay. *J Virol* 2009;83(8):3944–3955.

374. Hengrung N, El Omari K, Serna Martin I, et al. Crystal structure of the RNA-dependent RNA polymerase from influenza C virus. *Nature* 2015;527(7576):114–117.

375. Henkel M, Mitzner D, Henklein P, et al. The proapoptotic influenza A virus protein PB1-F2 forms a nonselective ion channel. *PLoS One* 2010;5(6):e11112.

376. Henry Dunand CJ, Leon PE, Kaur K, et al. Preexisting human antibodies neutralize recently emerged H7N9 influenza strains. *J Clin Invest* 2015;125(3):1255–1268.

377. Herberg JA, Kaforou M, Gormley S, et al. Transcriptomic profiling in childhood H1N1/09 influenza reveals reduced expression of protein synthesis genes. *J Infect Dis* 2013;208(10):1664–1668.

378. Herlocher ML, Truscon R, Elias S, et al. Influenza viruses resistant to the antiviral drug oseltamivir: transmission studies in ferrets. *J Infect Dis* 2004;190(9):1627–1630.

379. Herrler G, Durkop I, Becht H, et al. The glycoprotein of influenza C virus is the haemagglutinin, esterase and fusion factor. *J Gen Virol* 1988;69:839–846.

380. Herrler G, Rott R, Klenk HD, et al. The receptor-destroying enzyme of influenza C virus is neuraminate-O-acetylesterase. *EMBO J* 1985;4(6):1503–1506.

381. Hickman HD, Mays JW, Gibbs J, et al. Influenza A virus negative strand RNA is translated for CD8. *J Immunol* 2018;201(4):1222–1228.

382. Hillaire ML, Nieuwkoop NJ, Boon AC, et al. Binding of DC-SIGN to the hemagglutinin of influenza A viruses supports virus replication in DC-SIGN expressing cells. *PLoS One* 2013;8(2):e56164.

383. Hilsch M, Goldenbogen B, Sieben C, et al. Influenza A matrix protein M1 multimerizes upon binding to lipid membranes. *Biophys J* 2014;107(4):912–923.

384. Hirayama E, Atagi H, Hiraki A, et al. Heat shock protein 70 is related to thermal inhibition of nuclear export of the influenza virus ribonucleoprotein complex. *J Virol* 2004;78(3):1263–1270.

385. Hirst GK. The quantitative determination of influenza virus and antibodies by means of red cell agglutination. *J Exp Med* 1942;75(1):49–64.

386. Hoffman LR, Kuntz ID, White JM. Structure-based identification of an inducer of the low-pH conformational change in the influenza virus hemagglutinin: irreversible inhibition of infectivity. *J Virol* 1997;71(11):8808–8820.

387. Hoffmann HH, Kunz A, Simon VA, et al. Broad-spectrum antiviral that interferes with de novo pyrimidine biosynthesis. *Proc Natl Acad Sci U S A* 2011;108(14):5777–5782.

388. Hoffmann E, Mahmood K, Yang CF, et al. Rescue of influenza B virus from eight plasmids. *Proc Natl Acad Sci U S A* 2002;99(17):11411–11416.

389. Hoffmann E, Neumann G, Hobom G, et al. "Ambisense" approach for the generation of influenza A virus: vRNA and mRNA synthesis from one template. *Virology* 2000;267(2):310–317.

390. Hoffmann E, Neumann G, Kawaoka Y, et al. A DNA transfection system for generation of influenza A virus from eight plasmids. *Proc Natl Acad Sci U S A* 2000;97(11):6108–6113.

391. Holsinger LJ, Nichani D, Pinto LH, et al. Influenza A virus M2 ion channel protein: a structure-function analysis. *J Virol* 1994;68(3):1551–1563.

392. Honda A, Ueda K, Nagata K, et al. Identification of the RNA polymerase-binding site on genome RNA of influenza virus. *J Biochem (Tokyo)* 1987;102(5):1241–1249.

393. Hongo S, Ishii K, Mori K, et al. Detection of ion channel activity in Xenopus laevis oocytes expressing Influenza C virus CM2 protein. *Arch Virol* 2004;149(1):35–50.

394. Hongo S, Kitame F, Sugawara K, et al. Cloning and sequencing of influenza C/Yamagata/1/88 virus NS gene. *Arch Virol* 1992;126(1–4):343–349.

395. Hooper KA, Bloom JD. A mutant influenza virus that uses an N1 neuraminidase as the receptor-binding protein. *J Virol* 2013;87(23):12531–12540.

396. Hooper KA, Crowe JE, Bloom JD. Influenza viruses with receptor-binding N1 neuraminidases occur sporadically in several lineages and show no attenuation in cell culture or mice. *J Virol* 2015;89(7):3737–3745.

397. Horimoto T, Iwatsuki-Horimoto K, Hatta M, et al. Influenza A viruses possessing type B hemagglutinin and neuraminidase: potential as vaccine components. *Microbes Infect* 2004;6(6):579–583.

398. Horimoto T, Kawaoka Y. Designing vaccines for pandemic influenza. *Curr Top Microbiol Immunol* 2009;333:165–176.

399. Horimoto T, Takada A, Iwatsuki-Horimoto K, et al. Generation of influenza A viruses with chimeric (type A/B) hemagglutinins. *J Virol* 2003;77(14):8031–8038.

400. Horvath CM, Williams MA, Lamb RA. Eukaryotic coupled translation of tandem cistrons: identification of the influenza B virus BM2 polypeptide. *EMBO J* 1990;9(8):2639–2647.

401. Hrincius ER, Wixler V, Wolff T, et al. CRK adaptor protein expression is required for efficient replication of avian influenza A viruses and controls JNK-mediated apoptotic responses. *Cell Microbiol* 2010;12(6):831–843.

402. Hsu M-T, Parvin JD, Gupta S, et al. Genomic RNAs of influenza viruses are held in a circular conformation in virions and in infected cells by a terminal panhandle. *Proc Natl Acad Sci U S A* 1987;84(22):8140–8144.

403. Hu Y, Liu X, Zhang A, et al. CHD3 facilitates vRNP nuclear export by interacting with NES1 of influenza A virus NS2. *Cell Mol Life Sci* 2015;72(5):971–982.

404. Hu Y, Lu S, Song Z, et al. Association between adverse clinical outcome in human disease caused by novel influenza A H7N9 virus and sustained viral shedding and emergence of antiviral resistance. *Lancet* 2013;381(9885):2273–2279.

405. Hu F, Luo W, Hong M. Mechanisms of proton conduction and gating in influenza M2 proton channels from solid-state NMR. *Science* 2010;330(6003):505–508.
406. Hu Y, Sneyd H, Dekant R, et al. Influenza A virus nucleoprotein: a highly conserved multi-functional viral protein as a hot antiviral drug target. *Curr Top Med Chem* 2017;17(20):2271–2285.
407. Huang S, Chen J, Chen Q, et al. A second CRM1-dependent nuclear export signal in the influenza A virus NS2 protein contributes to the nuclear export of viral ribonucleoproteins. *J Virol* 2013;87(2):767–778.
408. Huang F, Chen J, Zhang J, et al. Identification of a novel compound targeting the nuclear export of influenza A virus nucleoprotein. *J Cell Mol Med* 2018;22(3):1826–1839.
409. Huang X, Liu T, Muller J, et al. Effect of influenza virus matrix protein and viral RNA on ribonucleoprotein formation and nuclear export. *Virology* 2001;287(2):405–416.
410. Huarte M, Falcón A, Nakaya Y, et al. Threonine 157 of influenza virus PA polymerase subunit modulates RNA replication in infectious viruses. *J Virol* 2003;77(10):6007–6013.
411. Hughey PG, Compans RW, Zebedee SL, et al. Expression of the influenza A virus M2 protein is restricted to apical surfaces of polarized epithelial cells. *J Virol* 1992;66(9):5542–5552.
412. Hurt AC, Holien JK, Parker MW, et al. Oseltamivir resistance and the H274Y neuraminidase mutation in seasonal, pandemic and highly pathogenic influenza viruses. *Drugs* 2009;69(18):2523–2531.
413. Hussain S, Turnbull ML, Wise HM, et al. Mutation of influenza A virus PA-X decreases pathogenicity in chicken embryos and can increase the yield of reassortant candidate vaccine viruses. *J Virol* 2019;93(2):e01551–e01518.
414. Hutchinson EC, Charles PD, Hester SS, et al. Conserved and host-specific features of influenza virion architecture. *Nat Commun* 2014;5:4816.
415. Hutchinson EC, Curran MD, Read EK, et al. Mutational analysis of cis-acting RNA signals in segment 7 of influenza A virus. *J Virol* 2008;82(23):11869–11879.
416. Hutchinson EC, Fodor E. Transport of the influenza virus genome from nucleus to nucleus. *Viruses* 2013;5(10):2424–2446.
417. Hutchinson EC, Wise HM, Kudryavtseva K, et al. Characterisation of influenza A viruses with mutations in segment 5 packaging signals. *Vaccine* 2009;27(45):6270–6275.
418. Ichinohe T, Pang IK, Iwasaki A. Influenza virus activates inflammasomes via its intracellular M2 ion channel. *Nat Immunol* 2010;11(5):404–410.
419. Imai M, Watanabe S, Ninomiya A, et al. Influenza B virus BM2 protein is a crucial component for incorporation of viral ribonucleoprotein complex into virions during virus assembly. *J Virol* 2004;78(20):11007–11015.
420. Imai M, Watanabe S, Odagiri T. Influenza B virus NS2, a nuclear export protein, directly associates with the viral ribonucleoprotein complex. *Arch Virol* 2003;148(10):1873–1884.
421. Inagaki A, Goto H, Kakugawa S, et al. Competitive incorporation of homologous gene segments of influenza A virus into virions. *J Virol* 2012;86(18):10200–10202.
422. Isaacs A, Lindenmann J. Virus interference. I. The interferon. *Proc R Soc Lond B Biol Sci* 1957;147(927):258–267.
423. Ison MG, Hayden FG. Therapeutic options for the management of influenza. *Curr Opin Pharmacol* 2001;1(5):482–490.
424. Ito T, Couceiro JN, Kelm S, et al. Molecular basis for the generation in pigs of influenza A viruses with pandemic potential. *J Virol* 1998;72(9):7367–7373.
425. Ives JA, Carr JA, Mendel DB, et al. The H274Y mutation in the influenza A/H1N1 neuraminidase active site following oseltamivir phosphate treatment leave virus severely compromised both in vitro and in vivo. *Antiviral Res* 2002;55(2):307–317.
426. Iwatsuki-Horimoto K, Horimoto T, Fujii Y, et al. Generation of influenza A virus NS2 (NEP) mutants with an altered nuclear export signal sequence. *J Virol* 2004;78(18):10149–10155.
427. Iwatsuki-Horimoto K, Horimoto T, Noda T, et al. The cytoplasmic tail of the influenza A virus M2 protein plays a role in viral assembly. *J Virol* 2006;80(11):5233–5240.
428. Jackson D, Barclay W, Zürcher T. Characterization of recombinant influenza B viruses with key neuraminidase inhibitor resistance mutations. *J Antimicrob Chemother* 2005;55(2):162–169.
429. Jackson D, Cadman A, Zurcher T, et al. A reverse genetics approach for recovery of recombinant influenza B viruses entirely from cDNA. *J Virol* 2002;76(22):11744–11747.
430. Jackson RJ, Cooper KL, Tappenden P, et al. Oseltamivir, zanamivir and amantadine in the prevention of influenza: a systematic review. *J Infect* 2011;62(1):14–25.
431. Jackson D, Elderfield RA, Barclay WS. Molecular studies of influenza B virus in the reverse genetics era. *J Gen Virol* 2011;92(Pt 1):1–17.
432. Jackson D, Killip MJ, Galloway CS, et al. Loss of function of the influenza A virus NS1 protein promotes apoptosis but this is not due to a failure to activate phosphatidylinositol 3-kinase (PI3K). *Virology* 2010;396(1):94–105.
433. Jagger B, Wise H, Kash J, et al. An overlapping protein-coding region in influenza A virus segment 3 modulates the host response. *Science* 2012;337(6091):199–204.
434. Jennings S, Martinez-Sobrido L, Garcia-Sastre A, et al. Thogoto virus ML protein suppresses IRF3 function. *Virology* 2005;331(1):63–72.
435. Jiang Y, Wang X. Structural insights into the species preference of the influenza B virus NS1 protein in ISG15 binding. *Protein Cell* 2018:1–7.
436. Jin H, Leser GP, Zhang J, et al. Influenza virus hemagglutinin and neuraminidase cytoplasmic tails control particle shape. *EMBO J* 1997;16(6):1236–1247.
437. Jin H, Subbarao K, Bagai S, et al. Palmitylation of the influenza virus hemagglutinin (H3) is not essential for virus assembly or infectivity. *J Virol* 1996;70(3):1406–1414.
438. Johnson NP, Mueller J. Updating the accounts: global mortality of the 1918–1920 "Spanish" influenza pandemic. *Bull Hist Med* 2002;76(1):105–115.
439. Jones LV, Compans RW, Davis AR, et al. Surface expression of influenza virus neuraminidase, an amino-terminally anchored viral membrane glycoprotein, in polarized epithelial cells. *Mol Cell Biol* 1985;5(9):2181–2189.
440. Jones IM, Reay PA, Philpott KL. Nuclear location of all three influenza polymerase proteins and a nuclear signal in polymerase PB2. *EMBO J* 1986;5(9):2371–2376.
441. Jorba N, Coloma R, Ortin J. Genetic trans-complementation establishes a new model for influenza virus RNA transcription and replication. *PLoS Pathog* 2009;5(5):e1000462.
442. Jorba N, Juarez S, Torreira E, et al. Analysis of the interaction of influenza virus polymerase complex with human cell factors. *Proteomics* 2008;8(10):2077–2088.
443. Jordan PC, Stevens SK, Deval J. Nucleosides for the treatment of respiratory RNA virus infections. *Antivir Chem Chemother* 2018;26:2040206618764483.
444. Joyce MG, Wheatley AK, Thomas PV, et al. Vaccine-induced antibodies that neutralize group 1 and group 2 influenza A viruses. *Cell* 2016;166(3):609–623.
445. Ju X, Yan Y, Liu Q, et al. Neuraminidase of influenza A virus binds lysosome-associated membrane proteins directly and induces lysosome rupture. *J Virol* 2015;89(20):10347–10358.
446. Kadam RU, Wilson IA. Structural basis of influenza virus fusion inhibition by the antiviral drug Arbidol. *Proc Natl Acad Sci U S A* 2017;114(2):206–214.
447. Kakisaka M, Yamada K, Yamaji-Hasegawa A, et al. Intrinsically disordered region of influenza A NP regulates viral genome packaging via interactions with viral RNA and host PI(4,5)P2. *Virology* 2016;496:116–126.
448. Kamal R, Alymova I, York I. Evolution and virulence of influenza A virus protein PB1-F2. *Int J Mol Sci* 2017;19(1):96.
449. Kao RY, Yang D, Lau LS, et al. Identification of influenza A nucleoprotein as an antiviral target. *Nat Biotechnol* 2010;28(6):600–605.
450. Karakus U, Thamamongood T, Ciminski K, et al. MHC class II proteins mediate cross-species entry of bat influenza viruses. *Nature* 2019;567(7746):109–112.
451. Karlas A, Machuy N, Shin Y, et al. Genome-wide RNAi screen identifies human host factors crucial for influenza virus replication. *Nature* 2010;463(7282):818–822.
452. Karlsson EA, Meliopoulos VA, Savage C, et al. Visualizing real-time influenza virus infection, transmission and protection in ferrets. *Nat Commun* 2015;6:6378.
453. Karlsson EA, Meliopoulos VA, Tran V, et al. Measuring influenza virus infection using bioluminescent reporter viruses for in vivo imaging and in vitro replication assays. *Methods Mol Biol* 2018;1836:431–459.
454. Kash JC, Cunningham DM, Smit MW, et al. Selective translation of eukaryotic mRNAs: functional molecular analysis of GRSF-1, a positive regulator of influenza virus protein synthesis. *J Virol* 2002;76(20):10417–10426.
455. Kashyap AK, Steel J, Rubrum A, et al. Protection from the 2009 H1N1 pandemic influenza by an antibody from combinatorial survivor-based libraries. *PLoS Pathog* 2010;6(7):e1000990.
456. Katoh K, Standley DM. MAFFT multiple sequence alignment software version 7: improvements in performance and usability. *Mol Biol Evol* 2013;30(4):772–780.
457. Kawaguchi A, Matsumoto K, Nagata K. YB-1 functions as a porter to lead influenza virus ribonucleoprotein complexes to microtubules. *J Virol* 2012;86(20):11086–11095.
458. Kerry PS, Ayllon J, Taylor MA, et al. A transient homotypic interaction model for the influenza A virus NS1 protein effector domain. *PLoS One* 2011;6(3):e17946.
459. Kerry PS, Long E, Taylor MA, et al. Conservation of a crystallographic interface suggests a role for beta-sheet augmentation in influenza virus NS1 multifunctionality. *Acta Crystallogr Sect F Struct Biol Cryst Commun* 2011;67(Pt 8):858–861.
460. Kesinger E, Liu J, Jensen A, et al. Influenza D virus M2 protein exhibits ion channel activity in Xenopus laevis oocytes. *PLoS One* 2018;13(6):e0199227.
461. Khaperskyy DA, Emara MM, Johnston BP, et al. Influenza a virus host shutoff disables antiviral stress-induced translation arrest. *PLoS Pathog* 2014;10(7):e1004217.
462. Khaperskyy DA, Schmaling S, Larkins-Ford J, et al. Selective degradation of host RNA polymerase II transcripts by influenza A virus PA-X host shutoff protein. *PLoS Pathog* 2016;12(2):e1005427.
463. Kilbourne ED, Pokorny BA, Johansson B, et al. Protection of mice with recombinant influenza virus neuraminidase. *J Infect Dis* 2004;189(3):459–461.
464. Kilby JM, Hopkins S, Venetta TM, et al. Potent suppression of HIV-1 replication in humans by T-20, a peptide inhibitor of gp41-mediated virus entry. *Nat Med* 1998;4(11):1302–1307.
465. Kirkpatrick E, Qiu X, Wilson PC, et al. The influenza virus hemagglutinin head evolves faster than the stalk domain. *Sci Rep* 2018;8(1):10432.
466. Kiso M, Mitamura K, Sakai-Tagawa Y, et al. Resistant influenza A viruses in children treated with oseltamivir: descriptive study. *Lancet* 2004;364(9436):759–765.
467. Kiso M, Takahashi K, Sakai-Tagawa Y, et al. T-705 (favipiravir) activity against lethal H5N1 influenza A viruses. *Proc Natl Acad Sci U S A* 2010;107(2):882–887.
468. Klemm C, Boergeling Y, Ludwig S, et al. Immunomodulatory nonstructural proteins of influenza A viruses. *Trends Microbiol* 2018;26(7):624–636.
469. Klenk HD, Rott R, Orlich M, et al. Activation of influenza A viruses by trypsin treatment. *Virology* 1975;68(2):426–439.
470. Klumpp K, Ruigrok RW, Baudin F. Roles of the influenza virus polymerase and nucleoprotein in forming a functional RNP structure. *EMBO J* 1997;16(6):1248–1257.
471. Knossow M, Gaudier M, Douglas A, et al. Mechanism of neutralization of influenza virus infectivity by antibodies. *Virology* 2002;302(2):294–298.
472. Kochs G, Bauer S, Vogt C, et al. Thogoto virus infection induces sustained type I interferon responses that depend on RIG-I-like helicase signaling of conventional dendritic cells. *J Virol* 2010;84(23):12344–12350.
473. Kochs G, Garcia-Sastre A, Martinez-Sobrido L. Multiple anti-interferon actions of the influenza A virus NS1 protein. *J Virol* 2007;81(13):7011–7021.
474. Kochs G, Weber F, Gruber S, et al. Thogoto virus matrix protein is encoded by a spliced mRNA. *J Virol* 2000;74(22):10785–10789.
475. Koday MT, Nelson J, Chevalier A, et al. A computationally designed hemagglutinin stem-binding protein provides in vivo protection from influenza independent of a host immune response. *PLoS Pathog* 2016;12(2):e1005409.
476. Kohno S, Kida H, Mizuguchi M, et al. Intravenous peramivir for treatment of influenza A and B virus infection in high-risk patients. *Antimicrob Agents Chemother* 2011;55(6):2803–2812.
477. Kolesnikova L, Heck S, Matrosovich T, et al. Influenza virus budding from the tips of cellular microvilli in differentiated human airway epithelial cells. *J Gen Virol* 2013;94(Pt 5):971–976.
478. König R, Stertz S, Zhou Y, et al. Human host factors required for influenza virus replication. *Nature* 2010;463(7282):813–817.
479. Koppstein D, Ashour J, Bartel DP. Sequencing the cap-snatching repertoire of H1N1 influenza provides insight into the mechanism of viral transcription initiation. *Nucleic Acids Res* 2015;43(10):5052–5064.

480. Košík I, Hollý J, Russ G. PB1-F2 expedition from the whole protein through the domain to aa residue function. *Acta Virol* 2013;57(2):138–148.
481. Koszalka P, Tilmanis D, Hurt AC. Influenza antivirals currently in late-phase clinical trial. *Influenza Other Respir Viruses* 2017;11(3):240–246.
482. Kozakov D, Chuang GY, Beglov D, et al. Where does amantadine bind to the influenza virus M2 proton channel? *Trends Biochem Sci* 2010;35(9):471–475.
483. Krammer F. The human antibody response to influenza A virus infection and vaccination. *Nat Rev Immunol* 2019;19(6):383–397.
484. Krammer F, Fouchier RAM, Eichelberger MC, et al. NAction! How can neuraminidase-based immunity contribute to better influenza virus vaccines? *MBio* 2018;9(2).
485. Krammer F, Palese P. Advances in the development of influenza virus vaccines. *Nat Rev Drug Discov* 2015;14(3):167–182.
486. Krammer F, Smith GJD, Fouchier RAM, et al. Influenza. *Nat Rev Dis Primers* 2018;4(1):3.
487. Kretzschmar E, Bui M, Rose JK. Membrane association of influenza virus matrix protein does not require specific hydrophobic domains or the viral glycoproteins. *Virology* 1996;220(1):37–45.
488. Krug RM. Functions of the influenza A virus NS1 protein in antiviral defense. *Curr Opin Virol* 2015;12:1–6.
489. Krug RM, Ueda M, Palese P. Temperature-sensitive mutants of influenza WSN virus defective in virus-specific RNA synthesis. *J Virol* 1975;16(4):790–796.
490. Krug RM, Yuan W, Noah DL, et al. Intracellular warfare between human influenza viruses and human cells: the roles of the viral NS1 protein. *Virology* 2003;309(2):181–189.
491. Krumm SA, Ndungu JM, Yoon JJ, et al. Potent host-directed small-molecule inhibitors of myxovirus RNA-dependent RNA-polymerases. *PLoS One* 2011;6(5):e20069.
492. Kumakura M, Kawaguchi A, Nagata K. Actin-myosin network is required for proper assembly of influenza virus particles. *Virology* 2015;476:141–150.
493. Kumar N, Liang Y, Parslow TG. Receptor tyrosine kinase inhibitors block multiple steps of influenza a virus replication. *J Virol* 2011;85(6):2818–2827.
494. Kumar N, Sharma NR, Ly H, et al. Receptor tyrosine kinase inhibitors that block replication of influenza a and other viruses. *Antimicrob Agents Chemother* 2011;55(12):5553–5559.
495. Kundu A, Avalos RT, Sanderson CM, et al. Transmembrane domain of influenza virus neuraminidase, a type II protein, possesses an apical sorting signal in polarized MDCK cells. *J Virol* 1996;70(9):6508–6515.
496. Lai JC, Chan WW, Kien F, et al. Formation of virus-like particles from human cell lines exclusively expressing influenza neuraminidase. *J Gen Virol* 2010;91(Pt 9):2322–2330.
497. Lai AL, Tamm LK. Shallow boomerang-shaped influenza hemagglutinin G13A mutant structure promotes leaky membrane fusion. *J Biol Chem* 2010;285(48):37467–37475.
498. Lakadamyali M, Rust MJ, Babcock HP, et al. Visualizing infection of individual influenza viruses. *Proc Natl Acad Sci U S A* 2003;100(16):9280–9285.
499. Lakdawala SS, Fodor E, Subbarao K. Moving on out: transport and packaging of influenza viral RNA into virions. *Annu Rev Virol* 2016;3(1):411–427.
500. Lakdawala SS, Wu Y, Wawrzusin P, et al. Influenza a virus assembly intermediates fuse in the cytoplasm. *PLoS Pathog* 2014;10(3):e1003971.
501. Lamb RA, Choppin PW. Segment 8 of the influenza virus genome is unique in coding for two polypeptides. *Proc Natl Acad Sci U S A* 1979;76(10):4908–4912.
502. Lamb RA, Choppin PW. Identification of a second protein (M2) encoded by RNA segment 7 of influenza virus. *Virology* 1981;112(2):729–737.
503. Lamb RA, Choppin PW, Chanock RM, et al. Mapping of the two overlapping genes for polypeptides NS1 and NS2 on RNA segment 8 of influenza virus genome. *Proc Natl Acad Sci U S A* 1980;77(4):1857–1861.
504. Lamb RA, Lai CJ. Sequence of interrupted and uninterrupted mRNAs and cloned DNA coding for the two overlapping nonstructural proteins of influenza virus. *Cell* 1980;21(2):475–485.
505. Lamb RA, Lai CJ. Spliced and unspliced messenger RNAs synthesized from cloned influenza virus M DNA in an SV40 vector: expression of the influenza virus membrane protein (M1). *Virology* 1982;123(2):237–256.
506. Lamb RA, Lai CJ. Expression of unspliced NS1 mRNA, spliced NS2 mRNA, and a spliced chimera mRNA from cloned influenza virus NS DNA in an SV40 vector. *Virology* 1984;135(1):139–147.
507. Lamb RA, Lai CJ, Choppin PW. Sequences of mRNAs derived from genome RNA segment 7 of influenza virus: colinear and interrupted mRNAs code for overlapping proteins. *Proc Natl Acad Sci U S A* 1981;78(7):4170–4174.
508. Lambert AJ, Velez JO, Brault AC, et al. Molecular, serological and in vitro culture-based characterization of Bourbon virus, a newly described human pathogen of the genus Thogotovirus. *J Clin Virol* 2015;73:127–132.
509. Landeras-Bueno S, Jorba N, Pérez-Cidoncha M, et al. The splicing factor proline-glutamine rich (SFPQ/PSF) is involved in influenza virus transcription. *PLoS Pathog* 2011;7(11):e1002397.
510. Larson JL, Kang SK, Choi BI, et al. A safety evaluation of DAS181, a sialidase fusion protein, in rodents. *Toxicol Sci* 2011;122(2):567–578.
511. Laursen NS, Friesen RHE, Zhu X, et al. Universal protection against influenza infection by a multidomain antibody to influenza hemagglutinin. *Science* 2018;362(6414):598–602.
512. Laver WG. Influenza virus surface glycoproteins, haemagglutinin and neuraminidase: a personal account. In: Potter CW, ed. *Influenza*, vol. 7. Amsterdam: Elsevier Science B.V.; 2002.
513. Lazarowitz SG, Choppin PW. Enhancement of the infectivity of influenza A and B viruses by proteolytic cleavage of the hemagglutinin polypeptide. *Virology* 1975;68(2):440–454.
514. Le Sage V, Nanni AV, Bhagwat AR, et al. Non-uniform and non-random binding of nucleoprotein to influenza A and B viral RNA. *Viruses* 2018;10(10).
515. Leahy MB, Zecchin G, Brownlee GG. Differential activation of influenza A virus endonuclease activity is dependent on multiple sequence differences between the virion RNA and cRNA promoters. *J Virol* 2002;76(4):2019–2023.
516. Lee MK, Bae SH, Park CJ, et al. A single-nucleotide natural variation (U4 to C4) in an influenza A virus promoter exhibits a large structural change: implications for differential viral RNA synthesis by RNA-dependent RNA polymerase. *Nucleic Acids Res* 2003;31(4):1216–1223.
517. Lee J, Boutz DR, Chromikova V, et al. Molecular-level analysis of the serum antibody repertoire in young adults before and after seasonal influenza vaccination. *Nat Med* 2016;22(12):1456–1464.
518. Lee MG, Kim KH, Park KY, et al. Evaluation of anti-influenza effects of camostat in mice infected with non-adapted human influenza viruses. *Arch Virol* 1996;141(10):1979–1989.
519. Lee J, Kim J, Son K, et al. Acid phosphatase 2 (ACP2) is required for membrane fusion during influenza virus entry. *Sci Rep* 2017;7:43893.
520. Lee MTM, Klumpp K, Digard P, et al. Activation of influenza virus RNA polymerase by the 5′ and 3′ terminal duplex of genomic RNA. *Nucleic Acids Res* 2003;31(6):1624–1632.
521. Lee N, Le Sage V, Nanni AV, et al. Genome-wide analysis of influenza viral RNA and nucleoprotein association. *Nucleic Acids Res* 2017;45(15):8968–8977.
522. Lee JH, Oh JY, Pascua PN, et al. Impairment of the Staufen1-NS1 interaction reduces influenza viral replication. *Biochem Biophys Res Commun* 2011;414(1):153–158.
523. Lee KH, Seong BL. The position 4 nucleotide at the 3′ end of the influenza virus neuraminidase vRNA is involved in temporal regulation of transcription and replication of neuraminidase RNAs and affects the repertoire of influenza virus surface antigens. *J Gen Virol* 1998;79:1923–1934.
524. Lee CW, Suarez DL. Reverse genetics of the avian influenza virus. *Methods Mol Biol* 2008;436:99–111.
525. Leibbrandt A, Meier C, König-Schuster M, et al. Iota-carrageenan is a potent inhibitor of influenza A virus infection. *PLoS One* 2010;5(12):e14320.
526. Leser GP, Lamb RA. Lateral organization of influenza virus proteins in the budozone region of the plasma membrane. *J Virol* 2017;91(9).
527. Leung HS, Li OT, Chan RW, et al. Entry of influenza A virus with a α2,6-linked sialic acid binding preference requires host fibronectin. *J Virol* 2012;86(19):10704–10713.
528. Levental I, Veatch S. The continuing mystery of lipid rafts. *J Mol Biol* 2016;428(24 Pt A):4749–4764.
529. Leyssen P, De Clercq E, Neyts J. Molecular strategies to inhibit the replication of RNA viruses. *Antiviral Res* 2008;78(1):9–25.
530. Li Y, Anderson DH, Liu Q, et al. Mechanism of influenza A virus NS1 protein interaction with the p85beta, but not the p85alpha, subunit of phosphatidylinositol 3-kinase (PI3K) and up-regulation of PI3K activity. *J Biol Chem* 2008;283(34):23397–23409.
531. Li Y, Cao H, Dao N, et al. High-throughput neuraminidase substrate specificity study of human and avian influenza A viruses. *Virology* 2011;415(1):12–19.
532. Li Y, Chen ZY, Wang W, et al. The 3′-end-processing factor CPSF is required for the splicing of single-intron pre-mRNAs in vivo. *RNA* 2001;7(6):920–931.
533. Li W, Escarpe PA, Eisenberg EJ, et al. Identification of GS 4104 as an orally bioavailable prodrug of the influenza virus neuraminidase inhibitor GS 4071. *Antimicrob Agents Chemother* 1998;42(3):647–653.
534. Li ZN, Mueller SN, Ye L, et al. Chimeric influenza virus hemagglutinin proteins containing large domains of the Bacillus anthracis protective antigen: protein characterization, incorporation into infectious influenza viruses, and antigenicity. *J Virol* 2005;79(15):10003–10012.
535. Li X, Palese P. Characterization of the polyadenylation signal of influenza virus RNA. *J Virol* 1994;68(2):1245–1249.
536. Li S, Polonis V, Isobe H, et al. Chimeric influenza virus induces neutralizing antibodies and cytotoxic T cells against human immunodeficiency virus type 1. *J Virol* 1993;67(11):6659–6666.
537. Li ML, Ramirez BC, Krug RM. RNA-dependent activation of primer RNA production by influenza virus polymerase: different regions of the same protein subunit constitute the two required RNA-binding sites. *EMBO J* 1998;17(19):5844–5852.
538. Li S, Rodrigues M, Rodriguez D, et al. Priming with recombinant influenza virus followed by administration of recombinant vaccinia virus induces CD8+ T-cell-mediated protective immunity against malaria. *Proc Natl Acad Sci U S A* 1993;90(11):5214–5218.
539. Li Z, Watanabe T, Hatta M, et al. Mutational analysis of conserved amino acids in the influenza A virus nucleoprotein. *J Virol* 2009;83(9):4153–4162.
540. Liang Y, Hong Y, Parslow TG. cis-Acting packaging signals in the influenza virus PB1, PB2, and PA genomic RNA segments. *J Virol* 2005;79(16):10348–10355.
541. Liang Y, Huang T, Ly H, et al. Mutational analyses of packaging signals in influenza virus PA, PB1, and PB2 genomic RNA segments. *J Virol* 2008;82(1):229–236.
542. Liao TL, Wu CY, Su WC, et al. Ubiquitination and deubiquitination of NP protein regulates influenza A virus RNA replication. *EMBO J* 2010;29(22):3879–3890.
543. Lietzén N, Ohman T, Rintahaka J, et al. Quantitative subcellular proteome and secretome profiling of influenza A virus-infected human primary macrophages. *PLoS Pathog* 2011;7(5):e1001340.
544. Lin S, Naim HY, Rodriguez AC, et al. Mutations in the middle of the transmembrane domain reverse the polarity of transport of the influenza virus hemagglutinin in MDCK epithelial cells. *J Cell Biol* 1998;142(1):51–57.
545. Lindenmann J. [Interferon and inverse interference]. *Zeitschr f Hygiene* 1960;146:287–309.
546. Liu C, Eichelberger MC, Compans RW, et al. Influenza type A virus neuraminidase does not play a role in viral entry, replication, assembly, or budding. *J Virol* 1995;69(2):1099–1106.
547. Liu H, Golebiewski L, Dow EC, et al. The ESEV PDZ-binding motif of the avian influenza A virus NS1 protein protects infected cells from apoptosis by directly targeting Scribble. *J Virol* 2010;84(21):11164–11174.
548. Liu J, Lynch PA, Chien CY, et al. Crystal structure of the unique RNA-binding domain of the influenza virus NS1 protein. *Nat Struct Biol* 1997;4(11):896–899.
549. Londrigan SL, Turville SG, Tate MD, et al. N-linked glycosylation facilitates sialic acid-independent attachment and entry of influenza A viruses into cells expressing DC-SIGN or L-SIGN. *J Virol* 2011;85(6):2990–3000.
550. Long JS, Giotis ES, Moncorgé O, et al. Species difference in ANP32A underlies influenza A virus polymerase host restriction. *Nature* 2016;529(7584):101–104.
551. Lorieau JL, Louis JM, Bax A. The complete influenza hemagglutinin fusion domain adopts a tight helical hairpin arrangement at the lipid:water interface. *Proc Natl Acad Sci U S A* 2010;107(25):11341–11346.
552. Lu Y, Qian XY, Krug RM. The influenza virus NS1 protein: a novel inhibitor of pre-mRNA splicing. *Genes Dev* 1994;8(15):1817–1828.

553. Ludwig S. Disruption of virus-host cell interactions and cell signaling pathways as an antiviral approach against influenza virus infections. *Biol Chem* 2011;392(10):837–847.
554. Ludwig S, Wang X, Ehrhardt C, et al. The influenza A virus NS1 protein inhibits activation of Jun N-terminal kinase and AP-1 transcription factors. *J Virol* 2002;76(21):11166–11171.
555. Lukarska M, Fournier G, Pflug A, et al. Structural basis of an essential interaction between influenza polymerase and Pol II CTD. *Nature* 2017;541(7635):117–121.
556. Luo G, Cianci C, Harte W, et al. Conquering influenza: recent advances in anti-influenza drug discovery. *IDrugs* 1999;2(7):671–685.
557. Luo G, Luytjes W, Enami M, et al. The polyadenylation signal of influenza virus RNA involves a stretch of uridines followed by the RNA duplex of the panhandle structure. *J Virol* 1991;65(6):2861–2867.
558. Luo C, Nobusawa E, Nakajima K. An analysis of the role of neuraminidase in the receptor-binding activity of influenza B virus: the inhibitory effect of Zanamivir on haemadsorption. *J Gen Virol* 1999;80(Pt 11):2969–2976.
559. Luo C, Nobusawa E, Nakajima K. Analysis of the desialidation process of the haemagglutinin protein of influenza B virus: the host-dependent desialidation step. *J Gen Virol* 2002;83(Pt 7):1729–1734.
560. Luytjes W, Krystal M, Enami M, et al. Amplification, expression, and packaging of foreign gene by influenza virus. *Cell* 1989;59(6):1107–1113.
561. Ma K, Roy AM, Whittaker GR. Nuclear export of influenza virus ribonucleoproteins: identification of an export intermediate at the nuclear periphery. *Virology* 2001;282(2):215–220.
562. Ma X, Xie L, Wartchow C, et al. Structural basis for therapeutic inhibition of influenza A polymerase PB2 subunit. *Sci Rep* 2017;7(1):9385.
563. Magadán JG, Khurana S, Das SR, et al. Influenza A virus hemagglutinin trimerization completes monomer folding and antigenicity. *J Virol* 2013;87(17):9742–9753.
564. Maier HJ, Kashiwagi T, Hara K, et al. Differential role of the influenza A virus polymerase PA subunit for vRNA and cRNA promoter binding. *Virology* 2008;370(1):194–204.
565. Malakhova OA, Yan M, Malakhov MP, et al. Protein ISGylation modulates the JAK-STAT signaling pathway. *Genes Dev* 2003;17(4):455–460.
566. Manicassamy B, Manicassamy S, Belicha-Villanueva A, et al. Analysis of in vivo dynamics of influenza virus infection in mice using a GFP reporter virus. *Proc Natl Acad Sci U S A* 2010;107(25):11531–11536.
567. Manzoor R, Igarashi M, Takada A. Influenza A virus M2 protein: roles from ingress to egress. *Int J Mol Sci* 2017;18(12).
568. Mar KB, Rinkenberger NR, Boys IN, et al. LY6E mediates an evolutionarily conserved enhancement of virus infection by targeting a late entry step. *Nat Commun* 2018;9(1):3603.
569. Marazzi I, Ho JS, Kim J, et al. Suppression of the antiviral response by an influenza histone mimic. *Nature* 2012;483(7390):428–433.
570. Marc D. Influenza virus non-structural protein NS1: interferon antagonism and beyond. *J Gen Virol* 2014;95(Pt 12):2594–2611.
571. Marcos-Villar L, Pazo A, Nieto A. Influenza virus and chromatin: role of the CHD1 chromatin remodeler in the virus life cycle. *J Virol* 2016;90(7):3694–3707.
572. Marsh GA, Hatami R, Palese P. Specific residues of the influenza A virus hemagglutinin viral RNA are important for efficient packaging into budding virions. *J Virol* 2007;81(18):9727–9736.
573. Marsh M, Helenius A. Virus entry into animal cells. *Adv Virus Res* 1989;36:107–151.
574. Marsh GA, Rabadán R, Levine AJ, et al. Highly conserved regions of influenza a virus polymerase gene segments are critical for efficient viral RNA packaging. *J Virol* 2008;82(5):2295–2304.
575. Martin K, Helenius A. Transport of incoming influenza virus nucleocapsids into the nucleus. *J Virol* 1991;65(1):232–244.
576. Martin K, Helenius A. Nuclear transport of influenza virus ribonucleoproteins: the viral matrix protein (M1) promotes export and inhibits import. *Cell* 1991;67(1):117–130.
577. Martin-Benito J, Area E, Ortega J, et al. Three-dimensional reconstruction of a recombinant influenza virus ribonucleoprotein particle. *EMBO Rep* 2001;2(4):313–317.
578. Martinez-Sobrido L, Garcia-Sastre A. Generation of recombinant influenza virus from plasmid DNA. *J Vis Exp* 2010;42:2057.
579. Martyna A, Bahsoun B, Badham MD, et al. Membrane remodeling by the M2 amphipathic helix drives influenza virus membrane scission. *Sci Rep* 2017;7:44695.
580. Mata MA, Satterly N, Versteeg GA, et al. Chemical inhibition of RNA viruses reveals REDD1 as a host defense factor. *Nat Chem Biol* 2011;7(10):712–719.
581. Matlin KS, Reggio H, Helenius A, et al. Infectious entry pathway of influenza virus in a canine kidney cell line. *J Cell Biol* 1981;91(3 Pt 1):601–613.
582. Matrosovich MN, Matrosovich TY, Gray T, et al. Human and avian influenza viruses target different cell types in cultures of human airway epithelium. *Proc Natl Acad Sci U S A* 2004;101(13):4620–4624.
583. Matrosovich MN, Matrosovich TY, Gray T, et al. Neuraminidase is important for the initiation of influenza virus infection in human airway epithelium. *J Virol* 2004;78(22):12665–12667.
584. Mayer D, Molawi K, Martínez-Sobrido L, et al. Identification of cellular interaction partners of the influenza virus ribonucleoprotein complex and polymerase complex using proteomic-based approaches. *J Proteome Res* 2007;6(2):672–682.
585. McAuley JL, Chipuk JE, Boyd KL, et al. PB1-F2 proteins from H5N1 and 20 century pandemic influenza viruses cause immunopathology. *PLoS Pathog* 2010;6(7):e1001014.
586. McAuley JL, Hornung F, Boyd KL, et al. Expression of the 1918 influenza A virus PB1-F2 enhances the pathogenesis of viral and secondary bacterial pneumonia. *Cell Host Microbe* 2007;2(4):240–249.
587. McCown MF, Pekosz A. The influenza A virus M2 cytoplasmic tail is required for infectious virus production and efficient genome packaging. *J Virol* 2005;79(6):3595–3605.
588. McCown MF, Pekosz A. Distinct domains of the influenza a virus M2 protein cytoplasmic tail mediate binding to the M1 protein and facilitate infectious virus production. *J Virol* 2006;80(16):8178–8189.
589. McDonald SM, Patton JT. Assortment and packaging of the segmented rotavirus genome. *Trends Microbiol* 2011;19(3):136–144.
590. McKimm-Breschkin JL. Management of influenza virus infections with neuraminidase inhibitors: detection, incidence, and implications of drug resistance. *Treat Respir Med* 2005;4(2):107–116.
591. Medcalf L, Poole E, Elton D, et al. Temperature-sensitive lesions in two influenza A viruses defective for replicative transcription disrupt RNA binding by the nucleoprotein. *J Virol* 1999;73(9):7349–7356.
592. Medina RA, Stertz S, Manicassamy B, et al. Glycosylations in the globular head of the hemagglutinin protein modulate the virulence and antigenic properties of the H1N1 influenza viruses. *Sci Transl Med* 2013;5(187):187ra170.
593. Meindl P, Bodo G, Palese P, et al. Inhibition of neuraminidase activity by derivatives of 2-deoxy-2,3-dehydro-N-acetylneuraminic acid. *Virology* 1974;58(2):457–463.
594. Meineke R, Rimmelzwaan GF, Elbahesh H. Influenza virus infections and cellular kinases. *Viruses* 2019;11(2).
595. Melen K, Fagerlund R, Franke J, et al. Importin alpha nuclear localization signal binding sites for STAT1, STAT2, and influenza A virus nucleoprotein. *J Biol Chem* 2003;278(30):28193–28200.
596. Melen K, Kinnunen L, Fagerlund R, et al. Nuclear and nucleolar targeting of influenza A virus NS1 protein: striking differences between different virus subtypes. *J Virol* 2007;81(11):5995–6006.
597. Memoli MJ, Davis AS, Proudfoot K, et al. Multidrug-resistant 2009 pandemic influenza A(H1N1) viruses maintain fitness and transmissibility in ferrets. *J Infect Dis* 2011;203(3):348–357.
598. Memoli MJ, Hrabal RJ, Hassantoufighi A, et al. Rapid selection of a transmissible multidrug-resistant influenza A/H3N2 virus in an immunocompromised host. *J Infect Dis* 2010;201(9):1397–1403.
599. Memoli MJ, Hrabal RJ, Hassantoufighi A, et al. Rapid selection of oseltamivir- and peramivir-resistant pandemic H1N1 virus during therapy in 2 immunocompromised hosts. *Clin Infect Dis* 2010;50(9):1252–1255.
600. Mercer J, Schelhaas M, Helenius A. Virus entry by endocytosis. *Annu Rev Biochem* 2010;79:803–833.
601. Mibayashi M, Martinez-Sobrido L, Loo YM, et al. Inhibition of retinoic acid-inducible gene I-mediated induction of beta interferon by the NS1 protein of influenza A virus. *J Virol* 2007;81(2):514–524.
602. Mindich L. Packaging, replication and recombination of the segmented genome of bacteriophage Phi6 and its relatives. *Virus Res* 2004;101(1):83–92.
603. Miyake Y, Keusch JJ, Decamps L, et al. Influenza virus uses transportin 1 for vRNP debundling during cell entry. *Nat Microbiol* 2019;4(4):578–586.
604. Mjaaland S, Rimstad E, Falk K, et al. Genomic characterization of the virus causing infectious salmon anemia in Atlantic salmon (*Salmo salar* L.): an orthomyxo-like virus in a teleost. *J Virol* 1997;71(10):7681–7686.
605. Mochalova L, Gambaryan A, Romanova J, et al. Receptor-binding properties of modern human influenza viruses primarily isolated in Vero and MDCK cells and chicken embryonated eggs. *Virology* 2003;313(2):473–480.
606. Moeller A, Kirchdoerfer RN, Potter CS, et al. Organization of the influenza virus replication machinery. *Science* 2012;338(6114):1631–1634.
607. Momose F, Basler CF, O'Neill RE, et al. Cellular splicing factor RAF-2p48/NPI-5/BAT1/UAP56 interacts with the influenza virus nucleoprotein and enhances viral RNA synthesis. *J Virol* 2001;75(4):1899–1908.
608. Momose F, Kikuchi Y, Komase K, et al. Visualization of microtubule-mediated transport of influenza viral progeny ribonucleoprotein. *Microbes Infect* 2007;9(12–13):1422–1433.
609. Momose F, Naito T, Yano K, et al. Identification of Hsp90 as a stimulatory host factor involved in influenza virus RNA synthesis. *J Biol Chem* 2002;277(47):45306–45314.
610. Momose F, Sekimoto T, Ohkura T, et al. Apical transport of influenza A virus ribonucleoprotein requires Rab11-positive recycling endosome. *PLoS One* 2011;6(6):e21123.
611. Mondal A, Dawson AR, Potts GK, et al. Influenza virus recruits host protein kinase C to control assembly and activity of its replication machinery. *Elife* 2017;6:e26910.
612. Mondal A, Potts GK, Dawson AR, et al. Phosphorylation at the homotypic interface regulates nucleoprotein oligomerization and assembly of the influenza virus replication machinery. *PLoS Pathog* 2015;11(4):e1004826.
613. Monto AS. The role of antivirals in the control of influenza. *Vaccine* 2003;21(16):1796–1800.
614. Monto AS, Petrie JG, Cross RT, et al. Antibody to influenza virus neuraminidase: an independent correlate of protection. *J Infect Dis* 2015;212(8):1191–1199.
615. Moreira ÉA, Weber A, Bolte H, et al. A conserved influenza A virus nucleoprotein code controls specific viral genome packaging. *Nat Commun* 2016;7:12861.
616. Morgan R, Klein SL. The intersection of sex and gender in the treatment of influenza. *Curr Opin Virol* 2019;35:35–41.
617. Morokutti-Kurz M, König-Schuster M, Koller C, et al. The intranasal application of zanamivir and carrageenan is synergistically active against influenza A virus in the murine model. *PLoS One* 2015;10(6):e0128794.
618. Mould JA, Drury JE, Frings SM, et al. Permeation and activation of the M2 ion channel of influenza A virus. *J Biol Chem* 2000;275(40):31038–31050.
619. Mould JA, Li HC, Dudlak CS, et al. Mechanism for proton conduction of the M(2) ion channel of influenza A virus. *J Biol Chem* 2000;275(12):8592–8599.
620. Mould JA, Paterson RG, Takeda M, et al. Influenza B virus BM2 protein has ion channel activity that conducts protons across membranes. *Dev Cell* 2003;5(1):175–184.
621. Mühlbauer D, Dzieciolowski J, Hardt M, et al. Influenza virus-induced caspase-dependent enlargement of nuclear pores promotes nuclear export of viral ribonucleoprotein complexes. *J Virol* 2015;89(11):6009–6021.
622. Mukaigawa J, Nayak DP. Two signals mediate nuclear localization of influenza virus (A/WSN/33) polymerase basic protein 2. *J Virol* 1991;65(1):245–253.
623. Müller A, Solem ST, Karlsen CR, et al. Heterologous expression and purification of the infectious salmon anemia virus hemagglutinin esterase. *Protein Expr Purif* 2008;62(2):206–215.
624. Mullin AE, Dalton RM, Amorim MJ, et al. Increased amounts of the influenza virus nucleoprotein do not promote higher levels of viral genome replication. *J Gen Virol* 2004;85:3689–3698.

625. Muraki Y, Furukawa T, Kohno Y, et al. Influenza C virus NS1 protein upregulates the splicing of viral mRNAs. *J Virol* 2010;84(4):1957–1966.

626. Muraki Y, Hongo S. The molecular virology and reverse genetics of influenza C virus. *Jpn J Infect Dis* 2010;63(3):157–165.

627. Muraki Y, Murata T, Takashita E, et al. A mutation on influenza C virus M1 protein affects virion morphology by altering the membrane affinity of the protein. *J Virol* 2007;81(16):8766–8773.

628. Muraki Y, Washioka H, Sugawara K, et al. Identification of an amino acid residue on influenza C virus M1 protein responsible for formation of the cord-like structures of the virus. *J Gen Virol* 2004;85(Pt 7):1885–1893.

629. Muramoto Y, Noda T, Kawakami E, et al. Identification of novel influenza A virus proteins translated from PA mRNA. *J Virol* 2013;87(5):2455–2462.

630. Muramoto Y, Takada A, Fujii K, et al. Hierarchy among viral RNA (vRNA) segments in their role in vRNA incorporation into influenza A virions. *J Virol* 2006;80(5):2318–2325.

631. Murayama R, Harada Y, Shibata T, et al. Influenza A virus non-structural protein 1 (NS1) interacts with cellular multifunctional protein nucleolin during infection. *Biochem Biophys Res Commun* 2007;362(4):880–885.

632. Murti KG, Webster RG, Jones IM. Localization of RNA polymerases on influenza viral ribonucleoproteins by immunogold labeling. *Virology* 1988;164(2):562–566.

633. Musiol A, Gran S, Ehrhardt C, et al. Annexin A6-balanced late endosomal cholesterol controls influenza A replication and propagation. *MBio* 2013;4(6):e00608–e00613.

634. Nachbagauer R, Krammer F. Universal influenza virus vaccines and therapeutic antibodies. *Clin Microbiol Infect* 2017;23(4):222–228.

635. Nachbagauer R, Palese P. Development of next generation hemagglutinin-based broadly protective influenza virus vaccines. *Curr Opin Immunol* 2018;53:51–57.

636. Nakada S, Creager RS, Krystal M, et al. Influenza C virus hemagglutinin: comparison with influenza A and B virus hemagglutinins. *J Virol* 1984;50(1):118–124.

637. Nakada S, Graves PN, Desselberger U, et al. Influenza C virus RNA 7 codes for a nonstructural protein. *J Virol* 1985;56(1):221–226.

638. Nakada S, Graves PN, Palese P. The influenza C virus NS gene: evidence for a spliced mRNA and a second NS gene product (NS2 protein). *Virus Res* 1986;4(3):263–273.

639. Nakada R, Hirano H, Matsuura Y. Structure of importin-α bound to a non-classical nuclear localization signal of the influenza A virus nucleoprotein. *Sci Rep* 2015;5:15055.

640. Nakagawa S, Umehara T, Matsuda C, et al. Hsp90 inhibitors suppress HCV replication in replicon cells and humanized liver mice. *Biochem Biophys Res Commun* 2007;353(4):882–888.

641. Nakamura S, Miyazaki T, Izumikawa K, et al. Efficacy and safety of intravenous peramivir compared with oseltamivir in high-risk patients infected with influenza A and B viruses: a multicenter randomized controlled study. *Open Forum Infect Dis* 2017;4(3):ofx129.

642. Nakatsu S, Murakami S, Shindo K, et al. Influenza C and D viruses package eight organized ribonucleoprotein complexes. *J Virol* 2018;92(6):e02084.

643. Nakatsu S, Sagara H, Sakai-Tagawa Y, et al. Complete and incomplete genome packaging of influenza A and B viruses. *MBio* 2016;7(5).

644. Nath ST, Nayak DP. Function of two discrete regions is required for nuclear localization of polymerase basic protein 1 of A/WSN/33 influenza virus (H1 N1). *Mol Cell Biol* 1990;10(8):4139–4145.

645. Nayak D, Hui E, Barman S. Assembly and budding of influenza virus. *Virus Res* 2004;106(2):147–165.

646. Nedland H, Wollman J, Sreenivasan C, et al. Serological evidence for the co-circulation of two lineages of influenza D viruses in equine populations of the Midwest United States. *Zoonoses Public Health* 2018;65(1):e148–e154.

647. Nemeroff ME, Barabino SM, Li Y, et al. Influenza virus NS1 protein interacts with the cellular 30 kDa subunit of CPSF and inhibits 3′ end formation of cellular pre-mRNAs. *Mol Cell* 1998;1(7):991–1000.

648. Nemeroff ME, Utans U, Kramer A, et al. Identification of cis-acting intron and exon regions in influenza virus NS1 mRNA that inhibit splicing and cause the formation of aberrantly sedimenting presplicing complexes. *Mol Cell Biol* 1992;12(3):962–970.

649. Neumann G, Brownlee G, Fodor E, et al. Orthomyxovirus replication, transcription, and polyadenylation. In: Kawaoka Y, ed. *Biology of Negative Strand Rna Viruses: The Power of Reverse Genetics*. Berlin/Heidelberg: Springer; 2004:121–143.

650. Neumann G, Fujii K, Kino Y, et al. An improved reverse genetics system for influenza A virus generation and its implications for vaccine production. *Proc Natl Acad Sci U S A* 2005;102(46):16825–16829.

651. Neumann G, Hughes MT, Kawaoka Y. Influenza A virus NS2 protein mediates vRNP nuclear export through NES-independent interaction with hCRM1. *EMBO J* 2000;19(24):6751–6758.

652. Neumann G, Kawaoka Y. Reverse genetics systems for the generation of segmented negative-sense RNA viruses entirely from cloned cDNA. *Curr Top Microbiol Immunol* 2004;283:43–60.

653. Neumann G, Watanabe T, Ito H, et al. Generation of influenza A viruses entirely from cloned cDNAs. *Proc Natl Acad Sci U S A* 1999;96(16):9345–9350.

654. Neumann G, Zobel A, Hobom G. RNA polymerase I-mediated expression of influenza viral RNA molecules. *Virology* 1994;202(1):477–479.

655. Ng WC, Londrigan SL, Nasr N, et al. The C-type lectin Langerin functions as a receptor for attachment and infectious entry of influenza A virus. *J Virol* 2016;90(1):206–221.

656. Ng AK-L, Zhang H, Tan K, et al. Structure of the influenza virus A H5N1 nucleoprotein: implications for RNA binding, oligomerization, and vaccine design. *FASEB J* 2008;22(10):3638–3647.

657. Nguyen PA, Soto CS, Polishchuk A, et al. pH-induced conformational change of the influenza M2 protein C-terminal domain. *Biochemistry* 2008;47(38):9934–9936.

658. Nguyen-Van-Tam JS, Venkatesan S, Muthuri SG, et al. Neuraminidase inhibitors: who, when, where? *Clin Microbiol Infect* 2015;21(3):222–225.

659. Nishimura H, Hara M, Sugawara K, et al. Characterization of the cord-like structures emerging from the surface of influenza C virus-infected cells. *Virology* 1990;179(1):179–188.

660. Nishimura K, Kim S, Zhang L, et al. The closed state of a H+ channel helical bundle combining precise orientational and distance restraints from solid state NMR. *Biochemistry* 2002;41(44):13170–13177.

661. Noah DL, Twu KY, Krug RM. Cellular antiviral responses against influenza A virus are countered at the posttranscriptional level by the viral NS1A protein via its binding to a cellular protein required for the 3′ end processing of cellular pre-mRNAS. *Virology* 2003;307(2):386–395.

662. Noble E, Mathews DH, Chen JL, et al. Biophysical analysis of influenza A virus RNA promoter at physiological temperatures. *J Biol Chem* 2011;286(26):22965–22970.

663. Noda T, Murakami S, Nakatsu S, et al. Importance of the 1+7 configuration of ribonucleoprotein complexes for influenza A virus genome packaging. *Nat Commun* 2018;9(1):54.

664. Noda T, Sagara H, Yen A, et al. Architecture of ribonucleoprotein complexes in influenza A virus particles. *Nature* 2006;439(7075):490–492.

665. Noda T, Sugita Y, Aoyama K, et al. Three-dimensional analysis of ribonucleoprotein complexes in influenza A virus. *Nat Commun* 2012;3:639.

666. Nogales A, Martínez-Sobrido L. Reverse genetics approaches for the development of influenza vaccines. *Int J Mol Sci* 2016;18(1):20.

667. Nogales A, Martinez-Sobrido L, Topham DJ, et al. NS1 protein amino acid changes D189N and V194I affect interferon responses, thermosensitivity, and virulence of circulating H3N2 human influenza A viruses. *J Virol* 2017;91(5):e01930.

668. Nogales A, Martinez-Sobrido L, Topham D, et al. Modulation of innate immune responses by the influenza A NS1 and PA-X proteins. *Viruses* 2018;10(12):708.

669. O'Neill RE, Jaskunas R, Blobel G, et al. Nuclear import of influenza virus RNA can be mediated by viral nucleoprotein and transport factors required for protein import. *J Biol Chem* 1995;270(39):22701–22704.

670. O'Neill R, Talon J, Palese P. The influenza virus NEP (NS2 protein) mediates the nuclear export of viral ribonucleoproteins. *EMBO J* 1998;17(1):288–296.

671. Odagiri T, Hong J, Ohara Y. The BM2 protein of influenza B virus is synthesized in the late phase of infection and incorporated into virions as a subviral component. *J Gen Virol* 1999;80(Pt 10):2573–2581.

672. Oguin TH, Sharma S, Stuart AD, et al. Phospholipase D facilitates efficient entry of influenza virus, allowing escape from innate immune inhibition. *J Biol Chem* 2014;289(37):25405–25417.

673. Ohkura T, Momose F, Ichikawa R, et al. Influenza A virus hemagglutinin and neuraminidase mutually accelerate their apical targeting through clustering of lipid rafts. *J Virol* 2014;88(17):10039–10055.

674. Ohuchi M, Asaoka N, Sakai T, et al. Roles of neuraminidase in the initial stage of influenza virus infection. *Microbes Infect* 2006;8(5):1287–1293.

675. Oishi K, Yamayoshi S, Kawaoka Y. Mapping of a region of the PA-X protein of influenza A virus that is important for its shutoff activity. *J Virol* 2015;89(16):8661–8665.

676. Oishi K, Yamayoshi S, Kawaoka Y. Identification of novel amino acid residues of influenza virus PA-X that are important for PA-X shutoff activity by using yeast. *Virology* 2018;516:71–75.

677. Okomo-Adhiambo M, Demmler-Harrison GJ, Deyde VM, et al. Detection of E119V and E119I mutations in influenza A (H3N2) viruses isolated from an immunocompromised patient: challenges in diagnosis of oseltamivir resistance. *Antimicrob Agents Chemother* 2010;54(5):1834–1841.

678. Okuno Y, Isegawa Y, Sasao F, et al. A common neutralizing epitope conserved between the hemagglutinins of influenza A virus H1 and H2 strains. *J Virol* 1993;67(5):2552–2558.

679. Operario DJ, Moser MJ, St George K. Highly sensitive and quantitative detection of the H274Y oseltamivir resistance mutation in seasonal A/H1N1 influenza virus. *J Clin Microbiol* 2010;48(10):3517–3524.

680. Opitz B, Rejaibi A, Dauber B, et al. IFNbeta induction by influenza A virus is mediated by RIG-I which is regulated by the viral NS1 protein. *Cell Microbiol* 2007;9(4):930–938.

681. Ortega J, Martin-Benito J, Zurcher T, et al. Ultrastructural and functional analyses of recombinant influenza virus ribonucleoproteins suggest dimerization of nucleoprotein during virus amplification. *J Virol* 2000;74(1):156–163.

682. Ozawa M, Fujii K, Muramoto Y, et al. Contributions of two nuclear localization signals of influenza A virus nucleoprotein to viral replication. *J Virol* 2007;81(1):30–41.

683. Ozawa M, Goto H, Horimoto T, et al. An adenovirus vector-mediated reverse genetics system for influenza A virus generation. *J Virol* 2007;81(17):9556–9559.

684. Ozawa M, Maeda J, Iwatsuki-Horimoto K, et al. Nucleotide sequence requirements at the 5′ end of the influenza A virus M RNA segment for efficient virus replication. *J Virol* 2009;83(7):3384–3388.

685. Pachler K, Mayr J, Vlasak R. A seven plasmid-based system for the rescue of influenza C virus. *J Mol Genet Med* 2010;4:239–246.

686. Pachler K, Vlasak R. Influenza C virus NS1 protein counteracts RIG-I-mediated IFN signalling. *Virol J* 2011;8:48.

687. Palese P. The genes of influenza virus. *Cell* 1977;10(1):1–10.

688. Palese P, Compans RW. Inhibition of influenza virus replication in tissue culture by 2-deoxy-2,3-dehydro-N-trifluoroacetylneuraminic acid (FANA): mechanism of action. *J Gen Virol* 1976;33(1):159–163.

689. Palese P, Garcia-Sastre A. Influenza vaccines: present and future. *J Clin Invest* 2002;110(1):9–13.

690. Palese P, Muster T, Zheng H, et al. Learning from our foes: a novel vaccine concept for influenza virus. *Arch Virol Suppl* 1999;15:131–138.

691. Palese P, Racaniello VR, Desselberger U, et al. Genetic structure and genetic variation of influenza viruses [and Discussion]. *Philos Trans R Soc Lond Ser B Biol Sci* 1980;288(1029):299–305.

692. Palese P, Schulman JL, Bodo G, et al. Inhibition of influenza and parainfluenza virus replication in tissue culture by 2-deoxy-2,3-dehydro-N-trifluoroacetylneuraminic acid (FANA). *Virology* 1974;59(2):490–498.

693. Palese P, Tobita K, Ueda M, et al. Characterization of temperature sensitive influenza virus mutants defective in neuraminidase. *Virology* 1974;61(2):397–410.

694. Pan W, Dong Z, Li F, et al. Visualizing influenza virus infection in living mice. *Nat Commun* 2013;4:2369.

695. Pappas C, Aguilar PV, Basler CF, et al. Single gene reassortants identify a critical role for PB1, HA, and NA in the high virulence of the 1918 pandemic influenza virus. *Proc Natl Acad Sci U S A* 2008;105(8):3064–3069.

696. Paragas J, Talon J, O'Neill RE, et al. Influenza B and C virus NEP (NS2) proteins possess nuclear export activities. *J Virol* 2001;75(16):7375–7383.
697. Park CJ, Bae SH, Lee MK, et al. Solution structure of the influenza A virus cRNA promoter: implications for differential recognition of viral promoter structures by RNA-dependent RNA polymerase. *Nucleic Acids Res* 2003;31(11):2824–2832.
698. Park YW, Katze MG. Translational control by influenza virus. Identification of cis-acting sequences and trans-acting factors which may regulate selective viral mRNA translation. *J Biol Chem* 1995;270(47):28433–28439.
699. Park YW, Wilusz J, Katze MG. Regulation of eukaryotic protein synthesis: selective influenza viral mRNA translation is mediated by the cellular RNA-binding protein GRSF-1. *Proc Natl Acad Sci U S A* 1999;96(12):6694–6699.
700. Parvin JD, Palese P, Honda A, et al. Promoter analysis of influenza virus RNA polymerase. *J Virol* 1989;63(12):5142–5152.
701. Pascua PN, Marathe BM, Burnham AJ, et al. Competitive fitness of influenza B viruses possessing E119A and H274Y neuraminidase inhibitor resistance-associated substitutions in ferrets. *PLoS One* 2016;11(7):e0159847.
702. Pautus S, Sehr P, Lewis J, et al. New 7-methylguanine derivatives targeting the influenza polymerase PB2 cap-binding domain. *J Med Chem* 2013;56(21):8915–8930.
703. Pekosz A, He B, Lamb RA. Reverse genetics of negative-strand RNA viruses: closing the circle. *Proc Natl Acad Sci U S A* 1999;96(16):8804–8806.
704. Pekosz A, Lamb RA. The CM2 protein of influenza C virus is an oligomeric integral membrane glycoprotein structurally analogous to influenza A virus M2 and influenza B virus NB proteins. *Virology* 1997;237(2):439–451.
705. Pena L, Sutton T, Chockalingam A, et al. Influenza viruses with rearranged genomes as live-attenuated vaccines. *J Virol* 2013;87(9):5118–5127.
706. Peng W, de Vries RP, Grant OC, et al. Recent H3N2 viruses have evolved specificity for extended, branched human-type receptors, conferring potential for increased avidity. *Cell Host Microbe* 2017;21(1):23–34.
707. Perez DR, Donis RO. The matrix 1 protein of influenza A virus inhibits the transcriptase activity of a model influenza reporter genome in vivo. *Virology* 1998;249(1):52–61.
708. Perez D, Rimstad E, Smith G, et al. Orthomyxoviridae. In: King AMQ, Adams MJ, Carstens EB, et al., eds. *Virus Taxonomy*. Oxford: Elsevier; 2011:749–762.
709. Perez JT, Varble A, Sachidanandam R, et al. Influenza A virus-generated small RNAs regulate the switch from transcription to replication. *Proc Natl Acad Sci U S A* 2010;107(25):11525–11530.
710. Perreira JM, Aker AM, Savidis G, et al. RNASEK is a V-ATPase-associated factor required for endocytosis and the replication of rhinovirus, influenza A virus, and dengue virus. *Cell Rep* 2015;12(5):850–863.
711. Pflug A, Gaudon S, Resa-Infante P, et al. Capped RNA primer binding to influenza polymerase and implications for the mechanism of cap-binding inhibitors. *Nucleic Acids Res* 2018;46(2):956–971.
712. Pflug A, Guilligay D, Reich S, et al. Structure of influenza A polymerase bound to the viral RNA promoter. *Nature* 2014;516(7531):355–360.
713. Pflug A, Lukarska M, Resa-Infante P, et al. Structural insights into RNA synthesis by the influenza virus transcription-replication machine. *Virus Res* 2017;234:103–117.
714. Pichlmair A, Buse J, Jennings S, et al. Thogoto virus lacking interferon-antagonistic protein ML is strongly attenuated in newborn Mx1-positive but not Mx1-negative mice. *J Virol* 2004;78(20):11422–11424.
715. Pichlmair A, Schulz O, Tan CP, et al. RIG-I-mediated antiviral responses to single-stranded RNA bearing 5′-phosphates. *Science* 2006;314(5801):997–1001.
716. Pinto LH, Holsinger LJ, Lamb RA. Influenza virus M2 protein has ion channel activity. *Cell* 1992;69(3):517–528.
717. Pinto LH, Lamb RA. The M2 proton channels of influenza A and B viruses. *J Biol Chem* 2006;281(14):8997–9000.
718. Pinto LH, Lamb RA. Controlling influenza virus replication by inhibiting its proton channel. *Mol Biosyst* 2007;3(1):18–23.
719. Pleschka S, Jaskunas R, Engelhardt OG, et al. A plasmid-based reverse genetics system for influenza A virus. *J Virol* 1996;70(6):4188–4192.
720. Pleschka S, Wolff T, Ehrhardt C, et al. Influenza virus propagation is impaired by inhibition of the Raf/MEK/ERK signalling cascade. *Nat Cell Biol* 2001;3(3):301–305.
721. Plotch SJ, Bouloy M, Ulmanen I, et al. A unique cap (m7GpppXm)-dependent influenza virion endonuclease cleaves capped RNAs to generate the primers that initiate viral RNA transcription. *Cell* 1981;23(3):847–858.
722. Pohl MO, Edinger TO, Stertz S. Prolidase is required for early trafficking events during influenza A virus entry. *J Virol* 2014;88(19):11271–11283.
723. Pons MW, Schulze IT, Hirst GK, et al. Isolation and characterization of the ribonucleoprotein of influenza virus. *Virology* 1969;39(2):250–259.
724. Poon LL, Fodor E, Brownlee GG. Polyuridylated mRNA synthesized by a recombinant influenza virus is defective in nuclear export. *J Virol* 2000;74(1):418–427.
725. Poon LL, Pritlove DC, Sharps J, et al. The RNA polymerase of influenza virus, bound to the 5′ end of virion RNA, acts in cis to polyadenylate mRNA. *J Virol* 1998;72(10):8214–8219.
726. Portela A, Digard P. The influenza virus nucleoprotein: a multifunctional RNA-binding protein pivotal to virus replication. *J Gen Virol* 2002;83:723–734.
727. Porter AG, Barber C, Carey NH, et al. Complete nucleotide sequence of an influenza virus haemagglutinin gene from cloned DNA. *Nature* 1979;282(5738):471–477.
728. Pourceau G, Chevolot Y, Goudot A, et al. Measurement of enzymatic activity and specificity of human and avian influenza neuraminidases from whole virus by glycoarray and MALDI-TOF mass spectrometry. *Chembiochem* 2011;12(13):2071–2080.
729. Prabhu SS, Chakraborty TT, Kumar N, et al. Association between IFITM3 rs12252 polymorphism and influenza susceptibility and severity: a meta-analysis. *Gene* 2018;674:70–79.
730. Predicala R, Zhou Y. The role of Ran-binding protein 3 during influenza A virus replication. *J Gen Virol* 2013;94(Pt 5):977–984.
731. Presti RM, Zhao G, Beatty WL, et al. Quaranfil, Johnston Atoll, and Lake Chad viruses are novel members of the family Orthomyxoviridae. *J Virol* 2009;83(22):11599–11606.
732. Pritlove DC, Poon LL, Devenish LJ, et al. A hairpin loop at the 5′ end of influenza A virus virion RNA is required for synthesis of poly(A)+ mRNA in vitro. *J Virol* 1999;73(3):2109–2114.
733. Pritlove DC, Poon LL, Fodor E, et al. Polyadenylation of influenza virus mRNA transcribed in vitro from model virion RNA templates: requirement for 5′ conserved sequences. *J Virol* 1998;72(2):1280–1286.
734. Prokudina-Kantorovich EN, Semenova NP. Intracellular oligomerization of influenza virus nucleoprotein. *Virology* 1996;223(1):51–56.
735. Qian XY, Chien CY, Lu Y, et al. An amino-terminal polypeptide fragment of the influenza virus NS1 protein possesses specific RNA-binding activity and largely helical backbone structure. *RNA* 1995;1(9):948–956.
736. Qin C, Li W, Li Q, et al. Real-time dissection of dynamic uncoating of individual influenza viruses. *Proc Natl Acad Sci U S A* 2019;116(7):2577–2582.
737. Quinlivan M, Zamarin D, Garcia-Sastre A, et al. Attenuation of equine influenza viruses through truncations of the NS1 protein. *J Virol* 2005;79(13):8431–8439.
738. Racaniello VR, Palese P. Influenza B virus genome: assignment of viral polypeptides to RNA segments. *J Virol* 1979;29(1):361–373.
739. Rajendran M, Nachbagauer R, Ermler ME, et al. Analysis of anti-influenza virus neuraminidase antibodies in children, adults, and the elderly by ELISA and enzyme inhibition: evidence for original antigenic sin. *MBio* 2017;8(2).
740. Rajsbaum R, Albrecht RA, Wang MK, et al. Species-specific inhibition of RIG-I ubiquitination and IFN induction by the influenza A virus NS1 protein. *PLoS Pathog* 2012;8(11):e1003059.
741. Randolph AG, Yip WK, Allen EK, et al. Evaluation of IFITM3 rs12252 association with severe pediatric influenza infection. *J Infect Dis* 2017;216(1):14–21.
742. Reece PA. Treatment options for H5N1: lessons learned from the H1N1 pandemic. *Postgrad Med* 2010;122(5):134–141.
743. Reich S, Guilligay D, Pflug A, et al. Structural insight into cap-snatching and RNA synthesis by influenza polymerase. *Nature* 2014;516(7531):361–366.
744. Reinhardt J, Wolff T. The influenza A virus M1 protein interacts with the cellular receptor of activated C kinase (RACK) 1 and can be phosphorylated by protein kinase C. *Vet Microbiol* 2000;74(1–2):87–100.
745. Resa-Infante P, Jorba N, Coloma R, et al. The influenza virus RNA synthesis machine: advances in its structure and function. *RNA Biol* 2011;8(2):207–215.
746. Rialdi A, Hultquist J, Jimenez-Morales D, et al. The RNA exosome syncs IAV-RNAPII transcription to promote viral ribogenesis and infectivity. *Cell* 2017;169(4):679–692.e614.
747. Richardson JC, Akkina RK. NS2 protein of influenza virus is found in purified virus and phosphorylated in infected cells. *Arch Virol* 1991;116(1–4):69–80.
748. Richt JA, Garcia-Sastre A. Attenuated influenza virus vaccines with modified NS1 proteins. *Curr Top Microbiol Immunol* 2009;333:177–195.
749. Rinkenberger N, Schoggins JW. Mucolipin-2 cation channel increases trafficking efficiency of endocytosed viruses. *MBio* 2018;9(1).
750. Ritchie KJ, Hahn CS, Kim KI, et al. Role of ISG15 protease UBP43 (USP18) in innate immunity to viral infection. *Nat Med* 2004;10(12):1374–1378.
751. Robb NC, Jackson D, Vreede FT, et al. Splicing of influenza A virus NS1 mRNA is independent of the viral NS1 protein. *J Gen Virol* 2010;91(Pt 9):2331–2340.
752. Robb NC, Smith M, Vreede FT, et al. NS2/NEP protein regulates transcription and replication of the influenza virus RNA genome. *J Gen Virol* 2009;90(Pt 6):1398–1407.
753. Robb NC, Te Velthuis AJ, Wieneke R, et al. Single-molecule FRET reveals the pre-initiation and initiation conformations of influenza virus promoter RNA. *Nucleic Acids Res* 2016;44(21):10304–10315.
754. Roberts NA. Treatment of influenza with neuraminidase inhibitors: virological implications. *Philos Trans R Soc Lond B Biol Sci* 2001;356(1416):1895–1897.
755. Roberts P, Compans R. Host cell dependence of viral morphology. *Proc Natl Acad Sci U S A* 1998;95(10):5746–5751.
756. Roberts PC, Lamb RA, Compans RW. The M1 and M2 proteins of influenza A virus are important determinants in filamentous particle formation. *Virology* 1998;240(1):127–137.
757. Roberts KL, Leser GP, Ma C, et al. The amphipathic helix of influenza A virus M2 protein is required for filamentous bud formation and scission of filamentous and spherical particles. *J Virol* 2013;87(18):9973–9982.
758. Robertson JS. 5′ and 3′ terminal nucleotide sequences of the RNA genome segments of influenza virus. *Nucleic Acids Res* 1979;6(12):3745–3758.
759. Robertson JS, Schubert M, Lazzarini RA. Polyadenylation sites for influenza virus mRNA. *J Virol* 1981;38(1):157–163.
760. Rockman S, Lowther S, Camuglia S, et al. Intravenous immunoglobulin protects against severe pandemic influenza infection. *EBioMedicine* 2017;19:119–127.
761. Rodriguez Boulan E, Sabatini DD. Asymmetric budding of viruses in epithelial monolayers: a model system for study of epithelial polarity. *Proc Natl Acad Sci U S A* 1978;75(10):5071–5075.
762. Rodriguez A, Perez-Gonzalez A, Hossain MJ, et al. Attenuated strains of influenza A viruses do not induce degradation of RNA polymerase II. *J Virol* 2009;83(21):11166–11174.
763. Rodriguez A, Perez-Gonzalez A, Nieto A. Influenza virus infection causes specific degradation of the largest subunit of cellular RNA polymerase II. *J Virol* 2007;81(10):5315–5324.
764. Rodriguez A, Pérez-González A, Nieto A. Cellular human CLE/C14orf166 protein interacts with influenza virus polymerase and is required for viral replication. *J Virol* 2011;85(22):12062–12066.
765. Rogers GN, Paulson JC, Daniels RS, et al. Single amino acid substitutions in influenza haemagglutinin change receptor binding specificity. *Nature* 1983;304(5921):76–78.
766. Rosenthal PB, Zhang X, Formanowski F, et al. Structure of the haemagglutinin-esterase-fusion glycoprotein of influenza C virus. *Nature* 1998;396(6706):92–96.
767. Rossignol JF, La Frazia S, Chiappa L, et al. Thiazolides, a new class of anti-influenza molecules targeting viral hemagglutinin at the post-translational level. *J Biol Chem* 2009;284(43):29798–29808.
768. Rossman JS, Jing X, Leser GP, et al. Influenza virus m2 ion channel protein is necessary for filamentous virion formation. *J Virol* 2010;84(10):5078–5088.
769. Rossman JS, Jing X, Leser GP, et al. Influenza virus M2 protein mediates ESCRT-independent membrane scission. *Cell* 2010;142(6):902–913.
770. Rossman JS, Lamb RA. Influenza virus assembly and budding. *Virology* 2011;411(2):229–236.
771. Rossman JS, Leser GP, Lamb RA. Filamentous influenza virus enters cells via macropinocytosis. *J Virol* 2012;86(20):10950–10960.

772. Roth MG, Compans RW, Giusti L, et al. Influenza virus hemagglutinin expression is polarized in cells infected with recombinant SV40 viruses carrying cloned hemagglutinin DNA. *Cell* 1983;33(2):435–443.
773. Roy AM, Parker JS, Parrish CR, et al. Early stages of influenza virus entry into Mv-1 lung cells: involvement of dynamin. *Virology* 2000;267(1):17–28.
774. Ruigrok RW, Barge A, Durrer P, et al. Membrane interaction of influenza virus M1 protein. *Virology* 2000;267(2):289–298.
775. Ruigrok RW, Baudin F. Structure of influenza virus ribonucleoprotein particles. II. Purified RNA-free influenza virus ribonucleoprotein forms structures that are indistinguishable from the intact influenza virus ribonucleoprotein particles. *J Gen Virol* 1995;76:1009–1014.
776. Ruigrok RW, Calder LJ, Wharton SA. Electron microscopy of the influenza virus submembranal structure. *Virology* 1989;173(1):311–316.
777. Russell CJ, Hu M, Okda FA. Influenza hemagglutinin protein stability, activation, and pandemic risk. *Trends Microbiol* 2018;26(10):841–853.
778. Sabath N, Morris JS, Graur D. Is there a twelfth protein-coding gene in the genome of influenza A? A selection-based approach to the detection of overlapping genes in closely related sequences. *J Mol Evol* 2011;73(5–6):305–315.
779. Saha RK, Takahashi T, Kurebayashi Y, et al. Antiviral effect of strictinin on influenza virus replication. *Antiviral Res* 2010;88(1):10–18.
780. Sakaguchi A, Hirayama E, Hiraki A, et al. Nuclear export of influenza viral ribonucleoprotein is temperature-dependently inhibited by dissociation of viral matrix protein. *Virology* 2003;306(2):244–253.
781. Salvatore M, Basler CF, Parisien JP, et al. Effects of influenza A virus NS1 protein on protein expression: the NS1 protein enhances translation and is not required for shutoff of host protein synthesis. *J Virol* 2002;76(3):1206–1212.
782. Sandbulte MR, Westgeest KB, Gao J, et al. Discordant antigenic drift of neuraminidase and hemagglutinin in H1N1 and H3N2 influenza viruses. *Proc Natl Acad Sci U S A* 2011;108(51):20748–20753.
783. Satterly N, Tsai PL, van Deursen J, et al. Influenza virus targets the mRNA export machinery and the nuclear pore complex. *Proc Natl Acad Sci U S A* 2007;104(6):1853–1858.
784. Scheiffele P, Rietveld A, Wilk T, et al. Influenza viruses select ordered lipid domains during budding from the plasma membrane. *J Biol Chem* 1999;274(4):2038–2044.
785. Scheiffele P, Roth MG, Simons K. Interaction of influenza virus haemagglutinin with sphingolipid-cholesterol membrane domains via its transmembrane domain. *EMBO J* 1997;16(18):5501–5508.
786. Schepens B, De Vlieger D, Saelens X. Vaccine options for influenza: thinking small. *Curr Opin Immunol* 2018;53:22–29.
787. Schmitt AP, Lamb RA. Influenza virus assembly and budding at the viral budozone. *Adv Virus Res* 2005;64:383–416.
788. Schmolke M, Viemann D, Roth J, et al. Essential impact of NF-kappaB signaling on the H5N1 influenza A virus-induced transcriptome. *J Immunol* 2009;183(8):5180–5189.
789. Schneider J, Dauber B, Melen K, et al. Analysis of influenza B Virus NS1 protein trafficking reveals a novel interaction with nuclear speckle domains. *J Virol* 2009;83(2):701–711.
790. Schnell JR, Chou JJ. Structure and mechanism of the M2 proton channel of influenza A virus. *Nature* 2008;451(7178):591–595.
791. Schroeder C, Heider H, Möncke-Buchner E, et al. The influenza virus ion channel and maturation cofactor M2 is a cholesterol-binding protein. *Eur Biophys J* 2005;34(1):52–66.
792. Schultz-Cherry S, Dybdahl-Sissoko N, Neumann G, et al. Influenza virus NS1 protein induces apoptosis in cultured cells. *J Virol* 2001;75(17):7875–7881.
793. Schultz-Cherry S, Hinshaw VS. Influenza virus neuraminidase activates latent transforming growth factor beta. *J Virol* 1996;70(12):8624–8629.
794. Scott C, Griffin S. Viroporins: structure, function and potential as antiviral targets. *J Gen Virol* 2015;96(8):2000–2027.
795. Seibert CW, Kaminski M, Philipp J, et al. Oseltamivir-resistant variants of the 2009 pandemic H1N1 influenza A virus are not attenuated in the guinea pig and ferret transmission models. *J Virol* 2010;84(21):11219–11226.
796. Selman M, Dankar SK, Forbes NE, et al. Adaptive mutation in influenza A virus non-structural gene is linked to host switching and induces a novel protein by alternative splicing. *Emerg Microbes Infect* 2012;1(11):e42.
797. Seo YJ, Pritzl CJ, Vijayan M, et al. Sphingosine kinase 1 serves as a pro-viral factor by regulating viral RNA synthesis and nuclear export of viral ribonucleoprotein complex upon influenza virus infection. *PLoS One* 2013;8(8):e75005.
798. Sezgin E, Levental I, Mayor S, et al. The mystery of membrane organization: composition, regulation and roles of lipid rafts. *Nat Rev Mol Cell Biol* 2017;18(6):361–374.
799. Sha B, Luo M. Structure of a bifunctional membrane-RNA binding protein, influenza virus matrix protein M1. *Nat Struct Biol* 1997;4(3):239–244.
800. Shapira SD, Gat-Viks I, Shum BO, et al. A physical and regulatory map of host-influenza interactions reveals pathways in H1N1 infection. *Cell* 2009;139(7):1255–1267.
801. Shapiro GI, Gurney T Jr, Krug RM. Influenza virus gene expression: control mechanisms at early and late times of infection and nuclear-cytoplasmic transport of virus-specific RNAs. *J Virol* 1987;61(3):764–773.
802. Shapiro GI, Krug RM. Influenza virus RNA replication in vitro: synthesis of viral template RNAs and virion RNAs in the absence of an added primer. *J Virol* 1988;62(7): 2285–2290.
803. Sharma M, Yi M, Dong H, et al. Insight into the mechanism of the influenza A proton channel from a structure in a lipid bilayer. *Science* 2010;330(6003):509–512.
804. Shaw ML. The host interactome of influenza virus presents new potential targets for antiviral drugs. *Rev Med Virol* 2011;21(6):358–369.
805. Shaw ML. The next wave of influenza drugs. *ACS Infect Dis* 2017;3(10):691–694.
806. Shaw MW, Choppin PW, Lamb RA. A previously unrecognized influenza B virus glycoprotein from a bicistronic mRNA that also encodes the viral neuraminidase. *Proc Natl Acad Sci U S A* 1983;80(16):4879–4883.
807. Shaw ML, Stertz S. Role of host genes in influenza virus replication. *Curr Top Microbiol Immunol* 2018;419:151–189.
808. Shaw M, Stone K, Colangelo C, et al. Cellular proteins in influenza virus particles. *PLoS Pathog* 2008;4(6):e1000085.
809. Sherry L, Punovuori K, Wallace LE, et al. Identification of cis-acting packaging signals in the coding regions of the influenza B virus HA gene segment. *J Gen Virol* 2016;97(2):306–315.
810. Shi M, Jagger BW, Wise HM, et al. Evolutionary conservation of the PA-X open reading frame in segment 3 of influenza A virus. *J Virol* 2012;86(22):12411–12413.
811. Shih SR, Krug RM. Novel exploitation of a nuclear function by influenza virus: the cellular SF2/ASF splicing factor controls the amount of the essential viral M2 ion channel protein in infected cells. *EMBO J* 1996;15(19):5415–5427.
812. Shih SR, Krug RM. Surprising function of the three influenza viral polymerase proteins: selective protection of viral mRNAs against the cap-snatching reaction catalyzed by the same polymerase proteins. *Virology* 1996;226(2):430–435.
813. Shih SR, Nemeroff ME, Krug RM. The choice of alternative 5′ splice sites in influenza virus M1 mRNA is regulated by the viral polymerase complex. *Proc Natl Acad Sci U S A* 1995;92(14):6324–6328.
814. Shih SR, Suen PC, Chen YS, et al. A novel spliced transcript of influenza A/WSN/33 virus. *Virus Genes* 1998;17(2):179–183.
815. Shimizu K, Iguchi A, Gomyou R, et al. Influenza virus inhibits cleavage of the HSP70 pre-mRNAs at the polyadenylation site. *Virology* 1999;254(2):213–219.
816. Shimizu T, Takizawa N, Watanabe K, et al. Crucial role of the influenza virus NS2 (NEP) C-terminal domain in M1 binding and nuclear export of vRNP. *FEBS Lett* 2011;585(1):41–46.
817. Shin YK, Li Y, Liu Q, et al. SH3 binding motif 1 in influenza A virus NS1 protein is essential for PI3K/Akt signaling pathway activation. *J Virol* 2007;81(23):12730–12739.
818. Shin YK, Liu Q, Tikoo SK, et al. Influenza A virus NS1 protein activates the phosphatidylinositol 3-kinase (PI3K)/Akt pathway by direct interaction with the p85 subunit of PI3K. *J Gen Virol* 2007;88(Pt 1):13–18.
819. Shinya K, Ebina M, Yamada S, et al. Avian flu: influenza virus receptors in the human airway. *Nature* 2006;440(7083):435–436.
820. Sieczkarski SB, Brown HA, Whittaker GR. Role of protein kinase C betaII in influenza virus entry via late endosomes. *J Virol* 2003;77(1):460–469.
821. Sieczkarski SB, Whittaker GR. Influenza virus can enter and infect cells in the absence of clathrin-mediated endocytosis. *J Virol* 2002;76(20):10455–10464.
822. Sieczkarski SB, Whittaker GR. Differential requirements of Rab5 and Rab7 for endocytosis of influenza and other enveloped viruses. *Traffic* 2003;4(5):333–343.
823. Simpson-Holley M, Ellis D, Fisher D, et al. A functional link between the actin cytoskeleton and lipid rafts during budding of filamentous influenza virions. *Virology* 2002;301(2):212–225.
824. Skehel JJ, Bayley PM, Brown EB, et al. Changes in the conformation of influenza virus hemagglutinin at the pH optimum of virus-mediated membrane fusion. *Proc Natl Acad Sci U S A* 1982;79(4):968–972.
825. Skehel JJ, Bizebard T, Bullough PA, et al. Membrane fusion by influenza hemagglutinin. *Cold Spring Harb Symp Quant Biol* 1995;60:573–580.
826. Skehel JJ, Hay AJ, Armstrong JA. On the mechanism of inhibition of influenza virus replication by amantadine hydrochloride. *J Gen Virol* 1978;38(1):97–110.
827. Smee DF, Bailey KW, Wong MH, et al. Treatment of influenza A (H1N1) virus infections in mice and ferrets with cyanovirin-N. *Antiviral Res* 2008;80(3):266–271.
828. Smirnov YuA, Kuznetsova MA, Kaverin NV. The genetic aspects of influenza virus filamentous particle formation. *Arch Virol* 1991;118(3–4):279–284.
829. Smith GL, Hay AJ. Replication of the influenza virus genome. *Virology* 1982;118(1):96–108.
830. Smith GL, Levin JZ, Palese P, et al. Synthesis and cellular location of the ten influenza polypeptides individually expressed by recombinant vaccinia viruses. *Virology* 1987;160(2):336–345.
831. Smith DR, McCarthy S, Chrovian A, et al. Inhibition of heat-shock protein 90 reduces Ebola virus replication. *Antiviral Res* 2010;87(2):187–194.
832. Söderholm S, Kainov DE, Öhman T, et al. Phosphoproteomics to characterize host response during influenza A virus infection of human macrophages. *Mol Cell Proteomics* 2016;15(10):3203–3219.
833. Solorzano A, Webby RJ, Lager KM, et al. Mutations in the NS1 protein of swine influenza virus impair anti-interferon activity and confer attenuation in pigs. *J Virol* 2005;79(12):7535–7543.
834. Song H, Qi J, Khedri Z, et al. An open receptor-binding cavity of hemagglutinin-esterase-fusion glycoprotein from newly-identified influenza D virus: basis for its broad cell tropism. *PLoS Pathog* 2016;12(1):e1005411.
835. Sonnino S, Prinetti A. Membrane domains and the "lipid raft" concept. *Curr Med Chem* 2013;20(1):4–21.
836. Sridharan H, Zhao C, Krug RM. Species specificity of the NS1 protein of influenza B virus: NS1 binds only human and non-human primate ubiquitin-like ISG15 proteins. *J Biol Chem* 2010;285(11):7852–7856.
837. Sriwilaijaroen N, Nakakita SI, Kondo S, et al. N-glycan structures of human alveoli provide insight into influenza A virus infection and pathogenesis. *FEBS J* 2018;285(9):1611–1634.
838. Sriwilaijaroen N, Wilairat P, Hiramatsu H, et al. Mechanisms of the action of povidone-iodine against human and avian influenza A viruses: its effects on hemagglutination and sialidase activities. *Virol J* 2009;6:124.
839. Staschke KA, Hatch SD, Tang JC, et al. Inhibition of influenza virus hemagglutinin-mediated membrane fusion by a compound related to podocarpic acid. *Virology* 1998;248(2):264–274.
840. Stauffer S, Feng Y, Nebioglu F, et al. Stepwise priming by acidic pH and a high K+ concentration is required for efficient uncoating of influenza A virus cores after penetration. *J Virol* 2014;88(22):13029–13046.
841. Steinhauer DA, Wharton SA, Skehel JJ, et al. Amantadine selection of a mutant influenza virus containing an acid-stable hemagglutinin glycoprotein: evidence for virus-specific regulation of the pH of glycoprotein transport vesicles. *Proc Natl Acad Sci U S A* 1991;88(24):11525–11529.
842. Steinhauer DA, Wharton SA, Wiley DC, et al. Deacylation of the hemagglutinin of influenza A/Aichi/2/68 has no effect on membrane fusion properties. *Virology* 1991;184(1):445–448.

843. Stertz S, Shaw ML. Uncovering the global host cell requirements for influenza virus replication via RNAi screening. *Microbes Infect* 2011;13(5):516–525.

844. Stevens J, Blixt O, Glaser L, et al. Glycan microarray analysis of the hemagglutinins from modern and pandemic influenza viruses reveals different receptor specificities. *J Mol Biol* 2006;355(5):1143–1155.

845. Stevens J, Blixt O, Paulson JC, et al. Glycan microarray technologies: tools to survey host specificity of influenza viruses. *Nat Rev Microbiol* 2006;4(11):857–864.

846. Stevens J, Chen LM, Carney PJ, et al. Receptor specificity of influenza A H3N2 viruses isolated in mammalian cells and embryonated chicken eggs. *J Virol* 2010;84(16):8287–8299.

847. Stevens J, Corper AL, Basler CF, et al. Structure of the uncleaved human H1 hemagglutinin from the extinct 1918 influenza virus. *Science* 2004;303(5665):1866–1870.

848. Stewart SM, Wu WH, Lalime EN, et al. The cholesterol recognition/interaction amino acid consensus motif of the influenza A virus M2 protein is not required for virus replication but contributes to virulence. *Virology* 2010;405(2):530–538.

849. Stieneke-Gröber A, Vey M, Angliker H, et al. Influenza virus hemagglutinin with multibasic cleavage site is activated by furin, a subtilisin-like endoprotease. *EMBO J* 1992;11(7):2407–2414.

850. Stouffer AL, Acharya R, Salom D, et al. Structural basis for the function and inhibition of an influenza virus proton channel. *Nature* 2008;451(7178):596–599.

851. Strasser P, Unger U, Strobl B, et al. Recombinant viral sialate-O-acetylesterases. *Glycoconj J* 2004;20(9):551–561.

852. Strauch EM, Bernard SM, La D, et al. Computational design of trimeric influenza-neutralizing proteins targeting the hemagglutinin receptor binding site. *Nat Biotechnol* 2017;35(7):667–671.

853. Su WC, Chen YC, Tseng CH, et al. Pooled RNAi screen identifies ubiquitin ligase Itch as crucial for influenza A virus release from the endosome during virus entry. *Proc Natl Acad Sci U S A* 2013;110(43):17516–17521.

854. Su CY, Cheng TJ, Lin MI, et al. High-throughput identification of compounds targeting influenza RNA-dependent RNA polymerase activity. *Proc Natl Acad Sci U S A* 2010;107(45):19151–19156.

855. Su S, Fu X, Li G, et al. Novel influenza D virus: epidemiology, pathology, evolution and biological characteristics. *Virulence* 2017;8(8):1580–1591.

856. Su WC, Hsu SF, Lee YY, et al. A nucleolar protein, ribosomal RNA processing 1 Homolog B (RRP1B), enhances the recruitment of cellular mRNA in influenza virus transcription. *J Virol* 2015;89(22):11245–11255.

857. Su WC, Yu WY, Huang SH, et al. Ubiquitination of the cytoplasmic domain of influenza A virus M2 protein is crucial for production of infectious virus particles. *J Virol* 2018;92(4).

858. Sugita Y, Sagara H, Noda T, et al. Configuration of viral ribonucleoprotein complexes within the influenza A virion. *J Virol* 2013;87(23):12879–12884.

859. Sugiyama K, Kawaguchi A, Okuwaki M, et al. pp32 and APRIL are host cell-derived regulators of influenza virus RNA synthesis from cRNA. *Elife* 2015;4.

860. Sugiyama K, Obayashi E, Kawaguchi A, et al. Structural insight into the essential PB1-PB2 subunit contact of the influenza virus RNA polymerase. *EMBO J* 2009;28(12):1803–1811.

861. Sugrue RJ, Belshe RB, Hay AJ. Palmitoylation of the influenza A virus M2 protein. *Virology* 1990;179(1):51–56.

862. Sugrue RJ, Hay AJ. Structural characteristics of the M2 protein of influenza A viruses: evidence that it forms a tetrameric channel. *Virology* 1991;180(2):617–624.

863. Sui J, Hwang WC, Perez S, et al. Structural and functional bases for broad-spectrum neutralization of avian and human influenza A viruses. *Nat Struct Mol Biol* 2009;16(3):265–273.

864. Sun E, He J, Zhuang X. Dissecting the role of COPI complexes in influenza virus infection. *J Virol* 2013;87(5):2673–2685.

865. Sun X, Shi Y, Lu X, et al. Bat-derived influenza hemagglutinin H17 does not bind canonical avian or human receptors and most likely uses a unique entry mechanism. *Cell Rep* 2013;3(3):769–778.

866. Sun X, Whittaker GR. Role of the actin cytoskeleton during influenza virus internalization into polarized epithelial cells. *Cell Microbiol* 2007;9(7):1672–1682.

867. Suzuki Y, Nei M. Origin and evolution of influenza virus hemagglutinin genes. *Mol Biol Evol* 2002;19(4):501–509.

868. Suzuki T, Takahashi T, Guo CT, et al. Sialidase activity of influenza A virus in an endocytic pathway enhances viral replication. *J Virol* 2005;79(18):11705–11715.

869. Takeda M, Leser GP, Russell CJ, et al. Influenza virus hemagglutinin concentrates in lipid raft microdomains for efficient viral fusion. *Proc Natl Acad Sci U S A* 2003;100(25):14610–14617.

870. Talon J, Horvath CM, Polley R, et al. Activation of interferon regulatory factor 3 is inhibited by the influenza A virus NS1 protein. *J Virol* 2000;74(17):7989–7996.

871. Talon J, Salvatore M, O'Neill RE, et al. Influenza A and B viruses expressing altered NS1 proteins: a vaccine approach. *Proc Natl Acad Sci U S A* 2000;97(8):4309–4314.

872. Tan J, Asthagiri Arunkumar G, Krammer F. Universal influenza virus vaccines and therapeutics: where do we stand with influenza B virus? *Curr Opin Immunol* 2018;53:45–50.

873. Tan GS, Krammer F, Eggink D, et al. A pan-h1 anti-hemagglutinin monoclonal antibody with potent broad-spectrum efficacy in vivo. *J Virol* 2012;86(11):6179–6188.

874. Tan GS, Lee PS, Hoffman RM, et al. Characterization of a broadly neutralizing monoclonal antibody that targets the fusion domain of group 2 influenza a virus hemagglutinin. *J Virol* 2014;88(23):13580–13592.

875. Tang Y, Zhong G, Zhu L, et al. Herc5 attenuates influenza A virus by catalyzing ISGylation of viral NS1 protein. *J Immunol* 2010;184(10):5777–5790.

876. Tauber S, Ligertwood Y, Quigg-Nicol M, et al. Behaviour of influenza A viruses differentially expressing segment 2 gene products in vitro and in vivo. *J Gen Virol* 2012;93(Pt 4):840–849.

877. Te Velthuis AJ, Fodor E. Influenza virus RNA polymerase: insights into the mechanisms of viral RNA synthesis. *Nat Rev Microbiol* 2016;14(8):479–493.

878. Terrier O, Carron C, De Chassey B, et al. Nucleolin interacts with influenza A nucleoprotein and contributes to viral ribonucleoprotein complexes nuclear trafficking and efficient influenza viral replication. *Sci Rep* 2016;6:29006.

879. Thaa B, Levental I, Herrmann A, et al. Intrinsic membrane association of the cytoplasmic tail of influenza virus M2 protein and lateral membrane sorting regulated by cholesterol binding and palmitoylation. *Biochem J* 2011;437(3):389–397.

880. Thaa B, Siche S, Herrmann A, et al. Acylation and cholesterol binding are not required for targeting of influenza A virus M2 protein to the hemagglutinin-defined budozone. *FEBS Lett* 2014;588(6):1031–1036.

881. Thaa B, Tielesch C, Möller L, et al. Growth of influenza A virus is not impeded by simultaneous removal of the cholesterol-binding and acylation sites in the M2 protein. *J Gen Virol* 2012;93(Pt 2):282–292.

882. Thierry E, Guilligay D, Kosinski J, et al. Influenza polymerase can adopt an alternative configuration involving a radical repacking of PB2 domains. *Mol Cell* 2016;61(1):125–137.

883. Thomaston JL, Alfonso-Prieto M, Woldeyes RA, et al. High-resolution structures of the M2 channel from influenza A virus reveal dynamic pathways for proton stabilization and transduction. *Proc Natl Acad Sci U S A* 2015;112(46):14260–14265.

884. Thompson MG, Muñoz-Moreno R, Bhat P, et al. Co-regulatory activity of hnRNP K and NS1-BP in influenza and human mRNA splicing. *Nat Commun* 2018;9(1):2407.

885. Throsby M, van den Brink E, Jongeneelen M, et al. Heterosubtypic neutralizing monoclonal antibodies cross-protective against H5N1 and H1N1 recovered from human IgM+ memory B cells. *PLoS One* 2008;3(12):e3942.

886. Thukral V, Varshney B, Ramly RB, et al. s8ORF2 protein of infectious salmon anaemia virus is a RNA-silencing suppressor and interacts with Salmon salar Mov10 (SsMov10) of the host RNAi machinery. *Virus Genes* 2018;54(2):199–214.

887. Tiley LS, Hagen M, Matthews JT, et al. Sequence-specific binding of the influenza virus RNA polymerase to sequences located at the 5′ ends of the viral RNAs. *J Virol* 1994;68(8):5108–5116.

888. Tomassini JE, Davies ME, Hastings JC, et al. A novel antiviral agent which inhibits the endonuclease of influenza viruses. *Antimicrob Agents Chemother* 1996;40(5):1189–1193.

889. Tomassini J, Selnick H, Davies ME, et al. Inhibition of cap (m7GpppXm)-dependent endonuclease of influenza virus by 4–substituted 2,4-dioxobutanoic acid compounds. *Antimicrob Agents Chemother* 1994;38(12):2827–2837.

890. Tome-Amat J, Ramos I, Amanor F, et al Influenza a virus utilizes low-affinity, high-avidity interactions with the nuclear import machinery to ensure infection and immune evasion. *J Virol* 2019;93(1).

891. Tomescu AI, Robb NC, Hengrung N, et al. Single-molecule FRET reveals a corkscrew RNA structure for the polymerase-bound influenza virus promoter. *Proc Natl Acad Sci U S A* 2014;111(32):E3335–E3342.

892. Tong S, Zhu X, Li Y, et al. New world bats harbor diverse influenza A viruses. *PLoS Pathog* 2013;9(10):e1003657.

893. Toro-Ascuy D, Cortez-San Martín M. Rescue of infectious salmon anemia virus (ISAV) from cloned cDNA. In: Perez DR, ed. *Reverse Genetics of RNA Viruses*. New York: Springer/Humana Press; 2017:239–250.

894. Toro-Ascuy D, Tambley C, Beltran C, et al. Development of a reverse genetic system for infectious salmon anemia virus: rescue of recombinant fluorescent virus by using salmon internal transcribed spacer region 1 as a novel promoter. *Appl Environ Microbiol* 2015;81(4):1210–1224.

895. Torreira E, Schoehn G, Fernandez Y, et al. Three-dimensional model for the isolated recombinant influenza virus polymerase heterotrimer. *Nucleic Acids Res* 2007;35(11):3774–3783.

896. Tran V, Moser LA, Poole DS, et al. Highly sensitive real-time in vivo imaging of an influenza reporter virus reveals dynamics of replication and spread. *J Virol* 2013;87(24):13321–13329.

897. Tran V, Poole DS, Jeffery JJ, et al. Multi-modal imaging with a toolbox of influenza A reporter viruses. *Viruses* 2015;7(10):5319–5327.

898. Tripathi S, Pohl MO, Zhou Y, et al. Meta- and orthogonal integration of influenza "OMICs" data defines a role for UBR4 in virus budding. *Cell Host Microbe* 2015;18(6):723–735.

899. Tsai PL, Chiou NT, Kuss S, et al. Cellular RNA binding proteins NS1-BP and hnRNP K regulate influenza A virus RNA splicing. *PLoS Pathog* 2013;9(6):e1003460.

900. Tsfasman T, Kost V, Markushin S, et al. Amphipathic alpha-helices and putative cholesterol binding domains of the influenza virus matrix M1 protein are crucial for virion structure organisation. *Virus Res* 2015;210:114–118.

901. Tumpey TM, Basler CF, Aguilar PV, et al. Characterization of the reconstructed 1918 Spanish influenza pandemic virus. *Science* 2005;310(5745):77–80.

902. Tumpey TM, García-Sastre A, Mikulasova A, et al. Existing antivirals are effective against influenza viruses with genes from the 1918 pandemic virus. *Proc Natl Acad Sci U S A* 2002;99(21):13849–13854.

903. Uhlendorff J, Matrosovich T, Klenk HD, et al. Functional significance of the hemadsorption activity of influenza virus neuraminidase and its alteration in pandemic viruses. *Arch Virol* 2009;154(6):945–957.

904. Ulmanen I, Broni BA, Krug RM. Role of two of the influenza virus core P proteins in recognizing cap 1 structures (m7GpppNm) on RNAs and in initiating viral RNA transcription. *Proc Natl Acad Sci U S A* 1981;78(12):7355–7359.

905. Vahey MD, Fletcher DA. Low-fidelity assembly of influenza A virus promotes escape from host cells. *Cell* 2019;176(3):678.

906. Valcarcel J, Fortes P, Ortin J. Splicing of influenza virus matrix protein mRNA expressed from a simian virus 40 recombinant. *J Gen Virol* 1993;74(Pt 7):1317–1326.

907. Vale-Costa S, Amorim MJ. Recycling endosomes and viral infection. *Viruses* 2016;8(3):64.

908. Varga ZT, Palese P. The influenza A virus protein PB1-F2: killing two birds with one stone? *Virulence* 2011;2(6).

909. Varga ZT, Ramos I, Hai R, et al. The influenza virus protein PB1-F2 inhibits the induction of type i interferon at the level of the MAVS adaptor protein. *PLoS Pathog* 2011;7(6):e1002067.

910. Varghese JN, Colman PM, van Donkelaar A, et al. Structural evidence for a second sialic acid binding site in avian influenza virus neuraminidases. *Proc Natl Acad Sci U S A* 1997;94(22):11808–11812.

911. Varghese JN, Laver WG, Colman PM. Structure of the influenza virus glycoprotein antigen neuraminidase at 2.9 A resolution. *Nature* 1983;303(5912):35–40.

912. Vasin AV, Temkina OA, Egorov VV, et al. Molecular mechanisms enhancing the proteome of influenza A viruses: an overview of recently discovered proteins. *Virus Res* 2014;185:53–63.

913. Veit M, Klenk HD, Kendal A, et al. The M2 protein of influenza A virus is acylated. *J Gen Virol* 1991;72(Pt 6):1461–1465.

914. Veit M, Kretzschmar E, Kuroda K, et al. Site-specific mutagenesis identifies three cysteine residues in the cytoplasmic tail as acylation sites of influenza virus hemagglutinin. *J Virol* 1991;65(5):2491–2500.

915. Veit M, Schmidt MF. Timing of palmitoylation of influenza virus hemagglutinin. *FEBS Lett* 1993;336(2):243–247.

916. Ver LS, Marcos-Villar L, Landeras-Bueno S, et al. The cellular factor NXP2/MORC3 is a positive regulator of influenza virus multiplication. *J Virol* 2015;89(19):10023–10030.

917. Versteeg GA, Hale BG, van Boheemen S, et al. Species-specific antagonism of host ISGylation by the influenza B virus NS1 protein. *J Virol* 2010;84(10):5423–5430.

918. Vlasak R, Krystal M, Nacht M, et al. The influenza C virus glycoprotein (HE) exhibits receptor-binding (hemagglutinin) and receptor-destroying (esterase) activities. *Virology* 1987;160(2):419–425.

919. Vlasak R, Luytjes W, Spaan W, et al. Human and bovine coronaviruses recognize sialic acid-containing receptors similar to those of influenza C viruses. *Proc Natl Acad Sci U S A* 1988;85(12):4526–4529.

920. Vlasak R, Muster T, Lauro AM, et al. Influenza C virus esterase: analysis of catalytic site, inhibition, and possible function. *J Virol* 1989;63(5):2056–2062.

921. von Itzstein M, Wu WY, Kok GB, et al. Rational design of potent sialidase-based inhibitors of influenza virus replication. *Nature* 1993;363(6428):418–423.

922. Vreede FT, Brownlee GG. Influenza virion-derived viral ribonucleoproteins synthesize both mRNA and cRNA in vitro. *J Virol* 2007;81(5):2196–2204.

923. Vreede FT, Chan AY, Sharps J, et al. Mechanisms and functional implications of the degradation of host RNA polymerase II in influenza virus infected cells. *Virology* 2010;396(1):125–134.

924. Vreede FT, Fodor E. The role of the influenza virus RNA polymerase in host shut-off. *Virulence* 2010;1(5):436–439.

925. Vreede FT, Gifford H, Brownlee GG. Role of initiating nucleoside triphosphate concentrations in the regulation of influenza virus replication and transcription. *J Virol* 2008;82(14):6902–6910.

926. Vreede FT, Jung TE, Brownlee GG. Model suggesting that replication of influenza virus is regulated by stabilization of replicative intermediates. *J Virol* 2004;78(17):9568–9572.

927. Wagner E, Engelhardt OG, Gruber S, et al. Rescue of recombinant Thogoto virus from cloned cDNA. *J Virol* 2001;75(19):9282–9286.

928. Wagner R, Herwig A, Azzouz N, et al. Acylation-mediated membrane anchoring of avian influenza virus hemagglutinin is essential for fusion pore formation and virus infectivity. *J Virol* 2005;79(10):6449–6458.

929. Wagner R, Matrosovich M, Klenk HD. Functional balance between haemagglutinin and neuraminidase in influenza virus infections. *Rev Med Virol* 2002;12(3):159–166.

930. Walker AP, Fodor E. Interplay between influenza virus and the host RNA polymerase II transcriptional machinery. *Trends Microbiol* 2019;27(5):398–407.

931. Walther T, Karamanska R, Chan RW, et al. Glycomic analysis of human respiratory tract tissues and correlation with influenza virus infection. *PLoS Pathog* 2013;9(3):e1003223.

932. Wang X, Basler CF, Williams BR, et al. Functional replacement of the carboxy-terminal two-thirds of the influenza A virus NS1 protein with short heterologous dimerization domains. *J Virol* 2002;76(24):12951–12962.

933. Wang QY, Bushell S, Qing M, et al. Inhibition of dengue virus through suppression of host pyrimidine biosynthesis. *J Virol* 2011;85(13):6548–6556.

934. Wang Q, Cheng F, Lu M, et al. Crystal structure of unliganded influenza B virus hemagglutinin. *J Virol* 2008;82(6):3011–3020.

935. Wang D, Harmon A, Jin J, et al. The lack of an inherent membrane targeting signal is responsible for the failure of the matrix (M1) protein of influenza A virus to bud into virus-like particles. *J Virol* 2010;84(9):4673–4681.

936. Wang W, Krug RM. The RNA-binding and effector domains of the viral NS1 protein are conserved to different extents among influenza A and B viruses. *Virology* 1996;223(1):41–50.

937. Wang S, Li H, Chen Y, et al. Transport of influenza virus neuraminidase (NA) to host cell surface is regulated by ARHGAP21 and Cdc42 proteins. *J Biol Chem* 2012;287(13):9804–9816.

938. Wang X, Li M, Zheng H, et al. Influenza A virus NS1 protein prevents activation of NF-kappaB and induction of alpha/beta interferon. *J Virol* 2000;74(24):11566–11573.

939. Wang P, Palese P, O'Neill RE. The NPI-1/NPI-3 (karyopherin alpha) binding site on the influenza A virus nucleoprotein NP is a nonconventional nuclear localization signal. *J Virol* 1997;71(3):1850–1856.

940. Wang J, Pielak RM, McClintock MA, et al. Solution structure and functional analysis of the influenza B proton channel. *Nat Struct Mol Biol* 2009;16(12):1267–1271.

941. Wang W, Riedel K, Lynch P, et al. RNA binding by the novel helical domain of the influenza virus NS1 protein requires its dimer structure and a small number of specific basic amino acids. *RNA* 1999;5(2):195–205.

942. Wang C, Takeuchi K, Pinto LH, et al. Ion channel activity of influenza A virus M2 protein: characterization of the amantadine block. *J Virol* 1993;67(9):5585–5594.

943. Wang TT, Tan GS, Hai R, et al. Broadly protective monoclonal antibodies against H3 influenza viruses following sequential immunization with different hemagglutinins. *PLoS Pathog* 2010;6(2):e1000796.

944. Wang Q, Tian X, Chen X, et al. Structural basis for receptor specificity of influenza B virus hemagglutinin. *Proc Natl Acad Sci U S A* 2007;104(43):16874–16879.

945. Wanitchang A, Wongthida P, Jongkaewwattana A. Influenza B virus M2 protein can functionally replace its influenza A virus counterpart in promoting virus replication. *Virology* 2016;498:99–108.

946. Wasilewski S, Calder LJ, Grant T, et al. Distribution of surface glycoproteins on influenza A virus determined by electron cryotomography. *Vaccine* 2012;30(51):7368–7373.

947. Watanabe K, Handa H, Mizumoto K, et al. Mechanism for inhibition of influenza virus RNA polymerase activity by matrix protein. *J Virol* 1996;70(1):241–247.

948. Watanabe T, Kawakami E, Shoemaker JE, et al. Influenza virus-host interactome screen as a platform for antiviral drug development. *Cell Host Microbe* 2014;16(6):795–805.

949. Watanabe R, Lamb RA. Influenza virus budding does not require a functional AAA+ ATPase, VPS4. *Virus Res* 2010;153(1):58–63.

950. Watanabe R, Leser GP, Lamb RA. Influenza virus is not restricted by tetherin whereas influenza VLP production is restricted by tetherin. *Virology* 2011;417(1):50–56.

951. Watanabe K, Shimizu T, Noda S, et al. Nuclear export of the influenza virus ribonucleoprotein complex: interaction of Hsc70 with viral proteins M1 and NS2. *FEBS Open Bio* 2014;4:683–688.

952. Watanabe K, Takizawa N, Katoh M, et al. Inhibition of nuclear export of ribonucleoprotein complexes of influenza virus by leptomycin B. *Virus Res* 2001;77(1):31–42.

953. Watanabe T, Watanabe S, Kawaoka Y. Cellular networks involved in the influenza virus life cycle. *Cell Host Microbe* 2010;7(6):427–439.

954. Watanabe T, Watanabe S, Noda T, et al. Exploitation of nucleic acid packaging signals to generate a novel influenza virus-based vector stably expressing two foreign genes. *J Virol* 2003;77(19):10575–10583.

955. Weber F, Haller O, Kochs G. Nucleoprotein viral RNA and mRNA of Thogoto virus: a novel "cap-stealing" mechanism in tick-borne orthomyxoviruses? *J Virol* 1996;70(12):8361–8367.

956. Weber F, Kochs G, Gruber S, et al. A classical bipartite nuclear localization signal on Thogoto and influenza A virus nucleoproteins. *Virology* 1998;250(1):9–18.

957. Weis W, Brown JH, Cusack S, et al. Structure of the influenza virus haemagglutinin complexed with its receptor, sialic acid. *Nature* 1988;333(6172):426–431.

958. Wharton SA, Belshe RB, Skehel JJ, et al. Role of virion M2 protein in influenza virus uncoating: specific reduction in the rate of membrane fusion between virus and liposomes by amantadine. *J Gen Virol* 1994;75(Pt 4):945–948.

959. White KM, Abreu P, Wang H, et al. Broad spectrum inhibitor of influenza A and B viruses targeting the viral nucleoprotein. *ACS Infect Dis* 2018;4(2):146–157.

960. White KM, De Jesus P, Chen Z, et al. A potent anti-influenza compound blocks fusion through stabilization of the prefusion conformation of the hemagglutinin protein. *ACS Infect Dis* 2015;1(2):98–109.

961. White MC, Lowen AC. Implications of segment mismatch for influenza A virus evolution. *J Gen Virol* 2018;99(1):3–16.

962. White MC, Steel J, Lowen AC. Heterologous packaging signals on segment 4, but not segment 6 or segment 8, limit influenza A virus reassortment. *J Virol* 2017;91(11).

963. White JM, Whittaker GR. Fusion of enveloped viruses in endosomes. *Traffic* 2016;17(6):593–614.

964. Whitehead TA, Chevalier A, Song Y, et al. Optimization of affinity, specificity and function of designed influenza inhibitors using deep sequencing. *Nat Biotechnol* 2012;30(6):543–548.

965. Whittaker G, Bui M, Helenius A. Nuclear trafficking of influenza virus ribonuleoproteins in heterokaryons. *J Virol* 1996;70(5):2743–2756.

966. Whittaker G, Kemler I, Helenius A. Hyperphosphorylation of mutant influenza virus matrix protein, M1, causes its retention in the nucleus. *J Virol* 1995;69(1):439–445.

967. Williams GD, Townsend D, Wylie KM, et al. Nucleotide resolution mapping of influenza A virus nucleoprotein-RNA interactions reveals RNA features required for replication. *Nat Commun* 2018;9(1):465.

968. Wilson RL, Frisz JF, Klitzing HA, et al. Hemagglutinin clusters in the plasma membrane are not enriched with cholesterol and sphingolipids. *Biophys J* 2015;108(7):1652–1659.

969. Wilson IA, Skehel JJ, Wiley DC. Structure of the haemagglutinin membrane glycoprotein of influenza virus at 3 A resolution. *Nature* 1981;289(5796):366–373.

970. Wise HM, Foeglein A, Sun J, et al. A complicated message: identification of a novel PB1-related protein translated from influenza A virus segment 2 mRNA. *J Virol* 2009;83(16):8021–8031.

971. Wise HM, Hutchinson EC, Jagger BW, et al. Identification of a novel splice variant form of the influenza A virus M2 ion channel with an antigenically distinct ectodomain. *PLoS Pathog* 2012;8(11):e1002998.

972. Wohlbold TJ, Chromikova V, Tan GS, et al. Hemagglutinin stalk- and neuraminidase-specific monoclonal antibodies protect against lethal H10N8 influenza virus infection in mice. *J Virol* 2015;90(2):851–861.

973. Wohlbold TJ, Krammer F. In the shadow of hemagglutinin: a growing interest in influenza viral neuraminidase and its role as a vaccine antigen. *Viruses* 2014;6(6):2465–2494.

974. Wohlbold TJ, Nachbagauer R, Xu H, et al. Vaccination with adjuvanted recombinant neuraminidase induces broad heterologous, but not heterosubtypic, cross-protection against influenza virus infection in mice. *MBio* 2015;6(2).

975. Wohlbold TJ, Podolsky KA, Chromikova V, et al. Broadly protective murine monoclonal antibodies against influenza B virus target highly conserved neuraminidase epitopes. *Nat Microbiol* 2017;2(10):1415–1424.

976. Wohlgemuth N, Lane AP, Pekosz A. Influenza A virus M2 protein apical targeting is required for efficient virus replication. *J Virol* 2018;92(22).

977. Wolff T, Ludwig S. Influenza viruses control the vertebrate type I interferon system: factors, mechanisms, and consequences. *J Interferon Cytokine Res* 2009;29(9):549–557.

978. Wolff T, O'Neill RE, Palese P. Interaction cloning of NS1-I, a human protein that binds to the nonstructural NS1 proteins of influenza A and B viruses. *J Virol* 1996;70(8):5363–5372.

979. Wolff T, O'Neill RE, Palese P. NS1-Binding protein (NS1-BP): a novel human protein that interacts with the influenza A virus nonstructural NS1 protein is relocalized in the nuclei of infected cells. *J Virol* 1998;72(9):7170–7180.

980. Worch R. Structural biology of the influenza virus fusion peptide. *Acta Biochim Pol* 2014;61(3):421–426.

981. Wressnigg N, Voss D, Wolff T, et al. Development of a live-attenuated influenza B DeltaNS1 intranasal vaccine candidate. *Vaccine* 2009;27(21):2851–2857.

982. Wu Y, Cho M, Shore D, et al. A potent broad-spectrum protective human monoclonal antibody crosslinking two haemagglutinin monomers of influenza A virus. *Nat Commun* 2015;6:7708.

983. Wu CY, Jeng KS, Lai MM. The SUMOylation of matrix protein M1 modulates the assembly and morphogenesis of influenza A virus. *J Virol* 2011;85(13):6618–6628.

984. Wu NC, Wilson IA. A perspective on the structural and functional constraints for immune evasion: insights from influenza virus. *J Mol Biol* 2017;429(17):2694–2709.

985. Wu NC, Wilson IA. Structural insights into the design of novel anti-influenza therapies. *Nat Struct Mol Biol* 2018;25(2):115–121.

986. Wurzer WJ, Planz O, Ehrhardt C, et al. Caspase 3 activation is essential for efficient influenza virus propagation. *EMBO J* 2003;22(11):2717–2728.

987. Xia S, Monzingo AF, Robertus JD. Structure of NS1A effector domain from the influenza A/Udorn/72 virus. *Acta Crystallogr D Biol Crystallogr* 2009;65(Pt 1):11–17.

988. Xia S, Robertus JD. X-ray structures of NS1 effector domain mutants. *Arch Biochem Biophys* 2010;494(2):198–204.

989. Xu R, Ekiert DC, Krause JC, et al. Structural basis of preexisting immunity to the 2009 H1N1 pandemic influenza virus. *Science* 2010;328(5976):357–360.

990. Xu R, McBride R, Paulson JC, et al. Structure, receptor binding, and antigenicity of influenza virus hemagglutinins from the 1957 H2N2 pandemic. *J Virol* 2010;84(4):1715–1721.

991. Xu R, Wilson IA. Structural characterization of an early fusion intermediate of influenza virus hemagglutinin. *J Virol* 2011;85(10):5172–5182.

992. Xu X, Zhu X, Dwek RA, et al. Structural characterization of the 1918 influenza virus H1N1 neuraminidase. *J Virol* 2008;82(21):10493–10501.

993. Yamashita M. Laninamivir and its prodrug, CS-8958: long-acting neuraminidase inhibitors for the treatment of influenza. *Antivir Chem Chemother* 2010;21(2):71–84.

994. Yamashita M, Krystal M, Palese P. Evidence that the matrix protein of influenza C virus is coded for by a spliced mRNA. *J Virol* 1988;62(9):3348–3355.

995. Yamashita M, Krystal M, Palese P. Comparison of the three large polymerase proteins of influenza A, B, and C viruses. *Virology* 1989;171(2):458–466.

996. Yamauchi Y, Boukari H, Banerjee I, et al. Histone deacetylase 8 is required for centrosome cohesion and influenza A virus entry. *PLoS Pathog* 2011;7(10):e1002316.

997. Yamauchi Y, Helenius A. Virus entry at a glance. *J Cell Sci* 2013;126(Pt 6):1289–1295.

998. Yamayoshi S, Watanabe M, Goto H, et al. Identification of a novel viral protein expressed from the PB2 segment of influenza A virus. *J Virol* 2016;90(1):444–456.

999. Yang T. Baloxavir marboxil: the first cap-dependent endonuclease inhibitor for the treatment of influenza. *Ann Pharmacother* 2019;53(7):754–759.

1000. Yang X, Steukers L, Forier K, et al. A beneficiary role for neuraminidase in influenza virus penetration through the respiratory mucus. *PLoS One* 2014;9(10):e110026.

1001. Yanguez E, Castello A, Welnowska E, et al. Functional impairment of eIF4A and eIF4G factors correlates with inhibition of influenza virus mRNA translation. *Virology* 2011;413(1):93–102.

1002. Yánguez E, Hunziker A, Dobay MP, et al. Phosphoproteomic-based kinase profiling early in influenza virus infection identifies GRK2 as antiviral drug target. *Nat Commun* 2018;9(1):3679.

1003. Yanguez E, Nieto A. So similar, yet so different: selective translation of capped and polyadenylated viral mRNAs in the influenza virus infected cell. *Virus Res* 2011;156(1–2):1–12.

1004. Yasuda J, Nakada S, Kato A, et al. Molecular assembly of influenza virus: association of the NS2 protein with virion matrix. *Virology* 1993;196(1):249–255.

1005. Ye Q, Krug RM, Tao YJ. The mechanism by which influenza A virus nucleoprotein forms oligomers and binds RNA. *Nature* 2006;444(7122):1078.

1006. Ye Z, Liu T, Offringa DP, et al. Association of influenza virus matrix protein with ribonucleoproteins. *J Virol* 1999;73(9):7467–7473.

1007. Yen HL, Herlocher LM, Hoffmann E, et al. Neuraminidase inhibitor-resistant influenza viruses may differ substantially in fitness and transmissibility. *Antimicrob Agents Chemother* 2005;49(10):4075–4084.

1008. Yen HL, Liang CH, Wu CY, et al. Hemagglutinin-neuraminidase balance confers respiratory-droplet transmissibility of the pandemic H1N1 influenza virus in ferrets. *Proc Natl Acad Sci U S A* 2011;108(34):14264–14269.

1009. Yin C, Khan JA, Swapna GV, et al. Conserved surface features form the double-stranded RNA binding site of non-structural protein 1 (NS1) from influenza A and B viruses. *J Biol Chem* 2007;282(28):20584–20592.

1010. Yip TF, Selim ASM, Lian I, et al. Advancements in host-based interventions for influenza treatment. *Front Immunol* 2018;9:1547.

1011. Yogaratnam J, Rito J, Kakuda TN, et al. Antiviral activity, safety, and pharmacokinetics of AL-794, a novel oral influenza endonuclease inhibitor: results of an influenza human challenge study. *J Infect Dis* 2019;219(2):177–185.

1012. Yondola MA, Fernandes F, Belicha-Villanueva A, et al. Budding capability of the influenza virus neuraminidase can be modulated by tetherin. *J Virol* 2011;85(6):2480–2491.

1013. York A, Hutchinson EC, Fodor E. Interactome analysis of the influenza A virus transcription/replication machinery identifies protein phosphatase 6 as a cellular factor required for efficient virus replication. *J Virol* 2014;88(22):13284–13299.

1014. Yu J, Hika B, Liu R, et al. The hemagglutinin-esterase fusion glycoprotein is a primary determinant of the exceptional thermal and acid stability of influenza D virus. *mSphere* 2017;2(4).

1015. Yu J, Li X, Wang Y, et al. PDlim2 selectively interacts with the PDZ binding motif of highly pathogenic avian H5N1 influenza A virus NS1. *PLoS One* 2011;6(5):e19511.

1016. Yuan W, Aramini JM, Montelione GT, et al. Structural basis for ubiquitin-like ISG 15 protein binding to the NS1 protein of influenza B virus: a protein-protein interaction function that is not shared by the corresponding N-terminal domain of the NS1 protein of influenza A virus. *Virology* 2002;304(2):291–301.

1017. Yuan P, Bartlam M, Lou Z, et al. Crystal structure of an avian influenza polymerase PA N reveals an endonuclease active site. *Nature* 2009;458(7240):909.

1018. Yuan W, Krug RM. Influenza B virus NS1 protein inhibits conjugation of the interferon (IFN)-induced ubiquitin-like ISG15 protein. *EMBO J* 2001;20(3):362–371.

1019. Zamarin D, Garcia-Sastre A, Xiao X, et al. Influenza virus PB1-F2 protein induces cell death through mitochondrial ANT3 and VDAC1. *PLoS Pathog* 2005;1(1):e4.

1020. Zamarin D, Ortigoza MB, Palese P. Influenza A virus PB1-F2 protein contributes to viral pathogenesis in mice. *J Virol* 2006;80(16):7976–7983.

1021. Zebedee SL, Lamb RA. Influenza A virus M2 protein: monoclonal antibody restriction of virus growth and detection of M2 in virions. *J Virol* 1988;62(8):2762–2772.

1022. Zeng Q, Langereis MA, van Vliet AL, et al. Structure of coronavirus hemagglutinin-esterase offers insight into corona and influenza virus evolution. *Proc Natl Acad Sci U S A* 2008;105(26):9065–9069.

1023. Zeng LY, Yang J, Liu S. Investigational hemagglutinin-targeted influenza virus inhibitors. *Expert Opin Investig Drugs* 2017;26(1):63–73.

1024. Zenilman JM, Fuchs EJ, Hendrix CW, et al. Phase 1 clinical trials of DAS181, an inhaled sialidase, in healthy adults. *Antiviral Res* 2015;123:114–119.

1025. Zhang J, Kong W, Ashraf S, et al. A one-plasmid system to generate influenza virus in cultured chicken cells for potential use in influenza vaccine. *J Virol* 2009;83(18):9296–9303.

1026. Zhang J, Lamb RA. Characterization of the membrane association of the influenza virus matrix protein in living cells. *Virology* 1996;225(2):255–266.

1027. Zhang J, Li G, Ye X. Cyclin T1/CDK9 interacts with influenza A virus polymerase and facilitates its association with cellular RNA polymerase II. *J Virol* 2010;84(24):12619–12627.

1028. Zhang J, Pekosz A, Lamb RA. Influenza virus assembly and lipid raft microdomains: a role for the cytoplasmic tails of the spike glycoproteins. *J Virol* 2000;74(10):4634–4644.

1029. Zhang K, Shang G, Padavannil A, et al. Structural–functional interactions of NS1-BP protein with the splicing and mRNA export machineries for viral and host gene expression. *Proc Natl Acad Sci U S A* 2018;115(52):E12218–E12227.

1030. Zhang K, Wang Z, Fan GZ, et al. Two polar residues within C-terminal domain of M1 are critical for the formation of influenza A Virions. *Cell Microbiol* 2015;17(11):1583–1593.

1031. Zhao C, Denison C, Huibregtse JM, et al. Human ISG15 conjugation targets both IFN-induced and constitutively expressed proteins functioning in diverse cellular pathways. *Proc Natl Acad Sci U S A* 2005;102(29):10200–10205.

1032. Zhao H, Ekström M, Garoff H. The M1 and NP proteins of influenza A virus form homo- but not heterooligomeric complexes when coexpressed in BHK-21 cells. *J Gen Virol* 1998;79(Pt 10):2435–2446.

1033. Zhao C, Hsiang TY, Kuo RL, et al. ISG15 conjugation system targets the viral NS1 protein in influenza A virus-infected cells. *Proc Natl Acad Sci U S A* 2010;107(5):2253–2258.

1034. Zhao N, Sebastiano V, Moshkina N, et al. Influenza virus infection causes global RNAPII termination defects. *Nat Struct Mol Biol* 2018;25(9):885–893.

1035. Zhao C, Sridharan H, Chen R, et al. Influenza B virus non-structural protein 1 counteracts ISG15 antiviral activity by sequestering ISGylated viral proteins. *Nat Commun* 2016;7:12754.

1036. Zheng H, Palese P, García-Sastre A. Nonconserved nucleotides at the 3′ and 5′ ends of an influenza A virus RNA play an important role in viral RNA replication. *Virology* 1996;217(1):242–251.

1037. Zhirnov OP, Grigoriev VB. Disassembly of influenza C viruses, distinct from that of influenza A and B viruses requires neutral-alkaline pH. *Virology* 1994;200(1):284–291.

1038. Zhirnov OP, Kirzhner LS, Ovcharenko AV, et al. [Clinical effectiveness of aprotinin aerosol in influenza and parainfluenza]. *Vestn Ross Akad Med Nauk* 1996;(5):26–31.

1039. Zhirnov OP, Klenk HD. Histones as a target for influenza virus matrix protein M1. *Virology* 1997;235(2):302–310.

1040. Zhirnov OP, Klenk HD, Wright PF. Aprotinin and similar protease inhibitors as drugs against influenza. *Antiviral Res* 2011;92(1):27–36.

1041. Zhirnov OP, Ovcharenko AV, Bukrinskaya AG. Suppression of influenza virus replication in infected mice by protease inhibitors. *J Gen Virol* 1984;65(Pt 1):191–196.

1042. Zhou B, Donnelly ME, Scholes DT, et al. Single-reaction genomic amplification accelerates sequencing and vaccine production for classical and Swine origin human influenza a viruses. *J Virol* 2009;83(19):10309–10313.

1043. Zhou B, Jerzak G, Scholes DT, et al. Reverse genetics plasmid for cloning unstable influenza A virus gene segments. *J Virol Methods* 2011;173(2):378–383.

1044. Zhu P, Liang L, Shao X, et al. Host cellular protein TRAPPC6AΔ interacts with influenza A virus M2 protein and regulates viral propagation by modulating M2 trafficking. *J Virol* 2017;91(1).

1045. Zhu L, Ly H, Liang Y. PLC-γ1 signaling plays a subtype-specific role in postbinding cell entry of influenza A virus. *J Virol* 2014;88(1):417–424.

1046. Zhu X, McBride R, Nycholat CM, et al. Influenza virus neuraminidases with reduced enzymatic activity that avidly bind sialic acid receptors. *J Virol* 2012;86(24):13371–13383.

1047. Zhu X, Yang H, Guo Z, et al. Crystal structures of two subtype N10 neuraminidase-like proteins from bat influenza A viruses reveal a diverged putative active site. *Proc Natl Acad Sci U S A* 2012;109(46):18903–18908.

1048. Zhu X, Yu W, McBride R, et al. Hemagglutinin homologue from H17N10 bat influenza virus exhibits divergent receptor-binding and pH-dependent fusion activities. *Proc Natl Acad Sci U S A* 2013;110(4):1458–1463.

1049. Zurcher T, Luo G, Palese P. Mutations at palmitylation sites of the influenza virus hemagglutinin affect virus formation. *J Virol* 1994;68(9):5748–5754.

Orthomyxoviruses

Gabriele Neumann • John J. Treanor • Yoshihiro Kawaoka

INTRODUCTION

Influenza viruses (family *Orthomyxoviridae*) cause highly contagious respiratory disease with potentially fatal outcomes. Symptoms include fever, headache, cough, sore throat, nasal congestion, sneezing, and body aches. Influenza viruses also cause local epidemics or pandemics (worldwide outbreaks) with significant infection rates. Although the economic burden of influenza is most prominent during pandemics, the combined annual costs of seasonal epidemics due to sick days, emergency room visits, and medications are significant. With the realization that avian influenza viruses can be directly transmitted to humans (Fig. 15.1), influenza viruses are now considered a major, global health threat.

Technologies such as reverse genetics[103] have allowed the routine manipulation of influenza viral genomes. In addition, a number of other technologies and approaches—including large-scale sequencing of viral genomes (through conventional Sanger sequencing and next-generation sequencing); improved computational tools for sequence analysis; small interfering RNA (siRNA)–mediated screens; transcriptomics, proteomics, metabolomics, and lipidomics studies; gene knockout technologies including CRISPR/Cas9–mediated gene knockout; and much-improved approaches for the production of human monoclonal antibodies—are being used to study the viral and cellular factors that control influenza virus replication, interspecies transmission, pathogenesis, and host immune responses to viral infections. Despite recent advances, much still needs to be learned about the molecular determinants of these events.

NOMENCLATURE

Influenza viruses belong to the *Orthomyxoviridae* family. This family comprises seven genera: *Alphainfluenzavirus* with the species *Influenza A virus*; *Betainfluenzavirus* with the species *Influenza B virus*; *Deltainfluenzavirus* with the species *Influenza D virus*; *Gammainfluenzavirus* with the species *Influenza C virus*; *Isavirus* with the species *Salmon isavirus*; *Quaranjavirus* with the species *Johnston Atoll quaranjavirus* and *Quaranfil quaranjavirus*; and *Thogotovirus* with the species *Dhori thogotovirus* and *Thogoto thogotovirus* (see the International Committee on Taxonomy of Viruses Web site: http://www.ictvonline.org). *Deltainfluenzavirus*, *Isavirus*, *Quaranjavirus*, and *Thogotovirus* do not circulate in humans and will not be discussed in this chapter. Influenza A viruses are further classified into subtypes based on the antigenicity of their hemagglutinin (HA) and neuraminidase (NA) proteins; currently, 18 HA subtypes (H1–H18) and 11 NA subtypes (N1–N11) are known. The present nomenclature system includes type of virus, host of origin (except for humans), geographic site of isolation, strain number, and year of isolation, followed by the antigenic description of the HA and NA subtypes in parenthesis: for viruses isolated before 2000, the year should be given as two digits; for viruses isolated in 2000 or later, the year should be given as four digits. For example, A/swine/Iowa/15/30 (H1N1) describes an influenza A virus isolated from a pig in Iowa in 1930 with a strain number of 15 and an H1N1 subtype. Antigenic subtypes have not been identified for influenza B and C viruses. Orthomyxoviruses of different genera do not cross-react antigenically.

Seroarcheology

Retrospective seroepidemiologic analysis, or seroarcheology, has provided information about influenza virus outbreaks that preceded the virologic techniques currently used to unequivocally identify infectious agents. Early studies suggested that the pandemic of 1889 to 1891 was caused by a virus of the H2N2 subtype, whereas that of 1900 had been attributed to an H3N8 strain. More recent reevaluation of the data indicates that the 1889 to 1891 pandemic was caused by an H3-like virus and there is no compelling evidence that links the H2 subtype to a pandemic other than that of 1957 (see The Pandemic of

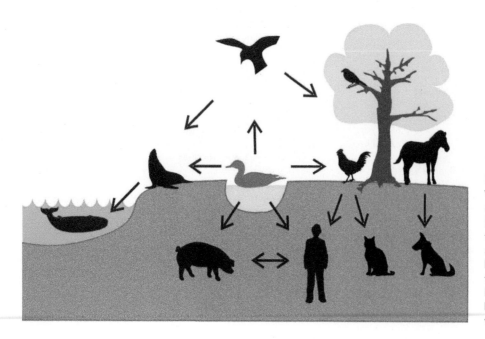

FIGURE 15.1 Influenza A virus reservoir. Wild aquatic birds are the main reservoir of influenza A viruses. Virus transmission has been reported from wild waterfowl to poultry, sea mammals, pigs, horses, and humans. Viruses are also transmitted between pigs and humans and from poultry to humans. Equine influenza viruses have been transmitted to dogs. Cats can be infected by avian, human, or canine viruses.

1957— Asian Influenza section). The latter conclusion is substantiated by the lack of protection among those who were at least 80 years old during the 1957 pandemic. Seroarcheology has also linked the 1918/1919 pandemic to an H1 virus, a finding that has been confirmed by sequence determination of influenza viral RNA (vRNA) from the lung tissues of victims[117] (see also The Pandemic of 1918/1919—Spanish Influenza [H1N1] section). Studies using antibodies to the NA protein suggest that in the late 1800s, viruses of the N8 subtype were circulating and were later replaced by N1 and N2 subtype viruses. Thus, during the 1900s, only a limited number of virus subtypes (H1N1, H2N2, H3N2, H3N8) were established in humans. Reassortant H1N2 viruses emerged in humans in 2001 and circulated in 2002 and 2003 but have not been isolated from humans since early 2004.

Virus Isolation

In 1930, the first swine influenza virus, A/swine/Iowa/30, was isolated, but it was not until 1933 that the first human virus was isolated by Wilson Smith, Sir Christopher Andrewes, and Sir Patrick Laidlaw of the National Institute for Medical Research in London, England. These investigators inoculated ferrets intranasally with human nasopharyngeal washes from an influenza patient. The animals exhibited an influenza-like disease, and the virus was transmitted to cage mates. One of their junior colleagues (later Sir Charles Stuart-Harris) became infected by these experimentally infected animals, and the virus was subsequently isolated from him. Because it was the first human influenza virus, it was named influenza A virus. In 1940, an antigenically distinct virus was isolated and named type B virus (B/Lee/40). The first influenza C virus was isolated in 1947. "Fowl plague" was first described in 1878 as a disease that affected chickens in Italy. The causative agent was isolated in 1902 (A/chicken/Brescia/1902 [H7N7]); however, it was not until 1955 that Schafer recognized fowl plague virus as an influenza virus.

Virus Propagation

Influenza viruses were first propagated in embryonated hens' eggs, which continue to be the most widely used system for vaccine production, although cell culture systems are now also in use (see later discussion). Avian and equine strains of influenza A viruses can be isolated from the allantoic cavity of 10- to 11-day-old embryonated eggs after 2 to 3 days of incubation at 33°C to 37°C. Human influenza A and B viruses have also been isolated from clinical samples inoculated into the allantoic or amniotic cavity of eggs and incubation at 33°C to 34°C. However, recent human influenza viruses of the H3N2 subtype are difficult to isolate from embryonated eggs because of mutations in HA that alter the receptor-binding specificity. Influenza virus growth in embryonated eggs leads to the selection of antigenic variants that are characterized by mutations in the HA protein[9] (see also Host Cell–Mediated Selection of Antigenic Variants section). Influenza C viruses amplify in the amniotic, but not allantoic, cavity of eggs and are usually grown for 5 days in 7- to 8-day-old embryonated eggs.

Influenza viruses can also be propagated in cell culture. Madin-Darby canine kidney (MDCK) cells support the efficient replication of many influenza A and B viruses and are used to isolate viruses from human samples. Recent human H3N2 viruses do not efficiently grow in MDCK cells and are often amplified in modified MDCK cells overexpressing Siaα2,6Gal (i.e., human-type receptors; see Receptor Specificity of Influenza Viruses section). Although many influenza viruses can grow in African green monkey kidney (Vero) cells, they do so less efficiently than in MDCK cells. Cell culture systems based on MDCK, Vero, and PER.C6 (human primary embryonic retinoblast) cells have been developed for influenza virus vaccine production, and MDCK and Vero cell–based vaccines are approved in Europe for use in humans; MDCK cell–based vaccines are now also approved in the United States. Influenza viruses also replicate in a number of primary cell cultures, including monkey, calf, hamster, and chicken kidney cells, as well as in chicken embryo fibroblasts and primary human epithelial cells. With the exception of primary human airway epithelium and kidney cells, most cell culture systems require the addition of trypsin to cleave the HA protein of human viruses (except highly pathogenic H5 and H7 viruses), a prerequisite for efficient replication (see HA Cleavage section).

Replication of influenza viruses in eggs or cell culture is measured by using conventional plaque assays, hemagglutination assays that measure the viruses' ability to agglutinate erythrocytes (note that recent human H3N2 viruses have lost the ability to agglutinate commonly used erythrocyte species), or molecular biology techniques, such as reverse transcriptase (RT)–polymerase chain reaction (PCR).

EVOLUTION OF INFLUENZA VIRUSES

Influenza viruses evolve via a complex process that involves the accumulation of mutations over time and the rearrangement of vRNA segments in cells infected with two (or more) different viruses (known as "reassortment"). In wild aquatic birds, avian influenza viruses evolve slowly; while mutations occur, most are not sustained in viral populations because they do not provide an evolutionary advantage. The exceptions are avian viruses in terrestrial poultry, including highly pathogenic H5 viruses, which evolve rapidly (see Infections of Humans with H5 Viruses of the A/goose/Guangdong/1/1996 Lineage section). In contrast to most avian influenza viruses, human influenza viruses show detectable net evolution over time.

Evolutionary Rates of Influenza A Viruses

The mutation rate (i.e., the rate at which mutations occur during viral replication) is higher for RNA viruses than for DNA viruses. For influenza viruses, the reported mutation rates range from approximately 10^{-6} to approximately 10^{-4} substitutions per nucleotide site per cell infection (s/n/c). Not all mutations occur at the same frequency: for example, transitions are detected more frequently than transversions, and G-to-A mutations occur more frequently than other transitions. These differences in mutation rates affect the probability with which particular amino acid changes can be expected. In contrast to the mutation rate, the evolutionary rate describes the rate at which mutations are fixed in a population. The evolutionary rate is affected by multiple factors including the mutation rate; the fitness effect of mutations (mutations can be deleterious, neutral, or beneficial); clonal interference (i.e., the competition among different lineages with beneficial mutations); epistatic effects (in which the effect of one mutation is dependent on another mutation); and population and within-host dynamics (including population sizes and host immune selective pressure). For influenza viruses, the reported evolutionary rates range from approximately 5×10^{-4} to approximately 8×10^{-3} substitutions per nucleotide site per year (s/n/y).[155]

At the amino acid level, viruses from wild aquatic birds evolve slower than those from terrestrial poultry, swine, or humans.[155] The fact that in wild aquatic birds, most avian influenza A viruses seem to evolve slowly suggests that they are well adapted to their hosts. Thus, although mutations may occur with similar frequency to that in other hosts, they do not result in many amino acid changes. Among avian influenza A viruses, the evolutionary rates are highest for the HA, NA, and NS1 proteins, possibly reflecting their immunogenic or immunomodulatory functions.

Proteins of mammalian and terrestrial poultry viruses continuously accumulate amino acid substitutions. For human influenza A viruses, the evolutionary rates differ among the proteins, likely reflecting differences in the selective pressure of the host. For example, the HA protein has a higher evolutionary rate than the other viral proteins, reflecting host immune pressure acting on HA. This is further supported by the finding that the HA head region (in which the antigenic epitopes are located) has a higher evolutionary rate than that of the HA stalk region; moreover, the antigenic epitopes exhibit a higher rate of nonsynonymous nucleotide changes than do other regions of HA. The human M1 and M2 proteins, encoded by overlapping reading frames, are under different selective pressures: for the M1 protein, a higher percentage of changes is silent than for the M2 protein. The M1 protein thus appears to be well adapted to its mammalian hosts, whereas the M2 protein is under stronger selective pressure. The biologic reason for the selective pressure on the M2 protein is unknown. The two proteins encoded by the NS vRNA segment also differ in their evolutionary rates, with NS1 showing more variation between alleles than NS2. High evolutionary rates have been reported during the establishment of new virus lineages, for example, the introduction of avian H1N1 influenza viruses into European pigs in 1977, the emergence of highly pathogenic avian H5N2 influenza viruses in poultry in Mexico in 1993/1994, and the emergence of highly pathogenic avian H5N1 influenza viruses in Hong Kong in 1997, which may reflect preferential selection of mutants that provide an advantage in a new host.

Host-Specific Lineages, and Geographic Segregation of Influenza A Viruses

Extensive phylogenetic analyses have revealed host-specific virus lineages for several viral genes.[155] The phylogenetic trees of the PB2, PA, NP, M1/M2, and NS1/NS2 genes (which encode the viral polymerase subunits PB2 and PA, the nucleoprotein NP, the matrix protein M1, the ion channel protein M2, the interferon-antagonist protein NS1, and the nuclear export protein NS2 or NEP; see Chapter 14 for more information) are similar in that they can be divided into two major branches consisting of avian and avian-like swine, or classic swine and human influenza viruses, respectively.

The phylogenetic tree of the PB1 gene (which encodes one of the viral polymerase subunits) differs from those of other influenza virus genes. The PB1 genes of human H1N1 viruses cluster with classic swine viruses, whereas the PB1 genes of human H2N2 and H3N2 viruses form a different sublineage that reflects the introduction in 1957 and 1968 of avian virus PB1 genes into human influenza viruses.[67,123] The genes other than the HA and NA of equine H7N7 viruses do not cluster with avian, human, or swine influenza viruses, suggesting their early separation into a separate lineage.

The phylogenetic tree of the NS1 gene is divided into two alleles: A and B. All mammalian virus NS1 genes belong to allele A, whereas avian influenza virus NS1 genes can belong to allele A or B.

The H1 HA genes can be separated into a branch consisting of avian and avian-like swine influenza viruses versus a branch consisting of human and classic swine viruses. The phylogenetic tree of the H3 HA gene consists of two major branches: one branch splits into two major sub-branches that represent equine/canine and North American avian virus isolates. The second branch can be separated into Eurasian avian viruses and human and swine H3 HAs that separated from the avian viruses in the 1960s. The human H3 gene has evolved in a single lineage since its introduction into the human population in 1968.

The phylogenetic tree of N1 NA genes shows two major branches that separate into human and classic swine, or Eurasian swine and avian N1 NA genes, respectively. The phylogenetic tree of the N2 NA gene can be divided into a North American avian clade, and a second clade that evolved into Eurasian avian and human virus genes at the beginning of the last century.

The bat influenza virus PB2, PB1, PA, NP, M1/M2, and NS1/NS2 genes are ancestral to those of other influenza A viruses.[141,142] The bat influenza virus HA genes are more closely related to Group 1 HAs (i.e., H1, H2, H5, H6, H8, H9, H11, H12, H13, and H16 HAs) than to Group 2 HAs (i.e., H3, H4, H7, H10, H14, and H15 HAs).[141,142] The bat influenza virus NA genes are ancestral to the known influenza A and B virus NAs.[141,142]

These analyses also reveal that influenza virus genes can be separated by their geographic origin, with a North American and a Eurasian gene pool. These gene pools appear to evolve largely independently, although reassortment between North American and Eurasian viruses has been reported.

Host-Specific Amino Acids

Recent large-scale sequencing efforts have generated thousands of full-genome influenza viral sequences (https://www.ncbi.nlm.nih.gov/genomes/FLU/Database/nph-select.cgi?go=database; www.fludb.org; www.gisaid.org). The comparison of viral proteins derived from different host species and virus lineages has revealed signature amino acids at specific positions that distinguish viruses of different host origins and/or from different lineages. In particular, comparative studies have identified a number of mammalian-adapting signature amino acids in highly pathogenic avian H5 influenza viruses, H7N9 influenza viruses of low or high pathogenicity, the pandemic 1918 virus, and A(H1N1)pdm09 viruses that may play a role in adaptation to humans. For some of these signature amino acids, a role in pathogenicity has been demonstrated (see Molecular Determinants of Host-Range Restriction and Pathogenesis section).

Computational analyses of viral sequences have also identified differences in mutation patterns and codon usage between human and avian influenza viruses. Such approaches may improve our understanding of influenza virus evolution.

Quasispecies

The high error rate of the replication complex of RNA viruses results in the generation of different genetic variants within a host organism, referred to as quasispecies. In the event of host or environmental pressure (including innate and adaptive immune responses and selective pressure resulting from a host change or antiviral pressure), a quasispecies may become the dominant virus population. In the past, the detection of quasispecies was cumbersome due to the detection limits of conventional sequencing techniques. However, with robust deep-sequencing platforms, minor sequence variants can now be detected more easily. These techniques are used to assess the levels of minor variants encoding mammalian-adapting amino acid changes, mutations that confer resistance to antivirals, antigenic escape variants, and so forth. The increasing number of datasets on viral quasispecies may facilitate our understanding of mutational patterns, selective pressures, and evolutionary trends.

Evolution in Influenza B and C Viruses

Significant differences in evolutionary rates exist for influenza A, B, and C viruses. Type B viruses, and especially type C viruses, evolve more slowly than do influenza A viruses. Type B and C viruses seem to be near or at an evolutionary equilibrium in humans; in contrast, the genes of type A human viruses were introduced from birds and have not reached an equilibrium in humans. Influenza A viruses in humans evolve along single lineages, which suggests evolution by clonal selection and limited cocirculation of sublineages. Cocirculation of sublineages has been shown over only limited periods. In contrast, the evolution of influenza B and C viruses is characterized by the cocirculation of antigenically and genetically distinct lineages over extended periods of time. For influenza B viruses, two lineages—B/Victoria (represented by B/Victoria/2/87) and B/Yamagata (represented by B/Yamagata/16/88)—have been cocirculating for about 25 years with changing patterns of prevalence and geographic distribution.

INFLUENZA VIRUS GENETICS

Reassortment

Reassortment is the rearrangement of vRNA segments in cells infected with two (or more) different influenza viruses (Fig. 15.2). Reassortment between 2 viruses can theoretically result in 256 (2^8) different vRNA constellations (i.e., the 2 parental genotypes and 254 new vRNA combinations). Reassortment occurs for influenza A, B, and C viruses but has not been observed among the different types of influenza viruses.

The importance of reassortment to the generation of new influenza virus strains is highlighted by the last three pandemics, which resulted from reassortment[39,67,105,123,130] (see The Pandemic of 1957—Asian Influenza [H2N2]; The Pandemic of 1968—Hong Kong Influenza [H3N2]; and The H1N1 Pandemic in 2009 sections). In addition, the highly pathogenic H5 viruses currently circulating in Southeast Asia and other

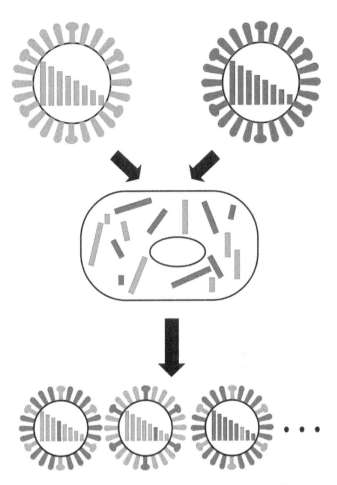

FIGURE 15.2 Reassortment. Coinfection of cells with 2 different influenza A viruses can theoretically result in 256 different genotypes (2^8, i.e., the two parental genotypes and 254 new genotypes). Reassortment is a major mechanism for the generation of pandemic influenza viruses, as demonstrated in 1957, 1968, and 2009.

parts of the world arose from multiple reassortment events among avian influenza viruses[12,46,78,82]; these viruses continue to undergo reassortment, including reassortment between the HA and NA vRNA segments of different subtypes (see Infections of Humans with H5 Viruses of the A/goose/Guangdong/1/1996 Lineage section). Similarly, the H7N9 viruses that emerged in China in 2013 resulted from reassortment among avian influenza viruses[37] and have undergone additional reassortment since their emergence (see Infections of Humans with Low and Highly Pathogenic H7N9 Viruses section).

In addition to reassortment events that create new pandemics, reassortment has also resulted in multiple novel influenza virus lineages in pigs and poultry. For human influenza viruses, intrasubtypic reassortment may be more important than previously thought and may have led to the epidemics observed with reassorted H1N1 viruses in 1947 and 1951, reassorted H2N2 viruses in 1967, and reassorted H3N2 viruses in 1997 and 2003.

In experimental settings, multiple reassortants can be generated between highly pathogenic avian H5N1 and human H3N2 or A(H1N1)pdm09 viruses; between A(H1N1)pdm09 and seasonal H1N1 or avian H9N2 viruses; between human H3N2 and genetically distant equine H7N7 viruses; and between avian H7N3 and A(H1N1)pdm09 viruses. However, not all vRNA segment combinations can be generated experimentally, and others may not be compatible in nature. Experimentally generated reassortant viruses have also been used to assess the virulence determinants of the 1918 pandemic virus and to study the determinants of influenza H5, H7, and H9 virus transmissibility in mammals.

Recombination

For negative-sense RNA viruses, homologous recombination is uncommon; however, recombination by "template switching" can occur and lead to increased biologic fitness of the virus. For example, the insertion of 54 nucleotides of 28S ribosomal RNA into the A/turkey/Oregon/71 HA gene increased HA cleavability.[68] Similarly, an A/seal/Massachusetts/1/80 variant contained a 60-nucleotide insertion (derived from the NP gene) in its HA gene, which also enhanced HA cleavability. Avian influenza viruses of low pathogenicity have converted to high pathogenicity following the insertion of 21 nucleotides of the M segment or 30 nucleotides of the NP segment into the HA segment. Serial egg passages of an A/WSN/33 virus containing a 24-amino-acid deletion in the NA stalk led to variants that replicated efficiently in eggs. The NA stalk of these variants contained sequences that originated from the PB1, PB2, and NP genes. In another example, a virus contained an NP gene that likely resulted from intracistronic recombination between two NP segments. In this case, it is unclear whether the recombination event provided a selective advantage to the virus.

Defective Interfering (DI) Viral RNAs and Particles

DI vRNAs possess large internal deletions in a viral genome segment, while the terminal regions of the vRNAs (which contain the viral promoters for replication and transcription) remain intact. The internal deletions result from replication errors in which the viral polymerase complex falls off the template and reinitiates replication at a downstream site. DI vRNAs have been reported for all influenza vRNAs but occur most frequently for the three largest vRNAs that encode the polymerase proteins. Due to their reduced length, DI vRNAs are replicated faster than the parent vRNA, resulting in "interference" with the replication of the parent vRNA. DI vRNAs can be packaged into virus particles; these DI particles are "defective" because they lack a full viral genome and cannot initiate a new round of replication and progeny virus generation. DI vRNAs are frequently detected under experimental conditions but are also found in clinical samples. Their role in the viral life cycle is not understood, although they may stimulate innate immune responses.

Reverse Genetics

Highly efficient systems are now in place for the artificial generation of influenza A,[29,103] B, and C viruses and of *Thogotovirus*. These systems rely on the intracellular synthesis of influenza vRNAs by a cellular enzyme, RNA polymerase I, that transcribes ribosomal RNA in the nucleus of eukaryotic cells. The influenza viral segments are encoded by cDNAs flanked by the RNA polymerase I promoter and the RNA polymerase I terminator or a ribozyme sequence. RNA polymerase I transcription in transfected cells results in the efficient synthesis of RNA transcripts with defined 5′ ends, whereas the integrity of the

3′ ends is achieved by using the nucleotide-specific RNA polymerase I terminator or a self-cleaving ribozyme. To generate influenza viruses, cells are transfected with RNA polymerase I plasmids to provide all eight vRNAs, as well as with up to four plasmids for the expression of the polymerase and NP proteins that are required to initiate viral replication. These systems have revolutionized influenza virus research in that they allow researchers to study the functions of viral proteins in the viral life cycle, as well as their roles in pathogenesis and hostrange restriction. Moreover, these systems are now used to generate recombinant influenza viruses expressing fluorescent proteins that can be used to monitor the infection process in live animals, thus providing novel insights into influenza target cells and the dynamics of virus spread.

Most importantly, reverse genetics systems are now invaluable tools for the generation of influenza virus vaccines and vaccine vectors. In fact, reverse genetics has permitted the generation of inactivated and live vaccine strains for H5 and H7 viruses that could not have been produced by conventional approaches because highly pathogenic viruses kill chicken embryo, resulting in low vaccine yield; this hurdle was overcome with genetically modified vaccine strains of low pathogenicity in eggs. In addition, reverse genetics systems have opened the door for conceptually novel vaccine candidates including vaccines with chimeric or headless HAs or single-cycle replication viruses (see Vaccines section).

INFLUENZA IN HUMANS—PAST PANDEMICS

Pandemics are outbreaks that impact large geographic areas and large portions of the population in a short period of time. Pandemics are the most dramatic manifestation of influenza, attacking 20% to 40% of the world population and causing significant mortality. Influenza pandemics have occurred in 10- to 40-year intervals, although reliable records only date back to the 1918/1919 pandemic (Fig. 15.3). The cumulative death toll of epidemics in interpandemic periods, although less dramatic, parallels those of pandemics.

The Pandemic of 1918/1919—Spanish Influenza (H1N1)

The pandemic of 1918/1919 remains unprecedented in its severity. It killed more people than World War I and reduced life expectancy in the United States by 10 years. AIDS has killed 25 million people in its first 25 years—the Spanish influenza killed an equal number in 25 weeks (from September 1918–March 1919). This pandemic occurred in three waves. In the spring of 1918, a mild respiratory disease started at Fort Funston, Kansas (now Fort Riley), attributed to a soldier who had been cleaning pig pens. There is no mention of the presence of poultry in the camp at that time. The disease spread among soldiers from Fort Funston along the rail lines to other military bases and cities in the United States and on troopships to Europe. This first wave was highly contagious but caused few deaths and received limited attention in most parts of the world. In Spain, a neutral country without news censorship, the outbreak was covered extensively by news media and was soon referred to as the "Spanish influenza." In late August, a second wave with a higher

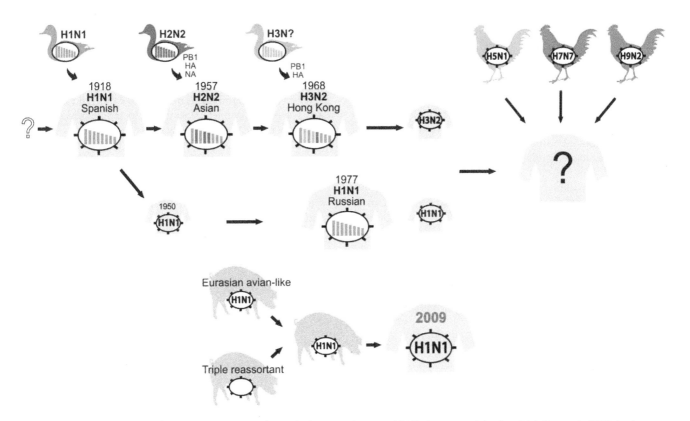

FIGURE 15.3 Evolution of influenza A viruses circulating in humans. An avian H1N1 virus caused the Spanish influenza in 1918. Its descendants circulated until the mid-1950s and reemerged in 1977, causing the Russian influenza. Viruses of this lineage continued to circulate in human populations until 2009. The 1957 pandemic was caused by an H2N2 virus that acquired its HA, NA, and PB1 vRNA segments from an avian H2N2 virus. A similar reassortment event in 1968 resulted in the introduction of avian virus HA and PB1 vRNA segments into the human population, causing the 1968 pandemic. H3N2 viruses circulate in humans to this day. In 2009, reassortment of triple reassortant swine viruses and Eurasian avian–like swine viruses (which donated the NA and M vRNA segments) resulted in the A(H1N1)pdm09 virus, which replaced the then-circulating H1N1 viruses. Sporadically, humans are infected by avian influenza viruses of the H5, H7, or H9N2 subtypes.

mortality rate started, probably in Western France, from where it spread around the world; this wave peaked between September and November. During that time, death tolls reached more than 10,000 people per week in some US cities. About one-third of the US population became sick, and the mortality rate was estimated to be over 2.5%, compared to less than 0.1% in typical influenza outbreaks. These figures reflect the impact of the pandemic on the developed world; death rates are believed to have been significantly higher in African and Asian countries. In some isolated populations, the mortality rate reached 70%, likely because of the lack of previous exposure to influenza virus. A third wave of similar impact to that of the second wave struck in late 1918/early 1919.

Typically, the onset of symptoms was sudden, with high fever, severe headache and myalgia, cough, pharyngitis, and coryza. Pathologic findings were mostly restricted to the respiratory tract; death was often due to secondary bacterial pneumonia and respiratory failure. There was no evidence of systemic viral infection. Most patients died of secondary bacterial pneumonia, but some showed massive acute pulmonary hemorrhage or pulmonary edema, indicating the extreme virulence of the virus. The high rate of bacterial complications may be attributed to the lack of antibiotics at that time.

Age-specific morbidity was similar to that of other pandemics, with children younger than 15 years experiencing the highest infection rates. The mortality pattern, however, differed

significantly from that of other influenza virus outbreaks. In typical influenza outbreaks, the highest death rates are observed in very young children and in the elderly. In 1918 and 1919, many deaths occurred among young, otherwise healthy adults. The death rate for the 15- to 35-year-old age group was 20 times higher in 1918 than in previous years, and persons younger than 65 years accounted for more than 99% of excess deaths. In particular, people born in 1889, the year of the outbreak of the then most recent pandemic (which, based on seroarcheological studies, was caused by an H3 virus), suffered from a high mortality rate. These findings suggested that prior exposures to influenza viruses shaped the immune response to infection with the 1918 pandemic virus.

The origin of the 1918/1919 virus remains an enigma. In 1927, E. Jordan published a comprehensive review of the origin of the pandemic. He found no evidence that the disease had originated in China. He also evaluated two reports that described local outbreaks of respiratory infections associated with high mortality and heliotrope cyanosis, which was observed during the 1918/1919 outbreak, in army camps in Étaples in Northern France in the winter of 1916 and in Aldershot barracks in March 1917. He dismissed both reports because the disease did not spread but disappeared after short episodes. The most likely origin of the pandemic was Haskell County, Kansas, where Dr. L. Miner noticed an outbreak of influenza in early February 1918 that differed from other influenza outbreaks in that it attacked young, healthy adults, who developed pneumonia that often led to sudden death. Dr. Miner's observations were published in *Public Health Reports* (now *Morbidity and Mortality Weekly Report*) and appear to be the first reference to the 1918/1919 pandemic. Men from Haskell County reported to Fort Funston for military training between February 26 and March 2, 1918. On March 4, the first soldier at the camp was reported ill; within a 3-week period, more than 1,100 soldiers at the camp required hospitalization.

Seroarcheology suggested that the causative agent was an H1N1 virus. This was confirmed by Taubenberger et al., who recovered vRNA from formalin-fixed, paraffin-embedded tissues from two soldiers who died in 1918 and from an Inuit female of unknown age whose body was exhumed from a mass grave in the permafrost of Alaska.[117,139] RT-PCR amplification of the vRNAs provided viral gene sequences. Phylogenetic analyses revealed that 1918 Spanish influenza virus proteins contain both "avian-like" and "human-like" signature amino acids (see Host-Specific Amino Acids section). Further analysis suggested that the 1918 virus genes were not directly transmitted from an avian species but likely circulated in a mammalian host for several years before causing the pandemic outbreak in 1918. Another study suggested that reassortment between human and avian influenza viruses created the 1918 pandemic virus.

Reconstitution of the 1918 Spanish influenza virus by use of reverse genetics demonstrated its high pathogenicity in mice, ferrets, and nonhuman primates.[72,143,144] In nonhuman primates, the virus caused severe respiratory disease with extensive edema and hemorrhagic exudates, similar to reports of human infections. Rapid recruitment of macrophages and neutrophils was observed in the lungs of infected mice, in line with findings of altered immune responses in infected mice and nonhuman primates. In both animal models, infection with 1918 virus resulted in dysregulated host responses to viral infection. In contrast to its high virulence in humans, mice, ferrets, and nonhuman primates, the 1918 virus is of low pathogenicity in pigs, guinea pigs, chickens, and mallard ducks. In one study, vRNA segments of naturally occurring viruses were identified that differed by a small number of mutations from those of the 1918 pandemic virus. A virus composed of these naturally occurring, "1918-like" avian vRNA segments was more pathogenic in mice and ferrets than a low pathogenic avian influenza virus. Consecutive passages in ferrets yielded an "1918-like" avian virus with seven amino acid mutations in HA and the polymerase complex that together conferred respiratory droplet transmissibility in ferrets. This study demonstrated that viruses with "1918-like" genes still circulate in nature.

Studies with reassortant and mutant 1918 viruses indicated a role in virulence for several viral proteins (see later discussion and Molecular Determinants of Host-Range Restriction and Pathogenesis section), in particular, HA and the polymerase proteins. Both HA and PB2 are critical for 1918 virus transmissibility in ferrets.[147] Reassortants possessing the 1918 HA, or HA and NA, vRNA segments are highly pathogenic in mice. Moreover, reassortant viruses containing the 1918 HA gene induce high levels of macrophage-derived cytokines and chemokines, which stimulate inflammatory cell infiltration and hemorrhage—hallmarks of Spanish influenza infection.

The amino acids at HA positions 190 and 225 determine the receptor-binding specificity of H1 HA proteins (see Receptor Specificity of Influenza Viruses section). The reconstituted A/South Carolina/1/1918 (SC18) virus encodes aspartic acid (i.e., "human-type") amino acids at both positions, conferring binding to Siaα2,6Gal and respiratory droplet transmission in ferrets. The reconstituted A/New York/1/1918 virus possesses HA-190D, but HA-225G (i.e., the "avian-type" residue), resulting in dual binding to Siaα2,6Gal and Siaα2,3Gal and less efficient respiratory droplet transmission in ferrets compared with the SC18 isolate. An artificially generated mutant 1918 virus encoding the "avian-type" residues (HA-190E and HA-225G) no longer bound to human-type receptors and did not transmit among ferrets, although the mutant virus maintained its lethal phenotype in infected animals.[144] Autopsy samples of people who succumbed to the 1918 pandemic revealed that samples from the spring of 1918 predominantly encoded HA-225G (i.e., the "avian-type" amino acid), whereas most samples from the fall of 1918 encoded HA-225D (i.e., the "human-type" amino acid); however, the distribution of viral antigen in respiratory tissues was not significantly different between autopsy samples harboring the HA-225G or HA-225D variants. The HA variants may reflect adaptation to humans, or they may reflect adaptation to specific cell types, as shown with the A(H1N1)pdm09 HA-225G variants found in human lungs.

The NS1 protein is an interferon antagonist and, as such, is considered a determinant of pathogenicity. The 1918 virus NS1 gene blocks the expression of interferon (IFN)-regulated genes more efficiently than does the parental A/WSN/33, and the PDZ ligand domain motif of the 1918 NS1 protein (formed by the four C-terminal amino acids of this protein; see The NS1 Protein section) increased the virulence in the background of A/WSN/33 virus. In addition, the PB1-F2 protein (see The PB1-F2 Protein section) of the 1918 virus contributes to virulence. Further studies using recombinant viruses found no significant contributions of the 1918 M and NP vRNA segments to viral pathogenicity.

The Pandemic of 1957—Asian Influenza (H2N2)

This pandemic originated in the Southern Chinese province of Guizhou in February 1957 and spread to Hunan Province and to Singapore and Hong Kong in March and April, respectively. In May 1957, the causative agent of the outbreak, an influenza A virus of the H2N2 subtype, was isolated in Japan. A first wave struck the United States and United Kingdom in October 1957 and was followed by a second wave in January 1958. The infection rate was highest in 5- to 19-year-olds, in whom it exceeded 50%. Both waves were characterized by heightened mortality, with about 70,000 deaths in the United States and more than 1 million deaths worldwide.

Genetic and biochemical analyses indicated that the 1957 pandemic virus originated from reassortment between human and avian viruses (Fig. 15.3). It contained H2 HA and N2 NA genes of avian virus origin.[123] Because the pandemic virus did not appear to be extraordinarily pathogenic, the increased mortality is attributed to the lack of preexisting immunity among humans to the new surface glycoproteins of this virus. In addition to avian virus HA and NA genes, the 1957 pandemic virus also possessed a PB1 gene of avian virus origin.[67] The contribution of this gene segment to the pathogenicity of the 1957 pandemic virus is unknown.

Influenza viruses of the H2 subtype continue to be isolated from avian species and were isolated from pigs in 2006.

A risk assessment of greater than 20 avian H2N2 viruses collected over 6 decades demonstrated binding to avian-type receptors (see Receptor Specificity of Influenza Viruses section), a lack of markers of adaptation to mammals, and antigenic properties similar to those of the prototype pandemic H2N2 virus. However, several viruses replicated in mice and/or ferrets, and three were transmitted to ferret cage mates. Since vaccination against H2N2 viruses was discontinued in the late 1960s, only individuals 50 years of age or older have protective antibodies against this subtype, suggesting that a new pandemic by an H2 virus would cause appreciable excess morbidity and mortality in a large section of the population. However, avian H2N2 viruses have evolved slowly, so the pandemic H2N2 vaccine from 1957 still protects mice against recently circulating avian or swine H2 strains; this vaccine may therefore provide a first line of defense in the event of an H2N2 pandemic.

The Pandemic of 1968—Hong Kong Influenza (H3N2)

Eleven years after their emergence, viruses of the H2N2 subtype were completely replaced by those of the H3N2 subtype (Fig. 15.3). The first signs of a new pandemic emerged in Southern Asia in the summer of 1968. A virus of the H3N2 subtype was isolated in Hong Kong in July 1968, which soon spread around the world. The attack rates reached 40% and were highest in 10- to 14-year-olds. The excess mortality was estimated to be 33,800 in the United States.

The 1968 pandemic virus contained an avian virus HA protein of the H3 subtype[123] that shared less than 30% sequence homology with its predecessor. However, preexisting antibodies to the N2 protein in human populations likely accounted for the moderate severity of the outbreak. In addition to an avian H3 gene, the 1968 pandemic strain also acquired an avian virus PB1 gene,[67] as did the 1957 pandemic strain. It is unknown whether the introduction of an avian virus PB1 gene into the human population contributed to the pathogenicity of the 1968 pandemic virus. The HA and PB1 genes originated from viruses of the Eurasian avian lineage, consistent with epidemiologic findings that Asia was the likely origin of the pandemic. Since the pandemic in 1968, H3N2 viruses have continued to circulate in humans and are now referred to as "seasonal" or "human" H3N2 influenza viruses.

The Reemergence of H1N1 Viruses in 1977—Russian Influenza

The first signs of a new influenza virus outbreak were noted in Tianjin, China, in May 1977. From November 1977 through the end of 1978, young adults around the world suffered from an influenza virus outbreak in the Union of Soviet Socialist Republics and in China. The United States experienced a similar outbreak in mid-January 1978, and outbreaks in other countries occurred during the following winter. Among school-age children, the attack rates were more than 50%. Morbidity was almost exclusively limited to persons younger than 25 years, suggesting that older individuals were protected by preexisting immunity. This assumption was proven when the causative agent was identified as an influenza H1N1 virus (A/USSR/77) closely related to strains that had circulated in the early 1950s (Fig. 15.3). This close relationship and the lack of mutations that are typically acquired during replication argued against maintenance of the virus in a nonhuman species.

It is now believed that accidental release of this virus or a vaccine trial with an insufficiently attenuated live virus started the pandemic. In contrast to 1968, when the newly emerging H3N2 viruses replaced the circulating H2N2 viruses, replacement of H3N2 viruses did not occur in 1977 with the reemergence of H1N1 viruses. Instead, both H1N1 and H3N2 viruses continue to circulate to this day.

The H1N1 Pandemic in 2009 [A(H1N1) pdm09]

The first reports of an influenza-like outbreak in a small Mexican town can be traced back to mid-February 2009. In mid-April, genetically similar swine-origin H1N1 influenza A viruses were detected in several specimens collected in Southern California and Mexico.[39,105] The novel virus spread rapidly among humans across different continents, prompting the World Health Organization (WHO) to declare Phase 6 (pandemic phase, which is characterized by community-level outbreaks with human-to-human spread in at least two countries in more than one WHO region) on June 12, 2009. The WHO suggested the name A(H1N1)pdm09 for the new virus. This outbreak marked the first pandemic in more than four decades. Viruses of the H1N1 subtype have circulated in humans since 1977; hence, pandemics are not limited to viruses with novel HA subtypes (i.e., those not recently circulating in humans) but can be caused by viruses possessing HA subtypes that are circulating in human populations, as long as the novel HA is antigenically distantly enough from its predecessor to escape human immune responses.

The pandemic virus spread rapidly and replaced the H1N1 viruses previously circulating in humans. The Southern Hemisphere (where the influenza season lasts from May–September) experienced significant pandemic influenza activity from May to mid-July of 2009; the United States experienced a first wave in May and June and a second wave that started in late August and peaked during the 2nd week of October. The Centers for Disease Control and Prevention (CDC) estimated that between 151,700 and 575,400 people died worldwide from A(H1N1)pdm09 infections during its 1st year of circulation (https://www.cdc.gov/flu/pandemic-resources/basics/past-pandemics.html). Morbidity and mortality rates differed significantly between age groups.[26] In contrast to seasonal influenza epidemics, the elderly experienced a low infection but high case fatality rate. The low infection rate among the elderly can be explained by serum cross-reactivity between A(H1N1)pdm09 viruses and close descendants of the pandemic 1918 virus,[39,58] which is a consequence of shared antigenic epitopes between the HA proteins of these two viruses. Those aged 5 to 59 years accounted for the highest absolute numbers of deaths and cases of pneumonia, in contrast to seasonal outbreaks. Epidemiologic data identified several factors associated with an increased risk of severe disease, including pregnancy (particularly in the last trimester), underlying chronic conditions, and obesity.

Human infections with A(H1N1)pdm09 viruses typically caused mild upper respiratory tract illnesses with fever, cough, sore throat, shortness of breath, headache, and rhinorrhea.[26,105,109] In addition, gastrointestinal symptoms (which are unusual with seasonal influenza infections) were reported in some cases. In some patients, respiratory and multiorgan failure occurred, leading to death. These severe infections caused diffuse alveolar damage, hemorrhagic interstitial pneumonitis, and peribronchiolar and perivascular lymphocytic infiltrates (Fig. 15.4), similar

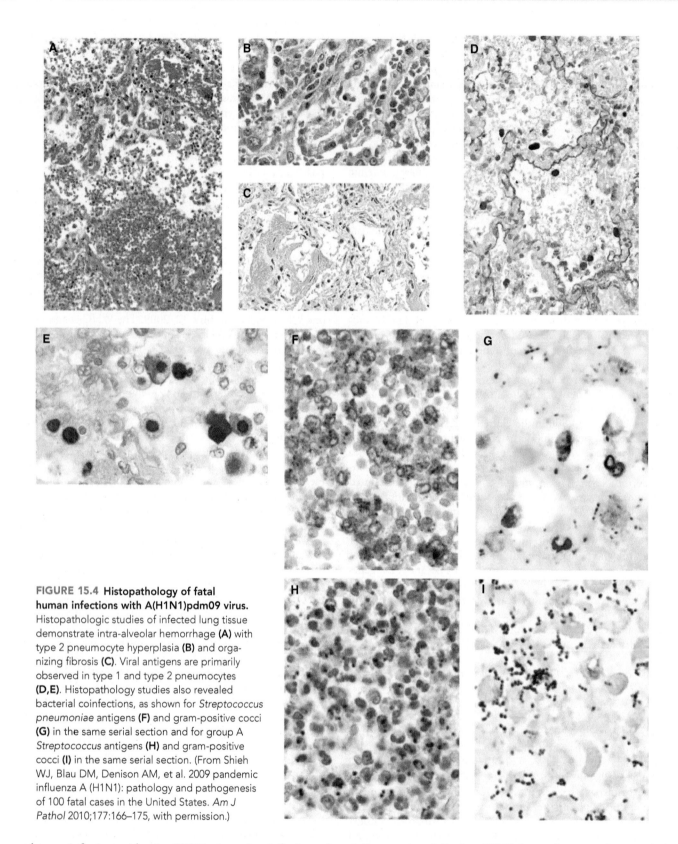

FIGURE 15.4 Histopathology of fatal human infections with A(H1N1)pdm09 virus. Histopathologic studies of infected lung tissue demonstrate intra-alveolar hemorrhage **(A)** with type 2 pneumocyte hyperplasia **(B)** and organizing fibrosis **(C)**. Viral antigens are primarily observed in type 1 and type 2 pneumocytes **(D,E)**. Histopathology studies also revealed bacterial coinfections, as shown for *Streptococcus pneumoniae* antigens **(F)** and gram-positive cocci **(G)** in the same serial section and for group A *Streptococcus* antigens **(H)** and gram-positive cocci **(I)** in the same serial section. (From Shieh WJ, Blau DM, Denison AM, et al. 2009 pandemic influenza A (H1N1): pathology and pathogenesis of 100 fatal cases in the United States. *Am J Pathol* 2010;177:166–175, with permission.)

to human infections with avian H5N1 viruses (see Infections of Humans with H5 Viruses of the A/goose/Guangdong/1/1996 Lineage section). These findings are in line with animal infection studies that demonstrated more severe lung lesions and higher lung virus titers in mice, ferrets, and nonhuman primates infected with A(H1N1)pdm09 virus compared with seasonal influenza virus infections.[58,88,101] In nonhuman primates, viral antigen was detected in type 1 and 2 pneumocytes, as has been reported for some human cases of A(H1N1)pdm09 infection and for nonhuman primates infected with avian H5N1 influenza virus. Efficient replication in type 1 and 2 pneumocytes in the infected lung (which likely contributes to the observed alveolar damage) may thus be a hallmark of severe influenza virus infections. In many human A(H1N1)pdm09 cases, bacterial coinfections were detected (Fig. 15.4), a finding that has rekindled interest in the contribution of bacterial infections to influenza-related morbidity and mortality.

Sequence and phylogenetic analyses revealed that the A(H1N1)pdm09 virus possesses PB2 and PA vRNA segments of North American avian virus origin; a PB1 vRNA segment of human H3N2 virus origin; HA (H1), NP, and NS vRNA segments of classic swine virus origin; and NA (N1) and M vRNA segments of Eurasian avian virus origin[39,105,130] (Fig. 15.3). In line with its presumed porcine origin, the virus replicates efficiently, but without symptoms, in experimentally infected miniature pigs and transmits efficiently among pigs. Other studies have demonstrated efficient transmission of A(H1N1)pdm09 viruses in ferrets. In nature, A(H1N1)pdm09 viruses have also infected turkeys, cats, dogs, and ferrets. The widespread circulation of A(H1N1)pdm09 viruses may lead to reassortment with other human, swine, or avian influenza viruses. In fact, the pandemic virus has infected pigs, and reassortment with swine influenza viruses has been reported. Experimental studies demonstrated ready reassortment of A(H1N1)pdm09 viruses with avian H5N1, avian H9N2, or contemporary human influenza viruses; some of these reassortants showed increased replicative ability compared with the A(H1N1)pdm09 parental viruses.

In the United States and Europe, the first vaccines to the novel virus were approved in September 2009 (after the first and second waves of the pandemic had already swept through many communities). A(H1N1)pdm09 viruses have now become seasonal influenza viruses and are part of annual trivalent and quadrivalent influenza vaccines (see also Vaccines section).

INFLUENZA IN HUMANS—EPIDEMIOLOGY

Since 1977, seasonal H1N1 and H3N2 viruses have been circulating together with influenza B viruses; in 2009, the seasonal H1N1 viruses were largely replaced by A(H1N1)pdm09 viruses. The prevalence of these groups of viruses varies geographically and temporally, making influenza virus epidemiology complex.

Several studies have assessed the global circulation patterns of influenza viruses; some analyses indicate that human H3N2 and H1N1 epidemic strains originate from Southeast Asia, from where they are seeded into temperate regions. Temporally overlapping epidemics in Southeast Asia result in continuous virus circulation. Even though influenza viruses circulate in tropical regions throughout the year, seasonality has been observed in these areas, although it is less pronounced than in temperate climates. In the temperate regions of North America and Europe, multiple variants may circulate during the early epidemic period, which are replaced by a dominant variant at the peak of an epidemic.

The epidemiology of human influenza viruses is defined by their constant antigenic variation to escape the host immune response. Unlike most other respiratory viruses, influenza viruses possess two different mechanisms that allow them to reinfect humans and cause disease—antigenic drift and antigenic shift.

Antigenic Drift

Antigenic drift describes gradual antigenic changes in the HA and/or NA proteins as a result of the accumulation of point mutations in the antigenic epitopes. In humans, antigenic drift variants result from the positive selection of mutants by neutralizing antibodies circulating in the infected individual. These variants can no longer be neutralized by antibodies to the "parental" strains. Antigenic drift variants cause epidemics and require the update of the vaccine strain; they typically prevail for 1 to 5 years before being replaced by a different variant. Antigenic drift has also been observed among influenza viruses in terrestrial poultry, pigs, and horses, although to a lesser extent than in humans.

Antigenic Drift of the HA Protein

The HA protein is the major antigenic component of the virus. Its function and structure are described in more detail in Chapter 14. The rate of antigenic drift of human H3 virus HAs has been faster than that of human H1 virus HAs, necessitating the update of the H3 vaccine component 19 times since 1968, whereas the H1 component has been replaced only nine times. The HA of A(H1N1)pdm09 viruses has undergone limited antigenic drift since its emergence, with one vaccine strain update in 2017.

Three major categories of HA epitopes have been identified as the following: (a) epitopes in the HA head with high sequence variability, which are immunodominant and primarily responsible for antigenic drift; (b) highly conserved epitopes in the HA stalk region, which do not play a role in antigenic drift but, instead, are attractive targets for the development of "universal" vaccines that elicit broadly protective antibodies that interact with HAs of various subtypes (see Vaccines section); and (c) conserved epitopes in the HA head, which are targeted by antibodies that confer various levels of cross protection (although not necessarily heterosubtypic cross protection).

For H3 HA, five immunodominant antigenic domains with high sequence variability have been identified[71,154,157,158] (Fig. 15.5A): site A is formed by a protruding loop (amino acids 140–146); site B is formed by another loop (amino acids 155–160) and an α-helix (amino acids 188–198) and is situated at the membrane distal end of HA; site C is located at the base of the globular domain in the antiparallel sheet of HA1; site D is situated near the trimeric interface of the globular head domains; and site E lies near the bottom of the globular distal domain between sites C and A. Based on limited experimental and computational modeling data, the immunodominant antigenic epitopes of H7 HAs are likely similar to those of H3 HAs, reflecting the phylogenetic relationship between these two subtypes.

For H1 viruses, the immunodominant antigenic sites are designated Ca1, Ca2, Cb, Sa, and Sb[40] (Fig. 15.5B). Some overlap exists among these sites. For H5 HAs, several x-ray crystallographic structures, some with monoclonal antibodies bound, have been resolved. Depending on the virus and antibodies used for the analysis, three to five immunodominant antigenic sites that confer neutralization have been identified, some of which overlap with antigenic sites in H3 or H1 HA proteins.

Numerous studies have analyzed antigenic drift in nature. In the laboratory, antigenic drift has historically been mimicked by virus propagation in the presence of monoclonal antibodies to a single site, with a low frequency of variant

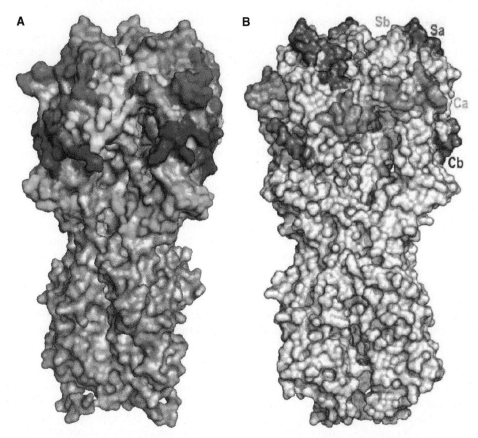

FIGURE 15.5 Crystallographic structures of influenza A virus H3 and H1 HA proteins.
A: Crystallographic structure of the trimeric complex of influenza A virus H3 HA protein (Protein Data Bank #1HGD) showing the locations of the five antigenic epitopes: antigenic site A (amino acids 122, 124, 126, 130–133, 135, 137, 138, 140, 142–146, 150, 152, 168), *red*; antigenic site B (amino acids 128, 129, 155–160, 163–165, 186–190, 196–198), *green*; antigenic site C (amino acids 44–48, 50, 51, 53, 54, 273, 275, 276, 278–280, 294, 297, 299, 300, 304, 305, 307–312), *blue*; antigenic site D (amino acids 96, 102, 103, 117, 121, 167, 170–177, 179, 182, 201, 203, 207–209, 212–219, 226–230, 238, 240, 242, 244, 246–248), *yellow*; and antigenic site E (amino acids 57, 59, 62, 63, 67, 75, 78, 80–83, 91, 92, 94, 109, 260–262, 265), *purple*. **B:** Crystallographic structure of the HA protein of A(H1N1)pdm09 virus. Shown is the trimeric complex with the antigenic sites Ca (amino acids 140–145, 169–173, 206–208, 224, 225, 238–240), *orange*; Cb (amino acids 79–84), *dark blue*; Sa (amino acids 128, 129, 156–160, 162–167), *red*; and Sb (amino acids 187–198), *light blue*. (**B:** Reproduced from Xu R, Ekiert DC, Krause JC, et al. Structural basis of preexisting immunity to the 2009 H1N1 pandemic influenza virus. *Science* 2010;328:357–360, with permission.)

selection. Over the past decade, novel molecular virology methods have been established in which reverse genetics-generated mutants have been tested for their antigenic properties. In other approaches, virus libraries comprising millions of mutant viruses with arbitrary or specific mutations at random or preselected amino acid positions have been generated and incubated with ferret sera and/or human sera to select potential antigenic escape variants. The selected variants are then tested for their antigenic properties by using hemagglutination-inhibition (HI) and/or focus reduction assays (FRA). The visualization and analysis of the resulting data can be achieved through antigenic cartography, a computational method based on HI or FRA data that provides an interpretation of antigenic clusters and their relationships, as well as the extent and directionality of the antigenic drift[129] (Fig. 15.6). Antigenic cartography is now routinely used by the WHO for the selection of vaccine strains.

The characterization of antigenic escape mutants has established that antigenic drift of human H3N2 viruses occurs in clusters: while nucleotide changes occur continually, clusters of antigenically similar variants exist for several years until they are replaced by a new cluster, founded by an antigenic variant that necessitates an update of the vaccine strain.[129] Hence, the genetic evolution of H3 HA genes is continuing, whereas their antigenic evolution is punctuated. Moreover, the major antigenic changes of human H3N2 viruses can be mapped to seven amino acid positions (in the known antigenic epitopes) located around the receptor-binding pocket.[74] Antigenic cluster changes that necessitate a replacement of the vaccine strain often result from single amino acid changes. Due to existing immunity in human populations, human H3 HAs evolve "away" from currently and previously circulating viruses. Thus, overall, human H3 HAs evolve in a single direction. A similar pattern of antigenic cluster transitions likely also exists for human H1 viruses.

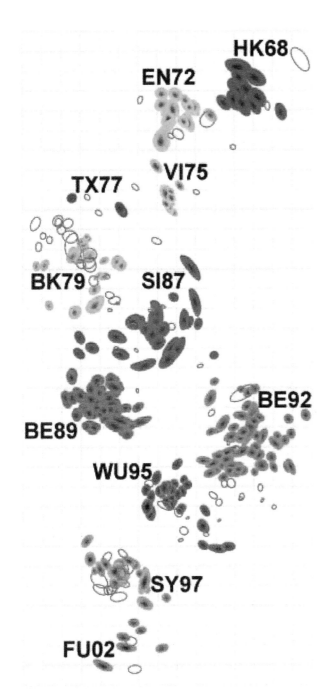

FIGURE 15.6 Antigenic cartography. The map shows seasonal H3N2 viruses from 1968 to 2003. Each *open circle* represents an antiserum used for analysis. Each *colored circle* represents an H3N2 strain tested by using the hemagglutination-inhibition assay against the selected antisera. The distances between strains and antisera are relative to their antigenic distances (in HI units). The spacing between the grid lines is equivalent to a twofold dilution of antiserum in the HI assay. Typically, fourfold changes in HI titers (i.e., two gridlines in the map) require an update of the vaccine. The different colors represent the antigenic clusters to which the strains belong (HK68, Hong Kong 1968; EN72, England 1972; VI75, Victoria 1975; TX77, Texas 1977; BK79, Bangkok 1979; SI87, Sichuan 1987; BE89, Beijing 1989; BE92, Beijing 1992; WU95, Wuhan 1995; SY97, Sydney 1997; FU02, Fujian 2002). (From Smith DJ, Lapedes AS, de Jong JC, et al. Mapping the antigenic and genetic evolution of influenza virus. *Science* 2004;305:371–376, with permission.)

H5 HA proteins of the lineage that emerged in Hong Kong in 1996 have also diversified into multiple antigenically and genetically distinguishable clades and subclades (see Infections of Humans with H5 Viruses of the A/goose/Guangdong/1/1996 Lineage section). Amino acid changes responsible for antigenic differences appear to be located around the receptor-binding site, similar to the antigenic cluster transitions described for human H3 HAs. Antigenic changes have also occurred among the H7N9 viruses that emerged in China in 2013 (see Infection of Humans with Low and Highly Pathogenic H7N9 Viruses). Based on limited data, the amino acids responsible for these changes appear to be located in the vicinity of the receptor-binding site.

Antigenic Drift of the NA Protein

The function and structure of this protein are discussed in detail in Chapter 14. In addition to HA, antigenic drift has also been reported for NA and correlated with amino acid differences in the molecule.[17,121] Studies with monoclonal antibodies and amino acid sequence analyses have revealed several antigenic sites. The NA of most influenza A virus subtypes and of influenza B viruses has been crystallized, and several structures are available for NA/antibody complexes. Two major antigenic sites of NA are located on the upper surface of the molecule, where they flank the sialic acid–binding site. A possible third antigenic site resides on the side of the head; some antibodies binding to this site provide protection via antibody-dependent cellular cytotoxicity (ADCC). A more detailed structural analysis of the Fab fragment of a monoclonal antibody to N9 NA showed that five peptide loops, located at the rim of the enzyme active site, constitute the epitope. The second epitope, characterized with monoclonal antibodies to N8 NA, is located at the interface of two adjacent monomers in the tetrameric NA protein and involves peptide loops on both monomers. Antibodies with this epitope bind only to NA tetramers. Another antibody makes contacts with two monomers of the A(H1N1)pdm09 N1 NA. Overall, our understanding of NA antigenic sites and epitopes remains limited.

The antigenic drift rates of human influenza virus NA proteins are lower than those of human influenza virus HA proteins. Antigenic changes can be conferred by single amino acid changes in NA, as has been reported for HA (see Antigenic Drift of the HA Protein section). Antigenic changes in HA and NA appear to occur independently from one another.

Antigenic Shift

Antigenic shift involves major antigenic changes in which an HA and/or NA that is antigenically distinct from the circulating variant is introduced into the human population. Infections with such viruses result in high infection rates in immunologically naïve populations, leading to pandemics. Typically, antigenic shift is caused by an HA of a new subtype, that is, one that did not circulate in humans prior to the pandemic; in addition, an NA of a novel subtype may be introduced into human populations. The H1N1 pandemic in 2009 was a notable exception because it was caused by a virus of the H1N1 subtype, even though viruses of this subtype had been circulating in humans since 1977.

Since the beginning of the last century, five antigenic shifts have occurred: in 1918, with the appearance of the H1N1 viruses that caused the Spanish influenza; in 1957, when the

H1N1 subtype was replaced with H2N2 viruses, causing the Asian influenza; in 1968, when H3N2 viruses replaced the H2N2 subtype, leading to the 1968 pandemic; in 1977, when H1N1 viruses similar to those circulating in humans in the 1950s reappeared and caused the Russian influenza; and in 2009, when a novel, antigenically distinct H1N1 virus caused a pandemic that largely replaced seasonal H1N1 viruses (see The H1N1 Pandemic in 2009 section). These new subtypes emerged suddenly and at irregular and unpredictable intervals.

Transmission Among Humans

Influenza viruses are transmitted from person-to-person via the respiratory tract, which could include small particle aerosols (<10 μm mass diameter) suspended in the air, larger particles or droplets, and indirect transmission via contaminated surfaces and fomites. The relative contributions of each of these routes have not been completely determined and could vary depending on the specific virus and levels of immunity in both the host and the recipient.

Small particle aerosols are generated by infected humans, and influenza genome can be detected in these small particles by PCR techniques. A significant portion of fine particle aerosols contain infectious virus,[160] and experimental studies in humans have shown that varying small amounts (~5 infectious particles) may be sufficient to infect humans by the aerosol route. Aerosol transmission has also been demonstrated in animal models in which infected and exposed ferrets or guinea pigs are separated by several meters, with transmission occurring in the direction of airflow.

Airborne transmission has also been implicated in outbreaks where an airborne route of transmission appears to be the most plausible explanation for the characteristics of the outbreak. The most often cited such outbreak occurred in a commercial airliner that was delayed for approximately 4½ hours with a poorly functioning ventilation system. The risk of transmission of influenza A from the index case to other passengers was related to the amount of time passengers spent on the aircraft, and not on their seating proximity to the index case. Since most of the passengers did not have direct contact with the index case, airborne transmission appears to be likely.[100] In hospital outbreaks, UV light and air handling procedures have been associated with decreased risks of transmission. In addition, in a study of zanamivir prophylaxis of influenza in families,[64] subjects who received short-term prophylaxis with inhaled zanamivir were protected compared to placebo recipients, but recipients of zanamivir administered by nasal spray were not.

In most of these scenarios, there were alternative explanations for the observations that could at least partially explain the epidemic behavior without requiring aerosol transmission, and the real role of aerosol transmission remains controversial. Several studies have attempted to evaluate the role of face masks in infection prevention in hospitals. In one large, randomized trial, nursing staff who were randomly assigned to wear N-95 respirators had the same rate of influenza as staff assigned to wear simple surgical masks while caring for patients with influenza.[83] This study suggests that airborne transmission does not play a major role at least in nosocomial influenza, although it has been pointed out that cases in the N-95 group could have been acquired outside the hospital and that compliance with these masks is frequently poor. In contrast, hand hygiene and simple surgical masks were reported to be modestly effective in the prevention of influenza transmission in households suggesting that in this setting, droplet spread was the predominant modality.

Seasonality

Influenza epidemiology is characterized by marked seasonality. In the Northern Hemisphere, epidemics generally peak between January and April but may flare up as early as December or as late as May, while in the Southern Hemisphere, seasonal epidemics typically occur between May and September. Seasonal periodicity is also observed in tropical climates, with increased activity during periods of low absolute humidity, although influenza can occur throughout the year and seasonal fluctuations are not as marked. The reasons for these seasonal changes are not entirely clear but might be the result of more favorable environmental conditions for virus survival. Using a statistical model called convergent cross mapping, temperature and absolute humidity were shown to be important drivers of seasonal epidemicity.[23] Studies in animal models have also supported a role for conditions of cold temperature and dry humidity in facilitating transmission.

Seasonality may also be associated with behavioral changes that may increase transmission, such as indoor crowding or school attendance. Possibly for this reason, the effects of weather variability may be greater in young children. Modeling studies based on medical claims data have suggested that winter holidays delay seasonal epidemic peaks and shift disease visits toward adults.

In contrast to seasonal influenza, novel influenza viruses can emerge at any time of the year. The occurrence of pandemics outside of the usual window of seasonality may be related to inherently greater transmissibility, allowing them to spread even under conditions that would not be favorable for transmission of seasonal influenza viruses.

Influenza Disease Burden

The impact of seasonal influenza on public health is generally measured in terms of excess deaths, hospitalizations, and illness associated with detectable influenza activity in the community, as compared to an expected seasonal baseline during periods of time when influenza is not present. As rapid and accurate diagnostic has become more widely available, these assessments have become more specifically based on testing results. It is important to recognize that in addition to these, influenza also causes prolonged negative impact on activities of daily living, absences from work or school, and significant resulting economic impact.

Mortality

The increase in mortality during pandemics and epidemics is a hallmark of influenza virus infection. Levels of excess mortality vary considerably from season to season depending on the extent of influenza activity and the specific types and subtypes of viruses circulating. In general, years with predominant H3N2 activity tend to be associated with the highest levels of excess mortality, partly because this subtype tends to be especially impactful in older populations. Years with predominant H1N1 or influenza B circulation are also associated with excess mortality but at substantially lower levels. Recent estimates of excess mortality associated with seasonal influenza in the

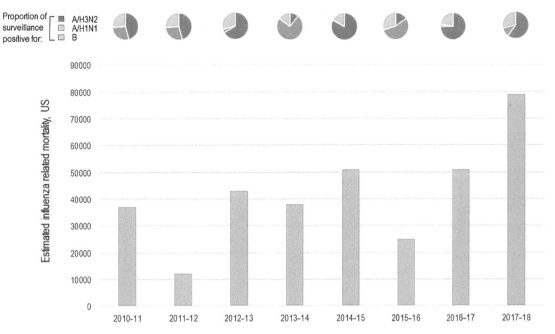

FIGURE 15.7 Influenza-related mortality is higher in years with predominant H3N2 viruses. Estimates of influenza-related mortality assessed using a mathematical model[115] as reported on the Centers for Disease Control and Prevention Web site (https://www.cdc.gov/flu/about/burden/past-seasons.html). The pie charts show the relative proportion of detected H3, H1, and B viruses in national surveillance conducted during that influenza season (https://www.cdc.gov/flu/weekly/fluviewinteractive.htm).

United States are shown in Figure 15.7. As many as 51,000 deaths annually in the United States can be attributed to influenza.[140] It is recognized that because not all influenza deaths are necessarily noted on death certificates as pneumonia or influenza related, these are generally underestimates of the overall impact. After correcting for under-reporting by assessing the fraction of cases with diagnostic testing, it has been estimated that there were between 155,000 and 624,000 hospitalizations, 18,000 and 95,000 ICU admissions, and 5,000 to 27,000 deaths per year in the United States attributable to influenza.[115]

Years in which pandemic influenza viruses emerge are usually associated with levels of excess mortality above those seen in seasonal influenza, because of general lack of immunity to these viruses. For example, excess mortality was estimated to be between 20 and 50 million deaths for the 1918 H1N1 pandemic worldwide, 70,000 excess deaths associated with the H2N2 pandemic of 1957, and 33,800 deaths associated with the H3N2 pandemic of 1968. In contrast, the recent emergence of the pandemic H1N1 virus in 2009 is estimated to have been associated with 12,470 deaths in the United States. However, a large proportion of deaths in the 2009 pandemic occurred in younger individuals, so that when evaluated in terms of years of life lost, this pandemic had significant impact. Although individual pandemics are associated with the largest numbers of excess deaths, the repetitive nature of seasonal epidemics results in a greater total overall mortality burden.

During seasonal epidemics, excess mortality tends to be highest in those older than 65 years, who account for approximately 90% of such excess mortalities, largely due to the presence of age-related concurrent medical conditions that increase the risk of influenza deaths. However, very different patterns of mortality may be seen during pandemics, where older age groups may be partially protected because of earlier exposures to antigenically related viruses, a phenomenon termed "antigenic recycling.[90]" For example, the highest mortality during the 1918 pandemic occurred in young adults, while older adults appeared to have been partially protected by exposure to previous H1N1 viruses circulating 50 years earlier. Similarly, older adults were relatively spared from the A(H1N1)pdm09 outbreak because of exposure to antigenically related viruses that circulated in the 1930s.

Morbidity

Mortality is only the most severe manifestation of influenza impact, and similar techniques can be used to estimate excess morbidity due to influenza epidemics. Influenza virus is estimated to cause about 50 million illnesses annually in the United States. Much of the impact of influenza is related to the malaise and consequent disability that it produces, even in young, healthy individuals. It has been estimated that a typical case of influenza, on average, is associated with 5 to 6 days of restricted activity, 3 to 4 days of bed disability, and about 3 days lost from work or school. Direct medical costs of illness account for only about 20% or the total expenses of a case of influenza, with a major proportion of the economic impact due to loss of productivity. Direct costs include hospitalizations, medical fees, drugs, and testing and were estimated in 1986 to be about $1 billion annually, while indirect costs such as loss of productivity reached $2 to $4 billion annually.

The impact of seasonal influenza is generally highest in identified high-risk groups such as young children and elders. Children younger than 2 years of age and the elderly have the highest hospitalization rates, reaching 1 per 270 for those older than 65 years, compared to 1 per 2,900 for the 1- to 44-year-old age group. Among children, 14% to 16% of those seeking medical care for acute respiratory illness or fever are infected with influenza virus.[113]

Surveillance

Surveillance efforts in humans are coordinated by the WHO through the Global Influenza Surveillance and Response System (GISRS). The system currently includes 6 Collaborating Centres (in Atlanta, Memphis, Beijing, London, Melbourne, and Tokyo), greater than 100 National Influenza Centres in greater than 100 countries, and several H5 Reference Laboratories and Essential Regulatory Laboratories. The National Influenza Centres collect samples each year from patients with influenza-like illness and submit representative samples per year to the Collaborating Centres for antigenic and genetic characterization. These data are used to monitor antigenic drift and resistance to antiviral compounds. Based on surveillance, antigenic, and genetic data, vaccine viruses are recommended by the WHO each February and September for the Northern and Southern Hemispheres, respectively.

Ongoing summaries of influenza activity in the United States, including the percent of influenza-like illness visits among all medical visits, proportions of positive diagnostic tests, genetic and antigenic characterization of selected viruses, and frequency of antiviral resistance, are maintained by the CDC and similar data worldwide by the WHO. In addition, these organizations collaborate to conduct intensive surveillance of zoonotic influenza viruses that could represent pandemic threats.

TRANSMISSION OF AVIAN AND SWINE INFLUENZA VIRUSES TO HUMANS

Infections of Humans with H5 Viruses of the A/goose/Guangdong/1/1996 Lineage

Outbreaks of highly pathogenic avian influenza (HPAI) occurred mainly in poultry until the emergence of HPAI H5 viruses of the A/goose/Guangdong/1/1996 lineage (H5/Gs/Gd) in 1996. Viruses of this lineage have infected many wild bird species, numerous mammalian species, and more than 860 people with a case fatality rate of approximately 53%.

H5 Virus Outbreaks of the A/goose/Guangdong/1/1996 Lineage Between 1996 and 2008

H5/Gs/Gd viruses were isolated from sick domestic geese in 1996 in Guangdong Province, followed by outbreaks in poultry in Hong Kong in 1997. The causative agent was identified as an H5N1 reassortant virus with an HA vRNA segment from an A/goose/Guangdong/1/96–like virus, an NA vRNA segment from another avian N1 virus, and the remaining six vRNA segments (i.e., PB2, PB1, PA, NP, M, and NS) from other avian viruses. The outbreaks in poultry were accompanied by the first transmissions of wholly avian influenza viruses to humans with fatal outcomes: in May 1997 in Hong Kong, a 3-year-old boy was infected with an H5N1 virus of the H5/Gs/Gd lineage and succumbed to the infection.[15,16,136] In November and December 1997, 17 additional cases were reported, 5 of which had fatal outcomes. The slaughter of poultry in Hong Kong in late December 1997/early January 1998 eliminated H5/Gs/

Gd viruses from the Hong Kong poultry markets at the time, but these viruses reappeared in poultry in Hong Kong in 2001. Waterfowl is usually resistant to HPAI viruses; however, in late 2002, waterfowl in Hong Kong succumbed to H5/Gs/Gd influenza virus infections. In February 2003, two Hong Kong residents were infected with H5/Gs/Gd virus, one of whom died.

In April/May 2005, more than 6,000 wild birds died from H5/Gs/Gd virus infection at the Qinghai Lake Nature Reserve in Gangcha County, Qinghai Province, China.[12,82] Although viruses of several genotypes were detected during the outbreak, one genotype was dominant. H5/Gs/Gd viruses closely related to the Qinghai Lake isolates have since spread through Russia, into Europe, the Middle East, and several African countries, most likely through migratory birds.

H5 Virus Outbreaks of the A/goose/Guangdong/1/1996 Lineage Since 2008

Since their reemergence in 2003, the H5/Gs/Gd viruses have undergone substantial evolution in their HA. A classification and nomenclature scheme based on the H5 HA nucleotide sequence has been established to describe the phylogenetic relationships of the H5/Gs/Gd viruses: currently 10 different clades (clades 0–9) are recognized, many of which have second-, third-, or fourth-tier subclades. Until 2008, frequent reassortment resulted in multiple genotypes that differed in the constellation of the internal vRNA segments; however, the HA/NA constellation was stable. This changed when H5N1/Gs/Gd viruses reassorted with different avian influenza viruses, resulting in viruses of the H5N2, H5N5, and H5N8 subtypes in 2008 to 2011 and the emergence of H5N6 viruses in 2013. These novel reassortant viruses possessed an HA of clade 2.3.4.4, which has since become dominant in several parts of the world; by 2012/2013, these viruses had further diversified into four genetically distinct groups (A–D).

The group A viruses caused an H5N8 virus outbreak in South Korea in 2014, and descendants of these viruses were detected in North America in late 2014, marking the first isolation of H5/Gs/Gd viruses on the American continent. These viruses underwent reassortment with North American avian viruses, resulting in novel H5/Gs/Gd viruses with NAs of different subtypes. Newly emerged North American H5N2 viruses of the H5/Gs/Gd lineage caused multiple outbreaks in commercial poultry operations in North America in the spring and summer of 2015 and were eradicated through rigorous control measures and the culling of approximately 48 million birds. No human infections were reported. Sister subgroups of the viruses that were introduced into North America caused outbreaks in South Korea during the following years and were introduced into Europe where they were primarily isolated from wild birds in 2014 to 2015. Group B viruses of the H5N8 subtype emerged in China in 2013 and caused outbreaks in the Republic of Korea. Descendants of these viruses moved westward and were isolated in Siberia, Europe, the Middle East, and Africa in the winter of 2016 to 2017. These novel H5N8 viruses caused multiple outbreaks in poultry farms in Europe, and more than 1,200 infected wild birds were reported in Germany alone. Group C viruses of the H5N6 subtype have been detected in China since 2013 and have spread to other Asian countries, but not to other continents. The H5N6 group C viruses have now replaced H5N1 as the most dominant subtype of H5/Gs/Gd viruses in Southern China. In contrast to H5N2 and H5N8 viruses, the H5N6 viruses have caused human infections[161]; to date, 28 confirmed cases (with most, but not all, viruses belonging to group C) with several fatalities have been reported. In addition, group C viruses have been isolated from pigs and cats. The infection of mammals with H5N6 group C viruses may be explained by the ability of the viruses to bind to human-type receptors, in addition to avian-type receptors. Consistent with this finding, these viruses bind to and replicate in *ex vivo* human organoids and transmit to cohoused ferrets (see Infections of Humans with H5 Viruses of the A/goose/Guangdong/1/1996 Lineage section). Group D viruses (mostly of the H5N6 subtype) were detected in China and Vietnam in 2013 to 2014.

As of September 2018, the majority of circulating H5/Gs/Gd viruses belonged to clade 2.3.4.4 with H5N8 viruses dominating in Europe and H5N6 viruses dominating in Southern China. In addition, viruses of clade 2.3.2.1a were circulating in parts of Asia, and viruses of clade 2.3.2.1c were circulating in parts of both Asia (including Indonesia) and Africa. In total, more than 70 countries have reported H5/Gs/Gd outbreaks to date.

Host Range of H5 Viruses of the A/goose/Guangdong/1/1996 Lineage

Since their emergence, H5/Gs/Gd viruses have become enzootic in poultry populations in different parts of the world. While HPAI outbreaks are typically limited to terrestrial poultry, the H5/Gs/Gd viruses have been isolated from a number of different wild birds including water birds (order Anseriformes) such as ducks, geese, and swans; shorebirds (order Charadriiformes) such as gulls and waders; small songbirds (order Passeriformes) such as sparrows and crows; large wading birds (order Ciconiiformes) such as herons, storks, and egrets; several *Ratites* species including ostriches, emu, and rhea; and species of several other bird orders. In addition, these viruses have been isolated from carnivores including dogs, cats, tigers, leopards, a stone marten, Owston civets, and raccoon dogs. Moreover, H5N1 and H5N6 viruses have been isolated from pigs on several occasions. No HPAI H5 infections have yet been reported in horses.

Virulence and Transmissibility of H5 Viruses of the A/goose/Guangdong/1/1996 Lineage

H5/Gs/Gd viruses have been extensively studied in primary human cells and in several animal models including mice, ferrets, guinea pigs, and nonhuman primates. In alveolar epithelial cells and macrophages, as well as in the lungs of infected mice, ferrets, and nonhuman primates, H5/Gs/Gd viruses typically elicit higher levels of proinflammatory cytokines than are observed upon infection with contemporary human viruses. In these animal models, the H5/Gs/Gd viruses are highly pathogenic and cause diffuse alveolar damage with massive infiltration of immune cells and infection of pneumocytes. In nonhuman primates, H5/Gs/Gd viruses cause severe pneumonia although the infections are usually not lethal. Two European H5N8 group B viruses were highly virulent in ducks and in mice but caused mild, nonlethal disease in ferrets.

The infection of more than 860 people with H5N1 and H5N6 viruses (no human infections have been reported with H5N2 and H5N8 viruses) has raised concern over a potential H5 pandemic. However, there are no reports of sustained human-to-human transmission of H5/Gs/Gd viruses. A number of studies have tested the transmissibility of H5/Gs/Gd viruses in ferrets, the most widely accepted mammalian model for influenza virus transmission studies. To date, no natural H5/Gs/Gd virus has been found to transmit among ferrets via respiratory droplets; however, several studies reported transmission of H5N6 viruses to cohoused ferrets (contact transmission). Several groups also tested the respiratory droplet transmissibility in ferrets of human/avian reassortant viruses bearing an H5 HA or of H5 viruses with mutations in HA known to increase the affinity for human-type receptors; no respiratory droplet transmission was detected in these studies. However, four studies[10,52,55,164] in 2012/2013 established that H5/Gs/Gd viruses can acquire respiratory droplet transmissibility in ferrets or guinea pigs. Although these studies used different H5/Gs/Gd viruses and different approaches (including reassortment, site-directed mutagenesis to introduce mammalian-adapting amino acid changes, and/or sequential passages in ferrets to acquire mutations that facilitate replication in mammals), common properties emerged that appear to be essential for respiratory droplet transmissibility in ferrets: HA binding to human-type receptors (see Receptor Specificity of Influenza Viruses); lack of a glycosylation site in HA, resulting in increased binding to human-type receptors; HA thermostability and fusogenicity at a relatively low pH; and highly efficient replication in mammalian cells, typically conferred by mutations in the PB2 polymerase protein (see The Replication Complex section).

Human Infections with H5 Viruses of the A/goose/Guangdong/1/1996 Lineage

As of January 21, 2019, 860 confirmed human infections have been reported since 2003 with H5N1/Gs/Gd viruses, resulting in 454 fatalities (https://www.who.int/influenza/human_animal_interface/2019_01_21_tableH5N1.pdf?ua=1). The largest numbers of human infections with H5N1 viruses have occurred in Indonesia, Vietnam, Egypt, and China. In Egypt in 2015, 136 people were infected with H5N1/Gs/Gd viruses; of those, 39 succumbed to their infections. The reasons for the large number of human H5N1 infections in Egypt in 2015 are not known. Since 2016, only a few human H5N1 infections have occurred, and they were limited to Egypt and Indonesia. Highly pathogenic H5N6/Gs/Gd viruses emerged in 2013 in China and have since infected 28 individuals, including several fatal cases. As stated earlier, there are no reports of sustained human-to-human transmissions of H5N1 or H5N6 viruses of the Gs/Gd lineage.

Although H5/Gs/Gd viruses have not acquired the ability to spread efficiently among humans, isolated cases of human-to-human transmission may have occurred. However, most of these clusters involved family members living in the same household, and infection may have occurred through exposure to a common source (such as sick or dead poultry), rather than human-to-human transmission. Overall, transmission of H5/Gs/Gd viruses to humans appears to be rare and primarily associated with contact with sick or dead poultry, although other modes of infection (e.g., through virus-contaminated feces or water) have also been considered.

During the 1997 and 2003 H5N1 outbreaks in Hong Kong, there was no evidence of systemic viral infection in infected individuals. However, after 2003, human infections with H5N1 viruses appear to be systemic[21]: virus has been recovered from not only respiratory organs but also stool and cerebrospinal fluid (CSF), while viral sequences and/or antigens have been detected in brain neurons; in epithelial cells of the intestinal tract; in the heart, spleen, kidney, and liver; and in the placenta and fetus of a pregnant women infected with an H5N1 virus. The detection of viral sequences and antigen in the intestinal tract is consistent with the expression of avian-like virus receptors in the human gut, the *ex vivo* infection of gut tissue with an H5N1 virus, and reports of gastrointestinal symptoms. In H5N1 virus–infected patients, acute respiratory distress syndrome (ARDS) with diffuse alveolar damage is common.[3] Virus and/or antigen binding has been detected to nonciliated epithelial cells in the bronchioles and type 2 pneumocytes and macrophages in the alveoli.[127,148] Type 2 pneumocytes differentiate to type 1 pneumocytes, which are critical for gas exchange in the alveoli; the infection of type 2 pneumocytes may therefore result in more severe lung damage. The levels of proinflammatory cytokines are higher in individuals infected with H5N1 viruses than in those infected with seasonal influenza virus and higher in fatal than in nonfatal cases of H5N1 infection.[21] The pathology in humans is in line with cell culture studies that demonstrate increased levels of proinflammatory cytokines upon H5N1 infection, animal infection studies that show increased pathology, viral targeting of type 2 pneumocytes,[148] and stronger innate immune responses upon H5N1 virus infection compared to infection with control viruses. Collectively, the available data suggest that the high mortality in humans results from a combination of high virus loads and the induction of high levels of proinflammatory pathways, which may culminate in extensive alveolar damage. Based on a small number of human H5N6 cases that have been studied in detail, H5N6 virus infection is comparable to H5N1 infections.

Some of the currently circulating H5N1 and H5N6 viruses are resistant to the antiviral drugs amantadine and rimantadine. Most H5N1 and H5N6 viruses are sensitive to the NA inhibitors (NAIs) oseltamivir and zanamivir; however, oseltamivir-resistant viruses have been isolated from H5N1 and H5N6 virus–infected patients treated with this drug. These viruses contain an amino acid substitution at position 274 or 294 (N2 NA numbering) of the NA protein.

Infections of Humans with Low and Highly Pathogenic H7N9 Viruses

On March 31, 2013, Chinese authorities announced three fatal human infections with novel H7N9 influenza viruses.[37] This marked the beginning of the first outbreak of novel H7N9 viruses in the spring of 2013, which was followed by a second outbreak in the winter of 2013/2014. In the following years, waves of human H7N9 virus infections occurred every winter until 2016/2017, with the fifth wave in 2016/2017 causing more human infections than the previous four waves combined. In the winter of 2017/2018, only three human cases were reported, presumably due to the use of an H5/H7N9 bivalent vaccine in poultry (see below). The first wave of human H7N9 infections in 2013/2014 was limited to provinces in the southeastern part of China, but the geographic range of human H7N9 infections expanded in the following years to southern, central, and western provinces of China.

To date, 1567 confirmed human infections with H7N9 viruses have occurred with a case fatality rate of 39%. Individuals with confirmed H7N9 virus infection typically develop a respiratory tract infection with fever and coughing, which may progress to severe pneumonia and ARDS, potentially with fatal outcome. In addition to the confirmed cases, a 10- to 100-fold higher number of asymptomatic or mild cases may have occurred. The case fatality rate of human H7N9 infections may therefore be lower than currently reported; however, appreciable numbers of unrecognized human H7N9 infections pose considerable challenges to the control of this virus.

Epidemiologic studies established an association between human H7N9 infections and exposure to poultry, typically in live-bird markets. Demographic studies revealed that the average age of H7N9-infected individuals is higher than that of people infected with H5/Gs/Gd viruses and that males have accounted for two-thirds of the human H7N9 cases, in contrast to a more balanced sex ratio among H5-infected people. One possible explanation is that elderly males spend more time in live-bird markets than females or younger people of both sexes. Several studies reported antibodies to H7N9 viruses in up to approximately 15% of the sera collected from workers in live-bird markets, and H7N9 viruses have been isolated repeatedly in live-bird markets in different provinces of China since 2013. Closures of live-bird markets or mandatory rest and cleaning days in various cities reduced the influenza virus load in these live-bird markets but did not eliminate the novel H7N9 viruses from Chinese poultry populations. In 2017, a poultry vaccination campaign with a recombinant bivalent inactivated vaccine against H5N1 (A/chicken/Guizhou/4/2013, clade 2.3.4.4) and H7N9 (A/pigeon/Shanghai/S1069/2013) viruses was implemented and reduced the seropositivity rate to the targeted virus in poultry by greater than 90%.[163] Importantly, only three human H7N9 cases have been reported since the implementation of the poultry vaccination campaign.[163] However, most poultry vaccines do not induce sterilizing immunity in the field, so the viruses targeted by the vaccine continued to circulate and evolve. It remains to be seen whether the inactivated H5N1/H7N9 vaccine recently used in China will eradicate the targeted viruses from Chinese poultry populations.

Soon after the first reports of fatal human H7N9 virus infections in China in 2013, the viral genomic sequences were determined and immediately made publicly available through GISAID, the Global Initiative on Sharing All Influenza Data (www.gisaid.org). Phylogenetic analyses suggested that the H7 HA segment originated from an H7N3 duck influenza virus, the N9 NA segment originated from an H7N9 virus from wild waterfowl, and the six remaining segments originated from H9N2 viruses circulating in poultry.[37,63,81] Since the emergence of the novel H7N9 viruses, reassortment has resulted in a number of constellations of the internal segments. Moreover, the HA genes of the H7N9 viruses have now evolved into two lineages, referred to as the "Yangtze River Delta" and "Pearl River Delta" lineages.

The HA of the H7N9 viruses circulating in 2013 to 2016 does not encode a multibasic sequence at the HA cleavage site (see HA Cleavage section), a hallmark of highly pathogenic influenza viruses. Based on the currently used Office International des Epizooties (OIE) criteria for the classification of influenza viruses, the H7N9 viruses that circulated between 2013 and 2016 are therefore low pathogenic avian influenza viruses (despite their appreciable mortality rate in humans). This is consistent with the lack of severe disease in H7N9-infected chickens and ducks. Prolonged circulation of low pathogenic H5 and H7 viruses in poultry can result in the emergence of highly pathogenic variants with multiple basic amino acids at the HA cleavage site (see HA Cleavage section). In fact, highly pathogenic H7N9 viruses emerged at the end of December 2016, and 32 human infections with highly pathogenic H7N9 viruses had been reported by September 2017. These viruses belong to the Yangtze River Delta lineage of H7N9 viruses and are characterized by an amino acid insertion of KRTA, resulting in the KRKRTAR/G or KGKRTAR/G sequence at the HA cleavage site (the backslash denotes the cleavage site between HA1 and HA2).

The H7N9 viruses replicate efficiently in cultured mammalian cells. In mice and ferrets, they replicate in the respiratory tract of infected animals but typically do not cause severe disease or death.[5,118,153] H7N9 viruses transmit to contact ferrets and, more importantly, to exposed ferrets via respiratory droplets; however, the transmission kinetics are delayed compared with seasonal human influenza viruses.[5,118,153] In contrast to H5/Gs/Gd viruses, H7N9 viruses therefore possess the intrinsic ability to transmit among mammals via respiratory droplets. A comparison of H7N9 viruses of low and high pathogenicity demonstrated that the highly pathogenic H7N9 virus was more pathogenic in mice and ferrets than the low pathogenic H7N9 isolate, killing some of the infected and exposed ferrets.

The replicative ability and transmissibility of H7N9 viruses in mammals likely result from several mammalian-adapting features of these viruses. H7N9 viruses bind to both human-type and avian-type receptors (see Receptor Specificity of Influenza Viruses), a property likely conferred by the HA-226L (H3 HA numbering) and HA-186V residues known to increase the affinity for human-type receptors, which are encoded by most H7N9 viruses. Interestingly, almost all highly pathogenic H7N9 viruses isolated to date encode HA-186V but possess the avian-type HA-226Q residue. In addition, the novel H7N9 viruses lack the glycosylation site at positions 158 to 160 of HA, which is important for the transmissibility of H5 viruses (see Glycosylation section). Moreover, most human (but not avian) H7N9 viruses encode PB2-627K or PB2-D701N, which facilitate the efficient replication of avian influenza viruses in mammals (see The Replication Complex section). During the fifth wave, the PB2-A588V mutation, which enhances the pathogenicity of avian influenza viruses in mice, was detected in most human H7N9 virus isolates.

The novel H7N9 viruses encode the M2-S31N mutation, which confers resistance to adamantanes. However, the circulating H7N9 viruses are sensitive to NA inhibitors, and early initiation of treatment with NA inhibitors has been shown to be beneficial. Treatment of H7N9-infected patients with NA inhibitors may result in the emergence of mutants that are resistant to the drug used for treatment. In fact, treatment of an H7N9-infected patient with oseltamivir resulted in the emergence of a virus resistant to both oseltamivir and zanamivir.

Infections of Humans with Other Avian Influenza Viruses

Prior to 1997, the direct transmission of avian influenza viruses to humans was not considered a serious human health threat. This assumption was based on findings that avian viruses do not replicate efficiently in experimentally infected humans and that no severe cases of human infections had been reported during any outbreaks of HPAI. The differences in receptor-binding specificities between human and avian viruses (for details, see Molecular Determinants of Host-Range Restriction and Pathogenesis section) were believed to provide a host-range barrier that limited the transmission of avian viruses to humans. Until 1997, only four cases of direct avian-to-human transmission of influenza viruses had been described: (a) an HPAI virus of the H7N7 subtype isolated from a patient with hepatitis in 1959; (b) an H7N7 HPAI virus isolated from a laboratory worker who developed conjunctivitis; (c) an H7N7 virus of low pathogenicity isolated from a woman who developed conjunctivitis and was likely infected from ducks she kept; and (d) an H7N7 virus isolated from a person in contact with a harbor seal experimentally infected with an H7N7 virus. With the emergence of the A/goose/Guangdong/1/1996-like H5 viruses in 1996 (see Infections of Humans with H5 Viruses of the A/goose/Guangdong/1/1996 Lineage section) and the novel H7N9 viruses in 2013 (see Infections of Human with Low and Highly Pathogenic H7N9 Viruses), the number of human infections with avian infections has increased considerably.

The vast majority of human infections with avian influenza viruses have been caused by viruses of the H5 and H7 subtypes. Human infections with H5/Gs/Gd viruses are described in the Infections of Humans with H5 Viruses of the A/goose/Guangdong/1/1996 Lineage section. Likewise, human infections with the novel H7N9 viruses are described in the Infections of Human with Low and Highly Pathogenic H7N9 Viruses section. In addition, during an outbreak of HPAI H7N7 viruses in poultry in the Netherlands in February/March 2003, 89 people were infected, 83 of whom developed conjunctivitis.[32,75] Most cases were mild and self-limiting, although a veterinarian developed acute respiratory distress and an ultimately fatal pneumonia. In three cases, human-to-human transmission was documented, and antibodies were detected in 59% of those who had contact with infected poultry workers. In November 2003, an H7N2 virus was isolated from an adult in New York who was hospitalized for upper and lower respiratory tract illness but eventually recovered. In 2004, two people developed conjunctivitis and mild respiratory symptoms after an outbreak of an HPAI H7N3 virus in poultry in Canada. Additional cases of human infection with avian influenza viruses were detected in the United Kingdom in 2006 and 2007, when H7N3 and H7N2 viruses caused conjunctivitis in one and four individuals, respectively, and in Mexico in 2013, when two poultry workers became infected with HPAI H7N3 viruses. In the winter of 2016/2017, a veterinarian who treated sick cats infected with novel H7N2 influenza viruses (see Influenza in Cats section) developed respiratory symptoms, and the novel feline H7N2 virus was isolated from the veterinarian. A low pathogenic avian H7N4 virus (A/Jiangsu/1/2018) was recently isolated from a person in China who was exposed to live poultry prior to the onset of symptoms. This individual was hospitalized with symptoms of severe pneumonia but recovered from the infection.

In addition to H5 and H7 viruses, avian H9N2 viruses have caused human infections (see Low Pathogenic H9N2 Avian Influenza Viruses section). In 1998 and 1999, H9N2 viruses transmitted from birds to pigs and humans. Five human infections were reported in Southern China, and, in March 1999, two children were infected in Hong Kong. Both presented with symptoms of typical influenza and recovered. The isolates were genetically similar to those from quail (A/quail/Hong Kong/G1/97 [H9N2]). In 2003, a young child in Hong Kong was infected with an H9N2 virus but recovered uneventfully. In Hong Kong in 2008 and 2009, genetically different H9N2 viruses were isolated from two immunocompromised patients. Additional human infections with H9N2 viruses have been reported in recent years, but the overall rate of reported human H9N2 viruses has not increased, perhaps because many of these infections are mild and not recognized as H9N2 virus infections.

In 2004, two cases of human infection with H10N7 virus were reported in Egypt (http://www.paho.org/english/ad/dpc/cd/eid-eer-07-may-2004.htm). In 2012, two Australian abattoir workers experienced conjunctivitis and mild respiratory systems after they processed chickens from a farm with an H10N7 poultry outbreak. Both workers tested positive for H10N7 virus. Influenza viruses of the H10N8 subtype caused three human infections in China in the winter of 2013/2014, two with fatal outcomes; the internal vRNA segments of these viruses originated from H9N2 influenza viruses (see Low Pathogenic H9N2 Avian Influenza Viruses section). A human H10N8 virus bound to avian- and human-type receptors, perhaps in part explaining its ability to replicate in humans. Moreover, an H10N8 virus isolated from an environmental sample replicated in mice without the need for prior adaptation and became lethal for mice after two passages. An avian H10N8 virus has also been isolated from dogs in live-bird markets in China. Collectively, these data indicate that H10N8 viruses are able to infect mammals.

In Taiwan in 2013, the first known human infection with an H6N1 virus occurred. Collectively, the number of reported human infections with avian influenza viruses has increased, most likely as a consequence of increased public awareness, increased surveillance, and frequent exposure of humans to animals at the human–animal interface.

Infections of Humans with Swine Influenza Viruses

In general, human infections with swine influenza viruses cause mild illness; however, several fatal cases have been reported. The most prominent example of swine influenza virus transmission to humans is the H1N1 pandemic of 2009[39,105] (see The H1N1 Pandemic in 2009 section) (Figs. 15.1 and 15.8). However, several other instances of human infection with swine influenza viruses have been reported. Human infections with H1N1 swine influenza viruses of different lineages occurred in North America, Europe, and Asia. Also, Eurasian reassortant human–like H3N2 swine viruses were transmitted to two children in The Netherlands in 1992/93 and to a child in Hong Kong in 1999. In North America in 2007, a number of people became infected with H1N1 viruses possessing an HA vRNA segment related to clade 1B.2 (see Influenza in Swine section) and internal vRNA segments derived from triple reassortant viruses (see The H1N1 Pandemic in 2009 section). North American H3N2 swine viruses (clade 3.1990.4; see Influenza in Swine section) with the M vRNA segment of H1N1pdm09 caused more than 300 human infections in 2011 to 2013, which were linked to exposure to swine at agricultural fairs. Most of the

infected individuals were small children, most likely because they lacked protective antibodies to the HA, which originated from human viruses circulating in the late 1990s. In subsequent years, the number of human infections with H3N2 swine viruses remained small but has increased again since 2016; these post-2016 viruses differ in their HA gene from those that caused human infections in 2011 to 2013.

EPIZOOLOGY AND PATHOGENESIS IN ANIMALS

Influenza A viruses infect a variety of animals, including humans, birds, swine, horses, and dogs (Fig. 15.1). Occasionally, influenza viruses have been isolated from cats, tigers and leopards, stone martens and Owston civets, whales, seals, mink, and camels. Serologic evidence also suggests exposure of bats, several ruminant, reptile, and amphibian species to immunogens related to influenza viruses.

Viruses of all known HA and NA subtypes are maintained in aquatic birds (with the exception of H17N10 and H18N11 viruses; see Influenza in Bats section),[155] generally without causing disease; therefore, aquatic birds are considered the natural reservoir of influenza A viruses. Nonpathogenic viruses of the H5 and H7 subtypes can evolve into highly pathogenic avian strains and cause significant losses to the poultry industry. Viruses of the H5, H7, and H9 subtypes have established lineages in terrestrial birds. Although human pandemics have been associated with viruses of the H1 to H3 subtypes, the ability of avian viruses of the H5, H7, and H9 subtypes to infect humans has flagged viruses of these subtypes as potential candidates for future influenza pandemics. Influenza B viruses typically replicate in humans but have been isolated from seals. Influenza C virus infects humans, swine, and dogs.

Influenza in Birds

The natural reservoir of influenza A viruses are the orders Anseriformes (ducks, geese, swans) and Charadriiformes (gulls, terns, shorebirds), although influenza A viruses have been isolated from at least 105 different avian species from 26 different families. Almost all HA and NA subtypes have been detected in dabbling ducks (*Anas* spp.), suggesting that these species are the major reservoir of influenza A viruses. In mallard ducks (*Anas platyrhynchos*), viruses of the H5, H3, H4, and H6 subtypes are isolated most frequently; the most prevalent subtypes are H5N1, H4N6, and H3N8. In addition, viruses of several HA subtypes (including H1, H2, H5, H7, and H9–H12), in combination with several NA subtypes, have been detected in waders of the Charadriidae family, suggesting a role for these species in the perpetuation of influenza A viruses. Viruses of the H13 and H16 subtypes appear to circulate only in Laridae (gull and tern) species. For the NA gene, N3, N4, N6, and N8 subtypes predominate in ducks, whereas N2 and N9 are most frequently detected in chickens. Poultry play a critical role in the perpetuation of influenza A viruses; in fact, most HA and NA subtypes can be isolated from poultry in live-bird markets.

Surveillance studies have demonstrated seasonal patterns in prevalence; the infection rate of mallard ducks reaches 60% before the autumn migration and declines to less than 10% in spring and summer. This pattern may represent the influx of immunologically naïve juveniles every summer and/or the high population density in marshalling areas before the migration. In contrast, in North American shorebirds, the infection rate is highest in late spring and early summer. Since the prevalence of infection declines along the migration route and is relatively low at the wintering grounds of mallard ducks, geographic patterns in prevalence can be observed (i.e., infection rates are higher at the marshalling areas in the north than at the wintering grounds in the south). Moreover, the prevalence of virus subtypes in the same species changes from year to year. In particular, cyclic patterns exist in which high rates of prevalence for one subtype in a certain population may be followed by low detection rates in this population in subsequent seasons, perhaps due to herd immunity to viruses of the respective subtype.

Reassortment plays a critical role in the evolution of avian influenza viruses with significant contributions of both intra-subtypic reassortment (i.e., reassortment between viruses of the same subtype) and intersubtypic reassortment (i.e., reassortment between viruses of different subtypes), as well as of reassortment between the North American and Eurasian gene pools, which evolve largely independently, as described earlier.

Based on their pathogenicity in chickens, avian influenza viruses are classified as HPAI or low pathogenicity avian influenza (LPAI) viruses. LPAI viruses cause mild respiratory disease, depression, and/or a decrease in egg production. For outbreak control purposes, the OIE classifies an avian influenza virus as HPAI if it is "lethal for six, seven, or eight of eight 4- to 8-week-old susceptible chickens within 10 days following intravenous inoculation with 0.2 mL of a 1/10 dilution of a bacteria-free, infective allantoic fluid" (OIE Manual of Diagnostic Tests and Vaccines for Terrestrial Animals 2010; accessible at: http://www.oie.int/en/international-standard-setting/terrestrial-manual/access-online/), or if it has an intravenous pathogenicity index (IVPI) greater than 1.2 (the IVPI is the mean clinical score of ten 6-week-old chickens intravenously infected).

The infection of aquatic birds with LPAI is typically asymptomatic, although even LPAI viruses can cause mild disease in mallards and swans. In ducks, avian viruses replicate in the epithelial cells in the intestinal tract and, to a substantially lesser extent, in cells of the respiratory tract. These viruses are resistant to the low pH environment they encounter during their passage through the digestive tract. Avian species shed influenza viruses in high concentrations in feces. The viruses are relatively stable in water and have been isolated from water samples of lakes where wild birds have nested or congregated before migration. Contaminated water and feces may, therefore, serve as major routes of transmission of LPAI among wild birds. By contrast, HPAI H5 viruses replicate efficiently in the upper respiratory tract of infected birds.

Typically, outbreaks of HPAI occur in poultry; historically, the resulting disease was called "fowl plague." Viruses that are highly pathogenic for chickens often cause high mortality in turkeys and Japanese quail but are usually nonpathogenic for ducks, geese, and other wild birds, with the exception of some of the recently circulating H5/Gs/Gd viruses (see Infections of Humans with H5 Viruses of the A/goose/Guangdong/1/1996 Lineage section). Infection of ducks with some H5/Gs/Gd viruses results in systemic infections with high virus titers in the respiratory organs; neurologic symptoms may also be observed. However, infected birds may die without clinical symptoms. In experimental infections of several bird species, H5/Gs/Gd viruses were not uniformly lethal, and infected animals shed

appreciable amounts of viruses, which could facilitate virus spread. A characteristic feature of H5/Gs/Gd infection in ducks is that virus titers in oropharyngeal swabs are higher than those in cloacal swabs.[135] In chickens, influenza virus infections with HPAI viruses can result in mortality rates of up to 100%. Historically, outbreaks of HPAI were controlled by depopulation and vaccination. While these and other control measures continue to be implemented, H5/Gs/Gd viruses have become enzootic in poultry populations in different parts of the world.

Most HPAI viruses have a series of basic amino acids at the HA cleavage site (see HA Cleavage section); however, exceptions exist in which viruses with multiple basic amino acids at this site are not highly pathogenic in chickens, or highly pathogenic viruses do not possess a conventional HA cleavage site. All HPAI viruses known to date belong to the H5 or H7 subtype; however, only a small proportion of all H5 and H7 viruses are highly pathogenic.

Occasionally, avian influenza viruses infect mammalian species (see Transmission of Avian and Swine Influenza Viruses to Humans section). Most of these infections are self-limiting, and stable lineages have emerged rarely, such as in pigs in 1979 with the introduction of an avian H1N1 virus. In mammals, LPAI viruses cause bronchitis, bronchiolitis, and pneumonia. A major exception is the H7N9 virus that emerged in China in 2013 (see Infections of Human with Low and Highly Pathogenic H7N9 Viruses section). Although most H7N9 viruses are of the low pathogenic type, they have infected 1567 people with a case fatality rate of 39%.

In the last 5 years, more than 7,100 outbreaks of HPAI viruses in domestic birds in 68 countries have been reported to the OIE (http://empres-i.fao.org/eipws3g/); most were caused by H5 viruses.

Non–Gs/Gd Lineage HPAI H5N2 Virus Outbreaks
Pennsylvania outbreak
In April 1983, a low virulent H5N2 virus (A/chicken/Pennsylvania/1/83) emerged in chickens in Pennsylvania. By October, this virus had mutated into a highly pathogenic variant (A/chicken/Pennsylvania/1370/83) causing a mortality rate of more than 80% in chickens. The virus was eventually eradicated by the slaughter of more than 17 million birds. The avirulent predecessor was unusual in that it had multiple basic amino acids at the HA cleavage site. The virulent strain differed from its predecessor by only a few nucleotides including one that caused the loss of an HA glycosylation site, thereby exposing the multiple basic HA cleavage site to the ubiquitous cellular proteases furin and PC6.

Mexican outbreak
In May 1994, a mildly pathogenic H5N2 virus was isolated from Mexican chickens (A/chicken/Mexico/26654-1374/94). This virus was not eradicated by mass slaughter because it had already spread widely. Stepwise accumulation of mutations over several months yielded moderately (A/chicken/Puebla/8624-602/94) and highly (A/chicken/Queretaro/14588-19/95) pathogenic strains with a series of basic residues at the HA cleavage site. Vaccination was implemented in 1995 and by 2001, more than 1 billion doses of inactivated vaccine had been used. Between 1998 and 2001, 459 million doses of recombinant fowlpox-vector vaccine were also administered. Low pathogenic H5N2 strains continue to circulate, as do genetically related viruses

in the neighboring countries of Guatemala and El Salvador. In 2005, an H5N2 virus with low pathogenicity emerged in chickens in Japan. This virus is a descendant of the virus responsible for the Mexican outbreak and is closely related to a virus isolated from Guatemala. The origin of the Japanese strain remains unknown.

H7N1 Outbreaks

In March 1999, an LPAI virus of the H7N1 subtype was isolated from a poultry farm in Italy. The virus was not eradicated and the infection spread, resulting, in December, in the emergence of a highly pathogenic isolate. More than 13 million birds were destroyed to control the outbreak. The reemergence of this LPAI in August 2000 was controlled by additional depopulation followed by a vaccination campaign from November 2000 to May 2002. The vaccine was based on an inactivated H7N3 virus to allow *d*ifferentiation of *i*nfected and *v*accinated *a*nimals (DIVA). Vaccination in combination with intensive monitoring led to the eradication of this H7N1 virus. Outbreaks of HPAI viruses of the H7N1 subtypes also occurred in ostriches in South Africa in 2012 and among wild water birds in Algeria in 2016. Both outbreaks were relatively small.

H7N2 Outbreak

Highly pathogenic H7N2 viruses killed more than 18,000 domestic chickens in a free-ranging and cage bird layer flock in Australia in 2013.

H7N3 Outbreaks

Several outbreaks of HPAI H7N3 viruses have occurred in poultry in Asia and in North and South America. During an outbreak in Canada in 2004, two workers developed symptoms of influenza virus infection. H7N3 viruses isolated from these individuals had increased affinity for human-type receptors (see Receptor Specificity of Influenza Viruses section). Both the Chilean and 2004 Canadian isolates arose from LPAI viruses through recombination events that inserted 10 amino acids from the NP protein (Chilean virus) or 7 amino acids from the M1 protein (Canadian virus) into the HA cleavage site.

In June 2012, an outbreak of HPAI H7N3 viruses (represented by A/chicken/Jalisco/CPA1/2012) started in commercial poultry farms in the Mexican state of Jalisco (a major egg production area), resulting in the death through disease or culling of more than 22 million poultry. During a second wave in the first half of 2013, the HPAI viruses spread to industrial and backyard poultry in neighboring states. Another large outbreak occurred in 2016 that led to greater than 250,000 poultry being culled.

Genetic and phylogenetic analysis revealed close similarity of the HPAI H7N3 Mexican viruses with North American avian viruses of different subtypes, suggesting that reassortment played a role in the generation of the Mexican H7H3 viruses. The HA gene of the Mexican HPAI H7N3 viruses possesses a 24-nucleotide insertion at the cleavage site, which was most likely derived from chicken 28S rRNA through nonhomologous recombination; this insertion encodes several basic amino acids. Interestingly, nonhomologous recombination of HA and 28S rRNA sequences had been reported previously, when sequential passages of A/turkey/Oregon/71 (H7N3) virus in embryonated chicken eggs resulted in the insertion of 54 nucleotides of 28S rRNA near the HA cleavage site.[68] The virus with the 28S rRNA insertion no longer required exogenous trypsin for HA cleavage (see HA Cleavage section) and was more pathogenic in chickens than the parent virus. Two human infections with the Mexican HPAI H7N3 viruses occurred among poultry workers; both developed conjunctivitis. The virus isolated from one of the infected people (A/Mexico/InDRE7218/2012) was lethal in mice. In ferrets infected with this virus, clinical signs of illness were observed; the virus replicated efficiently in the upper and lower respiratory tract and transmitted to naïve contact animals in the same cage.

H7N7 Outbreaks

In 2003, an HPAI of the H7N7 subtype caused outbreaks in layer farms in The Netherlands, resulting in the death or culling of more than 30 million birds. Experimental infection of chickens confirmed the highly pathogenic phenotype of the virus. The outbreak spread to Belgium and Germany but was brought under control by mass slaughtering. In The Netherlands, the outbreak was associated with one fatal human case, a veterinarian who contracted the disease, and with conjunctivitis in 78 individuals who either directly handled affected poultry or had family members who did.[32,75] These data suggest human-to-human transmission, and experimental infection of cats demonstrated that the virus isolated from the fatal case caused alveolar damage with infection of type 2 pneumocytes and non-ciliated bronchial cells, comparable to infection with an H5/Gs/Gd virus. The virus isolated from the fatal case differed by 14 amino acids from a virus isolated from another individual with conjunctivitis; the acquisition of PB2-627K (a known determinant of pathogenicity in mammals; see The Replication Complex section[48,137]) was pivotal for increased pathogenicity and tissue tropism. Depopulation of infected poultry and the treatment of at-risk individuals with NAIs likely prevented further spread of this virus.

In 2005, an outbreak of H7N7 HPAI occurred in chickens in the Democratic People's Republic of Korea. More than 200,000 chickens died from influenza virus infection or were destroyed. Further outbreaks of H7N7 HPAI occurred in several European countries including Spain, the United Kingdom, Italy, and Germany between 2008 and 2016, resulting in small to moderate numbers of poultry that succumbed to infection or were culled.

Non–Chinese Lineage H7N9 Outbreak

The H7N9 viruses that emerged in China in 2013 and caused human infections are discussed in the Infections of Humans with Low and Highly Pathogenic H7N9 Viruses section. In March of 2017, an outbreak of HPAI H7N9 viruses occurred in poultry farms in Tennessee. At the same time, LPAI H7N9 viruses were isolated in a neighboring county and later also in the neighboring states of Alabama, Kentucky, and Georgia. More than 100,000 animals were culled to stop the further spread of the viruses. The sequences of the LPAI and HPAI viruses were very similar, except for an 8-amino-acid insertion at the HPAI HA cleavage site that matched the sequence of chicken 28S rRNA. Interestingly, this insertion was almost identical to that detected in the 2012 Mexican HPAI H7N3 viruses. The American LPAI and HPAI H7N9 viruses were closely related to an American teal virus (A/blue-winged teal/Wyoming/AH0099021/2016; H7N9) but differed from the H7N9 viruses that emerged in China in 2013.

Low Pathogenic H9N2 Avian Influenza Viruses

Since the mid-1990s, LPAI viruses of the H9N2 subtype have become enzootic in poultry populations in many countries in Asia, the Middle East, and North Africa. H9N2 influenza viruses are currently the most prevalent LPAI in poultry in the world. Chickens infected with H9N2 viruses often experience respiratory distress with reduced egg production. In the field, mortality rates as high as 40% have been observed, which may be the consequence of coinfections with other pathogens. In contrast, H9N2 infections of specific pathogen-free chickens in laboratory settings are typically nonlethal with mild influenza-like symptoms. H9N2 influenza viruses are rarely detected in wild birds.

H9N2 influenza viruses can be separated into North American and Eurasian lineages. In Eurasia, several lineages are circulating, often referred to as the Y280-like lineage (named after A/duck/Hong Kong/Y280/97), the G1-like lineage (named after A/quail/Hong Kong/G1/97), the Korean or Y439-like lineage (named after A/duck/Hong Kong/Y439/97), the BJ/94–like lineage (named after A/chicken/Beijing/1/1994), and the F/98–like lineage (named after A/chicken/Shanghai/F/1998). Frequent reassortment has resulted in a large number of different genotypes within these lineages.

Since their introduction into poultry, the host range and virulence of H9N2 viruses have increased. Overall, early H9N2 virus isolates replicated less efficiently in poultry and were shed for shorter periods of time than more recent isolates. Since the early 2000s, many H9N2 viruses of the Y280 and G1 lineages have acquired an HA-Q226L (H3 numbering) mutation, which increases binding to human-type receptors (see Receptor Specificity of Influenza Viruses). The ability to efficiently bind to human-type receptors may explain the expanded host range of these H9N2 viruses, which have infected humans and other mammalian species including pigs, dogs, cats, weasels, and mink. In humans, H9N2 infections are typically mild, and serosurveillance studies suggest many unreported cases. All human H9N2 virus infections have been caused by viruses of the Y280 and G1 lineages, most of which encoded the mammalian-adapting HA-Q226L change. Since the late 1990s, H9N2 viruses have been isolated repeatedly from pigs; serosurveillance studies detected seroconversion rates of, for example, 16% in pigs in Southern China in 2010 to 2012. However, experimental infection of pigs with H9N2 viruses demonstrated that these viruses do not readily spread among pigs. H9N2 viruses replicate in mice and ferrets without the need for prior adaptation, and their virulence in mice differs, ranging from respiratory to systemic infection (with fatal outcome). In ferrets, H9N2 viruses replicate in the respiratory tract and transmit to cage mates. Importantly, six of nine H9N2 viruses isolated from chickens in China in 2010 to 2013 transmitted via respiratory droplets to exposed ferrets,[79] demonstrating that these viruses possess the ability to transmit among mammals via the airborne route.

Reassortment of H9N2 viruses with other avian influenza viruses has resulted in a number of viruses with all or some of their internal vRNA segments from H9N2 viruses, including viruses that have infected humans such as H5N1, H5N6, H7N9, and H10N8 viruses (see Transmission of Avian and Swine Influenza Viruses to Humans). The prevalence of H9N2 viruses in poultry and the donation of H9N2 internal vRNA segments to various subtypes that have caused human infections identify H9N2 influenza viruses as an important component of the influenza virus ecology.

Vaccines for Avian Influenza Viruses

The increasing number of outbreaks caused by H5 and H7 viruses, the fact that H5, H7, and H9 viruses are now enzootic in poultry populations in parts of the world, and the increasing number of human infections with these viruses have spurred the development of avian vaccines and the vaccination of poultry flocks. Most approved vaccines for H5, H7, and H9 viruses are based on inactivated whole-virus preparations, although some live recombinant vaccines based on Newcastle disease, fowl pox, and turkey herpesvirus are now available.

Official vaccination programs against H5 viruses have been carried out in several Asian and African countries but have failed to eradicate H5 viruses in most of these countries. Possible reasons include limited adoption of vaccination campaigns, failure to induce sterilizing immunity that may result in undetected virus spread and evolution, and limited cross-reactivity with viruses of different clades. In September of 2017, China implemented a vaccination campaign with a recombinant bivalent vaccine directed against H5 and H7 viruses. As a result, the isolation rate of H7N9 viruses from poultry dropped by greater than 90%, and only three human H7N9 virus infections were reported between October 1, 2017, and September 30, 2018.

Influenza in Swine

The first isolation of an influenza A virus from pigs dates to 1930 (A/swine/Iowa/15/30 [H1N1]). Swine influenza viruses are enzootic in swine populations around the world and cause a respiratory disease with high morbidity but low mortality in these animals. Signs of infection include inactivity, nasal discharge, coughing, fever, labored breathing, weight loss, and conjunctivitis. Infections are limited to the respiratory tract with tracheobronchial lesions. Avian and human viruses of several subtypes (or reassortants thereof) have caused local outbreaks or become enzootic in pigs. A novel H1N1 virus, which most likely originated from reassortment of different influenza viruses in pigs,[39,105,130] caused the 2009 H1N1 pandemic.

Collectively, the prominent role for pigs in the emergence of novel influenza viruses is supported by several findings: (a) pigs are sporadically infected with certain human seasonal influenza viruses and to a lesser extent avian influenza viruses, and swine influenza viruses have transmitted to humans; (b) epithelial cells in pig trachea contain both human- and avian-type receptors (i.e., Siaα2,6Gal and Siaα2,3Gal, respectively); and (c) frequent reassortment (both intra- and intersubtypic) occurs among swine influenza viruses, and reassortment has also been detected between swine and human influenza viruses and infrequently occurs between swine and avian viruses. These observations support the "mixing vessel" hypothesis that simultaneous infections of pigs with swine, avian, and human influenza viruses may result in the generation of reassortants capable of causing pandemics.

Over the last century, several major lineages of influenza A viruses of the H1 and H3 subtypes have circulated in swine populations in several continents (Fig. 15.8).

Swine H1 Viruses

Based on the phylogenetic relationships of swine influenza virus HA nucleotide sequences, a nomenclature system has been implemented that groups H1 swine influenza viruses into three major lineages, termed 1A, 1B, and 1C (Table 15.1). The 1A

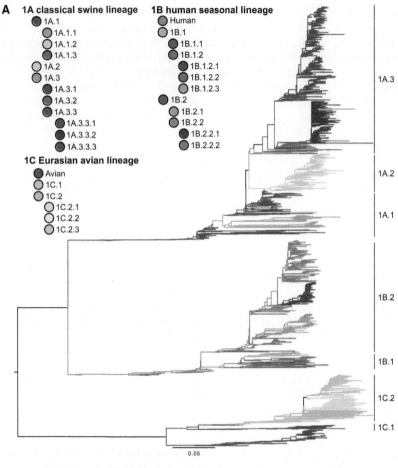

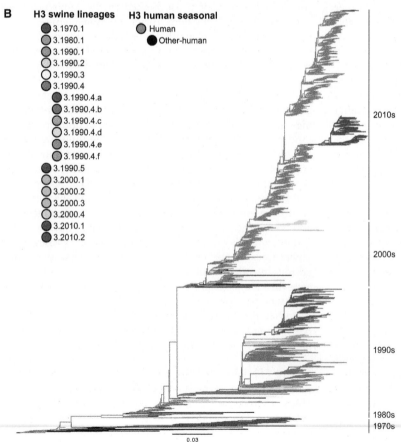

FIGURE 15.8 Phylogeny of swine H1 and H3 HA gene sequences. A: For swine H1 HA gene sequences, the phylogenetic tree was inferred by using maximum likelihood methods for 6296 H1 swine and 775 randomly sampled human and avian HA gene sequences demonstrating the three major lineages: 1A classical swine lineage, 1B human seasonal lineage, and 1C Eurasian avian lineage. **B:** For swine H3 HA gene sequences, 3507 swine HA gene sequences were combined with 5548 randomly sampled human seasonal HA gene sequences collected from 1968 to present. "Other-human" indicates seasonal H3 HA gene sequences detected in swine without evidence of sustained transmission. Branch color represents clade designations of currently circulating swine viruses. Each tree is midpoint rooted for clarity; all branch lengths are drawn to scale, and the scale bar indicates the number of nucleotide substitutions per site. Phylogenetic trees were generated by Tavis Anderson and Amy Vincent, U.S. Department of Agriculture (USDA). (**A** was adapted from Anderson TK, Macken CA, Lewis NS, et al. A phylogeny-based global nomenclature system and automated annotation tool for H1 hemagglutinin genes from swine influenza A viruses. *mSphere* 2016;1(6), pii: e00275-16; covered under an open access license.)

TABLE 15.1 Overview of major H1 swine virus lineages

Major Lineage	Clade	Geographic Distribution[a]	Comments
1A (formerly known as classical swine lineage)	1A.1	Americas, Europe, Asia	Descendants of 1918 pandemic virus; formerly called α-H1 viruses; 3 subclades (1A.1.1–1.3)
	1A.2	North America, (Asia)	Descendants of North American triple reassortant viruses; formerly called β-H1 viruses
	1A.3	Worldwide	Descendants of North American triple reassortant viruses; 3 subclades (1A.3.1–3.3); 1A.3.3 is further divided into 3 subclades: 1A.3.3.2 H1N1pdm09 viruses with worldwide distribution, and the numerically dominant 1A.3.3.3, formerly called γ-H1 viruses
1B (formerly known as human seasonal lineage)	1B.1	Europe	Descendants of human seasonal H1 viruses introduced into European pig populations in the 1990s; 2 subclades (1B.1.1–1.2); 1B.1.2 is further divided into 3 subclades
	1B.2	Americas	Descendants of human seasonal H1 viruses that were introduced into North American pig populations in the 2000s; 2 subclades (1B.2.1–2.2); 1B.2.1 and 1B.2.2 were formerly known as δ2- and δ1-H1 viruses, respectively; 1B.2.2 is further divided into 2 subclades
1C (formerly known as Eurasian avian lineage)	1C.1	Europe	Descendants of avian influenza viruses introduced into European pig populations in 1979
	1C.2	Europe, Asia, (North America)	Descendants of avian influenza viruses introduced into European pig populations in the late 1990s; 3 subclades (1C.2.1–2.3); subclade 1C.2.3 viruses originated in Europe but are now mostly detected in Hong Kong and mainland China

[a]Parenthesis indicates that only small proportions of viruses of the respective clade were detected in the indicated geographic location.

viruses were formerly known as "classical swine lineage"; they are descendants of the 1918 H1N1 pandemic virus and have been isolated in swine populations in North America, Europe, and parts of Asia.

In 1997 and 1998, H3N2 double human/swine reassortant and triple human/avian/swine reassortant viruses emerged in North America.[165] The double reassortant virus possessed human-like HA, NA, and PB1 genes, whereas the remaining genes were of classical swine virus origin, but this virus did not establish a stable lineage. The human/avian/swine triple reassortant viruses that contained HA, NA, and PB1 polymerase genes of human virus origin; PB2 and PA polymerase genes of avian virus origin; and NP, matrix (M), and nonstructural (NS) genes of classical H1N1 swine virus origin quickly became established throughout the North American swine population.[165] These viruses reassorted with enzootic classical H1N1 swine viruses, resulting in the diversification of H1 genes into the 1A.1, 1A.2, and 1A.3 subclades that have cocirculated in the United States and in parts of Asia. While reassortment has resulted in different HA/NA gene constellations, the constellation of the internal genes (i.e., PB2, PB1, PA, NP, M, and NS) was relatively stable for several years and became known as the TRIG (*t*riple *r*eassortant *i*nternal gene) cassette. The combination of the NA and M segments of a European avian–like swine virus with the remaining six segments from a triple reassortant virus resulted in the emergence of the H1N1pdm09 virus (subclade 1A3.3.2) in 2009.[39,105,130] This virus caused a pandemic and has now established a stable lineage in humans. Multiple "reverse zoonosis" (anthroponosis) events have repeatedly reintroduced the H1N1pdm09 virus from humans to pigs, where it has since reassorted with enzootic swine viruses.

The 1B lineage (formerly known as "human seasonal lineage") resulted from the introduction of human influenza viruses into pigs. Clade 1B.1 includes European human–like reassortant H1N2 viruses with an HA of human virus origin and the remaining genes from Eurasian reassortant human–like swine H3N2 viruses. The clade 1B.1 viruses have been limited to European swine populations. Clade 1B.2 viruses were detected globally in the early 2000s, with two separate introductions of human influenza viruses into pig populations in North America forming subclades 1B.2.1 and 1B.2.2.

The 1C lineage viruses were colloquially known as "Eurasian avian lineage" swine viruses. The 1C.1 H1N1 clade was founded by transmission of avian H1 influenza viruses into pigs in Europe in the late 1970s. Viruses of this clade caused multiple outbreaks throughout European pig populations, diverged, and formed a new clade 1C.2 in the late 1990s. Most 1C.2 viruses have been isolated in Europe, but viruses of the 1C.2.3 clade (which emerged in France in 1999) spread to Hong Kong and mainland China.

Swine H3 Viruses

Human H3N2 viruses have been transmitted to pigs multiple times in different locations and have founded several swine virus lineages. A new nomenclature for swine H3 similar to that developed for H1 viruses was proposed by the OIE and FAO influenza network (OFFLU) swine working group and is currently in development (T.K. Anderson, personal communication); it separates the currently circulating swine virus lineages based on the decade of their introduction into swine populations. For example, the human H3N2 viruses that were introduced into the European pig population in the early 1970s

TABLE 15.2 Overview of major, currently circulating H3 swine virus lineages

Major Lineage	Clade	Geographic Distribution[a]	Comments
1970s human-to-swine transmissions	3.1970.1	Europe, Asia	Formerly called A/Port Chalmers/1/73–like swine H3N2 viruses
1980s human-to-swine transmissions	3.1980.1	Taiwan	
1990s human-to-swine transmissions	3.1990.1	North America	Descendants of triple reassortant H3N2 viruses
	3.1990.2	Korea, United States, Mexico	Descendants of triple reassortant H3N2 viruses (formerly called cluster I)
	3.1990.3	Asia	
	3.1990.4	North America, (Korea, Vietnam)	Descendants of triple reassortant H3N2 viruses (formerly called cluster IV); 6 subclades (3.1990.4.a–f; formerly called clusters IV-A through IV-F)
	3.1990.5	Brazil	
2000s human-to-swine transmissions	3.2000.1	Argentina	
	3.2000.2	Asia	
	3.2000.3	Europe	
	3.2000.4	China, Hong Kong, Vietnam	
2010s human-to-swine transmissions	3.2010.1	North America	Formerly called US 2010 human-like
	3.2010.2	North America	

[a]Parenthesis indicates that only small proportions of viruses of the respective clade were detected in the indicated geographic location.

similar to A/Port Chalmers/1/73 are referred to as lineage 3.1970.1 (Table 15.2). In 1984, severe disease among Italian and French pigs was traced to a novel reassortant H3N2 strain that possessed human virus–like HA and NA genes from the 1970s introduction, but its internal genes were derived from Eurasian avian–like H1N1 swine viruses. This virus (referred to as Eurasian reassortant human–like swine H3N2 virus) soon became enzootic and replaced the human-like swine H3N2 viruses.

Viruses of the H3 subtype did not circulate widely in North American swine populations until the late 1990s, although low rates of seropositive samples were reported. As discussed with the swine H1 viruses, this changed in 1997/1998 with the introduction of double and triple reassortant H3N2 influenza viruses into North American pig populations. The triple reassortant H3N2 viruses evolved into five HA clades and the major HA clade (3.1990.4) has further diversified into several subclades. Viruses from clade 3.1990.4 have also infected humans (see Infections of Humans with Swine Influenza Viruses section). In the 2000s and 2010s, several independent introductions of human H3N2 viruses into pigs, followed by reassortment with enzootic swine viruses, resulted in new swine virus lineages in different continents. An introduction from the 2010/2011 influenza season led to a new stable lineage in the United States, 3.2010.1, that is now the dominant swine H3 lineage detected in this country and has caused a number of human infections.[114,162]

Genetic Diversity of Swine Influenza Viruses

In the 20th century, a limited number of swine influenza virus genotypes were known, some of which (such as the classical H1N1 viruses) circulated for several decades. Over the last few decades, changes in the epizoology of swine influenza viruses

(such as increased swine movement), and increased surveillance in pigs, have resulted in the detection of multiple novel genotypes. As described above, multiple clades and subclades of H1 and H3 viruses are now (co)circulating in several parts of the world. In addition, NAs of several major genetic lineages are (co)circulating in swine populations worldwide. The remaining viral segments typically originate from classical H1-1A, the TRIG cassette, H1-1C Eurasian avian, or H1N1pdm09 viruses.

Establishment of avian viruses in swine has been infrequent, although there is serologic and virologic evidence demonstrating that transmission events occur. In 1998, avian H9N2 viruses were first detected in swine in Hong Kong but did not establish a stable lineage. Based on their HA sequences, some of the swine H9N2 viruses may bind to human-type receptors. HPAI H5N1 viruses have been isolated from pigs in Asia on several occasions, although the prevalence of HPAI H5N1 viruses in pigs appears to be low. Moreover, H9N2 viruses with HPAI H5N1–like sequences have been described, suggesting reassortment between H5N1 and H9N2 viruses. To date, no H7N9 influenza viruses (see Infections of Humans with Low and Highly Pathogenic H7N9 Viruses) have been isolated from pigs. Viruses of other subtypes including H2N3, H3N1, H3N3, H3N8, H4N6, H4N8, H5N2, H6N6, H7N2, and H11N6 have been isolated from pigs, but these viruses have not established stable lines in swine populations.

Influenza in Horses

Two different subtypes of influenza A viruses are recognized in horses: H7N7, historically referred to as equine-1, and H3N8, referred to as equine-2. Equine influenza is typically associated with fever, nasal discharge, dry hacking cough, loss of appetite, muscular soreness, and tracheobronchitis. The disease is usually more severe with equine-2 (i.e., H3N8) viruses and can include inflammation of the heart muscle. Secondary bacterial infections can be fatal. Equine H3N8 influenza virus was the parent of the canine H3N8 influenza virus that emerged in 2004. Prior to the 20th century, equine and human or avian "influenza" epidemics were often temporally associated. Serum antibodies to influenza D virus have been detected in horses although as yet no virus isolation or clinical disease has been reported. Equine influenza viruses cause disease in experimentally infected mice and ferrets.

The first equine influenza virus (A/equine/Prague/56 [H7N7]) was isolated in 1956 during a widespread enzootic of respiratory disease among horses in Eastern Europe. The last confirmed outbreak of this subtype occurred in 1979. It is believed to be extinct; however anecdotal reports of equine H7N7 outbreaks in Egypt and India, and the sporadic detection of H7-specific antibodies in reportedly unvaccinated horses, suggest the possibility that the viruses still circulate in small geographic pockets or in a subclinical form since their last isolation. In 1963, an equine influenza virus of the H3N8 subtype (A/equine/Miami/63 [H3N8]) was isolated in the United States and caused a major epidemic. It was later found to have been introduced into North American horses via the importation of horses from Argentina. Several studies suggested reassortment between the equine H7N7 and H3N8 viruses while they were cocirculating. Another enzootic with an H3N8 virus occurred in China in 1989. This virus caused morbidity rates of up to 80% and mortality rates of up to 20%. Based on sequence analysis, the virus was of avian origin and unrelated to the H3N8 virus already established in horse populations. It remained confined to the Chinese horse population and was not isolated after the mid-1990s.

Phylogenetic separation of Eurasian and American lineages has been observed in the equine H3 HA proteins since 1987; within the American lineage, three sublineages (South American/Argentinian, Kentucky, and Florida) are recognized. The Florida sublineage has evolved into two clades (Florida clade 1 and Florida clade 2); viruses of these two clades have caused the major recent equine influenza virus outbreaks in horses around the world since 2003. For the other viral gene segments, phylogenetic lineages have been described corresponding to the Florida clade 1 and clade 2 lineages in HA.

Inactivated vaccines of the H3N8 subtype have been widely used. Studies suggest that the immunity conferred by inactivated vaccines is short-lived (<6 months in young horses); therefore, outbreaks of equine influenza can affect vaccinated horses as well. Outbreaks of equine H3N8 continue to occur throughout the world, probably supported by the international transportation of vaccinated horses, in which virus replicates in a subclinical form. For example, international transportation of vaccinated horses likely led to the introduction of equine influenza into Australia in 2007. Several equine influenza vaccines are now commercially available including inactivated vaccines (some of which are adjuvanted with immune-stimulating complexes); cold-adapted, temperature-sensitive, modified live equine influenza virus vaccine; and recombinant canarypox-vectored vaccine. Some of these vaccines do not provide sterilizing immunity, so the vaccinated horses continue to shed virus.

Influenza in Dogs

In 2004, outbreaks of respiratory disease occurred in racing greyhounds in Florida. The causative agent was an influenza A virus (A/canine/Florida/43/2004 [H3N8]) closely related to contemporary H3N8 equine viruses, suggesting interspecies transmission. The virus spread among the greyhound populations, indicating that the equine influenza viruses replicated in and transmitted among these dogs. This virus soon spread to other dog breeds but was largely maintained in large animal shelters in the United States, where the turnover of dogs and introduction of new susceptibles allowed the virus to be maintained for several years, although since 2016 the virus has only been detected at low levels and may have died out. The H3N8 viruses that circulated in horses and dogs in North America became genetically distinguishable and no additional interspecies transmission from horses to dogs or back to horses has been reported. Infection of individual dogs with an equine H3N8 virus was also reported in Australia in 2007, and a retrospective study showed that an outbreak of respiratory disease in English foxhounds in the United Kingdom in 2002 was also caused by an equine H3N8 virus. In experimental studies, horses infected with the canine virus seroconverted but showed little signs of disease. The infection of dogs with equine influenza viruses may be facilitated by the presence on canine respiratory epithelial cells of Siaα2,3Gal receptors, which are preferentially bound by equine influenza viruses.

In 2006, an avian H3N2 influenza–derived virus was isolated in Korea from domestic dogs with respiratory symptoms. Experimental testing showed that this virus caused tracheobronchitis and bronchiolitis in dogs and was transmitted to contact animals. While it is not clear where this virus first emerged, it was widespread in China and also isolated from an outbreak in Thailand. The virus may be maintained in farmed dogs, but seroprevalence studies have also detected it in household dogs. In 2015, the canine H3N2 virus was introduced into the United States from Korea, and in 2017 and 2018, there were multiple epidemics that spread through many US states; these epidemics mostly stemmed from the new introductions of viruses from Asia, although there was some long-term transmission.

Seroprevalence studies detected antibodies to human H1 and H3 viruses in dogs in China. Moreover, reassortants between canine H3N2 and human influenza viruses have been isolated from dogs. Several cases of canine infections with highly pathogenic H5 viruses have also been reported although without significant transmission, and experimental studies have confirmed the susceptibility of dogs to H5N1 viruses. Under experimental conditions, dogs are also susceptible to H9N2 influenza viruses. Collectively, these data demonstrate the susceptibility of dogs to human and avian influenza viruses. Inactivated vaccines are available against the canine H3N2 and H3N8 viruses.

Influenza in Cats

Cats are susceptible to both human and avian influenza viruses. In Italy in 2009, an outbreak of A(H1N1)pdm09 viruses occurred in a colony of approximately 90 cats; half of the animals exhibited disease symptoms and 25 cats died. Serum samples were collected from 38 animals; more than half were seropositive. Infections of cats with A(H1N1)pdm09 viruses have also been reported in the United States and Canada.

In 2016, approximately 500 cats in large shelters in New York City became infected with an H7N2 low pathogenic influenza virus similar to viruses circulating in live-bird markets in the New York area in the late 1990s to the early 2000s. A veterinarian who treated sick cats became infected with the virus and experienced respiratory symptoms. A retrospective serosurvey demonstrated that 1 of 121 shelter workers tested was seropositive for H7N2 influenza virus. The novel feline virus and the virus isolated from the infected veterinarian replicated in the respiratory organs of mice and ferrets but did not cause severe disease. The feline H7N2 virus transmitted via respiratory droplets to exposed ferrets; in an independent experiment carried out by a different research group, the H7N2 virus isolated from the veterinarian did not transmit to cohoused ferrets.

In addition to the outbreaks described above, transmission of canine H3N2 viruses (see Influenza in Dogs section) to cats resulted in an outbreak in an animal shelter in Seoul, South Korea, with 100% morbidity and 40% mortality. Infections of cats with highly pathogenic H5 viruses have been reported in China and South Korea; and zoo tigers died after eating poultry infected with highly pathogenic H5N1 viruses, with probable virus transmission among the tigers. The experimental infection of cats with two low pathogenic North American avian viruses resulted in virus replication in the respiratory tract of cats; no signs of disease were observed. Seroprevalence studies in various cat populations in North America showed low rates of exposure to highly pathogenic H5 viruses but appreciable rates of seropositivity to human influenza viruses. The susceptibility of cats to human and avian influenza viruses may, in part, be explained by the expression of both $Sia\alpha2,6Gal$ and $Sia\alpha2,3Gal$ in the respiratory tract of these animals.

Influenza in Seals and Whales

A significant epizootic in seals occurred in 1979 and 1980, when approximately 20% of the harbor seal (*Phoca vitulina*) population of the northeast coast of the United States died of a severe respiratory infection with consolidation of the lungs typical of primary viral pneumonia. Antigenic and genetic analyses revealed that the influenza virus isolated from the lungs and brains of dead animals (A/seal/Massachusetts/1/80 [H7N7]) was of avian origin. This virus replicated to high titers in ferrets, cats, and pigs and caused conjunctivitis in humans. From June 1982 to March 1983, harbor seals along the New England coastline again died of viral pneumonia, which was caused by an avian H4N5 virus that replicated in the intestinal tracts of ducks. Harbor seals along the New England coast experienced another outbreak of pneumonia in September through December of 2011, when more than 160 animals died. The causative agent was an avian H3N8 virus that possessed mammalian-adapting features, such as the ability to transmit among ferrets via respiratory droplets and the PB1-D701N mutation, which facilitates the replication of avian influenza viruses in mammals (see The Replication Complex section). In the second half of 2014, thousands of seals died along the coast of Sweden, Denmark, Germany, and The Netherlands due to infection with an H10N7 influenza virus (closely related to avian H10N7 viruses from wild birds) and secondary bacterial infections. Ferrets infected with the seal H10N7 virus displayed mild disease signs. Serology studies and direct virus isolation have also revealed infection of several seal species with different influenza A and B viruses.

Influenza viruses of the H13N2 and H13N9 subtypes were isolated from the lungs and hilar nodes of a stranded pilot whale. It is not known whether the influenza virus infection caused or contributed to the stranding of this whale. In addition, H1N3 viruses have been isolated from lung and liver samples of whales from the South Pacific.

Influenza in Mink

Mink are naturally susceptible to infection with human and avian influenza viruses. Avian influenza viruses of the H10N4 subtype killed mink in Sweden and spread to contact animals. In 2006, respiratory problems were noticed among mink in mink farms in Canada; subsequently, an influenza A virus was isolated from one animal with clinical signs. Further analysis identified the virus as a swine triple reassortant H3N2 virus. Another outbreak in a mink farm in the United States in 2010 was caused by a reassortant H1N2 virus. Moreover, HPAI H5N1 viruses have been isolated from dead mink in China; these viruses were also pathogenic in experimentally infected mice. Seroprevalence studies indicate high levels of exposure to avian H9N2 influenza viruses in Chinese mink populations. Two different H9N2 influenza viruses isolated from a Chinese mink farm in 2014 were tested in mice: one virus caused weight loss and 20% mortality in experimentally infected mice, whereas the other virus did not cause disease in infected mice. The virulent H9N2 virus encoded PB2-701N, a mammalian-adapted marker (see The Replication Complex section). Seroprevalence studies also indicate exposure of free-ranging mink in Spain to influenza viruses. Influenza viruses of human, swine, avian, and equine origin replicate in experimentally infected mink, and transmission to cage mates has been observed for some of these viruses.

Influenza in Bats

In 2012 and 2013, two new influenza virus genomic sequences were identified in yellow-shouldered bats in Guatemala and in flat-faced fruit bats in Peru, respectively.[141,142] Based on sequence and phylogenetic analyses, the viral sequences were provisionally designated as H17N10 and H18N11 subtypes, respectively. Serologic studies demonstrated antibodies to H17N10 and H18N11 viruses in bat populations; however, to date, no H17N10 or H18N11 live virus has been isolated from bats.

Initial attempts to generate live bat influenza viruses by employing reverse genetics failed. However, the *in vitro* characterization of bat influenza virus proteins and the characterization of reassortant viruses possessing one or several bat influenza virus genomic segments combined with the remaining genomic segments of conventional influenza viruses revealed that the polymerase complex of bat influenza viruses can catalyze the replication of vRNAs of conventional influenza A virus and that the bat influenza NS1 protein possesses RNA-binding and interferon-inhibiting activity similar to that of conventional influenza A viruses. The studies with reassortant viruses also revealed an incompatibility between conventional influenza A and bat influenza viruses at the level of vRNA packaging into new virions. The N10 and N11 NA proteins bear structural similarity with the NA proteins of conventional influenza A viruses, but the putative active site is wider than that of conventional NA proteins and lacks sialidase activity. Currently, the role of the bat influenza NA–like protein in the viral life cycle is not known. The H17 and H18 HA proteins are structurally similar to H1 to H16 HA proteins but lack the amino acids known to determine the receptor-binding specificity of conventional influenza A viruses. In fact, microarrays with hundreds of different glycans did not identify sialylglycopolymers that bind to the H17 and H18 HAs. The cellular receptor of bat influenza viruses may therefore differ from the sialic acids to which conventional influenza A viruses bind. In line with these findings, H17 and H18 HAs do not bind efficiently to MDCK cells, which are routinely used for the propagation of conventional influenza A viruses. However, the H17 and H18 HAs bind efficiently to MDCKII cells, which are derived from MDCK cells but differ from them in their passage history. With the identification of a cell line that supported H17 and H18 HA binding, both viruses were generated by reverse genetics. Further studies revealed that the bat influenza viruses infected MDCKII cells via the basolateral site, whereas conventional influenza A viruses infect polarized cells from the apical site. Recently, the MHC-II HLA-DR complex has been identified as the cellular receptor of bat influenza viruses; this finding will open the door for additional studies on the host range of bat influenza viruses.

Experimental Infections

Mice

Although mice are not naturally infected, they can be experimentally infected with influenza A or B viruses. Most human influenza viruses cause indiscernible infection of the upper and lower respiratory tract and do not cause lethal disease without adaptation, although A(H1N1)pdm09 viruses are more pathogenic than other human viruses.[58,88] Recent human H3N2 and influenza B viruses do not replicate efficiently in mice. Most avian influenza viruses will replicate in respiratory organs (but not cause lethal infections) without prior adaptation, most likely because of the presence of Siaα2,3Gal receptors in murine respiratory tissues. Notable exceptions include the highly pathogenic H5 and H7N9 viruses, which can cause lethal infections without prior adaptation. Most laboratory mouse strains are susceptible to infection with influenza A viruses and have been used widely to study the pathogenesis of and the immune response to influenza viruses. However, most laboratory strains lack the Mx gene, which plays a role in the innate host defense (see Mx Proteins section), and data obtained from laboratory strains may not therefore be strictly comparable to natural virus infections. Knockout mice are useful tools for deciphering the molecular basis of virus–host interactions. In addition, two genetically diverse groups of mice are now available to correlate phenotypes with genotypes. Based on eight genetically diverse founder strains, several carefully designed rounds of breeding between founder strains, and between their offspring, were carried out to increase the genetic diversity among these mice. Genetically diverse mice are available as Diversity Outbred (DO) or inbred (Collaborative Cross, CC) mice. These resources are now used to study the susceptibility of mice to various pathogens and the contribution of host genetics to the outcome of infection.

Guinea Pigs

Influenza virus propagation in guinea pigs was first reported in 1938 and then in the 1970s. Recently, guinea pigs have been established as a transmission model for influenza viruses.

Human, swine, and avian influenza viruses can be isolated from the lungs and nasal turbinates of infected animals, suggesting efficient virus replication; however, signs of disease such as weight loss and increased temperature are largely lacking, and no mortality was observed upon infection with H5/Gs/Gd or pandemic 1918 virus. The nasal tract and trachea of guinea pigs possess both avian-type (Siaα2,3Gal) and human-type (Siaα2,6Gal; see Receptor Specificity of Influenza Viruses section) receptors, whereas the lungs contain predominately avian-type receptors.

Syrian Hamsters

Syrian hamsters are susceptible to infection with human influenza A and B viruses. Importantly, recent human H3N2 viruses, which are restricted in their growth in mice, replicate in Syrian hamsters without prior adaptation. Human H3N2 viruses replicated in the respiratory tract of animals and caused pathologic effects, although no clinical signs of influenza virus infection were observed. Human influenza H3N2, A(H1N1)pdm09, and influenza B viruses are transmitted to exposed hamsters via respiratory droplets. Lectin binding studies have shown that the distribution in the respiratory organs of Siaα2,6Gal (i.e., human-type receptors, see Receptor Specificity of Influenza Viruses section) and Siaα2,3Gal (i.e., avian-type receptors) is identical to that of humans; that is, abundant human- and avian-type receptors were detected in the upper respiratory tract. In the lungs, human-type receptors were expressed on type 1 pneumocytes, whereas avian-type receptors were detected on type 2 pneumocytes.

Ferrets

Ferrets infected with influenza A or B viruses develop a febrile rhinitis. Upon infection with human influenza viruses, the lesions are usually confined to the nasal mucosa, but infection of the lower respiratory tract has been demonstrated. The pathologic changes of bronchitis and pneumonia resemble those seen in humans, which makes ferrets a valuable animal model to study various aspects of influenza virus infection. Unlike mice, ferrets can also be used to study the transmissibility of influenza viruses. The high susceptibility of ferrets to human influenza viruses may be due to the predominance of Siaα2,6Gal receptors in their upper respiratory tract. The genome of domestic ferrets has now been sequenced, which may aid in the characterization of the host responses to influenza virus infection.

Nonhuman Primates

Nonhuman primates can experience natural infections with influenza viruses. The rates of seropositive animals can be substantial among captive primates, most likely resulting from exposure to infected humans. Experimental infections with influenza viruses have been conducted with various old-world (e.g., rhesus and cynomolgus macaques, African green, chimpanzees, baboons, gibbons) and new-world (e.g., squirrel monkeys, tamarins, marmosets, capuchins) primates; rhesus and cynomolgus macaques are the most frequently used nonhuman primate species for influenza virus infection studies. Nonhuman primates have been infected with various human influenza A and B viruses, pandemic 1918 virus (or reassortants thereof), several avian influenza viruses including highly pathogenic H5N1 and H7N7 viruses, and the H7N9 viruses that emerged in China in 2013. These studies assessed the pathogenicity of influenza viruses in nonhuman primates, the effect of antivirals, the protective efficacy of approved or experimental vaccines, and the host responses to infection. In addition, immunosuppression models have been established to mimic the effect of immunosuppression on influenza virus infections. In general, influenza virus replication is confined to the respiratory tract. Infections with seasonal human influenza viruses typically cause few, mild signs of disease, whereas infection with A(H1N1)pdm09 viruses can result in high fever. Infection with pandemic 1918 virus resulted in severe disease that required euthanasia. Primates infected with highly pathogenic H5N1 viruses typically develop fever and visible signs of disease, and subsets of animal succumb to the infection. The severity of H7N9 virus infection ranges between that of infection with H5N1 and seasonal human influenza viruses.

MOLECULAR DETERMINANTS OF HOST-RANGE RESTRICTION AND PATHOGENESIS

Four influenza virus proteins—HA, PB2, NS1, and PB1-F2—are known determinants of host-range restriction and pathogenicity. Other viral proteins also participate in these events.

The HA Protein

The HA protein is responsible for virus attachment and the subsequent fusion of viral and cellular membranes. It is synthesized as a single polypeptide chain (HA0) that undergoes post-translational cleavage by cellular proteases. This cleavage is essential for infectivity because it exposes the hydrophobic N-terminus of HA2, which mediates fusion between the viral envelope and the endosomal membrane.[70]

HA Cleavage

HA is a critical determinant of the pathogenicity of avian influenza viruses, with a clear link between HA cleavability and virulence.[54] The HA proteins of highly pathogenic H5 and H7 viruses contain multiple basic amino acids at the cleavage site, which are recognized by ubiquitous proteases such as furin, PC6, mosaic serine protease large (MSPL), and transmembrane protease serine 13 (TMPRSS13). For this reason, these viruses can cause systemic infections in poultry. In cell culture, the HAs of these viruses do not need exogenous proteases to form plaques. In contrast, the HA proteins of low pathogenic avian and nonavian influenza A viruses, with the exception of H7N7 equine influenza viruses, contain a single arginine residue at the HA cleavage site and are cleaved in only a few organs. These viruses, therefore, produce localized infection of the respiratory and/or intestinal tract that is usually asymptomatic or mild. The tissue tropism of viruses is thus partly determined by the availability of host proteases to recognize and cleave the two types of amino acid sequences found at the HA cleavage site. The significance of HA cleavability for pathogenicity of avian influenza viruses is underscored by the finding that the acquisition of an amino acid sequence with multiple basic amino acids can convert low pathogenic strains to highly pathogenic strains, as occurred in Mexico in 1994 (H5N2), in Italy in 1999 (H7N1), in Chile in 2002 (H7N3), in Canada in 2004 (H7N3), in Mexico in 2012 (H7N3), and in China in 2016 (H7N9). Highly pathogenic

viruses can also emerge if avirulent viruses with a multibasic cleavage site lose a nearby glycosylation site, so that the cleavage site becomes accessible to proteases; this scenario resulted in the emergence of HPAI H5N2 viruses in Pennsylvania in 1983.

Two groups of proteases are responsible for HA cleavage. The first group recognizes a single arginine and cleaves all HAs. Members of this group include plasmin; blood-clotting factor X–like proteases; tryptase Clara; mast-cell tryptase; ectopic anionic trypsin I; tryptase TC30; miniplasmin; HAT (human airway trypsin–like protease); TMPRSS2 and TMPRSS4 (transmembrane protease serine S1 members 2 and 4, respectively); matriptase (a type II transmembrane serine protease); kallikrein-related peptidases 1, 5, and 12 (KLK1, 5, and 12, respectively; which are secreted serine proteases); and bacterial proteases. *In ovo*, a protease similar to the blood-clotting factor Xa that is present in allantoic fluid cleaves HA, which explains why influenza viruses grow efficiently in eggs. Tryptase Clara is secreted from specialized respiratory epithelial cells in rats and mice; mast-cell tryptase is found in mast cells, whereas ectopic anionic trypsin I is present is stromal cells in the peribronchiolar region. Tryptase TC30 has been isolated from mammalian airways. Similarly, the type II transmembrane serine proteases HAT, TMPRSS2, TMPRSS4, and matriptase localize to human airways and support influenza virus replication *in vitro* and/or *in vivo*. In TMPRSS2 knockout mice, H1 virus replication is substantially reduced, whereas smaller effects were observed for H3 viruses. Knockout of TMPRSS4 did not affect the body weight loss or survival of mice infected with an H3N2 virus. However, H3N2 virus titers and symptoms of disease were substantially reduced in double knockout mice lacking TMPRSS2 and TMPRSS4. The kallikrein-related peptidases 1, 5, and 12 are expressed in the human respiratory tract. These three peptidases differ in their preferred cleavage sequence: KLK1 cleaves H1, H2, and H3 HAs; KLK5 preferentially cleaves H1 and H3 HAs, whereas KLK12 cleaves H1 and H2 HAs most efficiently. Miniplasmin is a trypsin-type serine protease in the epithelial cells of the bronchia that cleaves HA downstream of the consensus motif Gln(Glu)-X-Arg. Cleavage of HA by plasmin can be augmented by the ability of the A/WSN/33 (H1N1) NA protein to sequester its protease precursor, plasminogen. Bacterial proteases can also activate HA, either directly or indirectly by activating plasminogen, a property that may explain the development of pneumonia after mixed infections with viruses and bacteria.

The second group of proteases that cleaves HA proteins comprises the ubiquitous intracellular subtilisin-related endoprotease furin and PC6. These enzymes are calcium-dependent, have an acidic pH optimum, and are located in the Golgi and/or *trans*-Golgi network. Two other ubiquitous type II membrane serine proteases (mosaic serine protease large [MSPL] form and transmembrane protease serine 13 [TMPRSS13]) have been identified that do not require calcium for enzymatic activity and support the replication of an H5/Gs/Gd virus in cell culture. The cleavage efficiency of these ubiquitous proteases is determined by the sequence at the cleavage site and absence or presence of a nearby carbohydrate chain on the HA molecule. The sequence required for the cleavage of HPAI HA is Q-R/K-X-R/K-R (X, nonbasic amino acid) in the absence of a nearby carbohydrate chain. The presence of a nearby carbohydrate chain requires insertion of two additional residues,

Q-X-X-R-X-R/K-R, or alteration of the conserved glutamine at position 5 or the proline at position 6, B(X)-X(B)-R/K-X-R/K-R (B, basic residue).

Introduction of multibasic HA cleavage sites into low pathogenic avian H6N1 or H9N2 viruses creates highly pathogenic variants. However, this finding is not universally applicable, as the introduction of multibasic HA cleavage sites into low pathogenic H5N1 or H3N8 viruses or into a human H3N2 virus did not create highly pathogenic viruses. Thus, a multibasic HA cleavage site seems to be necessary, but not always sufficient, for high pathogenicity.

Sialic Acid Receptors

Influenza viruses bind to sialic acids, that is, negatively charged 9-carbon sugars that typically occupy the terminal positions of glycoproteins or glycolipids. N-Acetylneuraminic acid (NeuAc) and N-glycolylneuraminic acid (NeuGc) are prevalent in many animal species, but notably humans and ferrets lack the latter. Influenza viruses differ in their recognition of these two sialic acid species. Most sialic acids are linked to galactose (Gal) or N-acetylgalactosamine (GalNAc) by α2,3- or α2,6-linkages (Siaα2,3/6Gal, Siaα2,3/6GalNAc) or to N-acetylglucosamine (GlcNAc) by α2,6-linkages (Siaα2,6GlcNAc).

Sialic acid receptors in humans

Early studies demonstrated that epithelial cells in the human trachea contain Siaα2,6Gal sialyloligosaccharides on their cell surface but lack those with α2,3-linkages.[20] Consequently, viruses with Siaα2,6Gal specificity (i.e., human viruses, which preferentially bind to Siaα2,6Gal), but not those with Siaα2,3Gal specificity (i.e., avian viruses, which preferentially bind to Siaα2,3Gal), bind to the epithelial cells lining the human trachea.[20] Data obtained with in vitro differentiated human epithelial cells from tracheal/bronchial tissues, as well as data obtained with "natural shotgun glycomics" (in which the glycans released from glycoproteins and glycolipids are separated by multidimensional HPLC to assess the natural sialylglycopolymers of the respective tissue), revealed a more detailed influenza virus receptor environment: Siaα2,6Gal

oligosaccharides are dominant on epithelial cells in nasal mucosa, paranasal sinuses, pharynx, trachea, and bronchi. Siaα2,3Gal oligosaccharides (in addition to Siaα2,6Gal) are found on nonciliated cuboidal bronchiolar cells at the junction between the respiratory bronchiole and alveolus and on type 2 pneumocytes lining the alveolar wall (Fig. 15.9).[127,148] Nonciliated epithelial cells express more Siaα2,6Gal oligosaccharides than do ciliated cells, which contain predominantly Siaα2,3Gal.[91] Collectively, these findings offer an explanation for the severe pneumonia observed after infection of humans with some avian influenza viruses and suggest that the limited human-to-human transmission of H5/Gs/Gd viruses likely reflects the restrictive replicative efficiency of these viruses in the upper portion of the respiratory tract, where transmission could occur via droplets generated by coughing and sneezing. Moreover, avian influenza viruses may be trapped by mucins secreted by goblet cells in the nasal passage, which are rich in glycans containing Siaα2,3Gal. Conversion to preferential recognition of the human-type receptor is required for efficient human-to-human transmission, an assumption supported by the finding that the earliest isolates of pandemic viruses preferentially recognized Siaα2,6Gal, rather than Siaα2,3Gal, sialyloligosaccharides.[92] One study found higher amounts of Siaα2,3Gal in the respiratory tract of children compared with adults, a finding that may suggest higher susceptibility of children to infection with avian influenza viruses. Another study reported predominant expression of Siaα2,3Gal in epithelial cells of the human eye, which may explain the conjunctivitis associated with H7 influenza virus infections.

Sialic acid receptors in other mammals

Epithelial cells in pig trachea contain both Siaα2,3Gal and Siaα2,6Gal (with the latter predominating), which may explain why this species can be infected by both avian and human influenza viruses. Moreover, NeuGc is found in pigs (but not in humans). For mice, one study reported the expression of both types of receptors in the trachea, lung, and other organs, whereas another study did not detect human-type receptors in these animals. Ferrets express predominantly Siaα2,6Gal

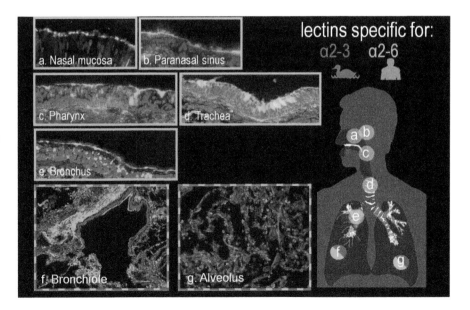

FIGURE 15.9 Expression of human virus (Siaα2,6Gal) and avian virus (Siaα2,3Gal) receptors in human respiratory tissue. The indicated tissues were tested with *Sambucus nigra* lectin (*green*), indicating the presence of sialic acid linked to galactose by an α2,6-linkage (Siaα2,6Gal), or with *Maackia amurensis* lectin (*red*), indicating the presence of Siaα2,3Gal. Cells were counterstained with DAPI (4,6-diamidino-2-phenylindole; *blue*). In the nasal mucosa, paranasal sinuses, pharynx, trachea, and bronchus, Siaα2,6Gal dominated. In the bronchiole and alveolus, both Siaα2,6Gal and Siaα2,3Gal were detected. The letters a–g refer to the respective area of the human respiratory tract. (From Shinya K, Ebina M, Yamada S, et al. Avian flu: influenza virus receptors in the human airway. *Nature* 2006;440:435–436, with permission.)

on cells of the upper respiratory tract. In the alveoli, both Siaα2,3Gal and Siaα2,6Gal were detected. In Syrian hamsters, the distribution of Siaα2,3Gal and Siaα2,6Gal is similar to that in humans with, for example, Siaα2,3Gal being expressed on type 2 pneumocytes in the lungs. The nasal tract and trachea of guinea pigs possess avian-type (Siaα2,3Gal) and human-type (Siaα2,6Gal) receptors, whereas the lungs contain predominately avian-type receptors. Equine viruses preferentially bind to Siaα2,3Gal sialyloligosaccharides, which predominate in horse trachea. These studies also demonstrated that epithelial cells in horse trachea express NeuGc in addition to NeuAc and that influenza viruses isolated from horses bind to oligosaccharides possessing NeuGc. Siaα2,3Gal is also found on epithelial cells in the respiratory tract of dogs and in the lungs of seals and whales.

Sialic acid receptors in avian species

The epithelial cells of duck intestine (where avian influenza viruses replicate) express predominantly Siaα2,3Gal,[57] although Siaα2,6Gal has also been detected. Likewise, both Siaα2,3Gal and Siaα2,6Gal have been detected in the respiratory tract of ducks, although Siaα2,3Gal predominates. The duck intestinal tract also possesses NeuGc, which appears to be absent in chickens. In the respiratory and intestinal tract of chickens, Siaα2,6Gal and Siaα2,3Gal are expressed. Similarly, both Siaα2,3Gal and Siaα2,6Gal are expressed on tracheal and intestinal cells of quail, turkey, pheasant, and guinea fowl, that is, species that may play a role in the adaptation of avian influenza viruses to mammalian species (see Role of Terrestrial

Poultry in the Emergence of New Influenza Viruses section). However, differences exist among poultry species in the relative abundances of influenza virus receptors in the different organs and cell types tested. Substantial amounts of Siaα2,6Gal were detected in the respiratory tract of pigeons, which are not known to play a significant role in influenza virus ecology.

Receptor Specificity of Influenza Viruses

The specificity of HA for the different sialyloligosaccharides is responsible for the host-range restriction of influenza virus. Human and classical H1N1 swine influenza viruses bind preferentially to Siaα2,6Gal, whereas most avian and equine viruses have higher affinity for Siaα2,3Gal.[19,35,92,120]

Receptor specificity is determined by the amino acids that surround the receptor-binding site. For H2 and H3 HAs, glutamine at position 226 and glycine at position 228 (H3 numbering; found in avian viruses) determine the specificity for Siaα2,3Gal oligosaccharides, whereas leucine and serine at these positions (found in human viruses) confer Siaα2,6Gal specificity[19,92,120,144] (Fig. 15.10). For H1 viruses, aspartate at positions 190 and 225 (H3 numbering; found in human viruses) confers binding to Siaα2,6Gal, whereas aspartate and glycine at these positions (found in swine viruses) allow binding to both α2,6 and α2,3 linkages; glutamate and glycine at positions 190 and 225 (found in avian viruses) are responsible for the interaction with α2,3-linked sialic acids.[36,73,92,134] In addition to these key residues, the amino acids at several other positions also affect receptor-binding properties. X-ray crystallographic structures of HA proteins in complex with receptor analogs are available

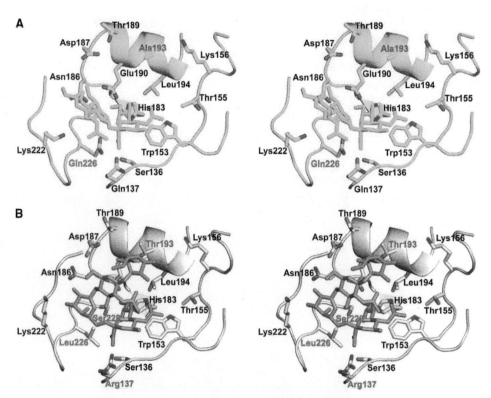

FIGURE 15.10 Structural models of HA–glycan receptor complexes. A: Interaction of avian H2 HA receptor–binding site (*magenta*) with avian-type receptor (*green*). **B:** Interaction of human H2 HA receptor–binding site (*gray*) with human-type receptor (*orange*). (From Viswanathan K, Koh X, Chandrasekaran A, et al. Determinants of glycan receptor specificity of H2N2 Influenza A virus hemagglutinin. *PLoS One* 2010;5:e13768, with permission.)

for human H1 to H3 HAs, avian H1 to H3 and H5 HAs, swine H1 and H9 HAs, H7 HA, and an avian H10 HA isolated from a person infected with an H10N8 virus; these structures provide detailed insights into the role of individual HA amino acids in receptor binding.

With the use of synthetic sialylglycopolymers and glycan arrays that allow the simultaneous testing of hundreds of carbohydrates and glycoproteins, a more complex picture of influenza viral receptor specificities has emerged. These studies have been complemented by approaches to catalogue the sialylglycopolymers in the lungs and/or respiratory organs of pigs and humans, including surface plasmon resonance, mass spectrometry, and natural shotgun glycomics. Collectively, these studies revealed that binding of influenza viruses to their receptors is not only determined by the linkage between the sialic acid and the penultimate sugar residue ($\alpha2,3$ vs. $\alpha2,6$) but also by the nature of the penultimate sugar (Gal, GalNAc, or GlcNAc), the length of the carbohydrate chain, and the inner core of the carbohydrate (such as the linkage between the second and third sugar residue, modifications such as sulfation, or other sugar residues such as fucose). Noteworthy differences exist between human and avian influenza viruses and among avian viruses. For example, viruses isolated from ducks, chickens, and gulls differ in their preference for the inner core structure of the receptor. Avian influenza viruses favor NeuAc$\alpha2,3$ attached to shorter carbohydrate chains over the same sialic acid attached to a longer chain; by contrast, human-adapted H1 and H3 influenza viruses bind to $\alpha2,6$ linkages preferentially in the context of long oligosaccharides. Avian virus HAs bind to their receptors in a narrow cone-like topology, whereas human virus HAs bind in a more flexible umbrella-like topology. Moreover, bi- and multiantennary glycans are bound by some viruses, most likely by two HA molecules within the trimer, which could increase the binding avidity. As a consequence of the steric differences between Sia$\alpha2,3$Gal and Sia$\alpha2,6$Gal linkages, biantennary binding is only possible with Sia$\alpha2,6$Gal, and not with Sia$\alpha2,3$Gal.[62] It has been speculated that biantennary binding could offset the reduced avidity of recent H3N2 viruses to Sia$\alpha2,6$, resulting from antigenic drift mutations near the receptor-binding site, which have weakened the interaction between the virus and the cellular receptor.

Receptor specificity of avian influenza viruses
H5/Gs/Gd viruses bind efficiently to Sia$\alpha2,3$Gal. Experimentally introduced mutations at position 190 or 225 (H3 numbering) that change the receptor-binding specificity of H1 HAs do not confer H5N1 virus binding to Sia$\alpha2,6$Gal; however, the introduction of human-type amino acids at positions 226 and 228 (H3 numbering) increase binding to Sia$\alpha2,6$Gal while retaining substantial binding to Sia$\alpha2,3$Gal.[133] The combination of the HA-Q226L and HA-G228S mutations with mutations detected in wild-type H5N1 viruses (such as HA-N186K or HA-S227N) results in even stronger binding to human-type receptors.

H5/Gs/Gd viruses isolated from infected individuals typically retain specificity for Sia$\alpha2,3$Gal. However, several H5/Gs/Gd viruses have been isolated that recognize Sia$\alpha2,6$Gal and Sia$\alpha2,3$Gal. This change in binding properties can be linked to several specific amino acid changes in HA.

All three ferret-transmissible H5 viruses described to date possess amino acid changes in HA that confer binding

to Sia$\alpha2,6$Gal. The experimentally introduced or *in vitro* selected sets of mutations differed (HA-N224K/HA-Q226L[55]; HA-Q226L/HA-G228S[52]; HA-Q196R/HA-Q226L/HA-G228S[10]; all H3 numbering) but shared the HA-Q226L mutation, which increases Sia$\alpha2,6$Gal binding for the HAs of other subtypes. Collectively, these findings indicate that the amino acid at position 226 of HA plays an important role in HA receptor–binding specificity.

Most of the H7N9 influenza viruses that emerged in China in 2013 encode the HA-Q226L (H3 numbering) mutation that increases binding to Sia$\alpha2,6$Gal; however, these viruses retained their ability to interact with Sia$\alpha2,3$Gal. One of the human H7N9 virus isolates, A/Anhui/1/2013, was extensively tested for its receptor-binding specificity and found to bind to biantennary sialic acids (see above). Typically, the H7N9 viruses that emerged in China in 2013 bind to cells in the upper and lower respiratory tract of humans and to type 1 and 2 pneumocytes. Three mutations in an H7N9 virus–derived HA (HA-V186K/G, HA-K193T, and HA-G228S; all H3 numbering) switched the receptor-binding specificity from Sia$\alpha2,3$Gal to Sia$\alpha2,6$Gal, resulting in a receptor-binding profile very similar to that of the prototype H1N1pdm09 virus, A/California/04/2009.

Poultry H9N2 viruses isolated in China in 1999 possessed mutations at positions 190 and 226 (H3 numbering) that conferred binding to Sia$\alpha2,6$Gal. Several low pathogenic H7 viruses isolated from avian species and humans in the United States in 2002 to 2003 and in Canada in 2004 showed increased binding to Sia$\alpha2,6$Gal, although they retained their ability to bind to avian-type receptors. In contrast, two highly pathogenic H7N7 viruses isolated from humans during the poultry outbreak in The Netherlands in 2003 bound to Sia$\alpha2,3$Gal.

Receptor specificity of human influenza viruses
The HA proteins of the pandemic 1918, 1957, and 1968 viruses originated from avian influenza viruses; nonetheless, the earliest available human isolates of these pandemic viruses already possessed Sia$\alpha2,6$Gal receptor–binding specificity,[19,41,92] indicative of strong selective pressure. However, early pandemic H3N2 viruses differ from more recent isolates in their amino acid sequence and their binding affinity for nonciliated cells.

For the pandemic 1918 virus, two variants have been identified that differ at amino acids 190 and 225 (H3 numbering): A/South Carolina/1/18 (possessing aspartate at positions 190 and 225, as is typically found in human influenza viruses) binds to Sia$\alpha2,6$Gal and transmits efficiently among ferrets, whereas A/New York/1/18 (possessing aspartate at position 190 but glycine at position 225) binds to both Sia$\alpha2,6$Gal and Sia$\alpha2,3$Gal and transmits with reduced efficiency compared with A/South Carolina/1/18.[41,144] Replacement of aspartate at positions 190 and 225 with the avian-like amino acids at these position—that is, glutamate and glycine—abolishes binding to Sia$\alpha2,6$Gal and transmission in ferrets.[144] The x-ray crystallographic structure of a 1918 HA protein in complex with receptor analogs demonstrates how this overall avian-like protein interacts with human-type receptors.[36]

The A(H1N1)pdm09 viruses possess aspartate at positions 190 and 225 (H3 numbering) and bind efficiently to Sia$\alpha2,6$Gal,[88] although one study reported dual recognition of both Sia$\alpha2,6$Gal and Sia$\alpha2,3$Gal. Molecular dynamic simulations of the H1 proteins of the 1918 pandemic virus, a swine virus from 1930, a seasonal human H1N1 virus from 2005, and the A(H1N1)pdm09 virus showed that lysine at position 145 and glutamate at position 227 (H3 numbering; found in the A(H1N1)pdm09 virus) increased the binding affinity for a human-type receptor and that aspartate 225 increased the number of hydrogen-bonding interactions compared with glycine at this position. An aspartate-to-glycine change at position 225 (H3 numbering) has been found in some A(H1N1) pdm09 viruses and appears to correlate with more severe disease outcomes in humans.[69] Few transmission events have been reported for this variant, suggesting that it does not transmit efficiently among humans. The aspartate-to-glycine change at position 225 arises during passage in eggs or adaptation to mice and increases virulence in mice. Experimental infection of pigs with a mixed population of viruses encoding glycine or glutamate at position 225 resulted in the selection of glutamate in viruses isolated from nasal secretions but glycine in viruses isolated from the lower respiratory tract.

As stated above, the receptor-binding specificity of human H2N2 and H3N2 viruses is determined by the amino acid residues at positions HA-226 and HA-228, with HA-226Q/ HA-228G conferring avian-type binding specificity, and HA-226L/HA-228S conferring human-type binding specificity (all H3 numbering). Glycan arrays in combination with x-ray crystallographic structures of 1957 pandemic H2 HA highlighted the significance of position 226 for H2 HA receptor–binding specificity. This was further supported by the finding that A/El Salvador/2/57, which possesses glutamine and glycine at positions 226 and 228, respectively, preferentially binds avian-type receptors and transmits poorly among ferrets, whereas A/Albany/6/58, which possesses leucine and serine at position 226 and 228, respectively, recognizes human- and avian-type receptors and transmits efficiently in ferrets. Moreover, a mutational study demonstrated a critical role for the amino acids at positions 226 and 228 in converting an avian H2N2 virus into one that binds human-type receptors. The amino acids at positions 137 and 193 also contributed to receptor-binding specificity.

Human H3N2 viruses encode HA-226L/HA-228S, which confer binding to Siaα2,6Gal. Viruses isolated in the 2000s have reduced affinity for both human- and avian-type receptors, which may be a consequence of an HA-L226V mutation, followed a few years later by the HA-V226I mutation. Thus, the currently circulating human H3N2 viruses encode an isoleucine at position HA-226. In addition, mutations have occurred at the surrounding residues (i.e., positions 222, 225, and 193), and crystal structures demonstrated that these amino acid changes affect the interaction between HA and the receptor. The changes in receptor-binding affinity are paralleled by altered binding patterns to red blood cells: essentially, human H3N2 viruses first lost their ability to agglutinate chicken red blood cells, followed by a loss of agglutination of turkey red blood cells. Recent human H3N2 viruses do not efficiently agglutinate any of the red blood cell species routinely used for hemagglutination assays, greatly affecting the characterization of these viruses. Concomitantly, human H3N2 viruses lost their ability to replicate efficiently in embryonated chicken eggs, followed by a loss of efficient replication in commonly used MDCK cells. Recent human H3N2 viruses are now typically propagated in MDCK cells

that have been modified to overexpress human-type receptors (see Virus Propagation section).

Glycosylation

Influenza virulence and host range are also affected by the number and location of oligosaccharide side chains, which are not conserved among strains or subtypes. HAs typically contain 5 to 11 glycosylation sites that affect receptor-binding affinity and/or specificity, antigenicity, innate immune responses, replication, fusion activity, virulence, and host range. For H1N1 and H3N2 viruses, the numbers of N-glycosylation sites have increased since they were introduced into human populations, most likely to shield the HA from antibodies. Also, H5 and H7 viruses isolated from terrestrial birds have more HA glycosylation sites than viruses isolated from wild birds. Two of the H5 viruses that acquired respiratory droplet transmissibility in ferrets lost the glycosylation site at HA-158 to HA-160 (H3 numbering) during passages in ferrets[52,55]; the third ferret-transmissible H5 virus naturally lacks this glycosylation site. The lack of HA-158 to HA-160 glycosylation affected the receptor-binding specificity and was critical for respiratory transmissibility in ferrets. The H7N9 viruses that emerged in China in 2013 naturally lack the glycosylation site at HA-158 to HA-160. HA glycosylation may also hamper the development of broadly protective influenza vaccines that elicit antibodies to conserved regions in the HA stalk. Several broadly reactive antibodies react with influenza viruses of group A, but not with viruses of group B, perhaps because of N-linked glycosylation at HA-38N in Group 2 HAs.

The NA protein is also glycosylated, but the number of glycosylation sites on human N1 and N2 NAs has remained relatively stable. For efficient virus replication, a functional balance between HA and NA is critical.

Role of Terrestrial Poultry in the Emergence of New Influenza Viruses

Terrestrial poultry, such as chickens and quail, are susceptible to infection with influenza viruses. Most influenza viruses circulating in wild birds are asymptomatic in poultry, but their continued circulation among terrestrial poultry can lead to viruses with increased virulence in these birds.

Adaptation of waterfowl viruses in terrestrial poultry may lead to the emergence of viruses that are better able to replicate in humans or pigs than their original counterparts due to altered receptor specificity. Support for this hypothesis comes from the finding that viruses isolated from terrestrial poultry resemble human viruses in their low affinity for Siaα2,3Gal relative to viruses isolated from wild birds. In addition, many of the H9N2 and H7N9 viruses isolated from terrestrial poultry bind to human-type receptors to some extent. The H5N1 viruses isolated from terrestrial poultry may possess an additional glycosylation site in HA that reduces the affinity for the receptor and a deletion in the NA stalk that reduces NA functionality and balances the functions of the HA and NA proteins. The presence of additional glycosylation sites and a deletion in the NA stalk are typical for human viruses and have also been found in different virus subtypes isolated from terrestrial poultry. Collectively, these data suggest that waterfowl viruses acquire certain mutations in terrestrial poultry, such as NA stalk deletions and additional HA glycosylation sites that may facilitate their transmission to humans or other mammals such as pigs.

Host Cell–Mediated Selection of Antigenic Variants

Historically, human influenza viruses have been isolated by virus amplification in the allantoic cavity of embryonated chicken eggs or by inoculation of samples into the amniotic cavity, followed by amplification in the allantoic cavity. In 1942, Burnet and Clarke first described "O" (original) and "D" (derived) variants that differed in their ability to agglutinate human or guinea pig erythrocytes after passage in eggs. The mutations acquired during egg passages typically cluster around the receptor-binding pocket of HA, resulting in reduced binding to Siaα2,6 and increased binding to Siaα2,3. This change in receptor-binding specificity likely reflects adaptation to the selective pressure in eggs with allantoic cells expressing Siaα2,3.

Subsequent studies established that the egg-adapting mutations in HA may also affect the antigenicity of viruses.[122] In fact, the low vaccine effectiveness of some H3N2 influenza vaccines has been linked to egg-adapting changes in HA. This is supported by findings that some vaccine recipients possess higher antibody titers to egg-adapted vaccine strains than to the circulating wild-type virus. Most influenza vaccine viruses are currently propagated in embryonated chicken eggs, requiring close monitoring of the potential antigenic effects of egg-adapting mutations in HA. Cell culture–based influenza vaccines are now available in several countries. Influenza virus amplification in these cell lines does not result in HA mutations that alter antigenicity; influenza vaccine production in cell culture may, therefore, be preferable to virus amplification in embryonated chicken eggs.

The NS1 Protein

The NS1 protein functions as an IFN antagonist that allows efficient virus replication in IFN-competent hosts,[38] in addition to having roles in the splicing and nuclear export of viral mRNAs and the enhancement of viral mRNA translation. NS1 interferes with type I IFN (IFN-α, IFN-β) synthesis and with the activation of IFN-induced antiviral factors. These functions are described in the Innate Immune Responses section.

The Replication Complex

The influenza viral replication complex comprises the three polymerase proteins—PB2, PB1, and PA—and the nucleoprotein NP (for a more detailed description of the functions of these proteins, see Chapter 14). The PB2 protein recognizes and binds to type I cap structures of cellular mRNAs. It has emerged as an important determinant of virulence and host-range restriction. Early studies suggested that the PB2 segment, in particular the amino acid at position 627, was involved in host-range restriction.[137] The significance of this finding in the context of interspecies transmission was not recognized, however, until 2001, when a substitution at position 627 of PB2 from glutamic acid (found in most avian isolates) to lysine (found in most human isolates with the exception of the A(H1N1)pdm09 viruses; see below) was shown to enhance the pathogenicity of an H5/Gs/Gd virus in mice.[48]

Multiple lines of evidence now suggest that PB2-627K is a major determinant of pathogenicity in mammals: (a)

PB2-627K leads to increased virulence of H5/Gs/Gd viruses[48]; (b) PB2-627K is critical for the respiratory droplet transmissibility of recombinant H5/Gs/Gd viruses in ferrets[52,80]; (c) PB2-627K is selected during the replication of avian H5/Gs/Gd, avian H7N9, and avian H7N7 viruses in humans; (d) H5/Gs/Gd viruses with PB2-627K have been isolated from mammalian species including tigers and cats; (e) viruses possessing PB2-627K were isolated after the adaptation of avian influenza viruses to mice, including HPAI H5, H7N7, and H9N2 viruses, and after virus replication in pigs; (f) PB2-627K has been found in viruses isolated from chickens and quail, suggesting that PB2-627K selection can occur in some avian species, which may facilitate the adaptation of avian influenza viruses to mammals (see Role of Terrestrial Poultry in the Emergence of New Influenza Viruses section); and (g) PB2-627K increases replicative ability in mammalian cells, particularly at the lower temperatures of the upper respiratory tract. Collectively, these findings suggest that PB2-627K provides a replicative advantage in mammals and is hence selected in these species. In particular, PB2-627K may facilitate PB2 adaptation to the mammalian form of ANP32A (acidic nuclear phosphoprotein 32 kDa); the differences between mammalian and avian ANP32A proteins were recently identified as a major host restriction factor of influenza viruses.[85] However, PB2-627K also emerged in H5/Gs/Gd viruses isolated from wild waterfowl at Qinghai Lake in 2005[12,82] (see Infections of Humans with H5 Viruses of the A/goose/Guangdong/1/1996 Lineage) and is maintained in descendants of the Qinghai Lake viruses to this day.

Considering the significance of PB2-627K for influenza virus replication in humans, the finding of PB2-627E (i.e., the avian-type amino acid) in A(H1N1)pdm09 viruses was unexpected; however, the lack of PB2-627K is compensated for by a basic amino acid at position 591.[96] In fact, PB2-627K does not provide a replicative advantage in the background of A(H1N1)pdm09 viruses. Structural analyses demonstrated that positions 591 and 627 are in close proximity and that a basic amino acid at position 591 alters both the shape and charges on the surface of the protein, which may affect the interaction of PB2 with other host and/or viral factors.

A second amino acid in PB2—at position 701—was first identified as a virulence factor of H5/Gs/Gd viruses in mice[77] and is now known to facilitate viral adaptation to mammalian species. Replacement of aspartic acid (found in most avian influenza viruses) with asparagine at residue 701 enhances the binding of PB2 to the cellular nuclear import factor importin α and facilitates PB2 nuclear import and replicative ability in mammalian cells.[34] This amino acid change was found upon adaptation of an avian H7N7 virus to mice; it also proved to be critical for virus transmission in guinea pigs. Like PB2-627K, PB2-701N is selected during the replication of H5/Gs/Gd and H7N9 viruses in humans but does not provide a replicative advantage to A(H1N1)pdm09 viruses.

Replacement of the avian-type threonine residue at position 271 of PB2 with alanine (i.e., the residue typically found in human influenza viruses) increases virus replication in mammalian cells and mice. The PB2 protein of the A(H1N1) pdm09 virus (which is of avian virus origin) encodes alanine at position 271, suggestive of mammalian adaptation. Another study found that the combination of three amino acid changes in PB2 (I147T/K339T/A588T) increased the replicative ability of a H5/Gs/Gd virus in mammalian cells and its virulence in mice to a level comparable to that of H5/Gs/Gd viruses encoding 627K. The percentage of H5/Gs/Gd viruses encoding the 147T/339T/588T residues in PB2 increased substantially between 2009 and 2012, and many of the circulating H5/Gs/Gd viruses now encode these residues. The residue at position 588 of PB2 has also been implicated in the mammalian adaptation of H7N9, H9N2, and H10N8 viruses.

The PB1 protein possesses conserved motifs found in all RNA-dependent RNA polymerases and is considered critical for the polymerase enzymatic function. In a minireplicon system, reporter gene expression was more efficient with avian than with human virus PB1 protein. Avian virus PB1 protein may therefore provide a replicative advantage over its human counterpart, an attractive hypothesis since both the 1957 and 1968 pandemic strains contained avian PB1 vRNA segments (in combination with avian HA or HA and NA genes). Moreover, in reassortment studies between H5/Gs/Gd and human H3N2 viruses, one of the most pathogenic reassortants possessed the avian PB1 vRNA segment. Reassortment studies also demonstrated a critical role for the pandemic 1918 PB1 vRNA segment in virulence in animal models. Studies with a recombinant H5N1 virus that acquired respiratory droplet transmissibility in ferrets (see Virulence and Transmissibility of H5 Viruses of the A/goose/Guangdong/1/1996 Lineage section) identified an H99Y mutation in PB1, which emerged during virus passages in ferrets; this mutation increased the viral polymerase activity and was essential for respiratory droplet transmissibility in ferrets.

The PA protein is an integral part of the influenza viral replication complex with a role in the cap-snatching process. Recent studies now also suggest a role for PA in the host adaptation of avian influenza viruses in mammals. For example, replacement of an avian virus PA vRNA segment with a human virus PA vRNA segment increased viral polymerase activity and mouse pathogenicity; a single mutation of T552S in PA was responsible for this effect. In another example, the PA vRNA segment of a A(H1N1)pdm09 virus conferred respiratory droplet transmissibility in guinea pigs to an H5N1 virus that otherwise lacked this ability.

In addition to the polymerase genes, the NP gene plays a role in host-range restriction[22] (see Mx Proteins section).

A large body of information has thus demonstrated that the composition of the replication complex affects viral pathogenicity. As a general trend, more efficient replication in minireplicon assays translates into increased pathogenicity in animal models.

The PB1-F2 Protein

PB1-F2 is a short protein of 87 to 90 amino acids that was discovered in 2001.[11] It is expressed from the +1 reading frame of the PB1 gene of most avian and human influenza viruses; however, human H1N1 viruses isolated after 1950 encode a truncated version of 57 amino acids. Most swine virus isolates (particularly classical H1N1 swine influenza viruses) do not encode a functional PB1-F2 peptide, due to several in-frame stop codons. These stop codons are also found in the reading frames of A(H1N1)pdm09 virus PB1-F2s, which likely originated from pigs; therefore, A(H1N1)pdm09 viruses do not encode a functional PB1-F2 protein. Reconstitution of full-length PB1-F2 expression in the background of A(H1N1)

pdm09 viruses had only minor effects on replicative ability and virulence in mice and ferrets, suggesting that PB1-F2 is not critical for the pathogenicity of A(H1N1)pdm09 viruses. The role of PB1-F2 in viral pathogenicity is discussed in more detail in the Innate Immune Responses section.

The NA Protein

As stated earlier, the structure and function of NA are discussed in more detail in Chapter 15. The sialidase activity of the NA protein removes sialic acid from sialyloligosaccharides, thereby serving two functions: (1) the removal of sialic acid from HA, NA, and the cell surface, facilitating virus release, and (2) the removal of sialic acid from the mucin layer, which likely allows the virus to reach the surface of the epithelial cells. The NA protein also has a role in host-range restriction and pathogenicity. Multiple studies now indicate that the length of the NA stalk affects pathogenicity; in particular, deletions in the NA stalk have been observed after virus replication in eggs and in poultry.

Notably, the NA activity of some avian viruses is more resistant to the low pH of the upper digestive tract than that of human- or swine-derived NA, a feature that may contribute to host-range restriction. Interestingly, low pH stability has also been reported for the NA protein of the pandemic 1918 virus. The NA protein of A/WSN/33 (H1N1) virus is critical for plaque formation in Madin-Darby bovine kidney cells and for neurovirulence; these two phenotypes are linked to the loss of a carbohydrate chain on NA and the presence of a C-terminal lysine residue. The lack of the carbohydrate chain at position 146 of NA (N2 numbering) allows the NA protein to bind to and sequester plasminogen, a plasmin precursor. This function facilitates HA cleavage and, thereby, virus pathogenicity in mice.

Like HA, the NA protein shows preference for certain types of sialyloligosaccharides according to the host species. Avian virus NAs cleave α2,3-linked, but not α2,6-linked, sialic acids. After their introduction into the human population, N2 NAs acquired the ability to cleave α2,6-linked sialic acids in addition to α2,3-linked sialic acids; however, the enzymatic activity for α2,6-linked sialic acids is significantly lower than that for α2,3-linked sialic acids. This acquired ability likely represents adaptation to the respective recognition pattern of the HA protein. NA substrate specificity is determined by the amino acid at position 275. Some NA proteins also have receptor-binding properties, a function encoded by amino acids outside the enzymatic site.

Although not directly related to host-range restriction and pathogenesis, the NA protein has recently (re)gained increased attention as a viral antigen. When administered as purified protein, NA is as immunogenic as HA. However, upon natural infection, antibody responses to NA are typically weaker than those elicited by HA, most likely because of the larger amount of HA protein compared with NA protein on the virion surface. Current vaccine preparations do not possess standardized amounts of NA and elicit low levels of antibodies to NA; current live attenuated vaccines in particular do not elicit substantial amounts of antibodies to NA. However, the addition of recombinant NA protein to vaccine preparations increased the antibody titers to NA. Higher titers of NA-inhibiting antibodies correlate with higher vaccine effectiveness and reduced disease severity. In addition, NA antibodies can confer intrasubtypic protection. It is now generally accepted that HA-and NA-specific antibodies are independent correlates of protection against influenza.

CLINICAL FEATURES AND PATHOGENESIS IN HUMANS

Pattern of Virus Shedding

Human influenza viruses replicate almost exclusively in superficial cells of the respiratory tract and are released from the apical surface of the cell, facilitating respiratory transmission. Alveolar macrophages and dendritic cells can also be infected and serve as antigen presenting cells for recognition by the adaptive immune system. Influenza virus replicates throughout the respiratory tract, with virus being recoverable from the upper and lower tracts of people naturally or experimentally infected with virus. As discussed earlier, the site of optimal growth in the respiratory tract for influenza viruses is in part determined by the distribution of the Siaα2,3Gal or Siaα2,6Gal sialic acid receptors.

A representative example of the pattern of virus shedding and cytokine responses of healthy adults experimentally infected by intranasal inoculation with influenza virus is shown in Figure 15.11.[50] The patterns of virus shedding in naturally infected individuals have not been measured as precisely but follow the same general pattern. Virus is first detected just before the onset of illness (within 24 hours), rapidly rises to a peak of 3.0 to 7.0 $\log_{10}$ tissue culture infectious doses 50 (TCID$_{50}$)/mL of nasal wash, remains elevated for 24 to 48 hours, and then rapidly decreases to low titers. Usually, virus is no longer detectable after 5 to 10 days of virus shedding. However, because of the relative lack of immunity in the young, more prolonged shedding of higher titers of virus is seen in children. Children also appear to exhibit heterogeneous shedding, with the top 20% of shedders estimated to represent 90% of infectiousness. In children, virus can be found for up to 13 days after the onset of symptoms. The higher titers and more prolonged shedding in children contribute to the important role of this population in the spread of influenza. While virus is typically confined to the respiratory tract, genome can be detected by PCR in peripheral blood in immunocompromised patients and may be a marker for more severe outcomes.

Pathology and Pathophysiology

Influenza A virus induces changes throughout the respiratory tract, but the most clinically important pathology develops in the lower respiratory tract. Bronchoscopy of individuals with typical, uncomplicated acute influenza has revealed diffuse inflammation of the larynx, trachea, and bronchi, with mucosal injection and edema. Biopsy in these cases has revealed a range of histologic findings, from vacuolization of columnar cells with cell loss to extensive desquamation of the ciliated columnar epithelium down to the basal layer of cells. Individual cells show shrinkage, pyknotic nuclei, and a loss of cilia. Viral antigen can be demonstrated in epithelial cells. Generally, the tissue response becomes more prominent as one moves distally in the airway. Epithelial damage is accompanied by cellular infiltrates primarily composed of lymphocytes and histiocytes. In more severe primary viral pneumonia, there is an interstitial pneumonitis with marked hyperemia and broadening of the alveolar walls, with a predominantly mononuclear leukocyte infiltration and capillary dilation and thrombosis. Influenza virus–specific antigen is present in type 1 and 2 alveolar epithelial cells, as well as in intra-alveolar macrophages[126] (Fig. 15.4).

Influenza infection causes the release of potent cytokines, such as type I interferons, tumor necrosis factor, and interleukins (ILs), by infected cells and responding lymphocytes. In fact, it has been suggested that an overly vigorous cytokine response to infection may contribute to the high fatality rate seen with H5N1 influenza[21] (see Human Infections with H5 Viruses of the A/goose/Guangdong/1/1996 Lineage section), sometimes referred to as a cytokine storm. On the other hand, defects in the cytokine response may increase the risk of severe influenza. Single nucleotide polymorphisms (SNPs) in the gene for interferon-inducible transmembrane 3 (IFITM3) have been associated with cytokine dysfunction and increased severity of seasonal influenza (see Effect of Host Genetics on Susceptibility to Infection and Disease Outcome section). Similar SNPs have also been identified as associated with increased severity of human H7N9. Carriers of the risk allele were shown to have decreased levels of CD8+ T cells in their airways during influenza infection, suggesting a critical function of this protein may be to promote immune cell persistence at mucosal sites.[1] Interferon deficiency related to mutations in IRF7 has also been contributory to severe influenza in a human child.

FIGURE 15.11 **Time course of virus shedding, symptoms, and cytokine responses of healthy seronegative adults after experimental nasal inoculation with wild-type A/Texas/36/91 virus. A:** Level of virus recovered from nasal wash, clinical symptom scores, and nasal mucus weights. **B:** Nasal cytokine levels measured by enzyme-linked immunosorbent assay (ELISA). In both graphs, multiple measurements have been combined for illustration, so that the y-axes are relative values only. (Data from Hayden FG, Fritz R, Lobo MC, et al. Local and systemic cytokine responses during experimental human influenza A virus infection. Relation to symptom formation and host defense. *J Clin Invest* 1998;101:643–649, with permission.)

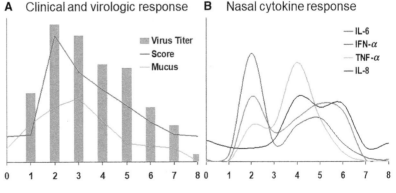

A Clinical and virologic response

B Nasal cytokine response

Day post inoculation with A/Texas/91 (H1N1) virus

A/Texas/36/91 10$^{5.0}$ TCID$_{50}$

Mutations in TLR3 and CD55 have also been associated with influenza hospitalizations or death.

Therapies designed to reduce the cytokine response have been beneficial in severe influenza in animal models, although this has not been tested rigorously in humans. However, a recent meta-analysis suggests that steroid therapy of severe influenza in humans is associated with increased mortality.[119] Commonly used statins also have anti-inflammatory properties, and an observational study has suggested that use prior or during hospitalization may be associated with decreased mortality. Because these drugs are very common, it has been suggested they may be useful in a pandemic response.

Clinical Features

Typical uncomplicated influenza often begins with an abrupt onset of symptoms after an incubation period of 1 to 2 days. The typical uncomplicated influenza syndrome is a tracheo-bronchitis with some involvement of small airways. The incubation period ranges from 1 to 5 days. The onset of illness is usually abrupt, with headache, chills, and dry cough, which are rapidly followed by high fever, myalgias, malaise, and anorexia, and many patients can pinpoint the hour of onset. The predominance of systemic symptoms is a major feature distinguishing influenza from other viral upper respiratory infections. Substernal tightness and soreness can accompany the cough. Fever is the most important physical finding. The temperature usually rises rapidly, concurrent with the development of systemic symptoms. Fever is usually continuous but may be intermittent. Typically, the duration of fever is 3 days, but it may last 4 to 8 days.

Physical findings in influenza are focused on the respiratory tract. Nasal obstruction, rhinorrhea, sneezing, and pharyngeal inflammation without exudate are common. Conjunctival inflammation and excessive tearing may occur. Small cervical nodes can be felt in a minority of cases. Chest radiograph and auscultatory findings are usually normal, although occasionally patchy rales and rhonchi are heard.

At the extremes of age, there are prominent differences in clinical presentation of influenza. Maximal temperatures tend to be higher among children, and cervical adenopathy is more frequent among children than among adults. Croup associated with influenza virus infection occurs only among children. Otitis media, croup, pneumonia, and myositis are also more frequent in children than in adults. Among older adults, fever remains a very frequent finding, although the height of the febrile response may be lower than among children and young adults. Pulmonary complications are far more frequent in older adults than in any other age group.

Lower Respiratory Tract Complications

Abnormalities of pulmonary function are frequently demonstrated in otherwise healthy, nonasthmatic young adults with uncomplicated (nonpneumonic) acute influenza. Demonstrated defects include diminished forced flow rates, increased total pulmonary resistance, and decreased density-dependent forced flow rates consistent with generalized increased resistance in airways less than 2 mm in diameter, as well as increased responses to bronchoprovocation. In addition, abnormalities of carbon monoxide diffusing capacity and increases in the alveolar–arterial oxygen gradient have been seen. Of note, pulmonary function defects can persist for weeks after clinical recovery.

Individuals with acute influenza may be more susceptible to bronchoconstriction from air pollutants such as nitrates.

Primary Viral Pneumonia

The syndrome of primary influenza viral pneumonia was first well documented in the H2N2 pandemic of 1957 to 1958. However, many of the deaths of young healthy adults in the 1918 to 1919 outbreak may have been were the result of this syndrome. In outbreaks since 1918, primary influenza viral pneumonia has occurred predominantly among persons with cardiovascular disease, especially rheumatic heart disease with mitral stenosis,[86] and to a lesser extent in others with chronic cardiovascular and pulmonary disorders and in pregnancy. The illness begins with a typical onset of influenza, followed by a rapid progression of fever, cough, dyspnea, and cyanosis. Physical examination and chest radiographs reveal bilateral findings consistent with the adult respiratory disease syndrome but no consolidation. Blood gas studies show marked hypoxia, gram stain of the sputum fails to reveal significant bacteria, and bacterial culture yields sparse growth of normal flora, whereas viral cultures yield high titers of influenza A virus. Such patients do not respond to antibiotics and mortality is high. At autopsy, findings consist of tracheitis, bronchitis, diffuse hemorrhagic pneumonia, hyaline membranes lining alveolar ducts and alveoli, and a paucity of inflammatory cells within the alveoli.

The trachea and bronchi contain bloody fluid, and the mucosa is hyperemic.[86] Tracheitis, bronchitis, and bronchiolitis are seen, with loss of normal ciliated epithelial cells. Submucosal hyperemia, focal hemorrhage, edema, and cellular infiltrate are present. The alveolar spaces contain varying numbers of neutrophils and mononuclear cells admixed with fibrin and edema fluid. The alveolar capillaries may be markedly hyperemic with intra-alveolar hemorrhage. Acellular hyaline membranes line many of the alveolar ducts and alveoli.

Secondary Bacterial Pneumonia

Secondary bacterial pneumonia is classically described as occurring as the patient is recovering from influenza. After a period of improvement lasting usually 4 to 14 days, fever recurs associated with symptoms and signs of bacterial pneumonia such as cough, sputum production, and lung consolidation. Secondary bacterial pneumonia was described following the 1957 H2N2[86] and 1968 H3N2 pandemics,[124] and available data suggests bacterial superinfections played a significant role in the mortality associated with the 1918 H1N1 pandemic. Bacterial superinfections were also frequently observed with A(H1N1)pdm09 infections, in particular with fatal cases[126] (Fig. 15.4).

The two pathogens that are currently most commonly associated with influenza are *Streptococcus pneumoniae* and *Staphylococcus aureus*, which is otherwise an uncommon cause of community-acquired pneumonia. Community-acquired, methicillin-resistant *S. aureus* has been seen in children following influenza, and recent study suggests that addition of a second active antibiotic may be important in children with MRSA complicating infection. *Haemophilus influenzae* and group A streptococci have also been associated with influenza.

Combined Viral–Bacterial Pneumonia

Clinically, this syndrome may be indistinguishable from primary viral pneumonia, except that the symptoms of pneumonia appear somewhat after the influenza symptoms and chest radiographs are more likely to show pleural effusions. Virus has been recovered from the lungs and pleural fluid. The case fatality rate for combined viral–bacterial pneumonia is 10% to 12%. Coinfection with influenza and *S. aureus* can have a fatality rate of up to 42%.

During an outbreak of influenza, many patients do not clearly fit into either of the aforementioned categories. The disease is not relentlessly progressive, and yet the fever pattern may not be biphasic. These patients may have primary viral, secondary bacterial, or mixed viral and bacterial infection of the lung. In addition, milder forms of influenza viral pneumonia involving only one lobe or segment have been described that do not invariably lead to death and that are more likely to be confused with pneumonia caused by *Mycoplasma pneumoniae* than to pneumonia produced by bacterial infection. Some studies have suggested that elevated levels of procalcitonin or C-reactive protein, as well as specific transcriptional profiles, can be helpful in distinguishing secondary bacterial from primary viral pneumonia.

The pathophysiology of bacterial superinfection has been studied intensively,[65] and a number of factors have been identified that could play a role. Uncomplicated influenza is associated with significant abnormalities in ciliary clearance mechanisms, resulting in reduced clearance of bacteria from epithelial surfaces. Alterations in polymorphonuclear neutrophils (PMNs) and mononuclear cells may also contribute to enhanced bacterial infection. In mouse models, the inflammatory response to influenza, particularly the type I interferon response, also contributes to the down-regulation of host antibacterial defense mechanisms. The cytokine IL-10 plays an important role in this regard. Influenza infection also reduces clearance by alveolar macrophages and weakens NK responses. In humans with H1N1 influenza, the development of pneumonia was associated with an early increase in regulatory T cells (Treg) in peripheral blood. All of these observations are consistent with the concept that the inflammatory response to influenza infection leads to disruption in the normal host defense against bacterial pathogens, although direct demonstration of this in humans is lacking.

Some bacterial infections could also increase the pathogenicity of influenza virus. There are strains of *S. aureus* that secrete proteases capable of activating the infectivity of influenza virus by proteolytic cleavage of the HA. These strains play a synergistic role in experimental pneumonia in mice. Such protease-secreting bacterial strains could be an added pathogenic factor in combined viral–staphylococcal pneumonias in humans. An apparent increase in combined viral–bacterial pneumonias was being noted with the 2003 to 2004 influenza A H3N2 epidemic, perhaps coincident with the rapidly increasing impact of staphylococcal disease and emergence of methicillin-resistant *S. aureus*.[61]

Other Pulmonary Complications

In addition to pneumonia, other pulmonary complications of influenza have been recognized. Bronchiolitis may also occur as a result of influenza A or B virus infection, but respiratory syncytial virus and parainfluenza virus type C are more important causes of bronchiolitis. Significant numbers of cases of croup occur in influenza A and B outbreaks. Croup associated with influenza A virus appears to be more severe but less frequent than that associated with parainfluenza virus types A or

C or respiratory syncytial virus infections. Acute exacerbation of chronic bronchitis is a common complication of influenza and may result in a permanent loss of pulmonary function. Exacerbations of asthma and worsening pulmonary function in children with cystic fibrosis may also occur.

Extrapulmonary Manifestations
Myositis

Myositis and myoglobinuria with tender leg muscles and elevated serum creatine phosphokinase (CPK) levels have been reported, mostly in children, but they can occur in adults as well. Symptoms may be sufficiently severe to interfere with walking. Although influenza virus has been recovered from muscle, the relation between the virus and myositis remains unclear. Onset of myositis occurs as respiratory illness wanes. The course is usually benign and reversible, and light microscopic changes of muscle necrosis and inflammatory cell infiltrates are seen.

Cardiac Involvement

Both myocarditis and pericarditis have been rarely associated with influenza A or B virus infection, although not observed at autopsy among those who died of primary influenza viral pneumonia. Myocardial infarction may also be triggered by influenza infection, possibly as an effect on platelet aggregation. Recent studies have showed a substantially increased risk of myocardial infarction in the 7 days following hospitalization for influenza.[76]

Reye Syndrome

Reye syndrome is a rapidly progressive noninflammatory encephalopathy and fatty infiltration of the viscera, especially the liver, which results in severe hepatic dysfunction with elevated serum transaminase and ammonia levels. This syndrome is seen following respiratory, varicella, and gastrointestinal viral infections. The onset of the central nervous system (CNS) and hepatic symptoms usually begins as respiratory tract symptoms wane. The etiology and pathogenesis of this syndrome are unknown; however salicylate administration is a critical cofactor. There has been a dramatic decrease in Reye syndrome cases in the United States associated with reduced use of salicylates, which are now widely recognized to be contraindicated in influenza virus infection. Children who require continuous aspirin therapy are an important target group for influenza vaccination to reduce the risks of Reye syndrome.

Central Nervous System Involvement

A wide spectrum of CNS disease has been observed during influenza A and B virus infections in humans, ranging from irritability, drowsiness, boisterousness, and confusion to serious manifestations such as psychosis, delirium, and coma. Febrile convulsions leading to hospitalization occur in children with and without underlying CNS abnormalities. The pathogenesis of these CNS symptoms is unclear. Nonspecific metabolic effects such as hypoxia resulting from severe pulmonary infection may contribute to the CNS signs and symptoms.

Encephalopathy can occur during influenza, typically at the height of illness and may be fatal. A subset of influenza encephalopathy has been described extensively in Japan and seen in other countries as an acute necrotizing encephalopathy with bilateral thalamic and cerebellar involvement.[106,156]

The syndrome of encephalitis lethargica followed by postinfluenzal encephalitic Parkinson disease was associated with the influenza epidemics of 1918 and the epidemics that followed. Experiments in animals suggest that avian H5N1 viruses can cause pathology similar to Parkinson disease.

Guillain-Barré syndrome has been reported to occur after influenza A infection, as it has after numerous other infections. In addition, cases of transverse myelitis and encephalitis have occurred rarely. Most cases occur in children, but associated morbidity is higher in adults.[106]

Toxic Shock Syndrome

Toxic shock has occurred in previously healthy children and adults during outbreaks of influenza A or B, presumably because viral infection changed colonization and replication characteristics of the toxin-producing staphylococcus.

Infection During Pregnancy

The increased risk of influenza during pregnancy was dramatically demonstrated during the 2009 pandemic. Previous studies had identified an increased risk of hospitalization associated with influenza epidemics during pregnancy, especially in the second and third trimester and in the immediate postpartum period. During the pandemic, women in each stage of pregnancy, or in the immediate postpartum period, were significantly over represented among those admitted to hospitals and ICUs. A recent meta-analysis has suggested that the overall risk of influenza related hospitalization was more than twice as great during pregnancy. The mechanism(s) by which pregnancy enhances the risk of influenza is not clear but might include the increased cardiovascular demands of pregnancy as well as hormonally mediated changes to the innate and adaptive immune response. Influenza virus itself has not been implicated as a cause of congenital defects and no consistent association between specific defects or malignancies and influenza epidemics has emerged.

Infection in Immunosuppressed Patients

Influenza has been noted to cause severe disease with an increased incidence of pneumonia in immunosuppressed children with cancer, particularly in bone marrow transplant recipients and leukemic patients. Relatively more immunosuppressed individuals early after transplantation appear to be at greater risk. Influenza virus shedding can be quite prolonged in immunosuppressed children, particularly those with HIV and low CD4+ counts. In general, T-cell defects appear to have a greater negative effect on recovery than do B-cell defects. Because of the prolonged, unchecked replication of influenza viruses in immunosuppressed individuals, resistance to antiviral drugs eventually occurs in many treated patients[56] (see Resistance to Neuraminidase Inhibitors section).

Influenza B and C Virus Infections

Influenza B virus causes the same spectrum of disease as influenza A, but the frequency of serious influenza B virus infections requiring hospitalization is about fourfold less than that of influenza A virus. Generally, years with predominant influenza B circulation are associated with lower rates of pneumonia- and influenza-associated hospitalizations and deaths. However, in children, myositis, Reye syndrome, and gastrointestinal symptoms appear to occur more commonly with influenza B than A virus infection.

Influenza C virus causes sporadic upper respiratory tract illness and is rarely associated with severe lower respiratory tract disease. By early adulthood, most individuals have antibody to influenza C virus, and most cases occur in children younger than 6 years of age. Although very young children may experience complications of bronchitis, bronchiolitis, and bronchopneumonia, overall influenza C virus is not a major cause of lower respiratory tract infection in children.

Innate Immune Responses

In vertebrates, innate immune responses are a vital first line of defense against microbes. Innate immune responses can broadly be divided into three steps: (1) microbe recognition by a pathogen recognition receptor (PRR), resulting in the production of type I IFN, chemokines, and cytokines; (2) activation of IFN-signaling pathways leading to the up-regulation of IFN-stimulated genes (ISGs), many of which have antimicrobial functions; and (3) the actions of cellular proteins with antimicrobial functions. Recent data also demonstrate high induction of IFN-λ upon influenza virus infection, suggesting a role for type III IFN in innate immune responses to influenza virus infections.

Microbes are recognized by PRRs, including toll-like receptors (TLRs), RIG-I–like receptors, and NOD-like receptors (NLRs). Recognition of pathogen-associated molecular patterns by PRRs results in the activation of signaling pathways that ultimately converge on the expression of antimicrobial genes. Influenza virus infection is sensed by TLR3 and TLR7, up-regulating their expression. RIG-I is activated by 5′-triphosphate groups on influenza vRNAs, resulting in the stimulation of IRF3, IRF7, and NF-κB activity. The inflammasome, a complex of a NLR and the ASC adaptor protein, is also activated by influenza virus infection. Inflammasome activation leads to the cleavage and activation of procaspase-1, which in turn cleaves and activates certain cytokines, particularly IL-18 and IL-1β.

Role of NS1 in the Modulation of Host Immune Responses to Viral Infection

Influenza viruses have evolved mechanisms to counteract the induction of antiviral responses, primarily through their NS1 protein.[38] NS1 interferes with antiviral responses through several mechanisms, including the following:

1. NS1 suppresses RIG-I activation[93,107,111,116] by interacting with it directly, by interacting with the RIG-I ligands TRIM25 and Riplet, and by sequestering double-stranded RNA.
2. NS1 expression prevents the activation of several transcription factors including IRF3, AP-1, and NF-κB, thus blocking IFN expression.
3. NS1 also controls IFN levels by blocking the splicing and polyadenylation of cellular premRNAs (including IFN-β mRNA). This function requires the interaction of NS1 with the 30-kDa subunit of the cleavage and polyadenylation specificity factor (CPSF). Two amino acids in NS1, at positions 103 and 106, are critical for CPSF30 binding and affect virulence.
4. NS1 directly binds to and blocks the antiviral factor protein kinase R (PKR), thereby preventing the phosphorylation of the translation initiation factor eIF2α, which is required for the translation of host proteins.

5. NS1 also binds to 2′–5′-oligoadenylate synthetase (OAS) and thus interferes with RNA degradation mediated by the OAS/RNase L complex.

6. NS1 interaction with NLRP3 prevents the activation of the inflammasome, hence preventing the activation of pro-inflammatory responses.

7. NS1 activates the PI3K/Akt pathway, which plays a role in the transcriptional regulation of ISGs and in the regulation of TLR-mediated cytokine production. The PI3K/Akt pathway is activated by the NS1 proteins of influenza A, but not by those of influenza B viruses.

8. The four C-terminal amino acids of some (but not all) NS1 proteins form a PDZ ligand domain motif, which is recognized by PDZ domain proteins. The amino acid sequence of the PDZ ligand domain motif can affect the virulence of influenza viruses, possibly because the proapoptotic function of some PDZ domain proteins is modulated by NS1 binding.

9. NS1 binds to several host proteins involved in the nuclear export of mRNA (including NXF1 and P15), a function that may contribute to the shutoff of host protein synthesis.

10. The amino acid at position 92 of NS1 affects the pathogenicity of H5 viruses in pigs (with aspartic acid conferring low pathogenicity and glutamic acid conferring high pathogenicity); the underlying mechanism and the potential involvement of innate immune responses are currently unknown.

11. Since 2000, most H5/Gs/Gd viruses possess a deletion of amino acids 80 to 84 in their NS1 proteins, which enhances virulence. Interestingly, H5/Gs/Gd viruses isolated in 2004 and 2005 in Thailand possessed both the 5-amino-acid deletion at positions 80 to 84 and the D92E mutation. In virus-infected cells, the 5-amino-acid deletion and the D92E mutation affect responses to TNF-α and the induction of IFN, respectively.

The PB1-F2 Protein

Depending on the virus strain and the length of the PB1-F2 protein, PB1-F2 increases viral pathogenicity, inflammation, and the frequency and severity of bacterial coinfections in mice.[11,93] These phenotypic differences likely result from the currently known functions of PB1-F2 in the modulation of host immune responses and the induction of apoptosis.

PB1-F2 modulates host immune responses by interacting with MAVS and other components of the RIG-I/MAVS signaling pathway, resulting in the inhibition of IRF3 and type I IFN induction. The PB1-F2/MAVS interaction may be regulated by CALCOCO2 (calcium-binding and coiled-coil domain-containing protein 2), which was recently identified as a binding partner of PB1-F2. In addition, PB1-F2 interferes with the activation of NF-κB–dependent signaling pathways.

PB1-F2 translocates into mitochondria via the Tom40 channel, the import channel of the mitochondrial outer membrane. PB1-F2 oligomers can form amyloid-like structures that disrupt membranes. Moreover, PB1-F2 interaction with the ANT3 (adenine nucleotide translocator 3) and VDAC1 (voltage-dependent anion channel 1) proteins induces the formation of membrane pores in mitochondrial membranes and subsequently changes mitochondrial permeability. The resulting induction of apoptosis, which is primarily observed in immune cells, may contribute to the increased virulence upon PB1-F2

expression. However, the induction of apoptosis may be strain specific and not the major function of PB1-F2.

PB1-F2 enhances inflammatory responses, as demonstrated by an increased influx of inflammatory cells into the lungs of mice infected with an influenza virus expressing the PB1-F2 protein derived from the 1918 pandemic influenza virus.[18] This PB1-F2 protein encodes serine at position 66, instead of the asparagine residue commonly found among human influenza viruses at this position. Serine at position 66 of PB1-F2 increases virus titers and pathogenicity, immunopathology, cytokine levels, and the severity of secondary bacterial pneumonia in mice, resulting in higher mortality. The virulence-enhancing effect of serine at this position has also been demonstrated for other influenza viruses, including H5/Gs/Gd viruses.

The PA-X Protein

The PA-X protein was discovered in 2012.[59] It is encoded by the PA vRNA segment and shares its first 191 amino acids with the PA protein before a ribosomal frameshift shifts the open reading frame into the +1 frame relative to PA. Consequently, PA-X has a unique C-terminus of 61 amino acids (the majority of PA-X proteins) or 41 amino acids (~25% of the PA-X proteins including those of the A(H1N1)pdm09 viruses). Only approximately 2% of PA mRNA transcripts undergo the ribosomal frameshift, resulting in low amounts of PA-X in influenza virus–infected cells.

The main function of PA-X is the degradation of host mRNAs, causing a shutoff of host protein expression. PA and PA-X share the endonuclease domain encoded in the N-terminal portion of PA (see The Replication Complex section); the endonucleolytic cleavage of host mRNAs contributes to the shutoff of host protein expression. However, the unique PA-X C-terminus in itself plays a major role in host RNA degradation, and several studies have implicated the first 15 and the last 20 amino acids of the unique PA-X C-terminus in this function.

PA-X acts as a modulator of innate immune responses. Loss of PA-X expression typically leads to increased viral replicative ability and apoptosis in cultured cells, increased induction of proinflammatory cytokines *in vitro* and *in vivo*, and increased virulence in animal models, although exceptions have been noted.

Host Defense Mechanisms

In addition to the host defense mechanisms that are counteracted by NS1 (see previous section), several other host defense mechanisms against influenza virus infections exist.

ISG15

Interferon-stimulated gene 15 (ISG15) conjugation to its target proteins is believed to alter the normal (enzymatic) function of those proteins. ISG15$^{-/-}$ mice are more susceptible to infection with influenza A and B viruses than are control mice. Mechanistically, conjugation of ISG15 to NS1 appears to impair the dimerization of the NS1 RNA–binding domain; disrupt NS1 binding to dsRNA, U6 snRNA, and PKR; interfere with NS1-mediated disruption of antiviral gene expression; and inhibit NS1 association with importin α. In contrast to the influenza A virus NS1 protein, the influenza B virus NS1 protein blocks the antiviral activity of ISG15 by interfering with the E1 ligase for ISG15.

Mx proteins

Mx proteins are IFN-induced GTPases of the dynamin superfamily. They have been identified in several mammalian and avian species; most, but not all, inhibit influenza viruses (e.g., the Mx proteins of chickens and ducks lack antiviral activity against influenza viruses) (reviewed in Reference[47]). Mx proteins confer resistance to influenza virus infections by interfering with viral replication. Murine Mx1 localizes to the nucleus and interferes with viral mRNA elongation, whereas the human Mx1 protein resides in the cytoplasm and blocks influenza virus replication through a mechanism that is not yet fully understood. Influenza viruses differ in their sensitivity to Mx proteins: in general, avian influenza viruses are more sensitive to inhibition by Mx proteins than are human influenza viruses. Mx1 binds to the influenza viral NP, and human influenza viruses have acquired mutations in NP that confer partial resistance to Mx1,[22] which explains the lower sensitivity of human influenza viruses to Mx1 inhibition. Most conventional laboratory mice lack a functional Mx gene. This fact should be taken into account when interpreting data obtained with such mice.

IFITM

The host interferon–inducible transmembrane (IFITM) proteins 1 to 3 localize to the plasma membranes and the membranes of lysosomes and endocytic vesicles. They block the cell entry step of a variety of enveloped viruses (including influenza viruses) by inhibiting the fusion of the viral and cellular membranes; the underlying mechanism is not fully understood.

MicroRNAs

MicroRNAs (miRNAs) are short, noncoding RNAs that modulate gene expression in eukaryotes by binding to their target mRNAs and destabilizing them and/or blocking their translation. Several studies have now been conducted to catalogue the miRNAs that are differentially regulated upon influenza virus infection and whose levels may correlate with the severity of disease. miRNAs can affect pathogen infections by modulating innate immune responses and/or by targeting pathogen mRNAs directly.

Several miRNAs bind to the influenza virus PB1 mRNA and regulate PB1 expression. Another miRNA targets the viral M1 mRNA. The expression levels of viral proteins can also be affected through indirect mechanisms: for example, one miRNA has been shown to affect the levels of two viral proteins by targeting the mRNA of a host protein (ARCN1) that plays a role in influenza virus entry and assembly.

A number of miRNAs modulate influenza virus-induced innate immune responses by regulating the activation of RIG-I, NF-κB, IFN-α/β, MAPK3, and IRF3/IRF7, among others. For example, infection with influenza viruses results in the up-regulation of several miRNAs that bind to the 3′-untranslated region of RIG-I, thus suppressing the activation of type I and II IFN and of ISGs. Currently, the mechanisms by which influenza virus infection modulates the levels of miRNAs are not understood.

Mitogen-activated protein kinase (MAPK) signaling pathways

Stimulation of PRRs activates the mitogen-activated protein kinase (MAPK) signaling cascades, which activate the expression of multiple genes, including factors involved in inflammatory responses. Several MAPK pathways have been extensively studied for their role in innate immunity, including the extracellular signal-regulated kinases 1/2 (ERK1/ERK2), the c-jun N-terminal kinase (JNK), and p38 pathways. These pathways are activated upon influenza virus infection and modulate viral infections through their roles in the expression of cytokines and chemokines. These effects differ depending on the influenza virus tested.

Effect of host genetics on susceptibility to infection and disease outcome

Genome-wide association studies (GWAS) based on the genomic data of groups of people have allowed the identification of single nucleotide polymorphisms (SNPs) that are associated with susceptibility to infection or the severity of disease. Alternatively, the genome of a single patient of interest (e.g., a person experiencing a severe infection) can be analyzed to identify rare mutations that may be correlated with the disease phenotype. These approaches have identified SNPs in IFITM3, IRF7 (IFN regulatory factor 7), and SFTPA/SFTPB (surfactant, pulmonary-associated proteins A and B) that are associated with the severity of influenza virus infections. SNPs in the carnitine palmitoyltransferase II (CPTII) gene are linked to influenza-associated encephalopathy.

Adaptive Immune Responses

Humoral Immunity

Infection with influenza virus results in the development of antibody to the influenza virus envelope glycoproteins HA and NA, as well as to the structural M and NP proteins. Some individuals may develop antibody to the M2 protein as well. As measured by enzyme-linked immunosorbent assay (ELISA), serum IgM, IgA, and IgG antibody to the HA appear simultaneously within 2 weeks of inoculation of virus. The antibody response is more rapid after reinfection. The development of anti-NA antibodies parallels that of hemagglutinin-inhibiting (HI) antibodies. Peak antibody responses are seen at 4 to 7 weeks after infection and decline slowly thereafter; titers can still be detected years after infection even without reexposure.[2]

Antibody to the HA can prevent attachment of the virus to the cell and neutralizes virus infectivity. A surrogate measurement of the neutralizing activity of serum is the hemagglutination-inhibition (HI) assay, in which sera is tested for the ability to prevent agglutination of red blood cells by a virus preparation. An increased risk of laboratory-documented influenza among those with the lowest titers of preexposure HI or neutralizing antibody is a consistent finding of most but not all studies. However, there is considerable uncertainty about the actual level of HA antibody that is the best predictor of protection, with estimates ranging from HI titers of 1:8 to 1:160 or higher.[8] Given the substantial variation from laboratory to laboratory in the estimation of the HI titer on the same set of samples, the inability to use an absolute value for protection is not unexpected. In addition, the amounts of antibody needed to mediate protection could vary by population, degree of exposure, age, and specific influenza type or subtype, although this has not been analyzed comprehensively. Most neutralizing antibodies are believed to bind conformational epitopes.

Studies evaluating the B-cell response of patients infected with novel influenza viruses, such as H5N1 or primary infections with pandemic H1N1, have identified B cells directed against epitopes on the stalk of the HA molecule.[66] The monoclonal antibodies produced by these B cells are typically highly cross-reactive among HA molecules within the same group, for example, group 1 specific antibodies reacting with H1, H2, and H5 viruses and group 2 specific antibodies reacting with H3 and H7 viruses. Some levels of stalk-specific antibody are present in the sera of most adults, and the role of these antibodies in protection in humans has not been defined. However, there is considerable interest in exploiting this observation in the development of broadly cross protective influenza vaccines.

Antibody to the NA can be measured by NA inhibition or ELISA. In contrast to anti-HA antibody, anti-NA antibody does not neutralize virus infectivity but instead reduces efficient release of virus from infected cells, resulting in decreased plaque size in *in vitro* assays and in reductions in the magnitude of virus shedding in infected animals. Observations on the relative protection of those with anti-N2 antibody during the 1968 pandemic,[97] as well as experimental challenge studies in humans, have shown that anti-NA antibody can be protective against disease and results in decreased virus shedding and severity of illness but that it is infection permissive.

Antibody to other influenza viral proteins has also been evaluated for potential protection. Antibody to M2 reduces plaque size *in vitro*, and passive transfer studies in mice have also suggested that antibody to the M2 protein of influenza A viruses may be partially protective if present in large enough amounts. The mechanism of protection *in vivo* is related to mediation of ADCC.[60] Antibody to internal viral proteins such as M or NP is also elicited by infection, but they are non-neutralizing. Studies in mice have suggested that such non-neutralizing but cross-reactive antibody may mediate protection under some circumstances. The mechanism by which antibody to viral proteins that are not exposed on the surface can mediate protection is unclear.

Infection with influenza virus is somewhat unique in that humans are repeatedly exposed throughout their lifetimes with influenza viruses that share many immunologic epitopes but differ in others. There is increasing evidence that the result of this repeated exposure is that the antibody response tends to be dominated by epitopes that are shared with the individuals' original exposure to influenza virus. This phenomenon of imprinting by prior exposure continues throughout life and impacts the susceptibility to infection and the response to vaccination.[99] For example, it has been suggested that the differential age-related impact of H7N9 and H5N1 may be related to prior exposures to group A (H1N1 and H5N1) or group B (H3N2 and H7N9) viruses, such that older individuals with childhood exposure to H1 are relatively more susceptible to H7 than H5, with the opposite effect is seen in individuals whose first exposures may have been to H3 viruses.[43]

Cellular Immunity

The induction of cellular immune response to influenza virus infection has been studied intensively in murine models, and such studies suggest that B-cell, CD4+ T-cell, and CD8+ T-cell responses all can play a role in protection against disease and recovery from infection. A large number of HLA class I restricted (CD8+ T-cell) and HLA class II restricted (CD4+ T-cell) epitopes have been described, and in situations where those epitopes are relatively well conserved on proteins such as

the polymerase, NP, and M proteins, the cellular responses are cross-reactive between subtypes, although not between types A and B.

Cellular immune responses to influenza vaccination and infection have not been studied as extensively in humans, but B-cell (memory B-cell and antibody secreting cell), CD4+ T-cell, and CD8+ T-cell responses in peripheral blood have been described after infection or vaccination. It can be difficult to capture the peak of the response as detectable increases in antigen-specific cells may only be seen in peripheral blood on a few days after exposure. Generally, the peak cellular response occurs somewhere between 5 and 14 days depending on the status of the subject and the nature of the response. As seen in murine models, a major component of the cellular response is directed at conserved peptides to which the subject has already been exposed during previous infections or vaccinations.

An important role of the cellular immune response in recovery from influenza infection in humans is strongly supported by the observation of prolonged illness and viral shedding in individuals who are lymphopenic as a result of disease or chemotherapy. However, it has been difficult to develop specific markers of T-cell immunity as correlates of protective immunity. Activated T cells, in the form of granzyme B–positive T cells, have been associated with protection in older subjects.[94] In the human challenge model, early studies identified virus-specific cytotoxic T cells as correlated with reductions in the duration and level of virus replication in adults.[95] In a subsequent study done many years later by the same group, pre-challenge CD4+ T cells, but not CD8+ T cells, correlated with relatively lower levels of viral shedding and symptoms following experimental infection.[159]

In community surveillance of healthy adults during the pandemic of 2009, and in a setting of low baseline antibody to the pandemic virus, CD8+ T cells were strongly correlated with protection against severe illness.[132] Under similar circumstances, the presence of NP-specific, predominantly CD8+ T cells was correlated with less symptomatic influenza.[51] In addition, an early CD8+ T-cell response is associated with successful recovery from severe H7N9 illness in humans.[152] The development of more sophisticated markers that can specifically identify reactive cells in peripheral blood will help to define the role of cellular immunity in protection, but the field remains limited by the lack of convenient access to compartments other than the peripheral blood in humans.

Mucosal Antibody Response

The majority of studies of mucosal responses to influenza in humans have concentrated on measurement of HA responses by ELISA or by neutralization tests, because nonspecific inhibitors of hemagglutination present in nasal mucus interfere with the standard HI test. These studies have demonstrated significant mucosal responses to infection with wild-type virus or live attenuated influenza vaccines. Both IgA and IgG are found in nasal secretions. Nasal HA-specific IgG is predominantly IgG$_1$, and its levels correlate well with serum levels of HA-specific IgG$_1$, suggesting that nasal IgG originates by passive diffusion from the systemic compartment. Nasal HA-specific IgA is predominantly polymeric and IgA$_1$, suggesting local synthesis. Local IgA antibody stimulated by natural infection is detectable for 3 to 5 months after infection, and there is local IgA memory for influenza antigen. After secondary infection, local antibody is also primarily of the IgA isotype, those with a local IgA response also have a serum IgA response, and the magnitude of the serum IgA HA antibody response correlates with that of the local response.

Studies in mice and ferrets have emphasized the importance of local IgA antibody in resistance to **infection**, particularly in protection of the upper respiratory tract. Polymeric IgA was shown to be specifically transported into the nasal secretions of mice and to protect against nasal challenge. Protection could be abrogated by intranasal administration of antiserum against IgA but not IgM or IgG. Local antibody has also been shown to play a role in protection against antigenic variants in mice. Studies in humans have also suggested that the resistance to reinfection induced by virus infection is mediated predominantly by local HA-specific IgA, whereas that induced by parenteral immunization with inactivated virus depends also on systemic IgG. Importantly, either mucosal or systemic antibody alone can be protective if present in high enough concentrations, and optimal protection occurs when both serum and nasal antibodies are present.

DIAGNOSIS

Clinical Diagnosis

Most cases of influenza are diagnosed based on compatible clinical symptoms and seasonal epidemiology. That is, when the presence of influenza virus is confirmed in a region or community, healthy adults with acute influenza–like illness most commonly have influenza. In fact, several studies have shown that the accuracy of a clinical diagnosis in healthy adults in the setting of an influenza outbreak is as high as 80% to 90%. In an analysis of symptoms in young adults being assessed for entry into studies of influenza virus treatment, the best multivariate predictors of laboratory-confirmed influenza virus infection were cough and fever,[98] with an increasing predictive value with increasing levels of fever. However, the predictive value of such a symptom complex may be less in older adults and in children.

Virus Isolation

Isolation of influenza virus in cell culture has traditionally been the definitive laboratory test to diagnose influenza infection. Virus can be isolated readily from nasal swab specimens, throat swab specimens, nasal washes, or combined nose and throat swab specimens or sputum samples. Over 90% of positive cultures can be detected within 3 days of inoculation and the remainder by 5 to 7 days. However, virus isolation requires specialized expertise and equipment and does not provide diagnosis within the timeframe of clinical decision-making. Thus, a wide variety of more rapid diagnostic approaches have been developed. Available diagnostic testing is updated frequently by the Centers for Disease Control and Prevention (CDC) on the Web site http://www.cdc.gov/flu/professionals/diagnosis/table-testing-methods.htm.

Rapid Influenza Diagnostic Tests (RIDT)

The most widely used rapid diagnostic tests are based on immunologic detection of viral antigen in respiratory secretions. In this approach, the sample is treated with a mucolytic agent and then tested with specific antibody that results in a color change or similar endpoint that is read visually. All of these rapid tests are relatively simple to perform and can provide results within 30 minutes, and many tests are eligible for Clinical Laboratory Improvement Amendments (CLIA) waiver and can be performed at the point of care (POC). The reported sensitivities of each test in comparison to cell culture have ranged between 40% and 80%, and they are somewhat dependent on the nature of the samples tested and the patients from whom they were derived. In general, sensitivities in adults and older adult patients tend to be lower than those reported in young children, who shed much larger quantities of virus in nasal secretions and therefore have much higher concentrations of antigen in their samples. Similarly, sensitivity is likely to be higher early in the course of illness, when viral shedding is maximal. Although all types of respiratory samples can be used in such tests, the sensitivity appears to be better with nasopharyngeal swabs and aspirates than with throat swabs or gargles. In some tests, the use of a digital readout can improve sensitivity compared to visual inspection. However, because of the relatively low sensitivities of these tests, their utility in clinical decision-making may be limited.

Polymerase Chain Reaction–Based Tests

PCR-based tests have the advantage of being potentially more sensitive than cell culture and allow detection in samples in which the virions have lost viability. In addition, it is possible to devise multiplex techniques so that a single test can detect a number of different agents, and many PCR methods allow rapid subtyping of the virus as well. For these reasons, real-time reverse transcriptase PCR (rtRT-PCR) has become the gold standard of influenza diagnostic testing and is generally available at clinical laboratories. Diagnostic sensitivities of the tests depend on the level of virus present in various specimens; generally, samples obtained by nasopharyngeal swabs have slightly higher sensitivity, similar to the findings with antigen detection tests. In some patients with lower respiratory tract disease, sputum samples or tracheal aspirates have been positive when nasal swabs were not. Swabs with wooden handles should be avoided for PCR diagnostic testing, as these can interfere with the chemistry of the assay.

Clinical laboratory–based PCR diagnostics will typically require transport of the specimen from the POC to the laboratory and typically take 3 to 4 hours to complete. Although highly accurate, this may not be useful for patient management, particularly in an outpatient setting. Therefore, there has been considerable effort to develop simple, rapid nucleic acid–based detection methods that could be utilized at the POC.

Rapid Nucleic Acid Amplification Tests (NAAT)

An alternative method of nucleic acid detection is isothermal amplification, which does not require a thermal cycler. A variety of isothermal amplification techniques have been developed, with the most frequently used approach being loop-mediated isothermal amplification (LAMP). These assays are highly accurate, on a par with PCR-based tests, and are rapid, giving results in less than 30 minutes.[4] Because they are simple to operate, they can be approved for use at the POC, therefore greatly improving their potential utility. However, these assays are currently expensive and not generally designed to identify other respiratory viruses.

Role of Viral Diagnosis in Clinical Decision-Making

Most cases of influenza, occurring in otherwise healthy individuals with typical symptoms during the course of a recognized influenza epidemic, do not need specific viral confirmation. However, diagnostic testing should be used if the results of the test will influence subsequent clinical management. This would include decisions regarding the use of antiviral agents, the need for antibacterial drugs, and considerations for infection control (reviewed in Reference[145]).

ANTIVIRALS

Several antiviral compounds—the M2 ion channel inhibitors amantadine and rimantadine; the NA inhibitors oseltamivir, zanamivir, peramivir, and laninamivir; and the viral polymerase inhibitors baloxavir marboxil and favipiravir—are currently approved in one or several countries for use in humans (for restrictions on favipiravir use, see below). Most influenza A and B viruses currently circulating in humans are sensitive to the NA and polymerase inhibitors. The currently circulating human influenza A viruses are resistant to the ion channel inhibitors, which are also not effective against influenza B viruses. Accordingly, ion channel inhibitors are no longer recommended for use in humans.

M2 Ion Channel Inhibitors

Amantadine hydrochloride and rimantadine, an analog of amantadine, were licensed for prophylactic and therapeutic use against influenza A virus in humans in the United States in the 1960s. These compounds are active against all subtypes of influenza A virus, but not against influenza B or C viruses. Amantadine and rimantadine are adamantane derivatives. They inhibit virus replication by blocking the acid-activated ion channel formed by the virion-associated M2 protein.[49] These compounds also inhibit the replication of viruses that have multiple basic amino acids at their HA cleavage site by inhibiting M2 ion channel activity in the *trans*-Golgi network, which prevents the premature low pH-induced conformational change of HAs cleaved by furin.

Until 2004, amantadine and rimantadine were used for prophylaxis and to treat infections caused by seasonal influenza A viruses. Before 2004, the rates of drug resistance among seasonal influenza viruses were low, although adamantane-resistant variants had been isolated from infected individuals. However, from 2003 to 2005, the rate of adamantane-resistant seasonal H3N2 viruses increased to more than 90%, typically conferred by a Ser-to-Asn mutation at position 31 of M2. At that time, many seasonal H1N1 viruses remained sensitive to ion channel inhibitors. In 2009, the seasonal H1N1 viruses were largely replaced by the novel A(H1N1)pdm09 viruses, which are resistant to adamantanes. Hence, the H1N1 and H3N2 viruses circulating in humans since 2009 are resistant to adamantanes, and the use of these compounds is no longer recommended.

Resistance to adamantanes is conferred by mutations at position 26, 27, 30, 31, 34, or 38 of M2, with mutations at position 27, 30, or 31 found most frequently. Structural studies of the M2 ion channel in the absence and presence of amantadine show that the channel is relatively narrow at position Val27 but opens into a wider cavity that is lined by Ala30 and Ser31 (among other amino acids), providing structural information on the effect of mutations at these key positions.

For H5/Gs/Gd viruses, the rate of adamantine resistance varies greatly depending on their geographic origin. With few exceptions, the H7N9 viruses that emerged in China in 2013 encode asparagine at position 31 of M2, resulting in resistance to adamantanes. Many European swine viruses of several lineages are resistant to adamantanes, likely because their M genes belong to the same phylogenetic lineage. The pandemic 1918 virus is sensitive to ion channel inhibitors.

Neuraminidase Inhibitors

The first NAIs included DANA (2-deoxy-2,3-dihydro-N-acetylneuraminic acid; Neu5Ac2en) and its N-trifluoroacetyl analog FANA, which were effective *in vitro* but did not inhibit replication of influenza viruses in animals. After resolution of the NA structure, DANA served as the lead compound in the rational design of drugs targeting the NA protein. All four currently approved NAIs bind to the catalytic site of NA and block its function. The compounds differ in their side chains, which affects their bioavailability, their binding kinetics to NA, and the rate with which resistant NA variants emerge.

Indications and Dosages

The NAI oseltamivir phosphate (US trade name Tamiflu®) was approved in the United States in 1999 and is also available in many other countries. It is effective against influenza A and B viruses and is currently approved in the United States for the "treatment of acute, uncomplicated influenza A and B in patients 2 weeks of age and older who have been symptomatic for no more than 48 hours" and for the "prophylaxis of influenza A and B in patients 1 year and older." It is available as capsules and for oral suspension. Tamiflu® is a prodrug that is converted in the liver into the active form, oseltamivir carboxylate. For therapeutic treatment, 5-day courses are recommended with 75 mg of Tamiflu® twice a day for patients 13 years and older; lower doses are recommended for pediatric patients. For prophylaxis, the therapeutic doses are recommended for at least 10 days; community outbreaks may require treatment for up to 6 weeks. Treatment with Tamiflu® may cause nausea and discomfort, and rare cases of serious skin reactions and neuropsychiatric events have occurred.

Zanamivir (US trade name Relenza®) was also approved in the United States in 1999 and is available in other countries as well. In the United States, it is indicated for the "treatment of acute, uncomplicated influenza type A and B infections in patients 7 years and older who have been symptomatic for no more than 2 days." The prophylactic indication is for patients 5 years and older. Relenza® is provided as a powder and administered by inhalation. For patients of all age groups, two daily inhalations (10 mg each) are recommended for the treatment of infections, whereas one daily inhalation of 10 mg for up to 28 days is recommended for prophylaxis. Because Relenza® is administered by oral inhalation, it is not recommended for patients with underlying airway diseases. In rare cases, Relenza® may cause bronchospasm, allergic reaction, or neuropsychiatric episodes.

Peramivir (US trade name Rapivab®) received emergency use authorization by the U.S. Food and Drug Administration from October 23, 2009, to June 23, 2010, during the 2009 H1N1 pandemic. It was permanently approved in the United

States in 2014 and is currently indicated for the "treatment of acute uncomplicated influenza in patients 2 years of age and older who have been symptomatic for no more than 2 days." Peramivir is also available in Japan, South Korea, and China. It is administered intravenously as a single dose of 600 mg for patients 13 years of age or older or 12 mg/kg (up to 600 mg) for pediatric patients 2 to 12 years of age. Patients treated with peramivir may experience diarrhea; in rare instances, serious skin reactions and neuropsychiatric events can occur.

Laninamivir octanoate (Japanese trade name Inavir®) was approved in Japan in 2010 for the treatment of patients over 10 years of age. In 2013, it was also approved for prophylactic use in Japan. It has completed phase III clinical trials in the United States. Patients 10 years of age or older receive a single inhaled dose of 40 mg, whereas younger patients are treated with 20 mg. For prophylaxis, a single inhalation of 20 mg is recommended for 2 days. Since Inavir® is effective in humans for several days, a single inhaled dose is sufficient to treat influenza virus infections. The prodrug laninamivir octanoate is converted to the active compound, laninamivir, in the respiratory tract. Gastrointestinal side effects, including vomiting and diarrhea, may occur.

Efficacy of Neuraminidase Inhibitors

The efficacy of NAIs in the treatment and prevention of influenza A and B virus infections has been assessed in a number of studies. In general, the initiation of treatment within 48 hours of the onset of symptoms is critical; however, treatment later in infection may still provide some benefit. For uncomplicated infections with human influenza viruses, these drugs reduce the duration of illness by about 1 day (if treatment is started early). In addition, the amount of virus shed appears to be reduced. Several studies suggest that treatment with NAIs also reduces the risk of severe complications.

The currently available NAIs are also effective against H7N9 and H5/Gs/Gd viruses. Clinical data from infected individuals suggest that treatment with NAI improves survival rates; early treatment was again noted as a critical factor. Based on these findings, NAIs are recommended by the WHO for the treatment for human H7N9 and H5/Gs/Gd virus infections. While treatment with NAIs improves the outcome of H7N9 or H5/Gs/Gd infections in humans, a significant percentage of individuals still succumb to the infection. One reason might be that treatment is not always started within 48 hours after the onset of symptoms. Higher doses and prolonged treatment with NAIs have shown additional benefits in animal studies and in infected individuals.

Treatment with NAIs does not appear to prevent the development of humoral antibodies, which is critical to protect against reinfection with antigenically similar viruses. Ferret studies have demonstrated protection against reinfection, and seroconversion has also been noted in individuals.

Resistance to Neuraminidase Inhibitors

Variants with reduced sensitivity to NAIs can be selected experimentally and have been isolated from patients treated with NAIs. Mutations that confer resistance to NAIs typically map to catalytic sites in NA (R118, D151, R152, R224, E276, R292, R371, and Y406; N2 numbering here and below) or to framework sites (E119, R156, W178, S179, D/N198, I222, E227, H274, E277, N294, and E425) that stabilize the active site.[149] NAI-resistant viruses have often been isolated from immunocompromised patients treated with a NA inhibitor. In this group of patients, delayed virus clearance results in prolonged virus replication and thus a higher risk for the emergence of drug-resistant mutants.

Among human H1N1 and H5N1 viruses, the most frequently detected resistance mutation is H274Y, which is primarily detected after treatment with oseltamivir. This mutation confers high resistance to oseltamivir and peramivir; however, zanamivir and laninamivir remain effective against H274Y mutants. Other oseltamivir-resistance mutations map to amino acid position 222; while these variants are sensitive to the other NAIs, double mutants possessing I222V/H274Y are moderately or highly resistant to all four NAIs. For human H3N2 viruses, frequently detected oseltamivir-resistant variants include those with R292K or E119A/V mutations. The R292K mutation confers resistance to oseltamivir, zanamivir, and peramivir, but not to laninamivir. The E119A mutation renders mutants resistant to oseltamivir and zanamivir, while the sensitivity to the other two NAI has not been tested. Variants encoding E119V are resistant to oseltamivir but can be controlled with the other three NAIs. Treatment with zanamivir or oseltamivir, respectively, resulted in the isolation of influenza B viruses with R152K and D198N mutations in NA; these mutants are resistant to oseltamivir, zanamivir, and peramivir.

Overall, resistance to oseltamivir is more frequently detected in treated patients than is resistance to zanamivir. This may be a consequence of the structural differences between zanamivir and oseltamivir, or it may result from the more frequent use of oseltamivir compared with zanamivir. However, several viruses have been isolated that are resistant to both oseltamivir and zanamivir.

The rate of resistance to oseltamivir among human influenza viruses remained relatively low until the influenza season of 2007/2008, when resistance was observed more often with H1N1 viruses than with H3N2 or influenza B viruses. During the 2007/2008 season, an increase in the number of oseltamivir-resistant H1N1 viruses was noted, and by March 2009, 1291 of 1362 seasonal H1N1 viruses analyzed had acquired resistance. Clinical data indicated that oseltamivir-resistant H1N1 viruses were comparable in their severity to oseltamivir-sensitive viruses, a finding that is consistent with studies in ferrets. In 2009, the oseltamivir-resistant H1N1 viruses were largely replaced by A(H1N1)pdm09 viruses. Among currently circulating H1N1, H3N2, and B viruses, approximately 1% are resistant to oseltamivir. Typically, these viruses are not transmitted efficiently, although small community clusters of oseltamivir-resistant viruses have been reported. Currently, most H7N9 and H5/Gs/Gd viruses are sensitive to NAIs, although several resistant variants have been isolated.

Early studies indicated that viruses resistant to oseltamivir are attenuated in animal models, so viruses resistant to NAIs were not expected to outcompete the viruses circulating at the time. Therefore, the rapid spread of oseltamivir-resistant seasonal H1N1 viruses in 2007/2008 was unexpected. However, these viruses possessed additional mutations in NA (V234M and R222Q) that compensated for the loss of viral fitness due to the H274Y mutation. Several pairs of NAI-resistant or NAI-sensitive viruses have now been compared in animal models: while most NAI-resistant viruses are attenuated, some are comparable in their pathogenicity and transmissibility to the respective NAI-sensitive variant.

Polymerase Inhibitors

Baloxavir Marboxil

Baloxavir marboxil (trade name Xofluza®) was approved in the United States and in Japan in 2018. It is indicated for the "treatment of acute uncomplicated influenza in patients 12 years of age and older who have been symptomatic for no more than 48 hours." It is available in tablet form and is administered at a single dose of 40 or 80 mg (for patients with a body weight of less than, or at least, 80 kg, respectively). The most common adverse reaction is diarrhea.

Baloxavir marboxil is a rationally designed prodrug that is metabolized to baloxavir acid, the active compound. It interacts with the PA subunit of the viral polymerase complex and blocks its endonuclease activity, which is critical to generate short, capped oligomers that serve as primers for influenza virus transcription[104] (see Chapter 14). In clinical trials, almost one-quarter of the drug recipients developed resistance to baloxavir acid, conferred by amino acid changes at position 38 of PA. Drug-resistant influenza A viruses were attenuated in their replicative ability compared to the drug-sensitive viruses, whereas drug-resistant influenza B viruses replicated to titers similar to those obtained with the drug-sensitive viruses.

Favipiravir

Favipiravir (T-705) is an antiviral compound that has completed a phase III clinical trial in the United States. In Japan, its use is highly restricted and limited to the treatment of "novel or reemerging influenza virus infections to which NAI or other antiviral agents could be ineffective." It has favorable pharmacokinetics and is recognized by RNA-dependent RNA polymerases as a purine analog. Consequently, it is effective against influenza viruses and a number of other RNA viruses. In contrast to ribavirin, favipiravir does not affect cellular DNA or RNA polymerases.

Combination Therapy

Several studies have assessed the potential benefits of combination therapies compared with monotherapies. In particular, the combination of inhibitors that target different steps in the viral life cycle could lead to synergistic beneficial effects and reduce the rate of emergence of resistant variants. Accordingly, combinations of NAIs and ion channel inhibitors have been tested for use against viruses that are sensitive to the latter category of compounds, such as H5/Gs/Gd viruses. The combination of amantadine and oseltamivir was well tolerated in volunteers and superior to monotherapy in terms of efficacy in mice. Similarly, the combination of rimantadine with oseltamivir, zanamivir, or peramivir provided additive effects in cell culture and mice. A triple combination regimen consisting of amantadine, oseltamivir, and ribavirin was superior to monotherapy or dual therapies in mice. Synergistic effects relative to monotherapy were also detected for several combinations of a polymerase inhibitor and a NA inhibitor including favipiravir/oseltamivir, favipiravir/peramivir, and baloxavir marboxil/oseltamivir.

Experimental Antivirals Against Influenza

Several compounds are in different stages of development as inhibitors of influenza viruses. Among them is FluDase (DAS181), a recombinant fusion protein of a bacterial sialidase with an anchor domain that mimics the sialidase activity of NA. In a phase II clinical trial, treatment with FluDase reduced virus load and shedding. Nitazoxanide (NT-300) is an approved antiparasitic agent that blocks HA maturation; it is currently being tested in a phase III clinical trial for its efficacy and safety in the treatment of uncomplicated influenza. JNJ63623872 (VX-787) inhibits the polymerase complex of influenza A viruses (but not that of influenza B viruses) by binding to the influenza A virus PB2 subunit. Phase II clinical trials demonstrated a reduction in virus shedding and a shorter duration of influenza symptoms relative to controls. Celecoxib, an approved COX-2 inhibitor, is undergoing phase III clinical trials in combination with oseltamivir for the treatment of patients with severe influenza virus infection. Monoclonal antibodies targeting the highly conserved stalk region of HA have gained attention because of their broadly protective potential; several candidates are now being evaluated in clinical trials. For two monoclonal antibodies, data from phase II clinical trials indicated a reduction in virus shedding following treatment.

VACCINES

Currently Available Vaccines

Multiple forms of influenza vaccine are currently available both in the United States and elsewhere, including virion- or protein-based inactivated influenza vaccines (IIV) administered intramuscularly and live attenuated influenza vaccines (LAIV) administered intranasally. Both types of vaccines are thought to work primarily by inducing antibody against the viral HA, although other mechanisms probably also play a role.

As described earlier, influenza viruses undergo continual antigenic evolution to escape from prior immunity. As a result, the match between the viruses chosen as components of the vaccine and the viruses that circulate during the season is an important determinant of the efficacy of that season's vaccine. Successfully matching the vaccine to epidemic requires a considerable effort devoted to worldwide surveillance and subsequent antigenic characterization of emerging new variants. A final decision regarding strain selection for next year's vaccine generally must be made at least 6 months before expected vaccination, for example, in February for the Northern Hemisphere and September for the Southern Hemisphere. The need to constantly update vaccine formulations, and readminister vaccine on a yearly basis, represents some of the biggest challenges in effectively controlling the impact of influenza.

The composition of the vaccine has changed over time to reflect changes in the epidemiology of influenza viruses. Since 1977, influenza vaccines have contained three strains representing the most up-to-date antigenic variants of A/H3N2, A/H1N1, and B viruses. Since approximately 2004, two antigenically distinct lineages of influenza B viruses, the Victoria lineage and the Yamagata lineage, have cocirculated. Therefore, quadrivalent formulations of vaccine containing both lineages were licensed beginning in the 2013 to 2014 influenza season. The nomenclature of influenza vaccines has changed to reflect this difference, with trivalent preparations now termed inactivated influenza vaccine-3 (IIV-3) and quadrivalent IIV-4.

Protein-Based or Inactivated Vaccines

The original influenza vaccine, which consisted of formalin-inactivated whole virions grown in embryonated chicken eggs, was demonstrated to have a protective efficacy of 70% in healthy adults[33] and licensed in 1945. Since then, although there have been several important advances in the techniques for producing vaccine, the basic vaccine strategy has remained the same. The development of the zonal gradient centrifuge allowed more efficient production and more highly purified vaccines from which reactogenic contaminants had been removed. Treatment of the whole virus with solvents to create "split" vaccines, or with detergents to create "subunit" vaccines, resulted in a vaccine with fewer adverse reactions, particularly fever, than the whole-cell vaccine. The efficiency of vaccine production was also improved through the development of techniques to create reassortant viruses adapted to provide high yield from hens' eggs. Since the late 1970s, egg-grown vaccines have been standardized to contain at least 15 μg of each HA antigen as assessed by single radial immunodiffusion (SRID) using antibody reagents prepared against the components of the vaccine. Embryonated hen's eggs are an extremely efficient substrate for the growth of most influenza viruses, and consequently egg production remains the primary mode of production for current influenza vaccines. However, while eggs are an efficient substrate for vaccine production, the process of adapting to growth in an avian substrate can result in mutations in the HA protein that result in significant antigenic differences from the original starting material and adversely affect vaccine performance in unpredictable ways[166] (see Host Cell–Mediated Selection of Antigenic Variants section).

One strategy to avoid the problems associated with egg-adaptation would be to produce the vaccine by propagating the viruses in mammalian cell culture. Currently, a vaccine produced in a qualified line of MDCK cells is licensed for use in individuals age 4 years and above in the United States. Other cell lines such as Vero cells and PerC.6 cells have also been explored for influenza vaccine production. Another alternative is to express the HA using an appropriate expression system. The expression of proteins in insect cells using recombinant baculovirus expression vectors can be achieved rapidly and results in proteins with mammalian-like glycosylation. A recombinantly expressed HA vaccine is currently licensed in the United States for ages 18 and above. This vaccine uses a higher dose of HA antigen per component (45 μg), although the reagents used for release criteria are different than those used for egg-derived vaccine.

Several attempts have been made to improve the performance of IIV in risk population such as older adults. A vaccine that uses four times the usual dose (60 μg per component) has been developed and shown to induce higher levels of antibody and improved protection against H3N2 viruses in older adults. The vaccine is produced in eggs and contains a single B virus lineage and is licensed for use in adults 65 and above. Another approach to improving vaccine performance is the use of adjuvants or immune stimulators designed to improve the response to a coadministered antigen. The squalene-based oil-in-water adjuvant MF59 has been shown to increase the immunogenicity of egg-derived influenza vaccine in older adults and has been licensed in the United States and elsewhere in this age group. MF59 adjuvanted vaccine is also currently being evaluated for potential improved efficacy in children.

Live Attenuated Influenza Vaccines

Live attenuated vaccines (LAIV) have a long track record of success against a wide variety of viral diseases, such as smallpox, measles, polio, and others, in part because they generate a diverse immune response that mimics the immune response to the pathogen. Developing live vaccines for influenza represents a special challenge because of the frequent antigenic changes in the virus. Creation of reproducibly attenuated antigenically variant LAIVs takes advantage of the principle of reassortment to generate attenuated vaccines for new antigenic variants using a vaccine master donor virus. The master donor viruses used in the LAIV currently licensed in the United States are the cold-adapted influenza A/Ann Arbor/6/60 (H2N2) and B/Ann Arbor/1/66 viruses. A quadrivalent formulation of these viruses (LAIV-4) is currently licensed in the United States and other countries for use in individuals ages 2 to 49. A second type of LAIV, based on the cold-adapted A/Leningrad/60 and B/Leningrad/66 master donor viruses, is also licensed in some countries.

Safety

Intramuscular Protein Vaccines

Hundreds of millions of doses of IIV are administered to adults, elders, and children each year, and the safety of these vaccines has been repeatedly confirmed. For example, no increase in clinically important medically attended events has been noted among over 251,000 children less than 18 years of age who were enrolled in 1 of 5 health maintenance organizations within the Vaccine Safety Datalink, the largest published postlicensure population–based study of vaccine safety. The most common adverse events reported following immunization with IIV are tenderness and/or pain at the injection site. Most injection site reactions are mild and rarely interfere with daily activities. Systemic reactions following immunization of adults with inactivated vaccine are uncommon. In placebo-controlled clinical trials in younger and elderly adults, rates of systemic reactions were similar among groups given inactivated vaccine or placebo.

Immediate hypersensitivity reactions (hives, wheezing, angioedema, or anaphylactic shock) following inactivated vaccine can also occur, and vaccine is considered contraindicated for persons who experienced a previous anaphylactic reaction following vaccine. However, recent studies support the safety of egg-derived IIV among persons who experience mild allergic reactions to eggs such as hives.[14] Current recommendations for persons with other forms of egg allergy such as history of angioedema or respiratory distress are that any inactivated vaccine may be used but that vaccine should be administered in a medical setting where emergent severe allergic reactions can be treated.

The Guillain-Barré syndrome (GBS), an acute inflammatory demyelinating polyneuropathy, was associated with the 1976 swine influenza vaccination campaign, with an increased risk of approximately 1 per 100,000 vaccinees. Subsequent studies have suggested a statistically significant but very slight increased relative risk of GBS within 7 weeks of influenza vaccination. A recent meta-analysis of 39 observational studies conducted from 1981 to 2014 confirmed a slightly increased risk of GBS following influenza vaccination.[89]

Pregnancy is recognized as a risk factor for more severe influenza, and pregnant women are an important target group for immunization. Most studies of pregnancy outcomes have found no association between vaccination and adverse pregnancy outcomes, although relatively less information is available regarding first trimester vaccination. Influenza vaccine is currently considered safe in all trimesters.

During the response to the 2009 pandemic, monovalent H1N1 inactivated vaccines were administered in several countries adjuvanted with the squalene-based adjuvant AS03. The use of the AS03 with A(H1N1)pdm09 vaccine was associated with an increased risk of narcolepsy during vaccine campaigns in Europe. Initially noted in Finland, this association has been established in multiple other locations where AS03-adjuvanted A(H1N1)pdm09 vaccines were used routinely in young children. The pathogenesis of this disorder involves presumably immune destruction of neurons in the hypothalamus responsible for synthesis of the neurotransmitter hypocretin. The mechanism that might link the use of influenza vaccine to the development of narcolepsy is unclear. An increased incidence of narcolepsy was also reported following H1N1 infection in China, suggesting that narcolepsy may be linked in some way to the specific antigen in the vaccine. Narcolepsy cases exhibited higher T-cell reactivity to a specific A(H1N1)pdm HA peptide and single-cell T-cell receptor sequencing has suggested that in some cases, narcolepsy may have been associated with molecular mimicry between H1 and the hypocretin protein.[87]

Live Attenuated Influenza Vaccines

LAIV based on the cold-adapted A/Ann Arbor and B/Ann Arbor viruses display three characteristic phenotypes: effective replication at low temperatures (25°C), reduced replication at high temperature (38°C–39°C), and attenuation in a variety of animal models. Multiple mutations in the internal gene segments contribute to these phenotypes. Studies using single-gene reassortants demonstrated that at least three of these gene segments (PB1, PB2, and PA) independently participate in attenuation in both animals and human subjects. For the influenza B/Ann Arbor virus, the PA, PB2, NP, and M gene segments contribute to the cold-adapted and attenuation phenotypes. The attenuated A/Leningrad/134/17/57 virus was developed through 17 sequential passages in embryonated chicken eggs at 25°C. It differs by eight amino acids from the parental virus, which map to the PB2, M1, M2, and NS2 proteins (one amino acid change each) and the PB1 and PA proteins (two amino acid changes each). The ts phenotype is conferred by mutations in the polymerase proteins. The ts phenotype of the attenuated B/USSR/60/69 virus is defined by mutations in the PB2 and PA genes. Because both donor viruses are attenuated at multiple sites, it would be predicted that the vaccines should be phenotypically stable even after prolonged replication in seronegative children, and this has been shown in clinical studies.

Cold-adapted LAIV based on the Ann Arbor master donor viruses have been well tolerated in adults and children, with mild nasal symptoms and sore throat occurring at rates slightly in excess of those in placebo recipients. However, wheezing has been consistently identified as a vaccine-associated side effect in young children, although occurring at low rates. In the largest trial, medically significant wheezing within 42 days of vaccination was reported in 3.8% of children less than 2 years old after receipt of LAIV compared to 2.1% in those who received IIV.[6] Wheezing generally occurs in the youngest, previously unvaccinated children following the first dose of vaccine. Because

of this observation, LAIV is currently approved for use in the United States for children ≥2 years old who do not have a history of asthma.

Safety of LAIV has also been demonstrated in some high-risk patient groups. No significant vaccine-related adverse events were seen in studies of children with cystic fibrosis or asthma, and vaccinated children with asthma did not experience significant changes in FEV_1, use of beta-adrenergic rescue medications or asthma symptom scores compared with placebo recipients. LAIV has also been well tolerated in adults with chronic obstructive airway disease and older adults although the vaccine is not recommended for use in these populations.

Transmission of LAIV to susceptible contacts does not appear to happen frequently. LAIV can be recovered from nasal secretions of about half of adult recipients, although generally shedding of LAIV by adults is of low titer and short duration. Transmission of LAIV from vaccine recipients to susceptible contacts has been rarely detected in studies of young children involved in day care–like settings. In the largest study, 197 children between 8 and 36 months of age in a day care setting were randomized to receive LAIV or placebo, and LAIV was detected in one placebo recipient. The estimate of transmissibility in this age group was 0.6% to 2.0%.[150] However, because of the possibility of transmission, LAIV is not recommended for close contacts of individuals who have levels of immunocompromised that require a protected environment.

Immune Responses to Vaccination

Intramuscular Protein Vaccines

Increases in serum HI antibody are seen in about 90% of healthy adult recipients of vaccine. Only a single dose of vaccine is required in individuals who were previously vaccinated or who experienced prior infection with a related subtype, but a two-dose schedule is required in unprimed individuals. Primed individuals also generally respond with antibody that recognizes a broader range of antigenic variants than do unprimed individuals. Serum antibodies peak between 2 and 4 weeks after vaccination but fall quickly, reaching near baseline before the next influenza season. Despite evidence that NA-specific antibody responses contribute to protection, neither the NA content nor the enzymatic activity of the vaccine is standardized, and NA-specific antibody responses are not routinely assessed.

Mucosal HA-specific antibody responses are generally not a major component of the response to parenterally administered inactivated vaccine. However, dose-related increases in mucosal HA-specific antibody responses have been observed following intramuscular immunization with increasing doses of a monovalent influenza A/H1N1 vaccine.

Cellular responses, including CD4+ T-cell responses are also noted after IIV, and there is a strong correlation between the CD4 T-cell response and the antibody response.[102] Baseline frequencies of influenza-specific, interferon γ–producing memory CD4+ T cells are higher in children who received more previous vaccinations. An increase in HA-specific CD8+ T cells on day 7 after vaccination has also been detected by tetramer staining in adults receiving IIV. While the induction of HI antibody is generally accepted as a correlate of vaccine protection, in some populations such as the elderly, it has been suggested that induction of cellular responses may also correlate with protection.[94]

Unimmunized young children generally require two doses of IIV given at least 4 weeks apart to generate substantial serum antibody responses. Once a child has been primed with two doses of vaccine, a single dose of vaccine is recommended in subsequent seasons regardless of age. While most children 6 months of age or older respond to vaccine after receiving the recommended number of doses, antibody responses in infants are reduced compared to older children. Reduced responses among very young children may be related to a combination of immaturity of the immune system and a lower degree of priming.

When compared with younger adults, the proportions of elderly subjects who achieve a putative protective HI antibody titer are lower. Both age and underlying conditions may contribute to these lowered responses. Unlike children, the administration of a second dose of vaccine in elders is not associated with improved responses. In some studies, the history of multiple prior vaccinations was better correlated to reduce vaccine responses than was age.[53] While the dose-response curve for seasonal influenza vaccine is rather flat, the administration of a fourfold higher dose (60 μg/HA) is associated with an improved serum HI response in elders and higher levels of antibody to the NA. The high-dose vaccine is licensed in the United States for use in adults over 65.

The MF59 adjuvant is also associated with improved antibody responses in older adults. While there is relatively little effect on the immune response to seasonal vaccines in healthy young adults, the oil-in-water emulsion results in an approximately 50% increase in antibody titers in older adults, and MF59 adjuvanted seasonal inactivated vaccines have been licensed for use in elders in Italy for several years. Recently, MF59 adjuvanted standard-dose inactivated vaccine was licensed for elders in the United States based on studies showing noninferiority of the immune response to that of standard-dose inactivated vaccine.

Individuals on immunosuppressive therapy, those with renal disease, and transplant recipients have impaired responses to vaccination. To be maximally effective, immunizations should be given before transplantation, should avoid the nadir of white counts, and should include vaccination of close contacts. Factors impacting the response in stem cell transplant recipients include the type of transplant, the time since transplantation, the use of myeloablative therapy as opposed to reduced intensity, the presence of graft versus host disease, and the specific immunosuppressive chemotherapy being used. In both allogeneic HSCT recipients and SOT types of transplant recipients, there is concern regarding whether the immune stimulus of vaccination, with or without an adjuvant, might nonspecifically stimulate increased severity of graft versus host disease or organ rejection. However, the weight of evidence does not support a significant association between vaccination and the development of autoimmune adverse events.

Live Attenuated Influenza Vaccines

Studies of the immunogenicity of cold-adapted reassortant vaccines have been carried out in children, adults, and older adults. The results of these studies are consistent with the hypothesis that the replication of cold-adapted vaccines in the upper respiratory tract, and hence their immunogenicity, is influenced by the susceptibility of the host at the time of vaccination. The frequency and magnitude of immune responses to vaccination are therefore highest in young children, intermediate in adults, and lowest in older adult subjects who have been repeatedly infected with influenza viruses throughout their lifetime. In addition, the mucosally administered LAIV is generally more effective than parenterally administered IIV at inducing nasal HA-specific IgA, whereas inactivated vaccine usually induces higher serum titers of HI and HA-specific IgG antibody.

Most susceptible children demonstrate measurable serum and mucosal HA-specific antibody responses. Mucosal responses have been demonstrated in up to 85% of young children after LAIV. In contrast, adults generally have a low rate of serum antibody response after LAIV and relatively lower rates of mucosal responses. Even in those prescreened to have low prevaccination vaccine–specific influenza antibody, the rates of serum antibody responses to intranasal LAIV in adults and older adults are low. Influenza-specific IgA and IgG antibody–secreting cells (ASC) peak on days 7 to 12 after either LAIV or IIV in both adults and older children and may be a more sensitive indicator of vaccine take after LAIV than antibody response. Influenza-specific interferon-gamma (IFNγ) producing CD4+ and CD8+ lymphocytes have also been detected following both LAIV or IIV.

The mechanism of protection induced by cold-adapted vaccine has mostly been evaluated in experimental infection studies. Cold-adapted vaccine is protective in these experiments in the absence of significant serum HI responses, suggesting that the main protective effect is induction of mucosal antibodies. Finally, an analysis of data collected during a large field trial evaluation of LAIV concluded that the postvaccination numbers of influenza virus–specific IFNγ producing T cells was the best correlate of vaccine-induced protection.[31] However, no definitive correlate of immune protection afforded by LAIV has been identified.

Efficacy (Results of Randomized Prospective Studies)

The ability of influenza vaccines to prevent influenza has been assessed in numerous clinical studies which vary greatly in design, populations, and endpoints. These studies have included prospective, randomized controlled studies, in which case they are referred to as efficacy studies, as well as a wide variety of nonrandomized cohort and retrospective study designs which assess vaccine effectiveness. Endpoints evaluated in these studies have included both laboratory confirmed influenza and nonlaboratory confirmed respiratory illnesses. In this regard, it has been recognized that studies that utilize a serologic definition of influenza infection may overestimate the efficacy of influenza vaccine, since it will be harder to demonstrate postvaccination to postseason antibody increases in the vaccinated group.[110]

Intramuscular Protein Vaccines

Randomized studies of inactivated vaccine efficacy against laboratory confirmed influenza have mostly been conducted in healthy adults. These studies have shown a wide range of efficacy, from approximately 40% to 80%, with lower levels of efficacy typically seen in years with apparent antigenic mismatch. For example, the efficacy of IIV for preventing culture-proven influenza A illness in adults was 76% (95% confidence interval [CI], 58%–87%) for H1N1 and 74% (95% CI, 52%–86%) for H3N2 in a controlled trial comparing live and inactivated vaccines.[27] Vaccination of adults is also associated with decreased absenteeism from work or school and is significantly cost-effective, but these benefits may not be seen in years when there is not a good match between vaccine and circulating viruses.

A recent meta-analysis of eight randomized, controlled trials in healthy adults during 2004 to 2008 estimated the pooled efficacy of trivalent inactivated vaccine (TIV) against culture-confirmed influenza to be 59% (95% CI, 51%–67%) among those aged 18 through 64 years.[108] The role of antigenic mismatch in the efficacy observed in these trials is unclear, and some studies in young adults have demonstrated high levels of efficacy despite a degree of antigenic mismatch. Recent studies using virus culture and/or PCR endpoints have demonstrated similar levels of efficacy for both egg-grown 78% and cell culture–grown TIVs (84%). The protective efficacy of the recombinant HA vaccine in healthy adults was approximately 47% in healthy adults in a study done in a single season with significant antigenic mismatch.

Although annual vaccination of elders and other high-risk persons has been recommended for many years, there are few randomized trials demonstrating absolute efficacy in these groups, in part because the existing vaccine recommendations make it difficult to do studies using a placebo group. In the most commonly referenced study, TIV was 52% (95% CI, 29%–67%) efficacious in preventing serologically documented influenza illness in a population of adults 60 years of age and older.[44] When the groups were further stratified by age, efficacy estimates against serologically documented influenza illness were 57% (95% CI, 33%–72%) in those 60 through 69 years and 23% (95% CI, 51%–61%) in those ≥70 years old. However, interpretation of this study is complicated by the use of postvaccination to postseason serologic response as definition of infection.

Using higher doses of vaccine induces a stronger antibody response in older subjects, and in a large randomized study, the relative efficacy of high-dose vaccine was 24% compared to standard-dose vaccine,[24] with reductions in small numbers of more severe endpoints as well. As described earlier, recombinant HA vaccine is also administered at a higher HA dose than standard-dose egg-vaccine and was also shown to have approximately 30% improved efficacy compared to standard-dose egg vaccine during a season with substantial H3N2 vaccine mismatch.[25] Standard-dose inactivated vaccine has been shown to be protective in limited studies in other high-risk groups, including those with HIV infection.

Relatively few prospective trials have assessed inactivated vaccine efficacy in children. In one randomized, controlled trial in healthy children aged 6 through 23 months, vaccine efficacy was 66% (95% CI, 34%–82%) in the 1st year, but efficacy could not be assessed in the 2nd year due to a very low influenza attack rate. In an early efficacy study comparing LAIV and TIV over 5 years in children, IIV-3 had 77% efficacy against culture-confirmed H3 and 91% efficacy against H1. In a large field trial conducted at multiple international sites in children 3 to 8 years old, IIV-4 was shown to have efficacy of 59% in prevention of PCR-confirmed influenza and 74% efficacy against moderate to severe influenza.

Two large studies have evaluated the addition of MF59 to inactivated vaccine in children. In the first randomized placebo-controlled study done in children 6 to 72 months of age, the efficacy of IIV-3 against PCR-confirmed influenza was 43% and that of the MF59 adjuvanted vaccine was 86%. In a second study done in a population in which most children had previously been vaccinated, MF59 adjuvanted vaccine efficacy was similar to that of unadjuvanted vaccine in the entire study population but was 31% better than standard vaccine in the subpopulation 6 to 23 months of age,[151] consistent with observations of greater adjuvant effect in immunologically naïve populations.

Live Attenuated Influenza Vaccine

LAIV was demonstrated to be efficacious in the prevention of influenza in a 2-year, randomized, placebo-controlled trial conducted in 1,314 children 15 to 74 months of age. Efficacy against culture-confirmed influenza illness in the 1st year of this trial was 95% against influenza A/H3N2 and 91% against influenza B. In the 2nd year of the trial, the H3 component of the vaccine (A/Wuhan/93) was not a close match with the predominant H3 virus that season, A/Sydney/95. However, the efficacy of LAIV against this variant was 86% (95% CI, 75%–92%),[7] suggesting that LAIV can induce protective immunity against drift variants. Overall, the efficacy of LAIV to prevent any influenza illness during the 2-year period of surveillance in this field study was 92% (95% CI, 88%–94%). The overall efficacy of LAIV against culture-confirmed influenza among children 6 to less than 36 months who were attending day care was shown to be 85% and 89% in the 1st and 2nd year of the study, respectively. Studies done in Asia have reached similar conclusions, with an efficacy of LAIV compared to placebo of between 64% and 84% over multiple seasons, depending on the antigenic match with the vaccine.

Relatively, few placebo-controlled trials of the efficacy of LAIV have been conducted in adults. In the human challenge model, cold-adapted and IIVs were of approximately equal efficacy in prevention of experimentally induced influenza A (H1N1), A (H3N2), and B. The combined efficacy in preventing laboratory-documented influenza illness due to the three wild-type influenza strains was 85% for LAIV. In a randomized, controlled study in healthy persons aged 1 through 64 years, of whom most of the participants were adults, the efficacy of a prelicensure, bivalent preparation of LAIV for preventing culture-confirmed influenza A illness in adults was 85% (95% CI, 70%–92%) for H1N1 and 58% (95% CI, 29%–75%) for H3N2. LAIV was also evaluated in a large study against clinical endpoints performed in 4,561 healthy working adults. In this study, the effectiveness of LAIV in preventing severe febrile respiratory illness of any cause during the influenza season was 29%.

Effectiveness (Results of Observational Studies)

Many recent studies have utilized a test-negative, case-control design, in which individuals meeting a particular case definition are tested for influenza using a highly sensitive and specific diagnostic test, and the vaccination exposure of test-positive cases and test-negative controls is determined. Large surveillance networks have been established in Canada, the United States, Europe, and Australia for purposes of making interim and end-of-season estimates of vaccine effectiveness. Studies using this design have shown variable results with estimates generally ranging from as low as 20%, or in some cases, no effectiveness, to as high as 60% to 70%. Updated results of vaccine effectiveness studies in the United States are available at https://www.cdc.gov/flu/professionals/vaccination/effectiveness-studies.htm.

While the various networks vary in their study design and the specific selection criteria for subject inclusion, a few overall generalizations can be stated. Failure to detect vaccine effectiveness has typically occurred in studies with very low prevalence of influenza in the study population, or in years with substantial antigenic mismatch between the vaccine and circulating strains but even in situations of antigenically matched viruses, vaccine effectiveness remains in the 50% to 60% range. In some cases, these viruses have been shown to have substantial changes on a HA sequence level despite appearing well matched by traditional HI tests.

Most studies have not enrolled enough subjects in a single season to make age-specific estimates of vaccine effectiveness. However, there is a trend toward decreased vaccine effectiveness in elderly, not surprising given their diminished immune response to vaccination. After accumulating cases over several seasons, it is possible to use the same test-negative case-control design to demonstrate vaccine effectiveness of approximately 60% against influenza-related hospitalization in a population of community-dwelling older adults. Among hospitalized patients, vaccinated individuals have lower rates of ICU admission and in-hospital deaths.

The ability to compare the effectiveness of different vaccines using observational approaches depends on the extent to which various vaccines are being used in the study population, so complete information is not always available. In a cohort study based on Medicare beneficiary data in the United States, the use of high-dose vaccine was associated with a significantly greater reduction in influenza-related deaths among seniors in a year in which H3N2 viruses predominated, but not in a year of primarily A(H1N1)pdm09 virus.[125] In a case–control study among elderly individuals in Canada, MF-59 adjuvanted vaccine also appeared to be more effective than standard-dose unadjuvanted vaccine.[146]

Effects of Prior Vaccination

Recent studies of influenza vaccine effectiveness using the test-negative design, as well as other study designs, have suggested that vaccine effectiveness is decreased in those who are yearly vaccine recipients, compared to those who receive vaccine for the first time this year. These findings would be consistent with very early observations made in a boy's boarding school, referred to as the "Hoskins effect." However, not all studies have shown a negative effect of prior vaccination. The effects seem to be greatest when this season and the previous season vaccine components are similar to each other but the circulating virus is a mismatch.[128]

The immunologic mechanisms that might be responsible for the negative effects of prior vaccination are not known. Individuals with higher prevaccination antibody levels tend to have lower magnitude responses to vaccination although still typically achieving very high levels of antibody. Prior vaccination might result in memory responses that preferentially recognize shared epitopes and not new epitopes that are present in antigenically drifted viruses, representing a form of back boosting.[30]

Because at least one component of the vaccine changes each year, there is not practical solution to influenza control using current vaccine strategies other than annual vaccination. Further research to understand the magnitude and mechanisms of putative negative effects of prior vaccination will clearly be important in improving influenza control.

Comparisons of Live and Inactivated Vaccines

While relatively few randomized direct comparisons of the efficacy of live and inactivated vaccines have been performed, the available studies are consistent with the observed effects of age and prior influenza experience on immunogenicity. When these vaccines have been compared in young children 12 months through 59 months of age, LAIV has shown consistently superior protection, with an approximately 50% greater protective efficacy than inactivated vaccine.

In contrast, studies that directly compared the vaccines in adults have suggested that the vaccines have similar efficacy or that IIV is slightly more efficacious than live vaccine. In one three-armed study, the efficacy of LAIV compared to placebo for prevention of laboratory-confirmed influenza in healthy adults was 57%, while the efficacy of the IIV was 77%, but the difference between the two vaccines was not statistically significant. In a subsequent season in the same population, the absolute efficacies of IIV and LAIV were 68% and 36%, respectively. In an effectiveness assessment in the US military, the effectiveness of IIV against medical visits for pneumonia or other influenza-related diagnoses was higher than that of LAIV, except for personnel who had not been vaccinated in previous years.

When the H1N1 component of LAIV was replaced by a virus with the HA and NA of an A/California/09 virus following the pandemic, there was a substantial decrease in effectiveness of LAIV, particularly against H1N1.[13] This poor effectiveness was repeatedly demonstrated in the United States and to a lesser extent in other countries. The reasons for the diminished effectiveness of this formulation are not completely known but may be related to the replication fitness of the specific H1N1 virus, increasing levels of background immunity in the vaccinated population, or other factors. However, as a result, use of LAIV in the United States was not recommended by the Advisory Committee on Immunization Practices (ACIP) for several years. Subsequently, the H1N1 component has been updated with a virus (A/Slovenia/2093/2015) that appears to generate stronger immune responses, and use of LAIV has resumed. No information is available regarding the efficacy or effectiveness of this new formulation at this time.

Secondary Protection

Generally, individuals at the highest risk for influenza complications may also be compromised in their ability to respond to vaccination. There has been considerable interest in potential strategies to protect such individuals indirectly by preventing illness and viral transmission within highly susceptible populations that probably play a role on community transmission, such as schoolchildren. Several studies have suggested that this may be possible. During the 1968 pandemic, it was observed that the incidence of respiratory illness during the period of influenza A circulation among unvaccinated adults was substantially lower in a community in which schoolchildren were immunized than in a community with no school immunization. Influenza B was not contained in the vaccine, and during a subsequent influenza B epidemic, there was no difference in adjusted respiratory illness rates in adults in the two communities. In a recent study, closed agricultural communities of Hutterites were randomized to vaccination of schoolchildren with influenza vaccine or with hepatitis A vaccine as a control. In the subsequent influenza A epidemic, the rate of laboratory-documented influenza A in unvaccinated adults residing in school-vaccinated communities was reduced by 61% (95% CI, 8%–83%) compared to adults in unvaccinated communities.[84] Vaccination of children in day care has been reported to reduce the rates of febrile respiratory illnesses in unvaccinated household contacts. Observations in Japan, where it appeared that substantial fluctuations in overall influenza-related mortality (occurring mostly in the elderly) were directly related to the rate of school-age influenza vaccination, also support a potential role for school vaccination in protection of elders. A retrospective study conducted in Japan demonstrated that universal vaccination of schoolchildren reduced the number of class cancellation days and absenteeism when compared with years during which the immunization program was abandoned.

A critical target group for vaccination is health care workers. At a minimum, universal vaccination of heath care workers will reduce workplace absences and prevent disruptions in care. In addition, there is supportive evidence that vaccination of health care workers reduces the risk of nosocomial influenza in hospitals. In nursing homes, vaccination of staff reduces mortality in residents independently of the vaccination status of the residents themselves.

Maternal Immunization

Infants less than 6 months of age are at substantial risk for influenza-related morbidity but are too young to receive influenza vaccine. One strategy to protect vulnerable infants is maternal immunization, with protection mediated by both transfer of maternal antibody as well as reduced potential for contact with an influenza-infected mother. In a multiple randomized studies of maternal immunization, infants born to mothers immunized with influenza vaccine have had substantially lower rates of laboratory-documented influenza in the first 6 months of life than did infants born to mothers immunized with control vaccine.[138] Similarly, in a retrospective case-control study, the frequency of influenza immunization was substantially lower in the mothers of infants hospitalized with PCR-confirmed influenza than in mothers of infants hospitalized who were PCR negative, with an estimated protective effect of 92%.

Recommendations for Vaccine Use

Current US recommendations are for routine annual influenza vaccination of all individuals aged 6 months and above. Ideally, vaccine should be administered by October, but later vaccination can still be beneficial if the seasonal epidemic has not yet occurred. Recommendations for influenza vaccine in the United Sates are updated annually by the Centers for Disease Control and Prevention.[45]

Vaccines for Pandemic Influenza

As described earlier, there have been multiple observations of human infection with avian or swine influenza viruses with novel HA and/or NA subtypes, and there continues to be concern regarding the potential of such viruses to acquire the ability to transmit efficiently from person to person and result in the next human influenza pandemic. In addition to active ongoing surveillance, there have been substantial efforts to prepare for such a pandemic by developing potential pandemic vaccines in advance. Because seasonal vaccines are licensed for use in all age groups and have substantial evidence of safety and efficacy, pandemic preparedness efforts have generally focused on development of pandemic formulations of seasonal vaccines, including inactivated and live varieties. Several of these have undergone advanced clinical development and have been licensed or approved for emergency use based on a favorable safety and immunogenicity profile.

A large number of inactivated H5 and H7 vaccines have been developed and tested in humans. These vaccines have included egg-derived, cell culture–grown, and recombinant HA vaccines similar to the approaches taken for seasonal influenza. Extensive clinical trials have generally shown that these vaccines are well tolerated but, when administered without an adjuvant, poorly immunogenic. Generation of potentially protective immunity, as measured by serum HI and neutralizing antibody responses, requires a two-dose schedule and the use of doses substantially higher than those used for seasonal vaccines. When responses are seen, they are typically limited in breadth and predominantly focused on the homologous antigen. Limited studies of whole virion vaccines have suggested slight improvements in immunogenicity.

Oil-in-water emulsions such as MF59 and AS03 have allowed much lower doses of pandemic vaccines to be used successfully. With these adjuvants, substantial immune responses have been seen at doses as low as 3.75 μg of antigen, compared to the need to use 45 or 90 μg of unadjuvanted vaccine, allowing for the generation of a much larger supply of vaccine in the event of a pandemic. In addition, responses after adjuvanted vaccine are typically more broad, with higher titers of antibody recognizing antigenic variants of the vaccine subtype. A number of other adjuvants have also been tested with pandemic vaccines and also show effective improvement in response. Limited studies have suggested that the use of an adjuvant is much more important with the first dose of vaccine. However, even with adjuvants, inactivated pandemic vaccination will likely require a two-dose schedule, imposing significant operational challenges to a pandemic response.

Despite the relatively poor immunogenicity of these vaccines, multiple studies have shown that even unadjuvanted pandemic vaccines may induce long-lasting immune memory, demonstrated by vigorous responses to subsequent booster doses many years later. Such responses can be demonstrated even in subjects who did not respond to the primary series. These studies have also suggested that priming and boosting with antigenically variant HAs can also generate strong responses to revaccination. Hence, prepandemic priming,[42] potentially limited to high-risk groups, could be considered to prepare for a possible H5N1 pandemic.

Live attenuated pandemic vaccines have also been evaluated in clinical trials. Evaluation of pandemic live vaccines is complicated by the concerns regarding potential transmission of the vaccine virus, possible reassortment with cocirculating human influenza viruses, and potential generation of virulent human viruses with novel HA or NA surface proteins. Therefore, these studies have been conducted under isolation conditions to prevent possible transmission outside the study and consequently have been somewhat limited in size.

Surprisingly, all of these studies have shown very limited replication of the pandemic vaccine viruses on either the A/Ann Arbor or the A/Leningrad backbone. Vaccine virus shedding occurs in a minority of susceptible recipients and, when it is detected, is almost invariably of limited magnitude and short duration. Because immune correlates of protection afforded by seasonal live vaccines have not been determined, it is not possible to draw definitive conclusions regarding the relevant immunogenicity of pandemic formulations of these vaccines. However, measurable serum or mucosal immune responses occur rarely.

Similar to the findings with inactivated vaccines, pandemic formulations of LAIV appear to induce long-lasting immune memory despite the lack of measureable immune response to the initial immunization.[112,131] These observations have caused some to suggest that the most effective use of vaccines for pandemic control would be prepandemic vaccination, in which the population would be vaccinated with a prototypic H5, H7, or other threat subtypes prior to a pandemic, and then boosted with an antigenically matched virus should a pandemic occur.

Strategies for More Broadly Protective Vaccines

For a variety of reasons previously outlined, there is considerable interest in the development of influenza vaccine approaches that could generate more broadly protective immunity, potentially providing protection against multiple antigenic variants within a subtype or possibly even providing protection against multiple subtypes. Several approaches have emerged in pursuit of this goal (for a recent review, see Reference[28]).

In contrast to the globular head of the HA, the stalk, or HA2 region, remains relatively conserved from season to season. Stalk-directed antibody or stalk-reactive B cells are seen most frequently when individuals are exposed to a novel influenza virus, such as after infection with H5N1 or A(H1N1) pdm09 viruses in 2009. Stalk-specific antibodies are capable of mediating virus neutralization by inhibiting HA-mediated fusion. In addition, these antibodies can mediate antibody-dependent cellular cytotoxicity. Therefore development of vaccines to induce stalk antibodies is one of the prime strategies for more broadly protective vaccines. Both chimeric approaches, where several doses of a vaccine in which the HA1 domain is derived from a novel subtype, and the stalk remain the same, and stalk-only constructs are in development.

The influenza NA has also been explored as a potential target for more broadly protective vaccines. The rate at which mutations accumulate in the NA appears to be less than that in the HA, suggesting that vaccines that induced substantial NA-specific immunity would continue to provide protection against drifted viruses and would need updating less often than HA-centric vaccines.

The third envelope protein, the M2, has also been identified as a potential target since the extracellular domain (M2e) is fairly well conserved among human influenza A viruses. The mechanism of protection by M2e antibodies also involves antibody-dependent cellular cytotoxicity in M2e antibody–mediated protection. Multiple platforms have been used to induce

antibody specific for M2e, which have induced variable levels of M2e antibodies in humans.

Vaccines designed primarily to elicit cellular antibodies often contain mixtures of peptides computationally identified as cellular target epitopes. Immunization of humans with a mixture of linear peptides has been reported to induce cellular immunity and prime for subsequent vaccine responses. Such epitopes could be delivered by mixtures of peptides or by live viral vectors, such as vaccinia. Virus-like particles and gamma-irradiated whole virus have also been evaluated for their ability to induce cellular immune responses.

PERSPECTIVES

Over the last decade, we have witnessed several important developments in influenza virology. HPAI viruses, which in the past caused transient, local outbreaks, have now expanded their geographic range and become enzootic in parts of Asia and the Middle East, with frequent introductions into Europe. In several studies, recombinant H5 viruses have been shown to acquire respiratory droplet transmissibility in ferrets; based on these results, the pandemic potential of these viruses should not be discounted. In 2013, novel influenza viruses of the H7N9 subtype emerged in China and have caused greater than 1,500 human infections with a case fatality rate of approximately 40%. The recent poultry vaccination campaigns in China may have controlled this outbreak. The last decade has also seen major efforts to improve influenza vaccine efficacy including the development of broadly protective ("universal") vaccines; several concepts are being pursued, and first candidates are now being tested in clinical trials. Moreover, we have witnessed the development and approval for human use of a novel class of antivirals to influenza, that is, inhibitors of the viral polymerase complex. While progress has been made in several areas of influenza virus research, key questions remain: How can we better predict the pandemic potential of newly emerging influenza viruses? And how can we better understand the antigenic evolution of human influenza viruses, so that vaccines can be ready before appreciable numbers of people get sick?

REFERENCES

1. Allen EK, Randolph AG, Bhangale T, et al. SNP-mediated disruption of CTCF binding at the IFITM3 promoter is associated with risk of severe influenza in humans. *Nat Med* 2017;23:975.
2. Babu TM, Perera RAPM, Wu JT, et al. Population serologic immunity to human and avian H2N2 viruses in the United States and Hong Kong for pandemic risk assessment. *J Infect Dis* 2018;218:1054–1060.
3. Beigel JH, Farrar J, Han AM, et al. Avian influenza A (H5N1) infection in humans. *N Engl J Med* 2005;353(13):1374–1385.
4. Bell J, Boner A, Cohen DM, et al. Multicenter clinical evaluation of the novel Alere™ i Influenza A&B isothermal nucleic acid amplification test. *J Clin Virol* 2014;61:81–86.
5. Belser JA, Gustin KM, Pearce MB, et al. Pathogenesis and transmission of avian influenza A (H7N9) virus in ferrets and mice. *Nature* 2013;501(7468):556–559.
6. Belshe RB, Edwards KM, Vesikari T, et al. Live attenuated versus inactivated influenza vaccine in infants and young children. *N Engl J Med* 2007;356(7):685–696.
7. Belshe RB, Gruber WC, Mendelman PM, et al. Efficacy of vaccination with live attenuated, cold-adapted, trivalent, intranasal influenza virus vaccine against a variant (A/Sydney) not contained in the vaccine. *J Pediatr* 2000;136(2):168–175.
8. Black S, Nicolay U, Mesikari T, et al. Hemagglutination inhibition antibody titers as a correlate of protection for inactivated influenza vaccines in children. *Pediatr Infect Dis J* 2011;30(12):1081–1085.
9. Burnet FM. Influenza virus on the developing egg. I. Changes associated with the development of an egg-passage strain of virus. *Br J Exp Pathol* 1936;17:282–293.
10. Chen LM, Blixt O, Stevens J, et al. In vitro evolution of H5N1 avian influenza virus toward human-type receptor specificity. *Virology* 2012;422(1):105–113.

11. Chen W, Calvo PA, Malide D, et al. A novel influenza A virus mitochondrial protein that induces cell death. *Nat Med* 2001;7(12):1306–1312.

12. Chen H, Smith GJ, Zhang SY, et al. Avian flu: H5N1 virus outbreak in migratory waterfowl. *Nature* 2005;436(7048):191–192.

13. Chung JR, Flannery B, Thompson MG, et al. Seasonal effectiveness of live attenuated and inactivated influenza vaccine. *Pediatrics* 2016;137(2):1–10.

14. Chung EY, Huang L, Schneider L. Safety of influenza vaccine administration in egg-allergic patients. *Pediatrics* 2010;125:e1024–e1030.

15. Claas EC, de Jong JC, van Beek R, et al. Human influenza virus A/HongKong/156/97 (H5N1) infection. *Vaccine* 1998;16(9–10):977–978.

16. Claas EC, Osterhaus AD, van Beek R, et al. Human influenza A H5N1 virus related to a highly pathogenic avian influenza virus. *Lancet* 1998;351(9101):472–477.

17. Colman PM, Ward CW. Structure and diversity of influenza virus neuraminidase. *Curr Top Microbiol Immunol* 1985;114:177–255.

18. Conenello GM, Tisoncik JR, Rosenzweig E, et al. A single N66S mutation in the PB1-F2 protein of influenza A virus increases virulence by inhibiting the early interferon response in vivo. *J Virol* 2011;85(2):652–662.

19. Connor RJ, Kawaoka Y, Webster RG, et al. Receptor specificity in human, avian, and equine H2 and H3 influenza virus isolates. *Virology* 1994;205(1):17–23.

20. Couceiro JN, Paulson JC, Baum LG. Influenza virus strains selectively recognize sialyloligosaccharides on human respiratory epithelium; the role of the host cell in selection of hemagglutinin receptor specificity. *Virus Res* 1993;29(2):155–165.

21. de Jong MD, Simmons CP, Thanh TT, et al. Fatal outcome of human influenza A (H5N1) is associated with high viral load and hypercytokinemia. *Nat Med* 2006;12(10):1203–1207.

22. Deeg CM, Hassan E, Mutz P, et al. In vivo evasion of MxA by avian influenza viruses requires human signature in the viral nucleoprotein. *J Exp Med* 2017;214(5):1239–1248.

23. Deyle ER, Maher MC, Hernandez RD, et al. Global environmental drivers of influenza. *Proc Natl Acad Sci U S A* 2016;113:13081–13086.

24. DiazGranados CA, Dunning AJ, Kimmel M, et al. Efficacy of high-dose versus standard-dose influenza vaccine in older adults. *N Engl J Med* 2014;371:635–645.

25. Dunkle LM, Izikson R, Patriarca P, et al. Efficacy of recombinant influenza vaccine in adults 50 years of age or older. *N Engl J Med* 2017;376:2427–2436.

26. Echevarria-Zuno S, Mejia-Arangure JM, Mar-Obeso AJ, et al. Infection and death from influenza A H1N1 virus in Mexico: a retrospective analysis. *Lancet* 2009;374(9707):2072–2079.

27. Edwards KM, Dupont WD, Westrich MK, et al. A randomized controlled trial of cold-adapted and inactivated vaccines for the prevention of influenza A disease. *J Infect Dis* 1994;169(1):68–76.

28. Epstein SL. Universal influenza vaccines: progress in achieving broad cross-protection in vivo. *Am J Epidemiol* 2018;187(12):2603–2614.

29. Fodor E, Devenish L, Engelhardt OG, et al. Rescue of influenza A virus from recombinant DNA. *J Virol* 1999;73(11):9679–9682.

30. Fonville JM, Wilks SH, James SL, et al. Antibody landscapes after influenza virus infection or vaccination. *Science* 2014;346(6212):996–1000.

31. Forrest BD, Pride MW, Dunning AJ, et al. Correlation of cellular immune responses with protection against culture-confirmed influenza virus in young children. *Clin Vaccine Immunol* 2008;15:1042–1053.

32. Fouchier RA, Schneeberger PM, Rozendaal FW, et al. Avian influenza A virus (H7N7) associated with human conjunctivitis and a fatal case of acute respiratory distress syndrome. *Proc Natl Acad Sci U S A* 2004;101(5):1356–1361.

33. Francis T Jr, Salk JE, Pearson HE, et al. Protective effect of vaccination against influenza A. *Proc Soc Exp Biol Med* 1944;55:104–105.

34. Gabriel G, Herwig A, Klenk HD. Interaction of polymerase subunit PB2 and NP with importin alpha1 is a determinant of host range of influenza A virus. *PLoS Pathog* 2008;4(2):e11.

35. Gambaryan AS, Tuzikov AB, Piskarev VE, et al. Specification of receptor-binding phenotypes of influenza virus isolates from different hosts using synthetic sialylglycopolymers: non-egg-adapted human H1 and H3 influenza A and influenza B viruses share a common high binding affinity for 6'-sialyl(N-acetyllactosamine). *Virology* 1997;232(2):345–350.

36. Gamblin SJ, Haire LF, Russell RJ, et al. The structure and receptor binding properties of the 1918 influenza hemagglutinin. *Science* 2004;303(5665):1838–1842.

37. Gao R, Cao B, Hu Y, et al. Human infection with a novel avian-origin influenza A (H7N9) virus. *N Engl J Med* 2013;368(20):1888–1897.

38. Garcia-Sastre A, Egorov A, Matassov D, et al. Influenza A virus lacking the NS1 gene replicates in interferon-deficient systems. *Virology* 1998;252(2):324–330.

39. Garten RJ, Davis CT, Russell CA, et al. Antigenic and genetic characteristics of swine-origin 2009 A(H1N1) influenza viruses circulating in humans. *Science* 2009;325(5937):197–201.

40. Gerhard W, Yewdell J, Frankel ME, et al. Antigenic structure of influenza virus haemagglutinin defined by hybridoma antibodies. *Nature* 1981;290(5808):713–717.

41. Glaser L, Stevens J, Zamarin D, et al. A single amino acid substitution in 1918 influenza virus hemagglutinin changes receptor binding specificity. *J Virol* 2005;79(17):11533–11536.

42. Goodman JL. Investing in immunity: pre-pandemic immunization to combat future influenza pandemics. *Clin Infect Dis* 2016;62(4):495–498.

43. Gostic KM, Ambrose M, Worobey M, et al. Potent protection against H5N1 and H7N9 influenza via childhood hemagglutinin imprinting. *Science* 2016;354(6313):722–726.

44. Govaert TM, Thijs CT, Masurel N, et al. The efficacy of influenza vaccination in elderly individuals. A randomized double-blind placebo-controlled trial. *JAMA* 1994;272(16):1956–1961.

45. Grohskopf LA, Sokolow LZ, Broder KR, et al. Prevention and control of seasonal influenza with vaccines: recommendations of the Advisory Committee on Immunization Practices—United States, 2018-19 influenza season. *MMWR Recomm Rep* 2018;67:1–20.

46. Guan Y, Peiris JS, Lipatov AS, et al. Emergence of multiple genotypes of H5N1 avian influenza viruses in Hong Kong SAR. *Proc Natl Acad Sci U S A* 2002;99(13):8950–8955.

47. Haller O, Arnheiter H, Pavlovic J, et al. The discovery of the antiviral resistance gene Mx: a story of great ideas, great failures, and some success. *Annu Rev Virol* 2018;5(1):33–51.

48. Hatta M, Gao P, Halfmann P, et al. Molecular basis for high virulence of Hong Kong H5N1 influenza A viruses. *Science* 2001;293(5536):1840–1842.

49. Hay AJ, Wolstenholme AJ, Skehel JJ, et al. The molecular basis of the specific anti-influenza action of amantadine. *EMBO J* 1985;4(11):3021–3024.

50. Hayden FG, Fritz R, Lobo MC, et al. Local and systemic cytokine responses during experimental human influenza A virus infection. Relation to symptom formation and host defense. *J Clin Investig* 1998;101(3):643–649.

51. Hayward AC, Wang L, Goonetilleke N, et al. Natural T cell-mediated protection against seasonal and pandemic influenza: results of the Flu Watch cohort study. *Am J Respir Crit Care Med* 2015;191:1422–1431.

52. Herfst S, Schrauwen EJ, Linster M, et al. Airborne transmission of influenza A/H5N1 virus between ferrets. *Science* 2012;336(6088):1534–1541.

53. Hopping AM, McElhaney JE, Fonville JM, et al. The confounded effects of age and exposure history in response to influenza vaccination. *Vaccine* 2016;34:540–546.

54. Horimoto T, Kawaoka Y. Pandemic threat posed by avian influenza A viruses. *Clin Microbiol Rev* 2001;14(1):129–149.

55. Imai M, Watanabe T, Hatta M, et al. Experimental adaptation of an influenza H5 HA confers respiratory droplet transmission to a reassortant H5 HA/H1N1 virus in ferrets. *Nature* 2012;486(7403):420–428.

56. Ison MG, Gubareva LV, Atmar RL, et al. Recovery of drug-resistant influenza virus from immunocompromised patients: a case series. *J Infect Dis* 2006;193(6):760–764.

57. Ito T, Suzuki Y, Suzuki T, et al. Recognition of N-glycolylneuraminic acid linked to galactose by the alpha2,3 linkage is associated with intestinal replication of influenza A virus in ducks. *J Virol* 2000;74(19):9300–9305.

58. Itoh Y, Shinya K, Kiso M, et al. In vitro and in vivo characterization of new swine-origin H1N1 influenza viruses. *Nature* 2009;460(7258):1021–1025.

59. Jagger BW, Wise HM, Kash JC, et al. An overlapping protein-coding region in influenza A virus segment 3 modulates the host response. *Science* 2012;337(6091):199–204.

60. Jegerlehner A, Schmitz N, Storni T, et al. Influenza A vaccine based on the extracellular domain of M2: weak protection mediated via antibody-dependent NK cell activity. *J Immunol* 2004;172:5598–5605.

61. Jernigan DB, Hageman JC, McDonald LC, et al. A national survey of severe influenza-associated complications among children and adults, 2003–2004. *Clin Infect Dis* 2005;40(11):1693–1696.

62. Ji Y, White YJ, Hadden JA, et al. New insights into influenza A specificity: an evolution of paradigms. *Curr Opin Struct Biol* 2017;44:219–231.

63. Kageyama T, Fujisaki S, Takashita E, et al. Genetic analysis of novel avian A(H7N9) influenza viruses isolated from patients in China, February to April 2013. *Euro Surveill* 2013;18(15):20453.

64. Kaiser L, Henry D, Flack NP, et al. Short-term treatment with zanamivir to prevent influenza: results of a placebo-controlled study. *Clin Infect Dis* 2000;30(3):587–589.

65. Kash JC, Taubenberger JK. The role of viral, host, and secondary bacterial factors in influenza pathogenesis. *Am J Pathol* 2015;185:1528–1536.

66. Kashyap AK, Steel J, Oner AF, et al. Combinatorial antibody libraries from survivors of the Turkish H5N1 avian influenza outbreak reveal virus neutralization strategies. *Proc Natl Acad Sci* 2008;105(16):5986–5991.

67. Kawaoka Y, Krauss S, Webster RG. Avian-to-human transmission of the PB1 gene of influenza A viruses in the 1957 and 1968 pandemics. *J Virol* 1989;63(11):4603–4608.

68. Khatchikian D, Orlich M, Rott R. Increased viral pathogenicity after insertion of a 28S ribosomal RNA sequence into the haemagglutinin gene of an influenza virus. *Nature* 1989;340(6229):156–157.

69. Kilander A, Rykkvin R, Dudman SG, et al. Observed association between the HA1 mutation D222G in the 2009 pandemic influenza A(H1N1) virus and severe clinical outcome, Norway 2009-2010. *Euro Surveill* 2010;15(9).

70. Klenk HD, Rott R, Orlich M, et al. Activation of influenza A viruses by trypsin treatment. *Virology* 1975;68(2):426–439.

71. Knossow M, Daniels RS, Douglas AR, et al. Three-dimensional structure of an antigenic mutant of the influenza virus haemagglutinin. *Nature* 1984;311(5987):678–680.

72. Kobasa D, Jones SM, Shinya K, et al. Aberrant innate immune response in lethal infection of macaques with the 1918 influenza virus. *Nature* 2007;445(7125):319–323.

73. Kobasa D, Takada A, Shinya K, et al. Enhanced virulence of influenza A viruses with the haemagglutinin of the 1918 pandemic virus. *Nature* 2004;431(7009):703–707.

74. Koel BF, Burke DF, Bestebroer TM, et al. Substitutions near the receptor binding site determine major antigenic change during influenza virus evolution. *Science* 2013;342(6161):976–979.

75. Koopmans M, Wilbrink B, Conyn M, et al. Transmission of H7N7 avian influenza A virus to human beings during a large outbreak in commercial poultry farms in the Netherlands. *Lancet* 2004;363(9409):587–593.

76. Kwong JC, Schwartz KL, Campitelli MA, et al. Acute myocardial infarction after laboratory-confirmed influenza infection. *N Engl J Med* 2018;378(4):345–353.

77. Li Z, Chen H, Jiao P, et al. Molecular basis of replication of duck H5N1 influenza viruses in a mammalian mouse model. *J Virol* 2005;79(18):12058–12064.

78. Li KS, Guan Y, Wang J, et al. Genesis of a highly pathogenic and potentially pandemic H5N1 influenza virus in eastern Asia. *Nature* 2004;430(6996):209–213.

79. Li X, Shi J, Guo J, et al. Genetics, receptor binding property, and transmissibility in mammals of naturally isolated H9N2 Avian Influenza viruses. *PLoS Pathog* 2014;10(11):e1004508.

80. Linster M, van Boheemen S, de Graaf M, et al. Identification, characterization, and natural selection of mutations driving airborne transmission of A/H5N1 virus. *Cell* 2014;157(2):329–339.

81. Liu Q, Lu L, Sun Z, et al. Genomic signature and protein sequence analysis of a novel influenza A (H7N9) virus that causes an outbreak in humans in China. *Microbes Infect* 2013;15(6–7):432–439.

82. Liu J, Xiao H, Lei F, et al. Highly pathogenic H5N1 influenza virus infection in migratory birds. *Science* 2005;309(5738):1206.

83. Loeb M, Dafoe N, Mahony J, et al. Surgical mask vs N95 respirators for preventing influenza among health care workers: a randomized trial. *JAMA* 2009;302:1865–1871.

84. Loeb M, Russell ML, Moss L, et al. Effect of influenza vaccination of children on infection rates in Hutterite communities: a randomized trial. *JAMA* 2010;303:943–950.

85. Long JS, Giotis ES, Moncorge O, et al. Species difference in ANP32A underlies influenza A virus polymerase host restriction. *Nature* 2016;529(7584):101–104.
86. Louria DB, Blumenfeld HL, Ellis JT, et al. Studies on influenza in the pandemic of 1957-1958. II. Pulmonary complications of influenza. *J Clin Investig* 1959;38:213–265.
87. Luo G, Ambati A, Lin L, et al. Autoimmunity to hypocretin and molecular mimicry to flu in type 1 narcolepsy. *Proc Natl Acad Sci U S A* 2019;115:e12323–e12332.
88. Maines TR, Jayaraman A, Belser JA, et al. Transmission and pathogenesis of swine-origin 2009 A(H1N1) influenza viruses in ferrets and mice. *Science* 2009;325(5939):484–487.
89. Martin Arias LH, Sanz R, Sainz M, et al. Guillain-Barré syndrome and influenza vaccines: a meta-analysis. *Vaccine* 2015;33:3773–3778.
90. Masurel N, Marine WM. Recycling of Asian and Hong Kong influenza A virus hemagglutinins in man. *Am J Epidemiol* 1973;97(1):44–49.
91. Matrosovich MN, Matrosovich TY, Gray T, et al. Human and avian influenza viruses target different cell types in cultures of human airway epithelium. *Proc Natl Acad Sci U S A* 2004;101(13):4620–4624.
92. Matrosovich M, Tuzikov A, Bovin N, et al. Early alterations of the receptor-binding properties of H1, H2, and H3 avian influenza virus hemagglutinins after their introduction into mammals. *J Virol* 2000;74(18):8502–8512.
93. McAuley JL, Hornung F, Boyd KL, et al. Expression of the 1918 influenza A virus PB1-F2 enhances the pathogenesis of viral and secondary bacterial pneumonia. *Cell Host Microbe* 2007;2(4):240–249.
94. McElhaney JE, Xie D, Hager WD, et al. T cell responses are better correlates of vaccine protection in the elderly. *J Immunol* 2006;176:6333–6339.
95. McMichael AJ, Gotch FM, Noble GR, et al. Cytotoxic T-cell immunity to influenza. *N Engl J Med* 1983;309:13–17.
96. Mehle A, Doudna JA. Adaptive strategies of the influenza virus polymerase for replication in humans. *Proc Natl Acad Sci U S A* 2009;106(50):21312–21316.
97. Monto AS, Kendal AP. Effect of neuraminidase antibody on Hong Kong influenza. *Lancet* 1973;7804(I):623–625.
98. Monto AS, Gravenstein S, Elliott M, et al. Clinical signs and symptoms predicting influenza infection. *Arch Intern Med* 2000;160(21):3243–3247.
99. Monto AS, Malosh RE, Petrie JG, et al. The doctrine of original antigenic sin: separating good from evil. *J Infect Dis* 2017;215:1782–1788.
100. Moser MR, Bender TR, Margolis HS, et al. An outbreak of influenza aboard a commercial airliner. *J Epidemiol* 1979;110:1–6.
101. Munster VJ, de Wit E, van den Brand JM, et al. Pathogenesis and transmission of swine-origin 2009 A(H1N1) influenza virus in ferrets. *Science* 2009;325(5939):481–483.
102. Nayak JL, Fitzgerald T, Richards KA, et al. CD4 T-cell expansion predicts neutralizing antibody responses to monovalent inactivated pandemic H1N1 influenza vaccine. *J Infect Dis* 2013;207:297–305.
103. Neumann G, Watanabe T, Ito H, et al. Generation of influenza A viruses entirely from cloned cDNAs. *Proc Natl Acad Sci U S A* 1999;96(16):9345–9350.
104. Noshi T, Kitano M, Taniguchi K, et al. In vitro characterization of baloxavir acid, a first-in-class cap-dependent endonuclease inhibitor of the influenza virus polymerase PA subunit. *Antiviral Res* 2018;160:109–117.
105. Novel Swine-Origin Influenza AVIT; Dawood FS, Jain S, et al. Emergence of a novel swine-origin influenza A (H1N1) virus in humans. *N Engl J Med* 2009;360(25):2605–2615.
106. Okuno H, Yahata Y, Tanaka-Taya K, et al. Characteristics and outcomes of influenza-associated encephalopathy cases among children and adults in Japan, 2010-2015. *Clin Infect Dis* 2018;66:1831–1837.
107. Opitz B, Rejaibi A, Dauber B, et al. IFNbeta induction by influenza A virus is mediated by RIG-I which is regulated by the viral NS1 protein. *Cell Microbiol* 2007;9(4):930–938.
108. Osterholm MT, Kelley NS, Sommer A, et al. Influenza vaccine efficacy and effectiveness: a new look at the evidence. *Lancet Infect Dis* 2012;12:36–44.
109. Perez-Padilla R, de la Rosa-Zamboni D, Ponce de Leon S, et al. Pneumonia and respiratory failure from swine-origin influenza A (H1N1) in Mexico. *N Engl J Med* 2009;361(7):680–689.
110. Petrie JG, Ohmit SE, Johnson E, et al. Efficacy studies of influenza vaccines: effect of end points used and characteristics of vaccine failures. *J Infect Dis* 2011;203(9):1309–1315.
111. Pichlmair A, Schulz O, Tan CP, et al. RIG-I-mediated antiviral responses to single-stranded RNA bearing 5′-phosphates. *Science* 2006;314(5801):997–1001.
112. Pitisuttithum P, Boonak K, Chamnanchanunt S, et al. Safety and immunogenicity of a live attenuated influenza H5 candidate vaccine strain A/17/turkey/Turkey/05/133 H5N2 and its priming effects for potential pre-pandemic use: a randomised, double-blind, placebo-controlled trial. *Lancet Infect Dis* 2017;17:833–842.
113. Poehling KA, Edwards KM, Weinberg GA, et al. The underrecognized burden of influenza in young children. *N Engl J Med* 2006;355:31–40.
114. Rajao DS, Gauger PC, Anderson TK, et al. Novel reassortant human-like H3N2 and H3N1 influenza A viruses detected in pigs are virulent and antigenically distinct from swine viruses endemic to the United States. *J Virol* 2015;89(22):11213–11222.
115. Reed C, Chaves SS, Daily Kirley P, et al. Estimating influenza disease burden from population-based surveillance data in the United States. *PLoS One* 2015;10(3):e0118369.
116. Rehwinkel J, Tan CP, Goubau D, et al. RIG-I detects viral genomic RNA during negative-strand RNA virus infection. *Cell* 2010;140(3):397–408.
117. Reid AH, Fanning TG, Hultin JV, et al. Origin and evolution of the 1918 "Spanish" influenza virus hemagglutinin gene. *Proc Natl Acad Sci U S A* 1999;96(4):1651–1656.
118. Richard M, Schrauwen EJ, de Graaf M, et al. Limited airborne transmission of H7N9 influenza A virus between ferrets. *Nature* 2013;501(7468):560–563.
119. Rodrigo C, Leonardi-Bee J, Nguyen-Van Tam JS, et al. Effect of corticosteroid therapy on influenza-related mortality: a systemic review and meta-analysis. *J Infect Dis* 2015;212:183–194.
120. Rogers GN, Paulson JC. Receptor determinants of human and animal influenza virus isolates: differences in receptor specificity of the H3 hemagglutinin based on species of origin. *Virology* 1983;127(2):361–373.
121. Sandbulte MR, Westgeest KB, Gao J, et al. Discordant antigenic drift of neuraminidase and hemagglutinin in H1N1 and H3N2 influenza viruses. *Proc Natl Acad Sci U S A* 2011;108(51):20748–20753.
122. Schild GC, Oxford JS, de Jong JC, et al. Evidence for host-cell selection of influenza virus antigenic variants. *Nature* 1983;303(5919):706–709.
123. Scholtissek C, Rohde W, Von Hoyningen V, et al. On the origin of the human influenza virus subtypes H2N2 and H3N2. *Virology* 1978;87(1):13–20.
124. Schwarzmann SW, Adler JL, Sullivan RFJ, et al. Bacterial pneumonia during the Hong Kong influenza epidemic of 1968-1969. *Arch Intern Med* 1971;127:1037–1041.
125. Shay DK, Chillarige Y, Kelman J, et al. Comparative effectiveness of high-dose versus standard-dose influenza vaccines among US Medicare beneficiaries in preventing postinfluenza deaths during 2012-2013 and 2013-2014. *J Infect Dis* 2017;215:510–517.
126. Shieh WJ, Blau DM, Denison AM, et al. 2009 pandemic influenza A (H1N1): pathology and pathogenesis of 100 fatal cases in the United States. *Am J Pathol* 2010;177:166–175.
127. Shinya K, Ebina M, Yamada S, et al. Avian flu: influenza virus receptors in the human airway. *Nature* 2006;440(7083):435–436.
128. Skowronski DM, Chambers C, Sabaiduc S, et al. A perfect storm: impact of genomic variation and serial vaccination on low influenza vaccine effectiveness during the 2014–2015 season. *Clin Infect Dis* 2016;63(1):21–32.
129. Smith DJ, Lapedes AS, de Jong JC, et al. Mapping the antigenic and genetic evolution of influenza virus. *Science* 2004;305(5682):371–376.
130. Smith GJ, Vijaykrishna D, Bahl J, et al. Origins and evolutionary genomics of the 2009 swine-origin H1N1 influenza A epidemic. *Nature* 2009;459(7250):1122–1125.
131. Sobhanie M, Matsuoka Y, Jegaskanda S, et al. Evaluation of the safety and immunogenicity of a candidate pandemic live attenuated influenza vaccine (pLAIV) against influenza A(H7N9). *J Infect Dis* 2016;213(6):922–929.
132. Sridhar S, Begom S, Bermingham A, et al. Cellular immune correlates of protection against symptomatic pandemic influenza. *Nat Med* 2013;19:1305–1312.
133. Stevens J, Blixt O, Tumpey TM, et al. Structure and receptor specificity of the hemagglutinin from an H5N1 influenza virus. *Science* 2006;312(5772):404–410.
134. Stevens J, Corper AL, Basler CF, et al. Structure of the uncleaved human H1 hemagglutinin from the extinct 1918 influenza virus. *Science* 2004;303(5665):1866–1870.
135. Sturm-Ramirez KM, Ellis T, Bousfield B, et al. Reemerging H5N1 influenza viruses in Hong Kong in 2002 are highly pathogenic to ducks. *J Virol* 2004;78(9):4892–4901.
136. Subbarao K, Klimov A, Katz J, et al. Characterization of an avian influenza A (H5N1) virus isolated from a child with a fatal respiratory illness. *Science* 1998;279(5349):393–396.
137. Subbarao EK, London W, Murphy BR. A single amino acid in the PB2 gene of influenza A virus is a determinant of host range. *J Virol* 1993;67(4):1761–1764.
138. Tapia MD, Sow SO, Tamboura B, et al. Maternal immunisation with trivalent inactivated influenza vaccine for prevention of influenza in infants in Mali: a prospective, active-controlled, observer-blind, randomised phase 4 trial. *Lancet Infect Dis* 2016;16(9):1026–1035.
139. Taubenberger JK, Reid AH, Krafft AE, et al. Initial genetic characterization of the 1918 "Spanish" influenza virus. *Science* 1997;275(5307):1793–1796.
140. Thompson WW, Shay DK, Weintraub E, et al. Mortality associated with influenza and respiratory syncytial virus in the United States. *JAMA* 2003;289(2):179–186.
141. Tong S, Li Y, Rivailler P, et al. A distinct lineage of influenza A virus from bats. *Proc Natl Acad Sci U S A* 2012;109(11):4269–4274.
142. Tong S, Zhu X, Li Y, et al. New world bats harbor diverse influenza A viruses. *PLoS Pathog* 2013;9(10):e1003657.
143. Tumpey TM, Basler CF, Aguilar PV, et al. Characterization of the reconstructed 1918 Spanish influenza pandemic virus. *Science* 2005;310(5745):77–80.
144. Tumpey TM, Maines TR, Van Hoeven N, et al. A two-amino acid change in the hemagglutinin of the 1918 influenza virus abolishes transmission. *Science* 2007;315(5812):655–659.
145. Uyeki TM, Bernstein HH, Bradley JS, et al. Clinical practice guidelines by the infectious diseases Society of America: 2018 update on diagnosis, treatment, chemoprophylaxis, and institutional outbreak management of seasonal influenzaa. *Clin Infect Dis* 2019;68(6):895–902.
146. Van Buynder PG, Konrad S, Van Buynder JL, et al. The comparative effectiveness of adjuvanted and unadjuvanted trivalent inactivated influenza vaccine (TIV) in the elderly. *Vaccine* 2013;31(51):6122–6128.
147. Van Hoeven N, Pappas C, Belser JA, et al. Human HA and polymerase subunit PB2 proteins confer transmission of an avian influenza virus through the air. *Proc Natl Acad Sci U S A* 2009;106(9):3366–3371.
148. van Riel D, Munster VJ, de Wit E, et al. H5N1 virus attachment to lower respiratory tract. *Science* 2006;312(5772):399.
149. Varghese JN, Laver WG, Colman PM. Structure of the influenza virus glycoprotein antigen neuraminidase at 2.9 A resolution. *Nature* 1983;303(5912):35–40.
150. Vesikari T, Karvonen A, Korhonen T, et al. A randomized, double-blind study of the safety, transmissibility, and phenotypic and genotypic stability of cold-adapted influenza virus vaccine. *Pediatr Infect Dis J* 2006;25:590–597.
151. Vesikari T, Kirstein J, Devota Go G, et al. Efficacy, immunogenicity, and safety evaluation of an MF59-adjuvanted quadrivalent influenza virus vaccine compared with non-adjuvanted influenza vaccine in children: a multicentre, randomised controlled, observer-blinded, phase 3 trial. *Lancet Respir Med* 2018;6(5):345–356.
152. Wang Z, Wan Y, Qiu C, et al. Recovery from severe H7N9 disease is associated with diverse response mechanisms dominated by CD8+ T cells. *Nat Commun* 2015;6:6833.
153. Watanabe T, Kiso M, Fukuyama S, et al. Characterization of H7N9 influenza A viruses isolated from humans. *Nature* 2013;501(7468):551–555.
154. Webster RG, Laver WG. Determination of the number of nonoverlapping antigenic areas on Hong Kong (H3N2) influenza virus hemagglutinin with monoclonal antibodies and the selection of variants with potential epidemiological significance. *Virology* 1980;104(1):139–148.
155. Webster RG, Bean WJ, Gorman OT, et al. Evolution and ecology of influenza A viruses. *Microbiol Rev* 1992;56(1):152–179.
156. Weitkamp JH, Spring MD, Brogan T, et al. Influenza A virus-associated acute necrotizing encephalopathy in the United States. *Pediatr Infect Dis J* 2004;23(3):259–263.

157. Wiley DC, Skehel JJ. The structure and function of the hemagglutinin membrane glycoprotein of influenza virus. *Annu Rev Biochem* 1987;56:365–394.

158. Wiley DC, Wilson IA, Skehel JJ. Structural identification of the antibody-binding sites of Hong Kong influenza haemagglutinin and their involvement in antigenic variation. *Nature* 1981;289(5796):373–378.

159. Wilkinson TM, Li CKF, Chui CSC, et al. Preexisting influenza-specific CD4+ T cells correlate with disease protection against influenza challenge in humans. *Nat Med* 2012;18:274–280.

160. Yan J, Grantham M, Pantelic J, et al. Infectious virus in exhaled breath of symptomatic seasonal influenza cases from a college community. *Proc Natl Acad Sci U S A* 2018;115:1081–1086.

161. Yang ZF, Mok CK, Peiris JS, et al. Human infection with a novel avian influenza A(H5N6) virus. *N Engl J Med* 2015;373(5):487–489.

162. Zeller MA, Anderson TK, Walia RW, et al. ISU FLUture: a veterinary diagnostic laboratory web-based platform to monitor the temporal genetic patterns of Influenza A virus in swine. *BMC Bioinformatics* 2018;19(1):397.

163. Zeng X, Tian G, Shi J, et al. Vaccination of poultry successfully eliminated human infection with H7N9 virus in China. *Sci China Life Sci* 2018;61(12):1465–1473.

164. Zhang Y, Zhang Q, Kong H, et al. H5N1 hybrid viruses bearing 2009/H1N1 virus genes transmit in guinea pigs by respiratory droplet. *Science* 2013;340(6139):1459–1463.

165. Zhou NN, Senne DA, Landgraf JS, et al. Genetic reassortment of avian, swine, and human influenza A viruses in American pigs. *J Virol* 1999;73(10):8851–8856.

166. Zost SJ, Parkhouse K, Gumina ME, et al. Contemporary H3N2 influenza viruses have a glycosylation site that alters binding of antibodies elicited by egg-adapted vaccine strains. *Proc Natl Acad Sci U S A* 2017;114:12578–12583.

Bunyavirales: The Viruses and Their Replication

John N. Barr • Friedemann Weber • Connie S. Schmaljohn

INTRODUCTION

The *Bunyavirales* order includes 12 families of single-strand RNA viruses with genomes that are typically composed of two or three (but sometimes even up to eight) segments with negative sense or ambisense coding strategies. The families are *Arenaviridae, Cruliviridae, Fimoviridae, Hantaviridae, Leishbuviridae, Mypoviridae, Nairoviridae, Peribunyaviridae, Phasmaviridae, Phenuiviridae, Tospoviridae,* and *Wupedeviridae* families. This large and diverse group of viruses, generically termed "bunyaviruses," infect a broad range of natural hosts including mammals, reptiles, birds, plants, and arthropods. Certain bunyaviruses are pathogenic for humans, but most are not known to infect or cause disease in humans. Bunyaviruses have numerous characteristics consistent with those required for emerging pathogens, such as error-prone polymerases, segmented genomes, persistent infection cycles in the vector organism, and widespread host distribution, which provide opportunities for genetic drift and shift and spillover to new hosts. In this chapter, we describe characteristics of the four traditional virus families within the *Bunyavirales* order that include important human pathogens. We briefly describe

characteristics of the other families, with the exception of the Family *Arenaviridae*, which is addressed in a separate chapter.

HISTORY AND CLASSIFICATION

The order takes its name from Bunyamwera virus (BUNV), which was isolated originally from *Aedes* mosquitoes in the Semliki Forest, Uganda, during a yellow fever study in 1943[414] and which was subsequently associated with a mild febrile illness in humans known as Bunyamwera fever. BUNV is the prototype of the order, and remains an important research model; it was the first bunyavirus whose genome was completely sequenced,[106,247] and was the first segmented genome negative-sense RNA virus that was generated entirely from cloned DNA.[54,367] From these beginnings, the *Bunyavirales* order now contains approximately 500 named viruses aligned to almost 300 species and as such is one of the largest of all virus taxonomic groupings.

At the time of the isolation of BUNV, arboviruses were categorized according to their serological characteristics, which led to the establishment of classical arbovirus groups A, B and C. While viruses within groups A and B were later included in the *Flaviviridae* and *Togaviridae* families, further virus discovery along with detailed serological analyses[294] led to the expansion of group C arboviruses into the Bunyamwera supergroup,[69] which consisted of viruses that could be linked by repeatable serologic cross-reactions.[61]

The family *Bunyaviridae* was formally established in 1975,[339] and in 1980 the International Committee on Taxonomy of Viruses (ICTV) approved the creation of the *Bunyavirus* genus, along with *Uukuvirus, Phlebovirus,* and *Nairovirus* genera that contained viruses morphologically and biochemically similar but antigenically distinct.[42] The discovery of a novel group of rodent-borne viruses and another group of plant-infecting viruses with conforming molecular properties, respectively, led to the creation of the *Hantavirus* genus in 1985, and the *Tospovirus* genus in 1991, and in the same year, further studies demonstrated a close biochemical similarity between uukuviruses and phleboviruses, resulting in their combination into the *Phlebovirus* genus.[60] The *Bunyavirus* genus was renamed *Orthobunyavirus* in 1995, to provide distinction between members of the respective genus and family taxa,[107] and thus a taxonomic structure with five distinctive genera was established.

TABLE 16.1 Representative sizes of viral structural proteins from within selected families of the *Bunyavirales* order

	Peribunyaviridae (*Orthobunyavirus* Genus)	Hantaviridae (*Orthohantavirus* Genus)	Nairoviridae (*Orthonairovirus* Genus)	Phenuiviridae (*Phlebovirus* Genus)	Tospoviridae
L	260	250	460	250	330
Gc	110	55	75	65	75
Gn	35	70	35	55–70	50
N	25	50	50	30	30

Sizes given in kD.

Assignment of species to one of these genera was based upon multiple factors; a lack of serologic cross-reactivity with members of other genera, the patterns of sizes of virion proteins (Table 16.1) and genome segments (Table 16.2), gene expression strategy (Fig. 16.1), and conserved terminal nucleotide sequences of the genomic RNAs (Table 16.3).

However, both further virus isolations as well as implementation of large-scale meta-transcriptomic sequencing projects[257,403,464] have dramatically increased the membership of the family, and revealed the previously unseen scope of bunyaviral genetic diversity. A measure of this diversity is that the previous and defining bunyavirus characteristic of a trisegmented, single-stranded RNA genome of negative- or ambisense polarity is no longer a distinctive property shared by all members of this order, with members of the newly-incorporated *Tenuivirus* genus (*Phenuiviridae* family) possessing up to 6 RNA segments, and members of the *Emaravirus* genus (*Fimoviridae* family) possessing up to eight. Instead, taxonomic assignments can be made solely based on viral nucleotide sequences, and in the case of bunyaviruses, their current phylogeny is primarily based on the sequence of conserved motifs within the viral RNA dependent RNA polymerase (RdRp). It should be noted that many of these newly classified viruses have not been isolated, and thus biochemical and molecular characteristics, as well as information about their natural history and pathogenesis are as yet unknown.

Consequently, in 2016, the ICTV *Bunyaviridae* study group initiated a taxonomic revision to incorporate the many unclassified bunyavirus-like species that could not be assimilated within the established five genera scheme, and to place all related viruses within a new high level overarching taxon, namely the *Bunyavirales* order. This involved the renaming and expansion of previous genera into family taxa, creation of four additional families containing newly identified species

with invertebrate and plant hosts, as well as inclusion of the *Arenaviridae* family. Of these 12 families, 5 represent vertebrate-infecting bunyaviruses: the *Hantaviridae*, *Nairoviridae*, *Peribunyaviridae*, *Phenuiviridae*, and *Arenaviridae* families. The first four of these will be discussed in this chapter, as these groupings contain the vast majority of bunyavirales members for which molecular and biochemical information has been gathered. For historical reasons, the *Arenaviridae* family will be discussed separately in Chapter 18.

These taxonomic assignments should be regarded as being in a state of flux. Implementation of further large-scale sequencing projects involving diverse vertebrate, invertebrate, and plant hosts will aid in deciphering the complex evolutionary relationships between the bunyaviruses to fill the gaps that currently exist in the phylogenetic tree, and it is certain that further changes will be made to their taxonomy.[56,305,315,316]

Table 16.4 lists notable members in the families within the *Bunyavirales* order and includes the traditional bunyaviruses. A brief description of the genera within the four families follows.

Hantaviridae Family

More than 100 small mammal species, to include rodents, shrews, moles and bats, have been found to host hantaviruses in nature.[283] Very recently, using a large-scale meta-transcriptomic approach, hantavirus-related gene sequences were also identified in reptiles, ray-finned fish, and jawless fish.[220] To date, all human pathogens in this family are carried by rodents and transmitted through aerosol exposure and occasionally by bite. The current taxonomy of the trisegmented negative-sense RNA virus family *Hantaviridae* includes 4 subfamilies (*Actantavirinae*, *Agantavirinae*, *Mammantavirinae*, *Repantavirinae*), 7 genera, approximately 50 viral species, and 70 named viruses.

TABLE 16.2 Representative sizes of the L, M and S genome segments from within selected families of the *Bunyavirales* order

	Peribunyaviridae (*Orthobunyavirus* Genus)	Hantaviridae (*Orthohantavirus* Genus)	Nairoviridae (*Orthonairovirus* Genus)	Phenuiviridae (*Phlebovirus* Genus)	Tospoviridae
L	6.9	6.5	12.2	6.4	8.9
M	4.5	3.6	5.3	3.5	4.8
S	1.0	1.7	1.7	1.7	2.9
Total	12.4	11.8	19.2	11.6	16.6

Sizes given in kb.

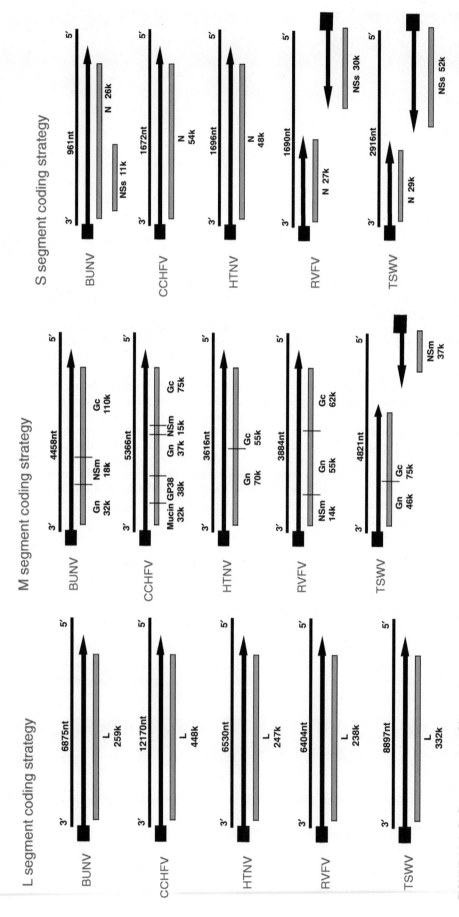

FIGURE 16.1 Coding strategies of bunyavirus genome segments. Genomic RNAs are represented by *thin lines* (the length in nucleotides is given above each segment) and the mRNAs are shown as *arrows* (■ indicates host-derived sequences at 5′ end). Gene products, with their apparent M_n are represented by colored boxes. BUNV, Bunyamwera orthobunyavirus; CCHFV, Crimean–Congo hemorrhagic fever nairovirus; HTNV, Hantaan hantavirus; RVFV, Rift Valley fever phlebovirus; TSWV, tomato spotted wilt tospovirus. In the CCHFV M segment, mucin represents the mucin-like region.

TABLE 16.3   Consensus 3′ and 5′ terminal nucleotide sequences of genome RNAs of representative viruses from within selected families of the *Bunyavirales* order

Peribunyaviridae (*Orthobunyavirus* genus)	3′ UCAUCACAUGA ... ... UCGUGUGAUGA 5′
Hantaviridae (*Orthohantavirus* genus)	3′ AUCAUCAUCUG ... ...AUGAUGAU 5′
Nairoviridae (*Orthonairovirus* genus)	3′ AGAGUUUCU ... . AGAAACUCU 5′
Phenuiviridae (*Phlebovirus* genus)	3′ UGUGUUUC ... . .GAAACACA 5′
Tospoviridae	3′ UCUCGUUAG ... . CUAACGAGA 5′

TABLE 16.4   Mammal- or plant-infecting species in the order *Bunyavirales*

Genus	Species	Notable Virus	Geographic Distribution	Principal Vector	Disease
Orthobunyavirus	Acara virus	Acara virus	SA/NA	Mosquitoes	
	Akabane virus	Akabane virus	Africa, Asia, Australia	Mosquitoes, culicoid flies	Cattle
	Alajuela virus	Alajuela virus	NA	Mosquitoes	
	Anopheles A virus	Anopheles A virus	SA	Mosquitoes	
	Anopheles B virus	Anopheles B virus	SA	Mosquitoes	
	Bakau virus	Bakau virus	Asia	Mosquitoes	
	Batama virus	Batama virus	Africa	N.D.	
	Benevides virus	Benevides virus	SA	Mosquitoes	
	Bertioga virus	Bertioga virus	SA	N.D.	
	Bimiti virus	Bimiti virus	SA	Mosquitoes	
	Botambi virus	Botambi virus	Africa	Mosquitoes	
	Bunyamwera virus	Bunyamwera virus	Africa	Mosquitoes	Human
		Batai virus	Asia, Europe	Mosquitoes	Human
		Cache Valley virus	NA	Mosquitoes	Sheep, Cattle, Human
		Fort Sherman virus	SA	Mosquitoes	Human
		Germiston virus	Africa	Mosquitoes	Human
		Ilesha virus	Africa	Mosquitoes	Human
		Ngari virus	Africa	Mosquitoes	Human
		Shokwe virus	Africa	Mosquitoes	Human
		Xingu virus	SA	Mosquitoes	Human
	Bushbush virus	Bushbush virus	SA	Mosquitoes	
	Bwamba virus	Bwamba virus	Africa	Mosquitoes	Human
		Pongola virus	Africa	Mosquitoes	Human
	California encephalitis virus	California encephalitis virus	NA	Mosquitoes	Human
		Inkoo virus	Europe	Mosquitoes	Human
		Jamestown Canyon virus	NA	Mosquitoes	Human
		La Crosse virus	NA	Mosquitoes	Human
		Lumbo virus	Africa	Mosquitoes	Human
		Snowshoe hare virus	NA	Mosquitoes	Human
		Tahyna virus	Europe	Mosquitoes	Human
	Capim virus	Capim virus	SA	Mosquitoes	
	Caraparu virus	Caraparu virus	SA, NA	Mosquitoes	Human

(continued)

TABLE 16.4 Mammal- or plant-infecting species in the order *Bunyavirales* (*Continued*)

Genus	Species	Notable Virus	Geographic Distribution	Principal Vector	Disease
		Apeu virus	SA	Mosquitoes	Human
		Ossa virus	NA	Mosquitoes	Human
	Catu virus	Catu virus	SA	Mosquitoes	Human
	Estero Real virus	Estero Real virus	NA	Ticks	
	Gamboa virus	Gamboa virus	NA	Mosquitoes	
	Guajara virus	Guajara virus	SA, NA	Mosquitoes	
	Guama virus	Guama virus	SA, NA	Mosquitoes	Human
	Guaroa virus	Guaroa virus	SA, NA	Mosquitoes	Human
	Kairi virus	Kairi virus	SA	Mosquitoes	Horse
	Kaeng Khoi virus	Kaeng Khoi virus	Asia	Nest bugs	
	Koongol virus	Koongol virus	Australia	Mosquitoes	
	Madrid virus	Madrid virus	NA	Mosquitoes	Human
	Main Drain virus	Main Drain virus	NA	Mosquitoes, culicoid flies	Horse
	Manzanilla virus	Ingwavuma virus	Africa, Asia	Mosquitoes	Pig
	Marituba virus	Marituba virus	SA	Mosquitoes	Human
		Murutucu virus	SA	Mosquitoes	Human
		Nepuyo virus	SA, NA	Mosquitoes	Human
		Restan virus	SA	Mosquitoes	Human
	Minatitlan virus	Minatitlan virus	NA	Mosquitoes	
	M'Poko virus	M'Poko virus	Africa	Mosquitoes	
	Nyando virus	Nyando virus	Africa	Mosquitoes	Human
	Olifantsvlei virus	Olifantsvlei virus	Africa	Mosquitoes	
	Oriboca virus	Oriboca virus	SA	Mosquitoes	Human
		Itaqui virus	SA	Mosquitoes	Human
	Oropouche virus	Oropouche virus	SA	Mosquitoes, culicoid flies	Human
	Patois virus	Patois virus	NA	Mosquitoes	
	Schmallenberg virus	Schmallenberg virus	Europe	Culicoid flies	Sheep, cattle
		Sathuperi virus	Africa, Asia	Mosquitoes, culicoid flies	
		Shamonda virus	Africa	Culicoid flies	
	Simbu virus	Simbu virus	Africa	Mosquitoes, culicoid flies	
	Shuni virus	Shuni virus	Africa	Mosquitoes, culicoid flies	
	Tacaiuma virus	Tacaiuma virus	SA	Mosquitoes	Human
	Tete virus	Tete virus	Africa	N.D.	
		Weldona virus	NA	culicoid flies	
	Thimiri virus	Thimiri virus	Africa, Asia	N.D.	
	Timboteua virus	Timboteua virus	SA	Mosquitoes	
	Turlock virus	Turlock virus	NA, SA	Mosquitoes	
	Wyeomyia virus	Wyeomyia virus	SA	Mosquitoes	Human
	Zegla virus	Zegla virus	NA	N.D.	

Genus	Species	Notable Virus	Geographic Distribution	Principal Vector	Disease
Orthohantavirus	*Andes virus*	Andes virus	SA	*Oligoryzomys longicaudatus*	Human
		Bermejo virus	SA	*Oligoryzomys chacoensis*	Human
		Lechiguanas virus	SA	*Oligoryzomys flavescens*	Human
		Maciel virus	SA	*Bolomys obscurus*	
		Oran virus	SA	*Oligoryzomys longicaudatus*	Human
		Pergamino virus	SA	*Akadon azarae*	
	Bayou virus	Bayou virus	NA	*Oryzomys palustris*	Human
	Black Creek Canal virus	Black Creek Canal virus	NA	*Sigmodon hispidus*	Human
	Cano Delgadito virus	Cano Delgadito virus	SA	*Sigmodon alstoni*	
	Dobrava-Belgrade virus	Dobrava virus	Europe	*Apodemus flavicollis*	Human
	El Moro Canyon virus	El Moro Canyon virus	NA	*Reithrodontomys megalotis*	
	Hantaan virus	Hantaan virus	Asia	*Apodemus agrarius coreae*	Human
	Isla Vista virus	Isla Vista virus	NA	*Microtus californicus*	
	Khabarovsk virus	Khabarovsk virus	Asia	*Microtus maximowiczii, Microtus fortis*	
	Laguna Negra virus	Laguna Negra virus	SA	*Calomys laucha*	Human
	Muleshoe virus	Muleshoe virus	NA	*Sigmodon hispidus*	
	New York virus	New York virus	NA	*Peromyscus leucopus*	Human
	Prospect Hill virus	Bloodland Lake virus	NA	*Microtus ochrogaster*	
		Prospect Hill virus	NA	*Microtus pennsylvanicus*	
	Puumala virus	Puumala virus	Europe, Asia	*Myodes glareolus*	Human
	Rio Mamore virus	Rio Mamore virus	SA	*Oligoryzomys microtis*	
	Rio Segundo virus	Rio Segundo virus	NA, SA	*Reithrodontomys mexicanus*	
	Saaremaa virus	Saaremaa virus	Europe	*Apodemus agrarius agrarius*	Human
	Seoul virus	Seoul virus	Worldwide	*Rattus norvegicus*	Human
	Sin Nombre virus	Blue River virus	NA	*Peromyscus leucopus*	
		Monongahela virus	NA	*Peromyscus maniculatus*	Human
		Sin Nombre virus	NA	*Peromyscus maniculatus*	Human
	Thailand virus	Thailand virus	Asia	*Bandicota indica*	
	Thottapalayam virus	Thottapalayam virus	India	*Suncus murinus*	
	Topografov virus	Topografov virus	Asia, Europe	*Lemmus sibiricus*	
	Tula virus	Tula virus	Europe	*Microtus arvalis, M. rossiaemeridionalis*	

(continued)

TABLE 16.4   Mammal- or plant-infecting species in the order _Bunyavirales_ (_Continued_)

Genus	Species	Notable Virus	Geographic Distribution	Principal Vector	Disease
Orthonairovirus	Crimean–Congo hemorrhagic fever virus	Crimean–Congo hemorrhagic fever virus	Africa, Asia, Europe	Culicoid flies, ticks	Human
		Hazara virus	Asia	Ticks	
	Dera Ghazi Khan virus	Dera Ghazi Khan virus	Asia	Ticks	
	Dugbe virus	Dugbe virus	Africa	Ticks	Human, cattle
		Nairobi sheep disease virus (Ganjam virus)	Africa, Asia	Ticks, culicoid flies, mosquitoes	Human, cattle
	Hughes virus	Hughes virus	NA, SA	Ticks	Seabirds
	Qalyub virus	Qalyub virus		Ticks	
	Sakhalin virus	Sakhalin virus	Asia	Ticks	
	Thiafora virus	Erve virus	Europe	N.D.	Human
Phlebovirus	Bujaru virus	Bujaru virus	SA	**N.D.**	
	Candiru virus	Alenquer virus	SA	**N.D.**	Human
		Candiru virus	SA	**N.D.**	Human
	Chilibre virus	Chilibre virus		Phlebotomines	
	Frijoles virus	Frijoles virus		Phlebotomines	
	Punta Toro virus	Punta Toro virus	NA, SA	Phlebotomines	Human
	Rift Valley fever virus	Rift Valley fever virus	Africa	Mosquitoes	Human, cattle
	Salehabad virus	Salehabad virus	Asia	Phlebotomines	
	Sandfly fever Naples virus	Sandfly fever Naples virus	Europe, Africa, Asia	Phlebotomines	Human
		Sandfly fever Sicilian virus	Europe	Phlebotomines	Human
		Toscana virus	Europe	Phlebotomines	Human
	Uukuniemi virus	Uukuniemi virus	Europe	Ticks	Seabirds
Banyangvirus	Huaiyangshan banyangvirus (= Severe fever with thrombocytopenia syndrome virus)	Severe fever with thrombocytopenia syndrome virus	Asia	Ticks	Human
		Heartland virus	USA	Ticks	Human
Tospovirus	Groundnut bud necrosis virus	Groundnut bud necrosis virus (Peanut bud necrosis virus)	Asia	_Frankliniella schultzei_, _Thrips palmi_	Plant
	Groundnut ringspot virus	Groundnut ringspot virus	SA, Africa	_F. occidentalis_, _F. schultzei_, _F. gemina_	Plant
	Groundnut yellow spot virus	Groundnut yellow spot virus (Peanut yellow spot virus)	Asia	N.D.	
	Impatiens necrotic spot virus	Impatiens necrotic spot virus	NA, Europe	_F. occidentalis_	Plant
	Tomato spotted wilt virus	Tomato spotted wilt virus	Worldwide	_F. bispinosa_, _F. cephalica_ _F. gemina_, _F. fusca_, _F. intonsa_, _F. occidentalis_, _F. schultzei_, _F. setosus_, _T. tabaci_	Plant
	Watermelon silver mottle virus	Watermelon silver mottle virus	Asia	_T. palmi_	Plant
	Zucchini lethal chlorosis virus	Zucchini lethal chlorosis virus	SA	_F. zucchini_	Plant

NA, North America; SA, South America; N.D., not determined.

Orthohantavirus Genus

Hantaviruses infecting mammals are included into the *Mammantavirinae* subfamily, with the *Orthohantavirus* genus (family *Hantaviridae*, order *Bunyavirales*) constituting all of the important rodent-borne human pathogens. The type species of the *Orthohantavirus* genus is Hantaan virus (HTNV), which was named after a small river close to the location where the virus was first identified.[245] The discovery of hantaviruses traces back to the early 1950s when United Nations troops were deployed during the border conflict between North and South Korea. More than 3,000 cases of an acute febrile illness were seen among the troops, about one third of which exhibited hemorrhagic manifestations, with an overall mortality of 5% to 10%.[102,245] The disease was initially termed Korean hemorrhagic fever but is now referred to as hemorrhagic fever with renal syndrome (HFRS). Despite considerable effort, it took about 25 years until the field mouse, *Apodemus agrarius*, was identified as the rodent reservoir, and HTNV was eventually isolated from the lungs of this animal.

During the course of the early studies in Korea, it became clear that HFRS cases were also occurring in urban areas. Years of investigation finally demonstrated that the urban cases in Korea, China, and Japan were associated with infection with Seoul virus (SEOV), which is hosted by the rats *Rattus norvegicus* and *R. rattus*.[243,245,426] For more than 50 years, a similar, but generally milder, disease termed nephropathia epidemica (NE) was described in various parts of Scandinavia.[298] Following the isolation of HTNV, the virus was shown to react with sera from patients with convalescent phase NE.[298] This led to the discovery of Puumala virus (PUUV) as the cause of this form of HFRS and the bank vole, *Myodes glareolus*, as the virus host. A fourth pathogenic hantavirus, Dobrava virus, was isolated from *Apodemus flavicollis* in Slovenia and causes severe HFRS in central and southeastern Europe and in European Russia.[317]

The most recent major event in the history of hantaviruses was the discovery of hantavirus pulmonary syndrome (HPS) in the southwestern United States in 1993.[297] A cluster of cases was first identified in New Mexico, which presented with a "flu-like illness" (i.e., fever, headache, muscle aches, chills, and so on), but rapidly progressed to a more severe respiratory disease with bilateral pulmonary infiltrates, respiratory failure, shock, and death, occurring approximately 2 to 10 days after onset of illness in almost 50% of the cases.[213] Within a couple of weeks of the initial outbreak, a newly identified virus, Sin Nombre virus (SNV), was shown to be the cause of HPS, and the rodent reservoir was shown to be the common deer mouse, *Peromyscus maniculatus*.[76,297] Within the next several years, HPS was shown to occur throughout the Americas from Canada to Patagonia, and was found to be caused by numerous hantaviruses, associated with various diverse rodent species.

Further Genera of the Mammantavirinae Subfamily

The genus *Thottimvirus* contains two shrew-borne viruses. Thottapalayam virus was isolated from an Asian house shrew (*Suncus murinus)* in Southern India although it was not recognized as a hantavirus until several years later.[65] Imjin virus was isolated from a musk shrew (*Crocidura lasiura*) shrews in the demilitarized zone of Korea.[350] Neither of these shrew-borne hantaviruses are known to be pathogenic to humans.

The name of the genus *Mobatvirus* is an amalgamation derived from "moles" and "bats." The prototype virus, Nova virus, was first detected in 2009 in archival liver tissue of the European mole (*Talpa europaea*) in Hungary.[202] Complete L-, M- and S- segment nucleotide sequences of a Nova virus strain circulating in Belgium demonstrated that this virus was related to, but highly divergent from, the orthohantaviruses and thus was placed into a new genus of the family.[236] The other two viruses in the genus, Laibin and Quezon viruses, have been detected in bats, and complete genome sequences have been determined.[18,470]

The *Loanvirus* genus contains currently a single virus, Longquan virus. The virus was detected in intermediate horseshoe bats (*Rhinolophus affinis*) in China. Although it is phylogenetically distinct from other hantaviruses, it has not yet been isolated or characterized.[151]

Nairoviridae Family

The *Nairoviridae* family comprises trisegmented negative-sense RNA viruses grouped into *Orthonairovirus*, *Shaspivirus*, and *Striwavirus* genera. Of these, the *Orthonairovirus* genus is the largest with 15 discrete species that are mostly maintained in tick hosts, but isolations have also been made from mosquitoes and midges. In contrast, the members of the *Shaspivirus* and *Striwavirus* genera were identified in spiders and water striders, respectively (Table 16.4). Information of these viruses outside of nucleotide sequence data is currently lacking, and consequently this text will focus on viruses within the *Orthonairovirus* genus.

The *Orthonairovirus* genus was named after Nairobi sheep disease virus (NSDV), which was originally isolated in Nairobi, Kenya, in 1910 by inoculation of sheep with the blood of sheep with acute gastroenteritis.[289] The virus causes fatal disease in sheep and goats and is present throughout various parts of Africa, and also India where it is known as Ganjam virus. The most important orthonairovirus from a human health perspective is Crimean–Congo hemorrhagic fever virus (CCHFV), which was first recognized in the Crimean peninsula in the mid-1940s, when a large outbreak of severe hemorrhagic fever among agricultural workers was identified. The outbreak included more than 200 cases with a case/fatality of about 10%.[78] Cases exhibiting similar disease were later reported throughout the European and central Asian republics of the former Soviet Union, to include Romania, and Bulgaria. However, the virus was first isolated in 1956 from a patient with a 1-day fever in Kisangani, Democratic Republic of Congo.[411] It was some years before the connection was established, but subsequent serologic studies and virus isolations from Asia and Europe revealed that the viruses from the different outbreaks and geographic regions were essentially the same virus, which then became named CCHFV.[70,79] CCHFV is now endemic in over 30 countries across Africa, Asia, Europe and the Middle East,[38] with outbreaks centered around southeastern regions exhibiting highly variable case/fatality rates of up to 30%.

Peribunyaviridae Family

The *Peribunyaviridae* family is the largest within the *Bunyavirales* order and includes four genera of tri-segmented negative-sense RNA viruses: the *Orthobunyavirus*, *Herbevirus*, *Pacuvirus*, and *Shangavirus* genera. Of these, 82 of the 89 species belong to the *Orthobunyavirus* genus, which is the only genus in this family to include animal and human pathogens, with select members associated with arthropod-borne hemorrhagic fevers with severe or fatal disease potential.

The Orthobunyavirus Genus

The largest genus of bunyaviruses is the *Orthobunyavirus* genus (family *Peribunyaviridae*, order *Bunyavirales*), which contains almost 200 named viruses that are found throughout the world.[3,391] Almost all of these viruses are transmitted by mosquitoes and have amplification cycles in a variety of vertebrate hosts.[61] Among important orthobunyavirus human pathogens are La Crosse virus (LACV), which causes pediatric encephalitis; Oropouche virus (OROV), which causes a debilitating febrile illness; and Ngari virus, which causes hemorrhagic fever. In contrast, Aino, Akabane, Cache Valley, and Schmallenberg viruses are examples of viruses causing disease in domestic animals (Table 16.4).

Classification of orthobunyaviruses has proven to be complex. The majority of viruses have been placed in one of 20 serogroups based on serologic relatedness of complement-fixing antibodies (mediated by the N protein) and hemagglutinating and neutralizing antibodies (mediated by the glycoproteins), although a number of viruses classified into the *Orthobunyavirus* genus are currently not assigned to any of these serogroups.[3,391] The 20 serogroups are Anopheles A, Anopheles B, Bakau, Bunyamwera, Bwamba, California, Capim, Gamboa, Group C, Guama, Koongol, Mapputta, Minatitlan, Nyando, Olifanstlei, Patois, Simbu, Tete, Turlock, and Wyeomyia. Serologic relatedness varies within a serogroup and is further complicated by the occurrence of natural reassortant viruses (Fig. 16.2), such that viruses may be more related to members of one group or another depending on the assay used.[59]

Molecular genetic studies comprising all three genome segments of the orthobunyaviruses have been conducted on viruses in 13 of the serogroups, namely Anopheles A,

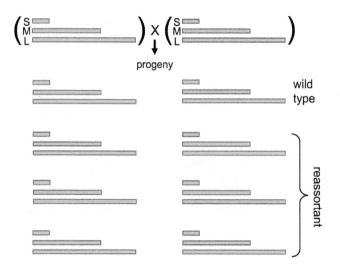

progeny

wild type

reassortant

FIGURE 16.2 Reassortment of bunyavirus genome segments. When a cell is coinfected with two genetically compatible bunyavirus strains (parent 1 and parent 2), eight different genotypes can be represented in progeny virus: the two parental genotypes and six reassortant genotypes, each with two segments from one parent and one segment from the other parent.

Bunyamwera, California, Capim, Gamboa, Group C, Guama, Koongol, Mapputta, Nyando, Simbu, Tete, and Turlock,[52,99,132,150,304,305,374,391] as well as several ungrouped orthobunyaviruses.[260,365] In many cases the S genome segment encodes two proteins, N and, in an overlapping reading frame, a small nonstructural protein termed NSs. N and NSs proteins are translated from the same viral messenger RNA (mRNA) molecule as the result of alternate AUG-initiation codon selection.[43,109] However, viruses in the Anopheles A, Anopheles B, Capim, Guama, Koogol, Mapputta, Tete, and Turlock serogroups as well some ungrouped orthobunyaviruses do not show evidence of having an NSs ORF.[132,391]

Phenuiviridae Family

The *Phenuiviridae* family comprises a diverse collection of viruses grouped into 15 genera that infect vertebrates, invertebrates, and plants. Of these 15 genera, only 2 contain viruses known to be associated with significant human and animal disease, namely the *Phlebovirus* and *Banyangvirus* genera. These viruses possess trisegmented, partially ambisense RNA genomes and have been the primary focus of phenuivirus research to date. The other 13 genera comprise plant and arthropod viruses for which biochemical and molecular data are currently lacking.

Phlebovirus Genus

The *Phlebovirus* genus (family *Phenuiviridae*, order *Bunyavirales*) contains more than 80 viruses, classified into 10 species. Phleboviruses orginated in ticks, and evolved into tick-borne and dipteran-borne viruses that are present throughout the world.[276] Most dipteran-borne species are associated with phlebotomine sandflies, hence the genus name *Phlebovirus* (see Table 16.4). However, there are prominent exceptions, such as Rift Valley fever virus (RVFV), a medically and agriculturally important virus in Africa, which is primarily associated with *Aedes* species mosquitoes, and the tick-borne apathogenic Uukuniemi virus (UUKV).[277]

RVFV, the type species, was first isolated in 1930 by Daubney et al. from an infected newborn lamb as part of an investigation of a large epizootic of disease causing abortion and high mortality in sheep.[90] Large RVFV epizootics in various areas of sub-Saharan Africa have been noted since that time, and clinically compatible outbreaks have been retrospectively identified as far back as 1912.[103] Several decades passed before serologic and molecular similarities to phlebotomine fever viruses were noted. Sandfly fever Sicilian virus (SFSV), one of the most widespread phleboviruses, and Sandfly fever Naples virus (SFNV) were first isolated from American troops with febrile illness in the Palermo region of Sicily, Italy in 1943 and Naples, Italy in 1944, respectively, by inoculation of acute-phase sera into human volunteers and passage in newborn mice.[373] Outbreaks of compatible human illness in the Mediterranean region date back to the time of the Napoleonic Wars, and association of the disease with sandflies was suggested as early as 1905.[171]

Banyangvirus Genus

The *Banyangvirus* genus (family *Phenuiviridae*, order *Bunyavirales*) contains the type species Huaiyangshan banyangvirus (better known as severe fever with thrombocytopenia syndrome virus (SFTSV) or Henan fever virus (HNFV),[469,472] which is prevalent in East Asia. The related Heartland virus (HRTV) is endemic in the United States.[281] Both viruses are tick-borne and are highly pathogenic.

Tospoviridae Family

The Family *Tospoviridae* has only one genus, the *Orthotospovirus* genus, which includes 18 species of plant-infecting trisegmented ambisense RNA viruses[168,271] that are transmitted propagatively by at least 15 different species of thrips[461] of the *Thysanoptera* order[309,457] with the western flower thrip *Frankliniella occidentalis* identified as the primary vector. Several tospoviruses are now recognized as being of significant agricultural importance, inflicting massive losses in economically important crops, in major part due to the wide plant host range of *F. occidentalis* as well as the broad distribution of this vector across North and South America, Australia, Europe, and the Middle East.[142,342]

The history of the tospoviruses goes back to 1915, with the recognition of a spotted wilt of tomatoes in Australia,[57] and then the subsequent isolation in 1930 of tomato spotted wilt virus (TSWV), from which the genus gained its name[230] and which remains the prototype of the genus. By the late 1940s, TSWV infections were greatly reduced in the United States and Western Europe due to pesticide use controlling the onion thrips, *Thrips tabaci*, which was likely the primary vector at that time. The geographic spread during the 1960s and 1970s of *F. occidentalis* led to a rapid expansion of TSWV[457] which is now known to be global in distribution, and it is found throughout agricultural areas in warmer climate zones and prevalent in greenhouse cultivations in more temperate areas. In contrast to the other genus members, TSWV has an unusually wide host range, with more than 925 plant species, including 82 botanical families, reported to be susceptible to infection. These include several important crops such as peanuts, peppers, tobacco, potatoes, peas, tomatoes, celery, lettuce, and ornamental flowers, with annual crop losses amounting to more than a billion dollars.[318]

VIRION STRUCTURE

Under the electron microscope, negatively stained bunyaviruses appear in most cases spherical to pleomorphic, 80 to 120 nm in diameter, and display surface glycoprotein (GP) projections of 5 to 10 nm, which are embedded in a lipid bilayered envelope approximately 5 to 7 nm thick (Fig. 16.3). Cryo-electron microscopic and tomographic techniques combined with computational three-dimensional reconstruction revealed the structures of virions at a resolution of about 2 to 3 nm (Fig. 16.4). Virions of BUNV orthobunyavirus (family *Peribunyaviridae*) are pleomorphic and approximately 108 nm in diameter.[51]

Although several studies reported hantaviruses to be highly pleomorphic with spherical particles of 135 nm median diameter and tubular particles up to 350 nm long and approximately 80 nm in diameter, more recent EM and cryo-EM observations reveal a mostly spherical morphology, suggesting that mechanical stress likely contributed to earlier reports of pleomorphism.[35,170,180]

Virions of RVFV and UUKV phleboviruses (family *Phenuiviridae*) are distinct from all other bunyaviruses thus far characterized in that they are not pleomorphic but instead possess T = 12 icosahedral symmetry with mean diameters

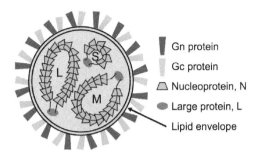

FIGURE 16.3 Schematic of a bunyavirus virion. The genome segments (commonly *S*, *M*, and *L*) are encapsidated by nucleocapsid protein (*N*) to form ribonucleoprotein complexes (RNPs), and together with the viral *L* protein (RNA dependent RNA polymerase, RdRp) are packaged within a host cell–derived lipid envelope modified by insertion of the viral glycoproteins Gn and Gc. Note that there is no matrix protein.

of approximately 100 and 125 nm, respectively.[122,181,313] The surface projections are thought to consist of equimolar heterodimers of the two viral GPs. They interact with each other to form family-specific surface morphologic units, namely 110 hexameric and 12 pentameric rings that form the well-defined and symmetric virions characteristic of this genus.[163,181,313,392] Whether this icosahedral symmetry is also a property of members of the other genera within the *Phenuiviridae* family is unknown, although electron microscopic images of SFTSV and HRTV (*Banyangvirus* genus) particles show regular, uniformly sized particles with similarity to phleboviruses.[281,472]

Orthobunyavirus virions (*Peribunyaviridae* family) have tripod-like GP spikes arranged with threefold symmetry in patches with gaps in between.[51] The surfaces of HTNV and Tula hantavirus (TULV) display spike projections with fourfold symmetry, and each spike contains four molecules of both glycoproteins. The fourfold symmetry is proposed to be maintained by homo-oligomerization of Gn and by interactions between Gn tetramers that interconnect to Gc dimers with one dimer at each face of the square-like spike.[35,170,180]

This localized architecture is also seen in the nairoviruses, with patches of spikes exhibiting fourfold symmetry and extending in a discontinuous manner over the virion surface.[35,180,256,343]

To date, structural analyses of viruses within the *Tospoviridae* family to a similar resolution have not yet been reported, although negative-stain EM has confirmed the presence of GP projections, which are observed as a characteristic fringe.[284]

The viral GP spikes represent both the cell attachment and membrane fusion machinery, responsible for the merging of viral and cellular envelopes during the entry process (see later) and these must be active only at the appropriate stage of the virus multiplication cycle. Stage-specific activation is achieved by the induction of GP conformational changes that are both pH dependent and ion dependent and are driven by the biochemical properties of the milieu present within various cellular compartments through which viruses must pass during entry. pH- and ion-dependent conformational changes have been visualized for orthobunyaviruses, phleboviruses, and nairoviruses,[51,163,313,343] and it is suggested that such changes expose

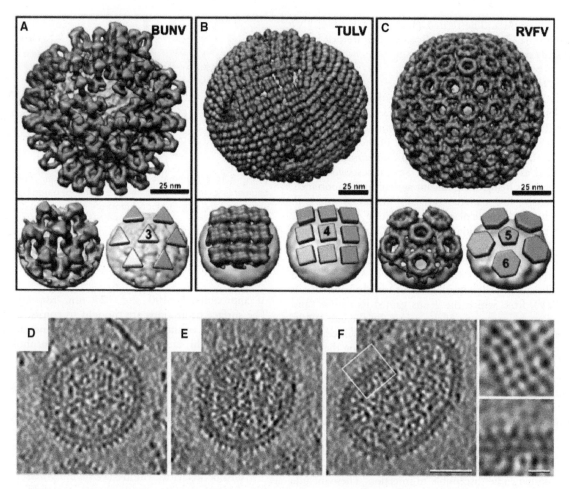

FIGURE 16.4 Structural diversity of bunyavirus surface glycoprotein architectures. A–C: Structures of Gn–Gc glycoprotein spikes (*orange*) are shown mapped onto the membrane surface (*cyan*) of **(A)** an orthobunyavirus (Bunyamwera virus; BUNV), **(B)** a hantavirus (Tula virus; TULV; EMD-170411), and **(C)** a phlebovirus (Rift Valley fever virus; RVFV; EMD-15507). At the bottom of each panel, a close-up view of a glycoprotein spike cluster (*left*) and a schematic representation of the spike arrangement (*right*) is shown. Symmetries of individual spikes are annotated. **D–F:** Central tomographic sections of three Hazara nairovirus (HAZV) virions, with fourfold symmetry of spikes shown in a tangential section. Scale bars represent 50 nm. (**Panels A–C** from Bowden TA, Bitto D, McLees A, et al. Orthobunyavirus ultrastructure and the curious tripodal glycoprotein spike. *PLoS Pathog* 2013;9(5):e1003374. **Panels D–F** from Punch EK, Hover S, Blest HTW, et al. Potassium is a trigger for conformational change in the fusion spike of an enveloped RNA virus. *J Biol Chem* 2018;293(26):9937–9944.)

hydrophobic regions on Gc that facilitate fusion between the viral and endosomal membranes during viral entry, a mechanism observed for other enveloped viruses that enter cells via the endocytic pathway. In addition, specific lateral interactions between spike complexes are thought to induce membrane curvature during the budding process.

In contrast to the features on the virion exterior, the content of the virion interior is poorly resolved. Cryo-electron tomography reveals the presence of electron density consistent with the filamentous RNA segments in the form of ribonucleoprotein (RNP) complexes[51,97,181,256] and the proximity of this density located very close to the inner face of the viral envelope suggests a possible interaction with the cytoplasmic tails of one or both of the glycoproteins.[35,180,181,313,355] The precise architecture of bunyaviral RNPs within virions remains unclear, presumably due to their flexibility that complicates subtomogram averaging.

GENOME STRUCTURE AND ORGANIZATION

Viral Genome

The bunyavirus genome comprises two to eight single-stranded RNA segments, and at all stages of the multiplication cycle, these RNAs are enwrapped in the cognate N protein to form an N-RNA complex known as an RNP. For the classical trisegmented bunyaviruses within *Hantaviridae*, *Nairoviridae*, *Peribunyaviridae*, *Phenuiviridae*, and *Tospoviridae* families, these segments are designated according to their relative sizes: large (L), medium (M), and small (S). In contrast, for viruses with more than three segments, a numerical system is used. All segments sequenced to date possess a short stretch of up to 9 contiguous complementary nucleotides at their extreme 3′ and 5′ termini, with these being highly conserved among viruses within a family, but being distinct from those of viruses in different families (Table 16.3). Some degree of interterminal base pairing of these nucleotides is predicted to allow formation of stable panhandle structures, possibly driving the circularization of bunyaviral RNAs, and this suggestion is supported by direct visualization of purified RNPs by electron microscopy, as well as biochemical and genetic evidence (see later section).

Electron microscopic analysis of segments released from phlebovirus, orthobunyavirus, and nairovirus virions reveal pseudocircular structures,[332] again consistent with 3' and 5' terminal interactions, described above. These RNPs do not exhibit obvious helical symmetry, which is in stark contrast to those belonging to members of the *Mononegavirales* order for which their RNPs form compact and often rigid helices that assemble into rod-like structures.[370] Instead, bunyaviral RNPs appear highly flexible and with diameters on the order of 10 nm. In some instances the RNPs appear as "beads on a string," implying N protein monomers contact adjacent monomers only. In other instances, localized regions of compact helical symmetry are evident, suggestive of interactions between N monomers on successive turns of an ordered helix.[20,118,355,358,450]

At least one each of the individual RNPs must be contained in a virion for infectivity; however, equal numbers of nucleocapsids may not always be packaged in mature virions, as suggested by various reports of nonequimolar ratios of L, M, and S RNAs in natural virions or of elevated segment numbers in recombinant virions containing additional, artificial segments.[44,182,459,460] Unequal complements of the RNPs may contribute to the size differences of virions observed by electron microscopy[35,431] and also argues against a selective packaging mechanism that several segmented RNA viruses from other taxonomic orders (like influenza viruses) appear to possess.[47,301] Whether a segment selection mechanism exists for other newly classified bunyaviruses with as many as eight segments remains to be determined.

In addition to RNPs containing virion-sense RNA (vRNA), certain viruses in the *Phlebovirus* genera and *Tospoviridae* family encapsidate small amounts of complementary sense (cRNA or antigenome). The phlebovirus UUKV was found to contain S- but not M-segment cRNA, and the tospovirus TSWV had both M and S cRNAs in virions.[228,408] For the orthobunyavirus LACV, S-segment cRNA was detected in virions synthesized in insect cells, but not in mammalian cells.[348] Interestingly, the phlebovirus RVFV encapsidated all three cRNA gene segments, and, as will be described later (see "S-segment products"), at least one of the cRNA genes may have a role in early replication processes.[187]

Coding Strategies of Viral Genes

All bunyaviruses follow a common strategy in which mRNAs for their structural proteins (N, Gn/Gc, and L) are transcribed from their vRNA, whereas their nonstructural protein mRNAs can be transcribed from either their cRNA or vRNA strands. Therefore, some viruses in the order *Bunyavirales* use only a negative-sense coding strategy, while others use a combination of negative-sense and also ambisense coding strategies (Fig. 16.1). For either of these strategies, the bunyaviral RdRp is capable of transcribing only one mRNA molecule from each cRNA or vRNA template, and the ability to alternatively promote either negative-sense or ambisense transcription is dictated by specific

3' and 5' terminal nucleotides that constitute the transcription promoter[29] such that viruses that utilize an ambisense transcription strategy possess transcription promoters in both vRNA and cRNA strands. For all bunyaviruses studied to date, their vRNA segments conform to a common arrangement in which nontranslated sequences containing transcription and replication promoters flank one or more open reading frames (ORFs) within a single transcriptional unit. In the following section, the coding strategies of only bunyaviruses that possess trisegmented genomes (S, M, and L) will be described, due to the current lack of detailed information concerning the strategies of bunyaviruses with more than three segments.

S-Segment Strategies

Without exception, the S segment of all bunyaviruses encodes the corresponding viral nucleocapsid protein (N). While the S segment of some bunyaviruses expresses only the N protein,[287] in many instances, the S segment also has the capacity to express a second protein, known as NSs (nonstructural, S), either from an alternative ORF[43] (Fig. 16.1), or from an ORF accessed by ambisense transcription. The various bunyavirus NSs proteins exhibit low sequence similarity, but all have common functions relating to the mitigation of host innate immunity and apoptosis (see below). The presence of NSs in virus-infected cells was demonstrated for several members of the *Orthobunyavirus* genus[105] and, as only one S segment mRNA species is transcribed in orthobunyavirus-infected cells,[71] it was deduced that N and NSs were generated by alternative start codon recognition by leaky ribosome scanning[99,109] confirmed by rescue of NSs knock out BUNV from cDNAs.[55] In general, the S segments of members of the *Peribunyaviridae* family are the shortest within the order, although there are exceptions; Brazoran orthobunyavirus has a long S segment corresponding to its uncharacteristically large N protein[237] with a long C-terminal extension of unknown function.

Hantaviruses and nairoviruses encode larger N proteins than do viruses in other families, and so their S segments are also correspondingly larger (Table 16.1; Fig. 16.1).[275,385] Some hantaviruses (e.g., SNV, PUUV, TULV, Prospect Hill virus [PHV] and Andes virus [ANDV]), have second ORFs within their cRNAs, and a corresponding NSs protein has been detected in PUUV-, ANDV-, and TULV-infected cells.[189] For ANDV, expression of NSs was proposed to result from leaky scanning of the translation initiation codon for N.[441] An NSs protein has also been detected in CCHF orthonairovirus-infected cells[27] and it is thought to be translated from an NSs-specific mRNA generated by ambisense transcription, and to induce apoptosis.

The S segments of phleboviruses, banyangviruses, and tospoviruses are ambisense, with N mRNAs transcribed from the genomic vRNA strand, and NSs mRNAs transcribed from the complementary cRNA strand (Fig. 16.1).[91,183,469,472] This dictates that expression of NSs relies on the presence of cRNA within cells, and it was first postulated that replication of the infecting S-segment vRNA was required to provide this cRNA template. Consistent with this, for the phlebovirus UUKV, N was detected at 4 to 6 hours after infection, whereas NSs did not appear until 2 hours later.[409,436] Likewise, the mRNA for NSs of the tospovirus TSWV was detected in infected plant cells 15 hours later than for N.[418] In addition, and consistent with a need for vRNA replication prior to NSs expression, studies with the phlebovirus Punta Toro virus (PTV) demonstrated that protein synthesis inhibitors arrest production of NSs mRNA, but not N mRNA.[185] In contrast, studies with the phlebovirus RVFV demonstrated the presence of cRNAs of all three RNA segments in purified virions, removing the need for a replication step prior to the access of ambisense ORFs. Moreover, mRNA for the NSs protein was detected as early as 20 minutes after infection, concomitant with the appearance of mRNA for N, suggesting that for RVFV the ambisense-encoded NSs mRNA is transcribed from incoming cRNA strands.[187]

M-Segment Strategies

Sizes of bunyavirus M segments range from approximately 3,600 to 5,300 nucleotides (Table 16.2). All bunyavirus M segments encode a single polyprotein precursor from a single ORF that is subsequently processed by cellular peptidases to yield at least two envelope GPs (Fig. 16.1) These GPs were previously designated G1 and G2 based on relative migration of the glycoproteins in polyacrylamide gels, but are now named Gn and Gc, referring to the amino-terminal or carboxy-terminal position of the proteins within the precursor.[238] As described below, it is becoming increasingly clearer that the functions of the Gn and Gc proteins are conserved among the bunyaviruses.

Some, but not all, bunyaviruses encode additional polypeptides from their M segments. For orthobunyaviruses, nairoviruses, and phleboviruses a nonstructural protein known as NSm is cleaved from the M-segment polyprotein precursor during the processing of Gn and Gc.

The roles of these NSm proteins are not yet clearly defined; genetically engineered RVFV lacking NSm was found to induce more extensive apoptosis than did one with NSm, and the expression of NSm significantly inhibited the cleavage of caspase 8 and 9 induced by staurosporine, indicating that the NSm protein suppresses apoptosis.[465] In addition, the detection of BUNV NSm in the proximity of virus assembly sites within the Golgi apparatus, as well as the activity of NSm knock out BUNV mutants, suggests the orthobunyavirus NSm may play a role in altering local cellular architecture to establish replication factories.[121]

In contrast, members of the plant-infecting *Tospoviridae* family express an NSm protein using an ambisense transcription strategy in which a subgenomic mRNA is transcribed from the cRNA template.[227,240] The tospovirus NSm protein is readily detected in infected plants and is the only M-segment nonstructural protein in the *Bunyavirales* order to have a clearly defined role, which is as a movement protein (see "M-Segment Products," below).

L-Segment Strategies

Without exception, the bunyavirus L segment encodes the RdRp, or L protein. The L segments of hantaviruses, orthobunyaviruses, phleboviruses, and banyangviruses are of similar size (~6,500 nucleotides), whereas those of tospoviruses and nairoviruses are considerably larger (~9,000 and 12,000 nucleotides, respectively; Table 16.2). All L segments of viruses in the order, except for arenaviruses, which are not discussed in this chapter, use conventional negative-sense coding strategies (Fig. 16.1) and there is no evidence for additional coding regions in either the cRNA or vRNA.[106,108,177,229,292,382]

STAGES OF REPLICATION

The principal stages of the replication process for viruses in the *Bunyavirales* order are illustrated in Figure 16.5 and are summarized in the following:

1. Attachment, mediated by an interaction of viral proteins and host receptors
2. Entry, predominantly by receptor-mediated endocytosis
3. Uncoating, by acidification of endocytic vesicles, and fusion of viral membranes with endosomal membranes
4. Primary transcription of viral-complementary mRNA species from genome templates using host-cell–derived primers and the virion-associated polymerase
5. Translation of S-, M- and L-segment mRNAs
   - cotranslational cleavage of M-segment polyprotein and postranslational cleavage of precursors for some viruses
   - dimerization of Gn and Gc in the endoplasmic reticulum (ER)
6. Membrane-associated RNA replication
   - synthesis and encapsidation of cRNA to serve as templates for vRNA or, for ambisense genes, templates for subgenomic mRNA
   - genome replication
7. Morphogenesis
   - localization of N in budding compartments
   - transport of dimerized Gn and Gc to the Golgi
   - glycosylation
   - acquisition of modified host membranes, generally by budding into the Golgi cisternae
8. Fusion of cytoplasmic vesicles containing viruses with the plasma membrane and release of mature virions
   - More rarely, some viruses in some cell types have been observed to bud directly from the host cell plasma membrane.

Attachment and Entry

Viral Attachment Proteins and Cellular Receptors

The mechanisms by which bunyaviruses gain access to the host cell cytoplasm appear similar to those reported for many other enveloped viruses. The first step involves an interaction between cell surface exposed receptors, and the bunyaviral Gn and/or Gc glycoproteins. The presence of neutralizing and hemagglutination-inhibiting sites on both the Gn and Gc proteins of phleboviruses and hantaviruses[19,209] suggests that both proteins may be involved in attachment. However, it is more likely that both are needed due to conformational requirements that depend on dimerization of Gn and Gc.

In general, Gc appears to be the primary attachment protein for orthobunyaviruses in mammalian cells, mosquito cells, and mosquitoes.[160,216,427] Consistent with this view, expression of M-segment products of three orthobunyaviruses demonstrated that Gc, but not Gn, could affect attachment and entry when tested in a cell-to-cell fusion assay and a pseudotype transduction assay.[335] However, the amino terminal half of BUNV Gc ectodomain is not required for infection of cultured mammalian cells,[399] and this region can be replaced by green fluorescent protein (GFP) allowing the creation of viable viruses expressing chimeric Gc-GFP in their virions.[404]

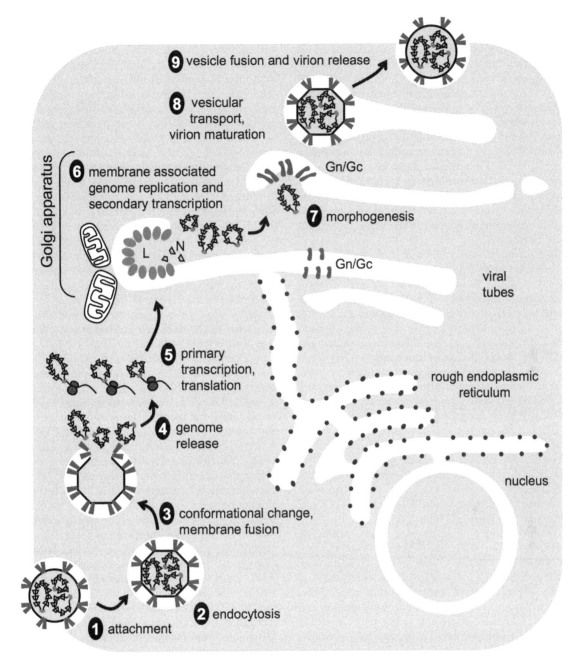

FIGURE 16.5 General virus multiplication scheme for members of the order *Bunyavirales*. Steps in the replication cycle are the following: *1*. Attachment, mediated by an interaction of viral proteins and host receptors; *2*. Receptor-mediated endocytosis; *3*. Uncoating, by acidification of endocytic vesicles, and fusion of viral membranes with endosomal membranes; *4*. Primary transcription of viral-complementary messenger RNA (mRNA) species from genome templates using host-cell–derived primers and the virion-associated polymerase; *5*. Translation of L, M, and S mRNAs, cotranslational cleavage of the M-segment polyprotein, dimerization of Gn and Gc in the endoplasmic reticulum (ER); *6*. Membrane-associated RNA replication, synthesis, and encapsidation of cRNA to serve as templates for vRNA or, for ambisense genes, templates for subgenomic mRNA, genome replication; *7*. Morphogenesis including transport of the structural proteins to the Golgi, glycosylation of Gn and Gc, budding into the Golgi cisternae; *8*. Migration of Golgi vesicles containing viruses to the cell surface, fusion of vesicular membranes with the plasma membrane, and *9*, release of infectious virions. Some viruses in some cell types can bud both into intracellular vesicles and also from the plasma membrane.

For tospoviruses, the envelope GPs are required only for infection of their arthropod vectors, as evidenced by the ability of envelope-deficient mutants to replicate in plants after mechanical transmission but their inability to infect thrips.[362] In addition, analysis of reassortant viruses demonstrated that mutations that disrupted the Gn-Gc ORF of TSWV ablated transmissibility by thrips.[412] These studies provide indirect evidence that the L-polymerase protein remains associated with ribonucleocapsids and is active despite the absence of intact virions.

Although there are no specific reports of Gc being the attachment protein of tospoviruses, functional homology to the Gc proteins of other bunyaviruses was proposed based on amino acid sequence homologies detected for iris yellow spot virus.[84] In contrast, however, a study with a soluble, truncated form of TSWV Gn produced by recombinant baculoviruses showed binding of this protein to epithelial cells in the midguts of thrips, suggesting that Gn could mediate attachment in these hosts.[456] Similar results were reported earlier with the orthobunyavirus LACV, in that virions treated with a protease that cleaved Gc but not Gn exhibited increased binding to the insect vector midgut but reduced binding to cultured mammalian or mosquito cells.[267] Given that both of these systems use a Gn protein in the absence of Gc, it remains to be determined whether Gn functions for attachment when in its native conformation on virions.

Host cell receptors have not been identified for most viruses in the order; however, pathogenic and nonpathogenic hantaviruses were shown to use $\beta 3$ and $\beta 1$ integrins, respectively, to enter endothelial cells.[133] This finding was suggested to relate to pathogenesis, in that binding of hantaviruses to integrins might disrupt their ability to regulate cell-to-cell adhesion and result in the vascular permeability characteristic of hantaviral diseases.[134] For two HPS-causing hantaviruses, ANDV and SNV, the human asthma-associated gene protocadherin-1 was identified as an essential determinant of entry and infection in pulmonary endothelial cells. Hamsters genetically engineered to remove the gene were resistant to a normally fatal infection by ANDV.[193] In addition to these entry determinants, decay accelerating factor (DAF)/CD55, a glycosylphosphatidylinositol (GPI)-anchored protein, has been shown to mediate HTNV and PUUV entry across the apical membrane of polarized epithelial cells,[232] and gC1qR/p32, a 32-kD glycoprotein that interacts with complement protein C1q, binds HTNV and mediates infection of cultured A549 lung cells.[77]

Several phleboviruses and banyangviruses, including RVFV, UUKV, SFSTV, PTV, and Toscana virus (TOSV), have been shown to use the C-type lectins DC-SIGN or L-SIGN (also known as DC-SIGNR) as receptors for infecting dendritic cells or liver sinusoidal endothelial cells, respectively. DC-SIGN was also found to be required for both binding and internalization of UUKV, whereas L-SIGN only promoted binding.[8,174,248,265] In addition, DC-SIGN has been implicated as a receptor for CCHFV and LACV.[174,425] Other factors identified to promote bunyavirus infection include heparan sulfate for RVFV and TOSV, nucleolin for CCHFV, and a thrips midgut 50-kDa protein for TSWV.[8]

Aside from the requirement of specific host gene products, many bunyaviruses have been shown to be highly sensitive to perturbation of cholesterol biosynthesis pathways for their entry,[218,330,407] and it has been postulated that cholesterol modulates virus entry by facilitating the interaction of the viral fusion machinery with target endosomal membranes.[437]

Entry of the Viral Genome into the Host Cytoplasm

Shortly after attachment, viruses in the *Phlebovirus* and *Orthonairovirus* genera were observed in phagocytic vacuoles.[110,372] This suggested a mode of viral entry similar to that first described for alphaviruses in which the virus is endocytosed in coated vesicles, and inhibitor studies have confirmed this to

be so for the animal-infecting bunyaviruses. Orthobunyaviruses, hantaviruses, and nairoviruses enter by clathrin-mediated endocytosis,[130,199,381,407] and HTNV proteins were shown to colocalize with clathrin in confocal immunofluorescence studies.[199] Although clathrin-mediated endocytosis appears to be most common for bunyaviruses, other entry mechanisms have been reported, to include caveolae-mediated endoctytosis and macropinocytosis for RVFV,[167] and undefined nonclathrin as well as clathrin-mediated entry routes for the hantaviruses SNV and ANDV.[75] Likewise, UUKV phlebovirus has been found to enter cells predominantly in a clathrin-independent manner.[266]

After endocytosis, acidification of the endocytic vesicles is thought to promote a conformational change in Gn and/or Gc that facilitates fusion of the viral and cellular membranes, thereby allowing the viral genome in the form of an RNP with its associated polymerase access to the cytoplasm. Consistent with pH-dependent fusion and entry, infection by several bunyaviruses was shown to be blocked by treatment with ammonium chloride to prevent endosomal acidification.[191,335,381,401] Additional indirect support for membrane fusion as a mode of entry came from experiments demonstrating the ability of viruses in the family to mediate syncytia formation at low pH.[119,145,191,308,335,401,458]

Of the bunyaviruses studied to date, most appear to traffic through the early endosomes (EE) to the more acidic late endosomes (LE) where fusion is triggered.[264] Infection by CCHFV, as well as UUKV and certain hantaviruses, have been reported to use functional microtubules, which are known to be required for directing LE toward the nucleus.[406] CCHFV and LACV, however, have both been found to infect cells in the absence of Rab7, a critical component of LE fusion, indicating that the viruses do not traffic to LE.[130,175] Instead, CCHFV was found to enter the cytosol via multivesicular bodies just prior to transitioning from EE to LE.[405] In addition to a role for low pH in virus entry, the use of inhibitors of specific cellular ion channels has shown that the concentration of potassium ions within specific cellular compartments also influences bunyavirus entry[179] (Fig. 16.6). Biochemical analyses suggest that the escape of RNPs from endosomes requires an influx of potassium ions that depends on the activity of cellular potassium ion channels, located within endosomal membranes. Structural studies show that elevated levels of potassium ions directly influence the conformation of the viral Gn/Gc spikes, activating their fusogenic properties, which likely promotes fusion between virion and endosomal membranes.[343] Potassium channel blockade prevents virus escape, and virions are trafficked to later compartments within the endosomal pathway, or lysosomes, where they are inactivated by low pH.[179]

High-resolution structural studies (see below) have revealed that the bunyaviral Gc proteins have characteristics similar to those of class II fusion proteins identified for positive-sense RNA viruses in the *Flaviviridae* and *Togaviridae* families,[131] raising interesting questions concerning the evolution of these virus groups. Such proteins have internal fusion domains known as fusion loops, as opposed to terminal fusion peptides found for the class I fusion proteins. Experimental support for this finding was obtained by demonstrating interaction of the fusion loop postulated for the Gc protein of the hantavirus, ANDV, with artificial membranes.[435] In addition, several lines of evidence indicate that the Gc of orthobunyaviruses is involved in membrane fusion. Protease sensitivity assays,

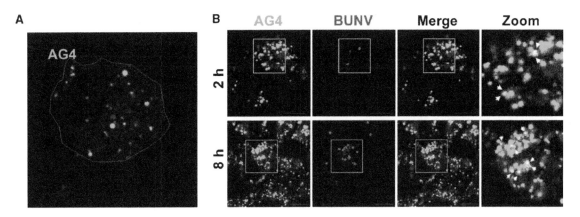

FIGURE 16.6 BUNV traffics through endosomes containing K⁺ ions. A: K⁺-containing vesicles can be labeled with the membrane-impermeable K⁺-specific fluorescent probe Asante potassium green-4 (AG4), the membrane-permeable form of which has previously been used to monitor cytoplasmic [K⁺]. AG4 (10 μM) was added to A549 cells for 40 minutes to allow endosomal uptake, and live cells were imaged. Representative images are shown ($n \geq 100$ cells). Scale bar = 10 μM. **B:** A549 cells were infected with a fluorescently labeled BUNV in the presence of AG4 (10 μM) to allow virus penetration into cells, and live cells were imaged 2 or 8 hours postinfection. Images are representative of ≥50 cells. (Taken from Hover S, Foster B, Fontana J, et al. Bunyavirus requirement for endosomal K+ reveals new roles of cellular ion channels during infection. *PLOS Pathog* 2018;14(1):e1006845.)

detergent partitioning experiments, and antibody-binding studies suggest that Gc undergoes a conformational change at pH conditions where fusion is observed.[144] Mutational analyses of a hydrophobic region (residues 1,066–1,087) of LACV Gc that is well conserved among different orthobunyaviruses[84] supported this notion,[191,336] and the residues flanking the predicted fusion peptide in BUNV Gc (residues 1,058–1,079) were shown to be structurally critical for the conformational change in Gc that occurs during the fusion process.[399] LACV Gc alone, however, when expressed from recombinant vaccinia viruses, could not cause cell fusion, suggesting that an association of the two GPs may be needed for activation of the fusion machinery,[191] and mutations in the cytoplasmic tail of BUNV Gn severely affected fusion activity indicating that Gn must also play an important role in this process.[401] Likewise for HTNV, both Gn and Gc were required to achieve surface expression and cell-to-cell fusion activity.[308] Recombinant LACV carrying mutations in the Gc fusion peptide was impaired for growth in both mammalian and insect cells but were still neurotoxic to neuronal cells, implying that the fusion peptide is a determinate of neuroinvasiveness but not necessarily neurovirulence.[415]

Transcription and Replication

After release of the virion-associated segments from within the virus particle, the initial RNA synthetic event is primary transcription in which each vRNA is transcribed as a complementary mRNA by the RNP-associated RdRp. *In vitro* experiments showing transcriptional activity of permeabilized purified virions as well as atomic structures show that the RdRp is located at the vRNA termini of each RNP segment while still inside the infecting particle, positioned alongside the transcription promoter.[138,323] Thus, it can commence primary transcription upon release into the cytosol.

Studies with hantavirus N protein suggest that N participates in transcription initiation by facilitating dissociation of the RNA panhandle and by subsequently remaining attached to the 5′ terminus of the RNA, thereby freeing the 3′ terminus for RdRp interactions. Furthermore, N was suggested to be important for replication by acting as an RNA chaperone and transiently and continuously unfolding the RNA to allow it to form more stable structures.[285] A role for N in both transcription and replication is also evident by analysis of the behavior of BUNV N proteins carrying specific mutations, either in a minigenome assay or in the context of virus infection.[20,104,448] BUNV N mutants could be divided into two groups, those that were defective in antigenome synthesis but not mRNA transcription, and those that were replication defective but transcription competent, suggesting that different domains within N are associated with different RNA synthesis activities.[104] The mechanism by which residues in N modulate template activity requires elucidation; one possibility is that transcription and replication require different binding partners that interact with distinct regions on the N protein, or alternatively that these mutations result in subtle conformational changes in N that modulate its function.

Genome Promoters

The template for bunyavirus transcription and replication is not naked RNA but instead is an RNP in which the RNA is enwrapped with the corresponding N protein to form a flexible assembly that is resistant to RNase digestion.[100,262,288,356] Extensive analysis of the RNA synthesis activity of model RNA segments from members of the *Phlebovirus* and *Orthobunyavirus* genera have revealed that nucleotides within the 3′ and 5′ nontranslated regions of these RNPs contain signals for both mRNA transcription and genome replication. Furthermore, targeted mutagenesis of these regions has helped define the roles of individual nucleotides in promoting these activities. For the phleboviruses RVFV and UUKV, the first 13 or the first 10 nucleotides, respectively, of the 3′ end of the genome are sufficient for RNA synthesis activity,[120,340] whereas for the orthobunyavirus BUNV, at least 17 nucleotides at each of the termini are required for detectable levels of RNA replication.[288]

For BUNV, studies have suggested that at the extreme 3′ and 5′ termini, precise nucleotide sequence rather than complementarity is required to form the RNA synthesis promoters.

A striking example is in the role of the conserved nucleotide mismatch located among a run of otherwise perfect complementary residues, which is a common feature of many bunyaviruses. Saturation mutagenesis showed that this 3′ position 9 must be a U residue in order to signal maximal transcription, and this signaling ability was completely independent of the corresponding 5′ position 9[32]; thus, arguing against the need for interterminal cooperation within these initial nucleotides.

However, for BUNV and other orthobunyaviruses, there is considerable evidence in support of a counterargument, suggesting 3′ and 5′ terminal interactions are important; Firstly, the precise nucleotides that form the BUNV transcription promoter have been identified and shown to constitute nucleotides within both 3′ and 5′ termini,[29] a finding that implies the polymerase must contact both termini during transcription initiation.[31,223] Secondly, genetic manipulation of model BUNV segments revealed RNA synthesis was promoted only when potential interterminal interactions within terminal-distal nucleotides (residues 12–15) were maintained, independent of specific nucleotide sequences.[31] In addition, inter-terminal secondary structures were identified in virion-associated RNAs following psoralen cross-linking.[172,348]

Interestingly, the recently solved crystal structure of the orthobunyavirus LACV RdRp in complex with 3′ and 5′ terminal RNAs suggested that the termini interact with separate sites on the polymerase surface. Nucleotides 1 to 8 of the 3′ end bind as a single extended strand whereas 5′ nucleotides 1 to 10 form an intraterminal stem-loop "hook" structure,[138] suggesting that interaction between the two termini may not actually be due to interterminal base pairing, but instead mediated by the polymerase (see below). However, it is possible that the existence of inter- and intraterminal interactions are not mutually exclusive, and both forms may be required at different stages of the virus replication cycle. Thus, it is likely that some regions of the 3′ and 5′ termini form sequence specific signals, whereas other sequences form signals based on structure. Moreover, by setting progressive terminal deletions it was found that the minimal BUNV RNA replication promoters comprise 17 nucleotides from each end,[288] but that production of infectious virus also requires additional segment-specific sequences in the untranslated regions (UTRs),[263] presumably for activities other than RNA synthesis such as virus assembly.

The *in vivo* importance of intact termini was also suggested by a study in which terminally deleted RNAs were shown to accumulate during the establishment of persistent infections with the hantavirus, SEOV. It was hypothesized that as deletions accrued, fewer replication-competent genomes were present, leading to a down-regulation of the replication processes, and possibly to persistence.[282] Similar deletions were found on the termini of ANDV M and L, but not S genes, leading to a speculation that differences observed in the relative abundance of Gn and Gc compared to N could reflect down-regulation of M-segment expression from genes without intact termini.[314]

Primed mRNA Synthesis (Cap Snatching)

Like influenza viruses, viruses in the *Bunyavirales* order prime mRNA synthesis with capped oligoribonucleotides that are scavenged from host mRNAs (Fig. 16.7). However, unlike influenza viruses, which take primers from newly synthesized mRNAs in the host cell nucleus, members of the order *Bunyavirales* use primers cleaved from host cell mRNAs in the cytoplasm.

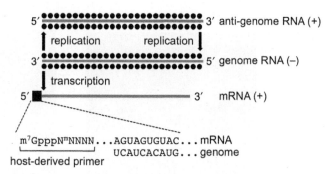

FIGURE 16.7 Transcription and replication scheme of negative-sense bunyavirus genome segments. The genome RNA and the positive-sense complementary RNA known as the antigenome RNA are found only as ribonucleoprotein complexes and are encapsidated by N protein (●). Segments are shown as linear RNA molecules for simplicity, whereas all available evidence suggests the active templates for RNA synthesis are circularized by noncovalent terminal interactions. The messenger RNA (mRNA) species contain host-derived primer sequences at their 5′ ends (■) and are truncated at the 3′ end relative to the virion RNA (vRNA) template; the mRNAs are neither polyadenylated nor encapsidated by N protein. The sequence at the 5′ end of an orthobunyavirus mRNA is shown.

Work with influenza virus has shown that cap snatching requires both cap-binding and endonuclease activities, which are encoded within different polymerase subunits. For bunyaviruses, generation of the capped primers is accomplished by an endonuclease domain belonging to the PD-D/ExK superfamily of cation-dependent nucleases[95,117,176,219,290,323,357,359,368,446] and in all bunyavirales members examined thus far, the endonuclease domain resides within the N-terminus of the respective proteins. Comparison of endonuclease domains from segmented negative-stranded RNA viruses revealed them all to possess structural similarity, but two distinct classes were apparent: one with a canonical catalytic histidine (His+) as exemplified by influenza virus and bunyaviruses and another class in which this histidine is replaced by an acidic residue (His-), typified by the arenaviruses.[117,176,357] In contrast to the endonuclease domain, no cap-binding domain has yet been identified for any bunyavirales member, although comparison between the segmented architecture of the influenza virus RdRp alongside the monomeric bunyavirales L protein suggests it is likely to reside within the C terminus. It is also thought that the distance between the cap-binding and endonuclease domains dictates the length of the snatched primer. In the case of the bunyaviruses, this appears to fall within a characteristic range for viruses within the different families, with mean lengths of between 10 and 20 nucleotides.[50,74,98,129,197,338,410] In the case of influenza virus, the endonuclease is sequence specific, with the RNA cleavage event preferentially occurring between 10 and 13 nucleotides downstream of the cap, at a G residue.[89] There is some evidence to suggest that the site of bunyaviral primer cleavage may also be sequence dependent, with certain snatched primer sequences being selected over others. During TSWV transcription, the TSWV mRNAs acquired 5′ extensions with a preference for cleavage at an A residue.[98] It was suggested that this preference was due to a need for base pairing at the ultimate U residue of the TSWV gene segments. Consistent with this, later studies indicated that double- and triple-base complementarity to nucleotides at the ends of the tospovirus gene segments were preferred, even more than the single complementary residue.[439]

Other viruses in the order also have nucleotide or nucleotide motif preferences for endonuclease cleavage of capped primers. These preferences vary among the families and genera, and sometimes even among viruses within a genus. A preferred primer sequence, or a favored nucleotide at the site of cleavage due to a need for limited base pairing with the viral genome, appears to be a common feature of primed transcription for bunyaviruses. In one study, the 3'-terminal nucleotides of the scavenged host primers often were similar to the 5'-terminal viral nucleotides.[197] It was proposed that after transcription of two or three nucleotides of the nascent mRNA, the viral polymerase slips backward on the template before further elongation, resulting in a partial reiteration of the 5'-terminal sequence. An extension of this concept, termed "prime and realign," was proposed for mRNA transcription of hantaviruses.[129] According to this model (Fig. 16.8), priming by host oligonucleotides with a terminal G residue would initiate transcription by aligning at the third nucleotide of the viral RNA template (C residue). After synthesis of a few oligonucleotides, the nascent RNA could realign by slipping backward two nucleotides on the repeated terminal sequences (AUCAUCAUC) (Table 16.3), such that the G becomes the first nucleotide of the nontemplated 5' extensions (Fig. 16.8). The frequent deletion of one or two of the triplet repeats in hantaviral mRNA supports this

sort of slippage mechanism and suggests that sometimes the initial priming might start at the C residue of the third triplet in the conserved sequence rather than at the C of the second triplet.[129]

A problem that the bunyaviruses must overcome is in locating sufficient capped mRNAs to support viral transcription. In the case of hantaviruses and phleboviruses, evidence has been presented that one such source may be cytoplasmic processing bodies (P bodies) that contain much of the RNA decay machinery where 5' caps are sequestered, including the canonical mRNA decapping enzyme Dcp2. In the case of RVFV, a genome-wide RNAi screen in insect cells identified Dcp2 as a viral restriction factor, possibly reducing the pool of available capped mRNA substrate and thus restricting RVFV gene expression.[178] In the case of hantaviruses, the N protein accumulates in P bodies where it is thought to bind to the 5' cap of cellular mRNAs to protect them from cell-mediated degradation, also maintaining the pool of cellular messages for subsequent use as cap substrate.[157]

Transcription Termination
The mRNAs transcribed by the nonsegmented negative-stranded RNA viruses resemble host cell mRNAs in that they are 5' capped and possess 3' poly(A) tails, and mRNAs generated by the segmented negative-stranded influenza virus also fit this description. However, this does not appear to be the case for most members of the *Bunyavirales* order; while their

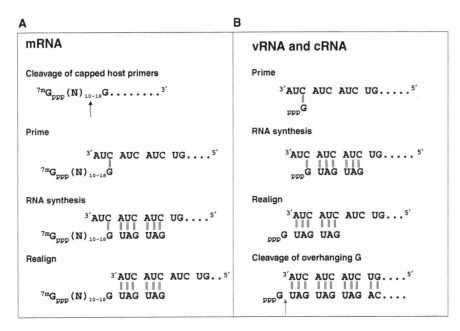

FIGURE 16.8 Prime- and- realign models for primary transcription and genome replication as illustrated to occur for a hantavirus.[129] **A:** Primed messenger RNA (mRNA) transcription. According to this model, priming by host oligonucleotides with a terminal G residue would initiate transcription by aligning at the third nucleotide of the viral RNA template (C residue). After synthesis of a few nucleotides, the nascent RNA realigns by slipping backward two nucleotides on the repeated terminal sequences (AUCAUCAUC), such that the G becomes the first nucleotide of the nontemplated 5' extension. **B:** Nonprimed transcription of vRNA and cRNA. In the model, transcription initiates with pppG aligned at the third nucleotide (C residue) of the template RNA. After synthesis of several nucleotides, polymerase slippage realigns the nascent RNA such that the initial priming G residue overhangs the template, but is subsequently removed (perhaps by nucleolytic activity of the L protein) leaving a monophosphorylated U residue at the nascent 5' end.

5′ ends are capped, their 3′ ends do not in general possess 3′ poly(A) tails.[1,325,436] The only instance where a poly(A) tail has been identified on a bunyavirales transcript is the M-segment mRNA from SNV hantavirus,[182] which also contains a U-tract that in nonsegmented negative-sense RNA viruses is the template for reiterative transcription coupled to termination.[33,389] In all other instances where bunyaviral mRNA ends have been identified, the 3′ end has mapped to either the vRNA 5′ end, indicating run-off transcription,[182] or alternatively, putative transcriptional termination signals.[7,30,188,239]

Transcription termination is well studied for members of the orthobunyavirus group, for which synthesis of M- and S-segment mRNAs terminates between 40 to 100 nucleotides before the end of the genome RNA template, and L-segment mRNAs thought to be terminated by run-off.[85,86,112,198,324] By using a system in which the RNAs generated from mutated S segments were directly visualized, the transcription termination signal for the orthobunyavirus BUNV was mapped to a 33-nucleotide region within the 5′ nontranslated region of the S segment[30] with a 6-nucleotide motif, 3′-GUCGAC-5′, being particularly critical for termination signaling. Interestingly, a second redundant termination signal was also identified further downstream, with the related sequence, 3′-UGUCG′-5′, and a similar motif was observed within the BUNV L, but not the M segment.[30] Detailed experimental mapping of BUNV M and L mRNA termination sites has not been reported. The finding that there were no U-rich regions in the transcription termination signal of BUNV was consistent with the absence of 3′ poly-A tails on the mRNAs.

Comparison of these S-segment sequences with those of other orthobunyaviruses revealed a high degree of conservation, suggesting that similar motifs may also function for transcription termination throughout the genus, at least for S segments. A cross-genus comparison of orthobunyaviral mRNA 3′ ends also revealed the presence of sequences with the potential to form short stem loop structures, outside of the conserved hexanucleotide sequence.

In contrast to the orthobunyaviruses that perform strictly negative-sense transcription, viruses that use an ambisense transcription strategy, such as the phleboviruses and tospoviruses (and also arenaviruses—see Chapter 18), possess segments with a different arrangement of *cis*-acting signals. One of these differences is a centrally located untranslated sequence known as the intergenic region (IGR). Although the IGR sequences are diverse across the various families, they mostly possesses the potential to form stem-loop secondary structures,[214] and previous work has suggested these structures may play a role in transcription termination.[80,91,111,148,149,410] However, the likelihood of hairpin formation in the IGRs of RVFV, TOSV, and SFTSV phleboviruses has been questioned[7] and detailed mapping of mRNA termination sites for the corresponding N and NSs mRNA showed that the 3′ ends contained most of the intergenic sequence and indeed overlapped each other.[7] Furthermore, termination occurred for both mRNAs at the same motif, 3′-C$_{1-3}$GUCG/A-5′, which was also identified as the termination signal in the negative stranded M segment. Two copies of this motif were identified in the ambisense S segment, one in vRNA (genome) and one in the cRNA (antigenome), and thus it was proposed that transcription termination was signaled by a specific sequence motif rather than a secondary structural element. The similarity between this phleboviral termination signal and that identified for orthobunyaviruses described above is striking and points toward a common mechanism.

Sequences within the 3′ nontranslated regions of bunyaviral mRNAs have been shown to enhance mRNA translatability,[46,442] possibly providing functions that are normally associated with the canonical mRNA poly(A) tail and its synergistic association with the 5′cap.[127] While the precise identity or function of this enhancing element are currently unknown, one possibility is that the secondary structures found within most bunyaviral mRNA 3′ ends are involved.[46]

Bunyavirus transcription is unique among negative-sense RNA viruses in that it requires ongoing protein synthesis,[28,325,346,347,349,444] a finding that at face value appears incompatible with the presence of a virion-associated transcriptase. In the absence of protein synthesis, only short transcripts are produced *in vivo* and *in vitro*, although if the *in vitro* reaction is supplemented with rabbit reticulocyte lysate, full-length RNAs are synthesized. The translational requirement is not at the level of mRNA initiation, but rather during elongation or, more precisely, to maintain transcriptase processivity. A model to account for these observations suggested that in the absence of ribosome binding and protein translation, the nascent mRNA chain and its template could base-pair, thereby preventing progression of the transcriptase.[37] The translational requirement (Fig 16.9) was formally proven using BUNV model templates containing translational stop codons[28] in which the presence of in-frame stop codons within the transcriptional unit reduced polymerase processivity, with termination events occurring at specific locations resembling transcription termination signals. In contrast, out of frame stop codons had no influence on polymerase processivity, and transcription termination signals placed immediately downstream of stop codons were unrecognized. Taken together, these observations are consistent with a model in which the translocation of a ribosome along the nascent mRNA alters RdRp processivity, in particular in the recognition of consensus or spurious transcription termination signals. Similar findings have been reported for RVFV[239] and thus orthobunyaviruses and possibly phleboviruses appear to have adopted a mechanism whereby transcription and translation are coupled, a feature commonly found in prokaryotes but rare in eukaryotic cells where these processes are compartmentalized. The dependence of transcription on translation has an important implication for the very first stages of the cytosolic phase of the virus replication cycle, as upon release from the infecting virion the bunyaviral RNP/polymerase complex must first sequester ribosomes in order to maintain polymerase processivity and commence primary transcription. How this is achieved is currently unknown.

Genome Replication

The first RNA synthesis activity performed within the infected cell by the bunyaviral RdRp is primary transcription, in which short capped RNA oligomers are used to prime mRNA synthesis. However, at a later stage of the infection, the RdRp must commence RNA replication, for which the RdRp is thought to initiate primer-independent RNA polymerization at the precise 3′ end of the template to produce a full-length copy of the template. The molecular mechanism that regulates this switch from primary transcription to genome replication has not been defined for any member of the *Bunyavirales* order, and other

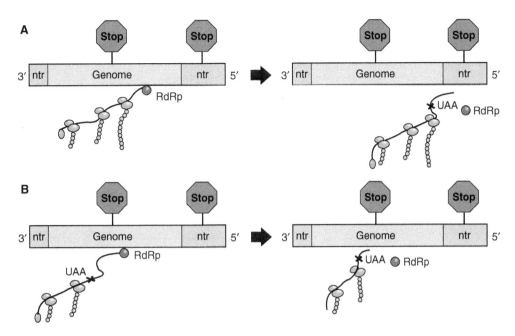

FIGURE 16.9 Model of obligatorily coupled bunyavirus transcription and translation.
A: Transcription of full length mRNAs requires on-going translation to allow translocation of ribosomes along the nascent mRNA. Transcription termination signals (shown as STOP signs) within coding regions (*green*) are not recognised by the RdRp, whereas transcription termination signals within the ntr (*blue*) are active, leading to generation of the mRNA 3′ end. **B:** When translation is prevented by the presence of in-frame stop codons within the mRNA, ribosome translocation is blocked and previously unrecognised transcription termination signals are now active. Ribosome translocation is proposed to suppress the activity of spurious or cryptic transcription termination signals. (Redrawn from Barr JN. Bunyavirus mRNA synthesis is coupled to translation to prevent premature transcription termination. *RNA* 2007;13:731–736.)

fundamental differences between replication and transcription actvities, such as the ability of the nascent strand to be encapsidated or terminated, remain unexplained. It is established that bunyavirus genome replication and subsequent secondary transcription prevented by translational inhibitors such as cycloheximide, which indicates that continuous protein synthesis is required for replication of the genome. Although not proven, it is likely that synthesis of N is required for genome replication, as described for other negative-strand RNA viruses such as the rhabdovirus, vesicular stomatitis virus, and the paramyxovirus Sendai virus. For these viruses, supply of N protein for encapsidation of new replication products was proposed as a critical component that mediates the transcription–replication switch, and other possibilities have now been suggested.[302]

A prime-and-realign model was also postulated for the nonprimed transcription of hantaviral vRNA and cRNA, except that transcription would initiate with pppG alignment at the third nucleotide (C residue) of the template RNA. After synthesis of several nucleotides, polymerase slipping would realign the nascent RNA such that the initial priming G residue would overhang the template. It was further theorized that nucleolytic activity of the L protein might remove the overhanging G, leaving a monophosphorylated U residue at the nascent 5′ end. The presence of the monophosphorylated U on HTNV RNA was experimentally demonstrated[129] (Fig. 16.8).

Indirect evidence suggesting that a prime-and-realign method of initiation is used by phleboviruses was obtained by using a reconstituted transcription system to study the polymerase recognition sequence at the 3′ termini of the ambisense

S-segment RNA of RVFV. In those studies, mutational analysis of the terminal nucleotides revealed that the first 13 nucleotides are required for polymerase recognition, but that one of the two terminal dinucleotides (UGUG) could be removed without deleterious effects on transcription.[340] These data also suggested that realignment is not a prerequisite for transcription initiation. In contrast, a recent study using the BUNV minigenome system showed that the viral polymerase was able to repair both insertions and deletions in model template RNAs, although this did not appear to involve the prime-and-realign mechanism.[447]

Schematics of transcription and replication based on information above are presented in Figures 16.7 and 16.10.

Encapsidation Signals
The existence of specific RNA signals that drive the formation of RNPs has been proposed only for hantaviruses, as described above. For all other bunyavirales members, RNA sequence signals that drive specific interaction between viral RNAs and the cognate N protein have been proposed based on secondary structure predictions, but not formally identified. The observation that BUNV RNPs functional for RNA replication can be assembled with as few as 17 nucleotides from each of the 3′ and 5′ termini argues that if RNP encapsidation signals existed they would reside within these short UTRs.[288] Interestingly, a stem loop structure comprising these nucleotides was predicted to form in the BUNV 5′ UTR, and proposed to bind N, as demonstrated by *in vitro* gel shift binding assays.[312] However, it is also plausible that no such encapsidation signals exist, and instead, selective encapsidation of viral templates is driven by

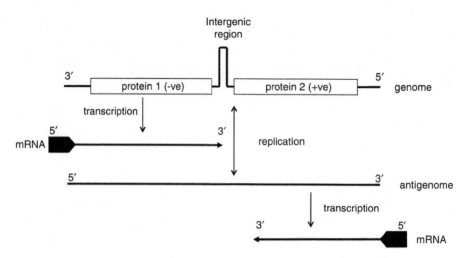

FIGURE 16.10 Transcription and replication scheme of ambisense-sense bunyavirus genome segments. The genome RNA encodes proteins in both negative- and positive-sense orientations, separated by an intergenic region that for some viruses has the potential to form a hairpin structure. The proteins are translated from specific subgenomic messenger RNAs (mRNAs), with the mRNA-encoding protein 2 transcribed from the antigenome RNA after the onset of genome replication.

proximity of solely these RNAs to N protein in viral replication factories, as well as the ability of the polymerase to interact with N,[104] thus, ensuring encapsidation occurs simultaneous with polymerization.[138] In support of this proposal, the recent high-resolution crystal structures of many bunyaviral N proteins do not provide any structural basis for sequence specificity that would favor the interaction between terminal sequences over any other. Work with BUNV has also suggested the terminal UTRs play an important role in segment packaging into virions, whereas the coding regions do not.[225] Mutational analysis of the BUNV M segment revealed a conserved sequence within nucleotides 20 to 33 of the 5′ end of vRNA that was critical for maintaining the segment during serial passage of virus-like particles (VLPs).[225] Variable packaging efficiencies were noted for the L-, M-, and S-segment–derived minireplicons, and packaging appeared to be independent for each.

Host Factors
Beyond the need for host-derived primers for initiating mRNA synthesis, little is known about the role that host factors might play in viral replication. One putative host transcription factor is an approximately 40-kD protein isolated from the main insect vector of TSWV, and it was shown to bind to the viral RdRp at its C-terminus and to the viral RNA at its N-terminus.[92] Both this protein and reticulocyte lysates were needed for RNA synthesis *in vitro*, indicating that other cellular factors are also required. Expression of this protein in mammalian cells rendered them permissive to TSWV replication.[92] As is the case for a number of other negative-strand RNA viruses, heat-shock protein 90 (Hsp90) appeared essential for LACV replication in that virus yields were diminished in cells treated with Hsp90 inhibitors like geldanamycin due to destabilization of the viral L protein.[82]

Translation and Processing of Viral Proteins
Viral polypeptides are synthesized shortly after infection, with S and L mRNAs translated on free ribosomes and M mRNAs translated on membrane-bound ribosomes. Expression products vary among the genera, and even within a genus.

S-Segment Products: N and NSs
The N protein is the most abundant viral product in virions and infected cells, and while the most prominent role of N is in the encapsidation of viral replication products, it is becoming clear that N plays several other important structural roles in the viral multiplication cycle. For example, N interacts with Gn and Gc, postulated to mediate virion assembly, and N interacts with L, possibly to drive formation of RNPs and mediate encapsidation. In addition, some of the larger N proteins of the hantaviral and nairovirus groups (Table 16.1) have been shown to possess activities unrelated to RNA binding, such as interaction with a diverse set of cellular proteins relating to translation,[165,195] protein folding[306,429,473] regulators of innate immunity,[13,432] and the cytoskeleton.[16,429]

The high-resolution crystal structures of N proteins from several members of the *Hantaviridae*,[156,310] *Peribunyaviridae*,[20,258,300,358] *Nairoviridae*[67,155,428,449,451] and *Phenuiviridae* families[118,311,354,355] have been solved, with a sole example solved for the tospoviruses (Fig. 16.11). In the case of orthobunyaviruses and phleboviruses (*Phenuiviridae* family), which possess N proteins within the smaller size range (Table 16.1), the solved structures are of both RNA-bound and RNA-unbound multimeric forms, which has revealed important information relating to the mechanism of RNA binding and N–N multimerization. BUNV, LACV, Schmallenberg virus (SBV) and Leanyer orthobunyavirus possess globular N proteins that are almost entirely alpha-helical in composition, with a positively charged RNA binding groove that bisects a bilobed globular core and primarily interacts with the phosphate backbone of RNA through electrostatic and polar interactions, with each N monomer contacting 10 to 11 nucleotides. Orthobunyavirus N proteins possess flexible N- and C-terminal arms that each contact one adjacent monomer, thus providing the basis for multimerization. The RNA is buried deep within

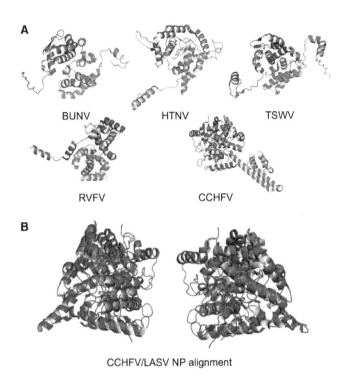

A

BUNV   HTNV   TSWV

RVFV   CCHFV

B

CCHFV/LASV NP alignment

FIGURE 16.11 Crystal structures of N proteins from prototypic members of five families within the *Bunyavirales* order. A and B: BUNV peribunyavirus, HTNV hantavirus, TSWV tospovirus, RVFV phenuivirus and CCHFV nairovirus structures shown as ribbons with the N terminal lobe in *pink* and C terminal lobe in *blue*. Enlarged structural alignments of CCHFV and Lassa arenavirus nucleoproteins, with one alignment rotated 180 degrees. Ribbon models drawn with Pymol using PDB codes as follows: BUNV 4IJS; HTNV 5FSG; TSWV 5IP1; RVFV 4H5M; CCHFV 3U3I. (Figure courtesy of Francis Hopkins, University of Leeds, UK.)

the binding cleft, on the inner face of the multimer forms, with the bases inaccessible from the outside, thus requiring transient dislocation of the RNA from N in order for the polymerase to copy the RNA template. The orthobunyaviral N proteins all have a tendency to form predominantly closed and planar tetrameric rings when generated in heterologous expression systems, with a diameter that closely matches that of the assembled RNP extracted from virions. However, the tetramer unit is unlikely to represent the RNP building block in this closed form, and the relevance, if any, of this multimer in the replication cycle is unclear. The extended N- and C-terminal arms permit considerable flexibility in the assembled N multimer, which is also seen in RNPs purified from viruses, that while being uniformly circular are heterogenous in their overall morphology (Fig. 16.12).

The members of the *Tospoviridae* family also possesses relatively small N proteins (Table 16.1), and the crystal structure of the type species TSWV reveals a very similar overall fold to that of the four orthobunyaviruses described above,[154,226] with somewhat reduced structural similarity with N from TOSV and RVFV phleboviruses, and SFTSV from the *Banyangvirus* genus, described below. As with orthobunyaviruses, N–N multimerization is mediated through extended and flexible N- and C-terminal arms that contact adjacent monomers, with a C-terminal helix providing additional interprotomer contact, suggested to make TSWV RNPs more stable during inter–plant

cell transport. Solution of the structure of the TSWV N cocrystalized with nucleic acids albeit at low resolution[226] revealed a high degree of similarity with the SBV orthobunyavirus RNA-binding groove.

The N proteins of phleboviruses RVFV and TOSV exhibit a tendency to form hexamers in solution, and structural analyses show both possess highly flexible N-terminal arms but a C terminus that lies against the globular body and not in contact with adjacent N molecules.[118,311,354,355] This different oligomerization strategy compared with orthobunyaviruses and tospoviruses may explain the different morphologies of the respective RNPs extracted from infected cells or virions, with phleboviral RNPs appearing more flexible (Fig. 16.12). In the case of apo-N from RVFV, the N-terminal arm lies on the monomer surface to sterically block the RNA-binding groove, and this interaction has been proposed to autoinhibit the interaction of monomeric N with RNA, possibly preventing its association with nonviral RNAs. However, upon N–N multimerization the N-terminal arm relocates to interact with an adjacent N monomer within a hydrophobic cleft, thus exposing the RNA binding groove and providing a mechanism where multimerization and RNA binding are mechanistically coupled. The TOSV N protein cocrystalized with RNA as a series of staggered hexamers, and it has been proposed that RNA binding induces an upward shift in the position of adjacent N monomers, transitioning a planar ring into one with proto-helical properties.[311] In yet another twist of the virus family tree, the phlebovirus N protein exhibits structural similarity to the RNA-binding capsid protein of positive sense RNA plant viruses from the potyvirus genus, implying a shared genetic origin, perhaps as a consequence of the shared arthropod phase of their respective replication cycles.[4]

Despite exhibiting little in the way of nucleotide sequence similarity, the crystal structures of the SNV, HTNV, and ANDV hantavirus N proteins reveal distant structural homology between orthobunyaviral and phleboviral N proteins, sharing the same gross structural architecture that constitutes a bi-lobed globular core that is bisected by an RNA binding groove[156] flanked by flexible N and C terminal arms,[310] with the N-terminal arm forming a coiled coil domain.[48] Interestingly, HTNV N shows partial but close structural homology with tumor suppressor PDCD4, which has been shown to interact with eIF4A,[72] possibly to promote preferential translation of hantaviral mRNAs.

The N proteins from members of the *Nairoviridae* family share no discernable structural homology to N from the orthobunyavirus, hantavirus or phlebovirus groups, and instead display considerable structural homology with N proteins from members of the *Arenaviridae* family,[67] recently incorporated into the *Bunyavirales* order. Rather than being bilobed, with flanking flexible arms, the nairovirus N proteins possess a globular core linked to a stalk (or arm) by a flexible loop. The N and C termini do not extend away from the globular core, and are instead located on its surface and thus are unlikely to mediate intersubunit interactions that drive assembly of RNPs. Instead, N–N multimerization is proposed to involve contact between the tip of the arm domain of one monomer and the base of the globular domain of a neighboring molecule. Interestingly, in the case of several nairoviruses, the residues that are involved in this interaction at the tip of the arm domain constitute a conserved caspase-3 cleavage site, at which site many of these N proteins are cleaved.[205,449]

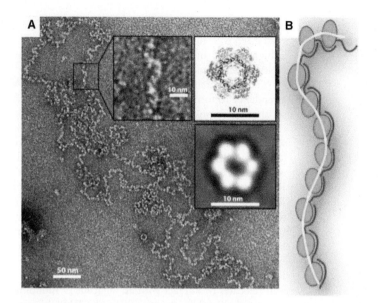

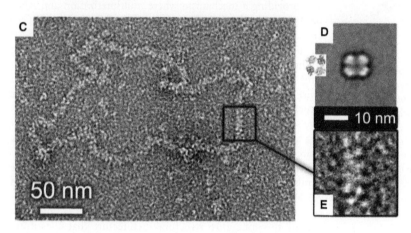

FIGURE 16.12 Bunyavirus RNPs adopt different morphologies. A: Rift Valley fever virus (RVFV) RNPs purified from infected cells and visualized by negative staining reveals a highly flexible morphology, represented in diagrammatic form **(B)** as a series of NP monomers that each only contacts one adjacent neighboring monomer through the N-terminal arm (*red*). The dimensions of the hexameric N ring are inconsistent with the monomer providing the RNP building block. **C:** A negatively stained Bunyamwera virus (BUNV) L-segment RNP purified from virions appears more rigid, with straight sections (one example is boxed). **D,E:** The diameter of the RNP is more similar to that of N tetramer rather than the monomer, suggesting differences between RVFV and BUNV RNP assembly strategies.

Recently, the rescue of CCHFV lacking this DEVD motif was shown to be highly attenuated in tick cells, although not in mammalian cell lines, suggesting an important role for this site in the context of infection.[376] As none of the nairoviral N proteins have been crystallized in complex with RNA, the location of the RNA binding surface is unclear, and no positively charged deep groove is evident. However, the above mentioned structural similarity with arenavirus N proteins, for which the RNA binding surface is known, suggests that RNA is bound within a positively charged crevice that extends from the beginning of the arm domain to the base of the globular domain.

How the crystal structures of N monomers or closed multimers relates to that of N in virion-associated RNPs is unclear. However, in LACV, N crystallized in a superhelical form, with a diameter in close agreement to that of assembled RNPs purified from virions, suggesting this structure may be physiologically relevant, revealing how N monomers interact to build an extended multimeric chain (Fig. 16.13). Similarly, the CCHFV N was crystallized as antiparallel superhelical chains, revealing N–N interfaces that may play important roles in assembly of native RNPs[449] (Fig. 16.13). Insight into the mechanism of orthohantaviral N–N multimerization and RNP formation was provided by the cryo-EM structure of full-length recombinant HTNV N, expressed in insect cells, which forms rigid helical filaments with a diameter similar to that of virion-associated RNPs[21] (Fig. 16.13). The terminal arms of each monomer contact each other through subdomain exchange, and also contact the core domains of neighboring monomers. While these terminal arms are connected to the globular core by flexible hinges, each monomer contacts a total of six other protomers within the helical assembly, contributing to the rigidity of the structure. In contrast, native hantaviral RNPs are circular, indicative of considerable flexibility and suggesting that N within such RNPs must undergo other conformational rearrangements absent in the recombinant filaments.

For all these bunyaviral N proteins, the mechanism of RNA encapsidation during genome replication is poorly understood, although the recent solution of crystal structures of many N proteins as well as the LACV RdRp[138] provide some important clues, from which an excellent working model has arisen. This model posits that the RNA template transiently dissociates from N during polymerization to expose the RNA bases for copying, and the nascent replication product is encapsidated as it emerges from the RdRp exit channel by addition of single N monomers.

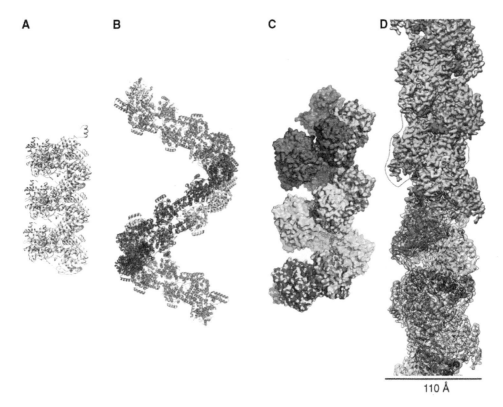

110 Å

FIGURE 16.13 Helical assemblies of bunyaviral N proteins. A: The P4₁ crystal of N from La Crosse orthobunyavirus (LACV). **B:** The P3121 crystal form of RNA-free CCHFV N, strain IbAr10200 (PDB code: 4aqf). **C:** The helical RNP model of Toscana phlebovirus, based on the crystal structures of RNA-free and RNA-bound N hexameric rings. **D:** Cryo-EM structure of the recombinant Hantaan virus N-RNA complex. (**A, B,** and **C** taken from Sun Y, Li J, Gao GF, et al. Bunyavirales ribonucleoproteins: the viral replication and transcription machinery. *Crit Rev Microbiol* 2018;44:5, 522–540. **D** taken from Arragain B, Reguera J, Desfosses A, et al. High resolution cryo-EM structure of the helical RNA-bound Hantaan virus nucleocapsid reveals its assembly mechanisms. *eLife* 2019;8:e43075.)

The S segments of viruses in the *Phlebovirus* and *Orthotospovirus* genera and some viruses in *Orthonairovirus*, *Orthobunyavirus*, and *Orthohantavirus* genera encode NSs proteins in addition to their N proteins. Sizes of NSs range from 10 kD for orthobunyaviruses and orthohantaviruses to more than 50 kD for orthotospoviruses (Fig. 16.1). As the name suggests, the various bunyaviral NSs proteins are nonstructural and possess diverse roles that can be broadly described as suppressors of innate immunity (see below), with the best-studied example being NSs from the phlebovirus RVFV. RVFV NSs is a major pathogenicity factor, with both naturally occurring and engineered variants of RVFV lacking NSs unable to inhibit interferon production and thus being apathogenic in mice. RVFV NSs accumulates in the nuclei of infected cells where it forms large and dense fibrillar structures (Fig. 16.14)[424] comprising NSs as well as multiple nuclear proteins including p44 and XPB of TFIIH, as well as SAP30 and YY1[241,242] although it is not clear whether filament formation is required for the NSs function.

The structure of a soluble core domain of RVFV NSs (NSs ΔN-ΔC) missing terminal residues 1 to 83 and 248 to 265 revealed a novel all-helical fold, which formed double helical fibrils within the crystal lattice, stabilized by multiple interfaces[34] (Fig. 16.14). The dimensions and architecture of these fibrils were comparable with fibril bundles that build up the

characteristic nuclear filaments, and structure-guided mutagenesis of NSs ΔN-ΔC multimer interfaces allowed critical residues in filament formation to be identified. The ability of NSs ΔN-ΔC to form filaments in virus-infected cells shows the termini are dispensable for this activity but conflicts with the finding that NSs binds p62 through a conserved C terminal ΩXaV motif (deleted in NSs ΔN-ΔC) that is also proposed to be required for filament formation.[88]

Comparing the deduced amino acid sequences of NSs for five different phleboviruses revealed similarities of only 17% to 30%.[143] However, comparison of the NSs gene sequences for a number of strains of a single phlebovirus, RVFV, showed that certain areas were highly conserved.[377] These data suggest that there may be a strong evolutionary pressure to maintain distinct portions of the NSs for individual viruses but that the remainder of the protein can diverge without affecting the function of NSs.

As RVFV NSs is expressed by ambisense transcription, it requires the cRNA template for protein production. Earlier work suggested that the NSs of phleboviruses and tospoviruses were only synthesized after onset of viral replication at later times of infection, required to generate the cRNA template. However, recent work with RVFV indicates that virions can encapsidate S-segment cRNAs and that these incoming cRNA RNPs can serve as templates for transcription of NSs mRNA.[187]

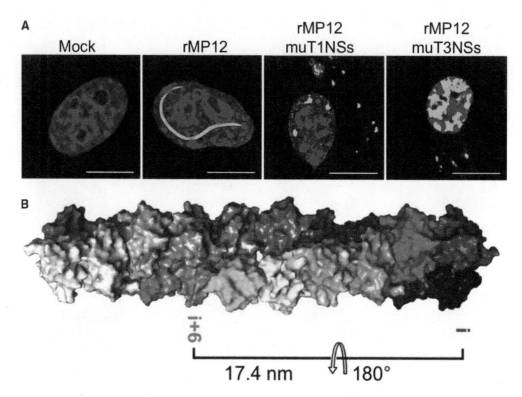

A

Mock   rMP12   rMP12 muT1NSs   rMP12 muT3NSs

B

i+6

17.4 nm   180°

FIGURE 16.14 Rift Valley fever virus NSs protein accumulates in the nucleus as an ultrastructural filament. A: BHK cells infected with Rift Valley fever virus (RVFV) were stained with an anti-NSs antibody showing fibrillar structures in the nucleus. NSs fibrils do not form during infection with recombinant RVFV expressing NSs with alterations at critical fibril interfaces. **B:** Surface rendered model of the double helical NSs filament, with individual monomers alternatively colored, and with 6 monomers per 180-degree turn. (Figures taken from Barski M, Brennan B, Miller OK, et al. Rift Valley fever phlebovirus NSs protein core domain structure suggests molecular basis for nuclear filaments. *eLife* 2017;6:e29236.)

The outcome of this is that NSs is expressed early in infection, in agreement with reports that innate immunity is activated upon entry of RNPs.[454] Also, the NSs of three orthobunyaviruses all inhibited BUNV RNA synthesis in a dose-dependent manner in a minireplicon system.[453] These results were suggested to indicate a function for NSs in regulating the activity of the RdRp, in addition to their role in interferon antagonism, apoptosis, host-range determination, and gene silencing described below.

M-Segment Products: Gn, Gc, and NSm

Without exception, the bunyaviral M segment encodes a glycoprotein precursor (GPC) that is cotranslationally cleaved by various proteases to generate two viral envelope glycoproteins (GPs), Gn and Gc, and following heterodimerization, these form the viral spikes involved in virus entry. However, there are significant differences among the bunyaviruses in the way the GPC is processed, and also in the GPC-derived products that are generated.

M-segment gene products have a high cysteine content of approximately 4% to 7%, with the positions of these residues being highly conserved within families, suggesting that extensive disulfide-bridge formation may occur and that the positions may be crucial for determining correct polypeptide folding. The secondary structure of the proteins is also involved in immunogenicity, as indicated by the finding that neutralizing or protective epitopes are often nonlinear.

All M-segment polyproteins display variable numbers of predicted transmembrane regions, and a hydrophobic sequence at the carboxy-terminus, indicative of a membrane anchor region. Therefore, the M-segment translation products of viruses in the order *Bunyavirales* are typical class 1 membrane proteins, with their N terminus exposed on the surface of the virion and a membrane anchor within the C terminus, with a small number of C-terminal residues potentially exposed within the virion interior.

The Gn and Gc proteins of all characterized bunyaviruses possess asparagine-linked oligosaccharides. Examination of the oligosaccharides attached to the Gn and Gc proteins of orthobunyaviruses revealed that Gc has mostly high-mannose glycans, whereas Gn contains both complex and a novel intermediate-type oligosaccharide.[269,303,395] In contrast, the GPs of hantaviruses were found to be mostly of the high-mannose type.[384] These findings indicate that the proteins are incompletely processed through the Golgi. This is likely related to retention of Gn and Gc in the Golgi, where assembly occurs, discussed more fully below.

In some orthobunyaviruses, nairoviruses, and phleboviruses, but not hantaviruses,[386] processing of the GPC generates an additional nonstructural protein known as NSm, and the characteristics and functions of this module are discussed below. In addition, some nairoviruses further process GPC to generate additional polypeptides that are proposed to have other nonstructural roles, also described below.

The GPC polyprotein of bunyaviruses is not seen in infected cells, and has been observed only by *in vitro* translation of RNA transcripts in the absence of microsomal membranes.[436] For orthobunyaviruses, hantaviruses,[261] and phleboviruses, both Gn and Gc are preceded by signal peptide (SP) sequences, and therefore, cleavage of the polyprotein precursor is likely mediated cotranslationally by host signal peptidase (SPase) in the ER.[114] In the case of BUNV orthobunyavirus, the GPC constitutes a single ORF with Gn, NSm, and Gc modules arranged in that order,[113] and being released by SPase cleavage at their respective N termini. Cleavage at the Gn/NSm boundary was shown to occur at an internal SPase cleavage site located within domain 1 of NSm, releasing pre-Gn in which the SP was still attached to the Gn C-terminus (Pre-Gn).[394] The SP was cleaved from the C terminus of pre-Gn to yield Gn by further processing by signal peptide peptidase (SPP) in the ER. The function of NSm remains unclear; its hydropathy profile suggests that it is a membrane-bound protein, and expression studies demonstrated that it localizes to the Golgi along with Gn and Gc.[246] Although a function for this protein has not been identified, localization studies suggest that it might be involved in facilitating virion assembly in the Golgi.[121,400]

Release of the Gn, Gc, and NSm proteins from the GPC of the insect-borne phleboviruses also involves SPase cleavage, although in the case of RVFV, the protein modules are arranged with the NSm module located at the N terminus of the GP, thus in the order NSm, Gn, Gc (Fig. 16.15). Nucleotide sequence studies revealed five in-frame translation initiation codons (AUG) upstream of the N-terminus of Gn. Mutational analysis of those codons indicated the fourth and the fifth AUGs to translate Gn and Gc. Whilst NSm was found to originate from the second AUG and a 78-kDa polypeptide, representing uncleaved NSm and Gn, was translated from the first AUG.[166] Pulse-chase experiments revealed no precursor–product relationship between the 78- and 14-kDa proteins; therefore, it appears that use of the first and second AUGs, respectively, is what dictates generation of these proteins.[63] Both the 14-kDa NSm and the 78-kDa polypeptide are found in abundance in RVFV-infected cells,[64] suggesting that they might play a role in replication or morphogenesis. A RVFV mutant rescued with M-segment mutations ablating NSm expression was indistinguishable to wild-type in its growth characteristics, suggesting NSm was dispensable for RVFV multiplication.[139]

An even larger NSm (~30 kDa) is cleaved from the amino terminus of the M-segment polyprotein of the phlebovirus, PTV (Fig. 16.15). *In vitro* expression studies indicated that both envelope GPs could be produced in the absence of the NSm coding region,[279] but other studies to evaluate the use of the 13 potential translation initiation codons present in the NSm coding information have not been reported. No homology between the NSm proteins of PTV and RVFV was apparent.[184]

In contrast to the mosquito-borne phleboviruses PTV and RVFV, the tick-borne phlebovirus UUKV does not produce an NSm (Fig. 16.15). The first (and only) initiation codon preceding sequences of the envelope GPs is located 17 amino acids upstream of the amino terminus of Gn[366]; hence, the Gn protein of UUKV appears to be analogous to the 78-kDa NSm–Gn fusion product produced by RVFV (although there is no obvious sequence homology of these predicted products). Until a function can be assigned to NSm, it is impossible to determine whether UUKV replicates in the absence of such a function or accomplishes whatever function is required without removal of a portion of the amino terminus of Gn.

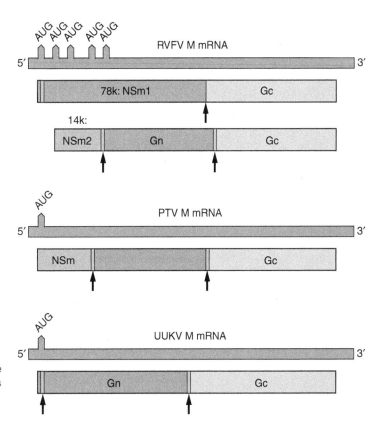

FIGURE 16.15 Expression of phlebovirus M-segment encoded gene products. Schematic representation of the gene products, AUG codons (*lollipops*), and proteolytic cleavage sites (*arrows*) of the M segments of Rift Valley fever virus (RVFV), Punta Toro virus (PTV), and Uukuniemi virus (UUKV).

Alternative GPC processing pathways have also been identified, with nairoviruses relying on proteases other than signalase for their GPC processing events (Fig. 16.16). The nucleotide sequences of Dugbe virus (DUGV), CCHFV, and NSDV M segments reveal the presence of characteristic Gn and Gc modules, as well as NSm.[274] However, studies using CCHFV demonstrate the Pre-Gn moiety is extremely large at approximately 140 kDa, suggesting additional coding capacity.[11,39,378,379,445] Studies show PreGn is further processed to the mature 37-kDa Gn by cleavage with a cellular secretory pathway protease, SKI-1, early in the secretory pathway at a consensus motif, RRLL.[378,445] SKI-1 cleavage generates a subprecursor of two other polypeptides that is cleaved by a furin-like protease at a later stage in the secretory pathway.[378] This cleavage site is completely conserved among several CCHFV strains, suggesting that it has importance for viral replication or pathogenicity.[378] The amino-terminal portion of this subprecursor is a highly variable (among CCHFV strains) polypeptide with mucin-like characteristics, including numerous serines, threonines, and prolines and predicted extensive O-linked glycosylation. The carboxy-terminal portion of the subprecursor is a 38-kDa nonstructural polypeptide. After furin cleavage, secreted proteins GP38, GP85, and GP160 and the mucin-like protein are produced, and it is presumed these products reflect extensive O-linked glycosylation differences. Although the PreGc precursor also possesses a SKI-1–like cleavage motif, SKI-1 cleavage could not be demonstrated for this protein, so it

is likely that a related enzyme is responsible for the processing to yield mature Gc.[378] The importance of furin cleavage in this processing pathway was confirmed by experiments with rescue of a CCHFV mutant lacking a functional furin site,[40] which was highly attenuated in infectious virus production. While the role of the mucin-like domain is unknown, GP38 appears in a secreted form and has been proposed to act as an immune decoy.[378]

Unlike all other viruses in the family, the NSm protein of tospoviruses is translated from an ambisense mRNA.[228] It is also the only NSm protein in the family to have a definitively assigned function. By subcellular fractionation of infected plants, or in thin-section immunoelectron microscopy studies, the NSm of TSWV was found to be present in cell wall–containing fractions or associated with aggregates of nucleocapsids and with the plasmodesmata.[230] Expression of the NSm protein in plant cells or insect cells revealed that the protein first appeared near the cell surface and later as tubular structures protruding from the cell surface. In infected leaf tissues, the tubules were observed only in the plasmodesmata.[420] These findings are characteristic of proteins able to aggregate into plasmodesmata-penetrating tubules that allow cell-to-cell movement of the virus across the cell walls in infected plants. In several other studies, the TSWV NSm protein was shown to have additional characteristics of plant movement proteins, including sequence similarity, expression during the early stages of infection, and RNA-binding activity. Formal proof

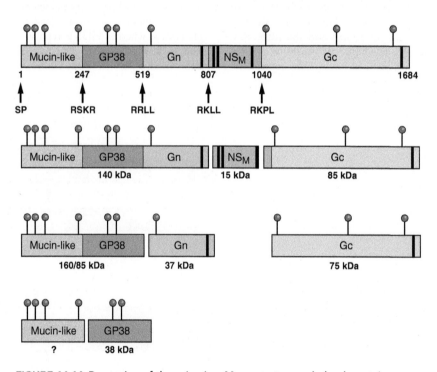

FIGURE 16.16 Processing of the nairovirus M-segment–encoded polyprotein. *Arrows* indicate the known and predicted cleavage site positions and their sequence motifs. *Lollipop shapes* represent predicted N-linked glycosylation sites. Cleavage events are represented sequentially, and the protein products and their sizes are indicated (*middle* and *bottom* panels). *Black bars* represent transmembrane (hydrophobic) regions. Amino acid positions are based on Crimean–Congo hemorrhagic fever virus (CCHFV) strain IbAr 10200. (Modified from Bergeron E, Vincent MJ, Nichol ST. Crimean-Congo hemorrhagic fever virus glycoprotein processing by the endoprotease SKI-1/S1P is critical for virus infectivity. *J Virol* 2007;81:13271–13276.)

of this function was obtained from experiments in which NSm of TSWV was able to complement cell-to-cell movement of a movement-defective tobacco mosaic virus vector.[251] This expression system was also used to show that NSm alone induced tubule formation in protoplasts and induced TSWV-like symptoms in *Nicotiana benthamiana*, and separate domains within NSm have been mapped for each of these functions.[254] More recently, the TSWV NSm protein has been shown to be physically associated with the endoplasmic reticulum (ER), which extends throughout plants via the ER-desmotubule, providing the basis for TSWV movement and dissemination.[116] NSm was found to be expressed in its natural thrip insect vector, but did not aggregate into tubules, leading to the suggestion that NSm might only have a role in the plant portion of the tospovirus replication cycle.[421]

As described above, the viral spikes must perform multiple roles including interaction with host entry factors during virus binding, as well as mediating the fusion of viral and endosomal membranes, thus releasing the RNPs into the cytosol (Fig. 16.17). Recent structural analyses of several bunyaviral Gn/Gc spikes using both crystallography and cryo-EM techniques has provided important insight into these critical virus activities, and has illuminated the molecular basis of these functions. The fusogenic component of all bunyaviral Gn/Gc heterodimer resides within Gc, all of which are class-II fusion proteins comprising predominantly beta-sheet secondary structural elements. Crystal structures of the phlebovirus RVFV and SFTSV Gc proteins in pre- and postfusion confirmations[94,162] characterized the conformational changes predicted to occur during pH triggered fusion, as well as identify the potential histidine residues involved in pH-sensing activities, and the hydrophobic fusion loops.

By solving the crystal structure of RVFV Gn and docking the resulting Gn/Gc structural model into a cryo-EM derived

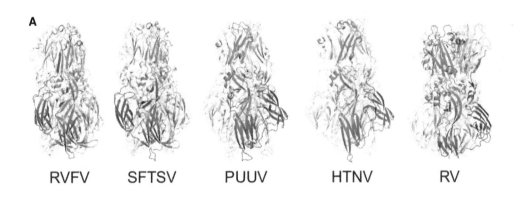

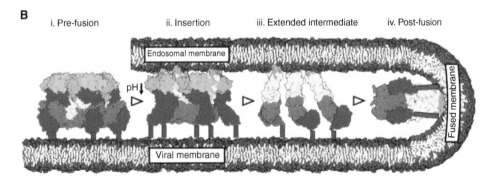

FIGURE 16.17 Structure and function of bunyavirus spikes. A: Crystal structures of Gc from RVFV, SFTSV and PUUV from the *Phlebovirus* genus, HTNV from the *Hantavirus* genus, and rubella virus from the *Togaviridae* family of positive-sense RNA viruses. Ribbon structural models drawn with Pymol using PDB codes as follows: RVFV 6EGU; STFSV 5G47; PUUV RJ81; HTNV 5LJZ; RV 4ADG. (Figure courtesy of Francis Hopkins, University of Leeds, UK.) **B:** Model for fusogenic activation of phleboviral Gn/Gc spikes in response to the lowered pH of endosomal compartments. In (*i*), Gn/Gc heterodimers on the virus surface, with Gn domains A, B and the beta-ribbon colored teal, green and purple, respectively located on top of Gc domains I, II, and III colored red, yellow, and blue respectively. The Gc fusion loops are buried and colored orange. In (*ii*), the biochemical changes that occur during transit through the endosome network induce conformational change, whereby Gn domains move to the side, as Gc domains extend exposing the fusion loops of each monomer at its apex, to insert into the target membrane. In (*iii*), the Gn/Gc moieties dissociate, allowing redistribution of Gc, leading to further conformational changes that culminate in formation of Gc trimers within the fused membrane. (Schematic taken from Halldorsson S, Li S, Li M, et al. Shielding and activation of a viral membrane fusion protein. *Nature Commun* 2018;9:349.)

structural model of the RVFV spike envelope, the location of Gn and Gc on the virion surface was determined, which confirmed the existence of Gn/Gc heterodimers, and defined their interacting interfaces.[163] By comparing the structures of Gn/Gc heterodimers with and without the provision of biochemically relevant lipids at low pH, the conformational changes associated with membrane interaction were observed, which revealed exposure and insertion of the Gc fusion loop in concert with a dramatic conformational shift of Gn. These findings suggested that in the prefusion state, Gn shields the hydrophobic fusion loop of Gc, blocking premature fusion until the appropriate cellular compartments are reached. Gn conformational changes allow extension of Gc and insertion of the fusion loop into target membranes, driving subsequent fusion events. The fusion event is facilitated by the ability of Gc to sequester glycerophospholipid head groups within a binding pocket under the fusion loop that participate in polar interactions, thus stabilizing the inserted fusion loop.[152]

Similar conformational changes in Gn and Gc structure have also been described for Hantaan and Puumala hantaviruses, which share significant structural similarity despite their different geographic origins.[8,153,364,463] As for phlebovirus Gn/Gc assemblies, lowered pH induces dramatic conformational changes, allowing dissociation of the Gn/Gc lattice that is proposed to stearically facilitate the extension and insertion of the Gc fusion loop into the host cell target membrane. As for phleboviruses, Gn has been proposed to provide a shielding role to Gc, with structural rearrangements of the hantaviral glycoprotein lattice in response to appropriate biochemical cues resulting in exposure of the fusion loop, and its availability for insertion into target endosomal membranes.

L Segment Product: L Polymerase Protein

As their name suggests, bunyavirus L proteins are large, with those of the *Peribunyaviridae*, *Hantaviridae*, and *Phenuiviridae* families possessing molecular weights around 240 kDa, whereas members of the *Tospoviridae* and *Nairoviridae* families are somewhat larger, around 330 to 450 kDa respectively (Fig. 16.1). To mediate both primed synthesis of mRNAs, as well as nonprimed synthesis of vRNA from cRNA templates, these RdRps must possess numerous enzymatic activities including endonuclease, transcriptase, replicase, and probably cap-binding.

All RdRps for which the structure has been solved adopt a canonical RdRp fold, often described as a right hand with a palm, fingers and thumb domains containing catalytic core motifs,[17,196,235,292] and the recently described crystal structure of a near full-length construct of LACV L (Fig. 16.18) (residues 1–1,750; 77%) is no exception to this.[138] The LACV RdRp possesses much structural similarity with the RdRp from the segmented negative stranded influenza virus, and alignment of the two molecules shows that the PA, PB1, and PB2 subunits can be mapped head-to-tail onto the LACV structure, in that order.[474] The central RdRp core domain of LACV L (residues 760–1,432) maps to IAV PB1 and constitutes the palm, fingers, fingertips, and thumb features. In LACV, this central RdRp core is buttressed by substantial extensions: on one side by a N-terminal region (residues 1–759) corresponding to PA, and on the opposite side by a C-terminal region that aligns with the N-terminus of PB2 (PB2-N) constituting LACV

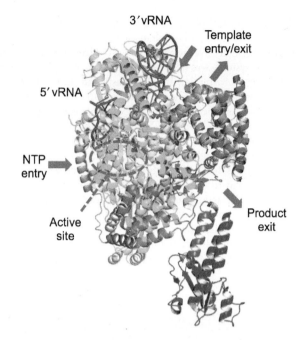

FIGURE 16.18 The crystal structure of the LACV RNA-dependant RNA polymerase (RdRp). The RdRp is shown bound to RNAs constituting 3′ and 5′ vRNA sequences, with *red arrows* showing entrances to tunnels that permit entry and exit of template, product, and NTP substrate, and the active site is marked with a *red dashed oval*. (Structural model drawn using Pymol from PDB code 5AMQ, and annotated with information from Gerlach P, Malet H, Cusack S, et al. Structural insights into Bunyavirus replication and its regulation by the vRNA promoter. *Cell* 2015;161(6):1267–1279. doi: 10.1016/j.cell.2015.05.006. Figure courtesy of Francis Hopkins, University of Leeds, UK.)

residues 1,433–1,750. The C terminal residues of the LACV L (1,751–2,263) were not represented in the LACV L expression construct, but likely correspond to the C terminal portion of PB2, which includes a cap-binding domain, although the existence of cap-binding activity or an associated domain in any bunyaviral RdRp has yet to be confirmed.

The N-terminus of the LACV L protein (residues 1–184) contains the endonuclease domain, responsible for generation of the capped RNA primers, and bears a high degree of structural similarity to the influenza virus endonuclease within PA.[96,474] Both endonucleases are members of the PD-(D/E) × K cation–dependent superfamily, and structural, bioinformatic, and functional analyses indicate that viruses in all the other *Bunyavirales* families contain a similar domain,[95,117,176,219,290,357,359,368,446] suggesting a common origin of the cap-snatching process of segmented negative sense viruses. The LACV endonuclease is linked to the rest of the PA-like region by an extended flexible linker (residues 185–270) that may permit significant mobility of this domain. Residues 271 to 759 can be divided into two lobes, one of which interacts in a sequence-specific manner with the two vRNA termini at separate binding sites, while the other buttresses the thumb and palm of the RdRp core. Within the central PB1-like RdRp core (residues 760–1,432), the palm domain comprises conserved polymerase motifs A-D, while the fingers represent motif F. Together, these regions build up the internal active site chamber, within which the active site is located and accessed by four solvent accessible tunnels. Two of these are assigned as template entry and exit tunnels, which are adjacent and force the template through an internal path approximately 20 nucleotides in length, passing alongside the active site. The confined dimensions of the polymerization chamber do not permit the formation of an extensive template/product hybrid, and instead the strands are forced to separate, with the nascent RNA product exiting the complex through the third tunnel, the product exit channel, with the fourth channel assigned to rNTP entry. The proximity of the template entry and exit channels potentially allows the RNA to be extracted and replaced within the N protein RNA binding groove within the RNP without breaking N–N interactions nor exposure of the RNA (Fig. 16.18). Access of the capped RNA oligomers to prime transcription are postulated to enter the active site through the product exit channel, as is the case for influenza virus, facilitated by the flexibility of the endonuclease linker.

This first high-resolution structure of the bunyavirus RdRp has allowed an elegant model to be proposed, which describes the concerted events involved in bunyavirus RNA replication (Fig. 16.19). Critical features of this model include transition of an inactive preinitiation RNA-L complex into an active form by relocation of the 3′ vRNA end, the ability of RNA to transiently dissociate from N without disruption of the N–N multimeric chain, and the association of the nascent replication product with a second polymerase with associated N, thus ensuring encapsidation of the newly synthesised RNA strand, and maintaining the replication competence of the subsequently formed RNP. Cap-dependant mRNA transcription will likely involve major mechanistic differences, allowing access of the capped oligoribonucleotide to the active site, preventing encapsidation of the nascent RNA and thus allowing recognition of transcription termination signals that are presumably within the nascent transcript.

The significantly larger L proteins of nairoviruses possess identifiable motifs of both the endonuclease and catalytic core domains, although these are located further toward the C terminus of the molecule than in the other bunyaviruses.[95,176] Bioinformatics analysis revealed that the N terminus of the DUGV L protein contained a motif characteristic of cysteine proteases of the ovarian tumor (OTU) protein superfamily,[272] which were also subsequently identified in CCHFV[177,217] along with a C2H2 zinc finger domain, and motifs corresponding to a leucine zipper and the active site of topoisomerase 1. The OTU domain acts to remove both ubiquitin (Ub) and also the Ub-like protein IFN-stimulated gene 15 (ISG15) from various cellular target substrates that serve as antiviral signaling platforms, thus it acts as both a deuquitinating enzyme (DUB) and also a de-ISGylase,[6,62,125,192,438] although sequence and structure variation is high and not always are both these activities realized.[101] The crystal structure of the CCHFV OTU revealed structural similarity to DUBs of both eukaryotic and viral origin, and revealed the molecular basis for Ub and ISG15 cross-substrate specificity. The catalytic activity of the OTU domain is not required for the RNA polymerase activity by CCHFV in a minigenome system[39]; however, it is essential for infectious virus production[388] with the catalytic knock out C40A mutant CCHFV being nonviable. In contrast, CCHFV mutants with reduced Ub or ISG15 binding were highly attenuated for growth in IFN-competent cell lines.

Morphogenesis

Transport of Viral Proteins

In contrast to other negative-strand RNA viruses, bunyaviruses usually mature within cells by budding at smooth membranes of the Golgi. The plant-infecting members of the family, the tospoviruses, also appear to assemble in the Golgi; however, it was suggested that instead of budding, there is a coalescence of Golgi membranes around the RNPs.[215] Budding at membranes other than those associated with the Golgi have been reported for some viruses; for example, the hantaviruses, SNV, and Black Creek Canal virus (BCCV), and the phlebovirus RVFV were found to bud from the plasma membrane as well as in the Golgi in some cells.[12,353] The reason(s) for maturation of bunyaviruses in the Golgi complex as opposed to the more usual mode of viral morphogenesis (budding at the plasma membrane) are not understood completely; however, important clues have been obtained by studying the viral proteins' transport to, and retention in, the Golgi.

Golgi Targeting and Retention

Expression of M gene segments of representative bunyaviruses demonstrated that Gn and Gc are targeted to the Golgi in the absence of other viral components. When expressed individually, Gn is able to exit the ER, but Gc remains in the ER for the orthobunyaviruses, phleboviruses, nairoviruses, and tospoviruses.[41,217,238,278] For hantaviruses, neither protein exits the ER when expressed separately.[371,396] For all studies to date, the signal for Golgi transport has been localized to Gn and complexing of Gn and Gc in the ER is necessary for efficient transport of Gc to the Golgi. Although ER retention signals have not been identified on Gc for most viruses, the phleboviruses have a characteristic carboxy-terminal ER retention motif (KKXX, where K = lysine and X = any amino acid).[140] Evidently, this signal can be overcome when Gn and Gc oligomerize. For BUNV, the Golgi localization and retention signal was mapped to the transmembrane domain of Gn.[402] The Golgi localization signal for the phleboviruses PTV and RVFV was identified within the transmembrane domain plus 10 (PTV) or 28 (RVFV) amino acids of the cytoplasmic tail.[140,278] The Golgi localization signal of another phlebovirus, UUKV, was found to be within a 30–amino acid peptide of the cytoplasmic tail.[15]

Similar expression studies with M-segment constructs of HTNV indicated that the ability of Gn to transport Gc to the Golgi requires the presence of the complete signal sequence of Gc. This suggests that the Gc signal peptide remains attached to the Gn cytoplasmic tail. This signal alone, however, is apparently not sufficient for Golgi targeting because M-segment constructs that maintained the Gc signal peptide but had other internal deletions in Gn or Gc failed to reach the Golgi. These results were interpreted to indicate that the correct conformation of the oligomerized Gn and Gc is also important for Golgi targeting.[386] Consistent with this is the observation that overexpression of SNV Gn resulted in the apparent accumulation of misfolded proteins in aggresomes.[417] In addition, the cytoplasmic tail of Gn was found to be polyubiquitinated when expressed alone, suggesting that it would undergo proteasomal degradation if not complexed with Gc.[135]

For the nairovirus, CCHFV, removal of the transmembrane domain and cytoplasmic tail of Gn did not prevent Golgi targeting, and this soluble truncated Gn was still able to

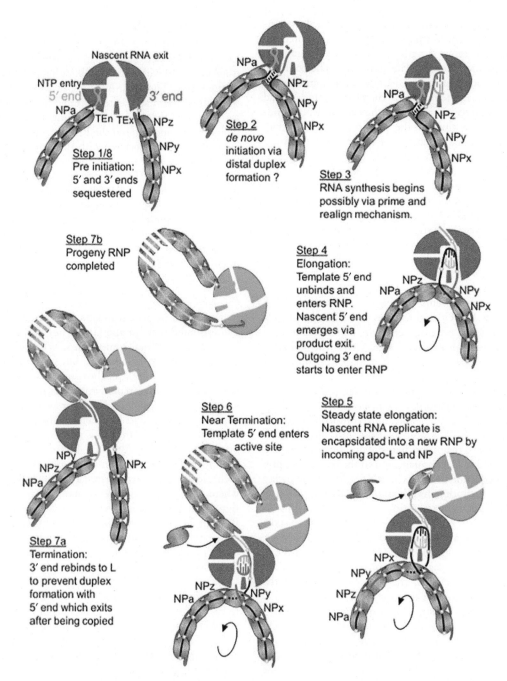

FIGURE 16.19 Model describing bunyavirus RNA replication. The initial RNP cartoon (step1/8) shows the resident polymerase (*purple*) in its preinitiation state with vRNA 3′ (*red*) and 5′ (*cyan*) sequences bound at sites on the polymerase surface. Tunnels for template entrance (TEn), template exit (TEx), nascent RNA, and NTP entry are marked. NP molecules are represented as circles with N- and C- terminal arms, bound to 11 nucleotides of RNA forming the RNP chain. In step 2, the 3′ vRNA end becomes relocated in the active site, and in step 3, cRNA synthesis begins, and in step 4, the nascent cRNA emerges from the RNA exit channel. The proximity of TEn and TEx allow only a short RNA sequence to enter the active site, and thus the disruption of the RNA-NP template is minimal and may affect only one or two NP monomers. In step 5, an apo-L (*green*) complete with bound NP recruits the newly synthesized 5′ end, allowing encapsidation to commence. Further NP molecules join the growing cRNA strand, until the 5′ end of the template passes through the active site, to rebind on the surface of the encapsidating (*green*) polymerase, shown in steps 6 and 7a. All 3′ and 5′ ends relocate to surface-bound locations, the newly name cRNA complete with resident RdRp can generate further vRNAs, and the cycle can begin again, step 7b. (Figure adapted from Gerlach P, Malet H, Cusack S, et al. Structural insights into Bunyavirus replication and its regulation by the vRNA promoter. *Cell* 2015;161(6):1267–1279. doi: 10.1016/j.cell.2015.05.006.)

dimerize with Gc and transport both proteins to the Golgi.[41] In another study, Golgi targeting was dependent on a signal found both in the hydrophobic region of the cytoplasmic tail as well as in the ectodomain[161]; therefore, unlike other bunyaviruses, nairoviruses appear to have at least part of their Golgi-targeting signal in the ectodomain, rather than only in the transmembrane or cytoplasmic tail regions of Gn.

Clearly, although there are definite signals targeting the viral glycoproteins to the Golgi, there is no consensus motif or even region of Gn conserved among viruses across the order.

Trafficking Through the Golgi

The Golgi complex consists of several subcompartments, including the cis-, medial-, and trans-Golgi.[221] By using the fungal antibacterial reagent Brefeldin A, which inhibits transport of proteins out of the ER and causes a redistribution of the Golgi component to the ER, the GPs of the phlebovirus PTV were found to be localized in the cis and medial Golgi membranes.[36] Similar redistribution of Gn and Gc from the Golgi to the ER were observed following Brefeldin A treatment of cells infected with vaccinia virus recombinants expressing the M segment of BUNV.[295] Immunohistochemical and electron microscopy studies of the phlebovirus UUKV demonstrated that budding may begin as early as the pre-Golgi intermediate compartment and that virus budding continues in the Golgi stack.[194,375]

Examination of the type and amount of oligosaccharides attached to viral proteins influences trafficking and provides clues regarding the transit of the proteins through the Golgi compartments. For example, shortly after primary glycosylation of nascent proteins at the ER, oligosaccharides are susceptible to cleavage by endoglycosidase H (endo-H), an enzyme that cleaves only high-mannose residues. Later, after removal of glucose residues at the rough ER, migration of the GPs to the smooth ER and Golgi, trimming of residues, and attachment of peripheral sugars, the oligosaccharides are no longer susceptible to endo-H cleavage. Therefore, acquired resistance to endo-H generally indicates that the proteins have been processed through specific Golgi compartments as described earlier (see "M-segment products"). For the nairovirus CCHFV and the hantavirus HTNV the GPs remain endo-H sensitive, suggesting that they have not been processed through the medial Golgi.[41,397] In contrast, the GPs of the orthobunyavirus, BUNV, become endo-H resistant, so they can be assumed to have moved through the trans-Golgi.[303]

To identify the roles of specific glycosylation sites on trafficking of HTNV GPs, a series of expression constructs were created in which each of the four glycosylation sites that are used on Gn and the single site used on Gc were mutated. Removal of the glycosylation site closest to the amino-terminus of Gn resulted in its inability to exit the ER and for a loss of reactivity with monoclonal antibodies to native Gn.[397] Mutating the third glycosylation site in Gn was also poorly tolerated, and resulted in inefficient Golgi targeting and loss of monoclonal antibody reactivity. In contrast, mutating the single site on Gc or two of the other three sites of Gn were well tolerated. A similar study with BUNV indicated that the single Gn glycosylation site is absolutely required for correct protein folding, trafficking, and infectivity.[395] These data are consistent with results from another study, which will be described below, indicating that the processing of sugars plays a key role in maturation of BUNV.[303]

The time required to convert between endo-H susceptibility and resistance correlates with the time needed for protein transport from the ER to the Golgi. For the phlebovirus PTV, heterodimerization occurred between newly synthesized Gn and Gc within 3 minutes after protein synthesis, and the dimers were found to be linked by disulfide bonds. The dimeric Gn–Gc proteins were observed both during transport and after accumulation in the Golgi complex.[36] For another phlebovirus, UUKV, it was found that the transport of Gn and Gc from their site of synthesis on the rough ER through the Golgi occurred at an estimated two to three times slower rate than that of most viral membrane GPs destined to be transported to the plasma membrane.[126] That is, endo-H resistance was achieved at 45 and 90 to 150 minutes for Gn and Gc of UUKV,[233] compared to 15 to 20 minutes for the hemagglutinin protein of influenza virus or the G protein of vesicular stomatitis virus. The finding that UUKV Gn and Gc have different transport kinetics (i.e., Gn is incorporated into virions 20 minutes faster than Gc) suggests that the dimers may arise from different precursor proteins, possibly because faster-folding Gn cannot dimerize with slower-folding Gc until Gc has reached its correct conformation.[462] In this same study, the Gn and Gc proteins of UUKV were found to exit the ER quickly, but did not enter the Golgi for 15 to 20 minutes. These findings suggest that the Gn and Gc proteins may dimerize in an intermediate compartment between the ER and Golgi.[462]

The NSm proteins are not known to play a role in transport or Golgi retention. For representative phleboviruses and orthobunyaviruses, expression of Gn and Gc in the absence of NSm had no effect on their transport to the Golgi; however, when the entire M segments were expressed, NSm co-localized to the Golgi with Gn and Gc, suggesting an interaction of these proteins before their exit from the ER.

Assembly

For assembly to occur, N, L as well as Gn and Gc must move to the same intracellular location. For the hantavirus, SEOV, N could first be observed approximately 2 hours after infection and accumulated as scattered granules in the cytoplasm. Although N was not observed in the Golgi, it could be observed to surround the Golgi by 24 hours after infection.[204] The N proteins of the nairovirus CCHFV and the hantavirus BCCV were both observed in the perinuclear region of infected cells, and both were found to bind to actin.[16,352] Disrupting the cellular actin network by treatment with cytochalasin D reduced the assembly of infectious CCHFV, suggesting a role for actin in transporting N to the site of virion assembly. For BCCV, the N protein was found to be peripherally associated with Golgi membranes, suggesting that the RNPs are recruited to the Golgi for assembly.[417] In contrast, the CCHFV N protein was not found in association with Golgi membranes; therefore, it is unclear where the actual assembly site is for nairoviruses, and it was suggested that some sort of novel structure close to the nucleus might be involved.[16] Immunofluorescence and cell fractionation studies showed the L protein of TULV associated with perinuclear membranes[234] with partial co-localization with Golgi matrix protein GM130. Similarly, an epitope-tagged L protein expressed from a recombinant BUNV was also identified within the perinuclear region, and cell fractionation studies showed L to be distributed in both cytosolic and microsomal fractions.[398] These studies pointed

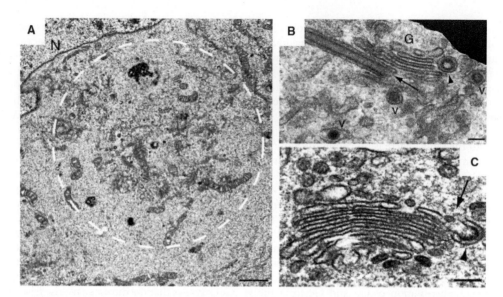

FIGURE 16.20 Visualization of viral factory in Bunyamwera virus (BUNV)-infected BHK cells by electron microscopy. A: Viral factory (*dashed white circle*) shows groups of organelles near the nucleus (N). **B:** Higher magnification shows longitudinal (*arrow*) and transverse (*arrowhead*) sections of tubular structures in Golgi stacks (G). Virus particles (V) are also seen. **C:** Tubular assembly with a bigger globular domain (*arrow*). N, nucleus; G, Golgi stack; V, virus particle; scale bar represents 1 μm in **(A)**. (Modified from Fontana J, Lopez-Montero N, Elliott RM, et al. The unique architecture of Bunyamwera virus factories around the Golgi complex. *Cell Microbiol* 2008;10:2012–2028.)

to bunyaviruses establishing membrane-associated virus factories, similar to those described for flaviviruses, and this was confirmed by detailed electron microscopic analysis of BUNV-infected cells, which identified viral replication occurring in membranous structures built around the Golgi complex (Fig. 16.20). These comprised repetitive units of Golgi stacks, mitochondria, components of the rough ER, and virus-derived tubular structures with a globular head.[375] The viral polymerase and N protein were found mainly in the globular head, and viral RNPs were released from disrupted, purified tubes.[121] Viral tubes contain cellular proteins such as actin and myosin I, and both tube assembly and viral morphogenesis were sensitive to drugs that affect actin. Advanced imaging and three-dimensional (3D) reconstruction of infected cells showed that the tubes link cellular organelles, for example, mitochondria, to the Golgi and interact with intracellular viral forms, thereby providing a route for cellular factors required for genome replication. Based on these observations a model has been proposed (Fig. 16.21) whereby viral RNPs are transported from sites of replication in the globular domain to the cytoplasm where they condense on Golgi membranes modified by the insertion of Gn and Gc, and promote budding of immature particles into Golgi-derived cisternae that separate from Golgi stacks. Further studies using the orthobunyavirus OROV showed that Golgi membranes become remodeled by using the cellular ESCRT (endosomal complex required for transport) machinery.[26] As already mentioned, localization studies with BUNV suggest that the nonstructural protein NSm might be involved in facilitating virion assembly in the Golgi.[121,400]

Unlike most other negative-strand RNA viruses, bunyaviruses do not have a matrix (M) protein to link the integral viral envelope proteins and their nucleocapsids and to act as the nucleating step for assembly. The absence of an M protein suggests a direct interaction between the ribonucleocapsids, which accumulate on the cytoplasmic side of vesicular membranes, and viral envelope proteins, which are displayed on the luminal side.[422] Electron microscopy of cells infected with the phleboviruses PTV or Karimabad virus revealed that RNPs and spike structures (i.e., viral envelope GPs) were present only in regions of Golgi membranes where budding appeared to be occurring, and not on adjacent areas of the same membrane, suggesting a transmembranal interaction of N with Gn or Gc.[413] Direct evidence for the requirement of the cytoplasmic tails of both glycoproteins has been obtained using VLP production assays.[401]

The signal directing the RNPs to the budding compartment has not been identified for most bunyaviruses. For hantaviruses, however, N was shown to interact with the cellular proteins, SUMO-1 (small ubiquitin-like modifier-1) and Ubc9 (SUMO-1 conjugating enzyme 9) in yeast two-hybrid systems.[208,246,270] For HTNV, the interaction occurred at a four–amino acid motif, MAKE, located at amino acid positions 188 and 189 of N, and mutation of this motif prevented transport of N to the perinuclear region, suggesting a role for this interaction in directing N to the site of assembly.

Excess RNPs of hantaviruses, tospoviruses, and nairoviruses were found to accumulate in large cytoplasmic inclusions, suggesting that only RNPs that interact with the envelope proteins are transported to the Golgi. Although not yet defined, it is likely that the transmembrane domains of Gn or Gc that are exposed on the cytoplasmic face of the membrane are involved in this interaction. Candidate transmembrane regions have been predicted from hydropathic characteristics of derived amino acid sequences representing the envelope proteins of all bunyaviruses examined to date. Direct examination

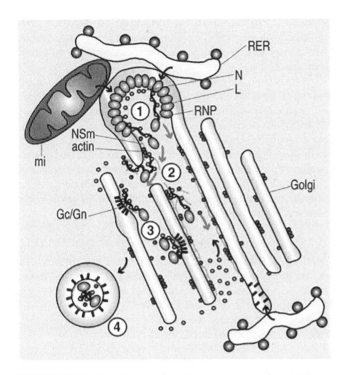

FIGURE 16.21 Model for the functional structure of viral tubes integrated in the Bunyamwera viral factory. Viral tubes assemble in association with Golgi membranes using endogenous actin and polymerized NSm as scaffold. Tubes attach to rough endoplasmic reticulum (*RER*) cisternae and mitochondria that provide cell factors needed for viral replication and assembly. Viral polymerase (*L*) concentrates in the globular domain. Replicated viral RNA (*1*) gets protected by interaction with N molecules, abundant around Golgi membranes and inside tubes. N molecules enter the tubes through their openings to the cytoplasm. With the help of actomyosin-based motors, assembled ribonucleoprotein complexes (*RNPs*) then travel toward the cytoplasm (*2*), where they bind to the cytoplasmic domains of viral glycoproteins (*Gc/Gn*) concentrated in the nearby Golgi membranes. Budding events (*3*) lead to new viral particles that incorporate some amounts of the scaffold NSm protein and actin inside. Assembled immature viral particles are then ready for maturation and secretion (*4*). (Redrawn from Fontana J, Lopez-Montero N, Elliott RM, et al. The unique architecture of Bunyamwera virus factories around the Golgi complex. *Cell Microbiol* 2008;10:2012–2028.)

of a phlebovirus by enzymatic digestion of exposed proteins embedded in intracellular membranes demonstrated that approximately 12% of Gn or Gc was exposed on the cytoplasmic face of membranes in infected cells and was accessible to digestion. A large protease-resistant fragment was identified, which was presumably sequestered in the membrane in a manner that rendered it safe from enzymatic digestion.[413] These enzyme-resistant fragments may therefore represent transmembrane regions of proteins, which could provide the interaction between RNPs and the cellular membranes required for envelopment. The predicted cytoplasmic tails on Gn have also been suggested to be logical candidates for interacting with the ribonucleocapsids.[361]

Tospovirus assembly and release in plants may differ from those processes of other viruses in the *Bunyavirales* order. A model was proposed in which Golgi membranes with integral viral envelope proteins wrap around RNPs. These particles may then fuse with each other or with ER membranes to release single enveloped particles into the cisternae.[215] Mature virions accumulated within the ER cisternae likely remain there until ingested by thrips.

Transport and Release

After budding into the Golgi cisternae, virions apparently are transported to the cell surface within vesicles analogous to those in the secretory pathway. The release of virus from infected cells presumably occurs when the virus-containing vesicles fuse with the cellular plasma membrane (i.e., by normal exocytosis). Numerous viruses in the family have been observed late in infection within vesicles or in the process of exocytosis by electron microscopy, and more recently by light microscopy of BUNV expressing a Gc-GFP fusion protein (Fig. 16.22). In polarized cells, the phleboviruses PTV and RVFV show differing release characteristics, in that no marked polarized release could be detected for RVFV whereas PTV was released primarily from the basolateral surfaces.[73,141] In contrast to these phleboviruses, the hantavirus BCCV was released from the apical surface.[353] Such polarized release of viruses might be important for disseminating virus during natural infection to produce a systemic disease. Release of tospoviruses from insect cells probably occurs via secretory exocytosis similar to that of animal-infecting members of the family.[461]

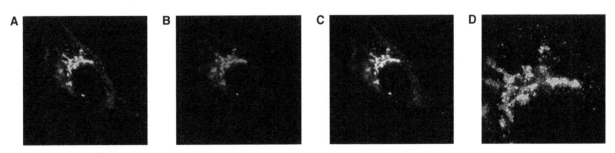

FIGURE 16.22 Bunyavirus budding at the Golgi. BSR-T7/5 cells, BHK-derived cells constitutively expressing T7 RNA polymerase, were infected with a recombinant Bunyamwera virus (BUNV) expressing a Gc-GFP (*green* fluorescent protein) fusion protein (*autofluorescence* shown in **A**) and co-stained with antibodies to the Golgi marker GM130 (in *red* in **B**). Colocalization between Gc proteins and the Golgi protein is shown in *yellow* in the merged images (**C**), and an enlarged image is shown in **D**. (From Shi X, van Mierlo JT, French A, et al. Visualizing the replication cycle of Bunyamwera orthobunyavirus expressing fluorescent protein-tagged Gc glycoprotein. *J Virol* 2010;84(17):8460–8469. doi: 10.1128/JVI.00902-10. Reproduced with permission from American Society for Microbiology.)

EFFECTS OF VIRAL REPLICATION ON HOST CELLS

Cytopathic Effects

The cytopathic effects observed in cultured cells infected with bunyaviruses vary widely, depending on both the virus and the type of host cell studied. Most bunyaviruses are capable of alternately replicating in vertebrates (or plants for tospoviruses) and arthropods, and generally they are cytolytic for their vertebrate/plant hosts but cause little or no cytopathogenicity in their invertebrate hosts. Hantaviruses have no known arthropod vector, and generally cause persistent infections in their hosts and in cultured cells. Little is known about hantaviruses from fish and reptiles, as only gene sequences have been detected for these thus far. Some bunyaviruses display a narrow host range, especially for arthropod vectors. Although the reason for this has not been defined completely, studies on variant and revertant LACV orthobunyaviruses have suggested that the specificity was related to Gc, probably at the level of viral attachment to susceptible cells.[427] In natural infections of mammals, viruses are often targeted to a particular organ or cell type. For example, orthobunyaviruses such as LACV appear to be neurotropic[321]; the phlebovirus RVFV is primarily hepatotropic[329]; and the hantavirus HTNV persists in rodent lungs.[244] It will be interesting to determine whether this targeting is due solely to host-cell receptors or to other factors such as differences in effects on host-cell metabolism in targeted cell types versus the unnatural situation in cultured vertebrate cell lines.

Host-Cell Metabolism

In vertebrate cells, orthobunyaviruses and some phleboviruses were found to cause a reduction in host-cell protein synthesis, which became more prominent as the infection progressed. For example, by 5 hours after infection, cells infected with BUNV at high multiplicity showed reduced levels of host protein synthesis, and by 7 hours there was almost no synthesis.[327] RVFV-infected cells displayed reduced host protein synthesis, which gradually became more pronounced from 4 to 20 hours after infection.[320] In contrast, a reduction in host protein synthesis did not occur, even late in infection, with another phlebovirus, UUKV, or with the nairovirus DUGV,[331,436] both of which are transmitted by ticks rather than mosquitoes. Hantaviruses not only cause no detectable reduction in host macromolecular synthesis[383] but routinely establish persistent, noncytolytic infections in susceptible mammalian host cells, a finding consistent with their nonpathogenic persistence in their natural rodent hosts.[244]

The arthropod-borne members of the family, like most other arboviruses, cause little detectable cytopathology in mosquito cell cultures, and viral persistence is readily established. Unlike cultured vertebrate cells, mosquito cells infected with the orthobunyavirus, Marituba virus, displayed no reduction in host macromolecular synthesis; therefore, viral infection apparently does not drastically interfere with normal cellular processes.[68] One suggested reason for this is that, in arthropod cells, excess viral proteins do not accumulate in the cells but rather are more efficiently processed into mature virions.[296] Another possibility is that viral transcriptase may be less active in arthropod cells than in mammalian cells and that the endonuclease activity of the polymerase (which is used to acquire transcriptional primers) is detrimental to host-cell messages. A reduced level of activity of the viral transcriptase would, therefore, produce less damage to host-cell messages and consequently to protein synthesis.[369]

Persistence, in both insect and mammalian cells, can be mediated by defective interfering (DI) viruses. Conventional DI particles, which displayed deletions only in L, were described for orthobunyaviruses and tospoviruses. The L deletions identified both in the TSWV and BUNV DI particles were in-frame, thus allowing translation of truncated L polypeptides.[93,322] Persistent infections of viruses in the family have also been described that do not involve typical DI particles, but instead are caused by infection with temperature-sensitive and plaque morphology mutants.

Host-Cell Responses and Viral Suppression

Interferon-Stimulated Genes and Gene Products

A first line of host defense against viruses is the innate immunity mechanism mediated by the type I interferon (IFN) pathway. Type I IFN (also called IFNα/β) is produced in, and secreted from, infected cells, and in neighboring cells activates the expression of hundreds of ISGs whose gene products directly or indirectly inhibit virus replication. IFN induction is mediated by the recognition of pathogen-associated molecular patterns (PAMPs) by cellular receptors.[333] Two RNA helicases, RIG-I and MDA5, are intracellular receptors that are activated by specific double-stranded RNA (dsRNA) PAMPs, though the dsRNA–binding protein kinase PKR may also assist.[207,334,351,360,390] RIG-I binds short dsRNAs with 5' triphosphate groups, whereas MDA5 recognizes any long dsRNA. Negative-sense RNA viruses do not produce much of long dsRNA[455] but are strong activators of RIG-I because of the 5' triphosphorylated dsRNA panhandle on their genome.[454] Activation of RIG-I by binding of RNA initiates a signaling cascade that leads to phosphorylation of the transcription factor IFN regulator factor 3 (IRF-3)[173]; phosphorylated IRF-3 dimerizes, enters the nucleus, and initiates IFN-β mRNA synthesis. Virus replication also activates other transcription factors such as IRF-7, NF-kB, and AP-1, which enhance IFN gene expression. IFN is then produced and secreted by the infected cells. After docking onto its cognate receptor in an autocrine or paracrine fashion, a signaling chain ensues that results in expression of ISG-encoded proteins. These newly made proteins have a myriad of functions, some of which have been characterized with respect to their specific antiviral activity. Major antiviral defense mechanisms concerning bunyaviruses are the Mx proteins, PKR, the 2'-5' oligoadenylate synthase (2'-5'-OAS)/RNaseL system, ISG20, IFITMs, tetherin, and viperin.

The Mx proteins are IFN-induced cytoplasmic proteins, which belong to a family of large GTPases that function in intracellular trafficking.[164] After viral infection and IFN induction, Mx proteins are rapidly induced and accumulate in the cytoplasm. Human MxA has been shown to inhibit the replication of representative members of the *Orthobunyavirus*, *Orthohantavirus*, *Orthonairovirus*, and *Phlebovirus* genera.[53,123,201,211] Both inhibition of primary transcription and genome replication have been observed.[123,158,361] The MxA protein was shown to bind to the N proteins of LACV, BUNV, RVFV, ANDV, and CCHFV[13,211,222,361] and in LACV-infected cells to redistribute it into membrane-associated perinuclear cytoplasmic complexes, thus removing the protein from use in viral replication.[222,361] For the orthobunyavirus LACV, MxA inhibits replication in mammalian cell cultures, in mosquito cells expressing the human MxA gene, and in MxA-transgenic mice that lack a functional IFN system.[123,169,286]

Inhibition of the replication of several hantaviruses by MxA protein has been described. ANDV infection of human vein endothelial cells (HUVECs) was found to up-regulate transcription of MxA RNA and expression of MxA protein. Virus replication was required for the induction of MxA, and the virus was found to replicate best in cells with low or no expressed MxA. Comparison of induction of MxA protein for pathogenic and nonpathogenic hantaviruses in HUVECs demonstrated that the nonpathogenic hantaviruses (PHV or TULV) induced an early and vigorous onset of MxA expression, whereas the pathogenic hantaviruses (ANDV or HTNV) induced MxA relatively late (48 hours) after infection.[137,231] In contrast, Vero E6 cells, which lack IFN genes, supported the growth of both viruses. These results suggest that pathogenic but not nonpathogenic hantaviruses can delay the IFN-β-induced antiviral MxA response and allow efficient viral replication early in infection.[231]

To determine whether MxA would be active against tospoviruses in plants, transgenic tobacco plants expressing MxA were created and then challenged with TSWV. No increased resistance to viral replication was observed in the transgenic plants, indicating that expression of human MxA alone is not sufficient to impart virus resistance to plants.[124]

In MxA-deficient systems bunyavirus replication can still be impaired, implying that other ISGs have anti-bunyaviral activity.[14,49,159,307] PKR is a dsRNA-activated inhibitor of translation that was shown to contribute to host resistance to BUNV, whereas the RNA-degrading 2′-5′ OAS/RNaseL system had no effect.[66,423] Moreover, RVFV lacking its NSs protein (see below) is highly sensitive to PKR *in vitro* and *in vivo*.[159,186] ISG20 (Interferon-stimulated gene 20 kDa protein) is a 3′-5′ exonuclease able to inhibit members of the *Peribunyaviridae*, *Hantaviridae*, and *Nairoviridae* families, whereas *Phenuiviridae* of the genus *Phlebovirus* (RVFV) and *Banyangvirus* (SFTSV, HRTV) were not affected.[115] Members of the IFN-induced transmembrane proteins (IFITMs) inhibit cytoplasmic entry of a broad range of viruses, including LACV (genus *Orthobunyavirus*, family *Peribunyaviridae*), RVFV (genus *Phlebovirus*, family *Phenuiviridae*), ANDV and HTNV (genus *Orthohantavirus*, family *Hantaviridae*), but not CCHFV (genus *Orthonairovirus*, family *Nairoviridae*).[291] Tetherin is a transmembrane protein that, different from the IFITMs, interferes with a late step in replication, the budding of enveloped virus particles from the cell. For orthobunyaviruses like, for example, SBV tetherin was shown to inhibit virus propagation by reducing the amount of GPs in viral particles.[440] Viperin is a member of the radical S-adenosylmethionine enzyme superfamily shown to inhibit BUNV multiplication by an unknown mechanism.[66]

Interferon Antagonism

Viruses encode IFN antagonistic proteins that allow them to overcome the antiviral effects of IFN. Evasion of the IFN response by viruses can occur by preventing IFN induction or by inhibiting IFN signaling and/or the activity of ISGs. IFN antagonism has been demonstrated for the NSs proteins of the phlebovirus RVFV, the orthobunyaviruses BUNV and LACV, and the

hantaviruses PUUV and TULV.[189,268,387,468] For the phleboviruses and orthobunyaviruses, NSs proteins were identified as IFN antagonists by comparing wild-type and mutant viruses that do not express NSs. An RVFV mutant, called Clone 13, was naturally occurring, whereas the BUNV and LACV mutants were created by reverse genetics.[45,55,293] The wild-type viruses induced little IFN and were virulent in mice, whereas the NSs-defective viruses were potent inducers of IFN and attenuated in mice. In genetically altered mice that are nonresponsive to type 1 IFN, the mutant viruses were just as virulent as the wild-type parents, indicating that type 1 IFN is the target of NSs.[46,55,452]

Although the orthobunyavirus and phlebovirus NSs have no sequence similarity and are expressed by different coding strategies, they both appear to antagonize host IFN at the level of cellular transcription. For BUNV and LACV, NSs was shown to interfere with the C-terminally hyperphosphorylated (i.e., elongating) state of the RNA polymerase II complex, leading to a down-regulation of host mRNA synthesis.[434,443] This effect was seen only in mammalian cells, not in insect cells, suggesting that IFN antagonism by NSs might be involved in the lytic infections observed in mammalian cells as opposed to viral persistence in insects.[224] BUNV NSs was shown to interact with the protein MED8, a component of the Mediator complex that is essential for mRNA synthesis.[249] LACV NSs selectively targets the RPB1 subunit of the elongating form of RNA polymerase II for proteasome-mediated degradation, an event similar to that seen during the cellular DNA damage response.[443] RVFV NSs inhibits transcription of IFN mRNA in several ways, firstly by sequestering the p44 subunit of the TFIIH general transcription factor,[241] secondly by proteasomally degrading the p44 subunit of TFIIH via the ubiquitin ligase FBXO3,[200] and thirdly by recruiting the SAP30 repressor factor to the IFN-β promoter.[242] RVFV NSs also interferes with host cell mRNA export from the nucleus, a mechanism most likely contributing to IFN antagonism.[83] The NSs proteins of several other pathogenic phleboviruses and banyangviruses including SFSV, TOSV, PTV, and SFTSV were also shown to efficiently block IFN induction.[146,147,159,299,328,344,363,380,466,467] The mechanisms, however, are quite different. Whereas SFSV NSs masks the DNA-binding domain of IRF-3 to hinder it from IFN promoter binding,[467] TOSV NSs interacts with RIG-I and triggers its proteasomal degradation.[147] PTV NSs affects neither IRF3 nor RIG-I but appears to act as a general host cell shutoff factor similar to RVFV NSs[259,467] SFTSV NSs sequesters a number of components of the RIG-I-dependent antiviral signaling chain (including RIG-I and the IRF-3 kinase TBK1) into inclusion bodies, thus disabling antiviral signaling.[299,380,466] Interestingly, the NSs of the avirulent phlebovirus UUKV is only a weak inhibitor of IFN induction.[363] A similar positive correlation between virulence and IFN antagonism was observed for the NSs-less orthobunyaviruses in the Anopheles A, Anopheles B, and Tete serogroups. The majority of them have not been associated with human disease, and failed to prevent induction of IFN-β mRNA. Tacaiuma virus (Anopheles A serogroup), causing a mild febrile disease in humans, was the exception as it was able to inhibit IFN induction, apparently in an NSs-independent manner.[287]

As described above, some hantaviruses have an additional ORF in the S segment,[337] and evidence for the expression of an NSs protein has been obtained for PUUV and TULV.[189] The NSs protein was shown to be weakly antagonistic to

IFN when overexpressed in cell culture, and the presence of a full-length NSs gave a growth advantage to TULV strains in IFN-competent cells.[190] Both hantaviruses and nairoviruses have 5′ monophosphorylated nucleotides on their genomes, thereby avoiding recognition by RIG-I and hence inducing IFN,[157] although the viruses also encode other countermeasures to innate immunity. The OTU domain in the nairovirus L protein deconjugates ubiquitin and ISG15 from cellular targets, thus antagonizing IFN induction.[25,63,125,192,388] Certain hantaviruses have also been shown to interfere with TNF-α induced activation of NF-κB signaling through an interaction between the viral N protein and karyopherin molecules that normally transport the NF-κB subunits from the cytoplasm to the nucleus, thus preventing their use to activate ISGs.[432]

It has been reported that pathogenic hantaviruses do not efficiently activate the IFN response as compared to nonpathogenic hantaviruses, suggesting the presence of an IFN antagonistic gene.[137] The cytoplasmic tail of the Gn glycoprotein (Gn-T) from pathogenic hantaviruses has been shown to down-regulate IFN induction by interacting with TNF receptor–associated factor 3 (TRAF3), an adaptor protein for IRF-3 and NF-kB signaling, whereas Gn-T from PHV fails to inhibit IFN induction.[9,10] However, a recent study showed that the Gn-T of nonpathogenic TULV can also down-regulate IFN induction, but does so in a manner not involving interaction with TRAF3.[280] These data suggest that the pathogenic potential of hantaviruses does not depend on their ability to down-regulate IFN alone. The situation is further complicated by the demonstration that for ANDV, IFN induction is inhibited by coexpression of the GPC and N protein, whereas downstream IFN signaling may be inhibited by either protein.[250] In addition, hantavirus infection of VeroE6 cells was reported to result in induction and secretion of type III IFN (IFN-γ).[341,419] Furthermore, the induction of ISGs in epithelial cell lines (e.g., A549 cells) infected with Vero cell grown virus was found to be due to the presence of IFN-γ rather than to virus infection.[341]

Cytokines/Chemokines/ITAMs

The host cells' responses to hantaviral infection have been studied in an attempt to understand the mechanism of disease. Hantaviruses cause two serious human disease syndromes: HFRS and HPS. Both HFRS and HPS are believed to result from host immune responses to viral infection, rather than damage caused by the viruses themselves.[212] In both syndromes, vascular endothelial cells show increased permeability, which is believed to contribute greatly to the diseases. Several studies have measured the types of cytokines and chemokines released in response to disease, and these are discussed in the context of viral pathogenesis below. Of note is the presence of immunoreceptor tyrosine-based activation motifs (ITAMs) within the cytoplasmic tails of the Gn protein of hantaviruses. ITAMS are cell-signaling elements involved in regulating endothelial cell function. The presence of these elements in hantaviruses has also been suggested to relate to the dysregulation of endothelial cells during hantaviral infection.[135,136]

Apoptosis

Apoptosis, a type of programmed cell death, has been described for orthobunyaviruses, phleboviruses, nairoviruses, and hantaviruses. Apoptosis usually results from activation of a proteolytic system involving caspases, a group of cysteine proteases that cleave cellular substrate proteins. The role of apoptosis in virus infection can be both supportive and suppressive, depending on the time point of its onset.

Apoptosis caused by a bunyavirus was first noted in cultured cells and brains of newborn mice infected with the orthobunyavirus LACV.[326] The NSs proteins of LACV and related viruses were found to have an amino acid sequence similar to that of a *Drosophila* protein, Reaper, which is involved in regulating caspase activity and can induce apoptosis.[81] Reaper is one of several proteins that are able to bind to a group of proteins, known as inhibitors of apoptosis, which function to control caspase activity.[393] Like Reaper, BUNV NSs proteins were shown to both inhibit cellular protein translation and activate caspase in cell-free extracts. To demonstrate *in vivo* apoptosis, a Sindbis virus replicon expressing NSs was injected into the brains of young mice. The mice developed neuronal apoptosis and died 6 days after infection. A similar mechanism of action for inducing apoptosis by Reaper and orthobunyavirus NSs was proposed because both were shown to bind to and counteract the effects of a protein known as Scythe, which is an apoptosis regulator.[81] Mosquito cells persistently infected by LACV do not undergo apoptosis.[45] The orthobunyavirus OROV induces apoptosis in HeLa cells that is dependent on virus uncoating and replication, but treatment of cells with a pan-caspase inhibitor did not affect virus production although apoptosis was prevented.[2] The results indicated that the intrinsic apoptosis pathway was triggered by virus replication but apoptosis was not necessary for efficient virus production in cell culture.

Apoptosis was also observed after infection with phleboviruses like RVFV or TOSV.[87] Similar to LACV NSs,[443] the nonstructural protein NSs of RVFV activates DNA damageresponse signaling in the nucleus and the apoptosis promoter[23] p53.[24] The nonstructural protein NSm of RVFV, however, suppresses apoptosis.[433,465] For the nairovirus CCHFV, the NSs protein was shown to trigger apoptosis by disrupting the mitochondrial membrane potential,[27] but at early stages of infection CCHFV inhibits apoptosis.[206]

For several hantaviruses, apoptosis was observed in infected cultured monkey kidney (Vero E6) cells,[203,252] in cultured human embryonic kidney cells (HEK-293),[273] and in lymphocytes of HFRS patients.[5] Unlike most infections with hantaviruses, which are generally noncytolytic and persistent, cytopathic effects were observed in the HEK-293 cells infected with hantaviruses, and apoptosis was observed almost entirely in cells adjacent to those actively infected with the hantavirus.[273] In another report, apoptosis was not seen in confluent Vero E6 cells infected with various hantaviruses, and only a few apoptotic cells could be seen when subconfluent cells were infected.[166] Likewise, infection of primary immature dendritic cells or HUVECs with HTNV did not induce cell lysis or apoptosis.[345] These differing results remain to be resolved, but it is likely that they can be attributed to differences in the cells or the condition and passage histories of the cells.

The factors triggering apoptosis for hantaviruses are not generally known. In TULV-infected Vero E6 cells, caspase 8 activation was observed and apoptosis could be inhibited with a caspase inhibitor.[252] Caspase 8 is one of several caspases that can be induced by the binding of a specific ligand to "death receptors," such as tumor necrosis factor 1 (TNF1) and Fas (also called CD95), which are found on certain cells.[22] Consistent with this, TNF1 was up-regulated at times when apoptosis was apparent in the TULV-infected cells and a Fas-mediated apoptosis enhancer, DAXX, was found to bind to PUUV N proteins.[255] However, in another study, no significant increase in the mRNAs of the TNF superfamily was observed in hantavirus-infected HEK-293 cells.[273]

Stress on the host cell ER is another cellular condition that can trigger apoptosis. TULV infection of Vero E6 cells was noted to activate markers of ER stress, including induction of the chaperone protein, Grp78/Bip, which was suggested to be induced by the accumulation of misfolded proteins in the ER.[253] Another cellular stress-response protein, heat shock protein 70, was found to be abundant in postmortem tissues of hantavirus-infected patients and to be up-regulated in VeroE6 cells infected with HTNV.[471] In this study, it was not clear what role the stress protein played in host-cell response to infection. Additional work is needed to identify the many possible factors that can contribute to cellular stress and apoptosis in Bunyavirus-infected cells.

As countermechanisms it was described that HTNV N protein stimulates the degradation of the apoptosis driver p53 via the E3 ubiquitin ligase MDM2,[319] and that HTNV and ANDV interferes with DAXX-mediated apoptosis by up-regulation of IFN-activated counterplayers like Sp100.[210]

RNA Silencing

RNA silencing, or RNA interference (RNAi) was first described for plants as a mechanism to defend against viral infection, but is now known to occur in most eukaryotes. The gene silencing is mediated by short interfering RNAs (siRNAs), which arise from cleavage of dsRNAs, including the replication intermediates of RNA viruses by a host enzyme known as Dicer. The 21 to 25 nucleotide siRNAs become part of a protein complex known as the RNA-induced silencing complex, which recognizes and degrades sequence-specific mRNAs. Some viruses have been shown to produce suppressors to counteract the gene silencing mechanism. In the family *Tospoviridae*, the NSs protein of TSWV was found to act as a suppressor of gene silencing.[58,430] In addition to the plant-infecting bunyaviruses, siRNA suppression has been observed with the orthobunyavirus LACV, in both mammalian and insect cells, and with the nairovirus Hazara virus (HAZV) in tick cells. As observed for the tospoviruses, the LACV-suppressing activity was localized to NSs, despite the completely different coding strategy used for this protein (i.e., ambisense vs. ORFs).[416] For HAZV, which does not produce an NSs protein, the activity was observed with the S-segment gene in either the sense or antisense orientation.[128]

REFERENCES

1. Abraham G, Pattnaik A. Early RNA synthesis in bunyamwera virus-infected cells. *J Gen Virol* 1983;64:1277–1290.
2. Acrani GO, Gomes R, Proenca-Modena JL, et al. Apoptosis induced by Oropouche virus infection in HeLa cells is dependent on virus protein expression. *Virus Res* 2010;149(1):56–63.
3. Adams MJ, Lefkowitz EJ, King AMQ, et al. Changes to taxonomy and the International Code of Virus Classification and Nomenclature ratified by the International Committee on Taxonomy of Viruses (2017). *Arch Virol* 2017;162(8):2505–2538.
4. Agirrezabala X, Méndez-López E, Lasso G, et al. The near-atomic cryoEM structure of a flexible filamentous plant virus shows homology of its coat protein with nucleoproteins of animal viruses. *Elife* 2015;4:e11795.
5. Akhmatova NK, Yusupova RS, Khaiboullina SF, et al. Lymphocyte apoptosis during hemorragic fever with renal syndrome. *Russ J Immunol* 2003;8(1):37–46.
6. Akutsu M, Ye Y, Virdee S, et al. Molecular basis for ubiquitin and ISG15 cross-reactivity in viral ovarian tumor domains. *Proc Natl Acad Sci U S A* 2011;108(6):2228–2233.
7. Albarino CG, Bird BH, Nichol ST. A shared transcription termination signal on negative and ambisense RNA genome segments of Rift Valley fever, sandfly fever Sicilian, and Toscana viruses. *J Virol* 2007;81(10):5246–5256.
8. Albornoz A, Hoffmann AB, Lozach PY, et al. Early Bunyavirus-host cell interactions. *Viruses* 2016;8(5).
9. Alff PJ, Gavrilovskaya IN, Gorbunova E, et al. The pathogenic NY-1 hantavirus G1 cytoplasmic tail inhibits RIG-I- and TBK-1-directed interferon responses. *J Virol* 2006;80(19):9676–9686.
10. Alff PJ, Sen N, Gorbunova E, et al. The NY-1 hantavirus Gn cytoplasmic tail coprecipitates TRAF3 and inhibits cellular interferon responses by disrupting TBK1-TRAF3 complex formation. *J Virol* 2008;82(18):9115–9122.
11. Altamura LA, Bertolotti-Ciarlet A, Teigler J, et al. Identification of a novel C-terminal cleavage of Crimean-Congo hemorrhagic fever virus PreGN that leads to generation of an NSM protein. *J Virol* 2007;81(12):6632–6642.
12. Anderson G, Smith J. Immunoelectron microscopy of Rift Valley morphogenesis in primary rat hepatocytes. *Virology* 1987;161:91–100.
13. Andersson I, Bladh L, Mousavi-Jazi M, et al. Human MxA protein inhibits the replication of Crimean-Congo hemorrhagic fever virus. *J Virol* 2004;78(8):4323–4329.
14. Andersson I, Lundkvist A, Haller O, et al. Type I interferon inhibits Crimean-Congo hemorrhagic fever virus in human target cells. *J Med Virol* 2006;78(2):216–222.
15. Andersson AM, Pettersson RF. Targeting of a short peptide derived from the cytoplasmic tail of the G1 membrane glycoprotein of Uukuniemi virus (Bunyaviridae) to the Golgi complex. *J Virol* 1998;72(12):9585–9596.
16. Andersson I, Simon M, Lundkvist A, et al. Role of actin filaments in targeting of Crimean Congo hemorrhagic fever virus nucleocapsid protein to perinuclear regions of mammalian cells. *J Med Virol* 2004;72(1):83–93.
17. Aquino VH, Moreli ML, Moraes Figueiredo LT. Analysis of oropouche virus L protein amino acid sequence showed the presence of an additional conserved region that could harbour an important role for the polymerase activity. *Arch Virol* 2003;148(1):19–28.
18. Arai S, Taniguchi S, Aoki K, et al. Molecular phylogeny of a genetically divergent hantavirus harbored by the Geoffroy's rousette (*Rousettus amplexicaudatus*), a frugivorous bat species in the Philippines. *Infect Genet Evol* 2016;45:26–32.
19. Arikawa J, Schmaljohn AL, Dalrymple JM, et al. Characterization of Hantaan virus envelope glycoprotein antigenic determinants defined by monoclonal antibodies. *J Gen Virol* 1989;70(Pt 3):615–624.
20. Ariza A, Tanner SJ, Walter CT, et al. Nucleocapsid protein structures from orthobunyaviruses reveal insight into ribonucleoprotein architecture and RNA polymerization. *Nucleic Acids Res* 2013;41(11):5912.
21. Arragain B, Reguera J, Desfosses A, et al. High resolution cryo-EM structure of the helical RNA-bound Hantaan virus nucleocapsid reveals its assembly mechanisms. *Elife* 2019;8:e43075.
22. Ashkenazi A, Dixit VM. Death receptors: signaling and modulation. *Science* 1998;281(5381):1305–1308.
23. Austin D, Baer A, Lundberg L, et al. p53 Activation following Rift Valley fever virus infection contributes to cell death and viral production. *PLoS One* 2012;7(5).
24. Baer A, Austin D, Narayanan A, et al. Induction of DNA damage signaling upon Rift Valley Fever virus infection results in cell cycle arrest and increased viral replication. *J Biol Chem* 2012;287(10):7399–7410.
25. Bakshi S, Holzer B, Bridgen A, et al. Dugbe virus ovarian tumour domain interferes with ubiquitin/ISG15-regulated innate immune cell signalling. *J Gen Virol* 2013;94:298–307.
26. Barbosa NS, Mendonca LR, Dias MVS, et al. ESCRT machinery components are required for Orthobunyavirus particle production in Golgi compartments. *PLoS Pathog* 2018;14(5).
27. Barnwal B, Karlberg H, Mirazimi A, et al. The non-structural protein of Crimean-Congo hemorrhagic fever virus disrupts the mitochondrial membrane potential and induces apoptosis. *J Biol Chem* 2016;291(2):582–592.
28. Barr JN. Bunyavirus mRNA synthesis is coupled to translation to prevent premature transcription termination. *RNA* 2007;13(5):731–736.
29. Barr JN, Rodgers JW, Wertz GW. The Bunyamwera virus mRNA transcription signal resides within both the 3′ and the 5′ terminal regions and allows ambisense transcription from a model RNA segment. *J Virol* 2005;79(19):12602–12607.
30. Barr JN, Rodgers JW, Wertz GW. Identification of the Bunyamwera bunyavirus transcription termination signal. *J Gen Virol* 2006;87:189–198.
31. Barr JN, Wertz GW. Bunyamwera bunyavirus RNA synthesis requires cooperation of 3′- and 5′-terminal sequences. *J Virol* 2004;78(3):1129–1138.
32. Barr JN, Wertz GW. Role of the conserved nucleotide mismatch within 3′- and 5′-terminal regions of Bunyamwera virus in signaling transcription. *J Virol* 2005;79(6):3586–3594.
33. Barr JN, Whelan SPJ, Wertz GW. cis-acting signals involved in termination of vesicular stomatitis virus mRNA synthesis include the conserved AUAC and the U7 signal for polyadenylation. *J Virol* 1997;71(11):8718–8725.
34. Barski M, Brennan B, Miller OK, et al. Rift Valley fever phlebovirus NSs protein core domain structure suggests molecular basis for nuclear filaments. *Elife* 2017;6.
35. Battisti AJ, Chu YK, Chipman PR, et al. Structural studies of Hantaan virus. *J Virol* 2011;85(2):835–841.
36. Becker C, Goubeaud G, Willems W. Hantaan virus infection (letter). *Dtsch Med Wochenschr* 1991;116(15):598.
37. Bellocq C, Kolakofsky D. Translational requirement for La Crosse virus S-mRNA synthesis: a possible mechanism. *J Virol* 1987;61(12):3960–3967.
38. Bente DA, Forrester NL, Watts DM, et al. Crimean-Congo hemorrhagic fever: history, epidemiology, pathogenesis, clinical syndrome and genetic diversity. *Antiviral Res* 2013;100(1):159–189.
39. Bergeron E, Albarino CG, Khristova ML, et al. Crimean-Congo hemorrhagic virus-encoded ovarian tumor protease activity is dispensable for virus RNA polymerase function. *J Virol* 2010;84(1):216–226.
40. Bergeron E, Zivcec M, Chakrabarti AK, et al. Recovery of recombinant Crimean Congo hemorrhagic fever virus reveals a function for non-structural glycoproteins cleavage by furin. *PLoS Pathog* 2015;11(5).

41. Bertolotti-Ciarlet A, Smith J, Strecker K, et al. Cellular localization and antigenic characterization of crimean-congo hemorrhagic fever virus glycoproteins. *J Virol* 2005;79(10): 6152–6161.
42. Bishop D, Calisher C, Casals J, et al. Bunyaviridae. *Intervirology* 1980;14(3–4):125–143.
43. Bishop D, Gould K, Akashi H, et al. The complete sequence and coding content of snowshoe hare bunyavirus small (S) viral RNA species. *Nucleic Acids Res* 1982;10(12):3703–3713.
44. Bishop D, Shope R. Bunyaviridae. In: Fraenkel-Conrat H, Wagner RR, eds. *Comprehensive Virology*. Vol. 14. 1979:1–156.
45. Blakqori G, Delhaye S, Habjan M, et al. La Crosse bunyavirus nonstructural protein NSs serves to suppress the type I interferon system of mammalian hosts. *J Virol* 2007;81(10):4991–4999.
46. Blakqori G, van Knippenberg I, Elliott RM. Bunyamwera orthobunyavirus S-segment untranslated regions mediate poly(A) tail-independent translation. *J Virol* 2009;83(8):3637–3646.
47. Bolte H, Rosu ME, Hagelauer E, et al. Packaging of the Influenza virus genome is governed by a plastic network of RNA- and nucleoprotein-mediated interactions. *J Virol* 2019;93(4).
48. Boudko SP, Kuhn RJ, Rossmann MG. The coiled-coil domain structure of the Sin Nombre virus nucleocapsid protein. *J Mol Biol* 2007;366(5):1538–1544.
49. Bouloy M, Janzen C, Vialat P, et al. Genetic evidence for an interferon-antagonistic function of rift valley fever virus nonstructural protein NSs. *J Virol* 2001;75(3):1371–1377.
50. Bouloy M, Pardigon N, Vialat P, et al. Characterization of the 5′ and 3′ ends of viral messenger RNAs Isolated from BHK21 cells infected with Germiston virus (Bunyavirus). *Virology* 1990;175:50–58.
51. Bowden TA, Bitto D, McLees A, et al. Orthobunyavirus ultrastructure and the curious tripodal glycoprotein spike. *PLoS Pathog* 2013;9(5):e1003374.
52. Bowen MD, Jackson AO, Bruns TD, et al. Determination and comparative analysis of the small RNA genomic sequences of California encephalitis, Jamestown Canyon, Jerry Slough, Melao, Keystone and Trivittatus viruses (Bunyaviridae, genus Bunyavirus, California serogroup). *J Gen Virol* 1995;76(Pt 3):559–572.
53. Bridgen A, Dalrymple DA, Weber F, et al. Inhibition of Dugbe nairovirus replication by human MxA protein. *Virus Res* 2004;99(1):47–50.
54. Bridgen A, Elliott RM. Rescue of a segmented negative-strand RNA virus entirely from cloned complementary DNAs. *Proc Natl Acad Sci U S A* 1996;93(26):15400–15404.
55. Bridgen A, Weber F, Fazakerley JK, et al. Bunyamwera bunyavirus nonstructural protein NSs is a nonessential gene product that contributes to viral pathogenesis. *Proc Natl Acad Sci U S A* 2001;98(2):664–669.
56. Briese T, Kapoor V, Lipkin WI. Natural M-segment reassortment in Potosi and Main Drain viruses: implications for the evolution of orthobunyaviruses. *Arch Virol* 2007;152(12):2237–2247.
57. Brittlebank CC. Tomato diseases. *J Agric* 1919;17:231–235.
58. Bucher E, Sijen T, De Haan P, et al. Negative-strand tospoviruses and tenuiviruses carry a gene for a suppressor of gene silencing at analogous genomic positions. *J Virol* 2003;77(2):1329–1336.
59. Calisher C. Evolutionary significance of the taxonomic data regarding bunyaviruses of the family Bunyaviridae. *Intervirology* 1988;29(5):268–276.
60. Calisher C. Classification and nomenclature of viruses. Fifth report of the international committeee on taxonomy of viruses. In: Francki RIB, Fauquet CM, Knudson DL, et al., eds. *Archives of Virology*. Vol Supplementum 2. New York: Springer Publishing Company; 1991:273–283.
61. Calisher CH. History, classification and taxonomy of viruses in the Family Bunyaviridae. In: Elliott RM, ed. *The Bunyaviridae*. New York: Plenum Press; 1996:1–17.
62. Capodagli GC, Deaton MK, Baker EA, et al. Diversity of Ubiquitin and ISG15 Specificity among Nairoviruses' Viral Ovarian Tumor Domain Proteases. *J Virol* 2013;87(7): 3815–3827.
63. Capodagli GC, McKercher MA, Baker EA, et al. Structural analysis of a viral ovarian tumor domain protease from the Crimean-Congo hemorrhagic fever virus in complex with covalently bonded ubiquitin. *J Virol* 2011;85(7):3621–3630.
64. Capstick PB, Gosden D. Neutralizing antibody response of sheep to pantropic and neurotropic Rift Valley fever virus. *Nature* 1962;195(4841):583–584.
65. Carey D, Reuben R, Panicker K, et al. Thottapalayam virus: a presumptive arbovirus isolated from a shrew in India. *Indian J Med Res* 1971;59:1758–1760.
66. Carlton-Smith C, Elliott RM. Viperin, MTAP44, and Protein kinase R contribute to the interferon-induced inhibition of Bunyamwera orthobunyavirus replication. *J Virol* 2012;86(21):11548–11557.
67. Carter SD, Surtees R, Walter CT, et al. Structure, function, and evolution of the Crimean-Congo hemorrhagic fever virus nucleocapsid protein. *J Virol* 2012;86(20):10914–10923.
68. Carvalho M, Frugulhetti I, Rebello M. Marituba (Bunyaviridae) virus replication in cultured Aedes albopictus cells and in L-A9 cells. *Arch Virol* 1986;90:325–335.
69. Casals J. Relationships among arthropod-borne animal viruses determined by cross-challenge tests. *Am J Trop Med Hyg* 1963;12:587–596.
70. Casals J. Antigenic similarity between the virus causing Crimean hemorrhagic fever and Congo virus. *Proc Soc Exp Biol Med* 1969;131(1):233–236.
71. Cash P, Vezza A, Gentsch J, et al. Genome complexities of the three mRNA species of Snowshoe hare bunyavirus and In vitro translation of S mRNA to viral N polypeptide. *J Virol* 1979;31(3):685–694.
72. Chang JH, Cho YH, Sohn SY, et al. Crystal structure of the eIF4A-PDCD4 complex. *Proc Natl Acad Sci U S A* 2009;106(9):3148–3153.
73. Chen S, Matsuoka Y, Compans R. Assembly and polarized release of Punta Toro virus and effects of Brefeldin A. *J Virol* 1991;65(3):1427–1439.
74. Cheng E, Mir MA. Signatures of host mRNA 5′ terminus for efficient Hantavirus cap snatching. *J Virol* 2012;86(18):10173–10185.
75. Chiang CF, Flint M, Lin JMS, et al. Endocytic pathways used by andes virus to enter primary human lung endothelial cells. *PLoS One* 2016;11(10).
76. Childs JE, Ksiazek TG, Spiropoulou CF, et al. Serologic and genetic identification of peromyscus maniculatus as the primary rodent reservoir for a new hantavirus in the southwestern united states. *J Infect Dis* 1994;169(6):1271–1280.
77. Choi Y, Kwon YC, Kim SI, et al. A hantavirus causing hemorrhagic fever with renal syndrome requires gC1qR/p32 for efficient cell binding and infection. *Virology* 2008;381(2):178–183.
78. Chumakov MP. Studies of virus haemorrhagic fevers. *J Hyg Epidemiol Microbiol Immunol* 1963;7:125–135.
79. Chumakov MP, Smirnova SE, Tkachenko EA. Relationship between strains of Crimean haemorrhagic fever and Congo viruses. *Acta Virol* 1970;14(1):82–85.
80. Collett MS. Messenger RNA of the M segment RNA of Rift Valley fever virus. *Virology* 1986;151(1):151–156.
81. Colon-Ramos DA, Irusta PM, Gan EC, et al. Inhibition of translation and induction of apoptosis by Bunyaviral nonstructural proteins bearing sequence similarity to reaper. *Mol Biol Cell* 2003;14(10):4162–4172.
82. Connor JH, McKenzie MO, Parks GD, et al. Antiviral activity and RNA polymerase degradation following Hsp90 inhibition in a range of negative strand viruses. *Virology* 2007;362(1):109–119.
83. Copeland AM, Van Deusen NM, Schmaljohn CS. Rift Valley fever virus NSS gene expression correlates with a defect in nuclear mRNA export. *Virology* 2015;486:88–93.
84. Cortez I, Aires A, Pereira AM, et al. Genetic organisation of Iris yellow spot virus M RNA: indications for functional homology between the G(C) glycoproteins of tospoviruses and animal-infecting bunyaviruses. *Arch Virol* 2002;147(12):2313–2325.
85. Coupeau D, Claine F, Wiggers L, et al. Characterization of messenger RNA termini in Schmallenberg virus and related Simbuviruses. *J Gen Virol* 2013;94:2399–2405.
86. Cunningham C, Szilagyi JF. Viral RNAs synthesized in cells infected with Germiston Bunyavirus. *Virology* 1987;157(2):431–439.
87. Cusi MG, Gori Savellini G, Terrosi C, et al. Development of a mouse model for the study of Toscana virus pathogenesis. *Virology* 2005;333(1):66–73.
88. Cyr N, de la Fuente C, Lecoq L, et al. A Omega XaV motif in the Rift Valley fever virus NSs protein is essential for degrading p62, forming nuclear filaments and virulence. *Proc Natl Acad Sci U S A* 2015;112(19):6021–6026.
89. Datta K, Wolkerstorfer A, Szolar OH, et al. Characterization of PA-N terminal domain of Influenza A polymerase reveals sequence specific RNA cleavage. *Nucleic Acids Res* 2013;41(17):8289–8299.
90. Daubney R, Hudson JR, Garnham PC. Enzootic hepatitis or Rift Valley fever. An undescribed virus disease of sheep cattle and man from East Africa. *J Pathol Bacteriol* 1931;34(2):545–579.
91. de Haan P, Wagemakers L, Peters D, et al. The S RNA segment of tomato spotted wilt virus has an ambisense character. *J Gen Virol* 1990;71(Pt 5):1001–1007.
92. de Medeiros RB, Figueiredo J, Resende Rde O, et al. Expression of a viral polymerase-bound host factor turns human cell lines permissive to a plant- and insect-infecting virus. *Proc Natl Acad Sci U S A* 2005;102(4):1175–1180.
93. de Oliveira Resende R, de Hann P, van de Vossen E, et al. Defective interfering L RNA segments of tomato spotted wilt virus retain both virus genome termini and have extensive internal deletions. *J Gen Virol* 1992;73:2509–2516.
94. Dessau M, Modis Y. Crystal structure of glycoprotein C from Rift Valley fever virus. *Proc Natl Acad Sci U S A* 2013;110(5):1696–1701.
95. Devignot S, Bergeron E, Nichol S, et al. A virus-like particle system identifies the endonuclease domain of Crimean-Congo hemorrhagic fever virus. *J Virol* 2015;89(11):5957–5967.
96. Dias A, Bouvier D, Crepin T, et al. The cap-snatching endonuclease of influenza virus polymerase resides in the PA subunit. *Nature* 2009;458(7240):914–918.
97. Donets MA, Chumakov MP, Korolev MB, et al. Physicochemical characteristics, morphology and morphogenesis of virions of the causative agent of Crimean hemorrhagic fever. *Intervirology* 1977;8:294–308.
98. Duijsings D, Kormelink R, Goldbach R. In vivo analysis of the TSWV cap-snatching mechanism: single base complementarity and primer length requirements. *EMBO J* 2001; 20(10):2545–2552.
99. Dunn EF, Pritlove DC, Elliott RM. The S RNA genome segments of Batai, Cache Valley, Guaroa, Kairi, Lumbo, Main Drain and Northway bunyaviruses: sequence determination and analysis. *J Gen Virol* 1994;75(Pt 3):597–608.
100. Dunn EF, Pritlove DC, Jin H, et al. Transcription of a recombinant bunyavirus RNA template by transiently expressed bunyavirus proteins. *Virology* 1995;211(1):133–143.
101. Dzimianski JV, Beldon BS, Daczkowski CM, et al. Probing the impact of nairovirus genomic diversity on viral ovarian tumor domain protease (vOTU) structure and deubiquitinase activity. *PLoS Pathog* 2019;15(1).
102. Earle D. Analysis of sequential physiologic derangements in epidemic hemorrhagic fever; with a commentary on management. *Am J Med* 1954;16:690–709.
103. Eddy GA, Peters CJ. The extended horizons of Rift Valley fever: current and projected immunogens. *Prog Clin Biol Res* 1980;47(7):179–191.
104. Eifan SA, Elliott RM. Mutational analysis of the Bunyamwera orthobunyavirus nucleocapsid protein gene. *J Virol* 2009;83(21):11307–11317.
105. Elliott RM. Identification of nonstructural proteins encoded by viruses of the Bunyamwera serogroup (family Bunyaviridae). *Virology* 1985;143(1):119–126.
106. Elliott RM. Nucleotide sequence analysis of the large (L) genomic RNA segment of Bunyamwera virus, the prototype of the family Bunyaviridae. *Virology* 1989;173(2):426–436.
107. Elliott RM, Bouloy M, Calisher CH. Family Bunyaviridae. In: van Regenmortel MHV, Fauquest CM, Bishop DHL, eds. *Virus Taxonomy: Classification and Nomenclature of Viruses. Seventh report of the International Committee on Taxonomy of Viruses*. San Diego: Academic Press; 2000.
108. Elliott RM, Dunn E, Simons JF, et al. Nucleotide sequence and coding strategy of the Uukuniemi virus L RNA segment. *J Gen Virol* 1992;73:1745–1752.
109. Elliott RM, McGregor A. Nucleotide sequence and expression of the small (S) RNA segment of Maguari bunyavirus. *Virology* 1989;171(2):516–524.
110. Ellis DS, Shirodaria PV, Fleming E, et al. Morphology and development of Rift Valley Fever virus in vero cell cultures. *J Med Virol* 1988;24:161–174.
111. Emery VC. Characterization of Punta Toro S mRNA species and identification of an inverted complementary sequence in the intergenic region of Punta Toro Phlebovirus Ambisense S RNA that is involved in mRNA transcription termination. *Virology* 1987;156:1–11.

112. Eshita Y, Ericson B, Romanowski V, et al. Analyses of the mRNA transcription processes of snowshoe hare bunyavirus S and M RNA species. *J Virol* 1985;55(3):681–689.
113. Fazakerley JK, Gonzalez-Scarano F, Strickler J, et al. Organization of the middle RNA segment of snowshoe hare Bunyavirus. *Virology* 1988;167(2):422–432.
114. Fazakerley JK, Ross AM. Computer analysis suggests a role for signal sequences in processing polyproteins of enveloped RNA viruses and as a mechanism of viral fusion. *Virus Genes* 1989;2(3):223–239.
115. Feng JJ, Wickenhagen A, Turnbull ML, et al. Interferon-stimulated gene (ISG)-expression screening reveals the specific antibunyaviral activity of ISG20. *J Virol* 2018;92(13).
116. Feng ZK, Xue F, Xu M, et al. The ER-membrane transport system is critical for intercellular trafficking of the NSm movement protein and tomato spotted wilt Tospovirus. *PLoS Pathog* 2016;12(2):e1005443.
117. Fernandez-Garcia Y, Reguera J, Busch C, et al. Atomic structure and biochemical characterization of an RNA endonuclease in the N terminus of Andes virus L protein. *PLoS Pathog* 2016;12(6):e1005635.
118. Ferron F, Li ZL, Danek EI, et al. The hexamer structure of the Rift Valley Fever Virus nucleoprotein suggests a mechanism for its assembly into ribonucleoprotein complexes. *PLoS Pathog* 2011;7(5):e1002030.
119. Filone CM, Heise M, Doms RW, et al. Development and characterization of a Rift Valley fever virus cell-cell fusion assay using alphavirus replicon vectors. *Virology* 2006;356(1–2):155–164.
120. Flick R, Elgh F, Pettersson RF. Mutational analysis of the Uukuniemi virus (Bunyaviridae family) promoter reveals two elements of functional importance. *J Virol* 2002;76(21):10849–10860.
121. Fontana J, Lopez-Montero N, Elliott RM, et al. The unique architecture of Bunyamwera virus factories around the Golgi complex. *Cell Microbiol* 2008;10(10):2012–2028.
122. Freiberg AN, Sherman MB, Morais MC, et al. Three-dimensional organization of Rift Valley Fever Virus revealed by cryoelectron tomography. *J Virol* 2008;82(21):10341–10348.
123. Frese M, Kochs G, Feldmann H, et al. Inhibition of bunyaviruses, phleboviruses, and hantaviruses by human MxA protein. *J Virol* 1996;70(2):915–923.
124. Frese M, Prins M, Ponten A, et al. Constitutive expression of interferon-induced human MxA protein in transgenic tobacco plants does not confer resistance to a variety of RNA viruses. *Transgenic Res* 2000;9(6):429–438.
125. Frias-Staheli N, Giannakopoulos NV, Kikkert M, et al. Ovarian tumor domain-containing viral proteases evade ubiquitin- and ISG15-dependent innate immune responses. *Cell Host Microbe* 2007;2(6):404–416.
126. Gahmberg N, Kuismanen E, Keranen S, et al. Uukuniemi virus glycoproteins accumulate in and cause morphological changes of the golgi complex in the absence of virus maturation. *J Virol* 1986;57(3):899–906.
127. Gallie DR. The cap and poly(A) tail function synergistically to regulate mRNA translational efficiency. *Genes Dev* 1991;5(11):2108–2116.
128. Garcia S, Billecocq A, Crance JM, et al. Nairovirus RNA sequences expressed by a Semliki Forest virus replicon induce RNA interference in tick cells. *J Virol* 2005;79(14):8942–8947.
129. Garcin D, Lezzi M, Dobbs M, et al. The 5′ ends of Hantaan virus (Bunyaviridae) RNAs suggest a prime-and-realign mechanism for the initiation of RNA synthesis. *J Virol* 1995;69(9):5754–5762.
130. Garrison AR, Radoshitzky SR, Kota KP, et al. Crimean-Congo hemorrhagic fever virus utilizes a clathrin- and early endosome-dependent entry pathway. *Virology* 2013;444(1–2):45–54.
131. Garry CE, Garry RF. Proteomics computational analyses suggest that the carboxyl terminal glycoproteins of Bunyaviruses are class II viral fusion protein (beta-penetrenes). *Theor Biol Med Model* 2004;1(1):10.
132. Gauci PJ, McAllister J, Mitchell IR, et al. Genomic characterisation of three Mapputta group viruses, a serogroup of Australian and Papua New Guinean bunyaviruses associated with human disease. *PLoS One* 2015;10(1):e0116561.
133. Gavrilovskaya IN, Brown EJ, Ginsberg MH, et al. Cellular entry of hantaviruses which cause hemorrhagic fever with renal syndrome is mediated by beta3 integrins. *J Virol* 1999;73(5):3951–3959.
134. Gavrilovskaya IN, Peresleni T, Geimonen E, et al. Pathogenic hantaviruses selectively inhibit beta3 integrin directed endothelial cell migration. *Arch Virol* 2002;147(10):1913–1931.
135. Geimonen E, Fernandez I, Gavrilovskaya IN, et al. Tyrosine residues direct the ubiquitination and degradation of the NY-1 hantavirus G1 cytoplasmic tail. *J Virol* 2003;77(20):10760–10868.
136. Geimonen E, LaMonica R, Springer K, et al. Hantavirus pulmonary syndrome-associated hantaviruses contain conserved and functional ITAM signaling elements. *J Virol* 2003;77(2):1638–1643.
137. Geimonen E, Neff S, Raymond T, et al. Pathogenic and nonpathogenic hantaviruses differentially regulate endothelial cell responses. *Proc Natl Acad Sci U S A* 2002; 99(21):13837–13842.
138. Gerlach P, Malet H, Cusack S, et al. Structural insights into Bunyavirus replication and its regulation by the vRNA promoter. *Cell* 2015;161(6):1267–1279.
139. Gerrard SR, Bird BH, Albarino CG, et al. The NSm proteins of Rift Valley fever virus are dispensable for maturation, replication and infection. *Virology* 2007;359(2):459–465.
140. Gerrard SR, Nichol ST. Characterization of the Golgi retention motif of Rift Valley fever virus G(N) glycoprotein. *J Virol* 2002;76(23):12200–12210.
141. Gerrard SR, Rollin PE, Nichol ST. Bidirectional infection and release of Rift Valley fever virus in polarized epithelial cells. *Virology* 2002;301(2):226–235.
142. Gilbertson RL, Batuman O, Webster CG, et al. Role of the insect supervectors *Bemisia tabaci* and *Frankliniella occidentalis* in the emergence and global spread of plant viruses. *Annu Rev Virol* 2015;2(1):67–93.
143. Giorgi C, Accardi L, Nicoletti L, et al. Sequences and coding strategies of the S RNAs of Toscana and Rift Valley fever viruses compared to those of Punta Toro, Sicilian Sandfly fever, and Uukuniemi viruses. *Virology* 1991;180(2):738–753.
144. Gonzalez-Scarano F, Janssen RS, Najjar JA, et al. An avirulent G1 glycoprotein variant of La Crosse Bunyavirus with defective fusion function. *J Virol* 1985;54(3):757–763.
145. Gonzalez-Scarano F, Pobjecky N, Nathanson N. LaCrosse bunyavirus can mediate pH-dependent fusion from without. *Virology* 1984;132:222–225.
146. Gori Savellini G, Weber F, Terrosi C, et al. Toscana virus induces interferon although its NSs protein reveals antagonistic activity. *J Gen Virol* 2011;92(Pt 1):71–79.
147. Gori-Savellini G, Valentini M, Cusi MG. Toscana virus NSs protein inhibits the induction of type I interferon by interacting with RIG-I. *J Virol* 2013;87(12):6660–6667.
148. Gro MC, Di Bonito P, Accardi L, et al. Analysis of 3′ and 5′ ends of N and NSs messenger RNAs of Toscana Phlebovirus. *Virology* 1992;191(1):435–438.
149. Gro MC, Di Bonito P, Fortini D, et al. Completion of molecular characterization of Toscana phlebovirus genome: nucleotide sequence, coding strategy of M genomic segment and its amino acid sequence comparison to other phleboviruses. *Virus Res* 1997;51(1):81–91.
150. Groseth A, Mampilli V, Weisend C, et al. Molecular characterization of human pathogenic bunyaviruses of the Nyando and Bwamba/Pongola virus groups leads to the genetic identification of Mojui dos Campos and Kaeng Khoi virus. *PLoS Negl Trop Dis* 2014;8(9):e3147.
151. Gu SH, Kumar M, Sikorska B, et al. Isolation and partial characterization of a highly divergent lineage of hantavirus from the European mole (Talpa europaea). *Sci Rep* 2016;6:21119.
152. Guardado-Calvo P, Atkovska K, Jeffers SA, et al. A glycerophospholipid-specific pocket in the RVFV class II fusion protein drives target membrane insertion. *Science* 2017;358(6363):663–667.
153. Guardado-Calvo P, Bignon EA, Stettner E, et al. Mechanistic insight into Bunyavirus-induced membrane fusion from structure-function analyses of the Hantavirus envelope glycoprotein Gc. *PLoS Pathog* 2016;12(10):e1005813.
154. Guo Y, Liu B, Ding Z, et al. Distinct mechanism for the formation of the ribonucleoprotein complex of tomato spotted wilt virus. *J Virol* 2017;91(23).
155. Guo Y, Wang WM, Ji W, et al. Crimean-Congo hemorrhagic fever virus nucleoprotein reveals endonuclease activity in bunyaviruses. *Proc Natl Acad Sci U S A* 2012;109(13): 5046–5051.
156. Guo Y, Wang WM, Sun Y, et al. Crystal structure of the core region of Hantavirus nucleocapsid protein reveals the mechanism for ribonucleoprotein complex formation. *J Virol* 2016;90(2):1048–1061.
157. Habjan M, Andersson I, Klingstrom J, et al. Processing of genome 5′ termini as a strategy of negative-strand RNA viruses to avoid RIG-I-dependent interferon induction. *PLoS One* 2008;3(4):e2032.
158. Habjan M, Penski N, Wagner V, et al. Efficient production of Rift Valley fever virus-like particles: the antiviral protein MxA can inhibit primary transcription of bunyaviruses. *Virology* 2009;385(2):400–408.
159. Habjan M, Pichlmair A, Elliott RM, et al. NSs protein of rift valley fever virus induces the specific degradation of the double-stranded RNA-dependent protein kinase. *J Virol* 2009;83(9):4365–4375.
160. Hacker JK, Volkman LE, Hardy JL. Requirement for the G1 protein of California encephalitis virus in infection in vitro and in vivo. *Virology* 1995;206(2):945–953.
161. Haferkamp S, Fernando L, Schwarz TF, et al. Intracellular localization of Crimean-Congo hemorrhagic fever (CCHF) virus glycoproteins. *Virol J* 2005;2(1):42.
162. Halldorsson S, Behrens AJ, Harlos K, et al. Structure of a phleboviral envelope glycoprotein reveals a consolidated model of membrane fusion. *Proc Natl Acad Sci U S A* 2016;113(26):7154–7159.
163. Halldorsson S, Li S, Li M, et al. Shielding and activation of a viral membrane fusion protein. *Nat Commun* 2018;9(1):349.
164. Haller O, Arnheiter H, Pavlovic J, et al. The discovery of the antiviral resistance gene Mx: a story of great ideas, great failures, and some success. *Annu Rev Virol* 2018;5(1):33–51.
165. Haque A, Mir MA. Interaction of hantavirus nucleocapsid protein with ribosomal protein S19. *J Virol* 2010;84(23):12450–12453.
166. Hardestam J, Klingstrom J, Mattsson K, et al. HFRS causing hantaviruses do not induce apoptosis in confluent Vero E6 and A-549 cells. *J Med Virol* 2005;76(2):234–240.
167. Harmon B, Schudel BR, Maar D, et al. Rift Valley Fever virus strain MP-12 enters mammalian host cells via caveola-mediated endocytosis. *J Virol* 2012;86(23):12954–12970.
168. Hassani-Mehraban A, Botermans M, Verhoeven JT, et al. A distinct tospovirus causing necrotic streak on Alstroemeria sp. in Colombia. *Arch Virol* 2010;155(3):423–428.
169. Hefti HP, Frese M, Landis H, et al. Human MxA protein protects mice lacking a functional alpha/beta interferon system against La crosse virus and other lethal viral infections. *J Virol* 1999;73(8):6984–6991.
170. Hepojoki J, Strandin T, Lankinen H, et al. Hantavirus structure—molecular interactions behind the scene. *J Gen Virol* 2012;93(Pt 8):1631–1644.
171. Hertig M, Sabin A. Sandfly fever (pappataci, phlebotomus, three-day fever) I. History of incidence, prevention and control. In: Coates J, Hoff E, Hoff P, eds. *Preventive Medicine in World War II.* Washington, DC: Office of the Surgeon General; 1964:109–174.
172. Hewlett MJ, Pettersson RF, Baltimore D. Circular forms of Uukuniemi virion RNA: an electron microscopic study. *J Virol* 1977;21(3):1085–1093.
173. Hiscott J, Pitha P, Genin P, et al. Triggering the interferon response: the role of IRF-3 transcription factor. *J Interferon Cytokine Res* 1999;19(1):1–13.
174. Hofmann H, Li XX, Zhang XA, et al. Severe fever with thrombocytopenia virus glycoproteins are targeted by neutralizing antibodies and can use DC-SIGN as a receptor for pH-dependent entry into human and animal cell lines. *J Virol* 2013;87(8):4384–4394.
175. Hollidge BS, Nedelsky NB, Salzano MV, et al. Orthobunyavirus entry into neurons and other mammalian cells occurs via Clathrin-mediated endocytosis and requires trafficking into early endosomes. *J Virol* 2012;86(15):7988–8001.
176. Holm T, Kopicki JD, Busch C, et al. Biochemical and structural studies reveal differences and commonalities among cap-snatching endonucleases from segmented negative-strand RNA viruses. *J Biol Chem* 2018;293(51):19686–19698.
177. Honig JE, Osborne JC, Nichol ST. Crimean-Congo hemorrhagic fever virus genome L RNA segment and encoded protein. *Virology* 2004;321(1):29–35.
178. Hopkins KC, McLane LM, Maqbool T, et al. A genome-wide RNAi screen reveals that mRNA decapping restricts bunyaviral replication by limiting the pools of Dcp2-accessible targets for cap-snatching. *Genes Dev* 2013;27(13):1511–1525.
179. Hover S, King B, Hall B, et al. Modulation of potassium channels inhibits Bunyavirus infection. *J Biol Chem* 2016;291(7):3411–3422.
180. Huiskonen JT, Hepojoki J, Laurinmaki P, et al. Electron cryotomography of Tula hantavirus suggests a unique assembly paradigm for enveloped viruses. *J Virol* 2010;84(10):4889–4897.
181. Huiskonen JT, Overby AK, Weber F, et al. Electron cryo-microscopy and single-particle averaging of Rift Valley fever virus: evidence for GN-GC glycoprotein heterodimers. *J Virol* 2009;83(8):3762–3769.

182. Hutchinson KL, Peters CJ, Nichol ST. Sin Nombre virus mRNA synthesis. *Virology* 1996;224(1):139–149.
183. Ihara T, Akashi H, Bishop DH. Novel coding strategy (ambisense genomic RNA) revealed by sequence analyses of Punta Toro Phlebovirus S RNA. *Virology* 1984;136(2):293–306.
184. Ihara T, Dalrymple JM, Bishop DHL. Complete sequences of the glycoprotein and M RNA of Punta Toro phlebovirus compared to those of Rift Valley fever virus. *Virology* 1985;144:246–259.
185. Ihara T, Matsuura Y, Bishop DH. Analyses of the mRNA transcription processes of Punta Toro phlebovirus (Bunyaviridae). *Virology* 1985;147(2):317–325.
186. Ikegami T, Narayanan K, Won S, et al. Rift Valley fever virus NSs protein promotes post-transcriptional downregulation of protein kinase PKR and inhibits eIF2alpha phosphorylation. *PLoS Pathog* 2009;5(2):e1000287.
187. Ikegami T, Won S, Peters CJ, et al. Rift Valley fever virus NSs mRNA is transcribed from an incoming anti-viral-sense S RNA segment. *J Virol* 2005;79(18):12106–12111.
188. Ikegami T, Won S, Peters CJ, et al. Characterization of rift valley fever virus transcriptional terminations. *J Virol* 2007;81(16):8421–8438.
189. Jaaskelainen KM, Kaukinen P, Minskaya ES, et al. Tula and Puumala hantavirus NSs ORFs are functional and the products inhibit activation of the interferon-beta promoter. *J Med Virol* 2007;79(10):1527–1536.
190. Jaaskelainen KM, Plyusnina A, Lundkvist A, et al. Tula hantavirus isolate with the full-length ORF for nonstructural protein NSs survives for more consequent passages in interferon-competent cells than the isolate having truncated NSs ORF. *Virol J* 2008;5:3.
191. Jacoby D, Cooke C, Prabakaran I, et al. Expression of the La Crosse M segment proteins in a recombinant vaccinia expression system mediates pH-dependent cellular fusion. *Virology* 1993;193:993–996.
192. James TW, Frias-Staheli N, Bacik JP, et al. Structural basis for the removal of ubiquitin and interferon-stimulated gene 15 by a viral ovarian tumor domain-containing protease. *Proc Natl Acad Sci U S A* 2011;108(6):2222–2227.
193. Jangra RK, Herbert AS, Li R, et al. Protocadherin-1 is essential for cell entry by New World hantaviruses. *Nature* 2018;563(7732):559.
194. Jantti J, Hilden P, Ronka H, et al. Immunocytochemical analysis of Uukuniemi virus budding compartments: role of the intermediate compartment and the Golgi stack in virus maturation. *J Virol* 1997;71(2):1162–1172.
195. Jeeva S, Cheng ED, Ganaie SS, et al. Crimean-Congo hemorrhagic fever virus nucleocapsid protein augments mRNA translation. *J Virol* 2017;91(15).
196. Jin H, Elliott RM. Mutagenesis of the L protein encoded by Bunyamwera virus and production of monospecific antibodies. *J Gen Virol* 1992;73(Pt 9):2235–2244.
197. Jin H, Elliott RM. Non-viral sequences at the 5′ ends of Dugbe nairovirus S mRNAs. *J Gen Virol* 1993;74:2293–2297.
198. Jin H, Elliott RM. Characterization of Bunyamwera virus S RNA that is transcribed and replicated by the L protein expressed from recombinant vaccinia virus. *J Virol* 1993;67(3):1396–1404.
199. Jin M, Park J, Lee S, et al. Hantaan virus enters cells by clathrin-dependent receptor-mediated endocytosis. *Virology* 2002;294(1):60–69.
200. Kainulainen M, Habjan M, Hubel P, et al. Virulence factor NSs of rift valley fever virus recruits the F-box protein FBXO3 to degrade subunit p62 of general transcription factor TFIIH. *J Virol* 2014;88(6):3464–3473.
201. Kanerva M, Melen K, Vaheri A, et al. Inhibition of puumala and tula hantaviruses in Vero cells by MxA protein. *Virology* 1996;224(1):55–62.
202. Kang HJ, Bennett SN, Sumibcay L, et al. Evolutionary insights from a genetically divergent hantavirus harbored by the European common mole (Talpa europaea). *PLoS One* 2009;4(7):e6149.
203. Kang JI, Park SH, Lee PW, et al. Apoptosis is induced by hantaviruses in cultured cells. *Virology* 1999;264(1):99–105.
204. Kariwa H, Tanabe H, Mizutani T, et al. Synthesis of Seoul virus RNA and structural proteins in cultured cells. *Arch Virol* 2003;148(9):1671–1685.
205. Karlberg H, Tan YJ, Mirazimi A. Induction of caspase activation and cleavage of the viral nucleocapsid protein in different cell types during Crimean-Congo hemorrhagic fever virus infection. *J Biol Chem* 2011;286(5):3227–3234.
206. Karlberg H, Tan YJ, Mirazimi A. Crimean-Congo haemorrhagic fever replication interplays with regulation mechanisms of apoptosis. *J Gen Virol* 2015;96(Pt 3):538–546.
207. Kato H, Oh SW, Fujita T. RIG-I-Like Receptors and Type I Interferonopathies. *J Interferon Cytokine Res* 2017;37(5):207–213.
208. Kaukinen P, Vaheri A, Plyusnin A. Non-covalent interaction between nucleocapsid protein of Tula hantavirus and small ubiquitin-related modifier-1, SUMO-1. *Virus Res* 2003;92(1):37–45.
209. Keegan K, Collett MS. Use of bacterial expression cloning to define the amino acid sequencins of antigenic dterminants on the G2 glycoprotein of Rift Valley fever Virus. *J Virol* 1986;58:263–270.
210. Khaiboullina SF, Morzunov SP, Boichuk SV, et al. Death-domain associated protein-6 (DAXX) mediated apoptosis in hantavirus infection is counter-balanced by activation of interferon-stimulated nuclear transcription factors. *Virology* 2013;443(2):338–348.
211. Khaiboullina SF, Rizvanov AA, Deyde VM, et al. Andes virus stimulates interferon-inducible MxA protein expression in endothelial cells. *J Med Virol* 2005;75(2):267–275.
212. Khaiboullina SF, St Jeor SC. Hantavirus immunology. *Viral Immunol* 2002;15(4):609–625.
213. Khan AS, Khabbaz RF, Armstrong LR, et al. Hantavirus pulmonary syndrome: the first 100 us cases. *J Infect Dis* 1996;173(6):1297–1303.
214. Kiening M, Weber F, Frishman D. Conserved RNA structures in the intergenic regions of ambisense viruses. *Sci Rep* 2017;7.
215. Kikkert M, Van Lent J, Storms M, et al. Tomato spotted wilt virus particle morphogenesis in plant cells. *J Virol* 1999;73(3):2288–2297.
216. Kingsford L, Ishizawa LD, Hill DW. Biological activities of monoclonal antibodies reactive with antigenic sites mapped on the G1 glycoprotein of La Crosse virus. *Virology* 1983;90:443–455.
217. Kinsella E, Martin SG, Grolla A, et al. Sequence determination of the Crimean-Congo hemorrhagic fever virus L segment. *Virology* 2004;321(1):23–28.
218. Kleinfelter LM, Jangra RK, Jae LT, et al. Haploid genetic screen reveals a profound and direct dependence on cholesterol for Hantavirus membrane fusion. *MBio* 2015;6(4):e00801.
219. Klemm C, Reguera J, Cusack S, et al. Systems to establish Bunyavirus genome replication in the absence of transcription. *J Virol* 2013;87(14):8205–8212.
220. Klempa B. Reassortment events in the evolution of hantaviruses. *Virus Genes* 2018; 54(5):638–646.
221. Klute MJ, Melancon P, Dacks JB. Evolution and diversity of the Golgi. *Cold Spring Harb Perspect Biol* 2011;3(8):a007849.
222. Kochs G, Janzen C, Hohenberg H, et al. Antivirally active MxA protein sequesters La Crosse virus nucleocapsid protein into perinuclear complexes. *Proc Natl Acad Sci U S A* 2002;99(5):3153–3158.
223. Kohl A, Dunn EF, Lowen AC, et al. Complementarity, sequence and structural elements within the 3′ and 5′ non-coding regions of the Bunyamwera orthobunyavirus S segment determine promoter strength. *J Gen Virol* 2004;85(Pt 11):3269–3278.
224. Kohl A, Hart TJ, Noonan C, et al. A bunyamwera virus minireplicon system in mosquito cells. *J Virol* 2004;78(11):5679–5685.
225. Kohl A, Lowen AC, Leonard VH, et al. Genetic elements regulating packaging of the Bunyamwera orthobunyavirus genome. *J Gen Virol* 2006;87(Pt 1):177–187.
226. Komoda K, Narita M, Yamashita K, et al. Asymmetric trimeric ring structure of the nucleocapsid protein of Tospovirus. *J Virol* 2017;91(20).
227. Kormelink R, de Haan P, Meurs C, et al. The nucleotide sequence of the M RNA segment of tomato spotted wilt virus, a bunyavirus with two ambisense RNA segments. *J Gen Virol* 1992;73:2795–2804.
228. Kormelink R, de Haan P, Peters D, et al. Viral RNA synthesis in tomato spotted wilt virus-infected Nicotiana rustica plants. *J Gen Virol* 1992;73(Pt 3):687–693.
229. Kormelink R, Kitajima EW, De Haan P, et al. The nonstructural protein (NSs) encoded by the ambisense S RNA segment of tomato spotted wilt virus is associated with fibrous structures in infected plant cells. *Virology* 1991;181(2):459–468.
230. Kormelink R, Storms M, Van Lent J, et al. Expression and subcellular location of the NSM protein of tomato spotted wilt virus (TSWV), a putative viral movement protein. *Virology* 1994;200(1):56–65.
231. Kraus AA, Raftery MJ, Giese T, et al. Differential antiviral response of endothelial cells after infection with pathogenic and nonpathogenic hantaviruses. *J Virol* 2004;78(12):6143–6150.
232. Krautkramer E, Zeier M. Hantavirus causing hemorrhagic fever with renal syndrome enters from the apical surface and requires decay-accelerating factor (DAF/CD55). *J Virol* 2008;82(9):4257–4264.
233. Kuismanen E. Posttranslational processing of uukuniemi virus glycoproteins G1 and G2. *J Virol* 1984;51:806–812.
234. Kukkonen SK, Vaheri A, Plyusnin A. Tula hantavirus L protein is a 250 kDa perinuclear membrane-associated protein. *J Gen Virol* 2004;85(Pt 5):1181–1189.
235. Kukkonen SK, Vaheri A, Plyusnin A. L protein, the RNA-dependent RNA polymerase of hantaviruses. *Arch Virol* 2005;150(3):533–556.
236. Laenen L, Vergote V, Nauwelaers I, et al. Complete genome sequence of Nova virus, a hantavirus circulating in the European mole in Belgium. *Genome Announc* 2015;3(4).
237. Lanciotti RS, Kosoy OI, Bosco-Lauth AM, et al. Isolation of a novel orthobunyavirus (Brazoran virus) with a 1.7 kb S segment that encodes a unique nucleocapsid protein possessing two putative functional domains. *Virology* 2013;444(1–2):55–63.
238. Lappin DF, Nakitare GW, Palfreyman JW, et al. Localization of Bunyamwera bunyavirus G1 glycoprotein to the Golgi requires association with G2 but not with NSm. *J Gen Virol* 1994;75(Pt 12):3441–3451.
239. Lara E, Billecocq A, Leger P, et al. Characterization of wild-type and alternate transcription termination signals in the Rift Valley Fever virus genome. *J Virol* 2011; 85(23):12134–12145.
240. Law MD, Speck J, Moyer JW. The M RNA of impatiens necrotic spot Tospovirus (Bunyaviridae) has an ambisense genomic organization. *Virology* 1992;188(2):732–741.
241. Le May N, Dubaele S, Proietti De Santis L, et al. TFIIH transcription factor, a target for the Rift Valley hemorrhagic fever virus. *Cell* 2004;116(4):541–550.
242. Le May N, Mansuroglu Z, Leger P, et al. A SAP30 complex inhibits IFN-beta expression in Rift Valley fever virus infected cells. *PLoS Pathog* 2008;4(1):e13.
243. LeDuc JW, Smith GA, Childs JE, et al. Global survey of antibody to Hantaan-related viruses among peridomestic rodents. *Bull World Health Organ* 1986;64(1):139–144.
244. Lee HW, French GR, Lee PW, et al. Observation on natural and laboratory infection of rodents with the etiologic agent of Korean hemorrhagic fever. *Am J Trop Med Hyg* 1981;30(2):477–482.
245. Lee HW, van der Groen G. Hemorrhagic fever with renal syndrome. *Prog Med Virol* 1989;36(6):62–102.
246. Lee BH, Yoshimatsu K, Maeda A, et al. Association of the nucleocapsid protein of the Seoul and Hantaan hantaviruses with small ubiquitin-like modifier-1-related molecules. *Virus Res* 2003;98(1):83–91.
247. Lees JF, Pringle CR, Elliot RM. Nucleotide sequence of the Bunyamwera virus M RNA segment: conservation of structural features in the Bunyavirus glycoprotein gene product. *Virology* 1986;148:1–14.
248. Leger P, Tetard M, Youness B, et al. Differential use of the C-type lectins L-SIGN and DC-SIGN for Phlebovirus endocytosis. *Traffic* 2016;17(6):639–656.
249. Leonard VH, Kohl A, Hart TJ, et al. Interaction of Bunyamwera orthobunyavirus NSs protein with mediator protein MED8: a mechanism for inhibiting the interferon response. *J Virol* 2006;80(19):9667–9675.
250. Levine JR, Prescott J, Brown KS, et al. Antagonism of type I interferon responses by new world hantaviruses. *J Virol* 2010;84(22):11790–11801.
251. Lewandowski DJ, Adkins S. The tubule-forming NSm protein from Tomato spotted wilt virus complements cell-to-cell and long-distance movement of Tobacco mosaic virus hybrids. *Virology* 2005;342(1):26–37.
252. Li XD, Kukkonen S, Vapalahti O, et al. Tula hantavirus infection of Vero E6 cells induces apoptosis involving caspase 8 activation. *J Gen Virol* 2004;85(Pt 11):3261–3268.
253. Li XD, Lankinen H, Putkuri N, et al. Tula hantavirus triggers pro-apoptotic signals of ER stress in Vero E6 cells. *Virology* 2005;333(1):180–189.
254. Li W, Lewandowski DJ, Hilf ME, et al. Identification of domains of the Tomato spotted wilt virus NSm protein involved in tubule formation, movement and symptomatology. *Virology* 2009;390(1):110–121.

255. Li XD, Makela TP, Guo D, et al. Hantavirus nucleocapsid protein interacts with the Fas-mediated apoptosis enhancer Daxx. *J Gen Virol* 2002;83(Pt 4):759–766.

256. Li S, Rissanen I, Zeltina A, et al. A Molecular-level account of the antigenic Hantaviral surface. *Cell Rep* 2016;15(5):959–967.

257. Li CX, Shi M, Tian JH, et al. Unprecedented genomic diversity of RNA viruses in arthropods reveals the ancestry of negative-sense RNA viruses. *Elife* 2015;4.

258. Li BB, Wang Q, Pan XJ, et al. Bunyamwera virus possesses a distinct nucleocapsid protein to facilitate genome encapsidation. *Proc Natl Acad Sci U S A* 2013;110(22):9048–9053.

259. Lihoradova OA, Indran SV, Kalveram B, et al. Characterization of Rift Valley fever virus MP-12 strain encoding NSs of Punta Toro virus or sandfly fever Sicilian virus. *PLoS Negl Trop Dis* 2013;7(4):e2181.

260. Liu R, Zhang G, Yang Y, et al. Genome sequence of abbey lake virus, a novel orthobunyavirus isolated from china. *Genome Announc* 2014;2(3).

261. Lober C, Anheier B, Lindow S, et al. The Hantaan virus glycoprotein precursor is cleaved at the conserved pentapeptide WAASA. *Virology* 2001;289(2):224–229.

262. Lopez N, Muller R, Prehaud C, et al. The L protein of Rift Valley fever virus can rescue viral ribonucleoproteins and transcribe synthetic genome-like RNA molecules. *J Virol* 1995;69(7):3972–3979.

263. Lowen AC, Elliott RM. Mutational analyses of the nonconserved sequences in the Bunyamwera orthobunyavirus S segment untranslated regions. *J Virol* 2005;79(20):12861–12870.

264. Lozach PY, Huotari J, Helenius A. Late-penetrating viruses. *Curr Opin Virol* 2011;1(1):35–43.

265. Lozach PY, Kuhbacher A, Meier R, et al. DC-SIGN as a Receptor for Phleboviruses. *Cell Host Microbe* 2011;10(1):75–88.

266. Lozach PY, Mancini R, Bitto D, et al. Entry of bunyaviruses into mammalian cells. *Cell Host Microbe* 2010;7(6):488–499.

267. Ludwig GV, Christensen BM, Yuill TM, et al. Enzyme processing of La Crosse virus glycoprotein G1: a bunyavirus-vector infection model. *Virology* 1989;171(1):108–113.

268. Ly HJ, Ikegami T. Rift Valley fever virus NSs protein functions and the similarity to other bunyavirus NSs proteins. *Virol J* 2016;13:118.

269. Madoff DH, Lenard J. A membrane glycoprotein that accumulates intracellularly: cellular processing of the large glycoprotein of LaCrosse virus. *Cell* 1982;28(4):821–829.

270. Maeda A, Lee BH, Yoshimatsu K, et al. The intracellular association of the nucleocapsid protein (NP) of hantaan virus (HTNV) with small ubiquitin-like modifier-1 (SUMO-1) conjugating enzyme 9 (Ubc9). *Virology* 2003;305(2):288–297.

271. Maes P, Adkins S, Alkhovsky SV, et al. Taxonomy of the order Bunyavirales: second update 2018. *Arch Virol* 2019;164(3):927–941.

272. Makarova KS, Aravind L, Koonin EV. A novel superfamily of predicted cysteine proteases from eukaryotes, viruses and Chlamydia pneumoniae. *Trends Biochem Sci* 2000;25(2):50–52.

273. Markotic A, Hensley L, Geisbert T, et al. Hantaviruses induce cytopathic effects and apoptosis in continuous human embryonic kidney cells. *J Gen Virol* 2003;84(Pt 8):2197–2202.

274. Marriott AC, el-Ghorr AA, Nuttall PA. Dugbe Nairovirus M RNA: nucleotide sequence and coding strategy. *Virology* 1992;190(2):606–615.

275. Marriott AC, Nuttall PA. Comparison of the S RNA segments and nucleoprotein sequences of Crimean-Congo hemorrhagic fever, Hazara, and Dugbe viruses. *Virology* 1992;189(2):795–799.

276. Matsuno K, Kajihara M, Nakao R, et al. The unique phylogenetic position of a novel Tick-Borne Phlebovirus ensures an ixodid origin of the genus Phlebovirus. *mSphere* 2018;3(3).

277. Matsuno K, Weisend C, Kajihara M, et al. Comprehensive molecular detection of tick-borne phleboviruses leads to the retrospective identification of taxonomically unassigned bunyaviruses and the discovery of a novel member of the genus phlebovirus. *J Virol* 2015;89(1):594–604.

278. Matsuoka Y, Chen SY, Compans RW. A signal for Golgi retention in the bunyavirus G1 glycoprotein. *J Biol Chem* 1994;269(36):22565–22573.

279. Matsuoka Y, Ihara T, Bishop DH, et al. Intracellular accumulation of Punta Toro virus glycoproteins expressed from cloned cDNA. *Virology* 1988;167(1):251–260.

280. Matthys V, Gorbunova EE, Gavrilovskaya IN, et al. The C-terminal 42 residues of the Tula virus Gn protein regulate interferon induction. *J Virol* 2011;85(10):4752–4760.

281. McMullan LK, Folk SM, Kelly AJ, et al. A new phlebovirus associated with severe febrile illness in Missouri. *N Engl J Med* 2012;367(9):834–841.

282. Meyer BJ, Schmaljohn CS. Persistent hantavirus infections: characteristics and mechanisms. *Trends Microbiol* 2000;8(2):61–67.

283. Milholland MT, Castro-Arellano I, Suzan G, et al. Global Diversity and Distribution of Hantaviruses and Their Hosts. *Ecohealth* 2018;15(1):163–208.

284. Milne RG, Francki RI. Should tomato spotted wilt virus be considered as a possible member of the family Bunyaviridae? *Intervirology* 1984;22(2):72–76.

285. Mir MA, Panganiban AT. The bunyavirus nucleocapsid protein is an RNA chaperone: possible roles in viral RNA panhandle formation and genome replication. *RNA* 2006;12(2):272–282.

286. Miura TA, Carlson JO, Beaty BJ, et al. Expression of human MxA protein in mosquito cells interferes with LaCrosse virus replication. *J Virol* 2001;75(6):3001–3003.

287. Mohamed M, McLees A, Elliott RM. Viruses in the Anopheles A, Anopheles B, and Tete serogroups in the Orthobunyavirus genus (family Bunyaviridae) do not encode an NSs protein. *J Virol* 2009;83(15):7612–7618.

288. Mohl BP, Barr JN. Investigating the specificity and stoichiometry of RNA binding by the nucleocapsid protein of Bunyamwera virus. *RNA* 2009;15(3):391–399.

289. Montgomery R. On a tick-borne gastro-enteritis of sheep and goats occurring in British East Africa. *J Comp Pathol* 1917;30:28–57.

290. Morin B, Coutard B, Lelke M, et al. The N-terminal domain of the Arenavirus L protein is an RNA endonuclease essential in mRNA transcription. *PLoS Pathog* 2010;6(9):e1001038.

291. Mudhasani R, Tran JP, Retterer C, et al. IFITM-2 and IFITM-3 but not IFITM-1 restrict Rift Valley fever virus. *J Virol* 2013;87(15):8451–8464.

292. Muller R, Argentini C, Bouloy M, et al. Completion of the genome sequence of Rift Valley fever phlebovirus indicates that the L RNA is negative sense or ambisense and codes for a putative transcriptase-replicase. *Nucleic Acids Res* 1991;19(19):5433.

293. Muller R, Saluzzo JF, Lopez N, et al. Characterization of clone 13, a naturally attenuated avirulent isolate of Rift Valley fever virus, which is altered in the small segment. *Am J Trop Med Hyg* 1995;53(4):405–411.

294. Murphy FA, Harrison AK, Whitfield SG. Bunyaviridae: morphologic and morphogenetic similarities of Bunyamwera serologic supergroup viruses and several other arthropod-borne viruses. *Intervirology* 1973;1(4):297–316.

295. Nakitare GW, Elliott RM. Expression of the Bunyamwera virus M genome segment and intracellular localization of NSm. *Virology* 1993;195:511–520.

296. Newton SE, Short NJ, Dalgarno L. Bunyamwera virus replication in cultured Aedes albopictus (mosquito) cells: establishment of a persistent viral infection. *J Virol* 1981;38(3):1015–1024.

297. Nichol ST, Spiropoulou CF, Morzunov S, et al. Genetic identification of a novel hantavirus associated with an outbreak of acute respiratory illness in the southwestern United States. *Science* 1993;262:914–917.

298. Niklasson B, Leduc J, Nystrom K, et al. Nephropathia epidemica: incidence of clinical cases and antibody prevalence in an endemic area of Sweden. *Epidemiol Infect* 1987;99(2):559–562.

299. Ning YJ, Wang ML, Deng MP, et al. Viral suppression of innate immunity via spatial isolation of TBK1/IKK epsilon from mitochondrial antiviral platform. *J Mol Cell Biol* 2014;6(4).

300. Niu FF, Shaw N, Wang YE, et al. Structure of the Leanyer orthobunyavirus nucleoprotein-RNA complex reveals unique architecture for RNA encapsidation. *Proc Natl Acad Sci U S A* 2013;110(22):9054–9059.

301. Noda T, Murakami S, Nakatsu S, et al. Importance of the 1+7 configuration of ribonucleoprotein complexes for influenza A virus genome packaging. *Nat Commun* 2018;9(1):54.

302. Noton SL, Fearns R. Initiation and regulation of paramyxovirus transcription and replication. *Virology* 2015;479:545–554.

303. Novoa RR, Calderita G, Cabezas P, et al. Key Golgi factors for structural and functional maturation of bunyamwera virus. *J Virol* 2005;79(17):10852–10863.

304. Nunes MR, Chiang JO, de Lima CP, et al. New genome sequences of gamboa viruses (family bunyaviridae, genus orthobunyavirus) isolated in panama and Argentina. *Genome Announc* 2014;2(6).

305. Nunes MR, Travassos da Rosa AP, Weaver SC, et al. Molecular epidemiology of group C viruses (Bunyaviridae, Orthobunyavirus) isolated in the Americas. *J Virol* 2005;79(16):10561–10570.

306. Nuss JE, Kehn-Hall K, Benedict A, et al. Multi-faceted proteomic characterization of host protein complement of Rift Valley Fever virus virions and identification of specific heat shock proteins, including HSP90, as important viral host factors. *PLoS One* 2014;9(5):e93483.

307. Oelschlegel R, Kruger DH, Rang A. MxA-independent inhibition of Hantaan virus replication induced by type I and type II interferon in vitro. *Virus Res* 2007;127(1):100–105.

308. Ogino M, Yoshimatsu K, Ebihara H, et al. Cell fusion activities of Hantaan virus envelope glycoproteins. *J Virol* 2004;78(19):10776–10782.

309. Ohnishi J, Katsuzaki H, Tsuda S, et al. *Frankliniella cephalica*, a New Vector for Tomato spotted wilt virus. *Plant Dis* 2006;90(5):685.

310. Olal D, Daumke O. Structure of the Hantavirus nucleoprotein provides insights into the mechanism of RNA encapsidation. *Cell Rep* 2016;14(9):2092–2099.

311. Olal D, Dick A, Woods VL, et al. Structural insights into RNA encapsidation and helical assembly of the Toscana virus nucleoprotein. *Nucleic Acids Res* 2014;42(9):6025–6037.

312. Osborne JC, Elliott RM. RNA binding properties of bunyamwera virus nucleocapsid protein and selective binding to an element in the 5′ terminus of the negative-sense S segment. *J Virol* 2000;74(21):9946–9952.

313. Overby AK, Pettersson RF, Grunewald K, et al. Insights into bunyavirus architecture from electron cryotomography of Uukuniemi virus. *Proc Natl Acad Sci U S A* 2008;105(7):2375–2379.

314. Padula PJ, Sanchez AJ, Edelstein A, et al. Complete nucleotide sequence of the M RNA segment of Andes virus and analysis of the variability of the termini of the virus S, M and L RNA segments. *J Gen Virol* 2002;83(Pt 9):2117–2122.

315. Palacios G, da Rosa AT, Savji N, et al. Aguacate virus, a new antigenic complex of the genus Phlebovirus (family Bunyaviridae). *J Gen Virol* 2011;92(Pt 6):1445–1453.

316. Palacios G, Tesh R, Travassos da Rosa A, et al. Characterization of the Candiru antigenic complex (Bunyaviridae: Phlebovirus), a highly diverse and reassorting group of viruses affecting humans in tropical America. *J Virol* 2011;85(8):3811–3820.

317. Papa A. Dobrava-Belgrade virus: phylogeny, epidemiology, disease. *Antiviral Res* 2012;95(2):104–117.

318. Pappu HR, Jones RA, Jain RK. Global status of tospovirus epidemics in diverse cropping systems: successes achieved and challenges ahead. *Virus Res* 2009;141(2):219–236.

319. Park SW, Han MG, Park C, et al. Hantaan virus nucleocapsid protein stimulates MDM2-dependent p53 degradation. *J Gen Virol* 2013;94:2424–2428.

320. Parker MD, Smith JF, Dalrymple JM. Rift Valley fever virus intracellular RNA: a functional analysis. In: Compans R, Bishop D, eds. *Segmented negative strand viruses*. Orlando: Academic Press; 1984:21–28.

321. Parsonson I, McPhee DA. Bunyavirus pathogenesis. *Adv Virus Res* 1985;30:279–316.

322. Patel AH, Elliott RM. Characterization of Bunyamwera virus defective interfering particles. *J Gen Virol* 1992;73:389–396.

323. Patterson JL, Holloway B, Kolakofsky D. La Crosse virions contain a primer-stimulated RNA polymerase and a methylated cap-dependent endonuclease. *J Virol* 1984;52:215–222.

324. Patterson JL, Kolakofsky D. Characterization of La Crosse virus small-genome segment transcripts. *J Virol* 1984;49:680–685.

325. Pattnaik AK, Abraham G. Identification of four complementary RNA species in Akabane virus-infected cells. *J Virol* 1983;47(3):452–462.

326. Pekosz A, Phillips J, Pleasure D, et al. Induction of apoptosis by La Crosse virus infection and role of neuronal differentiation and human bcl-2 expression in its prevention. *J Virol* 1996;70(8):5329–5335.

327. Pennington TH, Pringle CR, McCrae MA. Bunyamwera virus-induced polypeptide synthesis. *J Virol* 1977;24:397–400.

328. Perrone LA, Narayanan K, Worthy M, et al. The S segment of Punta Toro virus (Bunyaviridae, Phlebovirus) is a major determinant of lethality in the Syrian hamster and codes for a type I interferon antagonist. *J Virol* 2007;81(2):884–892.

329. Peters CJ, Liu CT, Anderson GW Jr, et al. Pathogenesis of viral hemorrhagic fevers: Rift Valley fever and Lassa fever contrasted. *Rev Infect Dis* 1989;11(1 Suppl 4):S743-S749.

330. Petersen J, Drake MJ, Bruce EA, et al. The major cellular sterol regulatory pathway is required for Andes virus infection. *PLoS Pathog* 2014;10(2):e1003911.
331. Pettersson RF. Effect of Uukuniemi virus infection on host cell macromolecule synthesis. *Med Biol* 1974;52:90–97.
332. Pettersson RF, Bonsdorf CH. Ribonucleoproteins of Uukuniemi virus are circular. *J Virol* 1975;15:386–392.
333. Pichlmair A, Reis e Sousa C. Innate recognition of viruses. *Immunity* 2007;27(3):370–383.
334. Pichlmair A, Schulz O, Tan CP, et al. Activation of MDA5 requires higher-order RNA structures generated during virus infection. *J Virol* 2009;83(20):10761–10769.
335. Plassmeyer ML, Soldan SS, Stachelek KM, et al. California serogroup Gc (G1) glycoprotein is the principal determinant of pH-dependent cell fusion and entry. *Virology* 2005;338(1):121–132.
336. Plassmeyer ML, Soldan SS, Stachelek KM, et al. Mutagenesis of the La Crosse virus glycoprotein supports a role for Gc (1066-1087) as the fusion peptide. *Virology* 2007; 358(2):273–282.
337. Plyusnin A. Genetics of hantaviruses: implications to taxonomy. *Arch Virol* 2002; 147(4):665–682.
338. Polyak SJ, Zheng S, Harnish DG. 5′ termini of Pichinde arenavirus S RNAs and mRNAs contain nontemplated nucleotides. *J Virol* 1995;69(5):3211–3215.
339. Porterfield JS, Casals J, Chumakov MP, et al. Bunyaviruses and Bunyaviridae. *Intervirology* 1975/76;6:13–24.
340. Prehaud C, Lopez N, Blok MJ, et al. Analysis of the 3′ terminal sequence recognized by the Rift Valley fever virus transcription complex in its ambisense S segment. *Virology* 1997;227(1):189–197.
341. Prescott J, Hall P, Acuna-Retamar M, et al. New World hantaviruses activate IFNlambda production in type I IFN-deficient vero E6 cells. *PLoS One* 2010;5(6):e11159.
342. Prins M, Goldbach R. The emerging problem of tospovirus infection and nonconventional methods of control. *Trends Microbiol* 1998;6(1):31–35.
343. Punch EK, Hover S, Blest HTW, et al. Potassium is a trigger for conformational change in the fusion spike of an enveloped RNA virus. *J Biol Chem* 2018;293(26):9937–9944.
344. Qu BQ, Qi X, Wu XD, et al. Suppression of the Interferon and NF-kappa B responses by severe fever with thrombocytopenia syndrome virus. *J Virol* 2012;86(16):8388–8401.
345. Raftery MJ, Kraus AA, Ulrich R, et al. Hantavirus infection of dendritic cells. *J Virol* 2002;76(21):10724–10733.
346. Raju R, Kolakofsky D. Inhibitors of protein synthesis inhibit both LaCrosse virus S-mRNA and S genome syntheses in vivo. *Virus Res* 1986;5:1–9.
347. Raju R, Kolakofsky D. Translational requirement of La Crosse virus S-mRNA synthesis. *J Virol* 1987;63:122–128.
348. Raju R, Kolakofsky D. The ends of La Crosse virus genome and antigenome RNAs within nucleocapsids are base paired. *J Virol* 1989;63(1):122–128.
349. Raju R, Raju L, Kolakofsky D. The translational requirement for complete La Crosse virus mRNA synthesis is cell-type dependent. *J Virol* 1989;63(12):5159–5165.
350. Ramsden C, Holmes EC, Charleston MA. Hantavirus evolution in relation to its rodent and insectivore hosts: no evidence for codivergence. *Mol Biol Evol* 2009;26(1):143–153.
351. Randall RE, Goodbourn S. Interferons and viruses: an interplay between induction, signalling, antiviral responses and virus countermeasures. *J Gen Virol* 2008;89(Pt 1):1–47.
352. Ravkov EV, Compans RW. Hantavirus nucleocapsid protein is expressed as a membrane-associated protein in the perinuclear region. *J Virol* 2001;75(4):1808–1815.
353. Ravkov EV, Nichol ST, Compans RW. Polarized entry and release in epithelial cells of Black Creek Canal virus, a New World hantavirus. *J Virol* 1997;71(2):1147–1154.
354. Raymond DD, Piper ME, Gerrard SR, et al. Phleboviruses encapsidate their genomes by sequestering RNA bases. *Proc Natl Acad Sci U S A* 2012;109(47):19208–19213.
355. Raymond DD, Piper ME, Gerrard SR, et al. Structure of the Rift Valley fever virus nucleocapsid protein reveals another architecture for RNA encapsidation. *Proc Natl Acad Sci U S A* 2010;107(26):11769–11774.
356. Reguera J, Cusack S, Kolakofsky D. Segmented negative strand RNA virus nucleoprotein structure. *Curr Opin Virol* 2014;5:7–15.
357. Reguera J, Gerlach P, Rosenthal M, et al. Comparative structural and functional analysis of Bunyavirus and Arenavirus cap-snatching endonucleases. *PLoS Pathog* 2016; 12(6):e1005636.
358. Reguera J, Malet H, Weber F, et al. Structural basis for encapsidation of genomic RNA by La Crosse Orthobunyavirus nucleoprotein. *Proc Natl Acad Sci U S A* 2013; 110(18):7246–7251.
359. Reguera J, Weber F, Cusack S. Bunyaviridae RNA polymerases (L-Protein) have an N-terminal, influenza-like endonuclease domain, essential for viral cap-dependent transcription. *PLoS Pathog* 2010;6(9):e1001101.
360. Rehwinkel J, Tan CP, Goubau D, et al. RIG-I detects viral genomic RNA during negative-strand RNA virus infection. *Cell* 2010;140(3):397–408.
361. Reichelt M, Stertz S, Krijnse-Locker J, et al. Missorting of LaCrosse virus nucleocapsid protein by the interferon-induced MxA GTPase involves smooth ER membranes. *Traffic* 2004;5(10):772–784.
362. Resende Rde O, de Haan P, de Avila AC, et al. Generation of envelope and defective interfering RNA mutants of tomato spotted wilt virus by mechanical passage. *J Gen Virol* 1991;72(Pt 10):2375–2383.
363. Rezelj VV, Li P, Chaudhary V, et al. Differential antagonism of human innate immune responses by tick-borne Phlebovirus nonstructural proteins. *mSphere* 2017;2(3).
364. Rissanen I, Stass R, Zeltina A, et al. Structural transitions of the conserved and metastable hantaviral glycoprotein envelope. *J Virol* 2017;91(21).
365. Rodrigues DS, Medeiros DB, Rodrigues SG, et al. Pacui Virus, Rio Preto da Eva Virus, and Tapirape Virus, three distinct viruses within the family Bunyaviridae. *Genome Announc* 2014;2(6).
366. Ronnholm R, Pettersson RF. Complete nucleotide sequence of the M RNA segment of Uukuniemi virus encoding the membrane glycoproteins G1 and G2. *Virology* 1987;160(1):191–202.
367. Rose JK. Positive strands to the rescue again: a segmented negative-strand RNA virus derived from cloned cDNAs. *Proc Natl Acad Sci U S A* 1996;93(26):14998–15000.
368. Rosenthal M, Gogrefe N, Vogel D, et al. Structural insights into reptarenavirus cap-snatching machinery. *PLoS Pathog* 2017;13(5):e1006400.
369. Rossier C, Raju R, Kolakofsky D. LaCrosse virus gene expression in mammalian and mosquito cells. *Virology* 1988;165(2):539–548.
370. Ruigrok RW, Crepin T, Kolakofsky D. Nucleoproteins and nucleocapsids of negative-strand RNA viruses. *Curr Opin Microbiol* 2011;14(4):504–510.
371. Ruusala A, Persson R, Schmaljohn CS, et al. Coexpression of the membrane glycoproteins G1 and G2 of Hantaan virus is required for targeting to the Golgi complex. *Virology* 1992;186(1):53–64.
372. Rwambo PM, Shaw MK, Rurangirwa FR, et al. Ultrastructural studies on the replication and morphogenesis of Nairobi sheep disease virus, a Nairovirus. *Arch Virol* 1996; 141(8):1479–1492.
373. Sabin AB. Experimental studies on Phlebotomus (Pappataci, Sandfly) fever during World War II. *Arch Gesamte Virusforsch* 1951;4:367–410.
374. Saeed MF, Li L, Wang H, et al. Phylogeny of the Simbu serogroup of the genus Bunyavirus. *J Gen Virol* 2001;82(Pt 9):2173–2181.
375. Salanueva IJ, Novoa RR, Cabezas P, et al. Polymorphism and structural maturation of bunyamwera virus in Golgi and post-Golgi compartments. *J Virol* 2003;77(2):1368–1381.
376. Salata C, Monteil V, Karlberg H, et al. The DEVD motif of Crimean-Congo hemorrhagic fever virus nucleoprotein is essential for viral replication in tick cells. *Emerg Microbes Infect* 2018;7:190.
377. Sall AA, de A Zanotto PM, Zeller HG, et al. Variability of the NS(S) protein among Rift Valley fever virus isolates. *J Gen Virol* 1997;78(Pt 11):2853–2858.
378. Sanchez AJ, Vincent MJ, Erickson BR, et al. Crimean-Congo hemorrhagic fever virus glycoprotein precursor is cleaved by Furin-Like and SKI-1 proteases to generate a novel 38-kilodalton glycoprotein. *J Virol* 2006;80(1):514–525.
379. Sanchez AJ, Vincent MJ, Nichol ST. Characterization of the glycoproteins of Crimean-Congo hemorrhagic fever virus. *J Virol* 2002;76(14):7263–7275.
380. Santiago FW, Covaleda LM, Sanchez-Aparicio MT, et al. Hijacking of RIG-I signaling proteins into virus-induced cytoplasmic structures correlates with the inhibition of type I interferon responses. *J Virol* 2014;88(8):4572–4585.
381. Santos RI, Rodrigues AH, Silva ML, et al. Oropouche virus entry into HeLa cells involves clathrin and requires endosomal acidification. *Virus Res* 2008;138(1–2):139–143.
382. Schmaljohn CS. Nucleotide sequence of the L genome segment of Hantaan virus. *Nucleic Acids Res* 1990;18(22):6728.
383. Schmaljohn CS, Dalrymple JM. Biochemical characterization of Hantaan virus. In: Compans RW, Bishop DHL, eds. *Segmented Negative Strand Viruses*. New York: Elsevier; 1984:117–124.
384. Schmaljohn CS, Hasty SE, Rasmussen L, et al. Hantaan virus replication: effects of monensin, tunicamycin and endoglycosidases on the structural glycoproteins. *J Gen Virol* 1986;67:707–717.
385. Schmaljohn CS, Jennings GB, Hay J, et al. Coding strategy of the S genome of Hantaan virus. *Virology* 1986;155:633–643.
386. Schmaljohn CS, Schmaljohn AL, Dalrymple JM. Hantaan virus M RNA: coding strategy, nucleotide sequence, and gene order. *Virology* 1987;157:31–39.
387. Schoen A, Weber F. Orthobunyaviruses and innate immunity induction: alieNSs vs PredatoRRs. *Eur J Cell Biol* 2015;94(7–9):384–390.
388. Scholte FEM, Zivcec M, Dzimianski JV, et al. Crimean-Congo hemorrhagic fever virus suppresses innate immune responses via a ubiquitin and ISG15 specific protease. *Cell Rep* 2017;20(10):2396–2407.
389. Schubert M, Keene JD, Herman RC, et al. Site on the vesicular stomatitis virus genome specifying polyadenylation and the end of the L gene mRNA. *J Virol* 1980;34(2):550–559.
390. Schulz O, Pichlmair A, Rehwinkel J, et al. Protein kinase R contributes to immunity against specific viruses by regulating interferon mRNA integrity. *Cell Host Microbe* 2010;7(5):354–361.
391. Shchetinin AM, Lvov DK, Deriabin PG, et al. Genetic and phylogenetic characterization of Tataguine and Witwatersrand viruses and other Orthobunyaviruses of the Anopheles A, Capim, Guama, Koongol, Mapputta, Tete, and Turlock Serogroups. *Viruses* 2015;7(11):5987–6008.
392. Sherman MB, Freiberg AN, Holbrook MR, et al. Single-particle cryo-electron microscopy of Rift Valley fever virus. *Virology* 2009;387(1):11–15.
393. Shi Y. Mechanisms of caspase activation and inhibition during apoptosis. *Mol Cell* 2002;9(3):459–470.
394. Shi X, Botting CH, Li P, et al. Bunyamwera orthobunyavirus glycoprotein precursor is processed by cellular signal peptidase and signal peptide peptidase. *Proc Natl Acad Sci U S A* 2016;113(31):8825–8830.
395. Shi X, Brauburger K, Elliott RM. Role of N-linked glycans on bunyamwera virus glycoproteins in intracellular trafficking, protein folding, and virus infectivity. *J Virol* 2005;79(21):13725–13734.
396. Shi X, Elliott RM. Golgi localization of Hantaan virus glycoproteins requires coexpression of G1 and G2. *Virology* 2002;300(1):31–38.
397. Shi X, Elliott RM. Analysis of N-linked glycosylation of hantaan virus glycoproteins and the role of oligosaccharide side chains in protein folding and intracellular trafficking. *J Virol* 2004;78(10):5414–5422.
398. Shi X, Elliott RM. Generation and analysis of recombinant Bunyamwera orthobunyaviruses expressing V5 epitope-tagged L proteins. *J Gen Virol* 2009;90(Pt 2):297–306.
399. Shi X, Goli J, Clark G, et al. Functional analysis of the Bunyamwera orthobunyavirus Gc glycoprotein. *J Gen Virol* 2009;90(Pt 10):2483–2492.
400. Shi X, Kohl A, Leonard VH, et al. Requirement of the N-terminal region of orthobunyavirus nonstructural protein NSm for virus assembly and morphogenesis. *J Virol* 2006; 80(16):8089–8099.
401. Shi X, Kohl A, Li P, et al. Role of the cytoplasmic tail domains of Bunyamwera orthobunyavirus glycoproteins Gn and Gc in virus assembly and morphogenesis. *J Virol* 2007; 81(18):10151–10160.
402. Shi X, Lappin DF, Elliott RM. Mapping the Golgi targeting and retention signal of Bunyamwera virus glycoproteins. *J Virol* 2004;78(19):10793–10802.

403. Shi M, Lin XD, Chen X, et al. The evolutionary history of vertebrate RNA viruses. *Nature* 2018;556(7700):197–202.

404. Shi X, van Mierlo JT, French A, et al. Visualizing the replication cycle of bunyamwera orthobunyavirus expressing fluorescent protein-tagged Gc glycoprotein. *J Virol* 2010; 84(17):8460–8469.

405. Shtanko O, Nikitina RA, Altuntas CZ, et al. Crimean-Congo hemorrhagic fever virus entry into host cells occurs through the multivesicular body and requires ESCRT regulators. *PLoS Pathog* 2014;10(9):e1004390.

406. Simon M, Johansson C, Lundkvist A, et al. Microtubule-dependent and microtubule-independent steps in Crimean-Congo hemorrhagic fever virus replication cycle. *Virology* 2009;385(2):313–322.

407. Simon M, Johansson C, Mirazimi A. Crimean-Congo hemorrhagic fever virus entry and replication is clathrin-, pH- and cholesterol-dependent. *J Gen Virol* 2009;90:210–215.

408. Simons JF, Hellman U, Pettersson RF. Uukuniemi virus S RNA segment: ambisense coding strategy, packaging of complementary strands into virions, and homology to members of the genus Phlebovirus. *J Virol* 1990;64(1):247–255.

409. Simons JF, Persson R, Pettersson RF. Association of the nonstructural protein NSs of Uukuniemi virus with the 40S ribosomal subunit. *J Virol* 1992;66(7):4233–4241.

410. Simons JF, Pettersson RF. Host-derived 5′ ends and overlapping complementary 3′ ends of the two mRNAs transcribed from the ambisense S segment of Uukuniemi virus. *J Virol* 1991;65(9):4741–4748.

411. Simpson DI, Knight EM, Courtois G, et al. Congo virus: a hitherto undescribed virus occurring in Africa. I. Human isolations—clinical notes. *East Afr Med J* 1967;44(2):86–92.

412. Sin SH, McNulty BC, Kennedy GG, et al. Viral genetic determinants for thrips transmission of Tomato spotted wilt virus. *Proc Natl Acad Sci U S A* 2005;102(14):5168–5173.

413. Smith JF, Pifat DY. Morphogenesis of sandfly viruses (Bunyaviridae family). *Virology* 1982;121(1):61–81.

414. Smithburn K, Haddow A, Mahaffy A. A neurotropic virus isolated from Aedes mosquitos caught in the Semliki Forest. *Am J Trop Med* 1946;26:189–208.

415. Soldan SS, Hollidge BS, Wagner V, et al. La Crosse virus (LACV) Gc fusion peptide mutants have impaired growth and fusion phenotypes, but remain neurotoxic. *Virology* 2010;404(2):139–147.

416. Soldan SS, Plassmeyer ML, Matukonis MK, et al. La Crosse virus nonstructural protein NSs counteracts the effects of short interfering RNA. *J Virol* 2005;79(1):234–244.

417. Spiropoulou CF, Goldsmith CS, Shoemaker TR, et al. Sin Nombre virus glycoprotein trafficking. *Virology* 2003;308(1):48–63.

418. Steinecke P, Heinze C, Oehmen E, et al. Early events of tomato spotted wilt transcription and replication in protoplasts. *New Microbiol* 1998;21(3):263–268.

419. Stoltz M, Klingstrom J. Alpha/beta interferon (IFN-alpha/beta)-independent induction of IFN-lambda1 (interleukin-29) in response to Hantaan virus infection. *J Virol* 2010;84(18):9140–9148.

420. Storms MM, Kormelink R, Peters D, et al. The nonstructural NSm protein of tomato spotted wilt virus induces tubular structures in plant and insect cells. *Virology* 1995;214(2):485–493.

421. Storms MM, Nagata T, Kormelink R, et al. Expression of the movement protein of tomato spotted wilt virus in its insect vector *Frankliniella occidentalis*. *Arch Virol* 2002;147(4):825–831.

422. Strandin T, Hepojoki J, Vaheri A. Cytoplasmic tails of bunyavirus Gn glycoproteins-Could they act as matrix protein surrogates? *Virology* 2013;437(2):73–80.

423. Streitenfeld H, Boyd A, Fazakerley JK, et al. Activation of PKR by Bunyamwera virus is independent of the viral interferon antagonist NSs. *J Virol* 2003;77(9):5507–5511.

424. Struthers JK, Swanepoel R. Identification of a major non-structural protein in the nuclei of Rift Valley fever virus-infected cells. *J Gen Virol* 1982;60(Pt 2):381–384.

425. Suda Y, Fukushi S, Tani H, et al. Analysis of the entry mechanism of Crimean-Congo hemorrhagic fever virus, using a vesicular stomatitis virus pseudotyping system. *Arch Virol* 2016;161(6):1447–1454.

426. Sugiyama K, Morikawa S, Matsuura Y, et al. Four serotypes of haemorrhagic fever with renal syndrome viruses identified by polyclonal and monoclonal antibodies. *J Gen Virol* 1987;68:979–987.

427. Sundin DR, Beaty BJ, Nathanson N, et al. A G1 glycoprotein epitope of La Crosse virus: a determinant of infection of Aedes triseriatus. *Science* 1987;235(4788):591–593.

428. Surtees R, Ariza A, Punch EK, et al. The crystal structure of the Hazara virus nucleocapsid protein. *BMC Struct Biol* 2015;15:24.

429. Surtees R, Dowall SD, Shaw A, et al. Heat shock protein 70 family members interact with Crimean-Congo hemorrhagic fever virus and Hazara virus nucleocapsid proteins and perform a functional role in the Nairovirus replication cycle. *J Virol* 2016;90(20):9305–9316.

430. Takeda A, Sugiyama K, Nagano H, et al. Identification of a novel RNA silencing suppressor, NSs protein of Tomato spotted wilt virus. *FEBS Lett* 2002;532(1–2):75–79.

431. Talmon Y, Prasad BV, Clerx JP, et al. Electron microscopy of vitrified-hydrated La Crosse virus. *J Virol* 1987;61(7):2319–2321.

432. Taylor SL, Frias-Staheli N, Garcia-Sastre A, et al. Hantaan virus nucleocapsid protein binds to importin alpha proteins and inhibits tumor necrosis factor alpha-induced activation of nuclear factor Kappa B. *J Virol* 2009;83(3):1271–1279.

433. Terasaki K, Won S, Makino S. The C-terminal region of Rift Valley Fever virus NSm protein targets the protein to the mitochondrial outer membrane and exerts antiapoptotic function. *J Virol* 2013;87(1):676–682.

434. Thomas D, Blakqori G, Wagner V, et al. Inhibition of RNA polymerase II phosphorylation by a viral interferon antagonist. *J Biol Chem* 2004;279(30):31471–31477.

435. Tischler ND, Gonzalez A, Perez-Acle T, et al. Hantavirus Gc glycoprotein: evidence for a class II fusion protein. *J Gen Virol* 2005;86(Pt 11):2937–2947.

436. Ulmanen I, Seppala P, Pettersson RF. In vitro translation of Uukuniemi virus-specific RNAs: identification of a nonstructural protein and a precursor to the membrane glycoproteins. *J Virol* 1981;37(1):72–79.

437. Umashankar M, Martin CSS, Liao M, et al. Differential cholesterol binding by class II fusion proteins determines membrane fusion properties. *J Virol* 2008;82(18):9245–9253.

438. van Kasteren PB, Beugeling C, Ninaber DK, et al. Arterivirus and Nairovirus ovarian tumor domain-containing deubiquitinases target activated RIG-I to control innate immune signaling. *J Virol* 2012;86(2):773–785.

439. van Knippenberg I, Lamine M, Goldbach R, et al. Tomato spotted wilt virus transcriptase in vitro displays a preference for cap donors with multiple base complementarity to the viral template. *Virology* 2005;335(1):122–130.

440. Varela M, Piras IM, Mullan C, et al. Sensitivity to BST-2 restriction correlates with Orthobunyavirus host range. *Virology* 2017;509:121–130.

441. Vera-Otarola J, Solis L, Soto-Rifo R, et al. The Andes Hantavirus NSs protein is expressed from the viral small mRNA by a leaky scanning mechanism. *J Virol* 2012;86(4):2176–2187.

442. Vera-Otarola J, Soto-Rifo R, Ricci EP, et al. The 3′ untranslated region of the Andes hantavirus small mRNA functionally replaces the poly(A) tail and stimulates cap-dependent translation initiation from the viral mRNA. *J Virol* 2010;84(19):10420–10424.

443. Verbruggen P, Ruf M, Blakqori G, et al. Interferon antagonist NSs of La Crosse virus triggers a DNA damage response-like degradation of transcribing RNA polymerase II. *J Biol Chem* 2011;286(5):3681–3692.

444. Vialat P, Bouloy M. Germiston virus transcriptase requires active 40S ribosomal subunits and utilizes capped cellular RNAs. *J Virol* 1992;66(2):685–693.

445. Vincent MJ, Sanchez AJ, Erickson BR, et al. Crimean-Congo hemorrhagic fever virus glycoprotein proteolytic processing by subtilase SKI-1. *J Virol* 2003;77(16):8640–8649.

446. Wallat GD, Huang QF, Wang WJ, et al. High-resolution structure of the N-terminal endonuclease domain of the Lassa virus L polymerase in complex with magnesium ions. *PLoS One* 2014;9(2):e87577.

447. Walter CT, Barr JN. Bunyamwera virus can repair both insertions and deletions during RNA replication. *RNA* 2010;16(6):1138–1145.

448. Walter CT, Bento DF, Alonso AG, et al. Amino acid changes within the Bunyamwera virus nucleocapsid protein differentially affect the mRNA transcription and RNA replication activities of assembled ribonucleoprotein templates. *J Gen Virol* 2011;92(Pt 1):80–84.

449. Wang Y, Dutta S, Karlberg H, et al. Structure of Crimean-Congo hemorrhagic fever virus nucleoprotein: superhelical homo-oligomers and the role of Caspase-3 cleavage. *J Virol* 2012;86(22):12294–12303.

450. Wang X, Li B, Guo Y, et al. Molecular basis for the formation of ribonucleoprotein complex of Crimean-Congo hemorrhagic fever virus. *J Struct Biol* 2016;196(3):455–465.

451. Wang WM, Liu X, Wang X, et al. Structural and functional diversity of Nairovirus-encoded nucleoproteins. *J Virol* 2015;89(23):11740–11749.

452. Weber F, Bridgen A, Fazakerley JK, et al. Bunyamwera bunyavirus nonstructural protein NSs counteracts the induction of alpha/beta interferon. *J Virol* 2002;76(16):7949–7955.

453. Weber F, Dunn EF, Bridgen A, et al. The Bunyamwera virus nonstructural protein NSs inhibits viral RNA synthesis in a minireplicon system. *Virology* 2001;281(1):67–74.

454. Weber M, Gawanbacht A, Habjan M, et al. Incoming RNA virus nucleocapsids containing a 5′-triphosphorylated genome activate RIG-I and antiviral signaling. *Cell Host Microbe* 2013;13(3):336–346.

455. Weber F, Wagner V, Rasmussen SB, et al. Double-stranded RNA is produced by positive-strand RNA viruses and DNA viruses but not in detectable amounts by negative-strand RNA viruses. *J Virol* 2006;80(10):5059–5064.

456. Whitfield AE, Ullman DE, German TL. Expression and characterization of a soluble form of tomato spotted wilt virus glycoprotein GN. *J Virol* 2004;78(23):13197–13206.

457. Whitfield AE, Ullman DE, German TL. Tospovirus-thrips interactions. *Annu Rev Phytopathol* 2005;43:459–489.

458. Whitfield AE, Ullman DE, German TL. Tomato spotted wilt virus glycoprotein G(C) is cleaved at acidic pH. *Virus Res* 2005;110(1–2):183–186.

459. Wichgers Schreur PJ, Kortekaas J. Single-molecule FISH reveals non-selective packaging of Rift Valley fever virus genome segments. *PLoS Pathog* 2016;12(8):e1005800.

460. Wichgers Schreur PJ, Oreshkova N, Moormann RJ, et al. Creation of Rift Valley fever viruses with four-segmented genomes reveals flexibility in bunyavirus genome packaging. *J Virol* 2014;88(18):10883–10893.

461. Wijkamp I, van Lent J, Kormelink R, et al. Multiplication of tomato spotted wilt virus in its insect vector, *Frankliniella occidentalis*. *J Gen Virol* 1993;74:341–349.

462. Wikstrom L, Persson R, Pettersson RF. Intracellular transport of the G1 and G2 membrane glycoproteins of Uukuniemi virus. In: Kolakosky D, Mahy B, eds. *Genetics and Pathogenicity of Negative Strand Viruses*. Amsterdam: Elsevier; 1989:33–41.

463. Willensky S, Bar-Rogovsky H, Bignon EA, et al. Crystal structure of glycoprotein C from a Hantavirus in the post-fusion conformation. *PLoS Pathog* 2016;12(10):e1005948.

464. Wolf YI, Kazlauskas D, Iranzo J, et al. Origins and Evolution of the Global RNA Virome. *MBio* 2018;9(6).

465. Won SY, Ikegami T, Peters CJ, et al. NSm protein of Rift Valley fever virus suppresses virus-induced apoptosis. *J Virol* 2007;81(24):13335–13345.

466. Wu XD, Qi X, Qu BQ, et al. Evasion of antiviral immunity through sequestering of TBK1/IKK epsilon/IRF3 into viral inclusion bodies. *J Virol* 2014;88(6):3067–3076.

467. Wuerth JD, Habjan M, Wulle J, et al. NSs protein of sandfly fever Sicilian Phlebovirus counteracts interferon (IFN) induction by masking the DNA-binding domain of IFN regulatory factor 3. *J Virol* 2018;92(23).

468. Wuerth JD, Weber F. Phleboviruses and the type I interferon response. *Viruses* 2016;8(6).

469. Xu B, Liu L, Huang X, et al. Metagenomic analysis of fever, thrombocytopenia and leukopenia syndrome (FTLS) in Henan Province, China: discovery of a new bunyavirus. *PLoS Pathog* 2011;7(11):e1002369.

470. Xu L, Wu J, He B, et al. Novel hantavirus identified in black-bearded tomb bats, China. *Infect Genet Evol* 2015;31:158–160.

471. Yoshimatsu K, Lee BH, Araki K, et al. The multimerization of hantavirus nucleocapsid protein depends on type-specific epitopes. *J Virol* 2003;77(2):943–952.

472. Yu XJ, Liang MF, Zhang SY, et al. Fever with thrombocytopenia associated with a novel bunyavirus in China. *N Engl J Med* 2011;364(16):1523–1532.

473. Yu L, Ye L, Zhao R, et al. HSP70 induced by Hantavirus infection interacts with viral nucleocapsid protein and its overexpression suppresses virus infection in Vero E6 cells. *Am J Transl Res* 2009;1(4):367–380.

474. Yuan PW, Bartlam M, Lou ZY, et al. Crystal structure of an avian influenza polymerase PA(N) reveals an endonuclease active site. *Nature* 2009;458(7240):909–912.

Orthohantavirus, Orthonairovirus, Orthobunyavirus and Phlebovirus

Christina F. Spiropoulou • Dennis A. Bente

INTRODUCTION

Among the approximately 500 identified viruses belonging to Bunyavirales order, at least 55 are known to cause disease in humans. Among them, Rift Valley fever virus (RVFV), Crimean-Congo hemorrhagic fever virus (CCHFV), severe fever with thrombocytopenia syndrome (SFTS) virus, Heartland virus (HRTV), and a number of hantaviruses and orthobunyaviruses present a significant public health concern due to varying properties, which may include potential for high morbidity and mortality, ability to transmit from person to person, or propensity to cause alarm to the public in outbreak settings. Fortunately, most bunyaviruses that cause human disease exhibit either no or low mortality rates, no human-to-human transmission, and usually restricted geographic distribution.

In this chapter, we review the emergence and reemergence of these high-consequence pathogens and their pathogenesis in both reservoirs and humans. We examine the clinical features of disease and highlight aspects of disease that warrant additional investigation. Viral epidemiology and ecology are summarized, focusing on viral maintenance and distribution in natural reservoirs and human disease incidence. The progress on diagnostics for these viruses is examined, and, finally, as no vaccines or antivirals are currently approved for prevention or treatment, the current state of experimental therapeutics and vaccines is discussed.

HANTAVIRIDAE, GENUS ORTHOHANTAVIRUS

Pathogenesis and Pathology
Reservoirs
Although a significant number of new hantaviruses has been recently discovered in insectivores and bats, all presently known pathogenic hantaviruses are harbored by rodents. Hantaviruses are horizontally transmitted among rodents, primarily through excreta and saliva. Infection of natural reservoirs results in an acute phase with high viremia, followed by prolonged or persistent infection with variable durations of virus shedding in the urine, feces, or saliva; persistent infection can last days to months, or even the rodent's lifespan.

Experimental infection of host rodents indicates that viremia peaks approximately 2 weeks post infection and results in dissemination of the virus throughout the animal. Hantaviruses appear to target primarily endothelial cells, with the highest concentrations of viral antigen observed in the lungs, heart, and kidneys.[52,280] Peak amounts of viral RNA in experimentally infected animals vary, with some animals exhibiting characteristics of super-shedders.[349] The end of viremia correlates with the induction of hantavirus-specific antibodies, which first become detectable around 14 days post infection, peak approximately 50 days post infection, and remain detectable throughout the rodent's lifespan.[228] Neutralizing antibodies are detected after 3 weeks post infection. Infection of the rodent host induces moderate inflammatory responses that are not harmful to the host and that contain the virus without clearing it. The infected endothelium and increased numbers of regulatory T cells (Tregs) that modulate the immune response allow the virus to establish persistence and periodic shedding.[109,110,347,348]

Although naturally infected rodent reservoirs do not display apparent disease symptoms, reduced winter survival and reduced body weights of infected rodents have been reported.[80,101,191] Aggressive behavior has been correlated with increased infection among rodents: older males and animals with more scars are more likely to be seropositive.[138]

Human Infections

In stark contrast to the asymptomatic infection of the primary rodent reservoir species, human hantavirus infection frequently results in hantavirus disease traditionally presenting as one of two main syndromes: hemorrhagic fever with renal syndrome (HFRS) caused by Old World hantaviruses, and hantavirus pulmonary syndrome (HPS) caused by New World hantaviruses. The pathogenesis of both HFRS and HPS is similar, although the disease manifests in different organs, primarily affecting the lungs in HPS and the kidneys in HFRS. Severe human disease has been attributed to microvascular leakage and inflammation. Humans are infected mainly by inhaling aerosols of the excreta of infected rodents or possibly through rodent bites. Human-to-human transmission can occur but is rare and has only been observed with Andes virus (ANDV) infection.

The cells initially infected by hantaviruses have not been identified, but the major target cells are microvascular (capillary) endothelial cells. Since inhalation of aerosols is the main route of infection in humans, it is tempting to assume that the virus first infects the upper respiratory epithelium or the macrophages and dendritic cells residing in the respiratory endothelium. How the virus passes through the respiratory epithelium to establish systemic infection is not clear, however. Studies in polarized epithelial cell cultures have shown an apical polarized entry and release of hantaviruses,[211,327] but experiments on entry and release of ANDV in primary hamster tracheal epithelial cells indicate bidirectional entry and release of this virus.[334] Apical release would facilitate virus spread into the respiratory tract, but such bidirectional infection and release may be an aspect unique to ANDV infection. In addition to the microvascular endothelium, epithelial cells, human dendritic cells, monocytes macrophages, and likely other cells are susceptible to hantavirus infection. Infected dendritic cells could disseminate the virus through the lymphatic system to lymph nodes and eventually to the vascular respiratory endothelium. As mentioned above, Old World hantaviruses preferentially affect kidney functions, while New World hantaviruses affect the lung. The mechanisms behind this preferential tissue tropism are currently unknown.

Immune response

Hantaviruses have developed multiple mechanisms to limit host cell immune responses early in infection (see details in Chapter 16). Although the extent to which pathogenic and nonpathogenic hantaviruses induce the interferon (IFN) response varies and pathogenic hantaviruses delay the induction of the innate immune responses, that delay alone is unlikely to be the source of differences in pathogenicity. All hantaviruses cause strong and long-lasting humoral immune responses in patients. Antibodies against the hantavirus N protein can be detected early after the onset of illness, and neutralizing antibodies directed against Gn and Gc develop soon after.[182] In general, generation of high levels of hantavirus-specific IgG early in the disease has been associated with increased chances of survival, and higher amounts of neutralizing antibodies correlate with milder disease.[37,246] Hantavirus infection of dendritic cells

in vitro induces their maturation, and mature dendritic cells can generate a strong adaptive immune response.[254,323]

Viral RNA is usually detectable in patients' blood during the early stages of disease, and viral load correlates with disease severity.[309,426] At the time of death, viral antigens are detectable in endothelial cell layers throughout the body, but predominantly in lung endothelial cells in HPS patients and in kidney endothelial cells in HFRS patients.[175,434] Interestingly, the numbers of monocytes and dendritic cells in the blood are reduced during the acute phase of hantavirus disease, likely not because of cell death but rather due to redistribution and migration of these cells to the infected tissues.[345] Additionally, soluble CD163, a biomarker of macrophage activation, is elevated in the sera of HFRS patients, correlating with disease severity.[413]

Neutrophils are the first immune cells recruited to the site of inflammation or infection, attracted by IL-8 released by hantavirus-infected endothelium. Activated neutrophils can release reactive oxygen species and serine proteases (degranulation) and form extracellular traps (NETosis). High levels of activated neutrophils and increased levels of histone/double-stranded DNA complexes have been observed in hantavirus patients.[324,346,371] Moreover, neutrophil activation has been correlated with kidney injury in Puumala virus (PUUV) infections in humans.[371]

A strong T-cell response followed by generation of long-lived memory T cells has been well documented in hantavirus infection.[232,252,326,398] CD4 and CD8 T cells obtained from blood samples of patients in the acute and convalescent phases of disease can recognize epitopes from viral N, Gn, and Gc proteins.[116,398] In cases of PUUV infection, proliferating, activated effector CD8 T cells can be seen in the peripheral blood and bronchoalveolar lavage early on the disease course.[232,326] High frequencies of virus-specific CD8 T cells have been linked to severe disease, suggesting the possibility of immune-mediated pathogenesis.[198,339,384] Early studies also indicate that severity of both HFRS and HPS in humans correlates with specific human lymphocyte antigen haplotypes.[249,278,400]

In general, very strong or very weak T-cell responses can lead to severe disease. The above studies suggest that strong cytotoxic T-cell responses contribute to the pathology of hantavirus disease. However, a protective role of T cells during hantavirus disease has also been reported, with Gn-specific effector memory T cells conferring protective immunity in ANDV-infected patients.[252] A strong CD4 T-cell response against Hantaan virus (HTNV) glycoproteins was also associated with controlling the virus and a better clinical outcome in HFRS cases.[244]

The expansion and long-term maintenance of natural killer (NK) cells has been reported in HFRS patients. NK cells become activated by IL-15 and IL-15Ra expressed by hantavirus-infected endothelial cells and can secrete proinflammatory cytokines such as tumor necrosis factor alpha (TNF-α) and interferon gamma (IFN-γ).[43,56] NK cells and cytotoxic T lymphocytes can eliminate infected target cells by inducing apoptosis. It is apparent, however, that they do not kill hantavirus-infected endothelial cells, since the microvascular endothelium remains undamaged. This is likely due to the antiapoptotic effects of hantaviruses, including the N protein, which protects infected endothelial cells from cytotoxic lymphocyte-induced apoptosis by inhibiting the function of granzyme B and caspase 3.[150,364]

Endothelial cell leakage

Hantavirus infection of the microvascular endothelium and immune cells does not result in a direct cytopathic effect.[434] The progression of the disease, with the associated increase in vascular permeability, is a complex process, with contributions directly from virus replication and from the induced immune responses to hantavirus infection. Studies using primary microvascular endothelial cells have indicated that hantavirus infection and replication alone can trigger pathways that lead to reduced endothelial integrity by down-regulating vascular endothelial cadherin (VE-cadherin or CD144), an essential component of adherence junctions, or ZO-1, an essential component of tight junctions.[210,356] Hantavirus N protein alone can influence vascular permeability of the endothelium by activating cellular RhoA GTPases.[144] The interaction between pathogenic hantaviruses and their cellular receptor $\beta 3$ integrin can also sensitize the endothelium and cause vascular hyperpermeability in response to added permeability factors like vascular endothelial growth factor (VEGF-A). The binding of VEGF-A to its receptor VEGF-R2 induces down-regulation of VE-cadherin, resulting in increased vascular permeability. Indeed, increased VEGF-A concentrations have been reported in serum, pulmonary edema fluid, and urine samples collected from patients.[136,245,295] Hantavirus infection can also activate the kallikrein–kinin system to release bradykinin, another potent permeability factor that can cause vascular leakage.[382]

A dysregulated immune response causing strong inflammation is believed to be another main contributor to hantavirus disease. The infected endothelium becomes activated and orchestrates a series of events by secreting various cytokines and chemokines and by up-regulating adhesion molecules that attract immune cells like neutrophils, NK cells, and CD8+ T cells that in turn can also produce high levels of proinflammatory cytokines.[375] Numerous *in vitro* experiments and studies of human infection have shown increased levels of proinflammatory cytokines and chemokines, including IL-6, IL-8, and IFN-γ, and permeability factors, such as TNF-α and VEGF.[136,194,268,295] High levels of cytokine production in specific tissues have been identified during hantavirus disease. For example, in HFRS, expression of TNF-α, TGF-β, and platelet-derived growth factor (PDGF) has been observed in the kidneys.[383] Similarly, high levels of cytokine production can be seen in the lungs (but not in kidneys and livers) of fatal HPS cases, suggesting that local cytokine production may play an important role in disease severity.[268] Among the induced cytokines, IL-6 strongly correlates with HPS severity.[13,250] The cytokine and chemokine profiles of HFRS and HPS cases are different, with proinflammatory responses in HPS found to be substantially stronger than in HFRS, likely reflecting the much higher case fatality rates (CFR) generally seen in HPS.[194]

In addition to endothelial cell activation and induction of proinflammatory cytokines, other factors that can contribute to the vascular leakage seen in hantavirus disease are complement activation and the coagulation system. Complement activation and elevated amounts of SC5B-9, a component of the complement cascade, have been associated with disease severity in HFRS patients.[359] Tissue-type plasminogen activator (tPA), but not its inhibitor PAI-1, is up-regulated in HFRS patients and is possibly responsible for stimulating fibrinolysis. The opposite is seen in severe HPS cases induced by Sin Nombre virus (SNV), in which a strong prothrombotic response with elevated PAI-1 levels has been reported, possibly explaining the absence of hemorrhagic symptoms in HPS.[30,46] Lastly, in addition to activated macrophages, T cells, and NK cells, neutrophils could play a role in vascular permeability by generating NETs and by secreting permeability factors like VEGF and TNF-α in the vicinity of the infected endothelium.[346] A proposed model for hantavirus disease is shown in Figure 17.1.

In addition to microvascular leakage, another prominent feature of hantavirus disease is induced thrombocytopenia (low number of blood platelets). The exact mechanism of this platelet deficiency is not known. However, the presence of normal or increased numbers of megakaryocytes in bone marrow of hantavirus disease patients indicates no deficiency in platelet production. In addition, evidence of fibrinolysis suggests that increased consumption or sequestration of platelets is the possible reason for hantavirus-induced thrombocytopenia.[137,220,221,226,434]

One enduring limitation to studying hantavirus pathogenesis has been the absence of suitable experimental animal models. The first breakthrough came with the discovery that Syrian golden hamsters infected with ANDV develop a disease with characteristics similar to those of human HPS, including interstitial pneumonitis, alveolar edema, mononuclear cell infiltrates in the lung, and high mortality rates.[166,411] However, only immunosuppressed Syrian golden hamsters infected with SNV and other New World hantaviruses can develop HPS-like disease.[60,404] The hamster animal model has been extensively used to study HPS pathogenesis. Depleting B cells, T cells, and alveolar macrophages does not affect the course of the disease in this model, indicating that these cells may not contribute to the induced pathogenesis. How much we can extrapolate from results in hamsters to human disease remains an open question. Non-human primate (NHP) animal models have been developed for PUUV-induced HFRS and, more recently, for SNV-induced HPS.[147,204,339] In the NHP model of HPS, thrombocytopenia, neutrophilia, eosinophilia, and monocytosis were noted, in addition to the development of an uncontrolled tissue-specific proinflammatory response.[339] Interestingly, depleting neutrophils in mice with severe combined immune deficiency (SCID) infected with HTNV suppresses hantavirus-induced pulmonary edema, highlighting a possible role of neutrophils in hantavirus pathogenesis.[207] Similarly, in a humanized mouse model, neutrophils and functional HLA-A2–restricted CD8 T cells were shown to play an important role in hantavirus-induced pathogenesis.[205]

Pathologic findings in biopsies of kidneys of HFRS patients include mild to moderate interstitial infiltration of lymphocytes, plasma cells, monocytes and macrophages, and polymorphonuclear leukocytes (mainly eosinophilic granulocytes and neutrophils), although the exact mechanism of kidney failure in HFRS patients is still unclear.[383] HPS patients usually develop pulmonary edema, plural effusions, interstitial mononuclear cell infiltrate, edema, and focal hyaline membranes[307,434] (Fig. 17.2).

Clinical Features

The main characteristics of hantavirus disease noted upon hospital admission are fever, thrombocytopenia, and acute kidney or lung injury followed by a number of abnormal clinical findings. Hemorrhage is not a common characteristic. Although here we present the clinical features of HFRS and HPS individually, this separation is based mainly on the distinct virus

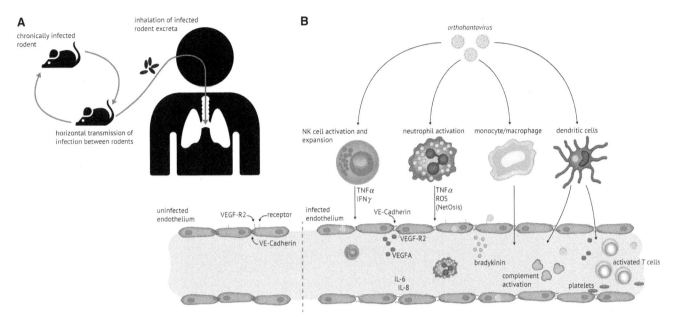

FIGURE 17.1 A: Hantavirus maintenance in the rodent reservoir in nature and transmission to humans. Humans acquire the virus by inhalation of aerosols or dust particles contaminated by excreta of infected rodents. **B:** Proposed model of the steps leading to hantavirus disease-induced vascular permeability. Orthohantaviruses gain access to the vascular endothelium through infected dendritic cells or infected macrophages. Hantavirus infection triggers both innate and adaptive immune responses. Infection of the endothelium can stimulate pathways that reduce endothelial integrity by down-regulating VE-cadherin and activating Rho GTPases. At the same time, hantavirus-infected endothelial cells produce proinflammatory cytokines and chemokines and up-regulate adhesion molecules on their cell surface, which in turn attract activated natural killer (NK) cells, neutrophils, and T cells to the infected area in addition to infected macrophages and dendritic cells. The activated immune cells secrete more chemokines, cytokines, and other proinflammatory molecules, like TNF-α and reactive oxygen species, resulting in a "cytokine storm." Secretion of potent permeability factors, such as VEGF and bradykinin, can directly disrupt the integrity of the endothelium. Additional factors, like complement activation, may also contribute to vascular leakage.

tropism in the 2 syndromes, kidneys in HFRS and lungs in HPS. We now know that pulmonary involvement can be seen in HFRS cases,[410] while petechia, hemorrhage, and renal signs can be observed in HPS cases.[74,161,195] The broad term "hantavirus disease" has therefore recently been proposed to describe the disease caused by hantaviruses.[299] A map of the distribu-

tion of pathogenic hantaviruses is presented in Figure 17.3, and a summary of symptoms of HFRS and HPS is presented in Figure 17.4.

The incubation period before the onset of HFRS symptoms typically lasts 2 to 3 weeks. Initial symptoms of severe HFRS are high fever, headache, malaise, chills, and prostration,

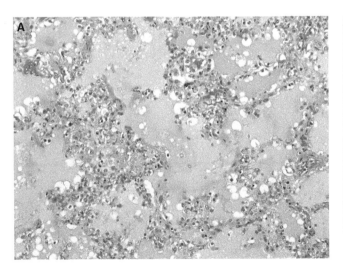
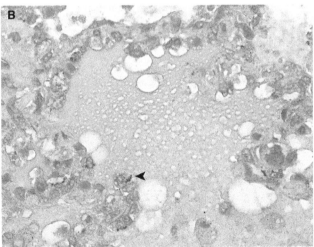

FIGURE 17.2 HPS is characterized by acute pulmonary edema and shock. A: Histological features of a lung section include interstitial pneumonitis and alveolar edema in a typical case. **B:** Immunostaining of hantavirus antigens in the lung shows that the viral antigen is localized mainly in pulmonary microvascular endothelial cells (in *red*, indicated by an *arrowhead*).

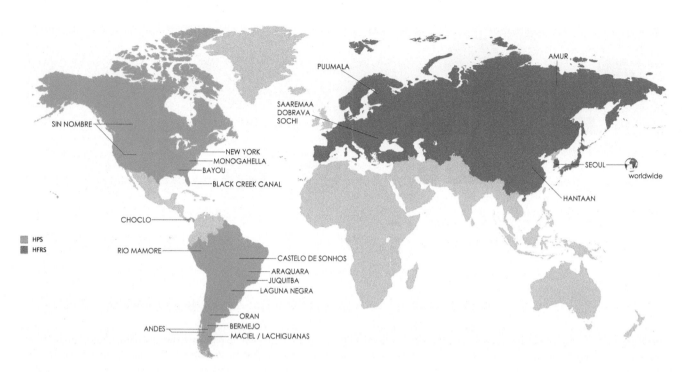

FIGURE 17.3 Global distribution of hantaviruses known to be pathogenic in humans. Hantaviruses cause two main clinical syndromes: hemorrhagic fever with renal syndrome (HFRS) and hantavirus pulmonary syndrome (HPS). HFRS is seen primarily in Europe and Asia, while HPS occurs mostly in the Americas.

which last 3 to 5 days. Flushing of the face and neck and conjunctival and pharyngeal injection (indicating capillary dilation) are frequently observed. Increased capillary permeability is likely responsible for the retroperitoneal edema and lower back pain often described. This febrile phase is followed by a hypotensive phase lasting several hours to days, characterized by marked thrombocytopenia and often by petechial hemorrhage. Many patients exhibit low-grade disseminated intravascular coagulation (DIC). Approximately 10% to 15% of patients show some degree of shock around this time, which improves

within 12 to 48 hours as blood pressure returns to normal, or as the patient becomes hypertensive. Oliguria may occur, and, historically, renal failure contributes to about half of all HFRS deaths. Recovering patients undergo a phase of diuresis that may last several months. Not all patients go through all the stages described; some rapidly progress to death within a few days, whereas others skip some phases of the disease or exhibit very mild symptoms that may not be recognized as HFRS. However, this progression tends to be seen with the most severe forms of HFRS caused by (HTNV) and Dobrava (DOBV)

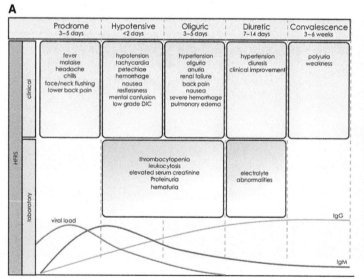

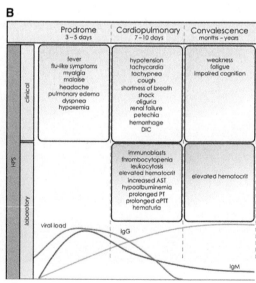

FIGURE 17.4 A: An outline of the main clinical manifestations and laboratory findings in severe HFRS. **B:** An outline of the main clinical manifestations and laboratory findings in severe HPS.

viruses, which are associated with 5% to 15% case fatality rate (CFR). HFRS associated with Seoul virus (SEOV) is usually milder, with a mortality rate of 1% to 2%.[199] HFRS associated with PUUV is the mildest form of the disease, with a mortality rate of less than 1%. In PUUV-associated HFRS, phases of the illness are generally less pronounced and symptoms are milder, with hypotension rather than shock, petechiae rather than frank hemorrhage, and relatively mild renal involvement.

Similarly to HFRS, HPS also begins with a 2- to 3-week incubation period (though longer incubation times have been documented) followed by rapid onset of acute disease. In SNV-caused HPS, the first 4 days often include fever, myalgia, malaise, headache, and gastrointestinal symptoms. Patients frequently present for medical attention with the onset of pulmonary edema, dyspnea, and hypoxemia. These features, together with the hemoconcentration that is frequently observed, are presumably linked to viral infection of the microvascular endothelial cells surrounding the lungs, which leads to increased permeability and fluid leakage into the lungs. Bilateral pulmonary infiltrates are often visible on chest x-rays. Deterioration of the patient's condition is often very rapid, with death occurring within 1 to 3 days of hospital admission in almost 40% of the cases. Clinical laboratory tests frequently reveal thrombocytopenia and prolonged partial thromboplastin time. Hypotension and shock can be prominent at this stage. A very similar clinical picture is seen in HPS cases caused by other viruses found in rodents of the *Sigmodontinae* subfamily. HPS cases have been associated with infection by Monongahela virus, which is related to SNV; New York virus; Bayou virus; Black Creek Canal virus (BCCV); and ANDV and the related Oran, Lechiguanas, Hu39694, Laguna Negra, Juquitiba, Araraquara, and Castelo dos Sonhos viruses. BCCV and Bayou virus infection generally leads to more renal involvement and elevated serum creatine phosphokinase. Renal failure also appears to be common with Oran virus-associated HPS in northern Argentina.[230] Flushing and petechiae, and frank hemorrhage, have been observed in some HPS patients infected with ANDV in Argentina and Chile, respectively.

Epidemiology and Ecology

The geographic distribution of hantaviruses and the epidemiologic patterns observed for HFRS and HPS reflect the distribution and natural history features of the rodent hosts of these viruses (Fig. 17.2). Epidemiologic data accumulated since the 1950s for a variety of hantaviruses, including HPS-associated hantaviruses, suggest that human-to-human virus transmission does not generally occur, and that virtually all human infections are acquired by exposure to infected rodent excreta. A notable exception is in ANDV-associated HPS, in which human-to-human transmissions have been demonstrated.[256,294,419]

In general, hantavirus disease incidence is higher in males than in females. However, a number of reports have shown that the CFR in females is higher than in males in particular age groups. The disease is rare in pediatric populations.[203,247,255] A short summary of each hantavirus family relative to epidemiology and ecology is described below.

HTNV and HTNV-like viruses (Amur/Soochong) are found in various parts of China, South Korea, and Far Eastern Russia, in *Apodemus agrarius mantchuricus*, a mouse common in the region's agricultural fields, and *Apodemus peninsulae*.[184] Adult humans in rural areas (e.g., farmers, forest workers, or troops stationed in the field) are the most at risk of infection.

HFRS cases peak in the fall, likely reflecting a mixture of factors, including increased abundance of virus-infected mice coinciding with increased human activity in the fields associated with harvest of crops, as well as movement of rodents into human dwellings as winter approaches.[225] Most HNTV HFRS patients are 20 to 50 years old, while cases in children younger than 10 are uncommon.[79,227] Males are more likely than females to become infected, consistent with predominant exposure being in the fields rather than in the homes. HTNV-related HFRS is most prevalent in China, where approximately 100,000 cases are reported each year; 300 to 900 HFRS cases are estimated to occur in Korea and in Far Eastern Russia annually.

SEOV is associated with the domestic rats, *Rattus norvegicus* and *Rattus rattus*,[227,372] and is distributed worldwide due to the recent global spread of rats to port cities and beyond through international shipping. A related virus, Thailand virus, is found in *Bandicota indica* rodents in Thailand but is not known to cause human disease. SEOV is the only hantavirus known to cause disease in urban areas, as other hantaviruses are associated with rodents that predominantly inhabit rural areas. Cases of SEOV contracted from pet rodents by humans are becoming more frequent in the last decade and have been reported both in Europe and North America.[127,193,380] SEOV-related HFRS cases in general tend to be more moderate than those associated with HTNV, with mortality rates approximately up to 1%.[83] Unlike HTNV-related HFRS, cases of SEOV-related HFRS occur year-round. The annual number of cases is unknown, as figures for SEOV- and HTNV-related HFRS are often not separated. However, Chinese reports suggest that SEOV-related HFRS cases in urban areas of several provinces have been growing since the discovery of the virus in 1981.

In Europe and Scandinavia, most cases of HFRS are caused by infection with PUUV. Particularly in Scandinavia, the disease is referred to as nephropathia epidemica (NE) and is usually milder than HTNV-associated HFRS. PUUV is hosted by the bank vole, *Myodes glareolus*. In Sweden and Finland, the number of cases in rural residents usually peaks in November and January, although cases in urban residents appear to peak in August, likely correlating with vacationing in summer cabins in rural areas. A male-to-female case ratio of approximately 2:1 is seen, and the disease is rare in children.[61] Local epidemics usually reflect increased local bank vole densities, which tend to cycle with a 3- to 4-year periodicity. Approximately 30% of PUUV infections result in reported disease, based on data from areas of Finland with high surveillance for disease.[61] In addition, antibody prevalence rates of up to 20% can be seen in known endemic areas in northern Sweden.[171] PUUV-associated disease in Belgium, northeastern France, and Germany occurs mainly in autumn and spring, and the extent of activity reflects the alterations in the size and structure of bank vole communities.[312] Large PUUV-associated HFRS outbreaks are periodically recorded in several areas of European Russia, particularly Udmurtia and Bashkortostan. A genetically distinct PUUV-like virus has also been identified in *Clethrionomys rufocanus* voles in Far Eastern Russia and on Hokkaido Island, Japan, but is not known to be associated with human disease.[192] Likewise, several additional hantaviruses are associated with other subfamily *Arvicolinae* rodents but are not known to cause human disease. For example, Topografov virus is present in lemmings in Arctic regions of Russia, and at least 5 hantaviruses are associated with various Old and New World rodents of the *Microtus* genus.

Dobrava virus (DOBV) also causes a considerable number of severe HFRS cases in Europe, particularly in the Balkan countries.[25,298] The primary rodent reservoir of DOBV is *Apodemus flavicollis*, which is widely abundant in this region. Variants of DOBV, such as Saaremaa and Kurkino viruses, can be found in *A. agrarius* (a subspecies distinct from that which carries HTNV in Asia), which is of greater abundance in more northern areas; Sochi virus is found in *Apodemus ponticus* in Southern Russia.[108,358] DOBV and Sochi genotypes cause severe illness with CFR of 9% to 15%.[212,296] Although *A. flavicollis* does not frequent houses and other man-made structures, it will often enter campsites or places where food may be present. Unlike HTNV-associated HFRS, most DOBV-associated HFRS cases occur in the late spring and summer months, when human activity in rural areas is greatest. Epidemics of disease are seen at times when rodent populations increase. Seroprevalence rates in humans can be high in rural areas; for instance, antibody positivity rates of up to 14% were seen in mountainous areas of northern and western Greece.[15]

Since the discovery of SNV and HPS in 1993,[283] numerous other hantaviruses have been detected in New World rodents of the *Sigmodontinae* subfamily. In North America, SNV is by far the most important cause of HPS[267] and is present in deer mice (*Peromyscus maniculatus*, grasslands form) throughout western and central United States and Canada.[267] The initially identified cluster of HPS cases occurred in the Four Corners region (meeting point of New Mexico, Arizona, Colorado, and Utah) in 1993; while the majority of subsequent cases have occurred in the southwestern United States, some have now been recorded in 32 states and 4 Canadian provinces. SNV-infected deer mice have been detected throughout most of this range, which stretches from the Yukon peninsula to Mexico and from California to the Appalachian mountains in the eastern United States and Canada.[265,267] A survey of 2,500 individuals in high-risk groups, such as persons with occupations that would bring them in close contact with rural rodents, found hantavirus-specific antibodies in only approximately 0.5% of those sampled,[409] suggesting that human SNV infections are rare.[435] Clusters of cases appear to be generally associated with local increases in infected deer mice populations. HPS cases peak in late spring and early summer. More cases in the United States have occurred in males, with a mean age of 37 years (range 6 to 83 years). Retrospective studies suggest that the disease had gone unrecognized since at least 1959.[129]

Through December 2018, 784 HPS cases have been reported in the United States, with a CFR around 35%. Since the Four Corners outbreak in 1993, the second largest SNV outbreak, with 10 cases and 3 deaths, was identified among overnight visitors at the Yosemite National park in 2012.[288] Several other hantaviruses are capable of causing HPS in the United States. The forest form of deer mice (*P. maniculatus nubiterrae*), found predominantly throughout the Appalachian mountain range extending from Georgia to eastern Canada, harbor a genetically distinct SNV-like virus referred to as Monongahela virus.[267,366] Monongahela virus has been associated with several HPS cases in the eastern United States. The white-footed mouse, *Peromyscus leucopus* (eastern haplotype), hosts another SNV-like virus, New York virus, responsible for some HPS cases in the northeastern United States.[160,172]

Other sigmodontines also harbor HPS-associated hantaviruses in the United States, such as BCCV, which was associated with a single HPS case in southern Florida and is hosted by the cotton rat, *Sigmodon hispidus* (eastern form).[328] The genetically distinct western form of *S. hispidus* hosts another hantavirus, Muleshoe virus.[329] Bayou virus was discovered in 1994, associated with a fatal HPS case in Louisiana,[273] and subsequently was shown to be hosted by the rice rat *Oligoryzomys palustris* and present throughout the range of the rodent.[394] Bayou virus was also associated with a nonfatal HPS case in Texas.[161] Although HPS associated with BCCV and Bayou virus is still predominantly a pulmonary disease, more renal involvement has been seen in those cases than in classic SNV-associated HPS.[161,196]

The confirmation of an HPS case in Brazil in late 1993 marked the beginning of a wave of discovery of HPS cases and associated hantaviruses throughout South and Central America.[188,241] In addition to Brazil, Argentina, Bolivia, Brazil, Chile, Ecuador, Paraguay, Panama, Uruguay, and Venezuela have also reported HPS cases. Rodents carrying viruses similar to SNV have been found in Colombia, Costa Rica, and Mexico but have not been associated with disease in humans.

The high prevalence of hantavirus-specific antibodies in the general population in some areas of South and Central America differs considerably from the epidemiologic picture seen in North America, where seropositivity rates of 0.2% or less are seen. For instance, high rates of hantavirus-specific antibodies have been detected on surveillance of general populations in regions of Paraguay (40%), Salta province in Argentina (17%), and Los Santos province in Panama (13%).[126,423] These data suggest more frequent exposure of people to hantaviruses in these areas and more asymptomatic or subclinical infections than seen with North American hantavirus infections.

Phylogenetic analysis of rodent-borne hantaviruses and their reservoir hosts indicated that their evolutionary trees largely overlapped, with a limited number of exceptions, suggesting that these viruses may have coevolved with their hosts over 20 to 30 million years.[317] The recent discoveries of hantaviruses in moles, shrews, and bats complicates the evolutionary history of hantaviruses. In addition to codivergence with their rodent hosts, cross-species transmission and geographic expansion could have also played an important role in hantavirus evolution, shifting the time frame of hantavirus–host coevolution to hundreds of millions of years.[163,318] Thus, while HPS and many hantaviruses have only recently been discovered, phylogenetic analysis clearly indicates that these viruses are of ancient origin.

Diagnosis

Clinical differential diagnosis of HFRS and HPS cases can be difficult due to the nonspecific early symptoms in both types of disease. Early signs of severe HFRS can be easily confused with those of leptospirosis, typhus, pyelonephritis, poststreptococcal glomerulonephritis, an acute abdominal emergency, or other hemorrhagic fevers.[227] In areas of China, Korea, Far Eastern Russia, Europe, and Scandinavia where HFRS is known to occur, a febrile patient presenting with thrombocytopenia and renal symptoms should be questioned about potential rodent exposure and tested for evidence of hantavirus infection. In the Americas, the early stages of HPS are easily confused with influenza and are thus extremely difficult to recognize. However, fever and myalgia and a history of potential rural rodent exposure together with the appearance of acute onset shortness of breath and findings of thrombocytopenia, leukocytosis with left shift (higher ratio of immature-to-mature neutrophils), and atypical lymphocytes would suggest HPS.[287] A peripheral rapid blood screening test has been developed and evaluated to quickly and inexpensively detect HPS based on five peripheral smear criteria, including thrombocytopenia, the presence of a left shift, hemoconcentration, lack of toxic changes, and the presence of immunoblasts.[106,209]

Laboratory diagnosis

Antibodies against hantaviruses are invariably seen in patient sera around the time of onset of illness. Laboratory analysis of the presence of virus-specific antibodies has historically included indirect fluorescent antibody testing. Serology is broadly used to detect hantavirus antibodies in patient sera. Acute diagnosis is best achieved by IgM capture enzyme-linked immunosorbent assay (ELISA) using either hantavirus-infected cell slurries or recombinant nucleocapsid proteins as antigen with appropriate negative controls.[115,124,214] Such assays have been shown to be highly sensitive, rapid, and inexpensive. Considerable cross-reactivity among related hantaviruses is seen, so inclusion of a limited number of antigens representative of various viruses (e.g., SNV, PUUV, and HTNV) allows detection of virtually all acute hantavirus infections. The disadvantage of the cross-reactivity of the assay is the inability to precisely identify the virus based on a positive result. Western blot assays utilizing recombinant nucleocapsid proteins or GPs have also been effectively used for acute diagnosis, particularly of New World hantaviruses and can provide additional insights into the identity of the virus.[162,182]

Virus isolation from acute clinical specimens is an almost impossible task, and only a few human virus isolates exist despite a plethora of newly discovered hantaviruses and available genome sequences. The exact reason for the difficulty of isolating hantaviruses is unknown but is likely related to the presence of a strong immune response at the time of disease onset, including serum-neutralizing antibodies. Given the frequent difficulties in obtaining infectious virus, reverse transcriptase-polymerase chain reaction (RT-PCR) assays have been used effectively to complement the serological assays. RT-PCR is used in acute diagnosis to detect viral RNA in the blood, serum, or tissue samples of patients and allows detailed genetic comparison of hantaviruses.[241,283,298] Given the potential for false positives due to cross-contamination, RT-PCR is not recommended as the sole means of establishing a hantavirus diagnosis, and a combination of RT-PCR and IgM/IgG ELISA is still the most appropriate way to establish for hantavirus diagnosis. Virus-specific real-time RT-PCR assays, in addition to microarrays and next-generation sequencing, are more expensive and complex techniques for laboratory diagnostics but are certainly gaining ground[407] (reviewed in Ref.[212]).

Immunohistochemistry on formalin-fixed or paraffin-embedded tissue samples from fatal cases can be useful in identifying hantavirus infection by detecting viral antigens.[434] Additionally, small fragments of virus genomic RNA can be detected by RT-PCT to establish a postmortem diagnosis of hantavirus infection.[157]

Prevention and Control

The primary means of preventing hantavirus infection is by reducing exposure to rodents. Effective measures include rodent-proofing homes, correctly storing food, airing seasonally closed cabins, and appropriately disinfecting and removing trapped rodents and rodent droppings.[139,170] In addition, public awareness and proactive public health educational efforts should target high-risk groups.[24,229] Yet for some occupations and for the residents of rural areas, avoiding rodent exposure is not an option. The lack of nosocomial and person-to-person transmission reported during virtually all hantavirus outbreaks (with the exception of ANDV) suggests that spread to medical personnel or case contacts is usually not a concern.

As for many viral infections, the development of a safe, effective, and inexpensive vaccine is needed.[344] However, the high genetic and antigenic diversity of hantaviruses poses a considerable challenge for the development of a multivalent, broadly protective vaccine that would be efficacious against most of the pathogenic hantaviruses. In addition, cross-protection vaccine studies are hard to perform, since currently animal models are available for only a few hantaviruses. A broad vaccine to prevent HFRS is needed purely because of the thousands of HFRS cases reported annually. Indeed, several different inactivated virus vaccines for HTNV and SEOV have been developed in Asia. These include antigens derived from virus-infected rodent brain and inactivated with formalin or beta-propiolactone. Upon vaccination, these antigens induce a weak neutralizing antibody response, and multiple booster doses are needed to elicit protective immunity.[167,367,427] Several monovalent and bivalent anti-HTNV and anti-SEOV tissue culture-derived inactivated vaccines have also been produced in China,[167] some of which may have high efficacy. In addition, a number of recombinant DNA approaches to vaccine development has been investigated.[343] The most advanced among them is a DNA vaccine composed of a mixture of HTNV and PUUV M segments; it was found to be safe and able to elicit neutralizing antibody responses in the majority of human participants in a phase I clinical trial.[168]

HPS caused by various hantaviruses remains a rare sporadic disease despite its high mortality rate. HPS vaccines can be useful against local epidemics but are unlikely to be broadly used because of the low frequency of HPS cases. This scenario could change in the future if the frequency of cases increases or if ANDV human-to-human transmission becomes more frequent. HPS prototype vaccines based on DNA and VSV platforms expressing the virus glycoproteins have shown promising results when tested in the hamster model.[59,319]

A neutralizing antibody response appears to be a strong correlate of protection from severe disease. Thus, passive immunotherapy has been tested as treatment for HFRS and acute HPS. Passive transfer of sera from convalescent patients has shown a modest survival benefit.[406] Recently, 2 potent neutralizing human monoclonal antibodies engineered from HPS patient sera have shown efficacy when administered as a monotherapy or as cocktail in the hamster model.[134] Similar results were also obtained using human polyclonal antibodies produced by DNA vaccination of transchromosomal bovines.[169] Antibody therapy could be developed as hantavirus disease treatment in the future.

Based on the hypothesis that HPS and HFRS are caused by an excessive host proinflammatory immune response, steroid treatments have been tested. However, in a double-blind, randomized controlled clinical trial in Chile, high concentration of methylprednisolone produced no significant clinical benefit in HPS patients in comparison to untreated controls, underscoring the complexity of this disease and the difficulty for successful immunotherapeutic intervention.[405] On the other hand, the immunotherapeutic icatibant, a bradykinin receptor antagonist, has been successfully used to treat 2 patients with severe PUUV infection.[14]

The only antiviral that has been used to treat hantavirus disease in humans is ribavirin. Ribavirin effectively suppressed HTNV replication in tissue culture and in animal models,[173] thereby promoting clinical trials in HFRS and HPS patients; promising results were reported in HFRS.[174,335] Although ribavirin treatment has shown activity against ANDV in an HPS animal model, no effect was seen in human trials in the United States and Chile when treatment was initiated during the symptomatic phase of infection.[78,264,338]

Current treatment of hantavirus disease is limited to intensive supportive care, including hemodialysis and mechanical ventilation. Extracorporeal membrane oxygenation, used in very severe cases of HPS in order to maintain a sufficient supply of oxygen, increased overall survival of patients.[420]

NAIROVIRIDAE

The most important human pathogen in the family Nairoviridae is CCHFV within the genus *Orthonairovirus*. Other Nairoviridae viruses of human concern are Dugbe virus (DUBV), Erve virus (ERVEV), and Nairobi sheep disease virus (NSDV). DUBV was first isolated in 1964 in Nigeria from *Amblyomma variegatum* ticks and causes a benign febrile illness in humans.[422] DUBV has been recovered from a wide range of ticks, domestic cattle, mosquitoes, and *Culicoides* in Western

Africa; however, serosurveys did not reveal wide spread human infections. ERVEV was isolated in 1982 from a white-toothed shrew (*Crocidura russula*) in the Erve river valley in northern France.[95] The virus has been found in Czech Republic, France, Germany, and the Netherlands. Very little is known about the involvement in human disease although it has been suspected to cause severe headache and intracerebral hemorrhage in humans. Nairobi sheep disease is a noncontagious, tick-borne infection of sheep and goats characterized by hemorrhagic gastroenteritis, abortion, and high mortality rates and is found in East and Central Africa. NSD virus has been isolated from sick patients in Uganda, as has the identical or closely related Ganjam virus from febrile patients in India, but their importance in terms of human disease is currently unclear.[253]

Crimean-Congo Hemorrhagic Fever Virus
Distribution and Significance

The human disease was first described as Crimean hemorrhagic fever (CHF) in 1944 in the Crimean peninsula, although the virus isolation took until 1967. In 1969, Jody Casals showed that an agent that had been isolated in the Belgian Congo (present Democratic Republic of the Congo, DRC) in 1956 and designated "Congo virus" was identical to CHF virus, leading to its current designation of CCHFV.[73] Today, we know that the virus is extensively distributed in wild and domestic animals, birds, and ticks through countries in Africa, Southeast Europe, the Middle East, Africa, and the Indian subcontinent (Fig. 17.5). As a result, CCHFV is the most widespread of all

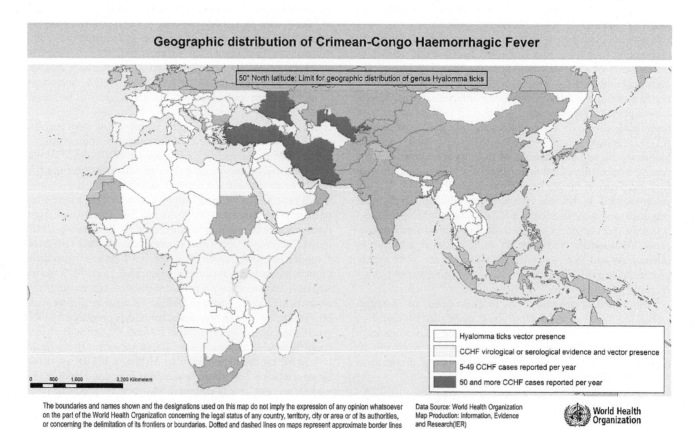

Geographic distribution of Crimean-Congo Haemorrhagic Fever

50° North latitude: Limit for geographic distribution of genus Hyalomma ticks

Hyalomma ticks vector presence

CCHF virological or serological evidence and vector presence

5-49 CCHF cases reported per year

50 and more CCHF cases reported per year

FIGURE 17.5 Geographic distribution of Crimean-Congo hemorrhagic fever virus (2017). (Figure © WHO 2017 All rights reserved.)

tick-borne viruses and second most widespread hemorrhagic fever virus after dengue virus. Nevertheless, human cases are typically sporadic and found in geographically circumscribed endemic foci within countries. The incidence of confirmed CCHF cases have markedly increased within the last two decades, Turkey, Iran, India, Southern Russia, and some Balkan countries. There is a concern about the increasing geographic spread of the disease illustrated by the recent report of CCHF cases in Spain.[370] It has been hypothesized that the increasing case numbers and geographic spread are a result of changes in environment and climate, land use/agricultural practices, and movement of livestock or migratory birds influencing the tick–virus–host dynamics ultimately changing the epidemiology of the disease.[35,120,121]

Epidemiology and Epizootiology

CCHFV transmitted to humans typically through tick bite or crushing of engorged tick and in some cases through direct contact with blood of viremic vertebrate hosts including livestock and humans (Fig. 17.6). In nature, CCHFV circulates in enzootic tick-vertebrate-tick cycle. Since neither the infected tick vector nor the infected vertebrate host show any signs of infection, this cycle perpetuates undetected. Ticks are virus vector and reservoir; once infected, they remain infected throughout their lifespans; the virus is maintained through transstadial (i.e., passing the virus through the various stages of the life

cycle, from larva to nymph to adult) and transovarial transmission (i.e., horizontal transmission to the next generation) in several species of ixodid (hard) ticks, accompanied by a seasonal bursts of amplification each spring and summer, when the ticks transmit the virus to mammals while taking the blood meals required for their maturation and for egg production (Fig. 17.6). The resulting viremia in mammalian animal hosts is transient. Humans are dead end hosts and the only host that shows overt signs of disease and human cases typically occur singly or sporadically in rural areas. The epidemiology of CCHFV reflects the complex ecology and geographic distribution of the ixodid tick hosts of the virus, particularly those of genus *Hyalomma*.[117,164] Although CCHFV has been isolated from approximately 30 different tick species, evidence is lacking as to whether they truly represent vectors or merely reflect the isolation of virus from engorged ticks that have fed on a viremic vertebrate host. Only some ticks of three genera, *Hyalomma, Dermacentor, and Rhipicephalus*, have actually been shown to be capable of transstadial transmission of CCHFV following feeding on a viremic host.[133] Transovarial transmission of CCHFV has also been shown to occur with some of the tick species in these genera. Moreover, the overall global pattern of geographic distribution of CCHFV cases corresponds most closely with the distribution of *Hyalomma* ticks, suggesting their principal role as vector.

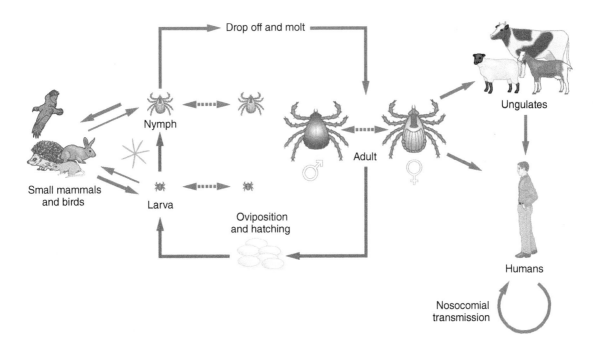

FIGURE 17.6 Life cycle of *Hyalomma* spp. ticks and vertical and horizontal transmission of CCHFV. The course of the tick life cycle is indicated with *blue arrows*. Upon hatching, larvae find a small animal host for their first blood meal (hematophagy). Depending on the tick species, the larvae either remain attached to their host following engorgement and molt in place (two-host ticks) or fall off and molt (three-host ticks); this transition is marked by an *asterisk*. The nymphs then either continue to feed on the animal on which they molted (two-host ticks) or attach to a new small animal (three-host ticks). Upon engorgement, nymphs of all species drop off their host and molt into adults. Adult ticks then find a large animal for hematophagy and mate while attached to the host. After taking a blood meal, the engorged females drop off and find a suitable location for ovipositing. During the tick life cycle, there are a number of opportunities for virus transmission between ticks and mammals (*solid red arrows*) and directly between ticks, through cofeeding (*dashed arrows*). For each form of virus transfer, the thickness of the *red arrow* indicates the efficiency of transmission. Infection of humans can occur through the bite of an infected tick or through exposure to the body fluids of a viremic animal or CCHF patient.

Reported CFR have been broad, ranging from 3% all the way to 100%. The variation in rates could be explained by differences in treatment, data sampling and diagnostics capabilities between outbreaks, as well as difference virulence of CCHFV strains. For instance, it has been suggested that the CCHFV strain AP92, originally isolated in and endemic in Greece, shows a lower virulence than other CCHFV strains due to the lack of clinical cases in Greece. Recently, strains very closely related to AP92 have been found in neighboring countries and have been detected in clinical cases. Turkey has overall the largest case numbers with a CFR just under 5%. CRFs in other countries for example Kosovo (34%) are higher. It is not known why this is the case.

Only limited information is available on CCHFV infections in special populations. CCHF appears to be associated with more severe disease in pregnant women with an overall CFR or 34%; however, the overall prevalence is very low and only few cases have been examined.[320] CCHFV infection of pregnant women can lead to spontaneous abortion, and the overall prognosis for the fetus is poor. The prevalence of CCHF in children is lower than in adults, and the disease is generally milder with lower fatality rates, although the full range of clinical features can be seen.[389] This might be due to the fact that the proinflammatory chemokine levels in children seemed to be not as often elevated as in adults.[18]

As one would expect based on the epidemiology, most cases are among individuals (e.g., shepherds, ranchers, and abattoir workers) living or working in close contact with livestock (e.g., sheep, goats, cattle, or ostriches) in endemic areas. Cases are usually start to occur in the early summer until early fall. Nosocomial outbreaks with cluster of cases have also been reported in several regions, with infection of medical personnel following treatment or surgery on an unsuspected CCHFV case.[35] This usually occurs when awareness of CCHF presents is low among medial personal not proper personal protective measures are taken.

Recent studies indicate that the human seroprevalence in enzootic areas of the disease can be as high as 90% with patients reporting no disease.[44,149,357] This could be an indicator for a much greater number of subclinical CCHFV infections as previously thought. A Russian study showed that one of every five infected people develops CCHF.[140]

The CCHFV genome has unique properties (see molecular chapter). For example, the M and L segment are significant larger than other bunyavirales and the function of many domains remains to be determined. CCHFV displays a great degree of sequence diversity among strains, with divergence of 20%, 22%, and 31% in the S, L, and M segments, respectively.[94] This suggests that significant genome and protein diversity is tolerated while maintaining fitness in the invertebrate vector and the vertebrate host. The sequence diversity is driven by genetic drift due to an error-prone polymerase as well as recombination and reassortment; although the latter two are considered rare events.[35,158] Reassortment and recombination could potentially have a significant influence on the virulence of CCHFV strains as described in a study from South Africa.[64] More subtle antigenic difference within the CCHFV group have been defined using monoclonal antibodies,[2] but it is unclear how such variation affect the virulence across or the cross-protection among viruses in vertebrate hosts.

Clinical Features

Although *Hyalomma* ticks feed on a range of vertebrate hosts, humans are the only species that have been described to show overt signs of disease. As discussed above, an indeterminate number of CCHFV infections in humans take their course asymptomatically or as a mild form.[44,149,357] Symptomatic CCHFV infections mostly take a characteristic course with four distinct phases: incubation, prehemorrhagic, hemorrhagic, and convalescence period (Fig. 17.7).[164] The incubation period likely depend on the mode of virus acquisition and viral dose and can range from 1 to 13 days. Following tick bite, the incubation period is usually short, up to 5 days.[35] However, determining the exact time when patient was bitten by a tick is difficult especially since tick saliva contains pharmacologically active substances that numb the bite site, and many tick bites go unnoticed. Humans can also become infected by crushing of engorged or semiengorged ticks percutaneously or through contact with mucous membranes. The incubation period following blood-borne transmissions from viremic animals or human patients most likely depends largely on the viral titers in the blood but is usually 5 to 7 days. No studies have defined the infectious dose or the stability of CCHFV in blood. Studies conducted in South Africa showed a time to onset of disease after exposure to tick bite was 3.2 days, 5 days following exposure to blood or tissue of livestock, and 5.6 days after exposure to blood of infected human beings.[378] The prehemorrhagic period is characterized by the sudden onset of fever (39°C–41°C), headache, malaise, myalgia, and dizziness, and in some patients nausea, diarrhea, and vomiting. Flushing of the face, neck, and chest, congested sclera, and conjunctivitis are also commonly noted.[197,274] Virus can be detected in the blood at this point. On average, the prehemorrhagic period lasts for 3 days (range: 1–7 days) and fever persists for 4 to 5 days.[117] The hemorrhagic period develops rapidly, usually begins between the 3 to 5 day of illness and is short (2–3 days). The first evidence is petechiae and ecchymosis in the skin and mucous membranes. Bleeding from other sites, including the vagina, gingival bleeding, and cerebral hemorrhage, have been reported.[197,378] The most common bleeding sites are the nose, gastrointestinal system (hematemesis, melena, and intra-abdominal), uterus (menometrorrhagia) and urinary tract (hematuria), and the respiratory tract (hemoptysis).[165,274] Atypical presentations of bleeding are also seen. Hepatomegaly and splenomegaly have been reported to be occurred in one-third of patients.[117,165] Several studies have shown that viral loads directly correlate with disease outcome and disease severity. Viral loads corresponding to greater than 10^8 genome equivalents/mL indicate a fatal outcome, while lower viral loads elicit a less severe disease course.[341] Deaths generally occur on day 5 to 14 of illness and are attributed to cardiovascular disturbances and multiorgan failure (MOF). The convalescence period usually begins in survivors about 10 to 20 days after the onset of illness and can take up to a year. During this period, generalized weakness, tachycardia, temporary hair loss, polyneuritis, difficulty breathing, xerostomia, impaired vision, hearing loss, and memory loss have been reported.[378] Thrombocytopenia, leukopenia and raised levels of aspartate aminotransferase (AST), alanine aminotransferase (ALT), lactate dehydrogenase (LDH) are hallmark features of CCHF infection. Furthermore, coagulation tests such as prothrombin time and activated partial thromboplastin (APTT)

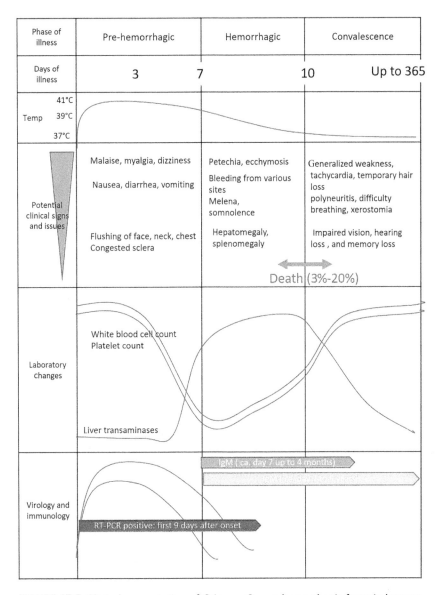

Phase of illness	Pre-hemorrhagic	Hemorrhagic	Convalescence

FIGURE 17.7 Clinical presentation of Crimean-Congo hemorrhagic fever in humans.
See text for detailed description.

time are prolonged. In some patients, DIC develops. In that case, platelet counts fall significant further and the level of fibrin degradation products and D-dimers increases. Clinical data indicate that viral load, thrombocytopenia, elevated prothrombin time ratio, and APTT likely play a central role in disease progression and severity.[104,341] No standardized case definition exists internationally and many countries have their own case definitions.[251]

Pathogenesis and Pathology

We only have a very limited understanding of the pathogenesis of the disease mainly due to sporadic nature of human cases, the requirement to work in maximum biocontainment with the virus, and the lack of suitable animal models. What is known is pieced together from a clinical pathology and biomarker studies in patients during the course of the disease and a very limited number of necropsies. Findings from cell culture studies and immunocompromised animal studies lend some support to the

findings and fill few knowledge gaps.[35] One of the big questions in CCHF research remains while in contrast to the inapparent infection characteristic of CCHFV infection of other vertebrate hosts, human infections often result in severe hemorrhagic fever. The sequence of events in those severe cases is largely as follows (Fig. 17.8). During attachment and feeding, the tick will introduce the virus into the skin. It is unknown when the tick after attachment will transmit the virus, and what virus titers are transmitted.[133] Studies with other tick-borne pathogens have shown that the immunomodulatory components in the tick saliva that facilitate tick attachment can be exploited by the pathogen to enhance infection.[289] This might explain a shorter incubation period after tick bite compared to human-to-human transmission; however, it remains to be determined for CCHFV as there are certain confounding factors, for example, tick bites go unnoticed sometimes. In addition to tick bite, CCHFV can also be transmitted from contact with the blood of infected animals during the slaughter process, through

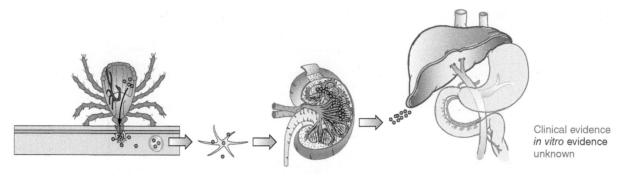

Clinical evidence
in vitro evidence
unknown

FIGURE 17.8 Transmission and dissemination of CCHFV after tick bite. CCHFV is introduced into the skin through tick bite. It is unclear at what time after tick attachment the virus is transmitted and how much virus is transmitted. Initial cell targets are most likely dermal dendritic cells, Langerhans cells, and in the skin residing macrophages in which the virus replicates. From here, the virus most likely spreads to the local draining lymph node; however, hematogenous spread is conceivable as well. The role of tick saliva in this process and if the dissemination occurs through free or cell bound virus remains unknown. Subsequent to local replication, the virus will spread systemically targeting cells in liver and spleen as well as myeloid cells in the blood where secondary replication occurs.

crushing of engorging ticks feeding on animals, or in a nosocomial setting.[117] On introduction of the virus into the dermis or mucosa, there is likely local primary replication mainly in resident mononuclear phagocytes followed by blood- and lymph-borne spread of the virus either in infected cells or not cell associated to the major organs where secondary replication occurs.[85,310,333] From there the virus is seeded back into the bloodstream to cause viremia. At this point, virus can also be shed from the blood into saliva and urine.[45] Little is known regarding host cell receptor use or factors driving cell and tissue tropism in the host. The systemic spread of CCHFV is aided by the virus ability to evade or suppress the innate immune response (see molecular chapter for more details).[417] The liver seems to be the main target organ in the systemic phase, where high levels of replication take place.[379] Histopathologic studies have been limited to a small number of human cases.[65,189] The most consistent microscopic changes in the liver tissues were eosinophilic necrosis, Councilman bodies, and Kupffer cell hyperplasia.[65,189] A spectrum of severity of hepatic damage was identified ranging from mild necrosis with occasional Councilman bodies to more severe necrosis with extensive damage of hepatic lobules (Fig. 17.9). Hepatic injury is also reflected by high levels of transaminases in the blood of patient during the hemorrhagic phase. Viral antigen could be detected focally in hepatocytes and Kupffer cells (Fig. 17.10). The main findings in other tissues included prominent splenic lymphoid apoptosis and depletion, and interstitial pneumonia. CCHFV was also detected in endothelial cells. Congestion, edema, and focal hemorrhage and necrosis are seen in most organs. Many of these findings have been supported by studies in immunocompromised mice, which model rather the most severe form of the disease.[34,36,442] Proinflammatory cytokines play a key role in the pathogenesis and severity of the disease. A range of clinical studies measured elevated levels of number of cytokines and chemokines in the blood of CCHF patients with TNF-α, IL-6, IL-8, and IL-10 being associated with severe disease.[300] These findings are by *in vitro* and *in vivo* studies. This suggests that a host-driven inflammatory response, mediated through an imbalance in cytokine and chemokine production, is the cause of severe disease progression. Proinflammatory cytokines, platelet aggregation, and activation of the intrinsic coagulation

cascade probably lead to an altered vascular function making bleeding in different organs common in CCHF patients. Increased levels of vascular adhesion markers such as ICAM-1 and VCAM-1 have been detected in cell culture studies as well as in clinical studies.[21,86] The humoral and cell-mediated immune responses to clear CCHFV infection remain poorly defined. One study showed higher levels of NK cells in CCHF patients with severe disease, whereas another study contradicted these findings and found higher levels of cytotoxic T cells instead.[4,428] Both IgM and IgG antibodies are usually detectable

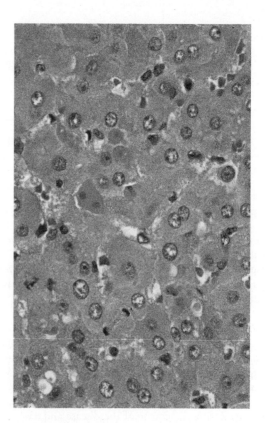

FIGURE 17.9 Multicellular hepatic necrosis. (Courtesy of Dr. Sherif Zaki, CDC, Atlanta.)

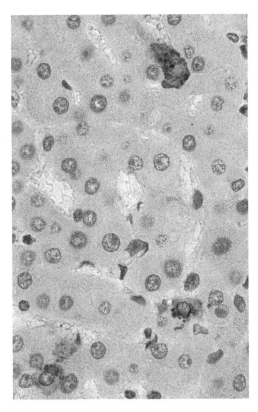

FIGURE 17.10 Immunohistochemistry of human liver. CCHFV antigen in hepatocytes in *red.* (Courtesy of Dr. Sherif Zaki, CDC, Atlanta.)

approximately 5 to 7 days after the onset of illness and reach maximum levels in survivors by the 2nd or the 3rd week after disease onset and are detectable until at least 3 years after infection.[35,76] Antibody responses are rarely detectable in fatal cases. Lastly, it has been suggested that genetic makeup such as HLA type or polymorphisms in TLR10 or IFNA expression could play a role in the disease severity.[3,114,202] Recently, an immunocompetent nonhuman primate model was reported in which cynomolgus macaques infected with CCHFV hallmark signs of human CCHF with remarkably similar viral dissemination, organ pathology, and disease progression as humans.[151] This model holds a lot of promise to fill knowledge gaps and needs to be further evaluated.

Diagnosis
Differential
Clinical differential diagnosis of CCHFV varies in the different regions where the disease is known to occur and can be difficult in early stages. In general, the disease can be suspected for patients presenting with a rapid onset of severe influenza-like symptoms and known exposure to tick bite or contact with blood or tissues of potentially infected livestock or humans. The early stages can be confused with sandfly fevers in regions where the diseases overlap, and leptospirosis, Omsk hemorrhagic fever, other viral hemorrhagic fevers (yellow fever, HFRS, Ebola), tick typhus, and mycotoxicoses can appear similar in the more advanced hemorrhagic phase of the illness. Although presentation is not pathognomonic, clinical values can be helpful in diagnosis when CCHF is suspected,

with leukopenia, thrombocytopenia, and elevated liver enzymes frequently being present early in the disease.[117,379]

Laboratory
Due to the requirement of high or maximum biocontainment laboratories to work with CCHFV, virus isolation is only used when facilities are available and is not the typical used to for the first-line diagnosis since it is also time consuming.[35] CCHFV antigen detection ELISAs from patient acute phase sera have been developed and are also performed.[35,62,117] For CCHFV isolation, i.c. or intraperitoneal inoculation of patient acute phase blood samples into newborn mice is probably most sensitive, although quicker results can be obtained by inoculation into susceptible tissue culture cells, such as Vero cells, followed by fluorescent antibody staining.[352] Rapid laboratory diagnosis of CCHFV can be achieved by nucleic acid detection and several RT-PCR, real-time RT-qPCRs, and Lamp assays have been developed.[47,63,103,135,240,293] Advantageous is that the sample can be inactivated before the assay is conducted. Commercial kits are used in some countries, but most countries rely on in-house established assays, and there is no internationally standardized nucleic acid test.[125] The virus, its genome, and antigen are usually detectable up to 1 to 2 weeks after onset of illness. Serological diagnostic is typically done by ELISA or indirect fluorescence assay (IFA), and several serological assays for human or animal sera have been developed.[125,297,340] Fatal cases rarely show significant antibody responses. However, in those destined to survive, IgM and IgG antibodies are frequently detectable after about a week of illness. Studies have shown that IgM can be detected up to 4 months and IgG is detectable for at least 3 years.[117]

Prevention and Control
Prevention
There is no vaccine against CCHF available for humans or animals, and anti-Hyalomma tick vaccine is currently available. Prevention therefore is to minimize exposure to the virus by avoiding tick exposure in endemic areas. Treatment of clothing with pyrethroid preparations, which repels and even kills ticks, is highly recommended for those persons likely to come into contact with CCHFV-infected ticks (e.g., slaughterhouse workers, sheep shearers, veterinarians, and others involved with livestock). In addition, habits that avoid virus-contaminated blood or tissues contacting the skin should be practiced (e.g., wearing of gloves and avoiding crushing ticks with fingers). Medical personnel should practice standard barrier-nursing techniques during care of suspected CCHFV patients.

Treatment
Most CCHF cases occur in rural areas often with low infrastructure. Treatment of those patients is by means of supportive and replacement therapy with blood products. When available, ribavirin treatment has been suggested and has been used to treat CCHF patients for more than three decades. Experimental tissue culture and mouse infections have shown that CCHFV susceptibility to ribavirin treatment. Studies have generally found that ribavirin is beneficial, so long as it is initiated early in the course of illness.[118,119,381] Nevertheless, recent meta-analysis studies question the therapeutic benefit of ribavirin creating uncertainty of its use as a treatment.[186,363] As a result, some investigators have called for randomized controlled

trials to be conducted. Two recent animal studies looked at Favipiravir (T-705) treatment and found it to be more efficient than ribavirin,[156,292] making it an interesting new candidate for treatment. There are limited reports on other experimental treatments such as ribavirin combined with plasma exchange transfusion, steroids, or double plasmapheresis with inconclusive results. Administration of immune plasma has been tried on numerous occasions, but its usefulness remains unclear.[148,179,215]

Vaccines

A chloroform-inactivated vaccine prepared from virus-infected suckling mouse brains was developed in the former Soviet Union in 1970 and was used in parts of Eastern Europe. The vaccine is currently licensed in Bulgaria and is given to high-risk personnel in endemic areas such as military personnel as well as medical and agricultural workers. Although the Bulgarian ministry of health reported a four-fold decrease in the incidence of the disease in two decades due to the vaccine, its efficacy remains still not well characterized. Furthermore, it requires a three booster vaccination, and a mouse brain-derived formulation raise concerns about side effects.[102] Multiple CCHFV vaccines have been developed experimentally, with vaccine types such as inactivated whole/purified virus, virus-like particles, vectored vaccines relying on vaccinia and adenovirus platforms, plasmid-based DNA vaccines, and subunit vaccines relying on either plant or insect produced antigens. With few exceptions, these vaccines have all been evaluated with a prime and boost (or multiboost) strategy along with the subunit and inactivated whole virus strategies containing adjuvants. Many of these listed vaccines have been evaluated in either BALB/c, STAT1 K/O, or IFNAR mice, though a consensus animal model for vaccine testing has not yet been established. Immune correlates of protection in these various vaccination strategies, antigenic targets, and animal models have not been uniform and therefore remains largely unknown. The predominant antigenic target has been whole or components of the glycoprotein precursor with 100% protection observed in vaccinia vectors, though a tandem nucleoprotein plus glycoprotein approach with DNA vaccines and an adenovirus vectored nucleoprotein only have both achieved >70% protection, suggesting both glycoprotein and nucleoprotein components are viable antigenic targets.[102] The lack of an immunocompetent animal model has made the assessment of vaccine candidates difficult. Moreover, immune correlates of protection not very well defined, and recent studies show that in addition to neutralizing, also non-neutralizing antibodies and the cellular response play a crucial role. The sporadic CCHF outbreaks in rural areas raises questions about the feasibility of a human vaccine. Therefore, One Health approaches using reservoir-targeted approaches through veterinary vaccines and acaricides have been suggested.

PERIBUNYAVIRIDAE, GENUS ORTHOBUNYAVIRUS

The *Orthobunyavirus* genus is a large genus containing 49 viral species based on the latest proposed taxonomy of the ICTV. However, the viruses can also be distinguished into 18 serogroups based on neutralization (NT), hemagglutination inhibition (HI), and complex fixation assays. Here, we group the viruses based on serogroups. Medically, the most important viruses such as Oropouche virus (OROV), La Crosse virus (LACV), and Jamestown Canyon virus (JCV) can be found in the Bunyamwera, California, and Simbu serogroups. This section will focus on these three serogroups since they contain members that medically most relevant.

Distribution and Significance

Most orthobunyaviruses are transmitted by mosquitoes, although a few have been isolated from tabanids, phlebotomines, ticks, and bedbugs, and have been found in every continent except Antarctica.[316]

Epidemiology

California Serogroup Viruses

LACV is the most significant of the California encephalitis serogroup viruses in terms of causing human disease in the United States, with 60 to 100 cases per year, predominantly in children younger than 15 years of age. There is, however, severe underreporting.[153,187] The primary vector is the forest-dwelling, tree-hole–breeding mosquito, *Aedes triseriatus*, although more recently, and concerning, the virus has also been isolated from the aggressive day-feeding Asian tiger-mosquito, *Aedes albopictus*.[224] *A. triseriatus* is found throughout the northern Midwestern and Northeastern United States, and LACV is maintained in these mosquitoes by transovarial transmission, which allows overwintering of the virus in mosquito eggs.[416] During the summer months, squirrels, chipmunks, foxes, and woodchucks become viremic following LACV infection and are important amplifying hosts.[391,433] The majority of La Crosse encephalitis cases occur in the summer and early fall months when risk of bite from infected female mosquitoes is highest. Historically, LACV infections mostly occurred in the Mississippi and Ohio river basins, with more than 90% of cases coming from Wisconsin, Minnesota, Iowa, Indiana, Ohio, and Illinois,[316] but since the 1980s, more cases have been reported from Appalachia and eastern Tennessee, and between 1987 and 2009, more than 30% of total cases in the United States were from West Virginia.[153] JCV (including the closely related Jerry Slough variety) is also associated with arboviral encephalitis in the United States. The virus is vectored by *Culex inornata* mosquitoes, and several species of Aedes mosquitoes, and is broadly distributed across much of North America. Vertical transmission of the virus has been demonstrated in several Aedes species mosquitoes.[154] White-tailed deer are the most likely vertebrate amplifying host.

Bunyamwera Serogroup Viruses

Bunyamwera virus is present throughout much of sub-Saharan Africa and appears to be an important cause of acute febrile illness in humans. The virus has been isolated from humans in Uganda, Nigeria, and South Africa.[142,206] More recently, Ngari virus has been identified as a reassortant BUNV. This reassortant virus has been associated with hemorrhagic fever cases in Somalia and Kenya and a large outbreak of acute febrile illness in Sudan.[53,57] In addition, human antibodies reactive with BUNV have been detected in most of sub-Saharan Africa, with high prevalence (up to 82%) being recorded in some locations.[361] Isolation of the virus from several Aedes species mosquitoes has implicated them as the primary vector.[206,361] Antibodies reactive with BUNV have been detected in domestic animals, nonhuman primates, rodents, and birds, and viremias capable of supporting mosquito transmission have been recorded in experimentally infected rodents, bats, and primates.[355,361] However, the role of a potential vertebrate amplifying host is currently unclear. Several additional Bunyamwera serogroup viruses are present in the Americas[281] and are infrequently reported to cause acute febrile illness in humans. Cache Valley virus is found throughout the United States, Canada, and Mexico and often infects sheep and possibly all ruminants; infections have been associated with embryonic and fetal death, stillbirths, and multiple congenital malformations in sheep.[112,258] The virus has caused a fatal encephalitis in a human.[350] It remains unclear whether Cache Valley and serologically closely related viruses may play a role in syndromes of congenital malformations and embryonic losses in humans in North America.[67]

Simbu Serogroup Viruses

Simbu serogroup viruses are global in distribution and are principally vectored by biting midges of the genus *Culicoides*. Since the original isolation of OROV from a febrile patient in Trinidad in the 1950s, the medical importance of the virus has become increasingly evident.[395] OROV has a wide geographic distribution in tropical regions of the Americas. It has been isolated from humans in Panama, Venezuela, Bolivia, and northern Argentina. It is probably much more common than reported, because of its similar clinical presentation to dengue, Zika, and other diseases causing acute nonspecific febrile illnesses. Between 1960 and 2009, at least 500,000 people are thought to have been infected in more than 30 outbreaks.[402] Most of these outbreaks were in relatively urban areas, leading to the suggestion that there are likely separate urban and sylvatic cycles.[97,332] The principal rural vector in Brazil appears to be the tiny biting midge, *Culicoides paraensis*,[313,332] which breeds in rotting vegetative matter, and seasonal populations can become high in agricultural areas, where build-up of debris such as banana tree stalks or cacao husks may occur (Fig. 17.11).[314]

These midges feed predominantly in the early evening hours and are quite anthropophilic. Infected humans develop viremia sufficiently high to transmit the virus to uninfected midges and appear capable of serving as the vertebrate amplifying host during urban epidemics.[314,395] Serologic data also suggest that primates or sloths, or even birds, may be potential hosts in the sylvatic cycle. There are well-documented outbreaks of OROV in urban areas associated with both *C. paraensis* and *Culex quinquefasciatus* (Fig. 17.11). The virus has

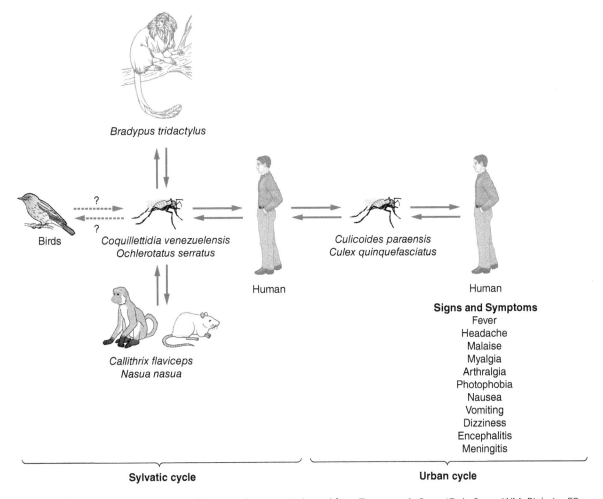

Bradypus tridactylus

Birds

Coquillettidia venezuelensis
Ochlerotatus serratus

Callithrix flaviceps
Nasua nasua

Human

Culicoides paraensis
Culex quinquefasciatus

Human

Signs and Symptoms
Fever
Headache
Malaise
Myalgia
Arthralgia
Photophobia
Nausea
Vomiting
Dizziness
Encephalitis
Meningitis

Sylvatic cycle   **Urban cycle**

FIGURE 17.11 Transmission cycles of Oropouche virus. (Adapted from Travassos da Rosa JF, de Souza WM, Pinheiro FP, et al. Oropouche virus: clinical, epidemiological, and molecular aspects of a neglected orthobunyavirus. *Am J Trop Med Hyg* 2017;96(5):1019–1030.)

been isolated repeatedly from *C. quinquefasciatus*, and experimental bite transmission has been demonstrated experimentally in this mosquito. Recent phylogenetic studies indicate that four distinct OROV lineages are present in different geographic areas, and that OROV emerged in Brazil in around 1790.[402]

Akabane virus (AKAV) is widely distributed throughout Australasia (Australia, Japan, Korea, Taiwan), the Middle East (occasionally extending as far north as Turkey), and sub-Saharan Africa.[5,11,91] The virus is an important cause of disease in livestock, with periodic outbreaks of abortions, stillbirths, and congenital malformations recorded in cattle, sheep, and goats in Australia, Japan, Korea, Taiwan, Israel, and Turkey, although intriguingly no disease outbreaks have been observed in Africa, despite the widespread presence of the virus.[5] The virus is vectored by midges of the genus *Culicoides*, and although *C. brevitarsis* is the primary vector in Australia,[277] different species are important in Asia and the Middle East.[6,183,217] Unlike LACV, which mainly causes encephalitis in children, JCV appears to predominantly cause disease in adults, although only 15 human cases have been reported since 2004.[330] No information on age depends is available for OROV.

Morbidity/Mortality

For most of the orthobunyavirus infections, no mortality has been reported. Nevertheless, due to the small case numbers, and for some with limited geographic range, under reporting is possible. Cases are usually sporadic. However, several thousand cases of acute febrile illness can occur during OROV epidemics observed throughout the Amazon basin regions of Brazil and Peru.

Clinical Features

The California serogroup viruses, LACV, Jamestown Canyon, and the prototype California encephalitis virus all cause a similar encephalitic disease in humans.[336] Indeed, due to serologic cross-reactivity, many of the early disease descriptions of California encephalitis cases were likely due to JCV or LACV rather than California encephalitis virus, which is now known to be less common.[69] The major difference between the viruses is in age dependence of the spectrum of clinical disease observed, in that LACV infections tend to be more severe in children, whereas JCV infection is more severe in adults. The spectrum of disease ranges from inapparent or mild febrile disease through to fatal encephalitis.[81,261,392] The incubation period is approximately 3 to 7 days. Most cases report sudden onset of fever, followed by stiff neck, lethargy, headache, and nausea and vomiting, and symptoms usually end within 7 days. Approximately half the cases exhibit seizures, and up to 30% develop coma and exhibit a longer disease course. About 65% of patients have meningitis on presentation, with both mononuclear and polymorphonuclear cells present in cerebrospinal fluid. Despite mild neurological symptoms often present at the time of patient discharge, surprisingly little residua is found. The most important sequela is epilepsy, which is observed in approximately 10% to 15% of children, and these are almost always patients who had seizures during acute phase of illness. In addition, about 2% of patients have persistent paresis.[81,152,261]

For OROV, the incubation period is approximately 4 to 8 days, followed by sudden onset of fever, with arthralgia, myalgia, severe headache, chills, photophobia, and prostration. Occasionally, rash, meningitis, or meningismus is seen.[275,315,395] Most of the symptoms resolve within 3 to 5 days, although the myalgia may last 1 or 2 weeks. Viremia is detectable in the majority of patients 2 to 3 days after onset of illness. Approximately half of the patients can exhibit recurrence of some disease symptoms 1 to 10 days after initial recovery.[315,395] OROV is also suspected to be infectious by aerosol, based on reported laboratory infections.[313]

Pathogenesis and Pathology

Human infections with California encephalitis, LACV, or JCV viruses are initiated by the bite of a virus-infected mosquito. The course of the infection has been extensively modeled in mice.[302] Similar to the human infection, the outcome of the infection in mice is dependent on the age of the animal and strain of virus used, with subcutaneous challenge of newborn mice most closely mimicking the natural human infection. The virus initially spreads from the site of inoculation into striated muscle, which is the major site of replication. It spreads to the plasma, presumably through the lymphatic channels, and the resulting high viremia allows the virus to cross the blood–brain barrier.[181] Mice inoculated intraperitoneally with LACV showed high levels of replication in nasal turbinates, suggesting the virus could enter the central nervous system (CNS) by olfactory neurons.[33] Once in the CNS, the virus replicates in neurons and glial cells, causing considerable neuronal necrosis. Death occurs 3 or 4 days postinfection. In contrast, although rhesus monkeys were highly susceptible to LACV infection, the animals remained asymptomatic and developed neutralizing antibodies.[33] High viremia is essential for neuroinvasion. A monoclonal antibody escape mutant of LACV (V22) showed decreased replication in striated muscle, and hence did not generate sufficient viremia to permit neuroinvasion, but V22 was as neurovirulent as wild-type LACV when inoculated intracranially.[143] A similar distinction between neurovirulence and neuroinvasiveness is implied from observations on recombinant LACV with mutations in the fusion peptide domain of Gc, which showed reduced replication in muscle cells but retained the ability to cause neuronal loss in culture.[365] The lesions observed in the brains of fatal La Crosse encephalitis cases differ from those in infected suckling mice. In humans, and to a large extent in adult mice infected intracerebrally, cerebral edema, perivascular cuffing, glial nodules, mild leptomeningitis, and occasional areas of focal necrosis that are typical of acute severe viral encephalitis are observed. Lesions are mostly in the cerebral cortex, with some in the brainstem.[190] Studies with Tahyna virus and JCV showed strain differences in neuroinvasiveness and neurovirulence in a Swiss Webster mouse model, whereas in rhesus monkeys, no clinical disease was observed but the animals mounted strong neutralizing antibody responses.[31,32]

Infection of natural vertebrate amplifying hosts of these viruses, such as adult chipmunks (LACV) or snowshoe hares (snowshoe hare virus), results in inapparent infection and viremia sufficient to infect mosquitoes.[351] *A. triseriatus* mosquitoes are the principal vector of LACV, and their experimental infection with California encephalitis serogroup viruses has been studied in detail.[29,386,390,415] Viruses ingested via a viremic bloodmeal infect the epithelial layer surrounding the mosquito midgut. Replication of the virus results in release of the virus across the basal lamina into the hemocele, allowing transport of the virus to tissues throughout the body. Virus infection of mosquitoes other than the principal vector species usually results in poor penetration of the virus across this midgut barrier. Experimental infections using reassortant viruses have shown that virus M genomic segment (encoding the glycoproteins and NSm protein) is an important component in the correct match between virus and host mosquito, which allows efficient transit across the midgut barrier.[29] Once across the barrier, virus replication occurs in a wide variety of tissues, including the ovaries and salivary glands.[386] Release of virus from the salivary glands allows virus transmission from the female mosquito to the vertebrate host during feeding. Mosquitoes begin to be infectious approximately 1 or 2 weeks after ingestion of virus, an interval referred to as the extrinsic incubation period.

The infection of the ovaries is thought to be crucial for virus maintenance in mosquito populations, in that it results in transovarial transmission of the virus from the female to the offspring and allows the virus to overwinter in infected eggs.[416] In addition, LACV-infected females appear to mate more efficiently than uninfected mosquitoes.[131] Male mosquitoes play no role in the vertical transovarial transmission of the virus, or in the horizontal transmission via amplifying vertebrate hosts, as they do not take a bloodmeal. However, the virus is detected in the gonads of transovarially infected males and can result in venereal transmission of the virus horizontally within the mosquito population.[390] This combination of transmission mechanisms allows efficient maintenance of the LACV in *A. triseriatus* populations. Similar processes are thought to function in host mosquito infections with other California serogroup viruses,[397] and results from studies with these viruses and their arthropod hosts serve as a model for understanding virus maintenance and transmission mechanisms for other Bunyavirales viruses.

Aino and AKAV are important causes of disease in livestock, causing epizootics of abortions and congenital defects in cattle, sheep, and goats.[200,201,396] Experimental infections of pregnant cattle or ewes with either virus have been shown to produce viremia, followed by virus replication in the placenta and fetal tissues, and resulting in congenital defects such as microencephaly and hydrocephalus.[201,303,396] Similarly, experimental infection of pregnant hamsters with AKAV results in death of the fetus.[12]

Natural reassortment among orthobunyaviruses is important as it confounds serology and classification of viruses in the genus.[58] A striking example is Ngari virus, a human pathogenic virus in Africa. Ngari virus was isolated during a large human hemorrhagic fever outbreak in 1997 in East Africa.[53] A genetic analysis revealed that Ngari virus is a naturally occurring reassortant between Bunyamwera virus (S and L segment) and Batai virus (M segment).[57] These two viruses do not cause a hemorrhagic disease in humans. As illustrated with Ngari, reassortants may be phylogenetically quite similar to other viruses but quite different phenotypically.

Diagnosis
Laboratory
A wide variety of assays have been used in the diagnosis of infections with viruses of the genus *Orthobunyavirus*, including complement fixation (CF), hemagglutination inhibition (HI), neutralization (NT), immunofluorescence assay, IgM capture ELISA, and RT-PCR.[66,107,146,216,223,321] Diagnosis of California serogroup virus infections relies on serologic methods, as the virus is generally absent from blood or secretions during the

phase of CNS disease. The HI test is considerably more sensitive for these viruses than CF, but NT assay or RT-PCR coupled with multiplex nucleotide sequencing is needed for confirmation and subtype identification.[222] The IgM capture ELISA works well for diagnosis of most infections by viruses of the genus *Orthobunyavirus* but has not been widely applied to date.[107,176,350] Virus isolation attempts complement serologic and genetic assays and is best achieved by intracerebral (i.c.) inoculation of suckling mice or infection of susceptible cells such as Vero cells.

Prevention and Control
Prevention and control is difficult for the mosquito-borne California and Bunyamwera serogroup viruses due to the widespread presence of the mosquito vector hosts and relatively sporadic nature of the associated human or livestock diseases. No vaccines are available for human-infecting orthobunyaviruses. Broad application of insecticides, as carried out in earlier decades, is no longer ecologically acceptable. Relative to human disease, use of fine mesh netting and personal protectants containing *N,N*-diethyl-meta-toluamide (DEET) are highly recommended in areas with high risk of people being bitten by virus-infected mosquitoes. Similar vector control challenges exist for the Simbu serogroup viruses vectored by *Culicoides* midges. With the OROV disease in Brazil and Peru, avoiding the build-up of rotting organic debris such as banana tree stalks or cacao husks in agricultural areas may help curtail population levels of *C. paraensis* and reduce the risk of seasonal epidemics.[314] Avoiding exposure (treated netting, DEET repellents) to these midges during their early evening feeding hours is also recommended. Similar protective measures are recommended for AKAV. In addition, a successful formalin-inactivated AKAV vaccine has been developed in Japan using virus-infected hamster lung cell cultures, and a trivalent-inactivated vaccine protective against AKAV, Aino virus (AINOV), and Chuzan orbivirus has been successfully trialed in Korea.[200] With knowledge of the distribution and seasonality of AKAV disease outbreaks, vaccination of at risk animals prior to pregnancy is feasible.

PHENUIVIRIDAE, GENUS PHLEBOVIRUS

Rift Valley Fever and Sandfly Group
Pathogenesis and Pathology
Sandfly fever disease is a febrile and occasionally encephalitic illness caused by viruses belonging to the *Phlebovirus* genus, family Phenuiviridae, which are harbored by phlebotomine sandflies. The main viruses currently known to cause sandfly fever are sandfly fever Sicilian virus (SFSV), sandfly fever Naples virus (SFNV), and Toscana virus (TOSV). Outbreaks of human disease have been identified as early as 1900s in the Mediterranean region. The only known reservoir of these viruses is the competent adult sandfly. There is no direct evidence of a vertebrate reservoir, although antibodies against all sandfly-borne phleboviruses have been detected in a number of animals in the Mediterranean region.[269] *In vitro* experiments have shown that human monocyte-derived dendritic cells and endothelial cells can be productively infected by TOSV and secrete proinflammatory cytokines.[90] Increased proinflammatory and

anti-inflammatory cytokine levels have been reported in cerebrospinal fluid of patients with TOSV encephalitic disease.[401] A specific antibody response develops rapidly in human infection and is long-lasting against TOSV. Moderate levels of neutralizing antibodies are maintained for more than a year.[311]

More is known about the pathogenesis and disease of another phlebovirus, mosquito-borne RVFV.[39,50,262] RVFV infections of livestock are often recognized by the onset of "abortion storms" that sweep through livestock-producing areas, with simultaneous acute febrile disease in humans. Humans are infected with RVFV either by mosquito bite or exposure to infected animals. Most RVFV infections in humans result in mild febrile illness, with about 1% to 2% of cases progressing to severe disease. Rift Valley fever (RVF) can present with varying degrees of symptoms, ranging from no symptoms or mild influenza-like illness to severe disease with hepatitis, retinitis, or encephalitis. Direct human-to-human transmission, including nosocomial transmission, has not been observed.[7]

Data from experimental infections and analogies from other arbovirus infections suggest that macrophages and dendritic cells are likely among the first cells infected by RVFV.[141,260] Subsequently, RVFV is transported by lymphatic drainage to the regional lymph node, where local viral replication takes place. The virus then enters the blood, causing primary viremia and spreading to the major organs. The main target organ of RVFV is the liver, and hepatic necrosis is prominent in severe cases. Replication in the lymph nodes, spleen, liver, adrenals, lungs, and kidneys results in high viremia. Viral load is prognostic of disease outcome: viral loads are 1 to 2 logs higher in patients who succumb to infection than in survivors.[38]

A small percentage of patients with severe disease develops retinitis and/or encephalitis 1 to 3 weeks after the onset of illness, and necrotic foci can be observed in the brain.[271] How RVFV reaches immune-privileged sites like the eye and brain is not known. One possible explanation is that the virus enters the peripheral nervous system and later replicates and spreads through either the systemic or neural route into the CNS, resulting in encephalitis. Disruption of the blood–brain barrier occurs in the late stages of infection, after the virus has been actively replicating inside the CNS.[412]

RVFV replication in cells is highly cytopathic, suggesting that most of the cellular destruction observed in acute illness is likely due to the virus directly killing host cells. In hemorrhagic RVF cases, a complex interaction exists between the virus and both fibrinolytic and coagulation pathways, with increased levels of tissue plasminogen and D-dimers indicative of ongoing fibrinolysis, and decreased levels of P-selectin, ADAMTS13, and fibrinogen during the acute phase of disease.[92] The RVFV NSs protein is a major virulence factor that allows the virus to escape the host innate immune response by down-regulating type I IFN response and shutting down host cell transcription.[243] In both animal models and human cases of RVF, failure to induce an early type I IFN immune response results in severe disease; in NHP models, survival is improved by administration of IFN-α.[270] Patients who succumb to disease often fail to generate RVFV-specific humoral immunity.[38] A strong innate immune response, followed by the generation of high-titer neutralizing antibodies, is currently considered to be a correlate of protection. The role of T cells during human RVFV infection is unclear. In experimental encephalitis in NHPs, survival correlated with higher numbers of activated CD4 and CD8 T cells.[424] Additionally, depleting T cells can worsen the development of RVF encephalitis.[98,155] However, dysregulation of the immune response may contribute to RVFV pathogenesis, and an uncontrolled inflammatory response to RVFV infection correlates with fatal outcome.[180,259,260]

As indicated above, clinical presentation of RVF varies greatly, likely due to a number of factors. The virus dose and route of exposure may contribute to the disease outcome. Epidemiological studies have shown that direct exposure to sick animals, which usually harbor high viral loads, could lead to severe disease with hemorrhage and encephalitis.[17,248] Experimental intranasal or aerosol infections lead to enhanced neurovirulence with a rapid replication of the virus in the CNS.[100,412]

Human genetic factors could also influence disease progression. Polymorphisms in human genes of the innate immune system have been shown to play a role in disease severity.[159,219] Other underlying conditions and coinfections, like HIV infection, have also been associated with disease severity and fatal outcome.[266]

Susceptibility of livestock to RVFV infection varies considerably depending on a variety of factors, including livestock species and age and the strain of the virus. Pathologic features of the disease in livestock also differ significantly. Leukopenia is frequently seen during the first 3 or 4 days of infection, when fever and viremia are usually highest. Altered serum enzyme levels (e.g., aspartate aminotransferase and sorbitol dehydrogenase), indicative of hepatocyte destruction, are often seen during the acute phase. Leukocytosis frequently occurs in the early phase of recovery. Thrombocytopenia and fibrin thrombi in several organs suggest that disseminated intravascular coagulopathy (DIC) may be a feature of severe disease in livestock, as seen in hemorrhagic infections in humans.[87,377]

RVFV infection of pregnant animals frequently results in abortion of the fetus, and the ability of the virus to cross the placenta to infect the fetus is well documented. Abortions early in the course of infection are probably the result of the high fever associated with the acute phase of illness; later abortions are more commonly the result of direct infection of the fetus, with resulting hepatic necrosis. Until recently, no clear correlation between RVFV infection and miscarriage has been noted in human infections. However, a recent cross-sectional study in hospitalized pregnant women in Sudan indicated a significant association between RVFV infection and miscarriage.[28] In humans, maternal transmission of RVFV to the fetus has only occasionally been documented.[1,20] This lack of widespread human fetal infection is in striking contrast to the classical abortifacient hallmarks of RVF in other vertebrate species.

Epidemiology and Ecology
Phlebovirus genus
The geographic distribution of SFSV and SFNV closely follows that of their sandfly host, *Phlebotomus pappataci*.[385] This distribution extends from the Mediterranean basin throughout the Middle East and the Arabian Peninsula, north up into areas around the Caucus Mountains, and as far east as Pakistan and India. Sandflies are most numerous in the warmer months, are found at ground level, and feed in the early evenings. Unfortunately, their small size allows them to pass through untreated mosquito netting.

A related phlebovirus, TOSV, is hosted by *Phlebotomus perniciosus* and is found in central Italy, Cyprus, Portugal, and

Spain. Relatively high (20%–25%) antibody prevalence rates suggest that human infections with TOSV are widespread and frequent in endemic areas.[54,113] In addition, many acute lymphocytic meningitis and meningoencephalitis cases occurring in the summer months, particularly in children, are attributable to TOSV infection.[55,113,285] SFSV, SFNV, TOSV, and related viruses replicate in their sandfly hosts, and transstadial and transovarial transmission of the virus has been demonstrated.[388] Sexual transmission of TOSV among sandflies has also been shown.[387] The relatively low efficiency of transovarial transmission demonstrated in experimental infections suggests that vertebrate amplifying hosts are required to maintain these viruses in endemic areas. However, although antibodies to TOSV are present in many domestic animals, virus isolation has been unsuccessful, suggesting that these animals do not act as reservoirs.[279] Thus, the identity of amplifying hosts remains uncertain. Data showing that viremic humans can infect *P. pappataci*, together with attack rates as high as 75% and urban outbreaks of sandfly fever, suggest that humans can on occasion serve as the amplifying vertebrate host of these viruses.[337]

The geographic distribution of RVFV covers much of Africa, including Madagascar and portions of the Arabian Peninsula, with most livestock epizootics reported in East and Southern Africa[218,219,304] (Fig. 17.12). *Aedes* sp. mosquitoes of the subgenera *Aedimorphus* and *Neomelaniconion* are likely the principal RVFV vectors and may maintain the virus in nature through vertical transmission.[233] The ecology of RVFV has been best studied in Kenya, Zimbabwe, and South Africa. In these regions, dambos or vleis, shallow depressions up to several hundred meters across, located near streams and fed by ground water, are thought to play a central role in RVFV epizootics. These dambos flood at times of unusually heavy rainfall, triggering a population explosion in floodwater *Aedes* sp. mosquitoes. RVFV epizootics have also been linked to periods of unusually high precipitation.[234]

Isolation of RVFV from unfed male and female *Aedes mcintoshi* mosquitoes hatched in a dambo in the endemic area of Kenya during an interepidemic period demonstrates maintenance of the virus between epidemics and transovarial transmission of the virus in these mosquitoes.[233] The transmission

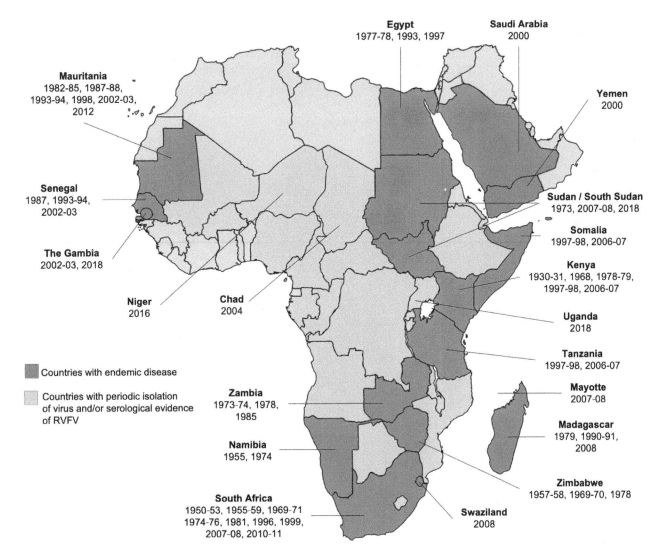

FIGURE 17.12 Geographic distribution of Rift Valley fever virus (RVFV). Countries in which Rift Valley fever (RVF) outbreaks have been identified are shown in *red*, with the dates of the major outbreaks noted. *Yellow* shows countries with indications of RVFV presence based on livestock serosurveys and identification of periodic cases.

cycle of the virus is summarized in Figure 17.13. *A. mcintoshi* is thought to be the principal RVFV maintenance vector in Kenya and Zimbabwe,[376] and these mosquitoes are among the earliest to hatch from eggs after flooding. If the eggs contain virus (passed via transovarial transmission), the hatching mosquitoes are infected and pass the virus on to nearby livestock during feeding, potentially initiating a local epizootic. Viremic livestock act as amplifying hosts that transmit RVFV to other floodwater *Aedes* sp. mosquitoes and to other species including culicines and anophelines, promoting further amplification and spread of the virus. Initiation of such mosquito-virus amplification cycles at dambos throughout a livestock-producing area could give rise to regional, relatively synchronous eruptions of RVFV activity with associated abortion storms across broad geographic areas. Indeed, such eruptions are observed at various intervals in livestock in East and Southern Africa.[304] Although such a scenario is an attractive explanation for the dynamics of explosive RVFV epizootics, longitudinal studies of the vector-virus ecology are necessary to confirm if these factors are solely responsible for the dramatic nature of RVF outbreaks.

Hemorrhagic fever cases in humans are usually seen 1 or 2 weeks after the appearance of abortions and disease in livestock. While humans are likely infected through bites from infected mosquitoes when vector densities are high, contact transmission from infected animals seems to be most important for human infections.[248,290] People involved in handling births or abortions of livestock and in butchering animals, such as farmers and abattoir workers, are at high risk of infection during epizootics.[77] RVFV is also highly infectious by aerosolization or mucosal exposure. Aerosolization resulted in many infections of laboratory personnel working with the virus before modern biosafety practices were developed,[130,362] but the relative contribution of infectious aerosols or fomites to transmission in natural settings is unclear. Although fewer than 2% of human infections result in serious disease, a substantial number of severe cases can occur given the large scale of some epizootics. For instance, an estimated 27,500 RVFV infections occurred during the 1997–1998 outbreak in the Garissa district of Kenya,[425] and approximately 200,000 human cases with 600 deaths were estimated to have occurred during the outbreak in Egypt in

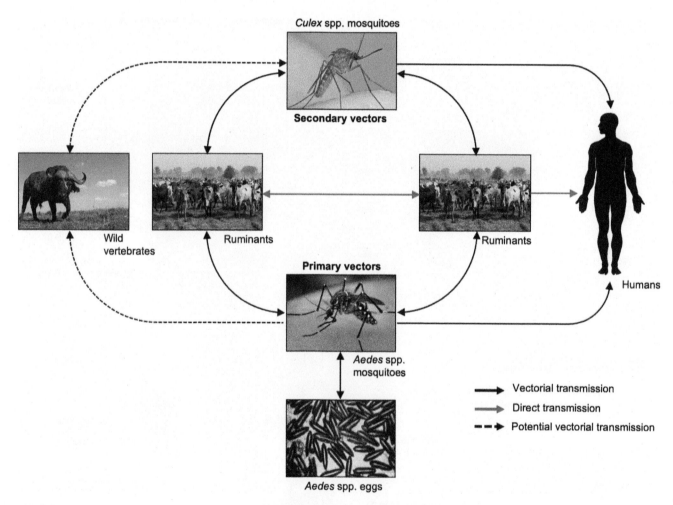

FIGURE 17.13 RVFV transmission cycle. In the enzootic cycle, primary vectors like *Aedes* species mosquitoes maintain RVFV in endemic areas during normal seasonal environmental conditions. The virus is vertically transmitted and can remain infectious in mosquito eggs for prolonged periods of time. During periods of unusual rainfall, secondary vectors, usually *Culex* mosquito species, are responsible for extended dissemination of the virus, causing broad epizootics. Humans become infected either through bites of infected mosquitoes or by exposure to tissues of infected animals. No human-to-human transmission of RVFV has been reported. Solid lines represent an experimentally established transmission route (*arrows* represent direction). *Dashed lines* represent potential vectorial transmission.

1977 and 1978. The 2008 RVFV outbreak in Sudan resulted in 698 human cases with 222 deaths, an unusually high CFR of 31.8%. Moreover, the economic effects of RVFV epidemics on animal keepers in endemic areas are devastating; for example, the 2006–2007 outbreak in Kenya resulted in over 7.6 million US dollars in losses from livestock deaths, and the overall monetary loss to the local economy was estimated to be up to 32 million US dollars.[331]

In contrast to the long history of periodic RVFV epizootics in East and Southern Africa, the large RVFV outbreaks in Egypt in 1977 and 1978 and in Mauritania and Senegal in 1987 were more isolated.[436] Retrospective studies showed that RVFV had not been enzootic in Egypt prior to 1977 and its activity disappeared after 1981, only to be reintroduced in 1993.[22] These data suggest that although mosquitoes capable of acting as epizootic vectors (e.g., *Culex* sp.) exist in Egypt, mosquitoes capable of transovarial RVFV transmission are probably absent. RVFV was most likely introduced into Egypt from enzootic areas in Sudan.

The first confirmed RVFV outbreak outside Africa was reported in September 2000, in the western coastal plains of Saudi Arabia and Yemen.[353] Unusually heavy rains and flooding of the foothills of the Asir Mountains appeared to cause increased mosquito populations and the explosive outbreak in naïve livestock. In Saudi Arabia, 884 hospitalized patients were identified, with 124 deaths.[248] In Yemen, 1,087 cases were estimated, with 121 deaths. The virus associated with this outbreak was almost identical to that associated with earlier RVFV epidemics in East Africa, consistent with the recent introduction of RVFV into the Arabian Peninsula from East Africa.[353] Outbreaks in Madagascar have also been linked to importation of infected animals from East Africa. Additional outbreaks have recently occurred in South Africa, Mauritania, Niger, South Sudan, Kenya, and Uganda.[19,354,369]

Despite its extensive geographic distribution, whole-genome sequencing and phylogenetic analyses indicate that RVFV is a highly conserved virus. Among all the RVFV stains circulating since 1970s, only 4% to 5% genetic diversity is observed at the nucleotide level.[41] Although accumulated mutations can be observed, especially in the virus surface glycoproteins, they do not seem to have resulted in increased RVFV virulence in human populations. Genetic reassortment of virus segments among co-circulating RVFV lineages occurs but is difficult to identify.[26]

Clinical Features

Human infections with sandfly fever viruses result in an acute febrile illness with rapid onset. The incubation period lasts 2 to 6 days and is followed by fever and general malaise, often accompanied by headache, vomiting, photophobia, and back and joint pain.[27,337] The disease is self-limiting, lasting 2 to 4 days before rapid and complete recovery. Leukopenia followed by protracted neutropenia is reported. TOSV infection can start as a mild illness but become neuroinvasive. In very severe cases, seizures, severe meningoencephalitis, deafness, personality changes, and encephalitis, including fatal cases, can be observed (reviewed in Ref.[9]).

Experimental RVFV infection of newborn lambs suggests that the incubation period is usually 24 to 36 hours but can be as short as 12 hours.[111] Fever, which is often biphasic, is accompanied by listlessness, lack of appetite, abdominal pain, increased respiration rate, and lack of movement. Mortality rates of over 90% can be seen in animals younger than 1 or 2 weeks of age, with animals rarely surviving beyond 24 to 36 hours after the onset of illness. Older animals are often less susceptible to RVFV infection, instead presenting peracute or inapparent infection. Mostly older animals develop a febrile acute illness similar to the disease seen in 1- to 2-week-old animals, but with lower mortality rates ranging from 5% to 60%. High and prolonged viremias, widespread tissue damage, vasculitis, hepatic necrosis, and acute renal injury are seen in the more severe cases.[291] Abortions in pregnant animals are frequently observed, with rates varying from 40% to 100%.

Human RVFV infections generally result in a self-limiting, influenza-like illness (Fig. 17.14). However, severe hemorrhagic fever occurs in approximately 2% of cases. In these patients, the reduction of the antithrombotic function of endothelial cells likely initiates intravascular coagulation. The release of procoagulants into the circulation, together with the extensive liver damage[259] (Fig. 17.15) that severely impairs synthesis of coagulation factors and removal of circulating activated coagulation factors, appears to be important factors resulting in DIC in hemorrhagic fever cases.[92,305,308] The mortality rate in hemorrhagic cases is up to 65%.

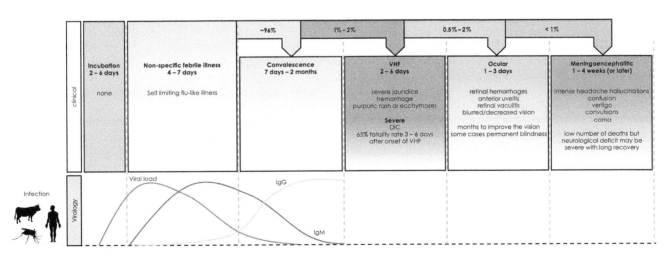

FIGURE 17.14 An outline of the main clinical manifestations and laboratory findings in RVFV human disease.

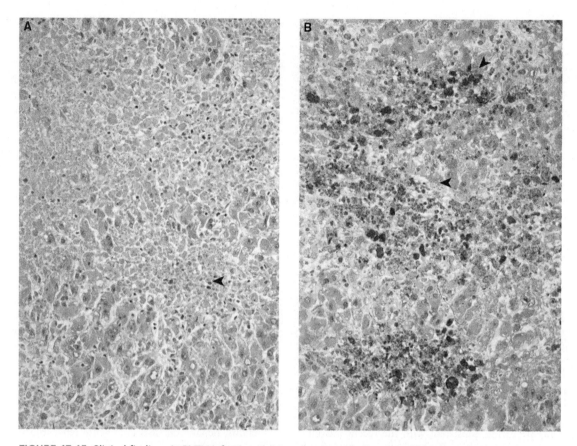

FIGURE 17.15 Clinical findings in RVFV infection. A: Histochemistry of a liver sample from a patient reveals extensive focal necrosis. **B:** Immunostaining of RVFV antigen (in *red*) indicates that the observed necrosis in the liver is mainly due to viral infection (arrowheads point to broader affected area).

In fewer than 0.5% of human RVFV infections, retinitis or encephalitis can be observed 1 to 4 weeks after recovery from the acute illness. Serious vision problems, blurred or decreased vision, or blindness can start developing at the end of either the febrile period or period of severe disease. Retinal hemorrhages, optic disc edema, anterior uveitis, and retinal vasculitis are common findings.[8] It takes several months after infection for vision to improve, and in many cases, it never completely recovers. Encephalitis begins with headache, meningismus, and confusion. Often fever reappears, and hallucinations, stupor, coma, and death may follow. Focal necrosis, which most likely involves direct cell destruction by RVFV, is seen in the brain. Patients may take months to recover from the neurological sequelae of RVF.[178,262]

Diagnosis

Sandfly fever should be suspected when patients present with a classic "3-day fever" in areas where phlebotomine sandflies are numerous.[113,337] Similarly, TOSV infection should be suspected in patients who develop acute CNS disease during the summer months in rural or semirural areas where phlebotomine sandflies are present.[54,285] Diagnostic confirmation using acute or early convalescent phase samples is readily achieved by virus isolation via intracranial inoculation into suckling mouse or susceptible tissue culture cells or by IgM capture ELISA. In human infections, specific antibody response develops rapidly and is long-lasting. During the acute phase of the disease,

RT-PCR or real-time RT-PCR can also be performed in blood or cerebrospinal fluid.[89,403]

Clinical differential diagnosis of RVF cases can be difficult due to the nonspecific early symptoms of disease. Severe cases can be confused with other cocirculating hemorrhagic fevers, including Ebola, Crimean-Congo hemorrhagic fever, dengue, and yellow fever, or with malaria, cholera, meningitis, and a number of other viral and bacterial diseases. Thus, differential clinical diagnosis of RVFV varies depending on the region in question. RVF disease should be suspected in RVFV-endemic regions following abnormally high precipitation, increased rates of abortions in livestock, and appearance of acute influenza-like illness in persons in close contact with potentially infected livestock (e.g., farmers, veterinarians, and abattoir workers). Virologic diagnosis is usually simple given the high-level viremia present throughout the acute phase of illness and the ease of growing the virus by intracranial inoculation into suckling mice or in a wide variety of susceptible tissue culture cells. Serologic testing is also straightforward, particularly if paired sera (one taken during acute illness and the other 1 or 2 weeks later) are available. IgM and IgG ELISAs using inactivated RVFV-infected cell lysates or slurries have proven particularly useful in outbreak investigations.[213,272,399,425] IgM and IgG ELISAs based on recombinant expressed nucleocapsid protein have also been developed.[432] Additionally, a number of sensitive nucleic acid-based assays exist, including RT-PCR, real-time quantitative RT-PCR, and a multiplex PCR-based macroarray assay.[38,418] Furthermore, immunohistology for detecting RVFV antigen and *in situ* hybridization for detecting RVFV genome in formaldehyde-fixed liver samples can also be used for establishing a RVF diagnosis.[325]

Prevention and Control

The sandfly hosts of SFSV, SFNV, and TOSV have a short flight range and often locomote by hopping, making localized use of insecticide sprays particularly effective around residences. In addition, the use of repellants and treated bed nets and screens is recommended in areas where sandflies are prominent.

No specific treatment is required for the majority of human cases of RVF, which are mild and self-limiting. For severe cases, treatment is currently limited to intensive supportive care, including monitoring fluid and electrolyte balance and renal function, blood pressure, and oxygenation. No effective therapeutics against RVFV have been approved for human use.[23] In experiments using animal models, the antiviral favipiravir has been shown to protect against clinical disease when given within the first 24 hours postinfection, but treatment at 48 hours can result in neurologic disease, with the virus escaping to the brain.[72] Similarly, ribavirin showed antiviral activity in early *in vitro* studies and some therapeutic effect in animal models, depending on the challenge route, but treated animals ultimately succumbed to late-onset encephalitis.[306,342] The combination of the two drugs in *in vivo* studies has shown some efficacy but neither is currently recommended for treating human infections. Studies have been initiated to generate strongly neutralizing monoclonal antibodies against RVFV, which could potentially be used as part of future therapeutic cocktails.[10]

Many human RVFV infections can be avoided by preventing mosquito bites through the use of insect repellents and insecticide-treated bed nets. Currently no vaccines against RVFV have been approved for people or for routine veterinary use outside the endemic areas. Based on the One Health approach, immunization of livestock remains the most effective way to prevent RVFV epizootics and human disease.[40,208] Several vaccines exist for use in livestock. Live attenuated viruses based on the mouse neuroadapted Smithburn RVFV strain are used in Kenya and South Africa.[70,360] Formalin-inactivated wild-type viruses have also been used in Egypt and South Africa. The modified live Smithburn vaccine produced in cell culture has been shown to be efficacious in sheep but not in cattle, with a single dose inducing lasting immunity in sheep 6 to 7 days after vaccination.[84] However, this vaccine appears to be only partially attenuated, causing abortions or teratology in some pregnant animals.[51,177] Formalin-inactivated vaccines are safer but are expensive, require multiple doses, and induce only short-lived immunity in sheep and cattle.[105] Other candidate live-attenuated vaccines, such as the mutagen-derived MP12 strain; the naturally occurring clone 13, which has a large deletion in the NSs gene; and genetically engineered recombinant viruses lacking NSs and/or NSm protein, or containing 4 instead of 3 genomic segments, have also been evaluated.[42,122,177,421] Other immunization approaches include vectored vaccines, DNA vaccines, non-replicating virus-like particles, and subunit vaccines.[99,123,414] The main problems for vaccinating livestock are the long periods between epizootics and their irregular appearance, which make convincing livestock owners to vaccinate regularly difficult. Recent advances in the use of satellite imagery

and surface ocean temperatures to predict regions at increased risk of RVFV activity may allow timely vaccination of animals prior to potential epizootics.[16,234,408]

In RVFV-endemic regions, humans are probably best protected by vaccination of livestock to prevent amplification of virus, thus limiting human exposure and epizootic potential. However, RVF outbreaks are often only detected after the diagnosis of human cases, due to weak animal disease surveillance in resource-poor regions of Africa. Human vaccines are needed for high-risk groups like veterinarians, farmers, and slaughterhouse workers, and for general naïve populations. RVFV is highly infectious by aerosol, as shown by numerous infections of laboratory personnel. To prevent infection, workers at risk of exposure should wear protective clothing to avoid contact with potentially infectious materials and aerosols. Neutralizing antibody response appears to be strongly associated with protection from infection, and since RVFV is highly conserved, a single vaccine should effectively protect against all or most RVFV strains.

SEVERE FEVER WITH THROMBOCYTOPENIA SYNDROME VIRUS GROUP

Severe Fever with Thrombocytopenia Syndrome Virus

Distribution and Significance

SFTS is an emerging tick-borne disease caused by SFTS virus (SFTSV), a novel member of *Phlebovirus* genus. The virus was first reported in the Hubei and Henan provinces of China in 2009. Since then, the virus has been detected in 23 provinces in China as well as South Korea and Japan in 2013 (Fig. 17.16).[430,437] The clinical symptoms were initially considered to resemble those of human anaplasmosis; however, no bacterial DNA was detected in blood samples and instead SFTSV was isolated.[322,430] Phylogenetic characterization of virus isolates revealed that SFTSV is in between from the Sandfly fever group and the Uukuniemi group, indicating that SFTSV forms of a third and novel group within the genus *Phlebovirus*.

Epidemiology

Following the identification of the human cases, SFTSV was detected in ixodid ticks of the species *Haemaphysalis longicornis* that were collected from domestic animals where the patients lived. Viral genome analysis revealed that the sequences from ticks were very closely related to those of SFTSV isolates from the patients, implicating this tick species as the main vector.[322,430] A recent study confirmed vector competence of this species and demonstrated its potential as a reservoir.[242] However, SFTSV has been detected in other ixodid tick species with typically lower prevalence levels, and it remains to be shown what role different tick species play in different geographic regions. SFTSV most likely circulates silently tick-vertebrate cycle in nature causing no overt signs of disease in the tick vector and the animal hosts, only human show signs of disease. To determine relevant animal hosts, studies surveyed SFTSV prevalence in animal hosts in endemic areas. SFTSV RNA or antibodies were found in multiple wild and domestic animals in China, Japan, and Korea including sheep, goats, cattle, pigs,

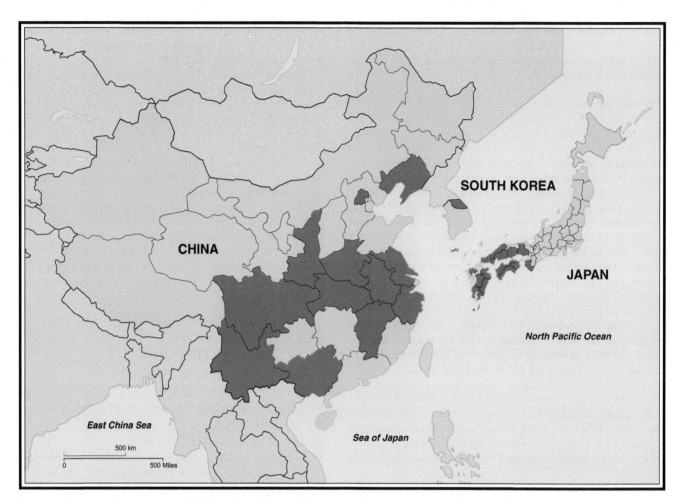

FIGURE 17.16 Distribution of severe fever with thrombocytopenia virus.

chicken dogs, hedgehogs and rodents.[282,286,438] Nevertheless, it still remains to be determined what animal host plays a crucial role in the perpetuation of the ticks and virus in nature. As a tick-borne disease, the human hospitalizations are linked to the seasonal activity of the tick vector, typically peaking between late spring to early fall. The majority of affected patients are farmers living in wooded and hilly areas working in the fields, demonstrating that agricultural work is a major risk factor. Between 2010 and 2016, the Chinese Disease Prevention and Control Information System reported SFTS cases in 23 provinces with 1,000 to 2,500 cases annually and a cumulative CFR of 5.3%. The highest numbers of reported cases occurred in Henan (37%), Shandong (26.6%), Anhui (14%), and Hubei (12.6%).[238,437] The disease occurs mainly in the elderly population, and death is most frequent in patients over 50 years of age.[238,441] In addition to the tick-borne transmission, human-to-human transmission has also been suggested.

Clinical Features

The incubation time has been reported to be 5 to 14 days, and there is some evidence that the incubation period after tick bite can be shorter versus human-to-human transmission. However, more studies need to be conducted to exclude confounding factors. Patient profiling has shown that the clinical progression of the disease occurs in three stages: fever stage, MOF stage,

and convalescent stage (Fig. 17.17).[88,93,132,322,439] The fever stage is characterized by a sudden onset of fever (>38°C), headache, fatigue, myalgia, as well as gastrointestinal symptoms, such as nausea, vomiting, and diarrhea. As the agent's names implies, this stage is also accompanied by marked thrombocytopenia (platelet count of <100,000 per cubic millimeter) as well as leukocytopenia and lymphadenopathy and lasts for up 5 to 11 days. A high viral load can be detected at this stage. The subsequent MOF stage lasts for 7 to 14 days and is defined by progressive worsening organ (liver, heart, lungs, and kidneys) functions all the way to failure in fatal cases or a self-limiting process in survivors.[93,132] In this stage, hemorrhagic presentations (bleeding from mouth mucosa, lungs, and gastrointestinal lumen) and/or CNS involvement (lethargy, convulsions, and coma) are present. This stage is also characterized by elevated levels of ALT, AST, CK, LDH, and CRP. Coagulation disturbances are also observed, which can lead to DIC. The viral load gradually falls in survivors but remains high in patients who succumb to the disease.[88,439] The key risk factors contributing to a patient's death have been identified as increased viremia, elevated AST, ALT, LDH, CK, and CK-MB levels past the fever stage, and the appearance of CNS symptoms, manifestation of hemorrhagic tendency, DIC and MOF. The convalescence stage in which surviving patients recover starts on average 13 days after disease onset in which clinical and laboratory

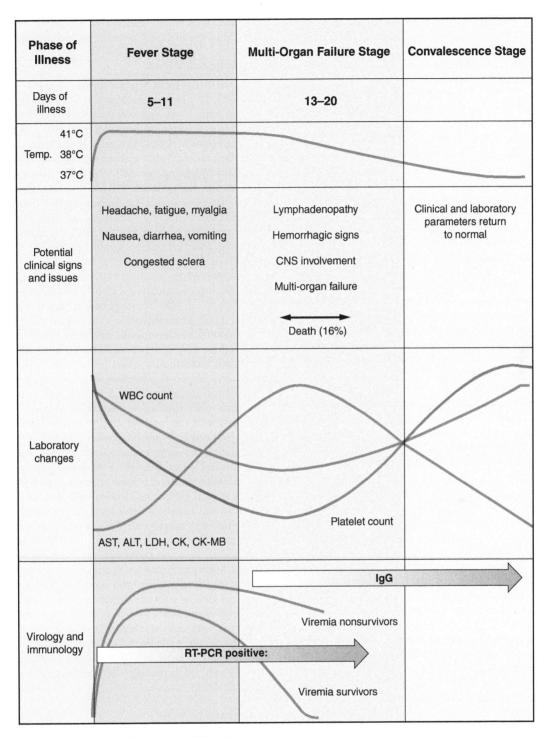

Phase of Illness	Fever Stage	Multi-Organ Failure Stage	Convalescence Stage
Days of illness	5–11	13–20	
Temp. 41°C 38°C 37°C			
Potential clinical signs and issues	Headache, fatigue, myalgia Nausea, diarrhea, vomiting Congested sclera	Lymphadenopathy Hemorrhagic signs CNS involvement Multi-organ failure ◄──► Death (16%)	Clinical and laboratory parameters return to normal
Laboratory changes	WBC count AST, ALT, LDH, CK, CK-MB		Platelet count
Virology and immunology	RT-PCR positive:	IgG Viremia nonsurvivors Viremia survivors	

FIGURE 17.17 Clinical findings in SFTSV infection.

parameters gradually revert to normal. Although the reported CFR ranges from 6% to 30%, a recent meta-analysis of confirmed patient case studies in China showed an pooled CFR of 16%.[235]

Pathogenesis and Pathology

Due to its recent discovery, little is known about the pathogenesis; however, certain aspects might be extrapolated from related viruses with similar disease presentation such as Crimean-Congo hemorrhagic fever. Upon introduction of the virus into the dermis or mucosa, there is likely local replication followed by blood- and lymph-borne spread of the virus to the major organs. A recent study detected SFTSV in multiple organs with the highest titer in the spleen, moderate titers in the kidney, and the lowest titers in lung and heart.[231] Several studies looked at serum levels of cytokines (TNF, IL-6, IL-8, IL-10) and chemokines (MCP-1, IP-10, MIP-1a, G-CSF) in mild and severe cases in a comparative fashion showing that more severe SFTS disease is associated with higher levels of cytokines and chemokines.[93,96,373] This suggests that a host-mediated inflammatory response, through an imbalance in cytokine and chemokine production, might result in a severe disease progression. Furthermore, studies have shown that decrease in leukocyte populations, specifically T cells and myeloid dendritic cells, may be associated with a more severe form of disease.[239,368] Although not thoroughly characterized, it was shown that SFTS survivors develop low level neutralizing antibodies that wane overtime; however, in some patients, they can be detected up to 4 years after SFTSV infection. The study of the SFTS pathogenesis has been hampered by the availability of a suitable animal model.[257] A number of laboratory animals including mice, rats, hamsters, and nonhuman primates have been evaluated in an attempt to model human disease. Immunocompetent animals typically do not show overt signs of disease. In one study, investigators showed thrombocytopenia, leukocytopenia, and elevated liver transaminases, hallmarks of human SFTS, in immunocompetent strain C57BL/6 mice. Viral RNA and histopathological changes were identified in the spleen, liver, and kidney. Consequently, this animal model mimics the aspects of a mild form of SFTS in humans.[440] When the same strain of mice was treated with mitomycin C in order to suppress the immune response, SFTSV challenge was lethal. Similarly, SFTSV challenge in immunocompromised mice (interferon-α or α/β receptor deficient mice) or hamsters (signal transducer and activator of transcription 2 knockout [STAT2 KO]) is typically lethal indicating the importance of the IFN response in controlling virus replication.[145,237,257] In IFN receptor deficient mice, high levels of SFTSV RNA were found in the brain, liver, kidney, and spleen, and major target tissues of SFTSV appear to be reticular cells in lymphoid tissues of lymph nodes and spleen. No specific cell receptor has been identified.

Diagnosis

The disease presentation is not pathognomonic and can be confused with other diseases. Although patient history such as time of the year, contact with ticks, and geographic location as well as blood chemistry can give clues. Direct diagnosis of the viral RNA in the patient sera can be conducted by conventional RT-PCR or quantitative real-time RT-PCR.[374,429] Infection with SFTSV can also be diagnosed in sera of patients either by detecting the presence of IgM during the acute phase or IgG in convalescent patients. Initially, an IFA was developed and was used for laboratory confirmation. Meanwhile, different ELISA kits have been developed in the effected countries and validated for sensitivity and specificity.[185,431] High levels of neutralizing antibodies are generated during convalescence phase, and virus neutralizations assays can be used to determine antibody titers and specificity.

Prevention and Control

Currently, there is no specific treatment available for SFTSV infection and treatment is symptomatic. Ribavirin has been suggested as a treatment; however, limited studies showed inconclusive effects on disease outcome.[236,301] Favipiravir has been suggested as a treatment, and its efficacy was demonstrated in STAT2 KO hamsters.[145] A clinical trial testing the efficacy of favipiravir is currently ongoing in Japan. No internationally or locally approved vaccines are available. Nevertheless, there has been an increasing number of preclinical studies have been conducted. Limiting tick exposure through individual protective

measures such as tick repellents or protective clothing or avoidance of where ticks are common are recommended.

Heartland Virus

Distribution and Significance

In 2009, two farmers in Missouri were independently hospitalized with fever, thrombocytopenia, and leukopenia. Both patients were bitten by ticks approximately 5 to 7 days prior to onset of signs of illness. Collected blood samples were negative for *Ehrlichia chaffeensis* and electron microscopy and next-generation sequencing revealed that the virus was a new members of the bunyavirales, HRTV.[263] Genome sequences from both patients were similar, indicating that both patients were infected independently with the same virus. Further, phylogenetic analysis identified that the HRTV is closely related to the recently identified tick-borne phlebovirus SFTSV in China.[322]

Epidemiology

The phylogenic proximity to SFTSV as well as the patient description of tick bite suggested a tick-borne transmission route. Pools of *Amblyomma americanum* ticks collected on a farm owned by the original case were positive for HRTV.[263] Since then, HRTV has been detected in *A. americanum* ticks in other locations in Missouri. Additionally, the virus has been detected in *A. americium* ticks over multiple years in the same location indicating that HRTV can persist in ticks.[284] As with other tick-borne diseases, human disease occurrence overlaps with the seasonal activity of the ticks, which is typically between late spring and early fall with the peak in June. Serosurveys of domestic and wild animals near the sites of where HRTV-positive ticks were found neutralizing antibodies in white-tail deer, horses, raccoons, opossums, and dogs.[48] Experimental infections of white-tail deer, raccoons, chicken, rabbits, and hamsters demonstrated that they seroconvert to the virus, yet, develop no viremia or signs of disease and are therefore not likely a reservoir for HRTV in nature.[49,82] As of September 2018, over 40 cases have been reported from states in the Midwestern and southern United States.[75] The median age of identified patient is 66 years.[413] The disease distribution overlaps closely with the distribution of *A. americanum* ticks, although some states in which *A. americanum* can be found have not reported the disease. Further studies need to be performed to determine the vector capacity of *A. americanum* and competence of other tick species and potential animal hosts of HRTV with high enough viremia levels to transmit the virus back to ticks.

Clinical Features

Since the initial two cases, eight additional cases have been reported.[71,128,276] All cases had a sudden onset of fever and the majority of cases presented with fever, fatigue, diarrhea, headache, myalgia, nausea, elevated hepatic aminotransferase levels, marked thrombocytopenia, and leukopenia. In some cases, neurological symptoms such as confusion were also reported. Three of the 10 cases, all male greater than 60 years, were fatal due to MOF. However, two of those three had preexisting comorbidities.

Pathogenesis and Pathology

Due to the limited number of cases and experimental studies, very little is known about the pathogenesis of HRTV and can only be extrapolated from closely related viruses. High levels of IgG antibodies were detected in serum of the initial two patients even up to 2 years.[263] A recent pathology case report from a fatal case detected HRTV antigen in the brain (thalamus), liver (Kupffer cells), pancreas, heart, lung, large bowel, small bowel, kidney, testes, bone marrow, lymph nodes, spleen, and muscle by immunohistochemistry. Evidence of lymphocytic myocarditis with viral antigens was present. In the liver, focal hepatocellular necrosis and Kupffer cell hyperplasia was detected. The kidneys demonstrated hemorrhage, interstitial inflammation, scattered glomerulosclerosis, and acute tubular necrosis with viral antigens present within scattered glomeruli.[128] Another limiting factor in understanding the HRTV pathogenesis is the lack of an immune competent animal model to study the disease seen in humans. Animal studies demonstrated that immunocompetent mice are not susceptible after peripheral or even intracranial or Cynomolgus macaques after peripheral HRTV inoculation.[49,257] A study showed that interferon-$\alpha/\beta/\gamma$ receptor-deficient mice are susceptible to HRTV and indicated the importance of the IFN response in controlling virus replication.[49]

Diagnostics

RT-PCR and serological assays for the detection of viral RNA and antibodies have been developed. Monoclonal antibodies developed against the nucleoprotein of HRTV are also available.[68,284,393]

Prevention and Control

No specific treatment or vaccines are currently available. The treatment remains symptomatic.

PERSPECTIVES

The degree of understanding of the various bunyaviruses and their ability to cause disease in humans varies greatly, depending on the severity of the resulting clinical illness and the impact of each virus to public health. Because of the high level of containment required to work with human pathogens and the stringent restrictions on sharing viruses and clinical specimens, studies of pathogenesis and the development of animal models remain limited. However, progress has been made in many areas, particularly virus detection using next-generation sequencing, outbreak investigations, and development of a number of experimental therapeutics and vaccines. Still, the extensive number of bunyaviruses pathogenic to humans presents multiple future research needs. To highlight just a few: (a) obtaining a better understanding of how bunyaviruses persist in either their arthropod or rodent hosts; (b) sequencing the viruses for analyzing phylogenetics, improving diagnostics, and studying virus evolution (e.g., adaptations resulting in increased virulence or the ability to spill over into new host species); (c) studying pathogenesis, especially in severe human disease; (d) determining how some viruses initially cause a self-limiting disease but eventually reach the brain to lead to severe neurologic disease; (e) characterizing the immune responses responsible for viral restriction and clearance, and determining whether these responses are regulated and protective or dysregulated and damaging to the host; and (f) identifying broad-spectrum antivirals or immunotherapeutics, and developing vaccines for higher incidence and morbidity-associated infections.

REFERENCES

1. Adam I, Karsany MS. Case report: Rift Valley fever with vertical transmission in a pregnant Sudanese woman. *J Med Virol* 2008;80:929.
2. Ahmed AA, et al. Presence of broadly reactive and group-specific neutralizing epitopes on newly described isolates of Crimean-Congo hemorrhagic fever virus. *J Gen Virol* 2005;86(Pt 12):3327–3336. doi: 10.1099/vir.0.81175-0.
3. Akinci E, Bodur H, Muşabak U, et al. The relationship between the human leukocyte antigen system and Crimean-Congo hemorrhagic fever in the Turkish population. *Int J Infect Dis* 2013;17(11):e1038–e1041. doi: 10.1016/j.ijid.2013.06.005.
4. Akinci E, et al. Analysis of lymphocyte subgroups in Crimean-Congo hemorrhagic fever. *Int J Infect Dis* 2009;13(5):560–563. doi: 10.1016/j.ijid.2008.08.027.
5. Al-Busaidy S, Hamblin C, Taylor WP. Neutralising antibodies to Akabane virus in free-living wild animals in Africa. *Trop Anim Health Prod* 1987;19(4):197–202. doi: 10.1007/BF02242116.
6. Al-Busaidy SM, Mellor PS. Isolation and identification of arboviruses from the Sultanate of Oman. *Epidemiol Infect* 1991;106(2):403–413. doi: 10.1017/S095026880004855X.
7. Al-Hamdan NA, et al. The risk of nosocomial transmission of Rift Valley fever. *PLoS Negl Trop Dis* 2015;9:e0004314.
8. Al-Hazmi A, et al. Ocular complications of Rift Valley fever outbreak in Saudi Arabia. *Ophthalmology* 2005;112:313–318.
9. Alkan C, et al. Sandfly-borne phleboviruses of Eurasia and Africa: epidemiology, genetic diversity, geographic range, control measures. *Antiviral Res* 2013;100:54–74.
10. Allen ER, et al. A protective monoclonal antibody targets a site of vulnerability on the surface of Rift Valley fever virus. *Cell Rep* 2018;25:3750–3758.e4.
11. An DJ, Yoon SH, Jeong WS, et al. Genetic analysis of Akabane virus isolates from cattle in Korea. *Vet Microbiol* 2010;140(1–2):49–55. doi: 10.1016/j.vetmic.2009.07.018.
12. Andersen AA, Campbell CH. Experimental placental transfer of Akabane virus in the hamster. *Am J Vet Res* 1978;39(2):301–304.
13. Angulo J, et al. Serum levels of interleukin-6 are linked to the severity of the disease caused by Andes virus. *PLoS Negl Trop Dis* 2017;11:e0005757.
14. Antonen J, et al. A severe case of Puumala hantavirus infection successfully treated with bradykinin receptor antagonist icatibant. *Scand J Infect Dis* 2013;45:494–496.
15. Antoniadis A, Le Duc JW, Daniel-Alexiou S. Clinical and epidemiological aspects of hemorrhagic fever with renal syndrome (HFRS) in Greece. *Eur J Epidemiol* 1987;3:295–301.
16. Anyamba A, et al. Prediction of a Rift Valley fever outbreak. *Proc Natl Acad Sci U S A* 2009;106:955–959.
17. Anyangu AS, et al. Risk factors for severe Rift Valley fever infection in Kenya, 2007. *Am J Trop Med Hyg* 2010;83:14–21.
18. Arasli M, et al. Elevated chemokine levels during adult but not pediatric crimean-congo hemorrhagic fever. *J Clin Virol* 2015;66:76–82. doi: 10.1016/j.jcv.2015.03.010.
19. Archer BN, et al. Epidemiologic investigations into outbreaks of Rift Valley fever in humans, South Africa, 2008–2011. *Emerg Infect Dis* 2013;19(12). doi: 10.3201/eid1912.121527.
20. Arishi HM, Aqeel AY, Al Hazmi MM. Vertical transmission of fatal Rift Valley fever in a newborn. *Ann Trop Paediatr* 2006;26:251–253.
21. Arslan M, et al. Importance of endothelial dysfunction biomarkers in patients with Crimean-Congo hemorrhagic fever. *J Med Virol* 2017;89(12):2084–2091. doi: 10.1002/jmv.24881.
22. Arthur RR, et al. Recurrence of Rift Valley fever in Egypt. *Lancet* 1993;342:1149–1150.
23. Atkins C, Freiberg AN. Recent advances in the development of antiviral therapeutics for Rift Valley fever virus infection. *Future Virol* 2017;12:651–665.
24. Avsic-Zupanc T, Saksida A, Korva M. Hantavirus infections. *Clin Microbiol Infect* 2019;21S:e6–e16. doi: 10.1111/1469-0691.12291.
25. Avsic-Zupanc T, Toney A, Anderson K, et al. Genetic and antigenic properties of Dobrava virus: a unique member of the Hantavirus genus, family Bunyaviridae. *J Gen Virol* 1995;76(Pt 11):2801–2808.
26. Baba M, Masiga DK, Sang R, et al. Has Rift Valley fever virus evolved with increasing severity in human populations in East Africa? *Emerg Microbes Infect* 2016;5:e58.
27. Bartelloni PJ, Tesh RB. Clinical and serologic responses of volunteers infected with phlebotomus fever virus (Sicilian type). *Am J Trop Med Hyg* 1976;25:456–462.
28. Baudin M, et al. Association of Rift Valley fever virus infection with miscarriage in Sudanese women: a cross-sectional study. *Lancet Glob Health* 2016;4:e864–e871.
29. Beaty BJ, Miller BR, Shope RE, et al. Molecular basis of bunyavirus per os infection of mosquitoes: role of the middle-sized RNA segment. *Proc Natl Acad Sci U S A* 1982;79(4):1295–1297. doi: 10.1073/pnas.79.4.1295.
30. Bellomo C, et al. Differential regulation of PAI-1 in hantavirus cardiopulmonary syndrome and hemorrhagic fever with renal syndrome. *Open Forum Infect Dis* 2018;5:ofy021.
31. Bennett RS, Gresko AK, Murphy BR, et al. Tahyna virus genetics, infectivity, and immunogenicity in mice and monkeys. *Virol J* 2011;8:135. doi: 10.1186/1743-422X-8-135.
32. Bennett RS, Nelson JT, Gresko AK, et al. The full genome sequence of three strains of Jamestown Canyon virus and their pathogenesis in mice or monkeys. *Virol J* 2011;8:136. doi: 10.1186/1743-422X-8-136.
33. Bennett RS, et al. La Crosse virus infectivity, pathogenesis, and immunogenicity in mice and monkeys. *Virol J* 2008;5:25. doi: 10.1186/1743-422X-5-25.
34. Bente DA, et al. Pathogenesis and immune response of Crimean-Congo hemorrhagic fever virus in a STAT-1 knockout mouse model. *J Virol* 2010;84(21):11089–11100. doi: 10.1128/JVI.01383-10.
35. Bente DA, et al. Crimean-Congo hemorrhagic fever: history, epidemiology, pathogenesis, clinical syndrome and genetic diversity. *Antiviral Res* 2013;100(1):159–189.
36. Bereczky S, et al. Crimean-Congo hemorrhagic fever virus infection is lethal for adult type I interferon receptor-knockout mice. *J Gen Virol* 2010;91(Pt 6):1473–1477. doi: 10.1099/vir.0.019034-0.
37. Bharadwaj M, Nofchissey R, Goade D, et al. Humoral immune responses in the hantavirus cardiopulmonary syndrome. *J Infect Dis* 2000;182:43–48.

38. Bird BH, Bawiec DA, Ksiazek TG, et al. Highly sensitive and broadly reactive quantitative reverse transcription-PCR assay for high-throughput detection of Rift Valley fever virus. *J Clin Microbiol* 2007;45:3506–3513.
39. Bird BH, McElroy AK. Rift Valley fever virus: unanswered questions. *Antiviral Res* 2016;132:274–280.
40. Bird BH, Nichol ST. Breaking the chain: Rift Valley fever virus control via livestock vaccination. *Curr Opin Virol* 2012;2:315–323.
41. Bird BH, et al. Multiple virus lineages sharing recent common ancestry were associated with a Large Rift Valley fever outbreak among livestock in Kenya during 2006–2007. *J Virol* 2008;82:11152–11166.
42. Bird BH, et al. Rift valley fever virus vaccine lacking the NSs and NSm genes is safe, nonteratogenic, and confers protection from viremia, pyrexia, and abortion following challenge in adult and pregnant sheep. *J Virol* 2011;85(24):12901–12909.
43. Bjorkstrom NK, et al. Rapid expansion and long-term persistence of elevated NK cell numbers in humans infected with hantavirus. *J Exp Med* 2011;208:13–21.
44. Bodur H, Akinci E, Ascioglu S, et al. Subclinical infections with Crimean-Congo hemorrhagic fever virus, Turkey. *Emerg Infect Dis* 2012;18(4):640–642. doi: 10.3201/eid1804.111374.
45. Bodur H, et al. Detection of Crimean-Congo hemorrhagic fever virus genome in saliva and urine. *Int J Infect Dis* 2010;14(3):e247–e249. doi: 10.1016/j.ijid.2009.04.018.
46. Bondu V, et al. Elevated cytokines, thrombin and PAI-1 in severe HCPS patients due to Sin Nombre virus. *Viruses* 2015;7:559–589.
47. Bonney LC, et al. A recombinase polymerase amplification assay for rapid detection of Crimean-Congo Haemorrhagic fever Virus infection. *PLoS Negl Trop Dis* 2017;11(10):e0006013. doi: 10.1371/journal.pntd.0006013.
48. Bosco-Lauth AM, et al. Serological investigation of Heartland virus (Bunyaviridae: *Phlebovirus*) exposure in wild and domestic animals adjacent to human case sites in Missouri 2012-2013. *Am J Trop Med Hyg* 2015;92(6):1163–1167. doi: 10.4269/ajtmh.14-0702.
49. Bosco-Lauth AM, et al. Vertebrate host susceptibility to Heartland virus. *Emerg Infect Dis* 2016;22(12):2070–2077. doi: 10.3201/eid2212.160472.
50. Boshra H, Lorenzo G, Busquets N, et al. Rift valley fever: recent insights into pathogenesis and prevention. *J Virol* 2011;85:6098–6105.
51. Botros B, et al. Adverse response of non-indigenous cattle of European breeds to live attenuated Smithburn Rift Valley fever vaccine. *J Med Virol* 2006;78:787–791.
52. Botten J, et al. Experimental infection model for Sin Nombre hantavirus in the deer mouse (*Peromyscus maniculatus*). *Proc Natl Acad Sci U S A* 2000;97:10578–10583.
53. Bowen MD, et al. A reassortant bunyavirus isolated from acute hemorrhagic fever cases in Kenya and Somalia. *Virology* 2001;291(2):185–190. doi: 10.1006/viro.2001.1201.
54. Braito A, et al. Evidence of Toscana virus infections without central nervous system involvement: a serological study. *Eur J Epidemiol* 1997;13:761–764.
55. Braito A, et al. Phlebotomus-transmitted toscana virus infections of the central nervous system: a seven-year experience in Tuscany. *Scand J Infect Dis* 1998;30:505–508.
56. Braun M, et al. NK cell activation in human hantavirus infection explained by virus-induced IL-15/IL15Ralpha expression. *PLoS Pathog* 2014;10:e1004521.
57. Briese T, Bird B, Kapoor V, et al. Batai and Ngari viruses: M segment reassortment and association with severe febrile disease outbreaks in East Africa. *J Virol* 2006;80(11):5627–5630. doi: 10.1128/JVI.02448-05.
58. Briese T, Calisher CH, Higgs S. Viruses of the family Bunyaviridae: are all available isolates reassortants? *Virology* 2013;446(1–2):207–216. doi: 10.1016/j.virol.2013.07.030.
59. Brocato RL, Josleyn MJ, Wahl-Jensen V, et al. Construction and nonclinical testing of a Puumala virus synthetic M gene-based DNA vaccine. *Clin Vaccine Immunol* 2013;20:218–226.
60. Brocato RL, et al. A lethal disease model for hantavirus pulmonary syndrome in immunosuppressed Syrian hamsters infected with Sin Nombre virus. *J Virol* 2014;88:811–819.
61. Brummer-Korvenkontio M, Henttonen H, Vaheri A. Hemorrhagic fever with renal syndrome in Finland: ecology and virology of nephropathia epidemica. *Scand J Infect Dis Suppl* 1982;36:88–91.
62. Burt FJ, Leman PA, Abbott JC, et al. Serodiagnosis of Crimean-Congo haemorrhagic fever. *Epidemiol Infect* 1994;113(3):551–562. doi: 10.1017/S0950268800068576.
63. Burt FJ, Leman PA, Smith JF, et al. The use of a reverse transcription-polymerase chain reaction for the detection of viral nucleic acid in the diagnosis of Crimean-Congo haemorrhagic fever. *J Virol Methods* 1998;70(2):129–137. doi: 10.1016/S0166-0934(97)00182-1.
64. Burt FJ, Paweska JT, Ashkettle B, et al. Genetic relationship in southern African Crimean-Congo haemorrhagic fever virus isolates: evidence for occurrence of reassortment. *Epidemiol Infect* 2009;137(9):1302–1308. doi: 10.1017/S0950268808001878.
65. Butt J, et al. Immunohistochemical and in situ localization of Crimean-Congo hemorrhagic fever (CCHF) virus in human tissues and implications for CCHF pathogenesis. *Arch Pathol Lab Med* 1997;121(8):839–846.
66. Calisher CH, Pretzman CI, Muth DJ, et al. Serodiagnosis of La Crosse virus infections in humans by detection of immunoglobulin M class antibodies. *J Clin Microbiol* 1986;23(4):667–671.
67. Calisher CH, Sever JL. Are North American Bunyamwera serogroup viruses etiologic agents of human congenital defects of the central nervous system? *Emerg Infect Dis* 1995;1(4):147–151. doi: 10.3201/eid0104.950409.
68. Calvert AE, Brault AC. Development and characterization of monoclonal antibodies directed against the nucleoprotein of Heartland virus. *Am J Trop Med Hyg* 2015;93(6):1338–1340. doi: 10.4269/ajtmh.15-0473.
69. Campbell GL, Reeves WC, Hardy JL, et al. Seroepidemiology of California and bunyamwera serogroup bunyavirus infections in humans in California. *Am J Epidemiol* 1992;136(3):308–319. doi: 10.1093/oxfordjournals.aje.a116496.
70. Capstick PB, Gosden D. Neutralizing antibody response of sheep to pantropic and neurotropic rift valley fever virus. *Nature* 1962;195:583–584.
71. Carlson AL, et al. Heartland virus and hemophagocytic lymphohistiocytosis in immunocompromised patient, Missouri, USA. *Emerg Infect Dis* 2018;24(5):893–897. doi: 10.3201/eid2405.171802.
72. Caroline AL, et al. Broad spectrum antiviral activity of favipiravir (T-705): protection from highly lethal inhalational Rift Valley fever. *PLoS Negl Trop Dis* 2014;8:e2790.
73. Casals J. Antigenic similarity between the virus causing Crimean hemorrhagic fever and Congo virus. *Exp Biol Med* 1969;131(1):233–236. doi: 10.3181/00379727-131-33847.
74. Castillo C, Naranjo J, Sepulveda A, et al. Hantavirus pulmonary syndrome due to Andes virus in Temuco, Chile: clinical experience with 16 adults. *Chest* 2001;120:548–554.
75. CDC. *Heartland Virus: Statistics & Maps.*
76. Çevik MA, et al. Clinical and laboratory features of Crimean-Congo hemorrhagic fever: predictors of fatality. *Int J Infect Dis* 2008;12(4):374–379. doi: 10.1016/j.ijid.2007.09.010.
77. Chambers PG, Swanepoel R. Rift Valley fever in abattoir workers. *Cent Afr J Med* 1980;26:122–126.
78. Chapman LE, et al. Intravenous ribavirin for hantavirus pulmonary syndrome: safety and tolerance during 1 year of open-label experience. Ribavirin Study Group. *Antivir Ther* 1999;4:211–219.
79. Chen HX, Qiu FX. Epidemiologic surveillance on the hemorrhagic fever with renal syndrome in China. *Chin Med J (Engl)* 1993;106:857–863.
80. Childs JE, Glass GE, Korch GW, et al. Effects of hantaviral infection on survival, growth and fertility in wild rat (*Rattus norvegicus*) populations of Baltimore, Maryland. *J Wildl Dis* 1989;25:469–476.
81. Chun R. Clinical aspects of LaCrosse encephalitis: neurological and psychological sequelae. In: Calisher CH, Thompson WH, eds. *California Serogroup Viruses.* 1983; 193–201.
82. Clarke LL, Ruder MG, Mead D, et al. Experimental infection of white-tailed deer (*Odocoileus virginanus*) with Heartland virus. *Am J Trop Med Hyg* 2018;98(4):1194–1196. doi: 10.4269/ajtmh.17-0963.
83. Clement J, et al. Clinical characteristics of Ratborne Seoul hantavirus disease. *Emerg Infect Dis* 2019;25:387–388.
84. Coackley W, Pini A, Gosden D. The immunity induced in cattle and sheep by inoculation of neurotropic or pantropic Rift Valley fever viruses. *Res Vet Sci* 1967; 8:406–414.
85. Connolly-Andersen AM, Douagi I, Kraus AA, et al. Crimean Congo hemorrhagic fever virus infects human monocyte-derived dendritic cells. *Virology* 2009;390(2):157–162. doi: 10.1016/j.virol.2009.06.010.
86. Connolly-Andersen AM, et al. Crimean-Congo hemorrhagic fever virus activates endothelial cells. *J Virol* 2011;85(15):7766–7774.
87. Cosgriff TM, et al. Hemostatic derangement produced by Rift Valley fever virus in rhesus monkeys. *Rev Infect Dis* 1989:11(Suppl 4):S807–S814.
88. Cui N, et al. Clinical progression and predictors of death in patients with severe fever with thrombocytopenia syndrome in China. *J Clin Virol* 2014;59(1):12–17. doi: 10.1016/j.jcv.2013.10.024.
89. Cusi MG, Savellini GG. Diagnostic tools for Toscana virus infection. *Expert Rev Anti Infect Ther* 2011;9:799–805.
90. Cusi MG, et al. Toscana virus infects dendritic and endothelial cells opening the way for the central nervous system. *J Neurovirol* 2016;22:307–315.
91. Cybinski DH, St George TD, Paull NI. Antibodies to Akabane virus in Australia. *Aust Vet J* 1978;54(1):1–3. doi: 10.1111/j.1751-0813.1978.tb00256.x.
92. de St Maurice A, et al. Rift valley fever viral load correlates with the human inflammatory response and coagulation pathway abnormalities in humans with hemorrhagic manifestations. *PLoS Negl Trop Dis* 2018;12:e0006460.
93. Deng B, et al. Clinical features and factors associated with severity and fatality among patients with severe fever with thrombocytopenia syndrome bunyavirus infection in Northeast China. *PLoS One* 2013; 8(11):e80802. doi: 10.1371/journal.pone.0080802.
94. Deyde VM, Nichol ST, Ksiazek TG, et al. Crimean-Congo hemorrhagic fever virus genomics and global diversity. *J Virol* 2006;80(17):8834–8842. doi: 10.1128/jvi.00752-06.
95. Dilcher M, et al. Genetic characterization of Erve virus, a European Nairovirus distantly related to Crimean-Congo hemorrhagic fever virus. *Virus Genes* 2012;45(3):426–432. doi: 10.1007/s11262-012-0796-8.
96. Ding YP, et al. Prognostic value of clinical and immunological markers in acute phase of SFTS virus infection. *Clin Microbiol Infect* 2014;20(11):O870–O878. doi: 10.1111/1469-0691.12636.
97. Dixon KE, Travassos da Rosa AP, Travassos da Rosa JF, et al. Oropouche virus. II. Epidemiological observations during an epidemic in Santarem, Para, Brazil in 1975. *Am J Trop Med Hyg* 1981;30(1):161–164.
98. Dodd KA, McElroy AK, Jones ME, et al. Rift Valley fever virus clearance and protection from neurologic disease are dependent on CD4+ T cell and virus-specific antibody responses. *J Virol* 2013;87(11):6161–6171.
99. Dodd KA, Bird BH, Metcalfe MG, et al. Single-dose immunization with virus replicon particles confers rapid robust protection against Rift Valley fever virus challenge. *J Virol* 2012;86:4204–4212.
100. Dodd KA, et al. Rift Valley fever virus encephalitis is associated with an ineffective systemic immune response and activated T cell infiltration into the CNS in an immunocompetent mouse model. *PLoS Negl Trop Dis* 2014;8(6):e2874.
101. Douglass RJ, Calisher CH, Wagoner KD, et al. Sin Nombre virus infection of deer mice in Montana: characteristics of newly infected mice, incidence, and temporal pattern of infection. *J Wildl Dis* 2007;43:12–22.
102. Dowall SD, Carroll MW, Hewson R. Development of vaccines against Crimean-Congo haemorrhagic fever virus. *Vaccine* 2017;35(44):6015–6023. doi: 10.1016/j.vaccine.2017.05.031.
103. Drosten C, Kümmerer BM, Schmitz H, et al. Molecular diagnostics of viral hemorrhagic fevers. *Antiviral Res* 2003;57(1–2):61–87. doi: 10.1016/S0166-3542(02)00201-2.
104. Duh D, et al. Viral load as predictor of Crimean-Congo hemorrhagic fever outcome. *Emerg Infect Dis* 2007;13(11):1769–1772. doi: 10.3201/eid1311.070222.
105. Dungu B, Lubisi BA, Ikegami T. Rift Valley fever vaccines: current and future needs. *Curr Opin Virol* 2018;29:8–15.
106. Dvorscak L, Czuchlewski DR. Successful triage of suspected hantavirus cardiopulmonary syndrome by peripheral blood smear review: a decade of experience in an endemic region. *Am J Clin Pathol* 2014;142:196–201.
107. Dykers TI, Brown KL, Gundersen CB, et al. Rapid diagnosis of LaCrosse encephalitis: detection of specific immunoglobulin M in cerebrospinal fluid. *J Clin Microbiol* 1985;22(5):740–744.

108. Dzagurova TK, et al. Isolation of sochi virus from a fatal case of hantavirus disease with fulminant clinical course. *Clin Infect Dis* 2012;54:e1-e4.
109. Easterbrook JD, Klein SL. Immunological mechanisms mediating hantavirus persistence in rodent reservoirs. *PLoS Pathog* 2008;4:e1000172.
110. Easterbrook JD, Zink MC, Klein SL. Regulatory T cells enhance persistence of the zoonotic pathogen Seoul virus in its reservoir host. *Proc Natl Acad Sci U S A* 2007;104:15502–15507.
111. Easterday BC. Rift Valley fever. *Adv Vet Sci* 1965;10:65–127.
112. Edwards JF, Livingston CW, Chung SI, et al. Ovine arthrogryposis and central nervous system malformations associated with in utero Cache Valley virus infection: spontaneous disease. *Vet Pathol* 1989;26(1):33–39. doi: 10.1177/030098588902600106.
113. Eitrem R, Stylianou M, Niklasson B. High prevalence rates of antibody to three sandfly fever viruses (Sicilian, Naples, and Toscana) among Cypriots. *Epidemiol Infect* 1991;107:685–691.
114. Elaldi N, et al. Relationship between IFNA1, IFNA5, IFNA10, and IFNA17 gene polymorphisms and Crimean-Congo hemorrhagic fever prognosis in a Turkish population range. *J Med Virol* 2016;88(7):1159–1167. doi: 10.1002/jmv.24456.
115. Elgh F, et al. Serological diagnosis of hantavirus infections by an enzyme-linked immunosorbent assay based on detection of immunoglobulin G and M responses to recombinant nucleocapsid proteins of five viral serotypes. *J Clin Microbiol* 1997;35:1122–1130.
116. Ennis FA, et al. Hantavirus pulmonary syndrome: CD8+ and CD4+ cytotoxic t lymphocytes to epitopes on Sin Nombre virus nucleocapsid protein isolated during acute illness. *Virology* 1997;238:380–390.
117. Ergönül Ö. Crimean-Congo haemorrhagic fever—review. *Lancet Infect Dis* 2006;6(4):203–214.
118. Ergonul O. Evidence supports ribavirin use in Crimean-Congo hemorrhagic fever. *Int J Infect Dis* 2014;29:296. doi: 10.1016/j.ijid.2014.08.016.
119. Ergonul O, Mirazimi A, Dimitrov DS. Treatment of Crimean-Congo hemorrhagic fever. In: *Crimean-Congo Hemorrhagic Fever: A Global Perspective*. 2007. doi: 10.1007/978-1-4020-6106-6_19.
120. Estrada-Peña A, Ruiz-Fons F, Acevedo P, et al. Factors driving the circulation and possible expansion of Crimean-Congo haemorrhagic fever virus in the western Palearctic. *J Appl Microbiol* 2013;114(1):278–286. doi: 10.1111/jam.12039.
121. Estrada-Peña A, Sánchez N, Estrada-Sánchez A. An assessment of the distribution and spread of the tick Hyalomma marginatum in the Western Palearctic under different climate scenarios. *Vector Borne Zoonotic Dis* 2012;12(9):758–768. doi: 10.1089/vbz.2011.0771.
122. Faburay B, LaBeaud AD, McVey DS, et al. Current status of Rift Valley fever vaccine development. *Vaccines (Basel)* 2017;5.
123. Faburay B, et al. A recombinant Rift Valley fever virus glycoprotein subunit vaccine confers full protection against Rift Valley Fever Challenge in Sheep. *Sci Rep* 2016;6:27719.
124. Feldmann H, et al. Utilization of autopsy RNA for the synthesis of the nucleocapsid antigen of a newly recognized virus associated with hantavirus pulmonary syndrome. *Virus Res* 1993;30(3):351–367.
125. Fernandez-García MD, et al. European survey on laboratory preparedness, response and diagnostic capacity for crimean-congo haemorrhagic fever, 2012. *Euro Surveill* 2014;19(26). doi: 10.2807/1560-7917.ES2014.19.26.20844.
126. Ferrer JF, et al. High prevalence of hantavirus infection in Indian communities of the Paraguayan and Argentinean Gran Chaco. *Am J Trop Med Hyg* 1998;59:438–444.
127. Fill MA, et al. Notes from the field: multiple cases of Seoul virus infection in a household with infected pet rats—Tennessee, December 2016–April 2017. *MMWR Morb Mortal Wkly Rep* 2017;66:1081–1082.
128. Fill MA, et al. Novel clinical and pathologic findings in a Heartland virus-associated death. *Clin Infect Dis* 2017;64(4):510–512. doi: 10.1093/cid/ciw766.
129. Frampton JW, Lanser S, Nichols C, et al. Sin Nombre virus infection in 1959. *Lancet* 1995;346:781–782.
130. Francis T, Magill TP. Rift Valley fever: a report of three cases of laboratory infection and the experimental transmission of the disease to ferrets. *J Exp Med* 1935;62:433–448.
131. Gabitzsch ES, Beaty MK, Blair CD, et al. *Aedes triseriatus* females transovarially infected with La Crosse virus mate more efficiently than uninfected mosquitoes. *J Med Entomol* 2009;46(5):1152–1158. doi: 10.1603/033.046.0524.
132. Gai ZT, et al. Clinical progress and risk factors for death in severe fever with thrombocytopenia syndrome patients. *J Infect Dis.* 2012;206(7):1095–1102. doi: 10.1093/infdis/jis472.
133. Gargili A, et al. The role of ticks in the maintenance and transmission of Crimean-Congo hemorrhagic fever virus: a review of published field and laboratory studies. *Antiviral Res* 2017;144:93–119.
134. Garrido JL, et al. Two recombinant human monoclonal antibodies that protect against lethal Andes hantavirus infection in vivo. *Sci Transl Med* 2018;10.
135. Garrison AR, et al. Development of a TaqMan®-minor groove binding protein assay for the detection and quantification of Crimean-Congo hemorrhagic fever virus. *Am J Trop Med Hyg* 2007;77(3):514–520.
136. Gavrilovskaya I, Gorbunova E, Koster F, et al. Elevated VEGF levels in pulmonary edema fluid and PBMCs from patients with acute hantavirus pulmonary syndrome. *Adv Virol* 2012;2012:674360.
137. Gavrilovskaya IN, Gorbunova EE, Mackow ER. Pathogenic hantaviruses direct the adherence of quiescent platelets to infected endothelial cells. *J Virol* 2010;84:4832–4839.
138. Glass GE, Childs JE, Korch GW, et al. Association of intraspecific wounding with hantaviral infection in wild rats (*Rattus norvegicus*). *Epidemiol Infect* 1988;101:459–472.
139. Glass GE, et al. Experimental evaluation of rodent exclusion methods to reduce hantavirus transmission to humans in rural housing. *Am J Trop Med Hyg* 1997;56:359–364.
140. Goldfarb LG, Chumakov MP, Myskin AA. An epidiomological model of Crimean hemorrhagic fever. *Am J Trop Med Hyg* 1980;29(2):260–264. doi: 10.4269/ajtmh.1980.29.260.
141. Gommet C, et al. Tissue tropism and target cells of NSs-deleted rift valley fever virus in live immunodeficient mice. *PLoS Negl Trop Dis* 2011;5:e1421.
142. Gonzalez JP, Georges AJ. Bunyaviral Fevers: Bunyamwera, Ilesha, Germiston, Bwamba, and Tataguine. In: Monath TP, ed. *The Arboviruses: Epidemiology and Ecology*. Boca Raton: 1988; 87–98.
143. Gonzalez-Scarano F, Janssen RS, Najjar JA, et al. An avirulent G1 glycoprotein variant of La Crosse bunyavirus with defective fusion function. *J Virol* 1985;54(3):757–763.
144. Gorbunova EE, Simons MJ, Gavrilovskaya IN, et al. The Andes Virus nucleocapsid protein directs basal endothelial cell permeability by activating RhoA. *MBio* 2016;7.
145. Gowen BB, et al. Modeling severe fever with Thrombocytopenia syndrome virus infection in Golden Syrian Hamsters: importance of STAT2 in preventing disease and effective treatment with favipiravir. *J Virol* 2017;91(3). doi: 10.1128/JVI.01942-16.
146. Grimstad PR, Artsob H, Karabatsos N, et al. Production and use of a hemagglutinin for detecting antibody to Jamestown Canyon virus. *J Clin Microbiol* 1987;25(8):1557–1559.
147. Groen J, et al. A macaque model for hantavirus infection. *J Infect Dis* 1995;172:38–44.
148. Guner R, et al. Case management and supportive treatment for patients with Crimean-Congo hemorrhagic fever. *Vector Borne Zoonotic Dis* 2012;12(9):805–811. doi: 10.1089/vbz.2011.0896.
149. Gunes T, et al. Crimean-congo hemorrhagic fever virus in high-risk population, Turkey. *Emerg Infect Dis* 2009;15:461–464.
150. Gupta S, et al. Hantavirus-infection confers resistance to cytotoxic lymphocyte-mediated apoptosis. *PLoS Pathog* 2013;9:e1003272.
151. Haddock E, et al. A cynomolgus macaque model for Crimean-Congo haemorrhagic fever. *Nat Microbiol* 2018;3(5):556–562. doi: 10.1038/s41564-018-0141-7.
152. Haddow AD, Bixler D, Odoi A. The spatial epidemiology and clinical features of reported cases of La Crosse Virus infection in West Virginia from 2003 to 2007. *BMC Infect Dis* 2011;11:29. doi: 10.1186/1471-2334-11-29.
153. Haddow AD, Odoi A. The incidence risk, clustering, and clinical presentation of La Crosse virus infections in the Eastern United States, 2003-2007. *PLoS One* 2009;4(7):e6145. doi: 10.1371/journal.pone.0006145.
154. Hardy JL, Eldridge BF, Reeves WC, et al. Isolations of Jamestown Canyon virus (Bunyaviridae: California serogroup) from mosquitoes (Diptera: Culicidae) in the western United States, 1990–1992. *J Med Entomol* 1993;30(6):1053–1059. doi: 10.1093/jmedent/30.6.1053.
155. Harmon JR, et al. CD4 T cells, CD8 T cells, and monocytes coordinate to prevent Rift Valley fever virus encephalitis. *J Virol* 2018;92(24). doi: 10.1128/jvi.01270-18.
156. Hawman DW, et al. Favipiravir (T-705) but not ribavirin is effective against two distinct strains of Crimean-Congo hemorrhagic fever virus in mice. *Antiviral Res* 2018;157:18–26. doi: 10.1016/j.antiviral.2018.06.013.
157. Heiske A, et al. Polymerase chain reaction detection of Puumala virus RNA in formaldehyde-fixed biopsy material. *Kidney Int* 1999;55:2062–2069.
158. Hewson R, et al. Evidence of segment reassortment in Crimean-Congo haemorrhagic fever virus. *J Gen Virol* 2004;85(Pt 10):3059–3070. doi: 10.1099/vir.0.80121-0.
159. Hise AG, et al. Association of symptoms and severity of rift valley fever with genetic polymorphisms in human innate immune pathways. *PLoS Negl Trop Dis* 2015;9:e0003584.
160. Hjelle B, et al. Molecular linkage of hantavirus pulmonary syndrome to the white-footed mouse, *Peromyscus leucopus*: genetic characterization of the M genome of New York virus. *J Virol* 1995;69:8137–8141.
161. Hjelle B, et al. Hantavirus pulmonary syndrome, renal insufficiency, and myositis associated with infection by Bayou hantavirus. *Clin Infect Dis* 1996;23:495–500.
162. Hjelle B, et al. Rapid and specific detection of Sin Nombre virus antibodies in patients with hantavirus pulmonary syndrome by a strip immunoblot assay suitable for field diagnosis. *J Clin Microbiol* 1997;35:600–608.
163. Holmes EC, Zhang YZ. The evolution and emergence of hantaviruses. *Curr Opin Virol* 2015;10:27–33.
164. Hoogstraal H. The epidemiology of tick-borne Crimean-Congo hemorrhagic fever in Asia, Europe, and Africa. *J Med Entomol* 1979;5:307–417.
165. Hoogstraal H. Review Article 1: The epidemiology of tick-borne Crimean-Congo hemorrhagic fever in Asia, Europe, and Africa. *J Med Entomol* 1979;15(4):307–417. doi: 10.1093/jmedent/15.4.307.
166. Hooper JW, Larsen T, Custer DM, et al. A lethal disease model for hantavirus pulmonary syndrome. *Virology* 2001;289:6–14.
167. Hooper JW, Li D. Vaccines against hantaviruses. *Curr Top Microbiol Immunol* 2001;256:171–191.
168. Hooper JW, et al. A Phase 1 clinical trial of Hantaan virus and Puumala virus M-segment DNA vaccines for haemorrhagic fever with renal syndrome delivered by intramuscular electroporation. *Clin Microbiol Infect* 2014;20(Suppl 5):110–117.
169. Hooper JW, et al. DNA vaccine-derived human IgG produced in transchromosomal bovines protect in lethal models of hantavirus pulmonary syndrome. *Sci Transl Med* 2014;6:264ra162.
170. Hopkins AS, et al. Experimental evaluation of rodent exclusion methods to reduce hantavirus transmission to residents in a Native American community in New Mexico. *Vector Borne Zoonotic Dis* 2002;2:61–68.
171. Horling J, Lundkvist A, Huggins JW, et al. Antibodies to Puumala virus in humans determined by neutralization test. *J Virol Methods* 1992;39:139–147.
172. Huang C, Campbell WP, Means R, et al. Hantavirus S RNA sequence from a fatal case of HPS in New York. *J Med Virol* 1996;50:5–8.
173. Huggins JW, Kim GR, Brand OM, et al. Ribavirin therapy for Hantaan virus infection in suckling mice. *J Infect Dis* 1986;153:489–497.
174. Huggins JW, et al. Prospective, double-blind, concurrent, placebo-controlled clinical trial of intravenous ribavirin therapy of hemorrhagic fever with renal syndrome. *J Infect Dis* 1991;164:1119–1127.
175. Hung T, et al. Identification of Hantaan virus-related structures in kidneys of cadavers with haemorrhagic fever with renal syndrome. *Arch Virol* 1992;122:187–199.
176. Ide S, et al. Detection of antibodies against Akabane virus in bovine sera by enzyme-linked immunosorbent assay. *Vet Microbiol* 1989;20(3):275–280. doi: 10.1016/0378-1135(89)90051-5.
177. Ikegami T. Rift Valley fever vaccines: an overview of the safety and efficacy of the live-attenuated MP-12 vaccine candidate. *Expert Rev Vaccines* 2017;16:601–611.
178. Ikegami T, Makino S. The pathogenesis of Rift Valley fever. *Viruses* 2011;3:493–519.

179. Ilhan O, et al. O-21 double filtration plasmapheresis in the management of a Crimean-Congo hemorrhagic fever case. *Transfus Apher Sci* 2012;47(Suppl 1):S11. doi: 10.1016/s1473-0502(12)70022-8.

180. Jansen van Vuren P, et al. Serum levels of inflammatory cytokines in Rift Valley fever patients are indicative of severe disease. *Virol J* 2015;12:159.

181. Janssen R, Gonzalez-Scarano F, Nathanson N. Mechanisms of bunyavirus virulence. Comparative pathogenesis of a virulent strain of La Crosse and an avirulent strain of Tahyna virus. *Lab Invest* 1984;50(4):447–455.

182. Jenison S, et al. Characterization of human antibody responses to four corners hantavirus infections among patients with hantavirus pulmonary syndrome. *J Virol* 1994;68:3000–3006.

183. Jennings M, Mellor PS. *Culicoides*: biological vectors of akabane virus. *Vet Microbiol* 1989;21(2):125–131. doi: 10.1016/0378-1135(89)90024-2.

184. Jiang JF, Zhang WY, Wu XM, et al. Soochong virus and Amur virus might be the same entities of hantavirus. *J Med Virol* 2007;79:1792–1795.

185. Jiao Y, et al. Preparation and evaluation of recombinant severe fever with thrombocytopenia syndrome virus nucleocapsid protein for detection of total antibodies in human and animal sera by double-antigen sandwich enzyme-linked immunosorbent assay. *J Clin Microbiol* 2012;50(2):372–377. doi: 10.1128/JCM.01319-11.

186. Johnson S, et al. Ribavirin for treating Crimean Congo haemorrhagic fever. *Cochrane Database Syst Rev* 2018;6:CD012713. doi: 10.1002/14651858.CD012713.pub2.

187. Jones TF, et al. Newly recognized focus of La Crosse encephalitis in Tennessee. *Clin Infect Dis* 1999;28(1):93–97.

188. Jonsson CB, Figueiredo LT, Vapalahti O. A global perspective on hantavirus ecology, epidemiology, and disease. *Clin Microbiol Rev* 2010;23:412–441.

189. Joubert JR, King JB, Rossouw DJ, et al. A nosocomial outbreak of Crimean-Congo haemorrhagic fever at Tygerberg Hospital Part III. Clinical pathology and pathogenesis. *S Afr Med J* 1985;68(10):722–728.

190. Kalfayan B. Pathology of La Crosse virus infection in humans. *Prog Clin Biol Res* 1983;123:179–186.

191. Kallio ER, et al. Endemic hantavirus infection impairs the winter survival of its rodent host. *Ecology* 2007;88:1911–1916.

192. Kariwa H, et al. Genetic diversities of hantaviruses among rodents in Hokkaido, Japan and Far East Russia. *Virus Res* 1999;59:219–228.

193. Kerins JL, et al. Outbreak of Seoul Virus among rats and rat owners—United States and Canada, 2017. *MMWR Morb Mortal Wkly Rep* 2018;67:131–134.

194. Khaiboullina SF, et al. Serum cytokine profiles differentiating hemorrhagic fever with renal syndrome and hantavirus pulmonary syndrome. *Front Immunol* 2017;8:567.

195. Khan AS, et al. Fatal illness associated with a new hantavirus in Louisiana. *J Med Virol* 1995;46:281–286.

196. Khan AS, et al. Hantavirus pulmonary syndrome in Florida: association with the newly identified Black Creek Canal virus. *Am J Med* 1996;100:46–48.

197. Kilinc C, et al. Examination of the specific clinical symptoms and laboratory findings of crimean-congo hemorrhagic fever. *J Vector Borne Dis* 2016;53(2):162–167.

198. Kilpatrick ED, et al. Role of specific CD8+ T cells in the severity of a fulminant zoonotic viral hemorrhagic fever, hantavirus pulmonary syndrome. *J Immunol* 2004;172:3297–3304.

199. Kim YS, et al. Hemorrhagic fever with renal syndrome caused by the Seoul virus. *Nephron* 1995;71:419–427.

200. Kim YH, et al. Development of inactivated trivalent vaccine for the teratogenic Aino, Akabane and Chuzan viruses. *Biologicals* 2011;39(3):152–157. doi: 10.1016/j.biologicals.2011.02.004.

201. Kirkland PD. Akabane disease. In: *Diseases of Sheep: Fourth Edition*. 2008. doi: 10.1002/9780470753316.ch63.

202. Kızıldağ S, Arslan S, Özbilüm N, et al. Effect of TLR10 (2322A/G, 720A/C, and 992T/A) polymorphisms on the pathogenesis of Crimean Congo hemorrhagic fever disease. *J Med Virol* 2018;90(1):19–25. doi: 10.1002/jmv.24924.

203. Klein SL, et al. Sex differences in the incidence and case fatality rates from hemorrhagic fever with renal syndrome in China, 2004-2008. *Clin Infect Dis* 2011;52:1414–1421.

204. Klingstrom J, Plyusnin A, Vaheri A, et al. Wild-type Puumala hantavirus infection induces cytokines, C-reactive protein, creatinine, and nitric oxide in cynomolgus macaques. *J Virol* 2002;76:444–449.

205. Kobak L, et al. Hantavirus-induced pathogenesis in mice with a humanized immune system. *J Gen Virol* 2015;96:1258–1263.

206. Kokernot RH, Smithburn KC, De Meillon B, et al. Isolation of Bunyamwera virus from a naturally infected human being and further isolations from Aedes (Banksinella) circumluteolus theo. *Am J Trop Med Hyg* 1958;7(6):579–584.

207. Koma T, et al. Neutrophil depletion suppresses pulmonary vascular hyperpermeability and occurrence of pulmonary edema caused by hantavirus infection in C.B-17 SCID mice. *J Virol* 2014;88:7178–7188.

208. Kortekaas J. One health approach to Rift Valley fever vaccine development. *Antiviral Res* 2014;106:24–32.

209. Koster F, et al. Rapid presumptive diagnosis of hantavirus cardiopulmonary syndrome by peripheral blood smear review. *Am J Clin Pathol* 2001;116:665–672.

210. Krautkramer E, Grouls S, Stein N, et al. Pathogenic old world hantaviruses infect renal glomerular and tubular cells and induce disassembling of cell-to-cell contacts. *J Virol* 2011;85:9811–9823.

211. Krautkramer E, Lehmann MJ, Bollinger V, et al. Polar release of pathogenic Old World hantaviruses from renal tubular epithelial cells. *Virol J* 2012;9:299.

212. Kruger DH, Figueiredo LT, Song JW, et al. Hantaviruses—globally emerging pathogens. *J Clin Virol* 2015;64:128–136.

213. Ksiazek TG, et al. Rift Valley fever among domestic animals in the recent West African outbreak. *Res Virol* 1989;140:67–77.

214. Ksiazek TG, et al. Identification of a new north American hantavirus that causes acute pulmonary insufficiency. *Am J Trop Med Hyg* 1995;52(2):117–123.

215. Kubar A, et al. Prompt administration of crimean-congo hemorrhagic fever (CCHF) virus hyperimmunoglobulin in patients diagnosed with CCHF and viral load monitorization by reverse transcriptase-PCR. *Jpn J Infect Dis* 2011;64(5):439–443.

216. Kuno G, Mitchell CJ, Chang GJ, et al. Detecting bunyaviruses of the Bunyamwera and California serogroups by a PCR technique. *J Clin Microbiol* 1996;34(5):1184–1188.

217. Kurogi H, Akiba K, Inaba Y, et al. Isolation of Akabane virus from the biting midge *Culicoides oxystoma* in Japan. *Vet Microbiol* 1987;15(3):243–248. doi: 10.1016/0378-1135(87)90078-2.

218. LaBeaud AD, Kazura JW, King CH. Advances in Rift Valley fever research: insights for disease prevention. *Curr Opin Infect Dis* 2010;23:403–408.

219. LaBeaud AD, et al. Factors associated with severe human Rift Valley fever in Sangailu, Garissa County, Kenya. *PLoS Negl Trop Dis* 2015;9:e0003548.

220. Laine O, et al. Enhanced thrombin formation and fibrinolysis during acute Puumala hantavirus infection. *Thromb Res* 2010;126:154–158.

221. Laine O, et al. Hantavirus infection-induced thrombocytopenia triggers increased production but associates with impaired aggregation of platelets except for collagen. *Thromb Res* 2015;136:1126–1132.

222. Lambert AJ, Lanciotti RS. Consensus amplification and novel multiplex sequencing method for S segment species identification of 47 viruses of the Orthobunyavirus, Phlebovirus, and Nairovirus genera of the family Bunyaviridae. *J Clin Microbiol* 2009;47(8):2398–2404. doi: 10.1128/JCM.00182-09.

223. Lambert AJ, et al. Nucleic acid amplification assays for detection of La Crosse virus RNA. *J Clin Microbiol* 2005;43(4):1885–1889. doi: 10.1128/JCM.43.4.1885-1889.2005.

224. Lambert AJ, et al. La Crosse virus in *Aedes albopictus* mosquitoes, Texas, USA, 2009. *Emerg Infect Dis* 2010;16(5):856–858. doi: 10.3201/eid1605.100170.

225. LeDuc JW. Epidemiology of Hantaan and related viruses. *Lab Anim Sci* 1987;37:413–418.

226. Lee HW. Hemorrhagic fever with renal syndrome in Korea. *Rev Infect Dis* 1989;11(Suppl 4):S864–S876.

227. Lee HW, van der Groen G. Hemorrhagic fever with renal syndrome. *Prog Med Virol* 1989;36:62–102.

228. Lee HW, et al. Observations on natural and laboratory infection of rodents with the etiologic agent of Korean hemorrhagic fever. *Am J Trop Med Hyg* 1981;30:477–482.

229. Levine JR, Fritz CL, Novak MG. Occupational risk of exposure to rodent-borne hantavirus at US forest service facilities in California. *Am J Trop Med Hyg* 2008;78:352–357.

230. Levis S, et al. Genetic diversity and epidemiology of hantaviruses in Argentina. *J Infect Dis* 1998;177:529–538.

231. Li S, et al. Multiple organ involvement in severe fever with thrombocytopenia syndrome: an immunohistochemical finding in a fatal case. *Virol J* 2018;15(1):97. doi: 10.1186/s12985-018-1006-7.

232. Lindgren T, et al. Longitudinal analysis of the human T cell response during acute hantavirus infection. *J Virol* 2011;85:10252–10260.

233. Linthicum KJ, Davies FG, Kairo A, et al. Rift Valley fever virus (family Bunyaviridae, genus *Phlebovirus*). Isolations from Diptera collected during an inter-epizootic period in Kenya. *J Hyg (Lond)* 1985;95:197–209.

234. Linthicum KJ, et al. Climate and satellite indicators to forecast Rift Valley fever epidemics in Kenya. *Science* 1999;285:397–400.

235. Liu MM, Lei XY, Yu XJ. Meta-analysis of the clinical and laboratory parameters of SFTS patients in China. *Virol J* 2016;13(1):198. doi: 10.1186/s12985-016-0661-9.

236. Liu W, et al. Case-Fatality ratio and effectiveness of ribavirin therapy among hospitalized patients in china who had severe fever with thrombocytopenia syndrome. *Clin Infect Dis* 2013;57(9):1292–1299. doi: 10.1093/cid/cit530.

237. Liu Y, et al. The pathogenesis of severe fever with thrombocytopenia syndrome virus infection in alpha/beta interferon knockout mice: insights into the pathologic mechanisms of a new viral hemorrhagic fever. *J Virol* 2014;88(3):1781–1786. doi: 10.1128/JVI.02277-13.

238. Liu K, et al. A national assessment of the epidemiology of severe fever with thrombocytopenia syndrome, China. *Sci Rep* 2015;5:9679. doi: 10.1038/srep09679.

239. Liu J, et al. Dynamic changes of laboratory parameters and peripheral blood lymphocyte subsets in severe fever with thrombocytopenia syndrome patients. *Int J Infect Dis* 2017;58:45–51. doi: 10.1016/j.ijid.2017.02.017.

240. Logue CH, et al. Development of a real-time RT-PCR assay for the detection of Crimean-Congo hemorrhagic fever virus. *Vector Borne Zoonotic Dis* 2012;12(9):786–793. doi: 10.1089/vbz.2011.0770.

241. Lopez N, Padula P, Rossi C, et al. Genetic identification of a new hantavirus causing severe pulmonary syndrome in Argentina. *Virology* 1996;220:223–226.

242. Luo LM, et al. *Haemaphysalis longicornis* ticks as reservoir and vector of severe fever with thrombocytopenia syndrome virus in China. *Emerg Infect Dis* 2015;21(10):1770–1776. doi: 10.3201/eid2110.150126.

243. Ly HJ, Ikegami T. Rift Valley fever virus NSs protein functions and the similarity to other bunyavirus NSs proteins. *Virol J* 2016;13:118.

244. Ma Y, et al. Hantaan virus infection induces both Th1 and ThGranzyme B+ cell immune responses that associated with viral control and clinical outcome in humans. *PLoS Pathog* 2015;11:e1004788.

245. Mackow ER, Gorbunova EE, Gavrilovskaya IN. Endothelial cell dysfunction in viral hemorrhage and edema. *Front Microbiol* 2014;5:733.

246. MacNeil A, Comer JA, Ksiazek TG, et al. Sin Nombre virus-specific immunoglobulin M and G kinetics in hantavirus pulmonary syndrome and the role played by serologic responses in predicting disease outcome. *J Infect Dis* 2010;202:242–246.

247. MacNeil A, Nichol, ST, Spiropoulou CF. Hantavirus pulmonary syndrome. *Virus Res* 2011;162(1–2):138–147.

248. Madani TA, et al. Rift Valley fever epidemic in Saudi Arabia: epidemiological, clinical, and laboratory characteristics. *Clin Infect Dis* 2003;37:1084–1092.

249. Makela S, et al. Human leukocyte antigen-B8-DR3 is a more important risk factor for severe Puumala hantavirus infection than the tumor necrosis factor-alpha(-308) G/A polymorphism. *J Infect Dis* 2002;186:843–846.

250. Maleki KT, et al. Severity and outcome of hantavirus pulmonary syndrome marked by increased serum levels of IL-6 and intestinal fatty acid-binding protein. *J Infect Dis* 2019. doi: 10.1093/infdis/jiz005.

251. Maltezou HC, et al. Crimean-congo hemorrhagic fever in Europe: current situation calls for preparedness. *Euro Surveill* 2010;15(10):19504.

252. Manigold T, et al. Highly differentiated, resting gn-specific memory CD8+ T cells persist years after infection by Andes hantavirus. *PLoS Pathog* 2010;6:e1000779.
253. Marczinke BI, Nichol ST. Nairobi sheep disease virus, an important tick-borne pathogen of sheep and goats in Africa, is also present in Asia. *Virology* 2002;303(1):146–151. doi: 10.1006/viro.2002.1514.
254. Marsac D, et al. Infection of human monocyte-derived dendritic cells by ANDES hantavirus enhances pro-inflammatory state, the secretion of active MMP-9 and indirectly enhances endothelial permeability. *Virol J* 2011;8:223.
255. Martinez VP, et al. Hantavirus pulmonary syndrome in Argentina, 1995–2008. *Emerg Infect Dis* 2010;16:1853–1860.
256. Martinez-Valdebenito C, et al. Person-to-person household and nosocomial transmission of Andes hantavirus, Southern Chile, 2011. *Emerg Infect Dis* 2014;20:1629–1636.
257. Matsuno K, et al. Animal models of emerging tick-borne phleboviruses: determining target cells in a lethal model of SFTSV infection. *Front Microbiol* 2017;8:104. doi: 10.3389/fmicb.2017.00104.
258. McConnell S, Livingston C, Calisher CH, et al. Isolations of cache valley virus in Texas, 1981. *Vet Microbiol* 1987;13(1):11–18. doi: 10.1016/0378-1135(87)90093-9.
259. McElroy AK, Harmon JR, Flietstra T, et al. Human biomarkers of outcome following Rift Valley fever virus infection. *J Infect Dis* 2018;218:1847–1851.
260. McElroy AK, Nichol ST. Rift Valley fever virus inhibits a pro-inflammatory response in experimentally infected human monocyte derived macrophages and a pro-inflammatory cytokine response may be associated with patient survival during natural infection. *Virology* 2012;422:6–12.
261. McJunkin JE, Khan RR, Tsai TF. California-La Crosse encephalitis. *Infect Dis Clin North Am* 1998;12(1):83–93. doi: 10.1016/S0891-5520(05)70410-4.
262. McMillen CM, Hartman AL. Rift Valley fever in animals and humans: current perspectives. *Antiviral Res* 2018;156:29–37.
263. McMullan LK, et al. A new Phlebovirus associated with severe febrile illness in Missouri. *N Engl J Med* 2012;367(9):834–841. doi: 10.1056/NEJMoa1203378.
264. Mertz GJ, et al. Placebo-controlled, double-blind trial of intravenous ribavirin for the treatment of hantavirus cardiopulmonary syndrome in North America. *Clin Infect Dis* 2004;39:1307–1313.
265. Mills JN, et al. A survey of hantavirus antibody in small-mammal populations in selected United States National Parks. *Am J Trop Med Hyg* 1998;58:525–532.
266. Mohamed M, et al. Epidemiologic and clinical aspects of a Rift Valley fever outbreak in humans in Tanzania, 2007. *Am J Trop Med Hyg* 2010;83:22–27.
267. Monroe MC, et al. Genetic diversity and distribution of Peromyscus-borne hantaviruses in North America. *Emerg Infect Dis* 1999;5:75–86.
268. Mori M, et al. High levels of cytokine-producing cells in the lung tissues of patients with fatal hantavirus pulmonary syndrome. *J Infect Dis* 1999;179:295–302.
269. Moriconi M, et al. Phlebotomine sand fly-borne pathogens in the Mediterranean Basin: Human leishmaniasis and phlebovirus infections. *PLoS Negl Trop Dis* 2017;11:e0005660.
270. Morrill JC, Jennings GB, Cosgriff TM, et al. Prevention of Rift Valley fever in rhesus monkeys with interferon-alpha. *Rev Infect Dis* 1989;11:S815–S825.
271. Morrill JC, et al. Pathogenesis of Rift Valley fever in rhesus monkeys: role of interferon response. *Arch Virol* 1990;110:195–212.
272. Morvan J, Rollin PE, Laventure S, et al. Rift Valley fever epizootic in the central highlands of Madagascar. *Res Virol* 1992;143:407–415.
273. Morzunov SP, et al. A newly recognized virus associated with a fatal case of hantavirus pulmonary syndrome in Louisiana. *J Virol* 1995;69(3):1980–1983.
274. Mostafavi E, Pourhossein B, Chinikar S. Clinical symptoms and laboratory findings supporting early diagnosis of Crimean-Congo hemorrhagic fever in Iran. *J Med Virol* 2014;86(7):1188–1192. doi: 10.1002/jmv.23922.
275. Mourão MP, et al. Oropouche fever outbreak, Manaus, Brazil, 2007–2008. *Emerg Infect Dis* 2009;15(12):2063–2064. doi: 10.3201/eid1512.090917.
276. Muehlenbachs A, et al. Heartland virus-associated death in Tennessee. *Clin Infect Dis* 2014;59(6):845–850. doi: 10.1093/cid/ciu434.
277. Murray MD. Akabane epizootics in New South Wales: evidence for long-distance dispersal of the biting midge *Culicoides brevitarsis*. *Aust Vet J* 1987;64(10):305–308. doi: 10.1111/j.1751-0813.1987.tb07332.x.
278. Mustonen J, et al. Human leukocyte antigens B8-DRB1*03 in pediatric patients with nephropathia epidemica caused by Puumala hantavirus. *Pediatr Infect Dis J* 2004;23:959–961.
279. Navarro-Marí JM, Palop-Borrás B, Pérez-Ruiz M, et al. Serosurvey study of Toscana virus in domestic animals, Granada, Spain. *Vector Borne Zoonotic Dis* 2011;11:583–587.
280. Netski D, Thran BH, St Jeor SC. Sin Nombre virus pathogenesis in *Peromyscus maniculatus*. *J Virol* 1999;73:585–591.
281. Ngo KA, et al. Isolation of Bunyamwera serogroup viruses (Bunyaviridae, Orthobunyavirus) in New York State. *J Med Entomol* 2006;43(5):1004–1009. doi: 10.1603/0022-2585(2006)43[1004:iobsvb]2.0.co;2.
282. Ni H, et al. *Apodemus agrarius* is a potential natural host of severe fever with thrombocytopenia syndrome (SFTS)-causing novel bunyavirus. *J Clin Virol* 2015;71:82–88. doi: 10.1016/j.jcv.2015.08.006.
283. Nichol ST, et al. Genetic identification of a hantavirus associated with an outbreak of acute respiratory illness. *Science* 1993;262(5135):914–917.
284. Nicholson WL, et al. Surveillance for Heartland virus (Bunyaviridae: *Phlebovirus*) in Missouri during 2013: first detection of virus in adults of *Amblyomma americanum* (Acari: Ixodidae). *J Med Entomol* 2016;53(3):607–612. doi: 10.1093/jme/tjw028.
285. Nicoletti L, et al. Central nervous system involvement during infection by Phlebovirus toscana of residents in natural foci in central Italy (1977–1988). *Am J Trop Med Hyg* 1991;45:429–434.
286. Niu G, et al. Severe fever with thrombocytopenia syndrome virus among domesticated animals, China. *Emerg Infect Dis* 2013;19(5):756–763. doi: 10.3201/eid1905.120245.
287. Nolte KB, et al. Hantavirus pulmonary syndrome in the United States: a pathological description of a disease caused by a new agent. *Hum Pathol* 1995;26:110–120.
288. Nunez JJ, et al. Hantavirus infections among overnight visitors to Yosemite National Park, California, USA, 2012. *Emerg Infect Dis* 2014;20:386–393.
289. Nuttall PA, Labuda M. Tick-host interactions: saliva-activated transmission. *Parasitology* 2004;129(Suppl):S177–S189. doi: 10.1017/S0031182004005633.
290. Nyakarahuka L, et al. Prevalence and risk factors of Rift Valley fever in humans and animals from Kabale district in Southwestern Uganda, 2016. *PLoS Negl Trop Dis* 2018;12:e0006412.
291. Odendaal L, Clift SJ, Fosgate GT, et al. Lesions and cellular tropism of natural Rift Valley fever virus infection in adult sheep. *Vet Pathol* 2019;56:61–77.
292. Oestereich L, et al. Evaluation of antiviral efficacy of Ribavirin, Arbidol, and T-705 (Favipiravir) in a mouse model for Crimean-Congo hemorrhagic fever. *PLoS Negl Trop Dis* 2014;8(5):e2804. doi: 10.1371/journal.pntd.0002804.
293. Osman HAM, et al. Development and evaluation of loop-mediated isothermal amplification assay for detection of Crimean Congo hemorrhagic fever virus in Sudan. *J Virol Methods* 2013;190(1–2):4–10. doi: 10.1016/j.jviromet.2013.03.004.
294. Padula PJ, et al. Hantavirus pulmonary syndrome outbreak in Argentina: molecular evidence for person-to-person transmission of Andes virus. *Virology* 1998;241:323–330.
295. Pal E, et al. Relationship between circulating vascular endothelial growth factor and its soluble receptor in patients with hemorrhagic fever with renal syndrome. *Emerg Microbes Infect* 2018;7:89.
296. Papa A. Dobrava-Belgrade virus: phylogeny, epidemiology, disease. *Antiviral Res* 2012;95:104–117.
297. Papa A, Mirazimi A, Köksal I, et al. Recent advances in research on Crimean-Congo hemorrhagic fever. *J Clin Virol* 2015;64:137–143. doi: 10.1016/j.jcv.2014.08.029.
298. Papa A, et al. Retrospective serological and genetic study of the distribution of hantaviruses in Greece. *J Med Virol* 1998;55(4):321–327.
299. Papa A, et al. Meeting report: tenth international conference on hantaviruses. *Antiviral Res* 2016;133:234–241.
300. Papa A, et al. Cytokines as biomarkers of Crimean-Congo hemorrhagic fever. *J Med Virol* 2016;88(1):21–27. doi: 10.1002/jmv.24312.
301. Park I, Kim HI, Kwon KT. Two treatment cases of severe fever and thrombocytopenia syndrome with oral ribavirin and plasma exchange. *Infect Chemother* 2017;49(1):72–77. doi: 10.3947/ic.2017.49.1.72.
302. Parsonson IM, McPhee DA. Bunyavirus pathogenesis. *Adv Virus Res* 1985;30:279–316. doi: 10.1016/S0065-3527(08)60453-4.
303. Parsonson IM, Della Porta AJ, Snowdon WA. Congenital abnormalities in newborn lambs after infection of pregnant sheep with Akabane virus. *Infect Immun* 1977;15(1):254–262.
304. Pepin M, Bouloy M, Bird BH, et al. Rift Valley fever virus (Bunyaviridae: *Phlebovirus*): an update on pathogenesis, molecular epidemiology, vectors, diagnostics and prevention. *Vet Res* 2010;41:61.
305. Peters CJ, Liu CT, Anderson GW Jr, et al. Pathogenesis of viral hemorrhagic fevers: Rift Valley fever and Lassa fever contrasted. *Rev Infect Dis* 1989;11:S743–S749.
306. Peters CJ, Reynolds JA, Slone TW, et al. Prophylaxis of Rift Valley fever with antiviral drugs, immune serum, an interferon inducer, and a macrophage activator. *Antiviral Res* 1986;6:285–297.
307. Peters CJ, Simpson GL, Levy H. Spectrum of hantavirus infection: hemorrhagic fever with renal syndrome and hantavirus pulmonary syndrome. *Annu Rev Med* 1999;50:531–545.
308. Peters CJ, et al. Experimental Rift Valley fever in rhesus macaques. *Arch Virol* 1988;99:31–44.
309. Pettersson L, et al. Viral load and humoral immune response in association with disease severity in Puumala hantavirus-infected patients—implications for treatment. *Clin Microbiol Infect* 2014;20:235–241.
310. Peyrefitte CN, et al. Differential activation profiles of Crimean-Congo hemorrhagic fever virus- and Dugbe virus-infected antigen-presenting cells. *J Gen Virol* 2010;91(Pt 1):189–198. doi: 10.1099/vir.0.015701-0.
311. Pierro A, et al. Characterization of antibody response in neuroinvasive infection caused by Toscana virus. *Clin Microbiol Infect* 2017;23:868–873.
312. Pilaski J, et al. Genetic identification of a new Puumala virus strain causing severe hemorrhagic fever with renal syndrome in Germany. *J Infect Dis* 1994;170:1456–1462.
313. Pinheiro FP, Hoch AL, Gomes ML, et al. Oropouche virus. IV. Laboratory transmission by *Culicoides paraensis*. *Am J Trop Med Hyg* 1981;30(1):172–176. doi: 10.4269/ajtmh.1981.30.172.
314. Pinheiro FP, Travassos Da Rosa AP, Gomes ML, et al. Transmission of Oropouche virus from man to hamster by the midge *Culicoides paraensis*. *Science* 1982;215(4537):1251–1253. doi: 10.1126/science.6800036.
315. Pinheiro FP, et al. [Meningitis associated with Oropouche virus infections]. *Rev Inst Med Trop Sao Paulo* 1982;24(4):246–251.
316. Plyusnin A, Elliott RM. *Bunyaviridae: Molecular and Cellular Biology*. Caister Academic Press: Oxford, United Kingdom; 2011.
317. Plyusnin A, Morzunov SP. Virus evolution and genetic diversity of hantaviruses and their rodent hosts. *Curr Top Microbiol Immunol* 2001;256:47–75.
318. Plyusnin A, Sironen T. Evolution of hantaviruses: co-speciation with reservoir hosts for more than 100 MYR. *Virus Res* 2014;187:22–26.
319. Prescott J, DeBuysscher BL, Brown KS, et al. Long-term single-dose efficacy of a vesicular stomatitis virus-based Andes virus vaccine in Syrian hamsters. *Viruses* 2014;6:516–523.
320. Pshenichnaya NY, et al. Crimean-Congo hemorrhagic fever in pregnancy: a systematic review and case series from Russia, Kazakhstan and Turkey. *Int J Infect Dis* 2017;58:58–64. doi: 10.1016/j.ijid.2017.02.019.
321. Putkuri N, Vaheri A, Vapalahti O. Prevalence and protein specificity of human antibodies to Inkoo virus infection. *Clin Vaccine Immunol* 2007;14(12):1555–1562. doi: 10.1128/CVI.00288-07.
322. Qu J, et al. Fever with thrombocytopenia associated with a novel bunyavirus in China. *N Engl J Med* 2011;364:1523–1532. doi: 10.1056/nejmoa1010095.
323. Raftery MJ, Kraus AA, Ulrich R, et al. Hantavirus infection of dendritic cells. *J Virol* 2002;76:10724–10733.
324. Raftery MJ, et al. $\beta 2$ integrin mediates hantavirus-induced release of neutrophil extracellular traps. *J Exp Med* 2014;211:1485–1497.

325. Ragan IK, et al. Rift Valley fever viral RNA detection by in situ hybridization in formalin-fixed, paraffin-embedded tissues. *Vector Borne Zoonotic Dis* 2019;19(7):553–556. doi: 10.1089/vbz.2018.2383.

326. Rasmuson J, et al. Presence of activated airway T lymphocytes in human puumala hantavirus disease. *Chest* 2011;140:715–722.

327. Ravkov EV, Nichol ST, Compans RW. Polarized entry and release in epithelial cells of Black Creek Canal virus, a New World hantavirus. *J Virol* 1997;71:1147–1154.

328. Ravkov EV, Rollin PE, Ksiazek TG, et al. Genetic and serologic analysis of Black Creek Canal virus and its association with human disease and *Sigmodon hispidus* infection. *Virology* 1995;210:482–489.

329. Rawlings JA, et al. Cocirculation of multiple hantaviruses in Texas, with characterization of the small (S) genome of a previously undescribed virus of cotton rats (*Sigmodon hispidus*). *Am J Trop Med Hyg* 1996;55:672–679.

330. Report C. Human Jamestown canyon virus infection—Montana, 2009. *Morb Mortal Wkly Rep* 2011;60(20):652–655.

331. Rich KM, Wanyoike F. An assessment of the regional and national socio-economic impacts of the 2007 Rift Valley fever outbreak in Kenya. *Am J Trop Med Hyg* 2010;83:52–57.

332. Roberts DR, Hoch AL, Dixon KE, et al. Oropouche virus. III. Entomological observations from three epidemics in Para, Brazil, 1975. *Am J Trop Med Hyg* 1981;30(1):165–171. doi: 10.4269/ajtmh.1981.30.165.

333. Rodriguez SE, McAuley AJ, Gargili A, et al. Interactions of human dermal dendritic cells and langerhans cells treated with Hyalomma tick saliva with Crimean-Congo hemorrhagic fever virus. *Viruses* 2018;10(7). doi: 10.3390/v10070381.

334. Rowe RK, Pekosz A. Bidirectional virus secretion and nonciliated cell tropism following Andes virus infection of primary airway epithelial cell cultures. *J Virol* 2006;80:1087–1097.

335. Rusnak JM, et al. Experience with intravenous ribavirin in the treatment of hemorrhagic fever with renal syndrome in Korea. *Antiviral Res* 2009;81:68–76.

336. Rust RS, Thompson WH, Matthews CG, et al. La crosse and other forms of California encephalitis. *J Child Neurol* 1999;14(1):1–14. doi: 10.1177/088307389901400101.

337. Sabin AB. Experimental studies on Phlebotomus (Pappataci, Sandfly) fever during World War II. *Arch Gesamte Virusforsch* 1951;4:367–410.

338. Safronetz D, Haddock E, Feldmann F, et al. In vitro and in vivo activity of ribavirin against Andes virus infection. *PLoS One* 2011;6:e23560.

339. Safronetz D, et al. Pathophysiology of hantavirus pulmonary syndrome in rhesus macaques. *Proc Natl Acad Sci U S A* 2014;111:7114–7119.

340. Saijo M, et al. Recombinant nucleoprotein-based enzyme-linked immunosorbent assay for detection of immunoglobulin G antibodies to Crimean-Congo hemorrhagic fever virus. *J Clin Microbiol* 2002;40(5):1587–1591. doi: 10.1128/JCM.40.5.1587-1591.2002.

341. Saksida A, et al. Interacting roles of immune mechanisms and viral load in the pathogenesis of Crimean-Congo hemorrhagic fever. *Clin Vaccine Immunol* 2010;17(7):1086–1093. doi: 10.1128/CVI.00530-09.

342. Scharton D, et al. Favipiravir (T-705) protects against peracute Rift Valley fever virus infection and reduces delayed-onset neurologic disease observed with ribavirin treatment. *Antiviral Res* 2014;104:84–92.

343. Schmaljohn C. Vaccines for hantaviruses. *Vaccine* 2009;27(Suppl 4):D61–D64.

344. Schmaljohn CS. Vaccines for hantaviruses: progress and issues. *Expert Rev Vaccines* 2012;11:511–513.

345. Scholz S, et al. Human hantavirus infection elicits pronounced redistribution of mononuclear phagocytes in peripheral blood and airways. *PLoS Pathog* 2017;13:e1006462.

346. Schonrich G, Kruger DH, Raftery MJ. Hantavirus-induced disruption of the endothelial barrier: neutrophils are on the payroll. *Front Microbiol* 2015;6:222.

347. Schountz T, Prescott J. Hantavirus immunology of rodent reservoirs: current status and future directions. *Viruses* 2014;6:1317–1335.

348. Schountz T, et al. Regulatory T cell-like responses in deer mice persistently infected with Sin Nombre virus. *Proc Natl Acad Sci U S A* 2007;104:15496–15501.

349. Schountz T, et al. Kinetics of immune responses in deer mice experimentally infected with Sin Nombre virus. *J Virol* 2012;86:10015–10027.

350. Sexton DJ, et al. Life-threatening Cache Valley virus infection. *N Engl J Med* 1997;336(8):547–549.

351. Seymour C, Amundson TE, Yuill TM, et al. Experimental infection of chipmunks and snowshoe hares with La Crosse and snowshoe hare viruses and four of their reassortants. *Am J Trop Med Hyg* 1983;32(5):1147–1153. doi: 10.4269/ajtmh.1983.32.1147.

352. Shepherd AJ, Swanepoel R, Leman PA, et al. Comparison of methods for isolation and titration of Crimean-Congo hemorrhagic fever virus. *J Clin Microbiol* 1986;24(4):654–656.

353. Shoemaker T, et al. Genetic analysis of viruses associated with emergence of Rift Valley fever in Saudi Arabia and Yemen, 2000–01. *Emerg Infect Dis* 2002;8:1415–1420.

354. Shoemaker TR, et al. First laboratory-confirmed outbreak of human and animal Rift Valley fever virus in Uganda in 48 Years. *Am J Trop Med Hyg* 2019;100(3):659–671. doi: 10.4269/ajtmh.18-0732.

355. Shope RE, Whitman L. The California complex of arthropod-borne viruses and its relationship to the Bunyamwera group through Guaroa virus. *Am J Trop Med Hyg* 2017;11:691–696. doi: 10.4269/ajtmh.1962.11.691.

356. Shrivastava-Ranjan P, Rollin PE, Spiropoulou CF. Andes virus disrupts the endothelial cell barrier by induction of vascular endothelial growth factor and downregulation of VE-cadherin. *J Virol* 2010;84:11227–11234.

357. Sidira P, Maltezou HC, Haidich AB, et al. Seroepidemiological study of Crimean-Congo haemorrhagic fever in Greece, 2009–2010. *Clin Microbiol Infect* 2012;18(2):E16–E19. doi: 10.1111/j.1469-0691.2011.03718.x.

358. Sironen T, Vaheri A, Plyusnin A. Phylogenetic evidence for the distinction of Saaremaa and Dobrava hantaviruses. *Virol J* 2005;2:90.

359. Sironen T, et al. Fatal Puumala hantavirus disease: involvement of complement activation and vascular leakage in the pathobiology. *Open Forum Infect Dis* 2017;4:ofx229.

360. Smithburn KC. Rift Valley fever; the neurotropic adaptation of the virus and the experimental use of this modified virus as a vaccine. *Br J Exp Pathol* 1949;30:1–16.

361. Smithburn KC, Haddow AJ, Mahaffy AF. A neurotropic virus isolated from Aedes mosquitoes caught in the Semliki forest. *Am J Trop Med Hyg* 1946;26:189–208.

362. Smithburn KC, Mahaffy AF. Rift Valley fever; accidental infections among laboratory workers. *J Immunol* 1949;62:213–227.

363. Soares-Weiser K, Thomas S, Thomson G, et al. Ribavirin for Crimean-Congo hemorrhagic fever: systematic review and meta-analysis. *BMC Infect Dis* 2010;10:207. doi: 10.1186/1471-2334-10-207.

364. Sola-Riera C, Gupta S, Ljunggren HG, et al. Orthohantaviruses belonging to three phylogroups all inhibit apoptosis in infected target cells. *Sci Rep* 2019;9:834.

365. Soldan SS, Hollidge BS, Wagner V, et al. La Crosse virus (LACV) Gc fusion peptide mutants have impaired growth and fusion phenotypes, but remain neurotoxic. *Virology* 2010;404(2):139–147. doi: 10.1016/j.virol.2010.04.012.

366. Song JW, Baek LJ, Nagle JW, et al. Genetic and phylogenetic analyses of hantaviral sequences amplified from archival tissues of deer mice (*Peromyscus maniculatus nubiterrae*) captured in the eastern United States. *Arch Virol* 1996;141:959–967.

367. Song JY, et al. Long-term immunogenicity and safety of inactivated Hantaan virus vaccine (Hantavax) in healthy adults. *Vaccine* 2016;34:1289–1295.

368. Song P, et al. Downregulation of Interferon-β and Inhibition of TLR3 expression are associated with fatal outcome of severe fever with Thrombocytopenia syndrome. *Sci Rep* 2017;7(1):6532. doi: 10.1038/s41598-017-06921-6.

369. Sow A, et al. Widespread Rift Valley fever emergence in Senegal in 2013–2014. *Open Forum Infect Dis* 2016;3:ofw149.

370. Spengler JR, Bente DA. Crimean–Congo hemorrhagic fever in Spain—New arrival or silent resident? *N Engl J Med* 2017;377(2):106–108. doi: 10.1056/nejmp1707436.

371. Strandin T, Makela S, Mustonen J, et al. Neutrophil activation in acute hemorrhagic fever with renal syndrome is mediated by hantavirus-infected microvascular endothelial cells. *Front Immunol* 2018;9:2098.

372. Sugiyama K, et al. Four serotypes of haemorrhagic fever with renal syndrome viruses identified by polyclonal and monoclonal antibodies. *J Gen Virol* 1987;68(Pt 4):979–987.

373. Sun Y, et al. Host cytokine storm is associated with disease severity of severe fever with thrombocytopenia syndrome. *J Infect Dis* 2012;206(7):1085–1094. doi: 10.1093/infdis/jis452.

374. Sun Y, et al. Early diagnosis of novel SFTS bunyavirus infection by quantitative real-time RT-PCR assay. *J Clin Virol* 2012;53(1):48–53. doi: 10.1016/j.jcv.2011.09.031.

375. Sundstrom JB, et al. Hantavirus infection induces the expression of RANTES and IP-10 without causing increased permeability in human lung microvascular endothelial cells. *J Virol* 2001;75:6070–6085.

376. Swanepoel R, Coetzer JA. Rift Valley fever. In: Coetzer JA, Thomson GR, Tustin RC, eds. *Infectious Diseases of Livestock with Special Reference to South Africa*. Oxford University Press; 1994:688–717.

377. Swanepoel R, et al. Comparative pathogenicity and antigenic cross-reactivity of rift valley fever and other african phleboviruses in sheep. *J Hyg (Lond)* 1986;97:331–346.

378. Swanepoel R, et al. Epidemiologic and clinical features of Crimean-Congo hemorrhagic fever in Southern Africa. *Am J Trop Med Hyg* 1987;36(1):120–132.

379. Swanepoel R, et al. The clinical pathology of Crimean-Congo hemorrhagic fever. *Rev Infect Dis* 1989;11(Suppl 4):S794–S800. doi: 10.1093/clinids/11.Supplement_4.S794.

380. Taori SK, et al. UK hantavirus, renal failure, and pet rats. *Lancet* 2013;381:1070.

381. Tasdelen Fisgin N, Ergonul O, Doganci L, et al. The role of ribavirin in the therapy of crimean-congo hemorrhagic fever: early use is promising. *Eur J Clin Microbiol Infect Dis* 2009;28(8):929–933. doi: 10.1007/s10096-009-0728-2.

382. Taylor SL, Wahl-Jensen V, Copeland AM, et al. Endothelial cell permeability during hantavirus infection involves factor XII-dependent increased activation of the kallikrein-kinin system. *PLoS Pathog* 2013;9:e1003470.

383. Temonen M, et al. Cytokines, adhesion molecules, and cellular infiltration in nephropathia epidemica kidneys: an immunohistochemical study. *Clin Immunol Immunopathol* 1996;78:47–55.

384. Terajima M, Ennis FA. T cells and pathogenesis of hantavirus cardiopulmonary syndrome and hemorrhagic fever with renal syndrome. *Viruses* 2011;3:1059–1073.

385. Tesh RB. The genus Phlebovirus and its vectors. *Annu Rev Entomol* 1988;33:169–181.

386. Tesh RB, Beaty BJ. Localization of California serogroup viruses in mosquitoes. *Prog Clin Biol Res* 1983;123:67–75.

387. Tesh RB, Lubroth J, Guzman H. Simulation of arbovirus overwintering: survival of Toscana virus (Bunyaviridae: *Phlebovirus*) in its natural sand fly vector *Phlebotomus perniciosus*. *Am J Trop Med Hyg* 1992;47:574–581.

388. Tesh RB, Modi GB. Maintenance of Toscana virus in *Phlebotomus perniciosus* by vertical transmission. *Am J Trop Med Hyg* 1987;36:189–193.

389. Tezer H, et al. Crimean-Congo hemorrhagic fever in children. *J Clin Virol* 2010;48(3):184–186. doi: 10.1016/j.jcv.2010.04.001.

390. Thompson WH, Beaty BJ. Venereal transmission of La Crosse virus from male to female *Aedes triseriatus*. *Am J Trop Med Hyg* 1978;27(1 Pt 1):187–196.

391. Thompson WH. Vector-virus relationships. In: Calisher CH, Thompson WH, eds. *California Serogroup Viruses*. 1983; 57–63.

392. Thompson WH, Kalfayan B, Anslow RO. Isolation of California encephalitis group virus from a fatal human illness. *Am J Epidemiol* 1965;81:245–253. doi: 10.1093/oxfordjournals.aje.a120512.

393. Tokarz R, et al. A multiplex serologic platform for diagnosis of tick-borne diseases. *Sci Rep* 2018;8(1):3158. doi: 10.1038/s41598-018-21349-2.

394. Torrez-Martinez N, et al. Bayou virus-associated hantavirus pulmonary syndrome in Eastern Texas: identification of the rice rat, Oryzomys palustris, as reservoir host. *Emerg Infect Dis* 1998;4:105–111.

395. Travassos Da Rosa JF, et al. Oropouche virus: clinical, epidemiological, and molecular aspects of a neglected orthobunyavirus. *Am J Trop Med Hyg* 2017;96(5):1019–1030. doi: 10.4269/ajtmh.16-0672.

396. Tsuda T, et al. Arthrogryposis, hydranencephaly and cerebellar hypoplasia syndrome in neonatal calves resulting from intrauterine infection with Aino virus. *Vet Res* 2004;35(5):531–538. doi: 10.1051/vetres:2004029.

397. Turell MJ, Hardy JL, Reeves WC. Stabilized infection of California encephalitis virus in Aedes dorsalis, and its implications for viral maintenance in nature. *Am J Trop Med Hyg* 1982;31(6):1252–1259. doi: 10.4269/ajtmh.1982.31.1252.

398. Van Epps HL, et al. Long-lived memory T lymphocyte responses after hantavirus infection. *J Exp Med* 2002;196:579–588.

399. van Vuren PJ, Paweska JT. Comparison of enzyme-linked immunosorbent assay-based techniques for the detection of antibody to Rift Valley fever virus in thermochemically inactivated sheep sera. *Vector Borne Zoonotic Dis* 2010;10:697–699.

400. Vapalahti O, Lundkvist A, Vaheri A. Human immune response, host genetics, and severity of disease. *Curr Top Microbiol Immunol* 2001;256:153–169.

401. Varani S, et al. Meningitis caused by Toscana Virus is associated with strong antiviral response in the CNS and altered frequency of blood antigen-presenting cells. *Viruses* 2015;7:5831–5843.

402. Vasconcelos HB, et al. Molecular epidemiology of Oropouche virus, Brazil. *Emerg Infect Dis* 2011;17(5):800–806. doi: 10.3201/eid1705.101333.

403. Veater J, et al. Toscana virus meningo-encephalitis: an important differential diagnosis for elderly travellers returning from Mediterranean countries. *BMC Geriatr* 2017;17:193.

404. Vergote V, et al. A lethal disease model for New World hantaviruses using immunosuppressed Syrian hamsters. *PLoS Negl Trop Dis* 2017;11:e0006042.

405. Vial PA, et al. High-dose intravenous methylprednisolone for hantavirus cardiopulmonary syndrome in Chile: a double-blind, randomized controlled clinical trial. *Clin Infect Dis* 2013;57:943–951.

406. Vial PA, et al. A non-randomized multicentre trial of human immune plasma for treatment of hantavirus cardiopulmonary syndrome caused by Andes virus. *Antivir Ther* 2015;20:377–386.

407. Vial C, et al. Molecular method for the detection of Andes hantavirus infection: validation for clinical diagnostics. *Diagn Microbiol Infect Dis* 2016;84:36–39.

408. Vignolles C, Tourre YM, Mora O, et al. TerraSAR-X high-resolution radar remote sensing: an operational warning system for Rift Valley fever risk. *Geospat Health* 2010;5:23–31.

409. Vitek CR, Ksiazek TG, Peters CJ, et al. Evidence against infection with hantaviruses among forest and park workers in the southwestern United States. *Clin Infect Dis* 1996;23:283–285.

410. Vollmar P, et al. Hantavirus cardiopulmonary syndrome due to Puumala virus in Germany. *J Clin Virol* 2016;84:42–47.

411. Wahl-Jensen V, et al. Temporal analysis of Andes virus and Sin Nombre virus infections of Syrian hamsters. *J Virol* 2007;81:7449–7462.

412. Walters AW, et al. Vascular permeability in the brain is a late pathogenic event during Rift Valley fever virus encephalitis in rats. *Virology* 2019;526:173–179.

413. Wang J, et al. Elevated soluble CD163 plasma levels are associated with disease severity in patients with hemorrhagic fever with renal syndrome. *PLoS One* 2014;9:e112127.

414. Warimwe GM, et al. Chimpanzee Adenovirus vaccine provides multispecies protection against Rift Valley Fever. *Sci Rep* 2016;6:20617.

415. Watts DM, Pantuwatana S, Defoliart GR, et al. Transovarial transmission of LaCrosse virus (California Encephalitis Group) in the mosquito, *Aedes triseriatus*. *Science* 1973;182(4117):1140–1141. doi: 10.1126/science.182.4117.1140.

416. Watts DM, Thompson WH, Yuill TM, et al. Overwintering of La Crosse virus in *Aedes triseriatus*. *Am J Trop Med Hyg* 1974;23(4):694–700.

417. Weber F, Mirazimi A. Interferon and cytokine responses to Crimean Congo hemorrhagic fever virus; an emerging and neglected viral zoonosis. *Cytokine Growth Factor Rev* 2008;19(5–6):395–404. doi: 10.1016/j.cytogfr.2008.11.001.

418. Weidmann M, et al. Rapid detection of important human pathogenic Phleboviruses. *J Clin Virol* 2008;41:138–142.

419. Wells RM, et al. An unusual hantavirus outbreak in southern Argentina: person-to-person transmission? Hantavirus pulmonary syndrome study group for patagonia. *Emerg Infect Dis* 1997;3:171–174.

420. Wernly JA, et al. Extracorporeal membrane oxygenation support improves survival of patients with Hantavirus cardiopulmonary syndrome refractory to medical treatment. *Eur J Cardiothorac Surg* 2011;40:1334–1340.

421. Wichgers Schreur PJ, van Keulen L, Kant J, et al. Four-segmented Rift Valley fever virus-based vaccines can be applied safely in ewes during pregnancy. *Vaccine* 2017;35:3123–3128.

422. Williams RW, Causey OR, Kemp GE. Ixodid ticks from domestic livestock in Ibadan, Nigeria as carriers of viral agents. *J Med Entomol* 1972;9(5):443–445. doi: 10.1093/jmedent/9.5.443.

423. Williams RJ, et al. An outbreak of hantavirus pulmonary syndrome in western Paraguay. *Am J Trop Med Hyg* 1997;57:274–282.

424. Wonderlich ER, et al. Peripheral blood biomarkers of disease outcome in a monkey model of Rift Valley fever encephalitis. *J Virol* 2018;92(3).

425. Woods CW, et al. An outbreak of Rift Valley fever in Northeastern Kenya, 1997–98. *Emerg Infect Dis* 2002;8:138–144.

426. Xiao R, et al. Sin Nombre viral RNA load in patients with hantavirus cardiopulmonary syndrome. *J Infect Dis* 2006;194:1403–1409.

427. Yamanishi K, et al. Development of inactivated vaccine against virus causing haemorrhagic fever with renal syndrome. *Vaccine* 1988;6:278–282.

428. Yilmaz M, et al. Peripheral blood natural killer cells in Crimean-Congo hemorrhagic fever. *J Clin Virol* 2008;42(4):415–417. doi: 10.1016/j.jcv.2008.03.003.

429. Yoshikawa T, et al. Sensitive and specific PCR systems for detection of both Chinese and Japanese severe fever with thrombocytopenia syndrome virus strains and prediction of patient survival based on viral load. *J Clin Microbiol* 2014;52(9):3325–3333. doi: 10.1128/JCM.00742-14.

430. Yoshikawa T, et al. Phylogenetic and geographic relationships of severe fever with thrombocytopenia syndrome virus in China, South Korea, and Japan. *J Infect Dis* 2015;212(6):889–898. doi: 10.1093/infdis/jiv144.

431. Yu F, et al. Application of recombinant severe fever with thrombocytopenia syndrome virus nucleocapsid protein for the detection of SFTSV-specific human IgG and IgM antibodies by indirect ELISA. *Virol J* 2015;12:117. doi: 10.1186/s12985-015-0350-0.

432. Yu F, et al. Comparison of enzyme-linked immunosorbent assay systems using rift valley fever virus nucleocapsid protein and inactivated virus as antigens. *Virol J* 2018;15:178.

433. Yuill T. The role of mammals in the maintenance and dissemination of La Crosse virus. In: Calisher CH, Thompson WH, eds. *California Serogroup Viruses*. 1983: 77–88.

434. Zaki SR, et al. Hantavirus pulmonary syndrome. Pathogenesis of an emerging infectious disease. *Am J Pathol* 1995;146:552–579.

435. Zeitz PS, et al. Assessment of occupational risk for hantavirus infection in Arizona and New Mexico. *J Occup Environ Med* 1997;39:463–467.

436. Zeller HG, Fontenille D, Traore-Lamizana M, et al. Enzootic activity of Rift Valley fever virus in Senegal. *Am J Trop Med Hyg* 1997;56:265–272.

437. Zhan J, et al. Current status of severe fever with thrombocytopenia syndrome in China. *Virol Sin* 2017;32(1):51–62. doi: 10.1007/s12250-016-3931-1.

438. Zhang YZ, Xu J. The emergence and cross species transmission of newly discovered tick-borne Bunyavirus in China. *Curr Opin Virol* 2016;16:126–131. doi: 10.1016/j.coviro.2016.02.006.

439. Zhang YZ, et al. Hemorrhagic fever caused by a novel Bunyavirus in china: pathogenesis and correlates of fatal outcome. *Clin Infect Dis* 2012;54(4):527–533. doi: 10.1093/cid/cir804.

440. Zhang S, et al. Pathogenesis of emerging severe fever with thrombocytopenia syndrome virus in C57/BL6 mouse model. *Proc Natl Acad Sci* 2012;109(25):10053–10058. doi: 10.1073/pnas.1120246109.

441. Zhang XS, et al. An emerging hemorrhagic fever in China caused by a novel bunyavirus SFTSV. *Sci China Life Sci* 2013;56(8):697–700. doi: 10.1007/s11427-013-4518-9.

442. Zivcec M, et al. Lethal Crimean-Congo hemorrhagic fever virus infection in interferon α/β receptor knockout mice is associated with high viral loads, proinflammatory responses, and coagulopathy. *J Infect Dis* 2013;207(12):1909–1921. doi: 10.1093/infdis/jit061.

Arenaviridae: The Viruses and Their Replication

Sheli R. Radoshitzky • Michael J. Buchmeier • Juan Carlos de la Torre

HISTORY

The first arenavirus, lymphocytic choriomeningitis virus (LCMV), was isolated over 80 years ago from samples from a St. Louis encephalitis epidemic.[330] LCMV was found to be a cause of an aseptic meningitis in humans,[354] and the house mouse (*Mus musculus* Linnaeus, 1758) was identified as the virus's natural reservoir host.[381] By the 1960s, several other viruses had been discovered that shared common morphology,[285]

serology,[336] biochemical features, and a natural history of chronic infection of rodent reservoirs, leading to the recognition of the family *Arenaviridae*, named after the granular or sandy (Latin, *arenosus*) appearance of thin sections of virions examined by electron microscopy (EM).[336] In 1956, Tacaribe virus (TCRV) was isolated from phyllostomid Jamaican fruit-eating bats (*Artibeus jamaicensis trinitatis* K. Andersen, 1906) in Trinidad and Tobago, but the virus was not associated with virulence in humans.[92] The discoveries of Junín virus (JUNV) in the late 1950s as the causative agent of Argentinian hemorrhagic fever (AHF),[295] of Machupo virus (MACV) in 1962 as the etiologic agent of Bolivian hemorrhagic fever (BHF),[193] and of Lassa virus (LASV) in 1969 from Lassa fever (LF) patients in Nigeria[125] underscored the pathogenic potential of arenavirus infections of humans (Table 18.1). In the following years, additional pathogenic arenaviruses have been discovered, including Guanarito virus (GTOV),[346] Sabiá virus (SBAV),[69] and Chapare virus (CHAPV) in South America,[86] and Lujo virus (LUJV) in Africa.[37] As a result of new technologies of deep-sequencing and genome discovery, many new arenaviruses were uncovered in the last decade in mammals. Notably, arenaviruses were also discovered in reptiles (snakes) and fish, representing a significant expansion of the host range of arenaviruses.[168,359,366]

CLASSIFICATION OF VIRUSES WITHIN THE FAMILY *ARENAVIRIDAE*

Based on phylogenetic analyses of RNA-directed RNA polymerase (L) and nucleoprotein (NP) sequences, members of the family *Arenaviridae* are classified into four genera: *Antennavirus*, *Hartmanivirus*, *Mammarenavirus*, and *Reptarenavirus* (Fig. 18.1). The genus *Mammarenavirus* includes 35 species for 42 viruses. The genus *Reptarenavirus* currently includes five species for eight viruses; the genus *Hartmanivirus* includes one species for one virus (Haartman Institute snake virus 1); and the genus *Antennavirus* currently includes two species for two viruses. The hosts of mammarenaviruses are mainly rodents (with the exception of TCRV), and infection is generally asymptomatic. Some mammarenaviruses, such as LASV, LCMV, and several viruses of South American origin, can also infect humans and cause severe and sometimes fatal disease. Reptarenaviruses and hartmaniviruses infect (captive) snakes, some of which develop boid inclusion body disease

TABLE 18.1 Arenaviruses that are known to be human pathogens

Virus	Abbreviation	Reservoir Host	Geographic Distribution	Disease[a]
Lymphocytic choriomeningitis virus	LCMV	House mouse (*Mus musculus* Linnaeus, 1758)	Worldwide	Lymphocytic choriomeningitis (1C8F)
Lassa virus	LASV	Natal mastomys (*Mastomys natalensis* Smith, 1834)	Western Africa	Lassa fever (1D61.2)
Lujo virus	LUJV	Unknown	Zambia	Other specified arenavirus disease (1D61.Y)
Junín virus	JUNV	Drylands laucha (*Calomys musculinus* Thomas, 1913)	Argentina	Argentinian hemorrhagic fever (1D61.0)
Machupo virus	MACV	Big laucha (*Calomys callosus* Rengger, 1830)	Bolivia	Bolivian hemorrhagic fever (1D61.1)
Guanarito virus	GTOV	Short-tailed zygodont (*Zygodontomys brevicauda* J. A. Allen and Chapman, 1893)	Venezuela	Venezuelan hemorrhagic fever (1D61.3)
Sabiá virus	SBAV	Unknown	Brazil	Other specified arenavirus disease (1D61.Y)
Chapare virus	CHAPV	Unknown	Bolivia	Other specified arenavirus disease (1D61.Y)

[a]According to the World Health Organization's International Classification of Diseases revision 11 (ICD-11).

(BIBD). Reptarenaviruses are notable for their surface glycoproteins (GPs), which are more closely related to that of Ebola virus than to those of hartmaniviruses or mammarenaviruses. Hartmaniviruses do not encode the matrix (Z) protein, which is encoded by all known mammarenaviruses and reptarenaviruses. Antennaviruses were discovered in actinopterygian fish and have genomes consisting of three, rather than two, segments. Like hartmaniviruses, antennaviruses do not encode Z.[359]

Based on antigenic properties, mammarenaviruses have been divided traditionally into two distinct groups. Old World (OW) mammarenaviruses ("Lassa–lymphocytic choriomeningitis serocomplex") include viruses indigenous to Africa and the ubiquitous LCMV, whereas New World (NW) mammarenaviruses ("Tacaribe serocomplex") include viruses indigenous to the Americas.[47,100,143] This classification is largely consistent with phylogenetic data and muroid rodent host phylogeny, with OW mammarenaviruses infecting murid rodents primarily in Africa and NW mammarenaviruses infecting cricetid rodents primarily in the Americas. This clear-cut dichotomy is under assessment, however, since yet unclassified mammarenaviruses have been discovered in northern three-toed jerboas (Dipodoidea: Dipodidae, *Dipus sagitta* Pallas, 1773) in Mongolia.[320,321,408]

VIRION STRUCTURE

Arenavirions are pleomorphic, ranging in size from 40 to more than 200 nm in diameter[58,187] (Fig. 18.2). The virion's surface is studded with evenly spaced spike projections composed of complexes of the viral glycoproteins GP1 and GP2. The surface glycoproteins are aligned with subjacent Z and ribonucleoprotein (RNP) densities, which are packed into a two-dimensional lattice at the inner surface of the viral membrane.[187,286]

Virions contain the L and S genomic RNAs in helical nucleocapsid structures that are organized in circular configurations, with lengths ranging from 400 to 1,300 nm.[417] The L and S genomic RNAs are not present in equimolar amounts within virions (L:S ratios ~1:2), and low numbers of both L and S antigenomic RNAs are also present within virions. In addition, host ribosomes are documented to be incorporated into virions, but the biological significance of this incorporation remains uncertain.[43,284]

GENOME STRUCTURE AND ORGANIZATION

Arenavirus Genomic Organization

Arenaviruses produce enveloped particles with bisegmented (genera *Hartmanivirus*, *Mammarenavirus*, and *Reptarenavirus*) or trisegmented (genus *Antennavirus*) negative-sense (NS), single-stranded RNA genomes. The overall genome organization is well conserved across mammarenaviruses and reptarenaviruses. An ambisense coding strategy is used for the synthesis of two nonoverlapping polypeptides from each of the two genomic RNAs (Fig. 18.3). The term "ambisense" was coined to reflect that both genomic and antigenomic RNAs encode for proteins. This ambisense coding strategy might facilitate temporal control of gene expression of the two genes within an ambisense RNA genome segment. The open reading frames of these viruses are also separated by a noncoding intergenic region (IGR) with folding predicted to form a stable hairpin structure. The S RNA encodes the viral NP and glycoprotein precursor (GPC). The L RNA encodes the viral RdRp (or L polymerase) and Z.[301,371,382] However, the genomic S and L RNAs do not function as mRNAs and cannot direct translation of GPC and Z,

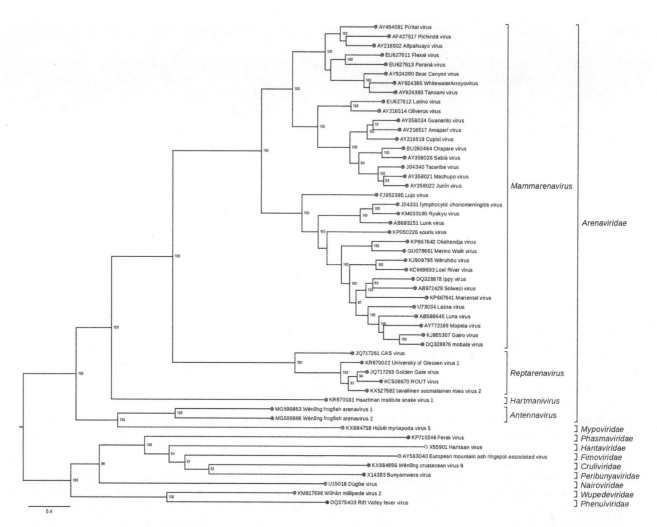

FIGURE 18.1 Phylogenetic relationships of arenaviruses. Maximum likelihood phylogenetic tree was inferred from probabilistic alignment kit (PRANK) alignment of the complete L amino acid sequences of 43 arenaviruses (*red dots*) assigned to four genera. Representative viruses of other bunyavirus families were also included (*dots in colors other than red*). The best-fit model of protein evolution (LG + G model) was selected using ProtTest 3 (v. 3.4.2). The maximum likelihood tree with 1,000 bootstrap replicates was produced using Randomized Axelerated Maximum Likelihood RAxML (v. 8). The percentage of replicate trees in which the associated taxa clustered together in the bootstrap is shown next to branch nodes (when ≥70%). The tree was visualized using FigTree (http://tree.bio.ed.ac.uk) and is rooted at the midpoint. (Courtesy of Manuela Sironi, Scientific Institute IRCCS E. MEDEA, BosisioParini (LC), Italy.)

respectively. Unlike other arenaviruses, antennaviruses have a trisegmented (L, M, and S) genome with the M segment coding GPC and an additional hypothetical protein of unknown function. Furthermore, the L segment of hartmaniviruses and antennaviruses lacks the Z open reading frame.

Arenaviruses have highly conserved sequences at the 3′ end of the L and S RNA genome segments, and genome and antigenome RNAs are highly complementary between their 5′ and 3′ termini. This complementarity predicts that both L and S genome segments form panhandle structures.[45] This prediction is supported by EM data showing the existence of circular RNP complexes within arenavirions.[417] This terminal complementarity has been proposed to favor the formation of both intra- and intermolecular L and S duplexes that might be part of the replication initiation complex.[348] For several arenaviruses, a nontemplated G residue has been detected at the 5′ end of progeny genomic RNAs during replication.[136,137]

Arenavirus IGRs are predicted to fold into a stable hairpin structure. Transcription termination of the S-derived NP and GP mRNAs occurs at multiple sites within the predicted stem of the IGR, supporting the view that a structural motif rather than a sequence-specific signal promotes the release of the arenavirus polymerase from the template RNA. There are significant differences in sequence and predicted folded structure between the S and L IGRs, but among isolates and strains of the same arenavirus, the S and L IGR sequences are highly conserved. Some arenaviruses contain one single predicted stem loop within the S IGR, whereas the S IGRs of other arenaviruses are predicted to contain two distinct stem–loop structures.[45]

Arenavirus Proteins

GPC is a class I fusion protein that is cotranslationally cleaved by cellular signal peptidases to generate a 58–amino acid-long stable signal peptide (SSP) and the immature GP1/2 precursor.

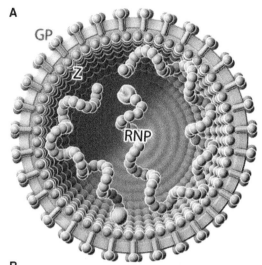

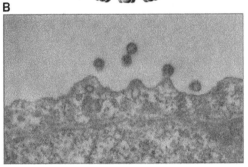

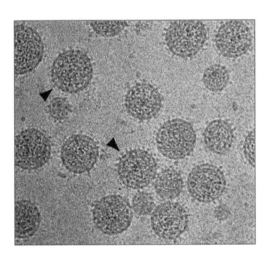

FIGURE 18.2 Arenavirion structure. A: Schematic illustration of an arenavirus particle. Shown is the spherical and enveloped (*gray*) particle that is spiked with GPs (glycoproteins; *gold*) around a layer of Zs (zinc-finger matrix proteins, *brown*; missing in hartmaniviruses). The small (S) and large (L) ribonucleoprotein (RNP) complexes inside the particle consist of genomic RNA, nucleoprotein (NP, *blue*) and RNA-directed RNA polymerase (L; *green*). (Courtesy of Fabian de Kok-Mercado and Jiro Wada, IRF-Frederick, Fort Detrick, MD, USA.) **B:** *Top panel:* LCMV strain Armstrong release from Vero cells in culture. Particles are visible at several stages of budding and release. Magnification 25,000 times. *Lower panel:* LCMV Armstrong strain, purified and prepared for cryo-electron microscopy. Nominally spherical virions of variable diameter are evident with surface "spikes" that are the glycoprotein complexes (*black arrowheads*). Original magnification ≈ 35,000 times.

The immature GP1/2 precursor is then posttranslationally processed by the cellular protease subtilisin kexin isozyme-1 (SKI-1)/site-1 protease (S1P) to generate the mature virion surface glycoproteins GP1 and GP2. GP1, GP2, and SSP form a tripartite heterotrimeric GP complex that mediates virion receptor recognition and cell entry.[24,310] The SSP has been implicated in the trafficking and processing of the viral envelope glycoproteins and in the GP2-mediated pH-dependent fusion process.[23,350,412–415] GP1 mediates virion interaction with host cell-surface receptors. GP1 is located at the top of the spike away from the membrane and held in place by ionic interactions with the N-terminus of transmembrane GP2.[46,49,319,322] GP2 directs fusion of virus and host cell membranes, a process that depends on low pH-driven conformational change of GP2 from a metastable prefusion structure to a more stable postfusion six-helix bundle.[106,174,296] GP2 has similarities with fusion-active domains of other viral envelope proteins.[132,411] Crystal structures of the prefusion GP complex of LASV and LCMV[155,159] revealed that compared to other class I viral glycoproteins, LASV GP has some unique structural features with implications for vaccine design.[158]

NP is the most abundant viral polypeptide in both infected cells and virions and the main structural component of the viral RNP responsible for directing RNA genome replication and gene transcription. The C-terminus of NP also counteracts type I interferon (IFN-I).[250–252] Crystallographic studies identified distinct N- and C-terminal domains within NP of the OW arenaviruses LASV[41,156,317] and LCMV,[403] and similar findings were subsequently documented for the NW arenaviruses JUNV[422] and TCRV.[189] The N-terminal domain contains an RNA-binding site[157] and was proposed to have potential cap-binding activity that could provide the host-derived primers to initiate transcription by the virus polymerase.[317] However, the cap-binding activity of NP remains to be proven. The folding of the C-terminal domain of NP mimics that of the DEDDH family of 3′ to 5′ exoribonucleases similar to the one described for the nonstructural protein 14 of severe acute respiratory syndrome (SARS) coronavirus.[95] Functional studies confirmed the 3′ to 5′ exoribonuclease (exo) activity of LASV NP. The exo activity of NP was proposed to be critical for its anti-IFN activity. However, subsequent studies demonstrated that the exo activity of NP plays critical roles in additional aspects of mammarenavirus multiplication that are yet to be elucidated.[172,250]

Arenavirus L has a central region of conserved motifs characteristically found in the RdRp domains of negative-sense RNA viruses.[313] However, the N- and C-terminal regions do not allow easy identification of RNA helicase or methyltransferase (RNA capping) functions.[387] Residues critical for LASV L function are located both within and outside the predicted RdRp domain.[153,219,221] Mutagenesis of evolutionarily conserved acidic (Asp and Glu) and basic (Lys and Arg) residues within LASV L's C-terminus revealed residues that play a critical role in mRNA synthesis without significantly affecting RNA replication.[221] Bioinformatic analysis revealed that the N-terminus of LASV L has a distant similarity to type II endonucleases.[221] Crystal structures of the N-terminal region of LCMV[283] and LASV L uncovered an endonuclease domain of similar structure to the cap-snatching endonuclease domains of influenza A virus polymerase acidic (PA) and La Crosse virus L. LASV L is organized into three distinct structural domains. At specific amino acid positions, LASV L can be split into N- and C-regions that are

A   **Genome organization**

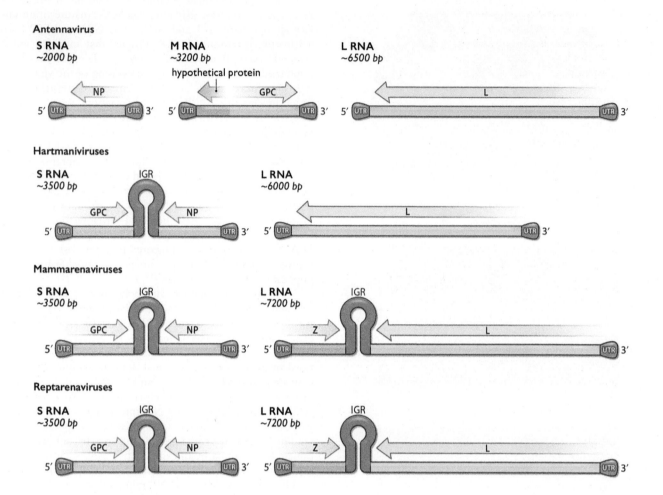

B   **RNA replication / gene transcription**

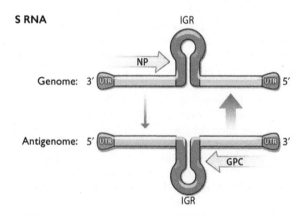

FIGURE 18.3 Arenavirus genome organization. A: Schematic representation of the bi- or trisegmented arenavirus genome organization. The 5' and 3' ends of all segments (S, [M], and L) are complementary at their termini, likely promoting the formation of circular ribonucleoprotein complexes within the virion (not shown). GPC, glycoprotein precursor; L, RNA-directed RNA polymerase; NP, nucleoprotein; Z, zinc-finger matrix protein. Open reading frames are separated by noncoding intergenic regions (IGRs), with predicted hairpin structures. **B:** RNA replication and gene transcription of the S segment. The NP gene is transcribed and translated first directly from the negative-sense viral genome. GPC is expressed later, after the S segment has undergone at least one round of replication, from the viral antigenome. A similar strategy is used for transcription and replication of the L segment. There are no direct experimental data examining these steps for antennaviruses and hartmaniviruses. (Courtesy of Fabian de Kok-Mercado and Jiro Wada, IRF-Frederick, Fort Detrick, MD, USA.)

able to functionally *trans*-complement each other.[42] In addition, EM characterization of a functional MACV L has revealed a core ring-domain decorated by appendages, which likely reflects a modular organization of the arenavirus polymerase.[207,209]

Mammarenavirus Zs are modestly conserved (below 20%); this similarity is even lower when Z sequences of the recently identified reptarenaviruses are included in alignments. However, three regions within Z have a higher degree of conservation: (a) an N-terminal myristoylation site marked by a highly conserved G motif that is critical for membrane anchoring[303,372] and interaction with other viral proteins,[50,51] (b) a RING domain that binds two zinc ions through three conserved motifs,[31] and (c) a C-terminal region containing proline-rich motifs that constitute, in most cases, functional late-budding motifs. These motifs are similar to those identified in the matrix proteins of many enveloped RNA viruses and in the group antigen (Gag) proteins of a number of retroviruses. Late-budding motifs mediate protein–protein interactions between viral proteins and components of the endosomal sorting complexes required for transport (ESCRT) within the vacuolar protein sorting (Vps) pathway.[128] Mammarenavirus Zs contain P[T/S]AP- and/or PPPY late-budding motifs in their C-terminal regions, whereas reptarenavirus Zs lack typical canonical motifs. In addition, mammarenavirus Zs contain a highly conserved YxxL motif located within the central RING domain. This motif is not present in reptarenaviruses.

The structure of LASV Z was solved in complex with eukaryotic translation initiation factor 4E (eIF4E) by nuclear magnetic resonance.[392] The N- (residues 1–29) and the C-terminal (residues 77–99) arms flanking the RING domain are disordered, and only the central RING domain is structured. The disordered regions may enable Z to recruit a variety of partners, including promyelocytic leukemia protein (PML), eIF4E, proline-rich homeodomain (PRH) protein, ribosomal P proteins, retinoic acid–inducible gene I protein (RIG-I), and caspases. The interactions of Z with PML protein and eIF4E have been proposed to contribute to the noncytolytic nature of LCMV infection and repression of cap-dependent translation, respectively.[88,392]

Under crystallographic conditions, Z assembles in a dodecameric manner through a head-to-tail dimerization of the RING domain.[160] This assembly involves conformational changes thought to be required for a stable oligomerization, leading to the viral matrix formation. The N- and C-terminal disordered regions do not appear to contribute to the assembly of the oligomeric Z structure, which is consistent with the N-terminus anchoring Z to the membrane and the C-terminus mediating Z's interaction with endosomal components required for moving the maturing virion toward the cell surface. These findings are consistent with Z playing a key role in virion assembly, which is further supported by EM studies indicating that Z bridges the viral RNP to the viral envelope. Z has been also involved in suppression of the host cell type I IFN response via its interaction with RIG-I–like receptors.[108,410]

STAGES OF REPLICATION

Knowledge about the molecular and cell biology of reptarenaviruses, hartmaniviruses, and antennaviruses is rather limited, and therefore the presentation of the arenavirus life cycle is based on information obtained from studies with mammarenaviruses.

However, many of the basic principles established for mammarenaviruses will likely also apply for members of the other genera.

Cell Attachment and Entry

Receptor-mediated endocytosis is the main cell entry pathway used by mammarenaviruses (Fig. 18.4). The acidic environment of the late endosome facilitates a pH-dependent conformational change in the GP complex that induces a GP2-mediated fusion step between viral and cell membranes. Following fusion, the viral RNP is released into the cytoplasm where it directs both replication and transcription of the viral genome.[106] α-Dystroglycan (aDG), a highly conserved and widely expressed cell-surface receptor for extracellular matrix proteins, is a main receptor for LCMV, LASV, and several other mammarenaviruses.[49,211] In mammals, aDG undergoes complex *O*-glycosylation posttranslational modifications, including the incorporation of a negatively charged sugar polymer called "matriglycan" as a result of the activities of the like-acetylglucosaminyltransferase (LARGE).[416] LARGE-dependent glycosylation is critical for aDG's function as a mammarenavirus receptor.[335] Intriguingly, specific LARGE alleles are positively selected among the Yoruba of Western Africa where LASV is endemic.[341] Pathogenic and nonpathogenic mammarenaviruses use aDG-mediated cell entry, indicating that aDG does not play a direct role in mammarenavirus pathogenesis.

aDG-mediated LASV entry into human epithelial cells and rapid virus internalization involve macropinocytosis.[178,291] Internalization is independent of dynamin, is dependent on sodium–hydrogen exchangers, and requires the dynamics of the actin cytoskeleton. LASV and LCMV pass through the multivesicular endosome, where the virion–receptor complex undergoes sorting by ESCRT, delivering the viruses to late endosomes.[297] LCMV and LASV GPs have a high binding affinity for aDG, and therefore the unusual endocytotic pathway used by these viruses may reflect the natural cellular trafficking of aDG. Alternatively, binding of GP to aDG could trigger a novel endocytic route for aDG that benefits virion cell entry as previously documented for other pathogens.[32]

The cellular tropism of LASV and LCMV does not always correlate with the presence of fully glycosylated aDG,[110,393] which may be explained by the cellular expression of secondary alternative receptors, including members of the Tyro3/Axl/Mer and T-cell immunoglobulin (TIM) and mucin receptor families. These receptors can facilitate cell entry by apoptotic mimicry via recognition of phosphatidylserine in the outer leaflet of the virion envelope.[39,111,265] In addition, C-type lectins have been also implicated in LASV cell entry into specific cell types such as dendritic cells (DCs).[140,360,361]

Human transferrin receptor 1 (TfR1) is the main cellular receptor used for cell entry of pathogenic NW mammarenaviruses such as JUNV and MACV.[319,323] Consistent with the use of TfR1 as a primary receptor for cell entry, JUNV enters cells through clathrin-mediated endocytosis.[319] Although TfR1 is internalized and recycled through early endosomes (pH ≈ 6), optimal fusion activity of JUNV GP requires a significantly lower (<5.5) pH. Perhaps, JUNV may redirect TfR1 from its normal recycling pathway into the late endosomes, a process likely influenced by the multivalent nature of the virus particle.

Cell entry of the OW HF mammarenavirus, LUJV, was found to be independent of aDG and TfR1[374] and mediated by neuropilin (NRP)-2, a cell-surface receptor for semaphorins and the tetraspanin protein CD63.[318] Interestingly, NRP-2 is highly expressed on microvascular endothelial cells, and the consequent high susceptibility of the microvasculature to LUJV may explain the extent of coagulopathy observed in LUJV-induced clinical disease.[355] Likewise, expression of NRP-2 on alveolar macrophages may facilitate aerosol transmission of LUJV.[355]

Completion of the cell entry process for some mammarenaviruses involves a late endosomal receptor switch mechanism. For LASV[67,68,179,180] and LUJV,[318] the late endosomal resident proteins LAMP1 and CD36, respectively, are required for cell entry.

Expression and Replication of the Viral Genome

NP and L coding regions are transcribed into a genomic complementary mRNA (Fig. 18.4). However, the GPC and Z coding regions are not translated directly from genomic RNA but rather from genomic sense mRNAs. These genomic sense mRNAs are transcribed from templates of the corresponding antigenome RNA, which also function as replicative intermediates (Fig. 18.3).

Activation of L's RNA synthesis activity is mediated by (i) structured (double-stranded) 5′ viral RNAs corresponding to the termini of genomic and antigenomic RNAs of both S and L in conjunction with a specific promoter and (ii) the nontemplated G at the 5′-end of the viral genome. Dinucleotide primers also enhance RNA synthesis by MACV, but not LASV, L, illustrating that polymerase complexes from different mammarenaviruses may have some unique features.[207,316,393]

Transcription initiation is performed through a unique mechanism shared by all polyploviricotine viruses called cap-snatching. Short fragments of 5′-capped primers composed of four to five nucleotides are "stolen" by the virus polymerase complex from host-cell mRNAs to prime the synthesis of viral mRNAs. This process is thought to be initiated by cleavage of cytoplasmic cellular mRNAs by the endonuclease activity associated with the N-terminus of L that generates 5′-capped primers.[221,327,395] However, the endonuclease activity of any arenavirus L has yet to be experimentally validated. Transcription of NP mRNA was detected in TCRV-infected cells at early times of infection and in the presence of inhibitors of protein synthesis, suggesting that, unlike closely related bunyaviruses, but similarly to orthomyxoviruses, rhabdoviruses, and paramyxoviruses, primary transcription directed by the incoming TCRV RNP can proceed in the absence of translation.[127] The 5′ ends of arenavirus genome and antigenome RNAs each contain a nontemplated G residue that has been proposed to reflect a prime-and-realign mechanism for RNA replication mediated by L.[136,137,324] Recent studies provided biochemical evidence for initiation of arenavirus replication through this mechanism.[393] This prime-and-realign mechanism assumes that arenavirus polymerases initiate, like many other viral RdRps, RNA synthesis *de novo* only with GTP. Accordingly, arenavirus RNA initiation would take place from an internal templated cytidylate. Once the first phosphodiester bond has been formed, the pppGpC$_{OH}$, an uncapped primer, will slip backward on the template and realign, creating a nascent chain whose 5′ end is at position 1 with respect to the template, before the polymerase resumes downstream synthesis. To maintain a constant length of the genome RNA despite addition of a nontemplated nucleotide at the 5′ end, the polymerase terminates RNA synthesis by removing the last base at the 5′ end of the nascent chain. Arenavirus genome, and antigenome, sequence terminal complementarity combined with the prime-and-realign

mechanism for replication initiation generates double-stranded RNAs with overhanging 5′-ppp nucleotides. These structures can escape RIG-I recognition[247] and act as RIG-I decoys,[246] thereby diminishing RIG-I–mediated interferon induction.[149]

Transcription termination occurs within the distal side of the IGR and generates nonpolyadenylated viral mRNAs.[269] The IGR acts as a *bona fide* transcription termination signal for the virus polymerase.[309] Virus replication proceeds in two steps: first the *de novo* (primer-independent) synthesis of an intermediate RNA with positive polarity (cRNA) and second, using this cRNA as template, the synthesis of progeny genomic vRNA with negative polarity.

Using cell-based minigenome (MG) assays for LCMV, LASV,[152] JUNV,[3] TCRV,[228] and Pichindé virus (PICHV),[212] NP and L have been identified as the minimal viral *trans*-acting factors required for efficient RNA synthesis mediated by the virus polymerase. In the case of LCMV, both genetic and biochemical evidence indicate that oligomerization of L is required for polymerase activity.[349] Z is not required for intracellular transcription and replication of an LCMV MG, but rather Z has a dose-dependent inhibitory effect on both transcription and replication of LCMV MG.[70–72] This inhibitory effect of Z has also been reported for TCRV[228] and LASV.[152] Consistent with these findings, studies using *in vitro* reconstitution of RNA synthesis directed by MACV polymerase have provided evidence that Z, via direct interaction with the polymerase, is able to lock the polymerase in a promoter-bound, catalytically inactive state.[208,209] Transcription of Z mRNA starts at the 3′ end of the L RNA antigenomic segment, once the L antigenomic RNAs have been produced. Low expression levels of Z early during the virus replication cycle facilitate viral RNA replication and gene transcription,[208,209] whereas increased Z expression levels at later times during the arenavirus replication cycle will inhibit viral RNA synthesis and promote virus assembly and budding.[301,371]

Mutation-function analysis of the genome 5′ and 3′ termini using the MG-based assays for LCMV, LASV, and MACV indicates that the activity of the arenavirus genomic promoter requires both sequence specificity within the highly conserved 3′-terminal 19 nt of arenavirus genomes and the integrity of the predicted panhandle structure. This panhandle is formed via sequence complementarity between the 5′ and 3′ termini of viral genome RNAs.[154,302] Mammarenavirus RNA replication and gene transcription are NP dependent, but NP levels do not affect the balance between replication and transcription.[308] MG-based assays confirmed the IGR role as a *bona fide* transcription termination signal, but synthesis of translation-competent viral mRNAs does not strictly require the presence of the IGR.[309]

Assembly and Budding

Assembly and cell release of infectious mammarenavirus progeny require both Z and GPC and the correct processing of GPC into GP1 and GP2 (Fig. 18.4).[222,223,310] Colocalization of all viral proteins for assembly is mediated by Z–L,[208] Z–NP,[362] and Z–GP[51,383] interactions. Mammarenavirus Z is a structural component of the virion, and cryoelectron microscopy structural studies reveal a location of LCMV Z within virions consistent with its role as a matrix protein.[286] In accordance, functional studies have shown LASV and LCMV Zs to be the main driving force of arenavirus budding,[301,371] a process mediated by the interaction of Z's late-budding motifs, PTAP and/or PPPY, with components of the cellular ESCRT complexes.[128] Targeting of Z to the plasma membrane, the location

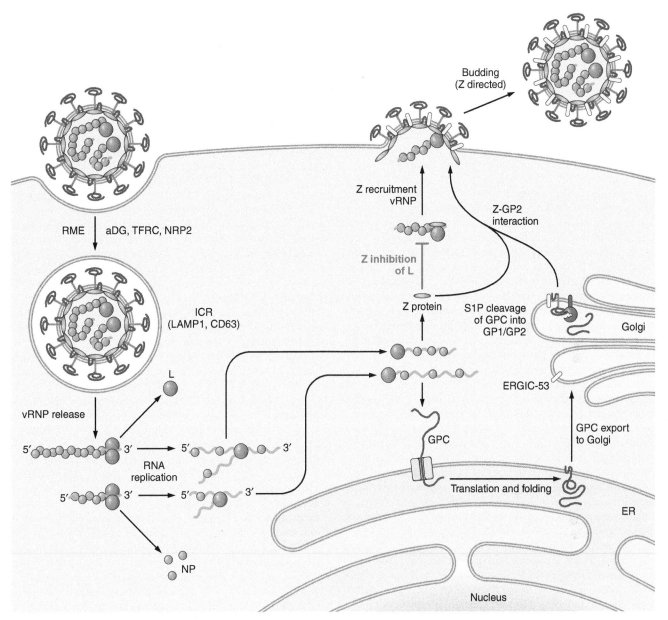

FIGURE 18.4 Mammarenavirus life cycle. Mammarenaviruses enter cells via receptor-mediated endocytosis (RME). Many Old World mammarenaviruses use α-dystroglycan (aDG) as the main receptor. Neuropilin (NRP)-2 is the cell-surface receptor used by the disease-causing Old World mammarenavirus LUJV. Clade B New World arenaviruses use transferrin receptor 1 (TfR1) as cellular receptor. The acidic environment of the endosome triggers a pH-dependent membrane fusion step that results in the release of the viral RNP into the cell cytoplasm where viral RNA genome replication and gene transcription take place. For some arenaviruses, completion of the entry process involves a late endosomal receptor switch mechanism. The late endosomal resident proteins LAMP1 and CD36 are required for LASV and LUJV cell entry, respectively. Transcription by the viral polymerase complex is initiated at promoters on each 3' end of the RNA segments, transcribing mRNA encoding NP and L (not shown). Transcription is terminated by structural motifs within the IGR. The virus polymerase complex switches from a transcriptase to a replicase mode and moves across the IGR, generating full-length antigenome (ag) RNAs that serve as templates for the synthesis of the GPC and Z mRNAs. The complete viral genome is also amplified from the agRNA templates. Arenavirus infection induces discrete cytosolic structures for RNA replication. Production of infectious progeny requires that assembled viral RNPs associate at the cell surface with membranes that are enriched in mature viral GP. It is also dependent on the host lectin ERGIC-53, which associates with viral GP and is incorporated into virions. Z plays critical roles in virion assembly and budding. Incorporation of arenavirus GPs into virion particles depends on the interaction of GP with Z. Canonical late-budding motifs found in most mammarenavirus Zs recruit components of ESCRT to promote virion budding.

of arenavirus budding, strictly requires myristoylation.[303,372] The cellular cargo receptor endoplasmic reticulum (ER)-Golgi intermediate compartment 53-kDa protein (ERGIC-53) is required for infectious arenavirion production. ERGIC-53 binds to arenavirus GPs, traffics to arenavirus budding sites, and is incorporated into virions. In the absence of ERGIC-53, GP-containing virus particles still form, but they are noninfectious, partially due to their inability to attach to and enter host cells.[204]

PATHOGENESIS AND PATHOLOGY

Pathogenesis of mammarenaviral disease is not well understood. The pathological findings (gross and light microscopic lesions) found postmortem in patients rarely account for the relative high case-fatality rate (CFR) and severity of disease.[61,98,346,393] Mammarenaviruses typically enter humans in an aerosolized form and are deposited in the lung, where initial viral replication occurs.[80] Antigen-presenting cells (APCs), DCs and macrophages, are prominent targets in the initial stages of infection. The abundance of these cells in the mucosal tissues and skin results in their early infection and amplification of the viruses. The mobility and wide distribution of APCs most likely facilitate mammarenavirus entry into the lymphoid system and their systematic spread to other organs and tissues.[5,142,167,256] Principal target organs, based on virus titers, EM, or viral antigen accumulation at death, include the lymphoid tissue, liver, kidneys, lungs, adrenal glands, and heart. In the case of LASV, the virus has also been recovered from the placenta, mammary glands, and aborted fetal tissues. In the case of AHF, virion-like particles were also observed in the central nervous system (CNS), ovaries, and testes.[73,142,167,256,393] In the case of LCMV, the virus eventually reaches the meninges, choroid plexus, and ventricular ependymal linings, where it replicates to high titers and where the inflammatory response produces the characteristic lymphocytic choriomeningitis (LCM) pathology and signs of meningitis.[30]

In most cases of congenital LCMV infection, the fetus becomes infected transplacentally. After reaching the fetus, the virus exhibits a strong tropism for the fetal brain, where the infection produces its most common and severe pathologic effects, including microencephaly, periventricular calcifications, hydrocephalus, cerebellar hypoplasia, focal cerebral destruction, and gyral dysplasia.[30]

Coagulopathy and Vascular Dysfunction
The extent of hemorrhagic and coagulopathy manifestations differs between pathogenic mammarenaviruses. Hemorrhages are uncommon in LF patients and are primarily limited to mucosal surfaces.[254] In AHF patients, hemorrhage is much more common. Bleeding is typically associated with coagulopathy including thrombocytopenia and platelet dysfunction.[81,120,163] The platelet malfunction may be associated with a yet unidentified plasma inhibitor of platelet aggregation.[76,78] There is no evidence that coagulation dysfunctions such as disseminated intravascular coagulation or complement activation play a role in mammarenavirus pathogenesis.[81] A recent metabolomics study found that levels of platelet-activating factor (PAF) and PAF-like molecules are lower in the serum of patients with fatal LF than in patients with nonfatal LF. The hemoglobin breakdown products D-urobilinogen and I-urobilin are also reduced in LF patients.[131]

Impairment of vascular function is most likely central for the pathology observed in LASV- and JUNV-infected patients. Edema and pleural and pericardial effusions that are associated with fatal LF cases are most likely due to increased vascular permeability. In both experimentally infected animals and LF patients, the disruption of vascular endothelium function is closely followed by shock and death.[121,234,393] In AHF patients, hemorrhagic disease manifestations are believed to be associated with vascular dysfunction.[210] However, only minimal vascular lesions are detected in fatal human LF and AHF cases and infected nonhuman primates (NHPs).[98] This discrepancy is probably because LASV and JUNV are nonlytic viruses and, as such, do not cause cytopathic effects or cellular damage in infected monocytes, macrophages, and endothelial cells.[139,234]

The mechanism of LASV-induced increase in vascular permeability is yet to be uncovered. A common hypothesis is that virus infection of the endothelium might cause changes in cellular function leading to increased fluid flow and subsequent edema. Infection with other hemorrhage-inducing viruses (e.g., Ebola virus) results in a "cytokine storm" that interferes with the integrity of the vascular endothelium. However, LASV-infected macrophages are not activated and proinflammatory cytokines are not released.[234,240] Recent studies with JUNV-infected endothelial cells reveal perturbation of specific endothelial cell functions, including increased expression of cell adhesion molecules (ICAM-1 and VCAM-1), coagulation factors (von Willebrand factor), and release of vasoactive mediators (nitric oxide and prostaglandin PGI_2) as a consequence of productive viral infection.[139] These studies provide the first possible links to the increased vascular permeability observed in AHF patients, but their relevance *in vivo* remains to be investigated.

Pathology
Macroscopic abnormalities in LF patients include gastric mucosal, renal, and subconjunctival hemorrhages, petechiae, and evidence of increased vascular permeability, such as pleural and pericardial effusions, ascites, and facial, intestinal, and laryngeal edema.[125,328] Microscopic findings reported in patients and in NHPs include multifocal hepatocellular necrosis with weak inflammatory cell involvement, splenic necrosis, necrosis of renal tubular cells, adrenocortical cell necrosis, focal renal interstitial lymphocytic infiltrates, mild mononuclear interstitial myocarditis, alveolar edema with capillary congestion, interstitial pneumonitis, and rhabdomyositis.[125,256,328,393]

The most consistent pathological hallmark of LF in humans is multifocal hepatocellular necrosis. In fatal cases, the extent of necrosis can range from 1% up to 50%. High virus titers in liver tissue correlate with severe hepatitis.[256] However, the degree of hepatic tissue damage is insufficient to cause hepatic failure. In addition, there is no correlation between the degree of hepatic necrosis and chemical indicators of liver damage, such as elevated concentrations of aspartate aminotransferase (AST), alanine transaminase (ALT), and lactate dehydrogenase (LDH) in serum.[256,393] Therefore, LASV-induced hepatitis is not the primary cause of death in fatal cases.

The most common macroscopic abnormality in severe cases of NW mammarenaviral disease is widespread hemorrhage, particularly in the skin and mucous membranes (gastrointestinal [GI] tract), intracranium (Virchow-Robin space), kidneys, pericardium, spleen, adrenal glands, and lungs. Microscopic lesions include acidophilic bodies and focal necroses in the liver, acute tubular and papillary necrosis in the kidneys, and reticular hyperplasia of the spleen and lymph nodes. In cases of BHF, hepatic petechiae are common and the number and size of Kupffer cells are also increased. Interstitial pneumonia has been observed in cases of BHF or Venezuelan hemorrhagic fever (VeHF). In cases of AHF, secondary bacterial lung infections (acute bronchitis and bronchopneumonia, myocardial and lung abscesses) have been observed.[61,98,150,346]

Patterns of clinical AHF illness are JUNV strain specific and can be "hemorrhagic" (Espindola strain), "neurologic" (Ledesma strain), "mixed" (P-3551 strain), and "common" (Romero strain).[146,259,260] In animal models of AHF, each isolate induces a disease syndrome that replicates the clinical variant of the disease in the human from whom the viral strain was obtained. Animals infected with JUNV Espindola strain ("hemorrhagic") demonstrate a pronounced bleeding tendency with disseminated cutaneous and mucous membrane hemorrhage. In guinea pigs, the Espindola strain replicates predominantly in the spleen, lymph nodes, and bone marrow, the major sites of necroses, whereas lower virus loads are present in the blood and brain. In contrast, animals infected with JUNV Ledesma strain ("neurologic") show little or no hemorrhagic manifestations but develop overt and generally progressive signs of neurologic dysfunction: limb paresis, ataxia, tremulousness, and hyperactive startle reflexes. The Ledesma strain is found predominantly in the brain, where moderate polioencephalitis is observed, and only low amounts of virus are recovered from the spleen and lymph nodes.

A single well-studied LCM encephalitis case showed mononuclear cell infiltrates in the meninges and around vessels and glial nodules in the deeper structures.[397] Fluorescent antibodies detected viral antigen in meninges and in cortical neurons. During the CNS disease, there is no viremia, but virus is still detectable in cerebrospinal fluid (CSF), and the pathogenesis is believed to be immunopathological. An animal model of congenital LCMV infection has demonstrated the very strong tropism of LCMV for neuroblasts and that infection disturbs neuron migration. These findings explain, respectively, the location of periventricular calcifications and the gyral malformations in children with congenital LCMV.[30] Studies with this model have also shown that the age of the developing host at the time of infection profoundly affects the patterns of infection and pathology within the brain.

Immune Responses

T-cell responses play a crucial role in the control of LASV infection in both *in vitro* and *in vivo* animal models. Severe or fatal LASV infection seems to be associated with defective T-cell responses (low and delayed T-cell activation), whereas the effective control of LF seems to be mediated by robust and efficient responses. In hospitalized patients and NHP models of LF, strong (IgG and IgM) antibody responses are not correlated with the outcome of disease; however, high viral loads are associated with a poor prognosis. Therefore, humoral responses are not effective in controlling LASV replication and the resulting pathology.[192,338] Unlike LF, humoral immunity plays an important role in controlling AHF. In both humans and animal models, immune plasma treatment from previously exposed individuals is efficacious in treating AHF if administered early during infection. The efficacy of the treatment appears to be due to the ability of the antibodies to neutralize virus, as viral loads are reduced after transfusion with immune plasma.[242]

A recent study suggests that the number of *N*-glycosylation sites on the arenaviral GPs is inversely correlated with the protective efficacy of neutralizing antibodies.[365]

Mammarenavirus infections cause immunosuppression in humans and other animals. The hallmark of LASV infection is generalized immunosuppression. In accordance, LASV-infected APCs do not mature or become activated; elevated levels of activation markers (CD80, CD86, CD40, CD54, and HLAs) or cytokines (tumor necrosis factor [TNF-α], interleukin [IL]-1β, IL-6, and IL-12) and increased phagocytic activity are not observed following infection.[263] Furthermore, in LF patients, fatal outcome correlates with absence or minimal levels of IL-8 and interferon-inducible protein 10 (IP-10) in serum.[240] In recent studies, however, human LF survival was correlated with low levels of IL-6, IL-8, IL-10, macrophage inflammatory protein (MIP1β), and CD40L.[35]

In AHF patients, immunosuppression is not generalized. Decreases in the number of T and B lymphocytes, lower ratio of CD4 to CD8 T cells, and diminished response to mitogens are reported in acute AHF patients. However, JUNV-infected patients have elevated proinflammatory cytokine (TNF-α, IFN-α, IL-6, and IL-10) levels. In fact, the severity of disease is consistently associated with elevated levels of TNF-α and IFN-α.[164,224,248]

In vitro studies suggest that macrophages are not responsible for the increased cytokine production as IFN-α, IFN-β, TNF-α, IL-10, IL-6, and IL-12 levels do not increase in these cells following inoculation with JUNV. In contrast to LASV, both JUNV and MACV can readily induce IFN production in cultured human primary DCs.[145,171,263] The exact role of cytokines in the pathogenesis of NW arenavirus disease is yet to be determined, but a common hypothesis is that cytokines may be important in controlling virus replication in the early stages of infection, whereas a delayed response could contribute to pathogenesis as seen in patients with severe disease and high levels of cytokines.

Congenital LCMV infection in animals triggers a robust inflammatory response, driven by cytotoxic T lymphocytes. This finding explains the lymphocytic pleocytosis in patients with LCM and the inflammation-induced destructive cerebral lesions in children with congenital LCMV.[30]

Mammarenavirus RNA can activate the RIG-I/melanoma differentiation–associated protein 5 (MDA5)-mitochondrial antiviral signaling (MAVS)-dependent signaling pathway to induce the IFN-I response.[423] However, mammarenaviral NP is a potent inhibitor of IFN-I. Specifically, NP (with the exception of TCRV NP) expression blocks phosphorylation and prevents the nuclear translocation of interferon regulatory factor 3 (IRF3).[251,316] NP (with the exception of TCRV NP) also inhibits the nuclear translocation and transcriptional activity of the nuclear factor kappa B (NF-κB).[332] NP interacts with RIG-I and MDA5[423] and prevents potentiation of RIG-I function by the cellular protein PACT. The exo activity of NP is required for this function.[357] The C-terminus (exoribonuclease domain) of LCMV NP also binds the kinase domain of cellular protein kinase IKKε, thereby blocking its autocatalytic activity and its ability to phosphorylate IRF3.[316]

In addition to NP, mammarenaviral Z suppresses IFN-I response. According to one study, pathogenic mammarenavirus Z binds to the CARD domains of RIG-I–like receptors and disrupts their interactions with MAVS, thereby leading to down-regulation of the IFN-β response.[410] Another study reported similar finding with the exception that Z of NW, but not OW, mammarenaviruses was found to interact with RIG-I and interfere with the interaction between RIG-I and MAVS.[108]

EPIDEMIOLOGY

Arenaviruses are ecologically diverse and have been found in rodents, bats, and ticks (mammarenaviruses)[92,320,351] snakes (reptarenaviruses, hartmaniviruses),[168–170,366] and fish (antennaviruses).[359] Most mammarenaviruses infect muroid rodents of only one or a few species and, therefore, are geographically constrained (Fig. 18.5). However, LCMV, which infects the ubiquitous house mouse, is distributed globally.[62,347] Within these host ranges, the prevalence of each virus may be spatially or temporally patchy. One mammarenavirus, TCRV, was found in phyllostomid bats and lone star ticks (*Amblyomma americanum* Linnaeus, 1758).[92,351] The natural distribution of reptilian and fish arenaviruses is unknown thus far.[168–170,366]

Typically, mammarenaviruses cause persistent, frequently asymptomatic infections in their reservoir hosts, which are characterized by virus multiplication in many different tissues and chronic viremia and viruria. Chronic infections are suspected to be caused by suppressed host immunity. The chronic carrier state in rodents usually results from vertical transmission (exposure to infectious virus early in ontogeny) or horizontal transmission (exposure to virus later in life through aggressive or venereal behavior).[30,114,271,339,394,398]

Mammarenaviruses do not normally infect mammals other than their immediate reservoir hosts. However, some viruses are pathogenic and are often highly virulent for humans. Human

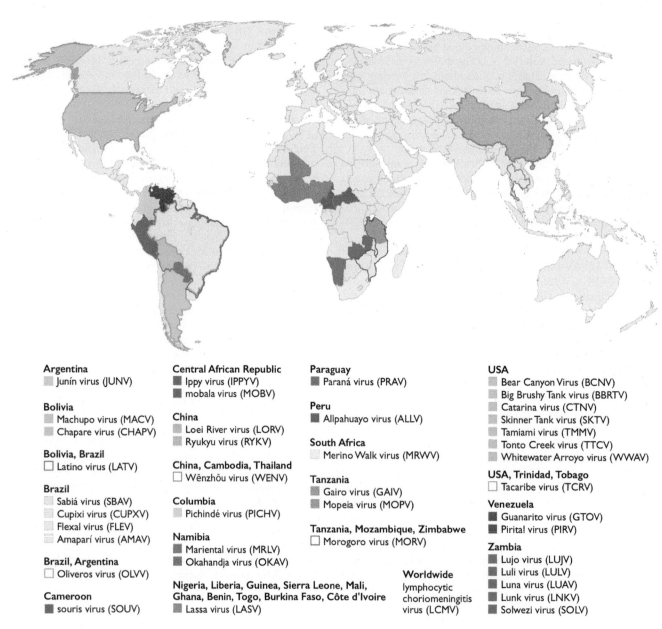

Argentina
Junín virus (JUNV)

Bolivia
Machupo virus (MACV)
Chapare virus (CHAPV)

Bolivia, Brazil
Latino virus (LATV)

Brazil
Sabiá virus (SBAV)
Cupixi virus (CUPXV)
Flexal virus (FLEV)
Amaparí virus (AMAV)

Brazil, Argentina
Oliveros virus (OLVV)

Cameroon
souris virus (SOUV)

Central African Republic
Ippy virus (IPPYV)
mobala virus (MOBV)

China
Loei River virus (LORV)
Ryukyu virus (RYKV)

China, Cambodia, Thailand
Wēnzhōu virus (WENV)

Columbia
Pichindé virus (PICHV)

Namibia
Mariental virus (MRLV)
Okahandja virus (OKAV)

Nigeria, Liberia, Guinea, Sierra Leone, Mali, Ghana, Benin, Togo, Burkina Faso, Côte d'Ivoire
Lassa virus (LASV)

Paraguay
Paraná virus (PRAV)

Peru
Allpahuayo virus (ALLV)

South Africa
Merino Walk virus (MRWV)

Tanzania
Gairo virus (GAIV)
Mopeia virus (MOPV)

Tanzania, Mozambique, Zimbabwe
Morogoro virus (MORV)

Worldwide
lymphocytic choriomeningitis virus (LCMV)

USA
Bear Canyon Virus (BCNV)
Big Brushy Tank virus (BBRTV)
Catarina virus (CTNV)
Skinner Tank virus (SKTV)
Tamiami virus (TMMV)
Tonto Creek virus (TTCV)
Whitewater Arroyo virus (WWAV)

USA, Trinidad, Tobago
Tacaribe virus (TCRV)

Venezuela
Guanarito virus (GTOV)
Pirital virus (PIRV)

Zambia
Lujo virus (LUJV)
Luli virus (LULV)
Luna virus (LUAV)
Lunk virus (LNKV)
Solwezi virus (SOLV)

FIGURE 18.5 Global mammarenavirus distribution. Human arenavirus infections are indicated on a global map by colors. (Courtesy of Jiro Wada, IRF-Frederick, Fort Detrick, MD, USA.)

infections occur via exposure to rodent fomites, ingestion of contaminated food, exposure to broken skin or mucous membranes, or inhalation of aerosolized virions from contaminated material.[25,73,104,253,276,375]

Lassa Fever

LF is endemic in areas of western sub-Saharan Africa: Nigeria, Liberia, Guinea, and Sierra Leone (Fig. 18.5). Recent data also indicate the presence of circulating strains in the surrounding countries of Mali,[342,345] Ghana,[94] Benin (http://www.who.int/csr/don/13-june-2016-lassa-fever-benin/en/), Togo,[299,404] Burkina Faso,[373] and Côte d'Ivoire.[364] Imported cases of LF have been reported in the United States, Canada, the United Kingdom, Japan, Germany, the Netherlands, and Israel.[147,236] The etiologic agent of LF is LASV.[125] The CFR of LF is about 1% to 2% in the endemic areas, with estimated 300,000 infections annually.[257] Most LASV infections in Africa are asymptomatic, mild, or subclinical, but the CFR in hospitalized confirmed cases of LF can be as high as 69%.[44,175,356] The CFR increases with age, and patients aged 50 years and older are more likely to die.[9,44,288] High CFR for children aged 9 years or younger and adolescents and adults less than 29 years of age has also been reported.[44,124,356] The disease is especially severe late in pregnancy with fetal death, miscarriage, or spontaneous abortion occurring in nearly all cases.[124,255,314,356] Most LF cases recorded during recent outbreaks were in the older age group of ≥20 years.[175,356]

The Natal mastomys (*Mastomys natalensis* Smith, 1834) is the main reservoir host of LASV.[215,279] Experimental LASV infection of adult and neonatal Natal mastomys and field studies support the notion that these rodents are not adversely affected by LASV infection. However, some infected adult rodents develop mild meningoencephalitis.[245,394] Maintenance of LASV in Natal mastomys is thought to occur via vertical transmission (*in utero* or postnatal transmission).[394] However, recent studies suggest the existence of an additional horizontal transmission mechanism.[114] Other rodents might also serve as LASV hosts or have roles in LASV transmission.[114,257,290,409] Humans become infected with LASV through direct contact with infected rodent excreta, tissues, or blood or via inhalation of aerosolized virus.[192,276,375] Accordingly, poor sanitation and housing conditions correlate with greatest risk of infection.[29] In Western Africa, peridomestic rodents are also part of the diet in certain populations. Consequently, infected meat could be another route of virus transmission.[199] Person-to-person transmission of LASV can occur in nosocomial settings via direct contact with body fluids from symptomatically infected individuals or corpses and is estimated to occur in ≈20% of LF cases.[122,227,276] Human infections tend to be more common in the dry season, between November and April,[97,175,356] which may reflect a higher prevalence of Natal mastomys inside houses.[115]

LASV prevalence is focal and varies greatly between geographical regions. In Guinea, the reported seroprevalence varies from 4% to 55% (with the highest prevalence in forested Guinea).[20,233] In Sierra Leone, seroprevalence ranges from 8% to 52%[257] and in Nigeria from 13% to 37%.[379] Prevalence of LASV IgG antibodies is 26% in Côte d'Ivoire.[2] At least in Nigeria, the occurrence of LF seems to drift from rural to predominantly urban residential areas.[358]

A striking feature of LASV is the high level of genetic diversity between strains; nucleotide differences can reach up to 32% and 25% for the L and S segments, respectively.[7,33,97] The diversity among LASV strains correlates with geographic location rather than time, and no evidence of a "molecular clock" has been found. Six major LASV clades have been reported thus far based on sequencing data: I–III in Nigeria; IV covering the countries of Sierra Leone, Guinea, and Liberia; V covering southern Mali and Côte d'Ivoire, and the recently recognized clade VI from Togo.[7,244,404] The high diversity of LASV might explain the observed variability of LF's clinical presentation and possible regional differences.

Lymphocytic Choriomeningitis

Mounting evidence indicates that LCMV is a neglected human pathogen. The disease burden in humans is unknown.[18] The primary host of LCMV is the house mouse, but other rodents, such as pet hamsters[26] and domesticated guinea pigs (*Cavia porcellus* Linnaeus, 1758), can become infected and transmit the virus to humans.[117] Infected rodents shed the virus in their urine, saliva, nasal secretions, and droppings throughout life.[30] LCMV is transferred vertically from one generation to the next via intrauterine infection within the mouse host. Offspring of rodents that acquire LCMV transplacentally are persistently infected and may have high viremia. However, these offspring often remain asymptomatic.[30]

Humans become infected with LCMV through close contact with infected rodents, through solid organ transplantation,[56,116] or by vertical transmission. Congenital LCMV infection occurs when a woman acquires a primary LCMV infection during pregnancy and the virus is passed to the fetus transplacentally or is acquired during the intrapartum period.[206] Human-to-human horizontal transmission of LCMV has not been documented (with the exception of transplantation).[26] Humans can acquire LCMV during any season, but most LCMV infections occur during the late autumn and early winter months, when house mice move into human dwellings during the cold season.[30] Human LCMV infections involve all age groups, and generally occur sporadically.[304] LCMV can also cause callitrichid hepatitis in New World primates. These primates develop hepatitis after contact with LCMV-infected house mice.[10,282,369]

The prevalence of LCMV within house mouse populations and in humans is highly variable, even within the same geographic region, resulting in the focal and uneven spatial distribution of the virus. For example, a study in Baltimore, MD, USA, found that the prevalence of LCMV antibody varied from 3.9% to 13.4% in house mice from inner-city locations. Study results provided evidence that infections were clustered within residential blocks and even within households.[63] In humans, LCMV prevalence in the USA and Argentina is estimated at ≈2% to 5%.[6,64,292,329,368] This prevalence suggests that the risk of infection has decreased since the 1940–1950s when the prevalence of LCMV infection was 8% to 11%.[1,270,326]

LCMV strains have been divided into four different lineages.[4] Most of the US strains, including the classic laboratory strains, WE and Armstrong, and virus strains from France, Germany, and Slovakia, are located within lineage I. Lineage II appears to contain only viruses from Europe. An LCMV 1984 isolate from the state of Georgia (USA) is the sole member of lineage III. Lineage IV consists of viruses isolated in Spain from wild-caught long-tailed field mice (*Apodemus sylvaticus* Linnaeus, 1758).[216] LCMV exhibits high genetic diversity, comparable to that of LASV.[4] Up to 18% and 25% nucleotide divergence was observed within the S and L segment lineages, respectively. The high genetic diversity of LCMV and the lack of clear correlation of virus genetic lineages to particular geographic locations likely reflect the long and complex phylogeographic history of the common house mouse host.[4]

Argentinian Hemorrhagic Fever

JUNV, the etiologic agent of AHF, is estimated to have caused around 30,000 cases. In the absence of treatment, the CFR can reach 20% to 30%. Pregnant women have an increased CFR and many miscarry, especially during the third trimester.[38] The AHF-endemic region has expanded progressively into north central Argentina to the extent that currently 3 million people are considered to be at risk of infection (Fig. 18.5).[104] AHF is typically a seasonal disease, with a peak of frequency occurring during the corn-harvesting season (March–June). Infected cases are primarily rural male agricultural workers, aged 15 to 55 years.[73] The drylands laucha (*Calomys musculinus* Thomas, 1913) is the main reservoir of JUNV.[339,340] However, other animals can become infected.[271,272] The drylands laucha inhabits crop fields, pastures and adjacent roadsides, and fence lines. It is rarely captured in or around human dwellings. The patchy spatial distribution of this rodent has been suggested to account for the focal distribution of AHF. Furthermore, annual increase in the number of drylands laucha coincides with the corn-harvesting season providing opportunities for rodent-to-man transmission. Transmission to humans is believed to occur predominantly by inhaling aerosolized viral particles from contaminated soil and plant litter, which are disturbed during the mechanized harvesting process, or by exposure to primary aerosols of rodent urine or contact with contaminated nesting materials in border habitats.[73,104]

Results from field and laboratory studies suggest that horizontal transmission via aggressive encounters among adult, male rodents is the primary mode of viral persistence in nature.[271,273] The high rate of JUNV production in salivary glands and virus isolation from saliva of drylands lauchas[271,300,339] make JUNV transmission following a bite highly likely. Vertical transmission has also been reported as possible maintenance mechanism of JUNV.[339] However, the virus cannot transgress the placenta,[391] and rodents infected at birth (during lactation) exhibit decreased survival, body growth, and fertility. In contrast, rodents infected as adults are usually asymptomatic.[388,389,391] Half of infected adult rodents develop persistent infection with virus isolated from the urine, saliva, blood, or brain, whereas the remainder develop serum antibodies and appear to clear the virus within 21 days.[391] Vertical transmission might contribute, to some extent, to the maintenance of infection, if not via transfer to the next generation, then via intragenerational infection by horizontal transmission when population numbers are reduced.[339,388,390]

Serological studies in Argentina found prevalence of JUNV-neutralizing antibodies to range from 4.7% to 12.3% in AHF-endemic areas.[82,400,401] In nonendemic areas, the prevalence is significantly lower (0.44%).[399] Clinically apparent disease occurs in nearly two-thirds of those infected. In rodents,

prevalence of infection can be as high as 10.9% with highest prevalence observed in current epidemic areas and lowest (0.2%) in nonendemic areas.[271–273,399]

Nucleotide similarity between JUNV strains is high and can reach up to 94.5% and 95.4% for GP and NP, respectively.[135,141]

Bolivian Hemorrhagic Fever

MACV is the etiological agent of BHF.[193] The CFR of BHF is approximately 5% to 30% with the highest rates occurring among those under 5 and over 55 years of age. BHF cases are more common during the dry season, at the peak of agricultural activity, with males over 15 years of age more frequently affected.[238] The big laucha (*Calomys callosus* Rengger, 1830), a small pastoral and peridomestic rodent, is the reservoir host of MACV.[191] Suckling big lauchas infected with MACV develop viremia but are "immunotolerant." In animals more than 9 days of age, a split response is observed following MACV infection (similarly to JUNV). "Immunocompetent" big lauchas (about 50%) develop circulating neutralizing antibodies and clear viremia and have minimal or absent viruria, whereas "immunotolerant" mice develop persistent viremia, viruria, and little or no neutralizing antibodies. MACV antigen can be detected in most tissues of the latter animals, including the reproductive organs. Long-term effects of tolerant infection include mild runting, reduced survival rate, and almost total sterility among females, largely caused by virus infection of embryos.[195,398] Both horizontal and vertical transmissions have been shown as possible maintenance mechanism of the virus within its reservoir rodent. Infection of newborn mice can occur neonatally through the milk and of adult mice can occur via venereal encounters.[398]

Person-to-person transmission of MACV is not frequent but possible by direct contact with body fluids or excreta of infected patients. Transmission by intimate contact during convalescence is also feasible.[91,190] Such transmission is probably not the principal mode of disease dissemination. In fact, the frequency of MACV isolation from human blood or from throat and oral swabs of infected patients is low, and only small quantities of the virus have been detected in successful isolation attempts.[193]

Venezuelan Hemorrhagic Fever

GTOV emerged in 1989 as the cause of VeHF. This severe hemorrhagic illness has focal distribution in the southern and southwestern portions of Portuguesa state and in adjacent areas of Barinas state (Fig. 18.5). VeHF cases peak between November and January, during the period of agricultural activity in the regions. Similar to AHF, the majority of cases have involved male agricultural workers. The CFR is ≈30%.[83,129,346,376] The short-tailed zygodont (*Zygodontomys brevicauda* J. A. Allen and Chapman, 1893) is the main reservoir host of GTOV. The virus is also commonly found in Alston's cotton rats (*Sigmodon alstoni* Thomas, 1880). These rodents are most abundant in tall grass along roadsides and fence lines, on the edges of cultivated fields, and in the naturally occurring savanna that dominates the landscape of the VeHF-endemic regions.[377] These hosts have not been reported within houses or farm building. Therefore, similar to JUNV, GTOV infections are assumed to occur outdoors and in rural areas, and persons that have frequent contact with rodent-infested grassland habitats are at higher risk.[83] Unlike, MACV and JUNV, newborn short-tailed zygodonts inoculated with GTOV develop chronic infection with no effect on growth and shed the virus in urine and saliva. Similarly to MACV and JUNV, GTOV infection of adult animals results in the typical split response: most animals produce chronic viremia characterized by persistent shedding of infectious virus in oral secretions and urine, whereas the rest develop neutralizing antibodies and clear viremia. Findings from experimentally GTOV-infected female zygodonts include a negative effect on reproductive fitness and evidence of vertical transmission to pups.[130]

CLINICAL FEATURES

Lassa Fever and Other Old World Mammarenaviral Diseases

The signs and symptoms of LF vary depending on the severity of the disease. The disease is mild or asymptomatic in about 80% of infected individuals, but 20% develop acute LF. The incubation period can range from 5 to 21 days but is typically 10 to 14 days. Disease onset is insidious with progressive fever, weakness, and general malaise (Fig. 18.6). Within 2 to 4 days, many patients experience an array of symptoms and signs including headache; myalgia; arthralgia; lower back, abdominal, and/or retrosternal chest pain; dizziness; nausea; tinnitus; or sore throat. Signs such as cough, vomiting, diarrhea, and/or constipation are also common. Lymphadenopathy (particularly cervical), oliguria, tachycardia, vertigo, splenomegaly, hepatomegaly, and jaundice have been reported occasionally. Pharyngitis, conjunctivitis, signs of respiratory distress (rales, wheezing, and rhonchi), pleural and pericardial effusions, or facial and neck edema can occur as the disease progresses.[20,75,123–125,198,205,255,267,277,281,288] The majority of patients begin to recover 8 to 10 days after disease onset, and virus is cleared from the blood 4 to 11 days later.[9,192,278] In severe cases, however, the illness worsens with respiratory distress and hemorrhagic and/or neurologic manifestations. Hemorrhagic manifestations can include skin and mucosal petechiae, mucosal bleeding (gums, vagina), epistaxis, hematuria, hemoptysis, bleeding from needle puncture sites, or conjunctival and GI bleeding (melena, hematemesis). Neuroglial findings such as moderate-to-severe diffuse encephalopathy, confusion, tremors, coma, and/or convulsions are common just prior to shock and death.[20,75,123–125,198,205,255,267,277,281,288] In children, edema of the neck and face may progress to widespread edema, abdominal distension, and bleeding (termed "swollen baby syndrome") that typically result in death.[280]

Common clinical findings include proteinuria, albuminuria, and elevated AST levels (at least mildly).[20,125,192,198,255,267,277,281,288] Moderate leukopenia, particularly in the initial phase of illness, has been reported in some, but not all, patients.[125,198,205,255,267,277,281] In some cases, hypotension has been described,[20,198,255,267] and even less frequently mild thrombocytopenia has been noted.[124,205,281]

Survivors of LASV infection often recover without sequelae. However, unilateral or bilateral sensorineural deafness, which may develop during disease, may persist permanently in ≈13% to 30% of survivors. The auditory patterns and clinical course resemble idiopathic sudden hearing loss.[77,226,289] In addition, pericarditis has been documented (particularly in males) as well as hair loss.[123,125,255]

LF presents with symptoms and signs indistinguishable from those of other febrile illnesses such as malaria, typhoid fever, gastroenteritis, pneumonia, and other severe viral infections. Therefore, LF is difficult to diagnose clinically but should be suspected in patients with fever (≥38°C) not responding to antimalarial and antibiotic drugs.[124,255,281] Past studies show that the most useful clinical predictors for diagnosis of LF are fever, pharyngitis, retrosternal pain, and proteinuria.[255] Fever, sore throat, vomiting, edema, and bleeding are the best predictors for negative outcome.[9,20,124,255,277] Disease outcome is also correlated to the degree of blood viremia; in fatal cases, viremia usually persists uncontrolled until death, and high LASV titers are found in visceral tissues at autopsy.[9,192] Recently, severe and nonsevere CNS signs, face and neck edema, jaundice, bleeding, hematuria, and proteinuria were shown to be more significantly associated with death.[288] Several laboratory-tested biomarkers had even greater association with increased CFR than did clinical features; these include raised concentrations of blood urea nitrogen and creatinine (biomarkers for kidney function), of serum AST (consistent with known liver malfunction), and of the serum electrolyte potassium. These results highlight the role of liver and renal dysfunction and electrolyte disturbance in the severity of LF.[9,125,288]

Patients infected with LUJV initially present with symptoms and signs of nonspecific febrile illness such as severe headache, malaise, vomiting, fever, retrosternal pain, or myalgia. Disease manifestations increase in severity over 7 days with the development of diarrhea and pharyngitis. In some patients, morbilliform rash or facial edema is evident. Terminal features are acute respiratory distress syndrome, cerebral edema, neurologic signs, deteriorating renal function, or circulatory collapse. In some patients, no overt hemorrhage is observed besides gingival bleeding, petechial rash, or oozing from injection sites.[37] However, the clinical description of disease caused by LUJV infection is currently based on the observation of only five patients.

Lymphocytic Choriomeningitis

Postnatal infections in persons with an intact immune system are often asymptomatic/subclinical or result in a mild febrile illness. Following 1 to 2 weeks of incubation, infected individuals develop flu-like illness with malaise and weakness, fever, myalgia, headache, and/or photophobia. Gastrointestinal (GI) symptoms and signs such as anorexia, nausea, and vomiting are also common, and in some cases, diarrhea has been reported. Sore throat, cough, pharyngitis, and other symptoms of respiratory tract involvement are less common. Lymphadenopathy, dysesthesia, conjunctivitis, arthralgia, arthritis, rash, testicular or parotid pain, and abdominal, back, and chest pain have been reported but occur infrequently. Typically, the disease lasts 5 to 15 days, and virus can be isolated from the blood. Clinical findings may include leukopenia, moderate thrombocytopenia, mild elevations of AST levels, and infiltrates on chest radiographs. However, these findings are not present in all patients.

CNS viral invasion is seen only in a minority of patients either after an initial prodromal febrile illness (as described above), defervescence, or, less commonly, without any early symptoms. During this neurologic phase, most patients

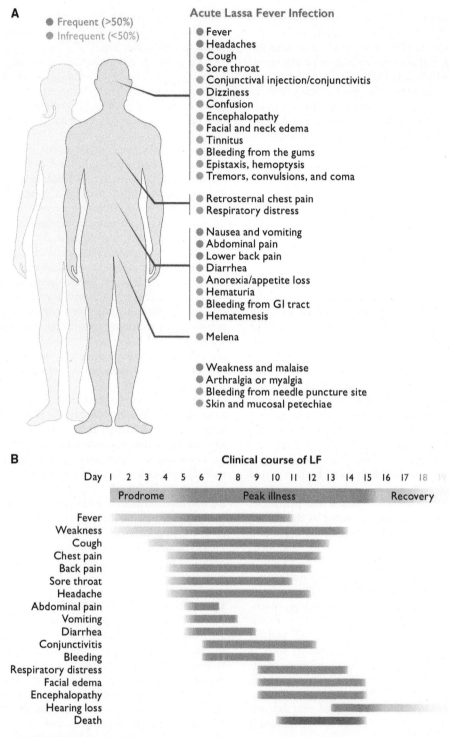

A

Frequent (>50%)
Infrequent (<50%)

Acute Lassa Fever Infection

Fever
Headaches
Cough
Sore throat
Conjunctival injection/conjunctivitis
Dizziness
Confusion
Encephalopathy
Facial and neck edema
Tinnitus
Bleeding from the gums
Epistaxis, hemoptysis
Tremors, convulsions, and coma

Retrosternal chest pain
Respiratory distress

Nausea and vomiting
Abdominal pain
Lower back pain
Diarrhea
Anorexia/appetite loss
Hematuria
Bleeding from GI tract
Hematemesis

Melena

Weakness and malaise
Arthralgia or myalgia
Bleeding from needle puncture site
Skin and mucosal petechiae

B

Clinical course of LF

Day 1 2 3 4 5 6 7 8 9 10 11 12 13 14 15 16 17 18 19

Prodrome   Peak illness   Recovery

Fever
Weakness
Cough
Chest pain
Back pain
Sore throat
Headache
Abdominal pain
Vomiting
Diarrhea
Conjunctivitis
Bleeding
Respiratory distress
Facial edema
Encephalopathy
Hearing loss
Death

FIGURE 18.6 Lassa fever clinical presentation. **A:** Listed are typical symptoms and clinical signs of LASV-infected adults. **B:** Idealized progression of key clinical signs in Lassa fever. (Courtesy of Jiro Wada, IRF-Frederick, Fort Detrick, MD, USA.)

experience symptoms/signs of classic aseptic meningitis that include fever, severe headache, vomiting, nuchal rigidity, and/or photophobia. In some cases, encephalitis, encephalomyelitis, meningoencephalitis, acute hydrocephalus, ascending or bulbar paralysis, or transverse myelitis may develop. The hallmark laboratory abnormality during this CNS phase of illness is a CSF pleocytosis. CSF leukocyte cell counts often exceed 1,000/μL.

Hypoglycorrhachia and mild elevations of CSF protein have also been reported. Virus can be isolated from the spinal fluid.[1,19,25,40,93,109,213,270,378,386,397] Infections are rarely fatal, and most patients survive without sequelae. However, some might experience asthenia, headaches, confusion, and difficulty in concentration. Alopecia, arthralgia, arthritis, orchitis, dysesthesias, and vertigo have also been reported infrequently.[1,19,386]

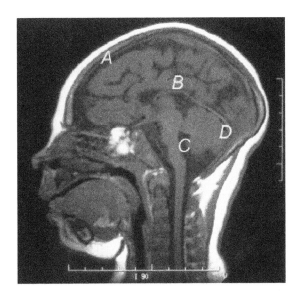

FIGURE 18.7 T1-weighted magnetic resonance imaging (MRI) scan of the brain of a 10-month-old child with congenital LCMV infection. The child had severe developmental delays, spastic quadriparesis, and medically intractable epilepsy. The MRI scan reveals microcephaly, a lissencephalic frontal lobe (*A*), and hypoplasia of the corpus callosum (*B*), the brainstem (*C*), and the cerebellum (*D*). (Courtesy of D. Bonthius, University of Iowa.)

Infection during pregnancy increases the risk for miscarriage (especially during the first trimester of pregnancy), *in utero* fetal death, fetopathy, and severe neurologic sequelae. Congenital LCMV can result in severe CNS or ocular malformations (Fig. 18.7), including chorioretinopathy, congenital hydrocephalus, macrocephaly, or microcephaly, and can mimic the signs/symptoms of classic TORCH (toxoplasmosis/*Toxoplasma gondii*, other infections, rubella, cytomegalovirus, herpes simplex virus) syndrome. Neurologic sequelae include spastic quadriparesis, mental retardation, seizures, and visual impairment.[17,407]

In immunosuppressed organ recipients, LCMV infection can be fatal.[56,57,116,239] Of 17 recipients described to date, 13 died of multisystem organ failure with LCMV-associated hepatitis as a prominent feature. Two surviving patients were treated with ribavirin. Initial illness in immunosuppressed patients is similar to the disease observed in immunocompetent patients (as described above): fatigue, headache, and GI-associated signs/symptoms (abdominal pain, anorexia, nausea, vomiting, diarrhea). However, in most immunosuppressed patients, the disease progresses to include CNS manifestations (meningoencephalitis, encephalopathy, encephalitis, confusion, seizures with myoclonus), hepatitis, and multisystem organ failure. Hypoxia and respiratory distress with pulmonary infiltrates have been reported in some cases as well as atrial fibrillation. Clinical findings include elevated transaminase (AST and ALT) levels, leukopenia, and/or thrombocytopenia. Elevated creatinine levels and hypotension are seen in some patients. Similarly to immunocompetent patients with CNS invasion with LCMV, CSF of immunosuppressed cases contains elevated protein levels, low glucose levels, and increased leukocyte numbers.

New World Mammarenaviral Hemorrhagic Fevers

Disease begins insidiously after an incubation period of 1 to 2 weeks. Initial symptoms/signs often include fever and malaise, headache, myalgia, epigastric pain, and anorexia. After 2 to 4 days, signs become increasingly severe with multisystem involvement: prostration and GI disturbances such as abdominal pain, nausea and vomiting, constipation, or mild diarrhea. In some cases, dizziness, photophobia, retro-orbital pain, or disorientation may also occur, and the earliest signs of vascular damage, such as conjunctival injection, skin petechiae, mild (postural) hypotension, or flushing over the head and upper torso, may appear. During the 2nd week of illness, about 20% to 30% of patients develop more severe hemorrhagic and/or prominent neurologic manifestations or secondary bacterial infections. Neurologic manifestations include seizures, convulsions, tremor of the hands and tongue, and, less frequently, delirium, coma, encephalitis, and meningoencephalitis. Typical hemorrhagic manifestations are bleeding from mucous membranes (gums, nose, vagina/uterus, GI tract) and ecchymoses at needle puncture sites. However, blood loss is minor overall. Following shock, death usually occurs 7 to 12 days after disease onset.

Typical clinical laboratory findings are leukopenia and thrombocytopenia. AST and ALT levels are usually normal or slightly elevated. The electrocardiogram may be nonspecifically abnormal, and chest radiography is usually normal in the absence of secondary infections.[8,82,151,275,311,337,353]

Patients who survive begin to improve during the 2nd week of disease onset as the appearance of neutralizing antibodies signals the beginning of the immune response.[81] Convalescence often lasts several weeks with polyuria, fatigue, alopecia, and dizziness.

NW mammarenaviral HF caused by CHAPV, GTOV, MACV, or SBAV is clinically similar to AHF.[69,83,86,238,370] In BHF patients (particularly severe cases), proteinuria and elevated hematocrit are typical during the peak of hemorrhagic manifestations. During convalescence, beau lines in digital nails are common.[238,370] In VeHF cases, pharyngitis is more prominent, and hearing loss in convalescence has been reported.[83,305,385] CNS manifestations, including encephalitis and convulsions, are associated with poor VeHF prognosis.[83] Furthermore, VeHF initially presents with symptoms and signs that are indistinguishable from dengue fever, also common in Venezuela, especially in urban areas.[83]

Only a single naturally acquired infection with SBAV has been identified, and the disease resembles other NW mammarenaviral HF except for extensive liver necrosis.[69]

DIAGNOSIS

Lassa Fever

LASV is readily isolated from blood during the febrile phase of LF disease up to 14 or more days after onset of disease. LASV can be detected in necropsy tissues or Vero cells infected with tissue homogenates.[126,192] LASV antigen can be detected by enzyme-linked immunosorbent assay (ELISA) capture in serum, and serum samples may become antigen negative with the appearance of IgM antibodies.[21] Detection of LASV antigen by ELISA is robust, is reliable, and can be completed in short time. LASV-specific antibodies can be detected by indirect immunofluorescence assay (IFA) using LASV-infected Vero cells, but the test is prone to discrepancies between laboratories. IFA IgG "seroreversion" has been reported and is thought to represent loss of antibody by previously seropositive individuals.[21,182,255] LASV-specific IgG and IgM can be detected by ELISA.[287] IgG ELISA antibody persists for long periods, whereas IFA antibody appears to wane below detectable limits within several years. ELISA IgM titers appear earlier and persist longer than IFA IgM titers.

Reverse transcriptase-PCR (RT-PCR) can detect virus RNA in blood with high sensitivity.[87,380] A recently available, recombinant Lassa virus (ReLASV) rapid diagnostic test (RDT)[27] is based on a lateral flow immunoassay using paired monoclonal antibodies to the Josiah strain of LASV (lineage IV). This test performed better than currently available RT-PCR detection assays, supporting the important role that recombinant antigen–based LASV immunoassays can play in the diagnosis of LASV infection.

Nanopore sequencing using the MinION device has been successfully used for genetic analysis of pathogens in field studies in regions with very limited resources[185] and was implemented to genetically characterize LASV isolates during the 2018 upsurge of LF cases in Nigeria.[196] The ability of this portable sequencing technology to genetically characterize *in situ* RNA viral samples will identify in real-time cases of LASV infection associated with disease symptoms. This approach, applicable to other arenaviruses, will represent a major breakthrough in the diagnosis of arenaviral HF.

Lymphocytic Choriomeningitis

During the acute febrile phase, LCMV can be isolated from blood. Viremia may also be detectable during meningitis symptoms, but CSF contains higher viral load.[109] Polymerase chain reaction (PCR) tests applied to CSF samples have been successfully used.[293] LCMV-specific IgM antibodies can be usually detected by ELISA and IFA in serum or CSF, or both, during acute cases.[84,85,113,220,225] As neutralizing antibodies appear late after onset of disease and are technically demanding to demonstrate, their value as a diagnostic tool is lessened.[220]

New World Mammarenaviral Hemorrhagic Fevers

Virus can be isolated from blood by inoculation of newborn hamsters or laboratory mice during the acute febrile phase up until 10 to 12 days after onset of symptoms.[34] Cocultivation of peripheral blood mononuclear cells with Vero cells seems to be more sensitive than suckling laboratory mouse or Vero cell inoculation for isolation of JUNV from AHF patients.[5] Virus can also be isolated from necropsy tissues, except from the brain. In rodent studies, virus is readily isolated from blood, urine, throat swabs, and autopsy tissue samples.[193,194] Antigen-capture ELISA detects viral antigen in blood and tissues from patients with JUNV, MACV, SBAV, or GOTV infection. Antigen detection is also possible in rodent urine, blood, and throat swabs during ecologic surveys.[271] Serologic diagnosis of AHF and BHF is usually made by complement fixation (CF)[237,405] and IFA,[249,307] but the limited specificity and sensitivity of these tests pose problems. The plaque neutralization test can

distinguish between antibodies to JUNV and MACV and has been used for evaluation of convalescent plasma units intended for therapeutic use in AHF.[103] The ELISA test is the most useful and practical for rapid detection of IgM and IgG antibodies in a clinical setting and sero-epidemiologic surveys.[134,176] Antibodies detected by ELISA can persist for ≥30 years in some cases.

PREVENTION AND CONTROL

Medical Management

Supportive therapy is important in the management of patients with arenaviral HF.[306] Avoidance of travel and general trauma, gentle sedation and pain relief with conservative doses of opiates, the usual precautions for patients with bleeding diatheses (e.g., avoiding intramuscular injections and acetylsalicylic acid), and careful maintenance of hydration are indicated. Bleeding can be managed by platelet transfusions and factor replacement as indicated by clinical judgment and laboratory studies. Management of patients that undergo shock is difficult. Hematocrit readouts suggest a generalized vascular permeability problem but of modest magnitude. Infusion of crystalloids should be carefully considered as it carries a high risk of pulmonary edema. The low cardiac output observed in animal models of AHF and clinical observations with human cases of AHF support the use of Swan-Ganz catheterization. The late neurological syndrome seen after immune plasma treatment of AHF is generally self-limited, and patient full recovery is accomplished with supportive therapy. LCMV ependymal infection and inflammation may cause acute hydrocephalus and a need for surgical shunting.[213] Steroids have not been evaluated in this condition.

Patients with arenaviral HF are considered to pose a minimal risk of contagion in the early stages of disease. Disease progression is associated with more extensive viral infection of target organs and increased viremia, which facilitate opportunities for dissemination. Nosocomial outbreaks and infection of multiple contacts have occurred when the index case corresponded to a severely ill patient, but they are uncommon.[52] The most dangerous exposure is parenteral and must be avoided through staff training. Protection to caregivers and other patients should be enhanced by implementing respiratory protection against small particle aerosols.[15] Special precautions are indicated when blood and other body fluids are handled in the clinical laboratory.

Close personal contacts should be monitored for fever for a period of 3 weeks. Patients may excrete virus in urine or semen for weeks after recovery from disease. Body fluids should be monitored for infectivity before the patient is released. In addition, counseling should be provided emphasizing protection of sexual partners and the use of disinfectant prior to use of toilets.

Antiviral Drugs

The prophylactic and therapeutic value of the nucleoside analog ribavirin (Rib) against several arenaviruses is well supported by results from both cell culture and all arenaviral HF animal models in which Rib has been studied.[79,181,200,203,352,363] Importantly, Rib has reduced both morbidity and lethality in human cases of LF. However, the need of intravenous administration for optimal efficacy, poor penetration into the CSF, and side effects, including anemia and congenital disorders, pose some limitations to the use of Rib. The mechanisms by which Rib exerts its antiarenaviral action are not fully understood but are likely to involve different steps of the virus life cycle.[294] Rib is efficacious against LF and remains the therapeutic agent of choice to treat cases of LF with a poor prognosis. Some evidence indicates that Rib is also efficacious against AHF,[105] and treatment with Rib of human MACV and SBAV infections has shown clinical benefits.[16,203]

Prophylaxis with Rib for 7 to 10 days delayed the onset of acute disease in guinea pigs experimentally infected with PICHV or LASV, whereas increasing Rib prophylactic treatment to 14 days prevented disease.[229,363,367] Rib prophylaxis for 14 to 21 days prevented acute disease in JUNV-infected domesticated guinea pigs, but it did not prevent JUNV entering the CNS and causing fatal encephalitis.[200] Thus, high-risk exposures to arenaviruses are probably best managed by implementing treatment at the first sign of fever, rather than dealing with the uncertainties of prophylaxis and its potential risks.

Besides Rib, several compounds have been reported to have antiarenaviral activity in cultured cells, but their safety and efficacy *in vivo* remain to be determined.[271] Recent high-throughput screening (HTS) identified a potent small molecule inhibitor of TCRV and several other NW arenaviruses.[28] Likewise, such cell-based screening using pseudotyped virion particles bearing the GP of highly virulent arenaviruses identified several small molecule inhibitors of virus cell entry mediated by LASV GP.[218] The broad-spectrum RdRp inhibitor favipiravir[144,264,344] and the GP-mediated fusion inhibitor ST-193[214] have shown promising results providing protection of domesticated guinea pigs from otherwise lethal LASV infection. Nevertheless, the identification and characterization of additional safe and effective antiviral drugs against human pathogenic arenaviruses can facilitate the implementation of combination therapy to combat human pathogenic arenaviruses. This approach is known to counteract the emergence of drug-resistant variants often observed with monotherapy strategies.[90]

Using arenavirus molecular genetics, investigators are developing screens to identify drugs targeting specific steps of the arenavirus life cycle. These drugs include direct-acting antivirals that target specific viral gene products and functions and drugs that target host cell factors required for the completion of virus replication cycle. Direct-acting antivirals are likely to be well tolerated by the infected host cell, but the rapid emergence of drug-resistant variants can compromise their use.[90] Combination therapy has proven effective to reduce and delay the selection of escape mutants, but does not entirely solve this problem, as illustrated by the selection of hepatitis C virus-resistant variants in patients who experienced virologic failure with asunaprevir and daclatasvir.[197] In contrast, intrahost virus evolution is unlikely to result in viral variants able to escape from host-targeting antivirals (HTAs). Moreover, related viruses are likely to rely on the same host machinery, thus providing an opportunity for the development of broad-spectrum antiviral therapeutics. HTAs can be associated with side effects that might be manageable during acute HF caused by arenaviruses, as the duration of the treatment would be rather short. An attractive host cell target for the development of broad-spectrum antiarenaviral drugs is SKI-1/S1P responsible for processing of arenavirus GPC into GP1 and GP2.[211,298,333,334,384] Several peptide-and non–peptide-based S1P inhibitors have been documented, but their lack of cell permeability would

pose severe limitations to their use as antiviral drugs. The small molecule PF-429242 is reported to be a potent S1P inhibitor both *in vitro* and in cell-based assays,[161,162] and PF-429242 efficiently inhibits S1P-mediated processing of arenavirus GPC, which correlated with the drug's ability to interfere with propagation of both LCMV and LASV in cultured cells.[384]

Advances in arenavirus molecular genetics have also enabled the generation of recombinant arenaviruses expressing a variety of reporter genes that can be used in high-throughput screens to rapidly identify drugs that inhibit arenavirus multiplication, including LASV and JUNV.[48,99,101,274,402] These cell-based infection screens can be used for drug repurposing approaches[186,266] with the appeal that significantly less time and resources are required to advance a candidate drug to the clinic.

Antibody Therapy

Treatment of JUNV infections with convalescent plasma has been studied in humans and experimental animals and is quite effective, with reduction of mortality from 15% to 30% to 1% to 2% if initiated within the first 8 days of illness.[103,242] About 10% of patients treated with convalescent plasma may later (3–6 weeks) exhibit neurologic signs including fever, headache, cerebellar tremor, and cranial nerve palsies. This late neurological syndrome is usually self-limited. These patients exhibit higher and later peaks of serum antibody titers, and increased serum/CSF antibody ratios, compared to treated patients who do not develop neurologic symptoms, suggesting the prior invasion of the CNS by virus.

Studies in animals suggest that passive antibody therapy would probably be useful to treat MACV and GOTV infections.[96,201] Early studies in animal models of LF required higher titers of virus-specific antibodies than MACV and GTOV infections, and treatment feasibility was contingent on availability of highly active preparations.[183,184] Experimental studies of passive protection by monoclonal antibodies have been successful in LCMV infection models.[13,14,406] Importantly, LASV GPC-specific recombinant human monoclonal antibodies derived from survivors of LF with strong neutralization profiles in cell-based assays exhibited robust therapeutic efficacy in a domesticated guinea pig model of LASV infection. These data support the feasibility of antibody-based therapy against LF.[74] Interestingly, the characterization of these antibodies revealed that most of them target quaternary epitopes that are displayed only in the context of the prefusion GPC trimer.[331] In contrast, in NW mammarenavirus infections, the GP1 subunit alone is the main target of neutralizing antibodies that act by blocking GP1 binding to TfR1.[241,420,421] Immune plasma therapy of LF is known to be complicated by a high prevalence of HIV-1 and *Plasmodium* spp. in the Western African population.[89]

Vaccines

The JUNV live attenuated Candid #1 strain was generated by serial passages of the JUNV XJ strain in laboratory mouse brains. The safety, immunogenicity, and protective efficacy of Candid #1 were demonstrated in preclinical studies in both domesticated guinea pigs and rhesus monkeys (*Macaca mulatta* Zimmermann, 1780).[261,262] Vaccination campaigns targeting agricultural workers in the JUNV-endemic area have shown Candid #1 to be an effective and safe vaccine in humans,[243,258] and it was licensed in 2006 for use exclusively in Argentina. Some concerns about the Candid #1 vaccine are the limited information about the viral determinants and mechanisms of Candid#1 attenuation and its potential genetic instability illustrated by a 1,000-fold range of virulence among Candid #1 clone isolates from blood of vaccinated rhesus monkeys.[102]

Among known mammarenaviruses, LASV poses the most concern to human health due to morbidity and lethality associated with LF together with the vast LASV-endemic regions and size of the population at risk in Western Africa. Accordingly, LF has been included on the revised list of priority diseases of the WHO R&D Blueprint, and therefore, accelerated research and development for LASV vaccine is encouraged.[22,356] The target product profile from WHO seeks a preventive LASV vaccine for healthy adults and children that would protect against strains from major lineages I to IV of LASV.[33] In addition, the vaccine should meet WHO prequalification criteria, including low cost, high efficacy, and thermostability, and be environmentally and user-friendly.

Studies involving LF survivors and animals experimentally infected with LASV indicate that early and robust virus-specific CD4+ and CD8+ T-cell responses,[12,118,148] rather than the presence of neutralizing antibodies, which appear late after infection and at low titers,[338] are the best correlates of recovery and protection. Accordingly, in experimentally vaccinated and exposed crab-eating macaques (*Macaca fascicularis* Raffles, 1821), depletion of CD8+ T cells abolished protection of vaccinated monkeys, whereas CD4+ T-cell depletion resulted in partial protection.[112] LASV-specific antibodies can be detected in individuals shortly after recovery from LF, but become undetectable after several months,[119] whereas these LF survivors retain robust LASV-specific CD4+ T-cell responses.[148] Although antibodies do not appear to contribute to viral control and recovery during acute LASV infection, neutralizing monoclonal antibodies genetically engineered from B cells of LF survivors can be successfully used for immunotherapy.[74,331] These data suggest that an ideal LASV vaccine should trigger both long-term robust cell-mediated immunity (CMI) and humoral responses following a single immunization. These responses are often induced by live attenuated vaccines (LAV); LAV, therefore, represent a highly promising approach to control LF.

LASV LAV candidates based on vaccinia virus,[11,66,118] vesicular stomatitis Indiana virus (VSIV),[133,138] Mopeia virus (MOPV),[53,202] ML29,[230,235] and yellow fever virus 17D[36,188] vectors and alphavirus replicons[315,396] have been tested in NHPs.[107,231,232] The Coalition for Epidemic Preparedness Innovations (CEPI) (http://cepi.net) was created as a nonprofit organization to accelerate vaccine development against emerging epidemic infections when the commercial market is insufficient to justify private investment.[312] One of the LASV vaccine candidates supported by CEPI is based on a measles virus vector that has shown promising results in human clinical trials providing antibody-based protection.[325] Whether this platform would be effective for development of a vaccine against LASV with predominant T cell–mediated mechanism of protection remains to be determined. Another CEPI-supported platform is DNA-based immunization, an approach that is efficacious in the crab-eating macaque model of LF.[55] However, it may take years for the advances in plasmid formulations and subsequent delivery required for licensure of the first DNA vaccine against LF.

Two additional CEPI-supported platforms are recombinant VSIV (rVSIV)-based LASV vaccines. The first one, "rVSVΔG/

LASV-GPC," uses the same concept behind the design of the "rVSVΔG/ZEBOV-GP" vaccine that showed promise in a ring vaccination trial against Ebola virus disease in Guinea. The vaccine's detailed efficacy profile remains to be determined.[165,166,268] A single injection of "rVSV/LASV-GPC" experimental vaccine, in which VSIV G was replaced with LASV-GPC, fully protected guinea pigs and NHPs against LASV strains from the same clade.[138,343] The "rVSVΔG/LASV-GPC" immunization did not induce detectable T-cell responses before virus exposure, and low IgG humoral responses detected by ELISA were found in three of four vaccinated animals. After LASV exposure, neutralizing antibodies were detected in all four macaques. Despite these promising results, there are still some safety concerns because of reported side effects in individuals vaccinated with "rVSVΔG/ZEBOV-GP." These side effects included postvaccination arthritis, vector RNAemia, and detection of infectious vaccine virus in the skin of vaccinated individuals.[173] The other rVSIV-based LASV vaccine candidate is based on the VesiculoVax platform licensed by Profectus BioSciences. This platform was developed to further improve safety of rVSIV vector by N gene translocation and truncation of the VSIV G cytoplasmic tail (CT1). The attenuated rVSV-N4CT1 vector is immunogenic in NHPs and induces only mild inflammatory response after intrathalamic inoculation.[65]

A number of other LASV vaccine platforms are in preclinical development. The reassortant ML29, an LAV vaccine, carries the L segment from nonpathogenic MOPV and the S segment from LASV strain Josiah. This vaccine induces, after single immunization in domesticated guinea pigs, a robust cross-reacting and protective, sterilizing cell-mediated immune response against strains from distantly related LASV lineages.[54,235] In addition, ML29 is highly stable and safe in animal models of LF, including immunocompromised NHPs.[418,419] This finding is relevant because the LASV vaccine target population will likely include individuals with some degree of undiagnosed immunosuppression due to the high prevalence of malaria and HIV-1 infections in Western Africa. The use of a trisegmented (r3) mammarenavirus platform[99] would allow the incorporation into attenuated forms of ML29 of additional antigens from distantly related LASV strains to expand the cross-protection range. Progress in arenavirus molecular genetics can also facilitate the incorporation of additional safety measures into LASV LAVs, including the use of codon deoptimization[60] and reorganization of the coding[59] and noncoding IGRs.[177] These strategies result in the generation of highly attenuated and stable versions of LCMV that are able to induce protective immunity against otherwise lethal exposure with wild-type LCMV.

PERSPECTIVE

Since the fortuitous discovery of LCMV more than 70 years ago, arenaviruses have served as important model systems for the study of host–virus interactions. These studies illuminate a wide range of principles, including persistent infection, virus-induced immunopathological disease, cytotoxic T-cell recognition, and immunologic memory. Despite this wealth of knowledge, arenavirus infections of humans remain a significant public health risk in much of the world. Prospects for control of these diseases remain remote due to poor diagnostic protocols and sparse resource allocation for vaccine development and other control measures. Recent laboratory developments have advanced our understanding of arenavirus structure and biology. New vistas have been opened into arenavirus prevalence and distribution as a result of the application of deep-sequencing protocols applied to this interesting group of viruses. As the application of new approaches to antivirals and vaccines targeting arenaviruses continues, the lessons learned may provide a useful model for other geographically localized viral diseases where the knowledge exists, but where the financial resources for control or eradication are limited.

ACKNOWLEDGMENTS

We thank Laura Bollinger and Jiro Wada (NIH/NIAID Integrated Research Facility at Fort Detrick, Frederick, MD, USA) for critically editing the chapter and figure creation, respectively.

DISCLAIMER

The views and conclusions contained in this document are those of the authors and should not be interpreted as necessarily representing the official policies, either expressed or implied, of the U.S. Department of the Army, the U.S. Department of Defense, the U.S. Department of Health and Human Services, or the institutions and companies affiliated with the authors.

REFERENCES

1. Adair CV, Gauld RL, Smadel JE. Aseptic meningitis, a disease of diverse etiology: clinical and etiologic studies on 854 cases. *Ann Intern Med* 1953;39(4):675–704.
2. Akoua-Koffi C, Ter Meulen J, Legros D, et al. Détection des anticorps anti-virus de Lassa dans l 'Ouest forestier de la Côte d'Ivoire. *Méd Trop (Mars)* 2006;66(5):465–468.
3. Albariño CG, Bergeron É, Erickson BR, et al. Efficient reverse genetics generation of infectious junin viruses differing in glycoprotein processing. *J Virol* 2009;83(11):5606–5614.
4. Albariño CG, Palacios G, Khristova ML, et al. High diversity and ancient common ancestry of lymphocytic choriomeningitis virus. *Emerg Infect Dis* 2010;16(7):1093–1100.
5. Ambrosio AM, Enria DA, Maiztegui JI. Junin virus isolation from lympho-mononuclear cells of patients with Argentine hemorrhagic fever. *Intervirology* 1986;25(2):97–102.
6. Ambrosio AM, Feuillade MR, Gamboa GS, et al. Prevalence of lymphocytic choriomeningitis virus infection in a human population of Argentina. *Am J Trop Med Hyg* 1994;50(3):381–386.
7. Andersen KG, Shapiro BJ, Matranga CB, et al. Clinical sequencing uncovers origins and evolution of Lassa virus. *Cell* 2015;162(4):738–750.
8. Arribalzaga RA. Una nueva enfermedad epidémica a germen desconocido: hipertermia nefrotóxica, leucopénica y enantemática. *Día Méd* 1955;27(40):1204–1210.
9. Asogun DA, Adomeh DI, Ehimuan J, et al. Molecular diagnostics for Lassa fever at Irrua specialist teaching hospital, Nigeria: lessons learnt from two years of laboratory operation. *PLoS Negl Trop Dis* 2012;6(9):e1839.
10. Asper M, Hofmann P, Osmann C, et al. First outbreak of callitrichid hepatitis in Germany: genetic characterization of the causative lymphocytic choriomeningitis virus strains. *Virology* 2001;284(2):203–213.
11. Auperin DD, Esposito JJ, Lange JV, et al. Construction of a recombinant vaccinia virus expressing the Lassa virus glycoprotein gene and protection of guinea pigs from a lethal Lassa virus infection. *Virus Res* 1988;9(2–3):233–248.
12. Baize S, Marianneau P, Loth P, et al. Early and strong immune responses are associated with control of viral replication and recovery in Lassa virus-infected cynomolgus monkeys. *J Virol* 2009;83(11):5890–5903.
13. Baldridge JR, Buchmeier MJ. Mechanisms of antibody-mediated protection against lymphocytic choriomeningitis virus infection: mother-to-baby transfer of humoral protection. *J Virol* 1992;66(7):4252–4257.
14. Baldridge JR, McGraw TS, Paoletti A, et al. Antibody prevents the establishment of persistent arenavirus infection in synergy with endogenous T cells. *J Virol* 1997;71(1):755–758.
15. Bannister BA. Stringent precautions are advisable when caring for patients with viral haemorrhagic fevers. *Rev Med Virol* 1993;3:3–6.
16. Barry M, Russi M, Armstrong L, et al. Treatment of a laboratory-acquired Sabiá virus infection. *N Engl J Med* 1995;333(5):294–296.
17. Barton LL, Mets MB. Lymphocytic choriomeningitis virus: pediatric pathogen and fetal teratogen. *Pediatr Infect Dis J* 1999;18(6):540–541.
18. Barton LL, Mets MB. Congenital lymphocytic choriomeningitis virus infection: decade of rediscovery. *Clin Infect Dis* 2001;33(3):370–374.
19. Baum SG, Lewis AM Jr, Rowe WP, et al. Epidemic nonmeningitic lymphocytic-choriomeningitis-virus infection. An outbreak in a population of laboratory personnel. *N Engl J Med* 1966;274(17):934–936.
20. Bausch DG, Demby AH, Coulibaly M, et al. Lassa fever in Guinea: I. Epidemiology of human disease and clinical observations. *Vector Borne Zoonotic Dis* 2001;1(4):269–281.
21. Bausch DG, Rollin PE, Demby AH, et al. Diagnosis and clinical virology of Lassa fever as evaluated by enzyme-linked immunosorbent assay, indirect fluorescent-antibody test, and virus isolation. *J Clin Microbiol* 2000;38(7):2670–2677.
22. Bausch DG, Sesay SSS, Oshin B. On the front lines of Lassa fever. *Emerg Infect Dis* 2004;10(10):1889–1890.
23. Bederka LH, Bonhomme CJ, Ling EL, et al. Arenavirus stable signal peptide is the keystone subunit for glycoprotein complex organization. *MBio* 2014;5(6):e02063.
24. Beyer WR, Pöpplau D, Garten W, et al. Endoproteolytic processing of the lymphocytic choriomeningitis virus glycoprotein by the subtilase SKI-1/S1P. *J Virol* 2003;77(5):2866–2872.
25. Biggar RJ, Douglas RG, Hotchin J. Lymphocytic choriomeningitis associated with hamsters. *Lancet* 1975;305/i(7911):856–857.
26. Biggar RJ, Woodall JP, Walter PD, et al. Lymphocytic choriomeningitis outbreak associated with pet hamsters. Fifty-seven cases from New York State. *JAMA* 1975;232(5):494–500.
27. Boisen ML, Hartnett JN, Shaffer JG, et al. Field validation of recombinant antigen immunoassays for diagnosis of Lassa fever. *Sci Rep* 2018;8(1):5939.
28. Bolken TC, Laquerre S, Zhang Y, et al. Identification and characterization of potent small molecule inhibitor of hemorrhagic fever New World arenaviruses. *Antiviral Res* 2006;69(2):86–97.
29. Bonner PC, Schmidt W-P, Belmain SR, et al. Poor housing quality increases risk of rodent infestation and Lassa fever in refugee camps of Sierra Leone. *Am J Trop Med Hyg* 2007;77(1):169–175.
30. Bonthius DJ. Lymphocytic choriomeningitis virus: an underrecognized cause of neurologic disease in the fetus, child, and adult. *Semin Pediatr Neurol* 2012;19(3):89–95.
31. Borden KL, Campbell Dwyer EJ, Salvato MS. An arenavirus RING (zinc-binding) protein binds the oncoprotein promyelocyte leukemia protein (PML) and relocates PML nuclear bodies to the cytoplasm. *J Virol* 1998;72(1):758–766.
32. Boulant S, Stanifer M, Lozach PY. Dynamics of virus-receptor interactions in virus binding, signaling, and endocytosis. *Viruses* 2015;7(6):2794–2815.
33. Bowen MD, Rollin PE, Ksiazek TG, et al. Genetic diversity among Lassa virus strains. *J Virol* 2000;74(15):6992–7004.
34. Boxaca MC, Guerrero LB, Parodi AS, et al. Viremia en enfermos de fiebre hemorrágica argentina. *Rev Asoc Med Argent* 1965;79:230–238.
35. Branco LM, Grove JN, Boisen ML, et al. Emerging trends in Lassa fever: redefining the role of immunoglobulin M and inflammation in diagnosing acute infection. *Virol J* 2011;8:478.
36. Bredenbeek PJ, Molenkamp R, Spaan WJM, et al. A recombinant Yellow Fever 17D vaccine expressing Lassa virus glycoproteins. *Virology* 2006;345(2):299–304.
37. Briese T, Paweska JT, McMullan LK, et al. Genetic detection and characterization of Lujo virus, a new hemorrhagic fever-associated arenavirus from southern Africa. *PLoS Pathog* 2009;5(5):e1000455.
38. Briggiler AM, Levis S, Enria DA, et al. Fiebre hemorrágica argentina (FHA) en la mujer embarazada. *Medicina (B Aires)* 1990;50:443.
39. Brouillette RB, Phillips EK, Patel R, et al. TIM-1 mediates dystroglycan-independent entry of Lassa virus. *J Virol* 2018;92(16):e00093-18.
40. Brouqui P, Rousseau MC, Saron MF, et al. Meningitis due to lymphocytic choriomeningitis virus: four cases in France. *Clin Infect Dis* 1995;20(4):1082–1083.
41. Brunotte L, Kerber R, Shang W, et al. Structure of the Lassa virus nucleoprotein revealed by X-ray crystallography, small-angle X-ray scattering, and electron microscopy. *J Biol Chem* 2011;286(44):38748–38756.
42. Brunotte L, Lelke M, Hass M, et al. Domain structure of Lassa virus L protein. *J Virol* 2011;85(1):324–333.
43. Bruns M, Cihak J, Müller G, et al. Lymphocytic choriomeningitis virus. VI. Isolation of a glycoprotein mediating neutralization. *Virology* 1983;130(1):247–251.
44. Buba MI, Dalhat MM, Nguku PM, et al. Mortality among confirmed Lassa fever cases during the 2015-2016 outbreak in Nigeria. *Am J Public Health* 2018;108(2):262–264.
45. Buchmeier MJ, Peters CJ, de la Torre JC. *Arenaviridae*: the virus and their replication. In: Fields BN, Knipe DM, Howley PM, eds. *Fields Virology*, vol. 2. 5th ed. Philadelphia, PA: Wolters Kluwer Health/Lippincott Williams & Wilkins; 2007:1792–1827.
46. Burri DJ, da Palma JR, Kunz S, et al. Envelope glycoprotein of arenaviruses. *Viruses* 2012;4(10):2162–2181.
47. Burri DJ, da Palma JR, Seidah NG, et al. Differential recognition of Old World and New World arenavirus envelope glycoproteins by subtilisin kexin isozyme 1 (SKI-1)/site 1 protease (S1P). *J Virol* 2013;87(11):6406–6414.
48. Caì Y, Iwasaki M, Beitzel BF, et al. Recombinant Lassa virus expressing green fluorescent protein as a tool for high-throughput drug screens and neutralizing antibody assays. *Viruses* 2018;10(11):655.
49. Cao W, Henry MD, Borrow P, et al. Identification of α-dystroglycan as a receptor for lymphocytic choriomeningitis virus and Lassa fever virus. *Science* 1998;282(5396):2079–2081.
50. Capul AA, de la Torre JC, Buchmeier MJ. Conserved residues in Lassa fever virus Z protein modulate viral infectivity at the level of the ribonucleoprotein. *J Virol* 2011;85(7):3172–3178.
51. Capul AA, Perez M, Burke E, et al. Arenavirus Z-glycoprotein association requires Z myristoylation but not functional RING or late domains. *J Virol* 2007;81(17):9451–9460.
52. Carey DE, Kemp GE, White HA, et al. Lassa fever. Epidemiological aspects of the 1970 epidemic, Jos, Nigeria. *Trans R Soc Trop Med Hyg* 1972;66(3):402–408.
53. Carnec X, Mateo M, Page A, et al. A vaccine platform against arenaviruses based on a recombinant hyperattenuated Mopeia virus expressing heterologous glycoproteins. *J Virol* 2018;92(12):e02230-17.

54. Carrion R Jr, Patterson JL, Johnson C, et al. A ML29 reassortant virus protects guinea pigs against a distantly related Nigerian strain of Lassa virus and can provide sterilizing immunity. *Vaccine* 2007;25(20):4093–4102.
55. Cashman KA, Wilkinson ER, Shaia CI, et al. A DNA vaccine delivered by dermal electroporation fully protects cynomolgus macaques against Lassa fever. *Hum Vaccin Immunother* 2017;13(12):2902–2911.
56. Centers for Disease Control and Prevention. Lymphocytic choriomeningitis virus infection in organ transplant recipients—Massachusetts, Rhode Island, 2005. *MMWR Morb Mortal Wkly Rep* 2005;54(21):537–539.
57. Centers for Disease Control and Prevention. Lymphocytic choriomeningitis virus transmitted through solid organ transplantation—Massachusetts, 2008. *MMWR Morb Mortal Wkly Rep* 2008;57(29):799–801.
58. Charrel RN, de Lamballerie X, Emonet S. Phylogeny of the genus *Arenavirus*. *Curr Opin Microbiol* 2008;11(4):362–368.
59. Cheng BY, Ortiz-Riaño E, de la Torre JC, et al. Arenavirus genome rearrangement for the development of live attenuated vaccines. *J Virol* 2015;89(14):7373–7384.
60. Cheng BY, Ortiz-Riaño E, Nogales A, et al. Development of live-attenuated arenavirus vaccines based on codon deoptimization. *J Virol* 2015;89(7):3523–3533.
61. Child PL, MacKenzie RB, Valverde LR, et al. Bolivian hemorrhagic fever. A pathologic description. *Arch Pathol* 1967;83(5):434–445.
62. Childs JE. Ecology and epidemiology of arenaviruses and their hosts. In: Salvato MS, ed. *The Arenaviridae*. New York: Springer Science+Business; 1993:331–401.
63. Childs JE, Glass GE, Korch GW, et al. Lymphocytic choriomeningitis virus infection and house mouse (*Mus musculus*) distribution in urban Baltimore. *Am J Trop Med Hyg* 1992;47(1):27–34.
64. Childs JE, Glass GE, Ksiazek TG, et al. Human-rodent contact and infection with lymphocytic choriomeningitis and Seoul viruses in an inner-city population. *Am J Trop Med Hyg* 1991;44(2):117–121.
65. Clarke DK, Nasar F, Chong S, et al. Neurovirulence and immunogenicity of attenuated recombinant vesicular stomatitis viruses in nonhuman primates. *J Virol* 2014;88(12):6690–6701.
66. Clegg JCS, Lloyd G. Vaccinia recombinant expressing Lassa-virus internal nucleocapsid protein protects guineapigs against Lassa fever. *Lancet* 1987;330/ii(8552):186–188.
67. Cohen-Dvashi H, Cohen N, Israeli H, et al. Molecular mechanism for LAMP1 recognition by Lassa virus. *J Virol* 2015;89(15):7584–7592.
68. Cohen-Dvashi H, Israeli H, Shani O, et al. Role of LAMP1 binding and pH sensing by the spike complex of Lassa virus. *J Virol* 2016;90(22):10329–10338.
69. Coimbra TLM, Nassar ES, Burattini MN, et al. New arenavirus isolated in Brazil. *Lancet* 1994;343(8894):391–392.
70. Cornu TI, de la Torre JC. RING finger Z protein of lymphocytic choriomeningitis virus (LCMV) inhibits transcription and RNA replication of an LCMV S-segment minigenome. *J Virol* 2001;75(19):9415–9426.
71. Cornu TI, de la Torre JC. Characterization of the arenavirus RING finger Z protein regions required for Z-mediated inhibition of viral RNA synthesis. *J Virol* 2002;76(13):6678–6688.
72. Cornu TI, Feldmann H, de la Torre JC. Cells expressing the RING finger Z protein are resistant to arenavirus infection. *J Virol* 2004;78(6):2979–2983.
73. Cossio P, Laguens R, Arana R, et al. Ultrastructural and immunohistochemical study of the human kidney in Argentine haemorrhagic fever. *Virchows Arch A Pathol Anat Histol* 1975;368(1):1–9.
74. Cross RW, Mire CE, Branco LM, et al. Treatment of Lassa virus infection in outbred guinea pigs with first-in-class human monoclonal antibodies. *Antiviral Res* 2016;133:218–222.
75. Cummins D, Bennett D, Fisher-Hoch SP, et al. Lassa fever encephalopathy: clinical and laboratory findings. *J Trop Med Hyg* 1992;95(3):197–201.
76. Cummins D, Fisher-Hoch SP, Walshe KJ, et al. A plasma inhibitor of platelet aggregation in patients with Lassa fever. *Br J Haematol* 1989;72(4):543–548.
77. Cummins D, McCormick JB, Bennett D, et al. Acute sensorineural deafness in Lassa fever. *JAMA* 1990;264(16):2093–2096.
78. Cummins D, Molinas FC, Lerer G, et al. A plasma inhibitor of platelet aggregation in patients with Argentine hemorrhagic fever. *Am J Trop Med Hyg* 1990;42(5):470–475.
79. Damonte EB, Coto CE. Treatment of arenavirus infections: from basic studies to the challenge of antiviral therapy. *Adv Virus Res* 2002;58:125–155.
80. Daneš L, Benda R, Fuchsová M. Experimentální inhalační nákaza opic druhů Macacus cynomolgus a Macacus rhesus virem lymfocitární choriomeningitidy (knenem WE). *Bratisl Lek Listy* 1963;2:71–79.
81. de Bracco MM, Rimoldi MT, Cossio PM, et al. Argentine hemorrhagic fever. Alterations of the complement system and anti-Junin-virus humoral response. *N Engl J Med* 1978;299(5):216–221.
82. de Guerrero LB, Avila MM, Milani HL, et al. Prevalencia de infección subclinica por virus Junin en una población seleccionada del área endémica de Fiebre hemorrágica Argentina. *Medicina (B Aires)* 1982;42(1):110.
83. de Manzione N, Salas RA, Paredes H, et al. Venezuelan hemorrhagic fever: clinical and epidemiological studies of 165 cases. *Clin Infect Dis* 1998;26(2):308–313.
84. Deibel R, Schryver GD. Viral antibody in the cerebrospinal fluid of patients with acute central nervous system infections. *J Clin Microbiol* 1976;3(4):397–401.
85. Deibel R, Woodall JP, Decher WJ, et al. Lymphocytic choriomeningitis virus in man. Serologic evidence of association with pet hamsters. *JAMA* 1975;232(5):501–504.
86. Delgado S, Erickson BR, Agudo R, et al. Chapare virus, a newly discovered arenavirus isolated from a fatal hemorrhagic fever case in Bolivia. *PLoS Pathog* 2008;4(4):e1000047.
87. Demby AH, Chamberlain J, Brown DW, et al. Early diagnosis of Lassa fever by reverse transcription-PCR. *J Clin Microbiol* 1994;32(12):2898–2903.
88. Djavani M, Rodas J, Lukashevich IS, et al. Role of the promyelocytic leukemia protein PML in the interferon sensitivity of lymphocytic choriomeningitis virus. *J Virol* 2001;75(13):6204–6208.
89. Djomand G, Quaye S, Sullivan PS. HIV epidemic among key populations in west Africa. *Curr Opin HIV AIDS* 2014;9(5):506–513.
90. Domingo E, Martin V, Perales C, et al. Viruses as quasispecies: biological implications. *Curr Top Microbiol Immunol* 2006;299:51–82.
91. Douglas RG, Wiebenga NH, Couch RB. Bolivian hemorrhagic-fever probably transmitted by personal contact. *Am J Epidemiol* 1965;82(1):85–91.
92. Downs WG, Anderson CR, Spence L, et al. Tacaribe virus, a new agent isolated from Artibeus bats and mosquitoes in Trinidad, West Indies. *Am J Trop Med Hyg* 1963;12:640–646.
93. Dykewicz CA, Dato VM, Fisher-Hoch SP, et al. Lymphocytic choriomeningitis outbreak associated with nude mice in a research institute. *JAMA* 1992;267(10):1349–1353.
94. Dzotsi EK, Ohene S-A, Asiedu-Bekoe F, et al. The first cases of Lassa fever in Ghana. *Ghana Med J* 2012;46(3):166–170.
95. Eckerle LD, Becker MM, Halpin RA, et al. Infidelity of SARS-CoV Nsp14-exonuclease mutant virus replication is revealed by complete genome sequencing. *PLoS Pathog* 2010;6(5):e1000896.
96. Eddy GA, Wagner FS, Scott SK, et al. Protection of monkeys against Machupo virus by the passive administration of Bolivian haemorrhagic fever immunoglobulin (human origin). *Bull World Health Organ* 1975;52(4–6):723–727.
97. Ehichioya DU, Hass M, Becker-Ziaja B, et al. Current molecular epidemiology of Lassa virus in Nigeria. *J Clin Microbiol* 2011;49(3):1157–1161.
98. Elsner B, Schwarz E, Mando OG, et al. Pathology of 12 fatal cases of Argentine hemorrhagic fever. *Am J Trop Med Hyg* 1973;22(2):229–236.
99. Emonet SF, Garidou L, McGavern DB, et al. Generation of recombinant lymphocytic choriomeningitis viruses with trisegmented genomes stably expressing two additional genes of interest. *Proc Natl Acad Sci U S A* 2009;106(9):3473–3478.
100. Emonet S, Lemasson J-J, Gonzalez J-P, et al. Phylogeny and evolution of old world arenaviruses. *Virology* 2006;350(2):251–257.
101. Emonet SF, Seregin AV, Yun NE, et al. Rescue from cloned cDNAs and *in vivo* characterization of recombinant pathogenic Romero and live-attenuated Candid #1 strains of Junin virus, the causative agent of Argentine hemorrhagic fever disease. *J Virol* 2011;85(4):1473–1483.
102. Enria DA, Barrera Oro JG. Junin virus vaccines. *Curr Top Microbiol Immunol* 2002;263:239–261.
103. Enria DA, Briggiler AM, Fernandez NJ, et al. Importance of dose of neutralising antibodies in treatment of Argentine haemorrhagic fever with immune plasma. *Lancet* 1984;324/ii(8397):255–256.
104. Enria DA, Feuillade MR. Argentine haemorrhagic fever (Junin virus, Arenaviridae): a review on a clinical, epidemiological, ecological, treatment and preventive aspects of the disease. In: Travassos da Rosa APA, Vasconcelos PFC, Traavassos da Rosa JFS, eds. *An Overview of Arbovirology in Brazil and Neighboring Countries*. Belem, Brazil: InstitutoEvandroChagas; 1998:219–232.
105. Enria DA, Maiztegui JI. Antiviral treatment of Argentine hemorrhagic fever. *Antiviral Res* 1994;23(1):23–31.
106. Eschli B, Quirin K, Wepf A, et al. Identification of an N-terminal trimeric coiled-coil core within arenavirus glycoprotein 2 permits assignment to class I viral fusion proteins. *J Virol* 2006;80(12):5897–5907.
107. Falzarano D, Feldmann H. Vaccines for viral hemorrhagic fevers—progress and shortcomings. *Curr Opin Virol* 2013;3(3):343–351.
108. Fan L, Briese T, Lipkin WI. Z proteins of New World arenaviruses bind RIG-I and interfere with type I interferon induction. *J Virol* 2010;84(4):1785–1791.
109. Farmer TW, Janeway CA. Infections with the virus of lymphocytic choriomeningitis. Medicine 1942;21:1–63.
110. Fazakerley JK, Southern P, Bloom F, et al. High resolution *in situ* hybridization to determine the cellular distribution of lymphocytic choriomeningitis virus RNA in the tissues of persistently infected mice: relevance to arenavirus disease and mechanisms of viral persistence. *J Gen Virol* 1991;72(Pt 7):1611–1625.
111. Fedeli C, Torriani G, Galan-Navarro C, et al. Axl can serve as entry factor for Lassa virus depending on the functional glycosylation of dystroglycan. *J Virol* 2018;92(5):e01613–01617.
112. Feldmann H. Lassa rVSV Vaccines. *Keystone Symposia on Hemorrhagic Fever Viruses*. 2016.
113. Ferencz A, Binder L, Telegdy L, et al. Felnőtt betegeink lymphocytás choriomeningitis vírus fertőzésének gyakorisága 1971–1976 között. *Orv Hetil* 1979;120(26):1563–1567.
114. Fichet-Calvet E, Becker-Ziaja B, Koivogui L, et al. Lassa serology in natural populations of rodents and horizontal transmission. *Vector Borne Zoonotic Dis* 2014;14(9):665–674.
115. Fichet-Calvet E, Lecompte E, Koivogui L, et al. Fluctuation of abundance and Lassa virus prevalence in Mastomys natalensis in Guinea, West Africa. *Vector Borne Zoonotic Dis* 2007;7(2):119–128.
116. Fischer SA, Graham MB, Kuehnert MJ, et al. Transmission of lymphocytic choriomeningitis virus by organ transplantation. *N Engl J Med* 2006;354(21):2235–2249.
117. Fisher-Hoch S. Arenavirus pathophysiology. In: Salvato MS, ed. *The Arenaviridae*. New York: Springer Science+Business; 1993:299–323.
118. Fisher-Hoch SP, Hutwagner L, Brown B, et al. Effective vaccine for Lassa fever. *J Virol* 2000;74(15):6777–6783.
119. Fisher-Hoch SP, McCormick JB. Lassa fever vaccine. *Expert Rev Vaccines* 2004;3(2):189–197.
120. Fisher-Hoch S, McCormick JB, Sasso D, et al. Hematologic dysfunction in Lassa fever. *J Med Virol* 1988;26(2):127–135.
121. Fisher-Hoch SP, Mitchell SW, Sasso DR, et al. Physiological and immunologic disturbances associated with shock in a primate model of Lassa fever. *J Infect Dis* 1987;155(3):465–474.
122. Fisher-Hoch SP, Tomori O, Nasidi A, et al. Review of cases of nosocomial Lassa fever in Nigeria: the high price of poor medical practice. *BMJ* 1995;311(7009):857–859.
123. Frame JD. Surveillance of Lassa fever in missionaries stationed in West Africa. *Bull World Health Organ* 1975;52(4–6):593–598.
124. Frame JD. Clinical features of Lassa fever in Liberia. *Rev Infect Dis* 1989;11(Suppl 4):S783–S789.
125. Frame JD, Baldwin JM Jr, Gocke DJ, et al. Lassa fever, a new virus disease of man from West Africa. I. Clinical description and pathological findings. *Am J Trop Med Hyg* 1970;19(4):670–676.
126. Frame JD, Yalley-Ogunro JE, Hanson AP. Endemic Lassa fever in Liberia. V. Distribution of Lassa virus activity in Liberia: hospital staff surveys. *Trans R Soc Trop Med Hyg* 1984;78(6):761–763.

127. Franze-Fernandez MT, Zetina C, Iapalucci S, et al. Molecular structure and early events in the replication of Tacaribe arenavirus S RNA. *Virus Res* 1987;7(4):309–324.

128. Freed EO. Viral late domains. *J Virol* 2002;76(10):4679–4687.

129. Fulhorst CF, Cajimat MNB, Milazzo ML, et al. Genetic diversity between and within the arenavirus species indigenous to western Venezuela. *Virology* 2008;378(2):205–213.

130. Fulhorst CF, Ksiazek TG, Peters CJ, et al. Experimental infection of the cane mouse *Zygodontomys brevicauda* (family Muridae) with guanarito virus (Arenaviridae), the etiologic agent of Venezuelan hemorrhagic fever. *J Infect Dis* 1999;180(4):966–969.

131. Gale TV, Horton TM, Grant DS, et al. Metabolomics analyses identify platelet activating factors and heme breakdown products as Lassa fever biomarkers. *PLoS Negl Trop Dis* 2017;11(9):e0005943.

132. Gallaher WR, DiSimone C, Buchmeier MJ. The viral transmembrane superfamily: possible divergence of Arenavirus and Filovirus glycoproteins from a common RNA virus ancestor. *BMC Microbiol* 2001;1:1.

133. Garbutt M, Liebscher R, Wahl-Jensen V, et al. Properties of replication-competent vesicular stomatitis virus vectors expressing glycoproteins of filoviruses and arenaviruses. *J Virol* 2004;78(10):5458–5465.

134. García Franco S, Ambrosio AM, Feuillade MR, et al. Evaluation of an enzyme-linked immunosorbent assay for quantitation of antibodies to Junin virus in human sera. *J Virol Methods* 1988;19(3–4):299–305.

135. García JB, Morzunov SP, Levis S, et al. Genetic diversity of the Junin virus in Argentina: geographic and temporal patterns. *Virology* 2000;272(1):127–136.

136. Garcin D, Kolakofsky D. A novel mechanism for the initiation of Tacaribe arenavirus genome replication. *J Virol* 1990;64(12):6196–6203.

137. Garcin D, Kolakofsky D. Tacaribe arenavirus RNA synthesis in vitro is primer dependent and suggests an unusual model for the initiation of genome replication. *J Virol* 1992;66(3):1370–1376.

138. Geisbert TW, Jones S, Fritz EA, et al. Development of a new vaccine for the prevention of Lassa fever. *PLoS Med* 2005;2(6):e183.

139. Gomez RM, Pozner RG, Lazzari MA, et al. Endothelial cell function alteration after Junin virus infection. *Thromb Haemost* 2003;90(2):326–333.

140. Goncalves AR, Moraz M-L, Pasquato A, et al. Role of DC-SIGN in Lassa virus entry into human dendritic cells. *J Virol* 2013;87(21):11504–11515.

141. Goñi SE, Stephan BI, Iserte JA, et al. Viral diversity of Junín virus field strains. *Virus Res* 2011;160(1–2):150–158.

142. González PH, Cossio PM, Arana R, et al. Lymphatic tissue in Argentine hemorrhagic fever. Pathologic features. *Arch Pathol Lab Med* 1980;104(5):250–254.

143. Gonzalez J-P, Georges AJ, Kiley MP, et al. Evolutionary biology of a Lassa virus complex. *Med Microbiol Immunol* 1986;175(2–3):157–159.

144. Gowen BB, Juelich TL, Sefing EJ, et al. Favipiravir (T-705) inhibits Junin virus infection and reduces mortality in a guinea pig model of Argentine hemorrhagic fever. *PLoS Negl Trop Dis* 2013;7(12):e2614.

145. Grant A, Seregin A, Huang C, et al. Junín virus pathogenesis and virus replication. *Viruses* 2012;4(10):2317–2339.

146. Green DE, Mahlandt BG, McKee KT Jr. Experimental Argentine hemorrhagic fever in rhesus macaques: virus-specific variations in pathology. *J Med Virol* 1987;22(2):113–133.

147. Greenky D, Knust B, Dziuban EJ. What pediatricians should know about Lassa virus. *JAMA Pediatr* 2018;172(5):407–408.

148. Günther S, Lenz O. Lassa virus. *Crit Rev Clin Lab Sci* 2004;41(4):339–390.

149. Habjan M, Andersson I, Klingström J, et al. Processing of genome 5' termini as a strategy of negative-strand RNA viruses to avoid RIG-I-dependent interferon induction. *PLoS One* 2008;3(4):e2032.

150. Hall WC, Geisbert TW, Huggins JW, et al. Experimental infection of guinea pigs with Venezuelan hemorrhagic fever virus (Guanarito): a model of human disease. *Am J Trop Med Hyg* 1996;55(1):81–88.

151. Harrison LH, Halsey NA, McKee KT Jr, et al. Clinical case definitions for Argentine hemorrhagic fever. *Clin Infect Dis* 1999;28(5):1091–1094.

152. Hass M, Gölnitz U, Müller S, et al. Replicon system for Lassa virus. *J Virol* 2004;78(24):13793–13803.

153. Hass M, Lelke M, Busch C, et al. Mutational evidence for a structural model of the Lassa virus RNA polymerase domain and identification of two residues, Gly1394 and Asp1395, that are critical for transcription but not replication of the genome. *J Virol* 2008;82(20):10207–10217.

154. Hass M, Westerkofsky M, Müller S, et al. Mutational analysis of the Lassa virus promoter. *J Virol* 2006;80(24):12414–12419.

155. Hastie KM, Igonet S, Sullivan BM, et al. Crystal structure of the prefusion surface glycoprotein of the prototypic arenavirus LCMV. *Nat Struct Mol Biol* 2016;23(6):513–521.

156. Hastie KM, Kimberlin CR, Zandonatti MA, et al. Structure of the Lassa virus nucleoprotein reveals a dsRNA-specific 3' to 5' exonuclease activity essential for immune suppression. *Proc Natl Acad Sci U S A* 2011;108(6):2396–2401.

157. Hastie KM, Liu T, Li S, et al. Crystal structure of the Lassa virus nucleoprotein-RNA complex reveals a gating mechanism for RNA binding. *Proc Natl Acad Sci U S A* 2011;108(48):19365–19370.

158. Hastie KM, Saphire EO. Lassa virus glycoprotein: stopping a moving target. *Curr Opin Virol* 2018;31:52–58.

159. Hastie KM, Zandonatti MA, Kleinfelter LM, et al. Structural basis for antibody-mediated neutralization of Lassa virus. *Science* 2017;356(6341):923–928.

160. Hastie KM, Zandonatti M, Liu T, et al. Crystal structure of the oligomeric form of Lassa virus matrix protein Z. *J Virol* 2016;90(9):4556–4562.

161. Hawkins JL, Robbins MD, Warren LC, et al. Pharmacologic inhibition of site 1 protease activity inhibits sterol regulatory element-binding protein processing and reduces lipogenic enzyme gene expression and lipid synthesis in cultured cells and experimental animals. *J Pharmacol Exp Ther* 2008;326(3):801–808.

162. Hay BA, Abrams B, Zumbrunn AY, et al. Aminopyrrolidineamide inhibitors of site-1 protease. *Bioorg Med Chem Lett* 2007;17(16):4411–4414.

163. Heller MV, Marta RF, Sturk A, et al. Early markers of blood coagulation and fibrinolysis activation in Argentine hemorrhagic fever. *Thromb Haemost* 1995;73(3):368–373.

164. Heller MV, Saavedra MC, Falcoff R, et al. Increased tumor necrosis factor-α levels in Argentine hemorrhagic fever. *J Infect Dis* 1992;166(5):1203–1204.

165. Henao-Restrepo AM, Camacho A, Longini IM, et al. Efficacy and effectiveness of an rVSV-vectored vaccine in preventing Ebola virus disease: final results from the Guinea ring vaccination, open-label, cluster-randomised trial (Ebola Ça Suffit!). *Lancet* 2017;389(10068):505–518.

166. Henao-Restrepo AM, Longini IM, Egger M, et al. Efficacy and effectiveness of an rVSV-vectored vaccine expressing Ebola surface glycoprotein: interim results from the Guinea ring vaccination cluster-randomised trial. *Lancet* 2015;386(9996):857–866.

167. Hensley LE, Smith MA, Geisbert JB, et al. Pathogenesis of Lassa fever in cynomolgus macaques. *Virol J* 2011;8:205.

168. Hepojoki J, Hepojoki S, Smura T, et al. Characterization of Haartman Institute snake virus 1 (HISV-1) and HISV-like viruses—the representatives of genus *Hartmanivirus*, family *Arenaviridae*. *PLoS Pathog* 2018;14(11):e1007415.

169. Hepojoki J, Salmenperä P, Sironen T, et al. Arenavirus coinfections are common in snakes with boid inclusion body disease. *J Virol* 2015;89(16):8657–8660.

170. Hetzel U, Sironen T, Laurinmäki P, et al. Isolation, identification, and characterization of novel arenaviruses, the etiological agents of boid inclusion body disease. *J Virol* 2013;87(20):10918–10935.

171. Huang C, Kolokoltsova OA, Yun NE, et al. Highly pathogenic New World and Old World human arenaviruses induce distinct interferon responses in human cells. *J Virol* 2015;89(14):7079–7088.

172. Huang Q, Shao J, Lan S, et al. *In vitro* and *in vivo* characterizations of Pichinde viral nucleoprotein exoribonuclease functions. *J Virol* 2015;89(13):6595–6607.

173. Huttner A, Combescure C, Grillet S, et al. A dose-dependent plasma signature of the safety and immunogenicity of the rVSV-Ebola vaccine in Europe and Africa. *Sci Transl Med* 2017;9:385.

174. Igonet S, Vaney M-C, Vonrhein C, et al. X-ray structure of the arenavirus glycoprotein GP2 in its postfusion hairpin conformation. *Proc Natl Acad Sci U S A* 2011;108(50):19967–19972.

175. Isere EE, Fatiregun AA, Ilesanmi O, et al. Lessons learnt from epidemiological investigation of Lassa fever outbreak in a Southwest State of Nigeria December 2015 to April 2016. *PLoS Curr* 2018;10.

176. Ivanov AP, Rezapkin GV, Dzagurova TK, et al. Indirect solid-phase immunosorbent assay for detection of arenavirus antigens and antibodies. *Acta Virol* 1984;28(3):240–245.

177. Iwasaki M, Ngo N, Cubitt B, et al. General molecular strategy for development of arenavirus live-attenuated vaccines. *J Virol* 2015;89(23):12166–12177.

178. Iwasaki M, Ngo N, de la Torre JC. Sodium hydrogen exchangers contribute to arenavirus cell entry. *J Virol* 2014;88(1):643–654.

179. Jae LT, Brummelkamp TR. Emerging intracellular receptors for hemorrhagic fever viruses. *Trends Microbiol* 2015;23(7):392–400.

180. Jae LT, Raaben M, Herbert AS, et al. Lassa virus entry requires a trigger-induced receptor switch. *Science* 2014;344(6191):1506–1510.

181. Jahrling PB, Hesse RA, Eddy GA, et al. Lassa virus infection of rhesus monkeys: pathogenesis and treatment with ribavirin. *J Infect Dis* 1980;141(5):580–589.

182. Jahrling PB, Niklasson BS, McCormick JB. Early diagnosis of human Lassa fever by ELISA detection of antigen and antibody. *Lancet* 1985;325/i(8423):250–252.

183. Jahrling PB, Peters CJ. Passive antibody therapy of Lassa fever in cynomolgus monkeys: importance of neutralizing antibody and Lassa virus strain. *Infect Immun* 1984;44(2):528–533.

184. Jahrling PB, Peters CJ, Stephen EL. Enhanced treatment of Lassa fever by immune plasma combined with ribavirin in cynomolgus monkeys. *J Infect Dis* 1984;149(3):420–427.

185. Jain M, Olsen HE, Paten B, et al. The Oxford Nanopore MinION: delivery of nanopore sequencing to the genomics community. *Genome Biol* 2016;17(1):239.

186. Janes J, Young ME, Chen E, et al. The ReFRAME library as a comprehensive drug repurposing library and its application to the treatment of cryptosporidiosis. *Proc Natl Acad Sci U S A* 2018;115(42):10750–10755.

187. Jasenosky LD, Neumann G, Lukashevich I, et al. Ebola virus VP40-induced particle formation and association with the lipid bilayer. *J Virol* 2001;75(11):5205–5214.

188. Jiang X, Dalebout TJ, Bredenbeek PJ, et al. Yellow fever 17D-vectored vaccines expressing Lassa virus GP1 and GP2 glycoproteins provide protection against fatal disease in guinea pigs. *Vaccine* 2011;29(6):1248–1257.

189. Jiang X, Huang Q, Wang W, et al. Structures of arenaviral nucleoproteins with triphosphate dsRNA reveal a unique mechanism of immune suppression. *J Biol Chem* 2013;288(23):16949–16959.

190. Johnson KM. Epidemiology of Machupo virus infection. III. Significance of virological observations in man and animals. *Am J Trop Med Hyg* 1965;14(5):816–818.

191. Johnson KM, Kuns ML, Mackenzie RB, et al. Isolation of Machupo virus from wild rodent *Calomys callosus*. *Am J Trop Med Hyg* 1966;15(1):103–106.

192. Johnson KM, McCormick JB, Webb PA, et al. Clinical virology of Lassa fever in hospitalized patients. *J Infect Dis* 1987;155(3):456–464.

193. Johnson KM, Wiebenga NH, Mackenzie RB, et al. Virus isolations from human cases of hemorrhagic fever in Bolivia. *Proc Soc Exp Biol Med* 1965;118:113–118.

194. Justines G, Johnson KM. Use of oral swabs for detection of Machupo-virus infection in rodents. *Am J Trop Med Hyg* 1968;17(5):788–790.

195. Justines G, Johnson KM. Immune tolerance in *Calomys callosus* infected with Machupo virus. *Nature* 1969;222(5198):1090–1091.

196. Kafetzopoulou LE, Pullan ST, Lemey P, et al. Metagenomic sequencing at the epicenter of the Nigeria 2018 Lassa fever outbreak. *Science* 2019;363(6422):74–77.

197. Kai Y, Hikita H, Morishita N, et al. Baseline quasispecies selection and novel mutations contribute to emerging resistance-associated substitutions in hepatitis C virus after direct-acting antiviral treatment. *Sci Rep* 2017;7:41660.

198. Keane E, Gilles HM. Lassa fever in Panguma Hospital, Sierra Leone, 1973-6. *Br Med J* 1977;1(6073):1399–1402.

199. Keenlyside RA, McCormick JB, Webb PA, et al. Case-control study of Mastomys natalensis and humans in Lassa virus-infected households in Sierra Leone. *Am J Trop Med Hyg* 1983;32(4):829–837.
200. Kenyon RH, Canonico PG, Green DE, et al. Effect of ribavirin and tributylribavirin on argentine hemorrhagic fever (Junin virus) in guinea pigs. *Antimicrob Agents Chemother* 1986;29(3):521–523.
201. Kenyon RH, Green DE, Eddy GA, et al. Treatment of Junin virus-infected guinea pigs with immune serum: development of late neurological disease. *J Med Virol* 1986;20(3):207–218.
202. Kiley MP, Lange JV, Johnson KM. Protection of rhesus monkeys from Lassa virus by immunisation with closely related arenavirus. *Lancet* 1979;314/ii(8145):738.
203. Kilgore PE, Ksiazek TG, Rollin PE, et al. Treatment of Bolivian hemorrhagic fever with intravenous ribavirin. *Clin Infect Dis* 1997;24(4):718–722.
204. Klaus JP, Eisenhauer P, Russo J, et al. The intracellular cargo receptor ERGIC-53 is required for the production of infectious arenavirus, coronavirus, and filovirus particles. *Cell Host Microbe* 2013;14(5):522–534.
205. Knobloch J, McCormick JB, Webb PA, et al. Clinical observations in 42 patients with Lassa fever. *Tropenmed Parasitol* 1980;31(4):389–398.
206. Komrower GM, Williams BL, Stones PB. Lymphocytic choriomeningitis in the newborn; probable transplacental infection. *Lancet* 1955;268(6866):697–698.
207. Kranzusch PJ, Schenk AD, Rahmeh AA, et al. Assembly of a functional Machupo virus polymerase complex. *Proc Natl Acad Sci U S A* 2010;107(46):20069–20074.
208. Kranzusch PJ, Whelan SPJ. Arenavirus Z protein controls viral RNA synthesis by locking a polymerase-promoter complex. *Proc Natl Acad Sci U S A* 2011;108(49):19743–19748.
209. Kranzusch PJ, Whelan SP. Architecture and regulation of negative-strand viral enzymatic machinery. *RNA Biol* 2012;9(7):941–948.
210. Kunz S. The role of the vascular endothelium in arenavirus haemorrhagic fevers. *Thromb Haemost* 2009;102(6):1024–1029.
211. Kunz S, Borrow P, Oldstone MB. Receptor structure, binding, and cell entry of arenaviruses. *Curr Top Microbiol Immunol* 2002;262:111–137.
212. Lan S, McLay Schelde L, Wang J, et al. Development of infectious clones for virulent and avirulent Pichinde viruses: a model virus to study arenavirus-induced hemorrhagic fevers. *J Virol* 2009;83(13):6357–6362.
213. Larsen PD, Chartrand SA, Tomashek KM, et al. Hydrocephalus complicating lymphocytic choriomeningitis virus infection. *Pediatr Infect Dis J* 1993;12(6):528–531.
214. Larson RA, Dai D, Hosack VT, et al. Identification of a broad-spectrum arenavirus entry inhibitor. *J Virol* 2008;82(21):10768–10775.
215. Lecompte E, Fichet-Calvet E, Daffis S, et al. *Mastomys natalensis* and Lassa fever, West Africa. *Emerg Infect Dis* 2006;12(12):1971–1974.
216. Ledesma J, Fedele CG, Carro F, et al. Independent lineage of lymphocytic choriomeningitis virus in wood mice (*Apodemus sylvaticus*), Spain. *Emerg Infect Dis* 2009;15(10):1677–1680.
217. Lee AM, Pasquato A, Kunz S. Novel approaches in anti-arenaviral drug development. *Virology* 2011;411(2):163–169.
218. Lee AM, Rojek JM, Spiropoulou CF, et al. Unique small molecule entry inhibitors of hemorrhagic fever arenaviruses. *J Biol Chem* 2008;283(27):18734–18742.
219. Lehmann M, Pahlmann M, Jérôme H, et al. Role of the C terminus of Lassa virus L protein in viral mRNA synthesis. *J Virol* 2014;88(15):8713–8717.
220. Lehmann-Grube F, Kallay M, Ibscher B, et al. Serologic diagnosis of human infections with lymphocytic choriomeningitis virus: comparative evaluation of seven methods. *J Med Virol* 1979;4(2):125–136.
221. Lelke M, Brunotte L, Busch C, et al. An N-terminal region of Lassa virus L protein plays a critical role in transcription but not replication of the virus genome. *J Virol* 2010;84(4):1934–1944.
222. Lenz O, ter Meulen J, Feldmann H, et al. Identification of a novel consensus sequence at the cleavage site of the Lassa virus glycoprotein. *J Virol* 2000;74(23):11418–11421.
223. Lenz O, ter Meulen J, Klenk H-D, et al. The Lassa virus glycoprotein precursor GP-C is proteolytically processed by subtilase SKI-1/S1P. *Proc Natl Acad Sci U S A* 2001;98(22):12701–12705.
224. Levis SC, Saavedra MC, Ceccoli C, et al. Correlation between endogenous interferon and the clinical evolution of patients with Argentine hemorrhagic fever. *J Interferon Res* 1985;5(3):383–389.
225. Lewis VJ, Walter PD, Thacker WL, et al. Comparison of three tests for the serological diagnosis of lymphocytic choriomeningitis virus infection. *J Clin Microbiol* 1975;2(3):193–197.
226. Liao BS, Byl FM, Adour KK. Audiometric comparison of Lassa fever hearing loss and idiopathic sudden hearing loss: evidence for viral cause. *Otolaryngol Head Neck Surg* 1992;106(3):226–229.
227. Lo Iacono G, Cunningham AA, Fichet-Calvet E, et al. Using modelling to disentangle the relative contributions of zoonotic and anthroponotic transmission: the case of Lassa fever. *PLoS Negl Trop Dis* 2015;9(1):e3398.
228. López N, Jácamo R, Franze-Fernández MT. Transcription and RNA replication of Tacaribe virus genome and antigenome analogs require N and L proteins: Z protein is an inhibitor of these processes. *J Virol* 2001;75(24):12241–12251.
229. Lucia HL, Coppenhaver DH, Baron S. Arenavirus infection in the guinea pig model: antiviral therapy with recombinant interferon-alpha, the immunomodulator CL246,738 and ribavirin. *Antiviral Res* 1989;12(5-6):279–292.
230. Lukashevich I. Generation of reassortants between African arenaviruses. *Virology* 1992;188:600–605.
231. Lukashevich IS. Advanced vaccine candidates for Lassa fever. *Viruses* 2012;4(11):2514–2557.
232. Lukashevich IS. The search for animal models for Lassa fever vaccine development. *Expert Rev Vaccines* 2013;12(1):71–86.
233. Lukashevich IS, Clegg JCS, Sidibe K. Lassa virus activity in Guinea: distribution of human antiviral antibody defined using enzyme-linked immunosorbent assay with recombinant antigen. *J Med Virol* 1993;40(3):210–217.
234. Lukashevich IS, Maryankova R, Vladyko AS, et al. Lassa and Mopeia virus replication in human monocytes/macrophages and in endothelial cells: different effects on IL-8 and TNF-alpha gene expression. *J Med Virol* 1999;59(4):552–560.
235. Lukashevich IS, Patterson J, Carrion R, et al. A live attenuated vaccine for Lassa fever made by reassortment of Lassa and Mopeia viruses. *J Virol* 2005;79(22):13934–13942.
236. Macher AM, Wolfe MS. Historical Lassa fever reports and 30-year clinical update. *Emerg Infect Dis* 2006;12(5):835–837.
237. Mackenzie RB. Epidemiology of Machupo virus infection. I. Pattern of human infection, San Joaquín, Bolivia, 1962-1964. *Am J Trop Med Hyg* 1965;14(5):808–813.
238. Mackenzie RB, Beye HK, Valverde Ch L, et al. Epidemic hemorrhagic fever in Bolivia. I. A preliminary report of the epidemiologic and clinical findings in a new epidemic area of South America. *Am J Trop Med Hyg* 1964;13:620–625.
239. Macneil A, Ströher U, Farnon E, et al. Solid organ transplant-associated lymphocytic choriomeningitis, United States, 2011. *Emerg Infect Dis* 2012;18(8):1256–1262.
240. Mahanty S, Bausch DG, Thomas RL, et al. Low levels of interleukin-8 and interferon-inducible protein-10 in serum are associated with fatal infections in acute Lassa fever. *J Infect Dis* 2001;183(12):1713–1721.
241. Mahmutovic S, Clark L, Levis SC, et al. Molecular basis for antibody-mediated neutralization of New World hemorrhagic fever mammarenaviruses. *Cell Host Microbe* 2015;18(6):705–713.
242. Maiztegui JI, Fernandez NJ, de Damilano AJ. Efficacy of immune plasma in treatment of Argentine haemorrhagic fever and association between treatment and a late neurological syndrome. *Lancet* 1979;314/ii(8154):1216–1217.
243. Maiztegui JI, McKee KT Jr, Barrera Oro JG, et al. Protective efficacy of a live attenuated vaccine against Argentine hemorrhagic fever. *J Infect Dis* 1998;177(2):277–283.
244. Manning JT, Forrester N, Paessler S. Lassa virus isolates from Mali and the Ivory Coast represent an emerging fifth lineage. *Front Microbiol* 2015;6:1037.
245. Mariën J, Borremans B, Gryseels S, et al. No measurable adverse effects of Lassa, Morogoro and Gairo arenaviruses on their rodent reservoir host in natural conditions. *Parasit Vectors* 2017;10(1):210.
246. Marq J-B, Hausmann S, Veillard N, et al. Short double-stranded RNAs with an overhanging 5′ ppp-nucleotide, as found in arenavirus genomes, act as RIG-I decoys. *J Biol Chem* 2011;286(8):6108–6116.
247. Marq J-B, Kolakofsky D, Garcin D. Unpaired 5′ ppp-nucleotides, as found in arenavirus double-stranded RNA panhandles, are not recognized by RIG-I. *J Biol Chem* 2010;285(24):18208–18216.
248. Marta RF, Montero VS, Hack CE, et al. Proinflammatory cytokines and elastase-α-1-antitrypsin in Argentine hemorrhagic fever. *Am J Trop Med Hyg* 1999;60(1):85–89.
249. Martinez Segovia ZM, Grazioli F, de Garre MEG, et al. Aplicación de la inmunofluorescencia al diagnóstico de la fiebre hemorrágica argentina. *Ciencia Invest* 1966;22:316–319.
250. Martínez-Sobrido L, Emonet S, Giannakas P, et al. Identification of amino acid residues critical for the anti-interferon activity of the nucleoprotein of the prototypic arenavirus lymphocytic choriomeningitis virus. *J Virol* 2009;83(21):11330–11340.
251. Martínez-Sobrido L, Giannakas P, Cubitt B, et al. Differential inhibition of type I interferon induction by arenavirus nucleoproteins. *J Virol* 2007;81(22):12696–12703.
252. Martínez-Sobrido L, Zúñiga EI, Rosario D, et al. Inhibition of the type I interferon response by the nucleoprotein of the prototypic arenavirus lymphocytic choriomeningitis virus. *J Virol* 2006;80(18):9192–9199.
253. McCormick JB. Epidemiology and control of Lassa fever. *Curr Top Microbiol Immunol* 1987;134:69–78.
254. McCormick JB, Fisher-Hoch SP. Lassa fever. *Curr Top Microbiol Immunol* 2002;262:75–109.
255. McCormick JB, King IJ, Webb PA, et al. A case-control study of the clinical diagnosis and course of Lassa fever. *J Infect Dis* 1987;155(3):445–455.
256. McCormick JB, Walker DH, King IJ, et al. Lassa virus hepatitis: a study of fatal Lassa fever in humans. *Am J Trop Med Hyg* 1986;35(2):401–407.
257. McCormick JB, Webb PA, Krebs JW, et al. A prospective study of the epidemiology and ecology of Lassa fever. *J Infect Dis* 1987;155(3):437–444.
258. McKee KT Jr, Enria DA, Barerra Oro JG. Junin (Argentine hemorrhagic fever). In: Barett ADT, Stanberry LR, eds. *Vaccines for Biodefense and Emerging and Neglected Diseases.* Amsterdam, Netherlands: Elsevier; 2009:537–550.
259. McKee KT Jr, Mahlandt BG, Maiztegui JI, et al. Experimental Argentine hemorrhagic fever in rhesus macaques: viral strain-dependent clinical response. *J Infect Dis* 1985;152(1):218–221.
260. McKee KT Jr, Mahlandt BG, Maiztegui JI, et al. Virus-specific factors in experimental Argentine hemorrhagic fever in rhesus macaques. *J Med Virol* 1987;22(2):99–111.
261. McKee KT Jr, Oro JGB, Kuehne AI, et al. Candid No. 1 Argentine hemorrhagic fever vaccine protects against lethal Junin virus challenge in rhesus macaques. *Intervirology* 1992;34(3):154–163.
262. McKee KT Jr, Oro JGB, Kuehne AI, et al. Safety and immunogenicity of a live-attenuated Junin (Argentine hemorrhagic fever) vaccine in rhesus macaques. *Am J Trop Med Hyg* 1993;48(3):403–411.
263. McLay L, Liang Y, Ly H. Comparative analysis of disease pathogenesis and molecular mechanisms of New World and Old World arenavirus infections. *J Gen Virol* 2014;95(Pt 1):1–15.
264. Mendenhall M, Russell A, Smee DF, et al. Effective oral favipiravir (T-705) therapy initiated after the onset of clinical disease in a model of arenavirus hemorrhagic Fever. *PLoS Negl Trop Dis* 2011;5(10):e1342.
265. Mercer J, Helenius A. Vaccinia virus uses macropinocytosis and apoptotic mimicry to enter host cells. *Science* 2008;320(5875):531–535.
266. Mercorelli B, Palu G, Loregian A. Drug repurposing for viral infectious diseases: how far are we? *Trends Microbiol* 2018;26(10):865–876.
267. Mertens PE, Patton R, Baum JJ, et al. Clinical presentation of Lassa fever cases during the hospital epidemic at Zorzor, Liberia, March-April 1972. *Am J Trop Med Hyg* 1973;22(6):780–784.
268. Metzger WG, Vivas-Martínez S. Questionable efficacy of the rVSV-ZEBOV Ebola vaccine. *Lancet* 2018;391(10125):1021.
269. Meyer BJ, de la Torre JC, Southern PJ. Arenaviruses: genomic RNAs, transcription, and replication. *Curr Top Microbiol Immunol* 2002;262:139–157.

270. Meyer HM Jr, Johnson RT, Crawford IP, et al. Central nervous system syndromes of "vital" etiology. A study of 713 cases. *Am J Med* 1960;29:334–347.

271. Mills JN, Ellis BA, Childs JE, et al. Prevalence of infection with Junin virus in rodent populations in the epidemic area of Argentine hemorrhagic fever. *Am J Trop Med Hyg* 1994;51(5):554–562.

272. Mills JN, Ellis BA, McKee KT Jr, et al. Junin virus activity in rodents from endemic and nonendemic loci in central Argentina. *Am J Trop Med Hyg* 1991;44(6):589–597.

273. Mills JN, Ellis BA, McKee KT Jr, et al. A longitudinal study of Junin virus activity in the rodent reservoir of Argentine hemorrhagic fever. *Am J Trop Med Hyg* 1992;47(6):749–763.

274. Miranda PO, Cubitt B, Jacob NT, et al. Mining a Kröhnke pyridine library for anti-arenavirus activity. *ACS Infect Dis* 2018;4(5):815–824.

275. Molteni HD, Guarinos HC, Petrillo CO, et al. Estudio clínico estadístico sobre 338 pacientes afectados por la fiebre hemorrágica epidémica del noroeste de la provincia de Buenos Aires. *Sem Méd* 1961;118:839–855.

276. Monath TP. Lassa fever: review of epidemiology and epizootiology. *Bull World Health Organ* 1975;52(4–6):577–592.

277. Monath TP, Maher M, Casals J, et al. Lassa fever in the Eastern Province of Sierra Leone, 1970-1972. II. Clinical observations and virological studies on selected hospital cases. *Am J Trop Med Hyg* 1974;23(6):1140–1149.

278. Monath TP, Mertens PE, Patton R, et al. A hospital epidemic of Lassa fever in Zorzor, Liberia, March-April 1972. *Am J Trop Med Hyg* 1973;22(6):773–779.

279. Monath TP, Newhouse VF, Kemp GE, et al. Lassa virus isolation from Mastomys natalensis rodents during an epidemic in Sierra Leone. *Science* 1974;185(4147):263–265.

280. Monson MH, Cole AK, Frame JD, et al. Pediatric Lassa fever: a review of 33 Liberian cases. *Am J Trop Med Hyg* 1987;36(2):408–415.

281. Monson MH, Frame JD, Jahrling PB, et al. Endemic Lassa fever in Liberia. I. Clinical and epidemiological aspects at Curran Lutheran Hospital, Zorzor, Liberia. *Trans R Soc Trop Med Hyg* 1984;78(4):549–553.

282. Montali RJ, Scanga CA, Pernikoff D, et al. A common-source outbreak of callitrichid hepatitis in captive tamarins and marmosets. *J Infect Dis* 1993;167(4):946–950.

283. Morin B, Coutard B, Lelke M, et al. The N-terminal domain of the arenavirus L protein is an RNA endonuclease essential in mRNA transcription. *PLoS Pathog* 2010;6(9):e1001038.

284. Muller G, Bruns M, Martinez Peralta L, et al. Lymphocytic choriomeningitis virus. IV. Electron microscopic investigation of the virion. *Arch Virol* 1983;75(4):229–242.

285. Murphy FA, Webb PA, Johnson KM, et al. Arenaviruses in Vero cells: ultrastructural studies. *J Virol* 1970;6(4):507–518.

286. Neuman BW, Adair BD, Burns JW, et al. Complementarity in the supramolecular design of arenaviruses and retroviruses revealed by electron cryomicroscopy and image analysis. *J Virol* 2005;79(6):3822–3830.

287. Niklasson BS, Jahrling PB, Peters CJ. Detection of Lassa virus antigens and Lassa virus-specific immunoglobulins G and M by enzyme-linked immunosorbent assay. *J Clin Microbiol* 1984;20(2):239–244.

288. Okokhere P, Colubri A, Azubike C, et al. Clinical and laboratory predictors of Lassa fever outcome in a dedicated treatment facility in Nigeria: a retrospective, observational cohort study. *Lancet Infect Dis* 2018;18(6):684–695.

289. Okokhere PO, Ibekwe TS, Akpede GO. Sensorineural hearing loss in Lassa fever: two case reports. *J Med Case Rep* 2009;3:36.

290. Olayemi A, Cadar D, Magassouba NF, et al. New hosts of the Lassa virus. *Sci Rep* 2016;6:25280.

291. Oppliger J, Torriani G, Herrador A, et al. Lassa virus cell entry via dystroglycan involves an unusual pathway of macropinocytosis. *J Virol* 2016;90(14):6412–6429.

292. Park JY, Peters CJ, Rollin PE, et al. Age distribution of lymphocytic choriomeningitis virus serum antibody in Birmingham, Alabama: evidence of a decreased risk of infection. *Am J Trop Med Hyg* 1997;57(1):37–41.

293. Park JY, Peters CJ, Rollin PE, et al. Development of an RT-PCR assay for diagnosis of lymphocytic choriomeningitis virus (LCMV) infection and its use in a prospective surveillance study. *J Med Virol* 1997;1997:107–114.

294. Parker WB. Metabolism and antiviral activity of ribavirin. *Virus Res* 2005;107(2):165–171.

295. Parodi AS, Greenway DJ, Rugiero HR, et al. Sobre la etiología del brote epidémico de Junín. *Día Méd* 1958;30(62):2300–2301.

296. Parsy M-L, Harlos K, Huiskonen JT, et al. Crystal structure of Venezuelan hemorrhagic fever virus fusion glycoprotein reveals a class 1 postfusion architecture with extensive glycosylation. *J Virol* 2013;87(23):13070–13075.

297. Pasqual G, Rojek JM, Masin M, et al. Old world arenaviruses enter the host cell via the multivesicular body and depend on the endosomal sorting complex required for transport. *PLoS Pathog* 2011;7(9):e1002232.

298. Pasquato A, Rochat C, Burri DJ, et al. Evaluation of the anti-arenaviral activity of the subtilisin kexin isozyme-1/site-1 protease inhibitor PF-429242. *Virology* 2012;423(1):14–22.

299. Patassi AA, Landoh DE, Mebiny-Essoh Tchalla A, et al. Emergence of Lassa fever disease in Northern Togo: report of two cases in Oti District in 2016. *Case Rep Infect Dis* 2017;2017:8242313.

300. Peralta LAM, Laguens RP, Cossio PM, et al. Presence of viral particles in the salivary gland of *Calomys musculinus* infected with Junin virus by a natural route. *Intervirology* 1979;11(2):111–116.

301. Perez M, Craven RC, de la Torre JC. The small RING finger protein Z drives arenavirus budding: implications for antiviral strategies. *Proc Natl Acad Sci U S A* 2003;100(22):12978–12983.

302. Perez M, de la Torre JC. Characterization of the genomic promoter of the prototypic arenavirus lymphocytic choriomeningitis virus. *J Virol* 2003;77(2):1184–1194.

303. Perez M, Greenwald DL, de la Torre JC. Myristoylation of the RING finger Z protein is essential for arenavirus budding. *J Virol* 2004;78(20):11443–11448.

304. Peters CJ. Arenaviruses. In: Richman DD, Whitley RJ, Hayden FG, eds. *Clinical Virology*. 2nd ed. Washington, DC: ASM Press; 2002:949–969.

305. Peters CJ. Human infection with arenaviruses in the Americas. *Curr Top Microbiol Immunol* 2002;262:65–74.

306. Peters CJ, Shelokov A. Viral hemorrhagic fever. In: Kass EH, Platt R, eds. *Current Therapy in Infectious Disease*, vol. 3. Toronto: B.C. Decker, Inc.; 1990:355–360.

307. Peters CJ, Webb PA, Johnson KM. Measurement of antibodies to Machupo virus by the indirect fluorescent technique. *Proc Soc Exp Biol Med* 1973;142(2):526–531.

308. Pinschewer DD, Perez M, de la Torre JC. Role of the virus nucleoprotein in the regulation of lymphocytic choriomeningitis virus transcription and RNA replication. *J Virol* 2003;77(6):3882–3887.

309. Pinschewer DD, Perez M, de la Torre JC. Dual role of the lymphocytic choriomeningitis virus intergenic region in transcription termination and virus propagation. *J Virol* 2005;79(7):4519–4526.

310. Pinschewer DD, Perez M, Sanchez AB, et al. Recombinant lymphocytic choriomeningitis virus expressing vesicular stomatitis virus glycoprotein. *Proc Natl Acad Sci U S A* 2003;100(13):7895–7900.

311. Pirosky I, Zuccarini J, Molinelli EA, et al. Virosis hemorrágica del noroeste bonaerense (endemo-epidémica, febril, enantémática, y leucopenica). In: *Ministerio de Asistencia Social y Salud Pública*. Buenos Aires Instituto Nacional de Microbiologia; 1959.

312. Plotkin SA. Vaccines for epidemic infections and the role of CEPI. *Hum Vaccin Immunother* 2017;13(12):2755–2762.

313. Poch O, Sauvaget I, Delarue M, et al. Identification of four conserved motifs among the RNA-dependent polymerase encoding elements. *EMBO J* 1989;8(12):3867–3874.

314. Price ME, Fisher-Hoch SP, Craven RB, et al. A prospective study of maternal and fetal outcome in acute Lassa fever infection during pregnancy. *BMJ* 1988;297(6648):584–587.

315. Pushko P, Geisbert J, Parker M, et al. Individual and bivalent vaccines based on alphavirus replicons protect guinea pigs against infection with Lassa and Ebola viruses. *J Virol* 2001;75(23):11677–11685.

316. Pyle JD, Whelan SPJ. RNA ligands activate the Machupo virus polymerase and guide promoter usage. *Proc Natl Acad Sci U S A* 2019;116(21):10518–10524.

317. Pythoud C, Rodrigo WWSI, Pasqual G, et al. Arenavirus nucleoprotein targets interferon regulatory factor-activating kinase IKKε. *J Virol* 2012;86(15):7728–7738.

318. Qi X, Lan S, Wang W, et al. Cap binding and immune evasion revealed by Lassa nucleoprotein structure. *Nature* 2010;468(7325):779–783.

319. Raaben M, Jae LT, Herbert AS, et al. NRP2 and CD63 are host factors for Lujo virus cell entry. *Cell Host Microbe* 2017;22(5):688.e5–696.e5.

320. Radoshitzky SR, Abraham J, Spiropoulou CF, et al. Transferrin receptor 1 is a cellular receptor for New World haemorrhagic fever arenaviruses. *Nature* 2007;446(7131):92–96.

321. Radoshitzky SR, Bào Y, Buchmeier MJ, et al. Past, present, and future of arenavirus taxonomy. *Arch Virol* 2015;160(7):1851–1874.

322. Radoshitzky SR, Buchmeier MJ, Charrel RN, et al. ICTV virus taxonomy profile: Arenaviridae. *J Gen Virol* 2019;100(8):1200–1201.

323. Radoshitzky SR, Kuhn JH, Spiropoulou CF, et al. Receptor determinants of zoonotic transmission of New World hemorrhagic fever arenaviruses. *Proc Natl Acad Sci U S A* 2008;105(7):2664–2669.

324. Radoshitzky SR, Longobardi LE, Kuhn JH, et al. Machupo virus glycoprotein determinants for human transferrin receptor 1 binding and cell entry. *PLoS One* 2011;6(7):e21398.

325. Raju R, Raju L, Hacker D, et al. Nontemplated bases at the 5′ ends of Tacaribe virus mRNAs. *Virology* 1990;174(1):53–59.

326. Ramsauer K, Schwameis M, Firbas C, et al. Immunogenicity, safety, and tolerability of a recombinant measles-virus-based chikungunya vaccine: a randomised, double-blind, placebo-controlled, active-comparator, first-in-man trial. *Lancet Infect Dis* 2015;15(5):519–527.

327. Rasmussen AF. The laboratory diagnosis of lymphocytic choriomeningitis and mumps. Proceedings of the Rocky Mountain Conference on Infantile Paralysis, Denver, CO, USA, 1946; 1947.

328. Reguera J, Gerlach P, Rosenthal M, et al. Comparative structural and functional analysis of bunyavirus and arenavirus cap-snatching endonucleases. *PLoS Pathog* 2016;12(6):e1005636.

329. Richmond JK, Baglole DJ. Lassa fever: epidemiology, clinical features, and social consequences. *BMJ* 2003;327(7426):1271–1275.

330. Riera L, Castillo E, Del Carmen Saavedra M, et al. Serological study of the lymphochoriomeningitis virus (LCMV) in an inner city of Argentina. *J Med Virol* 2005;76(2):285–289.

331. Rivers TM, McNair Scott TF. Meningitis in man caused by a filterable virus. *Science* 1935;81(2105):439–440.

332. Robinson JE, Hastie KM, Cross RW, et al. Most neutralizing human monoclonal antibodies target novel epitopes requiring both Lassa virus glycoprotein subunits. *Nat Commun* 2016;7:11544.

333. Rodrigo WWSI, Ortiz-Riaño E, Pythoud C, et al. Arenavirus nucleoproteins prevent activation of nuclear factor kappa B. *J Virol* 2012;86(15):8185–8197.

334. Rojek JM, Lee AM, Nguyen N, et al. Site 1 protease is required for proteolytic processing of the glycoproteins of the South American hemorrhagic fever viruses Junin, Machupo, and Guanarito. *J Virol* 2008;82(12):6045–6051.

335. Rojek JM, Pasqual G, Sanchez AB, et al. Targeting the proteolytic processing of the viral glycoprotein precursor is a promising novel antiviral strategy against arenaviruses. *J Virol* 2010;84(1):573–584.

336. Rojek JM, Spiropoulou CF, Campbell KP, et al. Old World and clade C New World arenaviruses mimic the molecular mechanism of receptor recognition used by α-dystroglycan's host-derived ligands. *J Virol* 2007;81(11):5685–5695.

337. Rowe WP, Murphy FA, Bergold GH, et al. Arenaviruses: proposed name for a newly defined virus group. *J Virol* 1970;5(5):651–652.

338. Rugiero HR, Ruggiero H, González Cambaceres C, et al. Fiebre hemorrágica Argentina. II. Estudio clínico descriptivo. *Rev Asoc Med Argent* 1964;78:281–294.

339. Russier M, Pannetier D, Baize S. Immune responses and Lassa virus infection. *Viruses* 2012;4(11):2766–2785.

340. Sabattini MS, Gonzalez de Rios LE, Diaz G, et al. Infección natural y experimental de roedores con virus Junín. *Medicina (B Aires)* 1977;37(Suppl 3):149–161.

341. Sabattini MS, Gonzalez LE. Identificación directa de virus Junin en roedores silvestres infectados en la naturaleza. *Rev Soc Argent Biol* 1967;43(5):252–260.

342. Sabeti PC, Varilly P, Fry B, et al. Genome-wide detection and characterization of positive selection in human populations. *Nature* 2007;449(7164):913–918.
343. Safronetz D, Lopez JE, Sogoba N, et al. Detection of Lassa virus, Mali. *Emerg Infect Dis* 2010;16(7):1123–1126.
344. Safronetz D, Mire C, Rosenke K, et al. A recombinant vesicular stomatitis virus-based Lassa fever vaccine protects guinea pigs and macaques against challenge with geographically and genetically distinct Lassa viruses. *PLoS Negl Trop Dis* 2015;9(4):e0003736.
345. Safronetz D, Rosenke K, Westover JB, et al. The broad-spectrum antiviral favipiravir protects guinea pigs from lethal Lassa virus infection post-disease onset. *Sci Rep* 2015;5:14775.
346. Safronetz D, Sogoba N, Diawara SI, et al. Annual incidence of Lassa virus infection in southern Mali. *Am J Trop Med Hyg* 2017;96(4):944–946.
347. Salas R, de Manzione N, Tesh RB, et al. Venezuelan haemorrhagic fever. *Lancet* 1991;338(8774):1033–1036.
348. Salazar-Bravo J, Ruedas LA, Yates TL. Mammalian reservoirs of arenaviruses. *Curr Top Microbiol Immunol* 2002;262:25–63.
349. Salvato MS. Molecular biology of the prototype arenavirus, lymphocytic choriomeningitis virus. In: Salvato MS, ed. *The Arenaviridae*. New York: Springer Science+Business; 1993:133–156.
350. Sánchez AB, de la Torre JC. Genetic and biochemical evidence for an oligomeric structure of the functional L polymerase of the prototypic arenavirus lymphocytic choriomeningitis virus. *J Virol* 2005;79(11):7262–7268.
351. Saunders AA, Ting JPC, Meisner J, et al. Mapping the landscape of the lymphocytic choriomeningitis virus stable signal peptide reveals novel functional domains. *J Virol* 2007;81(11):5649–5657.
352. Sayler KA, Barbet AF, Chamberlain C, et al. Isolation of Tacaribe virus, a Caribbean arenavirus, from host-seeking Amblyomma americanum ticks in Florida. *PLoS One* 2014;9(12):e115769.
353. Schmitz H, Köhler B, Laue T, et al. Monitoring of clinical and laboratory data in two cases of imported Lassa fever. *Microbes Infect* 2002;4(1):43–50.
354. Schwarz ER, Mando OG, Maiztegui JI, et al. Síntomas y signos iniciales de mayor valor diagnóstico en la fiebre hemorrágica argentina. *Medicina (B Aires)* 1970;30(Suppl 1):8–14.
355. Scott TF, Rivers TM. Meningitis in man caused by a filterable virus. I. Two cases and the method of obtaining a virus from their spinal fluids. *J Exp Med* 1936;63(3):397–414.
356. Sewlall NH, Richards G, Duse A, et al. Clinical features and patient management of Lujo hemorrhagic fever. *PLoS Negl Trop Dis* 2014;8(11):e3233.
357. Shaffer JG, Grant DS, Schieffelin JS, et al. Lassa fever in post-conflict Sierra Leone. *PLoS Negl Trop Dis* 2014;8(3):e2748.
358. Shao J, Huang Q, Liu X, et al. Arenaviral nucleoproteins suppress PACT-induced augmentation of RIG-I function to inhibit type I interferon production. *J Virol* 2018;92(13): e00482-18.
359. Shehu NY, Gomerep SS, Isa SE, et al. Lassa fever 2016 outbreak in Plateau State, Nigeria—the changing epidemiology and clinical presentation. *Front Public Health* 2018;6:232.
360. Shi M, Lin X-D, Chen X, et al. The evolutionary history of vertebrate RNA viruses. *Nature* 2018;556(7700):197–202.
361. Shimojima M, Kawaoka Y. Cell surface molecules involved in infection mediated by lymphocytic choriomeningitis virus glycoprotein. *J Vet Med Sci* 2012;74(10):1363–1366.
362. Shimojima M, Ströher U, Ebihara H, et al. Identification of cell surface molecules involved in dystroglycan-independent Lassa virus cell entry. *J Virol* 2012;86(4):2067–2078.
363. Shtanko O, Imai M, Goto H, et al. A role for the C terminus of Mopeia virus nucleoprotein in its incorporation into Z protein-induced virus-like particles. *J Virol* 2010;84(10):5415–5422.
364. Smee DF, Gilbert J, Leonhardt JA, et al. Treatment of lethal Pichinde virus infections in weanling LVG/Lak hamsters with ribavirin, ribamidine, selenazofurin, and ampligen. *Antiviral Res* 1993;20(1):57–70.
365. Sogoba N, Feldmann H, Safronetz D. Lassa fever in West Africa: evidence for an expanded region of endemicity. *Zoonoses Public Health* 2012;59(Suppl 2):43–47.
366. Sommerstein R, Flatz L, Remy MM, et al. Arenavirus glycan shield promotes neutralizing antibody evasion and protracted infection. *PLoS Pathog* 2015;11(11):e1005276.
367. Stenglein MD, Sanders C, Kistler AL, et al. Identification, characterization, and *in vitro* culture of highly divergent arenaviruses from boa constrictors and annulated tree boas: candidate etiological agents for snake inclusion body disease. *MBio* 2012;3(4): e00180-12.
368. Stephen EL, Jones DE, Peters CJ, et al. Ribavirin treatment of toga-, arena-, bunyavirus infection in subhuman primates and other laboratory animal species. In: Smith RA, Kirkpatrick W, eds. *Ribavirin: A Broad Spectrum Antiviral Agent*. New York: Academic Press; 1980:169–183.
369. Stephensen CB, Blount SR, Lanford RE, et al. Prevalence of serum antibodies against lymphocytic choriomeningitis virus in selected populations from two U.S. cities. *J Med Virol* 1992;38(1):27–31.
370. Stephensen CB, Jacob JR, Montali RJ, et al. Isolation of an arenavirus from a marmoset with callitrichid hepatitis and its serologic association with disease. *J Virol* 1991;65(8):3995–4000.
371. Stinebaugh BJ, Schloeder FX, Johnson KM, et al. Bolivian hemorrhagic fever. A report of four cases. *Am J Med* 1966;40(2):217–230.
372. Strecker T, Eichler R, Meulen J, et al. Lassa virus Z protein is a matrix protein and sufficient for the release of virus-like particles [corrected]. *J Virol* 2003;77(19):10700–10705.
373. Strecker T, Maisa A, Daffis S, et al. The role of myristoylation in the membrane association of the Lassa virus matrix protein Z. *Virol J* 2006;3:93.
374. Swaan C-M, van den Broek P-J, Wijnands S, et al. Management of viral haemorrhagic fever in the Netherlands. *Euro Surveill* 2002;7(3):48–50.
375. Tani H, Iha K, Shimojima M, et al. Analysis of Lujo virus cell entry using pseudotype vesicular stomatitis virus. *J Virol* 2014;88(13):7317–7330.
376. Ter Meulen J, Lukashevich I, Sidibe K, et al. Hunting of peridomestic rodents and consumption of their meat as possible risk factors for rodent-to-human transmission of Lassa virus in the Republic of Guinea. *Am J Trop Med Hyg* 1996;55(6):661–666.
377. Tesh RB, Jahrling PB, Salas R, et al. Description of Guanarito virus (Arenaviridae: *Arenavirus*), the etiologic agent of Venezuelan hemorrhagic fever. *Am J Trop Med Hyg* 1994;50(4):452–459.
378. Tesh RB, Wilson ML, Salas R, et al. Field studies on the epidemiology of Venezuelan hemorrhagic fever: implication of the cotton rat *Sigmodon alstoni* as the probable rodent reservoir. *Am J Trop Med Hyg* 1993;49(2):227–235.
379. Tindall GT, Gladstone LA. Hydrocephalus as a sequel to lymphocytic choriomeningitis. *Neurology* 1957;7(7):516–518.
380. Tomori O, Fabiyi A, Sorungbe A, et al. Viral hemorrhagic fever antibodies in Nigerian populations. *Am J Trop Med Hyg* 1988;38(2):407–410.
381. Trappier SG, Conaty AL, Farrar BB, et al. Evaluation of the polymerase chain reaction for diagnosis of Lassa virus infection. *Am J Trop Med Hyg* 1993;49(2):214–221.
382. Traub E. A filterable virus recovered from white mice. *Science* 1935;81(2099):298–299.
383. Urata S, Noda T, Kawaoka Y, et al. Cellular factors required for Lassa virus budding. *J Virol* 2006;80(8):4191–4195.
384. Urata S, Yasuda J. *Cis*- and cell-type-dependent *trans*-requirements for Lassa virus-like particle production. *J Gen Virol* 2015;96(Pt 7):1626–1635.
385. Urata S, Yun N, Pasquato A, et al. Antiviral activity of a small-molecule inhibitor of arenavirus glycoprotein processing by the cellular site 1 protease. *J Virol* 2011;85(2):795–803.
386. Vainrub B, Salas R. Latin American hemorrhagic fever. *Infect Dis Clin North Am* 1994;8(1):47–59.
387. Vanzee BE, Douglas RG, Betts RF, et al. Lymphocytic choriomeningitis in university hospital personnel. Clinical features. *Am J Med* 1975;58(6):803–809.
388. Vieth S, Torda AE, Asper M, et al. Sequence analysis of L RNA of Lassa virus. *Virology* 2004;318(1):153–168.
389. Vitullo AD, Hodara VL, Merani MS. Effect of persistent infection with Junin virus on growth and reproduction of its natural reservoir, *Calomys musculinus*. *Am J Trop Med Hyg* 1987;37(3):663–669.
390. Vitullo AD, Marani MS. Mecanismos de transmisión del virus Junín en su resrvorio natural, *Calomys musculinus*. *Medicina (B Aires)* 1987;47:440.
391. Vitullo AD, Merani MS. Is vertical transmission sufficient to maintain Junin virus in nature? *J Gen Virol* 1988;69(Pt 6):1437–1440.
392. Vitullo AD, Merani MS. Vertical transmission of Junin virus in experimentally infected adult *Calomys musculinus*. *Intervirology* 1990;31(6):339–344.
393. Vogel D, Rosenthal M, Gogrefe N, et al. Biochemical characterization of the Lassa virus L protein. *J Biol Chem* 2019;294(20):8088–8100.
394. Volpon L, Osborne MJ, Capul AA, et al. Structural characterization of the Z RING-eIF4E complex reveals a distinct mode of control for eIF4E. *Proc Natl Acad Sci U S A* 2010;107(12):5441–5446.
395. Walker DH, McCormick JB, Johnson KM, et al. Pathologic and virologic study of fatal Lassa fever in man. *Am J Pathol* 1982;107(3):349–356.
396. Walker DH, Wulff H, Lange JV, et al. Comparative pathology of Lassa virus infection in monkeys, guinea-pigs, and *Mastomys natalensis*. *Bull World Health Organ* 1975;52(4–6):523–534.
397. Wallat GD, Huang Q, Wang W, et al. High-resolution structure of the N-terminal endonuclease domain of the Lassa virus L polymerase in complex with magnesium ions. *PLoS One* 2014;9(2):e87577.
398. Wang M, Jokinen J, Tretyakova I, et al. Alphavirus vector-based replicon particles expressing multivalent cross-protective Lassa virus glycoproteins. *Vaccine* 2018;36(5):683–690.
399. Warkel RL, Rinaldi CF, Bancroft WH, et al. Fatal acute meningoencephalitis due to lymphocytic choriomeningitis virus. *Neurology* 1973;23(2):198–203.
400. Webb PA, Justines G, Johnson KM. Infection of wild and laboratory animals with Machupo and Latino viruses. *Bull World Health Organ* 1975;52(4–6):493–499.
401. Weissenbacher MC, Calello MA, Carballal G, et al. Actividad del virus Junin en humanos y roedores de áreas no endémicas de la provincia de Buenos Aires. *Medicina (B Aires)* 1985;45(3):263–268.
402. Weissenbacher M, De Guerrero LB, Frigerio MJ. Infeccion subclinica, infeccion clinica y vacunacion con virus Junin. *Medicina (B Aires)* 1976;36(1):1–8.
403. Weissenbacher MC, Sabattini MS, Avila MM, et al. Junin virus activity in two rural populations of the Argentine hemorrhagic fever (AHF) endemic area. *J Med Virol* 1983;12(4):273–280.
404. Welch SR, Guerrero LW, Chakrabarti AK, et al. Lassa and Ebola virus inhibitors identified using minigenome and recombinant virus reporter systems. *Antiviral Res* 2016;136:9–18.
405. West BR, Hastie KM, Saphire EO. Structure of the LCMV nucleoprotein provides a template for understanding arenavirus replication and immunosuppression. *Acta Crystallogr D Biol Crystallogr* 2014;70(Pt 6):1764–1769.
406. Whitmer SLM, Strecker T, Cadar D, et al. New lineage of Lassa virus, Togo, 2016. *Emerg Infect Dis* 2018;24(3):599–602.
407. Wiebenga NH, Shelokov A, Gibbs CJ Jr, et al. Epidemic hemorrhagic fever in Bolivia. II. Demonstration of complement-fixing antibody in patients' sera with Junín virus antigen. *Am J Trop Med Hyg* 1964;13:626–628.
408. Wright KE, Buchmeier MJ. Antiviral antibodies attenuate T-cell-mediated immunopathology following acute lymphocytic choriomeningitis virus infection. *J Virol* 1991;65(6):3001–3006.
409. Wright R, Johnson D, Neumann M, et al. Congenital lymphocytic choriomeningitis virus syndrome: a disease that mimics congenital toxoplasmosis or Cytomegalovirus infection. *Pediatrics* 1997;100(1):E9.
410. Wu Z, Du J, Lu L, et al. Detection of hantaviruses and arenaviruses in three-toed jerboas from the Inner Mongolia Autonomous Region, China. *Emerg Microbes Infect* 2018;7(1):35.
411. Wulff H, Fabiyi A, Monath TP. Recent isolations of Lassa virus from Nigerian rodents. *Bull World Health Organ* 1975;52(4–6):609–613.
412. Xing J, Ly H, Liang Y. The Z proteins of pathogenic but not nonpathogenic arenaviruses inhibit RIG-i-like receptor-dependent interferon production. *J Virol* 2015;89(5):2944–2955.
413. York J, Agnihothram SS, Romanowski V, et al. Genetic analysis of heptad-repeat regions in the G2 fusion subunit of the Junin arenavirus envelope glycoprotein. *Virology* 2005;343(2):267–274.

414. York J, Nunberg JH. Role of the stable signal peptide of Junín arenavirus envelope glycoprotein in pH-dependent membrane fusion. *J Virol* 2006;80(15):7775–7780.

415. York J, Nunberg JH. Distinct requirements for signal peptidase processing and function in the stable signal peptide subunit of the Junin virus envelope glycoprotein. *Virology* 2007;359(1):72–81.

416. York J, Nunberg JH. Intersubunit interactions modulate pH-induced activation of membrane fusion by the Junin virus envelope glycoprotein GPC. *J Virol* 2009;83(9):4121–4126.

417. York J, Romanowski V, Lu M, et al. The signal peptide of the Junín arenavirus envelope glycoprotein is myristoylated and forms an essential subunit of the mature G1-G2 complex. *J Virol* 2004;78(19):10783–10792.

418. Yoshida-Moriguchi T, Campbell KP. Matriglycan: a novel polysaccharide that links dystroglycan to the basement membrane. *Glycobiology* 2015;25(7):702–713.

419. Young PR, Howard CR. Fine structure analysis of Pichinde virus nucleocapsids. *J Gen Virol* 1983;64(Pt 4):833–842.

420. Zapata JC, Goicochea M, Nadai Y, et al. Genetic variation *in vitro* and *in vivo* of an attenuated Lassa vaccine candidate. *J Virol* 2014;88(6):3058–3066.

421. Zapata JC, Poonia B, Bryant J, et al. An attenuated Lassa vaccine in SIV-infected rhesus macaques does not persist or cause arenavirus disease but does elicit Lassa virus-specific immunity. *Virol J* 2013;10:52.

422. Zeitlin L, Geisbert JB, Deer DJ, et al. Monoclonal antibody therapy for Junin virus infection. *Proc Natl Acad Sci U S A* 2016;113(16):4458–4463.

423. Zeltina A, Krumm SA, Sahin M, et al. Convergent immunological solutions to Argentine hemorrhagic fever virus neutralization. *Proc Natl Acad Sci U S A* 2017;114(27):7031–7036.

424. Zhang Y, Li L, Liu X, et al. Crystal structure of Junin virus nucleoprotein. *J Gen Virol* 2013;94(Pt 10):2175–2183.

425. Zhou S, Cerny AM, Zacharia A, et al. Induction and inhibition of type I interferon responses by distinct components of lymphocytic choriomeningitis virus. *J Virol* 2010;84(18):9452–9462.

Index